Stroke
Practical Management

THIRD EDITION

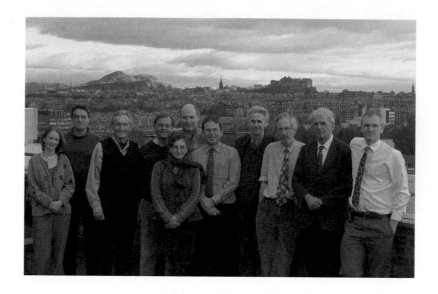

Dedication
To our many colleagues, young and old, with whom we have shared the care of so many stroke patients, and with whom we have discussed so many interesting ideas.

Acknowledgement
The authors of this book are particularly grateful to Joanna Warldlaw, who has drawn much of the line artwork throughout the three editions.

Stroke
Practical Management

THIRD EDITION

C. Warlow
J. van Gijn
M. Dennis
J. Wardlaw
J. Bamford
G. Hankey
P. Sandercock
G. Rinkel
P. Langhorne
C. Sudlow
P. Rothwell

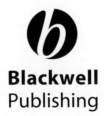

Blackwell
Publishing

© 2007 C. Warlow, J. van Gijn, M. Dennis, J. Wardlaw, J. Bamford, G. Hankey, P. Sandercock, G. Rinkel, P. Langhorne, C. Sudlow, P. Rothwell

Published by Blackwell Publishing
Blackwell Publishing, Inc., 350 Main Street, Malden, Massachusetts 02148-5020, USA
Blackwell Publishing Ltd, 9600 Garsington Road, Oxford OX4 2DQ, UK
Blackwell Publishing Asia Pty Ltd, 550 Swanston Street, Carlton, Victoria 3053, Australia

First edition published 1996
Second edition published 2001
Third edition published 2008

1   2008

Library of Congress Cataloging-in-Publication Data

Stroke : practical management / C. Warlow . . . [et al.]. – 3rd ed.
    p. ; cm.
  Includes bibliographical references and index.
  ISBN 978-1-4051-2766-0 (hardcover : alk. paper)
  1. Cerebrovascular disease.   2. Cerebrovascular disease – Treatment.   I. Warlow, Charles, 1934-
  [DNLM: 1. Cerebrovascular Accident – therapy.   2. Intracranial Hemorrhages – therapy.
3. Ischemic Attack, Transient – therapy. WL 355 S9208 2007]

  RC388.5.S847 2007
  616.8'1 – dc22

                                                                              2007022955

ISBN: 978-1-4051-2766-0

A catalogue record for this title is available from the British Library

Set in 9/12pt Stone Serif by Graphicraft Limited, Hong Kong
Printed and bound in Singapore by Markono Print Media Pte Ltd

Commissioning Editor: Martin Sugden
Editorial Assistant: Jennifer Seward
Development Editor: Lauren Brindley
Production Controller: Debbie Wyer

For further information on Blackwell Publishing, visit our website:
http://www.blackwellpublishing.com

The publisher's policy is to use permanent paper from mills that operate a sustainable forestry policy, and which has been manufactured from pulp processed using acid-free and elementary chlorine-free practices. Furthermore, the publisher ensures that the text paper and cover board used have met acceptable environmental accreditation standards.

Contents

Contributors

Charles Warlow
University of Edinburgh, Western General Hospital, Edinburgh, UK

Jan van Gijn
Utrecht University, Utrecht, the Netherlands

Martin Dennis
University of Edinburgh, Western General Hospital, Edinburgh, UK

Joanna Wardlaw
University of Edinburgh, Western General Hospital, Edinburgh, UK

John Bamford
St James' University Hospital, Leeds, West Yorkshire, UK

Graeme Hankey
Royal Perth Hospital, Stroke Unit, Perth WA, Australia

Peter Sandercock
University of Edinburgh, Western General Hospital, Edinburgh, UK

Gabriel Rinkel
Utrecht University, Utrecht, the Netherlands

Peter Langhorne
Academic Section of Geriatric Medicine, Royal Infirmary, Glasgow, UK

Cathie Sudlow
University of Edinburgh, Western General Hospital, Edinburgh, UK

Peter Rothwell
Department of Clinical Neurology, Radcliffe Infirmary, Oxford, UK

Acknowledgements

We have had invaluable help and advice from many people in the preparation of this third edition. So thank you all, including:

Sheena Borthwick
Judi Clarke
Carl Counsell
Ann Deary
Alice Emmott
Hazel Fraser
Paut Greebe
Gord Gubitz
Ingrid Kane
Sarah Keir
Alistair Lammie
Lynn Legg
Richard Lindley
Mike McDowell
Michael Mackie
Ian Marshall
Nick Morgan
Ross Naylor
Sarah Pendlebury
David Perry
Rustam Al-Shahi Salman
Cameron Sellers
Mark Smith
Ian Starkey
Stuart Taylor
Brenda Thomas
Theo vanVroonhoven
Nic Weir

Also, thank you to our teachers and colleagues from whom we have learned so many worthwhile things over the years:

Henry Barnett
Lou Caplan
David Chadwick
Iain Chalmers
Rory Collins
Hans van Crevel
Richard Doll
Geoff Donnan
Stuart Douglas
Shah Ebrahim
Rob Edis
Barbara Farrell
C. Miller Fisher
Chris Foote
John Fry
Mike Gent
Sonny Gubbay
Michael Harrison
Jim Heron
Steff Lewis
Bryan Matthews
Richard Peto
Alex Pollock
Geoffrey Rose
David Sackett
Robin Sellar
David Shepherd
Jim Slattery
Rien Vermeulen
Ted Stewart-Wynne
Derick Wade
Eelco Wijdicks

Abbreviations

We don't care much for abbreviations. They are not literate (Oliver Twist was not abbreviated to OT each time Dickens mentioned his name!), they don't look good on the printed page, and they make things more difficult to read and understand, particularly for non-experts. But they do save space and so we have to use them a bit. However, we will avoid them as far as we can in tables, figures and the practice points. We will try to define any abbreviations the first time they are used in each chapter, or even in each section if they are not very familiar. But, if we fail to be comprehensible, then here is a rather long list to refer to.

ACA	Anterior cerebral artery
ACE	Angiotensin converting enzyme
AChA	Anterior choroidal artery
ACoA	Anterior communicating artery
ACST	Asymptomatic Carotid Surgery Trial
ADC	Apparent diffusion coefficient
ADH	Antidiuretic hormone
ADL	Activities of daily living
ADP	Adenosine diphosphate
ADPKD	Autosomal dominant polycystic kidney disease
AF	Atrial fibrillation
AFx	Amaurosis fugax
AH	Ataxic hemiparesis
AICA	Anterior inferior cerebellar artery
AIDS	Acquired immune deficiency syndrome
AMI	Acute myocardial infarction
ANCA	Antineutrophil cytoplasmic antibody
ANF	Antinuclear factor
APS	Antiphospholipid syndrome
APT	Antiplatelet Trialists' Collaboration
APTT	Activated partial thromboplastin time
ARAS	Ascending reticular activating system
ARD	Absolute risk difference
ASA	Atrial septal aneurysm
ASD	Atrial septal defect
ATIII	Antithrombin III

ATP	Adenosine triphosphate
ATT	Antithrombotic Trialists' Collaboration
AVF	Arteriovenous fistula
AVM	Arteriovenous malformation
BA	Basilar artery
BIH	Benign intracranial hypertension
BMI	Body mass index
BP	Blood pressure
C	Celsius
CAA	Cerebral amyloid angiopathy
CADASIL	Cerebral autosomal dominant arteriopathy with subcortical infarcts and leukoencephalopathy
CAST	Chinese Acute Stroke Trial
CAVATAS	Carotid and Vertebral Artery Transluminal Angioplasty Study
CBF	Cerebral blood flow
CBFV	Cerebral blood flow velocity
CBV	Cerebral blood volume
CCA	Common carotid artery
CEA	Carotid endarterectomy
CHD	Coronary heart disease
CI	Confidence interval
CK	Creatine kinase
$CMRO_2$	Cerebral metabolic rate of oxygen
CMRglu	Cerebral metabolic rate of glucose
CNS	Central nervous system
CPP	Cerebral perfusion pressure
CPSP	Central post-stroke pain
CSF	Cerebrospinal fluid
CT	Computed tomography
CTA	Computed tomographic angiography
CVR	Cerebrovascular resistance
DBP	Diastolic blood pressure
DCHS	Dysarthria clumsy-hand syndrome
DIC	Disseminated intravascular coagulation
DNA	Deoxyribose nucleic acid
DSA	Digital subtraction angiography
DSM	Diagnostic and statistical manual of mental disorders

DVT	Deep venous thrombosis (in the legs or pelvis)
DWI	Diffusion weighted (MR) imaging
EACA	Epsilon-aminocaproic acid
EADL	Extended activities of daily living
EAFT	European Atrial Fibrillation Trial
ECA	External carotid artery
ECASS	European Cooperative Acute Stroke Study
ECG	Electrocardiogram
EC-IC	Extracranial-intracranial
ECST	European Carotid Surgery Trial
EEG	Electroencephalogram
EMG	Electromyography
ESR	Erythrocyte sedimentation rate
FDA	Food and Drug Administration
FIM	Functional independence measure
FLAIR	Fluid attenuated inversion recovery
FMD	Fibromuscular dysplasia
fMRI	Functional magnetic resonance imaging
FMZ	Flumazenil
GCS	Glasgow Coma Scale
GEF	Glucose extraction fraction
GKI	Glucose, potassium and insulin
HACP	Homolateral ataxia and crural paresis
Hg	Mercury
HITS	High intensity transient signals
HIV	Human immunodeficiency virus
HMPAO	Hexamethylpropyleneamine oxime
HTI	Haemorrhagic transformation of an infarct
HU	Hounsfield units
IAA	Internal auditory artery
IAA	Intra arterial angiography
ICA	Internal carotid artery
ICH	Intracerebral haemorrhage
ICIDH	International classification of impairments, disabilities and handicaps
ICP	Intracranial pressure
ICVT	Intracranial venous thrombosis
IADSA	Intra-arterial digital subtraction angiography
INR	International normalized ratio
IST	International Stroke Trial
IVDSA	Intravenous digital subtraction angiography
IVM	Intracranial vascular malformation
kPa	Kilopascals
L	Litre
LACI	Lacunar infarction
LACS	Lacunar syndrome
LGN	Lateral geniculate nucleus
LP	Lumbar puncture
LSA	Lenticulostriate artery
M	Molar
MAC	Mitral annulus calcification
MAOI	Monoamine oxidase inhibitor
MAST-I	Multicentre Acute Stroke Trial – Italy
MCA	Middle cerebral artery
MCTT	Mean cerebral transit time
MES	Microembolic signals
MI	Myocardial infarction
MLF	Medial longitudinal fasciculus
MLP	Mitral leaflet prolapse
MMSE	Mini mental state examination
MR	Magnetic resonance
MRA	Magnetic resonance angiography
MRC	Medical Research Council
MRI	Magnetic resonance imaging
MRS	Magnetic resonance spectroscopy
MRV	Magnetic resonance venogram
MTT	Mean transit time
NAA	N-acetylaspartate
NASCET	North American Symptomatic Carotid Endarterectomy Trial
NELH	National Electronic Library for Health
NG	Nasogastric
NIHSS	National Institute of Health Stroke Score
NINDS	National Institute of Neurological Disorders and Stroke
NNT	Number-needed-to-treat
NO	Nitric oxide
OCSP	Oxfordshire Community Stroke Project
OEF	Oxygen extraction fraction
OHS	Oxford Handicap Scale
OR	Odds ratio
PACI	Partial anterior circulation infarction
$PaCO_2$	Arterial partial pressure of carbon dioxide
PaO_2	Arterial partial pressure of oxygen
PACS	Partial anterior circulation syndrome
PCA	Posterior cerebral artery
PChA	Posterior choroidal artery
PCoA	Posterior communicating artery
PCV	Packed cell volume
PE	Pulmonary embolism
PEG	Percutaneous endoscopic gastrostomy
PET	Positron emission tomography
PFO	Patent foramen ovale
PICA	Posterior inferior cerebellar artery
PMS	Pure motor stroke
PNH	Paroxysmal nocturnal haemoglobinuria
POCI	Posterior circulation infarction
POCS	Posterior circulation syndrome
PD	Proton density
PSE	Present state examination
PSS	Pure sensory stroke
PT	Prothrombin time
PTA	Percutaneous transluminal angioplasty
PVD	Peripheral vascular disease

PWI	Perfusion weighted (MR) imaging	SLE	Systemic lupus erythematosus
QALYs	Quality adjusted life years	SMS	Sensorimotor stroke
RAH	Recurrent artery of Heubner	SPAF	Stroke prevention in atrial fibrillation (trial)
RCT	Randomized controlled trial	SPECT	Single photon emission computed
RIND	Reversible ischaemic neurological deficit		tomography
RNA	Ribonucleic acid	SVD	Small vessel disease
ROR	Relative odds reduction	TACI	Total anterior circulation infarction
RR	Relative risk	TACS	Total anterior circulation syndrome
RRR	Relative risk reduction	TCD	Transcranial Doppler
rt-PA	Recombinant tissue plasminogen activator	TEA	Tranexamic acid
SADS	Schedule for affective disorders and	TENS	Transcutaneous electrical nerve stimulation
	schizophrenia	TGA	Transient global amnesia
SAH	Subarachnoid haemorrhage	TIA	Transient ischaemic attack
SBP	Systolic blood pressure	TMB	Transient monocular blindness
SCA	Superior cerebellar artery	TOAST	Trial of ORG 10172 in Acute Stroke Therapy
SD	Standard deviation	TTP	Thrombotic thrombocytopenic purpura
SEPIVAC	Studio epidemiologico sulla incidenza delle	TTP	Time to peak
	vasculopathie acute cerebrali	US	Ultrasound
SF36	Short form 36	VA	Vertebral artery
SIADH	Syndrome of inappropriate secretion of	VB	Vertebrobasilar
	antidiuretic hormone	WHO	World Health Organization
SK	Streptokinase	WFNS	World Federation of Neurological Surgeons

1 Introduction

1.1 Introduction to the first edition

1.1.1 Aims and scope of the book

We, the authors of this book, regard ourselves as practising – and practical – doctors who look after stroke patients in very routine day-to-day practice. The book is for people like us: neurologists, geriatricians, stroke physicians, radiologists and general internal physicians. But it is not just for doctors. It is also for nurses, therapists, managers and anyone else who wants practical guidance about all and any of the problems to do with stroke – from aetiology to organization of services, from prevention to occupational therapy, and from any facet of cure to any facet of care. In other words, it is for anyone who has to deal with stroke in clinical practice. It is not a book for armchair theoreticians, who usually have no sense of proportion as well as difficulty in seeing the wood from the trees. Or, maybe, it is particularly for them so that they can be led back into the real world.

The book takes what is known as a problem-orientated approach. The problems posed by stroke patients are discussed in the sort of order that they are likely to present themselves. Is it a stroke? What sort of stroke is it? What caused it? What can be done about it? How can the patient and carer be supported in the short term and long term? How can any recurrence be prevented? How can stroke services be better organized? Unlike traditional textbooks, which linger on dusty shelves, there are no '-ology' chapters. Aetiology, epidemiology, pathology

Stroke: practical management, 3rd edition. C. Warlow, J. van Gijn, M. Dennis, J. Wardlaw, J. Bamford, G. Hankey, P. Sandercock, G. Rinkel, P. Langhorne, C. Sudlow and P. Rothwell. Published 2008 Blackwell Publishing. ISBN 978-1-4051-2766-0.

and the rest represent just the tools to solve the problems – so they are used when they are needed, and not discussed in isolation. For example, to prevent strokes one needs to know how frequent they are (epidemiology), what types of stroke there are (pathology), what causes them (aetiology) and what evidence there is to support therapeutic intervention (randomized controlled trials). Clinicians mostly operate on a need-to-know basis, and so when a problem arises they need the information to solve it at that moment, from inside their head, from a colleague – and we hope from a book like this.

1.1.2 General principles

To solve a problem one obviously needs relevant information. Clinicians, and others, should not be making decisions based on whim, dogma or the last case, although most do, at least some of the time – ourselves included. It is better to search out the reliable information based on some reasonable criterion for what is meant by reliable, get it into a sensible order, review it and make a summary that can be used at the bedside. If one does not have the time to do this – and who does for every problem? – then one has to search out someone else's systematic review. Or find the answer in this book. Good clinicians have always done all this intuitively, although recently the process has been blessed with the title of 'evidence-based medicine', and now even 'evidence-based patient-focused medicine'! In this book we have used the evidence-based approach, at least where it is possible to do so. Therefore, where a systematic review of a risk factor or a treatment is available we have cited it, and not just emphasized single studies done by us or our friends and with results to suit our prejudices. But so often there is no good evidence or even any evidence at all available, and certainly no systematic reviews. What to do then? Certainly not what most doctors are trained to do: 'Never be wrong, and if you are, never admit it!' If we do

1

not know something, we will say so. But, like other clinicians, we may have to make decisions even when we do not know what to do, and when nobody else does either. One cannot always adopt the policy of 'if you don't know what to do, don't do it'. Throughout the book we will try to indicate where there is no evidence, or feeble evidence, and describe what *we* do and will continue to do until better evidence becomes available; after all, it is these murky areas of practice that need to be flagged up as requiring further research. Moreover, in clinical practice, all of us ask respected colleagues for advice, not because they may know something that we do not but because we want to know what they would do in a difficult situation.

1.1.3 Methods

We were all taught to look at the 'methods' section of a scientific paper before anything else. If the methods are no good, then there is no point in wasting time and reading further. In passing, we do regard it as most peculiar that some medical journals still print the methods section in smaller letters than the rest of the paper. Therefore, before anyone reads further, perhaps we should describe the methods we have adopted.

It is now impossible for any single person to write a comprehensive book about stroke that has the feel of having been written by someone with hands-on experience of the whole subject. The range of problems is far too wide. Therefore, the sort of stroke book that we as practitioners want – and we hope others do too – has to be written by a group of people. Rather than putting together a huge multiauthor book, we thought it would be better and more informative, for ourselves as well as readers, to write a book together that would take a particular approach (evidence-based, if you will) and end up with a coherent message. After all, we have all worked together over many years, our views on stroke are more convergent than divergent, and so it should not be too terribly difficult to write a book together.

Like many things in medicine, and in life, this book started over a few drinks to provide the initial momentum to get going, on the occasion of a stroke conference in Geneva in 1993. At that time, we decided that the book was to be comprehensive (but not to the extent of citing every known reference), that all areas of stroke must be covered, and who was going to start writing which section. A few months later, the first drafts were then commented on in writing and in detail by all the authors before we got back together for a general discussion – again over a few drinks, but on this occasion at the Stockholm stroke conference in 1994. Momentum restored, we went home to improve what we had written,

and the second draft was sent round to everyone for comments in an attempt to improve the clarity, remove duplication, fill in gaps and expunge as much remaining neurodogma, neurofantasy and neuroastrology as possible. Our final discussion was held at the Bordeaux stroke meeting in 1995, and the drinks that time were more in relief and celebration that the end was in sight. Home we all went to update the manuscript and make final improvements before handing over the whole lot to the publisher in January 1996.

This process may well have taken longer than a conventional multiauthor book in which all the sections are written in isolation. But it was surely more fun, and hopefully the result will provide a uniform and coherent view of the subject. It is, we hope, a 'how to do it' book, or at least a 'how we do it' book.

1.1.4 Using the book

This is not a stroke encyclopaedia. Many very much more comprehensive books and monographs are available now, or soon will be. Nor is this really a book to be read from cover to cover. Rather, it is a book that we would like to be used on stroke units and in clinics to help illuminate stroke management at various different stages, both at the level of the individual patient and for patients in general. So we would like it to be kept handy and referred to when a problem crops up: how should swallowing difficulties be identified and managed? Should an angiogram be done? Is raised plasma fibrinogen a cause of stroke? How many beds should a stroke unit have? And so on. If a question is not addressed at all, then we would like to know about it so that it can be dealt with in the next edition, if there is to be one, which will clearly depend on sales, the publisher, and enough congenial European stroke conferences to keep us going.

It should be fairly easy to find one's way around the book from the chapter headings and the contents list at the beginning of each chapter. If that fails, then the index will do instead. We have used a lot of cross-referencing to guide the reader from any starting point and so avoid constant reference to the index.

As mentioned earlier, we have tried to be as selective as possible with the referencing. On the one hand, we want to allow readers access to the relevant literature, but on the other hand we do not want the text to be overwhelmed by references – particularly by references to unsound work. To be selective, we have tried to cite recent evidence-based systematic reviews and classic papers describing important work. Other references can probably mostly be found by those who want to dig deeper in the reference lists of the references we have cited.

Finally, we have liberally scattered what some would call practice points and other maxims throughout the book. These we are all prepared to sign up to, at least in early 1996. Of course, as more evidence becomes available, some of these practice points will become out of date.

1.1.5 Why a stroke book now?

Stroke has been somewhat of a Cinderella area of medicine, at least with respect to the other two of the three most common fatal disorders in the developed world – coronary heart disease and cancer. But times are gradually changing, particularly in the last decade when stroke has been moving up the political agenda, when research has been expanding perhaps in the slipstream of coronary heart disease research, when treatments to prevent, if not treat, stroke have become available and when the pharmaceutical industry has taken more notice. It seems that there is so much information about stroke that many practitioners are beginning to be overwhelmed. Therefore, now is a good time to try to capture all this information, digest it and then write down a practical approach to stroke management based on the best available evidence and research. This is our excuse for putting together what we know and what we do not know, what we do and why we do it.

1.2 Introduction to the second edition

Whether we enjoyed our annual 'stroke book' dinners at the European stroke conferences too much to abandon them, or whether we thought there really was a lot of updating to do, we found ourselves working on this second edition four short years after the first. It has certainly helped to have been so much encouraged by the many people who seemed to like the book, and find it useful. We have kept to the same format, authors, and principles outlined above in the introduction to the first edition. The first step was for all of us to read the whole book again and collect together any new comments and criticisms for each of the other authors. We then rewrote our respective sections and circulated them to all the other authors for their further comments (and they were not shy in giving them). We prepared our final words in early 2000.

A huge technical advance since writing the first edition has been the widespread availability of e-mail and the use of the Internet. Even more than before, we have genuinely been able to write material together; one author does a first draft, sends it as an attachment across the world in seconds, the other author appends ideas and e-mails the whole attachment back to the first author, copying to other authors for comments perhaps, and so on until it is perfect. Of course, we still do not all agree about absolutely everything all of the time. After all, we want readers to have a feel for the rough and ragged growing edge of stroke research, where there is bound to be disagreement. If we all knew what to do for stroke patients there would be no need for randomized controlled trials to help us do better – an unrealistic scenario if ever there was one. So where there is uncertainty, and where we disagree, we have tried to make that plain. But, on the whole, we are all still prepared to sign up to the practice points.

In this second edition, we have been able to correct the surprising number of minor typographical errors and hope not to have introduced any more, get all the X-rays the right way up, improve on some of the figures, remove some duplication, reorder a few sections, put in some more subheadings to guide the readers, make the section on acute ischaemic stroke more directive, improve the index, and generally tidy the whole thing up. It should now be easier to keep track of intracranial venous thrombosis and, in response to criticism, we have extended the section on leukoaraiosis, even though it is not strictly either a cause or a consequence of stroke. We have also introduced citations to what we have called 'floating references' – in other words, published work that is constantly being changed and updated as new information becomes available. An obvious example is the *Cochrane Library*, which is updated every 3 months and available on CD-ROM and through the Internet. There are no page numbers, and the year of publication is always the present one. We have therefore cited such 'floating references' as being in the present year, 2000. But we know that this book will not be read much until the year 2001 and subsequent years, when readers will have to look at the contemporary *Cochrane Library*, not the one published in 2000. The same applies to the new *British Medical Journal* series called 'Clinical Evidence' which is being updated every 6 months, and to any websites that may be updated at varying intervals and are still very much worth directing readers towards.

Rather to our surprise, there is a lot of new information to get across on stroke. Compared with 4 years ago, the concept of organized stroke services staffed by experts in stroke care has taken root and has allowed the increasingly rapid assessment of patients with 'brain attacks'. It is no longer good enough to sit around waiting 24 h or more to see if a patient is going to have a transient ischaemic attack or a stroke, and then another 24 h for a computed tomography brain scan to exclude intracerebral haemorrhage. These days we have to assess and scan stroke patients as soon as they arrive in hospital, perhaps give thrombolysis to a few, and enter many more into clinical trials, start aspirin in ischaemic stroke, and get the multidisciplinary team involved – and all of this well within 24 h of symptom onset. Through the *Cochrane Library*, which was in its infancy when the first edition was published, there is now easy, regularly updated electronic access to systematic reviews of most of the acute interventions and secondary prevention strategies for stroke, although the evidence base for rehabilitation techniques is lagging behind. Catheter angiography is giving way to non-invasive imaging. Magnetic resonance techniques are racing ahead of the evidence as to how they should be used in routine clinical practice. For better or worse, coiling cerebral aneurysms is replacing clipping. The pharmaceutical industry is still tenaciously hanging on to the hope of 'neuroprotection' in acute ischaemic stroke, despite numerous disappointments. Hyperhomocysteinaemia and infections are the presently fashionable risk factors for ischaemic stroke, and they may or may not stand the test of time. So, in this second edition, we have tried to capture all these advances – and retreats – and set them in the context of an up-to-date understanding of the pathophysiology of stroke and the best available evidence of how to manage it. Of course, it is an impossible task, because something new is always just around the corner. But then 'breakthroughs' in medicine take time to mature – maybe years until the evidence becomes unassailable and is gradually accepted by front-line clinicians. And then we can all sit back doing what we believe to be 'the right thing' for a few more years until the next 'breakthrough' changes our view of the world yet again.

We hope that the ideas and recommendations in this book will be sufficient 99% of the time – at least for the next 4 years, when we will have to see about a third edition.

1.3 Introduction to the third edition

Six years have gone quickly by since the second edition, much has happened in stroke research and practice in the meantime, and two of the authors are on the edge of retirement – so it is time for this third edition of what we fondly refer to as 'the book'. Maybe because the original authors were feeling tired, or increasingly unable to cover in depth all we wanted to, or perhaps because we wanted to ensure our succession, we have recruited four new and younger authors, all of whom have worked closely with us over many years, and whose help we acknowledged in the earlier editions – Gabriel Rinkel, Peter Langhorne, Cathie Sudlow and Peter Rothwell. But, even with their help, the rewriting has had to compete with all the far less interesting things which we have to do these days to satisfy managers, regulatory authorities and others keen to track and measure our every move. And maybe there is less imperative to write books like this which are out of date in at least some ways even before they are published. But then searching the Internet for 'stroke' does not come up with a coherent account of the whole subject of managing stroke patients using the best available evidence, which is what this book is all about. So, with the help and encouragement of Blackwell Publishing, here is the third edition of 'the book' at last.

We have written the book as before with most of the authors commenting on most of the chapters before all the chapters were finally written in the form you can read them in now. Again, you will have to guess who wrote what because we can all lay claim to most of the book in some sense or another. There has been a slight change in the arrangement of the chapters, but loyal readers of the earlier editions will not find this too upsetting – they will still find what they want in more or less its familiar place, and as ever we hope the index has been improved. The practice points we all sign up to and our day-to-day practice should reflect them. The uncertainties we all share – they will be gradually resolved as more research is done, and more uncertainties will then be revealed. The biggest change in this edition is succumbing to the space saving offered by a numbered reference system, and a change in the colour scheme from a pastel green to various shades of purple.

As with the second edition, much has changed and there has been more updating than we originally anticipated – what we know about stroke has moved on. Neuroprotection is even less likely to be an effective treatment for ischaemic stroke than it was in the 1990s, we still argue about thrombolysis, clopidogrel cannot very often be recommended, carotid stenting has still to prove its worth, routine evacuation of intracerebral haemorrhage is definitely not a good idea, and hormone replacement therapy far from protecting against vascular disease actually seems to increase the risk. But on the positive side, much has improved in brain and vessel imaging, it is now clear how much blood pressure lowering has to offer in secondary stroke prevention, and cholesterol lowering too. Carotid surgery can now be targeted on the few who really need it, not recommended for the greater number who may or may not need it.

Coiling has more or less replaced clipping of intracranial aneurysms, an astonishing change in practice brought about by a large trial energetically led by an interventional neuroradiologist and neurosurgeon. And it is not just acute stroke that needs urgent attention nowadays, transient ischaemic attacks must be assessed and managed very quickly to minimize the early high risk of stroke. Stroke services continue to improve all over the world, stroke has moved up the political agenda as we have managed to wrench it out of the rubric of 'cardiovascular' disease which always emphasized the cardiac rather than the cerebral, and more and more people are involved in stroke research, which is now a much more crowded and competitive field than it was when some of us started in the 1970s.

Will there be a fourth edition? We don't know; this will be in the hands of the remaining authors as Charles Warlow and Jan van Gijn dwindle into retirement of a sort, or at least a life that will not require the relentless battle to keep up with all the stroke literature, critique it, absorb anything that is worthwhile, and then put it into the context of active clinical practice. No one can write well about stroke unless they can connect research with their own active clinical practice – we are not, we hope, armchair theoreticians; we try to practise what we preach.

2 Development of knowledge about cerebrovascular disease

'Our knowledge of disorders of the cerebral circulation and its manifestations is deficient in all aspects' was the opening sentence of the chapter on cerebrovascular diseases in Oppenheim's textbook of neurology at the beginning of the 20th century.[1] More than 90 years later this still holds true, despite the considerable advances that have been made. In fact, the main reason for Oppenheim's lament, the limitations of pathological anatomy, is to some extent still valid. True, our methods of observation nowadays are no longer confined to the dead, as they were then. They have been greatly expanded, first by angiography, then by brain imaging and measurement of cerebral blood flow and metabolism, and most recently by non-invasive methods of vascular imaging such as ultrasound and magnetic resonance angiography. Yet, our observations are still mostly anatomical, and after the event. It is only in rare instances that are we able to reconstruct the dynamics of a stroke. At least in haemorrhagic stroke, brain computed tomography (CT) or magnetic resonance imaging (MRI) in the acute phase gives an approximate indication of where a blood vessel has ruptured (though not why exactly there and then) and how far the extravasated blood has invaded the brain parenchyma or the subarachnoid space. With ischaemic stroke, the growth of our understanding has been slower. The ubiquity of the term 'cerebral thrombosis' up to the 1970s exemplifies how deficient our understanding was even at that time.[2] Embolic occlusion, now known to result more often from arterial lesions than from the heart, can be detected in an early phase by non-invasive angiographic techniques or inferred by means of perfusion imaging, but so often the source of the clot is still elusive. We have also learned to distinguish many causes of cerebral infarction other than atherothrombosis, such as arterial dissection, mitochondrial cytopathies and moyamoya syndrome, but the precise pathogenesis of these conditions is still poorly understood.

So it is with humility, rather than in triumph, that we look back on the past. In each era the problems of stroke have been approached by the best minds, with the best tools available. Of course many ideas in the past were wrong, and so presumably are many of our own. Even though we are firm believers in evidence-based medicine, some – perhaps many or even most – of our own notions will not survive the test of time. Our knowledge may have vastly increased in the recent past but it is still a mere island in an ocean of ignorance.

Stroke: practical management, 3rd edition. C. Warlow, J. van Gijn, M. Dennis, J. Wardlaw, J. Bamford, G. Hankey, P. Sandercock, G. Rinkel, P. Langhorne, C. Sudlow and P. Rothwell. Published 2008 Blackwell Publishing. ISBN 978-1-4051-2766-0.

2.1 Ideas change slowly

The history of medicine, like that of kings and queens in world history, is usually described by a string of dates and names, by which we leapfrog from one discovery to another. The interval between such identifiable advances is measured in centuries when we describe the art of medicine at the beginning of civilization, but in mere years where our present times are chronicled. This leads to the impression that we are witnessing a dazzling explosion of knowledge. Some qualification of this view is needed, however. First of all, any generation of mankind takes a myopic view of history in that the importance of recent developments is overestimated. The Swedish Academy of Sciences therefore often waits for years, sometimes even decades, before awarding Nobel prizes, until scientific discoveries have withstood the test of time. When exceptions were made for the prize in medicine, the early accolades were not always borne out: Wagner-Jauregg's malaria treatment for neurosyphilis (1927) is no longer regarded as a landmark, while Moniz's prize (1949) for prefrontal leucotomy no longer seems justified; at least he also introduced contrast angiography of the brain, although this procedure may again not survive beyond the end of this century. We can only hope that the introduction of X-ray CT by Hounsfield (Nobel prize for medicine in 1979) will be judged equally momentous by future generations as by ourselves.

Another important caveat if one looks back on progress in medicine is that most discoveries gain ground only slowly. Even if new insights were quickly accepted by peer scientists, which was often not the case, it could still be decades before these had trickled down to the rank and file of medical practitioners. The mention of a certain date for a discovery may create the false impression that this change in medical thinking occurred almost overnight, like the introduction of the single European currency. In most instances, this was far from the truth. An apt example is the extremely slow rate at which the concept of lacunar infarction became accepted by the medical community, despite its potentially profound implications in terms of pathophysiology, treatment and prognosis. The first pathological descriptions date from around 1840,[3,4] but it took the clinicopathological correlations of C. Miller Fisher (Fig. 2.7) in the 1960s before the neurological community and its textbooks started to take any notice.[5–7] And it was not until new techniques for brain imaging in the 1980s provided instantaneous clinicoanatomical correlations that no practising neurologist could avoid knowing about lacunar infarcts – some 150 years after the first description! It is best to become reconciled to the idea that a slow rate of diffusion of new knowledge is unavoidable. The problem is one of all times. Franciscus Biumi, one of the early pathologists, lamented in 1765: *'Sed difficile est adultis novas opiniones inserere, evellere insitas'* (But it is difficult to insert new opinions in adults and to remove rooted ones).[8] How slowly new ideas were accepted and acted upon, against

the background of contemporary knowledge, can often be inferred from textbooks, particularly if written by full-time clinicians rather than by research-minded neurologists. Therefore we shall occasionally quote old textbooks to illustrate the development of thinking about stroke.

A reverse problem is that a new discovery or even a new fashion may be interpreted beyond its proper limits and linger on as a distorted idea for decades. Take the discovery of vitamin B_1 deficiency as the cause of a tropical polyneuropathy almost a century ago; the notion that a neurological condition, considered untreatable almost by definition, could be cured by a simple nutritional supplement made such an impact on the medical community that even in some industrialized countries vitamin B_1 is still widely used as a panacea for almost any neurological symptom.

So broadly speaking there are two kinds of medical history, that of the cutting edge of research and that of the medical profession as a whole. The landmarks are easy to identify only with the hindsight of present knowledge. In reality, new ideas often only gradually dawned on consecutive scientists, instead of the popular notion of a blinding flash of inspiration occurring in a single individual. For this reason, accounts of the history of stroke are not always identical.[9,10] Also many important primary sources are not easy to interpret – not only because they were written in Latin, but also because 'new observations' have sometimes been identified only by later historians, in retrospect, while the authors at the time attached no importance to them.[11]

2.2 The anatomy of the brain and its blood supply

From at least the time of Hippocrates (460–370 BC), the brain was credited with intelligence and thought, and also with movements of the opposite side of the body, through observation of unilateral convulsions after head wounds on the contralateral side.[12] Yet, stroke, or 'apoplexy' (Greek for 'being struck down'), was defined as a sudden but mostly general, rather than focal, disorder of the brain. The pathogenesis was explained according to the humoral theory, which assumed a delicate balance between the four humours: blood, phlegm, black bile and yellow bile. Anatomy played almost no part in these explanations. Apoplexy was often attributed to accumulation of black bile in the arteries of the brain, obstructing the passage of animated spirits from the ventricles.[13] Galenus of Pergamon (131–201), a prolific writer and animal experimenter whose views dominated medicine up to the 17th century,[14] distinguished 'karos' from 'apoplexy', in that respiration was unaffected in the former condition.[15] Leading Islamic physicians like Avicenna (980–1037) tried to reconcile Galenic tenets with the Aristotelian view of the heart as the seat of the mind.[16] In Western Europe, mostly deprived of Greek learning until the fall of Constantinople in 1453 prompted the Renaissance,[17] these Arabic texts were translated into Latin before those of Galen and Hippocrates.[18] All these theories had no anatomical counterpart; dissection of the human body was precluded by its divine connotations. Any illustrations of the human brain that are known before the 16th century are crude and schematic representations of Galenic theories, rather than attempts at copying the forms of nature. As a consequence, many non-neurological disease conditions with sudden onset must have been misclassified as 'apoplexy'.

In 1543 Andries van Wesele (1514–1564), the great Renaissance anatomist who Latinized his name to Andreas Vesalius, produced the first accurate drawings of the brain in his famous book *De humani corporis fabrica libri septem*, with the help of the draughtsman Johan Stephaan van Calcar and the printer Oporinus in Basle.[19] It was the same year in which Copernicus published *De revolutionibus*, proclaiming the sun and not the earth as the centre of the universe.[20] Vesalius largely ignored the blood vessels of the brain, although he retracted an earlier drawing (Fig. 2.1) depicting a '*rete mirabile*', a network of blood vessels at the base of the brain that

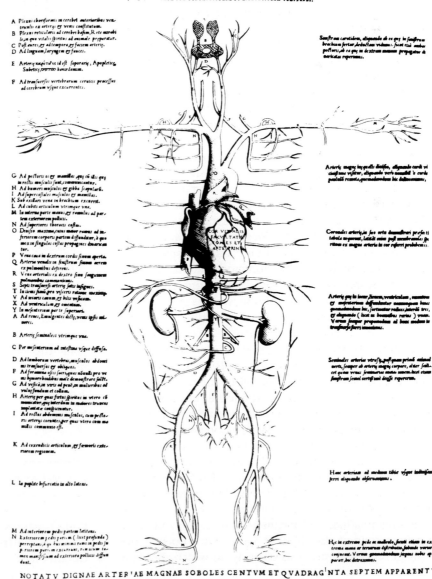

Fig. 2.1 Plate depicting the blood vessels, from Vesalius's *Tabulae Anatomicae Sex*, of 1538.[21] This shows the carotid arteries ending up in a network (b) at the base of the brain; the structures marked (a) represent the choroid plexus in the lateral ventricles. The network of blood vessels (*rete mirabile*) is found in oxen; Galen had assumed it was found also in the human brain, a belief perpetuated throughout the Dark and Middle Ages, up to the early Renaissance. Leonardo da Vinci had also drawn a (human?) brain with a '*rete mirabile*' at its base.[22] Vesalius retracted the existence of a network in his atlas of 1543.

Galen had found in pigs and oxen and that had been extrapolated to the human brain ever since.[21,22] Before him, Berengario da Carpi had also denied the existence of the *rete*.[23] Vesalius was vehemently attacked by traditionally minded contemporaries as an iconoclast of Galenic dogmas. Nevertheless, initially, he did not go as far as outright opposition to the central Galenic tenet that blood could pass through the septum between the right and left ventricle of the heart, allowing the mixture of blood and air and the elimination of 'soot'. Instead, he praised the creator for having made the openings so small that nobody could detect them, another striking example of how the power of theory may mislead even the most inquisitive minds. Only later, in the 1555 edition of his *De humani corporis fabrica*, did he firmly state that the interventricular septum was tightly closed. The decisive blow to the humoral theory came in 1628, through the description of the circulation by William Harvey (1578–1657);[24] it need no longer surprise us that it took many decades before these views were widely accepted. Harvey's work formed the foundation for the recognition of the role of blood vessels in the pathogenesis of stroke.

Thomas Willis (1641–1675) is remembered not so much for having coined the term 'neurology', or for his iatrochemical theories, a modernized version of humoral medicine, or for his part in the successful resuscitation of Ann Green after judicial hanging,[25] as he is for his work on the anatomy of the brain, first published in 1664,[26] especially for his description of the vascular interconnections at the base of the brain (Fig. 2.2).[27] Before him, Fallopius, Casserio, Vesling and Wepfer had all observed at least part of the circle,[28–31] in the case of Casserio and Vesling even with an illustration.[32] But undisputedly, it was Willis who grasped the functional implications of these anastomoses in a passage illustrating his proficiency in performing necropsies as well as postmortem experiments (from a posthumous translation):[33]

We have elsewhere shewed, that the *Cephalick* Arteries, viz. the *Carotides*, and the *Vertebrals*, do so communicate with one another, and all of them in different places, are so ingraffed one in another mutually, that if it happen, that many of them should be stopped or pressed together at once, yet the blood being admitted to the Head, by the passage of one Artery only, either the *Carotid* or the *Vertebral*, it would presently pass thorow all those parts exterior and interior: which indeed we have sufficiently proved by an experiment, for that Ink being squirted in the trunk of one Vessel, quickly filled all the sanguiferous passages, and every where stained the Brain it self. I once opened the dead Carcase of one wasted away, in which the right

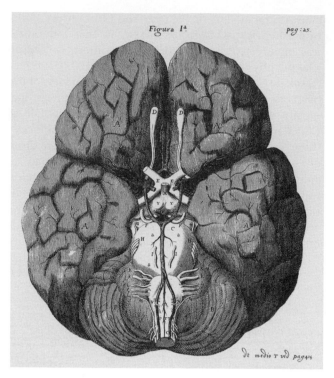

Fig. 2.2 Illustration of the base of the brain from Willis's *Cerebri Anatome* (1664),[26] showing the interconnections between the right and left carotid systems, and also between these two and the posterior circulation (drawing by Christopher Wren).

Arteries, both the *Carotid* and the *Vertebral*, within the Skull, were become bony and impervious, and did shut forth the blood from that side, notwithstanding the sick person was not troubled with the astonishing Disease.

It seems that the idea of infusing coloured liquids into blood vessels, practised from 1659 onwards and later perfected by Frederik Ruysch (1638–1731) and in the next century by John Hunter (1728–1793),[34,35] had come from Christopher Wren (1632–1723).[25] Wren also made the etchings for Willis's book (he is now mainly remembered as the architect of St Paul's Cathedral and many other churches built after the great fire of London in 1666).

2.3 What happens in 'apoplexy'?

Willis's 'astonishing Disease', apoplexy, had of old intuitively been attributed to some ill-defined obstruction, whether from want of 'animal spirits' via the nerves in the tradition of Greek medicine, or, after Harvey's time, by deprivation of blood flow. Yet, it should be remembered that the notion of an intrinsic 'nervous energy' only slowly lost ground. Even the great 18th-century physician Boerhaave, though clearly recognizing the role of blood vessels and the heart in the development of apoplexy, invoked obstruction of the cerebrospinal fluid.[36] In Table 2.1 we have provided a schematic representation of the development of ideas about apoplexy through the ages, together with its relationship to arterial lesions. That Willis had found 'bony' and 'impervious' arteries in patients who actually had not died from a stroke was probably the reason that he was not outspoken on the pathogenesis of apoplexy. His contemporaries, Wepfer (1620–1695) in Schaffhausen, and Bayle (1622–1709) in Toulouse, only tentatively associated apoplexy with 'corpora fibrosa',[31] or with calcification of cerebral arteries.[37]

Wepfer (Fig. 2.3) not only recognized arterial lesions, but he also prompted one of the great advances in the knowledge about stroke by distinguishing between, on the one hand, arterial obstruction preventing the influx of blood and, on the other, extravasation of blood into the substance of the brain or the ventricular cavities. His interpretation was, however, that blockage of arteries as well as extravasation of blood impeded the transmission of 'spiritus animalis' to the brain.[11] Accordingly, he regarded apoplexy as a process of global stunning of the brain, while the focal nature of the disease largely escaped him. The four cases of haemorrhage Wepfer described were massive, at the base of the brain or deep in the parenchyma. In cases with obvious hemiplegia, incidentally a term dating back to the Byzantine physician Paulus Aegineta (625–690),[38] Wepfer suspected dysfunction of the ipsilateral rather than the contralateral side. He also observed patients who had recovered from apoplectic attacks, and noted that those most liable to apoplexy were 'the obese, those whose face and hands are livid, and those whose pulse is constantly unequal'.

That the paralysis was on the opposite side of the apoplectic lesion was clearly predicted by Domenico Mistichelli (1675–1715) from Pisa on the basis of his observation of the decussation of the pyramids (Fig. 2.4).[39] A landmark in the recognition of the anatomical substrate of stroke – and of many other diseases – was the work of Morgagni (1682–1771), professor of medicine and subsequently of pathological anatomy in Padua. In 1761 Morgagni published an impressive series of clinico-pathological observations collected over a lifetime (he

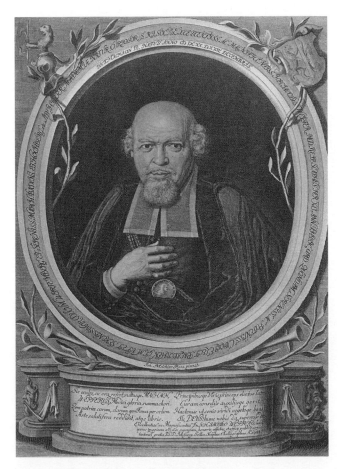

Fig. 2.3 Johann Jakob Wepfer (1620–1695).

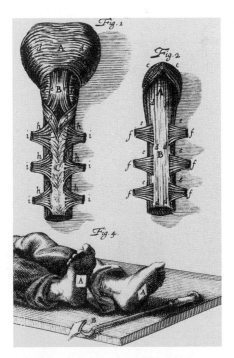

Fig. 2.4 Illustration from Mistichelli's book on apoplexy (1709) in which he shows the decussation of the pyramids and also the outward rotation of the leg on the paralysed side.[39]

Table 2.1 Development of ideas about 'apoplexy' and its relationship with arterial lesions.

Medical scientist	Ideas about 'apoplexy'		Medical scientist	Observations on arterial lesions	Historical events
	Haemorrhagic	Non-haemorrhagic			
Hippocrates (Kos) (460–370 BC)[13]	Sudden loss of consciousness, as a result of brain disease				0 Birth of Jesus Christ
Galenus (Pergamum and Rome) (131–201)[15]	Sudden loss of consciousness, as a result of brain disease				
Wepfer (Schaffhausen) (1620–1695)[31]	Extravasation of blood in brain tissue (1658)		Wepfer (1658)	'Corpora fibrosa'	1642 Rembrandt paints *Night Watch*
			Bayle (Toulouse) (1622–1709)[37]	Calcifications (1677)	1682 Peter I ascends Russian throne
Mistichelli (Pisa) (1675–1715)[39]		Paralysis is unilateral, and crossed with respect to lesion (1709)	Willis (Oxford) (1621–1675)[33]	'Bony, impervious arteries' (1684)	1707 Union between England and Scotland
Boerhaave (Leiden) (1668–1738)[36]	'Stoppage of the spirits'		Boerhaave	Narrowing due to cartilaginous change (1735)	1729 Bach writes *St Matthew Passion*
Morgagni (Padua) (1682–1771)[40]	'Sanguineous apoplexy' (1761)	'Serous apoplexy', extravasation of serum? (1761)	Baillie (London) (1761–1823)[42]	Hardening of arteries associated with haemorrhage? (1795)	1776 US Declaration of Independence
Rostan (Paris) (1790–1866)[57]		'Ramollissement' (1820): – softening more frequent than haemorrhage – condition not inflammatory?	Rostan	Ossification of cerebral arteries (1820)	1815 Battle of Waterloo; Schubert writes *Erlkönig*

Lallemand (Montpelier) (1790–1853)[58]	Cerebral softening is definitely inflammatory in nature (1824)	Lobstein (Strasbourg) (1777–1835)[67]	'Arteriosclerosis' (1829)	1829 Stephenson builds the railway engine called 'The Rocket'
Abercrombie (Edinburgh) (1780–1844)[60]	Cerebral softening analogous to gangrene of limb? (1836)	Abercrombie	Due to ossification of arteries?	1837 Queen Victoria ascends the throne of the British Empire
Carswell (London) (1793–1857)[62]	Cerebral softening caused by obliteration of arteries? (one of possible causes; 1838)			1848 Year of revolutions; Louis Napoleon elected president of France
Rokitansky (Vienna) (1804–1878)[219]	'Encephalomalacia' (1844): – white, or serous (congestion) – red (inflammatory) – yellow (frequent; unexplained)			1859 Darwin publishes *The Origin of Species* 1863 Manet paints *Le Déjeuner sur l'herbe*
Cruveilhier (Paris) (1791–1874)[63]	Cerebral softening caused by capillary congestion, secondary to 'irritation' (1842)	Virchow	Arteriosclerosis leads to thrombosis; thrombi may be torn off and lodge distally ('embolism') (1856)	1869 Opening of the Suez Canal 1871 Stanley meets Livingstone at Ujiji
Virchow (Berlin) (1821–1902)[66]	'Yellow softening' of the brain is secondary to arterial obliteration; any inflammation is secondary (1856)	Cohnheim	End-arteries most vulnerable; paradoxical embolism	1877 Bell invents telephone, Edison the phonograph
Cohnheim (Berlin) (1839–1884)[68]	'Infarction' (stuffing) is haemorrhagic by definition, as opposed to ischaemic necrosis (1872)	Chiari (Prague) (1851–1916)[70]	Thrombosis at the carotid bifurcation may cause secondary embolization to brain (1905)	1895 Röntgen discovers X-rays in Würzburg 1907 Ehrlich introduces arsphenamine as treatment for syphilis

was 79 at the time of publication), in which he firmly put an end to the era of systemic (humoral) theories of disease and replaced them by an organ-based approach, though he did not include even a single illustration; characteristically, the title of the book was *'De sedibus et causis morborum . . .'* (about the sites and causes of disease).[40] Morgagni not only confirmed the notion of crossed paralysis but also firmly divided apoplexy into 'sanguineous apoplexy' and 'serous apoplexy' (and a third form which was neither serous nor sanguineous). A decade later, Portal (1742–1832) rightly emphasized that it was impossible to distinguish between these two forms during life.[41] However, it would be a mistake to assume that 'serous' (non-haemorrhagic) apoplexy was recognized at that time as being the result of impaired blood flow, let alone of mechanical obstruction of blood vessels. Some even linked the arterial hardening with brain haemorrhages and not with the serous apoplexies.[42] Although we quoted 17th-century scientists such as Bayle and Wepfer in that they associated some non-haemorrhagic cases of apoplexy with obstruction of blood flow, in the 18th century medical opinion swayed towards 'vascular congestion', a kind of pre-haemorrhagic state. That explanation was propounded not only by Morgagni[40] but also by many of his contemporaries and followers.[41,43,44] John Cheyne (1777–1836) pointed out that autopsy in patients who had survived a 'stroke of apoplexy' for a considerable time might show a cavity filled with rusty serum that stained the adjacent brain tissue, but he may have been describing a residual lesion after cerebral haemorrhage rather than infarction.[45]

The anatomical, organ-based approach exemplified by Morgagni reflected the Italian practice, in which the separation between physicians and surgeons was much less strict than in northern Europe with its more theoretical framework of medicine. The protagonists of the Northern school of thinking were Herman Boerhaave (1668–1738) in Leiden and later William Cullen (1710–1790) in Edinburgh, the most influential clinical teachers of their time. They established a nosological classification that was based much more on holistic theory, in terms of a disturbed system, than on actual observations at the level of the organ, at least with 20th-century hindsight.[46] Probably our own time will be branded as the era of exaggerated reductionism! In the intellectual tradition of the Dutch-Scottish school, purely clinical classifications of apoplexy were proposed in the early 19th century by Serres (with and without paralysis),[47] by Abercrombie (primary apoplexy, with deprivation of sense and motion, and sometimes with convulsions, a second type beginning with headache, and a third type with loss of power on one side of the body and of speech, often with recovery),[48] and by Hope and Bennett (transient apoplexy, primary apoplexy with death or slow

recovery, ingravescent apoplexy with partial recovery and relapse, and paraplexic apoplexy with paralysis).[49]

There are several reasons why the brain lesion in what we now call cerebral infarction was not identified until the middle of the 19th century. First, it was impossible to recognize ischaemic softening in patients who had usually died not long after their stroke. Fixation methods were not available until the end of the 18th century; Vicq d'Azyr, Marie Antoinette's physician, was the first to use alcohol as a tissue fixative,[50] while formaldehyde fixation was not employed until a century later.[51] Second, it is probable that many patients diagnosed as having died from apoplexy in fact had suffered from other conditions. If in our time the diagnosis is wrong in 20–30% of patients referred with a presumed stroke,[52–54] the diagnostic accuracy was presumably no better in centuries past.

2.4 Cerebral infarction (ischaemic stroke)

After Morgagni's seminal book the organ-based approach to medicine quickly spread from Italy to other countries. In France, the first proponents were surgeons. After the French revolution the strict distinction between medicine and surgery disappeared, driven by the reorganization of hospital care (no longer managed by the church but by the state) and by the need to train a large number of new doctors, for military as well as civilian duties ('peu lire, beaucoup voir, beaucoup faire').[55,56] It was Leon Rostan (1790–1866; Fig. 2.5), a physician at the Salpêtrière in Paris, who clearly recognized softening of the brain as a separate lesion, distinct from haemorrhage, although the pathogenesis still escaped him. He published his findings in an unillustrated monograph, the first edition of which appeared in 1820.[57] The lesions were most commonly found in the corpus striatum, thalamus or centrum semiovale, but they also occurred in the cerebral cortex, brainstem and cerebellum. Old cases showed a yellowish-green discoloration, whereas if the patients had died soon after the event the colour of the lesion was chestnut or reddish. The softening might be so extreme as to lead to the formation of a cyst. In other patients it was difficult to detect any change in firmness or in colour. Rostan distinguished softening of the brain from 'apoplexy', a term he no longer used for stroke in general, but which he regarded as being synonymous with haemorrhagic stroke. He supposed that softening of the brain was more common than brain haemorrhage, although some haemorrhages were secondary to softening. The clinical manifestations were thought

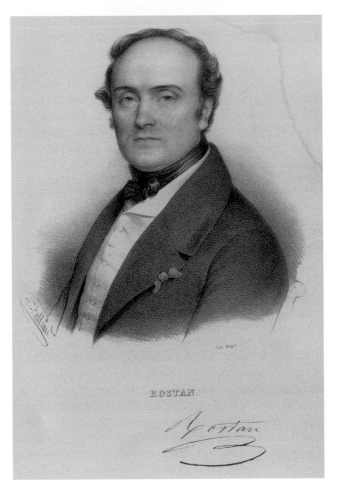

Fig. 2.5 Léon Rostan (1790–1866).

to occur in two stages: first 'fugitive' disturbances in the use of a limb, in speech or in visual or auditory perception, sooner or later followed by hemiplegia and coma, in a slowly progressive fashion.

Although Rostan recognized 'ossification' of the cerebral arteries, he did not associate these lesions with cerebral softening via obstruction of the arterial system. At any rate he doubted the prevailing opinion that the primary lesion was some kind of inflammatory response. After all, there was redness and swelling (*rubor*, *tumor*), if not warmth and pain (*calor*, *dolor*), to complete the cardinal signs of inflammation delineated by Celsus in the first century AD. Rostan's contemporary Lallemand (1790–1853) was much more outspoken and had little doubt that inflammation was at the root of cerebral softening.[58] Readers trained in the 21st century may find this difficult to understand but they should be aware that 'inflammation' was a rather common explanation for disease from the middle of the 18th century until some hundred years later.[46] Just as in our time some poorly understood medical conditions are often interpreted in terms of autoimmune disease, perhaps erroneously, inflammation

seemed for a long time the most logical 'paradigm' to fall back on to explain liquefaction of brain tissue.[59]

The first inkling of a relationship between arterial disease and 'ramollissement', as many English writers continued to call brain softening in deference to Rostan, was voiced by Abercrombie, in a later edition of his text-book.[60] He drew an analogy with gangrene, caused by 'failure of circulation', this in turn being secondary to 'ossification of arteries'. The role of arterial obstruction as a primary cause of softening of the brain was confirmed by others,[61,62] but the theory of inflammation continued to be defended by a few adherents.[63,64] Some were aware that apoplexy could be caused by 'cerebral anaemia' (as opposed to congestion), not only through loss of blood but also by a reduced vascular pressure, particularly in the case of heart disease.[44]

Other missing links in the understanding of cerebral infarction were clarified by Rokitansky (1804–1878) in Vienna and by Virchow (1821–1902) in Berlin. Rokitansky divided cerebral softening (which he termed encephalomalacia) into three varieties: red (haemorrhagic) softening, inflammatory in nature; white softening (synonymous with 'serous apoplexy') caused by congestion and oedema; and, the most common variety, yellow softening, of which the pathogenesis was unknown.[219] Virchow (Fig. 2.6) revolutionized medical thinking about vascular disease by firmly putting the

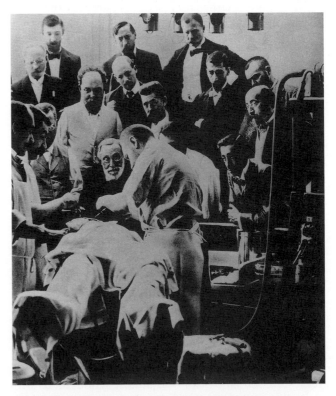

Fig. 2.6 Rudolph Virchow (1821–1902) teaching at a postmortem in the Charité Hospital in Berlin.

emphasis on changes in the vessel wall rather than in blood; Schiller called it the victory of 'solidism' over 'humoralism'.[9] Virchow also firmly established that thrombosis of arteries was caused not by inflammation but by fatty metamorphosis of the vessel wall, even if he had to found his own journal before his papers could be published.[65,66] To describe the changes in the arterial wall Virchow revived the term 'arteriosclerosis', first used by Lobstein.[67] Virchow's disciple Julius Cohnheim coined the culinary term 'infarction' (from the Latin verb *infarcire*, 'to stuff into'), but strictly reserved it for haemorrhagic necrosis ('stuffing', by seeping of blood into ischaemic tissue, through damaged walls of capillaries) as opposed to ischaemic necrosis.[68]

2.5 Thrombosis and embolism

Virchow observed thrombosis as the result of atherosclerosis, and also embolism, in patients with gangrene of the lower limbs caused by clots from the heart. The term 'embolism' was newly coined by him, at least in medical parlance. He extrapolated these events to the cause of cerebral softening:

> Here there is either no essential change in the vessel wall and its surroundings, or this is ostensibly secondary. I feel perfectly justified in claiming that these clots never originated in the local circulation but that they are torn off at a distance and carried along in the blood stream as far as they can go.[65]

The relationship between vegetations on the heart valves and stroke had in fact been suggested a century earlier by Boerhaave's pupil Gerard van Swieten, personal physician to the Austrian empress Maria Theresa and founder of the Viennese school of medicine:

> It has been established by many observations that these polyps occasionally attach themselves as excrescences to the columnae carneae of the heart, and perhaps then separate from it and are propelled, along with the blood, into the pulmonary artery or the aorta, and its branches . . . were they thrown into the carotid or vertebral arteries, could disturb – or if they completely blocked all approach of arterial blood to the brain – utterly abolish the functions of the brain.[69]

For more than a century after Virchow's accurate pathological descriptions of arterial occlusions, the term 'cerebral embolism' was almost synonymous with embolism from the heart (parenthetically, it still is, in many contemporary textbooks and papers – another

illustration of how slowly ideas change). Sources of embolism in the extracranial arteries were hardly considered until the 1960s, at least in teaching. By the same token, the term 'cerebral thrombosis' remained firmly entrenched in clinical thinking as being more or less synonymous with cerebral infarction without associated heart disease, the implication being that in these cases the site of the atheromatous occlusion was in the intracranial vessels. For example, this is what the sixth edition of Brain's *Diseases of the Nervous System* says on the subject in 1968:

> Progressive occlusion of cerebral blood vessels impairs the circulation in the regions they supply. The effects of this depend upon the size and situation of the vessel, and the rate of onset of the occlusion particularly in relation to the collateral circulation. Actual obstruction of an artery by atheroma, with or without subsequent thrombosis, causes softening of the region of the brain supplied by the vessel.[2]

That the notion of 'local thrombosis' persisted for such a long time must have been because of its appealing simplicity, not by lack of observations to the contrary. As long ago as 1905, Chiari drew attention to the frequency of atherosclerosis in the region of the carotid bifurcation and suggested that embolization of atheromatous material might be a cause of cerebral softening,[70] and not much later Hunt described the relationship between carotid occlusion and stroke.[71] The much later general acceptance of *extracranial* atherosclerosis as an important cause of cerebral ischaemia was prompted by two further developments. The first was the attention generated by Fisher's studies, in which he re-emphasized the role of atherosclerosis at the carotid bifurcation, at least in white patients.[72] He clinically correlated these lesions not only with contralateral hemiplegia but also with attacks of monocular blindness in the ipsilateral eye.[73] The second development was imaging. Cerebral angiography by direct puncture of the carotid artery had been introduced by Moniz in 1927,[74,75] but imaging of the carotid bifurcation in patients with stroke became common only after the advent of catheter angiography,[76] and later of ultrasound techniques. Now it is modern CT or MR angiography that often shows abnormalities of the internal carotid artery near its origin, at least in patients with transient or permanent deficits in the territory of the main trunk of the middle cerebral artery or one of its branches. The earlier patients are investigated, the greater the chance of detecting the site where the embolus has become impacted in the cerebral arterial tree. The therapeutic implications of identifying lesions in the carotid artery in symptomatic patients became clear through the two large randomized controlled trials of carotid endarterectomy in the 1980s and 1990s, which showed overall benefit from the operation for severe degrees of stenosis.[77]

In 25–30% of patients with temporary or permanent occlusion of large intracranial vessels no source of embolism can be found in the neck or in the heart.[78,79] Pathological observations suggesting that the aorta may harbour atherosclerotic lesions[80] have been confirmed in a large autopsy series and by transoesophageal echocardiography during life.[81,82] Of course, there is more to ischaemic stroke than embolism from large vessels, but the history of small vessel disease and non-atheromatous causes of ischaemia is rather more recent.

Before concluding the sections on cerebral infarction, thrombosis and embolism, we should like briefly to draw attention to the term 'cerebrovascular accident', which enjoyed some undeserved popularity in the middle half of the last century. The problem was that sometimes the term was used as a synonym for cerebral infarction, at other times to denote stroke in general. In this day and age the term is a highly specific sign of woolly thinking. We can do no better than quote Schiller:[9]

That rather blurry and pompous piece of nomenclature must have issued from the well-meant tendency to soften the blow to patients and their relatives, also from a desire to replace 'stroke', a pithy term that may sound unscientific and lacking gentility. 'Cerebrovascular accident (CVA)' can be traced to the early 1930s – between 1932, to be exact, when it was still absent from the 15th edition of *Dorland's Medical Dictionary*, and the following edition of 1936 where it first appeared.

The occasional medical student or junior doctor who still takes refuge in the term 'CVA' in an attempt to cover up ignorance about the precise type of cerebrovascular event in a given patient (while avoiding sharing the term 'stroke' with the laity) should either find out or come clean about not knowing.

2.6 Transient ischaemic attacks

It is difficult to trace the first descriptions of what we now call transient ischaemic attacks (TIAs) of the brain or eye, because symptoms representing focal deficits were not clearly distinguished from non-specific symptoms of a more global nature such as fainting or headache.[83] Wepfer recorded that he had seen patients who recovered from hemiplegia in one day or less.[31] An 18th-century account has been retrieved in the patient's own words, not muddled by medical interpretation, which makes it as lucid as it would have been today.

The subject is Jean Paul Grandjean de Fouchy, writing in 1783, at the age of 76 years:[84]

Toward the end of dinner, I felt a little increase of pain above the left eye and in that very instant I became unable to pronounce the words that I wanted. I heard what was said, and I thought of what I ought to reply, but I spoke other words than those which would express my thoughts, or if I began them I did not complete them, and I substituted other words for them. I had nevertheless all movements as freely as usual . . . I saw all objects clearly, I heard distinctly what was being said; and the organs of thought were, it seemed to me, in a natural state. This sort of paroxysm lasted almost a minute.

Once it had become established, in the middle of the 19th century, that cerebral softening was not caused by an inflammatory process but by occlusion of cerebral arteries, temporary episodes of ischaemia were recognized increasingly often in the next few decades.[1,85–89] In the course of time, three main theories have been invoked to explain the pathophysiology of TIAs, at least in relation to atherosclerosis: the vasospasm theory, the haemodynamic theory and the thromboembolic theory.[83]

2.6.1 The vasospasm theory

Arterial spasm as a cause of gangrene of the extremities was described by Raynaud (1834–1881) in his doctoral thesis of 1862.[90] Others extrapolated his theory of vasospasm to the cerebral circulation.[91,92] Russel, writing in 1909 about a 50-year-old farmer who had suffered three attacks of tingling and numbness in the right arm and the right side of the face, dismissed thrombosis ('Thrombus, once formed, does not break up and disappear in some mysterious way') and instead invoked a phenomenon of 'local syncope', analogous to Raynaud's disease or some cases of migraine: 'There must be some vessel constriction, local in site, varying in degree and in extent, coming and going, intermittent'.[92] Even the great Osler mounted the bandwagon of the vasospastic theory to explain transient attacks of aphasia and paralysis: 'We have plenty of evidence that arteries may pass into a state of spasm with obliteration of the lumen and loss of function in the parts supplied'.[89] Vasospasm remained the most popular theory to explain TIAs in the first half of the 20th century and provided the rationale for so-called cerebral vasodilators. Up to the 1980s these useless drugs were still widely prescribed in some European countries, not only for TIAs but for 'senility' in general; in France they were the third most commonly prescribed medication in 1982.[93]

In the front line of medicine, however, the vasospastic theory went into decline soon after World War II, firstly because the cerebral arteries are among the least reactive in the body,[94,95] and secondly because more plausible theories emerged (see below). Only under strictly defined conditions can vasospasm be a causal factor in the pathogenesis of cerebral ischaemia, that is, after subarachnoid haemorrhage or in association with migraine, and even in these conditions its role is contentious. Nevertheless, vasospasm has resurfaced as a possible cause of episodes of transient monocular blindness that are frequent and stereotyped and have no altitudinal distribution,[96] or even of transient motor or sensory deficits not related to migraine.[97] Such events must be extremely rare.

2.6.2 The haemodynamic theory

The notion of 'low flow' without *acute* vessel obstruction as a cause of cerebral ischaemia should perhaps be attributed to Ramsay Hunt, who drew an analogy between the symptoms of carotid stenosis or occlusion and the symptoms of intermittent claudication in patients with severe peripheral arterial disease.[71] But, it was especially after 1951, when Denny-Brown suggested that TIAs might be caused by 'episodic insufficiency in the circle of Willis',[95] that interest in the haemodynamic aspects of TIAs was fully aroused. Indeed, it was mainly the surgical community for which the concept of 'cerebral intermittent claudication' continued to have great appeal, despite the incongruity of the relatively constant blood flow to the brain and the large fluctuations in flow that occur in the legs, depending on their level of activity.

Clinical studies failed to support the notion of haemodynamic failure. After artificial lowering of the blood pressure by means of hexamethonium and postural tilting, in 35 patients who had either experienced TIAs or who had known carotid artery disease, only one of the patients developed symptoms of focal cerebral ischaemia before a syncopal attack which signified global rather than focal ischaemia of the brain.[98] Similarly, cerebral ischaemia with naturally occurring attacks of hypotension, such as cardiac arrhythmias, is almost always syncopal and not focal in nature,[99] and cardiac arrhythmias do not occur more often in patients with TIAs than in controls.[100] Once the first successful carotid reconstruction had been reported,[101] the intuitive belief in the haemodynamic theory led to an ever-increasing number of carotid endarterectomies being performed (indeed, often called 'carotid disobstruction') in patients with and even without TIAs, despite the absence of any formal proof of efficacy. These developments caused understandable concern in the neurological community.[102,103] Fortunately the controversy prompted well-designed clinical trials, which have served to define to a large extent the role of this operation.[77]

That the haemodynamic theory does not apply to most patients with TIAs is not to say that the exceptional patient cannot suffer from 'misery perfusion'.[104] In the presence of multiple occlusions or stenoses of the extracranial arteries, the haemodynamic reserve may be so poor that minor changes in systolic blood pressure cannot be compensated for. Such triggering events include a change from a sitting to a standing position, turning the head, heating of the face or looking into bright light.[105–107] Perhaps for this small group of patients extracranial-intracranial bypass surgery has something to offer after all, despite the negative results of the randomized trial in a large but relatively unselected group of patients with occlusion of the internal carotid or middle cerebral artery.[108]

2.6.3 The thromboembolic theory

In the 1950s C. Miller Fisher (Fig. 2.7) not only gave new impetus to some older observations about the relationship between stroke and atheromatous lesions of

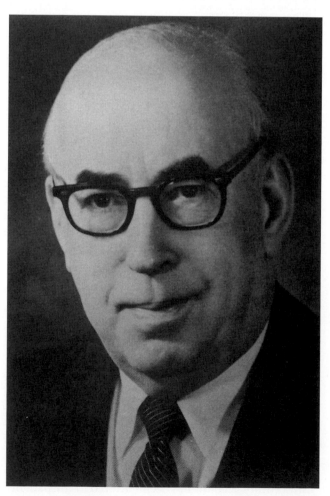

Fig. 2.7 C. Miller Fisher (1913–).

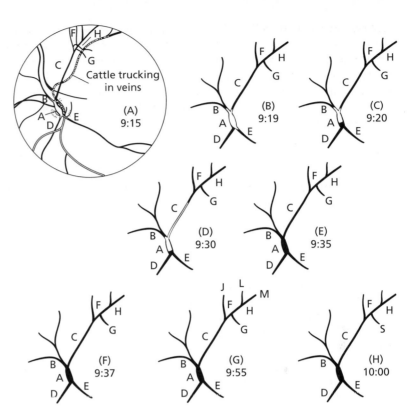

Fig. 2.8 Diagrams of observations in a patient with an attack of transient monocular blindness in the left eye (except the upper temporal quadrant); the attack had started at 8.55 am, 20 minutes before the beginning of the observations. The column of blood in the retinal arteries was in some places interrupted by white segments, initially at the stems of the superior and inferior retinal arteries (A); also the column of blood in at least six venous branches of the superior half of the retina was broken into transverse bands (so-called cattle trucking). The white segments in the retinal arteries slowly passed through the superior temporal artery (B–H). At (C) the vision in the upper half of the visual field had returned. At (D) a fine trickle of erythrocytes moved slowly along one side of white segment AB to the superior nasal artery, and at (E) vision had also returned in the inferior temporal quadrant. After (H), when the column of blood had been completely restored, vision returned to normal. (From Fisher, 1959;[109] by kind permission of the author and *Neurology*.)

the carotid bifurcation, but he also provided evidence that the pathogenesis was more complex than could be explained by fixed arterial narrowing. First, he saw a patient in whom hemiplegia had been preceded by attacks of transient monocular blindness in the contralateral eye, that is, 'the wrong eye'.[73] Second, through assiduous ophthalmoscopic observations, he saw white bodies passing slowly through the retinal arteries during an attack of transient monocular blindness (Fig. 2.8), the whitish appearance and friability of the moving material suggesting that these were emboli, largely made up of platelets.[109] These findings were confirmed by Ross Russell,[110] whilst others saw atheromatous emboli in the retinal vessels, which did not move but had become impacted.[111,112]

After these direct observations of the ocular fundus, additional – but more indirect – arguments corroborated the notion of artery-to-artery embolism as an important cause of TIAs.

- In many patients with attacks involving the cortical territory of the middle cerebral artery there is an associated lesion of the internal carotid artery, but in only very few of them is the stenosis severe enough, with a residual lumen of 1–2 mm, for blood flow to be impaired below critical levels, even assuming there is no collateral circulation.[113] In addition, the stenosis is constant but the episodes of ischaemia transient,

without evidence for cardiac arrhythmias as an additional factor.

- During carotid endarterectomy, fresh and friable thrombi are seen adherent to atheromatous plaques in the carotid bifurcation, especially in patients with recent attacks.[114]
- In patients with ocular as well as cerebral attacks, the two kinds of attack almost never occur at the same time.[114]
- Manual compression of the carotid artery may lead to dislodgement of atheromatous emboli to the cerebral circulation.[115]
- If patients continue to have TIAs after occlusion of the ipsilateral internal carotid artery, there is often an additional atheromatous lesion in the common carotid or external carotid artery, these vessels being important collateral channels, supplying the hemisphere via retrograde flow through the ophthalmic artery.[106]
- Asymptomatic emboli have been seen to flash up during angiography,[116] while fibrin thrombi have been seen to pass through a cortical artery during craniotomy for a bypass procedure.[117] Transcranial Doppler monitoring has uncovered an ongoing stream of high-intensity transient signals (HITS), probably small emboli, in patients with symptomatic carotid lesions.[118] The HITS disappear after carotid endarterectomy,[119] the rate depending on the interval since operation.[120]

Whilst artery-to-artery thromboembolism from atheromatous plaques may seem the most important factor in explaining TIAs and ischaemic strokes, it is not necessarily the only one, not even in a single individual patient. For example, it is probable that emboli have especially damaging effects in vascular beds that are chronically underperfused.

2.7 Intracerebral haemorrhage

Extravasation of blood into the brain parenchyma was recognized as early as 1658 by Wepfer,[31] although we commented above that he saw the clot as an obstruction of 'vital spirits' rather than as the disease in itself, and subsequently by Morgagni.[40] The cause remained obscure, and to a large extent it still is. In 1855, before blood pressure could be measured, Kirkes observed hypertrophy of the heart in 17 of 22 patients with fatal brain haemorrhage.[121] Charcot and Bouchard in 1868 examined the brains of patients who had died from intracerebral haemorrhage and immersed these in running water; they found multiple, minute outpouchings of small blood vessels, so-called miliary aneurysms.[122] The irony of these two names being joined is that Bouchard, once Charcot's pupil, in later years generated much hostility between himself and his former chief, because he wanted to found a school of his own and to be considered the most influential man in the faculty of

medicine.[123] It was in this adversarial atmosphere that in 1892 Bouchard, as president of the jury that had to judge the competition for the rank of *professeur agrégé*, did not admit Charcot's pupil Babinski.[124] Babinski subsequently left academic medicine by becoming chief of the Pitié hospital, where he devoted much time to the study of clinical signs, including the now famous 'toe sign'.[125] The aneurysms described by Charcot and Bouchard were white or brownish-coloured nodules about 0.5–2.0 mm in diameter, attached to a small arteriole, most often in the basal ganglia. At the beginning of the 20th century, Charcot and Bouchard's theory came under attack and some proposed that the primary lesion in intracerebral vessels was atherosclerosis, that most of these dilatations were not true aneurysms at all but false aneurysms caused by intramural dissection, while rupture could also occur by weakening of the vessel wall without previous aneurysm formation;[126] also some 'miliary aneurysms' may in fact have been clots in perivascular (Virchow-Robin) spaces.

Alternative explanations for the pathogenesis of primary intracerebral haemorrhage included primary necrosis of brain tissue or its vessels. Some assumed that arteries dilate and rupture only when a previous infarct had occurred, thus depriving the feeding vessel of its normal support.[127,128] The frequent coexistence of hypertension led to several theories other than plain rupture. Rosenblath postulated that a renal toxin caused necrosis of vessel walls,[129] Westphal that arterial spasm was an intermediate factor[130] and Schwartz that a multitude of terminal arterial branches became permeable.[224] In the 1960s injection techniques revived the notion

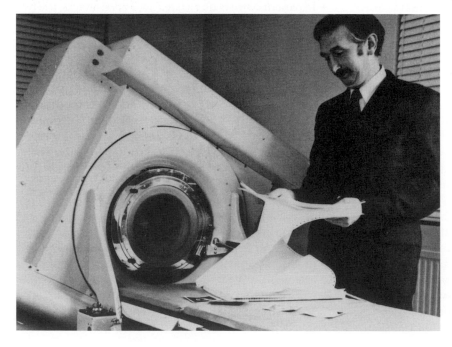

Fig. 2.9 Godfrey N. Hounsfield (1919– 2004), the British engineer who received the Nobel prize in medicine in 1979 for the development of computed tomography (together with the American physicist A.M. Cormack).

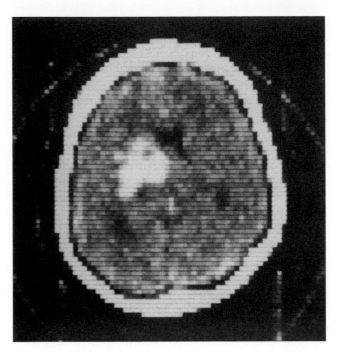

Fig. 2.10 CT scan of an intracerebral haemorrhage, from the early 1970s.[221]

of microaneurysms,[131,132] although some still suspect that the injection pressures can artifactually distend or rupture vessel walls.[133]

Amyloid angiopathy was first recognized as a cause of primary intracerebral haemorrhage in the first half of the 20th century.[134–136] This type of haemorrhage occurs especially at the border of white and grey matter and not in the deep regions of the brain that are the most common sites of haemorrhages associated with micro-aneurysms. The first series of such patients appeared in the 1970s.[137,138]

The invention of computed tomography by Hounsfield (1919–2004; Fig. 2.9) in the 1970s made it possible to distinguish intracerebral haemorrhage quickly and reliably from cerebral infarction (Fig. 2.10).[139,140]

2.8 Subarachnoid haemorrhage

The history of 'meningeal apoplexy' is relatively short. The disorder was not recognized until three years before the battle of Waterloo; in the following 125 years numerous accounts appeared that combined a few personal cases with attempts to review the entire world literature up to that time, the last being a heroic overview of 1125 patients.[141]

2.8.1 Diagnosis

The first unequivocal description of an aneurysm, though unruptured, was by Franciscus Biumi in 1765, who saw it not on the circle of Willis but in the cavernous sinus (at the time called Vieussens' receptacle).[8] Morgagni had also mentioned dilatations of arteries that may have been aneurysms.[40] In 1812 John Cheyne provided the first illustration of lethal subarachnoid haemorrhage at the base of the brain as a result of 'rupture of the anterior artery of the cerebrum' (Fig. 2.11), but the aneurysm that must have been the source of the haemorrhage was not recognized at the time.[45] One year later Blackall reported a postmortem observation in which the haemorrhage as well as the offending aneurysm (of the basilar artery) were identified in a 20-year-old woman.[142] The observation was coincidental, because Blackall was primarily interested in her 'anasarca' (generalized oedema, or 'dropsy'). The brain was also examined by Hodgson, who in his book on diseases of blood vessels

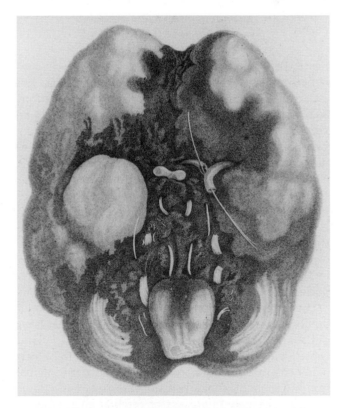

Fig. 2.11 The first anatomical illustration of subarachnoid haemorrhage, from Cheyne (1812).[45] A probe has been passed into the proximal end of the internal carotid artery and emerges at the presumed site of rupture; the offending aneurysm was not recognized at the time but presumably it was at the origin of the posterior communicating artery from the carotid artery, or at the anterior communicating artery complex.

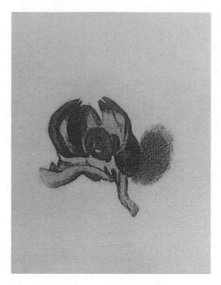

Fig. 2.12 Pea-sized aneurysmal dilatation of one of the branches of the middle cerebral artery (opened), containing a clot; the abnormality was surrounded by a large, fresh haemorrhage, which had caused the death of the 19-year-old patient, 8 days after a first episode with sudden headache (from Bright, 1831).[61]

made the point that the extravasated blood was contained under the arachnoid membrane.[143] Serres, not aware of these books, published two similar observations in a French periodical.[144] Parenthetically, it should be pointed out that medical journals, with articles about a variety of observations, did not emerge until the beginning of the 19th century, whereas the first scientific journals in general date from the middle of the 17th century.[145] In England, Richard Bright, one of the champions of the movement of 'organ-based medicine' that had started in Italy and France,[146] included an illustration of a pea-sized aneurysm on a branch of the middle cerebral artery in his richly illustrated book that appeared in 1831 (Fig. 2.12).[61] Series of other fatal cases were reported in the next few decades.[147–150]

The erroneous notion that aneurysms are congenital malformations, caused by a defect in the muscular layer of the arterial wall, was first put forward in 1887,[151] and subsequently adopted by other writers,[152,153] to be perpetuated into contemporaneous textbooks and students' minds. Turnbull also pointed out, correctly, that syphilis was an extremely rare cause of cerebral aneurysms.[153] Series of aneurysms diagnosed post mortem were often biased towards those measuring several cm,[154] or included septic aneurysms, associated with endocarditis.[155]

It took a long time before the clinical features were sorted out. In 1852 Brinton observed that fatal rupture was not the only possible presentation of aneurysms, and that other manifestations were local pressure,

convulsive attacks or 'inflammation' (a rather fuzzy notion at the time).[147] The sudden onset of the headache led Lebert and Bartholow to suppose, in the 1860s and 70s, that the diagnosis might be made during life.[149,150] Lebert also observed the characteristic paralysis of the oculomotor nerve in patients before they died from rupture of an aneurysm at the origin of the posterior communicating artery from the internal carotid artery.[149] Indeed the diagnosis of ruptured aneurysm was made on two occasions in a patient with sudden headache and oculomotor palsy, by Hutchinson in England and by Bull in Norway,[156,157] but apparently these two observations had little impact.

The introduction of lumbar puncture, in 1891 by Quincke,[158] initially only for therapeutic purposes in hydrocephalic patients, led to the diagnosis of 'meningeal apoplexy' in patients who survived a subarachnoid haemorrhage.[159–161] It took another three decades before the connection with rupture of a cerebral aneurysm was made. After all, the condition was supposed to be invariably fatal since it had been recognized only after death. The 'selection bias' seems obvious in retrospect, but in our own time the same error was made with intraventricular haemorrhage – until CT scanning showed it in those who survived.

That sudden headache and meningeal haemorrhage as diagnosed by lumbar puncture could be caused by a ruptured aneurysm without fatal outcome received widespread attention only after Charles Symonds (1890–1978; Fig. 2.13) had published two landmark articles about the subject in 1923 and 1924.[162,163] It had all started in 1920, when Symonds spent some time abroad as a temporary resident in the service of the neurosurgeon Harvey Cushing (1869–1939), who had moved not long before from Baltimore to Harvard University and the Peter Bent Brigham hospital in Boston. A 52-year-old woman had been admitted with repeated episodes of headache and unconsciousness; on examination she had a right oculomotor palsy and blurring of the optic discs. A right subtemporal decompression for a suspected tumour showed recently clotted blood extending over the entire hemisphere, apparently coming from the base of the skull.[162] Apparently Symonds suggested a ruptured aneurysm as the cause.[164] When the diagnosis was confirmed at autopsy (the patient had died the day after the operation) Cushing ordered Symonds to spend his remaining time in the library to review everything on the subject: 'Either this was a fluke or there was reason in it'.[165]

The next advances were neuroradiological. The first angiographic visualization of a cerebral aneurysm during life was reported by Egas Moniz in 1933,[166] six years after the technique had been first applied.[74] In those days angiography was a hazardous procedure (involving

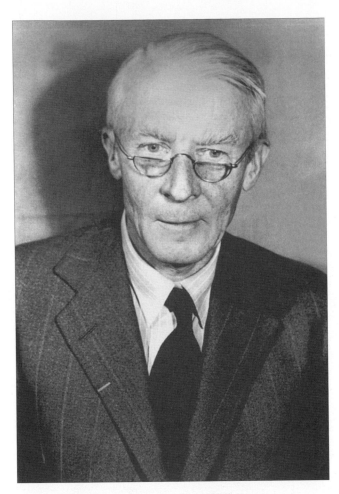

Fig. 2.13 Sir Charles Symonds (1890–1978).

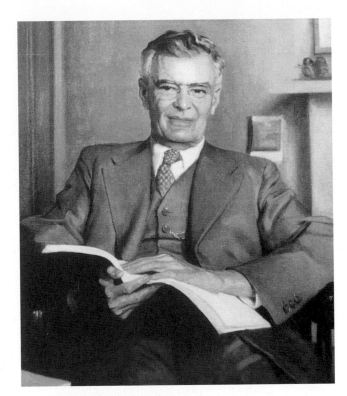

Fig. 2.14 Norman Dott (1897–1973).

surgical dissection of the carotid artery), to such an extent that someone like Cushing only rarely had his patients undergo it before neurosurgical exploration. Even today, in the era of selective catheterization, the risks are far from negligible. Fortunately, minimally or non-invasive techniques of angiography by means of computed tomography or magnetic resonance have largely replaced catheter angiography, at least for diagnostic purposes. The greatest leap forward in our times was the advent of computed tomography;[139] this technique made it possible to localize the extent of the haemorrhage in a precise fashion, to separate aneurysmal haemorrhage from non-aneurysmal haemorrhage and, by serial investigations, to detect and distinguish the most important complications: rebleeding, delayed ischaemia and hydrocephalus.

2.8.2 Surgical treatment

Ligation of the carotid artery has been practised since the times of Ambroise Paré (1510–1590) as a method to stop arterial bleeding in patients with neck wounds. Once

aneurysms were recognized as the cause of subarachnoid haemorrhage it was a logical step to consider this procedure as a method to decrease the risk of rebleeding.[157] Hutchinson would actually have carried out the operation in 1864 had the patient not declined at the last moment, going on to survive for another 11 years.[156] Around 1886 Horsley was one of the first who actually ligated the (common) carotid artery in the neck, for a tumorous aneurysm.[154] For decades carotid ligation remained the only surgical intervention possible, but most patients were managed conservatively because the complications of surgery were considerable.[167]

In 1931 the Edinburgh neurosurgeon Norman Dott (1897–1973; Fig. 2.14), at that time only 33 years old, carried out the first intracranial operation for a ruptured aneurysm.[168] It was a more or less desperate attempt because the aneurysm had already rebled twice, leaving the patient comatose for some hours after the last episode, also with some degree of right-sided hemiparesis and aphasia. To complicate matters further, the patient was a well-known Edinburgh solicitor, 53 years old and chairman of the board of governors of the Royal Hospital for Sick Children. But, both the patient and the young neurosurgeon were prepared to take the risk.[169] About the operation Dott wrote:[170]

A left frontal approach was employed and it was a difficult matter to elevate the tense and oedematous

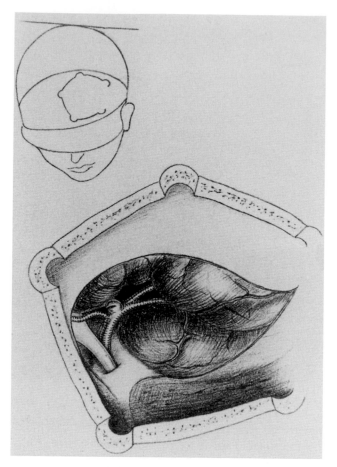

Fig. 2.15 Norman Dott's drawing of the first intracranial operation for aneurysm. The proximal middle cerebral artery aneurysm was exposed and wrapped with muscle through a left frontal flap. (From Todd *et al.*, 1990;[168] by kind permission of the authors and the *Journal of Neurology, Neurosurgery and Psychiatry*.)

brain and identify the basal structures, which were bloodstained and largely embedded in clot. The left optic nerve was found and the internal carotid artery was defined at its outer side. This vessel was closely followed upwards, outwards and backwards to its bifurcation into the middle and anterior cerebral arteries. As this point was being cleared of tenacious clot a formidable arterial haemorrhage filled the wound. With the aid of suction apparatus, held closely to the bleeding point, we were able to see the aneurysm. It sprang from the upper aspect of the bifurcation junction; it was about 3 mm in diameter; blood spurted freely from its semidetached fundus. Meanwhile a colleague was obtaining fresh muscle from the patient's leg. A small fragment of muscle was accurately applied to the bleeding point and held firmly in place so that it checked the bleeding and compressed the thin walled aneurysmal sac. Thus it was steadily maintained for

twelve minutes. As the retaining instrument was then cautiously withdrawn, no further bleeding occurred. The vessel was further cleared and thin strips of muscle were prepared and wound around it until a thick collar of muscle embedded the aneurysm and adjacent arterial trunks (Fig. 2.15).

The patient recovered well and a few weeks later Dott wrote, his sense of triumph carefully hidden: 'Mr Colin Black's tibialis anticus seems to have stuck well to his internal carotid – he has gone for a holiday'.[169] In later years Dott and his patient went fishing together on a number of occasions and Mr Black's neurological condition remained good until he died from myocardial infarction 11 years after the momentous operation. Unfortunately, on later occasions the outcome with a direct approach to the aneurysm was often disappointing, if not fatal, and Dott reverted to ligating the internal carotid artery in the neck or the proximal anterior cerebral artery intracranially.

In 1937 Dandy was the first to use a clip to occlude the neck of the aneurysm that had bled (Fig. 2.16).[171] Yet in some patients a clip could not be secured, and in those

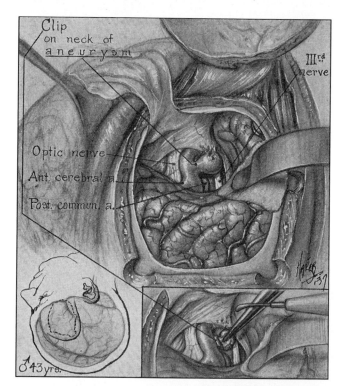

Fig. 2.16 Illustration from Dandy's 1944 monograph on intracerebral arterial aneurysms.[222] The legend is: 'Typical aneurysm of the intracranial internal carotid artery, showing the narrow neck of the sac and the bulging aneurysm; also the point of rupture. The inset shows the clip placed on the neck of the aneurysm, and the aneurysm itself shrivelled with the electric cautery.'

cases he often had to have recourse to so-called trapping, by clipping the parent vessel on either side of the aneurysm. Decades later, Drake devised a technique for approaching basilar artery aneurysms, notoriously difficult until then, and managed to apply clips to them.[172] In the 1960s, spring clips, which could be removed when placement was less than optimal, came into use and replaced the silver clips used by Dandy. Nevertheless, the direct operation of aneurysms remained dangerous and controlled trials of the efficacy of aneurysm operations were equivocal. Attempts to increase the safety of the operation included temporary cardiac arrest, hypotension and deep hypothermia, all without much success, although no formal trials were done.

In the 1980s, a consensus developed amongst neurosurgeons that direct operation of the aneurysm should best be delayed until 12–14 days after the initial haemorrhage. This regimen meant, of course, that a proportion of patients rebled or suffered other complications in the meantime. The gradual introduction of the operating microscope for aneurysm surgery in the 1970s made early operation (within 3 days) not only feasible but also fashionable, despite the dearth of evidence from controlled clinical trials. The medical management of patients with ruptured aneurysms has also improved in recent years, especially the prevention of delayed ischaemia.

In the 1980s the Italian neuroradiologist Guglielmi developed an endovascular method for occluding aneurysms by means of detachable platinum coils, initially only for aneurysms for which a surgical approach was hazardous or impossible.[173,174] In the last few years 'coiling' has largely replaced the surgical approach, provided the method is feasible for a particular aneurysm.

2.9 Treatment and its pitfalls

Doctoring has always implied treatment. In the past, medical management was almost invariably based on what later turned out to be erroneous pathophysiological concepts, and the treatments were almost invariably ineffective, if not actually harmful. Such pitiful situations are often repeated in present times, much more often than physicians and surgeons care to realize. Anyone who finds it amusing to read about 19th-century regimens, including measures such as bleeding, mustard poultices, castor oil and turpentine enemas as treatments for apoplexy, should read post-1950 treatises about the efficacy of vasodilator drugs or about transplantation

of omentum to the intracranial cavity, as a chastening experience.

2.9.1 The numerical method

Before different treatments could ever be compared, it was necessary to find methods for grouping patients together and also somehow to convert disease outcomes into numbers. The Paris physician Pierre Charles Alexandre Louis (1787–1872; he survives eponymously in the *angulus Ludovici* of the sternum) is generally credited with the introduction of the numerical method in medicine. In fact his contribution was more a credo than a practical method.[175] True enough, there is the famous example of his empirical criticism of bloodletting: of 47 patients with pneumonia treated with bloodletting 18 died, against only nine of the 36 patients in the untreated group.[176] But Louis did not have the mathematical training to estimate the likelihood that a difference of this magnitude might arise by chance. It was a mathematician, Jules Gavarret (1809–1890), who criticized the analysis and conclusions of Louis's studies, although he agreed with the design.[177] Even more purely mathematical was the notion of the 'average human', an approach proposed by Adolphe Quetelet (1796–1874).

Groups and averages, these were notions that evoked not merely resistance but outright revulsion in the ranks of the established medical professionals. How on earth could one ever ignore the unique characteristics of each single individual by forcing these together into an artificial 'mean'? And how could one ever believe in a standard treatment, any more than in a standard shoe? The advent of experimental physiology intensified the opposition. The famous Claude Bernard (1813–1878) warned that one will never encounter an 'average' in nature, and that grouping of observations will obscure the true relationships between natural phenomena.[178] And the equally legendary Lord Lister (1827–1912) relied more on the theoretical basis of his antiseptic method than on the actual death rates.[179]

Until the 20th century, counting disease events was limited to population studies.[180] The beginnings of epidemiology can be traced to Sir William Petty (1623–1687), one of the founders of the Royal Society, and John Graunt (1620–1674). They worked together in collecting numerical data to describe patterns of mortality. A century and a half later, E. Blackmore reported not only on deaths but also on incident cases of disease in Plymouth.[181,182] Victorian counterparts took this further. William Farr (1807–1883), who had trained under Louis in Paris, linked self-devised classifications of diseases and occupations to population statistics at the General Registry Office. John Snow (1813–1858) mapped the occurrence of cholera cases in the streets of London and related these to the positions of the local water pumps; these studies culminated in the famous act of Snow removing the handle from the pump in Broad Street, during the 1854 cholera epidemic. Incidentally, he later specialized in chloroform anaesthesia.[183]

The first epidemiological studies of stroke were not performed until after World War II. An early study of stroke incidence in the community was done in the UK.[184] Population-based studies addressing risk factors specifically for stroke were subsequently reported from the US (the Framingham cohort), Japan and Finland.[185–187]

2.9.2 Clinical trials

The introduction of the randomized controlled clinical trial heralded the era of 'evidence-based medicine' or rather 'organized empiricism', since medicine is not and probably will never be a positivist science like physics or chemistry.[188] Randomization in a therapeutic experiment slowly gained acceptance after the landmark UK Medical Research Council (MRC) trial of streptomycin in pulmonary tuberculosis with random assignment to treatment groups.[189] Some forerunners had already used parallel control groups. Louis (1787–1872) had been preceded by James Lind (1716–1794) in 1753 (lemons and oranges to prevent scurvy in sailors). A further step was the introduction of chance to obtain an equal balance between the experimental group and the control group. In 1898 Fibiger (1867–1928) used assignment on alternate days (injection of serum for diphtheria),[190,191] and in 1931 Amberson *et al.* flipped a coin to divide patients with pulmonary tuberculosis into those who received gold treatment and controls.[192] Blinding (or masking, as ophthalmologists prefer to say) of patients was also practised by Amberson's group, as had been done four years earlier by Ferguson *et al.* in a test of vaccines for the common cold.[193] Masking of those who were to assess outcome was advocated in 1944 by the pulmonary physicians Hinshaw and Feldman,[194] and eventually carried out in the MRC streptomycin trial of 1948. Allocation in that historic trial took place by means of randomization. An important advantage of random allocation, applied by R.A. Fisher in agriculture in the 1920s, is that it ensures equal and unbiased balancing between the two groups.[195] But the main reason why Sir Austin Bradford Hill (1897–1991), the trial's principal investigator, chose randomization is that at the same time it ensured concealment of the allocation schedule from those involved in entering patients in the trial.[196,197]

Clinical trials in cerebrovascular disease were no exception to the rule that most methodological errors have to be committed before they are recognized, as the correct solutions are often counter-intuitive. In the 1950s anticoagulant drugs seemed a rational form of treatment to prevent further strokes in survivors of (presumed) brain infarction. The same Bradford Hill who had pioneered the tuberculosis trial took the initiative for two such trials, the first in 142 and the second, with exclusion of hypertensives, in 131 patients.[198,199] There was no significant difference in the rate of non-fatal stroke between the treatment groups and controls, while there was some excess of fatal strokes, possibly haemorrhages, in patients on anticoagulants. From that time onwards anticoagulants were largely abandoned for the prevention of stroke, unless for specific indications such as a source of embolism in the heart. However, it took at least two decades before it dawned on the neurological community that the trials of anticoagulants in brain ischaemia had been too small, separately as well as collectively, to detect even large protective effects – apart from other shortcomings.[200] The same applied to an early secondary prevention trial with dipyridamole.[201]

The first intervention trial in acute stroke was with corticosteroids, by Dyken and White in 1956. They did not use randomization but stratified patients according to their clinical characteristics, and found a trend towards a higher death rate in the treated group (13/17 against 10/19 in controls), and ended up by identifying many of the methodological problems in this type of trial.[202] The first trial of carotid endarterectomy excluded surgical mishaps from the analysis;[203] subsequently the operation boomed to worrying levels, until checked by methodologically sound trials. The first large trial of aspirin in stroke prevention evoked much controversy,[204] for one thing because its initiators had chosen 'stroke or death' as the outcome event instead of stroke alone;[205] it took time for neurologists to realize that they treat whole patients rather than only their brains! Also, the initial conclusion that aspirin was ineffective for women is now a classical example of the dangers of subgroup analysis.

2.9.3 Measuring outcome: the ghost of Gall

One of the stumbling blocks in trials of acute stroke used to be the babel of tongues with regard to the measurement of outcome. Initially, so-called 'stroke scales' were applied for this aim, analogous to scales for other specific neurological conditions, such as Parkinson's disease or multiple sclerosis. Although the stated purpose of 'stroke scales' is to measure outcome, these scales are nothing but codifications of the neurological examination, while of course that examination has no other purpose than localizing lesions within the nervous system. With such a diagnostic approach, different functions of the nervous system are separately assessed: power of limbs, speech, visual fields, etc. This reductionist, mechanistic notion of brain function reflects the localizationists' position in the scientific battle that raged in the second half of the 19th century, the opposing party believing in so-called equipotentiality.

The 'equipotentialists' believed that the brain worked as a unitary system, brain tissue being omnipotent and flexible in its function. Consequently, brain damage would result in a decrease in the overall level of performance, but not in loss of specific functions. The champion of this camp was the French physiologist Flourens, who supported his views with experiments on dogs and pigeons.[206] The alternative notion, that of localization of specific functions, was propounded in a somewhat bizarre fashion by the anatomists Gall and Spurzheim.[207] They believed that every intellectual and moral property had its own position on the surface of the brain (Fig. 2.17) and that the degree of development of these dispositions could be identified by locating overlying protuberances on the skull (Fig. 2.18). However, the theory of localization gained respectability after the stimulation experiments of Fritsch and Hitzig on anaesthetized dogs, in which they found that weak electrical currents applied through platinum electrodes to the anterior regions of

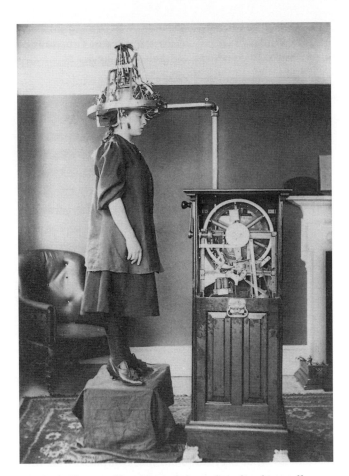

Fig. 2.18 The pseudo-science of phrenology lived on well beyond the 19th century. The Lavery Electric Phrenometer of 1907 was intended to lend modern accuracy to the measurements of bumps on the skull.[223] (Reproduced by kind permission of Cambridge University Press.)

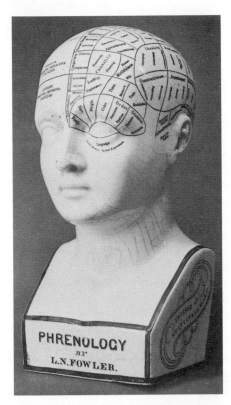

Fig. 2.17 Phrenology head (Fowler); each region of the skull is supposed to represent a mental faculty, such as 'mirthfulness', 'perception of form' or 'ideality'.

the brain surface produced muscle contractions in the opposite half of the body.[208,209] The clash between the two opposing factions culminated in 1881 at the Third International Congress of Medicine, held in London.[210] The equipotentialists were represented by the German physiologist Goltz, who showed the audience a dog in which a substantial portion of the brain had been removed by means of a hose, but who could still move all four limbs, trunk and tail, and who had retained all his senses. Later, it would turn out that the lesions were less extensive than had been claimed. On the same afternoon Ferrier showed two chimpanzees, one deaf after removal of the auditory cortex, the other limping with a hemiplegic gait after extirpation of the contralateral motor area (the sight of which led Charcot to jump up and exclaim: 'Mais c'est un patient!').

The localizationists had won the day, but they won too completely. The greater part of the brain has no 'primary' motor, sensory or cognitive tasks, and serves to

Table 2.2 The state of an individual cannot be constructed from separate components. Imagine that you met 'the boy next door' from your childhood days after an interval of 30 years, and that your question 'How are you?' was answered with a list of details, instead of by a general statement ('fine' for example).

Profession	dentist	for 15 years
Civil state	married	wife 1.68 m, 59 kg
Bank account	positive	€9634.92
Car	Volvo	240S
Holidays	Tuscany	3 weeks
Sport	golf	handicap 8
Total ?		

connect and integrate the separate 'functions'. Similarly, everyday life consists of a multitude of tasks that are integrated and difficult to separate. Mood, initiative and speed of thinking are some of the essential features of human life that can be severely affected by stroke but are sadly ignored in 'stroke scales'. It is therefore naive to try and rebuild an entire human being from separate 'building blocks' (Table 2.2; Fig. 2.19). Patients are more than the sum of their signs. A higher, more integrated level of measurement is needed; that is, scales should measure function not at the level of the organ but at the level of the person (disability scales), or even at the level of social interaction (handicap scales). What really counts for patients is what they can do in life, compared with what they want to do or were once able to do.

2.9.4 Meta-analysis and systematic reviews

In the last quarter of the 20th century, Richard Peto and his colleagues Tom Chalmers and Iain Chalmers developed a method to overcome the problem that single studies may or may not show a significant difference in treated patients compared with controls, but that the magnitude of the difference can only be expressed as a confidence interval, which is usually wide. They collated all related trials in a given field by which the differences between the treatment group and the control group in each trial could be combined.[211] The key assumption is that, if a given treatment has any material effect on the incidence or outcome of disease, then the direction, although not necessarily the size, of this effect tends to be similar in different circumstances. If all available studies are combined, the confidence interval can be narrowed considerably and reviewer bias is avoided. There clearly was a pressing need for up-to-date systematic reviews of all the available evidence regarding the various aspects of care of stroke patients – indeed, of all medical interventions. This need led to the Cochrane Collaboration, which includes a stroke review group.[212]

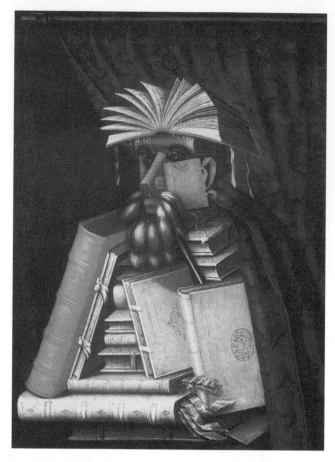

Fig. 2.19 The librarian (1566), by Giuseppe Arcimboldo (1530–1593). Oil on canvas, 97 × 71 cm. (By kind permission of Skokloster Castle, Sweden.)

The graphic representation of systematic reviews started in 1978, with simple lines to depict 95% confidence intervals.[213] In 1982 Lewis and Clarke had the idea to combine the separate estimates into an overall estimate, at the bottom of the figure.[214,215] Subsequently Richard Peto's group solved the paradox that small trials were most conspicuous because of their large confidence intervals, by putting a square at the site of the point estimate, the size of the square being proportional to the power of the trial (Fig. 2.20).[216] These graphs have since become known as 'forest plots', probably because the many lines might be seen as trees.[215]

2.10 Epilogue

Despite the many advances in the knowledge about stroke that we have highlighted, our story could not but

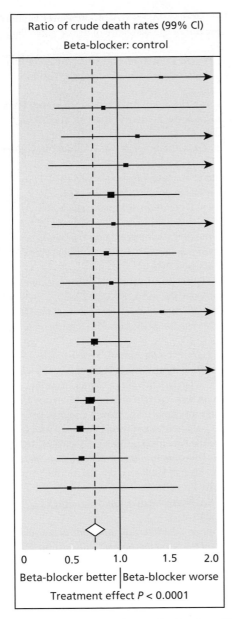

Fig. 2.20 'Forest plot'. Figure redrawn after Lewis and Ellis's original plot from 1982, which for the first time combined 99% confidence intervals of different placebo-controlled clinical trials of beta blockers after myocardial infarction.[214] This modern variant shows the results of each component study as a square centred on the point estimate of the result of each study; the size of each square is proportional to the amount of information provided in that trial. A horizontal line runs through the square to show its confidence interval (CI). The overall estimate from the meta-analysis and its confidence interval are put at the bottom, represented as a diamond.[215] (Reproduced by kind permission of the BMJ Publishing Group.)

remain anachronistic and fragmented. It is extremely difficult to try and stand in the shoes of one's forebears, because to achieve this the mind should be cleared from all knowledge obtained since their time.[217] For those of us who can think back as small a time span as three decades, what diagnosis did we make, in those times, in patients we now know to have survived carotid dissection or intracranial venous thrombosis, to name but two examples? Heaven only knows. In the same way, not so much longer ago, it was impossible to distinguish haemorrhage from infarction; or haemorrhage from some mysterious other condition that mimicked haemorrhage but in which the brain looked practically normal; or stroke from other brain diseases; or even stroke from heart disease. Necessarily our account has been anecdotal. In reality the progress of science is slow and continuous, not a succession of breakthroughs. This also applies to the few decades we have witnessed during our own careers. We do not expect a sensational novelty when we walk into hospital tomorrow, but a lot has changed since we were medical students. This refers not only to the body of medical knowledge but also to the methods of medical research. Empirical testing has gained ascendancy over pathophysiological theory, for the treatment as well as the prevention of disease. The rate of change is a bit like the shifting position of the sun across the sky: one cannot see it move, but there is a dramatic sweep between dawn and sunset. We expect to see many more dawns in stroke research.

References

1 Oppenheim H. *Lehrbuch der Nervenkrankheiten für Ärtzte und Studierende.* 6th ed. Berlin: S. Karger, 1913.
2 Brain WR. *Diseases of the Nervous System.* 6th ed. Oxford: Oxford University Press, 1968.
3 Dechambre A. Mémoire sur la curabilité du ramollissement cérébral. *Gaz Med Paris* 1838; 6:305–14.
4 Durand-Fardel CLM. Mémoire sur une altération particulière de la substance cérébrale. *Gaz Med Paris* 1842; 10:23–38.
5 Fisher CM. Lacunes: small, deep cerebral infarcts. *Neurology* 1965; 15:774–84.
6 Fisher CM, Curry HB. Pure motor hemiplegia of vascular origin. *Arch Neurol* 1965; 13:30–44.
7 Fisher CM. The arterial lesions underlying lacunes. *Acta Neuropathol (Berl)* 1969; 12:1–15.
8 Biumi F. Observatio V: Carotis ad receptaculum Vieusenii aneurysmatica etc. In: Sandifort E, editor. *Observationes anatomicae, scholiis illustratae (thesaurus dissertationum).* Leiden: S. & J. Lichtmans, 1765, pp. 373–9.

9 Schiller F. Concepts of stroke before and after Virchow. *Medical History* 1970; **14**:115–31.

10 McHenry LC. A history of stroke. *Int J Neurol* 1981; **15**:314–26.

11 Karenberg A. Johann Jakob Wepfers Buch uber die Apoplexie (1658). Kritische Anmerkungen zu einem Klassiker der Neurologie. *Nervenarzt* 1998; **69**:93–8.

12 McHenry LC. *Garrison's History of Neurology*. Springfield: Charles C. Thomas, 1969.

13 Clarke E. Apoplexy in the Hippocratic writings. *Bull Hist Med* 1963; **37**:301–14.

14 Karenberg A, Hort I. Medieval descriptions and doctrines of stroke: preliminary analysis of select sources. Part I: The struggle for terms and theories – late antiquity and early middle ages (300–800). *J Hist Neurosc* 1998; **7**:162–73.

15 Galenus. *Opera Omnia*. Leipzig: Cnobloch, 1824.

16 Karenberg A, Hort I. Medieval descriptions and doctrines of stroke: preliminary analysis of select sources. Part II: Between Galenism and Aristotelism – Islamic theories of apoplexy (800–1200). *J Hist Neurosc* 1998; **7**:174–85.

17 Jardine L. *Worldly Goods: a new history of the Renaissance*. London: Macmillan, 1996.

18 Karenberg A, Hort I. Medieval descriptions and doctrines of stroke: preliminary analysis of select sources. Part III: Multiplying speculations – the high and late middle ages (1000–1450). *J Hist Neurosc* 1998; **7**:186–200.

19 Vesalius A. *De humani corporis fabrica*. Basle: J. Oporini, 1543.

20 Copernicus N. *De revolutionibus orbium coelestium*. Nuremberg: J. Petreius, 1543.

21 Vesalius A. *Tabulae anatomicae*. Venice: D. Bernardini, 1538.

22 Clarke E, Dewhurst K. *An Illustrated History of Brain Function: imaging the brain from antiquity to the present*. 2nd ed. San Francisco: Norman, 1996.

23 Berengario da Carpi J. *Isagogae breves, perlucide ac uberrime, in anatomiam humani corporis etc*. Venice: Benedictum Hectoris, 1535.

24 Harvey W. *Exercitatio anatomica de motu cordis et sanguinis in animalibus*. Frankfurt: G. Fitzer, 1628.

25 Dewhurst K. *Thomas Willis's Oxford Lectures*. Oxford: Sandford Publications, 1980.

26 Willis T. *Cerebri Anatome*. London: Martyn & Allestry, 1664.

27 Meyer A, Hierons R. Observations on the history of the 'Circle of Willis'. *Medical History* 1962; **6**:119–30.

28 Fallopius G. *Observationes anatomicae*. Venice: Marcus Antonius Ulmus, 1561.

29 Casserio G. *Tabulae Anatomicae* (edited by D. Bucretius). Venice: E. Deuchinum, 1627.

30 Vesling J. *Syntagma anatomicum, locis pluribus actum, emendatum, novisque iconibus diligenter exornatum*. Patavii: Pauli Frombotti Bibliopolae, 1647.

31 Wepfer JJ. *Observationes anatomicae, ex cadaveribus eorum, quos sustulit apoplexia, cum exercitatione de ejus loco affecto*. Schaffhausen: J.C. Suteri, 1658.

32 Tatu L, Moulin T, Monnier G. The discovery of encephalic arteries. From Johann Jacob Wepfer to Charles Foix. *Cerebrovasc Dis* 2005; **20**:427–32.

33 Willis T. *Dr. Willis's Practice of Physick*. London: Dring, Harper & Leigh, 1684.

34 Kidd M, Modlin IM. Frederik Ruysch: master anatomist and depictor of the surreality of death. *J Med Biogr* 1999; **7**:69–77.

35 Moore W. *The Knife Man: the extraordinary life and times of John Hunter, father of modern surgery*. London: Bantam Press, 2005.

36 van Eems J. *Hermanni Boerhaave Praelectiones Academicae de Morbis Nervorum*. Leiden: Petrus van der Eijk and Cornelius de Pecker, 1761.

37 Bayle F. *Tractatus de apoplexia*. Toulouse: B. Guillemette, 1677.

38 Aegineta P. *The Seven Books* (translated by Francis Adams). London: The Sydenham Society, 1844.

39 Mistichelli D. *Trattato dell'apoplessia*. Roma: A. de Rossi, 1709.

40 Morgagni GB. *De sedibus et causis morborum per anatomen indigatis libri quinque*. Venice: ex typographica Remondiana, 1761.

41 Portal A. Observations sur l'apoplexie. *Histoire de l'Académie des Sciences* 1781; **83**:623–30.

42 Baillie M. *The Morbid Anatomy of Some of the Most Important Parts of the Human Body*. London: J. Johnson & G. Nicol, 1793.

43 Hall M. *Lectures on the Nervous System and its Diseases*. London: Sherwood, Gilbert & Piper, 1836.

44 Burrows G. *On Disorders of Cerebral Circulation and on the Connection between Affections of the Brain and Diseases of the Heart*. London: Longman, Brown, Green & Longmans, 1846.

45 Cheyne J. *Cases of Apoplexy and Lethargy with Observations on Comatose Patients*. London: Underwood, 1812.

46 King LS. *Transformations in American Medicine: from Benjamin Rush to William Osler*. Baltimore: Johns Hopkins University Press, 1991.

47 Serres ERA. Nouvelle division des apoplexies. *Ann Med Chir* 1819; **1**:246–363.

48 Abercrombie J. *Pathological and Clinical Researches on Diseases of the Brain and Spinal Cord*. Edinburgh: Waugh & Innes, 1828.

49 Hope J, Bennett JH, Pritchard JC, Taylor RH, Thomson T. Dissertations on nervous diseases. In: Tweedie A, editor. *Library of Practical Medicine*. Philadelphia: Lea & Blanchard, 1840.

50 Vicq d'Azyr F. *Traité d'anatomie et de physiologie*. Paris: F.A. Didot, 1786.

51 Blum F. Der Formaldehyd als Härtungsmittel: vorläufige Mitteilung. *Z wiss Mikr mikr Technik* 1893; **10**:314–5.

52 Harbison J, Hossain O, Jenkinson D, Davis J, Louw SJ, Ford GA. Diagnostic accuracy of stroke referrals from primary care, emergency room physicians, and ambulance staff using the face arm speech test. *Stroke* 2003; **34**:71–6.

53 Heckmann JG, Stadter M, Dutsch M, Handschu R, Rauch C, Neundorfer B. Einweisung von Nicht-Schlaganfallpatienten auf eine Stroke Unit [Hospitalization of non-stroke patients in a Stroke Unit]. *Dtsch Med Wochenschr* 2004; **129**:731–5.

54 Ronning OM, Thommessen B. Nar hjerneslagdiagnosen er feil [Stroke: when the diagnosis is wrong]. *Tidsskr Nor Laegeforen* 2005; **125**:1655–7.

55 Foucault M. *Naissance de la clinique*. Paris: Presses Universitaires de France, 1963.

56 Bynum WF. *Science and the Practice of Medicine in the Nineteenth Century*. Cambridge: Cambridge University Press, 1994.

57 Rostan L. *Recherches sur le ramollissement du cerveau. Ouvrage dans lequel on s'efforce de distinguer les diverses affections de ce viscère par des signes caractéristiques.* 1st ed. Paris: Béchet, 1820.

58 Lallemand F. *Recherches anatomo-pathologiques sur l'encéphale et ses dépendances*. Paris: Béchet, 1824.

59 Kuhn TS. *The Structure of Scientific Revolutions*. Chicago: Chicago University Press, 1962.

60 Abercrombie J. *Pathological and Practical Researches on Diseases of the Brain and Spinal Cord*. 2nd (from 3rd Brit.) ed. Philadelphia: Carey, Lea & Blanchard, 1836.

61 Bright R. *Reports of Medical Cases, selected with a view of illustrating the symptoms and cure of diseases by a reference to morbid anatomy*. London: Longman, Rees, Orme, Brown & Green, 1831.

62 Carswell R. *Pathological Anatomy: illustrations of the elementary forms of disease*. London: Longman & Co., 1838.

63 Cruveilhier J. *Anatomie pathologique du corps humain; descriptions avec figures lithographiés et coloriés; des diverses altérations morbides dont le corps humain est susceptible*. Paris: J.B. Baillière, 1842.

64 Durand-Fardel CLM. *Traité du ramollissement du cerveau*. Paris: J.-B. Baillière, 1843.

65 Virchow RLK. Ueber die akute Entzündung der Arterien. *Archiv Pathol Anat* 1847; **1**:272–378.

66 Virchow R. Thrombose und Embolie: Gefässentzündung und septische Infection. In: Virchow R, editor. *Gesammelte Abhandlungen zur wissenschaftlichen Medizin*. Frankfurt: Meidinger, 1856, pp. 219–732.

67 Lobstein JFM. *Traité d'anatomie pathologique*. Paris: Levrault, 1829.

68 Cohnheim J. *Untersuchungen ueber die embolischen Processe*. Berlin: Hirschwald, 1872.

69 van Swieten GLB. *Commentaria in Hermanni Boerhaave Aphorismos De Cognoscendis et Curandis Morbis*. Leiden: J. & H. Verbeek, 1755.

70 Chiari H. Über das Verhalten des Teilungswinkels des Carotis Communis bei der Endarteritis chronica deformans. *Verh Ddtsch path Ges* 1905; **9**:326–30.

71 Hunt JR. The role of the carotid arteries, in the causation of vascular lesions of the brain, with remarks on special features of the symptomatology. *Am J Med Sci* 1914; **147**:704–13.

72 Fisher CM. Occlusion of the internal carotid artery. *Arch Neurol Psych* 1951; **65**:346–77.

73 Fisher CM. Transient monocular blindness associated with hemiplegia. *Arch Ophthalmol* 1952; **47**:167–203.

74 Moniz E. L'encéphalographie artérielle, son importance dans la localisation des tumeurs cérébrales. *Rev Neurol (Paris)* 1927; **48**:72–90.

75 Moniz E. *Die cerebrale Arteriographie und Phlebographie*. Berlin: Julius Springer, 1940.

76 Seldinger SI. Catheter replacement of the needle in percutaneous arteriography. *Acta Radiol* 1953; **39**:368–78.

77 Rothwell PM, Eliasziw M, Gutnikov SA, Fox AJ, Taylor DW, Mayberg MR *et al.* Analysis of pooled data from the randomised controlled trials of endarterectomy for symptomatic carotid stenosis. *Lancet* 2003; **361**:107–16.

78 Sacco RL, Prabhakaran S, Thompson JL, Murphy A, Sciacca RR, Levin B *et al.* Comparison of warfarin versus aspirin for the prevention of recurrent stroke or death: subgroup analyses from the Warfarin-Aspirin Recurrent Stroke Study. *Cerebrovasc Dis* 2006; **22**:4–12.

79 Jood K, Ladenvall C, Rosengren A, Blomstrand C, Jern C. Family history in ischemic stroke before 70 years of age: the Sahlgrenska Academy Study on Ischemic Stroke. *Stroke* 2005; **36**:1383–7.

80 Soloway HB, Aronson SM. Atheromatous emboli to central nervous system. *Arch Neurol* 1964; **11**:657–67.

81 Amarenco P, Duyckaerts C, Tzourio C, Henin D, Bousser MG, Hauw JJ. The prevalence of ulcerated plaques in the aortic arch in patients with stroke. *N Engl J Med* 1992; **326**:221–5.

82 Amarenco P, Cohen A, Tzourio C, Bertrand B, Hommel M, Besson G *et al.* Atherosclerotic disease of the aortic arch and the risk of ischemic stroke. *N Engl J Med* 1994; **331**:1474–9.

83 Hachinski VM. Transient cerebral ischemia: a historical sketch. In: Clifford Rose F, Bynum WF, editors. *Historical Aspects of the Neurosciences (Festschrift for M. Critchley)*. New York: Raven Press, 1982, pp. 185–93.

84 Benton AL, Joynt RJ. Early descriptions of aphasia. *Arch Neurol* 1960; **3**:205–22.

85 Wood GB. *Treatise on the Practice of Medicine*. Philadelphia: Lippincott, 1852.

86 Jackson JH. A lecture on softening of the brain. *Lancet* 1875; **ii**:335–8.

87 Hammond WA. *Diseases of the Nervous System*. New York: D. Appleton, 1881.

88 Gowers WR. *A Manual of Diseases of the Nervous System*. 2 ed. London: J&A Churchill, 1893.

89 Osler W. Transient attacks of aphasia and paralysis in states of high blood pressure and arteriosclerosis. *Can Med Assoc J* 1911; **1**:919–26.

90 Raynaud M. *De l'asphyxie locale et de la gangrène symmétrique des extrémités*. Paris: L. Leclerc, 1862.

91 Peabody GL. Relation between arterial disease and visceral changes. *Trans Assoc Am Physicians* 1891; **6**:154–78.

92 Russel W. A post-graduate lecture on intermittent closing of the cerebral arteries: its relation to temporary and permanent paralysis. *Br Med J* 1909; **2**:1109–10.

93 Payer L. *Medicine and Culture: notions of health and sickness in Britain, the US, France and West Germany*. London: V. Gollancz, 1989.

94 Pickering GW. Transient cerebral paralysis in hypertension and in cerebral embolism with special reference to the pathogenesis of chronic hypertensive encephalopathy. *J Am Med Assoc* 1948; **137**:423–30.

95 Denny-Brown D. The treatment of recurrent cerebrovascular symptoms and the question of 'vasospasm'. *Med Clin North Am* 1951; **35**:1457–74.

96 Burger SK, Saul RF, Sclhorst JB, Thurston SE. Transient monocular blindness caused by vasospasm. *N Engl J Med* 1991; **325**:870–3.

97 Call GK, Fleming MC, Sealfon S, Levine H, Kistler JP, Fisher CM. Reversible cerebral segmental vasoconstriction. *Stroke* 1988; **19**:1159–70.

98 Kendell RE, Marshall J. Role of hypotension in the genesis of transient focal cerebral ischaemic attacks. *Br Med J* 1963; **2**:344–8.

99 Reed RL, Siekert RG, Merideth J. Rarity of transient focal cerebral ischemia in cardiac dysrhythmia. *J Am Med Assoc* 1973; **223**:893–5.

100 De Bono DP, Warlow CP. Potential sources of emboli in patients with presumed transient cerebral or retinal ischaemia. *Lancet* 1981; **i**:343–6.

101 Eastcott HHG, Pickering GW, Robb CG. Reconstruction of internal carotid artery in a patient with intermittent attacks of hemiplegia. *Lancet* 1954; **ii**:994–6.

102 Warlow C. Carotid endarterectomy: does it work? *Stroke* 1984; **15**:1068–76.

103 Barnett HJM, Plum F, Walton JN. Carotid endarterectomy: an expression of concern. *Stroke* 1984; **15**:941–3.

104 Klijn CJM, Kappelle LJ, Tulleken CAF, van Gijn J. Symptomatic carotid artery occlusion: A reappraisal of hemodynamic factors. *Stroke* 1997; **28**:2084–93.

105 Caplan LR, Sergay S. Positional cerebral ischaemia. *J Neurol Neurosurg Psychiatry* 1976; **39**:385–91.

106 Bogousslavsky J, Regli F. Delayed TIAs distal to bilateral occlusion of carotid arteries: evidence for embolic and hemodynamic mechanisms. *Stroke* 1983; **14**:58–61.

107 Ross Russell RW, Page NGR. Critical perfusion of brain and retina. *Brain* 1983; **106**:419–34.

108 The EC/IC Bypass Study Group. Failure of extracranial-intracranial arterial bypass to reduce the risk of ischemic stroke. Results of an international randomized trial. *N Engl J Med* 1985; **313**:1191–200.

109 Fisher CM. Observations on the fundus oculi in transient monocular blindness. *Neurology* 1959; **9**:333–47.

110 Ross Russell RW. Observations on the retinal blood-vessels in monocular blindness. *Lancet* 1961; **11**:1422–8.

111 Witmer R, Schmid A. Cholesterinkristall als retinaler arterieller Embolus. *Ophthalmologica* 1958; **135**:432–3.

112 Hollenhorst RW. Significance of bright plaques in the retinal arterioles. *J Am Med Assoc* 1961; **178**:23–9.

113 Archie JP, Feldtman JP. Critical stenosis of the internal carotid artery. *Surgery* 1981; **89**:67–70.

114 Gunning AJ, Pickering GW, Robb-Smith AHT, Ross Russell RW. Mural thrombosis of the internal carotid artery and subsequent embolism. *Q J Med* 1964; **33**:155–95.

115 Beal MF, Park TS, Fisher CM. Cerebral atheromatous embolism following carotid sinus pressure. *Arch Neurol* 1981; **38**:310–12.

116 Watts C. External carotid artery embolus from the internal carotid artery 'stump' during angiography: case report. *Stroke* 1982; **13**:515–17.

117 Barnett HJM. The pathophysiology of transient cerebral ischemic attacks: therapy with antiplatelet antiaggregants. *Med Clin North Am* 1979; **63**:649–80.

118 Markus H. Transcranial Doppler detection of circulating cerebral emboli. A review. *Stroke* 1993; **24**:1246–50.

119 Siebler M, Sitzer M, Rose G, Bendfeldt D, Steinmetz H. Silent cerebral embolism caused by neurologically symptomatic high-grade carotid stenosis. Event rates before and after carotid endarterectomy. *Brain* 1993; **116**:1005–15.

120 van Zuilen EV, Moll FL, Vermeulen FE, Mauser HW, van Gijn J, Ackerstaff RG. Detection of cerebral microemboli by means of transcranial Doppler monitoring before and after carotid endarterectomy. *Stroke* 1995; **26**:210–13.

121 Kirkes WS. On apoplexy in relation to chronic renal disease. *Med Times Gaz* 1855; **11**:515–16.

122 Charcot JM, Bouchard C. Nouvelles recherches sur la pathogénie de l'hémorrhagie cérébrale. *Arch Physiol norm pathol* 1868; **1**:110–27, 643–65, 725–34.

123 Iragui VJ. The Charcot-Bouchard controversy. *Arch Neurol* 1986; **43**:290–5.

124 Satran R. Joseph Babinski in the competitive examination (agrégation) of 1892. *Bull N Y Acad Med* 1974; **50**:626–35.

125 van Gijn J. The Babinski sign: the first hundred years. *J Neurol* 1996; **243**:675–83.

126 Ellis AG. The pathogenesis of spontaneous intracerebral hemorrhage. *Proc Pathol Soc Philadelphia* 1909; **12**:197–235.

127 Hiller F. Zirkulationsstörungen im Gehirn, eine klinische und pathologisch-anatomische Studie. *Arch Psychiat Nervenkr* 1935; **103**:1–53.

128 Globus JH, Epstein JA, Green MA, Marks M. Focal cerebral hemorrhage experimentally induced. *J Neuropathol Exp Neurol* 1949; **8**:113–16.

129 Rosenblath L. Über die Entstehung der Hirnblutung bei dem Schlaganfall. *Dtsch Z Nervenkr* 1918; **61**:10–143.

130 Westphal K. Über die Entstehung und Behandlung der Apoplexia sanguinea. *Dtsch med Wschr* 1932; **58**:685–90.

131 Ross Russell RW. Observations on intracerebral aneurysms. *Brain* 1963; **86**:425–42.

132 Cole FM, Yates PO. The occurrence and significance of intracerebral micro-aneurysms. *J Pathol Bacteriol* 1967; **93**:393–411.

133 Challa VL, Moody DM, Bell MA. The Charcot-Bouchard aneurysm controversy: impact of a new histologic technique. *J Neuropathol Exp Neurol* 1992; **51**:264–71.

134 Fischer O. Die presbyophrene Demenz, deren anatomische Grundlage und klinische Abgrenzung. *Z gesamte Neurol Psychiatr* 1910; **3**:371–471.

135 Scholz W. Studien zur Pathologie der Hirngefässe. II. Die drusige Entartung der Hirnarterien und -capillaren. *Z Gesamte Neurol Psychiatr* 1938; **162**:694–715.

136 Pantelakis S. Un type particulier d'angiopathie sénile du système nerveux central: l'angiopathie congophile: topographie et fréquence. *Monatsschr Psychiatr Neurol* 1954; **128**:219–56.

137 Torack RM. Congophilic angiopathy complicated by surgery and massive hemorrhage: a light and electron microscopic study. *Am J Pathol* 1975; **81**:349–65.

138 Jellinger K. Cerebrovascular amyloidosis with cerebral hemorrhage. *J Neurol* 1977; **214**:195–206.

139 Hounsfield GN. Computerised transverse axial scanning (tomography): I. Description of system. *Br J Radiol* 1973; **46**:1016–22.

140 Hayward RD, O'Reilly GV. Intracerebral haemorrhage. Accuracy of computerised transverse axial scanning in predicting the underlying aetiology. *Lancet* 1976; **1**:1–4.

141 McDonald CA, Korb M. Intracranial aneurysms. *Arch Neurol Psych* 1939; **42**:298–328.

142 Blackall J. *Observations on the Nature and Cure of Dropsies*. 5th ed. London: Longman & Co., 1813.

143 Hodgson J. *A Treatise on the Diseases of Arteries and Veins, containing the pathology and treatment of aneurisms and wounded arteries*. London: T. Underwood, 1815.

144 Serres ERA. Observations sur la rupture des anévrysmes des artères du cerveau. *Arch gén Méd* 1826; **10**:419–31.

145 Pyenson L, Sheets-Pyenson S. *Reading: Books and the Spread of Ideas. Servants of nature: a history of scientific institutions, enterprises, and sensibilities*. New York: W.W. Norton & Company, 1999: 211–35.

146 Berry D, Mackenzie C. *Richard Bright (1789–1858): physician in an age of revolution and reform*. London: Royal Society of Medicine Services Ltd., 1992.

147 Brinton W. Report on cases of cerebral aneurism. *Trans Pathol Soc London* 1852; **3**:47–9.

148 Gull W. Cases of aneurism of the cerebral vessels. *Guy's Hosp Rep* 1859; **5**:281–304.

149 Lebert H. Über die Aneurysmen der Hirnarterien. Eine Abhandlung in Briefen an Herrn Geheimrat Professor Dr. Frerichs. *Berl klin Wochenschr* 1866; **3**:209–405 (8 instalments).

150 Bartholow R. Aneurisms of the arteries at the base of the brain: their symptomatology, diagnosis and treatment. *Am J Med Sci* 1872; **44**:373–86.

151 Eppinger H. Pathogenesis (Histogenesis und Aetiologie) der Aneurysmen einschliesslich des Aneurysma equi verminosum. *Arch Klin Chir* 1887; **35** (suppl. 1):1–563.

152 Wichern H. Klinische Beiträge zur Kenntnis der Hirnaneurysmen. *Dtsch Zschr Nervenheilk* 1912; **44**:220–63.

153 Turnbull HM. Alterations in arterial structure, and their relation to syphilis. *Q J Med* 1914; **8**:201–54.

154 Beadles CF. Aneurisms of the larger cerebral arteries. *Brain* 1907; **30**:285–336.

155 Fearnsides EG. Intracranial aneurysms. *Brain* 1916; **39**:224–96.

156 Hutchinson J. Aneurism of the internal carotid artery within the skull diagnosed eleven years before the patient's death: spontaneous cure. *Trans Clin Soc London* 1875; **8**:127–31.

157 Bull E. Akut Hjerneaneurisma-Okulomotoriusparalyse-Meningealapoplexi. *Norsk Magasin for Laegevidenskapen* 1877; **7**:890–5.

158 Quincke H. Die Lumbalpunktion des Hydrocephalus. *Berl klin Wochenschr* 1891; **28**:929–33 and 965–8.

159 Froin G. *Les hémorrhagies sous-arachnoidiennes et le méchanisme de l'hématolyse en général*. Paris: G. Steinheil, 1904.

160 Guillain G. L'albuminurie massive dans le diagnostic des hémorrhagies méningées. *Presse Méd* 1915; **54**:441–2.

161 Goldflam S. Beiträge zur Aetiologie und Symptomatologie der spontanen subarachnoidalen Blutungen. *Dtsch Zschr Nervenheilk* 1923; **76**:158–82.

162 Symonds CP. Contributions to the clinical study of intracranial aneurysms. *Guy's Hosp Rep* 1923; **73**:139–58.

163 Symonds CP. Spontaneous subarachnoid haemorrhage. *Quart J Med* 1924; **18**:93–122.

164 Cushing H. Contributions to the clinical study of cerebral aneurisms. *Guy's Hosp Rep* 1923; **73**:159–63.

165 Symonds CP. Autobiographical introduction. In: Symonds CP, editor. *Studies in Neurology*. London: Oxford University Press, 1970, pp. 1–23.

166 Moniz E. Anévrysme intra-cranien de la carotide interne droite rendu visible par l'artériographie cérébrale. *Rev Oto-Neuro-Ophthal* 1933; **11**:198–203.

167 Schorstein J. Carotid ligation in saccular intracranial aneurisms. *Br J Surg* 1940; **28**:50–70.

168 Todd NV, Howie JE, Miller JD. Norman Dott's contribution to aneurysm surgery. *J Neurol Neurosurg Psychiatry* 1990; **53**:455–8.

169 Rush C, Shaw JF. *With Sharp Compassion: Norman Dott – freeman surgeon of Edinburgh*. Aberdeen: Aberdeen University Press, 1990.

170 Dott N. Intracranial aneurysms: cerebral arterio-radiography: surgical treatment. *Trans Med Chir Soc Edinb* 1932; **47**:219–40.

171 Dandy WE. Intracranial aneurysm of internal carotid artery, cured by operation. *Ann Surg* 1938; **107**:654–7.

172 Drake CG. Bleeding aneurysms of the basilar artery; direct surgical management in four cases. *J Neurosurg* 1961; **18**:230–8.

173 Guglielmi G, Vinuela F, Sepetka I, Macellari V. Electrothrombosis of saccular aneurysms via endovascular approach. Part 1: Electrochemical basis, technique, and experimental results. *J Neurosurg* 1991; **75**:1–7.

174 Guglielmi G, Vinuela F, Dion J, Duckwiler G. Electrothrombosis of saccular aneurysms via endovascular approach. Part 2: Preliminary clinical experience. *J Neurosurg* 1991; **75**:8–14.

175 Matthews JR. *Quantification and the Quest for Medical Certainty*. Princeton: Princeton University Press, 1995.

176 Louis PCA. *Recherches sur les effets de la saignée*. Paris: de Mignaret, 1835.

177 Gavarret J. *Principes généraux de statistique médicale*. Paris: Librairies de la Faculté de Médecine de Paris, 1840.

178 Bernard C. *Introduction à l'étude de la médecine expérimentale*. Paris: J.-B. Baillière, 1865.

179 Lister J. Effect of the antiseptic system of treatment on the salubrity of a surgical hospital. *Lancet* 1870; **i**:4–6; 40–2.

180 Stolley PD, Lasky T. *Investigating Disease Patterns: the science of epidemiology*. New York: W.H. Freeman & Company, 1995.

181 Blackmore E. Reports on the diseases of Plymouth I. *Edinburgh Medical and Surgical Journal* 1829; **31**:266–87.

182 Blackmore E. Reports on the diseases of Plymouth II. *Edinburgh Medical and Surgical Journal* 1829; **32**:1–20.

183 Snow SJ. *Operations Without Pain: the practice and science of anaesthesia in Victorian Britain*. Houndmills, Basingstoke: Palgrave Macmillan, 2006.

184 Acheson J, Acheson HW, Tellwright JM. The incidence and pattern of cerebrovascular disease in general practice. *J R Coll Gen Pract* 1968; **16**:428–36.

185 Kannel WB, Dawber TR, Cohen ME, McNamara PM. Vascular disease of the brain – epidemiological aspects: the Framingham study. *Am J Public Health* 1965; **55**:1355–66.

186 Hirota Y, Katsuki S, Asano C. A multivariate analysis of risk factors for cerebrovascular disease in Hisayama, Kyushu Island, Japan. *Behaviormetrika* 1975; **2**:1–11.

187 Salonen JT, Puska P, Mustaniemi H. Changes in morbidity and mortality during comprehensive community programme to control cardiovascular diseases during 1972–7 in North Karelia. *Br Med J* 1979; **2**:1178–83.

188 Montgomery M. *How Doctors Think: clinical judgment and the practice of medicine.* New York: Oxford University Press, 2005.

189 Medical Research Council. Streptomycin treatment of pulmonary tuberculosis. *Br Med J* 1948; **ii**:769–82.

190 Fibiger J. Om Serumbehandling af Difteri. *Hospitalstidende* 1898; **6**:309–25, 337–50.

191 Hróbjartsson A, Gøtzsche PC, Gluud C. The controlled clinical trial turns 100 years: Fibiger's trial of serum treatment of diphtheria. *Br Med J* 1998; **317**:1243–5.

192 Amberson JB, McMahon BT, Pinner M. A clinical trial of sanocrysin in pulmonary tuberculosis. *Am Rev Tuberc* 1931; **24**:401–35.

193 Ferguson FR, Davey AFC, Topley WWC. The value of mixed vaccines in the prevention of the common cold. *J Hyg* 1927; **26**:98–109.

194 Hinshaw HC, Feldman WH. Evaluation of chemotherapeutic agents in clinical tuberculosis. *Am Rev Tuberc* 1944; **50**:202–13.

195 Fisher RA. The arrangement of field experiments. *Journal of the Ministry of Agriculture* 1926; **33**:503–13.

196 Doll R. Controlled trials: the 1948 watershed. *Br Med J* 1998; **317**:1217–20.

197 Chalmers I. Why transition from alternation to randomisation in clinical trials was made. *Br Med J* 1999; **319**:1372.

198 Hill AB, Marshall J, Shaw DA. A controlled clinical trial of long-term anticoagulant therapy in cerebrovascular disease. *Quart J Med* 1960; **29**:597–609.

199 Hill AB, Marshall J, Shaw DA. Cerebrovascular disease: a trial of long-term anticoagulant tharapy. *Br Med J* 1962; **ii**:1003–6.

200 Jonas S. Anticoagulant therapy in cerebrovascular disease: a review and meta-analysis. *Stroke* 1988; **19**:1043–8.

201 Acheson J, Danta G, Hutchinson EC. Controlled trial of dipyridamole in cerebral vascular disease. *Br Med J* 1969; **1**:614–15.

202 Dyken ML, White PT. Evaluation of cortisone in treatment of cerebral infarction. *J Am Med Assoc* 1956; **162**:1531–4.

203 Fields WS, Maslenikov V, Meyer JS, Hass WK, Remington RD, Macdonald M. Joint study of extracranial arterial occlusion. V. Progress report of prognosis following surgery or nonsurgical treatment for transient ischemic attacks and cervical carotid artery lesions. *J Am Med Assoc* 1970; **211**:1993–2003.

204 Canadian Cooperative Study Group. A randomized trial of aspirin and sulfinpyrazone in threatened stroke. *N Engl J Med* 1978; **299**:53–9.

205 Kurtzke JF. Controversy in neurology: the Canadian study on TIA and aspirin – a critique of the Canadian TIA study. *Ann Neurol* 1979; **5**:597–9.

206 Flourens MJP. *Recherches expérimentales sur les propriétés et les fonctions du système nerveux, dans les animaux vertébrés.* Paris: Crevot, 1824.

207 Gall FJ, Spurzheim JC. *Anatomie et physiologie du système nerveux en général, et du cerveau en particulier, avec des observations sur la possibilité de reconnaître plusieurs dispositions intellectuelles et morales de l'homme et des animaux, par la configurations de leurs têtes.* Paris: Schoell, 1819.

208 Fritsch GT, Hitzig E. Ueber die elektrische Erregbarkeit des Grosshirns. *Arch Anat Physiol wiss Med* 1870; **37**:300–32.

209 Hitzig E. *Untersuchungen über das Gehirn.* Berlin: A. Hirschwald, 1874.

210 Thorwald J. *Das Weltreich der Chirurgen.* Stuttgart: Steingrüben, 1957.

211 Yusuf S, Peto R, Lewis J, Collins R, Sleight P. Beta blockade during and after myocardial infarction: an overview of the randomized trials. *Prog Cardiovasc Dis* 1985; **27**:335–71.

212 Counsell C, Warlow C, Sandercock P, Fraser H, van Gijn J. The Cochrane Collaboration Stroke Review Group. Meeting the need for systematic reviews in stroke care. *Stroke* 1995; **26**:498–502.

213 Freiman JA, Chalmers TC, Smith H, Jr., Kuebler RR. The importance of beta, the type II error and sample size in the design and interpretation of the randomized control trial. Survey of 71 'negative' trials. *N Engl J Med* 1978; **299**:690–4.

214 Lewis JA, Ellis SH. A statistical appraisal of postinfarction betablocker trials. *Prim Cardiol* 1982; suppl. 1:317.

215 Lewis S, Clarke M. Forest plots: trying to see the wood and the trees. *Br Med J* 2001; **322**:1479–80.

216 Antiplatelet Trialists' Collaboration. Secondary prevention of vascular disease by prolonged antiplatelet treatment. *Br Med J* 1988; **296**:320–31.

217 Temkin O. The historiography of ideas in medicine. In: Clarke E, editor. *Modern methods in the history of medicine.* London: The Athlone Press, 1971, pp. 1–21.

218 Hippocrates. *The Genuine Works of Hippocrates.* Baltimore: Williams & Wilkins, 1939.

219 Rokitansky C. *Handbuch der pathologischen Anatomie.* Wien: Braumüller und Seidel, 1842.

220 Todd EM. *The Neuroanatomy of Leonardo da Vinci.* Park Ridge: American Association of Neurological Surgeons, 1991.

221 New PJF, Scott WR. *Computed Tomography of the Brain and Orbit (EMI scanning).* Baltimore: Williams & Wilkins, 1975.

222 Dandy WE. *Intracranial Arterial Aneurysms.* Ithaca, New York: Comstock Publishing Company, 1944.

223 Blakemore C. *Mechanics of the Mind.* Cambridge: Cambridge University Press, 1977.

224 Schwartz P. Arten der Schlaganfälle des Gehirns. Berlin: Julius Springer, 1930.

3

Is it a vascular event and where is the lesion?

Identifying and interpreting the symptoms and signs of cerebrovascular disease

3.1 Introduction

This chapter deals with the first two of several questions that need to be answered in the assessment of patients

Table 3.1 The assessment process in the diagnosis and subsequent management of a vascular event of the brain or eye.

Is it a stroke, a transient ischaemic attack, or a brain attack?	Chapter 3
Which part of the brain has been affected?	Chapter 3
Which arterial territory has been affected?	Chapter 4
Is there a recognizable clinical syndrome?	Chapter 4
What pathological type of cerebrovascular event is it?	Chapter 5
What disease process caused the cerebrovascular event?	Chapters 6–9
What, if any, are the functional consequences?	Chapters 10,11
What treatment will improve survival free of handicap?	Chapters 12–16

Stroke: practical management, 3rd edition. C. Warlow, J. van Gijn, M. Dennis, J. Wardlaw, J. Bamford, G. Hankey, P. Sandercock, G. Rinkel, P. Langhorne, C. Sudlow and P. Rothwell. Published 2008 Blackwell Publishing. ISBN 978-1-4051-2766-0.

presenting with a suspected transient ischaemic attack of the brain or eye (TIA) or stroke – is it a vascular event, and where is the lesion? (Table 3.1). We will begin by defining what is meant by a TIA and stroke, and follow by describing our approach to distinguishing TIA and stroke from other differential diagnoses.

3.2 Definitions of transient ischaemic attack, stroke and acute stroke syndrome ('brain attack' or 'unstable brain ischaemia')

3.2.1 The definition of transient ischaemic attack

A standard definition of a TIA is 'a clinical syndrome characterized by an acute loss of focal cerebral or monocular function with *symptoms* lasting less than 24 h and which is thought to be due to inadequate cerebral or ocular blood supply as a result of low blood flow, thrombosis or embolism associated with disease of the arteries, heart or blood'.[1,2] By definition therefore, TIAs are caused by transient reduction in blood flow to a part of the brain as a result of thromboembolic disease of the arteries, heart and blood. However, it is conceivable that TIAs may also arise from disease of the *veins*, causing transient reduction in venous return from the brain or eye, but we are not aware of any patients with cerebral venous thrombosis who have presented with symptoms of TIA.[3,4] *The main features of TIAs are*:

- sudden onset;
- symptoms of loss of focal neurological function (Table 3.2);
- symptoms maximal at onset (more or less);
- symptoms resolve within 24 h;
- brain imaging (CT, MRI and DWI) may or may not show a relevant focal ischaemic lesion in the brain.

Focal neurological symptoms

Focal neurological symptoms are those that arise from a disturbance in an identifiable and localized area of the brain – for example, unilateral weakness from a lesion of the corticospinal tract (Table 3.2). However, there are some focal neurological symptoms which, when they occur *in isolation*, should *probably* not be considered as TIAs, because they occur more commonly in non-vascular conditions. Moreover, when present in isolation,

Table 3.2 Focal neurological and ocular symptoms.

Motor symptoms
Weakness or clumsiness of one side of the body, in whole or in part (hemiparesis, monoparesis and sometimes only just the hand)
Simultaneous bilateral weakness*
Difficulty in swallowing*
Imbalance*
Speech/language disturbances
Difficulty in understanding or expressing spoken language
Difficulty in reading (dyslexia) or writing
Difficulty in calculating
Slurred speech*
Sensory symptoms
Altered feeling on one side of the body, in whole or in part
Visual symptoms
Loss of vision in one eye, in whole or in part
Loss of vision in half or quarter of the visual field
Bilateral blindness
Double vision*
Vestibular symptoms
A sensation of movement*
Behavioural/cognitive symptoms
Difficulty in dressing, combing hair, cleaning teeth, geographical disorientation (visuospatial–perceptual dysfunction)
Forgetfulness*

*As an *isolated* symptom, this does not necessarily indicate focal cerebral ischaemia unless there is an appropriately sited acute infarct or haemorrhage, or there are additional definite focal symptoms.

they have not been shown to be associated with the high risk of future serious vascular events that characterizes TIAs. Such symptoms include rotational vertigo (caused by benign paroxysmal positional vertigo, vestibular neuritis, etc.), transient amnesia (transient global amnesia, psychogenic amnesia, etc.), and diplopia (myasthenia gravis, superior oblique myokymia, ocular myotonia, near-reflex accommodation spasm, etc.). Further research, based on imaging and long-term prognostic studies, of patients presenting with isolated focal neurological symptoms such as vertigo and dysarthria should help ascertain if, and how often, these symptoms are vascular in origin, and if so, what may help distinguish them from non-vascular causes (possibly older age and presence of other vascular risk factors).

> Some focal neurological symptoms should probably not be considered as transient ischaemic attacks if they occur in isolation (e.g. rotational vertigo, transient amnesia, and diplopia).

> Transient ischaemic attacks (and ischaemic stroke) are diagnosed with confidence only if the symptoms can be attributed to ischaemia of a focal brain area, and if there is no better explanation.

Non-focal neurological symptoms

Non-focal neurological symptoms (Table 3.3) are *not usually* caused by focal cerebral ischaemia; there are many other more common non-vascular neurological and non-neurological causes:

- Generalized weakness caused by depression, acute inflammatory demyelinating polyradiculoneuropathy, myasthenia gravis, botulism, periodic paralysis, tick paralysis, acute toxic motor neuropathy, porphyric polyneuropathy, Miller Fisher syndrome and acute myelopathy;
- Light-headedness caused by cardiac arrhythmias, aortic stenosis, cardiac tamponade, myocardial infarction, vasovagal syncope, reflex syncope and carotid sinus syncope;

Table 3.3 Non-focal neurological symptoms.

Generalized weakness and/or sensory disturbance
Light-headedness
Faintness
'Blackouts' with altered or loss of consciousness or fainting, with or without impaired vision in both eyes
Incontinence of urine or faeces
Confusion
Ringing in the ears (tinnitus)

(a)

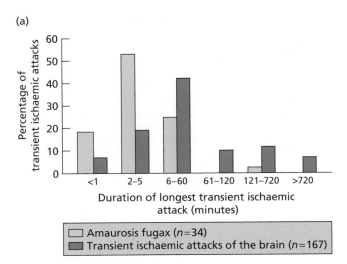

(b)

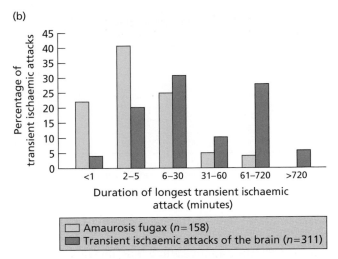

Fig. 3.1 Histogram showing the duration of the longest transient ischaemic attack (TIA) before presentation amongst (a) 184 TIA patients in the Oxfordshire Community Stroke Project;[6] (b) 469 TIA patients in a hospital-referred series (from Hankey & Warlow, 1994[2] by kind permission of the authors and W.B. Saunders Co Ltd).

- Postural hypotension secondary to dehydration, blood pressure-lowering drugs (e.g. antihypertensives, dopamine agonists) and autonomic neuropathy;
- Drop attacks (see below);
- Confusion/delirium caused by metabolic/toxic encephalopathy.

Therefore, non-focal symptoms should *not* be interpreted as being caused by a TIA or stroke unless accompanied by focal neurological symptoms. This is because – in isolation – they have other causes and do not seem to predict an increased risk of future serious vascular events.

> Non-focal symptoms such as faintness, dizziness or generalized weakness are seldom, if ever, likely to be due to focal cerebral ischaemia (i.e. seldom a transient ischaemic attack or stroke), but may be due to generalized brain ischaemia (e.g. syncope) as well as non-vascular neurological and non-neurological causes (e.g. hyperventilation or other manifestations of anxiety).

Neurological signs

The standard definition of TIA allows abnormal but functionally unimportant focal neurological signs such as reflex asymmetry or an extensor plantar response to persist for longer than 24 h, provided the *symptoms* have resolved within 24 hours; this occurs in about 5% of patients.[1,2]

Duration of symptoms

The upper limit for the duration of symptoms (24 h) has more to do with the earth's rotation than biology;

patients with focal ischaemic neurological symptoms lasting longer than 24 h (ischaemic stroke) have similar causes and prognosis for future vascular events as patients with focal ischaemic neurological symptoms lasting less than 24 h (TIA).[5] The duration of symptoms of TIA and ischaemic stroke are a continuum (Fig. 3.1);[2,6] the only 'relevance' of longer duration TIAs and minor ischaemic stroke is that a relevant ischaemic lesion is more likely to be demonstrated by brain imaging (Fig. 3.2)[7] and the risk of (recurrent) stroke increases.[8–11] Indeed, increasing duration of focal neurological symptoms is one of the five main predictors of early recurrent stroke, along with Age, Blood pressure, Clinical features and Diabetes (and Duration of symptoms) in the ABCD[2] prognostic model of early stroke risk after TIA[10] (section 16.2.1).

It has been suggested recently that the *lower* limit for the duration of symptoms should be 10 min.[8,12] We would agree that TIAs lasting less than 10 min are associated with a lower risk of stroke than longer duration TIAs,[10] and that focal neurological symptoms of the brain lasting seconds, and perhaps even a few minutes, are seldom likely to be TIAs of the brain (but TIAs of the eye – amaurosis fugax – may last only seconds). However, we remain uncertain just how short focal episodes can be and still be a TIA.

> It is not known how short a TIA can be (and still be a TIA).

Brain imaging

A substantial proportion of patients with cerebral TIA have evidence on brain imaging by CT or MRI of focal

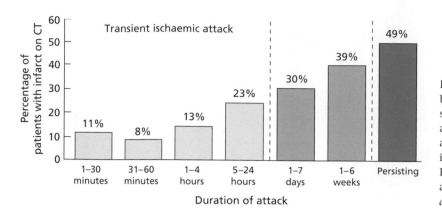

Fig. 3.2 Histogram showing the relationship between the duration of focal neurological symptoms due to TIA and ischaemic stroke and the percentage of patients with an appropriately sited abnormality on brain imaging with CT (from Koudstaal, van Gijn, Frenken *et al.*, 1992[7] by kind permission of the authors and *Journal of Neurology, Neurosurgery and Psychiatry*).

areas of altered signal intensity, suggestive of ischaemia, in an area of the brain relevant to the transient symptoms.[13–15] Diffusion-weighted MR imaging (DWI) is more sensitive than CT or MRI T2-weighted images, and identifies a relevant abnormality in up to two-thirds of patients with TIAs (Fig. 3.3).[14,16–20] As a result some have proposed a revised definition of TIA which is restricted to patients who experience a brief episode of focal neurological dysfunction, presumptively caused by focal brain ischaemia, but *without* neuroimaging evidence of acute ischaemia or infarction. It has been further proposed that all other episodes with transient focal neurological symptoms *with* relevant lesion(s) (presumed infarction) on brain imaging are called ischaemic stroke.[12,21–24] However, as stated in previous editions of this book, we do not accept such a definition, based on brain imaging, for the following reasons:

- A CT or MR (including DWI) scan then becomes essential for the diagnosis of TIA, precluding up to one-fifth of patients who cannot undergo brain imaging (e.g. because they have an intraocular or intracerebral metallic foreign body or pacemaker, or are claustrophobic). Further, as the time to scanning decreases, and technology advances, the definition of a TIA would be constantly changing.

- A positive CT, MRI or MRI-DWI may be a false positive (i.e. the 'relevant' abnormality on brain imaging may not represent recent infarction or ischaemia occurring at the time of the TIA (Table 3.4). Further, the limitations of DWI in diagnosing TIA cannot all be overcome (at present) by performing a complete stroke MRI examination, including T2-weighted imaging, angiography and perfusion imaging.[25]

- There is a gradual increase in the proportion of patients with a 'relevant' abnormality on brain imaging as the duration of symptoms increases, with no distinct change at 24 h[7,12,18,23,24] (Fig. 3.2). This argues against there being any significantly different underlying pathophysiology between TIA and minor ischaemic stroke. There are also no significant

Table 3.4 Causes of an inaccurate diffusion-weighted MRI (DWI) diagnosis of TIA.

False positive DWI diagnosis of TIA (at least 10%)
Non-ischaemic cause of DWI hyperintensity
Neurologically asymptomatic cause of DWI hyperintensity
Chronic, persistent cause of DWI hyperintensity (i.e. old lesion)

False negative DWI diagnosis of TIA (at least 10%)
Very early imaging after onset of ischaemia (i.e. too early)
Short-duration TIA (insufficient time to cause early ischaemic changes on DWI)
Penumbral ischaemia (ischaemia is sufficient to cause neurological symptoms but insufficient to cause failure of the sodium-potassium ATPase pump in the neuronal cell membranes)
Ischaemic region too small to image
Ischaemic region too difficult to image (e.g. in brainstem)
Confounding background lesion(s)
Late imaging after onset of ischaemia (e.g. > 2 weeks after resolution of symptoms)

differences in the clinical features and prevalence of vascular risk factors among TIA patients with and without a relevant infarct on brain imaging.[5] However, there may be a difference in prognosis if the results of initial studies showing the presence of such a 'TIA scar' on brain imaging is associated with an increased risk of future stroke are confirmed.[11,15,26]

- A new diagnostic category would have to be made for patients with a clinically definite stroke (i.e. symptoms for more than 24 h) but who have normal imaging, which could hardly be called a 'TIA'.

- There would be substantial implications of a tissue-based definition of TIA, in which patients with a TIA and a positive DWI would be reclassified as having a stroke, for epidemiological research and insurance policies.[27] For example, studies of secular trends in stroke incidence and outcome would be confounded by the inclusion of patients with 'TIA and brain imaging evidence of infarction' as a 'stroke', whereas they

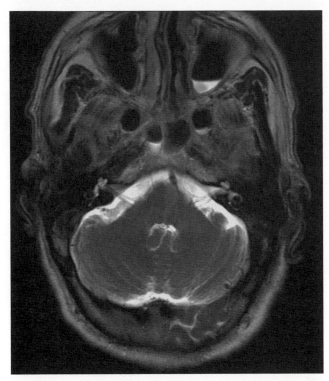

(a)

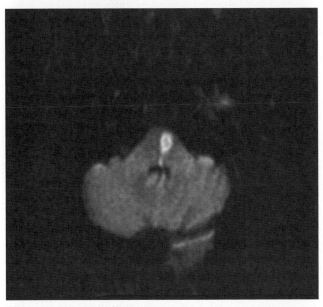

(b)

Fig. 3.3 (a) MRI (T$_2$ weighted) of the brainstem (pons) in a patient with a recent episode of transient hemiparesis (right face, arm and leg) and conjugate gaze palsy to the left showing a very subtle region of altered signal intensity in the left paramedian pons. (b) MRI (DWI) in the same patient showing a very obvious area of high signal intensity (so-called 'light bulb' sign), consistent with early ischaemic change, in the left paramedian pons which was relevant to the patient's focal neurological symptoms.

were previously considered a TIA and not included as stroke in earlier studies. Further, patients with TIA and brain imaging evidence of infarction may now not be able to obtain life insurance, or their premiums may increase substantially.[27] Critical illness insurance companies would even have to pay out for TIAs with DWI evidence of infarction that they would previously not have had to pay out for because the event would now be called a stroke; premiums would invariably rise to cover the new costs.

> At present there is no diagnostic test based on imaging or blood chemistry that is sufficiently sensitive, specific and widely available to reliably diagnose and exclude transient ischaemic attack and stroke.

We believe that patients with clinically definite TIAs (i.e. focal neurological symptoms lasting less than 24 hours with no other explanation other than a vascular origin), who have an appropriately sited and presumably ischaemic lesion on brain imaging, should have the fact noted (and considered to *possibly* be at increased risk of stroke).[11,15,26] However, they should still be classified as having had a TIA, or maybe a new term for short duration symptoms of focal brain or ocular ischaemia (less than 24 h) with a relevant lesion on MRI scan (e.g. transient symptoms associated with infarction [TSI]),[24] but definitely not a stroke. Our diagnostic criteria for TIA are summarized in Table 3.5.

> The presence of a presumed ischaemic lesion in the relevant part of the brain on CT or MR scan in a patient who presents with transient symptoms lasting less than 24 h should not change the diagnosis of a transient ischaemic attack (TIA) to a stroke.

> Although bright, high signal-intensity lesions ('light bulbs') on DWI and low apparent diffusion coefficient values have a high sensitivity (about 90%) and specificity (about 90%) for the diagnosis of acute focal cerebral ischaemia, the same findings have been reported in other diverse conditions such as focal brain haemorrhage, abscess and tumour (i.e. they are not 100% specific).

3.2.2 The definition of stroke

The most widely accepted definition of a stroke is 'a syndrome characterized by rapidly developing clinical symptoms and/or signs of focal, and at times global (applied to patients in deep coma and those with subarachnoid haemorrhage), loss of cerebral function, with symptoms lasting more than 24 h or leading to death,

Table 3.5 Diagnostic criteria for transient ischaemic attack (TIA).

Nature of symptoms
Focal neurological or monocular symptoms
Quality of symptoms
'Negative' symptoms, representing loss of focal neurological or monocular function (e.g. weakness, numbness, aphasia, loss of vision); rarely, 'positive' symptoms occur (e.g. pins and needles, limb shaking, scintillating visual field abnormality)
Time course of symptoms
Abrupt onset, starting in different parts of the body (e.g. face, arm, leg) at more or less the same time, without intensification or spread ('march'); deficit maximal usually within a few seconds; symptoms resolve more gradually but completely, usually within an hour and, by definition, always within 24 h. Very brief attacks, lasting only seconds, are unusual except for transient monocular blindness (TMB) (note: we do not know how brief an attack of TMB can be and still be classified as TMB due to transient ischaemia; perhaps 10 s or so?)
Associated symptoms
TIAs usually occur without warning
Antecedent symptoms are rare, but may reflect the cause (e.g. neck and face pain due to carotid dissection, headache due to giant-cell arteritis); otherwise, antecedent symptoms (e.g. headache, nausea or epigastric discomfort) usually suggest migraine or epilepsy
Headache may occur during and after a TIA; it is to be distinguished from migraine headache
Loss of consciousness is almost never due to a TIA; it usually suggests syncope or epilepsy
Neurological signs
Following symptomatic recovery, a few physical signs, such as reflex asymmetry or an extensor plantar response, which are not functionally significant, may be found
Brain CT or MR scan
The scan may show small areas of altered density, consistent with brain ischaemia or infarction, in a relevant part of the brain, or may have areas of hypodensity (on CT) or increased signal (on T2 weighted MR) remote from the symptomatic area
Frequency of attacks
TIAs often recur, but very frequent stereotyped attacks raise the possibility of partial epileptic seizures (sometimes due to an underlying structural abnormality such as an arteriovenous malformation, chronic subdural haematoma or cerebral tumour) or hypoglycaemia

with no apparent cause other than that of vascular origin'.[28] This definition embraces stroke due to cerebral infarction (ischaemic stroke), non-traumatic intracerebral haemorrhage, intraventricular haemorrhage and some cases of subarachnoid haemorrhage (SAH). By convention, this definition does not include retinal infarction, subdural haemorrhage, epidural haemorrhage, traumatic intracerebral haemorrhage or infarction, infection or tumour; nor does it embrace patients with intracranial venous thrombosis and SAH who are conscious and have a headache but no abnormal neurological signs. It is therefore important to be clear about what is, and what is not, included as 'stroke' in conversation, and in the literature.

Since the clinical features, aetiology, prognosis and treatment of SAH are, for the most part, quite distinct from those of other forms of stroke,[29,30] we think it is better to have a definition of stroke that does not include SAH, and so a completely separate definition for SAH. This is despite the fact that such a change in the definition of stroke would have implications for epidemiological studies of trends in incidence and outcome of stroke, just like changing the definition of TIA (see above), but in this instance would not be so dependent on the ever shifting sands of technology as changing the diagnosis of TIA to a tissue-based definition. Subarachnoid haemorrhage is therefore discussed separately below (section 3.7).

The revised definition of stroke which we propose is 'a clinical syndrome characterized by an acute loss of focal cerebral function with symptoms lasting more than 24 h or leading to death, and which is thought to be due to either spontaneous haemorrhage into the brain substance (haemorrhagic stroke) or inadequate cerebral blood supply to a part of the brain (ischaemic stroke) as a result of low blood flow, thrombosis or embolism associated with diseases of the blood vessels (arteries or veins), heart or blood'. Patients who are being assessed within 24 h of symptom onset and who still have focal neurological symptoms are temporarily classified as having a 'brain attack' (or something similar, such as an 'acute stroke syndrome' or 'unstable brain ischaemia').

In practice, the *absence* of an obvious focal neurological deficit in a patient with a suspected stroke does not necessarily exclude the diagnosis. It may simply be a consequence of a delay in presentation, so that the signs have resolved, or it may be that the signs are rather subtle (but nevertheless functionally important to the patient) and have been missed. Examples include:
- isolated dysphasia misinterpreted as confusion;
- isolated visuospatial or perceptual disorder (e.g. dressing apraxia, geographical disorientation) which may not be noticed at the bedside examination, at least to begin with;[31]
- isolated amnesia or other subtle form of cognitive dysfunction;[32]

- truncal and gait ataxia due to a cerebellar stroke which is only apparent (or elicitable) if the patient is asked to sit up, get out of bed and walk.[33]

These types of deficit may be missed (but should not be) in the emergency room, on busy ward rounds, during a hurried post-carotid endarterectomy or coronary artery bypass surgery assessment, and indeed any time.

3.2.3 The overlap between transient ischaemic attack and stroke, and the concept of an acute stroke syndrome ('brain attack' or 'unstable brain ischaemia')

There is a continuum from TIA to ischaemic stroke in terms of duration of symptoms (see above).[7] Moreover, patients with TIA and mild ischaemic stroke share a similar age and sex distribution, prevalence of vascular risk factors (and probably therefore pathogenesis) and *long*-term prognosis for serious vascular events although the short-term prognosis may differ.[5] Thus, from the point of view of pathogenesis and treatment (secondary prevention), there seems no pressing need to distinguish TIA from ischaemic stroke, and indeed many trials of secondary prevention have included patients with TIA and non-disabling, mild ischaemic stroke because they are essentially the same condition.

The problem in the era of increasingly rapid assessment and treatment of patients with acute cerebrovascular disease is how to use this time-based definition of TIA and stroke in patients who are being seen, and in some cases treated with potentially dangerous drugs (e.g. thrombolytics), within a few hours of the onset of symptoms. For example, if a hemiparetic patient is assessed 2 h after the onset of symptoms, an important question is whether this attack will recover and turn out to be a TIA, or not recover and become a stroke? There is no certain way of knowing, unless the patient is already recovering, but the longer the duration of symptoms of focal neurological dysfunction the more likely the deficit will persist,[24] and the greater the risk of subsequent early stroke.[9,10,34] Of course, for patients whose symptoms have resolved within 24 h of onset, they can be diagnosed retrospectively as having had a TIA. However, for those who still have symptoms within 24 h of onset, with or without relevant physical signs, it is appropriate to describe the acute presentation of focal cerebral ischaemia by a term such as a 'brain attack' or 'acute stroke syndrome' or 'unstable brain ischaemia'.[35] This emphasizes the need to rapidly exclude other differential diagnoses of TIA and stroke (e.g. hypoglycaemia, brain tumour), establish the pathological and aetiological subtype of the stroke and risk of recurrent stroke, and intervene with appropriate treatments that may include reperfusion therapy for focal brain ischaemia, maintenance of physiological homeostasis, prevention of complications of stroke, early prevention of recurrent stroke and other serious vascular events, and early rehabilitation.[36] 'Time is brain' in this setting.

> The anachronistic term 'cerebrovascular accident (CVA)' should be abandoned because it misleadingly implies that stroke is a chance event and that little can be done.

Reasons to distinguish TIA and minor ischaemic stroke

The are at least four reasons to distinguish TIA from minor ischaemic stroke.

First, when formulating a differential diagnosis in clinical practice the differential diagnosis of focal neurological symptoms lasting minutes (e.g. epileptic seizures, migraine) is somewhat different from that of attacks lasting several hours to days (e.g. intracranial tumour, intracerebral haemorrhage), and in any event the reliability of the clinical diagnosis of stroke is much better than for TIA (section 3.6).

Second, when conducting epidemiological studies of cerebrovascular disease consistency of diagnostic criteria is absolutely essential for comparing results over time and in different regions. Further, complete case ascertainment in incidence and prevalence studies is much less likely for TIA than stroke since patients who experience brief attacks are more likely to ignore or forget them, and are less likely to report them to a doctor than patients who suffer more prolonged or disabling events.

Third, for case–control studies, there is less change in 'acute phase' blood factors related to thrombosis and tissue infarction, and there is, by definition, no survival bias amongst TIA patients compared with stroke patients.

Fourth, distinguishing TIA from minor stroke can also aid assessment of case-mix in individual units and audits of management.

3.3 The diagnosis of a cerebrovascular event

The diagnosis of TIA and stroke is based on a constellation of clinical features that are thought to have a similar pathophysiology (i.e. caused by focal cerebral or ocular ischaemia or haemorrhage) (Table 3.2) and to be associated with similar outcomes (i.e. an increased risk of stroke and other major vascular events).

> TIA and stroke are clinical diagnoses, based on a history of rapidly developing symptoms and signs of focal, and at times global, loss of focal brain function lasting 24 h respectively with no apparent cause other than that of vascular origin. The absence of a persistent neurological deficit does not exclude the diagnosis of TIA or stroke; such 'negative' findings may represent a delay in presentation, signs that have resolved, or subtle signs that have been missed (e.g. visual-spatial-perceptual dysfunction). Similarly, the absence of a relevant acute lesion on brain imaging by CT, MRI or DWI does not exclude the diagnosis of TIA or stroke.

The assessment of patients with a suspected TIA or stroke depends on the *time* that has elapsed since the onset of symptoms. If the patient is assessed within 3–6 h of stroke onset, the main focus is to establish the diagnosis of stroke, the pathological type and severity, and whether early reperfusion, or antiplatelet therapy and/or carotid endarterectomy may be indicated. If the patient is assessed (or reassessed) after this time, the focus is not toward reperfusion therapy but to ascertaining and minimizing the risk of recurrent stroke and the adverse sequelae and complications of the stroke. The timing of the assessment may also influence the reliability of the clinical assessment and accuracy of the diagnosis;[37] focal neurological signs may resolve with time, which can make the diagnosis particularly difficult if the only signs were, for example, visual-spatial-perceptual dysfunction. But it can also make the diagnosis easier if neurological signs such as drowsiness and dysphasia recover, so more history can be obtained from the patient.

The first contact between clinician and patient is a crucial opportunity to conduct an appropriate history and physical examination, and obtain relevant information from any observers, family, friends, the patient's medical records and paramedical ambulance personnel (particularly when the patient is unable to communicate clearly due to dysphasia, depressed consciousness or knowledge only of a foreign language).[38] The prior probability of a stroke among unscreened patients with neurologically relevant symptoms transported to an emergency department is about 10%.[39] However, in some countries (e.g. Australia), paramedical ambulance personnel attend most patients admitted to hospital with stroke and they correctly identify about three-quarters of stroke patients.[40] However, because such personnel tend to overdiagnose stroke (not being aware of other conditions that mimic the symptoms of stroke) several prehospital screening tools have been developed, based on a few core clinical features (Tables 3.6, 3.7), to minimize the false positive diagnoses. These include:

- the Face Arm Speech Test (FAST);[41,42]
- the Cincinnati Prehospital Stroke Scale (CPSS);[43]
- the Los Angeles Paramedic Stroke Scale (LAPSS);[39]
- the Melbourne Ambulance Stroke Screen (MASS).[40]

These tools have proved particularly helpful in rapid assessment of stroke patients 'in the field', and in communicating to regional stroke centres the imminent arrival of a patient with probable acute stroke.

History

> When a patient presents with a suspected transient ischaemic attack, 'brain attack' or stroke, the first question to answer is whether it really is a vascular event or not. This begins with, and depends on, a sound, carefully taken clinical history.

Assessment	FAST	LAPSS	CPSS	MASS
History items				
Age > 45 years		X		X
Absent history of seizure or epilepsy		X		X
At baseline, not wheelchair bound or bedridden		X		X
Blood glucose concentration between 2.8 and 22.2 mmol/L		X		X
Physical assessment items				
Facial droop	X	X	X	X
Arm drift	X	X	X	X
Hand grip		X		X
Speech	X		X	X
Criteria for identifying stroke				
Presence of any physical assessment item	X	X	X	X
All history items answered yes		X		X

Table 3.6 Pre-hospital screening tools for the diagnosis of stroke: comparison of the Face Arm Speech Test (FAST), Los Angeles Paramedic Stroke Scale (LAPSS), Cincinnati Prehospital Stroke Scale (CPSS) and Melbourne Ambulance Stroke Screen (MASS).

Table 3.7 Motor and speech items assessed in several pre-hospital screening tools used for diagnosis of stroke.[39–42]

Assessment item	Normal response	Abnormal response
Facial droop Patient smiles or shows teeth	Both sides move equally	One side does not move
Arm drift Patient closes eyes and extends both arms for 10 s	Both arms move equally	One arm does not move or one arm drifts down, compared to the other
Hand grip Place a hand in each hand of the patient and ask him/her to squeeze hands	Both grip equally	Unilaterally weak or no grip
Speech Patient repeats a sentence	Normal language and articulation	Slurred or incorrect words, or unable to speak

When the patient is first assessed, take the patient and/or eyewitness back to the onset of symptoms, recording their own words and not just your interpretation of them. This can usually be achieved by asking the three questions:
- 'When did it happen?'
- 'Where were you when it happened?'
- 'What were you doing when it happened?'

For clarification, it is always worth asking patients to describe their symptoms in an alternative way, particularly if the terms they use are rather vague, e.g. 'dizziness' or 'heaviness'. Also it can sometimes be useful to ask patients whether they would have been able to do a specific task at the time of symptom onset; for example, if the patient describes an arm as being 'dead', asking whether they could lift the arm above their head would at least give a pointer as to whether the use of the word 'dead' was referring to a motor or just a sensory deficit.

> The use of certain terms is often culturally determined, and it must not be assumed that your interpretation of the term is the same as the patient's. The most appropriate response if you are unsure is 'what do you mean by that?' or 'try and describe what you mean in another way'.

The history should obtain information about the following.
- The nature of the symptoms and signs (sections 3.3.1–3.3.7):
  - which modalities were/are involved (e.g. motor, sensory, visual)?
  - which anatomical areas were/are involved (e.g. face, arm, leg, and was it the whole or part of the limb; one or both eyes)?
  - were/are the symptoms focal or non-focal (Tables 3.2 and 3.3)?
  - what was/is their quality (i.e. 'negative', causing loss of sensory, motor or visual function; or 'positive', causing limb jerking, tingling, hallucinations)?
  - what were/are the functional consequences (e.g. unable to stand, unable to lift arm)?
- The speed of onset and temporal course of the neurological symptoms (section 3.3.8):
  - what time of day did they begin?
  - was the onset sudden?
  - were the symptoms more or less maximal at onset; did they spread or progress in a stepwise, remitting, or progressive fashion over minutes/hours/days; or were there fluctuations between normal and abnormal function?
- Were there any possible precipitants (section 3.3.9)?
  - what was the patient doing at the time and immediately before the onset?
- Were there any accompanying symptoms (section 3.3.10), such as:
  - headache, epileptic seizures, panic and anxiety, vomiting, chest pain?
- Is there any relevant past or family history (section 3.3.11)?
  - have there been any previous TIAs or strokes?
  - is there a history of hypertension, hypercholesterolaemia, diabetes mellitus, angina, myocardial infarction, intermittent claudication, or arteritis?
  - is there a family history of vascular or thrombotic disorders?
- Are there any relevant lifestyle habits/behaviours (section 3.3.12)?
  - cigarette smoking, alcohol consumption, diet, physical activity, medications (especially the oral contraceptive pill, antithrombotic drugs, anticoagulants and recreational drugs such as amphetamines).

> A record in the notes such as 'no history available' probably reflects laziness on the part of a doctor who has not tried fully to obtain it, rather than the real lack of any information.

Examination

The examination aims to:
- confirm the presence of focal neurological signs, if any, anticipated from the history;
- discover possible aetiological explanations for the event (e.g. atrial fibrillation, carotid bruits, cardiac murmurs, etc.), some of which may not be anticipated (e.g. malignant hypertension);
- identify contraindications to investigation (e.g. a pacemaker – MR examination);

- anticipate nursing and rehabilitation needs (e.g. impaired swallowing, urinary incontinence, immobility, pre-existing reduced visual or auditory acuity).

A sophisticated knowledge of neurology is not needed to elicit and recognize the clinical features of a cerebrovascular event, as highlighted by the accurate paramedic and emergency room identification of stroke using simple stroke assessment tools (see above). However, a systematic approach is required as well as awareness of the discriminatory potential of symptoms and signs, in isolation and in groups (syndromes) (Table 3.8).[44,45]

Symptoms	% of patients		Odds ratio
	Stroke or TIA ($n = 176$)	Non-stroke ($n = 167$)	
Neurological symptoms			
Acute onset	96	47	27.6
Weakness			
Face	23	6	4.8
Arm	63	24	5.3
Leg	54	22	4.1
Incoordination			
Limb	5	2	2.2
Speech	53	22	4.0
Visual disturbance	11	7	1.7
Paraesthesia			
Face	9	7	1.3
Arm	20	16	1.4
Leg	17	11	1.6
Vertigo	6	5	1.2
Dizziness	13	33	0.3
Nausea	10	17	0.5
Vomiting	8	13	0.6
Headache	14	17	0.8
Confusion	5	25	0.2
Loss of consciousness	6	41	0.1
Convulsive seizures	1	10	0.1
Neurological signs			
Weakness			
Face	45	3	27.0
Arm	69	12	16.6
Leg	61	11	13.1
Visual field defect	24	2	12.8
Eye movement abnormality*	27	1	62.2
Dysphasia/dysarthria	57	8	15.6
Visuospatial neglect	23	5	5.8
Limb ataxia	4	2	2.3
Hemiparetic/ataxic gait	53	7	14.5
Sensory deficits			
Face	3	1	2.4
Arm	23	4	7.9
Leg	21	2	10.8

*Gaze palsy or opthalmoplegia. TIA, transient ischaemic attack.

Table 3.8 Neurological symptoms and signs amongst patients presenting with suspected transient ischaemic attack and stroke in the Recognition of Stroke in the Emergency Room (ROSIER) study, subdivided into those occurring in patients with stroke or TIA and those with non-stroke.[45]

The National Institutes of Health Stroke Scale (NIHSS) is a graded neurological examination which can be used as a template upon which to base a systematic neurological examination. It assesses neurological impairments such as level of consciousness, ocular gaze, visual fields, speech and language function, inattention, motor and sensory impairments, and ataxia, and thereby helps ensure that a reasonably thorough neurological examination is undertaken in the acute phase. It is quick to perform (taking less than a few minutes), is valid, and is reliable among neurologists, non-neurologist physicians, and non-physician coordinators in clinical trials for measuring neurological impairment and stroke severity.[46] However, the scale was originally developed for use in trials of treatments for patients who had already been diagnosed with stroke (to measure impairments and grade stroke severity); it was not designed for, and has limited application in, diagnosing stroke and differentiating stroke from its mimics.

> A sophisticated knowledge of neurology is not needed to elicit and recognize the clinical features of a cerebrovascular event, but physicians must continually make efforts to refine their clinical abilities if the symptoms and signs are to be documented accurately and the diagnosis of stroke and its localization are to be optimized.

3.3.1 The nature of the symptoms and signs

The symptoms and signs of TIA and stroke reflect the areas of the brain that are affected by the focal ischaemia or haemorrhage.[45] For short duration events, such as TIA, the symptoms also reflect the activities in which the patient was engaged during the attack. For example, if the patient was not speaking or did not try to speak or read during a brief ischaemic event, it is impossible to know whether aphasia or alexia were present or not. Similarly, a weak leg may well not be noticed if the patient was sitting down. As many hours of wakefulness are spent in an alert state with eyes open, an upright posture and often speaking or reading, it is not surprising that most of the symptoms that TIA patients experience are of motor, somatosensory, visual or language function (Table 3.9).[6,47,48] Other more transient activities such as swallowing and calculation are, not surprisingly, less frequently reported. Presumably TIAs, like strokes, can start during sleep, but the patient will be unaware of them if they have resolved before waking.

Among patients admitted to hospital with symptoms of brain attack (defined as 'apparently focal brain dysfunction of apparently abrupt onset'), only about two-thirds are subsequently diagnosed with stroke; one-third

Table 3.9 Neurological symptoms during transient ischaemic attacks.

	%
Unilateral weakness, heaviness or clumsiness	50
Unilateral sensory symptoms	35
Slurred speech (dysarthria)	23
Transient monocular blindness	18
Difficulty in speaking (aphasia)	18
Unsteadiness (ataxia)	12
Dizziness (vertigo)	5
Homonymous hemianopia	5
Double vision (diplopia)	5
Bilateral limb weakness	4
Difficulty in swallowing (dysphagia)	1
Crossed motor and sensory loss	1

From a series of 184 patients with a definite transient ischaemic attack (TIA) in the Oxfordshire Community Stroke Project.[6] Many patients had more than one symptom (e.g. weakness as well as sensory loss) and no patients had isolated dysarthria, ataxia, vertigo, diplopia or dysphagia. Lone bilateral blindness was excluded from this analysis but later considered to be a TIA.[48]

are a stroke mimic.[44] Clinical features that increase the odds of a final diagnosis of stroke include a definite history of focal neurological symptoms (odds ratio, OR = 7.2) and being able to determine the exact time of onset of symptoms (OR = 2.6) (Table 3.10).[44] This is consistent with the common clinical criteria for a cerebrovascular event (i.e. abrupt onset of focal neurological symptoms or signs of a presumed vascular aetiology). A logistic regression model (Table 3.10) based on eight independent and significant predictors of the diagnosis of stroke (vs non-stroke) resulted in 83% correct classifications in the data set from which it was derived (i.e. it was internally valid).[44] Other studies, using modern neuroimaging, have shown that the presence of acute facial weakness, arm drift and/or abnormal speech increased the likelihood of stroke, whereas the absence of all three decreased the odds.[49] The Recognition of Stroke in the Emergency Room (ROSIER) scale has been developed and validated as an effective instrument to differentiate stroke from its mimics in the emergency room.[45] It consists of seven items (total score from −2 to +5) comprising discriminating elements of the clinical history (loss of consciousness [score −1], convulsive seizures [score −1]) and neurological signs (face, arm, or leg weakness, speech disturbance, and visual field defect [each score +1]). A cut-off score >0 was associated with a sensitivity of 92%, specificity of 86%, positive predictive value of 88% and negative predictive value of 91% in the

Variable	OR	95% CI
Known cognitive impairment	0.33	(0.1–0.8)
An exact onset could be determined	2.59	(1.3–5.1)
Definite history of focal neurological symptoms	7.21	(2.5–20.9)
Any abnormal vascular findings*	2.54	(1.3–5.1)
Abnormal findings in any other system**	0.44	(0.2–0.8)
NIHSS = 0***		
NIHSS 1–4	1.92	(0.7–5.2)
NIHSS 5–10	3.14	(1.03–9.6)
NIHSS > 10	7.23	(2.2–24.0)
The signs could be lateralized to the left or right side of the brain	2.03	(0.9–4.5)
OCSP classification possible	5.09	(2.4–10.7)

Table 3.10 Logistic regression model for predicting the diagnosis of stroke.[44]

The model gives a predicted probability of stroke (ranging from 0 to 1).
*Systolic blood pressure > 150 mm Hg, atrial fibrillation, valvular heart disease, or absent peripheral pulses.
**Respiratory, abdominal or other abnormal signs.
***National Institute of Health Stroke Scale (NIHSS) = 0 was entered as the reference group (therefore it does not have a coefficient).
OCSP, Oxfordshire Community Stroke Project; OR, odds ratio; CI, confidence interval.

derivation data set (Table 3.8), and similar values in the test data set.[45]

> No one symptom or sign can rule in or rule out the diagnosis of stroke and transient ischaemic attack.

3.3.2 Disturbance of conscious level

Consciousness may be defined as 'the state of awareness of the self and the environment'. Coma is the total absence of such awareness. Vascular diseases are probably the second most common cause of non-traumatic coma after metabolic/toxic disorders; up to 20% of patients with stroke – but not TIAs – may have some impairment of consciousness.[44,45,47] (See also section 11.3.)

Clinical anatomy

Consciousness depends on the proper functioning of the ascending reticular activating system (ARAS). This is a complex functional, rather than anatomical, grouping of neural structures in the paramedian tegmentum of the upper brainstem, the subthalamic region and the thalamus (mainly the intralaminar nuclei). Focal lesions that impair consciousness tend to either disrupt the ARAS directly (i.e. mainly infratentorial lesions), or are large supratentorial lesions, which cause secondary brainstem compression or distortion (Table 3.11; Fig. 3.4).

Table 3.11 Causes of impaired consciousness after stroke.

Primary damage to subcortical structures (e.g. thalamus) or to the reticular activating system in the brainstem (e.g. brainstem haemorrhage)
Secondary damage to the reticular activating system in the brainstem (e.g. large supratentorial haemorrhage or infarct with transtentorial herniation and midline shift due to oedema)
Coexisting metabolic derangement (e.g. hypoglycaemia, hypoxia, renal or hepatic failure)
Drugs (e.g. sedatives)
To be distinguished from normal consciousness but with impaired responsiveness due to:
Locked-in syndrome
Akinetic mutism
Abulia
Severe extrapyramidal bradykinesia
Severe depression
Catatonia
Hysterical conversion syndrome
Paralysis from neuromuscular disorders

Clinical assessment

Conscious state is assessed by observing the patient's spontaneous activity and their response to verbal, painful and other stimuli. The Glasgow Coma Scale (GCS) provides a structured way of describing conscious level, and is usually part of the standard ambulance and nursing observation forms (Table 3.12). Because it was developed for patients with head injury and so for more

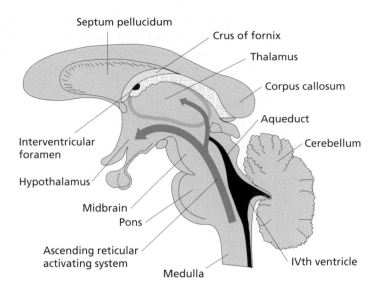

Fig. 3.4 Diagrammatic representation in the sagittal plane of the brainstem areas involved in consciousness (especially the ascending reticular activating system).

Table 3.12 The Glasgow Coma Scale.

Eye opening
E1	None
E2	To painful stimuli
E3	To command/voices
E4	Spontaneously with blinking

Motor response (best response in unaffected limb)
M1	None
M2	Arm extension to painful stimulus
M3	Arm flexion to painful stimulus
M4	Arm withdraws from painful stimulus
M5	Hand localizes painful stimulus in the face (reaches at least chin level).
M6	Obeys commands

Verbal response
V1	None
V2	Sounds but no recognizable words
V3	Inappropriate words/expletives
V4	Confused speech
V5	Normal

The score should be reported as: Ex, My, Vz, total score = $x + y + z / 15$.

diffuse rather than focal neurological deficits, care is needed when applying it to patients with stroke. The motor deficit must be assessed on the 'normal' side and not on the side with the motor deficit, and in the arm, not the leg, where the motor responses may be largely of spinal origin. The subscore of each item is probably more important than the total, since specific focal deficits, and particularly global aphasia, depress the overall score disproportionately to the level of alertness.

The GCS has value as an initial prognostic indicator in acute stroke.[50,51] It may also have value in monitoring the patient's neurological status over time. Any deterioration in the GCS is a prompt to consider whether it is because of the progression of the neurological deficit or because of non-vascular factors, such as infection, metabolic disturbance, or the effect of drugs (section 11.5). However, it is important not only to document the GCS scores (and over time), but to describe the patient's neurological impairments qualitatively and quantitatively (and over time) because the GCS measures only three of many important functions of the brain and frequently there is an obvious change in the patient on conventional neurological examination but not in the GCS.

> The Glasgow Coma Scale is an insensitive measure of neurological function and should not be the only measure to monitor the neurological status of the patient.

Clinical practice

Almost instantaneous loss of consciousness caused by a stroke suggests either a subarachnoid haemorrhage (section 3.7) or an intrinsic brainstem haemorrhage. Loss of consciousness within a few hours of onset is usually due to brainstem compression by a large intracerebral haematoma, or cerebellar haematoma or infarct. Early impairment of consciousness after supratentorial infarction is unusual. This is because the associated cerebral oedema responsible for the mass effect, and so the midline shift and brain herniation usually takes 1–3 days to develop, although some evidence of transtentorial herniation may be present within 24 h. Postmortem studies initially showed that infarction of the complete middle cerebral artery territory was needed before significant lateral and caudal (inferior) displacement of midline structures occurs. These findings have been confirmed in several imaging studies during life. Not surprisingly, level of consciousness is one of the best predictors of survival after stroke (section 10.2.7).

Loss of consciousness during a TIA is extremely unusual and should prompt a search for alternative explanations such as hypotension (e.g. vasovagal and reflex syncope, cardiac arrhythmia), systemic disorders (e.g. hypoglycaemia) and generalized epileptic seizures.[52,53] Even when transient loss of consciousness is followed by focal neurological signs, such as a hemiparesis, it is more commonly caused by an epileptic seizure resulting in a Todd's paresis[52] (section 3.4.2). When loss of consciousness does occur during a TIA, it seems to be associated with brainstem or bihemispheric ischaemia caused by either vertebrobasilar or bilateral carotid occlusive disease, respectively.[53,54] A few cases may be due to ischaemia in the territory of small, perforating arteries which supply the upper brainstem including components of the reticular activating system.

Impairment of consciousness must be distinguished from impaired responsiveness due to the following.

The 'locked-in' syndrome is a state of motor de-efferentation, where there is usually severe paralysis not only of the limbs but also of the neck, jaw and face. Indeed, the only muscles remaining under voluntary control may be those concerned with vertical eye movements and blinking. All this occurs with clear, and often extremely distressing, retention of awareness. The patient is unable to communicate by word or movement other than by blinking or moving their eyes up and down, but is fully aware of the surroundings and attempts to respond to them. Hearing, vision and often sensation are retained. There is usually an extensive, bilateral lesion in the ventral pons, which interrupts the descending motor tracts as well as the centre for horizontal eye movements in the pons, but the oculomotor nuclei and descending pathways for vertical eye movements are spared together with the ascending reticular activating system (Fig. 3.5). Cognitive functions are normal and so the patients must be given a full explanation of their predicament. Staff may need to be reminded to take appropriate account of the patient's normal cognition and sensation, since prolonged survival in this state is possible.[55,56]

> The relatives and staff caring for patients with the locked-in syndrome need reminding regularly that sensation, cognitive functions and awareness are all normal.

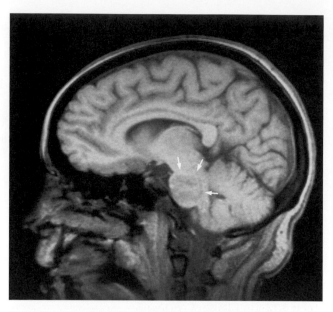

Fig. 3.5 A T1-weighted magnetic resonance (MR) image, sagittal plane, showing a ventral pontine infarct (*arrows*) in a patient with the locked-in syndrome.

Akinetic mutism and *abulia* are states where there is limited responsiveness to the environment, although the patients appear alert (or at least wakeful) in that their eyes are open and they follow objects. However, in contrast to the locked-in syndrome, the physical examination does not reveal evidence of a major lesion of the descending motor pathways. At its most extreme, patients with akinetic mutism may lie with open eyes, follow objects and become agitated or even say the occasional appropriate word following noxious stimuli (thus distinguishing this state from that of coma or the persistent vegetative state); but otherwise they do not respond to their environment. Occasionally, catatonic posturing may occur. If patients recover from this state, they have no recollection of it. 'Abulia' describes a less severe presentation of reduced spontaneous movement and speech. Such patients often appear to have a marked flatness of affect, but with adequate stimulation they can be shown to be conscious and have relatively preserved cognition. Both akinetic mutism and abulia occur with bilateral damage to the cingulate gyri, caudate nuclei and anterior limb of the internal capsules, but they can also occur with unilateral lesions of the caudate nucleus. Although these states are most commonly seen after head injury, following anterior communicating artery aneurysmal subarachnoid haemorrhage, or in multi-infarct states, they can occur with unilateral occlusion of the recurrent artery of Heubner.

3.3.3 Disturbance of higher cerebral function

Higher cerebral functions can be divided into those which are 'distributed' – i.e. involve several areas of the cortex, such as attention, concentration, memory and higher-order social behaviour – and those which are more 'localized', such as speech and language, visuo-spatial function and praxis.[32] Few tests are absolutely specific, however, for a single aspect of higher cerebral function. The nature of the cognitive assessment means that it is often appropriate to blend aspects of history taking with immediate confirmation by means of specific examination. Skilful examiners often weave their assessment into a relaxed conversation with the patients, making it more enjoyable for both. Many of the features of a brief cognitive assessment, an example of which is shown in Table 3.13,[32] can be modified to suit this style of assessment. It is important to determine the handedness of an individual patient to guide which hemisphere is dominant for language. The descriptions below assume left-hemisphere dominance.

Attention and concentration

Attention and concentration are the ability to maintain a coherent stream of thought or action. They are not synonymous with wakefulness.

CLINICAL ANATOMY

Attention and concentration are 'distributed functions' which depend on the integrated activity of the neocortex (predominantly the prefrontal, posterior parietal and ventral temporal lobes), the thalamus and brainstem. The reticular formation and other brainstem nuclei receive input from both ascending and descending pathways and there are then major ascending tracts to the thalamus, particularly its intralaminar nuclei.

CLINICAL ASSESSMENT

Failure of attention results in patients being unable to sustain concentration, and they are often reported to lack interest in things around them or to be tired or distractable. Another common complaint is that they have problems with memory. This may or may not be true, but from a practical point of view, if there is a significant disorder of attention, then extreme care is required when interpreting the results of tests of other higher-order functions such as memory. Attention and concentration can be assessed at the bedside (Table 3.14).

CLINICAL PRACTICE

Acute stroke patients who appear inattentive should be assessed carefully to exclude an underlying focal

Table 3.13 Features of the 12-minute cognitive assessment.[32]

Orientation
Time (day, date, month, season, year)
Place
Attention
Serial 7s, or
Months of the year backwards
Language
Engage in conversation and assess articulation, fluency, phonemic errors (e.g. 'the grass is greed' – Broca's area lesion) and semantic errors (e.g. 'the grass is blue' – posterior perisylvian lesion)
Naming of some low frequency items (e.g. stethoscope, nib, cufflinks, watch winder)
Comprehension (of both single words and sentences)
Repetition (e.g. emerald, aubergine, perimeter, hippopotamus; no ifs, ands or buts)
Reading
Writing
Memory
Anterograde: test recall of a name and address after 5 min
Retrograde: ask about recent sporting or personal events
Executive function
Letter (F) and category fluency (animals): e.g. name as many words beginning with the letter F or A or S (>15 words per minute is normal) and animals (15 is low average, 10 is definitely impaired)
Praxis
Meaningful gestures (e.g. wave, salute)
Luria three-step sequencing test (fist-edge-palm)
Visuospatial
Clock drawing, and overlapping pentagons
General neurological assessment with particular attention to:
Frontal lobe signs (grasp, pout, palmomental)
Eye movements
Presence of a movement disorder
Pyramidal signs
General impression
Slowness of thought
Inappropriateness
Mood

Table 3.14 Bedside testing of attention and concentration.

Digit span forwards and backwards*
Recite months of the year, or days of the week, backwards
Serial subtraction of 7s (although note that calculation ability needs to be intact)
*The normal range is forwards: 6 ± 1; backwards: 5 ± 1.

neurological disturbance such as aphasia, visuospatial or perceptual disturbance, hemianopia, or amnesia. If they really are inattentive they may have a metabolic/toxic encephalopathy, and an underlying treatable cause (e.g. hyponatraemia, hypoglycaemia, hypoxia, uraemia, dehydration, sepsis).

Memory

Memory function can be divided into 'explicit' memory (available to conscious access) and 'implicit' memory (relates to learned responses and conditioned reflexes). Explicit memory may be 'episodic' (dealing with specific events and episodes that have been personally experienced) or 'semantic' (dealing with knowledge of facts, concepts and the meaning of words, e.g. 'stroke is a clinical syndrome'). Episodic memory (personally experienced events) comprises anterograde (newly encountered information) and retrograde (past events) components.[32] Working memory refers to the very limited capacity which allows us to retain information for a few seconds.

> The terms 'short-term memory' and 'long-term memory' are used loosely by clinicians and often rather differently by neuropsychologists. In patients with stroke, in whom the time of onset is known, it may be easier to distinguish anterograde amnesia (failure to acquire new memories) from retrograde amnesia (failure to recall previously learnt material).

CLINICAL ANATOMY
Episodic memory depends on the hippocampal-diencephalic system, semantic memory on the anterior temporal lobe, and working memory on the dorsolateral prefrontal cortex.[32]

CLINICAL ASSESSMENT
Patients with stroke are generally of an age when there is a natural decline in memory anyway (or have coexistent Alzheimer's disease or vascular cognitive impairment). Therefore, many complain of memory problems before the stroke, and furthermore it is important to determine whether there really is a disturbance of memory (and not aphasia or disturbance of attention and concentration resulting in failure of registration of new information) and, if so, to identify what is a direct result of the stroke. A suggested method for assessing memory is set out in Table 3.15.

CLINICAL PRACTICE
Perhaps the most frequent stroke lesion causing amnesia is infarction of the medial temporal lobe (Fig. 3.6).

Table 3.15 Bedside testing of memory.

First check that patient is attentive (Table 3.14) and that language function is adequate (see below, and Table 3.16).
Anterograde verbal memory
  Ask the patient to name three distinct objects (e.g. 'Ball, Flag, Tree' or 'Boston, Car, Daisy')
  Ensure that the patient has registered the information (repeat up to three times if necessary)
  If the patient can immediately name the objects, ask the patient to repeat the three objects three minutes later
Anterograde visual memory
  Show the patient faces in a magazine
  Ensure they have recognized them
  Retest after 5 min
Retrograde memory
  Ask the patient to describe recent events on the ward, or visits from relatives
  Ask about important historical events and major events in the patient's life, e.g. date of marriage

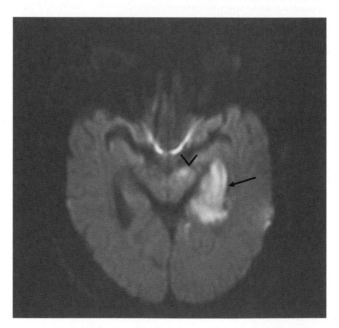

Fig. 3.6 MRI DWI showing area of high signal intensity, consistent with infarction, in the left medial temporal lobe (*arrow*) and cerebral peduncle (*arrowhead*), due to occlusion of the left posterior cerebral artery at its origin.

Because the cause is usually occlusion of the posterior cerebral artery or one of its branches, the patient may have a coexistent visual disorder (e.g. hemianopia or upper quadrantanopia, colour anomia, visual agnosia). A pure amnesic syndrome may be caused by a vascular lesion involving the mammillothalamic tract or anteriomedian territory of the thalamus (supplied by the polar

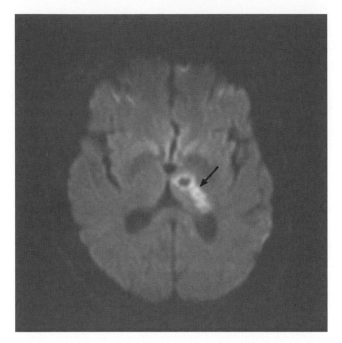

Fig. 3.7 MRI DWI showing area of altered signal intensity, consistent with haemorrhagic infarction, in the left thalamus (*arrow*).

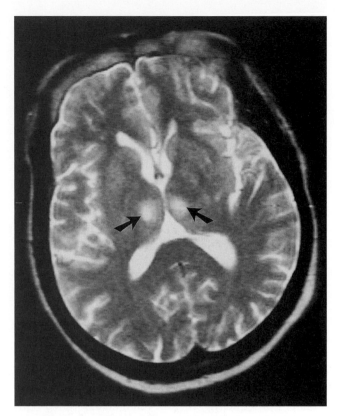

Fig. 3.8 A T2-weighted MR image, axial plane, showing bilateral thalamic infarction (*arrows*) in a patient with severe global amnesia.

and paramedian arteries) such as the anterior parts of the dorsomedian nucleus[57,58] (Fig. 3.7). In general, there is relative sparing of verbal memory with right thalamic lesions and visuospatial memory with left thalamic lesions, although the amnesia may be global with unilateral lesions. Particularly severe amnesia is more likely with paramedian thalamic infarction, which is frequently bilateral because the left and right paramedian arteries arise from one stem in many people (Fig. 3.8).[58] In most cases of thalamic amnesia there are also signs of upper midbrain dysfunction, such as somnolence, vertical gaze palsies and corticospinal and spinothalamic tract signs.

The syndrome of transient global amnesia is described in detail in section 3.4.3.

Speech and language

Language is difficult to define, but may be considered as a system for the expression of thoughts and feelings by the use of sounds and/or conventional symbols. It involves the production (or expression) and comprehension (or reception) of speech, as well as reading and writing.

- *Aphasia/dysphasia* is an acquired disorder of the production and/or comprehension of spoken and/or written language. Subtypes of aphasia include speech (verbal) apraxia, alexia, agraphia and anomia.

- *Speech apraxia/dyspraxia* is a syndrome in which there is variable misarticulation of single sounds, in the absence of dysarthria (in which there is constant misarticulation). This is because of impairment of planning of movements required for speech sounds and articulation, despite the ability to articulate speech being intact (e.g. similar to gait apraxia).

- *Alexia/dyslexia* is an inability to name or interpret previously learned printed symbols. The patient can see individual letters, but cannot decode a series of letters into a recognizable word. When it occurs in isolation, this is sometimes referred to as 'word blindness'.

- *Agraphia/dysgraphia* is an acquired disorder of writing, a subtype of aphasia.

- *Anomia/dysnomia* is an inability to generate a specific name. In the context of a vascular event, it is usually a manifestation of aphasia, but can be an amnesic disorder.

- *Anarthria/dysarthria* is a disorder of articulation of single sounds.

- *Dysphonia* is defined as a disorder of phonation of sounds.

> Disorders of speech and language are not synonymous; speech involves language and articulation, whereas language involves reading and writing as well as speech.

CLINICAL ANATOMY

In general, non-fluent (expressive, Broca's) aphasia is a syndrome with elements that range from initial mutism to speech apraxia and the classical pattern of agrammatism (inability to produce grammatical or intelligible speech, usually with simplified sentence structure – telegraphic speech – and errors in tense, number and gender). It is likely to be due to a lesion involving the posterior, inferior, dominant frontal lobe cortex and subcortex. The articulatory component (apraxia) is most heavily represented in the left insular region. Lesions of the dominant thalamus may also result in predominantly non-fluent aphasia. Fluent (receptive, Wernicke's) aphasia is commonly caused by a more posterior lesion involving the temporal lobe cortex and subcortex. Most patients with stroke have a combination referred to as 'mixed aphasia' (or, if severe, 'global aphasia'), due to more extensive lesions within the dominant hemisphere. Consequently, there is often an associated right hemiparesis and hemianopia.

Occasionally, patients with non-fluent aphasia have preserved repetition. This is termed *transcortical motor aphasia*, and it is usually caused by lesions restricted to the anterior cerebral artery territory and which spare the arcuate fasciculus, between Broca's area and Wernicke's area (section 4.2.2). Fluent aphasia with normal repetition (*transcortical sensory aphasia*) occurs with strokes in the left temporo-occipital region.

Dysarthria may be a result of cerebellar (ataxic), pyramidal (spastic), extrapyramidal (hypokinetic), or facial nerve (flaccid) dysfunction. Anarthria may occur as part of a pseudobulbar palsy caused by bilateral lesions of the internal capsule (not necessarily at the same time) or with a single lesion involving both sides of the brainstem.

Alexia, with or without agraphia, may result from strokes that involve the medial aspect of the left occipital lobe and the splenium of the corpus callosum. There is usually a right visual field defect but no hemiparesis, and it is thought that the lesion in the splenium interrupts the transfer of visual information from the normal left visual field (right occipital lobe) to the damaged left hemisphere language areas.

Gerstmann syndrome is the combination of aphasia, agraphia, right-left disorientation, and acalculia, due to a lesion in the region of the angular gyrus of the dominant hemisphere.[59]

CLINICAL ASSESSMENT

The first distinction to make is between *aphasia/dysphasia* (a disorder of language), *anarthria/dysarthria* (a disorder of articulation) and *dysphonia* (a disorder of phonation). If the patient's speech sounds 'like a drunk', and if the ability to understand and express spoken and written language is preserved, then the problem is dysarthria (or dysphonia). If the main difficulty is understanding or expressing spoken or written language – such as difficulty in reading (the patient can see the letters but cannot make sense of them); difficulty in writing, even though the use of the hand is otherwise normal (often not the case); or difficulty in producing sentences, with words not being in their proper place or even non-words being used – then the problem is aphasia. Table 3.16 sets out a scheme of bedside testing that will detect most speech and language problems. There is a general tendency in everyday clinical practice to underestimate the receptive component of aphasia, particularly if the examiner does not go beyond questions requiring a yes/no answer, or simple social conversation.

CLINICAL PRACTICE

> Beware labelling a patient as dysphasic when a lack of other symptoms and signs suggest isolated non-dominant hemisphere dysfunction.

'Crossed' aphasia is a disturbance of language which occurs from a right hemisphere lesion in a right-hand dominant patient and is seen in about 4% of such patients. It is presumed that some right-handed patients have mixed cerebral dominance for language, but other causes include bilateral strokes (including the thalamus) and previous strokes. It is worth noting that many right-handed patients with right hemisphere strokes show subtle alterations in the affective aspects of speech, such as intonation (aprosody).

Isolated dysarthria may be the only manifestation of a lacune at the genu of the internal capsule or in the corona radiata. In such cases, there is specific impairment of corticolingual fibres.[60]

Foreign accent syndrome is a rare, acquired disorder of speech in which native speakers listening to a patient speaking their language describe hearing a foreign-sounding accent – yet the patient may never have been exposed to any other language or dialect before the stroke. It is probably due to an inability to make the normal phonetic and phonemic contrasts of the native language. The syndrome has most often been associated with small, subcortical infarcts in the left cerebral hemisphere.

Table 3.16 Bedside testing of language function.

First ensure any hearing aid has a battery, is switched on and that appropriate, clean spectacles are worn

Also check that you are using the patient's native language – if not, use an interpreter

Spontaneous speech

Consider output (whether fluent or non-fluent), articulation and content: during history-taking and for a structured task (e.g. 'describe your surroundings')

Auditory comprehension

Simple yes/no questions (e.g. Is Russia the capital of Moscow? Can dogs fly? Do you put your shoes on before your socks?)

Give commands (being careful not to use non-verbal cues) of one, two and three steps using common objects, such as the manipulation of three different-coloured pens (care not to require the use of limbs with significant weakness or apraxia)

Naming

Ask the patient to name objects, parts of objects, colours, body parts, famous faces (certain groups, particularly the naming of people, may be more severely affected)

If visual agnosia is present, use auditory/tactile presentation, e.g. bunch of keys

Repetition

'West Register Street' (difficult if dysarthric)

'No ifs, ands or buts' (difficult if aphasic)

Reading

Aloud, e.g. from a book or newspaper

Comprehension of the same piece

Writing

Spontaneous ('why have you come into hospital?')

Dictation ('the quick brown fox jumped over the lazy black dog')

Copying

Articulation

Ask the patient to say:

p/p/p/p/p/p (labial sounds, which test the orbicularis oris)

t/t/t/t/t/t (lingual sounds, which test the anterior tongue)

k/k/k/k/k/k (palatal sounds, which test the posterior tongue and palate)

p/t/k/p/t/k (tests the overall coordination of sounds)

Visuospatial dysfunction

Many patients with stroke fail to respond to stimulation of, or to report information from, the side contralateral to the cerebral lesion. There are two broad categories of neglect: intrapersonal (i.e. with respect to the patient's own body) and extrapersonal or topographical (i.e. with respect to the surrounding environment). There are a number of different types and/or degrees of severity of neglect in patients with stroke, and in many, a combination of somatic sensory deficits and disturbed visual perception contribute to the clinically apparent 'neglect',

Table 3.17 Glossary of terms describing disorders of visuospatial function.

Hemi-inattention: where the patient's behaviour during examination suggests an inability to respond appropriately to environmental stimuli on one side, e.g. people approaching, noise, or activity in the ward

Sensory or tactile extinction: where the patient fails to register a tactile stimulus (light touch) of adequate intensity on one side of their body when both sides are stimulated simultaneously and adequately (i.e. double simultaneous stimulation) but where the stimulus has been registered when each side was stimulated separately

Visual inattention or extinction: where the patient fails to register a visual stimulus (e.g. finger movement) in one homonymous visual field (half field or quadrant) when the same stimulus is presented to both fields simultaneously, but where the patient had no field defect on normal testing

Allaesthesia: where the patient consistently attributes sensory stimulation on one side to stimulation of the other; this is related to right/left confusion, where the patient consistently moves the limbs on one side when requested to move the limbs on the other

Anosognosia: denial of a sensorimotor hemisyndrome

Anosodiaphoria: indifference to/unconcern about a sensorimotor hemisyndrome

Asomatognosia: lack of awareness of a body part

Somatoparaphrenia (non-belonging): lack of ownership of a paralysed limb

Experience of supernumary phantom limbs: reduplication of limbs on the affected side of the body

Personification: nicknaming a limb and giving it an identity of its own

Misoplegia: the morbid dislike or hatred of paralysed limbs in patients with hemiparesis[61]

Related phenomena seen in parietal lobe dysfunction:

Astereognosis: unable to recognize objects placed in the affected hand yet cutaneous sensation is preserved

Agraphaesthesia: unable to identify a number drawn on the palm of the affected hand yet cutaneous sensation is preserved

Geographical disorientation: where the patient becomes lost in familiar surroundings despite being able to see

Dressing apraxia: unable to dress, or dresses inappropriately, despite having no apparent weakness, sensory loss, visual or neglect problems; this is occasionally seen in an isolated form and probably occurs because of a combination of disordered body image, sensory and visual inattention rather than being a true apraxia

hence the use of the broader term 'visuospatial dysfunction'. Table 3.17 provides a glossary of the terms that are used,[61] Fig. 3.9 shows an example of anosognosia; this patient denies the presence of weakness of the left leg[62]

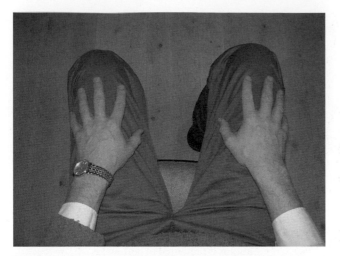 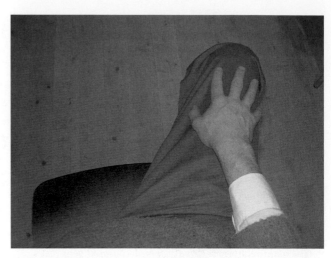

Fig. 3.9 Neglect and anosognosia: the photograph on the left shows how someone may normally view their hands and legs (before a stroke). The photograph on the right shows how the same person may view their hands and legs after a major right hemisphere stroke, causing neglect and anosognosia for the left hand and left leg.

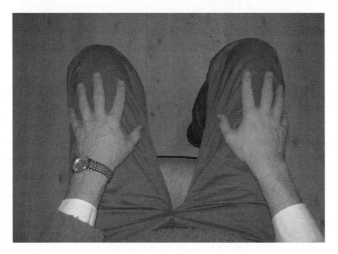 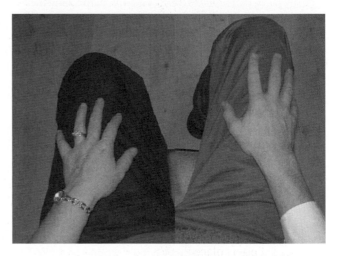

Fig. 3.10 Somatoparaphrenia (non-belonging): the photograph on the left shows how someone may normally view their hands and legs (before a stroke). The photograph on the right shows how the same person may view their hands and legs after a major right hemisphere stroke causing somatoparaphrenia (i.e. the man denies ownership of the paralysed arm and leg on the left side of the body, and even thinks the left arm and leg belong to another person, such as his wife – note the different left hand, wedding ring on the left hand, and the different left leg).

and Fig. 3.10 shows an example of somatoparaphrenia (non-belonging); this patient denies ownership of the paralysed leg on the left side of the body, and even attributes the left leg to another person.

CLINICAL ANATOMY

Visuospatial dysfunction is most severe with posterior parietal lesions of the non-dominant hemisphere, particularly those that extend to the visual association areas. Among patients with ischaemic stroke, the aetiology may be middle cerebral or posterior cerebral artery occlusion.[63] Although it can occur with dominant hemisphere lesions, when it does so detection is often hindered by coexistent language disturbance and inability to use the dominant hand.

CLINICAL ASSESSMENT

Relatives may report little more than 'confusion' or 'difficulty in dressing'. If visuospatial problems are suspected from the history, they should be carefully sought in the examination. Simply observing how patients respond to their environment and carry out tasks, such

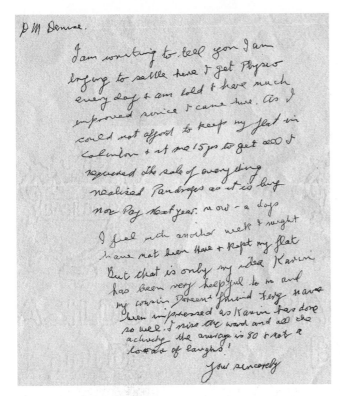

Fig. 3.11 A letter from a patient with left visual neglect, showing neglect of the left side of the page.

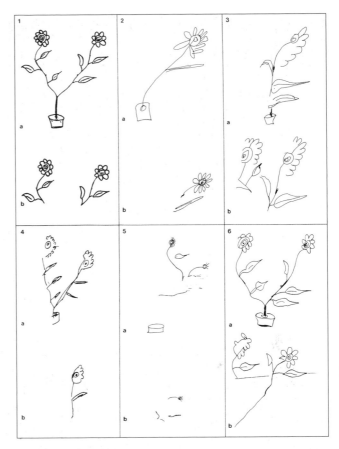

Fig. 3.12 Abnormalities of copying flowers. Five patients with right hemisphere lesions were asked to copy pictures (a) and (b) in panel 1. The figures illustrate the variation seen in copying tasks. Panel 2: this patient has mainly neglected the information on the left side of the page. Panel 3: this patient has omitted the left-hand components of the objects, but has shifted attention to the right-hand side of another object placed to the left of the neglected space. Panel 4: this patient has drawn the right side of both flowers in the pot, but has completely neglected the left of the two separate flowers. Panel 5: this patient has transposed objects in the left field to the right field, i.e. both flowers are drawn on a single stem. Panel 6: this patient has produced a 'hallucinatory' rabbit in the left field when copying the separate flowers; this has been termed 'metamorphopsia'.

as writing (Fig. 3.11), copying flowers (Fig. 3.12) and drawing a clock face (Fig. 3.13) can be revealing. An obvious example would be if a patient (without a hemianopia) does not register the doctor's presence when approached from one side, even when spoken to. Or they might be unable to find their way back to their hospital bed after being taken to the toilet, suggesting geographical disorientation. The nurses and therapists are often better placed than the doctor to identify visuospatial problems, so it is important that staff are trained to recognize and report them to other members of the team. Table 3.18 sets out a bedside examination that should detect significant visuospatial dysfunction.

Of the many cancellation tasks available, the star cancellation test is easy to use and probably the most sensitive (Fig. 3.14). Using two or three different tests increases the sensitivity of detecting visual neglect, but this may not always be practical in the setting of acute stroke.[64] Many aspects of these assessments of visuospatial function require subjective judgements to be made by the physician – which probably accounts for the relatively poor inter-observer reliability. Although many other tests to identify and quantify visuospatial dysfunction have been described, the 'gold standard' against which the tests are evaluated is often regarded as the functional assessment by an occupational therapist.

Table 3.18 Bedside tests of visuospatial function.

Is the patient aware, and reacting appropriately to their deficit?
Observe the patient's response to the environment
Observe the patient's ability to carry out a specific task
Check for sensory and visual extinction
Copy a simple picture, e.g. a flower (Fig. 3.12)
Draw a clock face and put the numbers in (Fig. 3.13); this may not be specific for visual neglect but rather reflect other cognitive problems, such as dementia
Perform the star cancellation test (Fig. 3.14)

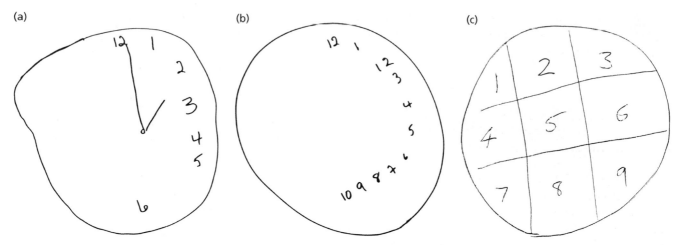

(a)   (b)   (c)

Fig. 3.13 (a) A drawing of a clock face by a patient with left visuospatial disturbance after a stroke, showing crowding of the digits on the right and neglect of the left side of the clock face. (b) A drawing of a clock face by a confused, elderly patient who has not had a stroke. The crowding of digits on the right occurs because of failure of planning. Many normal people insert 12, 3, 6 and 9 before other numbers. (c) Rather bizarre drawing of a clock face by a patient with strokes affecting both cerebral hemispheres.

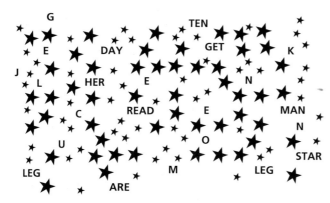

Fig. 3.14 Star cancellation test. The chart is placed in front of the patient, who is asked to cross out all the small stars while ignoring the large stars and letters (with permission from Thames Valley Test Company, 7–9 The Green, Flempton, Bury St Edmunds, Suffolk IP28 6EL, UK).

An elderly man who lived alone reported that he woke one morning and thought that there was 'something in bed with me'. He said it felt warm, and was pressing against the left side of his body. He thought his cat had got into bed with him, but when he touched it with his right hand he realized that it was his left arm. He had had a right parietal infarct during the night.

One can often deduce the presence of visuospatial problems by simply observing how the patient responds to the environment and carries out tasks around the ward.

CLINICAL PRACTICE

When there is an isolated problem with visuospatial function – i.e. when it is not accompanied by a more easily recognized 'stroke' deficit such as weakness – the patient's behaviour may seem extremely bizarre, and even be interpreted as psychiatric disease.

An elderly man was escorted to hospital by his concerned passenger after he drove his car along a street unaware that he was scraping along a whole row of other cars on the left-hand side. Examination revealed normal visual fields (when each eye was tested in turn) but visual inattention to the left (when the visual fields of each eye were tested simultaneously). There was also somatosensory extinction on the left when the arms were touched simultaneously. Brain CT scan showed a small right parietal haemorrhage.

A middle-aged single lady was flying home from holiday when she became 'confused'. On disembarking from the aircraft, she was staggering to the left, appeared unable to follow the signs to the customs point, and could not find her passport in her left-hand jacket pocket. She was held initially by the police on suspicion of alcohol or drug intoxication, but then admitted to a psychiatric hospital. It was only a week later, when she had a transient ischaemic attack affecting power in her left hand, that a right parietal infarct and severe stenosis of the right internal carotid artery were discovered.

Perhaps not surprisingly, there is some evidence that patients who have varying degrees of indifference to their stroke are more likely to delay seeking medical attention.[31,33] Visuospatial problems are a major cause of disability and handicap, and impede the patient's functional recovery (section 11.28).

Disorders of praxis

Apraxia is defined as inability to perform learned movements that cannot be explained by weakness, sensory loss, incoordination, inattention and other perceptual disorders, or by failure to understand the command. Dressing and constructional apraxias are best considered as disorders of visuospatial function rather than true apraxias (see above). Although the terms 'verbal apraxia' or 'speech apraxia' may be used by speech and language therapists when there are repeated phonemic substitutions, in practice such patients usually also have evidence of aphasia and/or dysarthria.

CLINICAL ANATOMY

It is thought that the programmes of learned movements (engrams) are maintained predominantly in the left temporoparietal cortex. Messages then pass to the left premotor frontal cortex and finally, via the anterior corpus callosum, to the right premotor frontal cortex (Fig. 3.15). Lesions in the posterior left hemisphere may result in bilateral apraxia (because the message is not transmitted); those in the premotor areas are usually associated with a hemiparesis and therefore apraxia may only be apparent in the non-paralysed limbs; and finally, a lesion of the corpus callosum may cause isolated apraxia of the left limbs, with normal function of the right limbs.

CLINICAL ASSESSMENT

Apraxia should always be considered as a potential explanation for disparity between the degree of deficit as tested at the bedside (when one often gives the patient relatively simple commands) and much more severely impaired functional abilities when the patient is observed around the ward (e.g. dressing, swallowing, speaking). Patients have difficulty with miming actions, imitating how an object is used, and even making symbolic gestures. However, at other times they may be observed making the individual movements that would be needed to perform the action. In general, they will have most difficulty in miming the action, less difficulty in imitating the examiner, and least difficulty when actually given the object to use. The more sequences there are to the action, the more difficult it is and so the more sensitive the test. These relatively common problems are sometimes referred to as 'ideomotor apraxias', and can be distinguished from ideational apraxias when the patient has difficulty in performing a sequence of

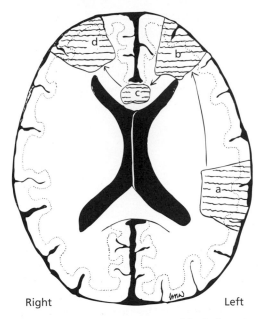

Right   Left

Fig. 3.15 Diagrammatic representation of the lesions that can result in apraxia. (a) The dominant temporoparietal cortex is probably the site of the programmes of learned movements (engrams). Lesions here result in bilateral apraxias, due to failure to transmit the information to both frontal lobes. The clinical signs may be difficult to identify because the interpretation of the command may be affected by receptive aphasia. (b) Although lesions of the dominant frontal lobe are often associated with expressive dysphasia, comprehension is usually relatively spared. The apraxia may only be apparent in the left limbs, since there will usually be a right hemiparesis. (c) Lesions in the anterior corpus callosum may result in isolated apraxia of the left limbs, because of failure of transmission of the motor information to the right frontal lobe, while the right arm and leg move normally. (d) Lesions of the non-dominant frontal lobe are not normally associated with clinically apparent apraxias, because there is usually a left hemiparesis.

movements even though the individual movements can be performed normally. However, the latter probably occurs very rarely in a pure form, and the distinction between ideomotor and ideational apraxias is of little value to clinicians. Table 3.19 suggests ways of screening for apraxia.

CLINICAL PRACTICE

In patients with stroke, the main problem is being sure that the patient has understood the command, because lesions of the relevant areas will often result in aphasia. Nevertheless, 80% of patients with aphasia also have evidence of apraxia with an imitation test (i.e. no verbal command). Because apraxic patients may perform actions reflexly that they are unable to do when asked, this should not be misinterpreted as a sign of a hysterical conversion disorder.

Table 3.19 Bedside testing of praxis.

Limbs
Ask the patient to:
    Mime the use of a pen, comb and toothbrush
    Imitate the examiner's use of the same objects
    Use the actual objects
Orofacial
Ask the patient to:
    Whistle
    Put tongue out
    Blow out cheeks
    Cough
Serial actions
Ask the patient to:
    Mime putting the address on a letter
    Then seal it
    Then put a stamp on it

3.3.4 Disturbance of the motor system

Clinical anatomy

Particular areas of the motor cortex, when stimulated, result in movement of a particular body part. This localization of function is traditionally portrayed by the homunculus (or manikin).[65] Although the absolute neuroanatomical relationships may be incorrect, it

is still useful as an aide-memoire (Fig. 3.16). The corticospinal tract (Fig. 3.17) descends from the primary and more anterior supplementary motor cortex, the fibres converging in the corona radiata. The fibres then pass through the internal capsule. The traditional view is that those relating to the head pass through the anterior limb; those relating to the mouth, larynx and pharynx are in the genu; those relating to the arm are in the anterior part of the posterior limb; while those relating to the leg lie more posteriorly. In fact, the fibres almost certainly follow an oblique course through the capsule, becoming progressively more posteriorly placed in the caudal (inferior) segments of the capsule. The fibres then pass into the brainstem. Here, the fibres that originate in the precentral gyrus lie in the cerebral peduncles of the midbrain and the base of the pons before entering the medullary pyramids (i.e. the pyramidal tracts).

The facial nerve nucleus in the pons has a rostral portion from which fibres innervate the muscles of the upper face, while the more caudal portion of the nucleus supplies fibres to the muscles of the lower face. The caudal loop of the fibres to the facial nerve descends as far as the medulla and explains why lesions of the medullary pyramid or medial medulla can be associated with contralateral upper motor neurone-type facial weakness.[66,67]

Most fibres in the corticospinal tract decussate in the lower medulla and come to lie in an anterolateral

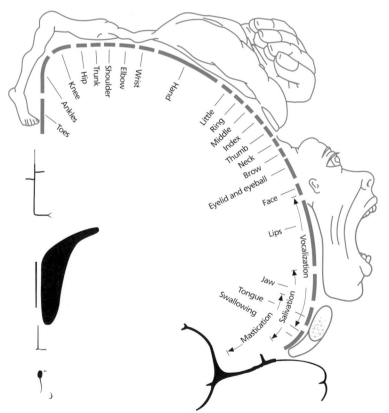

Fig. 3.16 Topographic organization of the motor cortex in the cerebral hemisphere, coronal view (after Penfield & Rasmussen, 1950[65]).

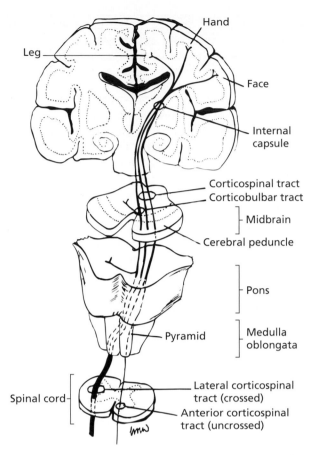

Fig. 3.17 Diagrammatic representation of the corticospinal and corticobulbar tracts.

position in the spinal cord, although a variable proportion remain uncrossed. These uncrossed fibres project to motor neurones in the medial part of the ventral horns, subserving axial and proximal muscles, corresponding with movements of the trunk, or of two limbs together. The uncrossed corticospinal fibres cannot be invoked to explain residual function in distal parts of an otherwise plegic limb, nor deficits in contralateral limbs.

Clinical assessment

Motor symptoms are usually described as 'weakness', 'heaviness' and 'clumsiness'. They are often accompanied by sensory symptoms of some sort, which can lead to diagnostic confusion because a purely weak limb may be described by the patient as 'numb' or 'dead'. Descriptions such as 'heaviness' and 'numbness' should not simply be accepted as evidence of motor and sensory disturbance, respectively. In our experience, the terms are used interchangeably (and are often culturally determined), and a little more questioning is often required.

> Patients use terms such as 'heaviness' and 'numbness' interchangeably; further questioning is needed to distinguish between motor and sensory deficits.

In patients with suspected TIA, unilateral facial weakness is probably under-reported, because they do not realize they have had facial weakness unless they have seen themselves in the mirror, or were seen by someone else. If there is a clear history of slurred speech, but no symptoms of cerebellar or bulbar dysfunction, it is reasonable to suspect facial weakness, because this may cause dysarthria. However, care should be taken before accepting a patient's or relative's description of the side of a facial weakness. They should be asked, 'Which side dropped?' and 'Did saliva trickle from one side of the mouth?' Upper motor neurone facial weakness affects the lower half of the face, while function of the forehead muscles is relatively preserved because of bilateral innervation of the forehead muscles. Mild weakness may only be apparent by observing asymmetry of the nasolabial folds. If the examiner is uncertain whether a facial weakness is present, or whether it is simply the normal side-to-side asymmetry, it may be useful to ask the patient to attempt to whistle, an action that requires fine control of the facial muscles. A mild upper motor neurone facial weakness can be overcome during emotionally generated movements, e.g. a smile.

Patients sometimes complain of being 'generally weak'. This should be viewed as a non-focal neurological symptom, as it is rarely described when they strictly mean motor weakness. It is sometimes used as a term for fatigue, tiredness, lethargy and just occasionally loss of balance.

For the clinician, the difficulties with the physical examination lie not with the densely hemiplegic patient with increased tone, brisk deep tendon reflexes and an extensor plantar response, but rather with the patient with a mild neurological deficit. Subtle abnormalities of motor function may be detectable in the hand at a time when there is no objective weakness. Impairment of fine finger movements (or rapid alternating hand movements) is a sensitive clinical test of corticospinal function. This equates with functional problems reported by patients who, in the presence of normal power, often have difficulty with delicate motor tasks such as doing up buttons or controlling a pen and so may describe the problem as 'clumsiness'. Of course, they are much more likely to notice this in their normally dominant hand.

> Impairment of fine finger or rapid hand movements is probably the most sensitive clinical test of corticospinal function.

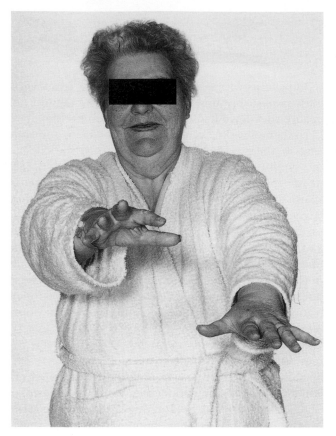

Fig. 3.18 Downward drift of the outstretched left arm in a patient with a right corticospinal tract motor deficit causing a mild left hemiparesis.

Drift of the outstretched pronated arm with the eyes closed is a good screening test of motor function (Fig. 3.18). However, there are several other potential causes including loss of proprioception, when the fingers tend to move independently – so-called 'piano-playing' or 'pseudoathetosis'; neglect, when there tend to be much larger-amplitude movements, including upwards; or cerebellar dysfunction, when there tend to be larger-amplitude oscillations, particularly if sharp downward pressure is applied to the arm. Thus, as a screening test for motor dysfunction, it is quite sensitive but not very specific and should be used in conjunction with the examination of fine finger movements. Some clinicians favour performing the test with the patient's palms facing upwards, and if asymmetrical internal rotation occurs without downward drift this is taken as a sign of very subtle motor dysfunction.

Minor motor deficits affecting the leg are probably best detected by drift of the leg (when flexed at the hip against gravity in a supine patient) and rapid tapping of the foot against the examiner's hand. Additionally, the patient's gait should be carefully observed.

Drift from the horizontal of the outstretched arm with the eyes closed, and rapid tapping of the foot against the examiner's hand, are both good screening tests of motor function in the arm and leg, respectively, but neither test is very specific.

The pattern of weakness within an individual limb is traditionally taught to be of localizing value. In particular, when the antigravity muscles (i.e. shoulder abductors; elbow, wrist, and finger extensors; hip and knee flexors; and ankle and toe dorsiflexors and ankle everters) are weaker than their counterparts (i.e. shoulder adductors; elbow, wrist, and finger flexors; hip and knee extensors; and ankle and toe flexors and ankle inverters), this is often described as a 'pyramidal distribution' of weakness. It has been suggested that this pattern is simply a function of the intrinsically greater strength in antigravity muscles together with the effects of hypertonia – the actual pattern of weakness being equally common in patients with central or peripheral lesions causing muscle weakness.[68] The deep tendon reflexes were considered of more value as a localizing feature,[68] although the inter-observer reliability of two standard scales for grading tendon reflexes is probably no better than 'fair' (kappa < 0.35).[69]

While the anatomical extent of the motor deficit is important for clinicoanatomical correlation, the severity is helpful in the acute phase for determining prognosis, the potential risks and benefits of interventions (such as thrombolysis) and the functional management and rehabilitation of the patient. There are several methods of quantifying the severity of motor weakness, such as the Medical Research Council (MRC) scale, NIHSS, and Scandinavian Neurological Stroke Scale which have an operational definition of the grades of weakness, and moderately good inter-observer reliability.[46] In addition a description of some actions the patient can and cannot perform (e.g. holding a cup of water, combing hair) is helpful when trying to understand the problems that the patient is having and for appropriate goal setting during rehabilitation. And, for assessing change, it can be helpful to ask the patient, or note, what they can *just* do (e.g. can *just* extend the fingers against gravity, walk 10 m in 15 s); and worsening or improvement can then be easily observed, even if the weakness appears to have the same MRC grade.

Attention should focus on the anatomical extent of the weakness and the functional consequences, rather than solely trying to grade the severity with a motor scale.

An extensor plantar response is only one part of a nociceptive spinal flexion reflex, which in its complete

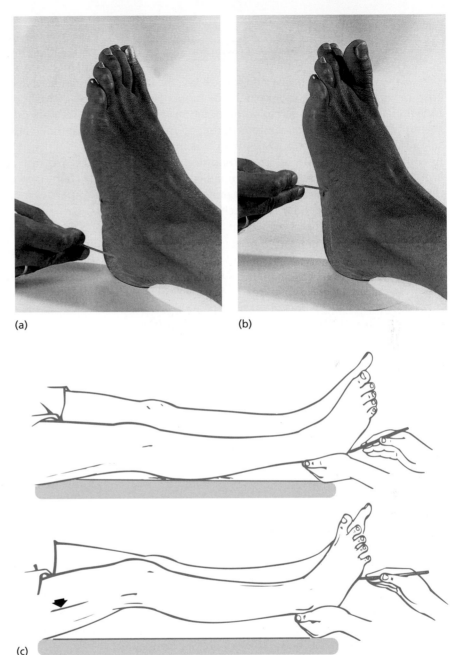

(a)   (b)

(c)

Fig. 3.19 The Babinski sign: (a,b) evoked in this case by stroking the lateral part of the dorsum, rather than the sole, of the foot, in order to avoid voluntary withdrawal. The Babinski sign (c) involves contraction of the extensor hallucis longus simultaneously with other muscles that shorten the leg: tibialis anterior, the hamstrings (*arrow*), and the tensor fasciae latae (from van Gijn, 1995[70], by kind permission of the author and *Postgraduate Medical Journal*).

form (the sign of Babinski) involves flexion at the hip, knee and ankle as well as extension of the great toe[70] (Fig. 3.19). Failure to appreciate this perhaps explains, in part, the rather poor reliability of the sign. While the presence of a Babinski response signifies a lesion of the corticospinal tract, it is not invariable, particularly if there is no weakness of the foot.

Although swallowing involves both the motor and sensory systems, mention will be made of it here. The gag reflex alone is not an adequate examination of the ninth and tenth cranial nerves, nor is it a good indicator of swallowing ability[71] (section 11.17). Sensation on the two sides of the soft palate should be tested separately with an orange-stick, elevation of the palate should be observed, and the patient should be asked to cough. Failure to oppose the vocal cords adequately will result in some air escaping, which should alert the physician that the patient may have swallowing difficulties.

Clinical practice

> Most patients with stroke have motor symptoms or signs.

Weakness usually affects one side of the body: the face, arm, or leg in isolation (monoparesis or monoplegia), each limb as a whole or in part, or a combination of these (hemiparesis or hemiplegia). Lesions in the internal capsule and ventral pons tend to result in a hemiparesis/hemiplegia that is equally severe (proportional) in the arm and leg and is seldom accompanied by other neurological symptoms and signs – a pure motor stroke (section 4.3.2). When there is a brachial monoparesis (isolated weakness of the arm), or the weakness affects predominantly the face, hand or fingers even, it is more likely to be due to a cortical (where function is distributed anatomically) rather than a subcortical (where function is concentrated) lesion.[72] When weakness involves the hand only, it is often referred to as a 'cortical hand'. This can be mistaken for a peripheral nerve lesion, but closer analysis reveals that this would require simultaneous involvement of the median, ulnar and radial nerves, a most unlikely occurrence. It is generally considered to occur because of the large cortical representation of the hand. Isolated upper motor neurone facial weakness, however, seems to be of less localizing value, and it can certainly occur with very small infarcts in the genu of the internal capsule and in the pons.

When weakness is confined to, or predominates in, the leg, the lesion is most likely to, but not invariably, involve the territory of the anterior cerebral artery or the sagittal venous sinus[73] (section 4.2.2). Crossed weakness (i.e. weakness of one side of the face and the contralateral limbs) indicates a brainstem lesion or bilateral lesions (e.g. both hemispheres, or one hemisphere and contralateral brainstem). Paraplegia, triplegia and tetraplegia all occur more commonly from spinal than brain disorders (although see 'locked-in syndrome', section 3.3.2).

When bilateral motor signs develop simultaneously – particularly if a cranial nerve palsy or crossed sensory disturbance (pointing to a brainstem lesion) are not present – and there is no sensory or reflex level to suggest a spinal cord lesion, cardiogenic embolism (i.e. causing two or more lesions), some kind of multifocal arteriopathy (such as vasculitis), abnormalities of the circle of Willis (section 4.2.2), or systemic hypotension (resulting in bilateral boundary-zone infarcts; section 4.2.4) must be considered. Very rarely hypotension results in paralysis predominantly of both arms (the 'man in the barrel' syndrome), with bilateral infarction in the boundary between the anterior and middle cerebral arteries.

Although most strokes causing facial weakness result in a typical upper motor neurone pattern, there are some exceptions, which can lead to the erroneous diagnosis of Bell's palsy if there is minimal associated limb weakness. The most obvious exception is that of a brainstem stroke affecting the facial nerve nucleus. Occasionally, patients with very severe lower facial weakness from a supranuclear lesion also have some weakness of the upper face as well, particularly in the first few days after a stroke. This may reflect individual variation in the bilateral innervation of the upper facial (forehead) muscles.

> Lesions of the seventh cranial nerve nucleus involve both the upper and lower parts of the face; this pattern is not always due to Bell's palsy.

Sometimes patients seem at one moment to have (or are reported to have) a dense hemiplegia (usually left-sided) and yet, very soon afterwards, move the 'paralysed' limbs. This may be misinterpreted as a hysterical conversion disorder.[74] However, this pattern can also be seen with the so-called capsular warning syndrome, or crescendo small vessel TIAs,[75] although in such cases the episodes seem much more discrete (section 6.7.3). It can also occur in patients with a haemodynamically significant internal carotid artery stenosis, presumably due to subtle changes in distal perfusion pressure. However, the majority are patients in whom this seems to be a manifestation of inattention/neglect, or even apraxia. In patients who are recovering from what appears to be an extensive non-dominant hemisphere stroke, what seems to be a dense hemiplegia may improve very rapidly as the inattention/neglect begins to resolve – a fact that needs to be borne in mind when predicting the eventual functional outcome.

> It is always important to see whether a patient can sit up, get off the bed and walk, provided there is no risk to the patient or physician, whatever the motor deficit when tested on the bed. A severe deficit may be due to neglect and not weakness, and profound ataxia of gait may be associated with no motor deficit at all.

Dysphagia is a common feature of acute stroke and an important cause of complications if not appropriately managed (section 11.17), but it is of limited neuro-anatomical localizing value.

Movement disorders such as hemiballismus, unilateral asterixis, hemichorea and focal dystonia occur in about 1% of patients with TIA and acute stroke due to contralateral, and rarely ipsilateral, small deep vascular lesions of the subthalamic nucleus, striatum or thalamus. Transient cerebral ischaemia may also masquerade as paroxysmal dyskinesia, and involuntary tonic limb spasms may arise contralateral to ventral pontine brainstem infarction. The abnormal movements usually regress spontaneously.

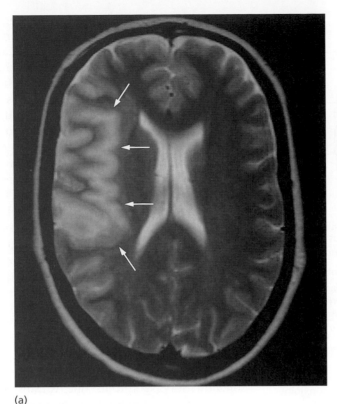

(a)

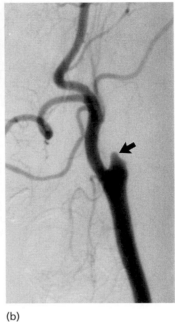

(b)

Fig. 3.20 (a) T2-weighted MR scan showing an extensive infarct in an area usually supplied by the middle cerebral artery (*arrows*) in a patient who initially presented with several episodes of jerking of the left arm (which were initially thought to be epileptic) and who awoke three days later with a left hemiparesis. (b) Catheter angiography showing occlusion of the ipsilateral internal carotid artery (*arrow*).

Occasionally, patients describe jerking movements of the limbs just before the onset of a stroke, or during a TIA. The distinction from focal motor epilepsy may be difficult (section 3.4.2).[52,76] However, in contrast to epileptic seizures, these attacks may be provoked by postural change (from lying to sitting or standing up), hyperextension of the neck, walking, coughing, or starting or increasing antihypertensive therapy, and they may be alleviated promptly by sitting or lying down, all of which suggest they are due to 'low flow' rather than embolism (section 6.7.5). There is an association with severe internal carotid artery stenosis or occlusion (Fig. 3.20),[76] and the attacks usually stop after carotid endarterectomy. This pattern has also been reported with internal boundary-zone infarcts (section 4.2.4).

Other disorders that sometimes need to be considered in the differential diagnosis of stroke are the Guillain-Barré syndrome, mononeuropathies, drop attacks, cataplexy and motor neurone disease (section 3.4.11).

3.3.5 Disturbance of the somatic sensory system

There are broadly two types of sensory message passing from the periphery to the brain. *Superficial sensation*

(also known as cutaneous or exteroceptive) includes light touch, pain and temperature modalities. *Deep and proprioceptive sensation* refers to deep pressure and joint position sense, respectively. Synthesis and appreciation of these sensory inputs occurs at a cortical level. *Discriminative sensation* refers to stereognosis, two-point discrimination and graphaesthesia. *Paraesthesiae* are positive sensory phenomena (e.g. pins and needles) that are presumed to occur because of partial damage to the sensory tracts or posterior horn cells, which become hyperexcitable (perhaps akin to brisk reflexes), such that ectopic impulses are generated either spontaneously or after a normal stimulus-evoked volley of impulses.

Clinical anatomy

The main sensory pathways are shown in Fig. 3.21. Impulses for superficial sensation are conveyed in the spinothalamic tracts, which synapse in the dorsal horn, cross the midline at about the same spinal level and then ascend through the lateral spinal cord and brainstem. Fibres carrying similar sensory impulses from the face enter the ipsilateral, descending (or spinal) trigeminal

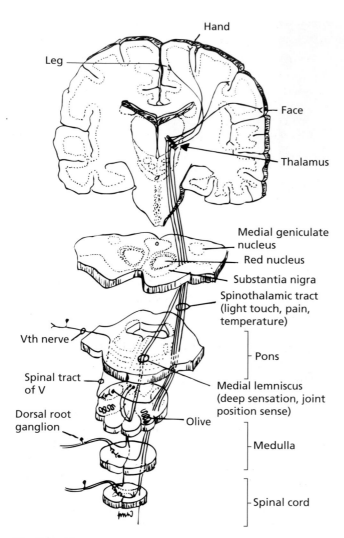

Fig. 3.21 Diagrammatic representation of the main sensory pathways between the entry of the dorsal root to the spinal cord and the sensory cortex.

postero-medial nuclei (face, tongue, fingers). Lesions of the thalamus often involve all sensory modalities, although deep sensation may be more affected than superficial sensation. From the thalamus there are probably two main projections. The first is to the postcentral or primary somatic cortex where there is somatotopic representation, with the leg uppermost and the face lowermost. The areas of sensory representation in the cortex match those of the motor homunculus (Fig. 3.16). A second projection is to the area adjacent to the upper part of the sylvian fissure and insula. Here there is less discrete localization, but in general, the face is rostral and the leg caudal. Interestingly, stimulation of this area may result in bilateral symptoms. Lesions confined to the parietal lobe generally affect higher-level 'discriminatory' functions (i.e. proprioception, two-point discrimination, astereognosis) rather than primary modalities of sensation (e.g. pain, temperature), but sometimes the primary modalities are affected, giving rise to a 'pseudothalamic' syndrome.

Clinical assessment

Somatosensory symptoms due to stroke are usually described by the patient as numbness ('like the numbness I have after going to the dentist'), tingling, or a dead sensation; occasionally as loss of temperature sensation when in the bath or shower; and very rarely as pain (at least at onset). Often, patients find it difficult to describe unusual sensations in a manner that allows accurate classification, and the descriptions seem to vary between cultures. Nevertheless, it is the distribution of the sensory disturbance, usually involving the face *and* arm, or hand *and* leg, or face *and* arm *and* leg, that stamp the disturbance as involving the central nervous rather than the peripheral nervous system. The difficulty lies with isolated sensory disturbances that are limited to a part of a limb or a part of the face, which can be central or peripheral in origin.

It is widely recognized that formal testing of the sensory system is one of the most unreliable parts of the neurological examination (see below). Quite frequently there is no detectable sensory loss. In general, therefore, sensory symptoms even in the absence of a deficit on examination should be noted. Indeed, on the assumption that the patients are able to communicate and do not have neglect, the only situation in which they will have sensory loss without sensory symptoms is when there is a restricted problem of discriminatory rather than primary sensory function (due to a parietal lesion), something that is uncommon in clinical practice. Conversely, care needs to be taken over the interpretation of very transient sensory symptoms, which can

nucleus and cross the midline in the upper cervical spinal cord. They then ascend through the medulla medially, close to the medial lemniscus, and separate to join the medial part of the spinothalamic tract in the pons. The relevant fibres for deep sensation are primarily in the ipsilateral posterior columns of the spinal cord. Decussation (crossing) occurs in the caudal medulla, after which the fibres ascend through the brainstem in the medial lemniscus. Fibres carrying similar sensory impulses from the face enter the primary trigeminal nucleus in the pons and cross the midline at this level to form the trigeminal lemniscus, which lies adjacent to the medial lemniscus.

All these ascending fibres converge towards the midbrain and project, in the main, to the posterior group of thalamic nuclei and in particular to the ventro-postero-lateral nuclei (trunk and legs) and ventro-

be within the range of normal experience, although the clinician should not accept uncritically the patients' common interpretation of sensory symptoms as being due to a 'trapped nerve' or 'lying in a draught'.

> Formal testing of the sensory system is the most unreliable part of the neurological examination. However, the physician should always take due note of sensory symptoms, even when there is no deficit on examination.

Superficial sensation should ideally be tested in the standard manner, using a wisp of cotton wool (light touch), the side of a tuning fork (cold temperature), and an appropriate pin (i.e. not a hat pin or hypodermic needle) or other sharp object that can be disposed of after it has been used (pain). Proprioception may be assessed with the patient's arms outstretched, the fingers spread and the eyes closed. Look for drift of the patient's arm in a 'pseudoathetoid' or 'piano-playing' manner. This can be amplified by asking the patient to touch the tip of his or her nose with the forefinger while the eyes remain closed; those with disturbed proprioception will repeatedly miss the target. This screening test will assess proprioception around proximal as well as distal joints, but drift can also be due to a motor deficit or neglect/inattention. Therefore, if possible, one should always attempt the traditional method of testing joint position sense of the distal interphalangeal joints. If there is expressive aphasia, it is sometimes worth asking the patient to indicate with gesture the direction of movement. Romberg's test can be useful to assess position sense in the legs if there are no other deficits affecting them (e.g. cerebellar ataxia).

Clinical practice

The lacunar syndrome of *pure sensory stroke* is typically caused by a lateral thalamic infarct or haemorrhage.[77] The deficit may involve all modalities, or may spare pain and temperature sensation. If there is extension to the internal capsule, a sensorimotor stroke may occur (section 4.3.2).

The *Déjerine–Roussy syndrome* is caused by more extensive lateral thalamic infarction, and consists of a mild contralateral hemiparesis, marked hemianaesthesia, hemiataxia, astereognosis and frequently paroxysmal pain/hyperaesthesia and choreoathetotic movements. The original cases had extension of the infarcts into the internal capsule and towards the putamen, although most of the features of this syndrome result from involvement of the ventroposterior nuclei of the thalamus[57] (section 4.2.3).

Central pain alone may be caused by lesions at any level of the somatosensory pathways. However, in our experience, most patients with a diffuse pain in the body at the *onset* of the event often turn out to have a non-organic/functional disorder, and patients with severe localized limb pain tend to have other disorders, such as nerve root compression in the neck or low back, or even myocardial infarction if the pain is down the arm or in the hand. Nevertheless, we have seen the occasional patient with thalamic infarction or haemorrhage develop unpleasant sensation in the contralateral limb within 2–3 days of onset.

Some patients have restricted sensory syndromes that affect unusual combinations of body parts. The most frequent is the *cheiro-oral syndrome*, where there is a sensory abnormality over the perioral area (sometimes bilaterally) and ipsilateral palm. In some patients, the foot may also be involved (the *cheiro-oral-pedal syndrome*) and, in both the hand and foot, certain digits may be affected while others are spared (a pseudoradicular distribution). Although lesions at most levels of the sensory pathways can give these patterns, lesions in the ventro-posterior nuclei of the thalamus are the most likely. It is thought that sensory projections from the face (with a particularly large representation for the lips), hand and foot are somatotopically arranged in the ventral portion of this nucleus, and the fingertips have particularly large representation areas, with that for the thumb more medial and the little finger more laterally. The projection areas for the trunk and proximal limbs are relatively small and sited more dorsally. However, a similar proximity of projection areas through the corona radiata and in the sensory cortex may also occur, and consequently lesions in these areas may also result in the cheiro-oral syndrome. An isolated deficit in a *pseudoradicular distribution* (most often involving the thumb and forefinger) is probably more often caused by a cortical lesion, because a stroke of any given size would there affect fibres from a more restricted anatomical area than in the thalamus. Bilateral symptoms may occur from midpontine lesions, because the sensory fibres from the mouth, arm and leg are once again arranged somatotopically in the medial lemnisci.

A defect of pain and temperature sensation below a certain level on the trunk on one side is usually a sign of spinal cord disease, but this may occur from ischaemic lesions in the lateral medulla on the contralateral side. This is thought to be due to the orientation of fibres from different body parts within the lateral spinothalamic tract. Although patients usually have contralateral facial sensory loss as well, during the recovery phase this can disappear, leaving only the pseudospinal sensory loss. It is also worth noting that infarction of the cervical spinal cord causing a partial Brown–Séquard syndrome can be due to bilateral vertebral artery dissection.[78]

3.3.6 Disturbance of the visual system

When trying to assess the visual disturbances that occur in patients with cerebrovascular disease, one needs to consider: the reception of visual stimuli by the eyes; the transmission of the visual information from the eyes to the occipital cortex and visual association areas; and the interpretation of the visual information in the occipital cortex. Additionally, we have included in this section information about pupillary reactions and eye movements.

Vision

CLINICAL ANATOMY

Lesions at different sites in the visual pathway give highly characteristic abnormalities (Fig. 3.22).

Amaurosis fugax (meaning literally 'fleeting blindness') and *transient monocular blindness* (TMB) are terms used interchangeably to describe temporary loss of vision in *one* eye. TMB may be caused by transient ischaemia in the distribution of the ophthalmic, posterior ciliary, or central retinal artery. Vascular lesions affecting the optic chiasm symmetrically (when one might detect a bi-temporal hemianopia) are rare. Indeed, the only vascular

lesion of note would be a large aneurysm of the circle of Willis.

Homonymous visual field deficits (i.e. loss of vision in the corresponding part of the visual fields in both eyes) signify a retrochiasmal lesion (Fig. 3.23). Lesions of the lateral geniculate nucleus may result in a homonymous horizontal sectoranopia (i.e. a segmental defect that respects the vertical but not the horizontal meridian) due to topographical organization within the lateral geniculate nucleus, but these rarely occur in isolation. The optic radiations pass from the lateral geniculate nucleus as the most posterior structures of the internal capsule. Involvement at this level is probably one of the causes of hemianopia in extensive middle cerebral artery territory infarction. The radiations do not seem to be affected by occlusion of a single perforating artery. Restricted lesions of the inferior optic radiation between the lateral geniculate nucleus and the calcarine cortex, where the fibres swing over the temporal horn of the lateral ventricle and deep into the temporal lobe (Meyer's loop), result in a homonymous superior quadrantanopia, while lesions of the superior optic radiation in the parietal lobe result in a homonymous inferior quadrantanopia. On purely anatomical grounds, one might anticipate encountering an inferior quadrantanopia fairly frequently, because the middle cerebral artery is traditionally considered to supply the area through which the superior but not the inferior optic

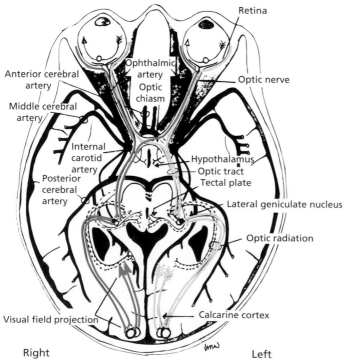

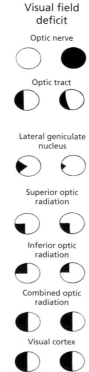

Visual field deficit

Optic nerve

Optic tract

Lateral geniculate nucleus

Superior optic radiation

Inferior optic radiation

Combined optic radiation

Visual cortex

Fig. 3.22 Diagram of the visual pathways and their vascular supply, and the visual field defects that may result from vascular lesions at various sites along the visual pathway. The visual fields represented by the arrows on the retina correspond with the arrowheads and tails superimposed on the visual cortex. The dark purple represents visual pathways carrying vision from the left homonymous half fields and the light purple those from the right homonymous half fields. Arteries are shown in solid black.

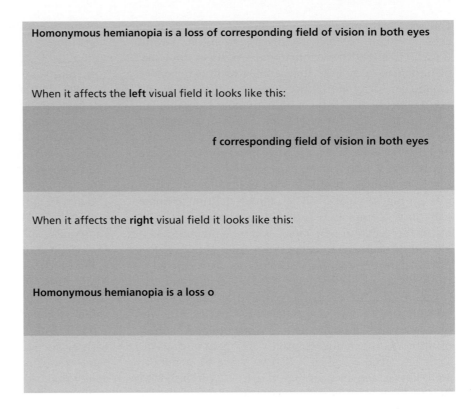

Homonymous hemianopia is a loss of corresponding field of vision in both eyes

When it affects the **left** visual field it looks like this:

f corresponding field of vision in both eyes

When it affects the **right** visual field it looks like this:

Homonymous hemianopia is a loss o

Fig. 3.23 Homonymous hemianopia.

radiation passes. However, in some patients, the area of supply of the middle cerebral artery extends much more posteriorly than is apparent on standard 'maps' (section 4.2.2), and an middle cerebral artery lesion thus produces a homonymous hemianopia by interrupting the optic radiations as they converge from the temporal and parietal lobe on their way to the occipital lobe.[79] Also, perforating arteries from the carotid system supply the optic tracts and lateral geniculate nucleus (section 4.2.2). In other patients, the posterior cerebral artery may derive its blood supply via the posterior communicating artery, and therefore, like the middle cerebral artery, be affected by embolism from the internal carotid artery. Perhaps the most likely explanation, however, is that in many patients there is a mixture of a true visual field loss and visual inattention.

If the entire calcarine cortex or optic tract on one side is damaged, there will be a complete homonymous hemianiopia, including macular vision. When this is an isolated feature, it is most likely due to a lesion in the occipital lobe, and when this is an infarct it will most often be due to occlusion of the posterior cerebral artery. Embolism is probably the most frequent cause, but giant-cell arteritis and migraine need to be considered. Sparing of macular vision with an otherwise complete hemianopia does occur in posterior cerebral artery territory infarction. The conventional explanation is that the infarction is confined to the lateral cortical surface and that the macular cortex is spared because it receives sufficient collateral supply from the terminal branches of the middle cerebral artery (section 4.2.2). In theory, if the deficit in the two eyes is incongruous, it is most likely to be due to a lesion of the optic tracts, whereas if the deficits are entirely congruous, the lesion is likely to be in the calcarine cortex. However, it can be difficult to make this distinction in routine clinical practice.

Visual agnosia is when primary visual perception is intact but the patient is unable to identify an object without resorting to the use of other sensory modalities such as touch. *Prosopagnosia* refers to the inability of patients to recognize familiar faces, even though they can describe them. In its pure form it is very rare, but it can result in enormous distress if patients deny recognizing their close family. Most lesions causing visual agnosia are in the anterior part of the dominant occipital lobe (the so-called visual association areas) and the angular gyrus, although most cases of prosopagnosia have occurred with bilateral lesions.

CLINICAL ASSESSMENT
Many patients have great difficulty in describing visual symptoms, particularly when they have resolved. It is therefore very important to be clear what a patient means. For example, the term 'blackout' may be used to mean bilateral blindness and also loss of consciousness,

and some patients who report 'blurred vision' in both eyes are actually trying to describe double vision. We find it useful to establish the functional severity of the visual disturbance – e.g. were they unable to find their way around, or to recognize faces (neither of which would occur with either TMB or an homonymous hemianopia).

In vascular TMB the symptoms usually occur without provocation, but they may occasionally be precipitated by bright or white light, a change in posture, exercise, a hot bath or a heavy meal, particularly in patients with severe ipsilateral carotid disease. Generally, the visual loss during vascular TMB is painless (although some patients do complain of a dull ache or numbness in or above the eye) and very rapid. It can be described as if a blind or shutter had come down from above or, less often, up from below. The visual loss may be restricted to either the upper or lower half of the visual field and, less frequently, to the peripheral nasal and/or temporal field (in which case, be suspicious that the visual loss is or was binocular; i.e. a homonymous hemianopia). A pattern of diffuse, constricting or patchy loss may also occur. TMB may recur, usually in a stereotyped fashion, but the area of visual impairment may vary from one episode to the next, depending on which part of the retina is ischaemic.

A frequent and, from a vascular anatomical point of view, very important clinical problem is trying to differentiate a transient homonymous hemianopia from TMB. The single most important question is to ask whether the patient covered each eye in turn during the episode. For patients without any residual visual disturbance, it can be useful to cover one eye and ask whether that reproduces the previously experienced effect. After covering the 'good eye', patients with TMB (of the 'bad eye') will have seen nothing, whereas patients with a homonymous hemianopia will have still seen something in the remaining half of the visual field. On the other hand, when patients cover the affected eye during TMB, they tend not to notice any visual disturbance because of normal vision from the other eye. In our experience, asking patients whether they saw half of everything often seems to cause confusion, and it may be better to ask them to look at your face and describe what they might have seen if they had been having an attack

When a patient complains of transient loss of vision in one eye, do not assume that the visual loss was monocular; it may have been a homonymous hemianopia. Ask the patient if they covered each eye in turn during the episode of loss of vision, and if so if the visual disturbance was present in both eyes or one (and if the latter, which eye).

Patients may not recognize an isolated homonymous hemianopia, or they may simply describe it as 'blurred vision' or 'a shadow'. Even if they covered each eye in turn during the symptoms, it still may not be possible to be really confident, because homonymous hemianopia does not necessarily split macular vision and may be interpreted by the patient as loss of vision in one eye only. The presence of other symptoms may be helpful – for example, if there are ipsilateral visual and brain symptoms the visual problem is likely to be a hemianopia, whereas if they are contralateral it points to TMB.

It may be difficult to test *visual acuity* formally (e.g. with a Snellen chart) in patients with acute stroke, because of drowsiness, aphasia, or the fact that they are bed-bound, but at least testing with a hand-held acuity chart or simply using everyday written material should be attempted. Many stroke patients are elderly, and concomitant eye diseases such as glaucoma, senile macular degeneration, cataracts and diabetic retinopathy are therefore common. It is important to identify these conditions at an early stage, because they may well make rehabilitation significantly more difficult. Indeed, the improved visual acuity that follows a cataract extraction may make the difference between being able to live independently (and safely) or not for a patient who has residual disability from a stroke. Because of the very large representation of the macula area in the occipital cortex, even patients who have a complete homonymous hemianopia do not have significantly reduced visual acuity per se.

Elderly patients rarely attempt, let alone accomplish, tests of visual acuity without their own clean spectacles.

If the visual loss is persistent (i.e. beyond several hours) and ophthalmoscopy reveals pallor of all or a section of the retina (due to cloudy swelling of the retinal ganglion cells), then the diagnosis is retinal infarction (Fig. 3.24). Additional findings may include an afferent pupillary defect, embolic material in the retinal arteries or arterioles, and a cherry-red spot over the fovea (due to accentuation of the normal fovea, which is devoid of ganglion cells, against the abnormally pale retina) in cases of central retinal artery occlusion (Fig. 3.25).

If the eye is red and painful with a fixed, semidilated, oval pupil and cloudy/steamy cornea, then acute glaucoma is the likely diagnosis (section 3.5.1) (Fig. 3.26). Episcleral vascular congestion, a cloudy cornea, neovascularization of the iris (rubeosis iridis) and a sluggishly reactive mid-dilated pupil indicate chronic anterior segment ocular ischaemia which may be due to carotid occlusive disease, or small vessel disease particularly in a diabetic. This is so-called *ischaemic oculopathy*

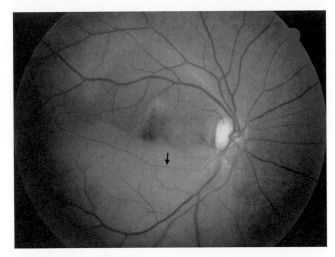

Fig. 3.24 An ocular fundus photograph of a patient with inferior temporal branch retinal artery occlusion, showing pallor of the inferior half of the retina due to cloudy swelling of the retinal ganglion cells caused by retinal infarction. The inferior temporal branch arteriole is attenuated and contains embolic material (*arrow*). Also reproduced in colour in the plate section.

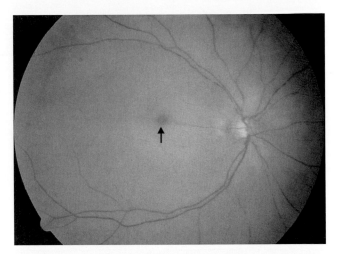

Fig. 3.25 An ocular fundus photograph of a patient with central retinal artery occlusion, showing a cherry-red spot over the fovea (*arrow*). The cherry red spot is the normal fovea (devoid of ganglion cells), which seems more obvious because the surrounding infarcted retina has lost its red colour and appears pale. Also reproduced in colour in the plate section.

(Fig. 3.27).[2] Because ischaemic oculopathy is a gradual, chronic process it is commonly also called *chronic ischaemic oculopathy*.

If there is a visual field defect of acute onset, such as an absolute or relative inferior altitudinal hemianopia, inferior nasal segmental loss, or central scotoma, and if ophthalmoscopy reveals swelling of a segment or all of the optic disc (which may be indistinguishable from that seen with raised intracranial pressure), flame-shaped haemorrhages near the disc and distended veins

(Fig. 3.28), then the diagnosis is likely to be *anterior ischaemic optic neuropathy* (section 3.5.2). Later the optic disc becomes pale.

Ophthalmoscopy may reveal retinal emboli but these are not necessarily symptomatic (up to 1–2% of the population over the age of 50 may have asymptomatic retinal emboli). The most common type are the bright orange or yellow crystals of cholesterol that originate from ulcerated atheroma in proximal arteries. Although cholesterol crystals are actually white, they appear orange

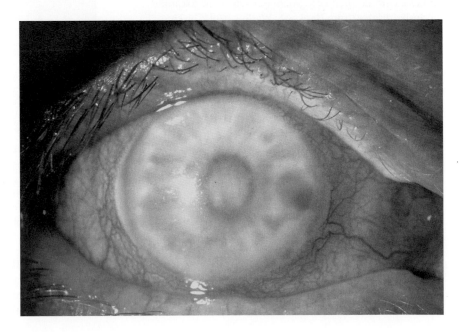

Fig. 3.26 A photograph of the eye of a patient with acute glaucoma, showing congested sclera, cloudy cornea and oval pupil. Also reproduced in colour in the plate section.

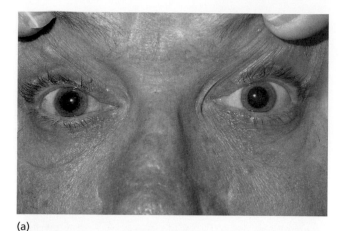

(a)

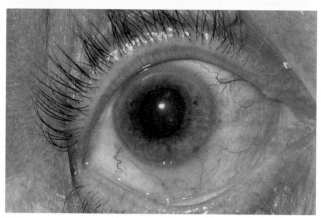

(b)

Fig. 3.27 (a) and (b) Ischaemic oculopathy of the right eye; note episcleral vascular congestion, cloudy cornea, neovascularization of the iris (rubeosis of the iris) and mid-dilated pupil on external examination of the eye, which indicate chronic anterior segment ischaemia due to carotid occlusive disease (from Hankey & Warlow, 1994[2] by kind permission of the authors and W.B. Saunders Co. Ltd). Also reproduced in colour in the plate section.

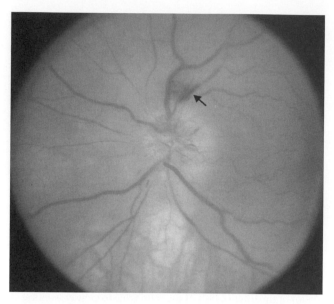

Fig. 3.28 An ocular fundus photograph of a patient with anterior ischaemic optic neuropathy due to occlusion of the posterior ciliary artery as a result of giant cell arteritis. Note the oedema of the optic disc and flame-shaped haemorrhages (*arrow*). Also reproduced in colour in the plate section.

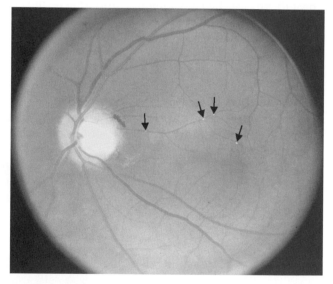

Fig. 3.29 An ocular fundus photograph showing golden orange cholesterol crystals (Hollenshorst plaques) in the cilioretinal artery (*arrows*). The cilioretinal artery is present in only about one-third of the population. It originates from a branch of the short posterior ciliary artery and supplies the macula. Also reproduced in colour in the plate section.

or golden because their thin, fish-scale contour permits blood to pass above and below them and thus produce their characteristic refractile appearance (Fig. 3.29). Most of the crystals, because of their small size, thin, flat structure and lack of adhesiveness, pass through the retinal arterioles rapidly and rarely occlude the larger vessels, although it is probable that large clumps of crystals briefly occlude the central artery of the retina, producing TMB, before breaking up and being flushed away.

White plugs of fibrin, platelets, or fatty material are less common. They occur in all sizes and are more likely to be symptomatic. Calcium emboli are chalky white angular crystals that tend to arise from calcific aortic stenosis, and they may permanently occlude the central retinal artery (behind the cribriform plate), or one of

the branch retinal arterioles near the optic disc. Other less common types of emboli include microorganisms (septic), fat and tumour cells. Roth spots, which are very small white infarcts encircled by haemorrhage, were

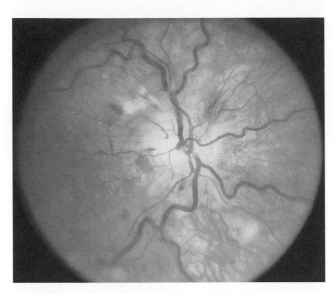

Fig. 3.30 An ocular fundus photograph showing narrowing and tortuosity of retinal arterioles, arteriovenous nipping, retinal haemorrhages and papilloedema. These are the features of hypertensive retinopathy seen in malignant hypertension. Also reproduced in colour in the plate section.

thought to be caused by septic emboli, but it now seems more likely that they are due to rupture of retinal capillaries and the extrusion of blood cells. Whilst the inter-observer and intra-observer agreement for the detection of retinal emboli is quite high (kappa = 0.73 and 0.63, respectively), agreement on a range of qualitative assessments of emboli type is much poorer.

Narrowing, focal irregularity/constriction and tortuosity of retinal arterioles, arteriovenous nipping and fluffy white patches of transudate ('cotton-wool patches' which are thought to represent small focal infarcts in the inner layers of the retina), indicate long-standing hypertension. If papilloedema and retinal haemorrhages are also present, this indicates malignant hypertension, but is now uncommon (Fig. 3.30).

Retinal haemorrhages without the other changes of hypertensive or diabetic retinopathy in a patient with a non-traumatic, acute neurological event is strong evidence of a haemorrhagic stroke. They are usually caused by a very sudden increase in intracranial pressure transmitted to the distal optic nerve sheath, where it causes a temporary obstruction of retinal venous outflow. The subsequent rise in retinal venous pressure leads to secondary bleeding from retinal veins and capillaries. The appearance of the haemorrhage depends on its site. Small dot and blot haemorrhages lie in the deep retinal layers; linear haemorrhages in the superficial (nerve fibre) layer; 'thumbprint' haemorrhages with frayed borders are preretinal or superficial retinal; and large subhyaloid haemorrhages (large round haemorrhages with a fluid level) lie between the retina and the internal limiting membrane. Subhyaloid haemorrhages and other types of retinal haemorrhage can be seen in about 20% of patients with subarachnoid haemorrhage (section 3.7).

Assessment of the visual fields must be tailored to the patient's overall condition. It is important that the physician has a repertoire of methods and does not give up simply because 'formal' testing by confrontation is impossible in a patient who is drowsy, aphasic, cognitively impaired, or just cannot sit up. Kinetic testing (i.e. using moving objects, waggling fingers, etc.) is a less sensitive way of detecting deficits than static methods such as counting fingers or comparing colours in each hemifield.

If the patients can understand and communicate, one should first ask them to describe what they see in front of them, perhaps using the same text as for testing visual acuity, and ideally testing each eye individually. After that, hold up fingers sequentially in each quadrant of vision in each eye and ask the patient to count them or, for greater sensitivity, use a pin with a red ball on its end. This will detect a hemianopia or quadrantanopia. Following this, perform bilateral, simultaneous finger movement to detect evidence of visual inattention. Testing of the visual fields with automated perimetry is extremely tiring and of little value in the acute situation. Indeed, it may produce bizarre deficits that are normally associated with non-organic disorders. However, it may be necessary later when there is doubt about eligibility for driving.

> Although testing the visual fields using conventional confrontation methods is often impossible because the patient is drowsy, dysphasic, cognitively impaired, or cannot sit up, one can usually use other methods to determine whether or not there is an abnormality.

If, for whatever reason, the patient cannot follow commands, one will need to use quite gross stimuli to be sure of eliciting and identifying a response if the visual fields are intact. Examples include observing if there is any response to moving a brightly coloured object in one hemifield, getting a colleague to approach the patient from one side, or seeing whether the patient blinks when a threatening stimulus (e.g. a quickly moving finger) is brought towards the eye (one needs to be careful that the associated air current is not simply stimulating a corneal reflex). A hemianopia is almost always associated with ipsilateral loss of this blink reflex, although the reverse is not always true. If the patient is not aphasic and there are members of the team around the bed, ask the patient to point to each one of the team in turn. An asymmetrical response to any of these tests suggests a field defect, inattention, neglect or a combination of these.

It is not surprising, given these difficulties, that the inter-observer reliability of the assessment of visual fields is relatively poor (Table 3.31).

CLINICAL PRACTICE

Some patients with severe stenosis or occlusion of one or both internal carotid arteries may experience a visual disturbance in one or both eyes on exposure to bright sunlight or white light. Blurring, dimming, or constriction of the visual field from the periphery to the centre of vision of the involved eye develops over minutes rather than seconds. Objects appear bleached like a photographic negative, or there may be a scotoma or complete visual loss; an altitudinal defect is most unusual. Such transient episodes of monocular or binocular blindness are presumed to be due to low flow in the choroidal circulation. They are typically less rapid in onset than the brief transient attacks of embolic origin, and sight returns more gradually. Sunglasses may be an effective symptomatic treatment.

Cortical blindness is a syndrome in which the patient has no vision despite normally functioning eyes and anterior visual pathways. Cases of sudden, spontaneous and simultaneous dimming or loss of vision in all of the visual field of both eyes are presumed to be due to bilateral occipital lobe (visual cortices and optic radiations) ischaemia/infarction due to occlusion of the top of the basilar artery or both posterior cerebral arteries. If the visual symptoms occur in isolation (without associated symptoms of focal cerebral ischaemia, seizures, or reduction in consciousness) in an elderly patient and if they resolve within 24 h, they are probably due to a TIA of the occipital lobes.[48] However, when the same symptom occurs in adolescents and young adults, investigations are unlikely to reveal a cause, and the long-term prognosis appears benign.

Occasionally, when the deficit persists, true cortical blindness has to be distinguished from non-organic visual loss. This is best detected with an optokinetic drum or a long piece of material with vertical stripes (e.g. a scarf or tape measure) because it is impossible to suppress nystagmus voluntarily if there is visual function. Sometimes, genuine bilateral blindness is denied by the patient (*Anton syndrome*) which signifies involvement of the association areas adjacent to the primary visual cortex, but otherwise the pathogenesis is as unclear as that of the denial of left hemiplegia or anosognosia in general. Perhaps the right hemisphere component is crucial.

Visual hallucinations can occur in patients with stroke involving the occipital, temporal and parietal cortices as well as the eye, optic pathways and cerebral peduncle (section 11.27.3). Those secondary to occipital lesions most commonly consist of elementary (unformed) visual perceptions, sensations of light and colours, simple geometric figures, and movements. Posterior temporal lesions, involving the association cortex, result in more complex (formed) visual hallucinations, consisting of faces and scenes that may include objects, pictures and people. Lesions in the high midbrain, particularly the pars reticulata of the substantia nigra, may give rise to the so-called 'peduncular hallucinosis' of Lhermitte, in which the hallucinations are purely visual, appear natural in form and colour, move about like an animated cartoon, and are usually considered to be unreal, abnormal phenomena (i.e. insight is preserved). More commonly, however, visual hallucinations are due to non-vascular disorders such as migraine or partial seizures (in which case, the hallucinations are usually unformed), psychosis, or an adverse effect of a drug such as levodopa. *Micropsia*, which is the illusion of objects appearing smaller than normal, and *palinopsia*, which is the persistence or recurrence of visual images after the stimulus has been removed, can occur with parietal lobe lesions.

Flashing lights, shooting stars, scintillations, or other positive phenomena in the area of impaired vision occasionally arise during retinal or optic nerve ischaemia, but are far more commonly features of migraine or glaucoma.

Pupils

CLINICAL ANATOMY

The size of the pupil is determined by the balance of tonic impulses from the pupillodilator fibres, which receive input from the sympathetic nervous system, and the pupilloconstrictor fibres, which receive input from the parasympathetic nervous system. The sympathetic fibres descend ipsilaterally from the hypothalamus, through the lateral brainstem adjacent to the spinothalamic tract. They occupy a more central position in the lateral grey column of the cervical spinal cord and exit via the first thoracic root. The fibres then pass across the apex of the lung to enter the sympathetic chain, which ascends through the neck in association with the carotid artery. The fibres associated with sweating separate in the superior cervical ganglion and then travel in association with branches of the external carotid artery. The other fibres enter the cranial cavity on the surface of the internal carotid artery. The fibres innervate the pupil via the long ciliary nerves, whilst those supplying the tarsal muscles are carried in the third cranial nerve.

Following reception of light by the retina, impulses are conveyed in the optic nerve. After the optic chiasm, they are conducted in both optic tracts to both Edinger–Westphal nuclei (a distinct part of the third nerve nuclear complex). The parasympathetic nerves exit

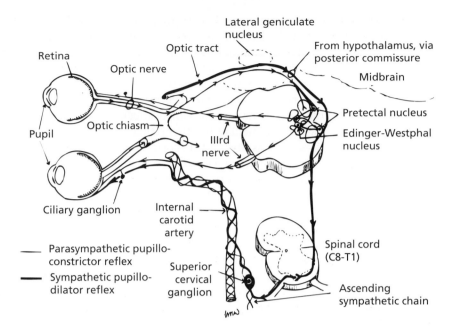

Fig. 3.31 The neurogenic control of pupil size: an outline of the parasympathetic and sympathetic pathways involved in pupil constriction (–) and pupil dilatation (–). The third cranial nerve nuclear complex consists of: the Edinger-Westphal nuclei concerned with parasympathetic innervation of the pupils; the midline nucleus of Perlia, concerned with convergence and accommodation; and the lateral nuclei, which innervate the levator palpebrae, superior recti, inferior oblique, medial recti and inferior recti muscles. It is possible for vascular lesions to cause ischaemia of the lateral nuclei (resulting in extraocular palsy) but spare the pupilloconstrictor fibres from the Edinger-Westphal nuclei.

alongside the third nerve and travel with it to the orbit (Fig. 3.31). There, they synapse in the ciliary ganglion, which gives rise to the short ciliary nerves that innervate the sphincter pupillae and the ciliary muscle. Lesions anterior to the lateral geniculate body result in loss of the pupillary light reflex.

CLINICAL ASSESSMENT

It is very uncommon for a patient to be aware of their own pupillary abnormalities, but others may notice. Just occasionally, patients notice that their pupils are unequal – they will usually think one is dilated, rather than the more common abnormality of one being constricted. With a truly dilated pupil, the patient may be distressed by abnormal brightness and difficulty focusing. The response of the pupils to light – both direct and consensual – should be tested, as well as accommodation, if possible.

Interruption of the descending sympathetic pathway in the brainstem and at other sites before the carotid bifurcation results in a complete ipsilateral *Horner syndrome*, i.e. miosis, ptosis and loss of sweating on the side of the face. Lesions of the internal carotid artery (e.g. carotid dissection; section 7.2.1) generally spare facial sweating. Sometimes a transient Horner syndrome is the only clue to a carotid dissection.

CLINICAL PRACTICE

There are many causes of *anisocoria* (unequal pupils) in the elderly, most are not vascular. Perhaps the commonest is the use of drops to treat glaucoma, but any local inflammatory condition (e.g. iritis) can be responsible. Furthermore, physiological anisocoria may occur in

up to 20% of the normal population. Therefore, anisocoria very much needs to be assessed in the context of any other signs (such as ptosis).

> Elderly patients with stroke may be using pupilloconstrictor drops for glaucoma, and this may cause unequal pupils.

Because of the functional separation of fibres within the third nerve nuclear complex, it is possible for third nerve palsies from midbrain vascular lesions to spare the pupillary reaction, which remains normal to light. On the other hand, in an unconscious patient with extensive damage to the midbrain (either due to intrinsic disease or secondary to pressure from above), the pupils will both be fixed and either dilated or in mid-position (4–5 mm), depending on whether the sympathetic as well as the parasympathetic fibres are involved. Bilateral 'pinpoint' pupils in an unconscious patient suggests an extensive lesion in the pons if there is no evidence of drug overdose (e.g. opiates). This is thought to be due to a combination of damage to the sympathetic fibres and irritation of the parasympathetic fibres (lesions solely of sympathetic fibres do not usually result in such intense pupilloconstriction). Despite this, the pupils react to a bright light, although this may be difficult to observe.

External ocular movements and eyelids

CLINICAL ANATOMY

The external ocular muscles maintain fusion of the images from each retina. The oculomotor (third nerve) complex in the midbrain innervates the medial, superior and inferior recti and inferior oblique muscles. The trochlear nerve (fourth nerve), also originating in the midbrain, innervates the superior oblique muscle, and the abducens nerve (sixth nerve) in the pons innervates the lateral rectus muscle. Other structures of importance include the medial longitudinal fasciculus (MLF) which effectively links the nuclei; the paramedian pontine reticular formation, sometimes known as the pontine lateral gaze centre; and the rostral interstitial nucleus of the MLF in the midbrain which generates the vertical and torsional components of eye movement (Fig. 3.32). The cerebellum and vestibular nuclei are also important for the control of eye movements.

The supranuclear control of conjugate eye movement is of relevance to patients with stroke. Voluntary eye movements are initiated in the frontal eye field, which is anterior to the precentral gyrus, whilst the reflex visual pursuit movements involve the occipital cortex and visual association areas. The fibres from these areas do not directly innervate the oculomotor nuclei, but rather their input is integrated by the MLF.

The levator palpebrae superioris is innervated by the superior division of the oculomotor nuclei in the midline, as are the superior rectus muscles. Because of this, movement of the eyelids is closely linked to vertical eye movements. The superior and inferior tarsal muscles receive sympathetic innervation via the third cranial nerve. They assist eye opening, and when they are paralysed (as in Horner syndrome), the palpebral fissure is narrowed (but there is not complete ptosis, as is seen with a third nerve palsy, or central nuclear third nerve palsy).

Nystagmus is an involuntary, biphasic ocular oscillation that occurs with lesions of the vestibular pathway and cerebellum. In patients with vascular disease, there may be either ischaemia of the labyrinth or of the vestibular nuclei in the brainstem, and the pattern of any associated signs may be of more use in localizing the lesions than attempts to analyse the nystagmus itself – i.e. with nuclear lesions, there are likely to be other signs of brainstem disturbance.

CLINICAL ASSESSMENT

Hemispheric stroke involving the frontal cortex results in a failure of voluntary conjugate gaze to the contralateral side. Because of the unopposed action of the intact frontal eye field of the hemisphere not affected by the stroke, there is conjugate deviation of gaze towards the side of the stroke lesion. This normally settles over a period of 1–2 weeks. The patients are usually drowsy so that reflex pursuit movements cannot be assessed, although if the lesion was confined to the frontal lobe one might expect such movements to be retained. If

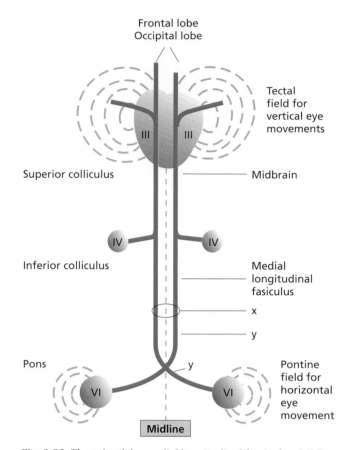

Fig. 3.32 The role of the medial longitudinal fasciculus (MLF) in the control of conjugate gaze. Conjugate gaze requires coordinated action of the third, fourth and sixth cranial nerve nuclei and nerves in the brainstem. The MLF links these nuclei and also provides a pathway for inputs from the frontal eye field (for voluntary eye movements – saccades) and the occipital lobe (for reflex movements), as well as the tectal field for vertical eye movements and the pontine field for horizontal eye movements. 'x' indicates the site of the lesion that results in the classical bilateral internuclear ophthalmoplegia often associated with multiple sclerosis. Vascular lesions ('y') more often result in unilateral internuclear ophthalmoplegia, presumably because they are more likely to respect the vascular territory of a paramedian pontine perforating artery, and thus the midline, than a plaque of demyelination. Conversely, a lesion of the lateral pons may prevent ipsilateral lateral gaze, and there may be a conjugate deviation of the eyes away from the side of the lesion.

patients have an acute pontine lesion, conjugate deviation away from the side of the lesion may occur, but this is less likely to recover.

When a patient complains of double vision, the following questions help to identify the site of the problem:
• is the double vision present when one eye is closed (monocular diplopia), or only when both eyes are open (binocular diplopia)?

- are the images separated side by side (horizontal), one above the other (vertical), or at an angle to one another (oblique)?
- and in which direction of gaze are the images separated maximally?

If the patient is conscious, communicative and cooperative, the eye movements can be tested in the normal way. However, it is difficult to do this if patients cannot follow commands. In such cases, spontaneous movements in each direction should be observed to confirm the absence of a gaze palsy. One can also stimulate patients to look in each direction by doing something 'interesting' in different fields of vision – so that they follow the examiner's face, for example, rather than a finger or a pen. This also has the advantage that the examiner can continually reinforce the command 'watch my nose'.

> The patient may be stimulated to look in each direction by doing something 'interesting' in different fields of vision – so that he or she follows the examiner's face, for example, rather than a finger or a pen.

Nystagmus of brainstem or cerebellar origin is probably best appreciated by asking the patient to fixate on, and then follow, a moving target. A few irregular 'jerks' of the eyes are often seen in normal people when they move their eyes, particularly at the extremes of lateral gaze. Acquired pendular nystagmus (i.e. where there is a sinusoidal waveform) is associated with lesions of the tegmentum of the pons and medulla. Upbeat nystagmus is associated with pontine or cerebellar lesions, and downbeat nystagmus with lesions in the medulla or at the craniocervical junction. A torsional or rotatory component can occur from both central and peripheral lesions. Convergence retraction nystagmus (rhythmic oscillation in which a slow abduction of the eyes in respect to each other is followed by a quick movement of adduction, and is usually accompanied by a quick rhythmic retraction of the eyes into the orbits) is considered indicative of midbrain disease; this is actually a disorder of horizontal eye movement rather than true nystagmus.

A number of related disorders, which are probably due to a disturbance of saccadic (voluntary) eye movements, are associated with cerebellar disease. These include ocular dysmetria (where there is overshoot of the eyes on attempted fixation), ocular flutter (where there are occasional bursts of rapid horizontal oscillations without an intersaccadic interval), and so-called square wave jerks.

CLINICAL PRACTICE

Transient diplopia in isolation may be an indication of a brainstem ischaemic event but can also be due to myasthenia gravis, for example. However, transient diplopia in association with other symptoms of brainstem or cerebellar dysfunction – such as unilateral or bilateral motor or sensory disturbances, vertigo, ataxia or dysarthria – usually signifies a TIA in the vertebrobasilar circulation.

Monocular diplopia is usually due to intraocular disease causing light rays to be dispersed onto the retina (e.g. corneal disease, cataract, vitreous haemorrhage) or to functional (non-neurological) disturbance. It has been reported rarely after occipital lesions but it is not due to paralysis of extraocular muscles.

Even though it is sometimes claimed to be a pathognomonic sign of multiple sclerosis, vascular disease can cause an *internuclear ophthalmoplegia* (failure of adduction in the adducting eye, with nystagmus in the abducting eye), due to involvement of the MLF on the side of the adducting eye (Fig. 3.32). A failure of conjugate horizontal gaze to one side can occur with ischaemia of the ipsilateral (the side to which the patient cannot look) paramedian pontine reticular formation. Additional involvement of the ipsilateral MLF (with failure of adduction of the ipsilateral eye on attempted gaze to the other side) may result in the so-called '*one-and-a-half syndrome*', where the only remaining horizontal eye movement is abduction of the contralateral eye.

An oculomotor (third cranial) nerve palsy at the onset of subarachnoid haemorrhage (SAH) frequently indicates a ruptured aneurysm at the origin of the posterior communicating artery from the internal carotid artery, less frequently an aneurysm of the carotid bifurcation, the posterior cerebral artery, the basilar bifurcation or the superior cerebellar artery. Third nerve palsy may also occur with unruptured aneurysms (presumably by expansion) or several days after SAH as a result of swelling of the ipsilateral cerebral hemisphere because of delayed cerebral ischaemia. Most often the pupil is dilated and unreactive, but in some patients it is spared.

Abducens (sixth cranial) nerve palsies, frequently bilateral in the acute stage, may develop after SAH as a false localizing sign of raised intracranial pressure, because of traction on the nerves against the petrous temporal bone, or by downward transtentorial herniation of the diencephalon. Occasionally, posterior circulation aneurysms may cause a sixth nerve palsy as a result of direct compression.

> If a patient presents following a sudden, severe headache and is found to have a third cranial nerve palsy, rupture of a posterior communicating artery aneurysm is highly likely.

Occasionally, one encounters patients who are unable to open their eyes. If *bilateral ptosis* is associated with a vertical gaze palsy and there is no suggestion of myasthenia gravis, then it is probably due to a nuclear third nerve palsy (dorsal part, in the midline) or a massive right hemisphere lesion ('cerebral ptosis').[80] 'Cerebral ptosis' must be distinguished from blepharospasm, and from apraxia of eyelid opening in which patients are unable to open their eyes on command but can do so spontaneously (i.e. the eyelid dysfunction is episodic and may be precipitated by eyelid closure, often in patients with extrapyramidal disorders).

Ocular bobbing is usually only present with an impaired conscious level and extensive pontine disease. The spontaneous rapid downward movement of the eyes is followed by a slow drift back to the original position. It is thought to occur because of the tendency of such patients to have roving eye movements but, without any horizontal gaze, the only possible movements are in the vertical plane.

Oscillopsia is an illusion of movement, or oscillation of the environment. The patient may complain that static objects are oscillating either from side to side or up and down. This can occur with nystagmus or any of the other tonic abnormalities of eye movement, but these can sometimes be difficult to demonstrate. This symptom, although uncommon, can be extremely distressing and disabling.

Tortopia is the illusion of transient tilting or inversion of the environment. This can occur with cerebellar ischaemia.

3.3.7 Disturbance of hearing, balance and coordination

Clinical anatomy

'*Dizziness*' may refer to light-headedness, imbalance, a feeling of faintness, a lack of mental clarity, or frank vertigo – the patient must be asked to explain exactly what he or she means by dizziness.

Vertigo is a subjective or objective illusion of motion (usually rotation) or position. It is a symptom of dysfunction of the peripheral or central vestibulocerebellar system.

Dysequilibrium is a sensation of imbalance when standing or walking due to impairment of vestibular, sensory, cerebellar, visual, or motor function, and consequently it may be due to lesions in many parts of the nervous system.

Ataxia (derived from the Greek meaning 'lack of order') is disordered coordination of the extremities (limb ataxia), and imbalance of sitting (truncal ataxia) or gait (gait ataxia). It is typically associated with disorders of the cerebellum or the cerebellar connections in the brainstem. However, lesions of the thalamus, particularly within the posterolateral territory supplied by the thalamogeniculate artery, may present with isolated contralateral ataxia – although more often there is an additional motor and/or sensory deficit.[57] The most likely explanation is that the ventrolateral nucleus receives input from the cerebellar, vestibular and spinothalamic systems (e.g. dentato-rubro-thalamic tract). A related condition in which patients are unable to stand or even sit unsupported, in the absence of marked motor deficit, has been termed *astasia* and is associated with lesions in the posterolateral thalamus.

Sudden unilateral hearing impairment, with or without ipsilateral tinnitus, is a symptom of dysfunction of the cochlea, vestibulocochlear nerve, or cochlear nucleus.

The relationship between the ascending and descending fibre tracts and the cranial nerve nuclei in the brainstem is shown in Fig. 3.33.

Clinical assessment

When patients complain of an illusory sense of movement, the first step is to distinguish rotatory vertigo or tilting of the visual axis from less specific symptoms such as faintness, and then to localize the disturbance to the brainstem (central) or to the vestibulocochlear nerve or labyrinth (peripheral).[81,82] To define as closely as possible the patient's actual sensations, direct questions often have to be asked; for example, 'is it a spinning feeling or just light-headedness?' Descriptions that include a subjective or objective illusion of motion, such as spinning or whirling, which is usually so unpleasant that it makes the patient feel nauseated and also unable to stand, denote what is meant by vertigo. Feelings of light-headedness, swaying, a swimming feeling, walking on air, queer head or faintness (often with accompanying feelings of panic, palpitations or breathlessness), without a feeling of motion, are non-specific and may be caused by a wide variety of systemic disturbances (usually hypotension, panic or overbreathing). Precipitating factors and premonitory symptoms may be of diagnostic value, as also may be the mode of onset (whether sudden or gradual), the duration, and the presence of any associated symptoms such as deafness, tinnitus and ear pain or fullness. Indeed, it is not so much the character of the vertigo that helps to localize the disorder as the associated features of the attacks. For example, vertigo accompanied by features of brainstem dysfunction such as diplopia and face and limb sensory disturbance, with normal hearing, points to a central cause; whereas vertigo triggered by sudden movements and positional

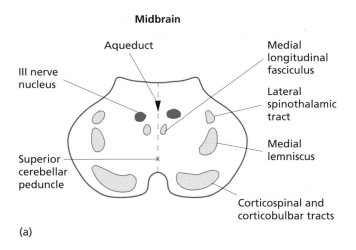

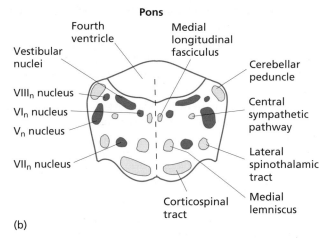

Fig. 3.33 Diagrammatic representation of the main anatomical structures within the brainstem: (a) midbrain; (b) pons; (c) medulla.

changes and associated with auditory or ear symptoms points to a peripheral cause.[53]

Unsteadiness is a fairly common symptom in stroke/ TIA patients, but unless it is associated with clearly focal symptoms or residual neurological signs of weakness or ataxia, it can be difficult to decide whether the patient means weakness, incoordination, vertigo, presyncope or anxiety, or indeed a combination of these. Sometimes it is helpful to ask patients whether they felt unsteady in the head or in the legs, or whether it was a visual problem. Patients often complain of being unsteady when they have rotational vertigo, but it is useful to ask quite specifically if there was persisting unsteadiness *after* the vertigo had stopped – a positive response suggesting a central rather than a peripheral problem.

The most common manifestation of cerebrovascular disease involving the cerebellum or its connections is truncal ataxia. Signs in the limbs are traditionally considered to need involvement of the ipsilateral cerebellar hemisphere rather than the midline structures, and thus there are often no cerebellar signs when the limbs are examined on the bed. Consequently, the problem may be overlooked if the patient's gait is not examined. If the disorder is mild, asking the patient to turn round quickly may be the most sensitive way of detecting an abnormality. It is also worth asking about the impact of loss of visual fixation, e.g. in the dark, in a shower, or performing Romberg's test. Most ataxic syndromes are somewhat worse when visual fixation is lost, but a marked loss of balance should make one think of disordered proprioception (i.e. sensory ataxia).

> Cerebellar disorders may be missed if the patient's gait is not examined.

Care must be taken when faced with a resolving hemiparesis, since at this time cerebellar-like signs can be elicited that are probably just a manifestation of impaired corticospinal control. This is most relevant when trying to distinguish the lacunar syndromes of pure motor stroke and ataxic hemiparesis from each other (section 4.3.2).

Clinical practice

Many patients complain of 'dizziness', either around the onset of a stroke or at other times, but this term alone is too imprecise to be of localizing value, even between carotid and vertebrobasilar territories, although it is probably more frequent in the latter. Other sensory experiences, such as giddiness, light-headedness, swimminess, or a feeling of passing out may be caused by diffuse cerebral ischaemia due to postural hypotension, vasoactive medication, cardiac dysrhythmias (all common in the elderly), and also with anxiety states, panic attacks and hyperventilation. These symptoms are of no localizing value and should not be considered to be indicative of a stroke/TIA.

The tendency to label any episode of 'dizziness', especially in the elderly, as vertebrobasilar ischaemia or – worse – insufficiency, should be strongly resisted.[53] All too frequently one sees patients who have complained of 'dizziness' when turning their neck, have then had a cervical spine X-ray that shows some degenerative changes (extremely common in the elderly population), and are then told that they are 'trapping the blood supply to the brain'. What little work there is to support this theory is mainly based on postmortem studies or dynamic arteriography in highly selected patients (section 7.1.5). Furthermore, many of the patients initially described under this banner had clear focal disturbances of brainstem and occipital lobe function. There is thought to be a considerable proprioceptive input from structures in and around the cervical spine to the vestibular system, and therefore for the vast majority of patients with these non-focal symptoms, the terms simply engender undue anxiety about impending strokes and divert attention from more likely and potentially treatable explanations of their dizziness.

When vertigo is an isolated phenomenon, and particularly when it is induced by head movement, severe, and short-lived, it is almost always a symptom of peripheral rather than central dysfunction. The relatively common condition of benign paroxysmal positional vertigo is described in section 3.4.7. Rarely, and most commonly in patients with diabetes, occlusion of a branch of the anterior cerebellar artery or the basilar artery supplying the inner ear can cause vertigo, unilateral hearing loss or both.[83] Some cerebellar strokes and lesions of more central vestibulocerebellar pathways may also mimic 'peripheral' symptoms. Multidirectional nystagmus that is not suppressed by visual fixation, an inability to stand without support and a negative 'head impulse test' in a patient with a first-ever attack of acute, spontaneous vertigo points to a central rather than a peripheral process.[81,82] The head impulse test is a simple clinical test comprising high acceleration head rotation;[84] with severe unilateral vestibular weakness the normal vestibuloocular reflex is replaced by a misalignment of the eyes followed by a series of corrective saccades which are evident to the examiner.[84]

Sudden hearing loss may be caused by trauma, tympanic membrane rupture, viral and other infections, toxic and metabolic disorders, and ischaemia.[85] How often sudden unilateral hearing loss in isolation (without vertigo or other brainstem dysfunction) is due to vascular disease is unknown, however, because histopathological examination of the temporal bone and labyrinth at postmortem is not performed routinely and, if it is, it is usually carried out so long after the onset of any hearing loss that the clinical details are unclear. Nevertheless, there is some histopathological evidence of labyrinthine infarction due to vascular disease. Even greater uncertainty prevails as to whether transient deafness in isolation is ever due to a TIA in the internal auditory artery territory, but we do not see why this should not sometimes be the case.

Acute cerebellar syndromes that can mimic strokes may be caused by drug toxicity, Wernicke's encephalopathy and Creutzfeldt–Jakob disease (sections 3.4.5 and 3.4.6).

3.3.8 The speed of onset of the symptoms and temporal course

Patients with a TIA or stroke usually describe their neurological symptoms as coming on abruptly, without warning, and as being more or less maximal at onset. However, patients are often frightened by their symptoms and are probably not very accurate about the exact time (seconds vs minutes) they take to develop. If several parts of the body (e.g. face, arm and leg) are affected, the symptoms usually start in each part almost simultaneously rather than intensifying or spreading ('marching') from one part to another – a pattern more typical of focal epilepsy[52] or a migrainous aura.[86] However, the simultaneous onset of a disturbance of several body parts may not be recognized, and the event misinterpreted as 'spread'. For example, a patient who is playing the piano at the time of a stroke will notice weakness of the hand but not weakness of the leg until he or she tries to stand up, or dysphasia until they try to speak.

> Because it is the suddenness of onset that stamps the event as vascular, it is useful to ask patients what they were doing at the time; if they were awake and do not remember, the onset was probably not all that sudden.

Less commonly, other patterns are encountered: the symptoms may evolve steadily over minutes or hours, they may develop in a stuttering/stepwise fashion over several hours, and occasionally they may continue to increase over a few days. In the last case, it can be virtually impossible to decide whether this is due to the primary condition continuing to evolve, or to other factors such as the development of cerebral oedema, infection, or metabolic upset. Not surprisingly, there is no agreed definition of the widely used term 'stroke-in-progression' (section 11.5).[87,88] Of course, in the face of a progressing deficit, it may not be possible to be absolutely certain whether the diagnosis is actually that of stroke/TIA at all, and the degree of diagnostic uncertainty will influence the extent of the investigations needed to firm up the clinical diagnosis.

3.3.9 Possible precipitants

In addition to giving an impression of the suddenness of onset of the symptoms, asking the patients (or witnesses) what they were doing at the time of symptom onset can also support a diagnosis of a vascular event.

- Vigorous physical activity and coitus have been associated with haemorrhagic stroke, particularly subarachnoid haemorrhage. However, apart from isolated case reports, there is no evidence that such activities precipitate TIAs and ischaemic stroke.
- A change in posture, neck turning (section 7.1.5), exposure to bright or white light, bending, straining, or sneezing, exercise, a hot bath, or a heavy meal, may provoke cerebral and ocular ischaemic symptoms in people with severe carotid and vertebrobasilar occlusive disease and a compromised collateral cerebral and ocular circulation. Of course, some of these stimuli may also provoke non-vascular symptoms, such as those due to hypoglycaemia (after a large carbohydrate meal) and seizures (after exposure to bright flashing lights).
- Certain circumstances may predispose to arterial dissection, such as neck manipulation, road traffic accidents and head injuries. There can often be a delay of days or weeks between the trauma and the first neurological symptoms (sections 7.2.1 and 8.2.13).
- Drug abuse is increasingly common, it is not confined to the very youngest age groups (section 7.15), and one should therefore have a relatively low threshold for specific questioning and toxicology screening.
- Symptoms beginning shortly after starting or increasing the dose of hypotensive drugs should raise the possibility of a so-called 'low-flow' stroke/TIA due to the combination of systemic hypotension, focal arterial stenosis/occlusion/compression and poor collateral circulation (section 6.7.5). A similar argument might also apply to symptoms present on waking from a general anaesthetic, although other factors such as intravascular thrombosis may be present, particularly if the symptoms are referable to the posterior circulation. Obviously, patients undergoing cardiac or carotid surgery are at special risk, and this should be explained to them prior to surgery (section 7.18).
- Pregnancy and the puerperium are times when otherwise healthy young women may be predisposed to stroke as a result of paradoxical embolism from the venous system of the legs or pelvis, intracranial haemorrhage due to eclampsia, or intracranial venous sinus thrombosis (section 7.14).
- There is a complex relationship between migraine and cerebrovascular disease, and this is discussed in detail in sections 3.4.1 and 7.8.
- There is some evidence that significant 'life events' in the preceding year may increase the risk of a stroke (section 6.6.18).

3.3.10 Accompanying symptoms

Any accompanying symptoms may be useful in sorting out whether the pathogenesis is vascular.

Headache

Headache occurs in about one-sixth of patients at the onset of a transient ischaemic attack of the brain or eye, about one-quarter of patients with acute ischaemic stroke, about one-half of patients with non-traumatic intracerebral haemorrhage, and nearly all patients with subarachnoid haemorrhage.[89–93]

Cortical ischaemia causes headache more often than small, deep, lacunar infarcts (section 6.7.6).[89,91,93] Given that ischaemic strokes are four times as common as haemorrhagic strokes, the predictive value of headache for the presence of haemorrhagic stroke is about 33%, while the predictive value of 'no headache' for ischaemic stroke is about 86%. The cause of the headache associated with ischaemic events is unknown. It has been suggested that it is due to the release of vasoactive substances such as serotonin and prostaglandins from activated platelets during cerebral ischaemia. Other possibilities include distortion or dilatation of collateral blood vessels, and mechanical stimulation of intracranial nociceptive afferents. Very occasionally, external carotid artery territory emboli can result in ischaemia of the scalp, and so pain. And, some headaches are probably due to anxiety and muscle tension.

Headache may not only be a consequence of the vascular event, but also a marker of the underlying cause of the event. Headache in anyone over the age of 50 or so presenting with ischaemia of the brain or eye demands immediate consideration of giant-cell arteritis (section 7.3.1). Similarly, severe pain on one side of the head, face, eye or neck before or around the time of onset is highly suggestive of carotid or vertebral arterial dissection,[94] and may even be the only symptom of carotid dissection[95] (section 7.2.1). Other causes of headache with focal neurological signs include carotidynia (secondary to carotid occlusion), migrainous stroke, meningitis and intracranial venous thrombosis, but usually there are other clues to these diagnoses.[96]

Epileptic seizures

About 2% of stroke patients have an epileptic seizure (sections 3.4.2, 6.7.6 and 11.8) at the onset; about half are generalized and half are partial seizures.[97] These are more common with intracerebral or subarachnoid haemorrhage than with arterial ischaemic stroke.[97] They are, however, a characteristic feature of intracranial venous infarction (section 7.21).[3] Onset seizures probably indicate irritation or damage to the cerebral cortex by the stroke, and are associated with an increased risk of further seizures.

Epileptic seizures may not only complicate stroke but also be a marker of increased risk of stroke. Looking forward, from the time of diagnosis of epilepsy, older people (>60 years of age) diagnosed with new-onset idiopathic epilepsy have an almost three-fold risk of subsequent stroke compared with others of the same age with no history of seizures.[98] Looking back, since the time of diagnosis of stroke, about 3% of patients with acute stroke have a past history of epileptic seizures, one-third of these occurring for the first time in the previous year.[97] Older people (>60 years of age) diagnosed with new-onset idiopathic epilepsy should therefore be screened for risk factors for stroke and treated appropriately.

Vomiting

Vomiting is very rare during TIA and is uncommon even in patients with stroke, at least near the onset. When it does occur, it suggests subarachnoid haemorrhage (see section 3.7.1), posterior fossa stroke (because of vertigo in some cases, and presumably because of direct involvement of the 'vomiting centre' in the area postrema in the floor of the fourth ventricle in others), or large supratentorial stroke causing raised intracranial pressure. Vomiting within 2 h of stroke onset is highly predictive of intracranial haemorrhage. Occasionally, patients with brainstem ischaemia can have profuse vomiting with little or no vertigo and few other clinical signs.

Neck stiffness

Meningism means painful resistance to passive or voluntary neck flexion because of irritation of the cervical meninges by subarachnoid blood, or by inflammation. Neck stiffness caused by meningism is a common symptom and sign of blood in the subarachnoid space, but it does not occur immediately; it takes some 3–12 h, and may not develop at all in deeply unconscious patients, or in patients with minor SAH (section 3.7.1).

Photophobia

Patients are often photophobic and irritable for several days after SAH, presumably as a result of meningeal irritation by the blood (section 3.7.1).

Hiccups and abdominal pain

Hiccups are brief bursts of intense inspiratory activity, involving the diaphragm and inspiratory intercostal muscles, with reciprocal inhibition of the expiratory intercostal muscles. Glottic closure occurs almost immediately after the onset of diaphragmatic contraction, generating the characteristic sound and sense of discomfort. Hiccups usually resolve spontaneously after a few minutes. If they persist for days, they may indicate underlying structural or functional disturbances of the medulla (in the region of the vagal nuclei and tractus solitarius), or of afferent or efferent nerves to the respiratory muscles, or diaphragmatic irritation. Hiccups are well recognized in patients with lateral medullary infarction, but may also occur with a lesion of any part of the medullary region that is associated with respiratory control. Neurogenic hiccup rarely occurs in isolation; usually there are associated brainstem or long tract signs (section 11.10).

If patients who have presented with a stroke also complain of abdominal pain, they may have ischaemia of the bowel or viscera – particularly if there are pointers to cardiogenic embolism being the underlying cause of the stroke (such as atrial fibrillation).

Chest pain, palpitations and shortness of breath

Chest pain and/or palpitations at the time of onset of the stroke/TIA suggest the possible coexistence of an acute coronary syndrome (due, among other things to simultaneous inflammation and rupture of cerebral and coronary atheromatous plaque) and cardiac dysrhythmias (as a consequence of cardiac ischaemia and as a possible source of embolism to the brain) (section 6.5). Other relevant causes of chest pain and/or shortness of breath include aortic dissection, pulmonary embolism and pneumonia.

Panic and anxiety

Sudden loss of limb power, speech or vision is a frightening experience which often evokes considerable anxiety and panic in patients and carers. Patients may consequently hyperventilate and in turn develop presyncopal or sensory symptoms including perioral and distal limb paraesthesia bilaterally, and even unilateral sensory symptoms. Under these circumstances, it is important to try to distinguish between the primary (stroke/TIA) and secondary (panic/anxiety) symptoms. It is also important to be clear about the timing of the symptoms; for example, palpitations occurring immediately before or concurrently with stroke/TIA are less likely to be a consequence of panic and anxiety than similar symptoms that clearly follow the onset of the neurological symptoms.

3.3.11 Past medical history

It is important to ask more than once about previous neurological symptoms. Many patients have told us several days after their transient ischaemic attack (TIA) or stroke about prior TIAs, having not recalled them for a number of reasons at the time of their first consultation. Sometimes this is because of anxiety, and of course a few patients are affected by altered awareness or amnesia during the event. Others may not wish to disclose such information for fear of potential repercussions for their employment or driving status. It is the doctor's responsibility to explore these possibilities with insight, sensitivity and confidentiality, using all available sources of information. Sometimes a detailed history of previous episodes helps confirm an alternative diagnosis such as focal epilepsy or migraine, while a detailed drug history may identify previous use of aspirin, or warfarin given after an otherwise forgotten event. We would recommend working through a checklist of focal neurological symptoms such as those in Table 3.20.

It is also important to ask specifically about:
- common vascular risk factors (e.g. hypertension, hyperlipidaemia, diabetes, smoking);
- other manifestations of vascular disease (e.g. angina, intermittent claudication of the legs);
- heart disease (e.g. valvular heart disease or cardiomyopathy – many lay people think a stroke is a form of heart attack);
- pointers to a thrombotic tendency (e.g. prior unexplained deep venous thrombosis);

Table 3.20 Checklist of symptoms of cerebrovascular disease.

Have you ever been told that you have had a stroke, ministroke, transient ischaemic attack or brain attack? If so, when did this occur and can you describe what happened?
Have you ever suddenly:
  Lost vision or gone blind in one eye?
  Had double vision for more than a few seconds?
  Had jumbled speech, slurred speech or difficulty in talking?
  Had weakness or loss of feeling in the face, arm or leg?
  Had clumsiness of an arm or leg?
  Had unsteadiness walking?
  Had a spinning (dizzy) sensation?
  Lost consciousness?
How long did the symptoms last?
Do you still have these symptoms?
Did you see a doctor about the episode and, if so, who was it and what were you told, and were you admitted to hospital?
What medications/drugs/tablets are you taking?
  (particularly aspirin, clopidogrel, dipyridamole, warfarin)

- and clues to vasculitis (e.g. arthralgia, skin rashes, renal problems (sections 6.7.6, 6.7.7 and 7.3).

3.3.12 Lifestyle, behaviour and family history

Relevant and potentially modifiable lifestyle factors include tobacco, alcohol, saturated fat, salt, recreational drug consumption and physical activity. A family history of stroke or myocardial infarction is a risk factor for ischaemic stroke, which is attributable, at least partly, to a familial predisposition to hypertension (section 6.6.3).[99,100]

3.4 Differential diagnosis of focal cerebral symptoms of sudden onset

There is a wide differential diagnosis of focal cerebral symptoms of rapid onset of short duration (Table 3.21) and long duration (Table 3.23). Tables 3.22 and 3.24 show the frequency of these possibilities in practice.

Because there is a continuum of the duration of neurological symptoms caused by focal neurological ischaemia,[7] patients who are being assessed within 24 hours of symptom onset and who still have focal neurological symptoms are temporarily classified as having a 'brain attack' ('acute stroke syndrome' or 'unstable brain ischaemia'; section 3.2.3). Another way of considering

Table 3.21 Differential diagnosis of transient ischaemic attack (in approximate order of frequency, depending on referral patterns).

Syncope
Migraine aura (with or without headache)
Labyrinthine disorders
Partial (focal) epileptic seizures
Hyperventilation, anxiety or panic attacks, somatization
    disorder
Intracranial structural lesion:
    meningioma
    tumour
    giant aneurysm
    arteriovenous malformation
    chronic subdural haematoma
Transient global amnesia
Acute demyelination (multiple sclerosis)
Drop attacks
Metabolic disorders: hypoglycaemia, hyperglycaemia,
    hypercalcaemia, hyponatraemia
Mononeuropathy/radiculopathy
Myasthenia gravis
Cataplexy

Table 3.22 Final diagnosis of all 512 patients with suspected transient ischaemic attacks notified to the Oxfordshire Community Stroke Project, modified from reference 6.

Confirmed transient ischaemic attacks:	209
Incident (i.e. first-ever)	184
Prevalent (i.e. had previous attacks)	11
Lone bilateral blindness*	14
Not transient ischaemic attacks:	303
Migraine	52
Syncope	48
Possible TIA†	46
'Funny turn'‡	45
Isolated vertigo	33
Epilepsy	29
Transient global amnesia	17
Isolated diplopia	4
Drop attack	3
Intracranial meningioma	2
Miscellaneous	24

*Lone bilateral blindness was later classified as a transient ischaemic attack after following up these patients and noting their similar prognosis to patients with definite transient ischaemic attack.[48]
†Possible transient ischaemic attack was diagnosed in patients with transient focal neurological symptoms in whom the clinical features were not sufficiently clear to make a diagnosis of definite transient ischaemic attack or of anything else.
‡'Funny turn' was used to describe transient episodes of only non-focal symptoms not due to any identifiable condition (e.g. isolated and transient confusion).

Table 3.23 Differential diagnosis of stroke (in approximate order of frequency, depending on referral patterns).

Systemic illness, or seizure, causing apparent deterioration
    of previous stroke
Epileptic seizure (postictal Todd's paresis) or non-convulsive
    seizures
Structural intracranial lesion:
    subdural haematoma
    brain tumour
    arteriovenous malformation
Metabolic/toxic encephalopathy:
    hypoglycaemia
    non-ketotic hyperglycaemia
    hyponatraemia
    Wernicke–Korsakoff syndrome
    hepatic encephalopathy
    alcohol and drug intoxication
    septicaemia
Functional/non-neurological (e.g. hysteria)
Hemiplegic migraine
Encephalitis (e.g. herpes simplex virus)/brain abscess
Head injury
Peripheral nerve lesion(s)
Hypertensive encephalopathy
Multiple sclerosis
Creutzfeldt–Jakob disease
Wilson's disease

the differential diagnoses according to duration of symptoms is outlined in Table 3.25.

> The top five differential diagnoses of brain attack (TIA and stroke) are the '5 Ss': seizures, syncope, sepsis, subdural haematoma and somatization.

The clinical diagnosis of stroke (differentiating 'stroke' from 'not stroke') is accurate more than 95% of the time if there is a clear history (from the patient or carer) of focal brain dysfunction of sudden onset (or first noticed on waking), with symptoms persisting for more than 24 h. This is particularly true if the patient is elderly or has other vascular diseases or risk factors, because the risk – i.e. the prior (or pretest) probability of stroke – is greater in elderly people with vascular disease than in younger people who have no evidence of vascular disease. However, the accuracy of the diagnosis of stroke is also influenced by the timing of the assessment, the experience and confidence of the examiner, and the likelihood of other differential diagnoses in the community[37,41,101–103] (Table 3.24). For example, the diagnosis of stroke (vs not stroke) can be quite difficult within the first few hours of symptom onset if it is not possible to obtain a clear history of the onset, or even the nature of the symptoms, because the patient is unconscious, confused, forgetful or dysphasic. In these patients in

Table 3.24 Final diagnosis in two recent studies of patients presenting with suspected TIA and stroke.[44,45]

Stroke 'mimic'	Nor et al.,[45] (n = 59)	Hand et al.,[44] (n = 109)
Seizure	8 (14%)	23 (21%)
Sepsis	8 (14%)	14 (13%)
Metabolic/toxic encephalopathy		12 (11%)
Space-occupying brain lesion	7 (12%)	10 (9%)
Tumour	4 (7%)	
Subdural haematoma	3 (5%)	
Syncope/presyncope	13 (22%)	10 (9%)
Acute confusional state		7 (6%)
Vestibular dysfunction (labyrinthitis)	3 (5%)	7 (6%)
Acute mononeuropathy		6 (5%)
Functional/somatization	7 (12%)	6 (5%)
Dementia		4 (4%)
Migraine		3 (3%)
Spinal cord lesion		3 (3%)
Other	13 (22%)	3 (3%)

particular, a persistent focal neurological deficit may not be due to stroke but to epileptic seizures (postictal), sepsis, encephalitis, brain abscess, brain tumour, head trauma, or a chronic subdural haematoma.[102]

Symptoms or signs that are unusual in uncomplicated stroke, such as papilloedema and unexplained fever, should also call into question the diagnosis. Further, a persistent focal neurological deficit may be due to a previous stroke, and the new clinical presentation may be caused by a non-vascular problem such as pneumonia (section 11.12). In the absence of information about the rate of onset and progression of symptoms, it is helpful to search for indirect clues to their cause in the past history and physical examination, and to continue to assess the patient over time for the development of new signs such as fever, and for the improvement that characterizes most non-fatal strokes.

> The diagnosis of a cerebrovascular event is usually made at the bedside, not in the laboratory or in the radiology department. It depends on the history of the sudden onset of focal neurological symptoms in the appropriate clinical setting (usually an older patient with vascular risk factors) and the exclusion of other conditions that can present in a similar way.

3.4.1 Migraine

Transient ischaemic attack

Migraines are not considered to be TIAs, because the clinical features (Table 3.26) and prognosis for serious vascular events are very different.[104] Classical migraine (migraine with aura) usually starts in younger patients who may have a family history of migraine. The attack begins with an aura that commonly consists of positive symptoms of focal cerebral dysfunction that develop gradually over 5–20 min and last less than 60 min.[86,105] The most common aura consists of homonymous, unilateral or central visual symptoms, such as flashes of light, zigzag lines, crescents, scintillations, or fortification spectra, which gradually 'build up', expand and migrate across the visual field. Somatosensory or motor disturbances, such as paraesthesiae or heaviness in one or more limbs, may also occur, evolving and spreading over a period of minutes in a 'marching' fashion (e.g. spread of tingling from hand to arm to face to tongue over several minutes). This serial progression from one accompaniment to another without delay, such as from visual symptoms to paraesthesiae and then to aphasia, is quite characteristic of migraine but can occur with cerebral ischaemia.[106] Sometimes, however, the symptoms are negative and consist of 'blind patches' (often a homonymous hemianopia) and, rarely, even loss of colour vision. Headache and nausea usually follow the focal neurological symptoms immediately or in less than an hour, but in some patients they precede the neurological symptoms and in others they occur simultaneously. Often there is associated photophobia and phonophobia, which clearly help distinguish migraine attacks from TIAs. The headache usually lasts 4–72 h.[86]

It is not unusual for patients who have experienced classical migraine to suffer identical auras, but without headache (acephalgic migraine aura), particularly as they get older (otherwise referred to as 'migraine aura without headache' or 'late-life migraine accompaniments').[107] This should not cause confusion with TIA. However, diagnostic difficulty arises when an older patient (over 40 years) with no previous history of classical migraine presents following a first-ever episode of transient symptoms of focal neurological dysfunction that are typical of a migraine aura, but without any associated headache.

Table 3.25 Differential diagnosis of sudden focal neurological symptoms by duration of symptoms.

	Transient ischaemic attack	Brain attack	Stroke
Migraine	+++	++	+
Epilepsy			
Partial seizures	+++	++	+
Todd's paresis	+++	++	+
Transient global amnesia	+++	++	–
Structural intracranial lesions			
Subdural haematoma	++	++	++
Tumour	+	++	++
Arteriovenous malformation/aneurysm	++	++	+
Metabolic/toxic disorders			
Hypoglycaemia	+++	++	+
Hyperglycaemia	+++	++	+
Hyponatraemia	++	++	+
Hypercalcaemia	++	++	+
Hepatic encephalopathy	+	++	++
Wernicke's encephalopathy	+	++	++
Hypertensive encephalopathy	+	++	++
Posterior reversible encephalopathy syndrome	+	++	++
CNS infections			
Encephalitis	+	++	++
Brain abscess	+	++	++
Subdural empyema	+	++	++
Creutzfeldt–Jakob disease	–	–	+
Progressive multifocal leukoencephalopathy	–	–	+
Labyrinthine disorders			
Vestibular neuronitis	+	++	++
Ménière's disease	++	–	–
Benign paroxysmal positional vertigo	++	–	–
Benign recurrent vertigo	++	+	–
Psychological disorders			
Hyperventilation	+++	–	
Panic attacks	+++	–	–
Somatization/conversion disorder	+++	++	++
Head injury	+	+	++
Multiple sclerosis	+	+	++
Neuromuscular disorders			
Mononeuropathy	++	++	++
Radiculopathy	++	++	++
Myasthenia gravis	++	++	+
Motor neurone disease	–	–	+

+++ Common or frequent; ++ encountered regularly in a busy practice or important, treatable condition; + infrequent; – rare.

Patients with these 'late-life migraine accompaniments' have a favourable prognosis with a lower risk of stroke and other serious vascular events compared with TIA patients.[104]

A 69-year-old former general practitioner was referred by a cardiologist for suspected ocular TIAs, a diagnosis that caused him some alarm. He had unexpectedly suffered a myocardial infarction at the age of 59, and had been receiving beta-blockers and aspirin since then. The attacks in question, of which he had now had nine, had first occurred more than 2 years previously, but had increased in frequency. Each attack began with a small, bright spot on the left or right side of the centre of vision. He verified that it occurred in both eyes by covering each eye in turn. In the course of 1–3 min, the bright spot would gradually enlarge and change

Table 3.26 Features of migraine aura that help distinguish it from TIA.

Gradual onset over minutes (usually)

Positive neurological symptoms such as visual scintillations, not blindness

Intensification and 'spread' of symptoms from point to point, or from one symptom to another symptom, over minutes

Gradual resolution of symptoms over 20–60 min

Headache (often unilateral and pulsatile) and nausea usually follow (but not always)

Onset in young and middle-aged adults

Family history of migraine is common

Recurrent attacks are usually stereotyped

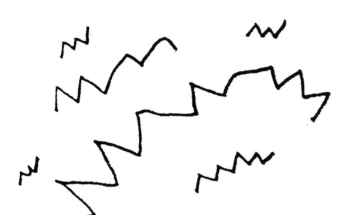

Fig. 3.34 A drawing by a physician who experienced 'late-life migraine accompaniments'. He wrote the following caption: 'These zigzag lines appear during an attack in both eyes, more often to the left than to the right of centre of vision, sometimes on both sides. The lines flicker on and off, about six times per second; they are colourless. Sometimes a dazzling white spot will appear within a line, which also turns on and off.'

into a cloudy area, until the centre of vision became obscured; the border of the opaque zone consisted of intensely bright and flickering shapes: zigzag lines, stars and sparks (Fig. 3.34). This phenomenon would remain for about 15 min; if he tried to read, he could not make out the words in the centre. Finally, the visual disturbance would disappear over a few minutes. He never had headache or other symptoms with the attacks, and was able to resume his normal activities afterwards. He could not recall that he had suffered similar attacks, or migraine, earlier in his life. This was migraine, not TIA.

A detailed history eliciting the slow onset, and spread and intensification of neurological symptoms – particularly if positive and visual or referable to more than one vascular territory during the same attack – points towards the diagnosis of migraine.[86,104] Careful questioning about childhood or menstruation-related headaches, and a family history of migraine, may suggest a predisposition to migraine. If the patient is young (i.e. less than about 40 years old), with a normal heart and no other clinical manifestations of arterial disease, it is most unlikely that the symptoms are those of a TIA caused by atherothrombosis. Perhaps this explains why young female patients with suspected TIA, with or without a family history of migraine, do not seem to have any higher risk of stroke than other women of the same age. In this group, there is a remote possibility of thrombophilic and vasculitic disorders but, for the most part, these patients can be reassured that they have not 'had a stroke'. Because the risks of stroke are very low in absolute terms in people with migraine, they do not require any potentially hazardous or costly investigations or prophylactic treatments[108,109] (section 7.8).

There is no convincing evidence that arteriovenous malformations or aneurysms occur more frequently than can be accounted for by chance in patients with migraine aura. There can, however, be particular concern about migraine occurring for the first time during pregnancy, because of the recognized propensity for meningiomas and possibly arteriovenous malformations to become symptomatic at this time.[110] In this group of patients, we would suggest careful clinical examination looking for residual focal signs following a single attack, and a low threshold for MR scanning after the baby has been born if the attacks are multiple and stereotyped, particularly if the same side of the brain is always involved.

In older patients, particularly those with their first attack of acephalgic migraine and if the neurological symptoms are other than positive visual ones, the distinction from TIAs can be much more difficult. From a purely pragmatic point of view, if there is a suspicion that the attack was a TIA, it seems prudent to modify any vascular risk factors and recommend aspirin. Although drugs used to lower blood pressure and cholesterol, and antiplatelet drugs such as aspirin, are not free of risk or expense, some of them (e.g. propranolol and aspirin) may also prevent migraines.

Stroke

Occasionally, the aura of a previously experienced and otherwise unremarkable attack of migraine persists for days or longer – a so-called migrainous stroke (section 7.8.1). The simultaneous occurrence of a stroke and a migraine attack may be:

- coincidental because, after all, both conditions are common, the prevalence of migraine in the general adult white population is about 10% and ischaemic cerebrovascular disease about 0.8%;

- causal, either migraine may predispose to cerebral ischaemia by leading to platelet activation, arteriolar constriction and dehydration, or cerebral ischaemia may trigger a migraine attack;
- a misdiagnosis (e.g. arterial dissection may cause headache and a neurological deficit due to thromboembolism that is misinterpreted as migraine); or
- both are a manifestation of a disorder such as a patent foramen ovale, an arteriovenous malformation, or a mitochondrial disorder[111-113] (sections 6.5.12, 7.19 and 8.2.4).

The 69-year-old wife of a general practitioner had suffered from classical migraine since she was a teenager. Her attacks always began with visual fortification spectra, progressing to a hemianopia (either left or right) over the next 10 min. The visual disturbance would resolve after about 30 min, and she would then get a severe throbbing headache, nausea and vomiting. She had always recognized bright light as a potential trigger factor. Because of a family history of glaucoma, an optician recommended that she have her visual fields tested using a Humphrey perimeter. She found the flashes of white light uncomfortable, and by the end of the examination she was aware that she had her typical migrainous visual disturbance in her right visual field. The headache was unusually severe and she went straight to bed. When she woke 6 h later, the headache had resolved but the right hemianopia was still present. A brain CT scan later that day showed a recent left occipital infarct. No other explanation for the stroke was found despite detailed investigation. The hemianopia persisted, and it was presumed that this had been a migrainous stroke.

3.4.2 Epilepsy

Transient ischaemic attack

Partial (focal) seizures can be distinguished from TIAs because they usually cause sudden positive sensory or motor symptoms that spread or 'march' fairly quickly to adjacent body parts (Table 3.27).[52] Although positive symptoms such as tingling and limb jerking can occur in TIAs,[76] they tend to arise in all affected body parts at the same time (i.e. in the face, arm and leg together), whereas the symptoms of partial seizures spread from one body part to another over a minute or so (cf. migraine aura, where any spread is usually over several minutes; section 3.4.1). Negative motor symptoms, such as postictal or Todd's paresis, are well recognized after a partial motor seizure or a generalized seizure with partial onset, but this should be obvious from the history unless

Table 3.27 Features of partial epileptic seizures that help distinguish them from TIAs.

Young and middle-aged adults commonly, but also patients with previous cortical stroke
Antecedent symptoms may occur (e.g. epigastric discomfort) which are the beginning of the seizure
Onset over several seconds or 1–2 min
Positive neurological symptoms usually
March or 'spread' of symptoms over seconds
Rapid resolution of symptoms over a few minutes
Amnesia for the event
Family history of epilepsy may be present
Recurrent attacks are usually stereotyped and reduced with antiepileptic treatment (if necessary)

the patient was asleep, or is aphasic and there is no witness (section 3.3.10).

Difficulty arises in the very rare patient in whom epileptic seizures actually cause transient 'negative' symptoms during the electrical discharge. One then has to rely on other factors, such as the patient's age, any past history of seizures and the nature of the symptoms. For example, transient speech arrest (as opposed to aphasia with muddled language output), which is characterized by the sudden onset of cessation of speech, often accompanied by aimless staring and subsequent amnesia for the details of the episode, is usually epileptic rather than ischaemic. Transient aphasia and rarely bilateral blindness or amnesia can also sometimes be epileptic.

Distinguishing between seizures and TIAs is occasionally very difficult.[76] Sometimes it requires prolonged and careful observation of, and interaction with, the patient (and witnesses) over several visits. The diagnosis should not be rushed, as patients may have several types of attack with different causes. Initially, it is important to explain the diagnostic uncertainty to the patient and why it is necessary to establish the precise diagnosis; to exclude a structural intracranial lesion (with brain imaging); and to advise the patient not to drive or put themselves in a position in which they would be a danger to themselves or others if they were to have another attack. Clues to the diagnosis of epilepsy can be obtained by taking a careful, targeted history, particularly with respect to previous epileptic seizures and any symptoms that immediately preceded the onset of the neurological deficit (e.g. epigastric discomfort and olfactory or gustatory hallucinations may be due to an initial partial sensory seizure involving the temporal or frontal lobes). The interictal electroencephalogram (EEG) can be normal but not usually in patients having several seizures a day. Ambulatory or telemetered EEG requires skilled and careful analysis because of the potential for a false positive diagnosis of epilepsy. Nevertheless, concomitant video recording of an attack can be very useful.

If recurrent partial seizures are suspected, brain MR should be performed to seek a focal structural lesion too small to be seen on CT, such as mesial temporal sclerosis, a hamartoma, or a tumour, usually in the frontal or temporal lobe. However, transient abnormalities that might be mistaken for areas of ischaemia on brain MR have been reported in patients with partial status epilepticus, although the abnormalities tend not to respect normal vascular distributions and to resolve with time.

A 64-year-old woman described about 20 attacks of pins and needles in her right arm and leg over a period of 6 weeks. Each attack lasted for about 5 min, and there were no associated symptoms. On closer interrogation, she said that the sensation started in the right foot and then over a period of about 1 min spread 'like water running up my leg' to involve the whole leg and arm. Each attack was identical. A brain CT scan showed a glioma in the left parietal lobe. A diagnosis of partial sensory seizures secondary to the glioma was made.

Stroke

An epileptic seizure is one of the most common reasons for the misdiagnosis of stroke.[41,44,45,103] The usual scenario is a patient with postictal confusion, stupor, coma or hemiparesis (Todd's paresis) where the preceding seizure was unwitnessed or unrecognized.[103] Todd's paresis refers to a focal deficit that may follow a focal motor seizure. In general, the deficit usually resolves very quickly (within minutes), but in patients with prior cerebral damage, e.g. an earlier stroke, the deficit can last for several days, or there may be permanent deterioration, making the distinction from a recurrent stroke very difficult.

It is noteworthy that involuntary convulsive-like movements sometimes occur in patients with brainstem strokes.[114] These movements vary in nature, frequency and triggers, including fasciculation-like, shivering, jerky, tonic-clonic and intermittent shaking movements. The episodes usually consist of brief clonic contractions of the proximal and distal upper extremities and occur in paroxysms lasting for 3–5 s.[114] Their pathogenesis is uncertain but may be related to ischaemia or haemorrhage in the corticospinal tracts. They should not be misinterpreted as decerebrate postures or seizures.

3.4.3 Transient global amnesia

Transient global amnesia (TGA) is not considered to be a TIA because its prognosis is so much better. It is a very characteristic clinical syndrome that typically occurs in a middle-aged or elderly person.[115] There is a sudden dis-

Table 3.28 Features of transient global amnesia that help distinguish it from TIAs.

Older adults
Sudden onset
Anterograde and retrograde memory disturbance
Repetitive questioning
Able to recognize familiar individuals and places with no loss of personal identity
Headache can occur
No focal neurological symptoms or signs
All but complete recovery within a few hours to a day or so, leaving a dense amnesic gap for the attack itself
Recurrent attacks are unusual, and if they occur may be due to migraine or partial seizures
Diagnosis is very difficult without a witness

order of memory, which is often reported as confusion.[116] For some hours, the patient cannot remember anything new (anterograde amnesia) and often cannot recall more distant events over the past weeks or years (retrograde amnesia). There is no loss of personal identity, personality, problem-solving, language or visuospatial function, and the patient can perform complex activities such as driving a car (Table 3.28). The patient seems healthy, but repetitively asks the same questions and has to be reminded continually of what he or she has just asked or done. There are no other symptoms, apart from perhaps headache (migraine is more common in TGA patients than in controls, and there are some theoretical reasons to implicate migraine in its pathogenesis).[117]

In women, episodes are mainly associated with an emotional precipitating event, a history of anxiety and a pathological personality. In men, they occur more frequently after a physical precipitating event, e.g. diving into a swimming pool.[115]

After the attack, anterograde memory returns to normal, but the patient cannot remember anything that happened during the amnesic period. The retrograde amnesia tends to diminish with recovery, but leaves a short retrograde gap for the period of the TGA. Recurrences are not very common, about 3% per year.

The early reports tended to view TGA as a type of TIA, and of course one does encounter patients with pure amnestic strokes (section 3.3.3). However, careful case–control studies have shown that both the prevalence of vascular risk factors and the rates of subsequent stroke or myocardial infarction are much lower in the TGA group and are indeed approximately similar to those in the age-matched general population.[115,118,119]

There is no overall difference in the prevalence of epilepsy between TGA patients and control groups, but an important minority (7%) of TGA patients go on to develop epilepsy, usually within a year of presentation. These patients tend to have had shorter attacks of 'TGA', lasting less than 1 h, and to have already experienced more than one attack at the time of presentation. It must be presumed that in this minority of cases with 'TGA', the cause was temporal lobe epileptic seizures from the beginning. Because of this, driving is generally allowed after a single episode of TGA but not after multiple attacks.

Functional imaging, such as perfusion CT, has shown transient bilateral hypoperfusion of the medial temporal lobes or basal ganglia, and unilateral left opercular and insular hypoperfusion, during the TGA attack.[120] However, it is not known whether this perfusion defect is a primary event or secondary to a reduction in cerebral metabolic activity in these areas, or due to other factors. Diffusion-weighted MRI during episodes of TGA shows transient signal abnormalities, consistent with oedema, in the uncal-hippocampal region unilaterally or bilaterally in a variable proportion of patients.[119,121,122] Ischaemia, due to arterial thromboemboli or venous stasis, has been proposed as a potential mechanism.[119,123,124] It has also been hypothesized that diverse stressful precipitants may trigger a release of an excitotoxic neurotransmitter (such as glutamate), which then temporarily shuts down normal memory function in the medial temporal regions via spreading depression, leading in turn to a fall in cerebral perfusion.

3.4.4 Structural intracranial lesions

Although structural intracranial lesions often cause focal brain dysfunction, the symptoms and signs generally progress over several days or weeks, or even months, they are not abrupt like strokes or TIAs. About 5–10% of patients who are initially diagnosed as having an acute stroke on the basis of the history and examination turn out to have a structural intracranial lesion on brain imaging, such as a subdural haematoma, tumour or arteriovenous malformation.[44,45] Possible explanations for transient neurological symptoms are listed in Table 3.29.

Non-traumatic intracerebral haemorrhage

Non-traumatic intracerebral haemorrhage almost invariably causes prolonged or permanent focal neurological dysfunction, although there are isolated reports of neurological deficits that have resolved within a few days, and even 24 h. However, one sometimes needs to probe quite hard to be sure about the duration of symptoms from the history. For example, 'I got better in 24 h' does not necessarily mean 'I got *completely* back to normal', which is what we are referring to when defining a TIA. Intracerebral haemorrhage can be misinterpreted as TIA, or

Table 3.29 Possible explanations for transient neurological symptoms in patients with a structural intracranial lesion.

Partial epileptic seizure
Spreading depression of Leao (as some suppose occurs in migraine)
Vascular 'steal', leading to focal brain ischaemia adjacent to the tumour
Vessel encasement or direct compression by the tumour mass
Indirect compression of vessels by herniating tissue or coning (usually a preterminal event)

ischaemic stroke, if CT brain imaging is not done early, and certainly within 10–14 days after the onset of symptoms by which time the characteristic changes will have resolved (section 5.4.1).[13] Fortunately, intracerebral haemorrhage is visible indefinitely on gradient echo MRI sequences as a low signal (black) ring or dot (section 5.5.1).

A 77-year-old man, whilst standing in his garden, suddenly developed weakness of the right arm and unsteadiness on walking. He had no headache or vomiting. He sat down and within 3 h was 'better', although on closer questioning it emerged that his arm had not returned to normal for about 3 days. A CT brain scan 8 days later showed a small resolving haemorrhage in the left putamen. This was not a TIA in either its duration or pathology.

Subdural haematoma

Transient focal neurological symptoms such as hemiparesis, hemisensory loss, aphasia and speech arrest may occur as a consequence of a chronic subdural haematoma (SDH)[125] (section 8.10). And SDH may rarely present with the abrupt onset of focal neurological signs, which then persist and so mimic a stroke.[45] Usually the patient has a confusional state and a history of minor neurological symptoms starting a few days to a few weeks previously. SDH should be suspected if there is any evidence of subacute onset of focal neurological symptoms and signs; persistent headache; more confusion and drowsiness than expected from the neurological deficit; or a progressive or fluctuating clinical course. Although SDH occurs in all age groups, it is more frequent among the elderly, alcoholics and patients receiving anticoagulants or who have a bleeding disorder. About 50% of patients recall sustaining a head injury, which may have been mild. SDH is a rare complication of lumbar puncture, and spontaneous or traumatic intracranial hypotension.

In the acute phase, the brain CT scan usually shows unilateral hyperdensity in the subdural space, ipsilateral effacement of sulci, and a mass effect causing shift of the midline and distortion of the ventricular system (Fig. 3.35). There is a transitional stage between 7 and 21 days, during which clotted blood evolves on the CT scan from a region of hyperintensity to one of isointensity. This can easily be missed, particularly if the subdural haematomas are bilateral, when there is little if any midline shift or asymmetrical ventricular compression. Thereafter, the haematoma becomes hypodense and thus more easily visible. MRI is more sensitive than CT for detecting subdural haematomas. In a few cases, a subdural haematoma may prove to be an incidental finding, and the TIA can be attributed to more commonly recognized factors such as carotid artery disease.

Tumour

Occasionally – perhaps if there is bleeding into a tumour – there can be a sudden focal neurological deficit caused by a brain tumour, although this usually lasts longer than 24 h.[126,127] Greater diagnostic difficulty arises when a structural lesion causes a partial and non-convulsive seizure, with or without postictal (Todd's) paresis, or intermittent focal neurological symptoms (so-called 'tumour attacks') that do not seem to be epileptic in origin.[44,45,49] The clinical features associated with these 'tumour attacks' are usually focal jerking or shaking, pure sensory phenomena, loss of consciousness and isolated aphasia or speech arrest.[126] With time, a more obvious epileptic syndrome often declares itself.

A 78-year-old woman complained of many attacks of weakness and clumsiness of the left arm over a period of 4 months. The weakness came on suddenly, lasted for between 10 and 45 min, and was not associated with any other symptoms. In between attacks, she had no symptoms. A diagnosis of transient ischaemic attack was made by both her general practitioner and the neurologist, and she was started on aspirin. A brain CT scan was performed later because the attacks continued, and this showed a meningioma involving the right frontal lobe (Fig. 3.36). A final diagnosis of 'tumour attacks' was made, but in view of the patient's age, the neurosurgeon thought an operation was not advisable.

Of course it is always important to consider intracranial tumours in the differential diagnosis of a patient with a progressing neurological deficit, particularly if the rate of progression is relatively slow (over days, weeks or months) and there is a history of recent headache or epileptic seizures, papilloedema, or any evidence of a primary extracranial source of malignancy. In practice, most patients with suspected stroke who turn out to have a cerebral tumour have actually had a focal neurological deficit (e.g. hemiparesis) gradually evolving over several weeks to several months.

> Papilloedema is very uncommon in acute stroke.

The brain tumours that tend to bleed are glioblastoma, choroid plexus papilloma, meningioma, neuroblastoma, melanoma, hypernephroma, lymphoma, endometrial carcincoma, bronchial carcinoma and choriocarcinoma (section 8.5.1). The CT scan may then disclose intracerebral haemorrhage in an unusual location or associated with considerable surrounding oedema, or multiple haemorrhages, or it may show other metastatic deposits (Fig. 3.37). If there has been no haemorrhage into the tumour, the CT scan usually shows a region of low attenuation (due to cerebral oedema) with imprecise boundaries and some mass effect, causing effacement of sulci or ventricular compression. If there is a breakdown of the blood–brain barrier, as commonly occurs in patients with cerebral tumours, then intravenous injection of iodinated contrast material leaks into the tumour and is seen on CT as an area of diffuse or peripheral enhancement (Fig. 3.38). A similar, but nevertheless distinctive, appearance of enhancement of the gyri, which may be seen within 1–2 weeks of a recent cerebral infarct, is also due to breakdown of the blood–brain barrier (Fig. 3.39). This can make interpretation difficult, particularly if only a contrast-enhanced scan is performed. If the clinical examination and CT are ambiguous, patients should be followed up clinically (because with a tumour they usually deteriorate), and a follow-up CT or MRI performed within a few weeks to a few months (depending on the patient's progress) to see if the lesion has resolved or, if it is a tumour, continued to grow.

Aneurysms and arteriovenous malformations

Intracranial aneurysms and cerebral arteriovenous malformations (sections 8.2.3, 8.2.4 and 9.1.1), and particularly cavernous malformations (section 8.2.5), can cause transient focal neurological deficits mimicking a TIA or ischaemic stroke, and even transient monocular blindness.[128,129] In the Scottish Intravascular Vascular Malformation Study, focal neurological deficits accounted for about 7% of presentations of symptomatic arteriovenous malformations (Rustam Al-Shahi Salman, personal communication). Possible explanations are embolization of thrombus from within an aneurysm (section 7.6), a partial seizure, a small intraparenchymal haemorrhage (e.g. from a cavernous malformation) and venous hypertension. Vascular steal around an arteriovenous malformation is not a certain mechanism. In many cavernoma cases it is impossible to identify the cause of some

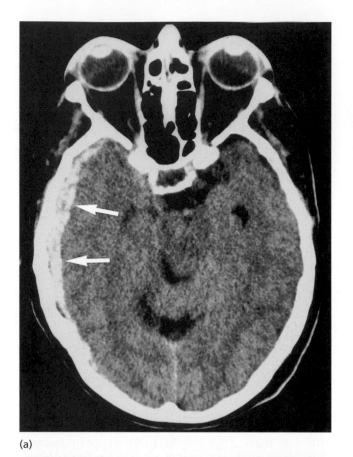

(a)

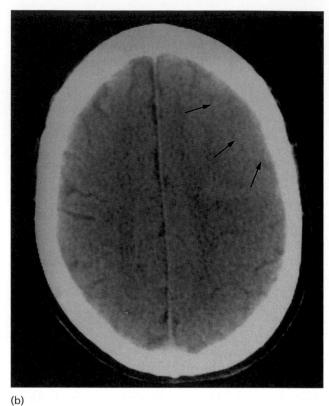

(b)

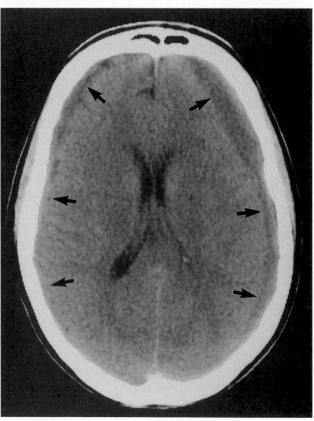

(c)

Fig. 3.35 (a) A plain CT brain scan showing *acute* right-sided subdural haematoma as an area of high density in the subural space (*arrows*). (b) A plain CT brain scan showing a *subacute* left frontal subdural haematoma (*arrows*) which is isodense, illustrating the difficulty of identifying subdural haematomas on CT at this stage of their evolution. (c) A plain CT brain scan showing *chronic* bilateral subdural haematomas as areas of low density in the subural space (*arrows*).

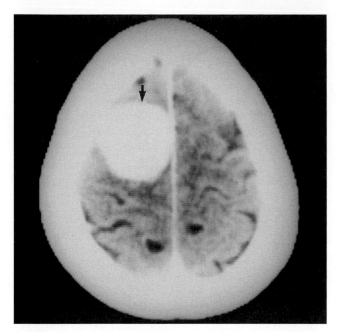

Fig. 3.36 A post-contrast CT brain scan showing a meningioma involving the posterior part of the right frontal lobe (*arrow*) in a patient who presented with a history suggesting transient ischaemic attacks; over 3 months, this elderly lady had eight attacks of sudden onset of weakness affecting the left arm, each lasting a few minutes. Between attacks the neurological examination was normal.

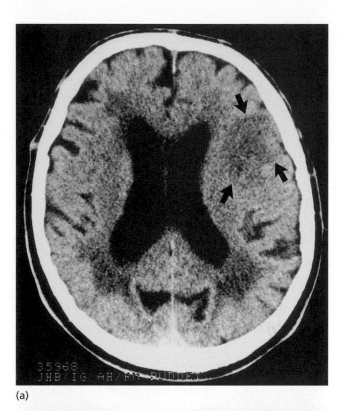

(a)

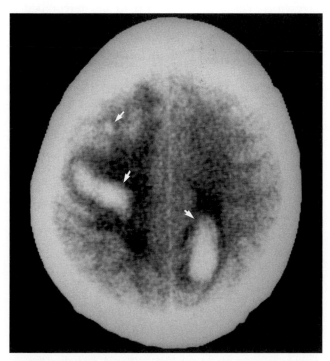

Fig. 3.37 A plain CT brain scan showing multiple areas of high density (*arrows*) due to spontaneous intracerebral haemorrhage in what turned out at postmortem to be metastases from choriocarcinoma.

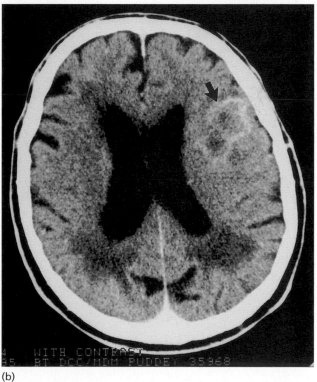

(b)

Fig. 3.38 A plain CT brain scan of a brain tumour showing (a) a region of low attenuation (due to cerebral oedema) with imprecise boundaries (arrows) and some mass effect, causing effacement of sulci. (b) After intravenous contrast injection there is enhancement (*arrow*) of the tumour.

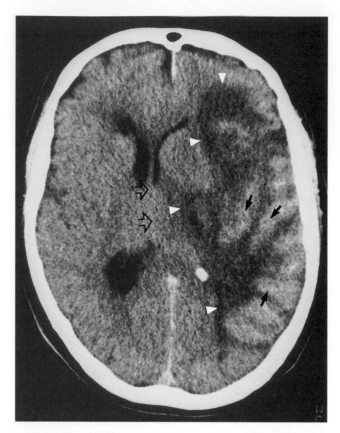

Fig. 3.39 A post-contrast CT brain scan 8 days after onset of ischaemic stroke showing a region of low attenuation consistent with infarction (*white arrowheads*) in the territory of the left middle cerebral artery, and a serpiginous gyral pattern of high attenuation due to breakdown of the blood–brain barrier (*black arrows*). There is considerable mass effect, with displacement of midline structures (*open arrows*), effacement of the lateral ventricle and obliteration of sulci.

transient focal neurological attacks which do not sound epileptic, and where early imaging shows no fresh blood or is done too late (or is not done at all in known cases); a psychogenic cause would not be surprising given the stress of knowing there is an intracranial lesion which might bleed.

Although aneurysms and arteriovenous malformations are one of the more common causes of intracerebral haemorrhage (sections 8.2.3 and 8.2.4), they may also cause focal neurological symptoms and signs as a direct consequence of their mass effect and compression of surrounding structures, e.g. a third cranial nerve palsy from a posterior communicating artery aneurysm.

Brain CT, with and without contrast, MRI or intraarterial cerebral angiography, may be required to make the diagnosis. Just occasionally, arteriovenous malformations can be suspected clinically, e.g. if there is cutaneous evidence of the Sturge–Weber syndrome or hereditary

haemorrhagic telangiectasia, a past history of subarachnoid haemorrhage, or, reputedly, a cranial bruit.[128]

3.4.5 Metabolic and toxic disorders

Encephalopathies due to metabolic or toxic disturbances generally present with epileptic seizures or a subacute alteration in consciousness, and few if any focal neurological signs (perhaps only generalized hyperreflexia, with or without extensor plantar responses). However, occasionally the presentation may be acute, with focal neurological symptoms and signs, which can therefore mimic a stroke or TIA.[44,45] The causes of the metabolic encephalopathy include hypoglycaemia, hyperglycaemia, hyponatraemia, hypercapnoea and hypoxia.

Hypoglycaemia

Hypoglycaemia may cause both transient and permanent focal neurological symptoms and signs, which can occur without any of the characteristic adrenergic symptoms[41,103,130,131] (section 7.16). The patient is almost always being treated with hypoglycaemic agents, but other possibilities include factitious hypoglycaemia, insulinoma, Addison's disease, hypopituitarism, hypothyroidism, sepsis, terminal malignancy, liver failure, starvation, or drugs whose adverse effects include hypoglycaemia. The symptoms tend to be stereotyped in an individual, and are most likely to occur before meals (i.e. before breakfast or during the night, after fasting for some time), after exercise, or 2–3 h after the ingestion of sugars and starch; they are relieved by glucose administration. The blood glucose is usually less than 2.5 mmol/L at the onset of an attack, but it may have normalized spontaneously or with glucose administration by the time the patient is seen. Particularly if a diabetic patient presents with a suspected stroke early in the morning, it is imperative that hypoglycaemia be considered and appropriate treatment given rapidly, although a blood glucose estimation should be mandatory for all patients with suspected stroke.

A 63-year-old man was admitted to a surgical ward because of abdominal pain, diarrhoea and signs of intestinal obstruction, 2 months after a partial gastrectomy for a gastric ulcer. He was treated with intravenous fluids and received nothing by mouth, whilst awaiting investigations. Five days after admission, he became restless and confused. Two hours later, left-sided weakness was noted. The neurology resident found a left hemiplegia and hypoaesthesia, including the face, with completely normal consciousness. The provisional diagnosis was ischaemic stroke, but the next morning the nurses found him unresponsive. On repeat examination, there was no eye opening to pain, extension of the arm was the best motor response, and there was no verbal response. The pupils were normal, but no oculocephalic responses could be elicited. The glucose level was 1.5 mmol/L. After administration of 100 mL of 50% glucose, he quickly recovered.

> The blood glucose concentration should be assessed in all patients with suspected stroke.

Hyperglycaemia

The hyperosmolarity of hyperglycaemia can itself cause regional reduction of cerebral blood flow, focal neurological deficits, focal epilepsy, stroke-like syndromes and cerebral infarction[132] (section 7.16). These deficits usually resolve as the blood glucose returns to normal.

Hyponatraemia

The most frequent neurological manifestation of hyponatraemia is reduced level of attention or consciousness. Long tract signs (6%), tremor (1%), hallucinations (0.5%), myoclonus and seizures (3%) may also occur. The reason for the appearance of focal symptoms, such as long tract signs, is unclear. The deficits usually respond to correction of the hyponatraemia, but this should be done cautiously to minimize the risk of developing central pontine myelinolysis. Of course, a stroke and in particular subarachnoid haemorrhage, may be the cause of hyponatraemia (section 11.18.2) and many cases are iatrogenic (e.g. use of intravenous fluids, diuretics and carbamazepine). Given that many patients with stroke have been smokers, a bronchial carcinoma should be considered if the pattern of serum and urine osmolalities suggests the syndrome of inappropriate ADH secretion.

Hypercalcaemia

The usual neurological manifestations of hypercalcaemia are either psychiatric symptoms or an encephalopathy, often accompanied by headache and sometimes seizures. Occasionally, cerebral infarction occurs. A proposed mechanism is vasospasm but this has not been established.

Hepatic encephalopathy

It is most unlikely that an acute or subacute portosystemic encephalopathy would be mistaken for a stroke or TIA. One case report in the literature describes a woman who developed a left hemiparesis following a general anaesthetic for manipulation of her left shoulder and at the time of transfer to the rehabilitation hospital was found to have a mild hepatic encephalopathy.[133] Acquired (non-Wilsonian) hepatocerebral degeneration can present with dysarthria, ataxia and intention tremor as well as upper motor neurone signs in the limbs, although there is usually a history of progressive deterioration. The catch is that routine liver function tests may be normal but the serum ammonia is raised and other tests of liver function may be abnormal (e.g. prothrombin time).

Wernicke's encephalopathy

Wernicke's encephalopathy can sometimes be mistaken for a stroke because of an unusually sudden onset of diplopia (due to abducens and conjugate gaze palsies and nystagmus), ataxia and mental confusion, either singly or, more often, in various combinations.[134] It is due to thiamine deficiency and is seen mainly, although not exclusively, in alcoholics and the malnourished elderly.

The diagnosis can be difficult because the history of symptom onset may be unclear due to recent alcohol intoxication or Korsakoff's psychosis, in which retentive memory is impaired out of all proportion to other cognitive functions in an otherwise alert and responsive patient. Pointers to the diagnosis on examination are signs of peripheral neuropathy (present in more than 80% of patients), postural hypotension (autonomic neuropathy), disordered cardiovascular function (tachycardia, exertional dyspnoea, minor ECG abnormalities), and impaired capacity to discriminate between odours (in the chronic stage of the disease due to a lesion of the medial dorsal nucleus of the thalamus). The diagnosis is supported by a marked reduction in red cell transketolase activity (one of the enzymes of the hexose monophosphate shunt that requires thiamine pyrophosphate as a cofactor) and striking improvement in the oculomotor disorder (but not other disorders such as amnesia, polyneuropathy and blindness) within hours of the administration of thiamine; completely normal values of transketolase are usually attained within 24 h. Failure of the ocular palsies to respond to thiamine within a few days should raise doubts about the diagnosis. The medial thalamic and periaqueductal lesions may be demonstrated on brain MRI.

> If Wernicke's encephalopathy is a diagnostic possibility, take blood (for red cell transketolase, thiamine and glucose levels) and then treat immediately with thiamine (100 mg IV or IM daily for 3–5 days, followed by 100 mg orally, daily) and a glucose infusion (since hypoglycaemia can precipitate Wernicke's disease); do not waste time waiting for the blood results to come back.

Hypertensive encephalopathy

Although encephalopathy caused by malignant or accelerated phase hypertension is now rare, it occurs most commonly in patients with an established history of hypertension, although only when the diastolic blood pressure exceeds about 150 mmHg. However, it is also seen in previously normotensive patients whose cerebral autoregulation is normal and so easily exceeded by a rapid rise in blood pressure, sometimes with a diastolic blood pressure of no more than 100 mmHg (i.e. associated with conditions such as pre-eclampsia, acute nephritis, phaeochromocytoma, renin-secreting tumour, ingestion of sympathomimetic drugs and tricyclic antidepressants, ingestion of tyramine in conjunction with a monoamine oxidase inhibitor, head injury, autonomic hyperactivity in patients with the Guillain–Barré syndrome or spinal cord disorders, and with baroreceptor reflex failure after bilateral carotid endarterectomy). The cause is thought to be widespread cerebral oedema resulting from a breakdown of cerebral blood flow autoregulation. The pathological hallmark is fibrinoid necrosis in resistance vessels in the retina and kidneys. The clinical picture is usually dominated by the subacute onset of headache, nausea, vomiting, confusion, declining conscious state, blurred vision, seizures and focal or generalized weakness. There may be focal neurological signs and hypertensive retinopathy (including papilloedema) (Fig. 3.30).

Hypertensive encephalopathy can sometimes be mistaken for intracranial venous thrombosis (particularly in pregnancy) or an arterial ischaemic stroke, especially if there is doubt about the onset of symptoms (i.e. if the patient is confused or obtunded) and if the blood pressure is only moderately elevated. Even a severely elevated blood pressure can be a consequence as well as a cause of stroke, but in these cases there is unlikely to be any evidence of end-organ damage such as retinopathy (section 11.7.1).

The aim of treatment should be a smooth reduction in blood pressure over hours rather than minutes; indeed precipitous falls in blood pressure can cause ischaemic stroke (section 4.2.4).

Posterior reversible encephalopathy syndrome

Posterior reversible encephalopathy syndrome (PRES), also called the reversible posterior leukoencephalopathy syndrome, is a fairly recently described clinico-neuroradiological syndrome that has many clinical and imaging similarities to hypertensive encephalopathy, and eclampsia, except there is usually no evidence of hypertensive end-organ damage, and the prognosis is generally very good.[135] Patients present with cortical blindness, headache, altered mental function (drowsiness, coma) and seizures, and brain MR usually shows very extensive white matter abnormalities, typical of oedema, in the posterior regions of both hemispheres (Fig. 3.40).

This syndrome has been associated with a number of immunosuppressive therapies (e.g. cyclosporin, cisplatinum, tacrolimus, and intravenous immunoglobulin therapy), vasculitis and drug withdrawal (e.g. clonidine). The pathophysiology is uncertain, but endothelial dysfunction (sometimes induced by cytotoxic therapies), breakdown of the blood–brain barrier and vasogenic oedema are thought to play a role, as in hypertensive encephalopathy. Indeed, PRES and hypertensive encephalopathy are probably the same syndrome, but with different causes.

There is usually, but not always, fairly rapid improvement of both the clinical and MR abnormalities with treatment that removes the cause (e.g. stopping cytotoxic drugs and lowering blood pressure) and controls the symptoms (antiepileptic drugs). However, the condition is not always reversible, confined to the posterior regions of the brain, or the white matter, and we agree with others that PRES is a misnomer.[135]

Wilson's disease

Wilson's disease may very rarely present as an acute stroke-like problem.[136]

3.4.6 Central nervous system infections

Encephalitis, brain abscess and subdural empyema

If a patient with a focal neurological deficit has an altered conscious state and a fever, then focal or multifocal infection of the brain (meningoencephalitis, brain abscess, progressive multifocal leucoencephalopathy, or subdural empyema) or elsewhere in the body (e.g. pneumonia, urinary tract infection, venous thrombophlebitis, septicaemia) needs to be considered (and perhaps even treated empirically), particularly if the prevalence of infection (e.g. HIV) in the community is high.[101,137] Indeed, among patients with a focal neurological deficit from a previous stroke, a subsequent systemic infection may lead to neurological decompensation and apparent worsening of the neurological deficit, prompting an incorrect diagnosis of recurrent stroke or 'extension' of the initial stroke. There may also be a history of subacute evolution of systemic upset (fever, malaise, lethargy) and focal neurological symptoms, as well as seizures, meningism or a predisposing

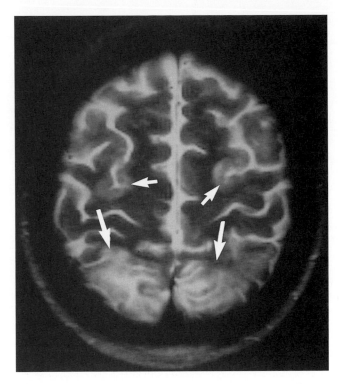

(a)

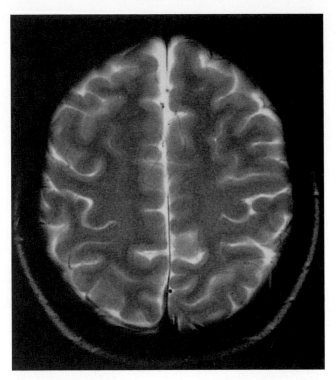

(b)

Fig. 3.40 (a) A T2-weighted MR scan of a patient with posterior leucoencephalopathy syndrome, which occurred following rapid blood transfusion after placental abruption. On the day of onset (a), the patient suddenly became cortically blind in association with a severe headache. She also had several seizures. On T2 MR, there were areas of increased signal in both occipital regions (*long arrows*). Note also the areas of increased cortical signal in the parietal regions (*short arrows*). All her symptoms resolved in 7 days. (b) Three months later, there was no residual visual field defect and the brain scan was normal.

condition such as sinusitis, mastoiditis, otitis, pneumonia, or congenital heart disease. Of course, it is conceivable that the diagnosis of stroke is correct, and the cause of the stroke is an infection (section 7.11).

The EEG, brain CT, MR scan and cerebrospinal fluid (CSF) are usually characteristically abnormal. For example, the parasitic infection cysticercosis may present like a stroke, but the patient will probably have lived in an endemic area and the CT scan often shows an area of calcification within a cyst, as well as scattered foci of parenchymal calcification. In unilateral subdural empyema, the EEG shows extensive unilateral depression of cortical activity and focal delta waves lasting up to 2 s, and the CT shows a non-homogeneous lenticular or semilunar extracerebral lesion with mass effect. However, CT can be normal early on, and MRI may be required to identify the subdural empyema. Likewise, brain CT or MRI of a cerebral abscess usually shows a low-density lesion that is not in a specific vascular territory and has peripheral ring enhancement following intravenous contrast; but sometimes the presentation

is acute and the typical CT findings of an abscess can be delayed for several weeks. It can also be difficult to distinguish radiologically between herpes simplex encephalitis of the frontotemporal lobes and a middle cerebral artery territory infarct (Fig. 3.41).

> If the patient has focal neurological signs, is systemically unwell with fever and has what looks like a normal CT scan, then an abscess, subdural empyema, and meningoencephalitis need to be excluded by MR scan, EEG and – if safe to do so – CSF examination.

Creutzfeldt–Jakob disease

Sporadic Creutzfeldt–Jakob disease (CJD) typically presents with a combination of rapidly progressive (over weeks) dementia and myoclonus, which may be accompanied by symptoms and signs of visual, pyramidal and cerebellar dysfunction. However, CJD may occasionally present acutely with a stroke-like syndrome.[138,139]

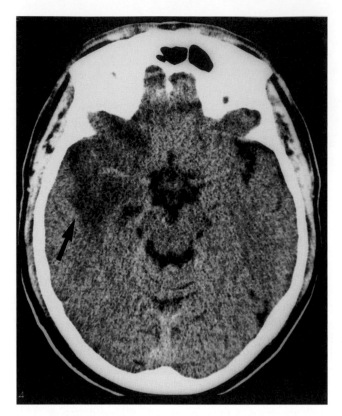

Fig. 3.41 A plain CT brain scan showing a region of low intensity in the right temporal lobe (*arrow*) due to herpes simplex encephalitis.

> If a 'stroke' patient deteriorates and develops myoclonus or dementia, think of sporadic Creutzfeldt–Jakob disease and order one or more EEGs (and MRIs).

3.4.7 Labyrinthine disorders

Vestibular neuronitis (labyrinthitis)

This is probably the commonest cause of severe acute vertigo.[140–143] There is associated nausea, vomiting, nystagmus and ataxia, but no deafness or tinnitus. The acute symptoms usually last for several days and may be followed by positional vertigo for some weeks or months. There is scant evidence for viral involvement of the superior part of the trunk of the vestibular nerve. A very similar, if not identical, clinical syndrome can clearly be caused by minor cerebellar strokes and multiple sclerosis, and the diagnosis is only revealed by MR imaging[144] (section 3.3.7). The arterial territory most commonly involved in cerebellar infarction causing vertigo is the medial branch of the posterior inferior cerebellar artery territory, followed by the anterior inferior cerebellar artery territory. Patients with infarcts in the territory of the superior cerebellar artery or multiple cerebellar arteries do not tend to have isolated spontaneous prolonged vertigo.[144]

Ménière's disease

Ménière's disease is characterized by repeated crises of quite severe rotatory or whirling vertigo, sometimes causing falling to one side, which can be sudden in onset and last from several minutes to a few days.[143] Varying degrees of nausea and vomiting, unilateral (initially) low-pitched tinnitus, sensorineural deafness and a feeling of fullness or pressure in the ear are almost always present as well. It usually begins in middle age. The diagnostic difficulty may come with the first attack, when the auditory symptoms may be mild or non-existent and caloric tests normal. In these cases, cerebellar infarction is a possible differential diagnosis (section 3.3.7).

Benign paroxysmal positional vertigo

Benign paroxysmal positional vertigo is characterized by recurrent episodes of vertigo and nystagmus that occur only after suddenly changing the position of the head – for example, when looking up, rolling over in bed and turning the head toward the affected ear, lying down, bending over and straightening up.[141] The vertigo is usually severe but very brief in duration, certainly less than 1 min, and usually less than 15 s. Hearing is normal. There may be a history of recent head trauma, viral illness, stapes surgery or chronic middle ear disease, but many cases are idiopathic. The cause in most cases is canalolithiasis – particles shed by the otolith membrane float freely in the endolymph of the posterior semicircular canal. A much less common cause is cupulolithiasis in which detritus gets caught on the cupula and causes positional vertigo due to excessive loading of the cupula. The diagnosis is established from the history and using the Dix–Hallpike manoeuvre.

Benign recurrent vertigo

Attacks of spontaneous vertigo not accompanied by cochlear or neurological symptoms in young or middle-aged adults, lasting from 20 min to a few hours, have been called 'benign recurrent vertigo'. The demographics and precipitants of this condition are very similar to those of migraine, and the attacks may respond to standard migraine prophylactic drugs, suggesting that it may be a migraine variant – but the exact pathophysiology remains uncertain.[145]

3.4.8 Psychological disorders

Psychological factors may give rise to subjective experiences (i.e. symptoms), such as hemiparaesthesiae during a panic attack, that commonly need to be differentiated from symptoms that arise from disease (e.g. TIA or stroke), physiological factors (e.g. physiological tremor), behaviours (e.g. excessive rest), and cultural or external factors (e.g. compensation and the welfare state). When there is no disease pathology it becomes tempting to suggest that the symptom must be 'not real' and that it is psychogenic and due to a conversion disorder. Conversion disorder is a psychoanalytic concept that describes the occurrence of motor or sensory neurological symptoms other than pain and fatigue that cause distress, are not explained by disease, not malingered (simulated for clear financial or material gain) and are thought to relate to psychological factors.[74] Whatever the cause of the symptoms, those unexplained by disease may be as or even more distressing than those caused by disease. The most common psychogenic symptoms mistaken for TIA and stroke are functional weakness and sensory loss.[103]

Functional weakness

Patients with functional weakness are likely to show *inconsistency* on observation of their behaviour. For example, their gait on entering the consulting room or at the beginning of the examination may differ from their gait when they leave the consulting room, or at the end of the examination. Further, their weakness when they have to take their clothes on or off may be inconsistent with their weakness when they do another functional task, such as when they have to get something from their bag.

If the patient complains of unilateral leg weakness, Hoover's sign of functional weakness is the only test that has been found in controlled studies to have good sensitivity and specificity.[146] It relies on the principle that we extend our hip when flexing our contralateral hip against resistance. It can be performed in two ways:

Hip extension: look for a discrepancy between voluntary hip extension (which is often weak) and involuntary hip extension (which should be normal) when the opposite hip is being flexed against resistance. It is important when testing involuntary hip extension to ask the patient to concentrate hard on their good leg.

Hip flexion: test hip flexion in the 'weak' leg while keeping your hand under the good heel. Feel for the absence of downward pressure in the good leg.

A similar principle can be used to examine weakness of hip abduction which may initially be weak but then come back to normal if tested simultaneously with the 'good side'.

These tests, although useful, should be interpreted cautiously because:

- pain in the affected hip may produce greater weakness on direct, compared with indirect, testing as a result of attentional phenomena (related to pain rather than weakness);
- cortical neglect can cause a positive Hoover's sign;
- the test may be mildly positive in normal individuals because of a splinting effect;
- none of the studies testing its utility were blinded and none mention the problem of neglect.

'Collapsing' and 'give-way' weakness are commonly present in patients with functional weakness: one moment the limb is strong, the next it is not. This should be not be described as 'intermittency of effort' since it is not possible to directly assess someone's effort. In this situation, normal power can often be achieved transiently with encouragement, for example by saying to the patient, 'At the count of three, stop me from pushing down . . . ' Alternatively, gradually increase the force applied to the limb, starting gently and building imperceptibly up to normal force. Inability to understand the instruction, pain in the relevant joint, being generally unwell, and a misguided eagerness of some patients to 'convince the doctor' may be problematic. These concerns have been vindicated in the small number of validity studies which have found that this sign is a rather poor discriminator between functional and disease-related symptoms.[74] However, it is our impression in daily practice that it is quite a good discriminating test, and more reliable than Hoover's sign.

Functional sensory disturbance

Functional sensory disturbance may be reported as a symptom, or detected first by the examiner. While a number of functional sensory signs have been described, none appear to be specific and they should not therefore be used carelessly to make a diagnosis.

- Patients may describe sensory loss that ends where the leg or arm ends, at the shoulder or groin.
- The hemisensory syndrome is a disturbance which is usually considered by the patient as 'something is not right down one side' or that they feel 'cut in half'. It is usually more patchy than complete, and of variable intensity. There are often accompanying symptoms of intermittent blurring of vision in the ipsilateral eye (asthenopia) and sometimes ipsilateral hearing problems.

- Exact splitting of sensation in the midline is said to be a functional sign because cutaneous branches of the intercostal nerves overlap from the contralateral side, so organic sensory loss should be 1 or 2 cm from the midline. However, midline splitting can also occur in thalamic stroke. Similarly, patients with disease should not report a difference in the sensation of a tuning fork placed over the left compared to the right side of the sternum or frontal bone, as these bones are a single unit and must vibrate as one. But these signs seem to be as common in patients with disease and so cannot be recommended.[74,147]

- Asking patients to 'Say yes when they feel touch and no when they don't', in order to see whether they say 'no' when the affected area is touched, is difficult to interpret because the patient may be saying 'no' to mean 'not as much'.

- Although often considered left-sided, a systematic review found only a slight left-sided preponderance for functional motor and sensory symptoms.[148]

- '*La belle indifférence*', an apparent lack of concern about the nature or implications of symptoms or disability, has no value in discriminating whether the patient is making an effort to appear cheerful in a conscious attempt to avoid being labelled as depressed, or factitious because he or she is deliberately making up the symptom and is not concerned about it.

> The diagnosis of functional motor and sensory symptoms depends on demonstrating positive functional signs as well as the absence of signs of disease. Most of these signs relate to inconsistency, either internal (for example, Hoover's sign reveals discrepancies in leg power) or external (for example, tubular field defect is inconsistent with the laws of optics). However, although inconsistency may be evidence that the signs are functional, it does not indicate whether they are consciously or unconsciously produced, and a positive functional sign does not exclude the possibility that the patient also has disease.

Dizziness

Panic attacks can present somatically with dizziness, a fear of embarrassment, and an inability to escape from situations in which they are likely to occur, such as supermarkets. However, anxiety and phobic avoidance of situations, or head positions, that bring on dizziness does not necessarily indicate a psychogenic aetiology. For example, physiological vestibular sensitivity to certain visual stimuli such as patterned lines or bright lights (sometimes called visual vertigo) may cause symptoms that also come on in crowded places. Asking the patient to hyperventilate to see if that reproduces the symptoms might appear straightforward, but this is often falsely positive in patients with dizziness caused by disease.

Depersonalization and derealization also may be described by the patient as 'dizziness'. If this sensation is there all the time, the patient may have depersonalization disorder (a chronic form of dissociation).

Speech and swallowing symptoms

Dysphonia is the most common functional speech complaint. Often the clinical presentation is of whispering or hoarse speech that is initially thought to be laryngitis by the patient, but then persists for months or years. The possibility of spasmodic adductor or abductor dysphonia must always be considered. Functional dysarthria typically resembles a stutter or is extremely slow with long hesitations that are hard to interrupt. The speech may be telegrammatic, consisting only of the main verbs and nouns in a sentence. In its extreme form the patient may become mute. However, these types of speech disturbance can also be seen in patients with disease.

Word-finding difficulty is a common symptom in anyone with significant fatigue or concentration problems and may compound any functional dysarthria. True dysphasia as a more severe functional symptom, however, is rare.

Globus pharyngis or functional dysphagia is also common. The patient normally complains of a sensation of a 'ball in the throat' and investigations do not reveal a cause.

Visual symptoms

Intermittent blurring of vision that returns to normal if the patient screws up their eyes tight and then relaxes them again is commonly reported. Some of these patients have convergence or accommodation spasm, with a tendency for the convergence reflex to be transiently overactive, either unilaterally or bilaterally. In this situation lateral gaze restriction can sometimes mimic a sixth nerve palsy, but miosis reveals the diagnosis. Voluntary nystagmus appears to be a 'talent' possessed by around 10% of the population.

Tests for functional visual acuity problems are described in detail elsewhere.[149] Simple bedside tests for a patient complaining of complete blindness are to ask them to sign their name or bring their fingers together in front of their eyes (which they should be able to do). They may have a normal response to menace and optokinetic nystagmus with a rotating drum. Decreased acuity in one eye can be assessed with a 'fogging test' in which plus lenses of increasing power are placed in front of the 'good' eye until the patient can only be using their 'bad' eye to see.

Spiral or tubular fields are common, and are often asymptomatic. Remember to test the fields at two distances when looking for a tubular field. Patients with functional hemianopia have been described who have homonymous hemianopia with both eyes open and then, inconsistent with this, a monocular hemianopia in one eye with a full field in the other eye. Monocular diplopia or polyopia may be functional but can be caused by ocular pathology.

3.4.9 Head injury

Head injury may cause a stroke, and a stroke may cause head injury. Without a detailed history of the onset from relevant people as well as the patient (witnesses, family members, ambulance officers, family doctor) it can be difficult to be sure what has happened. For example, head injury may cause intracranial haemorrhage, which can be mistaken for a primary stroke if the patient is amnesic for the injury and has no external scalp evidence of injury. Head injury can also cause ischaemic stroke as a result of arterial dissection (section 7.2). On the other hand, stroke can precipitate a fall, causing head injury and, if the CT scan shows intracranial haemorrhage, the primary stroke event may be missed. Brain imaging may shed some light on the cause; intracranial haemorrhage from head injury tends to be more common in the frontal and anterior temporal regions, superficial and multiple, and there may be accompanying extension into the subarachnoid space and associated skull fractures (Fig. 3.42) (section 9.1.4). One can often see soft tissue swelling of the scalp and brain contusions on the CT scan.

3.4.10 Multiple sclerosis

Patients with multiple sclerosis (MS) usually develop focal neurological symptoms in their third or fourth decade (as opposed to the seventh and eighth decades for stroke). The onset is typically subacute, with the symptoms coming on over days or even weeks. The diagnosis is seldom difficult because these patients are usually young without any vascular diseases or risk factors, the symptoms are as often positive as negative, there are usually more neurological signs than symptoms (compared with TIA and stroke, in which there are often more symptoms than signs), and some may have evidence of disease in other parts of the central nervous system that is asymptomatic but readily detected by clinical examination or brain/spinal cord MRI. Also, there may be a history of previous episodes that are typical of multiple

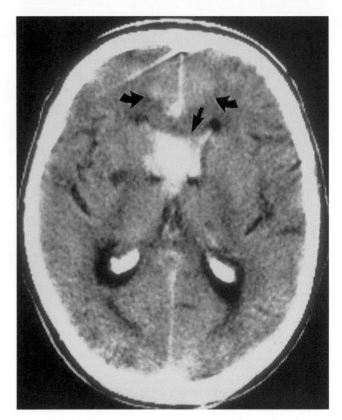

Fig. 3.42 A plain CT brain scan showing blood in the subarachnoid space in a patient who presented with confusion following a head injury. There is blood in the anterior interhemispheric fissure (*straight arrow*) in a pattern suggesting spontaneous subarachnoid haemorrhage. However, the presentation apparently followed a head injury and the suggestion of frontal haemorrhagic contusion (*curved arrows*) clouded the interpretation of the CT scan and delayed recognition of the true pathology (anterior communicating artery aneurysmal haemorrhage).

sclerosis, such as optic neuritis or transverse myelitis. However, sometimes symptoms do seem to start abruptly and so can mimic a TIA or stroke.[150]

The location and shape of the lesions on brain imaging are usually fairly characteristic (Fig. 3.43) (i.e. discrete round or oval lesions in the white matter of the cerebral or cerebellar hemispheres and brainstem, in the corpus callosum, and adjacent to the temporal horns of the lateral ventricles, not corresponding to territories supplied by specific cerebral arteries). In addition, the cerebrospinal fluid usually shows raised immunoglobulin (IgG) and oligoclonal bands, which are not present in the serum. However, none of these features is specific; for example, oligoclonal bands may be found in patients with acute stroke, particularly if due to vasculopathies associated with Behçet's disease, systemic lupus erythematosus and sarcoidosis, although in many of these cases oligoclonal bands are also present in the serum (section 7.3).

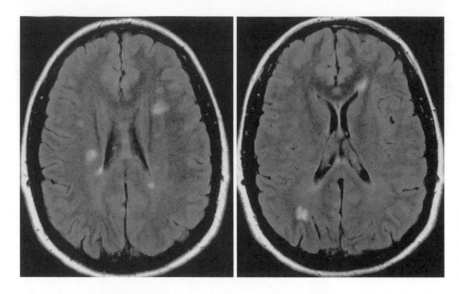

Fig. 3.43 A fluid-attenuated inversion recovery (FLAIR) MR brain scan showing typical 'flame-shaped' periventricular white matter lesions (*white areas*) in a patient with multiple sclerosis.

3.4.11 Neuromuscular disorders

Mononeuropathy and radiculopathy

It is not uncommon for TIA and stroke affecting just the hand or arm to have to be distinguished from a median neuropathy at the wrist (carpal tunnel syndrome), an ulnar neuropathy at the elbow, a radial nerve palsy, or cervical radiculopathy.[44,151] This is because peripheral nerve and nerve root lesions may occasionally cause sudden onset (or sudden awareness, perhaps waking up from sleep) of persisting focal sensory or motor symptoms, which can be confused with 'pseudoradicular' strokes (those due to small lesions in the contralateral precentral or postcentral gyrus, corona radiata, or thalamus) (section 3.3.5). Similarly, acute tetraparesis and cranial polyneuropathy associated with acute poly-radiculoneuropathy (e.g. Guillain-Barré syndrome and its Miller Fisher variant) can sometimes be mistaken for a brainstem stroke.[152–154] However, the physical signs (i.e. lower motor neurone signs and/or sensory loss to pain in a dermatomal or nerve distribution) are different from those of an intracranial cortical/subcortical lesion which tend to be associated with upper motor neurone signs and/or loss of discriminative/'cortical' sensations, such as joint position sense and two-point discrimination ability. Nevertheless, there are patients with the 'cortical hand syndrome' (section 3.3.4) in whom such distinguishing features are not present. Nerve conduction studies will usually identify a peripheral mononeuropathy unless the problem is very acute, but they are less helpful for more proximal radicular problems unless there are clearly absent F waves.

Myasthenia gravis

Although the symptoms of myasthenia gravis usually come on gradually, there are instances of fairly rapid development, sometimes precipitated by infection (usually respiratory), drugs, or emotional upset.[155,156] If the muscles of the eyes (levator palpebrae and extraocular muscles) and less often the face, jaw, throat and neck are the first to be affected (causing ptosis, diplopia, dysarthria or dysphagia), this can be mistaken for a brainstem vascular event, but the weakness tends to persist (if left untreated) and to fluctuate, increasing as the day wears on. Excess fatigability can be demonstrated by asking the patient to sustain the activity of the symptomatically involved muscles. Conversely, muscle power improves after a brief rest, or in response to 10 mg of edrophonium (tensilon) intravenously, or neostigmine (1.5 mg) intramuscularly. A preceding dose of atropine 0.5 mg IV not only counteracts parasympathetic over-stimulation but also serves as a placebo control for the motor effects. However, because false positive (e.g. motor neurone disease) and false negative (about 10% of cases) results are fairly common, and adverse reactions can occur rarely, the tensilon test is not used unless neurophysiological tests are unavailable or a rapid diagnosis is required. The presence of anti-acetylcholine receptor antibodies confirms the diagnosis in most patients but in those presenting acutely with a suspected 'stroke' the test result takes too long to obtain to be useful.

Motor neurone disease

It is surprising how often patients with bulbar motor neurone disease (MND) are said to have had a brainstem stroke. This is probably because MND symptoms sometimes seem to start surprisingly quickly and, early on, there may be little more than subtle dysarthria without any typical features of MND. What then tends to happen is that a brain CT or MRI is performed, and shows leukoaraiosis which is linked with 'stroke', despite this finding being quite common in the MND age group. The more useful investigation is electromyography which may reveal subclinical evidence of denervation which could not be caused by a stroke. Also, the MND patient continues to deteriorate, quite unlike a stroke patient.

3.4.12 Important non-focal disorders

Syncope

Syncope is probably the most important *non-focal* syndrome of impaired consciousness to distinguish from TIA and stroke, accounting for about one-fifth of patients presenting to the emergency room with a suspected brain attack in a recent study.[45] In another study, in which at least two neurologists aimed to validate the diagnosis of TIA made by general practitioners (GPs) and by hospital emergency physicians, the most frequent conditions misdiagnosed as TIAs were transient disturbances of consciousness, mental status and balance.[157] Compared with neurologists, GPs considered 'confusion' and 'unexplained fall' more often compatible with TIA and 'lower facial palsy' and 'monocular blindness' less often compatible with TIA.

Syncope is defined as a loss of consciousness and postural tone due to a sudden fall in blood flow to the brain.[158–161] Sometimes this may occur abruptly, without any warning (e.g. due to aortic stenosis, complete heart block), but more commonly there is a preceding feeling of light-headedness, faintness or 'dizziness' (not rotational vertigo), bilateral dimming or loss of vision (not to be confused with lone bilateral blindness), sounds seeming to be distant, generalized weakness, and symptoms of adrenergic activity such as nausea, hot and cold feelings and sweating.[52] During the attack, the patient is pale, sweaty, clammy and floppy, rather than cyanosed and rigid as in an epileptic seizure. The pulse is absent or difficult to feel (but this cannot be relied on) and the patient may be incontinent of urine. If the patient is lying flat and not held upright (by someone or by an obstacle), then consciousness is regained within seconds, and there is very little mental confusion or difficulty in recalling the warning symptoms (unless there has been head trauma). Additional features during unconsciousness may include multifocal, arrhythmic, myoclonic jerks (particularly in patients who are held upright), head turns, oral automatisms, righting movements (sustained head-raising or sitting up), eye movements (upward or lateral deviation of the eyes) and visual and auditory hallucinations, all of which are likely to lead to an erroneous diagnosis of epilepsy. There are usually no focal neurological symptoms unless the drop in blood pressure occurs in the presence of *severe* occlusive arterial disease in the neck, or impaired cerebral autoregulation due to a previous stroke. The key to the diagnosis is a sound history from a witness as well as the patient – use the telephone if necessary.[159–161] Making a correct diagnosis is important, because some causes are quite serious (e.g. Stokes–Adams attacks) and if misdiagnosed as a transient ischaemic attack may lead to the patient being denied an effective and possibly life-saving treatment (e.g. a pacemaker).

Drop attacks

'Drop attacks' are episodes of sudden loss of postural tone which cause the patient – usually a middle aged or elderly woman – to fall to the ground without apparent loss of consciousness, vertigo or other sensation. The attack occurs without warning and is not induced by a change of posture or movement of the head. The patient may be unable to rise immediately after the fall, despite being uninjured, perhaps because of the surprise. The most common differential diagnosis is vertebrobasilar ischaemia, but here there is usually some warning that the patient is going to fall, there are brainstem symptoms, such as vertigo or diplopia, and the limb weakness is persistent.[53,157] Not a single patient in the New England Medical Center Posterior Circulation Registry had a drop attack as the only symptom of posterior circulation ischaemia.[54]

Drop attacks have also been attributed to syncope, epilepsy, tumours in the region of the foramen magnum or third ventricle, vestibular disease, myxoedema, old age and even subconscious guilt. In the vast majority of cases no cause is found, and although the attacks may persist, the patients do not seem to have a high risk of stroke or other vascular events and so the episodes are called 'cryptogenic drop attacks'. Rarely the patient may have parasagittal motor cortex/subcortex ischaemia in the territory of both anterior cerebral arteries.[162]

Cataplexy

Cataplexy is characterized by transient episodes of sudden bilateral loss of muscle tone, weakness and areflexia provoked by emotions, and is highly specific to the narcolepsy syndrome.[163–165] Although excessive daytime sleepiness usually begins several months before the onset of cataplexy, up to 10% of patients have cataplexy first. Laughter is the most common precipitant, but other forms of emotion and athletic activities can induce cataplexy. The three typical situations that trigger cataplexy, and differentiate it from other types of muscle weakness, are 'when hearing and telling a joke', 'while laughing', and 'when angry'. Severe attacks cause complete paralysis except for the respiratory muscles, whereas the more common partial episodes cause patients to drop objects or to sit down or stop walking. Less than 1% of attacks cause unilateral weakness and so might be confused with a TIA. Momentary attacks are the usual pattern, and they generally last less than a minute. Prolonged episodes may be associated with hallucinations. Rarely, cataplexy can be almost continuous ('status cataplecticus'). Despite the recent discovery of hypocretin deficiency in the lateral hypothalamus as a cause of narcolepsy, the cause of cataplexy remains unclear.

Serotonin syndrome

The serotonin syndrome is a dose-related range of toxic symptoms caused by excessive stimulation of the central and peripheral nervous system serotonergic ($5\text{-}HT_{1A}$ and $5\text{-}HT_2$) receptors. It is a result of increased serotonin concentrations associated with serotinergic drug use (e.g. serotonin precursors, serotonin agonists, serotonin releasers, serotonin reuptake inhibitors, monoamine oxidase inhibitors, some herbal medicines, and anti-migraine medications such as sumatriptan and dihydro-ergotamine). The clinical picture includes mental-status changes, neuromuscular abnormalities and autonomic hyperactivity[166] which may be mistaken for stroke (with or without a complication such as infection) because the onset is quite rapid and patients have hyperreflexia and clonus (often greater in the legs than arms).

3.4.13 Neuroimaging in the diagnosis of focal neurological symptoms of sudden onset

Transient ischaemic attacks

The main purpose of brain imaging in patients with a suspected transient ischaemic attack (TIA) is to identify a relevant focal ischaemic lesion on MR DWI in cases in which the diagnosis of TIA is uncertain, and to exclude any underlying structural intracranial lesion and, rarely, an intracerebral haemorrhage which may present like a TIA.[13,167–169] Because the yield of CT for detecting structural lesions is only about 1% in patients with suspected TIA, the routine examination of every patient who has had a single TIA with CT is controversial (section 6.8.3).

We do not image the brain of patients with transient monocular blindness but do image patients with (potentially transient) 'brain attacks' with MR DWI. This is because DWI may not only help confirm the diagnosis,[169] but also helps localize the ischaemia to one or more arterial territories and so differentiate carotid from vertebrobasilar ischaemia, and sometimes cardiac embolism in clinically uncertain cases. This is particularly important when carotid surgery is being considered. However, there are limited data on the cost-effectiveness of brain imaging in TIA patients.[167,170]

Stroke

The diagnosis of stroke remains primarily clinical, and the main role of brain imaging is to exclude non-vascular structural pathology as the cause of the symptoms, and establish the underlying vascular pathology (Chapter 5) and aetiology (Chapters 6, 7 and 8). The choice of CT or MRI will depend on the question being asked of the test; local availability; how ill, confused or restless the patient is; and cost and effectiveness.

If CT is available, the imaging strategy producing the highest number of quality adjusted life years (QALYs) at lowest cost is to 'scan all patients immediately' with CT, because CT is practical, quick (a few minutes to scan the brain), widely available, easy to use in ill patients, affordable (£44–130), it accurately identifies intracranial haemorrhage as soon as it occurs (section 5.4.1) and it is essential to image suspected SAH (section 3.7.3).[13,167] Strategies that delay CT scanning reduce QALYs and increase cost. However, CT has limitations. Intracerebral haemorrhage will be misinterpreted as ischaemic stroke if CT is not done within 10–14 days after stroke;[167] delays in seeking medical attention or poor access to CT for stroke will result in failure to identify up to three-quarters of cases of intracerebral haemorrhage, and may lead to inappropriate treatment (e.g. antiplatelet drugs or carotid revascularization) for many.

Although CT shows positive features of ischaemic stroke in many patients with moderate and severe stroke scanned 2–7 days after the event, early signs of ischaemia, within 3–6 h, are difficult to recognize on CT (section 5.4.2). Furthermore, many patients with mild stroke never develop a visible infarct on CT, irrespective of when they are scanned.[167] The Acute Cerebral CT Evaluation of Stroke Study (ACCESS), in which as many doctors and radiologists as possible worldwide interpret typical CT scans of stroke over the Internet, aims to improve recognition of early signs of infarction (http://www.neuroimage.co.uk/access/).[171]

The advantage of MRI DWI is that it shows ischaemic changes as early as a few minutes after stroke as a bright white lesion ('light bulb'), and so shows more ischaemic strokes than CT or conventional MRI.[13,14,169,172,173] It also shows more ischaemic strokes several weeks later, and therefore is particularly useful for positive identification of an ischaemic stroke in patients presenting up to 8 weeks after stroke.[18] For patients presenting too late for CT to show intracerebral haemorrhage, gradient echo MR sequences reveal previous intracerebral haemorrhage indefinitely as a low signal (black) ring or dot, and can therefore distinguish previous haemorrhage from infarction. However, a limitation of MRI is that it may not identify hyperacute intracerebral haemorrhage correctly, and it can fail to detect subarachnoid haemorrhage. Further, it is difficult to use routinely in acute, particularly severe, stroke; it is less often available than CT; it requires more cooperation by the patient for a longer time; it is very noisy and it upsets confused patients. About one-fifth of patients cannot undergo MRI because they are too ill or confused, or have an intraocular or intracerebral metallic foreign body or pacemaker.

3.4.14 Electroencephalography in the diagnosis of focal neurological symptoms of sudden onset

With the increasing availability of neuroimaging, the indications for an EEG in patients with suspected TIA or stroke are now very limited. An EEG may be helpful when the clinical diagnosis of TIA is in doubt and partial (focal or localization-related) seizures are a possibility. However, while about one-third of all patients with clinically definite epilepsy consistently have epileptiform discharges on the waking interictal EEG, and about one-half do so on some occasions with repeated sleep-deprived recordings,[174] we know very little about the sensitivity and specificity of the test when the diagnosis is in doubt. Further difficulty arises as a result of the poor specificity of EEG abnormalities (all too frequently, patients with non-epileptic events such as TIAs are reported to have an abnormal EEG).

The role of the EEG in patients with persisting neurological signs is to help exclude a number of conditions that may mimic stroke, particularly when brain imaging is normal. For example, non-convulsive status epilepticus can present with a sudden confusional state, and in both Creutzfeldt–Jakob disease and herpes simplex encephalitis, where there can be clinical deterioration with new focal neurological signs, the EEG can have characteristic abnormalities (although not in all the patients all the time).

The usual abnormal EEG findings in acute stroke, at least in fairly large hemispherical cortical and subcortical stroke, are a localized reduction of normal cortical rhythms and presence of localized slow-wave abnormality.

Focal EEG slowing, however, is not specific, and only indicates the presence and side of the lesion. Although it has been suggested that the EEG may help distinguish between small deep (lacunar) and cortical infarction, the clinical features and brain CT or MRI scan are far more effective tools. A normal EEG may help to confirm the diagnosis of 'locked-in syndrome' caused by a lesion in the ventral pons (section 3.3.2), and can also lend some support to a diagnosis of a somatization disorder, at least if the clinical deficit is extensive.

3.5 Differential diagnosis of transient monocular blindness

Transient monocular blindness (TMB) and amaurosis fugax are two different terms for describing exactly the same symptom – blurring or loss of vision in the whole or part of the visual field of one eye. It is commonly caused by ischaemia of the retina (usually as a result of embolism from atherothrombosis of an artery between the heart and the eye, or from embolism form the heart), and sometimes by ischaemia of the anterior optic nerve (usually due to disease of the posterior ciliary artery, section 3.5.2).[175,176] However, there are other causes of TMB which are important to differentiate because the prognosis and treatments differ (Table 3.30). Many are uncommon and frequently go unrecognized if the patient is not examined during the acute episode (which of course is very difficult to achieve).

Patients with TMB should be considered for a competent ophthalmological examination to exclude primary disorders of the eye before concluding that the explanation is necessarily vascular disease.

3.5.1 Retinal disorders

Retinal migraine or 'vasospasm'

Migraine with aura (classical migraine) is usually ushered in by 'positive' binocular visual symptoms. However, transient monocular visual symptoms followed by pulsatile headache have occasionally been described in patients with known migraine, and classified as 'retinal migraine'.[177–183]

TMB as a result of thromboembolism is distinguished from retinal migraine on the basis of the symptoms; the former is characterized by the abrupt onset of 'negative' monocular visual phenomena (blindness), which is painless and usually lasts only a few minutes, while

Table 3.30 Causes of transient monocular blindness.

Retinal disorders (section 3.5.1)
Vascular
    Atherothromboembolism or other arterial disorders
      (e.g. dissection affecting the proximal internal carotid
      artery, and giant-cell arteritis affecting the posterior
      ciliary artery)
    Embolism from the heart (section 6.5)
    Low retinal artery perfusion pressure
    Retinal migraine
High resistance to retinal perfusion
    Intracranial vascular malformation
    Central or branch retinal vein thrombosis
    Raised intraocular pressure (glaucoma)
    Raised intracranial pressure
    Increased blood viscosity (section 7.9)
    Malignant arterial hypertension (section 3.4.5)
    Retinal haemorrhage
Retinal detachment
Paraneoplastic retinopathy
Phosphenes
Lightning streaks of Moore
Chorioretinitis
Optic nerve disorders (section 3.5.2)
Anterior ischaemic optic neuropathy
Malignant arterial hypertension (section 3.4.5)
Papilloedema
Optic neuritis and Uhthoff's symptom
Dysplastic coloboma
Eye/orbital disorders (section 3.5.3)
Vitreous haemorrhage
Reversible diabetic cataract
Lens subluxation
Orbital tumour (e.g. optic nerve-sheath meningioma)

the latter is characterized by the gradual build-up of transient monocular visual impairment (i.e. scotoma or blindness), which is usually incomplete and may be associated with 'positive' visual symptoms (e.g. scintillations) lasting for up to an hour, as well as a pulsatile headache or orbital pain. Sometimes, however, it can be very difficult to distinguish retinal ischaemia from retinal migraine, particularly in older patients without any headache. It has been suggested that non-invasive investigations, such as carotid ultrasound, may help distinguish between the two – i.e. tight stenosis of the internal carotid artery on the symptomatic side suggests retinal ischaemia (due to artery-to-artery embolism), and the absence of carotid disease favours retinal migraine. However, this is only circumstantial evidence.

Patients have been described with frequent (1–30 episodes per day), stereotyped episodes of brief (lasting less than 3 min) unilateral visual loss caused by presumed vasospasm. Fundus examination during the episodes shows constriction of the retinal arteries and segmentation in a thin and slowly moving column of blood. The calibre of the retinal vessels is restored with the return of vision. Occasional patients have responded to a calcium channel blocker. However, as there is really no proof of vasospasm, we have to be very cautious in the interpretation of these observations in what appear to be very rare patients.

Patients with TMB have a better prognosis than patients with TIA of the brain, despite similar degrees of carotid stenosis[184] (section 16.11.8). The reason remains uncertain, but is unlikely to be that some of the cases of TMB were really cases of retinal migraine.

The question therefore arises, how do we define retinal migraine? Is it a diagnosis based on the clinical symptoms and signs, the results of investigations, the response to treatment, or the prognosis? It has been traditionally diagnosed on the basis of the clinical history, but this may be non-specific, and it is seldom possible to examine the patient during the episode to see if 'vasospasm' is present. Any carotid disease may be coincidental, and of course the response to treatment and the prognosis are hardly helpful at the time the diagnosis has to be made. We cannot, therefore, provide any definitive answer.

Arteriovenous malformation

Anterior and middle fossa dural arteriovenous malformations very rarely cause TMB. When they do it is probably because of transient lowering of retinal arterial pressure associated with shunting of blood away from the ophthalmic artery.

Central or branch retinal vein thrombosis

Thrombosis of the central retinal vein, or branch retinal vein, sometimes presents with attacks of TMB.[175] The visual loss tends to be patchy rather than complete. The fundoscopic appearance is characteristic: engorged retinal veins and multiple retinal haemorrhages (Fig. 3.44).

Angle-closure glaucoma

This typically presents in people over the age of 50 years who are hypermetropic (long-sighted). Apposition of the peripheral iris to the trabecular meshwork decreases the outflow of the aqueous humour which in turn increases the intraocular pressure and reduces perfusion pressure to the choroid, retina and disc. Transient monocular visual disturbance may occur, particularly in poor light when the pupil is dilated. The onset is usually subacute. Vision may be decreased, blurred, foggy, or smoke-like, and the patient may see haloes around lights. Some patients complain of light sensitivity during the attack and most, but not all, have eye pain, which may radiate

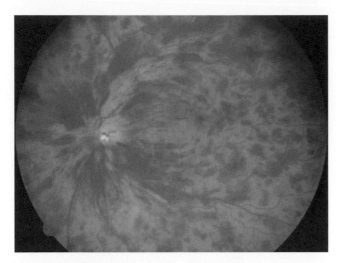

Fig. 3.44 An ocular fundus photograph showing engorged retinal veins and multiple retinal haemorrhages due to central retinal vein thrombosis. Also reproduced in colour in the plate section.

to the side of the head. The symptoms may last from a few minutes to hours. Eye pain and the stereotyped recurrence of attacks under certain lighting conditions are useful clues to the diagnosis, as are red eye, cloudy cornea and oval pupil (Fig. 3.27). The intraocular pressure should be checked in most, if not all, patients with TMB, but in those who have glaucoma it is not always raised between attacks.

Retinal and other intraocular haemorrhages

A small retinal haemorrhage may cause sudden reduced vision in one eye that resolves within hours. The diagnosis should be evident on ophthalmoscopy, particularly if the pupil is dilated. Similarly, vitreous and anterior chamber haemorrhage may cause TMB. The cause may be suspected from the history; for example, preretinal haemorrhage may occur during physical exertion, sexual activity, or Valsalva manoeuvre.

Paraneoplastic retinopathy

Transient episodes, lasting seconds to minutes, of painless monocular dimming of the central field of vision and overwhelming visual glare and photosensitivity when exposed to bright light suggests not only photoreceptor dysfunction due to transient retinal ischaemia, but also paraneoplastic retinopathy. Patients may also experience transient bizarre entoptic symptoms (alterations in normal light perception resulting from intraoptic phenomena, akin to the subjective perception of light resulting from mechanical compression of the eyeball – phosphenes). Ophthalmoscopy usually reveals

attenuated retinal arterioles, electroretinography demonstrates abnormal cone- and rod-mediated responses, and antiretinal antibodies may be identified in the serum. Over the subsequent months, progressive visual loss occurs, during which time a small-cell carcinoma of the lung often declares itself.

Phosphenes

Phosphenes are flashes of light and coloured spots that are induced by eye movement in a dark environment and occur in the absence of luminous stimuli. They may occur with disease of the visual system at many different sites, such as optic neuritis in the recovery phase, perhaps as a result of the mechanical effects of movement of the optic nerve. However, mechanical pressure from a sharp tap on the normal eyeball may also induce a phosphene, as every child discovers, by stimulating the retina. Phosphenes may also occur in a healthy dark-adapted closed eye after a saccade (flick phosphene).

Lightning streaks of Moore

In a dark environment, elderly people frequently experience recurrent, brief, stereotypic, vertical flashes of light in the temporal visual field of one eye, which are elicited by eye movement. These are known as Moore's lightning streaks and are benign. It is believed that, with advanced age, the posterior vitreous may collapse and detach from the retina, leading to persistent vitreoretinal adhesions. The mechanical forces associated with eye movement exert traction on the macula and retina, and induce the photopsias (subjective sensations of sparks or flashes of light).

Chorioretinitis

Macular disease due to chorioretinitis or retinal pigmentary degeneration can sometimes lead to loss of vision in bright light.

Central serous retinopathy

This typically affects young men. Over a period of hours to days, central vision becomes blurred associated with various degrees of metamorphopsia (defective, distorted vision), micropsia (objects appear smaller than their actual size due to segregation of the photoreceptors), chromatopsia (objects appear unnaturally coloured), central scotoma, and increasing hyperopia (far-sightedness). It lasts for days to weeks, usually resolving within 4–8 weeks.

Visual acuity in the acute stage ranges from 6/6 to 6/60 and averages 6/9. On fundoscopy, there is an accumulation of transparent fluid between the retinal pigment epithelium and the outer segments in the macular area, elevating the retina and causing a circumscribed area of retinal detachment at the posterior pole. The diagnosis is confirmed by fluorescein angiography. Typically the fluorescein enters into the blister and stains its contents, identifying one or more leakage points.

3.5.2 Optic nerve disorders

Anterior ischaemic optic neuropathy

Anterior ischaemic optic neuropathy (AION) is due to ischaemia in the territory of supply of the posterior ciliary arteries, which are branches of the ophthalmic artery, and which supply the anterior part of the optic nerve, the choroid and outer retina. Because the optic disc is close to an arterial border zone between the territories of the two major posterior ciliary arteries, it is particularly liable to ischaemia when the systemic blood pressure falls, when the intraocular pressure rises, or when there is occlusive disease of local small arteries. Less often, AION is caused by embolism from the heart or proximal arteries to, or *in situ* occlusion of, the posterior ciliary arteries or the arterioles feeding the anterior part of the optic nerve, e.g. by giant-cell arteritis (Fig. 3.45) and other types of vasculitis, such as polyarteritis nodosa (section 7.3). Atherosclerosis of the posterior ciliary artery is another presumed cause, given that patients with AION have an increased prevalence of hypertension and diabetes and an increased risk of subsequent cerebrovascular and cardiovascular events, but we are not aware of any histological proof of atheromatous occlusion of these arteries.

Ischaemia of the optic disc is characterized clinically by the sudden onset of painless visual loss in one eye.[185] This may involve the whole field, but it tends to be more severe in the lower half because the upper segment of the optic disc is more vulnerable to ischaemia. In the early stages, the circulation may be so precariously balanced that minor postural change may have profound effects on the degree of visual loss. The visual loss tends to be severe, non-progressive and prolonged, but it can be brief (and present as transient monocular blindness), or it can progress over several hours or days. In AION due to giant-cell arteritis, the visual loss may develop sequentially in both eyes within a few days and, rarely, almost simultaneously. Normal visual acuity does not exclude AION, and almost any part of the visual field can be affected.

The common patterns of visual loss are an altitudinal hemifield defect (loss of either the upper or, more frequently, the lower half of the field in one eye), an inferior nasal segmental loss, and a central scotoma. The disc may appear normal at first, but within a few days

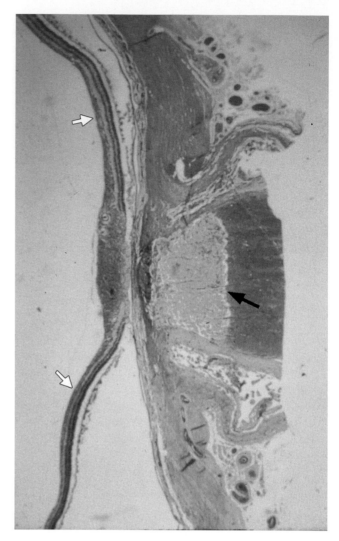

Fig. 3.45 A photomicrograph of anterior ischaemic optic neuropathy caused by giant-cell arteritis. The arrow indicates the infarcted optic nerve head (courtesy of Dr J.F. Cullen, Western General Hospital, Edinburgh). Also reproduced in colour in the plate section.

it becomes pale and swollen, often with small flame-shaped haemorrhages radiating from the disc margin (ischaemic papillopathy), distended veins and, occasionally, cotton-wool spots due to ischaemic change in the surrounding retina. The swelling may involve only one segment of the disc, or may be more marked in one segment than in another. The disc swelling is attributed partly to leakage of plasma from damaged blood vessels and partly to arrest of axoplasmic transport along damaged nerve fibres. The disc swelling itself may be indistinguishable from that seen with raised intracranial pressure, but the vision is usually normal in the latter. In about half of the eyes with AION due to giant-cell arteritis, the disc swelling has a chalky white appearance. Later, the swelling subsides, to be succeeded by optic atrophy with attenuation of the small blood vessels on the disc surface. The prognosis for recovery of vision is variable. Many patients recover good central vision, but are left with arcuate and sectorial visual field defects corresponding to loss of bundles of nerve fibres. In other patients, visual loss may be complete and permanent.

Malignant arterial hypertension

Some patients with malignant hypertension experience transient monocular blindness due to ischaemia of the optic nerve head. Associated headache, seizures, encephalopathy, renal impairment, high blood pressure and the characteristic ophthalmoscopic features of hypertension point to the diagnosis (Fig. 3.30).

Papilloedema

Patients with papilloedema (Fig. 3.46) from any cause may experience transient visual blurring or obscurations, with or without photopsias. The visual loss in chronic papilloedema is often postural, occurring as patients get up from a chair (or bend over), and may involve either eye alone, or both eyes together. The visual loss is typically 'grey' rather than 'black' and lasts for seconds rather than minutes.

The explanation may be transient optic nerve ischaemia secondary to a relative decrease in orbital blood flow, as a result of raised cerebrospinal fluid pressure in the subarachnoid space around the optic nerve, and so increased pressure in the veins draining the optic nerve head. Episodes of visual blurring or blindness in someone with papilloedema should lead to urgent investigation and appropriate action because permanent visual loss will eventually follow, gradually or suddenly.

Optic neuritis and Uhthoff's symptom

Patients with acute and chronic optic nerve demyelination due to multiple sclerosis may experience transiently decreased vision in one or both eyes during exercise (Uhthoff's symptom), or in association with other causes of increased temperature, emotional stress, increased illumination, eating, drinking, smoking and menstruation.[185,186] The pathophysiology is unknown, although reversible conduction block in demyelinated nerve fibres secondary to an increase in body temperature or to changes in blood electrolyte levels or pH are believed to play a role. Ophthalmoscopy may be normal, but if the optic nerve head is inflamed, the optic disc will be swollen and will look similar to papilloedema.

Optic disc anomalies

Transient monocular visual obscurations are occasionally associated with an elevated optic disc without increased intracranial pressure. Examples include congenital anomalies of the disc, such as drusen or posterior staphyloma.

3.5.3 Orbital disorders

Transient changes in the ocular media or intraocular pressure, such as vitreous floaters, vitreous haemorrhage, anterior chamber haemorrhage, lens subluxation, reversible cataract (in a diabetic) and glaucoma may cause transient monocular visual disturbance. Most of these conditions can be excluded by a competent ophthalmological examination.

An intraorbital mass, such as an optic nerve sheath meningioma, may produce gaze-evoked transient monocular blindness; the blindness is limited to the duration of gaze in the affected direction (usually abduction of the affected eye) and the visual acuity usually returns to normal about 30 s after the eye moves back to the primary position. The loss of vision is possibly caused by a reduction in flow to the blood vessels surrounding the optic nerve itself.

3.5.4 Corneal and eyelid disorders

Fuch's corneal endothelial dysfunction (corneal guttatae)

In the seventh and eighth decade, the corneal endothelial cells may become deficient and malfunction due to abnormal excrescences of the basement (Descemet's)

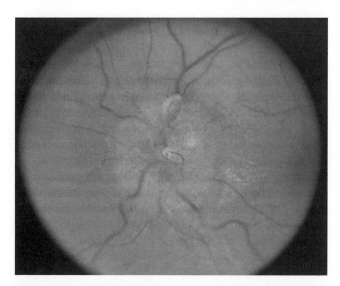

Fig. 3.46 An ocular fundus photograph showing papilloedema. Note the congested, swollen disc, with loss of the physiological cup, a blurred disc margin and congested retinal veins. Also reproduced in colour in the plate section.

membrane, called corneal guttatae. The corneal epithelium may then fail to pump fluid out of the cornea and patients complain of blurred vision (due to hydration of the cornea). It tends to occur in the morning and gradually clears as the day evolves, and as the cornea clears due to evaporation of tears. Similar symptoms can occur due to endothelial cell loss as a consequence of intraocular surgery.

Ptosis

Intermittent ptosis (e.g. myasthenia gravis) can cause transient monocular visual loss.

3.6 Improving the reliability of the clinical diagnosis

For every patient who presents to their family doctor with a definite transient ischaemic attack (TIA), there are many more who present with transient neurological symptoms due to other disorders. For example, in the Oxfordshire Community Stroke Project (OCSP), 512 patients were referred by their family doctor or a hospital doctor with a diagnosis of 'possible TIA', of whom 317 (62%) were considered by the OCSP neurologists *not* to have had a TIA (Table 3.22).[6] This problem is not unique to family doctors and junior hospital doctors. The inter-observer agreement for the diagnosis of TIA of the brain amongst eight senior and interested neurologists from the same department who interviewed 56 patients in alternating pairs revealed that both neurologists agreed that 36 patients had a TIA and 12 had not, but they disagreed about eight (kappa = 0.65; for perfect agreement kappa would be 1.0).[187]

> Even experienced neurologists with an interest in cerebrovascular disease show considerable inter-observer variability in the diagnosis of transient ischaemic attack. This does not imply lack of skill, but rather it is inherent in the clinical assessment of symptoms and signs. Sometimes the available information does not allow one to come to a 'right answer' as to whether the event was a transient ischaemic attack or not – in which case one ends up working on the basis of probability.

The inter-observer agreement for the diagnosis of stroke (vs not stroke) is made with moderate to good reliability (kappa = 0.77).[37]

The clinical features associated with high inter-observer agreement for the diagnosis of stroke or TIA versus no vascular event are a sudden change in speech, visual loss, diplopia, numbness or tingling, paralysis or weakness and nonorthostatic dizziness (kappa = 0.60).[49]

Several studies have shown that clinicians can differ in the interpretation of even isolated elements of the history, such as loss of power, loss of sensation, 'blurred or foggy vision', and headache.[37,188] When assessing patients with suspected stroke, the interobserver agreement for most items of the clinical history is moderate to good (kappa statistics for vascular risk factors range from 0.44 to 0.69) but there is much less inter-observer agreement for various features of the neurological examination (Table 3.31).[37,188,189]

3.6.1 Reasons for clinical disagreement

There are several factors that can increase the likelihood of clinical disagreement.

For patients with suspected TIA, the main problem is eliciting and interpreting the history of an event that has resolved by the time the history is taken. For example, since the symptoms of most TIAs resolve within about 15–60 min, the diagnosis is almost always based entirely on the clinical history, which for a number of reasons may not be very clear: the patient may have forgotten the symptoms (because of poor memory or delay in presenting to medical attention); the symptoms may have been remembered, but are difficult to describe (e.g. transient homonymous hemianopia); or the patient may have been so frightened by the attack that he or she was more preoccupied with the immediate outcome than the exact nature of the deficit. All of these problems are more common in the elderly. For patients with suspected stroke, the inter-observer reliability of the clinical assessment is affected by a variety of factors, such as the time since the onset of symptoms; there is a trend for worse inter-observer reliability among patients assessed very early and very late after symptom onset.[37]

Another problem is that the generally accepted definitions of stroke and TIA lack specific detail about which 'focal' symptoms are not acceptable (e.g. isolated vertigo or not?). In the context of TIAs, what is an acceptable lower time limit for the duration of symptoms? Is a sudden focal neurological deficit, particularly a sensory deficit, of less than 5 s duration a TIA?

Diagnostic conformity can only be achieved if precise criteria are available that are valid, reliable and generally accepted. In the particular case of TIA, it is difficult to determine the validity of any single diagnostic criterion, because there is no 'gold standard' against which to

Table 3.31 Inter-observer agreement for neurological signs in stroke patients.

Signs examined	Kappa value		
	Lindley *et al.*[189]	Shinar *et al.*[188]	Hand *et al.*[37]
Conscious level	0.60	0.38	0.70
Confusion	0.21	NS	0.45
Dementia	NS	0.34	NS
Weakness of arm	0.77	NS	0.65
Weakness of hand	0.68	0.58 (R) 0.49 (L)	0.72
Weakness of leg	0.64	NS	0.57
Weakness of face	0.63	0.51 (R) 0.66 (L)	0.50
Sensory loss on hand	0.19	0.50 (R) 0.32 (L)	0.49
Sensory loss on arm	0.15	NS	0.49
Aphasia/language problem	0.70	0.54	0.66
Dysarthria	0.51	0.53	0.41
Visuospatial dysfunction	0.44	NS	0.41
Hemianopia	0.39	0.40	0.46
Cerebellar signs/ataxia	0.46	0.45	NS
Cranial nerve palsy	0.34	NS	NS
Extraocular movement disorder	0.30	0.77	NS

NS, not stated.

judge it, other than perhaps the prognosis. For example, patients with lone bilateral blindness were followed up and found to have a similar prognosis to patients with TIA, implying that lone bilateral blindness is also a TIA.[48] Whether the prognosis of patients with isolated dysarthria or vertigo is similar is an important research question.

More widespread and consistent consideration, discussion and application of the diagnostic criteria could enhance diagnostic accuracy and inter-observer agreement, and might improve patient management and care.[188] However, as the diagnostic criteria become more specific, sensitivity is sacrificed and so an increasing number of genuine TIAs may be discarded and left untreated. Conversely, if the criteria become less specific, there may be a tendency to overdiagnose TIA, but this too can have adverse consequences such as the loss of a job, driver's or pilot's licence, money and self-esteem, as well as resulting in inappropriate investigation and the prescription of numerous unnecessary drugs.

The inter-observer reliability of the clinical assessment of stroke is also improved by the experience and confidence of the assessor.[37]

3.6.2 Strategies to reduce inter-observer variation

The clinical skills required to obtain an accurate and useful history are listed in Table 3.32, and strategies

Table 3.32 Clinical skills required to obtain an accurate and useful history.

The ability to:
   Establish understanding
   Establish information
   Interview logically
   Listen
   Interrupt only when necessary
   Observe non-verbal cues
   Establish a good relationship
   Interpret the interview
   Tell the story in plain language
   Tell the story in chronological order
   Make the story 'human'
Like this:
This 85-year-old widow was standing at the kitchen table peeling potatoes at 7 p.m. on 26 November 2006, with her daughter, when she suddenly stopped talking, dropped the potato peeler she was holding in her right hand and fell to the floor. She was unable to get up and has not been able to speak or move her right arm or leg since.
Not like this:
This lady developed sudden dysphasia and right hemiparesis.

for preventing or minimizing clinical disagreement in Table 3.33. If these principles are applied with a knowledge of the diagnostic criteria (Table 3.5), then diagnostic inconsistency should be minimized. If there is still uncertainty about the diagnosis at the end of the

Table 3.33 Strategies for preventing or minimizing clinical disagreement.

Assess the patient in a suitable consulting environment, i.e. quiet room, minimal interruptions if possible

Necessary equipment available: ophthalmoscope, sphygmomanometer, etc., telephone on desk to call witnesses (to clarify history) or colleagues (to obtain advice)

Clarify and confirm key points

Repeat key elements of the history or examination

Corroborate important findings with witnesses, documents and, if necessary, appropriate tests

Ask 'blinded' colleagues to see the patient also (e.g. at ward teaching sessions)

Record evidence as well as inference, making a clear distinction between the two, reporting exactly what the patient said and then your interpretation (e.g. 'the patient complained of heaviness of the right arm and leg' and not 'the patient complained of right-sided weakness' or 'the patient complained of right hemiparesis')

Apply the art and social sciences of medicine, as well as the biological sciences of medicine

Make sure you have enough time for the entire consultation

Table 3.34 Clinical features (i.e. the milieu) influencing the probability that the event was a stroke or transient ischaemic attack.

Very likely to be vascular, almost definite

Atrial fibrillation and rheumatic heart disease

Frequent carotid-distribution transient ischaemic attacks and focal, long, loud bruit over the carotid bifurcation on the symptomatic side

History and physical signs suggestive of infective endocarditis (i.e. fever, splinter haemorrhages, cardiac murmur)

Recent myocardial infarction (in last 3–4 weeks)

Likely to be vascular, but less definite

Atrial fibrillation and non-rheumatic valvular heart disease (but a few fibrillating stroke patients have primary intracerebral haemorrhage as the cause of the stroke)

Arterial bruits anywhere (e.g. carotid, orbital, aortic, femoral)

Prosthetic heart valve, taking anticoagulants (but some strokes are haemorrhagic, and some transient ischaemic attacks are related to coexistent carotid artery disease)

Unlikely to be vascular (particularly if neurological symptoms are transient)

Less than 40 years of age, no symptomatic vascular disease, no vascular risk factors, no family history of thrombosis or premature vascular disease, normal heart

history, then the general examination and special investigations aimed at detecting vascular diseases and risk factors may provide useful circumstantial evidence (Table 3.34).[44,45,49,190] The odds of an event being due to cerebrovascular disease are likely to be substantially less if the patient is young and has no vascular risk factors, compared with an elderly patient who has several vascular risk factors, clinical evidence of established vascular disease (e.g. carotid or femoral bruits, absent peripheral pulses) or symptomatic vascular disease elsewhere (e.g. angina, intermittent claudication)[190] – i.e. make sure that you use all the clinical evidence available to you.

> When coming to a view about whether an event was a transient ischaemic attack or stroke, make use of all the clinical evidence, both general and neurological, that is available after a detailed history and examination.

If the history is elicited independently by a second physician, a subsequent comparison of the symptoms as well as their interpretation may lead to a greatly increased reliability of the diagnosis. Teaching hospitals in particular are in a privileged position to apply this powerful but expensive diagnostic 'instrument', but even so, it is still unrealistic except for the occasional very difficult case. What is often available to those in

hospitals, however, is an account by the referring physician who saw the patient at an earlier time after the onset of symptoms – be sure to read it carefully and go over any symptoms described that were not reported to yourself by the patient. Implicit within this is the responsibility for all clinicians who take a history to document it in the patient's or witness's own words and not simply record their own interpretation.

The use of checklists written in simple language improves inter-observer reliability, and is likely to be useful for computer-aided diagnosis and further research studies.[191] However, although checklists may encourage more thorough history taking, the symptoms still have to be interpreted correctly. Very short checklists have been used successfully by paramedical personnel for diagnosing cerebrovascular events hyper-acutely (section 3.3, table 3.6).[39,40,42,43,49]

The relatively poor inter-observer agreement for physical signs (Table 3.31) is not peculiar to patients with stroke. The advent of MRI technologies such as DWI, which is becoming more widespread and can show what were hitherto unseen and yet recent relevant ischaemic lesions, has also improved the sensitivity, specificity and reliability of the diagnosis of TIA and minor ischaemic stroke[169] (section 3.2.1).

3.7 Is it a subarachnoid haemorrhage?

Subarachnoid haemorrhage (SAH) refers to the spontaneous extravasation of blood into the subarachnoid space when a blood vessel near the surface of the brain ruptures. It is a condition, not a disease, which has many causes (section 9.1).[29,30] Although, as we will see (section 5.3.1), the clinical distinction between ischaemic stroke and intracerebral haemorrhage is unreliable and we have to rely on imaging, the clinical features of SAH are reasonably distinct; at least this type of stroke can be diagnosed clinically with reasonable confidence. However, confirmatory investigations are needed in almost all cases.

3.7.1 Clinical features

Blood in the subarachnoid space is a meningeal irritant and incites a typical clinical response, regardless of the source. Patients usually complain of headache, photophobia, stiff neck and nausea, and they may also vomit. Confusion, restlessness and impaired consciousness are also frequent (Table 3.35).

Precipitating factors

More often than not, there is no obvious precipitating factor.[192] Among the 33 patients with SAH in the Oxford-

Table 3.35 Diagnosis of subarachnoid haemorrhage.

Principal symptoms
headache
– usually sudden, maximal in seconds, severe, and occipital or retro-orbital
– duration: hours (possibly minutes, we do not know) to weeks
nausea
vomiting
neck stiffness
photophobia
loss of consciousness
Neurological signs
none (very often)
meningism (after several hours)
focal neurological signs: third nerve palsy (mostly posterior communicating artery aneurysm), dysphasia, hemiparesis (arteriovenous malformation, intracerebral haemorrhage)
subhyaloid haemorrhages in optic fundi
fever
raised blood pressure
altered consciousness

shire Community Stroke Project, six (18%) occurred while resting (none occurred while asleep), 13 (39%) during moderate activity, and six (18%) during strenuous activity, such as weight-lifting and sexual intercourse; the activity at onset was not known in the other eight patients.[193] In a more recent series, higher proportions (up to 50%) of aneurysmal SAHs occurred during physical exertion.[194] Sexual activity may precipitate not only SAH,[195] but also – and more often – relatively harmless headaches, migrainous or not (section 3.7.2).[196]

Headache

Headache is the cardinal clinical feature of SAH. It is the *only* symptom in about one-third of patients,[194,197] but a symptom at some stage in almost every patient.[198,199] Conversely, in a prospective series of patients with sudden headache in general practice, SAH was the cause in one out of four patients, and only in one out of ten patients in whom sudden headache was the *only* symptom.[197]

> One out of every four patients with sudden, severe headache has a ruptured cerebral aneurysm, or one out of ten if sudden headache is the only symptom.

In SAH, the headache is generally diffuse and poorly localized but tends to spread over minutes to hours to the back of the head, neck and down the back as blood tracks into the spinal subarachnoid space. Sometimes the headache is maximal behind the eyes. The headache is often described by patients as the most severe headache they have ever had, but it can occasionally be milder. It is the suddenness of onset which is most characteristic.

Speed of onset and disappearance

The headache arises suddenly, classically in a *split second*, 'like a blow on the head' or 'an explosion inside the head', reaching a maximum within seconds. A potential pitfall is that patients may sometimes use the word 'sudden' to describe an episode of headache that came on over half an hour or longer, perhaps depending on the interval after which the history is taken. And even if the headache really comes on within seconds or minutes, this is not specific for ruptured aneurysms, or even for SAH in general. The reason is that in general practice, exceptional forms of common headaches outnumber common forms of a rare disease, in this case a ruptured aneurysm. This is one of the many examples of the risk paradox (section 18.5).[200] Another, more striking example is that most children with Down syndrome are born of mothers under 30 years old, despite older mothers being at higher risk. In the same way, most patients with ischaemic stroke are not severely hypertensive, etc. Given that the incidence of aneurysmal haemorrhage is about 10 per 100 000 population per year, a family physician with a practice of 2000 people will, on average, see only one such patient every five years.

Patients with rare manifestations of common headache syndromes (i.e. sudden onset of migraine) probably outnumber those with common manifestations of rare headache syndromes (i.e. sudden headache in subarachnoid haemorrhage).

> Patients with headache may present not only to general practitioners but also to an accident and emergency department where they make up around 1% of all attendances. The proportion with a serious neurological condition ranges from 16% for all patients with any headache, to 75% for those with sudden headache specifically referred to a neurologist.[201]

The exact speed of onset of 'sudden' headache, seconds or minutes, in patients without any other deficits, is of little help for the hospital physician in distinguishing aneurysmal haemorrhage from innocuous headaches, or from non-aneurysmal perimesencephalic haemorrhage (section 9.1.2). The predictive value of the speed of onset (seconds vs 1–5 min) can be calculated from two data sets. First, SAH from ruptured aneurysms is nine times as common as non-aneurysmal perimesencephalic haemorrhage[203] and in hospital series these two forms of SAH together are twice as common as innocuous headaches.[202] Second, headache develops almost instantaneously in 50% of patients with aneurysmal SAH, in 35% of patients with non-aneurysmal perimesencephalic haemorrhage, and in 68% of patients with benign 'thunderclap headaches'; for an onset within 1–5 min these proportions are 19%, 35% and 19%, respectively.[194] If, for the sake of simplicity, we ignore patients with sudden headache from other serious (non-haemorrhagic) brain disease, such as intracranial venous thrombosis,[204] a simple calculation leads to the disappointing conclusion that an onset within seconds correctly predicts aneurysmal haemorrhage in only 55%, and that headache onset in 5–10 min correctly predicts innocuous headache in only 30%.

The headache of SAH usually lasts 1–2 weeks, sometimes longer. We do not know exactly how short in duration a headache may be and still be due to SAH. However, we have not come across anyone with a headache due to proven SAH that resolved within 1 h. However, since there is no prospective study that has

addressed this question it is still conceivable that this may occur, so it is perhaps best to consider SAH in anyone with a sudden unusually severe headache that lasts longer than – shall we say – 1 h?

In brief, there are no single or combined features of the headache that distinguish reliably, and at an early stage, between SAH and innocuous types of sudden headache. The discomfort and cost of referring most patients for a brief consultation in hospital (which should include CT scanning and a delayed lumbar puncture if the scan is negative) is probably outweighed by avoidance of the potential disaster of missing a ruptured aneurysm and the patient later being admitted with rebleeding, or another secondary complication.

> There is no feature of the headache that distinguishes reliably, and at an early stage, between subarachnoid haemorrhage and innocuous types of sudden headache. Therefore, although most people with a sudden severe headache have not had a subarachnoid haemorrhage, they must all be investigated to exclude this diagnosis.

A biphasic headache may occur in patients whose SAH is due to dissection of a vertebral artery (section 9.1.3): first, a severe occipital headache radiating from the back of the neck, followed after an interval of hours or days by sudden exacerbation of the headache but of a more diffuse type.

A history of one or more previous episodes of sudden-onset headache ('sentinel headaches') is generally believed to be common in patients with aneurysmal SAH and these are often attributed to a 'warning leak' of the finally rupturing aneurysm. However, the notion of 'minor leaks' does not really hold up (section 9.2.4).

> It is doubtful if patients with aneurysmal subarachnoid haemorrhage often have preceding and unrecognized 'warning leaks'. Whatever the case, doctors must be educated to consider subarachnoid haemorrhage in any patient who reports a sudden severe headache.

Vomiting

Vomiting (and nausea) is common at the outset, in contrast to other differential diagnoses, such as migraine, in which vomiting more often comes after the headache starts.

Neck stiffness

Meningism refers to painful resistance to passive or voluntary neck flexion, mainly because of irritation of the cervical meninges by subarachnoid blood, or by inflammation. This sign can be elicited in the supine patient by placing both hands behind the patient's head and, as one attempts to lift the head up off the pillow the patient does not allow the neck to be flexed and so the examiner lifts the patient's head, neck and shoulders off the bed, as if the patient were like a board. In contrast, passive rotation of the neck is achieved with ease.

Neck stiffness is a common symptom and sign of blood in the subarachnoid space, but it does not occur immediately; it takes some 3–12 hours to appear and may not develop at all in deeply unconscious patients, or in patients with minor SAH.[205] Therefore, its absence cannot exclude the diagnosis of SAH in a patient with sudden headache. Brudzinski's sign (flexion at the hip and knee in response to forward flexion of the neck) is also associated with blood in the subarachnoid space but its sensitivity and specificity in this context are unknown.

Pain and stiffness in the back and legs may follow SAH after some hours or days because blood irritates the lumbosacral nerve roots. We know of one patient who was admitted during a weekend because of a sudden headache; on the following Monday, when seen by a new resident, he complained of pain in the back of his legs, but his notes could not be found (they were discovered only later, buried under a pile of X-rays). He was worked up for a back problem, but he suddenly died from what turned out to be rebleeding from a ruptured aneurysm.

Photophobia

Patients are often photophobic and irritable for several days after SAH.

Loss of consciousness

Loss of consciousness occurred in 50% of a large group of patients with presumed aneurysmal SAH who were well enough to be entered into a clinical trial of medical treatment.[206] As these figures did not include the 10% or so of patients with SAH who die at home or during transportation to hospital,[207] or the 20% who reach hospital and die within the first 24 h,[208] it is likely that at least 60% of all patients with SAH lose consciousness at, or soon after, onset. The patient may regain alertness and orientation or may remain with various degrees of lethargy, confusion, agitation or obtundation. An acute confusional state can occur and be misinterpreted as psychological in origin (grimacing, spitting, making sucking or kissing sounds, spluttering, singing, whistling, yelling and screaming).[209–211]

The impaired consciousness may be caused by the large amount of blood in the subarachnoid space, the reduced cerebral blood flow caused by the sudden increase in cerebrospinal fluid pressure, or by a complication of SAH such as brain displacement by haematoma or hydrocephalus, or a fall in systemic blood pressure or arterial oxygen concentration.

Epileptic seizures

Epileptic seizures (partial or generalized) may occasionally occur at onset or subsequently, as a result of irritation or damage to the cerebral cortex by the subarachnoid and any intracerebral blood. In the Oxfordshire Community Stroke Project, two of the 33 patients (6%) with SAH had an epileptic seizure at onset, but neither had later seizures.[97] Data from other series indicate that about 10% of patients with SAH develop epileptic seizures, most occurring on the first day of the SAH, but one-third not having their first seizure until 6 months later and one-third even more than a year later.[212–215] The only independent predictors of epilepsy after SAH are a large amount of cisternal blood on brain CT, and rebleeding.[213]

Subhyaloid haemorrhage

Intraocular haemorrhage develops in approximately 20% of patients with a ruptured aneurysm and may also complicate non-aneurysmal SAH, or intracranial haemorrhage in general. The haemorrhage is caused by a sustained increase in the pressure of the cerebrospinal fluid, with obstruction of the central retinal vein as it traverses the optic nerve sheath, in turn leading to congestion of the retinal veins.[216] Mostly, the haemorrhages appear at the time of aneurysmal rupture, but exceptionally later without evidence of aneurysmal rebleeding. Linear streaks of blood or flame-shaped haemorrhages appear in the pre-retinal layer (subhyaloid), usually near the optic disc (Fig. 3.47); one-third lie at the periphery.[217] If large, the pre-retinal haemorrhage may extend into the vitreous body (Terson syndrome; section 14.10.1). Patients may complain of large brown blobs obscuring their vision.

Focal neurological signs

Focal neurological signs may occur when an aneurysm has compressed a cranial nerve or has bled into the brain substance, causing an intracerebral haematoma (section 9.3.6). Sometimes, therefore, the clinical manifestations of a ruptured aneurysm may be indistinguishable from a stroke syndrome due to intracerebral haemorrhage or

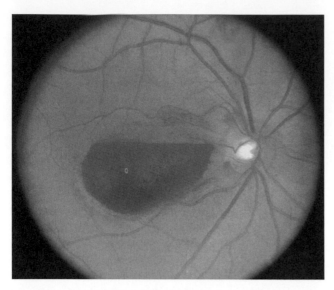

Fig. 3.47 Ocular fundus of a patient with subhyaloid haemorrhage, appearing as sharply demarcated linear streaks of brick red-coloured blood or flame-shaped haemorrhage in the preretinal layer, adjacent to the optic disc and spreading out from the optic disc. Also reproduced in colour in the plate section.

cerebral infarction, particularly if little or no blood has entered the subarachnoid space.

Systemic features

Fever, hypertension, albuminuria, glycosuria and electrocardiographic (ECG) changes may be present in the acute phase. Pyrexia rarely exceeds 38.5°C during the first 2–3 days, but thereafter it may rise to over 39°C, presumably due to accumulation of breakdown products of blood in the subarachnoid space; the pulse rate is not raised concomitantly.[218]

> The important distinguishing feature between pyrexia due to blood in the subarachnoid space and pyrexia due to intercurrent infection is the pulse rate; it remains disproportionately low in the former and rises with the latter.

Hypertension is a well-established risk factor for SAH;[219] a quarter to one-third of patients have a history of hypertension.[206,220] On admission, about 50% of patients with aneurysmal SAH have a markedly raised blood pressure. Unfortunately, high blood pressure is found in many patients presenting to an accident and emergency department for any reason, which makes the predictive value of blood pressure readings in that situation abysmally low. In many patients this raised blood pressure is a reactive phenomenon, and not a marker of long-standing hypertension; often the blood pressure

returns to normal within a few days. The blood pressure changes probably serve to counteract the decrease in cerebral perfusion resulting from increased cerebrospinal fluid pressure and later ischaemia (section 14.3.1).

Cardiac arrhythmias and ECG abnormalities are common after SAH (section 14.9.3).[221] The mechanism is unexplained but is thought to be sustained sympathetic stimulation, perhaps caused by dysfunction of the insular cortex, which results in reversible structural neurogenic damage to the myocardium, such as contraction bands, focal myocardial necrosis and subendocardial ischaemia.

3.7.2 Differential diagnosis

The abrupt onset of a severe headache may not only be caused by subarachnoid haemorrhage (SAH), but also by several other conditions, such as meningitis or encephalitis, intracerebral haemorrhage (particularly posterior fossa haemorrhage), obstruction of the cerebral ventricles, intracranial venous thrombosis, a rapid rise in blood pressure and, finally, a variety of alarming but innocuous conditions.[222] Associated features such as female sex, the presence of seizures, loss of consciousness or focal symptoms, vomiting, or exertion at onset increases the probability of aneurysmal SAH,[194] but the predictive value of these characteristics is far from helpful. Only a sudden headache during sleep should suggest hypnic headache (see below).

Acute painful neck conditions to be distinguished from meningism

Meningism may be a feature of SAH, meningitis, a posterior fossa mass and cerebellar tonsillar coning. However, it characteristically disappears as coma deepens. Other causes of a painful or stiff neck include bony lesions (i.e. trauma or arthritis) and ligamentous strain in the neck, extrapyramidal rigidity, systemic infections such as pneumonia, cervical lymphadenitis, parotitis, tonsillitis and upper lobe pneumonia. However, it is usually quite easy to distinguish meningism from these other acute painful neck conditions. For example, pain arising from the cervical spine may not only be felt in the neck and back of the head but also in the shoulder and arm, it is often evoked or exacerbated by certain movements or positions of the neck other than flexion, and there is usually tenderness to palpation over segments of the cervical spine.

Meningitis

Meningitis is an acute febrile illness that usually presents subacutely over 1 or 2 days with generalized headache, meningism, photophobia and fever. However, it can be difficult to distinguish from SAH if the patient is found confused or comatose, with marked neck stiffness and no available history. Clues to the diagnosis of meningitis include a high fever, tachycardia and a purpuric skin rash (meningococcal meningitis). If the patient is fully conscious and has no focal neurological signs and if meningitis is suspected, a lumbar puncture should be done immediately. But if the patient is very ill, antibiotics and steroids should be given at once, i.e. after venepuncture for blood cultures but before proceeding to brain CT and then, if no blood or intracranial mass is seen, a cerebrospinal fluid examination (section 3.7.3).

Cerebellar stroke

Cerebellar stroke often gives rise to sudden severe headache, particularly if it is haemorrhagic, and also to nausea and vomiting, but is usually accompanied by neurological symptoms and signs, such as vertigo, dysarthria and unsteadiness, which help distinguish it from SAH. However, if the lesion is large, the patient may present in coma due to direct brainstem compression or obstruction of cerebrospinal fluid flow from the fourth ventricle, causing hydrocephalus and raised intracranial pressure, or there may be meningism without signs of definite brainstem dysfunction. In a consecutive series of 100 patients with an initial diagnosis of subarachnoid haemorrhage, eight had a cerebellar haematoma (and another seven had supratentorial intracerebral haemorrhage).[223] Urgent brain CT is required to confirm the diagnosis of cerebellar haematoma, and lumbar puncture should certainly not be done; indeed, lumbar puncture should almost always be preceded by brain CT in unconscious patients, even if there are no focal signs of a mass lesion and no clinical evidence of raised intracranial pressure (such as papilloedema).

Intracerebral haemorrhage

More than 50% of patients with spontaneous intracerebral haemorrhage have headache at onset, particularly those with superficial lobar haemorrhages, but the headache is generally not as strikingly sudden in onset as SAH.[89] Furthermore, focal neurological deficits are almost always present, but they can also occur in about 20–30% of aneurysmal SAHs where there is intraparenchymal extension of the haemorrhage.[224] Conversely, some intracerebral haemorrhages, particularly those which are deep, have less prominent focal neurological signs and can easily be mistaken for SAH. CT brain scanning is always required.

Intraventricular haemorrhage

Intraventricular haemorrhage, which may arise within the ventricles or from immediately beneath the ependymal lining, or by extension from an intracerebral haemorrhage (i.e. from a caudate haemorrhage or ruptured subependymal vascular malformation into the intraventricular system), may mimic SAH (section 9.1.5). Also, intraventricular haemorrhage may occur together with SAH, usually from a ruptured aneurysm, most frequently at the anterior communicating artery complex. Patients present with sudden severe headache, confusion, vomiting or collapse with loss of consciousness.[225] Again, brain CT or MR scan is required for diagnosis during life.

Carotid or vertebral artery dissection

Dissection of the wall of the internal carotid artery may cause a fairly distinctive headache syndrome, which is ipsilateral, involving the forehead, periorbital region, face, teeth or neck, and has a burning or throbbing quality (section 7.2.1.). The headache may be associated with an ipsilateral Horner's syndrome or monocular blindness, and with contralateral focal neurological symptoms or signs. Dissection of the wall of the vertebral artery generally causes pain in the upper posterior neck and occiput, usually on one side, and may be associated with symptoms and signs of posterior circulation ischaemia, such as the lateral medullary syndrome. Transmural dissection of an intracranial artery can cause SAH (section 9.1.3).

Acute obstructive hydrocephalus

Any acute obstruction of the flow of cerebrospinal fluid causes headache through a rapid increase in intracranial pressure. The headache is commonly bilateral and exacerbated by coughing, sneezing, straining or head movement. Intermittent obstructive hydrocephalus may therefore cause severe paroxysmal headaches. A colloid cyst of the third ventricle is the classical cause of this syndrome; sometimes more than one family member is affected.[226] A decreased level of consciousness may follow the headache.[227] The outcome can be lethal if a diagnosis is not made.[228] Brain CT or MRI usually identifies the offending lesion (Fig. 3.48).

Migraine

Migraine headache can sometimes arise suddenly ('crash' migraine), be severe and prostrating, unilateral or generalized, and associated with photophobia, irritability,

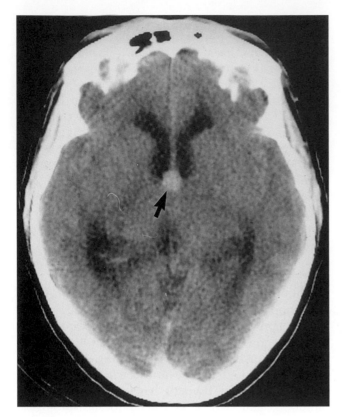

Fig. 3.48 CT brain scan showing a tumour in the third ventricle (*arrow*) at the foramen of Monro, causing obstructive hydrocephalus.

mild confusion, anorexia, mild fever, extraocular muscle palsy (ophthalmoplegic migraine) or symptoms of brainstem disturbance (basilar migraine) and thus be mistaken for SAH. However, migraineurs generally have a past or, less diagnostically helpful, a family history of migraine and the headache is commonly unilateral and throbbing, not so rapid in onset and of shorter duration than the headache of SAH.[86] Vomiting tends to start well into the migraine attack, in contrast to SAH, in which it commonly occurs at or soon after onset of the headache.

Idiopathic stabbing headache

Three specific varieties of sudden sharp stabbing headache have been described: ice-pick-like pains, 'jabs and jolts syndrome' and ophthalmodynia.[229,230] The pains are mostly at the temples or orbits but on occasion are elsewhere in the head.[231] Migraineurs are particularly susceptible.[231] Precipitants – which are seldom present – may be postural change, physical exercise, or head motion. As these pains are transient and lancinating, they are unlikely to be confused with the headache of SAH. The mechanism is unknown.

'Exploding head' syndrome

Clusters of attacks characterized by a sensation of sudden noise in the head and terror, rather than pain, can strike individuals over the age of 50 years, particularly during the twilight of sleep.[232,233] The cause is uncertain.

Cough headache

Idiopathic cough headache is defined as head pain brought on by coughing or other Valsalva manoeuvres, but not by prolonged physical exercise, in the absence of any intracranial disorder.[234,235] It is probably caused by distension of venous structures in the brain. It is a sudden-onset headache and lasts from 1 s to 30 min, tends to be bilateral and posterior, does not begin earlier than the fifth decade of life, is more frequent in men, is not accompanied by other neurological manifestations and often responds to indomethacin. These clinical characteristics allow its differential diagnosis from posterior fossa lesions, especially herniation of the cerebellar tonsils (Chiari-I malformation), even though a craniocervical magnetic resonance imaging study is useful to rule this out.

Hypnic headache

This type of headache has only been recognized recently.[236,237] It wakes patients up in the middle of the night, 2–6 h after sleep onset; it is usually diffuse and bilateral, or in the neck. It occurs almost exclusively in middle age, twice as often in women as in men. Patients usually get out of bed and walk around until the pain subsides, within 10 min to 3 h. Typically the attacks are recurrent, from once a week to 6 times per night. There are no known precipitating factors, there is no photophobia, phonophobia or nausea and there are no concomitant autonomic features, such as in cluster headache or chronic paroxysmal hemicrania.

Post-traumatic headache

Immediately after a head injury there is often headache; this may be pulsating and made worse by head movement, jolting, coughing, sneezing and straining.[229] Normally the headache gradually disappears as the soft and any bony tissue damage resolves. In a series of 200 patients admitted to hospital with head injury only 83 still had a headache by a day or so afterwards; only 22 of those 83 (11% of all patients) complained spontaneously, and only three required an analgesic.[238]

The diagnosis of post-traumatic headache should not be confused with SAH if there is a history of head injury, but the patient may be amnesic and there may be no witness, in which case acute head injury with secondary bleeding into the subarachnoid space can be confused with spontaneous SAH.

> If the circumstances of a traumatic head injury are unclear, and there is a reasonable chance that spontaneous intracranial haemorrhage was the cause of the accident and so the head injury, then brain CT should be done as soon as the patient's condition allows, regardless of the severity of the head injury.

Benign orgasmic cephalalgia and benign exertional headache

Acute, severe, explosive occipital or generalized headache, usually occurring at the moment of sexual orgasm or during strenuous exercise (benign orgasmic cephalalgia and benign exertional headache, respectively) may mimic SAH.[196,239,240] The history of onset during sexual intercourse (or masturbation) may not be forthcoming without specific and sensitive enquiry. Points in favour of the diagnosis are a history of similar previous sexual or exertional headaches, no alteration in consciousness, short duration of the headache (minutes to hours) and no signs of meningeal irritation such as neck stiffness, or low back pain, and nor sciatica in the ambulant patient. These headaches can occur at any time in life and do not necessarily occur every time the patient experiences orgasm, or exercises strenuously. If patients present soon after their first-ever sudden orgasmic headache, it is not possible to exclude SAH without brain CT and lumbar puncture. If a patient presents after recurrent attacks, and the history is characteristic, investigation is seldom necessary.

Reaction to monoamine oxidase inhibitor drugs

People taking classic monoamine oxidase inhibitors (MAOIs), of which phenelzine and tranylcypromine are the most commonly used, may experience sudden severe headache after ingesting sympathomimetic agents, red wine or foods with a high tyramine content, such as mature cheese, pickled herrings, game and yeast extract. This is because MAOIs irreversibly block the ability of both MAO isoforms (A and B) to metabolize dietary tyramine in the liver (A) and gut wall (B). The combination of a classic MAOI and oral tyramine can provoke dangerous hypertension. The headache tends to be over the occipital region of the head and is associated with a rapid rise in blood pressure. It can be relieved by the alpha noradrenergic blocking agent, phentolamine.

Phaeochromocytoma

Patients with a phaeochromocytoma experience acute pressor reactions; in about 80% of attacks they complain of headache[241,242] often in combination with palpitations or sweating.[243] The headache is usually of sudden onset, bilateral, severe and throbbing. It appears to be related to a rapid increase in blood pressure and lasts less than an hour in about 75% of patients, but it may last from a few minutes to a few hours. Some patients may collapse with loss of consciousness or develop focal neurological signs during the episode, as a result of cerebral oedema or sometimes haemorrhage. Attacks may be provoked by exertion, straining, emotional upset, worry or excitement.[242]

The diagnosis depends on clinical suspicion being aroused when the history is first taken (which can be difficult because the condition is so rare) and is confirmed by finding increased excretion of catecholamines (metanephrine and vanillylmandelic acid) in three 24-h specimens of urine, or raised plasma free metanephrine or normetanephrine levels during the attack.[244] The blood sugar is usually raised at the time of the attack, a useful distinction from hypoglycaemic attacks, which may simulate phaeochromocytoma because of secondary release of adrenaline in response to low blood sugar. The tumour may arise at any point along the line of development of the sympathetic chain from the neck to the pelvis and scrotum.

Headache may also reflect idiopathic surges of hypertension, not associated with phaechromocytoma or any other identifiable condition.[245]

Occipital neuralgia

Occipital neuralgia is characterized by an aching or paroxysmal jabbing pain in the posterior neck and occipital region in the distribution of the greater or lesser occipital nerves (Fig. 3.49). It may rarely present quite dramatically, like SAH,[246] but there is usually diminished sensation or dysaesthesiae of the affected area (C2 distribution), focal tenderness over the point where the greater occipital nerve trunk crosses the superior nuchal line, and a therapeutic response to infiltration of local anaesthetic near the tender area on the nerve trunk.

Benign 'thunderclap headache'

'Thunderclap headache' is not a true disease entity, but a convenient term to describe unclassifiable varieties of sudden-onset, severe, generalized pain in the head, sometimes with vomiting.[247] It may last up to a day or so. Clinically, the syndrome cannot be reliably distinguished

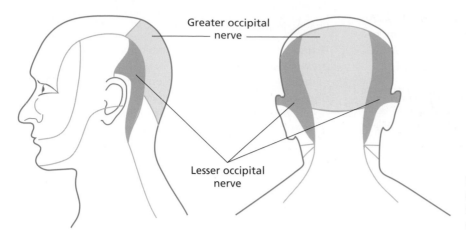

Fig. 3.49 Diagram showing the anatomical distribution of the sensory innervation of the greater and lesser occipital nerves.

from SAH, but the chances of aneurysmal SAH are increased in the presence of female gender, epileptic seizures, loss of consciousness at onset, focal neurological symptoms (e.g. diplopia), vomiting or exertion preceding the onset of headache.[194] The diagnosis is therefore made by exclusion, mainly of SAH. About 50% of these patients have a history of typical migraine or tension-type headache (with gradual onset).

The prognosis is benign; a 3-year follow-up of 71 patients seen in hospital found identical recurrences in 12, again without evidence of SAH, whereas nearly 50% developed episodes of more obvious migraine or tension headache.[248] Of 93 such patients identified in general practice and followed up for a median of 5 years, again none suffered SAH; recurrent attacks of 'thunderclap headache' occurred in eight patients, and 13 developed new tension headache or migraine.[249]

> Headache is common in clinical practice, but 'thunderclap' headache is not. No physical sign can definitely exclude subarachnoid haemorrhage if a sudden onset headache persists for a few hours.

3.7.3 Investigations to confirm the diagnosis of subarachnoid haemorrhage

Investigations are essential in making the diagnosis of subarachnoid haemorrhage (SAH), given the clinical features are relatively non-specific.[250]

Brain CT scan

All patients presenting with a suspected recent SAH (i.e. within the last few days) should initially have an urgent brain CT to determine:

• whether there is blood in the subarachnoid space;

• the site of any SAH or intracerebral or intraventricular haemorrhage and therefore the likely cause (section 9.4.1 and Fig. 3.50);

• the presence of any complications, such as hydrocephalus;

• any contraindications to lumbar puncture such as cerebral oedema or haematoma with brain shift, or a large cerebellar infarct, when there is no blood evident on CT;

• and whether there is any other intracranial abnormality that may account for the symptoms and signs.

The sensitivity of CT in SAH depends on the amount of subarachnoid blood, the resolution of the scanner, the skills of the radiologist and the timing of the CT after symptom onset. The sensitivity is greatest in the first few days and falls thereafter, as blood in the subarachnoid space is resorbed (Fig. 9.19). In fact, the term 'resorption' may not always be appropriate to describe this process, diffusion and sedimentation being other explanations. CT evidence of subarachnoid blood can disappear very rapidly. If brain CT is done within 1–2 days after SAH onset, extravasated blood will be demonstrated in more than 95% of patients.[202] But the chance of finding subarachnoid blood on brain CT then decreases sharply, to 50% on day 7, 20% on day 9, and almost nil after 10 days.[251,252]

> If brain CT is done within 1–2 days after subarachnoid haemorrhage onset, extravasated blood will be demonstrated in more than 95% of patients.

Of course, minute amounts of subarachnoid blood may be overlooked by the uninitiated (Fig. 3.51). Depending on the amount of blood in the cisterns and the delay before scanning, an 'absent' or 'missing' (isodense)

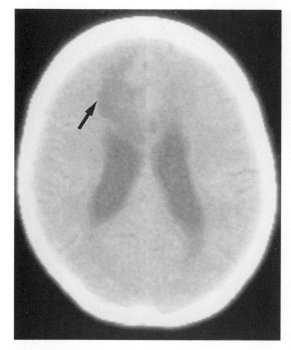

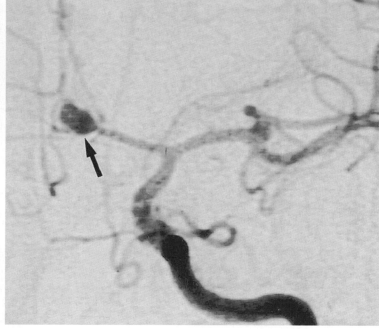

Fig. 3.50 Brain CT scan (a) showing a 2- or 3-week-old intracerebral haemorrhage in the frontal lobes (*arrow*) of a patient who presented with an acute behavioural disorder and was misdiagnosed as being a hysterical alcoholic. Subsequent catheter angiography (b) revealed an anterior communicating artery aneurysm (*arrow*) which had ruptured and bled into the frontal lobes.

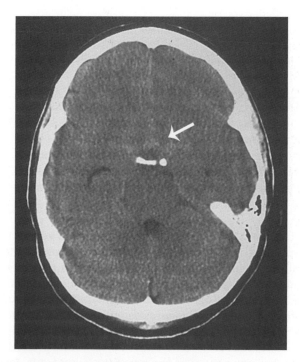

Fig. 3.51 CT brain scan showing a subtle amount of subarachnoid blood in the anterior part of the interhemispheric fissure (*arrow*), from a ruptured aneurysm of the anterior communicating artery.

cistern, or absent cortical sulci, may be the only clue to the presence of subarachnoid blood (Fig. 3.52).

> If subarachnoid haemorrhage is suspected and yet the brain CT scan appears normal, look carefully at the interpeduncular cistern, ambient cisterns, quadrigeminal cistern, the region of the anterior communicating artery and posterior inferior cerebellar artery, the posterior horns of the lateral ventricles and the cortical sulci. If blood is present in these sites, it may be isodense or slightly hyperdense, and hence the normally hypodense cisterns and sulci may be difficult to see and seem 'absent'.

Haemorrhage from an intracranial aneurysm can result not only in SAH but also in an intracerebral haemorrhage, which is easily seen on plain CT and generally persists for longer than subarachnoid blood, because the resorption of intraparenchymal blood, as seen on CT, occurs over several days to weeks rather than a few days.[251] However, small intracerebral haemorrhages can also resolve very quickly, within days (section 5.4.1). About one-quarter of unselected patients who reach hospital alive after aneurysmal haemorrhage have an intracerebral haemorrhage on CT.[224,251]

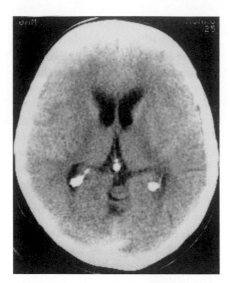

Fig. 3.52 Brain CT scan of a patient with subarachnoid haemorrhage showing isodense blood in the cortical sulci giving the appearance of 'absent' sulci. In particular, the sylvian fissures are not seen because they are filled with just enough blood to raise the density of the cerebrospinal fluid to that of brain parenchyma.

False positive evidence of SAH on CT scans

A false positive diagnosis of SAH may be made on the CT brain scan, for example in patients who are comatose and brain dead (i.e. have no cerebral blood flow at the time of the scan). The CT scan not only shows cerebral oedema, but hyperdense material in the subarachnoid space which represents blood in congested subarachnoid blood vessels[253–255](Fig. 3.53). Increased density of the tentorium and basal cisterns as a false positive sign of SAH on an unenhanced CT scan has also been described in polycythaemia,[256] purulent meningitis,[257] subdural haematoma,[258,259] gliomatosis cerebri[260] and spontaneous intracranial hypotension.[261]

Lumbar puncture

According to a consecutive series from the Netherlands, the negative predictive value of CT scanning performed within 12 h of onset of sudden headache is 97%.[202] In other words, there is an important small minority (of about 3%) with sudden headache and normal CT within 12 h who *do* have xanthochromia in the cerebrospinal fluid, and in whom angiography subsequently confirms a ruptured aneurysm. Therefore a lumbar puncture is necessary in any patient with sudden headache and a normal CT scan, even though the results will be normal in most patients.

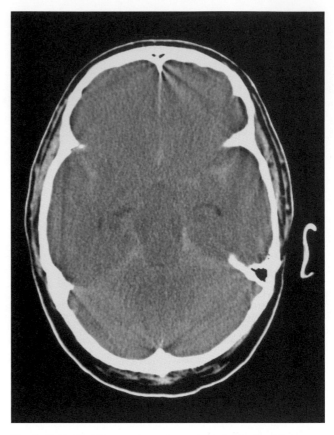

Fig. 3.53 Brain CT scan of a patient who is brain dead from general hypoxia. There is generalized oedema, with effacement of the cisternal cerebrospinal fluid spaces. These spaces appear hyperdense, through venous stasis, which may falsely suggest subarachnoid haemorrhage.

> Always do a lumbar puncture if the history is suggestive of subarachnoid haemorrhage and the CT scan (performed early, within a few days) is normal. Frequently, the cerebrospinal fluid will be normal too, but occasionally in this setting an abnormal cerebrospinal fluid will provide the only evidence of subarachnoid haemorrhage.

Lumbar puncture without prior brain CT is potentially dangerous in patients with an intracerebral haemorrhage.[262] Brain herniation may occur even in patients without focal signs or a decreased level of consciousness.[263]

Once the decision has been taken to do a lumbar puncture, the next requirement is to do it well. This is more difficult than it seems. Before drawing cerebrospinal fluid, the first rule is to wait until at least 6 and preferably 12 h have elapsed after the headache onset. This delay is absolutely essential because if cerebrospinal fluid obtained earlier turns out to be blood-stained, it is absolutely and irrevocably impossible to distinguish between blood that was there before (genuine SAH) and blood that was introduced by the needle (a bloody tap). With pre-existing blood in the cerebrospinal fluid, bilirubin will have been formed in the interval from SAH onset, from the breakdown of erythrocytes in the cerebrospinal fluid (see below), but of course not with a traumatic tap. A false positive diagnosis of SAH can be almost as damaging as a missed one, because insurance companies are bound to remain wary, despite negative investigations for an aneurysm. Never believe a colleague, however senior, who tells you that 'the tap went so smoothly, it is impossible that the blood was traumatic'. Even the smoothest puncture can hit a vein. Also the 'three-tube test' (a decrease in red blood cells in consecutive tubes) is notoriously unreliable.[264] Immediately proceeding with CT or MR angiography in all patients with bloodstained cerebrospinal fluid is not a good idea either, despite some people advocating this way of circumventing the 'bloody tap' problem: a small (<5 mm) unruptured aneurysm can be expected in every 50th adult and should in most cases be left untreated.

> It is a widely held myth that the distinction between subarachnoid haemorrhage and a traumatic 'bloody' tap can be made reliably by collecting the cerebrospinal fluid in three consecutive test tubes and counting the number of red cells in each tube.

Keeping patients in the emergency department or admitting them to hospital until 6–12 h after symptom onset may be a practical problem. However, there is no other option. If red cells have entered the cerebrospinal fluid during the headache episode, sufficient lysis will take place during that time for bilirubin and oxyhaemoglobin to be formed.[205] These pigments give the cerebrospinal fluid a yellow tinge after centrifugation (xanthochromia), a critical feature in the distinction from a traumatic tap; these pigments are almost invariably detectable until at least 2 weeks later.[265] Bilirubin is the most important pigment of the two, since it can be formed only *in vivo*, whereas haemoglobin can be broken down to oxyhaemoglobin in a test tube that has been left unattended for too long.

> Lumbar puncture should be done after a negative CT scan, but not until at least 6–12 h have elapsed since the onset of headache.

At least two test tubes should be filled with cerebrospinal fluid, with an extra tube for the microbiology laboratory if the fluid is not blood-stained but somewhat opaque (meningitis, after all?) while the tube is filling up. If the cerebrospinal fluid seems clear do not forget to measure the cerebrospinal fluid pressure, because sudden headache may be a first manifestation of intracranial venous thrombosis. After you have withdrawn the needle, had it properly disposed of and made sure your patient is comfortable, take a good look at the cerebrospinal fluid. There are roughly four possibilities:

- the cerebrospinal fluid is blood-stained;
- it is colourless but not clear;
- it is clear but there is some colour (mostly yellowish or pink);
- or it is crystal-clear.

So there are essentially two qualities to the fluid: colour and clarity. Clarity refers only to whether one can see through the tube, irrespective of the colour (a good glass of Bourgogne rouge is red but clear).

Each cerebrospinal fluid specimen should be sent to the clinical chemistry laboratory. If it is colourless, the cells should be counted. If there are no or only a few (<100) red cells, a recent SAH has been ruled out. And if there are no white cells and the pressure is normal, the patient can be sent home. If the cerebrospinal fluid is blood-stained, ask the laboratory to spin it down immediately at appropriate speed and to call you when they have done so. It is perhaps unconventional but absolutely essential that you go to the laboratory yourself to have a look at the supernatant after centrifugation and to compare it in bright light with water in a similar test tube, against a white background. If the supernatant is yellow, the diagnosis of subarachnoid haemorrhage is certain – though the cause of course still needs to be determined.

> Blood-stained cerebrospinal fluid should be immediately centrifuged; if the supernatant is yellow this proves haemorrhage. Xanthochromia is almost invariably found between 12 h and 2 weeks after subarachnoid haemorrhage.

Of course the presence of bilirubin can be confirmed by spectrophotometry the next day. This test should certainly be performed if one is in any doubt and perhaps even if the supernatant seems crystal-clear, although many neurologists can confidently exclude xanthochromia by visual inspection alone.[266] The specimen should be stored in darkness, preferably wrapped in tinfoil because the ultraviolet components of daylight can break down bilirubin – not only in icteric newborns but also in test tubes.

Spectrophotometry can confirm the presence of bilirubin.[267] In most cases this is accompanied by oxyhaemoglobin, but the presence of oxyhaemoglobin alone is irrelevant to the diagnosis of SAH. Although the sensitivity and specificity of spectrophotometry have not yet been confirmed in a series of patients with suspected SAH and a negative CT scan,[268] it is the best technique currently available.

Late presentation with a history of sudden headache

It is not uncommon in clinical practice to encounter patients who describe having had a severe headache of sudden onset 3 weeks (or more) ago, sounding very much like an SAH, which resolved after a few hours or days. If patients present 2 weeks or more after an episode of sudden headache, the diagnostic value of a normal CT scan is very limited. A lumbar puncture showing crystal-clear cerebrospinal fluid with no bilirubin on spectrophotometry will generally suffice to exclude SAH, provided the interval is not more than 1 week. With an initially positive CT scan, the cerebrospinal fluid is invariably xanthochromic for 2 weeks,[265] but the point has been made that xanthochromia may not last as long in the 5% of patients with SAH in whom early CT scanning is negative.[268] Indeed there is a report of a patient with aneurysmal rupture in whom not only CT scanning was normal on day 7, but also the cerebrospinal fluid, on the next day.[269]

In a patient presenting late, if there has been associated loss of consciousness, or if the patient has been severely ill for several days, the probability of a ruptured aneurysm is considerable, and there is a good case for angiography, at least CT angiography (section 9.4.4). The issue of distinguishing patients with non-haemorrhagic 'thunderclap headache' from those with ruptured aneurysms has been unnecessarily complicated by a few case reports of impressive but rare events. There is one report of fatal aneurysmal rupture in which the presence of iron-containing macrophages was interpreted as evidence of an earlier haemorrhage, in a patient with a preceding episode of headache.[270] This interpretation is questionable, as the patient survived the second episode for a few days. A second type of case report, exemplified by two patients from different sources, relates that an aneurysm can be found on cerebral angiography in patients with sudden headache and negative findings on CT as well as on lumbar puncture, accompanied by arterial narrowing.[271,272] At operation no evidence of haemorrhage around the aneurysm was found in either case, but it was claimed that the aneurysm had suddenly enlarged, without rupturing. Although a growing aneurysm may occasionally cause headache, a much more probable explanation is that in the course of life a few per cent of all adults develop asymptomatic aneurysms and that indiscriminate use of angiography is bound to reveal some of them (section 15.2.1). If it is assumed that the aneurysm was incidental in the two

case reports cited above, migraine might explain both the headache and the arterial narrowing ('vasospasm'). Segmental and fully reversible vasospasm has been demonstrated in patients with severe headache but without an aneurysm,[273] and even in a patient with benign exertional headache.[274] 'Thunderclap headache' does not warrant the potentially dangerous procedure of catheter angiography if both the CT scan and the cerebrospinal fluid are normal within 1 week of the event; CT angiography or MR angiography in 'late patients' should be reserved for those with a convincing history, e.g. having spent a few days in bed because of the headache.

> If a patient presents with a sudden severe headache and the CT scan and lumbar puncture are carried out in less than 1 week and are completely normal, with no evidence of intracranial haemorrhage, then cerebral catheter angiography is not indicated; CT or MR angiography should not be performed indiscriminately.

References

1 Hankey GJ, Slattery JM, Warlow CP. The prognosis of hospital-referred transient ischaemic attacks. *J Neurol Neurosurg Psychiatry* 1991; **54**(9):793–802.

2 Hankey GJ, Warlow CP. *Transient Ischaemic Attacks.* London: W.B. Saunders Company Ltd, 1994.

3 Ferro JM, Canhao P, Bousser MG, Stam J, Barinagarrementeria F. Cerebral vein and dural sinus thrombosis in elderly patients. *Stroke* 2005; **36**(9):1927–32.

4 van Gijn J. Cerebral venous thrombosis: pathogenesis, presentation and prognosis. *J R Soc Med* 2000; **93**(5):230–3.

5 Dennis MS, Bamford JM, Sandercock PA, Warlow CP. A comparison of risk factors and prognosis for transient ischemic attacks and minor ischemic strokes. The Oxfordshire Community Stroke Project. *Stroke* 1989; **20**(11):1494–9.

6 Dennis MS, Bamford JM, Sandercock PA, Warlow CP. Incidence of transient ischemic attacks in Oxfordshire, England. *Stroke* 1989; **20**(3):333–9.

7 Koudstaal PJ, van Gijn J, Frenken CW, Hijdra A, Lodder J, Vermeulen M *et al.* TIA, RIND, minor stroke: a continuum, or different subgroups? Dutch TIA Study Group. *J Neurol Neurosurg Psychiatry* 1992; **55**(2):95–7.

8 Johnston SC, Sidney S, Bernstein AL, Gress DR. A comparison of risk factors for recurrent TIA and stroke in patients diagnosed with TIA. *Neurology* 2003; **60**(2):280–5.

9 Rothwell PM, Buchan A, Johnston SC. Recent advances in management of transient ischaemic attacks and minor ischaemic strokes. *Lancet Neurol* 2006; **5**(4):323–31.

10 Johnston SC, Rothwell PM, Nguyen-Huynh MN, Giles MF, Elkins JS, Bernstein AL, Sidney S. Validation and refinement of scores to predict very early stroke risk after transient ischaemic attack. *Lancet* 2007; **369**:283–292.

11 Coutts SB, Simon JE, Eliasziw M, Sohn CH, Hill MD, Barber PA *et al.* Triaging transient ischemic attack and minor stroke patients using acute magnetic resonance imaging. *Ann Neurol* 2005; **57**(6):848–54.

12 Warach S, Kidwell CS. The redefinition of TIA: the uses and limitations of DWI in acute ischemic cerebrovascular syndromes. *Neurology* 2004; **62**(3):359–60.

13 Wardlaw JM, Farrall AJ. Diagnosis of stroke on neuroimaging. *Br Med J* 2004; **328**(7441):655–6.

14 Chalela JA, Kidwell CS, Nentwich LM, Luby M, Butman JA, Demchuk AM *et al.* Magnetic resonance imaging and computed tomography in emergency assessment of patients with suspected acute stroke: a prospective comparison. *Lancet* 2007; **369**:293–298.

15 Douglas VC, Johnston CM, Elkins J, Sidney S, Gress DR, Johnston SC. Head computed tomography findings predict short-term stroke risk after transient ischemic attack. *Stroke* 2003; **34**(12):2894–8.

16 Ay H, Oliveira-Filho J, Buonanno FS, Schaefer PW, Furie KL, Chang YC *et al.* 'Footprints' of transient ischemic attacks: a diffusion-weighted MRI study. *Cerebrovasc Dis* 2002; **14**(3–4):177–86.

17 Rovira A, Rovira-Gols A, Pedraza S, Grive E, Molina C, varez-Sabin J. Diffusion-weighted MR imaging in the acute phase of transient ischemic attacks. *Am J Neuroradiol* 2002; **23**(1):77–83.

18 Schulz UG, Briley D, Meagher T, Molyneux A, Rothwell PM. Diffusion-weighted MRI in 300 patients presenting late with subacute transient ischemic attack or minor stroke. *Stroke* 2004; **35**(11):2459–65.

19 Schulz UG, Briley D, Meagher T, Molyneux A, Rothwell PM. Abnormalities on diffusion weighted magnetic resonance imaging performed several weeks after a minor stroke or transient ischaemic attack. *J Neurol Neurosurg Psychiatry* 2003; **74**(6):734–8.

20 Lamy C, Oppenheim C, Calvet D, Domigo V, Naggara O, Meder JL *et al.* Diffusion-weighted MR imaging in transient ischaemic attacks. *Eur Radiol* 2006; **16**(5):1090–5.

21 Albers GW, Caplan LR, Easton JD, Fayad PB, Mohr JP, Saver JL *et al.* Transient ischemic attack: proposal for a new definition. *N Engl J Med* 2002; **347**(21):1713–16.

22 Easton JD, Albers GW, Caplan LR, Saver JL, Sherman DG. Discussion: Reconsideration of TIA terminology and definitions. *Neurology* 2004; **62**(8 Suppl 6):S29–S34.

23 Kidwell CS, Warach S. Acute ischemic cerebrovascular syndrome: diagnostic criteria. *Stroke* 2003; **34**(12):2995–8.

24 Ay H, Koroshetz WJ, Benner T, Vangel MG, Wu O, Schwamm LH *et al.* Transient ischemic attack with infarction: a unique syndrome? *Ann Neurol* 2005; **57**(5):679–86.

25 Saur D, Kucinski T, Grzyska U, Eckert B, Eggers C, Niesen W *et al.* Sensitivity and interrater agreement of CT and diffusion-weighted MR imaging in hyperacute stroke. *Am J Neuroradiol* 2003; **24**(5):878–85.

26 Purroy F, Montaner J, Rovira A, Delgado P, Quintana M, varez-Sabin J. Higher risk of further vascular events among transient ischemic attack patients with diffusion-weighted imaging acute ischemic lesions. *Stroke* 2004; **35**(10):2313–19.

27 Ovbiagele B, Kidwell CS, Saver JL. Epidemiological impact in the United States of a tissue-based definition of transient ischemic attack. *Stroke* 2003; **34**(4):919–24.

28 Hatano S. Experience from a multicentre stroke register: a preliminary report. *Bull World Health Organ* 1976; **54**(5):541–53.

29 Al-Shahi R, White PM, Davenport RJ, Lindsay KW. Subarachnoid haemorrhage. *Br Med J* 2006; **333**(7561):235–40.

30 Suarez JI, Tarr RW, Selman WR. Aneurysmal subarachnoid hemorrhage. *N Engl J Med* 2006; **354**(4):387–96.

31 Foerch C, Misselwitz B, Sitzer M, Berger K, Steinmetz H, Neumann-Haefelin T. Difference in recognition of right and left hemispheric stroke. *Lancet* 2005; **366**(9483):392–3.

32 Kipps CM, Hodges JR. Cognitive assessment for clinicians. *J Neurol Neurosurg Psychiatry* 2005; **76**(Suppl 1):i22–i30.

33 Fink JN. Underdiagnosis of right-brain stroke. *Lancet* 2005; **366**(9483):349–51.

34 Rothwell PM, Johnston SC. Transient ischemic attacks: stratifying risk. *Stroke* 2006; **37**(2):320–2.

35 Hankey GJ. Redefining risks after TIA and minor ischaemic stroke. *Lancet* 2005; **365**(9477):2065–6.

36 Johnston SC, Nguyen-Huynh MN, Schwarz ME, Fuller K, Williams CE, Josephson SA *et al.* National Stroke Association guidelines for the management of transient ischemic attacks. *Ann Neurol* 2006; **60**(3):301–13.

37 Hand PJ, Haisma JA, Kwan J, Lindley RI, Lamont B, Dennis MS *et al.* Interobserver agreement for the bedside clinical assessment of suspected stroke. *Stroke* 2006; **37**(3):776–80.

38 Caplan LR, Hon FK. Clinical diagnosis of patients with cerebrovascular disease. *Prim Care* 2004; **31**(1):95–109.

39 Kidwell CS, Starkman S, Eckstein M, Weems K, Saver JL. Identifying stroke in the field. Prospective validation of the Los Angeles prehospital stroke screen (LAPSS). *Stroke* 2000; **31**(1):71–6.

40 Bray JE, Martin J, Cooper G, Barger B, Bernard S, Bladin C. Paramedic identification of stroke: community validation of the melbourne ambulance stroke screen. *Cerebrovasc Dis* 2005; **20**(1):28–33.

41 Harbison J, Hossain O, Jenkinson D, Davis J, Louw SJ, Ford GA. Diagnostic accuracy of stroke referrals from primary care, emergency room physicians, and ambulance staff using the face arm speech test. *Stroke* 2003; **34**(1):71–6.

42 Nor AM, McAllister C, Louw SJ, Dyker AG, Davis M, Jenkinson D *et al.* Agreement between ambulance paramedic- and physician-recorded neurological signs with Face Arm Speech Test (FAST) in acute stroke patients. *Stroke* 2004; **35**(6):1355–9.

43 Kothari RU, Pancioli A, Liu T, Brott T, Broderick J. Cincinnati Prehospital Stroke Scale: reproducibility and validity. *Ann Emerg Med* 1999; **33**(4):373–8.

44 Hand PJ, Kwan J, Lindley RI, Dennis MS, Wardlaw JM. Distinguishing between stroke and mimic at the bedside: the brain attack study. *Stroke* 2006; **37**(3):769–75.

45 Nor AM, Davis J, Sen B, Shipsey D, Louw SJ, Dyker AG *et al.* The Recognition of Stroke in the Emergency Room (ROSIER) scale: development and validation of a stroke recognition instrument. *Lancet Neurol* 2005; **4**(11):727–34.

46 Dewey HM, Donnan GA, Freeman EJ, Sharples CM, Macdonell RA, McNeil JJ *et al.* Interrater reliability of the National Institutes of Health Stroke Scale: rating by neurologists and nurses in a community-based stroke incidence study. *Cerebrovasc Dis* 1999; **9**(6):323–7.

47 Rathore SS, Hinn AR, Cooper LS, Tyroler HA, Rosamond WD. Characterization of incident stroke signs and symptoms: findings from the atherosclerosis risk in communities study. *Stroke* 2002; **33**(11):2718–21.

48 Dennis MS, Bamford JM, Sandercock PA, Warlow CP. Lone bilateral blindness: a transient ischaemic attack. *Lancet* 1989; **1**(8631):185–8.

49 Goldstein LB, Simel DL. Is this patient having a stroke? *J Am Med Assoc* 2005; **293**(19):2391–402.

50 Prasad K, Menon GR. Comparison of the three strategies of verbal scoring of the Glasgow Coma Scale in patients with stroke. *Cerebrovasc Dis* 1998; **8**(2):79–85.

51 Weir CJ, Bradford AP, Lees KR. The prognostic value of the components of the Glasgow Coma Scale following acute stroke. *Q J Med* 2003; **96**(1):67–74.

52 McKeon A, Vaughan C, Delanty N. Seizure versus syncope. *Lancet Neurol* 2006; **5**(2):171–80.

53 Savitz SI, Caplan LR. Vertebrobasilar disease. *N Engl J Med* 2005; **352**(25):2618–26.

54 Caplan LR, Wityk RJ, Glass TA, Tapia J, Pazdera L, Chang HM *et al.* New England Medical Center Posterior Circulation registry. *Ann Neurol* 2004; **56**(3):389–98.

55 Smith E, Delargy M. Locked-in syndrome. *Br Med J* 2005; **330**(7488):406–9.

56 Chisholm N, Gillett G. The patient's journey: living with locked-in syndrome. *Br Med J* 2005; **331**(7508):94–7.

57 Carrera E, Michel P, Bogousslavsky J. Anteromedian, central, and posterolateral infarcts of the thalamus: three variant types. *Stroke* 2004; **35**(12):2826–31.

58 Perren F, Clarke S, Bogousslavsky J. The syndrome of combined polar and paramedian thalamic infarction. *Arch Neurol* 2005; **62**(8):1212–16.

59 Roux FE, Boetto S, Sacko O, Chollet F, Tremoulet M. Writing, calculating, and finger recognition in the region of the angular gyrus: a cortical stimulation study of Gerstmann syndrome. *J Neurosurg* 2003; **99**(4):716–27.

60 Urban PP, Wicht S, Hopf HC, Fleischer S, Nickel O. Isolated dysarthria due to extracerebellar lacunar stroke: a central monoparesis of the tongue. *J Neurol Neurosurg Psychiatry* 1999; **66**(4):495–501.

61 Loetscher T, Regard M, Brugger P. Misoplegia: a review of the literature and a case without hemiplegia. *J Neurol Neurosurg Psychiatry* 2006; **77**(9):1099–100.

62 Baier B, Karnath HO. Incidence and diagnosis of anosognosia for hemiparesis revisited. *J Neurol Neurosurg Psychiatry* 2005; **76**(3):358–61.

63 Bird CM, Malhotra P, Parton A, Coulthard E, Rushworth MF, Husain M. Visual neglect after right posterior cerebral artery infarction. *J Neurol Neurosurg Psychiatry* 2006; **77**(9):1008–12.

64 Jehkonen M, Ahonen JP, Dastidar P, Koivisto AM, Laippala P, Vilkki J. How to detect visual neglect in acute stroke. *Lancet* 1998; **351**(9104):727–8.

65 Penfield W, Rasmussen T. *The Cerebral Cortex of Man.* New York: Macmillan, 1950.

66 Terao S, Miura N, Takeda A, Takahashi A, Mitsuma T, Sobue G. Course and distribution of facial corticobulbar tract fibres in the lower brain stem. *J Neurol Neurosurg Psychiatry* 2000; **69**(2):262–5.

67 Urban PP, Wicht S, Fitzek S, Marx J, Thomke F, Fitzek C *et al.* Ipsilateral facial weakness in upper medullary infarction: supranuclear or infranuclear origin? *J Neurol* 1999; **246**(9):798–801.

68 Thijs RD, Notermans NC, Wokke JH, van der Graaf Y, van Gijn J. Distribution of muscle weakness of central and peripheral origin. *J Neurol Neurosurg Psychiatry* 1998; **65**(5):794–6.

69 Manschot S, van Passel L, Buskens E, Algra A, van Gijn J. Mayo and NINDS scales for assessment of tendon reflexes: between observer agreement and implications for communication. *J Neurol Neurosurg Psychiatry* 1998; **64**(2):253–5.

70 van Gijn J. The Babinski reflex. *Postgrad Med J* 1995; **71**(841):645–8.

71 Ramsey DJ, Smithard DG, Kalra L. Can pulse oximetry or a bedside swallowing assessment be used to detect aspiration after stroke? *Stroke* 2006; **37**(12):2984–8.

72 Ogino T, Hattori J, Abiru K, Nakano K, Ohtsuka Y. Left premotor lesion producing selective impairment of habitual finger movement. *Neurology* 2005; **64**(4):760–1.

73 Maeder-Ingvar M, van Melle G, Bogousslavsky J. Pure monoparesis: a particular stroke subgroup? *Arch Neurol* 2005; **62**(8):1221–4.

74 Stone J, Carson A, Sharpe M. Functional symptoms and signs in neurology: assessment and diagnosis. *J Neurol Neurosurg Psychiatry* 2005; **76**(Suppl 1):i2–12.

75 Donnan GA, O'Malley HM, Quang L, Hurley S, Bladin PF. The capsular warning syndrome: pathogenesis and clinical features. *Neurology* 1993; **43**(5):957–62.

76 Schulz UG, Rothwell PM. Transient ischaemic attacks mimicking focal motor seizures. *Postgrad Med J* 2002; **78**(918):246–7.

77 Wardlaw JM. What causes lacunar stroke? *J Neurol Neurosurg Psychiatry* 2005; **76**(5):617–19.

78 Novy J, Carruzzo A, Maeder P, Bogousslavsky J. Spinal cord ischemia: clinical and imaging patterns, pathogenesis, and outcomes in 27 patients. *Arch Neurol* 2006; **63**(8):1113–20.

79 Maulaz AB, Bezerra DC, Bogousslavsky J. Posterior cerebral artery infarction from middle cerebral artery infarction. *Arch Neurol* 2005; **62**(6):938–41.

80 Verbuch-Heller L, Leigh RJ, Mermelstein V, Zagalsky L, Streifler JY. Ptosis in patients with hemispheric strokes. *Neurology* 2002; **58**(4):620–4.

81 Halmagyi GM, Cremer PD. Assessment and treatment of dizziness. *J Neurol Neurosurg Psychiatry* 2000; **68**(2):129–34.

82 Halmagyi GM. Diagnosis and management of vertigo. *Clin Med* 2005; **5**(2):159–65.

83 Lee H, Cho YW. Auditory disturbance as a prodrome of anterior inferior cerebellar artery infarction. *J Neurol Neurosurg Psychiatry* 2003; **74**(12):1644–8.

84 Black RA, Halmagyi GM, Thurtell MJ, Todd MJ, Curthoys IS. The active head-impulse test in unilateral peripheral vestibulopathy. *Arch Neurol* 2005; **62**(2):290–3.

85 Rambold H, Boenki J, Stritzke G, Wisst F, Neppert B, Helmchen C. Differential vestibular dysfunction in sudden unilateral hearing loss. *Neurology* 2005; **64**(1):148–51.

86 Goadsby PJ. Recent advances in the diagnosis and management of migraine. *Br Med J* 2006; **332**(7532):25–9.

87 Birschel P, Ellul J, Barer D. Progressing stroke: towards an internationally agreed definition. *Cerebrovasc Dis* 2004; **17**(2–3):242–52.

88 Barber M, Stott DJ, Langhorne P. An internationally agreed definition of progressing stroke. *Cerebrovasc Dis* 2004; **18**(3):255–6.

89 Melo TP, Pinto AN, Ferro JM. Headache in intracerebral hematomas. *Neurology* 1996; **47**(2):494–500.

90 Ferro JM, Costa I, Melo TP, Canhao P, Oliveira V, Salgado AV *et al*. Headache associated with transient ischemic attacks. *Headache* 1995; **35**(9):544–8.

91 Salgado AV, Ferro JM. Headache in lacunar stroke. *Cephalalgia* 1995; **15**(5):410–13.

92 Ferro JM, Salgado AV, Oliveira V. Lacunar stroke associated headache is not related to intracranial large vessel disease. *Rev Neurol* 1995; **23**(122):741–2.

93 Schwedt TJ, Dodick DW. Thunderclap stroke: embolic cerebellar infarcts presenting as thunderclap headache. *Headache* 2006; **46**(3):520–2.

94 Razvi SS, Walker L, Teasdale E, Tyagi A, Muir KW. Cluster headache due to internal carotid artery dissection. *J Neurol* 2006; **253**(5):661–3.

95 Arnold M, Cumurciuc R, Stapf C, Favrole P, Berthet K, Bousser MG. Pain as the only symptom of cervical artery dissection. *J Neurol Neurosurg Psychiatry* 2006; **77**(9):1021–4.

96 Stang PE, Carson AP, Rose KM, Mo J, Ephross SA, Shahar E *et al*. Headache, cerebrovascular symptoms, and stroke: the Atherosclerosis Risk in Communities Study. *Neurology* 2005; **64**(9):1573–7.

97 Burn J, Dennis M, Bamford J, Sandercock P, Wade D, Warlow C. Epileptic seizures after a first stroke: the Oxfordshire Community Stroke Project. *Br Med J* 1997; **315**(7122):1582–7.

98 Sudlow CL. Epilepsy and stroke. *Lancet* 2004; **363**(9416):1175–6.

99 Flossmann E, Rothwell PM. Family history of stroke in patients with transient ischemic attack in relation to hypertension and other intermediate phenotypes. *Stroke* 2005; **36**(4):830–5.

100 Flossmann E, Rothwell PM. Family history of stroke does not predict risk of stroke after transient ischemic attack. *Stroke* 2006; **37**(2):544–6.

101 Kumwenda JJ, Mateyu G, Kampondeni S, van Dam AP, van Lieshout L, Zijlstra EE. Differential diagnosis of stroke in a setting of high HIV prevalence in Blantyre, Malawi. *Stroke* 2005; **36**(5):960–4.

102 Weir NU, Buchan AM. A study of the workload and effectiveness of a comprehensive acute stroke service. *J Neurol Neurosurg Psychiatry* 2005; **76**(6):863–5.

103 Scott PA, Silbergleit R. Misdiagnosis of stroke in tissue plasminogen activator-treated patients: characteristics and outcomes. *Ann Emerg Med* 2003; **42**(5):611–18.

104 Dennis M, Warlow C. Migraine aura without headache: transient ischaemic attack or not? *J Neurol Neurosurg Psychiatry* 1992; **55**(6):437–40.

105 Olesen J, Lipton RB. Headache classification update 2004. *Curr Opin Neurol* 2004; **17**(3):275–82.

106 Cohen SN, Muthukumaran A, Gasser H, el-Saden S. Symptom spread to contiguous body parts as a presentation of cerebral ischemia. *Cerebrovasc Dis* 2002; **14**(2):84–9.

107 Wijman CA, Wolf PA, Kase CS, Kelly-Hayes M, Beiser AS. Migrainous visual accompaniments are not rare in late life: the Framingham Study. *Stroke* 1998; **29**(8): 1539–43.

108 Etminan M, Takkouche B, Isorna FC, Samii A. Risk of ischaemic stroke in people with migraine: systematic review and meta-analysis of observational studies. *Br Med J* 2005; **330**(7482):63.

109 Kurth T, Slomke MA, Kase CS, Cook NR, Lee IM, Gaziano JM *et al*. Migraine, headache, and the risk of stroke in women: a prospective study. *Neurology* 2005; **64**(6):1020–6.

110 Dora B, Balkan S. Sporadic hemiplegic migraine and Sturge-Weber syndrome. *Headache* 2001; **41**(2):209–10.

111 Sztajzel R, Genoud D, Roth S, Mermillod B, Le Floch-Rohr J. Patent foramen ovale, a possible cause of symptomatic migraine: a study of 74 patients with acute ischemic stroke. *Cerebrovasc Dis* 2002; **13**(2):102–6.

112 Diener HC, Weimar C, Katsarava Z. Patent foramen ovale: paradoxical connection to migraine and stroke. *Curr Opin Neurol* 2005; **18**(3):299–304.

113 Schwedt TJ, Dodick DW. Patent foramen ovale and migraine: bringing closure to the subject. *Headache* 2006; **46**(4):663–71.

114 Saposnik G, Caplan LR. Convulsive-like movements in brainstem stroke. *Arch Neurol* 2001; **58**(4):654–7.

115 Quinette P, Guillery-Girard B, Dayan J, de la Sayette, V, Marquis S, Viader F *et al*. What does transient global amnesia really mean? Review of the literature and thorough study of 142 cases. *Brain* 2006; **129**(Pt 7):1640–58.

116 Quinette P, Guillery-Girard B, Noel A, de la Sayette, V, Viader F, Desgranges B *et al*. The relationship between working memory and episodic memory disorders in transient global amnesia. *Neuropsychologia* 2006; **44**(12): 2508–19.

117 Evans RW, Lewis SL. Transient global amnesia and migraine. *Headache* 2005; **45**(10):1408–10.

118 Pantoni L, Bertini E, Lamassa M, Pracucci G, Inzitari D. Clinical features, risk factors, and prognosis in transient

global amnesia: a follow-up study. *Eur J Neurol* 2005; **12**(5):350–6.

119 Winbeck K, Etgen T, von Einsiedel HG, Rottinger M, Sander D. DWI in transient global amnesia and TIA: proposal for an ischaemic origin of TGA. *J Neurol Neurosurg Psychiatry* 2005; **76**(3):438–41.

120 Sander K, Sander D. New insights into transient global amnesia: recent imaging and clinical findings. *Lancet Neurol* 2005; **4**(7):437–44.

121 Nakada T, Kwee IL, Fujii Y, Knight RT. High-field, T2 reversed MRI of the hippocampus in transient global amnesia. *Neurology* 2005; **64**(7):1170–4.

122 Cianfoni A, Tartaglione T, Gaudino S, Pilato F, Saturno E, Tonali PA *et al.* Hippocampal magnetic resonance imaging abnormalities in transient global amnesia. *Arch Neurol* 2005; **62**(9):1468–9.

123 Roach ES. Transient global amnesia: look at mechanisms not causes. *Arch Neurol* 2006; **63**(9):1338–9.

124 Bettermann K. Transient global amnesia: the continuing quest for a source. *Arch Neurol* 2006; **63**(9):1336–8.

125 Wilkinson CC, Multani J, Bailes JE. Chronic subdural hematoma presenting with symptoms of transient ischemic attack (TIA): a case report. *W V Med J* 2001; **97**(4):194–6.

126 Intracranial tumours that mimic transient cerebral ischaemia: lessons from a large multicentre trial. The UK TIA Study Group. *J Neurol Neurosurg Psychiatry* 1993; **56**(5):563–6.

127 Erten SF, Ertas E, Duygulu C, Aydin EN, Colak A. An unusual presentation of metastatic adenocarcinoma in the cerebellum associated with intratumoral hemorrhage mimicking a stroke. A case report. *Neurosurg Rev* 1998; **21**(1):69–71.

128 Jansen FE, van der Worp HB, van Huffelen A, van Niewenhuizen O. Sturge-Weber syndrome and paroxysmal hemiparesis: epilepsy or ischaemia? *Dev Med Child Neurol* 2004; **46**(11):783–6.

129 Herzig R, Bogousslavsky J, Maeder P, Maeder-Ingvar M, Reichhart M, Urbano LA *et al.* Intracranial arterial and arteriovenous malformations presenting with infarction. Lausanne Stroke Registry study. *Eur J Neurol* 2005; **12**(2):93–102.

130 Huff JS. Stroke mimics and chameleons. *Emerg Med Clin North Am* 2002; **20**(3):583–95.

131 Fagan M. [Hypoglycemic hemiparesis. A case report]. *Tidsskr Nor Laegeforen* 1989; **109**(27):2773–4.

132 Wintermark M, Fischbein NJ, Mukherjee P, Yuh EL, Dillon WP. Unilateral putaminal CT, MR, and diffusion abnormalities secondary to nonketotic hyperglycemia in the setting of acute neurologic symptoms mimicking stroke. *Am J Neuroradiol* 2004; **25**(6):975–6.

133 Atchison JW, Pellegrino M, Herbers P, Tipton B, Matkovic V. Hepatic encephalopathy mimicking stroke. A case report. *Am J Phys Med Rehabil* 1992; **71**(2):114–18.

134 Chang GY. Acute Wernicke's syndrome mimicking brainstem stroke. *Eur Neurol* 2000; **43**(4):246–7.

135 Stott VL, Hurrell MA, Anderson TJ. Reversible posterior leukoencephalopathy syndrome: a misnomer reviewed. *Intern Med J* 2005; **35**(2):83–90.

136 Pendlebury ST, Rothwell PM, Dalton A, Burton EA. Strokelike presentation of Wilson disease with homozygosity for a novel T766R mutation. *Neurology* 2004; **63**(10):1982–3.

137 McKellar MS, Mehta LR, Greenlee JE, Hale DC, Booton GC, Kelly DJ *et al.* Fatal granulomatous Acanthamoeba encephalitis mimicking a stroke, diagnosed by correlation of results of sequential magnetic resonance imaging, biopsy, in vitro culture, immunofluorescence analysis, and molecular analysis. *J Clin Microbiol* 2006; **44**(11):4265–9.

138 Hohler AD, Flynn FG. Onset of Creutzfeldt–Jakob disease mimicking an acute cerebrovascular event. *Neurology* 2006; **67**(3):538–9.

139 Szabo K, Achtnichts L, Grips E, Binder J, Gerigk L, Hennerici M *et al.* Stroke-like presentation in a case of Creutzfeldt–Jakob disease. *Cerebrovasc Dis* 2004; **18**(3):251–3.

140 Strupp M, Arbusow V. Acute vestibulopathy. *Curr Opin Neurol* 2001; **14**(1):11–20.

141 Dieterich M. Dizziness. *Neurologist* 2004; **10**(3):154–64.

142 Cesarani A, Alpini D, Monti B, Raponi G. The treatment of acute vertigo. *Neurol Sci* 2004; **25**(Suppl 1):S26–S30.

143 Magnusson M, Karlberg M. Peripheral vestibular disorders with acute onset of vertigo. *Curr Opin Neurol* 2002; **15**(1):5–10.

144 Lee H, Sohn SI, Cho YW, Lee SR, Ahn BH, Park BR *et al.* Cerebellar infarction presenting with isolated vertigo: frequency and vascular topographical patterns. *Neurology* 2006; **67**(7):1178–83.

145 Waterston J. Chronic migrainous vertigo. *J Clin Neurosci* 2004; **11**(4):384–8.

146 Ziv I, Djaldetti R, Zoldan Y, Avraham M, Melamed E. Diagnosis of 'non-organic' limb paresis by a novel objective motor assessment: the quantitative Hoover's test. *J Neurol* 1998; **245**(12):797–802.

147 Stone J, Carson A, Sharpe M. Functional symptoms in neurology: management. *J Neurol Neurosurg Psychiatry* 2005; **76**(Suppl 1):i13–i21.

148 Stone J, Sharpe M, Carson A, Lewis SC, Thomas B, Goldbeck R *et al.* Are functional motor and sensory symptoms really more frequent on the left? A systematic review. *J Neurol Neurosurg Psychiatry* 2002; **73**(5):578–81.

149 Beatty S. Non-organic visual loss. *Postgrad Med J* 1999; **75**(882):201–7.

150 Rosso C, Remy P, Creange A, Brugieres P, Cesaro P, Hosseini H. Diffusion-weighted MR imaging characteristics of an acute strokelike form of multiple sclerosis. *Am J Neuroradiol* 2006; **27**(5):1006–8.

151 Lampl Y, Gilad R, Eshel Y, Sarova-Pinhas I. Strokes mimicking peripheral nerve lesions. *Clin Neurol Neurosurg* 1995; **97**(3):203–7.

152 Cher LM, Merory JM. Miller Fisher syndrome mimicking stroke in immunosuppressed patient with rheumatoid arthritis responding to plasma exchange. *J Clin Neuroophthalmol* 1993; **13**(2):138–40.

153 Ikuta N, Koga M, Ogasawara J, Morimatsu M, Yuki N. [Anti-GD1b IgG antibody-related Guillain-Barre syndrome initially mimicking brainstem infarction]. *Rinsho Shinkeigaku* 2001; **41**(2–3):132–5.

154 Soler-Revert M, Galiano R, Bernacer-Alpera B, Pardo-Lillo M, Blanco-Hernandez T, Ortiz-Sanchez P. [Guillain-Barre syndrome mimicking a vertebrobasilar stroke]. *Rev Neurol* 2006; **42**(5):314–15.

155 Kleiner-Fisman G, Kott HS. Myasthenia gravis mimicking stroke in elderly patients. *Mayo Clin Proc* 1998; **73**(11):1077–8.

156 Libman R, Benson R, Einberg K. Myasthenia mimicking vertebrobasilar stroke. *J Neurol* 2002; **249**(11):1512–14.

157 Ferro JM, Falcao I, Rodrigues G, Canhao P, Melo TP, Oliveira V *et al*. Diagnosis of transient ischemic attack by the nonneurologist. A validation study. *Stroke* 1996; **27**(12):2225–9.

158 Thijs RD, Wieling W, Kaufmann H, van Dijk G. Defining and classifying syncope. *Clin Auton Res* 2004; **14**(Suppl 1):4–8.

159 Petkar S, Cooper P, Fitzpatrick AP. How to avoid a misdiagnosis in patients presenting with transient loss of consciousness. *Postgrad Med J* 2006; **82**(972):630–41.

160 Smars PA, Decker WW, Shen WK. Syncope evaluation in the emergency department. *Curr Opin Cardiol* 2007; **22**(1):44–8.

161 Brignole M. Diagnosis and treatment of syncope. *Heart* 2007; **93**(1):130–6.

162 Gerstner E, Liberato B, Wright CB. Bi-hemispheric anterior cerebral artery with drop attacks and limb shaking TIAs. *Neurology* 2005; **65**(1):174.

163 Guilleminault C, Gelb M. Clinical aspects and features of cataplexy. *Adv Neurol* 1995; **67**:65–77.

164 Krahn LE. Reevaluating spells initially identified as cataplexy. *Sleep Med* 2005; **6**(6):537–42.

165 Krahn LE, Lymp JF, Moore WR, Slocumb N, Silber MH. Characterizing the emotions that trigger cataplexy. *J Neuropsychiatry Clin Neurosci* 2005; **17**(1):45–50.

166 Boyer EW, Shannon M. The serotonin syndrome. *N Engl J Med* 2005; **352**(11):1112–20.

167 Wardlaw JM, Keir SL, Seymour J, Lewis S, Sandercock PA, Dennis MS *et al*. What is the best imaging strategy for acute stroke? *Health Technol Assess* 2004; **8**(1):iii, ix–iii, 180.

168 Muir KW, Santosh C. Imaging of acute stroke and transient ischaemic attack. *J Neurol Neurosurg Psychiatry* 2005; **76**(Suppl 3):iii19–iii28.

169 Muir KW, Buchan A, von KR, Rother J, Baron JC. Imaging of acute stroke. *Lancet Neurol* 2006; **5**(9):755–68.

170 Wardlaw JM, Seymour J, Cairns J, Keir S, Lewis S, Sandercock P. Immediate computed tomography scanning of acute stroke is cost-effective and improves quality of life. *Stroke* 2004; **35**(11):2477–83.

171 Wardlaw J. ACCESS: the acute cerebral CT evaluation stroke study. *Emerg Med J* 2004; **21**(6):666.

172 Rivers CS, Wardlaw JM, Armitage PA, Bastin ME, Carpenter TK, Cvoro V *et al*. Do acute diffusion- and perfusion-weighted MRI lesions identify final infarct volume in ischemic stroke? *Stroke* 2006; **37**(1):98–104.

173 Hjort N, Christensen S, Solling C, Ashkanian M, Wu O, Rohl L *et al*. Ischemic injury detected by diffusion imaging 11 minutes after stroke. *Ann Neurol* 2005; **58**(3):462–5.

174 Leach JP, Stephen LJ, Salveta C, Brodie MJ. Which electroencephalography (EEG) for epilepsy? The relative usefulness of different EEG protocols in patients with possible epilepsy. *J Neurol Neurosurg Psychiatry* 2006; **77**(9):1040–2.

175 Kappelle LJ, Donders RC, Algra A. Transient monocular blindness. *Clin Exp Hypertens* 2006; **28**(3–4):259–63.

176 Nakajima M, Kimura K, Minematsu K, Saito K, Takada T, Tanaka M. A case of frequently recurring amaurosis fugax with atherothrombotic ophthalmic artery occlusion. *Neurology* 2004; **62**(1):117–18.

177 Grosberg BM, Solomon S, Friedman DI, Lipton RB. Retinal migraine reappraised. *Cephalalgia* 2006; **26**(11):1275–86.

178 Grosberg BM, Solomon S. Retinal migraine: two cases of prolonged but reversible monocular visual defects. *Cephalalgia* 2006; **26**(6):754–7.

179 Gan KD, Mouradian MS, Weis E, Lewis JR. Transient monocular visual loss and retinal migraine. *Can Med Assoc J* 2005; **173**(12):1441–2.

180 Pradhan S, Chung SM. Retinal, ophthalmic, or ocular migraine. *Curr Neurol Neurosci Rep* 2004; **4**(5):391–7.

181 Doyle E, Vote BJ, Casswell AG. Retinal migraine: caught in the act. *Br J Ophthalmol* 2004; **88**(2):301–2.

182 Killer HE, Forrer A, Flammer J. Retinal vasospasm during an attack of migraine. *Retina* 2003; **23**(2):253–4.

183 Le FD, Safran AB, Picard F, Bouchardy I, Morris MA. Elicited repetitive daily blindness: a new familial disorder related to migraine and epilepsy. *Neurology* 2004; **63**(2):348–50.

184 Rothwell PM, Mehta Z, Howard SC, Gutnikov SA, Warlow CP. Treating individuals 3: from subgroups to individuals: general principles and the example of carotid endarterectomy. *Lancet* 2005; **365**(9455):256–65.

185 Purvin V, Kawasaki A. Neuro-ophthalmic emergencies for the neurologist. *Neurologist* 2005; **11**(4):195–233.

186 Balcer LJ. Clinical practice. Optic neuritis. *N Engl J Med* 2006; **354**(12):1273–80.

187 Kraaijeveld CL, van Gijn J, Schouten HJ, Staal A. Interobserver agreement for the diagnosis of transient ischemic attacks. *Stroke* 1984; **15**(4):723–5.

188 Shinar D, Gross CR, Mohr JP, Caplan LR, Price TR, Wolf PA *et al*. Interobserver variability in the assessment of neurologic history and examination in the Stroke Data Bank. *Arch Neurol* 1985; **42**(6):557–65.

189 Lindley RI, Warlow CP, Wardlaw JM, Dennis MS, Slattery J, Sandercock PA. Interobserver reliability of a clinical classification of acute cerebral infarction. *Stroke* 1993; **24**(12):1801–4.

190 Ferro JM, Pinto AN, Falcao I, Rodrigues G, Ferreira J, Falcao F *et al*. Diagnosis of stroke by the nonneurologist. A validation study. *Stroke* 1998; **29**(6):1106–9.

191 Koudstaal PJ, van Gijn J, Staal A, Duivenvoorden HJ, Gerritsma JG, Kraaijeveld CL. Diagnosis of transient ischemic attacks: improvement of interobserver agreement by a check-list in ordinary language. *Stroke* 1986; **17**(4):723–8.

192 Matsuda M, Ohashi M, Shiino A, Matsumura K, Handa J. Circumstances precipitating aneurysmal subarachnoid haemorrhage. *Cerebrovasc Dis* 1993; 3:285–8.

193 Wroe SJ, Sandercock P, Bamford J, Dennis M, Slattery J, Warlow C. Diurnal variation in incidence of stroke: Oxfordshire community stroke project. *Br Med J* 1992; **304**(6820):155–7.

194 Linn FH, Rinkel GJ, Algra A, van Gijn J. Headache characteristics in subarachnoid haemorrhage and benign thunderclap headache. *J Neurol Neurosurg Psychiatry* 1998; **65**(5):791–3.

195 Ferro JM, Pinto AN. Sexual activity is a common precipitant of subarachnoid haemorrhage. *Cerebrovasc Dis* 1994; 4:375.

196 Pascual J, Iglesias F, Oterino A, Vazquez-Barquero A, Berciano J. Cough, exertional, and sexual headaches: an analysis of 72 benign and symptomatic cases. *Neurology* 1996; **46**(6):1520–4.

197 Linn FH, Wijdicks EF, van der Graaf Y, Weerdesteyn-van Vliet FA, Bartelds AI, van Gijn J. Prospective study of sentinel headache in aneurysmal subarachnoid haemorrhage. *Lancet* 1994; **344**(8922):590–3.

198 Vestergaard K, Andersen G, Nielsen MI, Jensen TS. Headache in stroke. *Stroke* 1993; **24**(11):1621–4.

199 Kumral E, Bogousslavsky J, van Melle G, Regli F, Pierre P. Headache at stroke onset: the Lausanne Stroke Registry. *J Neurol Neurosurg Psychiatry* 1995; **58**(4):490–2.

200 Rose G. *The Strategy of Preventive Medicine*. Oxford: Oxford Medical Publications, 1992.

201 Fodden DI, Peatfield RC, Milsom PL. Beware the patient with a headache in the accident and emergency department. *Arch Emerg Med* 1989; **6**(1):7–12.

202 Van der Wee N, Rinkel GJ, Hasan D, van Gijn J. Detection of subarachnoid haemorrhage on early CT: is lumbar puncture still needed after a negative scan? *J Neurol Neurosurg Psychiatry* 1995; **58**(3):357–9.

203 Rinkel GJ, van Gijn J, Wijdicks EF. Subarachnoid hemorrhage without detectable aneurysm: a review of the causes. *Stroke* 1993; **24**(9):1403–9.

204 De Bruijn SF, Stam J, Kappelle LJ. Thunderclap headache as first symptom of cerebral venous sinus thrombosis. CVST Study Group. *Lancet* 1996; **348**(9042):1623–5.

205 Vermeulen M, van Gijn J. The diagnosis of subarachnoid haemorrhage. *J Neurol Neurosurg Psychiatry* 1990; **53**(5):365–72.

206 Vermeulen M, Lindsay KW, Murray GD, Cheah F, Hijdra A, Muizelaar JP *et al*. Antifibrinolytic treatment in subarachnoid hemorrhage. *N Engl J Med* 1984; **311**(7):432–7.

207 Schievink WI, Wijdicks EF, Parisi JE, Piepgras DG, Whisnant JP. Sudden death from aneurysmal subarachnoid hemorrhage. *Neurology* 1995; **45**(5):871–4.

208 Hijdra A, van Gijn J. Early death from rupture of an intracranial aneurysm. *J Neurosurg* 1982; **57**(6):765–8.

209 Fisher CM. Clinical syndromes in cerebral thrombosis, hypertensive hemorrhage, and ruptured saccular aneurysm. *Clin Neurosurg* 1975; **22**:117–47.

210 Reijneveld JC, Wermer M, Boonman Z, van Gijn J, Rinkel GJ. Acute confusional state as presenting feature in aneurysmal subarachnoid hemorrhage: frequency and characteristics. *J Neurol* 2000; **247**(2):112–16.

211 Caeiro L, Menger C, Ferro JM, Albuquerque R, Figueira ML. Delirium in acute subarachnoid haemorrhage. *Cerebrovasc Dis* 2005; **19**(1):31–8.

212 Hart RG, Byer JA, Slaughter JR, Hewett JE, Easton JD. Occurrence and implications of seizures in subarachnoid hemorrhage due to ruptured intracranial aneurysms. *Neurosurgery* 1981; **8**(4):417–21.

213 Hasan D, Schonck RS, Avezaat CJ, Tanghe HL, van Gijn J, van der Lugt PJ. Epileptic seizures after subarachnoid hemorrhage. *Ann Neurol* 1993; **33**(3):286–91.

214 Pinto AN, Canhao P, Ferro JM. Seizures at the onset of subarachnoid haemorrhage. *J Neurol* 1996; **243**(2):161–4.

215 Butzkueven H, Evans AH, Pitman A, Leopold C, Jolley DJ, Kaye AH *et al*. Onset seizures independently predict poor outcome after subarachnoid hemorrhage. *Neurology* 2000; **55**(9):1315–20.

216 Manschot WA. Subarachnoid hemorrhage; intraocular symptoms and their pathogenesis. *Am J Ophthalmol* 1954; **38**(4):501–5.

217 Fahmy JA. Fundal haemorrhages in ruptured intracranial aneurysms. I. Material, frequency and morphology. *Acta Ophthalmol (Copenh)* 1973; **51**(3):289–98.

218 Rousseaux P, Scherpereel B, Bernard MH, Graftieaux JP, Guyot JF. Fever and cerebral vasospasm in ruptured intracranial aneurysms. *Surg Neurol* 1980; **14**(6):459–65.

219 Feigin VL, Rinkel GJ, Lawes CM, Algra A, Bennett DA, van Gijn J *et al*. Risk factors for subarachnoid hemorrhage: an updated systematic review of epidemiological studies. *Stroke* 2005; **36**(12):2773–80.

220 Juvela S, Siironen J, Kuhmonen J. Hyperglycemia, excess weight, and history of hypertension as risk factors for poor outcome and cerebral infarction after aneurysmal subarachnoid hemorrhage. *J Neurosurg* 2005; **102**(6):998–1003.

221 Brouwers PJ, Wijdicks EF, Hasan D, Vermeulen M, Wever EF, Frericks H *et al*. Serial electrocardiographic recording in aneurysmal subarachnoid hemorrhage. *Stroke* 1989; **20**(9):1162–7.

222 Van Gijn J. Pitfalls in the diagnosis of sudden headache. *Proc R Coll Physicians Edinb* 1999; **29**:21–31.

223 Van Gijn J, van Dongen KJ. Computed tomography in the diagnosis of subarachnoid haemorrhage and ruptured aneurysm. *Clin Neurol Neurosurg* 1980; **82**(1):11–24.

224 Tokuda Y, Inagawa T, Katoh Y, Kumano K, Ohbayashi N, Yoshioka H. Intracerebral hematoma in patients with ruptured cerebral aneurysms. *Surg Neurol* 1995; **43**(3):272–7.

225 Darby DG, Donnan GA, Saling MA, Walsh KW, Bladin PF. Primary intraventricular hemorrhage: clinical and neuropsychological findings in a prospective stroke series. *Neurology* 1988; **38**(1):68–75.

226 Akins PT, Roberts R, Coxe WS, Kaufman BA. Familial colloid cyst of the third ventricle: case report and

review of associated conditions. *Neurosurgery* 1996; **38**(2):392–5.

227 Camacho A, Abernathey CD, Kelly PJ, Laws ER, Jr. Colloid cysts: experience with the management of 84 cases since the introduction of computed tomography. *Neurosurgery* 1989; **24**(5):693–700.

228 Skerbinjek KM, Kavalar R, Strokjnik T. A colloid cyst of the third ventricle: the cause of episodic headache and sudden unexpected death in an adolescent girl. *Wien Klin Wochenschr* 2006; **117**:837–40.

229 Lance JW. Current concepts of migraine pathogenesis. *Neurology* 1993; **43**(6 Suppl 3):S11–S15.

230 Raskin NH. Short-lived head pains. *Neurol Clin* 1997; **15**(1):143–52.

231 Raskin NH, Schwartz RK. Icepick-like pain. *Neurology* 1980; **30**(2):203–5.

232 Pearce JM. Clinical features of the exploding head syndrome. *J Neurol Neurosurg Psychiatry* 1989; **52**(7):907–10.

233 Green MW. The exploding head syndrome. *Curr Pain Headache Rep* 2001; **5**(3):279–80.

234 Boes CJ, Matharu MS, Goadsby PJ. Benign cough headache. *Cephalalgia* 2002; **22**(10):772–9.

235 Pascual J. Primary cough headache. *Curr Pain Headache Rep* 2005; **9**(4):272–6.

236 Raskin NH. The hypnic headache syndrome. *Headache* 1988; **28**(8):534–6.

237 Evers S, Goadsby PJ. Hypnic headache: clinical features, pathophysiology, and treatment. *Neurology* 2003; **60**(6):905–9.

238 Tubbs ON, Potter JM. Early post-concussional headache. *Lancet* 1970; **2**(7664):128–9.

239 Silbert PL, Edis RH, Stewart-Wynne EG, Gubbay SS. Benign vascular sexual headache and exertional headache: interrelationships and long term prognosis. *J Neurol Neurosurg Psychiatry* 1991; **54**(5):417–21.

240 Frese A, Evers S. [Unpleasant afterplay. Sex triggers a headache]. *MMW Fortschr Med* 2005; **147**(16):45–6.

241 Thomas JE, Rooke ED, Kvale WF. The neurologist's experience with pheochromocytoma: a review of 100 cases. *J Am Med Assoc* 1966; **197**(10):754–8.

242 Lance JW, Hinterberger H. Symptoms of pheochromocytoma, with particular reference to headache, correlated with catecholamine production. *Arch Neurol* 1976; **33**(4):281–8.

243 Baguet JP, Hammer L, Mazzuco TL, Chabre O, Mallion JM, Sturm N *et al.* Circumstances of discovery of phaeochromocytoma: a retrospective study of 41 consecutive patients. *Eur J Endocrinol* 2004; **150**(5):681–6.

244 Lenders JW, Keiser HR, Goldstein DS, Willemsen JJ, Friberg P, Jacobs MC *et al.* Plasma metanephrines in the diagnosis of pheochromocytoma. *Ann Intern Med* 1995; **123**(2):101–9.

245 Dodick DW. Recurrent short-lasting headache associated with paroxysmal hypertension: a clonidine-responsive syndrome. *Cephalalgia* 2000; **20**(5):509–14.

246 Pascual-Leone A, Pascual-Leone PA. Occipital neuralgia: another benign cause of 'thunderclap headache'. *J Neurol Neurosurg Psychiatry* 1992; **55**(5):411.

247 Schwedt TJ, Matharu MS, Dodick DW. Thunderclap headache. *Lancet Neurol* 2006; **5**(7):621–31.

248 Wijdicks EF, Kerkhoff H, van Gijn J. Long-term follow-up of 71 patients with thunderclap headache mimicking subarachnoid haemorrhage. *Lancet* 1988; **2**(8602):68–70.

249 Linn FH, Rinkel GJ, Algra A, van Gijn J. Follow-up of idiopathic thunderclap headache in general practice. *J Neurol* 1999; **246**(10):946–8.

250 Ramirez-Lassepas M, Espinosa CE, Cicero JJ, Johnston KL, Cipolle RJ, Barber DL. Predictors of intracranial pathologic findings in patients who seek emergency care because of headache. *Arch Neurol* 1997; **54**(12):1506–9.

251 Van Gijn J, van Dongen KJ. The time course of aneurysmal haemorrhage on computed tomograms. *Neuroradiology* 1982; **23**(3):153–6.

252 Brouwers PJ, Wijdicks EF, van Gijn J. Infarction after aneurysm rupture does not depend on distribution or clearance rate of blood. *Stroke* 1992; **23**(3):374–9.

253 Avrahami E, Katz R, Rabin A, Friedman V. CT diagnosis of non-traumatic subarachnoid haemorrhage in patients with brain edema. *Eur J Radiol* 1998; **28**(3):222–5.

254 Al-Yamany M, Deck J, Bernstein M. Pseudo-subarachnoid hemorrhage: a rare neuroimaging pitfall. *Can J Neurol Sci* 1999; **26**(1):57–9.

255 Phan TG, Wijdicks EF, Worrell GA, Fulgham JR. False subarachnoid hemorrhage in anoxic encephalopathy with brain swelling. *J Neuroimaging* 2000; **10**(4):236–8.

256 Javedan SP, Marciano F. Pseudo-enhancement from polycythemia. *Neurology* 2004; **62**(1):150.

257 Mendelsohn DB, Moss ML, Chason DP, Muphree S, Casey S. Acute purulent leptomeningitis mimicking subarachnoid hemorrhage on CT. *J Comput Assist Tomogr* 1994; **18**(1):126–8.

258 Huang D, Abe T, Ochiai S, Kojima K, Tanaka N, Zhang Y *et al.* False positive appearance of subarachnoid hemorrhage on CT with bilateral subdural hematomas. *Radiat Med* 1999; **17**(6):439–42.

259 Rabinstein AA, Pittock SJ, Miller GM, Schindler JJ, Wijdicks EF. Pseudosubarachnoid haemorrhage in subdural haematoma. *J Neurol Neurosurg Psychiatry* 2003; **74**(8):1131–2.

260 Belsare G, Lee AG, Maley J, Kirby P, St Louis EK, Follett K. Pseudo-subarachnoid hemorrhage and cortical visual impairment as the presenting sign of gliomatosis cerebri. *Semin Ophthalmol* 2004; **19**(3–4):78–80.

261 Schievink WI, Maya MM, Tourje J, Moser FG. Pseudo-subarachnoid hemorrhage: a CT-finding in spontaneous intracranial hypotension. *Neurology* 2005; **65**(1):135–7.

262 Duffy GP. Lumbar puncture in spontaneous subarachnoid haemorrhage. *Br Med J (Clin Res Ed)* 1982; **285**(6349):1163–4.

263 Hillman J. Should computed tomography scanning replace lumbar puncture in the diagnostic process in suspected subarachnoid hemorrhage? *Surg Neurol* 1986; **26**(6):547–50.

264 Buruma OJ, Janson HL, Den Bergh FA, Bots GT. Blood-stained cerebrospinal fluid: traumatic puncture

or haemorrhage? *J Neurol Neurosurg Psychiatry* 1981; **44**(2):144–7.

265 Vermeulen M, Hasan D, Blijenberg BG, Hijdra A, van Gijn J. Xanthochromia after subarachnoid haemorrhage needs no revisitation. *J Neurol Neurosurg Psychiatry* 1989; **52**(7):826–8.

266 Linn FH, Voorbij IIA, Rinkel GJ, Algra A, van Gijn J. Visual inspection versus spectrophotometry in detecting bilirubin in cerebrospinal fluid. *J Neurol Neurosurg Psychiatry* 2005; **76**(10):1452–4.

267 Beetham R. Recommendations for CSF analysis in subarachnoid haemorrhage. *J Neurol Neurosurg Psychiatry* 2004; **75**(4):528.

268 Beetham R, Fahie-Wilson MN, Park D. What is the role of CSF spectrophotometry in the diagnosis of subarachnoid haemorrhage? *Ann Clin Biochem* 1998; **35**(Pt 1):1–4.

269 McCarron MO, Choudhari KA. Aneurysmal subarachnoid leak with normal CT and CSF spectrophotometry. *Neurology* 2005; **64**(5):923.

270 Ball MJ. Pathogenesis of the 'sentinel headache' preceding berry aneurysm rupture. *Can Med Assoc J* 1975; **112**(1):78–9.

271 Day JW, Raskin NH. Thunderclap headache: symptom of unruptured cerebral aneurysm. *Lancet* 1986; **2**(8518):1247–8.

272 Clarke CE, Shepherd DI, Chishti K, Victoratos G. Thunderclap headache: symptom of unruptured cerebral aneurysm. *Lancet* 1988; **2**:625.

273 Call GK, Fleming MC, Sealfon S, Levine H, Kistler JP, Fisher CM. Reversible cerebral segmental vasoconstriction. *Stroke* 1988; **19**(9):1159–70.

274 Silbert PL, Hankey GJ, Prentice DA, Apsimon HT. Angiographically demonstrated arterial spasm in a case of benign sexual headache and benign exertional headache. *Aust N Z J Med* 1989; **19**(5):466–8.

Which arterial territory is involved?
Using arterial and brain anatomy to develop a clinically based method of subclassification

4.1 Introduction

Once the diagnosis of a cerebrovascular (vs non-vascular) event has been made in someone presenting with an acute stroke syndrome (Chapter 3), the clinician then needs a framework on which to base the further subclassification of that event. Although in the past, time-based schemes of subclassification were promoted, we have seen already that the distinction between stroke and transient ischaemic attack (TIA) is arbitrary, does not have any rational pathophysiological basis (section 3.2), and is of little value to the physician seeing a patient with persisting symptoms within minutes or hours after onset. Similarly, there is no evidence to suggest that a distinction between 'major stroke' and 'minor stroke' (defined as symptoms lasting more or less than 1 week respectively) or with reversible ischaemic neurological deficit (RIND) – variously defined as cases in which symptoms resolve in less than 1 week or 3 weeks – conveys any useful aetiological information. Indeed, the tendency for some physicians to use the terms 'minor' and 'major' as a type of shorthand to describe the level of residual disability simply leads to confusion.

Stroke: practical management, 3rd edition. C. Warlow, J. van Gijn, M. Dennis, J. Wardlaw, J. Bamford, G. Hankey, P. Sandercock, G. Rinkel, P. Langhorne, C. Sudlow and P. Rothwell. Published 2008 Blackwell Publishing. ISBN 978-1-4051-2766-0.

Much of the recent focus in the medical literature has been on classifications which depend on knowing the underlying cause of the stroke. While it is clearly logical to try to establish the cause of every individual stroke, since it is with this knowledge that rational treatments for limiting the acute damage and secondary prevention will be developed, tested and deployed, as will be seen, this is not always possible to achieve in a timely manner even in well-financed healthcare systems.

The subclassification of stroke has the potential to refine the practice of various different healthcare professionals, many of whom are more interested in the clinical deficits and functional consequences resulting from the brain lesion (e.g. nursing and rehabilitation) rather than the underlying cause. There are also many other reasons for subclassifying patients with strokes and TIAs which, while not all of immediate value to the individual patient or their relatives, may be helpful when considering the general management of cerebrovascular disease and the overall burden to the community (Table 4.1). This diversity of need perhaps explains why there is still no universal method of subclassification used equally by stroke physicians, therapists, health service managers and others.

If a method of subclassification is going to be applicable to all patients during life, irrespective of age, disability and geographical location, clinical data must be used as the core component because they are available to every clinician; subsequently obtained investigative data appropriate to the individual situation can then be used to refine that clinical subclassification. After the clinical

Table 4.1 Potential benefits of subclassifying patients with strokes and transient ischaemic attacks.

Aid cost-effective and timely search for the cause of the stroke or transient ischaemic attack

Aid planning of immediate supportive care and rehabilitation programme

Improve prognostication for survival, functional outcome, and recurrence

Stratify entry to clinical trials to reduce heterogeneity and therefore have the best chance of demonstrating treatment benefit in a subgroup if such a benefit is present

Help put the results of clinical trials into the context of an individual physician's own practice

Provide more sensitive assessment of case mix in individual units, for comparative audit and contracting purposes

Aid audit of management

history and examination, the clinician will have some information about the site of the brain lesion, the vascular territory affected and possibly some clues as to the potential aetiology (e.g. the presence of atrial fibrillation). This information needs to be organized in a manner that facilitates a modular and hierarchical approach to subclassification – i.e. additional but complementary levels of subclassification can be used in any particular situation to suit individual requirements and facilities. Thus, the basic scheme needs to provide a skeleton on which these fragments of information about an individual patient can be hung in an orderly manner so as to orientate further management. Ideally, such a 'core' clinical skeleton, usable in everyday practice, could be built on by both clinicians and researchers according to their access to, and the applicability of, various investigations. Used in this way, a system of classification should also facilitate the integration and application of research findings from the university centres into everyday practice.

Traditional neurological teaching has always focused on first determining the site of the lesion within the nervous system, since this nearly always narrows the range of possible underlying causes. It would seem logical, therefore, to attempt to identify groups of stroke patients with broadly similar brain and arterial lesions, since these are likely to be caused by broadly similar types of vascular disease. Following on from this, such groups might be expected to have certain nursing and rehabilitation needs, and also a distinctive prognosis. As will be seen, such an approach to subclassification, based initially on an analysis of the brain damage, is in fact entirely complementary to the aetiological classifications which usually have both clinical syndromes and the results of cross-sectional imaging as core components.

At the outset it is very important to recognize the limitations of both the clinical findings and the investigations that are used to subclassify patients; none will be

100% sensitive and specific, although there is a tendency for the results of investigations to be perceived, almost automatically, as the 'gold standard'. This fact may partially explain the trend for the literature to overemphasize the exceptions to general clinical rules, although even the most sophisticated images have to be interpreted (just like symptoms and signs) with the potential for both inter-observer and intra-observer variability and significant numbers of false positives and false negatives. There are always going to be exceptions to the rules, and one definition of clinical acumen is the ability to sense when such exceptions are likely. Thus, anyone using any system of classification must be blessed with a healthy dose of realism.

One should not presume that the results of investigations will necessarily be any more sensitive or specific than the clinical findings. Investigations contribute most to the diagnostic process when set in a proper clinical context and when they take the pre-test probability of the disorder to be diagnosed into account.

Many clinicians had anticipated that the advances in neuroimaging would have made any clinically based classification redundant long ago. Superficially, a method of subclassification based on the imaged site of brain damage (i.e. a topographical classification) and then describing this in terms of the likely vascular territory involved is attractive. Developments such as diffusion-weighted MR imaging (section 5.5.2) have certainly aided the identification of brain lesions; however, not all infarcts are visible even on DWI and the nature of the DWI 'lesion' does not appear to give additional prognostic information to clinical data.[1,2] There remains, therefore, an illogicality of basing a system on imaging 'holes in the brain', when the current thrust of acute treatments is to prevent such holes appearing by very early therapeutic intervention. So, although imaging has certainly been useful in the subclassification of intracerebral haemorrhage and subarachnoid haemorrhage (Chapters 5, 8 and 9), it has so far failed *on its own* to provide a useful framework for classification of ischaemic stroke and TIA, let alone the entity of 'brain attack'. The reasons for this include the following:

- the surprising inter-individual and intra-individual variability of the pattern of the vascular supply to the brain (section 4.2);
- the current limitations of even the most sophisticated imaging technology to produce reliable results in all patients with stroke – particularly within hours of onset (section 5.5);
- the variations in technology between centres and over time – even different researchers have different machines;

- the problems with generalizability of such a system, even if appropriate images were available (as they may well be in the future), given current problems with the funding of healthcare worldwide;
- the current lack of data correlating cross-sectional imaging with outcome.

In section 4.2, we will review the relevant vascular anatomy, and then in section 4.3 describe a system linking this with the features of the clinical examination of patients with 'brain attack' or stroke that assist lesion localization, as discussed in Chapter 3. Finally, in section 4.4 we will see how this provides a basis for a commonly used aetiological classification.

4.2 Cerebral arterial supply

4.2.1 Introduction

For the information from the clinical history and examination to be formulated in a manner that will have as much relevance as possible to the underlying vascular lesion, the clinician needs to have a working knowledge of the cerebral blood supply. This will also be required for planning and interpreting the results of investigations, and assessing the relevance of possible treatments. However, the general assumption that the vascular supply of the brain follows an entirely predictable pattern (as depicted in many textbooks) and that there are patterns of infarction which are 'typical' of a particular pathogenesis (e.g. embolism from the heart) should certainly not be accepted without closer scrutiny.

Many classifications refer to 'standard' maps of the areas of distribution of individual arteries, especially those that have been produced as cross-sectional templates to correspond with CT/MR sections (e.g. Damasio[3]). The theory goes that if one plots the site and size of the lesion on the scan onto these maps, then the occluded artery can be identified. Additionally, certain sites are identified as arterial boundary zones between the areas of supply of individual arteries, and further assumptions are then often made about the underlying pathophysiological process – e.g. low-flow haemodynamic ischaemic stroke rather than thromboembolism (sections 4.2.4 and 6.7.5). However, it is clear that the cerebral circulation is a dynamic system with large inter-individual and intra-individual variability (i.e. between hemispheres and even varying with time) and that atheroma or other arterial disease in one part of the system may have complex and relatively unpredictable effects on the patterns of vascular supply.[4–6] More recent publications dealing

with the localization of the arterial lesion have begun to take this variability into account.[7,8] But even then, there has to be a lesion on the scan to localize – this is something that is actually becoming less frequent with very early scanning, unless the latest MR techniques are used although these are not infallible; and even when lesions are visible, their size may change with time[9] (Fig. 4.1). Not surprisingly, this all means that attributing an infarct to a particular underlying pathogenesis on the basis of its site and size is often incorrect.[10–12] One important consequence of the above is that at the level of the individual patient, the occlusion of a specific artery may present clinically in different ways. Nevertheless, in this chapter, we have attempted to relate each part of the vascular anatomy to the symptoms and signs commonly, but not always, encountered in clinical practice.

> The pathogenesis of a cerebral infarct cannot be determined purely on the basis of its site and size.

The cerebral vascular anatomy can be described in two main parts: the anterior (carotid) and posterior (vertebrobasilar, VB) systems. With the exception of the basilar, anterior communicating and innominate arteries, the precerebral and intracerebral arteries are paired although only one artery will be described in each section unless there is significant side-to-side variation.

For each system, there are three components: the extracranial arteries, the major intracranial arteries and the small (in terms of diameter) superficial and deep perforating arteries. These component arteries have different structural and functional characteristics, which means that infarction within their territory of distribution is likely to be caused predominantly by different causes (Table 4.2):

Table 4.2 Functional characteristics of the intracranial arteries.

Main parent arteries (e.g. middle cerebral artery)
Anastomotic potential via circle of Willis, extracranial connections and pial collaterals
Thus, marked variability in the area of ischaemia as a result of occlusion
Embolism or *in situ* thrombosis is the most likely cause of occlusion

Cortical branch arteries
Anastomotic potential via pial collaterals
Thus, moderate variability in the area of ischaemia as a result of occlusion
Embolism is the most likely cause of occlusion

Deep perforating arteries
Limited anastomotic potential
Thus, very restricted areas of ischaemia as a result of occlusion
Intrinsic small vessel disease is the most likely cause of occlusion

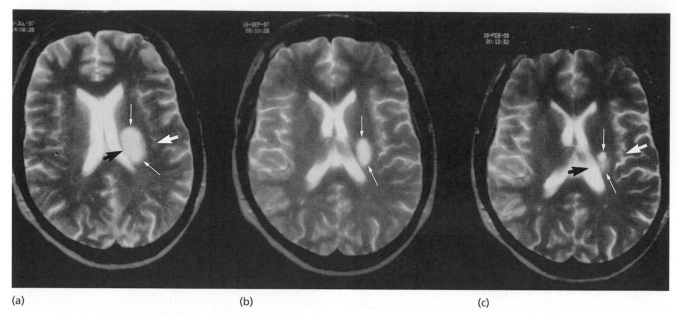

(a)   (b)   (c)

Fig. 4.1 Sequential T2-weighted MR brain scans of a patient with a pure motor stroke affecting the right arm and leg, showing the decreasing size of the small, left deep infarct over time (*thin white arrows*): (a) day 1, (b) 2 months, (c) 19 months post-stroke. Note that there is some swelling of the lesion in the acute phase.

There is slight compression of the adjacent left lateral ventricle (*black arrow*) and of the sylvian fissure (*thick white arrow*), which decreases with time, so that at 19 months, there is an *ex-vacuo* effect – the left lateral ventricle is now larger (*black arrow*) and the sylvian fissure more visible (*thick white arrow*).

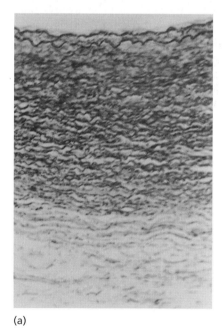
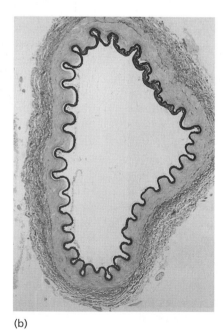
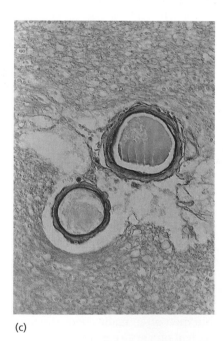

(a)   (b)   (c)

Fig. 4.2 (a) Internal carotid artery just above the common carotid bifurcation (elastic van Gieson (EVG) × 120). The intima at the top of the photograph is barely visible, lying inside an ill-defined internal elastic lamina. The relatively thick media is rich in elastic tissue. The adventitia is thin and poorly defined. (b) Cross-section of the middle cerebral artery (EVG × 50). The intima is barely visible, and lies internal to the folded internal elastic lamina, which shows mild focal reduplication. Both media and adventitia are thinner than in extracranial arteries

of comparable size. The media is virtually devoid of elastic tissue. There is no definite external elastic lamina. (c) A pair of basal ganglionic perforating vessels (EVG × 250). Each of these vessels has an indistinct internal elastic lamina, and a media composed of two to three layers of smooth muscle cells; arterioles are devoid of an internal elastic lamina. (Photographs courtesy of Dr Alistair Lammie, Department of Neuropathology, University of Wales College of Medicine.)

- The extracranial vessels (e.g. the common carotid artery) have a trilaminar structure (intima, media and adventitia) and act as capacitance vessels (Fig. 4.2a). There are a limited number of anastomotic channels between these arteries.

- The larger intracranial arteries (e.g. the middle cerebral artery) have potentially important anastomotic connections over the pial surface of the brain and at the skull base via the circle of Willis and choroidal circulation (see below).[13] The adventitia of these large intracranial arteries is thinner than that of the extracranial vessels, with little elastic tissue (Fig. 4.2b). The media is also thinner, although the internal elastic lamina is thicker (such changes occurring gradually as the arterial diameter decreases). Thus, these vessels are more rigid than extracranial vessels of similar size.

- The small, deep perforating (e.g. the lenticulostriate arteries) and superficial perforating arteries from the pial surface are predominantly end-arteries, with very limited anastomotic potential, and are primarily resistance vessels (Fig. 4.2c).

The overall resistance in any part of the arterial tree is inversely proportional to the vascular density, which, on average, is approximately four times greater in grey matter (cortical and subcortical) than in white matter.[6]

4.2.2 Anterior (carotid) system

Common carotid artery

The left common carotid artery (CCA) usually arises directly from the left side of the aortic arch, whereas the right CCA arises from the innominate (brachiocephalic) artery (Figs 4.3 and 6.2). The CCA ascends through the anterior triangle of the neck, and at the level of the thyroid cartilage divides into the internal carotid artery (ICA) and the external carotid artery (ECA). Throughout, the CCA is intimately associated with the ascending sympathetic nerve fibres. Thus, lesions of the CCA (trauma, dissection or sometimes thrombotic occlusion) may cause an ipsilateral oculosympathetic palsy (Horner's syndrome) with involvement of sudomotor fibres to the face. Damage to the CCA, or thrombus within it, may also result in carotidynia, a syndrome characterized by tenderness over the artery and pain referred to the ipsilateral frontotemporal region. It may also be the site of radiotherapy-induced damage (section 7.12).

> Lesions of the common carotid artery (trauma, dissection or sometimes thrombotic occlusion) may cause an ipsilateral oculosympathetic palsy (Horner's syndrome) with involvement of sudomotor fibres to the face because they are intimately associated with the ascending sympathetic nerve fibres.

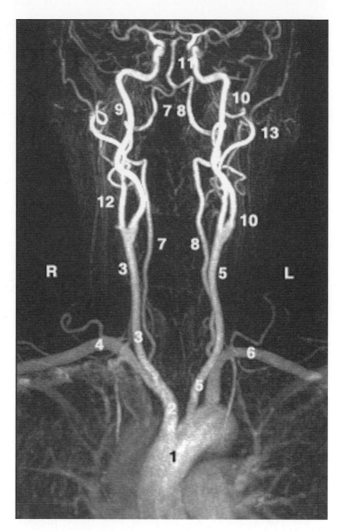

Fig. 4.3 (a) An anteroposterior projection of a contrast-enhanced MR angiogram, showing the origins of the major vessels from the aorta, the cervical course of the carotid and vertebral arteries, and the intracranial connections of anterior and posterior arterial systems. R right; L left; 1 aortic arch; 2 innominate artery; 3 right common carotid artery; 4 right subclavian artery; 5 left common carotid artery; 6 left subclavian artery; 7 right vertebral artery; 8 left vertebral artery; 9 right internal carotid artery; 10 left internal carotid artery; 11 basilar artery; 12 right external carotid artery; 13 left external carotid artery. (See also Fig. 6.2.)

Carotid bifurcation

The carotid bifurcation is usually at the level of the thyroid cartilage, but the exact site may vary by several centimetres (Fig. 4.4). It contains the carotid body (see below). The ICA is usually posterior to the ECA. The carotid body and carotid sinus nerve receive their blood supply from the ECA. The bifurcation is one of the most common sites for atheroma to develop in whites, and it is over this area that bruits can be heard (section 6.7.7). However, there is no way of telling on auscultation

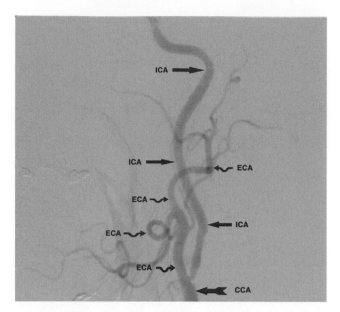

Fig. 4.4 Lateral view of catheter carotid angiogram. ECA external carotid artery and its branches (*curved arrows*); ICA internal carotid artery (*straight arrows*); CCA common carotid artery (*arrow with tail*).

whether a bruit arises from the ICA, ECA or both. One practical point relates to carotid duplex scanning; in most people this images the bifurcation and ICA/ECA for a few centimetres distal, so in patients with a high bifurcation only the CCA may be imaged.

The carotid body responds to increases in the arterial partial pressure of oxygen (PaO_2), blood flow and arterial pH, and to decreases in $PaCO_2$ and blood temperature. It has a modulatory role on pulse rate, blood pressure and hypoxic ventilatory drive.[14] Increased discharges in the carotid sinus nerve can be caused by stretching of its wall, and will increase the depth and rate of respiration and increase peripheral vascular resistance. Carotid sinus hypersensitivity is probably an under-recognized cause of collapse in the elderly, but is not necessarily associated with structural disease of the bifurcation.[15]

External carotid artery

The branches of the external carotid artery (ECA) (ascending pharyngeal, superior thyroid, lingual, occipital, facial, posterior auricular, internal maxillary and superficial temporal) are mainly of interest because of their potential for anastomoses with branches of the intracranial ICA (either spontaneously or by surgery) and their involvement in giant-cell arteritis (section 7.3.1). The presence of extracranial branches distinguishes the ECA from the ICA on arterial studies (Fig. 4.4). In the presence of an extracranial ICA occlusion or severe stenosis, blood flow may be maintained to the ipsilateral

intracranial circulation by ECA–ICA collaterals (see below). It has been suggested that transient monocular blindness can occur due to intermittent failure of perfusion through ECA–ICA collaterals because of stenosis of the ECA origin, particularly when there is ipsilateral ICA occlusion or severe stenosis. Palpable pulsation of the superficial temporal artery may be reduced or absent with ipsilateral CCA or ECA occlusion and, conversely, may be increased when there is ipsilateral ICA occlusion.

Extracranial internal carotid artery

The extracranial internal carotid artery (ICA) arises from the carotid bifurcation, ascends through the neck to the carotid canal of the petrous temporal bone, before passing through the foramen lacerum in the skull base. Along the petrosal section, it gives off small branches to the tympanic cavity and the artery of the pterygoid canal, which may anastomose with the internal maxillary artery, a branch of the ECA. When neurological symptoms occur from disease of the ICA, they may be due to artery-to-artery embolism, low distal flow, or occlusion due to local arterial thrombosis. The clinical picture may range from a transient disturbance of ipsilateral cortical or ocular function to the 'full house' of hemiplegia, hemianaesthesia, hemianopia and profound disturbance of higher cortical function. The variability in clinical presentation does not seem to depend on the presence of collateral flow, but the risk of stroke and TIA is increased when there is severely impaired cerebrovascular reactivity.[16,17] It is possible that the distal extent of any ICA thrombosis may be limited where there is retrograde filling of the ophthalmic artery.[18] Occlusion of the ICA is not always symptomatic; in a series of 994 consecutive autopsies, only 42 of 54 (78%) cases with an ICA occlusion had evidence of ipsilateral infarction, and in about 20% the occlusion had not caused any symptoms, at least as far as could be established from retrospective case note review.[19,20]

The proximal extracranial ICA just beyond the bifurcation is commonly affected by atheroma and when symptoms occur they are most often due to instability and rupture of an atherosclerotic plaque causing artery-to-artery embolism, or much less often low flow distal to an occlusion[21] (section 6.3.2). Other conditions involving the extracranial ICA include arterial dissection (traditionally associated with trauma but also recognized as occurring spontaneously, section 7.2.1) pseudo-aneurysms (caused by dissection) which may be a source of emboli (section 7.1.1); fibromuscular dysplasia (section 7.4.1) and a local arteritis secondary to paratonsillar infections (section 7.11).

The sympathetic nerve fibres lie on the surface of the ICA and can be affected by any of the above processes. The resulting oculosympathetic palsy should spare the sudomotor (sweating) fibres to the face because they are associated with the branches of the ECA. Around the origin of the ICA are the superior laryngeal and hypoglossal nerves, which may be affected by operative procedures and cause hoarseness and tongue weakness respectively (section 16.11.4 and Fig. 16.36).

Carotid siphon and cavernous sinus

After passing through the skull base, the next part of the ICA is the S-shaped carotid siphon which lies within the venous plexus of the cavernous sinus adjacent to cranial nerves III, IV, V_1, V_2 and VI, which run in the lateral wall of the sinus. There are several small branches (the most important of which is the meningo-hypophyseal trunk), which may anastomose with branches of the ECA. One congenital variant worth noting is the persistence of the trigeminal artery, which may arise from the ICA as it enters the cavernous sinus and links with the basilar artery, usually between the superior cerebellar artery and the anterior inferior cerebellar artery.

Atheroma may affect the ICA in the siphon but although this may be a source of embolism, flow restriction and, in a few cases, complete occlusion, the resulting symptoms are similar to those originating from more proximal ICA disease. The degree of atheroma is not necessarily related to that at the carotid bifurcation and when occlusion occurs in the siphon it is more likely to be due to impaction of an embolus from a proximal site than *in situ* thrombosis.[21]

Cavernous sinus thrombosis classically presents with varying degrees of ophthalmoplegia, eye swelling (chemosis) and proptosis (sometimes bilateral, because the venous plexus communicates across the midline) in a patient with facial or sinus infection (Fig. 4.5).[22] Aneurysms of the ICA at the level of the cavernous sinus are relatively common and may present with oculomotor nerve dysfunction. If there is rupture of the artery that is confined by the sinus, then a caroticocavernous fistula may develop. The typical picture is of pulsatile proptosis, with ophthalmoplegia and reduced visual acuity (section 8.2.14).

Supraclinoid internal carotid artery

The short supraclinoid part of the ICA lies in the subarachnoid space close to the oculomotor (III) cranial nerve. The most important branch from this part of the ICA is the ophthalmic artery, which enters the orbit through the optic foramen. Along with its branches

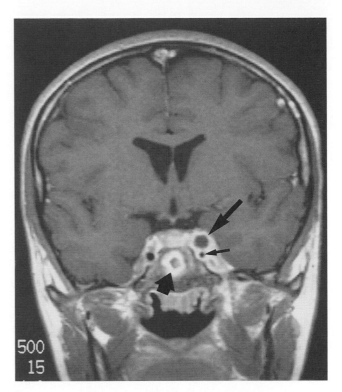

Fig. 4.5 A T1-weighted, gadolinium-enhanced, coronal MR scan, showing thrombosis within the left cavernous sinus. The thrombus (*long arrow*) is seen separate from the flow void in the left internal carotid artery (*short arrow*). Enhancement is seen in the sphenoid sinus (*broad arrow*), which is due to infection. The patient had a fever, chemosis and a partial third nerve palsy.

(lacrimal, supraorbital, ethmoidal, palpebral), the ophthalmic artery is probably the most important anastomotic link with the ECA (Fig. 4.6).

Transient monocular blindness (amaurosis fugax) may be due to emboli passing from the ICA to the ophthalmic artery[23] (section 3.3.6). However, a large proportion of such patients have no evidence of ICA disease, nor for that matter cardiac or aortic sources of embolism, and therefore local atheroma within the ophthalmic artery is presumed to be the cause in many cases. Fixed deficits come from retinal artery occlusion (usually considered to be embolic) and ischaemic optic neuropathy (section 3.5.2), although the latter is surprisingly infrequent with ICA occlusion, presumably because of adequate collateral flow.

The combination of ocular and cerebral hemisphere ischaemic attacks on the same side is a strong pointer towards severe ICA stenosis or occlusion, although the symptoms rarely occur simultaneously. When ICA occlusion occurs, the distal extent of the thrombus usually ends at the level of the ophthalmic artery.[18] The supraclinoid ICA may also be involved by inflammatory/infective processes, such as tuberculous meningitis,

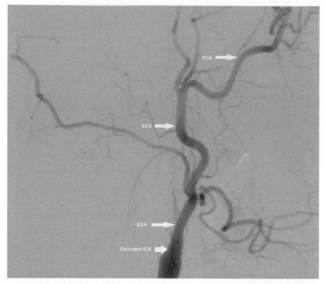

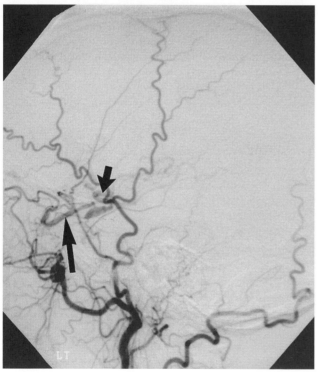

(a)

(b)

Fig. 4.6 (a) A selective intra-arterial catheter angiogram, lateral view, showing occlusion of the left internal carotid artery (ICA, *short arrow*) and filling of the external carotid artery (ECA, *long arrow*). (b) Intracranial views (lateral projection), showing retrograde filling of the ophthalmic artery (*long arrow*) from the ECA, which provides a collateral supply to the distal ICA (*short arrow*, showing the carotid siphon).

in the basal subarachnoid space. Severe stenosis or occlusion of the distal supraclinoid ICA is always present in the moyamoya syndrome (section 7.5).

> The combination of ocular and cerebral hemisphere ischaemic attacks on the same side is a strong pointer towards severe internal carotid artery stenosis or occlusion.

There are also a number of small perforating branches that supply the pituitary gland, hypothalamus and optic chiasm. Other branches may pass through the anterior perforated substance to supply the genu and part of the posterior limb of the internal capsule, and the globus pallidus.

Posterior communicating artery

The next branch of the ICA is usually the posterior communicating artery (PCoA). Arising from the dorsal aspect of the ICA, it runs back above the oculomotor (III) nerve to join the posterior cerebral artery (PCA) (Fig. 4.7). The PCoA may give off small branches which contribute to the blood supply of the basal ganglia.

Aneurysms at the origin of the PCoA may present with a painful oculomotor (III) nerve palsy usually but not always with a fixed, dilated pupil, or with subarachnoid haemorrhage (section 9.3.6). In a few patients, both PCoAs are absent which may result in much more

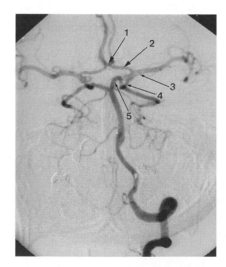

Fig. 4.7 Demonstration of the components of the circle of Willis by intra-arterial catheter angiography (anteroposterior projection). The whole of the circle is filled from a selective left vertebral artery injection in a patient who had bilateral internal carotid artery occlusions. The components are: 1 anterior communicating artery; 2 anterior cerebral artery; 3 middle cerebral artery; 4 posterior communicating artery; 5 posterior cerebral artery.

marked neurological deficits from lesions of the posterior circulation than in patients with a functionally intact circle of Willis (see below).

Anterior choroidal artery

Just before its terminal bifurcation into the anterior cerebral artery and middle cerebral artery (MCA), the ICA usually gives rise to the anterior choroidal artery (AChA) (Fig. 4.8), although occasionally the AChA arises from either the proximal stem of the MCA or the posterior communicating artery. It is a relatively small artery which gains its name because it supplies the choroid plexus. It may also supply the globus pallidus, anterior hippocampus, uncus, lower part of the posterior limb of the internal capsule and anterior part of the midbrain, including the cerebral peduncle.[24] It accompanies the

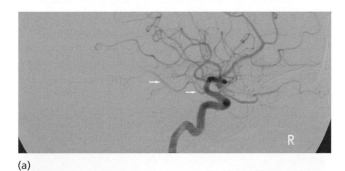

(a)

(b)

Fig. 4.8 Carotid catheter angiograms, showing the anterior choroidal artery (*arrows*): (a) lateral view, (b) anteroposterior view.

optic tract and sends branches to the lateral geniculate nucleus (LGN) and the anterior part of the optic radiation. It may anastomose with the posterior choroidal artery (a branch of the posterior cerebral artery).

The cause of occlusion of the AChA is very variable although when infarction is restricted to the internal capsule it is probably more often due to intrinsic disease of the artery complicated by *in situ* thrombosis than embolism from more proximal sources[25]. Also, the AChA may be particularly susceptible to the effects of intracarotid chemotherapy.[26] AChA territory infarcts typically produce a contralateral hemiparesis and hemisensory deficit, the latter often sparing proprioception. Language and visuospatial function may be affected, and are attributed to extension of the ischaemia to the lateral thalamus. Large AChA territory infarcts have an additional visual field defect. This can be a homonymous hemianopia (due to ischaemia of the optic tract) but the pathognomonic pattern is considered to be a homonymous horizontal sectoranopia due to involvement of the LGN.[27]

Distal internal carotid artery

At the bifurcation of the ICA, the main continuing branch is usually the middle cerebral artery, while the smaller anterior cerebral artery and the posterior communicating artery form the anterior portion of the circle of Willis (Fig. 4.7). This is not a common site for atheroma, but can be the superior extent of a carotid dissection (section 7.2.1). It is also a site of aneurysm formation (section 9.1.1).

Circle of Willis

In the embryo, a large branch from the ICA provides most of the blood supply to the occipital lobes. From this branch, the future posterior communicating artery (PCoA) and post-communicating (P2) segment of the posterior cerebral artery (PCA) will develop and these usually will link with the pre-communicating (P1) segment of the PCA, which develops from the basilar artery. The arterial components of the circle of Willis and the origins of its branches (i.e. the anterior cerebral arteries (ACAs), the PCAs, the anterior communicating artery (ACoA) and the PCoAs) are formed by 6–7 weeks of gestation.[28] At this stage, the PCoA and the P1 segment of the PCA are usually of approximately similar diameter and contribute equally to the supply of the P2 segment of the PCA. This 'transitional' configuration is present in nearly 80% of fetuses under 20 weeks gestation, but over the next 20 weeks (and particularly between the 21st and 29th weeks of gestation, which coincides with the period of most rapid growth of the occipital lobes) there is a change.[29] In the majority, the P1 segment of the PCA becomes larger than the PCoA, resulting in the 'adult' configuration, where the occipital lobes are supplied primarily by the posterior circulation. However, in a minority, the PCoA becomes larger and the occipital lobes then obtain most of their blood supply from the carotid circulation, a situation which is referred to as a 'fetal' configuration. The 'transitional configuration' persists in less than 10% of adults although the exact proportions of the different configurations are difficult to estimate from the literature, because of the very variable selection criteria that have been used.[29,30]

Anomalies of the circle of Willis are reported in between half and four-fifths of normal individuals, depending on selection criteria; for example, anomalies certainly seem to be more prevalent in patients with cerebrovascular disease.[30,31] The distribution of the abnormalities found in a study of 994 autopsies is shown in Fig. 4.9.[30] In this study, hypoplasia of part of the anterior part of the circle of Willis was found in 13%, of the posterior part in 32%, and of both parts in 36%. When there was maldevelopment of either the P1 segment of the PCA or

the pre-communicating (A1) segment of the ACA, there was usually an ectopic origin of the distal branches. Taken alongside the haemodynamic consequences of the hypoplastic segments of the circle of Willis, these anatomical factors result in considerable variation in the area of supply of the major intracerebral arteries and the ability of the cerebral circulation to respond to changes in perfusion pressure when more proximal arteries are diseased.[6,32] Not surprisingly, one cannot identify any particular clinical syndrome related to any specific anomalies of the circle of Willis.

Anterior cerebral artery

The anterior cerebral artery (ACA) arises as the medial branch of the bifurcation of the ICA, at the level of the anterior clinoid process and is traditionally divided into sections. The proximal (A1) sections of the ACAs pass medially and forward over the optic nerve or chiasm and corpus callosum to enter the inter-hemispheric fissure, where they are linked by the anterior communicating artery (ACoA) (Fig. 4.10). After the AChA the distal (A2) sections of the ACAs run together in the

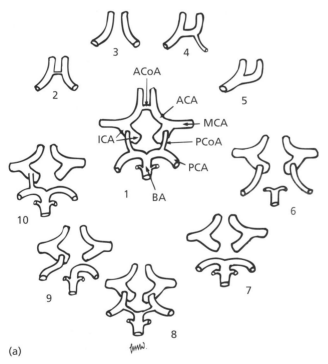

(a)

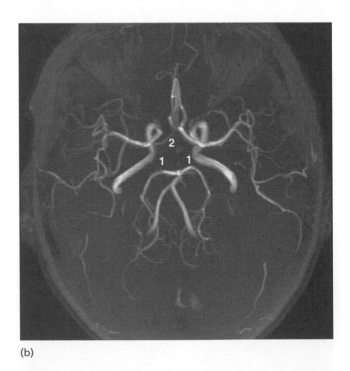

(b)

Fig. 4.9 Anomalies of the circle of Willis. (a) In the centre is a complete circle of Willis (1). There are 21 possible variants. Those involving the anterior cerebral arteries (ACA) and anterior communicating artery (ACoA) are shown at the top (2–5) and some of those involving the posterior communicating arteries (PCoA) below (6–10). The anterior part of the circle provides poor collateral supply in 24% of people

and no collateral supply in 7%. The most common anomaly of the PCoA is direct origin from the internal carotid artery (ICA) (6 and 9), which occurs in 30% of people (BA basilar artery; PCA posterior cerebral artery; MCA middle cerebral artery). (b) An MR angiogram of the circle of Willis demonstrating absence of both posterior communicating arteries (1) and hypoplasia of the left ACA (2).

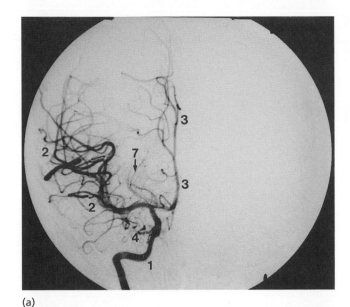

(a)

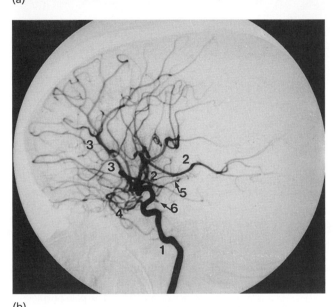

(b)

Fig. 4.10 Selective catheter carotid angiogram of the anterior intracranial circulation: (a) anteroposterior projection (b) lateral projection. 1 internal carotid artery; 2 middle cerebral artery and its branches; 3 anterior cerebral artery and its branches; 4 ophthalmic artery; 5 anterior choroidal artery; 6 vestigial stump of the posterior communicating artery (normal variant); 7 lenticulostriate arteries.

inter-hemispheric fissure and then continue backwards as the A3 sections, the anterior pericallosal and callosomarginal arteries. Other branches include the orbitofrontal, frontopolar, anterior, middle and posterior internal frontal, paracentral and superior and inferior parietal arteries. The anterior pericallosal arteries may form anastomoses with the posterior pericallosal

arteries from the posterior cerebral artery. The potential minimum and maximum areas of supply are shown in Fig. 4.11.[5]

Isolated infarction of the ACA territory is comparatively rare, other than when due to 'vasospasm' complicating subarachnoid haemorrhage (section 14.5.1). Part of the explanation may be that if the proximal ACA is occluded, the distal ACA obtains a blood supply from the other ACA, via the ACoA. Most cases of ACA territory infarction are probably due to either cardioembolism or artery-to-artery embolism from an occluded or stenosed internal carotid artery.[33] Bilateral ACA territory infarction should always prompt a search for an ACoA aneurysm which may have bled recently, although it may also be caused by thromboembolism in patients where both ACAs receive their supply from the same carotid artery via the ACoA, or more rarely when the distal branches cross the midline in the inter-hemispheric fissure.[34]

> Bilateral anterior cerebral artery territory infarction should always prompt a search for an anterior communicating artery aneurysm which may have bled recently.

The motor deficit in the leg usually predominates over that in the arm and is often most marked distally, in contrast to that from cortical middle cerebral artery infarcts.[35] When the arm is affected, this is usually attributed to extension of the ischaemic area to the internal capsule, although in some cases it may also be a form of motor 'neglect' through involvement of the supplementary motor area.[33] There is often no sensory deficit, but even when present it is usually mild. When the motor deficit is bilateral, ACA territory infarction needs to be distinguished from a lesion in the spinal cord or brainstem. Other frontal lobe features may be present, including urinary incontinence, lack of motivation or, paradoxically, agitation and social disinhibition. Abulia and akinetic mutism (section 3.3.2) may occur, usually with bilateral lesions. A grasp reflex may be elicited if the motor deficit in the hand is not too great. Various aphasic syndromes have been described, and these are usually attributed to involvement of the dominant supplementary motor area (rather than Broca's area). Typically, there will be reduced spontaneous output but preserved repetition. These patients may be mute immediately after the onset of the stroke. Occlusion of the ACA can result in apraxias and other disconnection syndromes[36] (section 3.3.3). Interruption of the frontocerebellar tracts can result in incoordination of the contralateral limbs which may mimic cerebellar dysfunction, a fact which in the pre-CT era occasionally resulted in suboccipital explorations looking for cerebellar tumours.[37] When

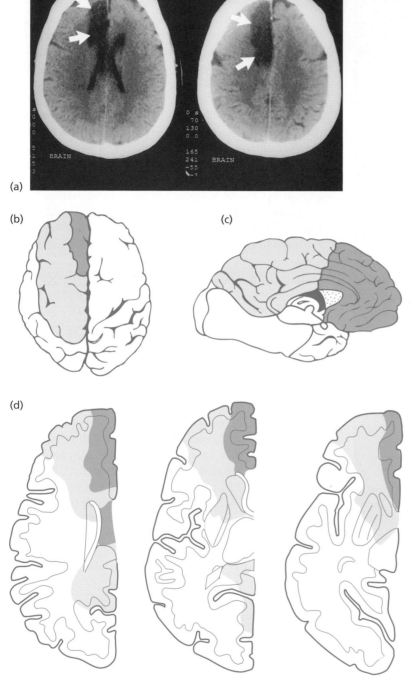

(a)

(b)

(c)

(d)

Fig. 4.11 Ischaemia in the territory of the anterior cerebral artery (ACA). (a) The typical appearance on an axial CT brain scan of ACA territory infarction (*arrows*). However, there is great inter-individual and inter-hemispheric variability in the area supplied by the ACA (b, c). The dark purple areas show the only part of the cortex on the superolateral surface (b) and the medial surface (c) of the hemisphere, which was *always* supplied by the ACA in a large pathological study.[230] (van der Zwan 1991). The pale purple represents the maximum extent of the area that may be supplied by the ACA in some patients. (d) There is a similar degree of variability for the intracerebral territory supplied by the ACA. The figure shows the minimum (dark purple) and maximum (pale purple) areas of supply at three levels in the same pathological study. (Reproduced with permission from Dr A. van der Zwan.)

there is also a corticospinal deficit, it may mimic the lacunar syndrome of homolateral ataxia and crural paresis (see below).[38] Amnesic disorders are also encountered, particularly after rupture of an ACoA aneurysm. The 'alien-hand sign' refers to a variety of dissociative movements between right and left hands due to a lesion of the medial frontal lobe and/or corpus callosum.[39,40]

Recurrent artery of Heubner

This artery is an inconstant branch of the ACA, which, if present, usually arises at the junction with or just beyond the level of the ACoA.[41] It may supply the head of the caudate, the inferior portion of the anterior limb of the internal capsule, and the hypothalamus (Fig. 4.12).

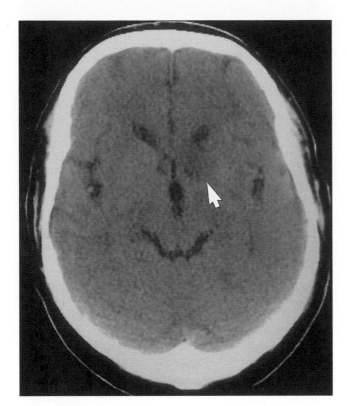

Fig. 4.12 A CT brain scan showing the typical area of infarction (*arrow*) resulting from occlusion of the recurrent artery of Heubner.

The characteristic deficit from unilateral occlusion was said to be weakness of the face and arm, often with dysarthria.[35] However, more recent work suggests that the motor deficit may actually be due to involvement of the medial striate arteries (see below).[42–44] The syndromes of akinetic mutism or abulia (section 3.3.2) may occur but are usually associated with bilateral lesions.

Anterior cerebral artery: deep perforating arteries (medial striate)

A variable number of small branches from the A1 segment of the ACA and ACoA enter the anterior perforated substance and may supply the anterior striatum, the superior anterior limb of the internal capsule and the anterior commissure. They may also supply the optic chiasm and tract.[45] Occlusion of the medial striate arteries cause weakness of the face and arm.

Middle cerebral artery: mainstem

The midle cerebral artery (MCA) is traditionally divided into sections. The first section (M1) passes laterally between the upper surface of the temporal lobe and the inferior surface of the frontal lobe until it reaches the lateral part of the Sylvian fissure (Fig. 4.10). The lenticulostriate arteries mostly arise from the proximal part of the MCA mainstem (see below).

Atheroma may develop *in situ*, but this is uncommon in whites but perhaps more frequent in people from east Asia (section 6.3.1). Therefore, in whites the mechanism of occlusion tends to be either impaction of an embolus, extension of a more proximal thrombus (e.g. from the internal carotid artery), or less commonly intracranial dissection.[46–48] As far as we know, occlusion of the MCA mainstem is nearly always symptomatic, although some young patients with very good cortical collateral supply may have remarkably few symptoms. In most cases, the occlusion occurs in the proximal mainstem, thereby involving the lenticulostriate arteries, and consequently there is ischaemia of both the deep and superficial territories of the MCA. Typically, this presents as a contralateral hemimotor and sensory deficit, with a homonymous hemianopia and aphasia or visuospatial disturbance depending on which hemisphere is affected. If the cortical collateral supply from the anterior cerebral artery (ACA) and posterior cerebral artery (PCA) is good, the brunt of the ischaemia tends to fall on the subcortical structures, resulting in a striatocapsular infarct (see below). If the occlusion is more distal in the mainstem and there is no ischaemia in the lenticulostriate territory, the leg may be relatively spared because most fibres to the leg originate in cortical areas usually supplied by the ACA and these descend medially in the corona radiata adjacent to the lateral ventricle.[49]

Middle cerebral artery: deep perforating arteries (lenticulostriate)

Arising from the main MCA mainstem, there are usually between 6 and 12 lenticulostriate arteries, most of which emerge at right angles to their parent artery to enter the anterior perforated substance. Three groups can be identified – medial, middle and lateral. These may supply the lentiform nucleus, lateral head of the caudate nucleus, anterior limb of the internal capsule, part of the globus pallidus and lower parts of the internal capsule (Fig. 4.13). Some, particularly those in the lateral group, have their origins from a cortical branch of the MCA, or from either the superior or inferior divisions of the MCA.[50]

When a thrombus or embolus in the MCA mainstem lies over the origins of all of the lenticulostriate arteries a 'comma'-shaped infarct (when viewed in the axial plane) may develop – a so-called striatocapsular infarct (Fig. 4.14 and see Fig. 6.20) (section 6.7.2). About one-third to one-half of cases will have a potential cardiac source of embolism, one-third stenotic or occlusive disease of the ICA, and one-third stenosis or occlusion

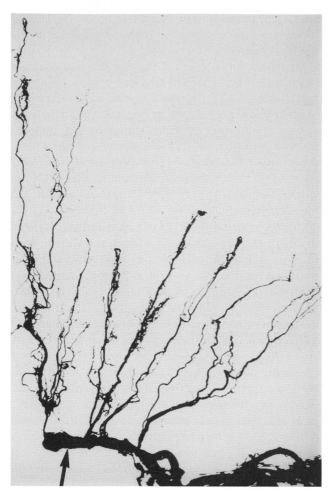

Fig. 4.13 Postmortem demonstration of the deep perforating arteries arising from the mainstem of the middle cerebral artery (*arrow*).

confined to the MCA mainstem.[51,52] Angiographic studies have shown that MCA mainstem occlusion of this type may be relatively short-lived, presumably due to fragmentation of the embolus.[46,47] The deficit in the limbs tends to be motor rather than sensory and is often similarly severe in the arm and leg. In about 70% there are symptoms of cortical dysfunction, although these may be mild and resolve rapidly. The pathogenesis of the cortical symptoms is much debated but seems most likely to be due to cortical ischaemia, which is not imaged by CT or MR, although it may be detected by functional imaging, such as position emission tomography (PET) and single-photon emission CT (SPECT).[51] The alternative explanations include deafferentation of the cortex, direct interruption of subcortical–cortical pathways, or involvement of subcortical structures which subserve language functions. Hemianopia is unusual.

Occlusion of a single lenticulostriate artery results in a 'lacunar infarct' (Fig. 4.15), there being no functional anastomoses between adjacent perforating arteries.[50]

It should be stressed that 'lacunar infarction' is a pathological term, and for clarity the radiological equivalent is best referred to as a 'small, deep infarct'.[53] Based on early pathological studies, most occlusions of single, deep perforating arteries from the MCA mainstem were thought to be caused by local *in situ* small-vessel disease rather than embolism, although the number of pathologically verified cases was very small. However, more recent pathological and radiological studies have suggested that at least some lacunar infarcts may be caused by a disturbance of blood–brain barrier permeability[54,55] (section 6.4). There is considerable inter-individual variation in the number of lenticulostriate arteries, and in general the largest area is supplied by the most lateral branch. Additionally, the volume of an individual infarct will depend on the actual site of occlusion, i.e. the more proximal the occlusion of the deep perforating artery, the larger the lacune. The tendency for studies not to consider small, deep infarcts greater than 1.5 m diameter as the radiological equivalent of lacunes probably leads to under-reporting, this cut-off size emanating originally from pathological studies.[56] When the results of acute imaging and subsequent autopsy have been compared directly, the lesion at autopsy was significantly smaller than that seen on brain imaging.[57] Single lacunes may present with one of the classical 'lacunar syndromes' (section 4.3.2) or, rarely, with isolated movement disorders, such as hemiballismus. However, the majority of lacunes (80%) are clinically silent (or at least clinically unrecognized), occurring most frequently in the lentiform nucleus.[56]

> Lacunar infarction is a pathological term, and for clarity the radiological equivalent should probably be referred to as a 'small, deep infarct'.

Multiple supratentorial lacunes, also referred to as *état lacunaire*, may present as a pseudobulbar palsy, with or without *marche à petits pas*. This abnormality of gait superficially resembles that of Parkinson's disease, but debate continues as to whether a true Parkinsonian syndrome can occur from lacunes in the basal ganglia.[58–62] It is important to distinguish *état lacunaire* from the dilatations of perivascular spaces (*état criblé*) that are often present in the basal ganglia of hypertensive individuals, and which may be difficult to differentiate on MR scans[63] (Fig. 4.16). These are not due to infarction and have not been convincingly associated with any particular clinical presentation.

Middle cerebral artery: cortical branches

In the sylvian fissure, the M2 section of the MCA usually bifurcates into superior and inferior divisions. The

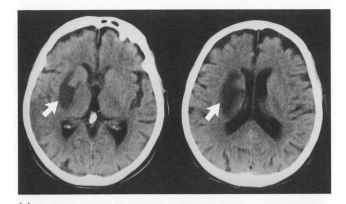

(a)

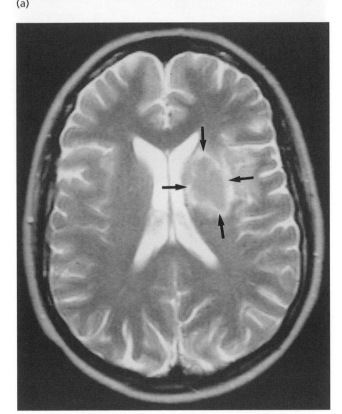

(b)

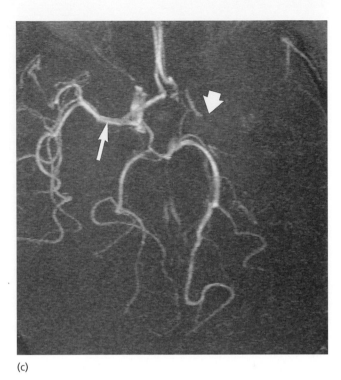

(c)

Fig. 4.14 Striatocapsular infarction. (a) The typical appearance of a right striatocapsular infarct on a CT brain scan, axial views (*arrows*). (b) A T2-weighted axial MR scan, showing a left striatocapsular infarct (*arrows*) and an MR angiogram (c) from the same patient, showing lack of flow in the proximal segment of the left middle cerebral artery (*broad arrow*). Normal flow is seen in the right middle cerebral artery (*narrow arrow*). The patient had had a recent anterior myocardial infarction, and it was presumed that an embolus had lodged in the proximal left middle cerebral artery. (See also Fig. 6.20e)

superior division generally gives rise to the orbitofrontal, prefrontal, pre-Rolandic, Rolandic, anterior parietal and posterior parietal branches, while the inferior division usually gives rise to the angular, temporo-occipital, posterior temporal, middle temporal, anterior temporal and temporopolar branches. However, there are many variations in this pattern. The potential minimum and maximum area of supply of these branches is shown in Fig. 4.17.[5] At their origins, the luminal diameter of these vessels is usually about 1 mm, but by the time they anastomose with the cortical branches of the anterior and posterior cerebral arteries, they are usually less than 0.2 mm in diameter.[13] There is almost no collateral connection between individual branches of the MCA.

The branches of the MCA are not often affected by local atherosclerotic disease although they can be affected by vasculitis, amyloid angiopathy and mycotic aneurysms. Therefore, the main causes of MCA branch ischaemia are probably embolism, or low flow, secondary to more proximal vascular lesions.[46,64] The usual clinical syndrome resulting from occlusion of the superior division is much the same as for the MCA mainstem, but in general the motor and sensory deficits are greater in the face and arm than in the leg. Occlusion of the inferior division usually causes a homonymous hemianopia or superior quadrantanopia and fluent aphasia (in the dominant hemisphere) but relatively mild problems in the limbs, although higher-level discriminatory sensory

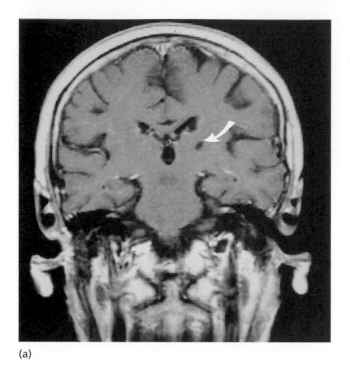

(a)

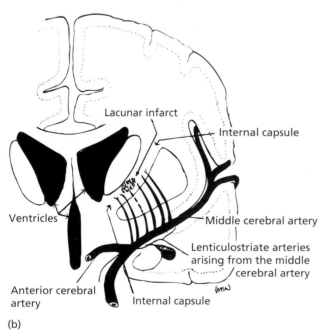

(b)

Fig. 4.15 Lacunar infarction. (a) The typical appearance of a small, deep infarct confined to the territory of a single, deep perforating artery on a T1-weighted, coronal MR scan (*curved arrow*). (b) A diagrammatic representation of the case, demonstrating the likely underlying vascular process (coronal brain section); one of the lenticulostriate arteries is occluded (*broken line*).

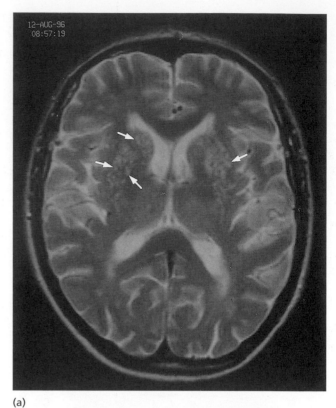

(a)

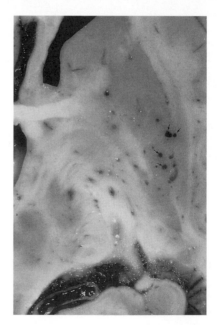

(b)

Fig. 4.16 The appearance of *état criblé*: (a) on a T2-weighted MR brain scan (*arrows*); (b) in a pathological specimen.

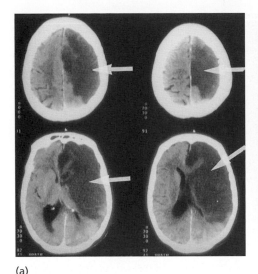

(a)

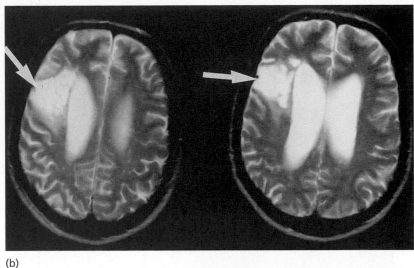

(b)

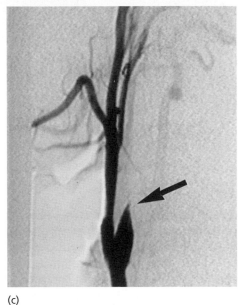

(c)

Fig. 4.17 Ischaemia in the territory of the middle cerebral artery (MCA). (a) The typical appearance on a CT brain scan of extensive MCA territory infarction (*arrows*) in a patient who had an occluded mainstem of the MCA. (b) The typical appearance on a T2-weighted MR scan of MCA branch occlusion (*arrows*). (c) The patient whose scan is shown in (b) was a young man with dissection of the proximal internal carotid artery (ICA) (*arrow*) in a road accident. The intra-arterial digital subtraction catheter angiogram shows a smooth, tapering, complete occlusion of the proximal ICA, typical of dissection.

functions may be affected. A similar pattern can, however, occur with occlusion of the posterior cerebral artery (section 4.2.3). The area of infarcted cortex may be very small, so small that the distinction on CT from cortical atrophy can be difficult (section 5.4.2). As a result, some very restricted clinical deficits occur. For example, it has been shown that isolated arm weakness is more likely to occur from a cortical than a subcortical lesion.[65–67]

Although there is a large volume of classical neurological literature correlating various restricted 'MCA' syndromes (most of which include some disturbance of higher cortical function) with ischaemia or haemorrhage in specific areas of brain parenchyma, the inter-individual variability of the vascular anatomy means that it is virtually impossible to link them reliably with occlusions of particular MCA branches.[68,69] Furthermore, many of the reports do not deal with deficits in the acute phase of stroke.

Middle cerebral artery: medullary perforating arteries

Medullary perforating arteries arise from distal branches of the middle cerebral artery (MCA) on the surface of the hemispheres. They are usually 20–50 mm in length and descend to supply the subcortical white matter (i.e. centrum semiovale), converging centripetally towards the lateral ventricle[70] (Fig. 4.18). These are functional end-arteries, and their distal fields are part of the internal boundary zone (section 4.2.4).

Isolated, acute infarcts of the centrum semiovale are thought to be uncommon but are probably being recognized more often with the greater use of MR

(d)

(e)

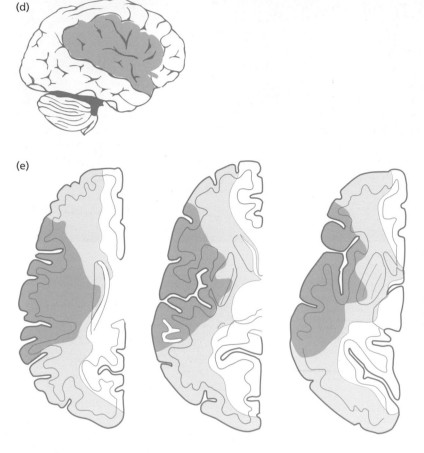

Fig. 4.17 (*continued*) (d) However, there is great inter-individual and inter-hemispheric variability in the area of brain supplied by the MCA. The dark purple area shows the only part of the cortex on the lateral surface of the hemisphere which was *always* supplied by the MCA in a large pathological study.[230] (e) There is a similar degree of variability for the intracerebral territory supplied by the MCA. The figure shows the minimum (dark purple) and maximum (light purple) areas of supply at three levels in the same pathological study. (Reproduced with permission of Dr A. van der Zwan.)

diffusion-weighted imaging.[71,72] The majority are small (<1.5 cm in diameter) and probably arise from occlusion of a single medullary perforating artery, although this has never been verified pathologically. The spectrum of clinical presentation is similar to that of single deep MCA perforating artery (i.e. lenticulostriate artery) occlusions, with the classical lacunar syndromes of pure motor stroke, sensorimotor stroke and ataxic hemiparesis predominating. In such cases, there is rarely evidence of large-vessel disease or cardioembolism. Larger infarcts in this area present with a syndrome similar to more extensive MCA cortical infarction, with weakness/sensory loss which is more marked in the face and arm than leg, aphasia or visuospatial disturbance and, if the optic radiation is involved, a visual field defect. These are more often associated with large-vessel disease (internal carotid artery/MCA occlusion or stenosis). However, such infarcts may in fact be in the internal boundary zone, particularly when there are multiple lesions.[72,73] The explanations for deficits of 'cortical' modalities are similar to those for striatocapsular infarction, i.e. ischaemia without necrosis, deafferentation of the cortex, or involvement of subcortical structures subserving 'cortical' functions, but there is little evidence to support any of them.

4.2.3 Posterior (vertebrobasilar) system

The vertebrobasilar (VB) system develops quite separately from the carotid system and is subject to many more changes during gestation. It is this that probably accounts for the much greater variation in arterial configuration within the VB than in the carotid system, and this may contribute to the development of ischaemia.[74]

Extracranial vertebral artery

The right vertebral artery (VA) arises as the first branch of the right subclavian artery (which arises from the innominate artery), while the left VA arises as the first branch of the left subclavian artery (which arises directly from the aortic arch) (Figs 4.3 and 4.19). The course of the VA is traditionally divided into sections. The V1 section is from the origin to the transverse foramen at either C5 or C6. The V2 section is within the transverse foramina from the C5/6 level to C2. The V3 section circles the arch of C1 and passes between the atlas and occiput. The major branch outside the skull is the single, midline anterior spinal artery, formed by a contribution from both VAs.

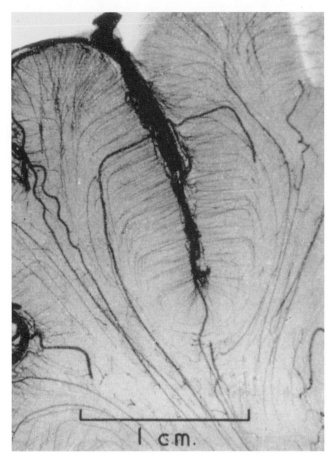

Fig. 4.18 Pathological demonstration of the medullary perforating arteries arising from the cortical surface (courtesy of Dr Nigel Hyman, Taunton, UK).

The origin of the VA can be affected by atheroma, either within the VA itself or by overlying plaque in the innominate or subclavian arteries, and may be the site of occlusion or a source of emboli.[75,76] It may also be involved in inflammatory disorders, such as Takayasu's arteritis (section 7.3.2) and be the site of arterial dissection) (section 7.2.1). Trapping of the VA by cervical spondylosis is frequently cited as a cause of symptoms attributed to 'vertebrobasilar insufficiency', but in reality, both the symptoms (which are generally non-focal) and the X-ray changes of cervical spondylosis are very common in older people, and rarely is there a convincing cause-and-effect relationship (section 7.1.5). However, thrombus may form in the VA after prolonged or unusual neck posturing.[77,78]

Intracranial vertebral artery

The V4 section of the vertebral artery (VA) is intracranial, until the two arteries unite to form the midline basilar artery at the pontomedullary junction (Fig. 4.19). As the VAs pierce the dura, there is a decrease in the thickness of the adventitial and medial layers, with marked reduction in both medial and external elastic laminae. There may be branches which supply the medulla.

As with the ICA, occlusion of a VA may be asymptomatic. At the other extreme, there may be extensive infarction of the lateral medulla and inferior cerebellar hemisphere. Atheroma is a common cause of stenosis or occlusion.[79] Dissection of the intracranial VA may present with subarachnoid haemorrhage (sections 7.2.2

Fig. 4.19 Angiographic demonstration of the vertebrobasilar arterial system. (a) Anteroposterior projection of an MR angiogram, showing the extracranial vertebral arteries. The numbers refer to the segments of the artery; (0) the origin; (1) the precanal portion; (2) the intracanalicular part; (3) the horizontal part. The large arrow shows an intravertebral disc. (b) Lateral projection of an intra-arterial catheter angiogram, showing (1) the distal vertebral artery; (2) the posterior inferior cerebellar artery; (3) the basilar artery; (4) the anterior inferior cerebellar artery; (5) the superior cerebellar artery; (6) the posterior cerebral artery.

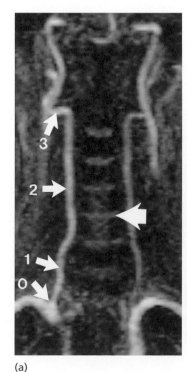

(a)

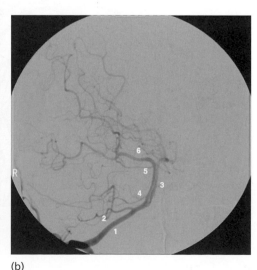

(b)

and 9.1.3). The subclavian steal syndrome, as memorable as it is rare, occurs when there is haemodynamically significant stenosis of the subclavian artery proximal to the origin of the VA. In this situation, the direction of blood flow is normal in the contralateral VA but reversed in the ipsilateral VA, with blood passing into the axillary artery from the VA. The blood pressure will be lower in the affected arm. Exercise of the ipsilateral arm increases the flow away from the brainstem, which may cause neurological symptoms. However, it is noteworthy that reversed flow in VA is a common finding on ultrasound and angiographic studies in patients with no neurological symptoms at all.[80]

> Reversed flow in one vertebral artery is a common finding in patients with no neurological symptoms – it is very rare to find a patient who has symptoms of the subclavian steal syndrome.

Posterior inferior cerebellar artery

The posterior inferior cerebellar arteries (PICAs) usually arise from the intracranial vertebral arteries (VA), although one may be absent in up to 25% of patients (Figs 4.19 and 4.20). Also, the VA may terminate in the PICA, i.e. there is no distal connection with the basilar artery. Small branches from the PICA may supply the lateral medulla, but more frequently it is supplied by direct branches from the VA originating between the origin of the PICA and the basilar artery.[81] There are medial and lateral branches of the PICA, the medial branch usually supplying the cerebellar vermis and adjacent cerebellar hemisphere and the lateral branch the cortical surface of the cerebellar tonsil and suboccipital cerebellar hemisphere.

Historically, occlusion of the PICA has been linked to lateral medullary infarcts, causing Wallenberg's syndrome. This consists of an ipsilateral Horner's syndrome (descending sympathetic fibres), loss of spinothalamic function over the contralateral limbs (spinothalamic tract) and ipsilateral face (descending trigeminal tract), vertigo, nausea, vomiting and nystagmus (vestibular nuclei), ipsilateral ataxia of limbs (inferior cerebellar peduncle) and ipsilateral paralysis of palate, larynx and pharynx (nucleus ambiguus), resulting in dysarthria, dysphonia and dysphagia. As with other 'classical' eponymous brainstem syndromes, the complete form of Wallenberg's syndrome is relatively infrequent in clinical practice. Indeed, syndromes which do not involve the lateral medulla but only the cerebellum are now recognized as being more frequent. These usually present with vertigo, ataxia (of gait and limbs), nystagmus and headache. Another striking symptom is ipsilateral axial lateropulsion, which seems to the patient like lateral displacement of their centre of gravity or being pushed to one side, although this can also

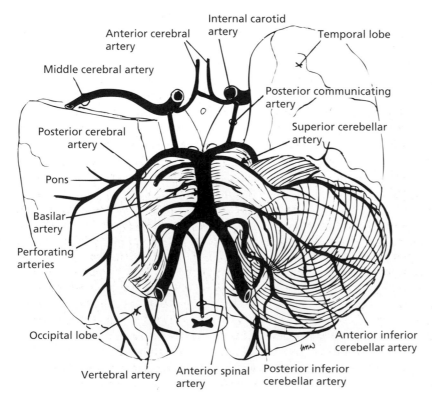

Fig. 4.20 Arterial supply of the cerebellum. The brainstem, cerebellum and inferior surface of the temporal and occipital lobes viewed from anteroinferiorly. The cerebellum, on the left-hand side of the drawing, has been cut away to reveal the inferior temporal and occipital lobes. Three major pairs of arteries supply the cerebellum: the superior cerebellar, the anterior inferior cerebellar (both branches of the basilar) and the posterior inferior cerebellar arteries (branch of the vertebral arteries). Perforating branches of the basilar artery supply the pons. The medial parts of the medulla are supplied by the anterior spinal artery and the lateral parts by branches of the vertebral arteries. The posterior cerebral arteries supply the posteromedial temporal lobes and the occipital lobes. The superior surface of the cerebellum (not shown) is predominantly supplied by the superior cerebellar arteries.

occur with ischaemia in the territories of the anterior inferior and superior cerebellar arteries.[82] Isolated vertigo has been reported in cases of PICA territory infarction but it is difficult if not impossible to distinguish the few cases of vertigo due to cerebellar stroke from the many more commoner causes of vestibular dysfunction unless the patient remains ataxic after any rotational component has settled, and there is an appropriate infarct on brain imaging[81,83,84] (section 3.3.7). Infarcts restricted to the territory of either the medial or lateral branches of the PICA usually cause less impairment.[82,85]

Basilar artery

The general pattern of branching from the basilar artery is of short paramedian (perforating) branches, which supply the base of the pons to either side of the midline and also the paramedian aspects of the pontine tegmentum. The lateral aspects of the base of the pons and the tegmentum are supplied by pairs of short and long circumferential arteries, which also supply the cerebellar hemispheres. The frequency of infarction from occlusion of such perforating arteries has probably been underestimated, partly because of the difficulty of imaging such infarcts in the pre-MRI era.

Occlusion of a single paramedian artery, resulting in a restricted infarct in the brainstem, can present with any of the classical lacunar syndromes (section 4.3.2). Disturbances of eye movement (either nuclear or internuclear) may also occur from such lesions, either in isolation or in addition to pure motor deficits (e.g. Weber's syndrome).[86,87] Unlike the anterior circulation, where intrinsic disease of the anterior cerebral or middle cerebral artery mainstem is uncommon, occlusion of the mouth of a single perforating artery by a plaque of atheroma in the parent basilar artery needs to be considered alongside intrinsic small-vessel disease as the underlying mechanism.[88] The 'locked-in syndrome' occurs with bilateral infarction, or haemorrhage, of the base of the pons (section 3.3.2).

The 'top of the basilar syndrome' is a constellation of symptoms and signs that may occur when an embolus impacts in the distal basilar artery, resulting in bilateral ischaemia of upper brainstem structures and of the posterior cerebral artery territories.[89] The syndrome consists of altered pupillary responses, supranuclear paresis of vertical gaze, ptosis or lid retraction, somnolence, hallucinations, involuntary movements such as hemiballismus, visual abnormalities such as cortical blindness (from involvement of the occipital lobes), and an amnesic state (from involvement of the temporal lobes or thalamus).

Sometimes the basilar artery becomes elongated (and therefore tortuous) and dilated (Figs 4.21 and 6.5). This is known as dolichoectasia, and its importance may have been underestimated[90–92] (sections 6.3.6 and 9.1.4). There are five potential consequences:

- the dilated artery may directly compress the brainstem, resulting in a mixture of cranial nerve and long tract signs;
- the disruption of laminar flow predisposes to *in situ* thrombosis, which may occlude the origins of the paramedian or long circumferential branches;
- there may be distal embolization from areas of *in situ* thrombosis;
- the changes in contour of the basilar artery may result in distortion around the origins of the perforating arteries;
- the artery may rupture causing a subarachnoid haemorrhage.

Anterior inferior cerebellar artery

The anterior inferior cerebellar arteries (AICAs) arise from the proximal basilar artery (Figs 4.19 and 4.20) and give off branches to the upper medulla and base of the pons before supplying the anterior cerebellar structures. In most people, they also give rise to the internal auditory arteries, but these may come directly from the basilar artery or, occasionally, the superior or posterior inferior cerebellar arteries. The internal auditory arteries are effectively end-arteries.

The internal auditory arteries supply the seventh and eighth cranial nerves within the auditory canal and, on entering the inner ear, divide into the common cochlear and anterior vestibular arteries. The common cochlear artery then divides into the main cochlear artery, which supplies the spiral ganglion, the basilar membrane structures and the stria vascularis, while the posterior vestibular artery supplies the inferior part of the saccule and the ampulla of the semicircular canal. The anterior vestibular artery supplies the utricle and ampulla of the anterior and horizontal semicircular canals.[93]

Isolated occlusion of the AICA is probably relatively uncommon, but when it does occur there is almost always infarction in both the cerebellum and pons.[94] Symptoms tend to be tinnitus, vertigo and nausea, with an ipsilateral Horner's syndrome, an ipsilateral nuclear facial palsy, dysarthria, nystagmus, ipsilateral trigeminal sensory loss, cerebellar ataxia (in the ipsilateral limbs) and sometimes a contralateral hemiparesis (i.e. similar to the lateral medullary syndrome with the seventh and eighth nerve lesions replacing those of the ninth and tenth nerves and a hemiparesis). Ischaemia in the territory of the internal auditory artery is probably an under-recognized cause of sudden unilateral deafness, which may occur in isolation, as may vertigo[95,96] (section 3.3.7). Occlusion of the AICA is probably most often secondary to atherothrombosis in the basilar artery.

Superior cerebellar artery

The superior cerebellar arteries (SCAs) arise from the basilar artery immediately before its terminal bifurcation (Figs 4.19 and 4.20). They usually supply the dorsolateral midbrain and have branches to the superior cerebellar peduncle and superior surface of the cerebellar hemispheres. The 'classical' syndrome of occlusion of the whole territory of the SCA includes an ipsilateral Horner's syndrome, limb ataxia and intention tremor, with contralateral spinothalamic sensory loss, contralateral upper motor neurone type facial palsy and sometimes a contralateral fourth nerve palsy. In its pure form, it is rare. However, it is often associated with other infarcts in the distal territory of the basilar artery, and may have a poor prognosis.[97] Infarcts that only involve the cerebellar territory of the SCA, on the other hand, have a better prognosis.[98,99] In these cases, headache, limb and gait ataxia, dysarthria, vertigo and vomiting are most prominent, but cases with some of these deficits in isolation have been reported, due to occlusion of the distal branches.[100] Vertigo is much less common in SCA than posterior or anterior inferior cerebellar artery territory infarction.[85] Embolism (either cardiac or artery-to-artery) is considered the most frequent cause of both complete and partial SCA territory infarcts.

The arterial supply of the cerebellum

The cerebellum is supplied by the three long circumferential arteries described above: posterior inferior cerebellar artery (PICA), anterior inferior cerebellar artery (AICA) and superior cerebellar artery (SCA). The PICA usually supplies the inferior surface, the AICA the anterior surface and the SCA the superior, tentorial surface (Fig. 4.20). Territorial infarction is considered most likely to be caused by thromboembolism, particularly from the heart or the basilar artery. However, these arterial systems also have perforating arteries. Cortical infarction in the cerebellum is of two types: infarction perpendicular to the cortical rim at the boundary zone between perforating arteries (which lack anastomoses); and infarction that parallels the cortical rim and is the boundary zone between the SCA and PICA. Small, deep infarcts occur within the deep white matter of the cerebellar hemispheres, usually around the deep boundary zones. Unlike other small, deep infarcts, the predominant cause may be low flow without acute occlusion as a result of large-vessel atherothrombosis[101] (Fig. 4.22).

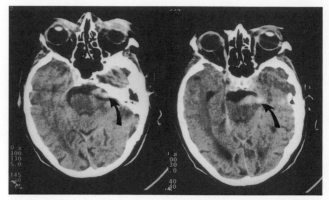

(a)

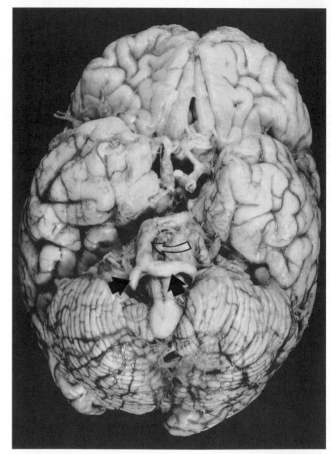

(b)

Fig. 4.21 (a) An axial CT brain scan, showing dolichoectasia of the basilar artery extending into the cerebellopontine angle (*curved arrow*). At this stage, the patient presented with trigeminal neuralgia. (b) Postmortem demonstration of the vertebral artery (*closed arrows*) and basilar artery (*open arrow*) in the same patient 2 years later, after massive infarction of the brainstem and cerebellum.

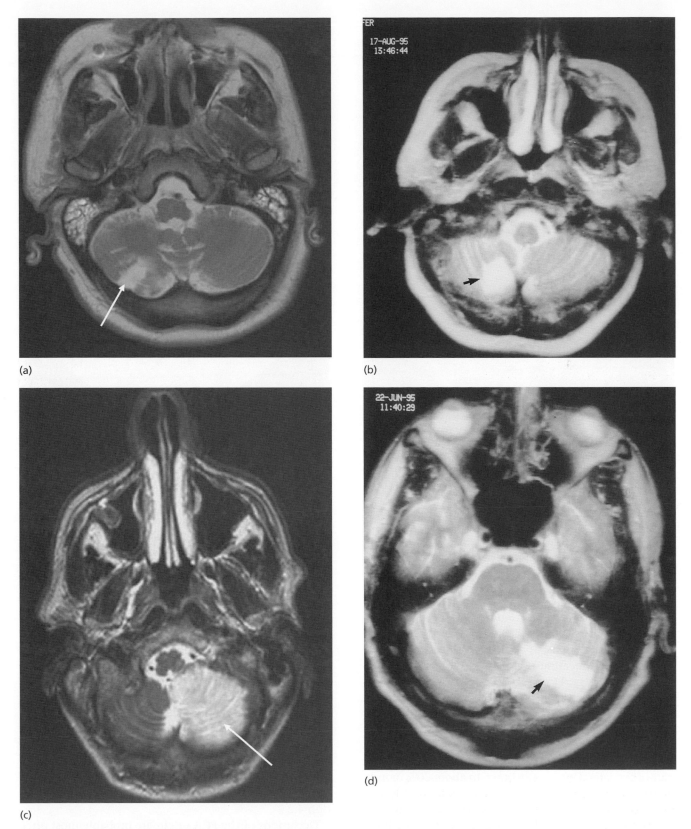

(a)

(b)

(c)

(d)

Fig. 4.22 A montage of MR scans and one CT scan, showing various cerebellar infarcts (*arrows*). (a) Small cerebellar cortical infarcts in the posterior inferior cerebellar artery (PICA) territories. (b) A unilateral small right cerebellar cortical infarct (medial branch of PICA). (c) A cortical infarct in the left PICA territory . (d) A left cerebellar cortical infarct (lateral branch of superior cerebellar artery).

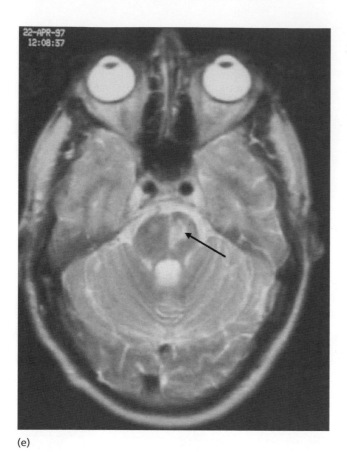

(e)

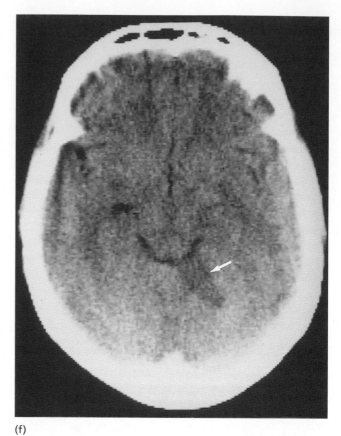

(f)

Fig. 4.22 (*continued*) (e) An infarct in the left brainstem just inferior to the pons (perforating branch of basilar artery). (f) A

CT scan, showing a left superior cerebellar infarct (medial branch of the superior cerebellar artery).

> Cerebellar infarction may be misdiagnosed as 'labyrinthitis', or even upper gastrointestinal disease if nausea and vomiting are prominent.

Posterior cerebral artery

The two posterior cerebral arteries (PCAs) are usually the terminal branches of the basilar artery (Figs 4.19 and 4.20) and their course is traditionally described in sections. The precommunicating (i.e. before the posterior communicating artery; PCoA) P1 section of the PCA passes around the cerebral peduncle and comes to lie between the medial surface of the temporal lobe and the upper brainstem. From this section, small paramedian mesencephalic arteries and the thalamic–subthalamic arteries arise to supply the medial midbrain, the thalamus and part of the lateral geniculate body. In about 30% of individuals, these vessels arise from a single pedicle and therefore bilateral midbrain infarction can result from a single PCA occlusion. After the PCoA (from which the polar arteries to the thalamus usually arise), there are usually the thalamogeniculate arteries and the posterior

choroidal artery (PChA), both of which supply the thalamus. Once the PCA has passed around the free medial edge of the tentorium, it usually divides into two, with a total of four main branches. The anterior division gives rise to the anterior and posterior temporal arteries, while from the posterior division the calcarine and parieto-occipital arteries arise. The posterior pericallosal arteries are usually branches of the parieto-occipital arteries, and pass anteriorly to form a potential anastomosis with the anterior pericallosal arteries from the anterior cerebral artery. The potential minimum and maximum areas of supply of these branches are shown in Fig. 4.23.[230] During early fetal development, the internal carotid artery (ICA) supplies most of the posterior aspect of the cerebral hemispheres and brainstem through the PCoA. In some adults this pattern persists, with only a vestigial basilar artery–PCA connection, and in about 30% one or both PCAs are supplied from the ICA, via the PCoA[29,30] (section 4.2.2).

Occlusions of the PCA origin are probably most often embolic from the heart or proximal arterial atheroma, and they are also due to the arrest of an embolus at the

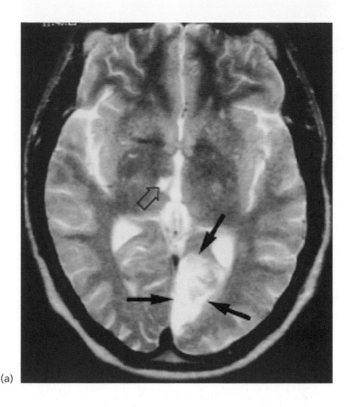

(a)

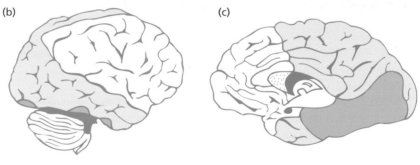

(b)

(c)

(d)

Fig. 4.23 Ischaemia in the territory of the posterior cerebral artery (PCA). (a) The typical appearance on a T2-weighted MR scan of PCA territory infarction (*arrows*). However, there is great inter-individual and inter-hemispheric variability in the area supplied by the PCA (b, c). The dark purple areas show the only part of the cortex on the lateral surface (b) and the medial surface (c) of the hemisphere, which was *always* supplied by the PCA in a large pathological study.[230] The pale purple represents the maximum extent of the area which may be supplied by the PCA in some patients. (d) There is a similar degree of variability for the intracerebral territory supplied by the PCA. The figure shows the minimum (dark purple) and maximum (pale green) areas of supply at three levels in the same pathological study. (Reproduced with permission of Dr A. van der Zwan.)

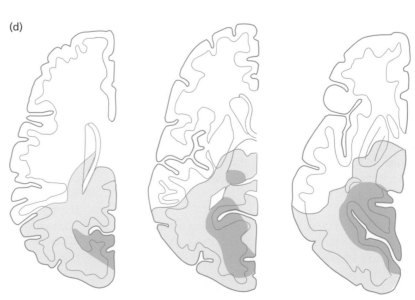

basilar bifurcation which then fragments.[89,102,103] As with occlusion of the mainstem of the middle cerebral artery (MCA), ischaemia can occur in both the deep and superficial territory of the PCA. Occlusion of the deep perforating branches results in ischaemia of the thalamus and upper brainstem, as described below. Such patients may have a hemiparesis in addition to their visual defects and so mimic extensive MCA territory infarction.[104–106] Visual field defects are the most commonly encountered syndrome from PCA infarction. A macular-sparing homonymous hemianopia is explained by collateral flow from the MCA supplying the occipital pole.[107] More restricted infarcts can result in small homonymous sectoranopias. Bilateral occipital infarction may result in cortical blindness. When visual function is less severely affected, disorders of colour vision (discrimination, naming) may be apparent. Transient ischaemia in the PCA territory may sometimes give 'positive' visual phenomena which are very similar to those of classical migraine.[108] Visual perseverations, such as seeing an object several times despite continued fixation, and continuing to see an object as an after-image (palinopsia) can also occur.[109] Disorders of language function can also arise from PCA territory infarction, probably due to involvement of the thalamus (see below) or its projection fibres. Alexia, with or without agraphia, results from a dominant hemisphere PCA occlusion (section 3.3.3). Amnesic disorders occur because of direct involvement of the temporal lobes, the thalamus, or the mamillothalamic tract[110] (section 3.3.3). Typically, there is marked amnesia for recent events. Non-dominant hemisphere PCA territory infarcts may result in disorders of visuospatial function.

Arterial supply of the thalamus

The thalamus is involved in about one-quarter of all posterior circulation ischaemic strokes, either in isolation following perforating artery occlusion, or in combination with other structures following large artery thrombosis or artery-to-artery embolism.[111] The blood supply to the thalamus comes from four groups of arteries, which over the years have, confusingly, been called by several different names[112] (Fig. 4.24). Unlike other lacunar infarcts, those in the thalamus are associated with a wide range of clinical syndromes, which can make clinical localization difficult.

THALAMIC–SUBTHALAMIC ARTERIES (ALSO KNOWN AS PARAMEDIAN, THALAMOPERFORATING AND POSTERIOR INTERNAL OPTIC ARTERIES)
These arise from the proximal posterior cerebral artery (PCA). They are usually 200–400 μm in luminal diameter.

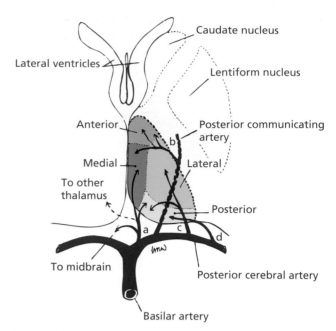

Fig. 4.24 Diagrammatic representation of the arterial supply of the thalamus, showing the anterior, medial, lateral and posterior nuclei. The branches are: (a) thalamic–subthalamic (paramedian, thalamoperforating, posterior internal optic) arteries (in addition to the thalamus, branches supply the midbrain, and in about 30% the branches to the thalamus in the other hemisphere arise from a common pedicle); (b) polar (tuberothalamic, anterior internal optic) arteries; (c) thalamogeniculate arteries; (d) posterior choroidal arteries.

In addition to supplying the thalamus, branches also go to the upper midbrain. In 30% of people, the branches to both sides of the thalamus have a common pedicle from just one PCA.[113] They supply the posteromedial thalamus, including the nucleus of the medial longitudinal fasciculus, the posterior dorsomedial nucleus and the intralaminar nuclei. The typical syndrome of unilateral infarction is of acute reduction of conscious level, neuropsychological disturbances such as apathy, disorientation and memory dysfunction, and impaired upgaze, with little or no motor or sensory disturbance. The neuropsychological abnormalities are difficult to distinguish from cortical syndromes and they also have a wide non-stroke differential diagnosis. The symptoms resulting from bilateral infarcts due to occlusion of a common vascular pedicle are similar to those from unilateral infarction, but are usually much more severe. Hypersomnolence can persist for many weeks, presumably due to involvement of the intralaminar nuclei and rostral fibres of the reticular activating system. Additionally, the syndrome of akinetic mutism can occur (section 3.3.2). Amnesic syndromes are most likely to occur when there is involvement of the dorsomedial nucleus, and mood disturbances may mimic frontal lobe syndromes. Thalamic dementia consists of impaired attention, slowed responses, apathy, poor motivation and amnesia.

> The neuropsychological abnormalities caused by ischaemia in the territory of the thalamic–subthalamic arteries are difficult to distinguish from cortical syndromes and they also have a wide non-stroke differential diagnosis.

POLAR ARTERIES (ALSO KNOWN AS TUBEROTHALAMIC AND ANTERIOR INTERNAL OPTIC ARTERIES)

These usually arise from the posterior communicating artery, although in about 30% of people the artery is absent and the blood supply comes from the thalamic–subthalamic arteries. The polar arteries supply the anteromedial and anterolateral areas, including the dorsomedial nucleus, the reticular nucleus, the mamillo-thalamic tract and part of the ventrolateral nucleus. These nuclei have substantial connections with the frontal lobes, and the dorsomedial nuclei link with medial temporal lobe structures. The deficits from polar infarcts are mainly neuropsychological; patients tend to be rather apathetic and lack spontaneity. Typically, left-sided infarcts result in an aphasia that is non-fluent, with poor naming but preserved comprehension and repetition, and impaired learning of verbal material.[114] Right-sided infarcts result in hemineglect syndromes and impaired visuospatial processing. Polar infarcts, particularly if bilateral, may result in acute amnesia.[115]

THALAMOGENICULATE ARTERIES

These are the five or six small branches arising from the more distal posterior cerebral artery, equivalent to the lenticulostriate arteries of the middle cerebral artery and are usually 400–800 μm in luminal diameter. They supply the ventrolateral thalamus, including the ventro-postero-lateral (VPL) and ventro-postero-medial (VPM) nuclei, i.e. the specific relay nuclei for motor and sensory functions. Pure sensory stroke is a typical lateral thalamic deficit due to ischaemia in the territory of a thalamogeniculate artery (section 4.3.2). There may be a full hemianaesthesia or partial syndromes such as hand and mouth (cheiro-oral), hand, foot and mouth (cheiro-podo-oral) and pseudoradicular sensory loss[116,117] (section 3.3.5). The deficit can involve all modalities, or spare pain and temperature sensation.[118] If there is extension to the internal capsule, a sensorimotor stroke occurs[119] (section 4.3.2). Hemiataxia is also a typical feature of involvement of the contralateral ventrolateral nucleus, because of interruption of fibres in the dentato-rubro-thalamic pathway. The clinical features are rather like cerebellar dysfunction and are not explained by

proprioceptive loss. The Déjerine–Roussy syndrome is caused by more extensive lateral thalamic infarction and is sometimes referred to as the syndrome of the thalamo-geniculate pedicle.[120,121] It consists of a mild hemipare-sis, marked hemianaesthesia, hemiataxia, astereognosis and frequently paroxysmal pain/hyperaesthesia (often of delayed onset) and choreoathetotic movements, all contralateral to the lesion. The original cases had extension of the infarcts into the internal capsule and towards the putamen, although most of the features of this syndrome result from involvement of the ventroposterior nucleus and ventrolateral nucleus of the thalamus.

Finally, there is the supply from the medial and lateral posterior choroidal arteries (PChAs), which also arise from the posterior cerebral artery. These supply the pulvinar and posterior thalamus, the geniculate bodies and the anterior nucleus. Involvement of the PChA presents typically with visual field deficits (upper or lower homonymous quadrantanopia, and rarely homonymous horizontal sectoranopia), with or without hemisensory loss. Some cases have associated neuropsychological deficits such as transcortical aphasia and disturbance of memory function.[122]

The thalamic arteries were traditionally considered to be end-arteries, but functional anastomoses probably do occur.[111] It is perhaps for this reason that the vascular pathology underlying thalamic infarcts is much more variable than that of other lacunar infarcts.

4.2.4 Arterial boundary zones

Arterial boundary zones may be defined as those areas of the brain where the distal fields of two or more adjacent arteries meet (section 6.7.5). The potential clinical relevance is that one might predict that these areas would be particularly vulnerable to haemodynamic stresses, such as hypotension and low focal or global cerebral perfusion pressure. There are two types of boundary zone:

- those where there are functional anastomoses between the two arterial systems, e.g. on the pial surface between the major cerebral arteries, and to a lesser extent at the base of the brain between the choroidal circulations;[13]
- those at the junction of the distal fields of two non-anastomosing arterial systems, e.g. deep perforating and pial medullary perforating arteries in the centrum semiovale.[123]

With the former, the boundary zone will occur at points of equal pressure between the two arterial systems. Consequently, changes in arterial pressure in one of the systems may result in a shift of the boundary zone towards the compromised artery (Figs 4.11, 4.17, 4.23). With the latter, the boundary zone is likely to be more or

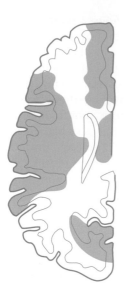
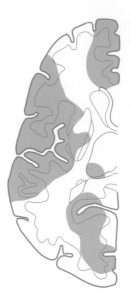
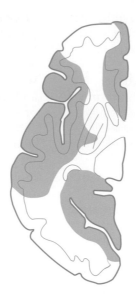

Fig. 4.25 Variability of the internal boundary zones. The purple shaded areas represent the minimum areas of intracerebral supply at three levels of the anterior, middle and posterior cerebral arteries in a large pathological study,[230] as shown individually in Figs 4.11d, 4.17e and 4.23d. The adjacent unshaded areas represent the areas of variation within which the boundaries between these territories were found. (Reproduced with permission of Dr A. van der Zwan.)

less fixed in the cerebral hemisphere (Fig. 4.25). Both types of boundary zone are present in the cerebellum.

The impression that might be gained from the clinico-radiological literature is that the major boundary zones occur at symmetrical, predictable sites in the hemispheres (e.g. Damasio[3]). Consequently, in some classifications of stroke, imaged infarcts in these areas are considered most likely to be haemodynamic rather than embolic in origin, i.e. due to low flow rather than acute arterial occlusion. But, as has been shown in Figs 4.11, 4.17, 4.23 and 4.25, for both types of boundary zone, there is considerable inter-individual and intra-individual variation.[5] More recent maps of arterial territories have taken account of this work.[8,10] Lang *et al.*[10] used the minimum and maximum areas of middle cerebral artery supply from van der Zwan *et al.*[5] to assess whether imaged areas of infarction distal to a haemodynamically significant internal carotid artery lesion should be regarded as being territorial infarcts or boundary zone infarcts. Using the minimum area of supply, two-thirds were considered as boundary zone infarcts, but when the maximum area of supply was considered only one-fifth were classified in the same way. We do not believe it is always possible to identify 'typical' CT or MR patterns associated with boundary zone infarction, given the very real difficulty of identifying where they are *in vivo* (section 6.7.5).

> We do not believe it always is possible to identify 'typical' CT or MR patterns associated with boundary zone infarction.

It has been suggested that while cortical boundary zone infarcts may have many causes (and not just low flow), it is in fact the deep or internal boundary zone that is most vulnerable to low blood flow.[123,124] However, whereas with cortical infarcts the differential diagnosis is from distal field embolism, in the subcortical region the differential is from intrinsic disease of the perforating arteries, and there are just as many problems with the anatomical localization of the boundary zones in individual patients.[5,72,73]

4.3 Clinical subclassification of stroke

4.3.1 Introduction

Having taken the history and performed a physical examination, the physician should have established which brain functions have been affected by the stroke (or, with more difficulty, the transient ischaemic attack). These clinical findings then need to be used to identify groups of patients in a manner which will bring together the brain and vascular anatomy. The traditional teaching of cerebrovascular neurology is based on the general assumption that particular symptoms and signs arise from restricted areas of damaged brain, which, in turn, receive their vascular supply in a reasonably predictable manner. This has its origins in the large classical literature describing patterns of neurological deficit which were linked (usually at a later postmortem) with particular vascular lesions, a process that produced a myriad of eponymous clinical syndromes. Although these were of value to those interested in exploring the subtleties of cerebral localization before the advent of PET and fMRI, and remain the stock in trade of many neurologists' clinical demonstrations, most of these 'classical' vascular syndromes occur infrequently (at least in their pure forms), and even when they do occur they rarely have a particularly distinctive cause. The sensitivity, specificity and generalizability of many of the clinico-anatomical correlations have rarely been tested on large, unselected groups of patients with stroke and they are of limited practical value to most clinicians. Additionally, the descriptions nearly always relate to ischaemic rather than haemorrhagic strokes and, although one might argue that this is perfectly acceptable in the context of a high proportion of patients having brain CT or MR scans, unfortunately there remain a large number of clinicians worldwide who do not have ready access to such technology to make the distinction with certainty.

> Despite being well known, many of the 'classical' vascular syndromes occur rather infrequently in routine clinical practice.

Early clinically based classifications distinguished anterior (carotid) circulation strokes and posterior (vertebrobasilar) circulation strokes.[125] It seems reasonable to retain this division, because certain investigations (e.g. carotid duplex) and treatments (e.g. carotid endarterectomy) are only appropriate to the carotid circulation – while recognizing that for a number of reasons there can be considerable overlap of symptoms between the two territories (Table 4.3). In terms of the intracranial circulation (both anterior and posterior), there are striking differences between the structure, anastomotic potential, vascular pathology and functional areas of the brain perfused by the main stems of the parent arteries, the

Table 4.3 Which arterial territory are the neurological problems in?

	Likely arterial territory		
	Anterior	Either	Posterior
Dysphasia	+		
Monocular visual loss	+		
Unilateral weakness*		+	
Unilateral sensory disturbance*		+	
Dysarthria†		+	
Ataxia†		+	
Dysphagia†			+
Diplopia†			+
Vertigo†			+
Bilateral simultaneous visual loss			+
Bilateral simultaneous weakness			+
Bilateral simultaneous sensory disturbance			+
Crossed sensory/motor loss			+

*Usually assumed to be 'anterior', but see under lacunar syndromes (section 4.3.2).

†In isolation, these symptoms are not normally regarded as indicating a cerebrovascular event (section 3.2.1)

Note: whether the neurological symptoms are transient or persistent, and irrespective of whether there are abnormal neurological signs, it can be all but impossible to be sure of which arterial territory is involved, because so often the symptoms are not entirely specific for one particular arterial territory. This is because of individual variation in arterial anatomy and the pattern of any arterial disease affecting the collateral circulation, and because one function can be distributed through both arterial territories (e.g. the corticospinal tract is supplied in the cerebral hemispheres by the anterior circulation and then, in the brainstem, by the posterior circulation). Sometimes brain imaging can help if one particularly recent lesion is found in a relevant place (e.g. if a patient with a hemiplegia has just one infarct in the contralateral pons on MRI, then it is more likely to have been due to posterior than anterior ischaemia, particularly if the infarct looks of an appropriate age). Arterial imaging is unhelpful, because so often a symptomatic lesion in one artery is associated with asymptomatic lesions in other arteries. Arterial bruits are unhelpful for the same reason.

cortical branch arteries and the small, deep perforating arteries (Table 4.2).

There is also good evidence that the prognosis of these groups differs (section 10.2). A case can therefore be made for further subdividing strokes into those that are:

- restricted to deep, subcortical areas (supplied by small perforating arteries);
- restricted to superficial cortical areas (supplied by small pial branch arteries); and finally
- those that involve both deep and cortical structures (implicating the whole area of supply of the parent cerebral artery).

However, this is likely to be easier and more robust for anterior than posterior circulation events. Next, one needs to consider whether these subgroups can be identified clinically with reasonable reliability. The greatest amount of information is available for the group of strokes due to ischaemia in the territory of a single, deep perforating artery, and these will be considered first.

4.3.2 Lacunar syndromes

The clinical syndrome

Ischaemia in the territory of a single, deep perforating artery can cause a restricted area of infarction known as a 'lacune' (section 6.4) (Fig. 4.26). Technically, it should be described as an ischaemic lacune because similar sized areas of tissue destruction can be caused by small haemorrhages.[126] The term 'lacune' is a pathological one and if only cross-sectional imaging is available, the term 'small, deep infarct' is preferred, with the presumption that the imaged area of infarction is within the territory of a single perforating artery.[53] In fact, most lacunes

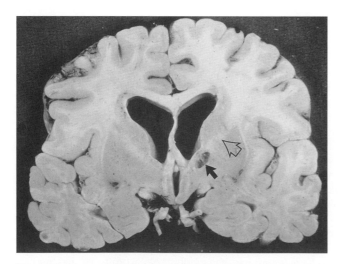

Fig. 4.26 Postmortem demonstration of a lacune (*closed arrow*) in the internal capsule (*open arrow*) of a coronal brain slice.

occur in areas such as the lentiform nucleus and do not present as stroke syndromes, but nonetheless are an important cause of cognitive decline.[127–130] Other lacunes, however, occur at strategic sites such as in the internal capsule and pons, where clinically 'eloquent' ascending and descending neural tracts are concentrated, with the result that an extensive clinical deficit can occur from an anatomically small lesion (sections 3.3.4 and 3.3.5). However, these lesions are much less likely to cause an acute disturbance of higher cognitive or visual function than those involving the cortex.

Initially, a small number of clinical syndromes were correlated with relevant lacunes at subsequent post-mortem.[131–134] These came to be regarded as the 'classical' lacunar syndromes, and to varying degrees the sensitivity and specificity of these relationships have been tested using CT/MRI. Since then many other syndromes have been reported in association with CT/MR imaged small, deep infarcts but rare associations, perhaps due to idiosyncratic individual variations in the vascular anatomy, are of little practical use to clinicians.[87,135] Consequently, the standard classification of subcortical infarction states that the term 'lacunar syndrome' should be restricted to a clinical situation in which the likely mechanism of infarction 'involves transient or permanent occlusion of a single perforating artery with a high degree of probability' – i.e. that this mechanism is the usual cause of a particular syndrome[53] (section 6.7.3).

PURE MOTOR STROKE

The association of pure motor deficits and lacunes was noted early in the 20th century.[63,136] Pure motor strike (PMS) will be described in detail since it is the most frequently encountered of all lacunar syndromes (LACS) and exemplifies many of their core features. The clinical 'rules' for diagnosing PMS were set out by Fisher and Curry who defined the syndrome as 'A paralysis complete or incomplete of the face, arm and leg on one side unaccompanied by sensory signs, visual field defect, aphasia, or apractagnosia. In the case of brainstem lesions the hemiplegia will be free of vertigo, deafness, tinnitus, diplopia, cerebellar ataxia, and gross nystagmus.'[131] This definition allowed sensory symptoms but not signs to be present. This puts into clinical terminology the fundamental neuroanatomical concepts of LACS (Table 4.4). For a patient to present with symptoms and signs that fulfil the above criteria, it is likely that the stroke has been caused by a lesion in an area where the motor tracts are closely packed together, since a lesion of the motor cortex sufficiently extensive to involve the face, arm and leg areas of the homunculus would almost certainly also affect neural pathways subserving higher cognitive or visual functions. It was stressed that the definition

Table 4.4 Lacunar syndromes.

Definition
Maximum deficit from a single vascular event
No visual field deficit
No new disturbance of higher cerebral function
No signs of brainstem disturbance*

Categories
Pure motor stroke
Pure sensory stroke
Ataxic hemiparesis (including dysarthria–clumsy hand
   syndrome and homolateral ataxia and crural paresis)
Sensorimotor stroke

To be acceptable as a pure motor, sensory or sensorimotor
   stroke, the relevant deficit must involve at least two out of
   three areas of the face, arm and leg, and, with particular
   reference to the arm, should involve the whole limb and
   not just the hand.

*Some brainstem syndromes may be caused by lacunar
infarcts.

applied to the maximum deficit in the acute phase of
a single stroke, a particularly important point in the
context of current hyperacute assessment, but also it did
not apply to less recent strokes where other signs were
present to begin with but had subsequently resolved.

Patients with lacunar syndromes should have no
aphasia, no visuospatial disturbance, no visual field
defect, no clear disturbance of brainstem function and
no drowsiness at any time after their stroke, unless
caused by a coexisting non-vascular condition.

In the original report of nine autopsied cases, six of the
lacunes were in the internal capsule and three in the
pons, which emphasizes the point that the same clinical
syndrome may occur with occlusion of a perforating
artery arising from the middle cerebral artery (anterior
circulation) or the basilar artery (posterior circulation).
Since then, cases of PMS have been reported with lacunes
at other sites along the cortico-spinal tract, including the
corona radiata, the cerebral peduncle and the medullary
pyramid.[137] Although the anatomical distribution of
lesions in large series is broadly similar to the original
pathological observations, diffusion tensor imaging is
beginning to provide more detailed information about
the impact and possibly prognosis of lacunar infarcts on
different parts of the corticospinal tract.[138,139]

In the early 1980s, series of cases with *slightly* more
restricted pure motor deficits (e.g. weakness of just the
face and arm, or arm and leg) associated with small, deep
infarcts on CT were reported – hence our preference
for the term PMS rather than the original pure motor

hemiplegia.[57,140] It should be stressed that the definitions
used stated that the *whole* of the arm or leg should be
affected, something one suspects is often overlooked.
The infarcts were in the corona radiata or the junctional
zone between it and the internal capsule, where nerve
fibres are relatively more dispersed than in the capsule or
pons.[57] Cases with these more restricted deficits are probably best described as 'partial' rather than 'classical'
LACS but they still seem most likely to be associated
with small, deep infarcts, although many large studies
that have reported on the sensitivity and specificity of
clinicoanatomical correlations have combined the two
groups.[135,141]

Although one might go even further and include any
case with a pure motor deficit no matter how anatomically restricted as a PMS, in practice the more restricted
a deficit, the more likely it is to arise from a cortical
lesion. In most studies of isolated upper or lower limb
motor deficit, less than a quarter were caused by lacunar
infarcts although lacunar infarcts may be more likely to
cause an isolated facial weakness.[65–67,142]

Only deficits involving the whole of the arm and face
(brachio-facial), or the whole of the arm and leg
(brachio-crural), should be accepted as partial lacunar
syndromes, not more restricted deficits (e.g. hand
only) that are more likely to be of cortical origin.

PURE SENSORY STROKE
Pure sensory stroke (PSS), the sensory counterpart of
pure motor stroke, in terms of the anatomical distribution of the deficit, is encountered much less frequently.
Although the definition in the original paper suggested
that there should be objective sensory loss, in a later
paper Fisher noted that there could be cases with persistent sensory symptoms in the absence of objective
signs.[132,143] A single case of a partial PSS has been verified
pathologically.[144] As noted in section 3.3.5, lesions
within the thalamus can give characteristic, restricted
syndromes such as hand and mouth (cheiro-oral), and
hand, mouth and foot (cheiro-oral-pedal), and although
the whole of the limb is not affected, these are most
often caused by lacunar infarcts. Overall, most lesions
causing PSS are in the thalamus, in keeping with the
original pathological studies and are the smallest of the
symptomatic small, deep infarcts.[145]

HOMOLATERAL ATAXIA AND CRURAL PARESIS,
DYSARTHRIA–CLUMSY HAND SYNDROME AND
ATAXIC HEMIPARESIS
These syndromes are less generally accepted as 'classical
LACS', unlike pure motor stroke and pure sensory stroke,
although they were all described at about the same time.

This may be because of the difficulty of interpreting some physical signs and the fact that the syndromes are less common. The original patients with homolateral ataxia and crural paresis were described as having weakness of the lower limb, especially the ankle and toes, a Babinski sign and 'striking dysmetria of the arm and leg on the same side'.[133] In the dysarthria–clumsy hand syndrome, although the deficit was described as being 'chiefly of dysarthria and clumsiness of one hand', two of the three original patients had signs suggestive of pyramidal dysfunction in the ipsilateral leg, and both had an ataxic gait.[134] In a later paper, Fisher reported three further patients who had prominent vertical nystagmus as well as pyramidal weakness and cerebellar signs, and suggested that a new term, 'ataxic hemiparesis', should be used for these cases and those with homolateral ataxia and crural paresis.[146] The relevant lacunes were all in the pons, and he attributed the variable distribution of the weakness in different cases to the involvement of motor fibres where they are relatively dispersed by the pontine nuclei. It has been reported that if 'rigid' clinical criteria for dysarthria–clumsy hand syndrome are used, the syndrome predicts a lesion in the contralateral pons but a more recent study which used MR as well as CT reported that 40% were in the internal capsule.[147,148] On the other hand, others have suggested that true homolateral ataxia and crural paresis may be caused most frequently by territorial infarcts in the anterior cerebral artery territory.[38] They also make the point that many other cases reported with similar-sized infarcts of the corona radiata on CT have had much more extensive deficits. Another possible explanation for the syndromes is that there is a second, non-imaged lesion. The data from detailed MRI studies argue against this being common. In one study, only 5 of 26 patients (19%) with ataxic hemiparesis had more than one small, deep infarct on imaging, but the figure for patients with PMS in the same study was similar, with 6 of 33 (18%).[86] Another study reported that 10% of patients with ataxic hemiparesis had a 'double lesion'.[149] Additionally, in the Stroke Data Bank study, a history of previous, clinically apparent stroke was no more common in the ataxic hemiparesis/dysarthria–clumsy hand syndrome group than in those with other LACS.[150] Sensory variants of ataxic hemiparesis have been reported, but there is no evidence that the anatomical and clinical issues raised are significantly different from those between PMS and sensorimotor stroke (see below).

> Limb ataxia does not necessarily imply a cerebellar stroke in the presence of ipsilateral pyramidal signs, but may be caused by a lacunar infarct or haemorrhage in the basal ganglia or pons.

SENSORIMOTOR STROKE

The inclusion of sensorimotor stroke (SMS) as a classical lacunar syndrome (LACS) is based on a single patient with a postmortem, reported almost a decade after the other classical LACS.[119] This case was due to a lacune in the ventroposterior nucleus of the thalamus, but there was also pallor of the adjacent internal capsule. Although there were marked sensory and motor signs which persisted, the onset of the sensory symptoms preceded the motor ones. There is also postmortem support for the view that an infarct primarily within the internal capsule can cause an SMS.[128] A similar syndrome was reported after a small haemorrhage in the same place.[151] These authors made the point that a sensory deficit can occur from lesions of the posterior limb of the internal capsule, presumably by interruption of the thalamocortical pathways. In an MR study, the infarcts in cases of SMS were larger than in other LACS, although they were still thought to be within the territory of a single perforating artery.[86] This supported an earlier CT study which reported that the infarcts in SMS were slightly larger and extended more medially than in patients with pure motor stroke (PMS), abutting the posterolateral aspect of the thalamus.[152] In the Stroke Data Bank, in which SMS was the second most frequent LACS after PMS, 31% had a lesion in the posterior limb of the internal capsule, 22% had a lesion in the corona radiata, 7% in the genu of the capsule, 6% in the anterior limb of the capsule and only 9% in the thalamus.[150] The lesions in the corona radiata were on average almost twice as large as those in the capsule, but both were larger than the corresponding lesions in the PMS group. MR scanning has disclosed that in some CT-negative cases the lesion can be in the medial part of the medulla.[153]

The brain lesion

Table 4.5 summarizes the large studies of the clinico-radiological correlations for the various lacunar syndromes (LACS) and imaged small, deep infarcts. Overall, it must be recognized that about 10% of patients presenting with a LACS will have a relevant lesion *other* than a small, deep infarct or haemorrhage on a scan, which might explain the neurological symptoms. The proportion of such 'atypical' patients does seem to be higher for SMS than for the other syndromes, and particular care should therefore be taken with this group. So most LACS are caused by small deep infarcts or haemorrhages, but not all of them. This inconsistency may be because additional deficits were not recognized by the clinicians (e.g. visual inattention, visuospatial disturbance) or had resolved by the time of assessment, or because the relevant lesion was misclassified on imaging, particularly in

Table 4.5 Clinicoradiological correlations of lacunar syndromes.

Syndrome, studies	Setting	Mean time to scan	Imaging	Number of patients	Non-lacunar infarct on imaging (n, %)	
Pure motor stroke						
Bamford et al.[214]	Community		CT	49	1	(2)
Hommel et al.[86]	Hospital		MR	35	0	(0)
Melo et al.[215]	Hospital		CT	121	6	(5)
Norrving & Staaf[216]*	Hospital		CT	123	0	(0)
Norrving & Staaf[216]†	Hospital		CT	52	5	(9)
Gan et al.[217]	Hospital		CT/MR	101	7	(7)
Arboix et al.[138]	Hospital		CT/MR	222	33 (15)	
Pure sensory stroke						
Bamford et al.[214]	Community		CT	7	0	(0)
Hommel et al.[86]	Hospital		MR	12	1	(8)
Gan et al.[217]	Hospital		CT/MR	15	0	(0)
Arboix et al.[145]	Hospital		CT/MR	99	7	(7)
Ataxic hemiparesis						
Bamford et al.[214]	Community		CT	9	0	(0)
Hommel et al.[86]	Hospital		MR	28	2	(7)
Gan et al.[217]	Hospital		CT/MR	41	1	(1)
Sensorimotor stroke						
Bamford et al.[214]	Community		CT	43	2	(5)
Huang et al.[229]	Hospital		CT	37	8 (21)	
Hommel et al.[86]	Hospital		MR	8	1 (12)	
Landi et al.[218]	Hospital		CT	34	3 (11)	
Lodder et al.[219]	Hospital		CT	47	5 (11)	
Arboix & Marti-Vilalta[220]	Hospital		CT/MR	42	8 (19)	
Gan et al.[217]	Hospital		CT/MR	46	1	(2)
All lacunar syndromes						
Wardlaw et al.[183]	Hospital		CT	19	2 (11)	
Boiten & Lodder[191]	Hospital		CT	109	11 (10)	
Ricci et al.[221]	Community		CT	56	2	(4)
Samuelsson et al.[222]	Hospital		MR	91	8 (11)	
Anderson et al.[179]‡	Community		CT	69	12 (17)	
Kappelle et al.[223]	Hospital		CT	78	5	(6)
All lacunar syndromes: studies using MR DWI						
Schonewille et al.[224]	Hospital	53 h	DWI	43	1	(2)
Lindgren et al.[225]	Hospital	33 h	DWI	23	2	(9)
Lee et al.[226]	Hospital	32 h	DWI/MRA	19	4 (21)	
Gerraty et al.[9]	Hospital	9 h	DWI/PWI/MRA	19	13 (68)	

*Classical or †partial pure motor stroke. ‡Retrospective classification from records.
MR, magnetic resonance; DWI, diffusion-weighted imaging; PWI, perfusion-weighted imaging.

studies performed without the benefit of MR diffusion-weighted imaging.

The vascular lesion

Any of the lacunar syndromes (LACS) may be caused by a small haemorrhage, and this accounts for about 5% of cases in community studies.[137] There is no direct information about the cause of the ischaemia in the territory of single perforating arteries, except in a handful of cases. Based on the results of postmortem studies, it has traditionally been considered that asymptomatic (smaller) lacunes are probably most often the consequence of occlusion by thickened vessel walls (lipohyalinosis), when the usual diameter of the vessel is less than 100 μm, while the larger symptomatic lacunes are probably most often the result of vessel occlusion due to complex small-vessel disease or microatheroma, when the vessel diameter is around 400 μm[127,154] (section 6.4). Some cases, particularly those in the pons with occlusion of a basilar perforating artery, may be caused by obstruction of the mouth of the perforating artery by an atheromatous plaque within the parent artery.[155] Although an embolic mechanism is possible, epidemiological evidence suggests that there is a low frequency of severe carotid stenosis or cardiac sources of embolism[156–164] (section 6.4). More recent pathology and MR studies have suggested that oedema secondary to endothelial dysfunction and the breakdown of the blood–brain barrier may also have a role.[54,55,165]

From the above, it can be seen that a LACS does not reliably distinguish whether the brain lesion relates to the anterior or posterior systems, although in older series and some schemes of classification it seems likely that it would always have been considered as an anterior circulation stroke (e.g. Rochester, Minnesota).[125,166] It has been recognized that small, deep infarcts are the usual cause of certain brainstem syndromes (usually a pure motor stroke plus a cranial nerve palsy or eye movement disorder) but before simply accepting these alongside the classical LACS, the even greater paucity of pathological studies should be recognized.[86] As noted above, the vascular lesion may be different, with atheroma overlying the mouth of the perforating artery being more frequent than in the anterior circulation.[155] Consequently, these types of deficit are not generally included in studies reporting the prognosis of patients with LACS, but this position may need to be reviewed in the light of future MR studies.

4.3.3 Posterior circulation syndromes

The clinical syndromes

Although there are some clinical syndromes due to well-localized lesions within the posterior circulation which, along with their eponymous names, are an integral part of 'classical neurology' (e.g. Weber, Millard–Gubler, Wallenberg), in practice such syndromes are rarely seen in their pure form. Indeed, the clinical consequences of a given vascular lesion are generally less predictable than for arteries in the anterior circulation because of the greater frequency of developmental vascular anomalies and the greater variability of the territory supplied by individual arteries. Additionally, until the advent of MRI, clinicoradiological correlation was difficult because of the poorer performance of CT in the posterior fossa compared with the supratentorial compartment, and catheter angiography was also performed much less frequently than for anterior circulation strokes because it rarely led to any change in management, such as

Table 4.6 Posterior circulation syndromes.

At time of maximum deficit, any of:
Ipsilateral cranial nerve (III–XII) palsy (single or multiple) with contralateral motor and/or sensory deficit
Bilateral motor and/or sensory deficit
Disorder of conjugate eye movement (horizontal or vertical)
Cerebellar dysfunction without ipsilateral long tract deficit (as seen in ataxic hemiparesis)
Isolated hemianopia or cortical blindness
Note that disorders of higher cerebral function (e.g. aphasia, agnosias) may be present in addition to the above features if the posterior cerebral artery territory is involved.

vascular surgery.[167] Consequently, at the present time, one must recognize that the posterior circulation syndromes (POCS) are a relatively crude grouping, which from both a topographic and aetiological perspective encompasses a heterogeneous group of strokes (section 6.7.4).

The clinical deficits that point to the lesion being in the distribution of the posterior circulation are shown in Table 4.6. Other symptoms and signs that may be present but are not of any particular localizing value include Horner's syndrome (which can occur in both carotid and vertebrobasilar strokes), nystagmus, vertigo (which in isolation is rarely due to a stroke), dysarthria (which can occur from lesions anywhere in the motor pathways) and hearing disturbance.[168,169] Occasionally, an otherwise typical POCS may be associated with disturbance of higher cerebral function, e.g. aphasia, agnosias. This should not come as a surprise, given the variable supratentorial territory supplied by the posterior cerebral arteries, and these cases should still be considered as POCS[104,105,170] (section 4.2.3).

When diagnosing POCS at the bedside it is useful to consider whether there is involvement of the:
- distal territory, i.e. beyond the top of the basilar artery (visual field defects, higher cerebral dysfunction);
- middle territory, i.e. the basilar artery (motor deficits, cranial nerves III–VII palsies);
- proximal territory, i.e. the vertebral arteries (crossed motor and sensory deficits, lower cranial nerve palsies),

since the mechanisms of stroke in the three areas may well differ.[79,170–173] The involvement of more than one territory, particularly if sequential and/or associated with fluctuating level of arousal, should raise the suspicion of occlusion of the basilar artery, which may in turn lead to consideration of thrombolytic therapy.[174–176] There is probably a tendency for POCS to be underdiagnosed in non-specialist centres. In our view, this most often results from a failure to appreciate that truncal or gait

Table 4.7 Clinicoradiological correlations of posterior circulation syndromes.

Study	Number	Appropriate infarct	No lesion	Inappropriate infarct
Bamford[177]*	81	19 (23%)	60 (74%)	2 (2%)
Lindgren et al.[178]*	32	12 (37%)	20 (62%)	0
Anderson et al.[179]*	36	16 (44%)	16 (44%)	4 (11%)
Wardlaw et al.[183]†	13	8 (62%)	5 (38%)	0
Al-Buhairi et al.[227]†	71	32 (45%)	39 (55%)	0
Mead et al.[228]†	212	105 (50%)	86 (41%)	21 (10%)

*Community-based study, first-ever strokes. †Hospital-based study, first-ever and recurrent strokes.

ataxia is present, because no one bothers to have the patient sit or stand up.

The brain lesion

In community-based studies between 10% and 18% of patients presenting with POCS had an intracerebral haemorrhage.[177–179] The correlation between the clinical syndrome and brain imaging in patients with ischaemic stroke is shown in Table 4.7. The 'inappropriate' lesions included a number of supratentorial small, deep infarcts. Given that most of the studies were based on CT, it is possible that these patients had a further and perhaps therefore relevant infarct in the brainstem that was not visible. With the increasing use of MRI, it has become clear that certain brainstem syndromes are usually associated with small, deep infarcts, compatible with ischaemia in the territory of a single basilar perforating artery.[86] Of 93 cases of isolated homonymous hemianopia associated with a vascular lesion, 80 (96%) were attributed to posterior cerebral artery occlusion.[180]

The vascular lesion

Traditionally, pathological series have suggested that within the anterior circulation the ratio of embolism to *in situ* thrombosis is about 3 : 1, while in the posterior circulation this ratio is reversed.[181] *In vivo* studies have questioned this, and it seems likely that at least some of the difference is the result of the inevitable selection bias that occurs in pathological series.[75,103,172,182] In a large hospital-based registry, 32% of posterior circulation infarcts were associated with large-artery occlusion, 14% were attributed to artery-to-artery emboli, 24% to embolism from the heart and 14% to perforating artery disease.[172] It is important to note that, in whites at least, atheroma of the intracranial portion of the vertebral arteries and the basilar artery is much more common than in the intracranial carotid or middle cerebral arteries. Thus, as noted above, while small deep infarcts

resulting from occlusion of a single perforating artery in the anterior circulation are most likely to be due to intrinsic disease of those vessels, in the posterior circulation atheromatous disease in the parent artery may cause a similar brain lesion by occluding the origin of a single perforating artery – a process referred to as 'basilar branch occlusion' (section 4.3.2). It seems likely that, because of the shape of the vertebrobasilar system, emboli are most likely to arrest either in the distal part of the vertebral artery or in the upper part of the basilar artery.

4.3.4 Total anterior circulation syndrome

The clinical syndrome

The clinical features of the total anterior circulation syndrome (TACS) (Table 4.8) are a hemiplegia (usually with an ipsilateral hemisensory loss), a visual field deficit on the same side and a new disturbance of higher cerebral function referable to the same cerebral hemisphere. 'Total' is used in this context to signify that all the major aspects of supratentorial cerebral function have been affected, and it does not imply necessarily that there has been infarction in the whole of the anterior circulation territory. TACS is very much the equivalent of the terms 'full house' and 'complete middle cerebral artery syndrome' which have been used in other classifications.[125,152] Some impairment of consciousness is often present, which can make formal testing of higher cortical and visual function difficult.

Table 4.8 Total anterior circulation syndrome.

At time of maximum deficit, all of:
  Hemiplegia or severe hemiparesis contralateral to the
    cerebral lesion
  Hemianopia contralateral to the cerebral lesion
  New disturbance of higher cerebral function (e.g.
    dysphasia, visuospatial disturbance)
+/– sensory deficit contralateral to the cerebral lesion

Study	Number	Appropriate infarct	No lesion	Inappropriate infarct
Bamford[177]*	55	52 (95%)	0	3 (5%)
Lindgren et al.[178]*	54	35 (65%)	15 (28%)	4 (7%)
Anderson et al.[179]*	68	44 (65%)	10 (15%)	12 (18%)
Wardlaw et al.[183]†	33	31 (94%)	0	2 (6%)
Al-Buhairi et al.[227]†	64	40 (62%)	15 (23%)	9 (14%)
Mead et al.[228]†	94	69 (73%)	7 (7%)	18 (19%)

Table 4.9 Clinicoradiological correlations of total anterior circulation syndromes.

*Community-based study, first-ever strokes. †Hospital-based study, first-ever and recurrent strokes.

The brain lesion

In community-based studies between 19% and 25% of patients presenting with TACS had an intracerebral haemorrhage.[177–179] The correlation between the clinical syndrome and brain imaging in patients with ischaemic stroke is shown in Table 4.9. Perhaps the biggest 'catch' is the well-described ability of posterior cerebral artery (PCA) territory ischaemia to produce a TACS;[104–106,183] the patients generally have a relatively mild hemiparesis but marked aphasia (not always fluent) and a visual field deficit. The motor deficit occurs because of involvement of the small, perforating arteries arising from the proximal PCA, which supply the upper midbrain (section 4.2.3). Although the original definition of TACS simply used the word 'hemiparesis', in fact the vast majority of patients in the Oxfordshire Community Stroke Project who were classified as having TACS were either hemiplegic or had a severe hemiparesis that would certainly have been incompatible with walking.[184] Therefore, it is worth bearing in mind the aphorism 'beware the walking TACS – the patient may have a posterior circulation syndrome'. The volume of infarction in patients with TACS, as judged by CT, is, not surprisingly, significantly greater than in patients with lesser deficits[152,178] (section 4.3.7).

> Occasionally, a total anterior circulation syndrome results from occlusion of the posterior cerebral artery. In such cases, there is often a relatively mild hemiparesis but marked aphasia and visual field loss – 'beware the walking TACS'.

The vascular lesion

From the early pathological studies, the TACS pattern of deficit was linked with occlusion of the proximal mainstem of the middle cerebral artery (MCA) and infarction in both the deep and superficial territories.[68] It was also recognized that, on occasion, the extent of infarction in the superficial territory was not as extensive, and this was presumed to be because of effective leptomeningeal collaterals (section 6.7.1). This is a similar argument to that relating to striatocapsular infarction (section 4.2.2). An early angiographic study reported that of 20 patients with extensive hemispheric infarction as judged by CT, 14 had MCA occlusion and the other 6 had either occlusion or more than 75% stenosis of the ipsilateral internal carotid artery (ICA).[46] Later studies of patients with non-haemorrhagic TACS who had an early carotid duplex examination reported that more than one-third had either occlusion or a high-grade stenosis of the ICA ipsilateral to the cerebral lesion, and many of the others had a major cardiac source of embolism.[160,164] In the Lausanne Stroke Registry, in which the topographically defined large MCA territory infarcts would be broadly equivalent to TACS, 41% of patients had occlusion of the ipsilateral ICA and 33% had a major source of cardiac embolism.[48]

4.3.5 Partial anterior circulation syndromes

The clinical syndrome

The final group of syndromes have less extensive deficits than a total anterior circulation syndrome and yet do not fulfil the specific criteria for a lacunar syndrome, either because of the presence of higher cortical deficits or because the motor/sensory deficit is too restricted in anatomical terms. These would be broadly similar to a combination of the superficial middle cerebral artery and anterior cerebral artery syndromes in other classifications.[125] The clinical features of partial anterior circulation syndromes (PACS) are set out in Table 4.10.

The brain lesion

In community-based studies between 6% and 13% of patients presenting with a partial anterior circulation syndrome had an intracerebral haemorrhage.[177–179] The correlation between the clinical syndrome and brain

Table 4.10 Partial anterior circulation syndromes.

At time of maximum deficit, any of:
  Motor/sensory deficit + hemianopia
  Motor/sensory deficit + new higher cerebral dysfunction
  New higher cerebral dysfunction + hemianopia
  Pure motor/sensory deficit less extensive than for lacunar
    syndromes (e.g. monoparesis)
  New higher cerebral dysfunction alone (e.g. aphasia)

When more than one type of deficit is present, they must all reflect damage in the same cerebral hemisphere.

imaging in patients with ischaemic stroke is shown in Table 4.11. Most of the patients with 'inappropriate' infarcts had either multiple small, deep infarcts, which may or may not have been relevant to the clinical syndrome, or what appeared to be isolated posterior cerebral artery (PCA) territory infarction. Although PCA territory infarction is usually considered to be due to embolism from the vertebrobasilar arteries, there will be up to 15% of patients whose PCAs are supplied by the carotid system, because of developmental variation in the circle of Willis (section 4.2.2).

The vascular lesion

In an angiographic study of 25 patients with medium (1.5–3.0 cm) areas of infarction on CT, 14 were found to have middle cerebral artery (MCA) occlusion, 6 had internal carotid artery (ICA) occlusion, and 5 had no significant angiographic lesion[46] (section 6.7.2). Later studies of patients with non-haemorrhagic partial anterior circulation syndromes (PACS) who had an early carotid duplex examination reported that about a quarter had either occlusion or high-grade stenosis of the ICA ipsilateral to the cerebral lesion, and up to half the other patients had a major cardiac source of embolism.[160,164] In the Lausanne Stroke Registry, in which the topographically defined limited superficial MCA territory infarcts would be broadly equivalent to the majority of

PACS (isolated anterior cerebral artery infarcts being relatively uncommon), 28% of patients had greater than 50% stenosis of the ipsilateral ICA, and 33% had a major source of cardiac embolism.[48]

4.3.6 Syndromes of uncertain origin

For a variety of reasons, the physician will occasionally have difficulty allocating cases with confidence on clinical grounds to one of the four stroke syndromes. For example, the patient may have had a previous stroke, be demented, or have had a limb amputated for peripheral vascular disease. In such cases, it may be unclear what new neurological deficits have arisen from the current stroke. There are also patients, who are often very elderly, in whom it can be difficult to decide whether they should be classified as having a partial anterior circulation syndrome (PACS) or a total anterior circulation syndrome (TACS), usually because of uncertainty about the presence of *new* higher cerebral dysfunction or a visual field deficit. If one is not certain about a deficit, it is usually best to consider it absent, and therefore the majority should be considered as having a PACS. The exception is if the patient is drowsy, which – if due to the cerebral lesion rather than any metabolic disturbance – would be indicative of an extensive supratentorial lesion with the patient being classified as having a TACS, or of a major brainstem stroke with the patient being classified as a posterior circulation syndrome. At the other end of the spectrum, one should be quite rigid about applying the rules describing the extent of a motor or sensory deficit which ought to be present before diagnosing LACS (i.e. only when there is involvement of the face, arm and leg; or the whole of the face and arm; or the whole of the arm and leg). At the end of the day, however, there is some evidence that making a 'best guess' on the basis of the evidence available to you is probably a reasonably accurate strategy.[185]

The results of any brain imaging may well assist the primary classification, i.e. point towards the most likely

Table 4.11 Clinicoradiological correlations of partial anterior circulation syndromes.

Study	Number	Appropriate infarct	No lesion	Inappropriate infarct
Bamford[177]*	106	47 (44%)	56 (53%)	3 (3%)
Lindgren *et al.*[178]*	61	21 (34%)	24 (39%)	16 (26%)
Anderson *et al.*[179]*	75	25 (33%)	31 (41%)	19 (25%)
Wardlaw *et al.*[183]†	43	29 (67%)	7 (16%)	7 (16%)
Al-Buhairi *et al.*[227]†	121	78 (64%)	39 (32%)	4 (3%)
Mead *et al.*[228]†	441	213 (48%)	143 (32%)	85 (19%)

*Community-based study, first-ever strokes. †Hospital-based study, first-ever and recurrent strokes.

clinical syndrome (section 4.3.7). This can be of value both in clinical practice and in research, where it will help minimize the risk of bias being introduced, particularly when considering the outcome of various groups of patients. Of course, on any imaging it is important to be sure that any 'infarct' is in an anatomically appropriate place to explain the symptoms and signs, and of the correct age to be compatible with the onset of the stroke.

4.3.7 The Oxfordshire Community Stroke Project (OCSP) classification and acute 'brain attacks'

The OCSP classification was developed primarily for epidemiological purposes from a data set that was based on the clinical examination of patients at a mean of 4 days post-stroke.[184] Furthermore, most of the other data referred to above have come from studies in which a substantial proportion of the patients were assessed more than 24 h after onset of symptoms. It is unlikely, therefore, that progression of the neurological deficit occurred in any significant proportion of the patients studied – thereby allowing a key feature of the syndromic diagnosis, i.e. the clinical pattern at the time of *maximum* deficit, to be assessed. We cannot assume, however, that the classification remains valid for the hyperacute examination of patients that is now becoming commonplace – i.e. those with brain attacks that started in the previous few hours. For example, in a study of 152 patients with supratentorial ischaemic stroke who were seen within 5 h of onset of symptoms, 39 (26%) had some neurological deterioration during the subsequent 4 days.[186–188] Most of these patients had extensive middle cerebral artery (MCA) territory infarction, and the results would be in keeping with those from the Lausanne Stroke Registry, in which only 159 of 208 (76%) patients with large MCA territory infarcts had a fixed neurological deficit 1 h after the onset of symptoms.[48] Table 4.12 shows the outcome for patients who presented with either a pure motor or sensorimotor stroke, i.e. lacunar syndromes (LACS), within 12 h of onset.[186] It is clear that one can see a patient very early who would be classified as having a lacunar syndrome (LACS), but who 24 h

later would be classified as having a total anterior circulation syndrome (TACS). Modern imaging techniques have now shown that those patients who present acutely with a lacunar syndrome but then progress have a visible deficit on perfusion MR imaging, something that is not seen after occlusion of a single deep perforating artery;[9] this is probably because occlusion of the proximal MCA causes symptoms (and in some cases changes on CT) that are first apparent in the territory of the lenticulostriate arteries before the cerebral cortex which may have a better collateral supply. However, there is another group of patients who present acutely with non-lacunar syndromes (principally, partial anterior circulation syndromes, PACS) who have small, deep infarcts (equivalent to lacunar infarcts) on the second CT scan.[186] Of these 47 patients, 23 (49%) improved over the following days with resolution of their 'cortical' symptoms and signs – i.e. if they had been examined a few days after the onset, and there had been no clear record or history of the clinical pattern at the time of maximum deficit, then they would have been classified (correctly) as having a LACS.

All this has led us to question the utility of using the OCSP classification alone as a method of stratifying subgroups of patients in hyperacute intervention trials, although it has been shown to be reasonably robust in less acute studies (Table 4.13).[189] As mentioned at the beginning of this chapter, one reason for having a clinically based method of classification is that if other information is available, then it can be used in a hierarchical manner and of course many patients will have some form of emergency cross-sectional imaging. We know that if patients present with a LACS but have evidence of new cortical infarction on CT in a potentially relevant place then they are more likely to have significant disease of the ipsilateral internal carotid artery (odds ratio 3.7) or a major source of cardioembolism (odds ratio 3.9) than those patients with small, deep infarcts on CT, i.e. from an aetiological perspective they are more like PACS.[190] Nevertheless, we think that the clinical classification may still be useful for identifying those patients most likely to have a particular vascular lesion of interest, who might then be targeted for further

Clinical syndrome at < 12 h	CT at 15 days compatible with lacunar infarction,* or postmortem	CT at 15 days not compatible with lacunar infarction,* or postmortem	Positive predictive value
Pure motor stroke	88	63	58%
Sensorimotor stroke	35	33	51%

*i.e. normal scan, or subcortical infarct < 1.5 cm diameter.

Table 4.12 Correlation of early diagnosis of lacunar syndromes with final lesion on CT scan.[186]

Table 4.13 Clinico-radiological correlation of Oxfordshire Community Stroke Project syndromes in the setting of an acute clinical trial.[189]

CT appearance	TACS		PACS		LACS		POCS	
Large cortical infarct	59	(50)	13	(5)	5	(3.5)	1	(2)
Medium or small cortical infarct or large subcortical MCA territory infarct	28	(24)	140	(58)	29	(20)	5	(9)
Small subcortical infarct	13	(11)	29	(12)	62	(44)	12	(22)
Cortical PCA territory, brainstem or cerebellar infarct	6	(5)	11	(4.5)	5	(3.5)	26	(47)
No recent infarct visible	12	(10)	50	(20.5)	41	(29)	11	(20)
Total	118	(100)	243	(100)	142	(100)	55	(100)

LACS lacunar syndrome; MCA middle cerebral artery; PACS partial anterior circulation syndrome; PCA posterior cerebral artery; POCS posterior circulation syndrome; TACS total anterior circulation syndrome

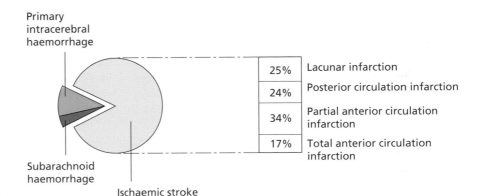

Fig. 4.27 The distribution of clinical subtypes of ischaemic stroke in the Oxfordshire Community Stroke Project.

emergency investigations – e.g. in trials of thrombolysis it may well be logical to distinguish TACS/PACS from LACS as a way of picking out those most likely to have large-vessel occlusion, or in clinical practice giving patients with PACS priority for carotid duplex because of the high proportion with surgically significant stenosis and at high risk of early recurrence.

4.3.8 Using the clinically based Oxfordshire Community Stroke Project (OCSP) classification

Any system of classification will not become widely accepted unless it is easy to use and conveys useful information to the clinician (Table 4.14). How do the clinical syndromes described above measure up to this challenge? The necessary information is, by and large, easy (and inexpensive) to collect from virtually all patients with stroke, and a checklist can be incorporated into stroke clerking or admission forms as an *aide-mémoire*. Each syndrome occurs sufficiently frequently in patients with stroke (Fig. 4.27) to promote pattern recognition, particularly by junior medical staff.

Moderately good inter-observer reliability (between a junior and a senior clinician) in the allocation of clinical

Table 4.14 Benefits of using the clinically based Oxfordshire Community Stroke Project classification.

Information is quick, easy and inexpensive to collect on virtually all patients

The syndromes occur frequently enough to promote pattern recognition

Reasonable inter-observer reliability

Some indication of the likelihood of the stroke being due to intracerebral haemorrhage in white northern European populations

Prediction of the volume of ischaemia on CT/MR scan and therefore at an early stage an indication of the risk of complications in the acute phase, and longer-term prognosis

An indication of the likely underlying vascular pathology and therefore a guide to appropriate investigations

In the era of acute 'brain attack', it could be used to predict where the 'hole' would have been without effective treatment

subtype (kappa = 0.54) has been reported.[185] Another study reported that the inter-observer agreement for the allocation of clinical subtypes between the initial 'routine' clinical examination (albeit using a clerking proforma) and another performed within 1 week by one of the authors was 92% (kappa = 0.89).[178] However, it is worth remembering that there is evidence of improved clinicoradiological correlation for lacunar syndromes (LACS), at least when the patients are seen by clinicians with a specific interest in stroke.[191,192] It is interesting that a recent community-based study reported better agreement between two neurologists (kappa = 0.53) than between the neurologists and trained nurses (although the agreement with the nurses was still fair to moderate).[193] Most difficulty is encountered in the interpretation of physical signs (e.g. hemianopia). A standard checklist can be usefully added to routine clerking proforma with algorithms to derive the OCSP classification, and the algorithm can be programmed into a hand-held computer (Table 4.15).[194]

The syndromes provide the clinician with some indication of the likelihood of a stroke being due to cerebral haemorrhage: unlikely (<5%) with LACS but more likely (25%) with total anterior circulation syndromes (TACS). This in no way obviates the need for CT scanning to make a definitive distinction between infarct and haemorrhage, but unfortunately, clinicians in some parts of the world continue to have restricted access to such facilities (section 5.3).

The syndromes predict the volume of cerebral infarction in patients with ischaemic stroke.[152,178] Thus, very rapidly, clinical staff can predict which patients are at greatest risk of developing impairment of conscious level and possible risk of aspiration (section 11.3). Consequently, the nursing staff and relatives can then be alerted to the possibility of aspiration and take appropriate action. In a study of patients with ischaemic strokes there was an impaired level of consciousness in 14% of those with TACS, 4% of those with partial anterior circulation syndromes (PACS), 5% of those with posterior circulation syndromes (POCS) and none of those with LACS.[195] Thus, impairment of consciousness developing in a patient with LACS should prompt a search for an alternative explanation (such as an infection) because these patients do not develop significant cerebral oedema. Patients with TACS are more likely to be admitted to hospital than those with LACS and also more likely to become febrile (often from urinary or respiratory infections), develop deep venous

Table 4.15 Algorithm employed by the International Stroke Trial randomization computer to assign Oxfordshire Community Stroke Project syndrome.

	Neurological deficit							
	1	2	3	4	5	6	7	8
Total anterior circulation syndrome	Y	Y	—	Y	Y	—	—	—
	—	Y	Y	Y	Y	—	—	—
	—	Y	Y	—	Y	Y	—	—
	Y	Y	—	—	Y	Y	—	—
	Y	Y	—	Y	O	—	—	—
	—	Y	Y	Y	O	—	—	—
	Y	Y	—	—	O	Y	—	—
	—	Y	Y	—	O	Y	—	—
	Y	Y	—	—	Y	O	—	—
	—	Y	Y	—	Y	O	—	—
	Y	Y	—	O	Y	—	—	—
	—	Y	Y	O	Y	—	—	—
Lacunar syndrome	Y	Y	—	N	N	N	N	N
	—	Y	Y	N	N	N	N	N
Posterior circulation syndrome	—	—	—	—	—	—	Y	—
	N	N	N	N	Y	N	N	N
Others	N	N	N	N	N	N	N	Y
Partial anterior circulation syndrome	Any other combination							

1 unilateral plegia and/or facial deficit
2 unilateral paresis and/or sensory deficit of upper limb
3 unilateral paresis and/or sensory deficit of lower limb
4 dysphasia
5 homonymous hemianopia
6 visuospatial deficit or neglect syndrome
7 brainstem or cerebellar signs
8 other symptoms

Y = yes, sign observed;   N = no, sign not observed   O = not assessable

Table 4.16 Carotid and cardiac findings by clinical subtype.[160]

	>80% stenosis or occlusion of the ipsilateral carotid artery	Major cardioembolic source
Total anterior circulation syndrome	43%	57%
Partial anterior circulation syndrome	19%	46%
Lacunar syndrome	5%	16%
Posterior circulation syndrome	10%	8%

Table 4.17 Carotid duplex findings by clinical subtype: degree of stenosis ipsilateral to the site of infarction.[164]

	Stenosis of ipsilateral internal carotid artery			
	0–49%	50–69%	70–99%	Occluded
Total anterior circulation syndrome (n = 117)	68 (58%)	6 (5%)	6 (5%)	33 (28%)
Partial anterior circulation syndrome (n = 128)	74 (58%)	9 (7%)	25 (20%)	17 (13%)
Lacunar syndrome (n = 108)	96 (89%)	8 (7%)	1 (1%)	3 (3%)
Posterior circulation syndrome (n = 27)	24 (89%)	2 (7%)	1 (4%)	0 (0%)

thrombosis, pulmonary embolism and possibly also hyponatraemia.[195,196]

Since the syndromes predict the volume of cerebral infarction, not surprisingly they also predict stroke outcome (section 10.2). Not only does this allow more accurate information to be given to the patients and their relatives, it also allows early, realistic discharge planning to begin. More research is required into whether given deficits occurring as part of different syndromes have different patterns of recovery, but certainly clear differences can be predicted for mobility milestones, as well as for the likely length of stay in hospital and utilization of resources.[195,197,198]

Finally, the syndromes provide the clinician with an indication of the most likely underlying vascular lesion, thereby linking with the aetiological schemes of subclassification (sections 6.7.1–6.7.4). TACS/PACS are most likely to be caused by occlusion of the larger cerebral arteries, and the clinician should therefore be thinking about cardiac sources of embolism or carotid and aortic atherosclerosis (Tables 4.16 and 4.17). If access to, for example, carotid duplex is restricted, one could argue that patients with PACS – in whom there is a significant chance of finding a more than 70% carotid stenosis in a patient who has a good chance of making an excellent physical recovery, and in whom the risk of early recurrence may be greatest – should take precedence over patients with LACS.[164,184,190,199] Conversely, if a patient presents with a LACS, the clinician should not be surprised if there is no lesion on the CT scan, carotid duplex or echocardiography, and should not 'chase' excessively rare causes of stroke without some good reason such as

the absence of any conventional risk factors for atherosclerosis.[200]

4.4 Subclassification based on aetiology

While there is a broad consensus about how the many underlying causes of cerebral infarction and cerebral haemorrhage should be grouped together and which investigations should be performed in order to identify the cause of the stroke (Chapters 6–8), even in the most sophisticated healthcare systems the allocation of individual patients to one of the groups poses an immense challenge. Several schemes based on the subclassification of cerebral infarcts according to the putative underlying causal mechanism, of which that for the Trial of Org 10172 in Acute Stroke Treatment (TOAST) remains the most well-known and widely used, were developed for specific research projects in specialist institutions, a quite different situation from routine clinical practice.[201–204] In these schemes the final aetiological classification of the ischaemic stroke is based on a combination of clinical features, the results of neuroimaging and of ancillary investigations (Table 4.18). Unfortunately, these classifications have only moderate inter-observer reliability and, even with the most intensive investigation protocols used in research environments, up to 40% of patients remain 'unclassifiable'.[160,205–208]

Table 4.18 The TOAST* classification of subtypes of acute ischaemic stroke (*Trial of Org 10172 in Acute Stroke Treatment).[204]

Large artery atherosclerosis	
Clinical	Cerebral cortical, brainstem or cerebellar symptoms, supported by history of intermittent claudication, transient ischemic attack in same vascular territory, carotid bruit or diminished pulses
Imaging	Cerebral cortical or cerebellar lesions or brainstem/subcortical lesions > 1.5 cm diameter on CT/MR
Tests	Stenosis > 50% of appropriate intracranial or extracranial artery on duplex or arteriography Potential sources of cardiac embolism should be excluded
Cardioembolism	
Clinical	Cerebral cortical, brainstem or cerebellar symptoms, supported by history of stroke or transient ischaemic attack in more than one vascular territory, or systemic embolism
Imaging	Cerebral cortical or cerebellar lesions or brainstem/subcortical lesions > 1.5 cm diameter on CT/MR
Tests	At least one cardiac source of embolism should be identified (from high-risk group for 'probable' or medium-risk group for 'possible' cardiac embolism) Potential large artery atherosclerosis sources of thrombosis or embolism should be excluded
Small artery disease	
Clinical	Patient should have one of the traditional clinical lacunar syndromes and no evidence of cerebral cortical dysfunction, supported by history of diabetes or hypertension
Imaging	Normal CT/MRI or relevant brainstem or subcortical hemispheric lesion < 1.5 cm diameter
Tests	Potential large artery atherosclerosis sources of thrombosis or embolism, and cardiac sources of embolism should be excluded
Other determined aetiologies	
Clinical	Any symptoms compatible with an acute stroke
Imaging	CT/MRI findings of acute ischaemic stroke regardless of the size or location
Tests	Includes patients with non-atherosclerotic vasculopathies, hypercoaguable states or haematological disorders Potential large artery atherosclerosis sources of thrombosis or embolism, and cardiac sources of embolism should be excluded
Undetermined aetiology	
Includes	No aetiology determined despite extensive evaluation No aetiology determined but cursory evaluation Patients with two or more potential causes of stroke

As with the OCSP syndromes, a further problem is that of trying to classify the mechanism of stroke when patients are assessed in the hyperacute phase. In a study using the detailed TOAST protocol, the initial (<24 hours from onset) impression of stroke subtype based on clinical, CT, electrocardiographic and initial laboratory results was confirmed in only 62% of cases when the classification was reviewed at 3 months in the light of all available investigational results.[209] Junior doctors are often the first to see an acute stroke patient but only half of their initial (<24 h) subclassifications based on clinical, CT and blood tests agreed with the final 'consensus' TOAST classification.[210] In the Erlangen study it was not possible to allocate a TOAST subtype in 9% of cases because the diagnostic procedures were incomplete and in a further 18% the diagnostic workup took more than a week.[211] Perhaps, not surprisingly, the unclassified patients were older and less likely to be admitted to hospital.

Thus, while clues about the likely cause of the cerebral event may be immediately apparent from the history and examination (e.g. the presence of atrial fibrillation), any classification that places an undue reliance on the results of investigations will be difficult to use for every patient in routine clinical practice (as opposed to research).[212] Factors that may influence the ability to classify in this way include:

- the variable availability of such investigations;
- the perceived appropriateness of using a particular investigation for an individual patient (e.g. because of the degree of pre-stroke or post-stroke disability, cost, etc.);
- the variability of the results, arising from both observer-dependent and technology-dependent factors;
- the speed with which any classification needs to be made (e.g. particularly now for acute treatments);
- the problem of identifying multiple potential causes of the stroke (e.g. atrial fibrillation and severe ipsilateral carotid stenosis).

> We still do not have the knowledge or the technology to determine the exact cause of stroke in every patient, certainly not within the first few hours of onset and very often even later.

In our view, the sequence of subclassification in the early phase of stroke should be first, in the vast majority of patients, a clinical (syndromic) diagnosis; followed where possible by a topographical (radiological) diagnosis if the imaging is abnormal and shows a recent, potentially relevant lesion; and then finally an aetiological diagnosis (Fig. 4.28). Such a three-step

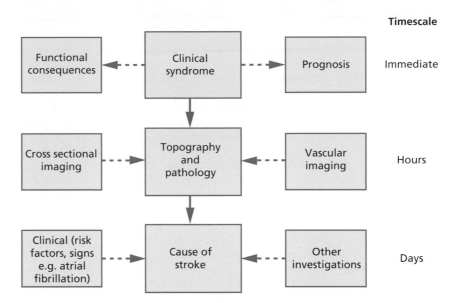

Timescale

Fig. 4.28 Diagram of the three-step model of acute diagnosis, i.e. syndrome --→ topography --→ cause.

Table 4.19 Correlation of clinical syndrome within first 24 hours after onset with CT/MR lesion.[213]

Syndrome	n	Cortical infarct	Boundary zone infarct	Lacunar infarct	Posterior circulation infarct	No lesion
Total anterior circulation infarction	55	53 (96%)	1 (2%)	0	1 (2%)	0
Partial anterior circulation infarction	49	36 (73%)	7 (14%)	2 (4%)	1 (2%)	3 (6%)
Lacunar infarction	103	11 (11%)	16 (16%)	70 (68%)	1 (1%)	5 (5%)
Posterior circulation infarction	43	2 (5%)	0	1 (2%)	37 (86%)	3 (6%)
Total	250	102	24	73	40	11

Table 4.20 Correlation of clinical syndrome within first 24hours after onset with final cause of infarction.[213]

Syndrome	n	Large artery atherosclerosis	Cardioembolic	Small artery disease	Other
Total anterior circulation infarction	55	11 (20%)	34 (62%)	0	10 (18%)
Partial anterior circulation infarction	49	20 (41%)	21 (43%)	0	8 (16%)
Lacunar infarction	103	30 (29%)	0	60 (58%)	13 (13%)
Posterior circulation	43	15 (35%)	9 (21%)	7 (15%)	12 (28%)
Total	250	76	64	67	43

model of subclassification has been reported:[213] 250 consecutive stroke patients aged 32–92 years who were seen within 24 h of the onset of symptoms were described. The first stage of their subclassification was to allocate them to one of the four clinically defined Oxfordshire Community Stroke Project subgroups. The second stage was to allocate patients to a radiological subgroup, based on brain CT or MR findings. Then, after completion of all relevant investigations, the patients were allocated to an aetiological subgroup. Table 4.19

shows the correlation between the clinical syndromes and the radiological diagnosis, and Table 4.20 the correlation between the clinical syndromes and the aetiological diagnosis. For both, the clinical syndrome performed moderately well.

Finally, it is important not to forget that running in parallel with this medically orientated diagnostic model will be a functional diagnosis (of impairment, disability and handicap) and finally a 'social' diagnosis (quality of life, reintegration, and so on; Chapter 10).

References

1 Wardlaw JM, Keir SL, Bastin ME, Armitage PA, Rana AK. Is diffusion imaging appearance an independent predictor of outcome after ischemic stroke? *Neurology* 2002; **59**(9):1381–7.

2 Hand PJ, Wardlaw JM, Rivers CS, Armitage PA, Bastin ME, Lindley RI *et al*. MR diffusion-weighted imaging and outcome prediction after ischemic stroke. *Neurology* 2006; **66**(8):1159–63.

3 Damasio H. A computed tomographic guide to the identification of cerebral vascular territories. *Arch Neurol* 1983; **40**(3):138–42.

4 Van der Zwan A, Hillen B. Review of the variability of the territories of the major cerebral arteries. *Stroke* 1991; **22**(8):1078–84.

5 Van der Zwan A, Hillen B, Tulleken CA, Dujovny M, Dragovic L. Variability of the territories of the major cerebral arteries. *J Neurosurg* 1992; **77**(6):927–40.

6 Van der Zwan A, Hillen B, Tulleken CA, Dujovny M. A quantitative investigation of the variability of the major cerebral arterial territories. *Stroke* 1993; **24**(12):1951–9.

7 Tatu L, Moulin T, Bogousslavsky J, Duvernoy H. Arterial territories of human brain: brainstem and cerebellum. *Neurology* 1996; **47**(5):1125–35.

8 Tatu L, Moulin T, Bogousslavsky J, Duvernoy H. Arterial territories of the human brain: cerebral hemispheres. *Neurology* 1998; **50**(6):1699–708.

9 Gerraty RP, Parsons MW, Barber PA, Darby DG, Desmond PM, Tress BM *et al*. Examining the lacunar hypothesis with diffusion and perfusion magnetic resonance imaging. *Stroke* 2002; **33**(8):2019–24.

10 Lang EW, Daffertshofer M, Daffertshofer A, Wirth SB, Chesnut RM, Hennerici M. Variability of vascular territory in stroke: pitfalls and failure of stroke pattern interpretation. *Stroke* 1995; **26**(6):942–5.

11 Hennerici MG, Schwartz A. Acute stroke subtypes: is there a need for reclassification? *Cerebrovasc Dis* 1998; **8** (Suppl 2):17–22.

12 Hennerici M, Daffertshofer M, Jakobs L. Failure to identify cerebral infarct mechanisms from topography of vascular territory lesions. *Am J Neuroradiol* 1998; **19**(6):1067–74.

13 Vander Eecken HM, Adams RD. The anatomy and functional significance of the meningeal arterial anastomoses of the human brain. *J Neuropathol Exp Neurol* 1953; **12**(2):132–57.

14 Calverley PM. Blood pressure, breathing, and the carotid body. *Lancet* 1999; **354**(9183):969–70.

15 Parry SW, Richardson DA, O'Shea D, Sen B, Kenny RA. Diagnosis of carotid sinus hypersensitivity in older adults: carotid sinus massage in the upright position is essential. *Heart* 2000; **83**(1):22–3.

16 Mead GE, Wardlaw JM, Lewis SC, Dennis MS. No evidence that severity of stroke in internal carotid occlusion is related to collateral arteries. *J Neurol Neurosurg Psychiatry* 2006; **77**(6):729–33.

17 Markus H, Cullinane M. Severely impaired cerebrovascular reactivity predicts stroke and TIA risk in patients with carotid artery stenosis and occlusion. *Brain* 2001; **124**(Pt 3):457–67.

18 Castaigne P, Lhermitte F, Gautier JC, Escourolle R, Derouesne C. Internal carotid artery occlusion: a study of 61 instances in 50 patients with post-mortem data. *Brain* 1970; **93**(2):231–58.

19 Torvik A, Jorgensen L. Thrombotic and embolic occlusions of the carotid arteries in an autopsy material. Part 1. Prevalence, location and associated diseases. *J Neurol Sci* 1964; **1**:24–39.

20 Torvik A, Jorgensen L. Thrombotic and embolic occlusions of the carotid arteries in an autopsy series. Part 2. Cerebral lesions and clinical course. *J Neurol Sci* 1966; **3**:410–32.

21 Lammie GA, Sandercock PA, Dennis MS. Recently occluded intracranial and extracranial carotid arteries: relevance of the unstable atherosclerotic plaque. *Stroke* 1999; **30**(7):1319–25.

22 Dinubile MJ. Septic thrombosis of the cavernous sinuses. *Arch Neurol* 1988; **45**(5):567–72.

23 Fisher CM. Observations of the fundus oculi in transient monocular blindness. *Neurology* 1959; **9**(5):333–47.

24 Marinkovic S, Gibo H, Brigante L, Nikodijevic I, Petrovic P. The surgical anatomy of the perforating branches of the anterior choroidal artery. *Surg Neurol* 1999; **52**(1):30–6.

25 Caplan LR. Anterior choroidal territory infarcts. In: Donnan G, Norrving B, Bamford J, Bogousslavsky J, eds. *Subcortical Stroke*. 2nd edn. Oxford: Oxford University Press, 2002, pp. 225–40.

26 Tamaki M, Ohno K, Niimi Y, Aoyagi M, Nagashima G, Ichimura K *et al*. Parenchymal damage in the territory of the anterior choroidal artery following supraophthalmic intracarotid administration of CDDP for treatment of malignant gliomas. *J Neurooncol* 1997; **35**(1):65–72.

27 Frisen L. Quadruple sectoranopia and sectorial optic atrophy: a syndrome of the distal anterior choroidal artery. *J Neurol Neurosurg Psychiatry* 1979; **42**(7):590–4.

28 Padget J. The development of the cranial arteries in the human embryo. *Contributions to Embryology* 1948; **32**:205–61.

29 Van Overbeeke JJ, Hillen B, Tulleken CA. A comparative study of the circle of Willis in fetal and adult life. The configuration of the posterior bifurcation of the posterior communicating artery. *J Anat* 1991; **176**:45–54.

30 Riggs HE, Rupp C. Variation in form of circle of Willis. The relation of the variations to collateral circulation: anatomic analysis. *Arch Neurol* 1963; **8**:8–14.

31 Alpers BJ, Berry RG. Circle of Willis in cerebral vascular disorders: the anatomical structure. *Arch Neurol* 1963; **8**:398–402.

32 Hillen B, Hoogstraten HW, Post L. A mathematical model of the flow in the circle of Willis. *J Biomech* 1986; **19**(3):187–94.

33 Bogousslavsky J, Regli F. Anterior cerebral artery territory infarction in the Lausanne Stroke Registry: clinical and etiologic patterns. *Arch Neurol* 1990; **47**(2):144–50.

34 Minagar A, David NJ. Bilateral infarction in the territory of the anterior cerebral arteries. *Neurology* 1999; **52**(4):886–8.

35 Critchley M. The anterior cerebral artery and its syndromes. *Brain* 1930; **53**:120–65.

36 Kazui S, Sawada T. Callosal apraxia without agraphia. *Ann Neurol* 1993; **33**(4):401–3.

37 Gado M, Hanaway J, Frank R. Functional anatomy of the cerebral cortex by computed tomography. *J Comput Assist Tomogr* 1979; **3**(1):1–19.

38 Bogousslavsky J, Martin R, Moulin T. Homolateral ataxia and crural paresis: a syndrome of anterior cerebral artery territory infarction. *J Neurol Neurosurg Psychiatry* 1992; **55**(12):1146–9.

39 McNabb AW, Carroll WM, Mastaglia FL. 'Alien hand' and loss of bimanual coordination after dominant anterior cerebral artery territory infarction. *J Neurol Neurosurg Psychiatry* 1988; **51**(2):218–22.

40 Josephs KA, Rossor MN. The alien limb. *Pract Neurol* 2004; **4**(1):44–5.

41 Loukas M, Louis RG, Jr., Childs RS. Anatomical examination of the recurrent artery of Heubner. *Clin Anat* 2006; **19**(1):25–31.

42 Dunker RO, Harris AB. Surgical anatomy of the proximal anterior cerebral artery. *J Neurosurg* 1976; **44**(3):359–67.

43 Feekes JA, Hsu SW, Chaloupka JC, Cassell MD. Tertiary microvascular territories define lacunar infarcts in the basal ganglia. *Ann Neurol* 2005; **58**(1):18–30.

44 Feekes JA, Cassell MD. The vascular supply of the functional compartments of the human striatum. *Brain* 2006; **129**(Pt 8):2189–201.

45 Perlmutter D, Rhoton AL, Jr. Microsurgical anatomy of anterior cerebral anterior communicating recurrent artery complex. *Surg Forum* 1976; **27**(62):464–5.

46 Olsen TS, Skriver EB, Herning M. Cause of cerebral infarction in the carotid territory: its relation to the size and the location of the infarct and to the underlying vascular lesion. *Stroke* 1985; **16**(3):459–66.

47 Fieschi C, Argentino C, Lenzi GL, Sacchetti ML, Toni D, Bozzao L. Clinical and instrumental evaluation of patients with ischemic stroke within the first six hours. *J Neurol Sci* 1989; **91**(3):311–21.

48 Heinsius T, Bogousslavsky J, Van Melle G. Large infarcts in the middle cerebral artery territory. Etiology and outcome patterns. *Neurology* 1998; **50**(2):341–50.

49 Ueda S, Fujitsu K, Inomori S, Kuwabara T. Thrombotic occlusion of the middle cerebral artery. *Stroke* 1992; **23**(12):1761–6.

50 Marinkovic SV, Milisavljevic MM, Kovacevic MS, Stevic ZD. Perforating branches of the middle cerebral artery: microanatomy and clinical significance of their intracerebral segments. *Stroke* 1985; **16**(6):1022–9.

51 Weiller C. Striatocapsular infarcts. In: Donnan G, Norrving B, Bamford J, Bogousslavsky J, eds. *Subcortical Stroke*. 2nd edn. Oxford: Oxford University Press, 2002, pp. 195–208.

52 Horowitz DR, Tuhrim S. Stroke mechanisms and clinical presentation in large subcortical infarctions. *Neurology* 1997; **49**(6):1538–41.

53 Donnan G, Norrving B, Bamford J, Bogousslavsky J. Classification of subcortical infarcts. In: Donnan G, Norrving B, Bamford J, Bogousslavsky J, eds. *Subcortical Stroke*. 2nd edn. Oxford: Oxford University Press, 2002, pp. 27–36.

54 Lammie A. The role of oedema in lacune formation. *Cerebrovasc Dis* 1998; **8**(4):246.

55 Wardlaw JM. What causes lacunar stroke? *J Neurol Neurosurg Psychiatry* 2005; **76**(5):617–9.

56 Fisher CM. Lacunes: small, deep cerebral infarcts. *Neurology* 1965; **15**:774–84.

57 Donnan GA, Tress BM, Bladin PF. A prospective study of lacunar infarction using computerized tomography. *Neurology* 1982; **32**(1):49–56.

58 Critchley M. Arteriosclerotic parkinsonism. *Brain* 1929; **52**:23–83.

59 Eadie MJ, Sutherland JM. Arteriosclerosis in parkinsonism. *J Neurol Neurosurg Psychiatry* 1964; **27**:237–40.

60 Parkes JD, Marsden CD, Rees JE, Curzon G, Kantamaneni BD, Knill-Jones R *et al*. Parkinson's disease, cerebral arteriosclerosis, and senile dementia: clinical features and response to levodopa. *Q J Med* 1974; **43**(169):49–61.

61 Friedman A, Kang UJ, Tatemichi TK, Burke RE. A case of parkinsonism following striatal lacunar infarction. *J Neurol Neurosurg Psychiatry* 1986; **49**(9):1087–8.

62 Ebersbach G, Sojer M, Valldeoriola F, Wissel J, Muller J, Tolosa E *et al*. Comparative analysis of gait in Parkinson's disease, cerebellar ataxia and subcortical arteriosclerotic encephalopathy. *Brain* 1999; **122** (Pt 7):1349–55.

63 Hauw JJ. The history of lacunes. In: Donnan G, Norrving B, Bamford J, Bogousslavsky J, eds. *Subcortical Stroke*. 2nd edn. Oxford: Oxford University Press, 2002, pp. 3–16.

64 Bogousslavsky J, Van Melle G, Regli F. Middle cerebral artery pial territory infarcts: a study of the Lausanne Stroke Registry. *Ann Neurol* 1989; **25**(6):555–60.

65 Boiten J, Lodder J. Isolated monoparesis is usually caused by superficial infarction. *Cerebrovasc Dis* 1991; **1**:337–40.

66 Isayev Y, Castaldo J, Rae-Grant A, Barbour P. Pure monoparesis: what makes it different. *Arch Neurol* 2006; **63**(5):786.

67 Maeder-Ingvar M, van Melle G, Bogousslavsky J. Pure monoparesis: a particular stroke subgroup? *Arch Neurol* 2005; **62**(8):1221–4.

68 Foix C, Levy M. Les ramollissements sylviens: syndromes des lésions en foyer du territoire de l'artère sylvienne et de ses branches. *Revue Neurologique (Paris)* 1927; **11**:1–51.

69 Waddington MM, Ring BA. Syndromes of occlusions of middle cerebral artery branches. *Brain* 1968; **91**(4):685–96.

70 De Reuck J. The human periventricular arterial blood supply and the anatomy of cerebral infarctions. *Eur Neurol* 1971; **5**(6):321–34.

71 Tsiskaridze A, de Freitas GR, Uldry P-A, Bogousslavsky J. Acute infarcts in the white matter medullary territory of the centrum ovale. In: Donnan G, Norrving B, Bamford J, Bogousslavsky J, eds. *Subcortical Stroke*. 2nd edn. Oxford: Oxford University Press, 2002, pp. 287–96.

72 Read SJ, Pettigrew L, Schimmel L, Levi CR, Bladin CF, Chambers BR *et al*. White matter medullary infarcts:

acute subcortical infarction in the centrum ovale. *Cerebrovasc Dis* 1998; **8**(5):289–95.

73 Lee PH, Oh SH, Bang OY, Joo IS, Huh K. Pathogenesis of deep white matter medullary infarcts: a diffusion-weighted magnetic resonance imaging study. *J Neurol Neurosurg Psychiatry* 2005; **76**(12):1659–63.

74 Chaturvedi S, Lukovits TG, Chen W, Gorelick PB. Ischemia in the territory of a hypoplastic vertebrobasilar system. *Neurology* 1999; **52**(5):980–3.

75 Caplan LR, Tettenborn B. Vertebrobasilar occlusive disease. Review of selected aspects, 2: posterior circulation embolism. *Cerebrovasc Dis* 1992; **2**:320–6.

76 Crawley F, Clifton A, Brown MM. Treatable lesions demonstrated on vertebral angiography for posterior circulation ischaemic events. *Br J Radiol* 1998; **71**(852):1266–70.

77 Caplan LR, Tettenborn B. Vertebrobasilar occlusive disease. Review of selected aspects, 1: spontaneous dissection of extracranial and intracranial posterior circulation arteries. *Cerebrovasc Dis* 1992; **2**:256–65.

78 Tettenborn B, Caplan LR, Sloan MA, Estol CJ, Pessin MS, DeWitt LD *et al*. Postoperative brainstem and cerebellar infarcts. *Neurology* 1993; **43**(3 Pt 1):471–7.

79 Shin HK, Yoo KM, Chang HM, Caplan LR. Bilateral intracranial vertebral artery disease in the New England Medical Center, Posterior Circulation Registry. *Arch Neurol* 1999; **56**(11):1353–8.

80 Hennerici M, Klemm C, Rautenberg W. The subclavian steal phenomenon: a common vascular disorder with rare neurologic deficits. *Neurology* 1988; **38**(5):669–73.

81 Duncan GW, Parker SW, Fisher CM. Acute cerebellar infarction in the PICA territory. *Arch Neurol* 1975; **32**(6):364–8.

82 Amarenco P. The spectrum of cerebellar infarctions. *Neurology* 1991; **41**(7):973–9.

83 Huang CY, Yu YL. Small cerebellar strokes may mimic labyrinthine lesions. *J Neurol Neurosurg Psychiatry* 1985; **48**(3):263–5.

84 Kerber KA, Brown DL, Lisabeth LD, Smith MA, Morgenstern LB. Stroke among patients with dizziness, vertigo, and imbalance in the emergency department: a population-based study. *Stroke* 2006; **37**(10):2484–7.

85 Kase CS, Norrving B, Levine SR, Babikian VL, Chodosh EH, Wolf PA *et al*. Cerebellar infarction. Clinical and anatomic observations in 66 cases. *Stroke* 1993; **24**(1):76–83.

86 Hommel M, Besson G, Le Bas JF, Gaio JM, Pollak P, Borgel F *et al*. Prospective study of lacunar infarction using magnetic resonance imaging. *Stroke* 1990; **21**(4):546–54.

87 Fisher CM. Lacunar infarcts: a review. *Cerebrovasc Dis* 1991; **1**:311–20.

88 Caplan LR. Intracranial branch atheromatous disease: a neglected, understudied, and underused concept. *Neurology* 1989; **39**(9):1246–50.

89 Caplan LR. 'Top of the basilar' syndrome. *Neurology* 1980; **30**(1):72–9.

90 Schwartz A, Rautenberg W, Hennerici M. Dolichoectatic intracranial arteries: review of selected aspects. *Cerebrovasc Dis* 1993; **3**:273–9.

91 Ince B, Petty GW, Brown RD, Jr., Chu CP, Sicks JD, Whisnant JP. Dolichoectasia of the intracranial arteries in patients with first ischemic stroke: a population-based study. *Neurology* 1998; **50**(6):1694–8.

92 Michel P, Lobrinus A, Wintermark M, Bogousslavsky J. Basilar dolichoectasia with clot formation and subarachnoid haemorrhage. *Pract Neurol* 2005; **5**(4):240–1.

93 Baloh RW. Stroke and vertigo. *Cerebrovasc Dis* 1992; **2**:3–10.

94 Amarenco P, Hauw JJ. Cerebellar infarction in the territory of the anterior and inferior cerebellar artery: a clinicopathological study of 20 cases. *Brain* 1990; **113**(Pt 1):139–55.

95 Amarenco P, Rosengart A, DeWitt LD, Pessin MS, Caplan LR. Anterior inferior cerebellar artery territory infarcts: mechanisms and clinical features. *Arch Neurol* 1993; **50**(2):154–61.

96 Kim JS, Lopez I, DiPatre PL, Liu F, Ishiyama A, Baloh RW. Internal auditory artery infarction: clinicopathologic correlation. *Neurology* 1999; **52**(1):40–4.

97 Amarenco P, Hauw JJ. Cerebellar infarction in the territory of the superior cerebellar artery: a clinicopathologic study of 33 cases. *Neurology* 1990; **40**(9):1383–90.

98 Amarenco P, Roullet E, Goujon C, Cheron F, Hauw JJ, Bousser MG. Infarction in the anterior rostral cerebellum (the territory of the lateral branch of the superior cerebellar artery). *Neurology* 1991; **41**(2 Pt 1):253–8.

99 Struck LK, Biller J, Bruno A. Superior cerebellar artery territory infarction. *Cerebrovasc Dis* 1991; **1**:71–5.

100 Amarenco P, Levy C, Cohen A, Touboul PJ, Roullet E, Bousser MG. Causes and mechanisms of territorial and nonterritorial cerebellar infarcts in 115 consecutive patients. *Stroke* 1994; **25**(1):105–12.

101 Amarenco P. Small, deep cerebellar infarcts. In: Donnan G, Norrving B, Bamford J, Bogousslavsky J, eds. *Lacunar and Other Subcortical Infarctions*. Oxford: Oxford University Press, 1995, pp. 208–13.

102 Koroshetz WJ, Ropper AH. Artery-to-artery embolism causing stroke in the posterior circulation. *Neurology* 1987; **37**(2):292–5.

103 Caplan LR. Brain embolism, revisited. *Neurology* 1993; **43**(7):1281–7.

104 Hommel M, Besson G, Pollak P, Kahane P, Le Bas JF, Perret J. Hemiplegia in posterior cerebral artery occlusion. *Neurology* 1990; **40**(10):1496–9.

105 Hommel M, Moreaud O, Besson G, Perret J. Site of arterial occlusion in the hemiplegic posterior cerebral artery syndrome. *Neurology* 1991; **41**(4):604–5.

106 Chambers BR, Brooder RJ, Donnan GA. Proximal posterior cerebral artery occlusion simulating middle cerebral artery occlusion. *Neurology* 1991; **41**(3):385–90.

107 Pessin MS, Lathi ES, Cohen MB, Kwan ES, Hedges TR, III, Caplan LR. Clinical features and mechanism of occipital infarction. *Ann Neurol* 1987; **21**(3):290–9.

108 Fisher CM. The posterior cerebral artery syndrome. *Can J Neurol Sci* 1986; **13**(3):232–9.

109 Critchley M. Types of visual perseveration: 'paliopsia' and 'illusory visual spread'. *Brain* 1951; **74**(3):267–99.

110 Clarke S, Assal G, Bogousslavsky J, Regli F, Townsend DW, Leenders KL *et al.* Pure amnesia after unilateral left polar thalamic infarct: topographic and sequential neuropsychological and metabolic (PET) correlations. *J Neurol Neurosurg Psychiatry* 1994; **57**(1):27–34.

111 De Freitas GR, Bogousslavsky J. Thalamic infarcts. In: Donnan G, Norrving B, Bamford J, Bogousslavsky J, eds. *Subcortical Stroke*. 2nd edn. Oxford: Oxford University Press, 2002, pp. 255–86.

112 Graff-Radford NR, Damasio H, Yamada T, Eslinger PJ, Damasio AR. Nonhaemorrhagic thalamic infarction. Clinical, neuropsychological and electrophysiological findings in four anatomical groups defined by computerized tomography. *Brain* 1985; **108**(Pt 2):485–516.

113 Castaigne P, Lhermitte F, Buge A, Escourolle R, Hauw JJ, Lyon-Caen O. Paramedian thalamic and midbrain infarct: clinical and neuropathological study. *Ann Neurol* 1981; **10**(2):127–48.

114 Bogousslavsky J, Regli F, Assal G. The syndrome of unilateral tuberothalamic artery territory infarction. *Stroke* 1986; **17**(3):434–41.

115 Von Cramon DY, Hebel N, Schuri U. A contribution to the anatomical basis of thalamic amnesia. *Brain* 1985; **108**(Pt 4):993–1008.

116 Kim JS. Restricted acral sensory syndrome following minor stroke: further observation with special reference to differential severity of symptoms among individual digits. *Stroke* 1994; **25**(12):2497–502.

117 Kim JS, Lee MC. Stroke and restricted sensory syndromes. *Neuroradiology* 1994; **36**(4):258–63.

118 Sacco RL, Bello JA, Traub R, Brust JC. Selective proprioceptive loss from a thalamic lacunar stroke. *Stroke* 1987; **18**(6):1160–3.

119 Mohr JP, Kase CS, Meckler RJ, Fisher CM. Sensorimotor stroke due to thalamocapsular ischemia. *Arch Neurol* 1977; **34**(12):739–41.

120 Dejerine J, Roussy G. Le syndrome thalamique. *Revue Neurologique (Paris)* 1906; **14**:521–32.

121 Caplan LR, DeWitt LD, Pessin MS, Gorelick PB, Adelman LS. Lateral thalamic infarcts. *Arch Neurol* 1988; **45**(9):959–64.

122 Neau JP, Bogousslavsky J. The syndrome of posterior choroidal artery territory infarction. *Ann Neurol* 1996; **39**(6):779–88.

123 Chambers BR, Bladin CF. Internal watershed infarction. In: Donnan G, Norrving B, Bamford J, Bogousslavsky J, eds. *Subcortical Stroke*. 2nd edn. Oxford: Oxford University Press, 2002, pp. 241–54.

124 Moriwaki H, Matsumoto M, Hashikawa K, Oku N, Ishida M, Seike Y *et al.* Hemodynamic aspect of cerebral watershed infarction: assessment of perfusion reserve using iodine-123-iodoamphetamine SPECT. *J Nucl Med* 1997; **38**(10):1556–62.

125 WHO Task Force on Stroke and other Cerebrovascular Disorders. Recommendations on stroke prevention, diagnosis, and therapy. Report of the WHO Task Force on Stroke and other Cerebrovascular Disorders. *Stroke* 1989; **20**:1407–31.

126 Poirier J, Derouesne C. Cerebral lacunae: a proposed new classification. *Clin Neuropathol* 1984; **3**(6):266.

127 Fisher CM. The arterial lesions underlying lacunes. *Acta Neuropathol (Berl)* 1969; **12**(1):1–15.

128 Tuszynski MH, Petito CK, Levy DE. Risk factors and clinical manifestations of pathologically verified lacunar infarctions. *Stroke* 1989; **20**(8):990–9.

129 Gold G, Kovari E, Herrmann FR, Canuto A, Hof PR, Michel JP *et al.* Cognitive consequences of thalamic, basal ganglia, and deep white matter lacunes in brain aging and dementia. *Stroke* 2005; **36**(6):1184–8.

130 Van der Flier WM, van Straaten ECW, Barkhof F, Verdelho A, Madureira S, Pantoni L *et al.* Small vessel disease and general cognitive function in nondisabled elderly: the LADIS Study. *Stroke* 2005; **36**(10):2116–20.

131 Fisher CM, Curry HB. Pure motor hemiplegia of vascular origin. *Arch Neurol* 1965; **13**:30–44.

132 Fisher CM. Pure sensory stroke involving face, arm, and leg. *Neurology* 1965; **15**:76–80.

133 Fisher CM, Cole M. Homolateral ataxia and crural paresis: a vascular syndrome. *J Neurol Neurosurg Psychiatry* 1965; **28**:48–55.

134 Fisher CM. A lacunar stroke: the dysarthria-clumsy hand syndrome. *Neurology* 1967; **17**(6):614–17.

135 Bamford J. Lacunar syndromes: are they still worth diagnosing? In: Donnan G, Norrving B, Bamford J, Bogousslavsky J, eds. *Subcortical Stroke*. 2nd edn. Oxford: Oxford University Press, 2002, pp. 161–74.

136 Besson G, Hommel M, Ferret J. Historical aspects of the lacunar concept. *Cerebrovasc Dis* 1991; **1**:306–10.

137 Bamford JM, Warlow CP. Evolution and testing of the lacunar hypothesis. *Stroke* 1988; **19**(9):1074–82.

138 Arboix A, Padilla I, Massons J, Garcia-Eroles L, Comes E, Targa C. Clinical study of 222 patients with pure motor stroke. *J Neurol Neurosurg Psychiatry* 2001; **71**(2):239–42.

139 Lie C, Hirsch JG, Rossmanith C, Hennerici MG, Gass A. Clinicotopographical correlation of corticospinal tract stroke: a color-coded diffusion tensor imaging study. *Stroke* 2004; **35**(1):86–92.

140 Rascol A, Clanet M, Manelfe C, Guiraud B, Bonafe A. Pure motor hemiplegia: CT study of 30 cases. *Stroke* 1982; **13**(1):11–17.

141 Fraix V, Besson G, Hommel M, Perret J. Brachiofacial pure motor stroke. *Cerebrovasc Dis* 2001; **12**(1):34–8.

142 Paciaroni M, Caso V, Milia P, Venti M, Silvestrelli G, Palmerini F *et al.* Isolated monoparesis following stroke. *J Neurol Neurosurg Psychiatry* 2005; **76**(6):805–7.

143 Fisher CM. Lacunar strokes and infarcts: a review. *Neurology* 1982; **32**(8):871–6.

144 Fisher CM. Thalamic pure sensory stroke: a pathologic study. *Neurology* 1978; **28**(11):1141–4.

145 Arboix A, Garcia-Plata C, Garcia-Eroles L, Massons J, Comes E, Oliveres M *et al.* Clinical study of 99 patients with pure sensory stroke. *J Neurol* 2005; **252**(2):156–62.

146 Fisher CM. Ataxic hemiparesis: a pathologic study. *Arch Neurol* 1978; **35**(3):126–8.

147 Glass JD, Levey AI, Rothstein JD. The dysarthria-clumsy hand syndrome: a distinct clinical entity related to pontine infarction. *Ann Neurol* 1990; **27**(5):487–94.

148 Arboix A, Bell Y, Garcia-Eroles L, Massons J, Comes E, Balcells M *et al.* Clinical study of 35 patients with dysarthria-clumsy hand syndrome. *J Neurol Neurosurg Psychiatry* 2004; **75**(2):231–4.

149 Moulin T, Bogousslavsky J, Chopard JL, Ghika J, Crepin-Leblond T, Martin V *et al.* Vascular ataxic hemiparesis: a re-evaluation. *J Neurol Neurosurg Psychiatry* 1995; **58**(4):422–7.

150 Chamorro A, Sacco RL, Mohr JP, Foulkes MA, Kase CS, Tatemichi TK *et al.* Clinical-computed tomographic correlations of lacunar infarction in the Stroke Data Bank. *Stroke* 1991; **22**(2):175–81.

151 Groothuis DR, Duncan GW, Fisher CM. The human thalamocortical sensory path in the internal capsule: evidence from a small capsular hemorrhage causing a pure sensory stroke. *Ann Neurol* 1977; **2**(4):328–31.

152 Allen CM, Hoare RD, Fowler CJ, Harrison MJ. Clinico-anatomical correlations in uncomplicated stroke. *J Neurol Neurosurg Psychiatry* 1984; **47**(11):1251–4.

153 Kim JS, Kim HG, Chung CS. Medial medullary syndrome: report of 18 new patients and a review of the literature. *Stroke* 1995; **26**(9):1548–52.

154 Fisher CM. Capsular infarcts: the underlying vascular lesions. *Arch Neurol* 1979; **36**(2):65–73.

155 Fisher CM, Caplan LR. Basilar artery branch occlusion: a cause of pontine infarction. *Neurology* 1971; **21**(9):900–5.

156 Millikan CH. About lacunes. In: Donnan G, Norrving B, Bamford J, Bogousslavsky J, eds. *Subcortical Stroke.* 2nd edn. Oxford: Oxford University Press, 2002, pp. 153–60.

157 Ay H, Oliveira-Filho J, Buonanno FS, Ezzeddine M, Schaefer PW, Rordorf G *et al.* Diffusion-weighted imaging identifies a subset of lacunar infarction associated with embolic source. *Stroke* 1999; **30**(12):2644–50.

158 Kappelle LJ, Koudstaal PJ, van Gijn J, Ramos LM, Keunen JE. Carotid angiography in patients with lacunar infarction: a prospective study. *Stroke* 1988; **19**(9):1093–6.

159 Norrving B, Cronqvist S. Clinical and radiologic features of lacunar versus nonlacunar minor stroke. *Stroke* 1989; **20**(1):59–64.

160 Lindgren A, Roijer A, Norrving B, Wallin L, Eskilsson J, Johansson BB. Carotid artery and heart disease in subtypes of cerebral infarction. *Stroke* 1994; **25**(12):2356–62.

161 Boiten J, Luijckx GJ, Kessels F, Lodder J. Risk factors for lacunes. *Neurology* 1996; **47**(4):1109–10.

162 Boiten J, Lodder J. Risk factors for lacunar infarction. In: Donnan G, Norrving B, Bamford J, Bogousslavsky J, eds. *Subcortical Stroke.* 2nd edn. Oxford: Oxford University Press, 2002, pp. 87–98.

163 Mead GE, Lewis SC, Wardlaw JM, Dennis MS, Warlow CP. Severe ipsilateral carotid stenosis and middle cerebral artery disease in lacunar ischaemic stroke: innocent bystanders? *J Neurol* 2002; **249**(3):266–71.

164 Mead GE, Murray H, Farrell A, O'Neill PA, McCollum CN. Pilot study of carotid surgery for acute stroke. *Br J Surg* 1997; **84**(7):990–2.

165 Lammie GA. Pathology of small vessel stroke. *Br Med Bull* 2000; **56**(2):296–306.

166 Turney TM, Garraway WM, Whisnant JP. The natural history of hemispheric and brainstem infarction in Rochester, Minnesota. *Stroke* 1984; **15**(5):790–4.

167 Barnett HJM. A modern approach to posterior circulation ischemic stroke. *Arch Neurol* 2002; **59**(3):359–60.

168 Kerber KA, Brown DL, Lisabeth LD, Smith MA, Morgenstern LB. Stroke among patients with dizziness, vertigo, and imbalance in the emergency department: a population-based study. *Stroke* 2006; **37**(10):2484–7.

169 Urban PP, Wicht S, Vukurevic G, Fitzek C, Fitzek S, Stoeter P *et al.* Dysarthria in acute ischemic stroke: lesion topography, clinicoradiologic correlation, and etiology. *Neurology* 2001; **56**(8):1021–7.

170 Brandt T, Steinke W, Thie A, Pessin MS, Caplan LR. Posterior cerebral artery territory infarcts: clinical features, infarct topography, causes and outcome. Multicenter results and a review of the literature. *Cerebrovasc Dis* 2000; **10**(3):170–82.

171 Bassetti C, Bogousslavsky J, Barth A, Regli F. Isolated infarcts of the pons. *Neurology* 1996; **46**(1):165–75.

172 Glass TA, Hennessey PM, Pazdera L, Chang HM, Wityk RJ, DeWitt LD *et al.* Outcome at 30 days in the New England Medical Center Posterior Circulation Registry. *Arch Neurol* 2002; **59**(3):369–76.

173 Voetsch B, DeWitt LD, Pessin MS, Caplan LR. Basilar artery occlusive disease in the New England Medical Center Posterior Circulation Registry. *Arch Neurol* 2004; **61**(4):496–504.

174 Von Campe G, Regli F, Bogousslavsky J. Heralding manifestations of basilar artery occlusion with lethal or severe stroke. *J Neurol Neurosurg Psychiatry* 2003; **74**(12):1621–6.

175 Lindsberg PJ, Mattle HP. Therapy of basilar artery occlusion: a systematic analysis comparing intra-arterial and intravenous thrombolysis. *Stroke* 2006; **37**(3):922–8.

176 Schonewille W, Wijman C, Michel P. Treatment and clinical outcome in patients with basilar artery occlusion. *Stroke* 2006; **37**(9):2206.

177 Bamford J. *The Classification and Natural History of Acute Cerebrovascular Disease.* Manchester University of Manchester; 1986.

178 Lindgren A, Norrving B, Rudling O, Johansson BB. Comparison of clinical and neuroradiological findings in first-ever stroke: a population-based study. *Stroke* 1994; **25**(7):1371–7.

179 Anderson CS, Taylor BV, Hankey GJ, Stewart-Wynne EG, Jamrozik KD. Validation of a clinical classification for subtypes of acute cerebral infarction. *J Neurol Neurosurg Psychiatry* 1994; **57**(10):1173–9.

180 Trobe JD, Lorber ML, Schlezinger NS. Isolated homonymous hemianopia: a review of 104 cases. *Arch Ophthalmol* 1973; **89**(5):377–81.

181 Escourolle R. *Manual of Basic Neuropathology.* Philadelphia: Saunders, 1978.

182 Caplan LR, Amarenco P, Rosengart A, Lafranchise EF, Teal PA, Belkin M *et al*. Embolism from vertebral artery origin occlusive disease. *Neurology* 1992; **42**(8):1505–12.

183 Wardlaw JM, Dennis MS, Lindley RI, Sellar RJ, Warlow CP. The validity of a simple clinical classification of acute ischaemic stroke. *J Neurol* 1996; **243**(3):274–9.

184 Bamford J, Sandercock P, Dennis M, Burn J, Warlow C. Classification and natural history of clinically identifiable subtypes of cerebral infarction. *Lancet* 1991; **337**(8756):1521–6.

185 Lindley RI, Warlow CP, Wardlaw JM, Dennis MS, Slattery J, Sandercock PA. Interobserver reliability of a clinical classification of acute cerebral infarction. *Stroke* 1993; **24**(12):1801–4.

186 Toni D, Del DR, Fiorelli M, Sacchetti ML, Bastianello S, Giubilei F *et al*. Pure motor hemiparesis and sensorimotor stroke. Accuracy of very early clinical diagnosis of lacunar strokes. *Stroke* 1994; **25**(1):92–6.

187 Toni D, Fiorelli M, Gentile M, Bastianello S, Sacchetti ML, Argentino C *et al*. Progressing neurological deficit secondary to acute ischemic stroke: a study on predictability, pathogenesis, and prognosis. *Arch Neurol* 1995; **52**(7):670–5.

188 Toni D. Hyperacute diagnosis of subcortical infarction. In: Donnan G, Norrving B, Bamford J, Bogousslavsky J, eds. *Subcortical Stroke*. 2nd edn. Oxford: Oxford University Press, 2002, pp. 185–94.

189 Wlodek A, Sarzynska-Dlugosz I, Sandercock PAG, Czlonkowska A. Agreement between the clinical Oxfordshire Community Stroke Project classification and CT findings in Poland. *Eur J Neurol* 2004; **11**(2):91–6.

190 Mead GE, Wardlaw JM, Lewis SC, McDowall M, Dennis MS. Can simple clinical features be used to identify patients with severe carotid stenosis on Doppler ultrasound? *J Neurol Neurosurg Psychiatry* 1999; **66**(1):16–19.

191 Boiten J, Lodder J. Lacunar infarcts: pathogenesis and validity of the clinical syndromes. *Stroke* 1991; **22**(11):1374–8.

192 Lodder J, Bamford J, Kappelle J, Boiten J. What causes false clinical prediction of small deep infarcts? *Stroke* 1994; **25**(1):86–91.

193 Dewey H, Macdonell R, Donnan G, McNeil J, Freeman E, Thrift A *et al*. Inter-rater reliability of stroke sub-type classification by neurologists and nurses within a community-based stroke incidence study. *J Clin Neurosci* 2001; **8**(1):14–17.

194 Aerden L, Luijckx GJ, Ricci S, Hilton A, Kessels F, Lodder J. Validation of the Oxfordshire Community Stroke Project syndrome diagnosis derived from a standard symptom list in acute stroke. *J Neurol Sci* 2004; **220**(1–2):55–8.

195 Pinto AN, Melo TP, Lourenco ME, Leandro MJ, Brazio A, Carvalho L *et al*. Can a clinical classification of stroke predict complications and treatments during hospitalization? *Cerebrovasc Dis* 1998; **8**(4):204–9.

196 Bamford J, Sandercock P, Warlow C, Gray M. Why are patients with acute stroke admitted to hospital? *Br Med J (Clin Res Ed)* 1986; **292**(6532):1369–72.

197 Smith MT, Baer GD. Achievement of simple mobility milestones after stroke. *Arch Phys Med Rehabil* 1999; **80**(4):442–7.

198 Di Carlo A, Lamassa M, Baldereschi M, Pracucci G, Consoli D, Wolfe CD *et al*. Risk factors and outcome of subtypes of ischemic stroke: data from a multicenter multinational hospital-based registry. The European Community Stroke Project. *J Neurol Sci* 2006; **244**(1–2):143–50.

199 Rothwell PM, Giles MF, Flossmann E, Lovelock CE, Redgrave JN, Warlow CP *et al*. A simple score (ABCD) to identify individuals at high early risk of stroke after transient ischaemic attack. *Lancet* 2005; **366**(9479):29–36.

200 De Jong S, Lodder J, Luijckx GJ. Is cerebral angiography redundant in undetermined cause of stroke in patients below 50 years when the stroke is lacunar? *J Neurol Sci* 2004; **222**(1–2):83–5.

201 Kunitz SC, Gross CR, Heyman A, Kase CS, Mohr JP, Price TR *et al*. The pilot Stroke Data Bank: definition, design, and data. *Stroke* 1984; **15**(4):740–6.

202 Bogousslavsky J, Van Melle G, Regli F. The Lausanne Stroke Registry: analysis of 1,000 consecutive patients with first stroke. *Stroke* 1988; **19**(9):1083–92.

203 Foulkes MA, Wolf PA, Price TR, Mohr JP, Hier DB. The Stroke Data Bank: design, methods, and baseline characteristics. *Stroke* 1988; **19**(5):547–54.

204 Adams HP, Jr., Bendixen BH, Kappelle LJ, Biller J, Love BB, Gordon DL *et al*. Classification of subtype of acute ischemic stroke. Definitions for use in a multicenter clinical trial. TOAST. Trial of Org 10172 in Acute Stroke Treatment. *Stroke* 1993; **24**(1):35–41.

205 Gross CR, Shinar D, Mohr JP, Hier DB, Caplan LR, Price TR *et al*. Interobserver agreement in the diagnosis of stroke type. *Arch Neurol* 1986; **43**(9):893–8.

206 Sacco RL, Ellenberg JH, Mohr JP, Tatemichi TK, Hier DB, Price TR *et al*. Infarcts of undetermined cause: the NINCDS Stroke Data Bank. *Ann Neurol* 1989; **25**(4):382–90.

207 Gordon DL, Bendixen BH, Adams HP, Jr., Clarke W, Kappelle LJ, Woolson RF. Interphysician agreement in the diagnosis of subtypes of acute ischemic stroke: implications for clinical trials. The TOAST Investigators. *Neurology* 1993; **43**(5):1021–7.

208 Berger K, Kase CS, Buring JE. Interobserver agreement in the classification of stroke in the physicians' health study. *Stroke* 1996; **27**(2):238–42.

209 Madden KP, Karanjia PN, Adams HP, Jr., Clarke WR. Accuracy of initial stroke subtype diagnosis in the TOAST study. Trial of ORG 10172 in Acute Stroke Treatment. *Neurology* 1995; **45**(11):1975–9.

210 Fure B, Wyller TB, Thommessen B. TOAST criteria applied in acute ischemic stroke. *Acta Neurol Scand* 2005; **112**(4):254–8.

211 Kolominsky-Rabas PL, Weber M, Gefeller O, Neundoerfer B, Heuschmann PU. Epidemiology of ischemic stroke subtypes according to TOAST criteria: incidence, recurrence, and long-term survival in ischemic stroke subtypes: a population-based study. *Stroke* 2001; **32**(12):2735–40.

212 Woo D, Gebel J, Miller R, Kothari R, Brott T, Khoury J, *et al.* Incidence rates of first-ever ischemic stroke subtypes among blacks: a population-based study. *Stroke* 1999; **30**(12):2517–22.

213 Tei H, Uchiyama S, Koshimizu K, Kobayashi M, Ohara K. Correlation between symptomatic, radiological and etiological diagnosis in acute ischemic stroke. *Acta Neurol Scand* 1999; **99**(3):192–5.

214 Bamford J, Sandercock P, Jones L, Warlow C. The natural history of lacunar infarction: the Oxfordshire Community Stroke Project. *Stroke* 1987; **18**(3):545–51.

215 Melo TP, Bogousslavsky J, Van Melle G, Regli F. Pure motor stroke: a reappraisal. *Neurology* 1992; **42**(4):789–95.

216 Norrving B, Staaf G. Pure motor stroke from presumed lacunar infarct: incidence, risk factors and initial course. *Cerebrovasc Dis* 1991; **1**:203–9.

217 Gan R, Sacco RL, Kargman DE, Roberts JK, Boden-Albala B, Gu Q. Testing the validity of the lacunar hypothesis: the Northern Manhattan Stroke Study experience. *Neurology* 1997; **48**(5):1204–11.

218 Landi G, Anzalone N, Cella E, Boccardi E, Musicco M. Are sensorimotor strokes lacunar strokes? A case-control study of lacunar and non-lacunar infarcts. *J Neurol Neurosurg Psychiatry* 1991; **54**(12):1063–8.

219 Lodder J, Boiten J, Heuts-van Raak L. Sensorimotor syndrome relates to lacunar rather than to non-lacunar cerebral infarction. *J Neurol Neurosurg Psychiatry* 1992; **55**(11):1097.

220 Arboix A, Marti-Vilalta JL. Lacunar syndromes not due to lacunar infarcts. *Cerebrovasc Dis* 1992; **2**:287–92.

221 Ricci S, Celani MG, La RF, Vitali R, Duca E, Ferraguzzi R, *et al.* SEPIVAC: a community-based study of stroke incidence in Umbria, Italy. *J Neurol Neurosurg Psychiatry* 1991; **54**(8):695–8.

222 Samuelsson M, Lindell D, Norrving B. Gadolinium-enhanced magnetic resonance imaging in patients with presumed lacunar infarcts. *Cerebrovasc Dis* 1994; **4**:12–19.

223 Kappelle LJ, Ramos LM, van Gijn J. The role of computed tomography in patients with lacunar stroke in the carotid territory. *Neuroradiology* 1989; **31**(4):316–19.

224 Schonewille WJ, Tuhrim S, Singer MB, Atlas SW. Diffusion-weighted MRI in acute lacunar syndromes : a clinical-radiological correlation study. *Stroke* 1999; **30**(10):2066–9.

225 Lindgren A, Staaf G, Geijer B, Brockstedt S, Stahlberg F, Holtas S *et al.* Clinical lacunar syndromes as predictors of lacunar infarcts: a comparison of acute clinical lacunar syndromes and findingson diffusion-weighted MRI. *Acta Neurol Scand* 2000; **101**(2):128–34.

226 Lee LJ, Kidwell CS, Alger J, Starkman S, Saver JL. Impact on stroke subtype diagnosis of early diffusion-weighted magnetic resonance imaging and magnetic resonance angiography. *Stroke* 2000; **31**(5):1081–9.

227 Al-Buhairi AR, Phillips SJ, Llewellyn G, January MMS. Prediction of infarct topography using the Oxfordshire Community Stroke Project classification of stroke subtypes. *J Stroke Cerebrovasc Dis* 1998; **7**:339–43.

228 Mead GE, Lewis SC, Wardlaw JM, Dennis MS, Warlow CP. How well does the Oxfordshire community stroke project classification predict the site and size of the infarct on brain imaging? *J Neurol Neurosurg Psychiatry* 2000; **68**(5):558–62.

229 Huang CY, Woo E, Yu YL, Chan FL. When is sensorimotor stroke a lacunar syndrome? *J Neurol Neurosurg Psychiatry* 1987; **50**:720–726.

230 Van der Zwan A. *The Variability of the Major Vascular Territories of the Human Brain.* MD dissertation, 1991. Utrecht: University of Utrecht.

5 What pathological type of stroke is it, cerebral ischaemia or haemorrhage?

5.1 Introduction

Having established the clinical diagnosis of stroke (Chapter 3) and determined clinically the part of the brain and vascular territory involved (Chapter 4), the next step is to identify the pathological type of the stroke, i.e. infarct or haemorrhage, arterial or venous, any other pathology which might be presenting with a stroke-like syndrome, and other conditions found on imaging (though not associated with specific focal neurology) such as micro-haemorrhages and leukoaraiosis. These are the subjects of this chapter. Diagnosis of the pathological type of stroke is clearly important because treatment, prognosis and secondary prevention differ for ischaemic and haemorrhagic (and arterial and venous) stroke.

In practical day-to-day terms, most patients have one of the common causes of stroke: ischaemic stroke caused by the complications of atherothrombosis (section 6.3), intracranial small vessel disease (section 6.4) or embolism from the heart (section 6.5); non-traumatic intracerebral haemorrhage (ICH) (Chapter 8); or sub-arachnoid haemorrhage (SAH, Chapter 9). A minority will have an unusual underlying cause of their ICH, an

odd presentation of SAH, a tumour presenting as a 'stroke' (section 3.4.4) or an unusual cause of ischaemic stroke such as venous infarction (section 7.21). Thus, while *most* strokes seen clinically, and on imaging, are caused by something which is common, it is important not to assume that *all* strokes are. Some strokes result from unusual causes. If there is something odd about either the clinical presentation or the imaging, then it is important to look for an explanation. This point will be illustrated with examples where appropriate.

> The clinician should look at both the patient and the brain imaging (ideally with the radiologist), not just a report of the imaging, because they are in the best position to identify discrepancies between the two. This comparison may alert them to a non-stroke diagnosis, or an unusual stroke.

5.2 Frequency of different pathological types of stroke

It is important to consider the frequency of a condition when evaluating a diagnostic method. The community-based studies of stroke incidence, described later in section 17.11.1, are mentioned here as background to the clinical and imaging diagnosis of stroke type. Two systematic reviews of stroke incidence studies[1,2] found that

Stroke: practical management, 3rd edition. C. Warlow, J. van Gijn, M. Dennis, J. Wardlaw, J. Bamford, G. Hankey, P. Sandercock, G. Rinkel, P. Langhorne, C. Sudlow and P. Rothwell. Published 2008 Blackwell Publishing. ISBN 978-1-4051-2766-0.

most strokes (about 80%) were said to be caused by cerebral infarction (Fig. 5.1), about 10% by intracerebral haemorrhage (ICH), 5% by subarachnoid haemorrhage (SAH) and in 5% the cause was uncertain or a result of non-vascular causes. There was, in general, reasonable agreement between these studies.

However, another systematic review – of the imaging used in stroke incidence studies[3] – found that in none were the investigators able to perform CT or MR scanning on *all* the patients soon enough to detect small haemorrhages reliably, i.e. within about a week of stroke onset (section 5.4.1). Furthermore, the reporting of scanning (type, timing, proportions scanned, those not scanned) was poor. In studies which did provide details, the median proportion scanned was 63% at a median of 18.5 days after stroke onset. Patients most likely not to be scanned were the elderly (over 75 years), those not admitted to hospital, and those who died soon after the stroke. The point estimate of the proportion of ICH in individual studies[3] varied from 6% to 24% (mean 11%), with a 'best case scenario' of 13% (assuming that patients with 'uncertain' cause *did not* have ICH) and a 'worst case scenario' of 25% (assuming that patients with uncertain cause *did* have ICH) (Fig. 5.1). Studies published since have still not achieved 100% scanning with CT,

supplemented by MR for patients presenting late, or post mortem for those who died before scanning.[4–8] It is likely therefore that the frequency of ICH has been underestimated, particularly in those aged over 75 years and in patients with mild strokes who may not have presented to medical services until some days after the stroke.[9]

It is generally considered that ICH is more frequent in patients with severe and moderate than with mild strokes. However, failure to diagnose small ICHs may have artifactually skewed the distribution curve of ICH towards the severe end of the stroke severity spectrum. Until a community-based incidence study achieves a 100% CT scanning rate within about 5 days of stroke, or uses appropriate MR sequences sensitive to haemorrhage in patients presenting after 5 days (section 5.5.1), or achieves a 100% postmortem rate (and even that may not be sensitive enough for small infarcts), the true incidence of ICH and its relationship with stroke severity and patient age will not be known. Support for this notion comes from the *apparent* increase in the proportion of patients admitted to hospital with ICH, in parallel with the increasing use of CT.[10] The increase in ICH was particularly striking for small ICHs, i.e. patients with milder strokes who otherwise would have been assumed to have had an ischaemic stroke on clinical grounds.

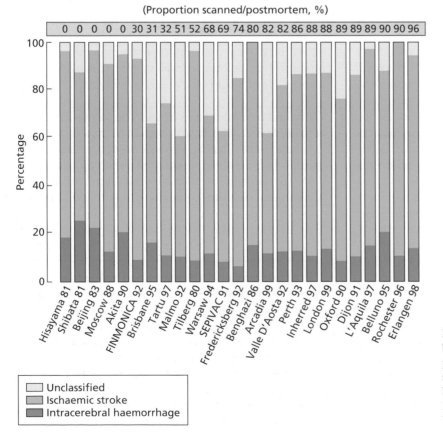

Fig. 5.1 Histogram of the cause of first stroke by pathological type ranked according to the proportion of patients who had a CT brain scan (or a postmortem) in the community-based studies (prepared by Dr Sarah Keir, Department of Clinical Neurosciences, Western General Hospital, Edinburgh, UK).

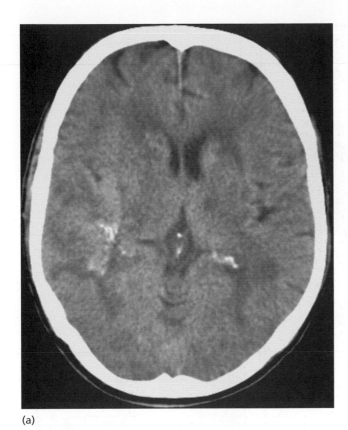

(a)

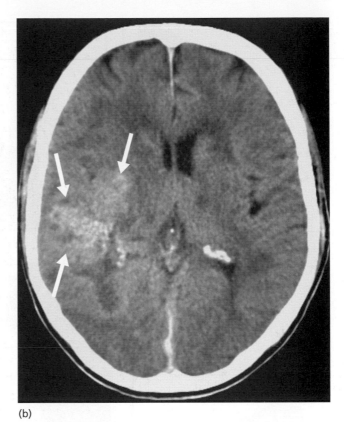

(b)

Fig. 5.2 CT brain scan (a) before and (b) after intravenous contrast from a patient who presented with a stroke (sudden-onset left hemiparesis), but whose scan shows a large enhancing (compare a with b) mixed attenuation primary brain tumour with considerable mass effect (probably a glioblastoma; *arrows*) to be the cause of the symptoms.

In both community- and hospital-based studies, a proportion of 'strokes' turn out to be caused by tumours, infections or some other non-vascular cause presenting as a 'stroke' (section 3.4). There may be clues to a non-vascular cause in that the history or examination is atypical. For example, a recent epileptic seizure, increasing headaches, stuttering onset, or previous malignant disease should all alert the clinician to possible non-vascular conditions. Fortunately, cross-sectional brain imaging can distinguish most of the structural alternatives (Fig. 5.2).

5.3 Differentiating ischaemic stroke from intracerebral haemorrhage

From a practical point of view, the first step in classification is the distinction of ischaemic stroke from intracerebral haemorrhage (ICH). This separates groups of stroke with different causes and different prospects for survival, and different medical and surgical treatments. The 'gold standard' for making the distinction is either CT or MR brain scanning, or postmortem (sections 5.4 and 5.5). There are three issues to be considered in assessing the reliability of the clinical diagnosis of stroke, namely:

- the diagnosis of stroke itself (i.e. is it a stroke or not?);
- whether the stroke is caused by an infarct or a haemorrhage;
- in ischaemic stroke, the site and size of the lesion (i.e. anterior vs posterior circulation, lacunar vs cortical, etc.), other features of the ischaemic lesion which might influence treatment decisions (e.g. 'is there salvageable tissue?'; 'is the artery still blocked or not?'), and other features of the appearance of the brain which might influence treatment decisions (e.g. presence of leukoaraiosis or microhaemorrhages).

The first and clinical aspects of the third of these have been discussed in Chapters 3 and 4, respectively, and will not be mentioned further here. The second and rest of the third are the basis for this chapter and require the use of CT or MR scanning.

However, before proceeding further, there is one key point worth emphasizing which underpins the use of

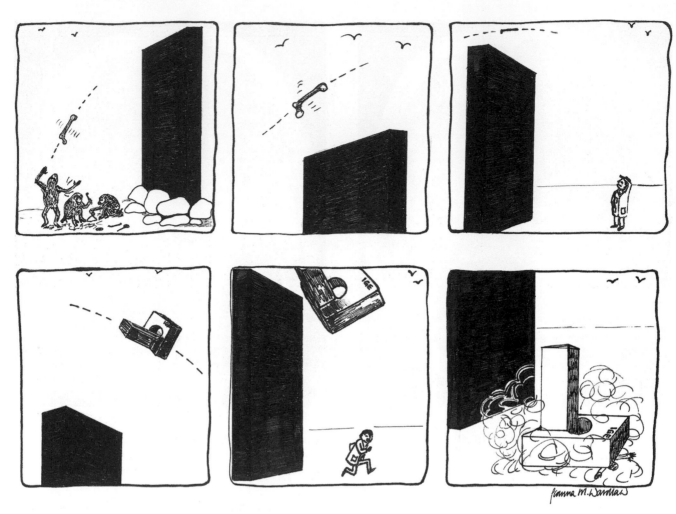

Fig. 5.3 'Beware the double-edged sword of technology.' The cartoon depicts the evolution of the use of 'tools' from the dawn of humankind (a simple bone hammer) to the present day (a CT scanner), but tools must be used with intelligence, otherwise our good intentions may backfire, a principle captured neatly in the acronym VOMIT – victim of modern imaging technology.[11] (Adapted from *2001: A Space Odyssey*, with apologies to Stanley Kubrick.)

imaging tests: it is essential for the correct conduct of the imaging investigation that the radiologist has all the relevant information, including time from symptom onset, relevant past history and current background information (such as use of anticoagulants, bleeding disorder, suspected malignancy, trauma). Otherwise the investigation may not be performed in the optimum way to obtain the information required, and misleading (or simply incorrect) reports may be issued (Fig. 5.3). Scanning can be difficult to interpret (especially with the increasingly complex MR sequences that are available), can be used in the wrong patients, or in the wrong way in the right patients and so identify coincidental and irrelevant findings or fail to identify important pathology – either scenario can lead to steps which are detrimental to the patient, waste staff time and potentially a lot of money, and turn the patient into a 'victim of modern imaging technology' ('VOMIT').[11] Technology is here to help us, not the other way round.

> For the correct conduct and interpretation of diagnostic imaging, the radiologist should receive all relevant information, especially how long ago the symptoms started, any previous strokes, the clinical features of this stroke, history of malignant disease, and any concurrent illnesses (e.g. renal failure, diabetes, infection).

Occasionally it is difficult to differentiate a tumour from an infarct or partially resolved ICH on the initial CT scan: ICHs may mimic tumours radiologically at certain phases in their evolution (section 5.4.1), and tumours may mimic infarcts (Fig. 5.4).[12] Therefore, it may be necessary to rescan the occasional patient after several

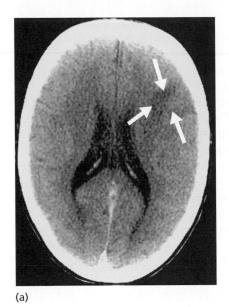
(a)

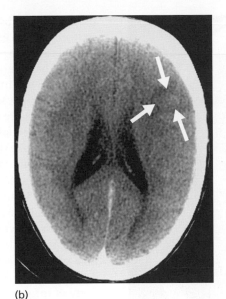
(b)

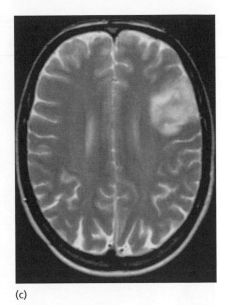
(c)

Fig. 5.4 CT brain scan of a patient with a tumour mimicking an infarct scanned within 12 h of a sudden right hemiparesis and dysphasia. (a) Non-contrast CT scan at 12 h after stroke. There is a wedge-shaped, relatively ill-defined, low-density area (*arrows*) involving grey and adjacent white matter, in a distribution consistent with a middle cerebral artery branch occlusion. (b) CT scan 6 weeks later fails to show any change in the appearance of the lesion. An infarct by this stage would have become atrophied and of the same density as cerebrospinal fluid. (c) T2-weighted MR scan 2 years later shows no change in the shape or size of the lesion, which is entirely consistent with a primary brain tumour. The patient had not received any specific treatment in the interim because her symptoms had not been troublesome.

weeks, when vascular lesions and tumours can usually be distinguished by the pattern of their evolution with time. Alternatively, an MR examination may help.

5.3.1 Clinical scoring methods

These are mentioned for historical reasons. It is important to remember that before the advent of CT scanning, attempts were made to correlate clinical findings with the pathological type of stroke at postmortem. Indeed, there are still large parts of the world where access to CT scanning is very restricted so clinical diagnosis remains important. In fatal ICH, mostly caused by very large intraparenchymal, intraventricular or subarachnoid haemorrhage, the common features were severe headache, vomiting and early reduction in the level of consciousness. When CT scanning became available, it was soon clear that many smaller ICHs were not associated with these 'typical' features. However, the several clinical scoring systems, devised specifically to differentiate ICH from infarction in the days when CT scanning was less readily available than it is now, are too unreliable: the Allen score,[13] the Siriraj score[14] and a further method.[15] Although these systems do increase clinical diagnostic accuracy, even some patients with a low probability of ICH on the basis of these scores actually have an ICH on CT: at least 7% with the Allen score and 5% with the Siriraj score.[16–19] For example, Fig. 5.5 shows a patient who had less than a 5% chance of haemorrhage according to the Siriraj score, but brain CT showed a thalamic ICH as the cause of the stroke. The proportion of ICHs misdiagnosed as infarct among patients with mild stroke may be even larger because the above results applied only to admitted patients (i.e. more likely to be moderate to severe strokes). As patients with ICH may even, very rarely, present with a transient ischaemic attack (TIA),[20–25] or recover very rapidly,[26] it is likely that the frequency of ICH as a cause of minor stroke, or even TIA, has been underestimated.[3]

> No clinical scoring method can differentiate, with absolute reliability, ischaemic stroke from intracerebral haemorrhage. To do this, brain CT (ideally within a week of stroke) or MRI is required.

Therefore CT and MR scanning are the only methods of distinguishing infarct from haemorrhage reliably, and even then only if they are used appropriately.

5.3.2 Cerebrospinal fluid examination

In the pre-CT era, cerebrospinal fluid (CSF) examination was more widely used in the diagnosis of all kinds of neurological diseases for which there are now much

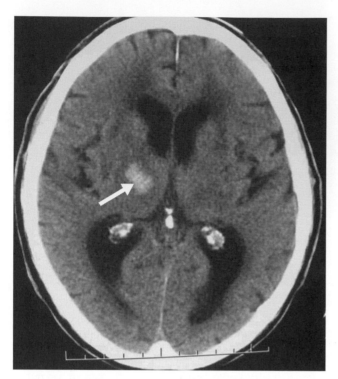

Fig. 5.5 CT brain scan of a patient presenting within 24 h of a stroke who had less than a 5% chance of having an intracerebral haemorrhage by the Siriraj score. The scan shows a primary thalamic haemorrhage (*arrow*).

better diagnostic tests. Abnormalities of the CSF cell and protein content do occur after ischaemic stroke and ICH, but they are so non-specific as to be probably even less reliable than the clinical features to make the distinction (section 6.8.11).[27] Examination of the CSF is clearly still important but only in selected patients with suspected subarachnoid haemorrhage in whom the CT scan is negative for subarachnoid blood (section 3.7.3), when the diagnosis of stroke is uncertain (e.g. could it be multiple sclerosis or encephalitis) or when an unusual cause is suspected (e.g. syphilis).

> Examination of the cerebrospinal fluid is useless and potentially hazardous to differentiate ischaemic stroke from intracerebral haemorrhage. But it still has an important role in the diagnosis of CT-negative suspected subarachnoid haemorrhage.

5.3.3 Biomarkers

Biomarkers are substances in the plasma which help to establish a diagnosis, or to determine the severity of a disease at an early stage, or to predict outcome. The term is also sometimes used for particular features seen on imaging which may have similar roles. Measuring

plasma troponin levels to diagnose acute myocardial ischaemia is an example of a plasma biomarker from the field of cardiology.

There has been a rapid increase in interest in the possibility of finding early diagnostic or prognostic biomarkers for stroke, mostly for ischaemic stroke. While initial results are interesting and promising, and indeed some commercial plasma assay kits are already available for acute stroke diagnosis, the research is still in a fairly early phase and much more information is needed before plasma biomarkers become an established part of acute stroke care. Similarly, there continues to be considerable interest in possible imaging biomarkers, such as the mismatch between magnetic resonance diffusion and perfusion imaging, or seeing a lesion in an appropriate area of brain on diffusion imaging in a patient with a TIA (section 5.5.2). However, despite a rather larger body of information being available for this and related imaging techniques, we are still some distance away from knowing what the day-to-day role of imaging biomarkers should be in routine stroke care, or even in stroke research.

Plasma biomarkers (for which the most information is presently available) that appear most promising for acute stroke diagnosis include S100-β (a glial cell protein),[28] D-Dimer (a fibrin degradation product),[29] C-reactive protein (CRP, an inflammatory marker)[30] and matrix metalloproteinase 9 (MMP-9, a proteolytic enzyme that degrades the extracellular matrix).[31] It is possible that not only might a combination of these tests allow early diagnosis of ischaemic stroke versus not stroke with confidence, but that CRP or MMP-9 levels might identify patients who are at high risk of serious haemorrhagic transformation if given thrombolysis.[32] However, the only data available to address the role of MMP-9 are from relatively small case series with non-random allocation of thrombolytic treatment. This area of knowledge is expected to change rapidly in the next few years.

5.4 CT scanning

After the earliest reports just over 30 years ago, CT scanning has revolutionized our understanding and treatment of cerebrovascular disease. The impact on acute treatment and secondary prevention has come particularly in the last 10 years. The earliest reports quickly demonstrated the value of CT for differentiating between intracerebral haemorrhage (ICH) and infarction (and other conditions, such as tumours) as the cause of acute focal neurological symptoms (Fig. 2.10). The first neuroradiologist to use CT, James Ambrose,[33] stated that 'in the overall investigation of cerebrovascular disease, computed tomography will, without doubt, come to be an invaluable means of distinguishing between haemorrhage and infarction'. There then followed reports of positive CT findings in patients with ICH and ischaemic stroke, and of density changes in the evolution of the infarcted brain tissue.[34–36] The quality of scans was poor by today's standards (Fig. 2.10): pixels were large, scan times long and processing algorithms less sophisticated, all of which limited the visualization of small infarcts and subtle changes in the early stages of larger infarcts. Other features were noted, such as mass effect in the early stages of large cerebral infarcts which could be confused with cerebral tumours. In almost half of the patients whose scan showed ICH, the clinical diagnosis had been acute ischaemic stroke and the haemorrhage would not have been diagnosed without CT,[35,36] one of the first indications of the unreliability of clinical criteria in differentiating infarct from haemorrhage.

Current routine CT brain scan technique for stroke

A standard brain CT consists of axial images through the whole brain, now usually obtained in a continuous spiral acquisition, starting at the skull base and ending at the vertex, reconstructed at 0.5 to 1-cm intervals through the cerebral hemispheres, and in thinner sections (0.25 to 0.5 cm) through the posterior fossa. This usually produces about 15–20 sequential axial images. The slices may be contiguous or overlapping, or leave gaps of a few millimetres in between, depending on the age of the scanner. A state-of-the-art mid-1980s scanner performed 10 slices through the whole brain and produced the images in about 10 min. A modern mid-2000s spiral CT scanner will produce the same set of images in about 10 s. Images can be acquired at narrower intervals to show fine detail, or in different planes of section to avoid bone artifacts, and at very fast scan speeds to reduce motion artifact (although this reduces image quality). With modern fast scanners, there is a great temptation to 'do a few extra slices', or to perform brain scans more readily, but a routine brain CT scan exposes the patient to the equivalent of 10 months of average background radiation.[37] For comparison, a chest X-ray is equivalent to about 2 days of background radiation. Pregnancy is a relative contraindication to brain CT, although it can be performed, when really necessary, with careful shielding of the abdomen.

As the purpose of CT in acute stroke is largely to differentiate haemorrhage from infarction, intravenous contrast is not usually required (see section 5.4.3 for details on CT perfusion imaging). Intravenous contrast may be given to help clarify some lesions (such as tumours from

infarcts, section 5.4.2), but generally is not used in the investigation of stroke, and may even cause diagnostic confusion. It is much better to perform a non-enhanced scan first; contrast may be given afterwards but only if necessary.

> A simple routine CT brain scan, i.e. about 20 slices through the whole brain at 0.5 to 1-cm intervals without intravenous contrast, is generally all that is required for acute stroke. This will exclude intracerebral haemorrhage, although it may not show the site of infarction.

Although CT scanning is more widely available than it once was, there are increasing pressures on imaging from all disease specialties. A few simple manoeuvres may help speed and smooth the path of the stroke patient to the CT scanner and maintain civilized relationships between clinicians and radiologists:

- Always make the request for the scan as soon as possible.
- If the patient is immobile, cannot transfer or stand, send him or her on a trolley.
- If dependent, and because most radiology department have few nurses (and the few nurses there are are increasingly tied up with interventional procedures), then send a nurse escort to look after the patient while in the scanning department.
- Good communication between clinician and radiologist helps this important relationship enormously, and so helps the patients.
- Feedback to the radiologist is always appreciated.
- A regular clinico-radiological conference (weekly or bi-weekly) is a very good way of building good communication channels and ensuring that all work together effectively to deliver best care for the patient.

> A few simple manoeuvres streamline CT access for stroke: make the request for the scan as soon as possible; if the patient is immobile, cannot transfer or stand, send him or her on a trolley; if dependent, then send a nurse escort to look after the patient while in the scanning department.

How quickly should patients with suspected stroke be (CT) scanned?

Ideally all patients with suspected stroke should be scanned as soon as they reach medical attention. Acute treatment of ischaemic stroke (whether with aspirin in the majority, or thrombolysis in a few) requires exclusion of haemorrhage and stroke mimics before starting treatment. Treatment of stroke mimics (abscess, tumour, subdural haematoma, etc.) also requires correct diagnosis. Secondary prevention of ischaemic stroke (whether with antithrombotic drugs or carotid endarterectomy) requires knowing that the stroke was ischaemic, not a haemorrhage or stroke mimic. Prevention of recurrent ICH requires knowing what caused the original ICH, and in general avoiding drugs which increase the risk of haemorrhage.

In the UK, a CT scan costs between about a sixth and a third of the cost of spending a day in an acute medical bed (depending on the type of hospital and time of day at which it was performed).[38] Patients who are independent in activities of daily living by 6 months after stroke spend on average only 14 days in hospital; patients who are dependent on others in activities of daily living spend on average 51 days in hospital; and patients who have died by 6 months spend on average 33 days in hospital.[38] These figures do not include any time spent in long-term care for those patients who do not return home after the stroke. Thus any action that improves outcome, even by a modest amount, can have a profound effect on reducing length of stay and therefore the cost of stroke. For example, for every 100 patients admitted to hospital with ischaemic stroke, aspirin might result in one or two more being independent.[39] The total number of bed-days for this group of patients without aspirin would be 3234 at a cost of about £740 586 at year 2000 UK prices; with aspirin the number of bed-days would be 3160 at a cost of about £723 640, a saving of nearly £17 000 just by improving outcome for a couple of patients. The average general hospital serving a population of about 500 000 would admit about 200 patients with ischaemic stroke per year, so it is not hard to see how rapidly the numbers add up.

Putting all this information together, and including several different strategies for prioritizing which patients might get scanned first and within what time all might be scanned, the most cost-effective strategy (most life years gained for least cost) is to 'scan all immediately'.[38,40] With all other strategies, the longer it takes to scan and the fewer scanned, the more the overall cost of stroke and the fewer benefits to the patient (Table 5.1).

5.4.1 The appearance of intracerebral haemorrhage on brain CT

Recent intracerebral haemorrhage

Acute ICH is of higher attenuation (whiteness) than normal brain parenchyma, typically about 80 Hounsfield units (HU) compared with 35 HU for normal brain (Figs 5.5 and 5.6). As far as we know, the attenuation increase occurs immediately and is thought to be caused

Table 5.1 Costs and quality adjusted life years (QALYs) for a cohort of 1000 patients aged 70–74 years, at year 2000 prices in UK £ of 12 different CT scanning strategies ranked by a combination of QALYs and least costs and compared to 'scan all patients within 48 h of stroke' (comparator).[38,40]

Strategies	Imaging strategies	QALYs	Costs (£)
S1	Scan all immediately	1982.4	9 993 676
S6	Scan patients on anticoagulants, in a life-threatening condition or who are candidates for thrombolysis immediately and scan all remaining patients within 24 h	1982.4	10 067 903
S2	Scan patients on anticoagulants or in a life-threatening condition immediately and scan all remaining patients within 24 h of admission to hospital	1982.4	10 072 294
S7	Scan patients on anticoagulants, in a life-threatening condition or who are candidates for thrombolysis immediately and scan all remaining patients within 48 h	1982.3	10 229 576
S3	Scan patients on anticoagulants or in a life-threatening condition immediately and scan all remaining patients within 48 h of admission to hospital	1982.3	10 241 793
Comparator	Scan all within 48 h of stroke	1982.3	10 279 728
S12	Do not scan anyone	1904.2	10 554 000
S11	Scan only patients with a life-threatening stroke or on anticoagulants within 7 days of admission to hospital	1899.0	10 786 817
S8	Scan patients on anticoagulants, in a life-threatening condition or who are candidates for thrombolysis immediately and scan all remaining patients within 7 days	1980.7	11 001 614
S4	Scan patients on anticoagulants or in a life-threatening condition immediately and scan all remaining patients within 7 days of admission to hospital	1980.7	11 050 666
S10	Scan only patients in atrial fibrillation, on anticoagulants or antiplatelet drugs within 7 days of admission to hospital	1944.0	11 443 623
S9	Scan patients on anticoagulants, in a life-threatening condition or who are candidates for thrombolysis immediately and scan all remaining patients within 14 days	1931.9	12 154 614
S5	Scan patients on anticoagulants or in a life-threatening condition immediately and scan all remaining patients within 14 days of admission to hospital	1931.8	12 592 666

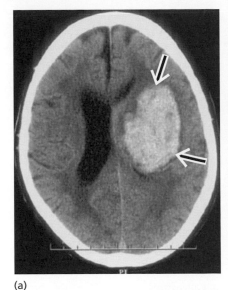
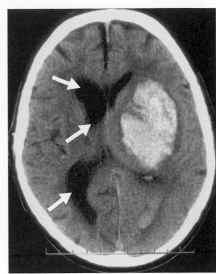

(a)   (b)

Fig. 5.6 CT brain scan showing a large left basal ganglia intracerebral haemorrhage (*open arrows*) with mass effect causing effacement of the left lateral ventricle (a) and shift of the midline structures to the right (a,b). There is also blood in the lateral ventricles (b). Note also the dilatation of the right lateral ventricle (*arrows*) (b) caused by obstruction of the foramen of Monro.

both by the haemoglobin content and the compactness of the static blood (or clot). A few reports of cerebral haemorrhage occurring while the patient was actually in the CT scanner confirm the immediacy of the change.[41,42] As soon as blood stops moving, its attenuation increases to appear 'whiter' on CT. This is true whether the blood is in the subarachnoid space, in the brain parenchyma, or in an embolus or thrombus blocking a large intracranial artery, cortical vein or venous sinus.

The area of high attenuation of a blood clot is usually well circumscribed (most often rounded or oval) and tends to be homogeneous (an exception being the appearance of a blood cell-fluid level in some large haematomas, see below). The ICH is surrounded by a variable amount of low attenuation, caused by a combination of oedema and ischaemic necrosis of compressed brain. As well as the increased density, ICHs exert mass effect, depending on their size and site, compressing and damaging adjacent structures. If they are large, supratentorial ICHs can cause herniation of the temporal lobe through the tentorial hiatus, with compression of vital brainstem structures, or of the ipsilateral parasagittal cortex under the falx, with compression of the ipsilateral – and dilatation of the contralateral – lateral ventricle (sections 11.5 and 12.1.5) (Fig. 5.6).

> Haemorrhage in the brain is visible on CT immediately. It does not take a few hours to develop its distinct appearance.

Change in appearance of intracerebral haemorrhage with time

The attenuation of the ICH decreases with time as the haemoglobin breaks down, and it can become isointense with brain and then hypoattenuated within only 5–7 days (Fig. 5.7); larger ICHs take longer to become isointense. But, even if isointense, the associated mass effect may still be evident, depending on haematoma size (Fig. 5.8). More often the ICH becomes hypoattenuated to normal brain between 1 and 3 weeks, so that, on CT it can look just like a hypoattenuated infarct (Fig. 5.8). Some ICHs at this stage have a thin hyperattenuated ring running round the rim of the lesion (Figs 5.7b, 5.11) which, if present, is a strong indication that the lesion is a resolving haemorrhage, not an infarct. We do not know how often the hyperattenuated ring remains visible, but in our experience, all of the lesions showing this feature on CT were confirmed as haematomas on MRI.

> Subacute haemorrhage is suggested on CT by the presence of a white (high attenuation) ring at the edge of the lesion.

Although large ICHs may remain visibly hyperattenuated for many weeks, small ones become hypoattenuated more quickly. To be sure of differentiating an ICH from an infarct, the CT scan should be performed as soon as possible, preferably within 1 week of onset, otherwise the small bleeds may be misinterpreted as infarcts.[9,43] This may be impossible if a patient delays seeking medical attention because their stroke was mild, and underscores the need for close liaison between clinical and radiological services to provide rapid stroke assessment facilities as soon as the patient does present. Patients who present too late for CT to differentiate small haemorrhages from infarcts may need MRI to determine the cause of the stroke (section 5.5.1). Indeed, for patients with mild stroke symptoms, there is little point in performing a CT scan after 2 weeks except to exclude

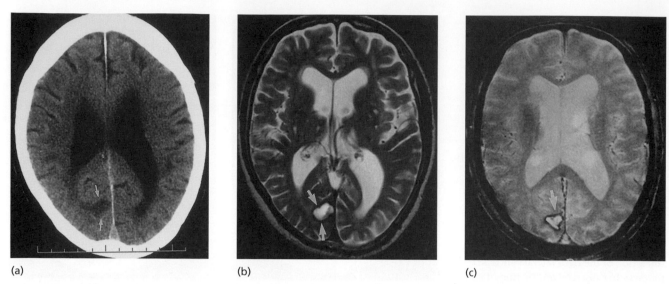

(a)   (b)   (c)

Fig. 5.7 (a) CT brain scan in an outpatient 8 days after stroke causing a left homonymous hemianopia. The arrows point to a low density in the right visual cortex which on CT looks just like a small infarct. (b) Fast spin echo T2 and (c) gradient echo T2 are the corresponding MR images obtained within 1 h of the CT, and which clearly show that the lesion (*arrows*) was in fact a haemorrhage. Note the dark haemosiderin ring around the edge of the hyperintense area.

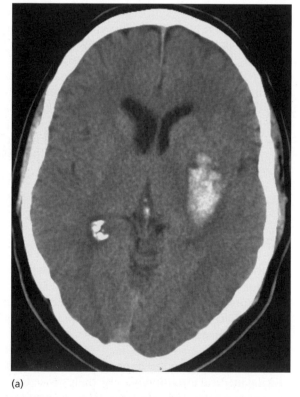

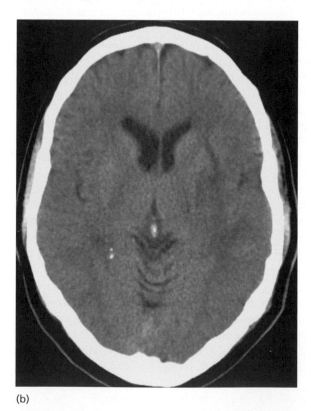

(a)   (b)

Fig. 5.8 Change in the appearance of haemorrhage on CT brain scan with time. (a) About 8 h after the stroke there is a hyperattenuated lesion (fresh blood) in the left basal ganglia (large white area). Very fresh haemorrhage is also seen in Figs 5.5 and 5.6. (b) About 3 weeks after the stroke the hyperattenuation has disappeared, leaving a hypoattenuated lesion with some persistent space-occupying effect (note slight effacement of left lateral ventricle) which could easily be mistaken for an infarct without the prior scan. The final diagnosis was intracerebral haemorrhage; CT angiography did not reveal any underlying structural cause. See Figs 5.9 and 5.10 for the appearance of 'months' old haemorrhage on CT, and Figs 5.11 and 5.12 for subacute ICH.

the rare case of tumour presenting as a stroke. Resources permitting, it is best to go straight to MR. Certainly, there is little point in performing both CT and MR. The additional problem of distinguishing intracerebral haemorrhage from haemorrhagic transformation of an infarct will be discussed in section 5.7.

> To have the maximum chance of excluding an intracerebral haemorrhage, brain CT should be performed within 1 week of the stroke, ideally within a few days, otherwise the characteristic 'whiteness' of the fresh haemorrhage will have disappeared.

Late appearance of the haematoma

After some weeks to months (depending on size), the process of ICH resorption is complete and all that may be left is a small slit-like cavity containing fluid of cerebrospinal fluid density, or there is no abnormality at all.[44–46] Small ICHs (less than 2 cm diameter) can disappear without trace.[45] Medium to large ICHs frequently leave an *ex vacuo* effect, such as enlargement of the lateral ventricle or sulci adjacent to the site of the original haemorrhage. In some patients an *ex vacuo* effect may be seen without any cavity.[44] At this late stage – in fact, at any stage beyond the time when the ICH becomes isointense – it may look identical to an old infarct.[9,43]

However, there are two features on CT which are strong indicators that an 'old vascular lesion' was probably a haemorrhage rather than an infarct: (1) the slit-like shape and (2) the thin rim of high attenuation at the edge of the lesion (Fig. 5.9), sometimes referred to as 'pseudocalcification'. The slit-like shape[45] is the result of the acute haemorrhage *pushing* the neuronal tracts apart – when the ICH resolves, the tracts collapse back towards their original position leaving a slit-like hole where the ICH was (Fig. 5.9), in contrast to an infarct which destroys most of the tracts passing through it and so leaves a more rounded hole. The thin high-attenuation (white) rim is haemosiderin or haematoidin[45] (Figs 5.9, 5.10) and is the CT equivalent of low signal on MR (section 5.5.1, Figs 5.7c, 5.33). In a small proportion of

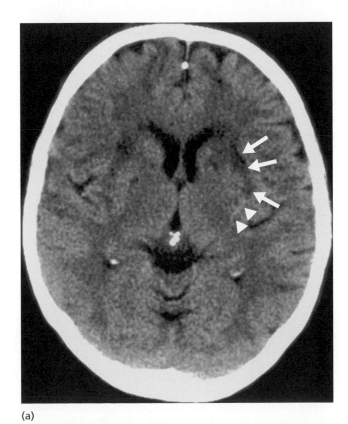

(a)

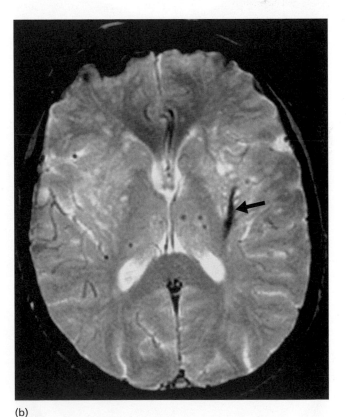

(b)

Fig. 5.9 Two examples showing the appearance of old ICH on CT. In case 1, an elderly lady with a right hemiparesis 3 months earlier, the scan (a) shows a linear slit-like low attenuation cavity in the left basal ganglia (*arrows*) with a linear high attenuation area posteriorly (*arrowheads*); the MR gradient echo image (b) shows low signal (dark line, *arrow*) in the posterior part of the lesion indicating haemosiderin (the high attenuation area on CT is the CT equivalent of haemosiderin) and that the lesion was therefore an ICH. Note in (b) that several microbleeds are also visible (black dots).

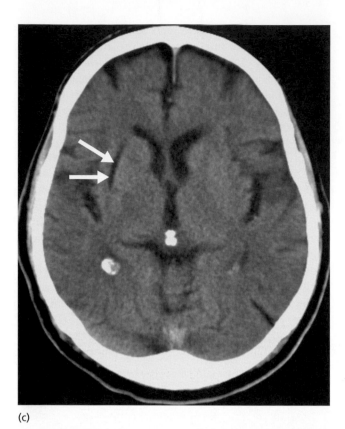

(c)

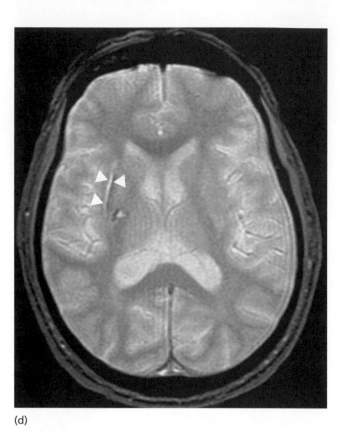

(d)

Fig. 5.9 (*continued*) In case 2, a patient with a left hemiparesis a year earlier, the CT (c) shows a low attenuation slit-like cavity in the right basal ganglia (*arrows*); the MR gradient echo image

(d) shows a low signal rim (*arrowheads*) indicating haemosiderin confirming that the lesion was an ICH.

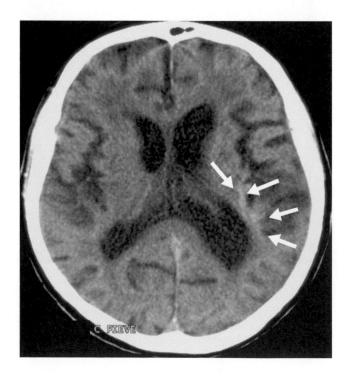

Fig. 5.10 Appearance of old haemorrhage on CT. This scan was taken 4 h after the onset of a sudden left hemiparesis. The patient had had a prior stroke (right hemiparesis) 10 years previously. Note the hyperattenuated (white) linear areas in the posterior part of the left sylvian fissure (*arrows*) and *ex vacuo* effect on the left lateral ventricle (left lateral ventricle is larger than the right). The hyperattenuated areas are haemosiderin, indicating that the prior stroke was an ICH. The new stroke lesion was in the right hemisphere (not shown on this section).

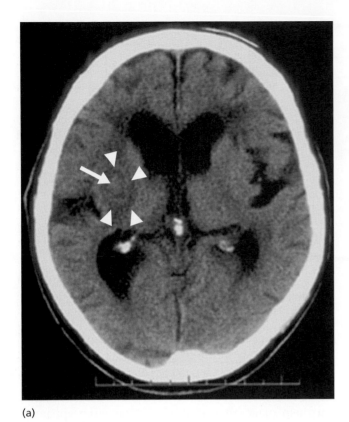

(a)

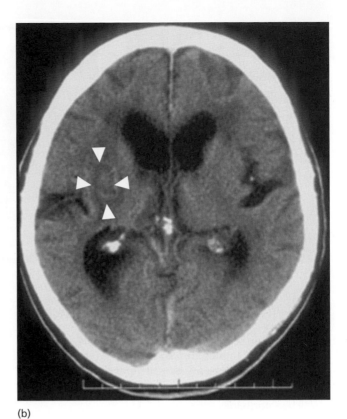

(b)

Fig. 5.11 Appearance of subacute haemorrhage on CT. This patient presented 7 days after a mild left hemiparesis. On the non-contrast CT scan at presentation (a) note the 2-cm diameter, rounded, low attenuation area (dark) in the right basal ganglia with a slightly hyperattenuated centre (white, *arrow*) and rim (white, *arrowheads*); (b) post-contrast CT scan on the same day shows only very slight enhancement of the hyperattenuated rim (*arrowheads*). This is a typical small subacute ICH.

patients, 'pseudocalcification' is the only visible evidence on late CT of previous haemorrhage. We do not know what proportion of old ICHs show this high-attenuation rim or the slit-like shape, but either of these appearances (but especially the high-attenuation rim) should be interpreted as 'old haemorrhage until proven otherwise' and an MRI obtained (section 5.5.1).

> Old haemorrhage on CT is suggested by a slit-like shape, *ex vacuo* effect or a thin high-attenuation rim. Any of these features, but especially the high-attenuation rim, should prompt the lesion to be treated as 'an old haemorrhage until proven otherwise'.

Does intravenous contrast help CT interpretation?

The use of intravenous contrast in the acute phase can complicate rather than clarify matters, although it may be necessary if an arteriovenous malformation (AVM) or a haemorrhagic metastasis is suspected. In the first few days, contrast has very little effect on the appearance of an ICH, even if an AVM is present, because the haemorrhage and its mass effect may obliterate all visible signs of abnormal vessel enhancement. Also contrast has little effect on the high-attenuation ring within the low density, if present, in subacute ICHs (Fig. 5.11). But contrast can be useful if haemorrhage into a metastasis is suspected, because it might show up small metastases elsewhere in the brain not visible on the unenhanced scan, thus establishing the diagnosis.

After about a week, enhancement at the edges of an ICH can be seen (sometimes ring enhancement), similar to the enhancement around tumours and abscesses (Fig. 5.12). Follow-up CT with contrast, preferably allowing a sufficient time delay (possibly several weeks or months depending on the size of the original ICH and the patient's individual circumstances) for any mass effect to settle, may be of value in revealing tumours or small vascular malformations (which may have been compressed by the acute ICH, so not visible initially), but MRI is more sensitive and specific (section 5.5.1).

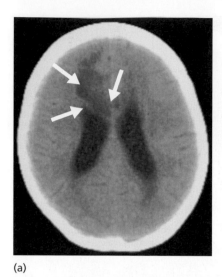
(a)

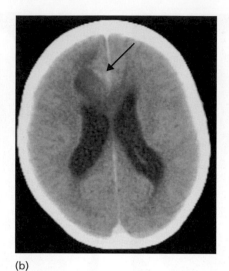
(b)

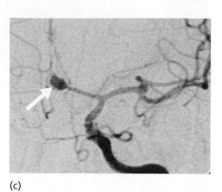
(c)

Fig. 5.12 CT brain scan of a patient who presented with a 2-week history of confusion and some headache. The scan shows a hypoattenuated mass in the right frontal lobe and corpus callosum (a, *white arrows*) with some enhancement after intravenous contrast (b, *black arrow*) interpreted as being a tumour. However, a biopsy showed only features of resolving haemorrhage and a subsequent angiogram (c) demonstrated the underlying anterior communicating artery aneurysm (*arrow*). The right frontal 'mass' was simply a 2-week-old ICH, showing how rapidly even quite sizeable ICHs can lose their 'whiteness' on CT.

Do all haemorrhages show up on CT?

Given a relatively artifact-free scan and an experienced viewer, all ICHs of sufficient volume to cause a clinically apparent stroke will be seen, assuming the CT scan was performed within the correct time frame, as discussed above. In a small series of anaemic patients, all ICHs were still readily visible despite the concern that they might not look 'white' on CT because of their reduced haemoglobin content.[47] There is just one case report of a patient whose CT scan 48 h after symptom onset appeared to show a recent infarct; the patient was given intravenous heparin, but an MR scan 3 h later showed a haemorrhage in place of the infarct.[48] This was interpreted as a 'CT-negative acute intracerebral haemorrhage' but the haemorrhage could actually have been much older than the symptoms suggested because it was in a relatively 'quiet' part of the brain, or this could have been an example of haemorrhagic transformation of the infarct (section 5.7).

A difficult area of the brain in which to see haemorrhage is in the posterior fossa, because of frequent artifacts caused by the dense surrounding bone, or patient movement. Additional thin sections at 2.5-cm slice intervals, or very rapid scan techniques available on most modern scanners, may help.

Another problem is the isodense subdural haematoma, especially if small and causing little mass effect (Fig. 5.13). Careful scrutiny of the margins of the cerebral cortex and whether they reach the inner skull or not, and are symmetrical between the two hemispheres, can help make an isodense subdural more apparent. And intravenous contrast may make the edge of the haematoma more obvious.

Viewer experience is very important. Substantial proportions of ICHs were overlooked or falsely diagnosed when CT scans of stroke patients were reviewed by doctors from different disciplines – admitting physicians only reliably detected 17%, neurologists 40% and general radiologists 52% compared with neuroradiologists.[49] Errors were to overlook some definite haemorrhages on some scans, and to mistake basal ganglia calcification (a quite frequent finding in the elderly) for haemorrhage.

Is there any underlying cause of the ICH?

The underlying cause of the haemorrhage may sometimes be inferred (traumatic, aneurysmal, vascular malformation, or into a tumour, or haemorrhagic transformation of an arterial or venous infarct) from the extent, site and distribution of blood and any associated features (section 8.9.2). Blood cell-fluid levels in an acute ICH on CT may be associated with a coagulopathy (including iatrogenic and alcohol-related), but the data for this statement are not very reliable and such levels may simply reflect the age of the ICH, because many large ICHs go through a phase where there is a fluid level.[50] Furthermore, fluid levels have been observed in ICHs associated with cerebral amyloid angiopathy.[51] Haemorrhage due to cerebral amyloid angiopathy is also

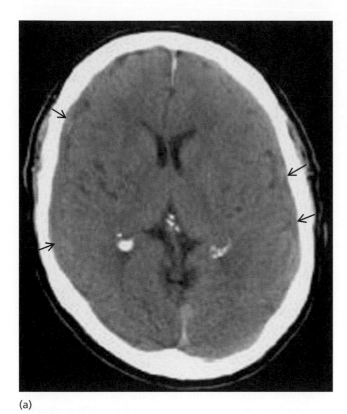

(a)

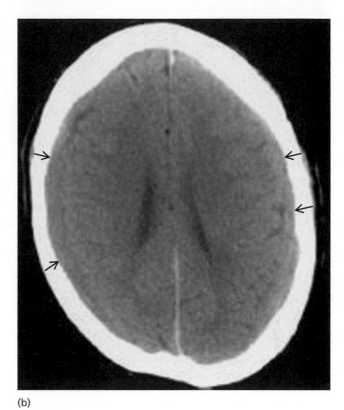

(b)

Fig. 5.13 Two adjacent slices (a,b) from a CT scan from an elderly patient who presented with a left hemiparesis starting several days previously. Note that the cortex does not extend completely to the inner skull on either side and there is a 'rind' of material between the cortex and skull (*arrows*). These are bilateral iso-attenuated subdural collections which are probably about 2 weeks old. There was no history of trauma.

associated with extension of the blood to the cortex and into the CSF, or rupture into the ventricles.

ICH due to aneurysmal rupture is discussed in greater detail in sections 9.1.1 and 9.4.1. It occurs in parts of the brain adjacent to the common sites of aneurysms, and sometimes without visible subarachnoid blood, but more often with subarachnoid blood visible in the sulci, fissures, basal cisterns or ventricles. If the patient was scanned several days after the ictus, then much of the blood may have cleared from the CSF but it is worth looking carefully for layering of small amounts of blood in the occipital horns of the lateral ventricles, and if any of the sulci and fissures are less clearly visible than they should be. Absence of visible subarachnoid blood might be because the patient was scanned late and the blood had cleared from the subarachnoid space, or because there was little leakage of blood into the subarachnoid space at the time of rupture. Typical sites of aneurysmal ICH include the inferomedial parts of the frontal lobes (anterior communicating artery aneurysm), the temporal or frontotemporal lobe (middle cerebral artery aneurysm), medial temporal lobe (internal carotid–

posterior communicating artery aneurysm), and lateral to or in the cerebellum (posterior inferior cerebellar artery aneurysm).

In patients with an underlying arteriovenous malformation (AVM) (section 8.2.4), abnormal arteries or areas of calcification close to, or in the ICH may be visible, although in the acute stage a large ICH can obliterate all signs of the underlying AVM on CT, MR and even catheter angiography. Follow-up imaging several weeks or months later (dynamic contrast CT angiography, MR angiography or catheter angiography, depending on the patient), once the ICH and its mass effect have resolved, is required to demonstrate small AVMs (section 8.9.4).

Haemorrhage into a tumour is unusual but may be the presenting feature (Fig. 5.14; section 8.5.1). Although the haemorrhage (if large) may obliterate any sign of the underlying tumour (if small), generally there is some evidence of the underlying tumour, for example more low-density areas than would be usual in an ICH of the same age without underlying tumour (Fig. 5.14). Primary brain tumours associated (occasionally) with haemorrhage include glioblastoma, oligodendroglioma,

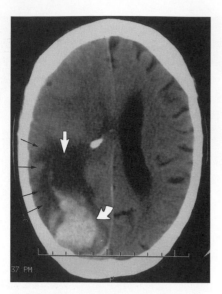

Fig. 5.14 (a) A 74-year-old lady who presented with a sudden left hemiparesis (total anterior circulation syndrome). CT scan at 12 h without contrast shows an extensive right occipitotemporal low density (*thick white arrow*) with some white matter oedema around it (*thin black arrows*) and high density of haemorrhage within it (*curved white arrow*), and much more mass effect than would be expected for a haemorrhage alone. There was little enhancement following intravenous contrast (not shown). At postmortem there was an underlying glioblastoma. Close questioning of relatives revealed that the patient had behaved increasingly oddly over the previous few months.

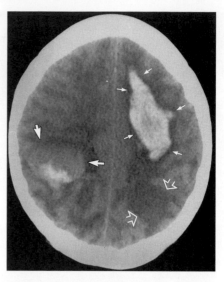

Fig. 5.15 CT brain scan showing typical features of cerebral amyloid angiopathy. There are at least three different ICHs in different parts of the brain (left frontoparietal, right parietal and left occipital lobes) all of different ages (*small arrows*, *thick arrows* and *open arrows*, respectively).

lymphoma, neuroblastoma, choroid plexus papilloma and meningioma. Secondary brain tumours presenting with haemorrhage are more frequent, although still relatively rare, and include melanoma, choriocarcinoma and thyroid, renal, lung and breast carcinoma. Multiple, mainly peripheral, or possibly recurrent haemorrhages in a patient with an appropriate past history (i.e. cancer), and with contrast enhancement, should suggest the diagnosis.

Multiple ICHs can also occur in cerebral amyloid angiopathy, intracranial venous thrombosis and after therapeutic thrombolysis. It seems that these causes of intracerebral haemorrhage are being increasingly recognized and, with more experience, more of these should be identified on imaging.

With *cerebral amyloid angiopathy* (section 8.2.2), the haemorrhage tends to be large, rather patchy and diffuse, may have a blood cell-fluid level and occurs in multiple sites, either simultaneously or sequentially (Fig. 5.15). The ICH is typically peripheral (i.e. involves the cortex), and may break through onto the surface of the brain.[51] If the ICH is large or deep in the brain, it frequently ruptures into the lateral ventricles. The amount

of amyloid deposition in the brain increases markedly between the seventh and tenth decades so the patients tend to be elderly, but pathologically proven cerebral amyloid angiopathy has been seen in patients in their 50s.

Intracranial venous thrombosis will be discussed in more detail in section 7.21. Patients can present with lesions which are mainly haemorrhagic (sections 5.8 and 8.2.10): deep bilateral haematomas occur in deep cerebral vein occlusion; cortical haematomas with a finger-like shape and surrounding low density with excessive mass effect occur in cortical vein thrombosis.[52] Both may occur with or without signs of sinus thrombosis, such as the 'hyper-attenuated sinus sign' (Fig. 5.62).

5.4.2 The appearance of ischaemic stroke on brain CT

Early CT signs of infarction

In the first decade in the development of CT, scanners had limited ability to detect infarction. Although occasionally ischaemic lesions could be seen as early as 3–6 h,[53,54] in general it was considered unusual to see signs of infarction on CT until 24–48 h after onset (indeed, some clinicians may have deliberately delayed CT scanning in order to 'see' the infarct). However, in the late 1980s and early 1990s, with improved CT technology, many subtle early signs of cerebral infarction were recognized (Fig. 5.16), namely:[55–58]

Fig. 5.16 Sequence of CT brain scans to demonstrate the evolution of the appearance of a left middle cerebral artery infarct with time. (a) At 3 h after the stroke onset there is loss of visibility of the normal basal ganglia and insular cortex (*thin arrows* indicate where the outline should be – compare with the right basal ganglia which are clearly seen) and some swelling is seen as slight compression of the frontal horn of the left lateral ventricle (*thick arrow*). (b) At 3 days after the stroke the infarct is more obviously hypoattenuated, demarcated and swollen. There is complete effacement of the left lateral ventricle (*thin arrow*) and small areas of increased density at the infarct margins suggest petechial haemorrhage (*small arrows*). The marginal petechial haemorrhage is not always seen – the infarct may simply appear uniformly hypoattenuated with very distinct sharp margins at this stage. Note that the infarct is wedge-shaped and involves cortex and adjacent white matter. (c) At 2 weeks after the stroke the swelling has subsided (the frontal horn of the lateral ventricle and the cortical sulci are clearly seen; *arrows*), the hypoattenuation has nearly gone and the lesion has similar density to normal brain as a result of the 'fogging' effect (see also Fig. 5.22). At this stage the lesion can be almost impossible to see despite being a sizeable infarct. Arrowheads indicate the margins of the infarct. (d) At 3 months the lesion is a shrunken, cerebrospinal fluid-containing hole (*thin arrows*). The surrounding normal structures show an *ex vacuo* effect; the frontal horn of the left lateral ventricle has expanded to take up space vacated by the damaged brain (*short arrow*).

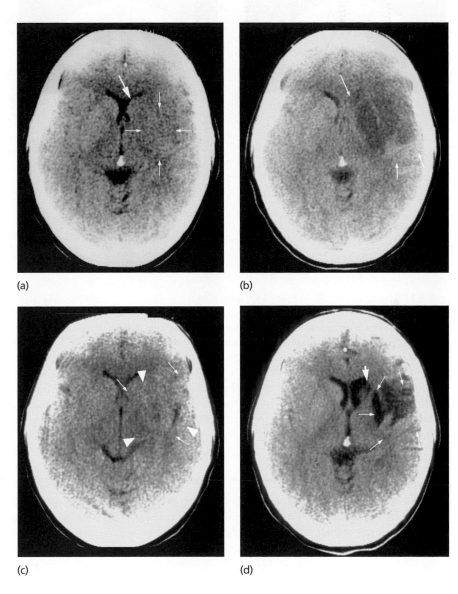

(a)   (b)   (c)   (d)

- loss of visualization of the insular ribbon;
- loss of outline of the lentiform nucleus;
- loss of normal grey–white matter differentiation (at the cortex–white matter and basal ganglia–white matter interfaces);
- effacement of the overlying cortical sulci and compression of the lateral ventricle;
- hypoattenuation, i.e. tissue of lower attenuation (darker) than the adjacent white and grey matter.

Our recent systematic review identified 17 individual early infarct signs, but most of them had not been defined by the authors.[59] Indeed, much confusion arose through use of multiple slightly different terms to describe a limited series of signs without good definitions.[59] In fact, all these multiple signs can be reduced to three basic groups: those that describe attenuation change, those that describe swelling and those that describe a hyper-attenuated artery.

ATTENUATION CHANGE

'Loss of grey–white matter definition', 'loss of basal ganglia outline' and 'loss of the insular ribbon' are all forms of hypoattenuation in which the ischaemic grey matter first becomes hypoattenuated with respect to normal grey matter and isointense with respect to normal white matter. That stage is followed by a greater degree of hypoattenuation in the infarct where the ischaemic white matter *also* becomes hypoattenuated with respect

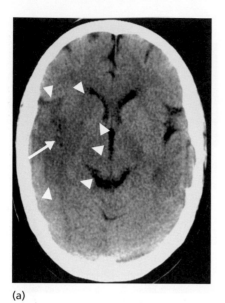

(a)

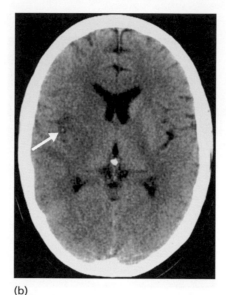

(b)

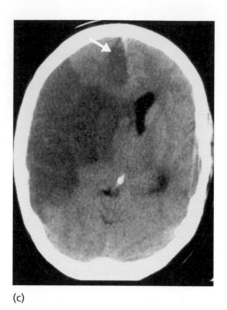

(c)

Fig. 5.17 Unenhanced CT brain scan 4 h after stroke onset (a,b). There is hypoattenuation of the right caudate and lentiform nuclei, insular and temporal cortex (*arrowheads*) and a hyperattenuated (blocked) sylvian branch of the right middle cerebral artery (MCA) (*arrow*). (c) Follow-up scan at 48 h shows an extensive, hypoattenuated, and swollen right hemisphere infarct involving most of the MCA territory and also the territory of the right anterior cerebral artery (*arrow*) (ACA). The ACA involvement is probably because of compression of the ACA by the infarct mass effect.

to normal white matter, as well as the abnormal grey matter becoming even more hypoattenuated, so that overall the whole lesion then appears darker than the surrounding brain (Fig. 5.17).

SWELLING

'Effacement of the cortical sulci' and 'effacement of the lateral ventricle' are both terms which describe swelling developing in the infarct, probably secondary to cellular oedema (but see below). Unfortunately, the terms 'hypoattenuation' and 'oedema', and 'swelling' and 'oedema', have all been used interchangeably with some confusion. To avoid confusion. it is preferable to use terms which describe what is actually seen on the scan (swelling or hypoattenuation) rather than terms which imply a particular pathological process (oedema).

Three methods for visually estimating the extent of the brain involved in the infarct have been described. Two of these, the '1/3 middle cerebral artery (MCA) sign'[60] and ASPECTS (Alberta Stroke Program Early CT Score[61]) refer only to infarcts in the MCA territory, whereas the third was developed to apply to any region in the brain.[62] Although the 1/3 MCA rule has been widely used, it was only clearly defined some time after it was originally introduced, and by a different group to those who originally described it.[63] Generally the 1/3 MCA and ASPECTS are understood to refer to density change rather than swelling, although that has never been explicitly mentioned. The third method[62] clearly distinguishes between the extent of any change in attenuation and swelling and codes these two features separately.

While hypoattenuation and swelling usually occur together, we have seen several cases where swelling occurred without hypoattenuation early after stroke, and the hypoattenuation developed later (Fig. 5.18). Studies in experimental ischaemic stroke have shown that there is a linear relationship between decreasing tissue attenuation and increasing tissue water content:[64] a 1% increase in tissue water content corresponds with a decrease of 1.8 HU. A typical early hypoattenuation is –3 HU or a 5–6% increase in tissue water content.[64] We believe that the swelling without attenuation change represents increased cerebral blood volume occurring by vasodilatation of the cerebral arterioles in response to falling cerebral blood flow (CBF)[65] before the CBF has fallen low enough to cause critical ischaemia, cell membrane failure, intracellular oedema and cell death.[66] These early infarct signs have not really been separated sufficiently in previous studies to test whether there is any prognostic relevance (however see section 5.5.4 on CT and MR in stroke).

HYPERATTENUATED ARTERY

The hyperattenuated artery sign is an early, but indirect, sign of ischaemic stroke (Figs 5.17, 5.19 and 5.20). It represents the visualization of the thrombus or embolus responsible for the acute arterial occlusion as increased attenuation (whiteness) in the artery.[67–69] It may be seen in any of the large basal intracranial arteries or their

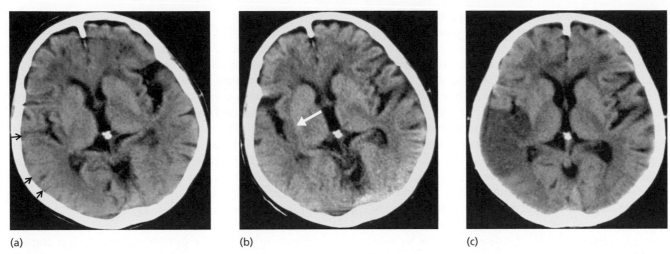

(a)

(b)

(c)

Fig. 5.18 Differential development of swelling and hypoattenuation in acute stroke. (a) CT scan of a patient at 2 h after onset of a left hemiparesis; there is swelling without any change in attenuation in the right posterior temporal cortex – note the thickened gyri (*arrows*). (b) At 5 h after onset some hypoattenuation is developing – note the cortex is now of similar attenuation to the white matter (*arrows*). (c) At 4 days after onset, there is a clearly demarcated right posterior temporoparietal infarct with swelling and hypoattenuation of both cortex and white matter.

Fig. 5.19 (a) Unenhanced CT brain scan from a patient 5 h after a sudden left hemiparesis showing a hyperattenuated middle cerebral artery branch in the right sylvian fissure (*thick arrow*). Note also the early signs of infarction (hypoattenuation) in the insular cortex and basal ganglia (*thin arrows*). (b) Unenhanced CT scan (different patient to a) of the foramen magnum showing a hyperattenuated right vertebral artery (*arrow*) in a patient with a brainstem stroke. (c) Same patient T2-weighted MR image 2 days later – increased signal and lack of flow void in the right vertebral artery (*arrow*) consistent with ongoing occlusion. (d) Same patient T2-weighted MR image of brainstem shows posterior high signal of recent infarct (*arrow*).

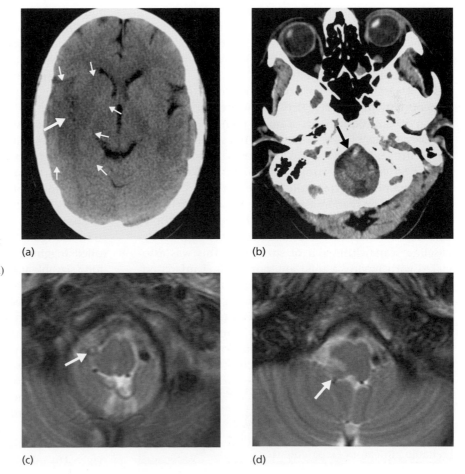

(a)

(b)

(c)

(d)

branches,[70,71] for example the MCA branches in the sylvian fissure[69] (Fig. 5.19), or the posterior cerebral[72] or basilar artery.[73] However, the reliability of this sign is uncertain. It may be a valid sign in young patients in whom the arteries tend to be less calcified, but elderly patients frequently have calcified artery walls, particularly around the carotid siphon, which can produce a similar appearance. Of course, calcification persists on rescanning, but the hyperattenuated artery sign mostly disappears in a few days.[68,71]

An absolute X-ray attenuation of > 43 HU, and a ratio of > 1.2 for the hyperattenuated MCA : normal MCA, improved identification of true hyperattenuated MCA signs[74] but needs to be confirmed in other studies.

A hyperattenuated MCA mimic has been reported in herpes simplex encephalitis, where the low attenuation of the temporal lobe adjacent to the MCA made the MCA look whiter than it actually was.[75] Increased haematocrit can also give the appearance of a hyperattenuated MCA, although usually bilateral, not unilateral.[76]

This sign was always related to occlusion of the MCA in patients who had angiography, giving a specificity of 100%.[68] But the hyperattenuated MCA sign was present in only about one-third of patients in the Prolyse in Acute Cerebral Thromboembolism (PROACT) trial on CT scanning within 6 h of stroke – as all had MCA main stem or major branch occlusion on angiography within 6 h of stroke as a trial inclusion criterion, providing a sensitivity of around 33%.[77]

The hyperattenuated artery sign is more frequent in patients with more severe strokes who are scanned early, e.g. in 50% of 36 patients scanned within 4 h of MCA territory stroke;[70] 18% of 620 patients scanned within 6 h of stroke;[78] and 41% of 620 patients scanned within 12 h of MCA territory stroke;[68] but in only 5% of a more general population of acute stroke patients.[79] In the first 500 patients randomized in the Third International Stroke Trial (IST3) of tissue plasminogen activator vs control, 41% had a hyperattenuated artery sign on the baseline scan within 6 h of stroke and this was associated with having a total anterior cerebral infarction, i.e. severe stroke. Of those with a hyperattenuated MCA sign on admission, the hyperattenuated artery was still visible on 24-h follow-up CT in 60% (personal data). Patients with the sign on baseline CT more frequently had more extensive tissue hypoattenuation and swelling, and a significantly worse ASPECTS score (5.6 vs 8.3).

> The hyperattenuated artery sign on CT is a reasonably reliable indicator of an occluded cerebral artery when the hyperattenuation is visible at a distance from the carotid siphon. An absent sign is certainly not a reliable indicator of a patent artery.

Evolution of the CT appearances of infarction

Evolution of the CT appearances of infarction is illustrated in Fig. 5.16. Initially, the lesion has ill-defined margins and slight swelling and is slightly hypoattenuated (dark) compared with normal brain. The infarct becomes more clearly demarcated and hypoattenuated during the first few days.[80,81] The swelling is usually maximal around the third to fifth days and gradually subsides during the second and third week.[82] Infarct swelling can occur very rapidly – within the first 24 h – to cause brain herniation, but generally only with large infarcts.

In general, swelling is most apparent in large infarcts but presumably also occurs in small ones, although it is difficult to see and is probably clinically less important. Extensive infarct swelling can compress adjacent normal brain and cause brain herniation (sections 11.5 and 12.1.5). It is an impression that younger patients are more prone to severe infarct swelling than older patients for a similar size of infarct, but perhaps older people – because of brain atrophy – simply have more space inside the cranial cavity to accommodate the swollen brain. The presence of recent haemorrhage in the infarct produces areas of increased density relative to both normal brain and the infarcted tissue, and further contributes to any swelling.

The amount of infarct swelling, and the rate at which it appears, varies between patients for reasons which are still not well understood. Limited data from observational studies[83] and thrombolysis trials[84] indicate that swelling is associated with large infarcts and is more severe in patients whose occluded artery fails to recanalize (spontaneously or pharmacologically) (Fig. 5.20). This notion is supported by very limited data that suggest that treatment with thrombolysis up to 6 h after stroke may reduce the risk of massive infarct oedema (Fig. 5.21).

During the second week, the infarct gradually increases in attenuation, sometimes becoming isointense and so indistinguishable from normal brain. This is the so-called 'fogging effect' and without close inspection even quite sizeable infarcts may be overlooked (Figs 5.16 and 5.22). Indeed, the 'fogging effect' may make the infarct impossible to see on CT scans performed at this time. This may lead to serious underestimation of infarct size. It does not occur in all infarcts and varies from 54% of patients scanned 10 days after onset[85] to all patients at some time examined with six consecutive CT scans within 42 days of stroke.[86] The 'fogging effect' may last up to 2 weeks and then the infarct becomes progressively more hypoattenuated (black).

Eventually, a sharply demarcated, atrophic, hypoattenuated (similar to cerebrospinal fluid) defect remains (Fig. 5.16). Although old infarcts usually have sharply

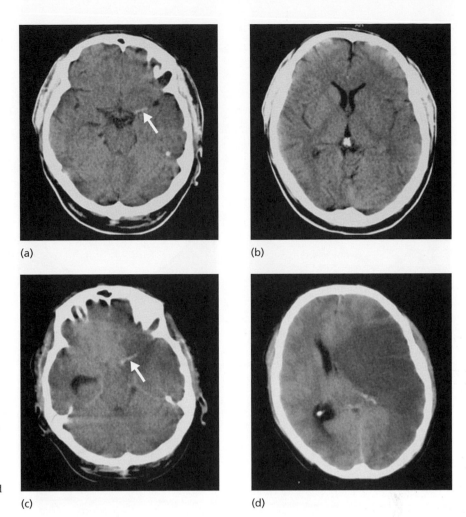

(a)

(b)

(c)

(d)

Fig. 5.20 An unenhanced CT brain scan from a patient at 4 h after sudden right hemiparesis showing (a) a hyperattenuated left middle cerebral artery (MCA) (*arrow*) and (b) early hypoattenuation of the left basal ganglia insular and temporal cortex. Twenty-four hours later, (c) the left MCA is still hyperattenuated (*arrow*) and (d) there is massive swelling of the infarct with midline shift to the right, obstruction and dilatation of the right lateral ventricle.

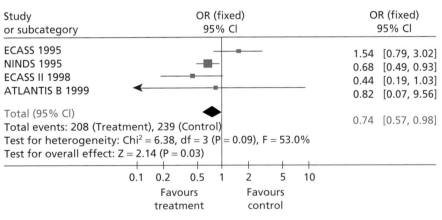

Study or subcategory	OR (fixed) 95% CI	OR (fixed) 95% CI
ECASS 1995		1.54 [0.79, 3.02]
NINDS 1995		0.68 [0.49, 0.93]
ECASS II 1998		0.44 [0.19, 1.03]
ATLANTIS B 1999		0.82 [0.07, 9.56]
Total (95% CI)		0.74 [0.57, 0.98]

Total events: 208 (Treatment), 239 (Control)
Test for heterogeneity: Chi² = 6.38, df = 3 (P = 0.09), F = 53.0%
Test for overall effect: Z = 2.14 (P = 0.03)

0.1 0.2 0.5 1 2 5 10

Favours treatment   Favours control

Fig. 5.21 Forest plot showing the limited data from the randomized controlled trials in acute ischaemic stroke of the effect of thrombolysis on major infarct swelling. The vertical line shows an odds ratio (OR) of 1.0 (no treatment effect), the horizontal lines represent the 95% confidence intervals around the point estimates of each trial, the boxes are the point estimates for each trial, their size being in proportion to the amount of information each contains, and the diamond represents the overall OR with its 95% confidence interval to the left of the vertical line of no effect, suggesting that thrombolysis reduces infarct swelling. Note the data for ATLANTIS B are only for the subgroup of patients randomized within 3 h of stroke onset (data for the whole trial are not available).

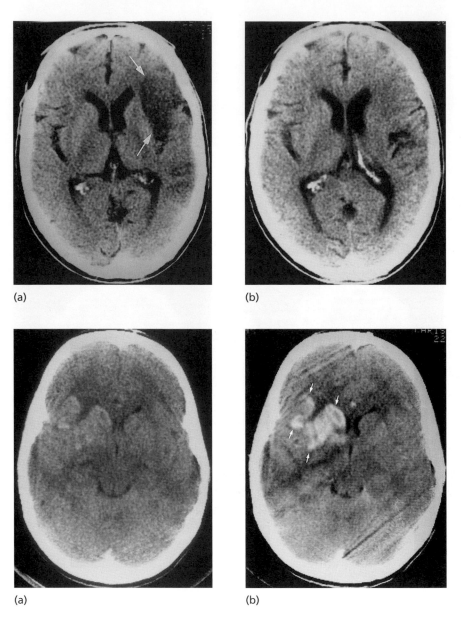

(a)

(b)

Fig. 5.22 CT brain scans to demonstrate 'fogging'. (a) Three days after onset of a right hemiparesis there is an obvious infarct (hypoattenuated area) in the left parietal cortex and adjacent white matter (*thin arrows*). (b) At 14 days after onset the recent infarct in the anterior left parietal region is almost invisible – it is now mainly iso-attenuated with normal brain and there is no mass effect – as a result of 'fogging'.

(a)

(b)

Fig. 5.23 CT brain scan (a) without and (b) with intravenous contrast at 10 days after a right basal ganglia infarct in a 10-year-old girl. There is marked serpiginous enhancement of the infarct (*arrows*) attributed to breakdown of the blood–brain barrier (sometimes also referred to previously as 'luxury perfusion').

demarcated borders, so making it possible to 'age' infarcts approximately, it is not always possible to tell with absolute certainty how old an infarct is, something that may be overlooked when ascribing particular clinical symptoms to lesions seen on CT.

> It is not always possible to tell the age of an infarct on CT, particularly in the case of small deep infarcts. Therefore, do not assume that a particular hypodense area on CT is necessarily relevant to a recent stroke – it could be old and irrelevant.

Effect of intravenous contrast

In the first week after stroke, intravenous X-ray contrast usually has little effect on the appearance of an infarct, although some enhancement of the gyri may be seen.[87,88] But, from the end of the first to the third week, more striking contrast enhancement occurs.[53,89] The likely cause is a combination of blood–brain barrier breakdown, neovascularization and impaired autoregulation, and the resulting appearance on CT was previously referred to as 'luxury perfusion' (because we seldom use contrast at this stage after stroke, this feature is rarely seen).[90] The enhancement can be very marked in children and young adults (Fig. 5.23). The tendency to enhance with contrast gradually resolves over the following few weeks.

It was suggested some years ago that stroke patients might deteriorate as a result of intravenous contrast.[91] It is certainly possible that extravasation of neurotoxic contrast agents could be harmful, but most patients described had large infarcts with a poor prognosis in any case. In recent years, contrast has been used much more frequently in patients with acute ischaemic stroke, although usually in the first few hours, for perfusion CT, CT angiography (section 5.4.3) or during catheter angiography prior to and during intra-arterial thrombolysis. However, the contrast used now is 'non-ionic' and considered to be much less toxic (including neurotoxic) than contrast agents available in the 1970s and 1980s which were 'ionic'.

Contrast extravasation into subdermal tissues at the time of intravenous injection certainly causes a nasty local tissue reaction and so contrast extravasating locally into the brain through the ischaemic arteriolar endothelium might also cause a nasty local tissue reaction and worsen outcome, but we have no information on whether this is likely to be relevant in practice. Another potential problem is that all non-ionic contrast agents so far tested significantly slow both spontaneous and thrombolysis-induced thrombus lysis,[92] prolonging the time to clot lysis threefold in a canine experimental model.[93,94] With the increasing use of CT perfusion prior to intravenous thrombolysis, and of intra-arterial thrombolysis, this delay in lysis time may increase the risk of a poor outcome (in addition to the delay to starting treatment caused by the time taken to do the extra procedure) which may inadvertently be causing more harm than good.

There is virtually no information on whether acute stroke patients given contrast (intravenously or intra-arterially) have a worse prognosis than those not given contrast. Many of these patients have severe strokes and without a randomized trial comparing patients who received contrast with those who did not (all other factors being equal) it would be difficult to detect whether contrast is harmful or not. Thus, until there is better evidence that the information provided by perfusion CT improves clinical outcome, or that intra-arterial thrombolysis is better than intravenous, the use of X-ray contrast in acute stroke should probably be avoided unless absolutely necessary.

> Intravenous contrast is rarely required to clarify the CT diagnosis in acute stroke, and should in general be avoided unless required for CT angiography or perfusion imaging. X-ray contrast agents interact with all thrombolytic drugs tested so far to significantly prolong the time to thrombus lysis, so should probably be avoided. Thus neither perfusion CT nor intra-arterial thrombolysis should be used routinely until there is good evidence to support this practice.

How often does the appropriate infarct become visible on CT?

In general, the more severe the stroke, the greater the volume of infarcted tissue, and so the more often the infarct is visible on CT scanning. Among 993 stroke patients scanned up to 99 days after stroke, 60% had a visible relevant infarct on CT within the first 24 h, rising to 70% by 72 h.[95] A greater proportion of the total anterior circulation infarction (TACI) patients had a visible infarct than those with small cortical, lacunar and posterior circulation infarcts, no matter how early or late they were scanned after the stroke. And among 13 000 patients randomized after CT scanning in the International Stroke Trial the highest proportion of patients with visible infarction was in the TACI group, the proportion increasing with time from onset to randomization in the first 48 h (Fig. 5.24).[96] Small infarcts

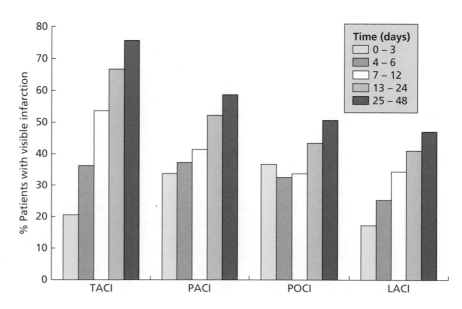

Fig. 5.24 Data from the First International Stroke Trial showing the effect of time and stroke clinical syndrome on the visibility of infarcts on CT brain scanning. The visibility of increases with time over the first 2 days from the onset of the stroke, and the larger the infarct the more often it is visible (i.e. total anterior circulation infarcts, TACIs, show up more than lacunar infarcts, LACIs, etc.). PACI, partial anterior circulation infarct; POCI, posterior circulation infarct.

appear later than large ones, because there is less tissue to alter their density. Therefore, lacunar infarcts are less likely to show up in the first 24 h and sometimes do not do so at all (Fig. 5.24).[95–100] Small infarcts in the brainstem and cerebellum are particularly difficult to visualize with CT because of artifacts arising from the petrous bones.

In any series, the proportion of patients with a visible infarct also depends on local factors, such as case mix, time to first scan, whether or not the scan is repeated, generation of CT scanner, etc. Not surprisingly, therefore, the proportion of TACI patients with a visible infarct is lower in some studies than others.[101–104]

It is uncertain just how many patients with a clinically definite stroke *never* have an appropriate infarct visible on brain CT, but the proportion is probably quite high (up to 50%) depending on the timing of the scan, the age of the scanner, the thickness of the slices, the cooperation of the patient, the size and age of the infarct, the location (e.g. the brainstem is a difficult area to visualize infarcts on CT), the vigilance of the radiologist, and possibly some pathophysiological characteristic of the lesion itself. However, the main clinical reason for performing the scan is to exclude haemorrhage (or tumour or infection) as the cause of the symptoms and, if the scan is normal, the presumptive diagnosis is of an ischaemic event if the clinical picture is compatible with a stroke. If, in a particular patient's case, it is absolutely critical to see positive evidence of an ischaemic stroke, then either the CT scan could be repeated at 3–4 days when the infarct is more likely to be visible, and certainly before 7–21 days when fogging is likely to obscure the infarct again.

> Brain CT only shows the appropriate infarct in about half of patients with an ischaemic stroke overall – those with symptoms of a more extensive stroke are more likely to have a visible relevant infarct than those with symptoms of a minor stroke. Therefore, absence of a visible infarct does not mean that the patient has not had a stroke; a patient with a clinical diagnosis of stroke, and an early CT scan which is normal, has still had an ischaemic stroke.

How well do the clinical and CT diagnosis of the site of the stroke lesion correspond?

The middle cerebral artery (MCA) territory is the most frequently affected on CT (60%), followed by the posterior cerebral artery (14%), the anterior cerebral artery (5%), the posterior fossa (5%) and the major artery territories combined or boundary zones (14%).[105] There is reasonable agreement between the stroke syndrome defined clinically using the Oxfordshire Community Stroke Project (OCSP) classification,[106] with the site of the infarct as demonstrated by cross-sectional imaging (sections 4.3.2, 4.3.3, 4.3.4 and 4.3.5). Of course, in all the studies which assessed this agreement, a proportion of the patients had 'normal' imaging – that is, the imaging did not show an appropriate recent infarct – but it is unlikely that any imaging technique, no matter how sophisticated, will ever be able to demonstrate *all* infarcts. One relatively common discrepancy between the clinical and radiological diagnosis of the ischaemic stroke subtype is that about 20% of patients thought to have a mild cortical infarct clinically actually had a recent and lacunar infarct on imaging in a relevant site, and about 15% of patients thought to have a lacunar stroke clinically actually had a small and relevant cortical infarct radiologically.[107,108] These patients behave epidemiologically more like the stroke type suggested by the imaging lesion than by the clinical syndrome, and so for them it is best to reclassify the stroke subtype from cortical to lacunar, and from lacunar to cortical on the basis of the imaging.[107]

The clinical diagnosis of lacunar stroke is particularly difficult in the first 12–24 h after onset.[109,110] This implies that about one-fifth of all lacunar or mild cortical strokes are misclassified clinically and that studies of pathogenesis, risk factors and prognosis for lacunar or mild cortical infarction have probably been 'clouded' by inadvertent inclusion of some lacunar infarcts in the mild cortical group and vice versa. Because MR diffusion-weighted imaging (DWI) is the most sensitive method of detecting infarcts underlying mild stroke syndromes (section 5.5.2), in future studies where it is necessary to distinguish lacunar from cortical ischaemic stroke this will be needed to establish the diagnosis with the best degree of reliability.[111]

In studies of stroke lesion site diagnosed clinically vs radiologically, which have used other more complex clinical classifications, the level of agreement between the clinician equipped with the traditional neurological tools of pin and tendon hammer, and the radiologist armed with a scanner, has been poorer.[112] Even the National Institute of Neurological Diseases and Stroke (NINDS) classification,[113] the Trial of ORG 10172 in Acute Stroke Therapy (TOAST) Trial classification,[114] the Stroke Data Bank classification,[115] all of which use risk-factor based classification and many investigations to apportion a cause of stroke, still find up to 40% of patients are unclassifiable. A further point to note is that classifications which use features other than simply the neurological symptoms and signs can introduce bias into studies of risk factors for stroke.[116]

Does infarct visibility on CT (early or established) have prognostic significance?

Among 3468 patients from 15 studies examining the relationship between infarct signs present on CT scanning within the first 6 h after stroke and functional clinical outcome (assessed at least 1 month or more after stroke), the presence of any early infarct sign increased the risk of poor functional outcome on univariate analyses (odds ratio for any early infarct sign 3.11, 95% CI 2.77–3.49).[59] This increased risk of poor functional outcome was present for all early infarct signs for which it was possible to extract data: any hypoattenuation vs no hypoattenuation (OR 2.73), more than 1/3 middle cerebral artery (MCA) territory affected vs less than 1/3 or normal (OR 6.44), less than 1/3 MCA vs normal CT (OR 2.66), and hyperattenuated artery vs no hyperattenuated artery (OR 2.09).[59] Studies comparing the ASPECTS CT rating score and outcome indicate that an ASPECTS score < 7 is associated with poor outcome.[61,117]

There is less information on whether thrombolysis alters the relationship between CT infarct signs and poor outcome. Two studies which sought an 'early infarct sign–thrombolysis' interaction found no evidence that thrombolysis given up to 3 h[118] or 6 h after stroke[119] in the presence of early infarct signs worsened the outcome over that due to early signs alone. The ASPECTS score applied to the PROACT II trial data showed improved functional outcome for those treated with thrombolysis compared with control in patients with ASPECTS > 7 (OR 5) but not in those with ASPECTS of 7 or less (OR 1).[120] When ASPECTS was applied to the NINDS, ECASS 2 and ATLANTIS B trials, there was also no association between an ASPECT score < 7 and worse outcome with thrombolysis,[121–123] although ECASS 2 patients with a low ASPECTS were at increased risk of haemorrhagic transformation after thrombolysis.[123]

Early infarct signs are subtle. They are therefore difficult to recognize and may have poor inter-observer reliability[59] (see below). Also CT technology has improved since the thrombolysis trials from which these data came (in the first half of the 1990s). Therefore, further data from current trials (e.g. the Third International Stroke Trial, www.ist3.com) are needed to determine whether thrombolysis does or does not modify the early infarct sign–poor prognosis relationship, and if so whether the treatment effect is different in patients with increasingly obvious early infarct signs.

> At present there is no evidence that patients with early CT signs of ischaemia are at increased risk of poor outcome if given thrombolysis.

Established visible infarction on CT has a clearer adverse independent relationship with prognosis than early infarct signs, it is easier to recognize, and there are more studies with larger sample sizes so the data are likely to be more robust[95,96] (note the the odds ratios for early infarct signs are mostly from univariate analyses which may be why they appear larger than those for established infarct signs). In the International Stroke Trial (IST), visible infarction on the CT scan within 48 h of the stroke onset was independently associated with increased death within 14 days (odds ratio (OR) 1.17), and of death or dependency at 6 months (OR 1.42), an absolute increase of 13%, or 130 per 1000 more dead or dependent patients with visible infarction than without it.[96] In our hospital stroke registry study, of 993 patients scanned mostly within the first week of stroke, the presence of a visible infarct was associated with an increased risk of poor functional outcome (OR 2.5; 95% CI 1.9–3.3) and death (OR 4.5; 95% CI 2.7–7.5) at 6 months, even after adjusting for time from stroke to scan, and important clinical prognostic variables.[95] Others have also found that established visible infarction conferred an adverse prognosis.[124–126] Therefore, it seems that a visible established infarct indicates a profound depth of ischaemia, which reflects a marked drop in blood flow to a largish area of brain, which suggests that the outcome will be poor.

> Visible infarction on CT, whether within the first 6 h or several days after the stroke, is independently associated with a poor functional outcome compared with no visible infarction. For patients scanned within the first 6 h, there is as yet no definite evidence that thrombolysis of those with early visible infarct signs either worsens their prognosis or is a clear contraindication to treatment.

Inter-observer reliability in the analysis of CT scans of stroke patients very early after the stroke, and in established infarction

Our systematic review of the inter-observer reliability of early infarct signs on CT scans up to 6 h after stroke (complete up to mid-2003) found 15 studies in which a median of 30 CT scans were rated by six observers.[59] Few studies gave any information on the demographics of the patients from whom the scans came. Between one and five early CT signs were analysed including: hypoattenuation, swelling, hyperattenuated middle cerebral artery sign, loss of grey and white matter definition, loss of basal ganglia outline, loss of the insular ribbon, infarction of more or less than one-third of the middle cerebral artery (MCA) territory, and cortical sulcal effacement. The reference standard was mostly a neuroradiologist with access to a follow-up CT scan. In the 15 studies, the mean prevalence of any early infarct sign was 61%. For *any* early CT sign, the inter-observer agreement ranged from 0.14 to 0.78 (kappa). The mean sensitivity and specificity (and range) for infarct sign detection were 66% (20–87%) and 87% (56–100%) respectively. Inter-observer agreement was worst for hypoattenuation and best for the hyperattenuated artery sign. The one study of inter-observer reliability of the ASPECTS scoring system available at the time of the study, which suggested very good inter-rater reliability of the scoring system, has since been replicated in other datasets with similar results.[127] The information, where given, suggested that experience improved detection, but knowledge of symptoms did not.[59] These rather limited data suggest that some early infarct signs are detected better than others (e.g. mass effect better than hypoattenuation) so there may be ways in which the inter-observer reliability for early infarct signs could be improved by focusing the observer's attention on specific features. Finding out specifically what makes more experienced observers more reliable would also help.

Our ACCESS Study (Acute Cerebral CT Scanning for Stroke, www.neuroimage.co.uk) was a very large inter-observer reliability study of early infarct signs on CT to see whether some signs were more reliably detected than others, whether scoring systems improved inter-rater reliability, whether 'distracters' on the scan (e.g. old infarcts) affected relability, and whether observer experience had any effect. We used a novel web-based method of showing digital scans to observers, recording some basic demographic information about the observers, and then their interpretation of each scan on a structured questionnaire via the same web page. The results to date, on 207 raters from 36 countries who read all 63 scans, and taking neuroradiologists as the reference standard, indicate that:

- hypoattenuation and swelling are recognized to an equal degree;
- hyperattenuated arteries are seen better than parenchymal hypoattenuation or swelling;
- any scoring system (whether 1/3 MCA,[63] ASPECTS[61] or our own method[62]) improves inter-rater reliability;
- distracters (e.g. old infarcts) worsen inter-rater reliability, particularly among less-experienced individuals.

> On CT scans up to 6 h after stroke, signs of hypoattenuation and swelling are detected equally reliably, using any scoring system helps improve inter-rater reliability for detection of early infarct signs, and any distracter (e.g. old infarcts, leukoaraiosis and atrophy) reduces early infarct detection.

The emphasis on detecting subtle early signs of ischaemia may have deflected attention away from looking for other important causes of the stroke which themselves may have only subtle CT signs. Worryingly, in a study of observer reliability of early infarct and haemorrhage detection on CT, only 17% of admitting physicians and 40% of neurologists were able to recognize intracranial haemorrhage with complete reliability.[49]

In *established* infarction, high levels of agreement (substantial to perfect) have been demonstrated.[128,129] However, where observers had free access to relevant clinical details, their interpretation of the scans may have been biased,[129] although there is little information about what effect this has on scan interpretation. When neurologists and radiologists reviewed the same two CT brain scans from patients with a lacunar stroke (camouflaged by an assortment of other scans), accompanied by misleading clinical information, the diagnosis of lacunar infarction did not appear to be biased by informing the observer that the patient was thought clinically to have had a stroke.[100] This lack of bias, even with knowledge of the clinical details, may have been because the study was small and may not have been a true reflection of the difficulties encountered in routine practice when faced with a CT scan showing multiple 'holes in the brain' and generalized atrophy. The former makes the diagnosis of recent lacunar infarction difficult, because it is impossible to decide which 'hole' is the relevant one unless serial scans show a new 'hole' developing, and the latter makes the diagnosis of a small cortical infarct difficult (when is a large sulcus actually an infarct?). In established infarction, the agreement as to the site of infarction, the amount of swelling, and haemorrhagic transformation was excellent between experienced neuroradiologists and good between trainee radiologists when using a simple stroke CT classification system.[62]

Online training in CT intepretation

As, in the interests of speed, most stroke CT scans in the very acute phase are likely to be read by the admitting neurologist or stroke physician (who are both probably less experienced than a dedicated neuroradiologist), methods of improving interpretation of CT scans from patients presenting with acute stroke are required. At the time of writing, there are two sources of scan examples for trainees available over the web, and more in development. At www.neuroimage.co.uk the reader can register to read CT scans from acute stroke patients over the web in their own time, and then obtain feedback comparing their performance with experts and observers from other specialties, as well as seeing what the follow-up scan showed. At www.ist3.com click on 'see BASP CT Training Series' for a demonstration of a variety of conditions presenting as acute stroke.

Appearances of the infarct: can we infer anything about its cause?

A typical established large artery infarct is wedge-shaped, of decreased attenuation compared with normal brain, sharply demarcated, and occupies a recognizable vascular territory (Fig. 6.20c).[105,130] It is usually due to embolism from a proximal arterial source or the heart.

Lacunar infarcts, thought to arise from occlusion of a single perforating artery (section 6.4), are arbitrarily less than 1.5 or 2 cm in diameter (section 4.3.2), usually rounded in shape, and sited in the deep white matter, basal ganglia and pons (Fig. 6.20d).[97,98]

Boundary zone infarcts lie in areas of brain at the edge of the large artery vascular territories, i.e. in the parieto-occipital region for the middle–posterior cerebral arteries and over the vertex for the anterior–middle cerebral arteries boundary zone, or in the internal boundary zone in the centrum semiovale at the junction of the deep and superficial arterial supply areas (section 4.2.4).[130–132] However, the boundary zone areas are potentially quite extensive, and vary between and within individuals (section 4.2.4 and Fig. 6.21),[133] so that in any one individual patient it can be very difficult to decide on the basis of brain imaging whether an infarct has arisen from occlusion of a cortical branch of the middle cerebral artery (MCA), which might be embolic, or from poor perfusion in the boundary zone as a result of established internal carotid artery occlusion (section 6.7.5).[132,134]

Striatocapsular infarcts are larger than lacunes and occur in the deep white matter and basal ganglia, with preservation of the overlying cortex (section 4.2.2). They are thought to arise from transient occlusion of the MCA mainstem, prolonged occlusion of the MCA mainstem with good cortical collaterals, or occlusion of multiple lenticulostriate artery origins from atheroma of the MCA.[135–137] This pattern is illustrated in Fig. 6.20e.

In our hospital-based stroke registry, we attempted to assign a cause of stroke in all patients admitted during one sample year.[138] Among 479 patients, those with large cortical infarcts had the greatest proportion of arterial (59%) or cardiac (29%) embolic sources, or both (15%), followed by small cortical infarcts (45%, 18% and 5%, respectively); lacunar infarcts (33%, 8% and 4%, respectively); and posterior circulation infarcts (32%, 9% and 4%, respectively) (Fig. 5.25). Thus, while patients with a cardiac source of embolism are at greater risk of having

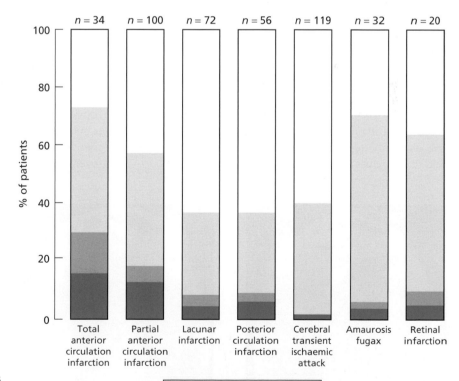

Fig. 5.25 The frequency of various sources of emboli in patients with different ischaemic stroke subtypes, ocular and hemispheric transient ischaemic attacks (prepared by Dr Stephanie Lewis, Edinburgh).[138]

a large cortical than any other type of infarct (if they have a stroke), 74% of the patients who *do* have a large cortical infarct have an arterial source of embolism. Patients with several recent infarcts in more than one vascular territory are more likely to have a proximal embolic source (e.g. myocardial mural thrombus, aortic atheroma), but in other circumstances, the use of a complex classification or multiple imaging modalities does not solve the problem of deciding what caused the stroke in patients with more than one possible cause.

> It is not valid to assume that a particular size, shape and position of an infarct on imaging was definitely caused by a particular embolic source or *in situ* thrombosis (and of course finding a potential source of embolism does not necessarily mean that it was the cause of the stroke). In up to 15% of patients (probably a greater proportion the harder one looks) there is more than one potential cause of the stroke.

As indicated above, about one-fifth of patients presenting with a cortical stroke syndrome (i.e. partial anterior circulation infarction) are found on brain imaging to have a recent lacunar infarct in the correct hemisphere without any sign of the expected cortical infarct. Equally, between one-sixth and one-fifth of patients with a lacunar infarct syndrome may have a recent cortical infarct on brain imaging with no hint of any subcortical lesion. This suggests that the syndrome (and so anatomical location of the brain lesion) attributed to an ischaemic stroke following clinical examination could and indeed should be modified by the position of any recent, and likely to be relevant, infarct on brain imaging, as this better reflects the underlying vascular lesion and so improves management and resource use.

> The anatomical location attributed to an ischaemic stroke following clinical examination may need to be modified if brain imaging shows a recent and probably relevant infarct in a different territory to that expected clinically. For example, a patient with a clinical lacunar syndrome, but whose CT scan shows a recent cortical infarct in the relevant hemisphere, should be regarded as being similar to a patient with a cortical syndrome (i.e. at high risk of early recurrent stroke, high probability of ipsilateral carotid stenosis or cardiac source of embolism).

Distinction of arterial infarcts from other conditions on CT

While many infarcts as a result of arterial occlusion are easy to diagnose on imaging from their site, shape, density and appropriate clinical features, other lesions occasionally produce very similar appearances, which can be confusing.

Viral encephalitis, if relatively focal in distribution, can appear exactly like an infarct, although this is rare. The typical appearance of herpes simplex encephalitis with involvement of the medial temporal lobes should not cause confusion, but we have seen patients with low-density areas in the temporoparietal region associated with rising viral titres, which resolved following treatment with aciclovir (Fig. 5.26). Encephalitis can also give the impression of a hyperattenuated middle cerebral artery,[75] possibly because the hypoattenuated temporal cortex (due to encephalitis) makes the adjacent middle cerebral artery look more hyperattenuated than it really is. As ever, it is vital that the imaging is reviewed with all the clinical information and, if there is any doubt (e.g. fever, subacute onset), other diagnostic tests must be

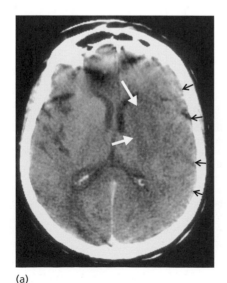

(a)

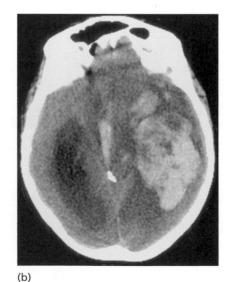

(b)

Fig. 5.26 Unenhanced CT brain scan (a) in a 70-year-old woman with a right hemiparesis, confusion and drowsiness for 6 h, showing an extensive area of low attenuation in the left temporoparietal region including the basal ganglia. There is loss of the outline of the normal basal ganglia (*thick arrows*) and loss of the overlying cortical sulci indicating slight swelling (compare with the easily seen right parietal sulci; *thin arrows*). The initial clinical diagnosis was of a stroke (infarct), but 1 week later (b) the patient deteriorated and the CT scan showed extensive haemorrhage in the left temporoparietal region. Subsequent postmortem confirmed the diagnosis of herpes simplex encephalitis.

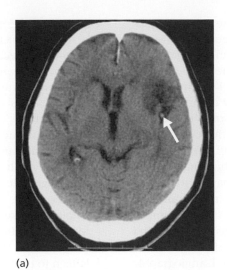

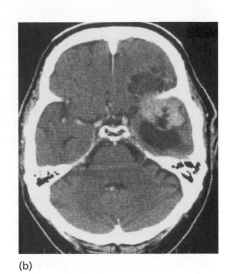

(a) (b)

Fig. 5.27 CT brain scan showing a tumour which initially looked like an infarct in a 60-year-old man who had presented with 'a stroke'. (a) The unenhanced scan shows a left temporal low attenuation area (the 'infarct') with a high attenuation dot in the sylvian fissure (the 'hyperattenuated artery'; *arrow*). This was misinterpreted as an acute left middle cerebral artery infarct. (b) Several weeks later a CT scan with intravenous contrast shows that the lesion had grown, with enhancement, consistent with a tumour. It was a secondary deposit from a colon primary.

carried out, including an electroencephalogram, MR scan and cerebrospinal fluid examination.

Purulent cerebritis can look like an infarct, although the lesion is usually not wedge-shaped, it involves more white matter than cortex, and the clinical picture should allow the distinction to be made.

Tumours: Occasionally, a peripheral metastasis with a large amount of white matter oedema can mimic an infarct on CT, although the density is usually lower than expected for an infarct, and administration of contrast may show up a cortical nodule (Fig. 5.27). If there is still doubt, either a repeat CT a few weeks later (because infarcts and tumours evolve differently, Fig. 5.4) or an MR examination (pinpoint metastases or a central tumour nodule may be detected) will usually determine the cause of the abnormality.

Venous infarction is not uncommonly mistaken for an arterial infarct. The difference between them is discussed in section 5.8.

> Time is a useful diagnostic tool, 'a chronogram'. If in doubt whether a lesion is a tumour or infarct on CT, repeat the scan in a few weeks. Infarcts get smaller (usually) due to *ex vacuo* effect, whereas tumours stay the same or get bigger.

5.4.3 CT perfusion imaging and CT angiography

Cerebral perfusion imaging with CT is a technique which has come to prominence in the last few years as the technology has improved, enabling rapid 'cine' scanning. At the time of writing, spiral and multislice scanners were able to provide sufficiently rapid data acquisition at four slices in the brain to enable the data to be processed to produce cerebral blood flow, cerebral blood volume and mean transit time maps.[139] This technique requires an intravenous bolus of about 50 mL of iodinated contrast

by pump injector and so exposes the patient to the lysis-retarding effects of the contrast agent described in section 5.4.2. The raw data then need to be processed, sometimes on a separate workstation, to produce the actual perfusion maps. This may take several minutes.

CT perfusion imaging is relatively more accessible than MR perfusion imaging, and can be performed during the same examination as the plain CT brain scan. Hence it provides limited data on cerebral perfusion to many who do not have access to MR perfusion imaging or other techniques.[139,140]

There is considerable interest in whether any lesion seen on the different forms of CT perfusion imaging indicates 'tissue at risk of infarction' and so helps guide thrombolytic treatment. However, so far, relatively few observational case series of patients undergoing CT perfusion have been published. All suggest that CT perfusion may improve outcome prediction over plain CT alone,[141] identify penumbral tissue[142,143] or thresholds of tissue viability,[144] but all used very early time points to assess 'final infarct extent' (2–7 days) and included a mixture of some thrombolysis-treated and some not thrombolysis treated patients. Larger studies[141–143] suggest that relative mean transit time (rMTT) maps predict final infarct extent in the absence of recanalization and that cerebral blood volume maps predict final infarct extent if there is early recanalization (i.e. *infarct core*),[143] although a combination of CBF and CBV may have highest sensitivity and specificity for predicting infarct core.[142] These results are preliminary and have yet to be tested in a prospective trial where patients are randomly allocated to thrombolysis vs control. Thus, more work is required to determine whether or not CT perfusion identifies a subset of patients who are more likely to benefit from thrombolysis than can be identified from plain CT alone, and if so which perfusion lesion is the best predictor, or whether the additional time taken to perform the CT perfusion and the thrombolysis-retarding properties of CT contrast agents negate the beneficial effects of the additional information gained.

CT angiography (CTA) has also become more practical and accurate with improvements in CT technology. It requires rapid scanning with a spiral or multislice scanner through the skull base and circle of Willis during an intravenous injection of about 50 mL of iodinated contrast, followed by reconstruction of the data into axial, coronal, sagittal or 3D 'angiographic' images of the arteries. This technique can identify major intracranial and branch artery occlusions, and so might improve selection of patients for thrombolysis if, for example, only patients with a visible arterial occlusion were found to benefit.[145] However, as with CT perfusion, it takes extra time to acquire and process the CT angiographic images, the contrast agent may delay thrombolysis, and it is unclear whether the additional information really does improve patient selection because there have been no randomized studies of thrombolysis vs control based on CTA. Indeed, the available evidence (*n* = 151 patients) suggests that CTA probably does not improve outcome prediction beyond that of clinical stroke severity alone and therefore may not aid decision making about thrombolysis treatment either.[146] It is useful to note that the NIHSS stroke severity score is closely related to the probability of having an arterial occlusion on angiography within the first 6 h of stroke – patients with proximal intracranial arterial occlusion have worse NIHSS scores.[147] Therefore, if it turns out that only patients with a large intracranial artery occlusion should be treated with thrombolysis, it may make sense to use the NIHSS score within 6 h of stroke as a surrogate for angiography-detected intracranial arterial occlusion. This would enable faster treatment delivery, avoid the cost of angiography (whether MRA, CTA or catheter) and the risk of catheter angiography, and minimize exposure to X-ray contrast agents. Until further reliable data are available, CTA is a useful diagnostic tool in occasional patients (but not for routine stroke investigation) but further research is needed to sort out its clinical application.

5.5 Magnetic resonance imaging

Historical note and practical points regarding use of MR

Magnetic resonance imaging (MRI) was first used as a clinical tool in the early 1980s. The equipment is more expensive than for CT scanning, both to purchase and to run, and MR was initially little used in acute stroke. It is not a practical technique for many acutely ill patients for the following reasons.

- The patient must be placed inside a tube-like structure, which creates difficulties for being able to see and communicate with the patient, and for access for monitoring and administration of anaesthetics.
- The patient must lie still, usually for at least 5 min at a time, although recent fast-scanning techniques mean that diagnostic images may be acquired in seconds.
- Because of the need to perform several sequences, the whole scan takes longer than a CT brain scan (i.e. longer to obtain a diagnosis), even with ultrafast scanners which are now becoming available.[148]
- Fifteen to twenty per cent of patients with *acute* stroke may not be suitable for MR on medical grounds because they are too ill, vomiting or unable to protect their airway, or because of a contraindication to MRI.[149–151]
- Many stroke patients are confused, restless and frightened by the noise and vibration of the scanner, and so move during the scan, which impairs the images.
- It is inadvisable for patients who cannot protect their airway to be placed supine for *any* length of time after stroke,[152] regardless of the value of the information so obtained.
- About 20% of patients with *acute* stroke become hypoxic while in the MR scanner.[150]
- In the only study which actually recorded it, about one-third of acute stroke patients required some form of physical intervention while in the scanner (reassurance, assistance while vomiting, administering oxygen, etc.), and 20% that started scanning did not complete all the sequences.[150]

In view of these constraints, patients with mild stroke (lacunar or small cortical) are more able to cooperate with scanning and a much larger proportion can be scanned (>95%).[153]

Given all these very real practical issues with MR, and until it is clear that the information gained from MR is so much better than from CT that it is worth the extra time, cost, risk to the patient from hypoxia, etc. and organizational difficulties, the first-line investigation for most stroke patients will probably continue to be CT in the immediate future,[154,155] reserving MR for 'difficult cases' with specific questions (see below), and for research.[156]

CT has enjoyed somewhat of a renaissance in the last few years with the advent of widely available multislice perfusion imaging[140] and rapid CT angiography with very good image reconstruction.[145] However, use of MR scanners may expand as their design evolves, the sequences become faster[148,157] and access to patients within the scanner becomes easier (e.g. wider bore), and therefore more user-friendly. The advantages of MR are not only its superior pathoanatomical cross-sectional imaging properties, but that the same machine can image vessels and assess cerebral blood flow non-invasively; provide diffusion imaging and spectroscopy to elucidate the pathogenesis of brain damage in ischaemia and how experimental treatments might modify it; and, by functional imaging, elucidate mechanisms of brain recovery.

Many of the general principles of recognizing an infarct by its shape and site, the correlations between clinical findings and infarct site, the time course of infarct swelling, fogging and haemorrhagic transformation as have been described for CT are equally relevant to MR and will not be repeated here. Rather, this section highlights where MR imaging provides different information to CT.

Routine MR brain imaging for suspected stroke

A routine MR brain scan for stroke should include a midline sagittal localizing view of the brain, usually T1-weighted, followed by axial diffusion-weighted images (DWI), a gradient echo (or T2*) sequence, axial T2-weighted images and/or a fluid attenuated inversion recovery (FLAIR) sequence – all covering the whole brain (Fig. 5.28). MR dynamic susceptibility perfusion imaging following an intravenous injection of a bolus of contrast, MR angiography and MR spectroscopy are also commonly available on modern MR scanners.

In simple terms, it is useful to think of:
- DWI showing as bright white (hyperintense) areas where water movement is restricted (i.e. intracellular oedema);
- FLAIR and T2-weighted images as showing brain water content (so areas of oedema will show up as hyperintense, i.e. white, with CSF also white on T2 and dark on FLAIR;
- gradient echo as being particularly sensitive to anything with paramagnetic effects, such as haemoglobin breakdown products, therefore being very good for showing new and old haemorrhage;
- T1-weighted images as showing brain structure.

Most scanners now use a 'fast spin echo' sequence for T2 which takes less time to acquire than the older 'spin echo' sequences. However, it is important to recognize that spin echo and fast spin echo do not produce the same images, the main difference being that fast spin echo is less sensitive to haemosiderin, a haemoglobin breakdown product.[158]

> A routine MR examination for stroke should include DWI, gradient echo and either T2 or FLAIR sequences.

Contraindications to MR

All patients should be screened for MR compatibility before they enter the magnetic field, but the key contraindications are mentioned here to help avoid inappropriate referrals: pacemakers, intracranial aneurysm clips (virtually all types), definite metallic intraocular foreign bodies, and cochlear implants (see www.mrisafety.com for details on specific manufacturers' devices and MRI compatibility). Intracranial aneurysm coils are not contraindications. Metallic prostheses, foreign bodies other than in the eyes or brain, some ventriculoperitoneal shunts, some artificial heart valves and first trimester of pregnancy are all relative contraindications which are useful for the MR department to know about well in advance, so that the individual patient's circumstances can be checked (to see whether MR scanning will be possible without undue risk) and to tailor the scan to the patient. Patients who are dysphasic may need to have their orbits and chest X-rayed prior to MR to exclude any intraocular metallic foreign body, and pacemakers (feeling the chest wall is probably not a sufficiently reliable substitute for chest X-ray for excluding a pacemaker).

5.5.1 The appearance of haemorrhage on MRI

The appearance of haemorrhage on MR is governed by the paramagnetic properties of haemoglobin breakdown products, and so it changes with time (Fig. 5.29).[46] Freshly extravasated red blood cells contain oxyhaemoglobin which does not have any paramagnetic properties. As soon as the blood becomes deoxygenated, the signal properties change, and this can be detected on sequences that are particularly sensitive to the oxygen state of haemoglobin, such as the echoplanar sequences used for diffusion-weighted imaging, or T2*-weighted gradient echo sequences. Thus, depending on the state of the oxygen in the intracerebral haemorrhage (ICH), there may be little immediate signal change and, although a lesion may be visible, the differentiation from infarction or some other mass lesion may be difficult within the first few hours, even when specific blood-sensitive sequences are used (Fig. 5.30). In some patients with ICHs scanned within the first few hours, there may be serpiginous low signal (dark) bands at the margins of the lesion on gradient echo (T2*) sequences and sometimes on DWI. However we have seen cases where low signal bands were minimal, only visible on the T2*-weighted gradient echo sequence, and which could easily have been overlooked if only the DWI had been done (Fig. 5.30). Thus, while several publications are optimistic about the ability of MR to detect parenchymal haemorrhage reliably within the first few hours of acute stroke,[159–162] we would

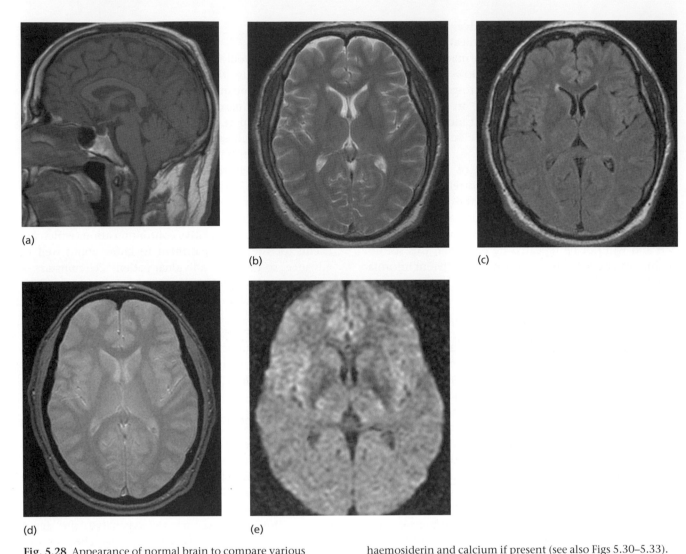

(a)

(b)

(c)

(d)

(e)

Fig. 5.28 Appearance of normal brain to compare various MR sequences. (a) T1-weighted midline sagittal – note the black CSF and little difference between grey and white matter. (b) T2-weighed fast spin echo axial – note CSF is very white (hyperintense), and grey matter is whiter (more intense) than white matter. (c) Fluid attenuated inversion recovery (FLAIR) axial – CSF is dark, grey and white matter are of similar intensity. (d) T2-weighted gradient echo axial – CSF is white, grey and white matter can be easily distinguished although the anatomical definition is not great – very sensitive to haemosiderin and calcium if present (see also Figs 5.30–5.33). (e) Diffusion-weighted axial imaging – poor anatomical detail, dark CSF – acute ischaemic lesions are bright white. Note that the CSF appears white on T2 and gradient echo imaging and dark on the other sequences. T2 and T1 provide the best anatomical detail, FLAIR is useful for seeing abnormal tissue near CSF interfaces (see Fig. 5.38), gradient echo is very sensitive to blood, metal and calcium, and diffusion imaging is very sensitive to acute ischaemia.

continue to urge caution – acute haemorrhage on MR in general is just not as easy to diagnose as CT acute haemorrhage, especially for the inexperienced or unwary. However, increasing use of MR in hyperacute stroke has raised confidence in distinguishing lesions which are primarily haemorrhagic from those which are ischaemic.

The time course of the change in appearance of an ICH on different sequences as it ages is now known to be much more variable than was originally thought.[163] In general, the pattern is as follows, but it will vary with the sequences used, and probably factors related to the patient and the ICH:

- Once enough deoxyhaemoglobin has formed the ICH shows a centrally hypointense (dark) area on T1-weighted imaging and a markedly hypointense (dark) area on T2-weighted imaging.
- As methaemoglobin is formed in the red cells, the lesion on the T1-weighted image becomes hyperintense (bright) while on the T2-weighted image it initially remains dark.

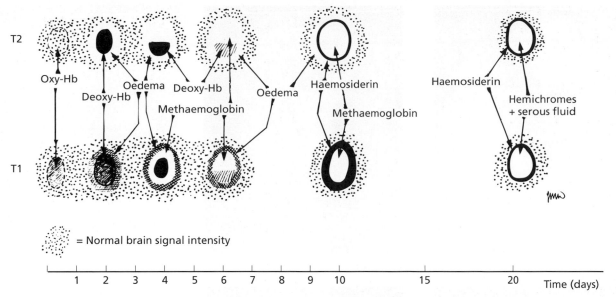

T2

Oxy-Hb

Deoxy-Hb

Oedema   Deoxy-Hb

Methaemoglobin   Oedema   Haemosiderin   Haemosiderin

Methaemoglobin   Hemichromes + serous fluid

T1

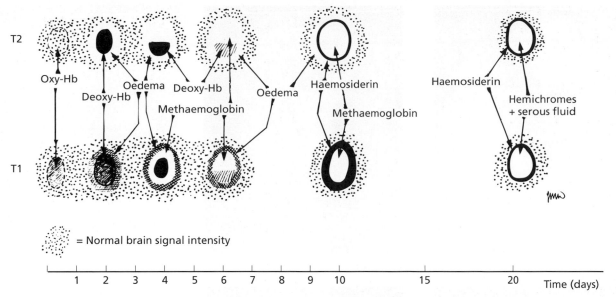
= Normal brain signal intensity

| 1 | 2 | 3 | 4 | 5 | 6 | 7 | 8 | 9 | 10 | 15 | 20 |

Time (days)

Fig. 5.29 Diagram of the change in the appearance of parenchymal brain haemorrhage on MRI. The top row shows the typical appearance on T2-, and the lower row on T1-weighted imaging. The normal brain is represented by the stippled background. To a certain extent, the exact appearance and timing of the changes depend on the field strength of the magnet. The most important things to remember are that intracellular deoxyhaemoglobin (deoxy-Hb) is dark on T1 and T2, methaemoglobin is bright on T1 and T2, and haemosiderin is dark on T1 and T2. Haemosiderin persists in the margins of a haematoma for years after the original haemorrhage. Oxy-Hb, oxyhaemoglobin.

- As the methaemoglobin becomes extracellular and the ICH liquefies, the lesion on the T2-weighted image becomes as hyperintense (bright) as on the T1-weighted image.
- After several weeks, lesions on T2-weighted images become bright in the centre with a very dark rim, and on T1-weighted images they are also bright centrally and moderately dark around the rim.
- Eventually the dark rim (haemosiderin) around a bright 'hole' on T2 is the only remaining feature.

The exact timing and degree of these signal changes depend on the strength of the magnet, which compartment of the brain the haemorrhage lies in, abnormal clotting, haematocrit, and the exact scan sequence used.[46] Some sequences are very sensitive to the presence of haemoglobin breakdown products, e.g. T2* (gradient echo T2)[164] and 'susceptibility-weighted imaging'[165] which show microhaemorrhages and petechial haemorrhage in infarcts, previously visible only to the pathologist (Fig. 5.31),[166] while other sequences are much less blood-sensitive (see below). The clinical utility of being able to see tiny amounts of petechial haemorrhage or chronic microhaemorrhages remains uncertain (see below), but it is certainly important to make sure that the routine MR imaging protocol for stroke (acute or chronic) includes sequences which can reliably detect blood of any age.

Does haemorrhage remain visible indefinitely on MR?

The MR features of haemosiderin may persist for life (Fig. 5.32) because, in general, old ICHs are visible pathologically as haemosiderin deposits at postmortem.[167] Haemosiderin is one of two major haemoglobin-derived pigments identifiable in tissue sections from around ICHs and represents aggregates of ferritin micelles within lysosomes of phagocytic cells. The other pigment is haematoidin, which is chemically identical to bilirubin, and forms locally as a result of haemoglobin breakdown in a milieu of reduced oxygen tension.[167] Haemosiderin is ferromagnetic and therefore visible on MR, whereas haematoidin has no particular magnetic properties and is not visible on MR.

We found that among 116 survivors of moderate to severe head injury of whom 78 had one or more parenchymal haemorrhages (total 106) at the time of injury, using a 1.0 Tesla MR scanner between 1 and 5 years after injury, 96 of the 106 (90%) haemorrhages were visible as haemosiderin on spin echo T2-weighted imaging. Of the ten haemorrhages without haemosiderin on MR (11% of patients), seven were in patients where another haemorrhage *with* haemosiderin was still visible elsewhere in the brain. There were no features of the haemorrhage (site, size, density, sharpness of edges) in the acute stage which correlated

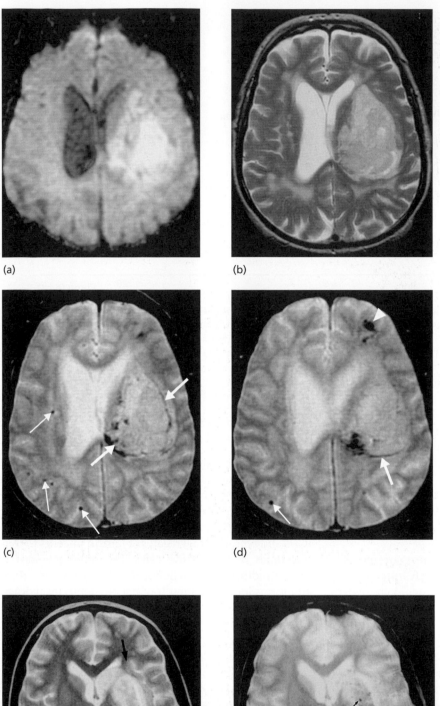

Fig. 5.30 MR brain scan at 4 h after sudden right hemiparesis: (a) diffusion-weighted; (b) T2-weighted; (c,d) gradient echo axial images. There is a large mass of increased signal on all sequences which could easily be mistaken for a tumour on T2 and an infarct on diffusion imaging. The clue that it was a haemorrhage is the hypointense (dark) wavy lines around the edges of the mass which represent blood products (thick *arrows*). Note that this patient has had an ICH previously (d) in the left frontal lobe (*arrowhead*) and has microhaemorrhages (c,d) (*thin arrows*). The CT scan from this patient is shown in Fig. 5.6.

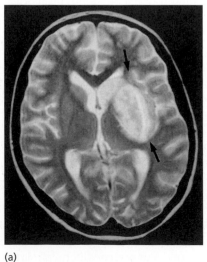
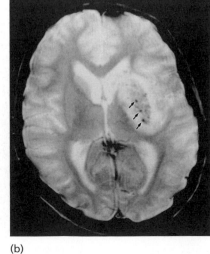

Fig. 5.31 MR scan of a 5-day-old left striatocapsular infarct to show the extreme sensitivity of appropriate MR sequences to tiny areas of petechial haemorrhage. (a) T2-weighted spin-echo sequence shows the infarct (*arrows*), but no haemorrhage. (b) T2-weighted gradient-echo 'haem' sequence shows tiny low-signal areas within the infarct caused by tiny amounts of petechial haemorrhage (*arrows*) which would previously have only been visible to the pathologist. The clinical relevance of this is uncertain.

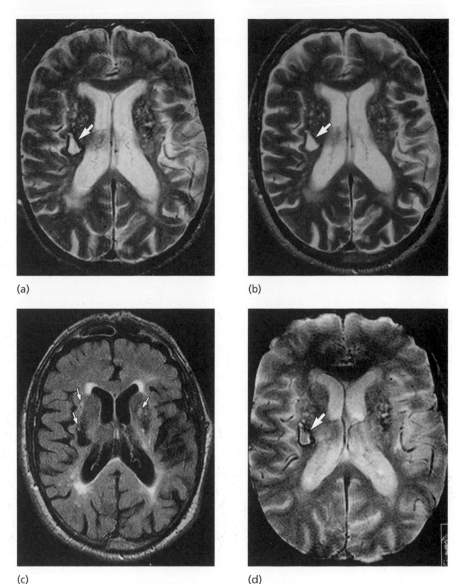

(a)　　　　　　　　(b)

(c)　　　　　　　　(d)

Fig. 5.32 MR scan showing an old ICH in the right basal ganglia. (a) T2 spin echo: the lesion has an obvious low signal (dark) area surrounding the high signal centre (*arrow*). (b) T2 fast spin echo: the lesion is more difficult to identify as an old haemorrhage as the low signal (dark) area is less obvious. (c) FLAIR: several small deep lesions shown (*arrows*), but no features to identify any of them as haemorrhage. (d) Gradient echo T2: the haemorrhage is obvious. Note the enlarged perivascular spaces (pinpoint high signal areas) best seen on T2 (b).

with the likelihood of haemosiderin being present at 1 year. Some quite large ICHs showed no trace of haemosiderin.[168]

Gradient echo (T2*-weighted) sequences are highly sensitive to deoxyhaemoglobin and haemosiderin (see above) but are still not routinely performed (in acute or chronic stroke) unless specifically requested, as they add an extra 2–5 min to the scanning time.[158,163,164,166] Furthermore, areas of calcification give a similar appearance to haemosiderin on gradient echo sequences, and so may cause confusion.[164] Fast spin echo T2-weighted and FLAIR sequences, particularly the latter, are too insensitive to deoxyhaemoglobin or haemosiderin to be reliable for identifying acute or old ICHs, or microhaemorrhages.[158]

In general, the characteristic signal changes of parenchymal haemorrhage on MRI persist indefinitely, but only if the appropriate imaging sequences are used; therefore, intracerebral haemorrhages can be identified even years after they have occurred. However, not all haemorrhages form haemosiderin during their resolution, therefore not all will be discernible as such on MR performed late after the event, even if the correct sequences are used.

Microhaemorrhages

More widespread use of MR in patients with stroke, dementia and normal older subjects has revealed that some patients, as well as occasional normal older people,

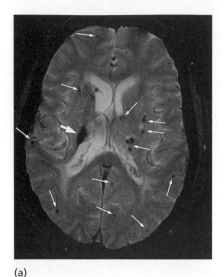

(a)

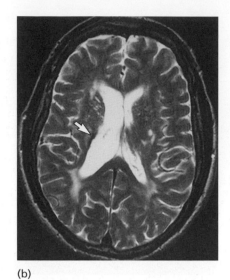

(b)

Fig. 5.33 MR image showing microhaemorrhages and an old ICH. (a) Gradient echo sequence shows the old symptomatic ICH was a right basal ganglia–thalamic haemorrhage measuring about 1 cm in diameter (*thick arrow*), with multiple small low signal dots (dark spots) indicating tiny microhaemorrhages (asymptomatic) that have occurred at some time throughout the brain (*thin arrows*). (b) Fast spin echo T2 demonstrates numerous small deep lesions, but even the old symptomatic right basal ganglia haemorrhage would be difficult to identify as haemorrhagic because of the lack of low signal (dark).

have solitary or multiple small (<5 mm diameter) dots of haemosiderin (low signal on T2*-weighted imaging) – so-called microhaemorrhages or microbleeds[169–171] – scattered throughout the brain without apparently having any previous relevant symptoms referable to them (Fig. 5.33).[172–174] For example, microhaemorrhages were present in 6.4% of community-dwelling neurologically normal individuals of mean age 60 (range 44–79) years in the Austrian Stroke Prevention Study[175] and 4.7% of community-dwelling neurologically normal individuals of mean age 64 (SD 12) years in the Framingham Study.[176] Microhaemorrhages occur most commonly at the cortico-subcortical junction, in the lentiform nuclei and thalami, and in the brainstem and cerebellum[177,178] and correspond with focal haemosiderin deposition on histopathology.[179] They are strongly associated with increasing age,[176] hypertension, and probably with other vascular risk factors.[169–171] They are also associated with old or recent ICHs[174,180] and leukoaraiosis[175,181] and tend to occur in similar parts of the brain as symptomatic ICHs.[182,183] They are also specifically associated with lacunar stroke (not just lacunes of uncertain clinical relevance seen on imaging),[184] suggesting that they may share a common vascular pathology. Although generally regarded as clinically 'silent' they are associated with cognitive impairment, even after adjusting for the amount of white matter lesions.[185] They likely indicate increased risk of intracerebral haemorrhage in patients with:[171]

• leukoaraiosis;[186]
• a past history of ischaemic stroke;[187,188]
• a past history of haemorrhagic stroke;[188]
• haemorrhagic transformation of cerebral infarction;[189]
• antithrombotic and possibly thrombolytic drugs,[190–192] although the data are conflicting.[171,193]

Microhaemorrhages may be related to fibrohyalinosis and amyloid angiopathy in the cerebral small vessels[179]

and some have suggested that microhaemorrhages are a diagnostic indicator of cerebral amyloid angiopathy,[194,195] although the reliability of this is uncertain.[171] Microhaemorrhages also occur in CADASIL (sections 7.20.1 and 8.2.1), a specific microvascular disorder, in a similar distribution to 'sporadic' microhaemorrhages.[196]

Whether or not the presence of microhaemorrhages should influence decisions regarding acute ischaemic stroke treatment or secondary prevention treatments, and therefore should routinely be sought in patients, is unclear.[171] However, microhaemorrhages do seem to indicate a generally increased bleeding tendency, so until further evidence is available, their presence should probably be considered (if known about) when planning acute or secondary treatment and in planning trials of new or multiple antiplatelet agents. Further study to determine their relationship with future haemorrhage risk, either spontaneously or in the presence of antithrombotic or thrombolytic drugs, is clearly required.

5.5.2 The appearance of ischaemic stroke on MRI

Early MR signs of infarction

It is essential to perform diffusion-weighted imaging (DWI) because it is the most sensitive sequence to early parenchymal ischaemic change, and much more sensitive than older sequences (T2-weighted fast spin echo or FLAIR) which are no better than CT. A typical sequence of change in the appearance of an infarct on DWI and T2 is shown in Fig. 5.34.

The perfect imaging technique for stroke would have most of the characteristics listed in Table 5.2. If, as in the case of DWI, the particular interest is in the use of the technique to accurately diagnose ischaemic stroke, to determine the extent of the lesion, the proportion of still

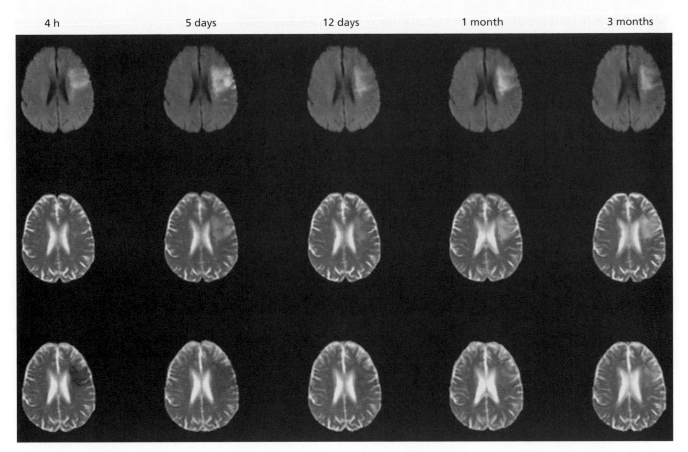

| 4 h | 5 days | 12 days | 1 month | 3 months |

Fig. 5.34 Appearance of infarction on MR imaging. Typical sequence of changes in appearance over time after right hemiparesis. Top row: diffusion-weighted imaging; middle row: T2-weighted imaging; bottom row: apparent diffusion coefficient (ADC) images. Note that the ischaemic lesion is hyperintense on diffusion imaging (hypointense on ADC) at 4 h but is not visible on T2 until 5 days. Note also that the 12-day scan suggests that the lesion is much smaller than its true extent at 3 months due to fogging (see also Figs 5.16, 5.22 for comparison with CT). (Figure prepared by Dr S. Munoz-Maniega, University of Edinburgh.)

Table 5.2 Brain imaging in acute stroke: what would be the properties of the ideal technique?

Widely available

Inexpensive

Fast, so as to obtain information quickly while not damaging the patient

Easy to observe the patient in the scanner

Easy to use in *all* severities of stroke, from mildest to most severe

Differentiate infarct from haemorrhage from non-vascular lesions, both early and late

Demonstrate the site of the infarct or haemorrhage at any time after the event

Differentiate irreparably damaged from salvageable tissue

Demonstrate features which might identify patients at risk of treatment complications

Demonstrate features which identify patients at risk of recurrent stroke

Be repeatable

Not harmful

viable brain and the likely clinical outcome, then a study to evaluate the technique would need the features or characteristics outlined in Table 5.3.

A great deal has been written about DWI and perfusion-weighted imaging (PWI) and the theory that the 'mismatch' between the two represents the ischaemic penumbra or 'tissue at risk' of infarction. Unfortunately most of this literature is of limited reliability because of problems with study methodology. The significance of the changes in relation to clinical outcome, the extent of the ischaemic penumbra, the influence of experimental treatments for ischaemic stroke and the effect of reperfusion, have all yet to be fully evaluated.[156,197–199] In the wave of enthusiasm for diffusion and perfusion MR imaging, it is worth pausing to take a critical look at what the studies have achieved so far, and reflect on the information that is still missing. The following is a distillate of the most clinically relevant and reliable information currently available on MR imaging in suspected acute ischaemic stroke.

Table 5.3 Brain imaging in acute stroke: what would be the ideal study to determine the 'best' imaging modality?

> Large sample size
> Prospective
> Patient population well characterized clinically
> Including a broad sample of the type of patients *relevant* to
>   the question being asked and at relevant time point(s)
>   and all *relevant to clinical practice*
> Blinded reading of imaging, to clinical and other imaging data
> Adequate description of the imaging to allow independent
>   confirmation
> Evaluation of complications or difficulties with imaging
> Clinical follow-up to relate imaging to long-term outcome

The thrombosed artery

A thrombosed artery may be seen as replacement of the normal flow void (within minutes of stroke onset) with high signal clot (either *in situ* thrombus or embolus) on FLAIR or proton density[200] sequences; this is the MR equivalent of the hyperdense artery sign on CT (section 5.4.2) and can be seen very early (Figs 5.19, 5.35, 5.52). Note T2-weighted imaging is relatively insensitive to early intravascular thrombus as fresh thrombus is of low signal and can easily be overlooked as a flow void (Fig. 5.35). Acute intravascular thrombus/embolus may also be detected as low signal on T2*-weighted (gradient echo or susceptibility-weighted) imaging.[201,202] The FLAIR sequence is very sensitive to intravascular thrombus/embolus as high signal, detecting all 25 occluded middle cerebral arteries in one study compared with 15/25 hyperdense arteries on CT and 22/25 low signal areas on T2* (gradient echo or susceptibility-weighted) imaging.[202] However, although intravascular thrombus/embolus may be visible commonly on T2*-weighted (gradient echo or

the susceptibility-weighted images obtained prior to the contrast bolus arrival on perfusion-weighted imaging), the hypointense signal was noted to fluctuate in one study,[202] i.e. it was sometimes present, sometimes not, in the same patient over the first few hours after stroke, which the authors interpreted as possible changes in the thrombus structure. Therefore, of the commonly used sequences, available data indicate that FLAIR is the most sensitive to acute intravascular thrombus/embolus by demonstrating increased signal in the clot.

Early ischaemic changes in the brain parenchyma

A brief description of the pathophysiological changes that create the signal changes on diffusion-weighted MRI (DWI) in acute ischaemia is relevant here. DWI exploits the Brownian motion of water molecules in the brain, largely in the extracellular space. In pure water with unrestricted movement, the free water molecule movement creates random phase shifts with loss of signal (dark) on the diffusion image. Where water movement is restricted, e.g. by cell membranes, there will be more retained signal proportionate to the degree and direction of restriction of movement, which can be used to build up a picture of the tissue structure. The parameter which expresses the amount by which water is free to move is known as the apparent diffusion coefficient (ADC). CSF has a high ADC (unrestricted water movement – bright signal) and different tissue structures have a lower ADC (restricted water movement – darker). Where there is a local change is diffusivity of tissue water, e.g. in an acute ischaemic stroke where one of the earliest changes is for water to enter the ischaemic cells thereby reducing the size of the extracellular space and restricting water movement, the tissue ADC falls (dark area on

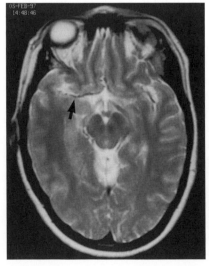

(a)

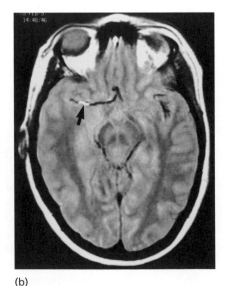

(b)

Fig. 5.35 MR image of a thrombosed right middle cerebral artery. Although there appears to be a flow void (dark) signal in the artery on T2 (a), on proton density (b) there is an obvious high signal area as a result of the fresh thrombus or embolus (*arrow*). FLAIR imaging would show a similar appearance to proton density. The examination was undertaken within 12 h of the stroke, but thrombus can appear dark on T2 up to 1–2 days after the stroke.

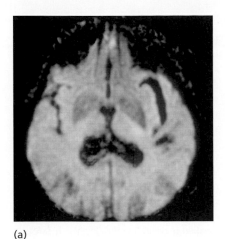

(a)

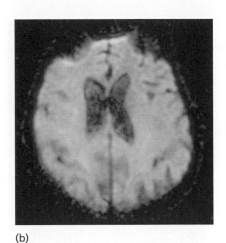

(b)

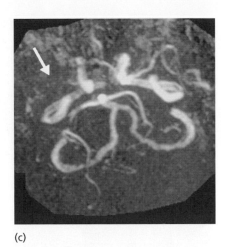

(c)

Fig. 5.36 MR images from a patient scanned at 4 hours after a sudden right hemisphere total anterior circulation infarct in whom (a,b) the diffusion weighted imaging did not show any acute ischaemic change despite there being severe symptoms, and (c) an occluded right middle cerebral artery (*arrow*) on MR angiography.

the ADC image) and the signal on the diffusion image increases (white). The white area stands out like a light bulb, making the acute ischaemic area much more obvious on DWI than on CT or other imaging techniques.

DWI shows abnormalities (increases in signal intensity) within minutes of vessel occlusion in experimental models,[203] and within 30 min of stroke in humans.[204] DWI is now available on most MR scanners and should be used if available when investigating suspected stroke. The acute DWI abnormality appears to represent *reversibly* as well as *irretrievably* damaged brain (see below)[205–207] and is also found in a proportion of patients with only TIA.[208] Also, not all patients, even those with severe stroke symptoms, have a DWI-visible ischaemic lesion (Fig. 5.36).[209]

Thus it is clear that diffusion imaging may demonstrate abnormalities in areas of brain which are not yet irreversibly damaged and may recover, and may never show abnormalities in areas of brain which, judging from the patient's symptoms, must be irreversibly damaged. The overall sensitivity and specificity of diffusion imaging (on its own or in combination with other MR techniques) has not yet been precisely defined.[198] That said, DWI shows a relevant ischaemic lesion far earlier and in a far greater proportion of patients of all stroke severities and at a range of times (up to several weeks after the event) than does any other MR or CT imaging technique. There are however a few caveats to that statement: for example, in patients with moderate to severe stroke presenting to hospital early after stroke, CT with a structured reading tool such as ASPECTS is as good as DWI at detecting the acute ischaemic lesion (section 5.5.4).

On FLAIR and T2-weighted imaging, large infarcts are often visible as areas of increased signal intensity corresponding with a vascular territory within 5 h,[210,211] but small cortical and subcortical infarcts may never become visible, rather as on CT (section 5.4.2 above), or are indistinguishable from background white matter changes (Fig. 5.37). FLAIR was slightly more sensitive to acute ischaemic change than T2, identifying more infarcts earlier (around 4 h), in several small retrospective analyses.[212–214] In our experience, FLAIR can demonstrate relevant infarcts days to weeks after the event, helping to locate the lesion in patients presenting late after their stroke. It can be particularly useful for differentiating small cortical and periventricular infarcts which might otherwise be difficult to distinguish from the adjacent cerebrospinal fluid (Fig. 5.38). However, FLAIR also shows more asymptomatic white matter lesions than does T2 or proton density MR, or CT, and this may be more confusing than helpful. Nonetheless, it may sometimes be possible to distinguish these old 'holes' from a new 'hole' caused by a lacunar stroke by the slightly less hyperintense (white) signal in the latter – both are hyperintense, but the old lesions are more hyperintense than the new.

Further points about the evolution of the appearance of infarction on MRI

The general principles of recognition of infarcts from their shape and site in the brain, and any relationship to the underlying cause, are the same as were described for CT scanning (section 5.4.2). Thus, the infarct swells and many of the other features change according to the same time frame.

On DWI, the initial hyperintense lesion (which may be quite subtle and ill-defined early on) (Fig. 5.39) becomes more hyperintense (white) with more sharply

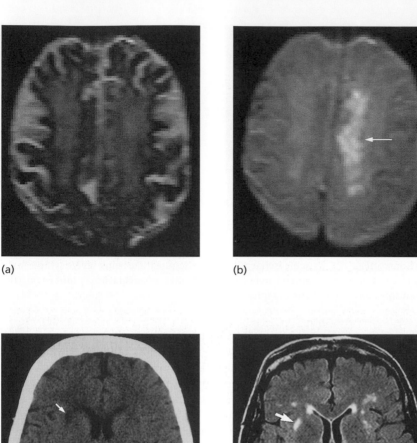

(a)   (b)

Fig. 5.37 (a) MR T2 and (b) diffusion images of an elderly patient with symptoms of a left cortical infarct. Although no definite recent lesion is visible on T2, and there is atrophy and white matter increased signal of small vessel disease, on diffusion there is an obvious area of high signal corresponding with the infarct (*arrow*). Note the 'fuzzyness' of the image is due to patient movement during the scan, which contributes to difficulty identifying any new lesion on T2. However, the marked increase in signal in the infarct on diffusion imaging is easily seen despite the movement.

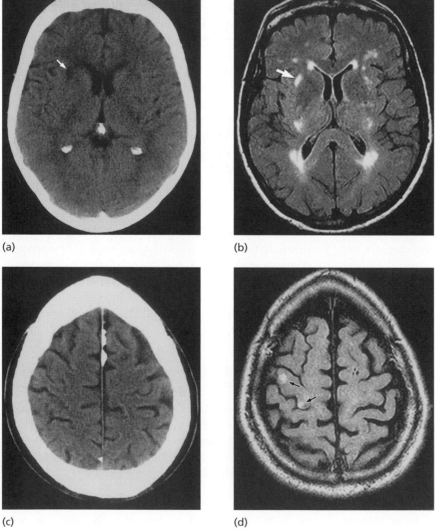

(a)   (b)

(c)   (d)

Fig. 5.38 Comparing CT with MR: examples from two patients. Patient 1: (a) on CT one small deep infarct (consistent with the symptoms) is visible in the anterior limb of the right internal capsule (*arrow*); (b) on MR FLAIR sequence not only is the symptomatic lesion visible (*arrow*), but numerous other areas of increased signal, a common finding with MR, which can confuse rather than clarify if MR is used indiscriminately. Patient 2 had symptoms of a small right cortical infarct: (c) CT was normal, but (d) FLAIR showed high signal in the right parietal cortex (*arrow*) consistent with a recent infarct (T2 was also normal).

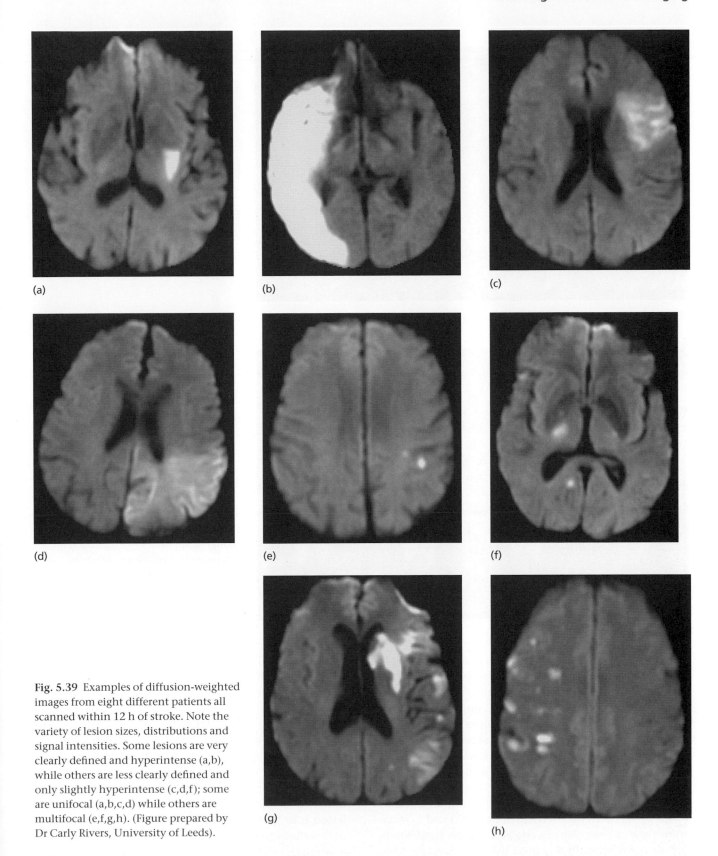

Fig. 5.39 Examples of diffusion-weighted images from eight different patients all scanned within 12 h of stroke. Note the variety of lesion sizes, distributions and signal intensities. Some lesions are very clearly defined and hyperintense (a,b), while others are less clearly defined and only slightly hyperintense (c,d,f); some are unifocal (a,b,c,d) while others are multifocal (e,f,g,h). (Figure prepared by Dr Carly Rivers, University of Leeds).

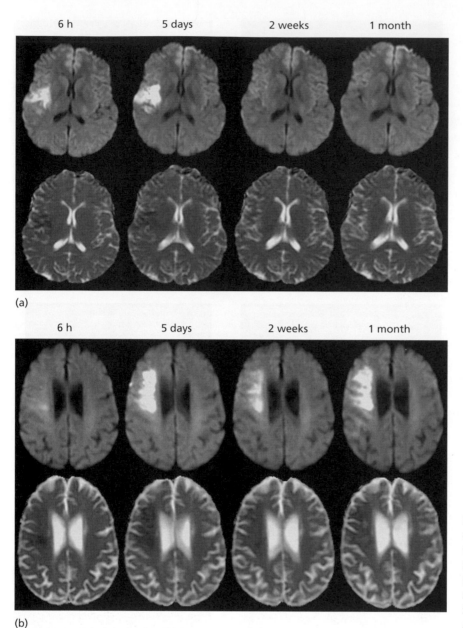

Fig. 5.40 Differences in the rate of change in appearance of infarction in two patients on diffusion-weighted imaging. (a) The diffusion hyperintensity (*top row*) and ADC hypointensity (*bottom row*) have resolved by 2 weeks, whereas in (b) both diffusion hyperintensity and ADC hypointensity are still present.

defined edges over the first few days and then begins to lose its hyperintensity until it becomes iso or hypodense to normal brain by 2 weeks or more (Fig. 5.34). The corresponding changes on the ADC image are that the initially dark lesion gradually becomes isointense and then possibly hyperintense to normal brain as the tissue is replaced with an area of cerebromalacea. The rate of change varies between infarcts and is much more variable than originally described. The overall infarct appearance on DWI at any one time is influenced mainly by the apparent diffusion coefficient (ADC) and T_2 relaxation time of the tissue. In the acute stage, hyperintensity on DWI is mainly caused by a decrease in ADC, while T_2 relaxation remains relatively normal.[215] In the subacute phase, the ADC gradually increases to or above

normal, generally by 2 weeks.[216,217] Hyperintensity seen thereafter on DWI has been attributed to increased T_2 relaxation of the tissue (T_2 'shine through').[215] However the speed with which the DWI and ADC signal changes evolve varies considerably (Fig. 5.40) and the DWI hyperintensity can become iso- or hypo-intense to normal tissue within 15, 57, and 72 days depending on the population studied.[217–220] The reasons for the variation in the appearance of infarct evolution are not fully understood, but are probably related to whether the lesion is in grey or white matter[221,222] and to the speed of reperfusion.[222,223]

A subset of patients have persistently reduced ADC, DWI hyperintensity and reduced perfusion at 1 or even 3 months after stroke, the reasons for which are as yet unclear, but this finding is associated with large infarcts and poor functional outcome.[222] This may be the MR equivalent of the 'no reflow' phenomenon (section 12.1.3)[224] and suggests that the delay in recovery of perfusion (i.e. reflow) is secondary to persistent intracellular oedema (i.e. persistent DWI hyperintensity/reduced ADC). Several other studies have found persistent hyperintensity on DWI many weeks after the stroke, frequently in small deep white matter lesions,[225–227] which taken with other work[222,228] suggests that there are important differences in the resistance to ischaemia and evolution of infarct over time between grey and white matter.

On DWI, many series have documented expansion of the acute ischaemic lesion between the admission scan and a scan days later. Partly this may be infarct oedema causing an apparent increase in volume and partly it may be genuine growth of the infarct.[229,230]

In the second week after stroke onset, diffuse increase in signal on T2-weighted images of gyri overlying the infarct is often visible. This is thought to be caused by neovascular capillary proliferation, or loss of autoregulation in leptomeningeal collaterals, and is visible for up to 8 weeks after onset.[231,232] It is mirrored by a similar appearance on CT scanning, attributed to areas of breakdown of the blood–brain barrier corresponding with the gyriform petechial haemorrhages seen at postmortem (Fig. 5.41).[53] In the second to third week after onset, some infarcts become isodense with normal brain on CT (fogging effect) and, as they may have lost most of their mass effect by that stage, are difficult to identify (section 5.4.2). A similar effect has been observed on T2-weighted MR imaging (5.34).[233–235] Changes in T1 (increased signal) and in T2 (decreased signal) suggesting diffuse haemorrhage occurs in the second to third week (Fig. 5.34 and

5.41), probably the result of leaky capillaries with diapedesis of red blood cells;[234,236] this fits with the 'fogging effect' on CT, as the red blood cells would cause a diffuse increase in Hounsfield numbers, raising the low attenuation of the lesion to that of normal brain parenchyma.

Infarcts do not usually enhance with intravenous gadolinium contrast until the first week after stroke onset. Thereafter, they generally show marked contrast enhancement around the edges (and within the infarct if enough contrast is administered) for several weeks.[237] The possible risks of gadolinium in ischaemic brain lesions have not been evaluated, although a widely used method of perfusion imaging requires an injection of gadolinium. Further information is required to determine whether gadolinium has any adverse effects on the acutely ischaemic brain, or interferes with thrombus lysis as do X-ray contrast media (section 5.4.2).

Late appearance of infarction on MRI

After several weeks the infarcted brain appears as an area with similar signal characteristics to cerebrospinal fluid, i.e. bright on T2 and dark on T1, with an *ex vacuo* effect in the surrounding brain. Other long-term effects of ischaemic stroke seen on MR include Wallerian degeneration, visible as atrophy and low intensity in the white matter of the brainstem, and the late effects of any haemorrhagic transformation (section 5.7).[232]

Differentiation of new from old infarcts, and detection of small cortical and subcortical infarcts

Magnetic resonance imaging is able to detect small infarcts well, especially lacunes.[236] Furthermore, in patients with numerous 'holes in the brain', DWI or

Fig. 5.41 MR T2-weighted images of petechial haemorrhage. (a) A patient with an extensive left middle cerebral artery infarct at 5 days after stroke, with a dark area of haemosiderin (petechial haemorrhage; *curved arrow*) at the medial margin of the infarcted area (*thin arrows*). (b) A patient with a left parieto-occipital infarct (*short arrows*) with tiny areas of dark serpiginous cortical signal caused by gyral petechial haemorrhage (*long arrow*).

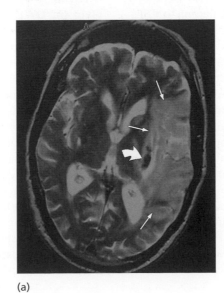

(a)

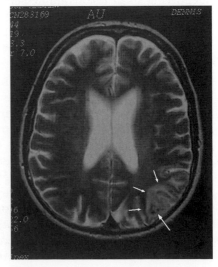

(b)

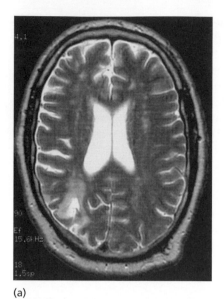

(a)

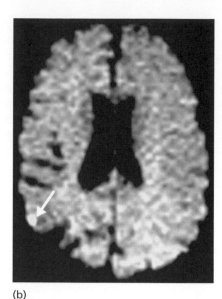

(b)

Fig. 5.42 MR imaging at 12 h in a patient with symptoms of a mild right cortical infarct. The patient had had a previous left hemiparesis some years earlier and it was unclear whether the recent symptoms indicated a new stroke or simply a worsening of the residual symptoms due to an intercurrent chest infection. (a) T2-weighted MR shows an established old infarct in the right posterior temporal cortex but does not clearly show any new lesion; (b) diffusion imaging shows a tiny area of high signal in the right parietal cortex (*arrow*) adjacent to the old infarct, corresponding with the patient's symptoms.

gadolinium-enhanced MRI can demonstrate which is the recent lacune. On DWI it will be hyperintense (often with reduced ADC depending on its age) and after gadolinium it will enhance whereas older lesions will not.[238,239] MRI is more sensitive to small lesions in the brainstem and posterior fossa than CT because there is less interference from bone artifacts (except for DWI sequences which may suffer image distortion near bone or air).[240]

DWI is particularly useful in locating the recent relevant infarct in patients with mild strokes. These patients are likely to have small lesions either in the cortex or subcortical white matter. A small cortical infarct may be difficult to identify on T2 or proton density MR, or on CT, but is often clearly seen as an area of increased signal on diffusion imaging up to several weeks after the stroke (Fig. 5.42).[226,227,241] The FLAIR sequence is also useful for identifying small lesions immediately adjacent to CSF, either in cortex or periventricular white matter. Patients with lacunar infarcts may already have multiple areas of increased signal in the periventricular white matter on T2 or FLAIR MR, or periventricular white matter lucencies on CT, which makes it difficult to identify a new lesion among established lesions. Diffusion imaging demonstrates the recent lesion as an area of increased signal (Fig. 5.43).[242–245] Similarly, in patients with old cortical infarcts, diffusion imaging can also be useful to determine whether there has been a new ischaemic lesion when it is not clear whether any neurological deterioration has been caused by a new ischaemic lesion, or an intercurrent illness such as pneumonia making a previous stroke deficit seem worse (Fig. 5.42) (section 11.4).[246–249] On other forms of MR imaging, or on CT, it may be difficult to determine whether a new

lesion has formed adjacent to an existing infarct as the cerebromalacic changes sometimes render interpretation difficult.

Is diffusion imaging specific for acute ischaemic stroke?

Diffusion imaging is not specific for acute ischaemia. Conditions such as encephalitis, migraine, vasculitis, brain tumours, following epileptic seizures, abscesses and multiple sclerosis (Fig. 5.44) can all show changes similar to acute ischaemic stroke.[209,250–252]

Can appropriate ischaemic lesions be seen on MR in patients with transient ischaemic attacks?

Several studies have documented acute hyperintense ischaemic lesions in clinically-appropriate areas of the brain on DWI within 24 h of symptom onset, in up to 50% of patients who on clinical follow-up turned out to have transient ischaemic attacks (TIAs), not strokes.[208,253–255] Thus early diffusion imaging cannot distinguish between patients having TIAs and those who will later turn out to have definite strokes, at least on the basis of symptoms lasting less than or more than 24 h. However, the abnormal areas on DWI in patients who had TIAs were generally smaller and less pronounced than the abnormal areas in patients who went on to have strokes.[253–255] Furthermore, the TIA patient with an acute DWI lesion tends to have symptoms that have lasted longer, and is more likely to have motor impairment or aphasia,[208,254] or an identified stroke mechanism such as a cardiac embolic source.[208] Moreover, compared with patients without DWI lesions, patients with TIA and an acute ischaemic lesion on DWI

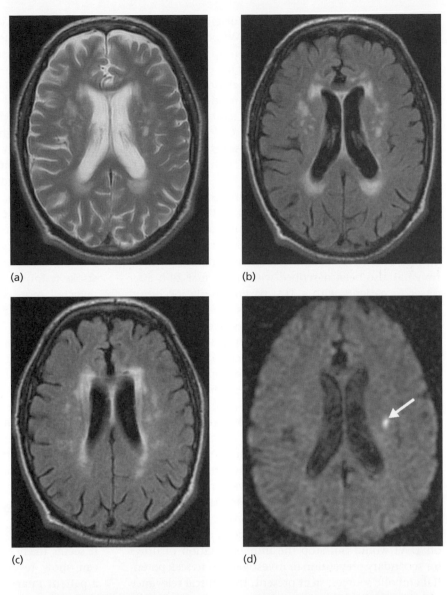

(a)

(b)

(c)

(d)

Fig. 5.43 MR images of a patient with a left hemisphere lacunar stroke. (a) T2-weighted, (b,c) adjacent FLAIR MR images show multiple areas of increased signal in the white matter adjacent to the lateral ventricles bilaterally (centrum semiovale). With so much white matter disease it is difficult to be sure which is the recent infarct. (d) But, on diffusion imaging, the recent infarct is obvious by its increased signal (*arrow*).

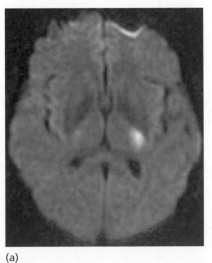

(a)

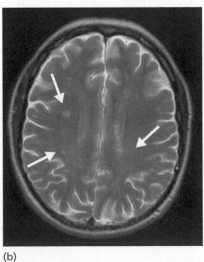

(b)

Fig. 5.44 An MR image from a 33-year-old patient 3 days after a right hemiparesis. Diffusion imaging a) shows a hyperintense lesion in the left centrum semiovale suggesting an infarct, but T2-weighted imaging shows several hyperintense areas (*arrows*) in the deep white matter consistent with multiple sclerosis.

are more likely to have an early recurrent stroke.[255–257] This has led some to suggest that DWI-positive TIAs are a clinically distinct important subgroup and that DWI could be used to triage TIA patients for early secondary prevention.[252,255,257] In fact, the association between TIA and a relevant ischaemic lesion on imaging with higher risk of recurrent stroke is not restricted to DWI. Similar findings have been reported using CT[258] although far fewer appropriate acute ischaemic lesions are seen on CT and it is harder to be certain with CT that the lesion is new rather than old.

FLAIR, T2- and T1-weighted MR imaging also detects signal changes in appropriate areas of the brain up to several days after TIAs,[259–261] about half as often as on DWI.[208,254] Pronounced brain parenchymal cortical enhancement following intravenous gadolinium injection has also been described within the first 24 h after onset in patients with a TIA, partial arterial occlusion and isolated boundary-zone infarcts.[211,259,262] However, even with DWI, the identification of these small acute ischaemic lesions is technique dependent, and false negatives and false positives can occur.[252] For example, low resolution DWI, either because of imaging too early or too late, acquisition in too few gradient directions, too thick slices or too wide a slice gap, could all miss a small acute lesion. Use of a higher resolution DWI sequence (thinner slices, no gap, averaging of more acquisitions) may show acute lesions in a higher proportion of patients.[252] Obviously, where possible, one should strive to use the most sensitive imaging available, but providing DWI for every TIA is impractical, even in well-resourced health care systems. Also, as far as stroke prevention is concerned, the absence of an acute lesion on DWI would not stop the implementation of drugs for secondary prevention or investigations to seek potential embolic sources, so at present, the clinical relevance of acute DWI visible lesions in patients with TIAs is uncertain. Possibly in occasional patients with carotid stenosis in whom there is uncertainty as to whether a TIA was in the anterior or posterior circulation, a DWI that showed where the lesion was might help in deciding whether an endarterectomy was needed (if the patient was one of the 50% or so of TIAs with a visible lesion and reached the scanner within a few days so that the lesion was still visible).

Are ischaemic lesions always visible on MR?

Some infarcts never become visible on DWI, FLAIR or T2,[263] although the actual proportion is not known, because most work with MR in stroke so far has focused on the detection of hyperacute ischaemia with DWI, rather neglecting the sensitivity and specificity of these techniques in a wider range of situations, and there are few comparisons with CT scanning in the generality of stroke. Diffusion imaging was negative in 20% of patients in one series when scanned within 24 h of stroke onset and about 10% of lesions were never visible (Fig. 5.36).[264–267]

Of patients who subsequently develop changes on routine T2-weighted MR, about 15% showed abnormalities within 8 h and 90% within 24 h of onset.[268] While it is likely that signal changes on FLAIR, T2- and proton density-weighted MR represent irreversibly damaged brain, this has not yet been conclusively established. We studied 230 patients presenting more than 5 days after a mild stroke (mostly as outpatients) with CT and MR T2-weighted fast spin echo, FLAIR and gradient echo.[38] MR with these sequences detected no more acute ischaemic stroke lesions than did CT, although MR gradient echo detected more small intracerebral haemorrhages (sections 5.4.1 and 5.5.1) which would have been mistaken for infarcts on CT. The reason for the failure of T2 and FLAIR sequences to detect small ischaemic lesions more reliably than CT is that these MR sequences also show more incidental white matter hyperintensities which obscure the new lesion. Also, on T2-weighted imaging, the cortex is often obscured by high signal in the adjacent CSF. The latter is less of a problem with FLAIR, but it can be hard to tell on FLAIR whether a small lesion is new or old, so the detection rate for small lesions is still much less than with DWI.[241]

Does DWI (or FLAIR or T2) only show changes in irreversibly damaged brain?

It seems likely that DWI and possibly other sequences can show reversible ischaemic change. For example, a patient imaged within 4 h of acute ischaemic stroke showed a lesion in the posterior limb of the internal capsule consistent with a lacunar infarct on diffusion and FLAIR MR imaging. However, by 24 h the patient had made a full neurological recovery and repeat MR imaging showed no trace of the lacunar lesion.[265] Further follow-up MR imaging at 7 and 30 days remained normal. Some patients imaged between 6 and 72 h of stroke and not treated with thrombolytic therapy[269] have abnormalities on DWI which do not go on to infarction (as demonstrated on follow-up CT or T2-weighted MR scanning) in one-quarter of ischaemic lesions (in the absence of clinical follow-up, it is possible that some of these patients actually had TIAs). An experimental model of cerebral infarction[270] showed abnormal diffusion in areas of brain when the cerebral blood flow fell below and between 34–41 mL/100 g brain/min, still well above the threshold considered to represent the ischaemic penumbra (10–20 mL/100 g brain/min) and of irreversible energy failure (below 9–20 mL/100 g brain/min). Note that a DWI lesion 'disappearing' after a few days does not mean that there is no permanent neurological damage (either on imaging or clinical examination). As detailed above, T2 or FLAIR imaging within the first 2 weeks or so is not a reliable indicator of final infarct damage, either because infarct swelling may cause overestimation of lesion size,[82,271] or fogging (see below) may obscure (sometimes totally) the true infarct extent.[233,235] Thus studies which compared early infarct appearance on DWI (or perfusion-weighted imaging) with a 'final infarct extent' at less than 1 month, of which there are many (e.g.[272–276]), may be unreliable in terms of identifying which tissue survived and which did not.

There have been few analyses of the stroke lesion by subregion to detect parts which might go on to infarct vs those that do not. Our own observations suggest that the DWI lesion is not 'one solid white blob' but rather often has an irregular pattern of increased signal, with some areas only marginally 'whiter' than normal tissue and other areas much more obviously 'whiter'. If the DWI signal reflects the degree of intracellular oedema, one would expect that minor degrees of oedema would produce minor degrees of 'whiteness' and more severe oedema would produce major 'whiteness'. Therefore minor 'whiteness' could resolve if the tissue recovered and major 'whiteness' probably would not.

Is there an apparent diffusion coefficient value that discriminates salvageable from dead tissue?

Many have hoped that the apparent diffusion coefficient (ADC) might provide an objective index of tissue viability. It is not too sensitive to individual scanner characteristics, it can be measured in an automated way allowing a threshold to be drawn on the lesion to indicate the area that was already infarcted/will infarct/will not infarct, and can be expressed as an absolute value. We have systematically reviewed the literature on DWI and perfusion weighted imaging (PWI) in acute ischaemic stroke; there are two studies with sufficient methodological reliability that identified ADC thresholds that predicted tissue infarction.[277,278] Although these proposed ADC ratio (of ischaemic to normal brain) thresholds of 0.53[277] and 0.85[278] (1.0 being normal), the authors were careful to point out the large overlap of ADC values between tissue that did and did not proceed to infarction, and that a single parameter was unlikely to sufficiently capture the complex ischaemic pathology to inform clinical decision making. A further systematic review has drawn similar conclusions.[279] Many studies have failed to find specific thresholds for infarction/survival.[276,280,281] Indeed,

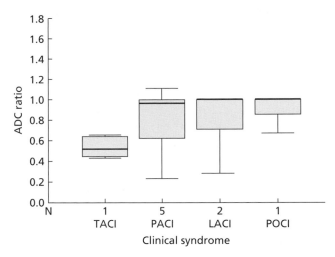

Fig. 5.45 Association between diffusion imaging parameters and clinical features. ADC ratio (ischaemic lesion/normal brain, mean and SD) and Oxfordshire Community Stroke Project classification – the more extensive the syndrome, the lower the ADC on admission. TACI, total anterior circulation infarct; PACI, partial anterior circulation infarct; LACI, lacunar infarct; POCI, posterior circulation infarct.[280,281] Reproduced with permission of *Neurology* © 2002 Lippincott Williams & Wilkins.

although we ourselves found an association between the ADC value in the ischaemic lesion within 24 h of stroke and the Oxfordshire Community Stroke Project classification (Fig. 5.45), we consistently found no relationship between ADC and functional outcome in two separate studies (Fig. 5.46).[280,281]

To find out more about the relationship between DWI lesion parameters and tissue state, we have also systematically reviewed the literature on DWI in experimental models of focal ischaemic stroke.[207] Our conclusions were limited because, of 141 potentially eligible papers, details of key experimental methods were unfortunately often omitted and anaesthesia and fixation techniques may inadvertently have affected the results. However, the consistent findings among the 13 high-quality studies (of which three had blinded analyses), included: neuronal damage persists or progresses despite early DWI lesion 'normalization'; the ADC is not very sensitive to the amount of neuronal damage; the 'brighter' the DWI lesion the greater the neuronal damage; and the DWI lesion may reflect glial more than neuronal changes. This, while frustrating, supports the findings of human studies to date by indicating that simply looking at the DWI lesion, without actually measuring anything (e.g. ADC), is as useful an indicator of the degree of tissue damage in the acute stage of stroke as can be obtained at present. Because this is fast (it does not introduce delays while the lesion is measured), it is clinically the most useful approach that could be hoped for.

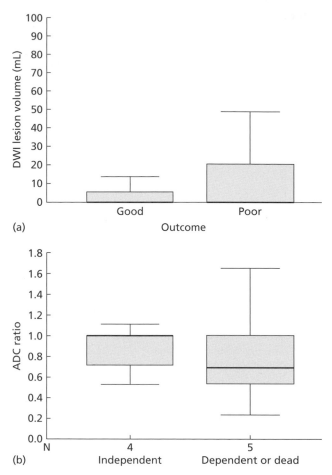

Fig. 5.46 Association between diffusion imaging parameters and clinical features. (a) Diffusion lesion volume (mean +/− SD) at baseline and death or dependency according to the Rankin score at 3 months – although larger lesion volumes are associated with more poor outcomes, there is considerable overlap and the association is not significant. (b) ADC (mean +/− SD) at baseline and death or dependency according to the Rankin score at 3 months – although there are more lower ADC values among those with poor outcomes, there is huge overlap and the association is not significant.[280,281]

Does diffusion imaging lesion appearance predict outcome?

The marked sensitivity of DWI to ischaemic lesions very early after the onset of stroke symptoms, coupled with the expense of large clinical trials, has provoked considerable interest in whether DWI might be a surrogate outcome marker in hyperacute stroke.[282,283] Several studies have found associations between the appearance of the ischaemic stroke at baseline on DWI (e.g. lesion volume or apparent diffusion coefficient – ADC) and functional outcome.[284–292] A 'three-item scale' incorporating DWI lesion volume, increasing time from symptom onset and

stroke severity independently predicted outcome in one retrospective study.[289] But others, conducted prospectively, with broad entry criteria, were unable to find any association between DWI lesion volume or ACD and outcome.[280,281,293] Few tested whether DWI was an *independent* outcome predictor.[280,288,289]

Accurate outcome prediction is difficult. Many predictive models (for many diseases) have been published but seldom translated into clinical practice[294] because of inadequate sample size, unrepresentative case mix, failure to blind outcome assessments to key baseline variables, lack of clinical credibility, lack of external validation, or impracticality.[295] If imaging features are to improve stroke outcome prediction, then this should be by adding to robust, proven, easy-to-elicit clinical variables such as age or stroke severity.[296] The disagreement between studies of DWI in outcome prediction means that these results may not be applicable to clinical practice, or of use as a surrogate outcome in trials.

We have evaluated DWI lesion volume and ADC as functional outcome predictors in a reasonably broad cross-section of strokes of all severities admitted to hospital and MR scanned within 24 h of stroke.[281] Among 82 patients, only patient age and stroke severity independently predicted functional outcome, and neither DWI lesion volume nor ADC ratio predicted outcome even on univariate analyses (Fig. 5.46). Nor were we able to replicate the predictive function of the 'three-item scale'.[289] Our study included a broader range of stroke severities than did those which found that DWI lesion volume predicted outcome. The studies where DWI lesion volume did predict outcome included patients with more severe strokes than the studies that did not. The interpretation of these findings is that among mild strokes, stroke severity is an overwhelmingly powerful outcome predictor, making it unlikely that other factors could add to outcome prediction. However, among more severe strokes, clinical severity is less powerful, making it possible that other factors could contribute to outcome prediction.[283] Clinical scales at baseline and for outcome assessment are very powerful, and should not be abandoned in favour of expensive, technologically dependent alternatives until the latter are proven to be better.

> Neither diffusion-weighted imaging lesion volume nor apparent diffusion coefficient values predict outcome in the generality of stroke. Clinical scales at baseline are reliable measures of severity and predictors of outcome, and should not be abandoned in favour of expensive technologically dependent alternatives until the latter are proven to be better.

In which patients does DWI (or MRI) influence clinical practice?

In what circumstances is DWI more likely to provide information that would influence clinical decision making than other techniques? Despite the huge literature on DWI, much of it is of limited generalizability. For example, many studies were small (mean sample size about 30), and few blinded the review of each imaging modality to other imaging results, and to clinical features and outcome. Most had very sketchy details of the clinical state of the patient, such as 'stroke' rather than more detail about the severity of the stroke or the part of the brain affected, making it difficult to know what type of patients they were describing. Few had any clinical follow-up. Many studies were conducted in well-resourced, highly specialized centres, making it difficult to extrapolate their results to the generality of ischaemic strokes.

In general, DWI is most likely to provide information not available from other imaging technique in several circumstances:

- Patients with milder strokes, including the ones who may have delayed seeking medical attention because their symptoms were so mild.[227,241,244,245,297] By the time they reach the clinic, their signs may have resolved, making it more difficult clinically to be certain that the event was a stroke or what part of the brain was affected.
- Compared with other MR sequences or CT, DWI is much more likely to demonstrate small acute ischaemic lesions, even several weeks after the event (Fig. 5.47).[226,227,241,297,298]
- DWI may show several acute lesions in different arterial territories, of which only one is symptomatic, and these patients are much more likely to have a cardiac embolic source which might otherwise have gone undetected for longer.[299,300]
- DWI can help distinguish mild cortical from subcortical infarction,[242,297,298,301–303] which might alter secondary prevention strategies.
- DWI can distinguish new from old infarcts in patients where it is unclear whether a deterioration in neurological state could be due to intercurrent illness or a recurrent stroke.[245,249]

In contrast, in patients with more severe strokes seen acutely, CT will often show the ischaemic lesion (see below) and can certainly exclude haemorrhage and most other causes of the symptoms, enabling appropriate treatment decisions to be made, and it is unclear whether demonstrating small ischaemic lesions in patients with TIAs should alter management (see above) – all TIAs need urgent investigation and implementation of rapid appropriate secondary prevention measures.

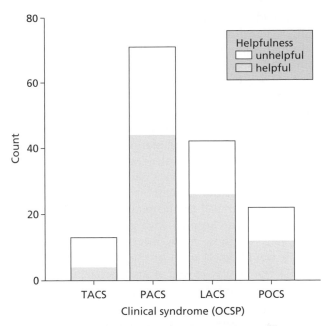

Fig. 5.47 The helpfulness of DWI compared with T2-weighted imaging in different clinical subtypes of ischaemic stroke. DWI scans were defined as 'helpful' if they distinguished a new from an old infarct or identified a new infarct not visible on T2-weighted imaging, and 'unhelpful' if recent infarction was visible on both DWI and T2-weighted imaging, or DWI did not demonstrate a recent lesion, or the scans were uninterpretable. 'Count' is number of scans considered helpful or unhelpful. The largest proportions of 'helpful' DWI scans are in the partial anterior circulation syndromes (PACS), lacunar syndromes (LACS) and posterior circulation syndromes (POCS) rather than total anterior circulation syndromes (TACS).[241] (Figure prepared by Dr S. Keir, Edinburgh. Reproduced with permission of *Journal of Neuroimaging*, © 2004 Blackwell Publishing.)

> In general, the patients in whom DWI is most likely to provide information not available from other imaging techniques are those with milder strokes, including the ones who may have delayed seeking medical attention because their symptoms were so mild.

Should the definition of stroke or TIA require a visible ischaemic lesion to be present on imaging? No

The increase in visibility of small ischaemic lesions made possible by DWI has led to recent suggestions that the definition of stroke and TIA should be changed from one which is clinically based to one which requires imaging demonstration of a visible ischaemic lesion in an appropriate area of the brain for the patient's symptoms.[252,304] Is this wise? This point has been discussed already (section 3.2), but we would just draw the reader's attention to a few further points about the imaging itself.

It should be readily apparent from all the discussion that *no* imaging technique will show an appropriate ischaemic lesion in *all* strokes (or all TIAs). In addition, minor adjustments in how a particular sequence is obtained (e.g. increasing the slice gap or using fewer averages) can alter the chances of detecting smaller lesions.[252] Scanning at different times, e.g. in one hospital stroke/TIA patients are scanned on arrival but in another hospital many patients are not scanned until the next day, would alter lesion detection – some lesions that were present at 6 h might have disappeared by 24 h, and some that were not present at 3 h might be visible by 24 h. And what if the hospital has a CT but not an MR scanner? The hospital with the MR scanner would on average diagnose many more strokes because with DWI it would detect most of the 50% of small lesions that CT would miss, as well as acute ischaemic lesions in TIA patients. Thus, by chance, a patient in a town with

several hospitals could end up diagnosed as a stroke in one, but not in the other, if the two hospitals had different imaging resources (or even if they had the same resources but the scanners were set up differently) and if undue reliance were placed on imaging. What about the patient with the absolutely 'barn door' stroke neurologically but with persistently negative imaging? Are they not a stroke? And what about the patient with no history of neurological disorder and no neurological signs but a subcortical or cortical infarct on imaging? Is this a stroke (Fig. 5.48)? This problem of shifting definition and consequence for clinical practice is not unlike the effect that measurement of plasma troponin has had on the diagnosis of myocardial infarction, except that troponins are measured by a standard laboratory assay on an easily transportable blood sample, and even if the assay is not available in a particular hospital, troponins can be assessed retrospectively from a stored sample taken at hospital

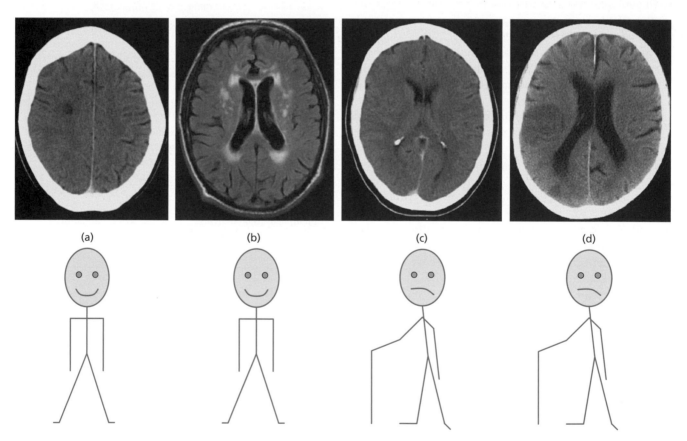

Fig. 5.48 A cartoon to illustrate the problem of increasing dependence on imaging to define stroke. (a) The patient has no symptoms of stroke but the brain CT to investigate chronic headache showed a small right hemisphere subcortical infarct – was this a 'stroke'? (b) At a nearby hospital MR is used routinely to investigate headache and commonly shows even more subcortical infarcts – the patient had no symptoms – should this be called a 'stroke'? (c) The patient had a definite right hemisphere lacunar stroke clinically but the brain CT was normal – overdependence on imaging might mean this case was inappropriately not regarded as a stroke, unless perhaps DWI was available and it showed a recent infarct. (d) This patient had a definite right hemisphere cortical stroke clinically and the CT scan shows an infarct in the right parietal cortex, so no argument here.

admission. Unfortunately, neither imaging technology nor whole patients are as easily stored or shipped.

The problem would be particularly dangerous if applied to TIAs – a patient with a TIA clinically but no lesion on imaging might be sent away without secondary preventive treatment or investigations to exclude carotid stenosis or cardiac source of embolism and remain at high risk of having a disabling stroke. We would have thrown away over 50 years of hard-won medical knowledge through the simple mistake of thinking that a TIA without an acute ischaemic lesion cannot be a TIA and therefore is not at risk of disabling stroke and does not need secondary prevention.

It is unlikely that imaging will ever be standardized to the point that we could overcome these sources of variation, or that imaging becomes so available that we could keep scanning the patient until a lesion showed up if the scan were initially negative. It would be much more sensible to stick with the definition that we have already, train physicians to apply it uniformly, and use imaging to answer specific questions that will guide medical management in an intelligent fashion.[305] All this will need to be worked out over the next few years to arrive at a happy medium. A definition written prior to the explosion in technology that we have witnessed over the last 30 years is bound to appear out of date, but we need to retain what is sensible in the old and add what is sensible from the new.

Perfusion-weighted MRI

Perfusion-weighted imaging (PWI) can be performed in two ways to examine the patency of the cerebral microcirculation:[306] either by using the magnetic properties of flowing blood ('arterial spin labelling')[307] or by injecting an intravenous contrast agent, such as gadolinium, to identify parts of the brain with reduced blood flow through the capillary microcirculation.[308] The former technique is still in development, because although the theory has been around for some time, there are still serious practical limitations to overcome (e.g. long acquisition time, and so the patient has to keep very still) and consequently there are very few reports of its use in stroke patients. The latter technique is more widely used, but requires an injection and takes additional time to set up the scan, although it only takes a few minutes to acquire the imaging data. There are concerns about the validity of the assumptions underlying the various processing methods required to extract accurate perfusion information,[308,309] and debate about how best to extract perfusion information from the concentration–time curve (Fig. 5.49),[144,310,311] and still most studies have included relatively small numbers of patients, making it difficult to draw generalizable conclusions.

Several parameters can be calculated from the concentration–time curve produced as the contrast passes through the brain (Fig. 5.49), some of which relate to cerebral blood volume, mean transit time or cerebral blood flow, or to combinations of these. Most of these parameters produce 'semi-quantitative' ($_{sq}$, relative), not 'quantitative' ($_q$, absolute) perfusion values. In general, 'semi-quantitative' measures require less intensive processing than 'quantitative' measures,[312,313] and include parameters such as:

- time-to-peak (TTP), which may be a good estimate of mean transit time (MTT),[314] but is difficult to compare between imaging episodes;[308]

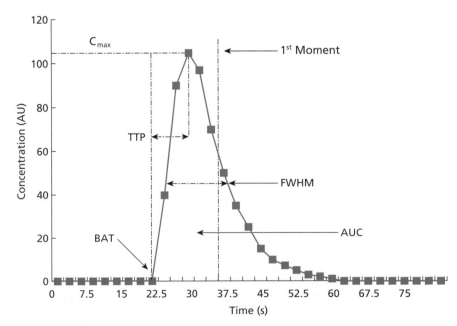

Fig. 5.49 Dynamic susceptibility-weighted perfusion imaging curve obtained from the passage of contrast through the brain showing the different parameters which may be extracted from the curve to estimate various aspects of cerebral perfusion. Full width half maximum (FWHM); 1st moment, 'balancing point' of curve along the time axis; C_{max}, maximum concentration value (also known as peak height); time to peak (TTP), time from arrival of contrast to C_{max} (also known as T_{max} after deconvolution); BAT, bolus arrival time; AUC, area under curve. AU, arbitrary units. (The figure was prepared by Dr Trevor Carpenter, Edinburgh.)

- cerebral blood volume (CBV$_{sq}$), calculated from the area under the curve;
- MTT$_{sq}$, calculated from the first moment of the concentration–time curve;[308]
- cerebral blood flow (CBF$_{sq}$), calculated as CBV$_{sq}$/MTT$_{sq}$.[315]

Colour-coded maps can be produced of each of these parameters to display the pattern of perfusion slice by slice through the brain (Fig. 5.50). 'Quantitative' perfusion (also called 'absolute') requires deconvolution of the concentration–time curve with an arterial input function:[308,312,313] CBFq may be calculated as the height, and CBVq as the area under, the deconvolved concentration–time curve; and MTTq as CBVq/CBFq.[308,312,313] CBV is not considered a good predictor of 'tissue-at-risk' due to its bimodal nature and insensitivity to bolus delay and dispersion.[316] Thus, parameters reflecting CBF and MTT have emerged as the most likely candidates for predicting final infarct extent.

If PWI were to be useful, it would be by identifying tissue, not visible by other means, that might go on to infarct without any intervention. Many studies have tried to identify a perfusion threshold that distinguished viable from infarcted tissue. Only 13 studies have assessed final infarct extent at 1 month or later and were sufficiently reliable for further consideration. These data are bedevilled by small sample sizes (average $n = 24$), different PWI lesion measurement methods, and inappropriate statistical tests (parametric instead of non-parametric). Of the 13 studies with adequate methodology, only three compared the size of the PWI lesion of quantitative CBF and MTT;[316–318] two found that quantitative CBF[316,318] and one that quantitative MTT[317] lesion size related best to final infarct volume. None directly compared lesion sizes produced by semi-quantitative CBF and MTT (more rapidly calculated than 'quantitative' data acutely). In the remainder, TTP lesion size correlated strongly with final infarct volume,[271,286] and both semi-quantitative and quantitative MTT and MTT lesions overestimated final infarct volume.[269,319–324] Only four studies included patients who did not receive thrombolysis or experimental agents.[269,316,317,323]

We have compared semi-quantitative CBF and MTT and DWI lesion size at baseline with final T2 infarct extent obtained at least 1 month after stroke in 46 acute stroke patients who did not receive thrombolysis.[311] The baseline DWI and semi-quantitative CBF lesion sizes were not significantly different from final T2-weighted lesion volume, but baseline semi-quantitative MTT lesions were significantly larger. The correlation with final T2-weighted lesion volume was strongest for DWI, intermediate for semi-quantitative CBF, and weakest for semi-quantitative MTT baseline lesion volumes. These results, in general agreement with previous studies, indicate that MTT lesions (semi-quantitative or quantitative) overestimate tissue at risk, and CBF provides a closer estimate of final infarct extent, although the DWI lesion itself is a reasonably good indicator.

Some have attempted to identify perfusion thresholds (rather than PWI lesions) that predict tissue infarction. Of these, the following studies were of reliable methodological design and found the following thresholds:

- Semi-quantitative perfusion thresholds for prediction of infarction included: CBF = 0.59, CBV = 0.85, and MTT = 1.63,[316] and CBF = 0.70 (quantitative CBF = 33.9 ± 9.7 mL/100 g brain min) and CBV = 1.20 (quantitative CBV = 4.2 ± 1.9 mL/100 g).[323]
- Quantitative perfusion thresholds included: an average MTT delay of 8.3 s in tissue that proceeded to infarction[321] but warned that MTT and CBF values overlapped significantly, and CBV values were not significantly different between infarcted and 'salvaged' tissue.
- The final study simply warned against using a single perfusion parameter threshold, because different perfusion parameters provide complementary information about the complex physiology of ischaemic tissue.[317]

Two recent systematic reviews identified wide variation in the methods used for processing PWI data with no common standard or agreement as to which parameter most closely predicted final clinical outcome or infarct size,[310] or agreement about thresholds that identified salvageable brain.[144] Processing the same MR perfusion data from 30 patients by 10 different methods (Fig. 5.50) resulted in considerable variation in the proportion of patients with any perfusion lesion, the size of any visible perfusion lesion, and the proportion of patients with diffusion/perfusion mismatch (see below). It is unclear at present which, if any, of these perfusion lesions should be used to guide clinical practice. Thus, on the information available to date, there does not appear to be an MR perfusion threshold that reliably distinguishes salvageable from dead tissue.

Diffusion-perfusion mismatch

As an alternative to measures of perfusion-weighted imaging (PWI) alone, it has been suggested that the difference between the extent of the lesion demonstrated on diffusion imaging and that on perfusion imaging may represent the reversibly damaged, potentially salvageable brain, or penumbra, so called 'diffusion-perfusion mismatch'. Knowledge of the extent of this salvageable brain might then be useful to guide the choice of acute stroke treatment, such as thrombolytic

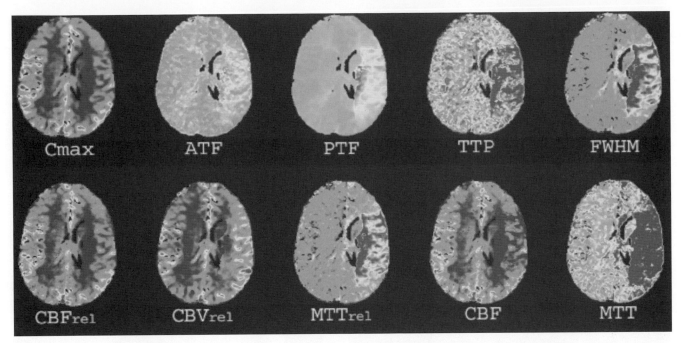

Fig. 5.50 The different perfusion maps generated from the ten different perfusion processing methods (from curve in Fig. 5.49) applied to the same perfusion data acquisition from one patient (same slice shown for each of the 10 methods). See Fig. 5.49 for abbreviations. Also reproduced in colour in the plate section. (Figure prepared by Dr Trevor Carpenter, Edinburgh.)

therapy.[325] However, this concept may be an over-simplification of the relatively complex processes taking place in the affected brain,[198] compounded by major uncertainties about how to extract the perfusion data. Nonetheless, there have been many studies of DWI and PWI suggesting that mismatch does predict infarct growth, and despite the absence of any randomized trials clearly showing it also predicts response to thrombolysis treatment, some clinicians are already using MR DWI/PWI to guide clinical decision making,[325] and to select patients for inclusion in randomized trials of new treatments.[326]

But how good is the evidence that mismatch predicts a group of patients with a different outcome, or who might benefit more from some treatments than patients without mismatch? In our recent systematic review of DWI/PWI mismatch and outcome, only 11 of 1652 papers initially identified were methodologically reliable, with a total sample of 641 patients.[310] However, less than half of these papers actually provided data on mismatch and outcome,[271,316,317] so the total amount of information available on this relationship is much less. There was wide variation in the definition of mismatch (the commonest being a PWI : DWI ratio of > 1.2) and in the PWI lesion used (although most tested a mean transit time derivative). The available data showed that mismatch (vs no mismatch) *without* thrombolysis was

associated with a non-significant twofold increase in the odds of infarct expansion (OR 2.2), which did not change *with* thrombolysis (OR 2.0). Half the patients without mismatch also had infarct growth, and thrombolysis did not change the odds ratio (Fig. 5.51).[310]

These data suggest that mismatch may be associated with an increased risk of infarct growth but are very unreliable, particularly on the question of whether thrombolysis changes infarct growth. A trial testing the mismatch hypothesis is ongoing (EPITHET).[327] About half of our own 46-patient cohort had mismatch on admission, and neither DWI/CBF nor DWI/MTT mismatch (both PWI parameters were semi-quantitative) predicted lesion growth; lesion growth was equally common in those *with and without* mismatch.[311] Thus although 'DWI/PWI mismatch' is being used to identify patients for inclusion in trials of stroke treatments,[326] our results imply that patients without 'mismatch' may also benefit and should not be denied that possibility by being excluded from acute stroke treatment trials.

It is conceivable that the mismatch approach could be used to extend the time window for treatment. There is increasing evidence of viable but at risk tissue up to 24 h after stroke, which might be amenable to thrombolytic or other treatment.[328] For example, thrombolysis is currently licensed for use within 3 h of stroke, but

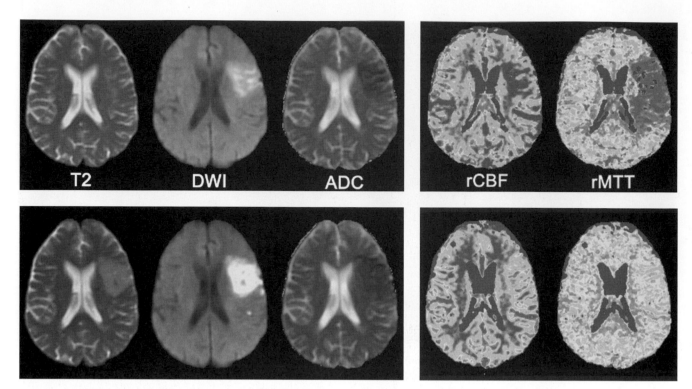

Fig. 5.51 An example of MR diffusion-perfusion mismatch. *Top row*: 4 h after onset of right hemiparesis shows T2, diffusion, ADC, relative CBF and mean transit time (relative MTT) maps. There is early ischaemic change on diffusion and ADC but not on T2; a perfusion deficit is visible on CBF and MTT, largest on MTT, but larger than the diffusion lesion on both CBF and MTT. The 'DWI/CBF mismatch' would be smaller than the 'DWI/MTT mismatch'. *Bottom row*: 7 days after stroke, the infarct is now visible on T2, diffusion and ADC and there is no longer any lesion on CBF or MTT which indicates reperfusion. The diffusion lesion does not seem to have grown particularly. This patient did not receive thrombolysis, so these perfusion changes were spontaneous. Also reproduced in colour in the plate section.

some clinicians use mismatch to decide whether to treat patients with thrombolysis between 3 and 6 h of stroke, and trials using DWI/PWI mismatch to select patients up to 9 h after stroke has recently finished (DIAS,[326] DEDAS and DIAS 2).

MR angiography

Magnetic resonance angiography allows the acquisition of images of blood vessels, without injection of contrast, by using the signal characteristics of flowing blood.[329–331] This technique can be used in acute ischaemic stroke, but the patient must keep very still for several minutes so it is not always of practical help (Fig. 5.52). It is used for the assessment of carotid stenosis in patients being considered for carotid endarterectomy (section 6.8.5)[332] and is also being evaluated for the detection of intracranial aneurysms (section 9.4.3). We do not use it routinely in acute stroke as there is no good evidence that routinely identifying the presence of arterial occlusion influences management in the majority of patients. We use it in specific

circumstances such as suspected arterial dissection or venous disease (sections 5.8 and 7.21.3).

5.5.3 Advanced magnetic resonance techniques

Magnetic resonance (MR) permits other useful methods of examining the brain, including MR spectroscopy to show the effect of ischaemia on brain metabolites, and functional MR to identify areas of the brain which control particular body and mind functions. The details of these techniques are beyond the scope of this chapter, but there are excellent reviews describing each technique, as detailed below.

Magnetic resonance spectroscopy

Magnetic resonance spectroscopy (MRS) can demonstrate metabolic changes in ischaemic tissue *in vivo*, particularly hydrogen, phosphate, carbon, fluorine and sodium metabolism.[329,333–335] *N*-acetyl aspartate (considered a marker of 'normal neurones'), creatine and phosphocreatine, choline-containing compounds, lactate

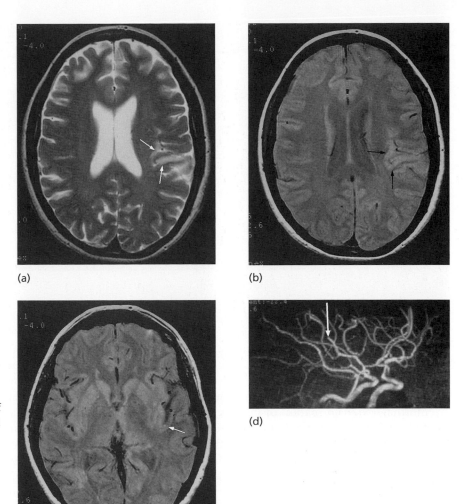

Fig. 5.52 MR imaging with (a) T2, (b,c) proton density and (d) MR angiography of a left middle cerebral artery (MCA) branch occlusion. Note the high signal of recent thrombus is visible on proton density (c, *arrow*) and the infarct in the insular cortex (a,b, *arrows*). (a) On T2 only dark signal mimicking a flow void is visible in the MCA branch so the thrombus might be overlooked. (d) The MR angiogram confirms the MCA branch occlusion (*arrow*). See also Fig. 5.36c.

(a)

(b)

(c)

(d)

and pH have all been measured in stroke patients, but it is still too early to be certain of the significance of the changes.[334,336–338] MRS can be performed by either the single voxel, in which a small cubic volume of brain – typically 8 cm³ – is sampled, or by chemical shift imaging techniques in which spectra from a whole slice of brain are obtained simultaneously (Fig. 5.53). Both scan techniques require the patient to keep still for up to 10 min and are not in routine use.

Functional MR imaging (fMRI)

When a part of the cerebral cortex becomes metabolically active its blood flow increases, thereby changing the MR signal obtained from this part of the brain. For example, if the subject is asked to undertake a task, such as wiggling a finger, while in the MR scanner, and the MR prior to the movement is compared with the image during the task, the difference between the two demonstrates the area of cortex activated by the function. It is thought that areas of the brain which may perhaps be 'taking over' – or at least influencing in some way – the function of damaged areas, can be identified by their activation on fMRI, and the pattern of brain compensation to injury studied during recovery from ischaemic stroke or head injury, or in patients with brain tumours. However, the technique is difficult and great care is required to obtain meaningful results. The subject must keep his or her head very still and only perform (and think about) the requested task, because inadvertent movement of other parts of the body will appear on MR and be misleading. Nonetheless, the technique shows promise by allowing insights into normal brain function as well as into recovery from injury.[339]

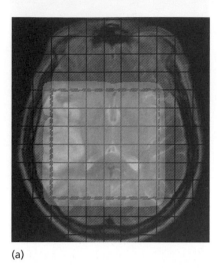
(a)

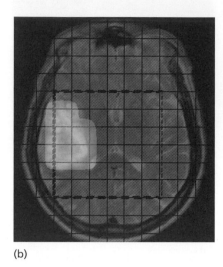
(b)

Fig. 5.53 MR spectroscopic chemical shift imaging at 1 day after stroke in a patient with a right middle cerebral artery infarct. The T2-weighted image is in the background and the spectroscopic colour maps of the distribution of (a) the normal neuronal metabolite *N*-acetyl aspartate (NAA) and (b) the marker of anaerobic metabolism lactate, are superimposed. Red indicates large amounts and blues and greens small amounts of the metabolites. You will need to see the colour plate section to appreciate the following. The area of increased T2 signal of the infarct corresponds with the area of blue on the NAA map (in keeping with neuronal loss) and red on the lactate map (indicating anaerobic metabolism taking place in the infarct). Also reproduced in colour in the plate section.

5.5.4 Comparative studies of CT and MRI in acute stroke

MR is more sensitive for detecting minor degrees of haemorrhagic transformation of infarcts during follow-up, but CT is better than MR (even with gradient echo imaging) for detecting acute intracerebral haemorrhage. Although MR may identify low signal areas indicating haemoglobin breakdown products, these can be quite subtle in the acute stage and CT is simply much easier to interpret.[340] Most studies of intracerebral haemorrhage on MR in hyperacute stroke report apparently high sensitivity for haemorrhage,[159] but in our experience acute haemorrhage can have few distinguishing features from an ischaemic lesion or other pathology and in some cases we have ended up doing a CT scan to make the diagnosis.

Most studies comparing the visibility of ischaemic lesions on brain CT and MRI in acute stroke performed MR after CT, making it likely that MR would be more often abnormal than CT. Some did not take account of the case mix of mild to severe strokes. Only one study apparently randomized the order of scanning,[341] but others found this to be impractical.[151] Several early studies suggested that in patients imaged within the first 6 h of stroke, DWI had a higher sensitivity and specificity and inter-rater reliability than CT.[342–345] All found excellent agreement between CT and DWI. DWI was performed on average 2–3 h after CT in all studies. None mentioned the proportion of patients who could not be scanned with either technique or in whom the images were not diagnostic.

A more recent and complete comparison of CT and MR in consecutive patients with moderate and severe strokes admitted hyperacutely and considered for thrombolysis found that MR could not be obtained in about one-third (patient too unwell, uncooperative, scanner unavailable despite '24-hour' availability) and when both modalities were interpreted using ASPECTS (a structured scoring system for scan interpretation) there was no difference between CT and DWI in the number of infarcts detected or in the inter-rater reliability.[151] Thus for patients admitted and scanned within 6 h of symptom onset, who are likely to have moderate to severe strokes, CT with a structured scoring system can detect as many early infarcts as DWI, detects haemorrhage better than MR, and can image all patients whereas the practical limitations of MR prevent imaging in up to one-third of patients. The situation is different for patients with mild strokes, including lacunar syndromes, and who present later, as discussed above. In this case, MR with DWI and gradient echo imaging is much more likely to show the acute ischaemic lesion (or old haemorrhage) than CT and this patient group is easier to scan with a much higher success rate.

> In patients with moderate to severe strokes, CT with a structured scoring system can detect as many early infarcts within 6 h as DWI, detects haemorrhage better than MR and can image all patients whereas the practical limitations of MR prevent imaging in up to one-third of patients. On the other hand, MRI with DWI is superior for lacunar, posterior fossa and small cortical and subcortical infarcts. Whether MRI is 'better' than CT depends on the question being asked of imaging. MRI is certainly less practical and takes longer.

5.6 Other 'sophisticated' methods of imaging cerebral ischaemia

Single-photon emission CT

Single-photon emission CT (SPECT) is a technique in which cross-sectional images of the brain are obtained by using either a rotating gamma-camera, or a dedicated SPECT scanner, and computerized reconstruction of the data from the emitted radiation following intravenous administration of a radioactive isotope. Various isotopes are available, such as hexamethyl propylene amine oxime (HMPAO) (Ceretec) which images regional perfusion and therefore can identify areas of abnormal perfusion early, or xenon-133, which can measure regional cerebral blood flow quantitatively.[346] However, the equipment for SPECT is not widely available, the scanning times are long (20 min or more) and so problems caused by movement artifacts can arise from restless stroke patients, and the isotopes are expensive. A potential source of error, which is particularly relevant to ischaemic stroke, is that blood–brain barrier breakdown alters the behaviour of the isotope and hence the accuracy and interpretation of the images.[347]

SPECT can demonstrate appropriate areas of low flow within a few hours of stroke onset, and even up to 60% of patients with a transient ischaemic attack have an appropriate abnormality within 24 h of onset.[348] In acute ischaemic stroke, SPECT demonstrates an area of relative hypoperfusion corresponding with the ischaemic tissue in most patients studied, although very few if any lacunar stroke patients were included in the studies.[348–353] Several studies have indicated that the size of the initial perfusion deficit on SPECT predicts the likely clinical outcome: the larger the deficit, the worse the outcome.[84,350–353] Also, evidence of reperfusion on SPECT is associated with improved clinical outcome both spontaneously[352,353] and in response to thrombolytic therapy.[84,354,355] In the first week after the stroke, the relative blood flow in the infarct may be increased or decreased, corresponding with luxury perfusion or persistent hypoperfusion, respectively.[356]

Abnormalities may be visible not only in the infarct itself, but also in remote parts of the brain, such as the opposite cerebral hemisphere or the contralateral cerebellum in patients with cerebral cortical infarcts.[357,358] This has given rise to the concept of 'diaschisis' or 'shutdown' of areas of the brain not directly involved in the infarct but whose function is in some way influenced, possibly through association fibres.[359] There is some evidence of clinical correlates of 'shutdown' of these areas in terms of symptoms and signs not fully explained by loss of the area of brain directly involved in the infarct.[358,359]

Positron emission tomography

Positron emission tomography (PET) can display a variety of physiological processes, from glucose metabolism to neuroreceptor density, thus allowing study of the normal workings of the brain, as well as the consequences of pathology.[360–362] The data, derived from collection and analysis of complicated signals from positron-emitting isotopes, may be shown as colour-coded tomographic pictures. PET has been available since the 1970s, but the imaging equipment and isotopes are extremely expensive, the scan times are prolonged and the patient must keep very still. Therefore PET is likely to remain a research tool with limited clinical applications, at least in stroke for the foreseeable future.[363,364]

PET studies in ischaemic stroke have provided evidence that the ischaemic penumbra really does exist in humans and that neural tissue in the penumbra may survive for up to 48 h.[328,361,365–368] They have also suggested that neurones in areas of the brain with cerebral blood flow below the threshold traditionally regarded as producing irreversible damage (<9 mL/100 g brain/min) may be able to recover after successful reperfusion with thrombolysis,[367,369,370] although probably not below 8.4 mL/100 g brain/min.[371] Use of tracers such as [^{18}F]fluoromisonidazole, a ligand binding to hypoxic but viable tissue, has shown that white matter may remain viable for longer than grey matter after a given ischaemic insult.[228] Comparison between PET and MR DWI/PWI in the same patients showed that the 'mismatch' area on DWI/PWI was viable (normal cerebral metabolic rate for oxygen) but had variable oxygen extraction fraction,[372] and in only half the patients did the mismatch volume correspond with the 'penumbra' (ischaemic but viable) volume defined by PET. This variability helps to explain the lack of a clear association between diffusion/perfusion mismatch and infarct growth (section 5.5.2).

5.7 Differentiating haemorrhagic transformation of an infarct from intracerebral haemorrhage

Haemorrhagic transformation of an infarct (HTI) is an aspect of stroke pathophysiology which has been difficult to assess and there are many misconceptions about its clinical relevance. The exact frequency is almost impossible to measure. Postmortem studies are biased towards severe strokes and only give a 'snapshot' of the brain at the point of death, leaving one to speculate on events earlier in the course of the stroke. Although imaging *in vivo* offers some improvement over autopsy, the studies have been small and there has never been a study where every patient had either a follow-up CT scan or a postmortem, so they have given a biased estimate of the frequency of HTI and its clinical associations (see below).

HTI can usefully be thought of as being either asymptomatic (i.e. picked up on repeat brain imaging but not associated with worsening of symptoms) or symptomatic (definite deterioration in symptoms associated with the appearance of new haemorrhage into an infarct on imaging). HTI is also described as 'petechial' (little areas of patchy haemorrhage without frank intracerebral haemorrhage) or as an intracerebral haemorrhage, although definitions vary which accounts for some of the variability of HTI frequency in published studies.

Appearance of haemorrhagic transformation of an infarct on CT or MR

Typically, HTI is distinguished from intracerebral haemorrhage (ICH) by the lack of homogeneity of the haemorrhagic area which lies within, or on the edge of, an area of low density confined to a single arterial territory, i.e. within a presumed infarct. However, it is clear that some cases which appear radiologically to be ICHs are actually caused by HTI occurring within hours of stroke onset, the so-called intra-infarct haematomas.[373] Indeed, the HTI can look so like an ICH on CT or MR that, without a prior scan showing no haemorrhage, the patient would have been labelled as ICH. The extent of this problem will become clearer with more experience of early scanning. Currently, however, there are no absolute rules for distinguishing those early HTIs which obliterate the infarct from a 'true' ICH.

> Haemorrhagic transformation of an infarct can occur very early after stroke onset and make the infarct look just like an intracerebral haemorrhage on brain CT or MR.

The more commonly seen forms of HTI consist of serpiginous areas of increased density (whiteness) on CT (or of appropriate signal characteristics on MR) at the margins of the infarct (Fig. 5.54); more obvious patchy areas of increased density throughout the infarct; or as

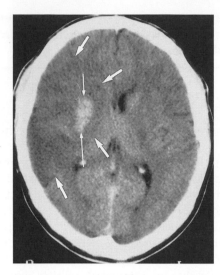

Fig. 5.54 CT brain scan showing petechial haemorrhage (*thin arrows*) into a right temporoparietal infarct (*thick arrows*) at 36 h after the stroke. The haemorrhage was not particularly dense, unlike a haematoma (see also Fig. 5.41).

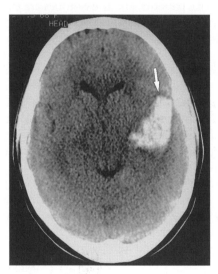

Fig. 5.55 CT brain scan showing very early haemorrhagic transformation of a left temporal arterial infarct. The scan was obtained within 3 h of onset of a right hemiparesis and shows a fairly dense haematoma in the left temporal region (*arrow*). Angiography immediately after the scan showed the proximal left middle cerebral artery (MCA) mainstem to be occluded by an embolus with dilated lenticulostriate arteries (collateral supply). The source of the embolus was never found. A repeat angiogram at 2 months showed that the left MCA had recanalized.

obvious haematomas exerting mass effect (Fig. 5.55). In large infarcts involving the cortex, curvilinear bands of increased density may be seen at the cortical edge, at the junction of the lesion with white matter and within the lesion, in the second and third weeks after the stroke. These areas also enhance markedly with X-ray and are thought to correspond with areas where the capillaries are leaky, where there is blood–brain barrier breakdown, and where there is frank petechial haemorrhage at postmortem.[53]

The influence of observer variability and visual perception

Some of the variability in the reported frequency of petechial haemorrhage must be a result of inter-observer variation, but this is less likely to apply to focal haematomas.[62,374,375] The visual perception of the density of normal brain is influenced by the density of adjacent tissue; normal brain next to the low density of an infarct looks of higher density than it really is, and so can be mistaken for areas of haemorrhage (Fig. 5.56). To avoid this mistake, the density of the brain can be measured on the CT console to distinguish petechial haemorrhage from normal brain. There are no data on observer variability in detection of HTI on MR.

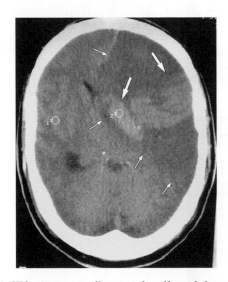

Fig. 5.56 CT brain scan to illustrate the effect of altered brain density on visual perception. The scan was from a 40-year-old man at 24 h after a left middle cerebral artery occlusion causing an extensive left hemispheric infarct (*thin arrows*). The areas of hyperattenuation (*thick arrows*) within the low density of the infarct were interpreted as being caused by haemorrhage by the clinician because of their apparent brightness. However, the actual density when measured on the CT scanning console was the same as normal grey matter, indicating that the areas of hyperattenuation were in fact islands of surviving, i.e. non-infarcted, brain and not haemorrhage at all. Area 1 (normal right insular cortex) was 51 Hounsfield units (HU: unit for measurement of density on CT) and area 2 (apparent increased density within the left infarct) was 46 HU. Blood generally registers at around 70–80 HU.

Frequency, risk factors and clinical relevance of haemorrhagic transformation of an infarct

Our systematic review of CT and MR scanning indicated that some degree of petechial haemorrhage occurs in 15–45% of patients and of symptomatic haematoma formation in 2.5–5%, at some point within 1–2 weeks after stroke.[374] This may be an under- or overestimate for the following reasons:

- the studies were generally small and few were of consecutive patients or prospective;
- not all patients were followed up, only survivors or those who remained in hospital for the study period;
- the definition of HTI was not stated in all the publications;
- the influence of inter-observer variability was not taken into account;
- the generation of scanner used varied and hence the sensitivity of the diagnosis of HTI;
- the number of patients given antithrombotic drugs was often not stated (the frequency of HTI generally increased with the amount of antithrombotic or thrombolytic drug given).

There was limited information suggesting that the major risk factors for HTI were large infarcts and increasing doses of antithrombotic or thrombolytic drugs, but we were not able to find an association with cardio-embolic stroke as has been previously suggested. We did not find any association with raised blood pressure.

The Multicentre rt-PA Acute Stroke Survey (MASS, an observational study of patients receiving open label thrombolysis) found associations between increased patient age, stroke severity, plasma glucose and falling platelet count with asymptomatic and symptomatic HTI.[376]

While minor degrees of HTI are regarded as asymptomatic, there is some evidence that any degree of bleeding inside the head may be associated with a worse outcome.[377,378] A combined analysis of all trials of plasminogen actvator showed that any asymptomatic intracranial haemorrhage reduced the probability of a good outcome by 30% (95% CI 60% reduction to 12% increase) – although not statistically significant, all the studies were underpowered to detect a statistically significant effect for which a trial of more than 4000 patients would be needed.[378]

Possible mechanisms of haemorrhagic transformation of an infarct

Traditionally, HTI was considered to occur when an arterial occlusion, usually embolic from the heart, resulted in ischaemia of the distal capillary bed and then, with fragmentation of the embolus, this ischaemic area was resubjected to arterial pressure, resulting in rupture of the necrotic arterioles and capillaries.[379] This notion arose from work with postmortem brains, but is clearly biased towards patients who die in the early stages of their stroke and who are therefore more likely to have had a large cerebral infarct. The signs of haemorrhage resolve with time so that, in patients dying weeks or months after their stroke, it may no longer be possible to distinguish the relative contribution of infarct and haemorrhage in the residual lesion.

The idea that embolism is the cause of HTI has become rather entrenched. However, closer examination of the literature shows that the situation is more complicated than the reperfusion–haemorrhagic transformation hypothesis would suggest.[380] Shortly before Fisher and Adam's (1951)[279] work became so widely publicized and accepted, Globus and Epstein[381] published the results of experimental cerebral infarction in monkeys and dogs and some observations on postmortem brains from stroke patients. They observed that haemorrhage into infarcted tissue was often worse when the occluded

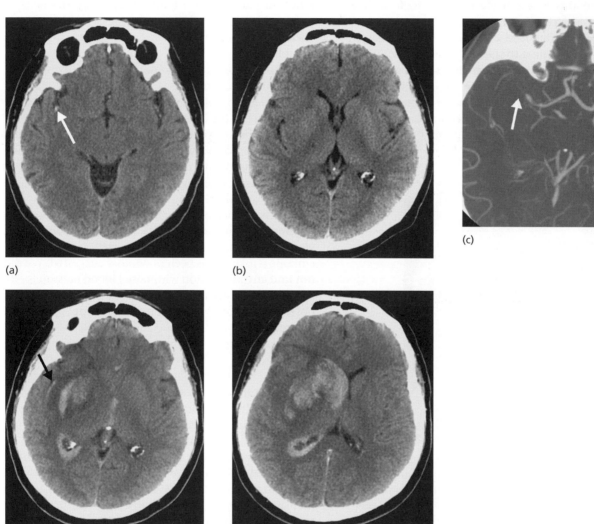

(a)   (b)   (c)

(d)   (e)

Fig. 5.57 Unenhanced CT brain scan at 2.5 h after onset of left hemiparesis. (a) The right middle cerebral artery (MCA) main stem is hyperattenuated (*arrow*) and (b) there is early parenchymal hypoattenuation in the right insular and posterior frontal cortex consistent with an early ischaemic stroke. (c) CT angiography confirmed the occluded right MCA (*arrow*). Intravenous thrombolysis was given immediately after the CT angiogram. (d,e) Eighteen hours later the patient deteriorated with worsening of the left hemiparesis and drowsiness, and repeat unenhanced CT showed extensive haemorrhagic transformation of the right MCA territory infarct with blood in the right lateral ventricle (d,e), and (d) persistent right MCA hyperattenuation (occlusion, *arrow*). There was also remote haemorrhage in the right cerebellum. In other words, haemorrhagic transformation is not simply a consequence of recanalization.

symptomatic artery *remained* occluded, and that the haemorrhage seemed to occur around the periphery of the infarct from collateral arterioles and postcapillary venules vasodilating to supply the ischaemic tissue and then leaking. They produced massive intracerebral haemorrhages in dogs by this means, although they noted differences between the species which seemed to depend on the adequacy of the collateral supply. This alternative, but possibly equally attractive, hypothesis has been all but forgotten, although it probably deserves further attention with increasing use of thrombolysis.

There is still debate about the effect of reperfusion of an infarct. Previously, it was thought that early recanalization, such as might occur with spontaneous lysis of an embolus, increased the risk of haemorrhagic transformation. However, several recent studies have contradicted this, suggesting that haemorrhage is more common into infarcts where the artery remains occluded, as shown by catheter angiography.[380,382–384] A substudy of 52 patients, randomized in the second European Cooperative Acute Stroke Study (ECASS II) of intravenous recombinant tissue plasminogen activator (rt-PA) using single-photon emission computed tomography (SPECT), found that patients with proximal middle cerebral artery occlusion and poor collaterals (i.e. very poor perfusion of the infarct) who did not reperfuse were the most likely to develop HTI; in the placebo group the haemorrhage was less extensive than in patients who received rt-PA; and patients with evidence of reperfusion of the infarct on SPECT were *less* likely to have haemorrhagic transformation.[84] Figure 5.57 shows a patient with a hyperattenuated middle cerebral artery (MCA) on admission who developed massive HTI 24 h later but the hyperattenuated MCA is still visible. Thus it would appear that, contrary to previous thinking, HTI is more likely to occur in the absence rather than the presence of reperfusion, but there are obviously still many unanswered questions about the causes, associated factors and clinical significance of HTI and the influence of commonly used treatments such as thrombolysis.

> Haemorrhagic transformation of an infarct is more likely in patients who do not recanalize the occluded artery, as opposed to those who do, contrary to previous thinking.

5.8 Imaging of intracranial venous thrombosis

(See also section 7.21)

Venous infarcts are probably more common than originally thought, but frequently misdiagnosed as arterial infarcts, intracerebral haemorrhages, or tumours on CT and MR. In our experience there are often clues on imaging which should point to the correct diagnosis. Many are overlooked simply because the possibility of venous infarction is not even considered (Table 5.4). In fact, intracranial venous thrombosis is a spectrum,

Table 5.4 Differentiation of arterial from venous infarcts.

	Arterial	Venous
Shape	Wedge or rounded	Usually wedge if cortical, rounded if deep
Number occurring simultaneously	Usually single	May be multiple
Margins	Indistinct early, distinct after several days	Distinct early
Swelling	Develops over days	Marked, appears usually very early
Haemorrhage	Infrequent, peripheral	Frequent, central, finger-like
Attenuation (CT)	Early: slightly hypoattenuated Later: more hypoattenuated	Early: obvious hypoattenuation
Signal (MR)	Early: increased on DWI Later: increased FLAIR, T2	Increased on FLAIR, T2
Additional signs (CT)	Hyperattenuated artery sign	Hyperattenuated sinus sign Empty delta sign (after contrast)
(MR)	Absent flow void; acute thrombus	Absent flow void; acute thrombus

varying from the effects of sinus thrombosis without any brain parenchymal change at one extreme, to purely parenchymal lesions, caused by cortical vein thrombosis (infarction with or without haemorrhage) without sinus thrombosis, at the other end. The clinical presentation and radiological appearance in any individual patient depend on where the patient lies on this spectrum.

Venous infarcts can usefully be thought of in two parts: the primary features of the parenchymal lesion, and the secondary features of sinus thrombosis, one or both of which may be present. Venous infarcts are typically of low attenuation on CT or high signal on MR DWI, FLAIR and T2-weighted imaging, and may be wedge-shaped, like arterial infarcts, but the key differentiating features are:

- not quite in the usual site of an arterial infarct;
- much more swelling than an equivalent-sized, equivalent-aged arterial infarct;

- swelling in the brain remote from the infarct;
- often haemorrhagic (Fig. 5.58),[52,385–387] the haemorrhage being typically in the centre of the low-attenuation area and patchy and finger-like in distribution, unlike arterial infarcts where the haemorrhage is usually around the edges.

Angiography for the veins and sinuses

Non-filling of a sinus, or part of it, on a catheter angiogram is in itself insufficient proof of venous thrombosis. Hypoplasia is an alternative explanation, especially in the case of the left lateral sinus or the anterior third of the superior sagittal sinus. To prove occlusion of a sinus, it is necessary to see delayed emptying or dilatation of collateral veins on the angiogram, or evidence of actual thrombus on CT scanning or MRI (see below and section 5.4.2). In most centres in the developed world,

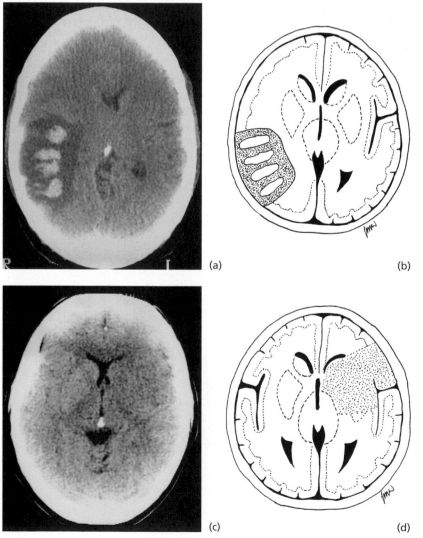

(a) (b) (c) (d)

Fig. 5.58 CT brain scans and diagrams to emphasize the differences between typical arterial and venous infarcts. (a) CT brain scan within 6 h of symptom onset showing a right parietal venous infarct. (b) Drawing of (a) to emphasize the key features: the margins are clearly seen and the lesion is very hypoattenuated even at such a short time after onset; there is marked swelling both within the infarct and within the rest of the hemisphere beyond the infarct; and there are central areas of haemorrhage. (c) CT brain scan within 6 h of symptom onset showing a left parietal arterial infarct. (d) Drawing of (c) to emphasize the key features: the margins are ill defined and the lesion is only slightly hypoattenuated compared with normal brain; there is only slight swelling within the infarct and none beyond it; and there is no haemorrhage.

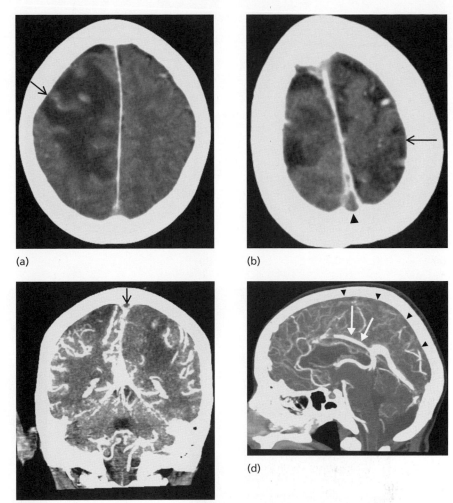

(a) (b)

(c) (d)

Fig. 5.59 CT brain scan and CT venography of intracranial venous thrombosis. (a,b) Post-contrast axial CT of the parietal lobes and sagittal sinus. Note the venous infarcts (bilateral, *arrows*) and the filling defect in the sagittal sinus due to thrombus (*arrowhead*). (c) Coronal CT venogram shows a filling defect in the sagittal sinus (*arrow*) due to thrombus. (d) Sagittal CT venogram showing prominent filling of the inferior sagittal sinus (*arrows*) but the virtual absence of the sagittal sinus (*arrowheads*) due to thrombus preventing contrast entering and outlining the sinus.

MR angiography (MRA) or CT angiography (CTA) has replaced catheter angiography, especially as CTA or MRA in combination with plain CT or other MR techniques respectively can show the thrombus itself (Fig. 5.59).[388]

CT scanning

Brain CT readily shows 'venous' infarcts: not corresponding with a known arterial territory (Figs 5.58, 5.60); commonly with haemorrhagic transformation; sometimes bilaterally, in the parasagittal area (Fig. 5.61) or in the deep regions of the brain (Fig. 5.62), or supra- as well as infratentorial.[52,385] After intravenous contrast, there may be serpiginous enhancement in the centre or at the edges of the infarct (Fig. 5.60). In addition, CT scanning often provides evidence of the underlying sinus thrombosis: the hyperattenuated sinus sign,[385,389,390] seen most clearly in the posterior part of the sagittal sinus ('dense triangle sign') or in the straight sinus (Fig. 5.62). The 'empty delta sign'[386,391] appears only after injection of intravenous contrast, through which enhancement

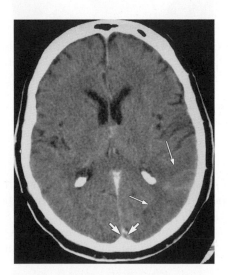

Fig. 5.60 CT brain scan (enhanced) showing a left occipital venous infarct (*thin arrows*) with thrombosis of the superior sagittal sinus as shown by the 'empty delta' sign (*thick arrow*) and serpiginous enhancement in the centre of the infarct (*open arrow*).

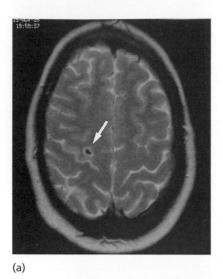

(a)

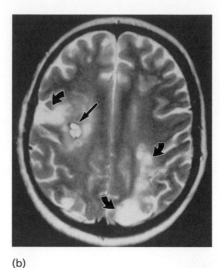

(b)

Fig. 5.61 T2-weighted MR images from two different patients to illustrate parasagittal haematomas found in venous sinus thrombosis. (a) A patient with sagittal sinus thrombosis and a small haemorrhage in the right parasagittal parietal cortex (*arrow*). (b) Another patient with sagittal sinus thrombosis with a right parasagittal haemorrhage (*arrow*) and infarcts in the left occipital and right parietal regions (*curved arrows*). Note that in neither case was there an obvious filling defect in the sagittal sinus on T2.

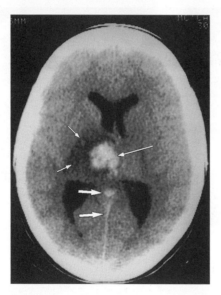

Fig. 5.62 CT brain scan (unenhanced) showing a right thalamic haematoma (*long thin arrow*) caused by infarction secondary to thrombosis of the deep cerebral veins. Note the increased density in the straight sinus (*thick arrows*) caused by the thrombus in the sinus (hyperattenuated sinus sign), the general brain swelling, and low density around the haemorrhage (*short small arrows*) indicating the venous infarct.

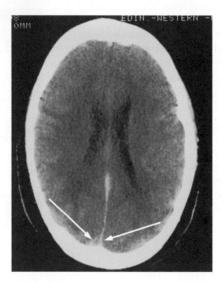

Fig. 5.63 CT brain scan with intravenous contrast shows a triangular filling defect outlined by contrast in the posterior sagittal sinus ('empty delta sign'; *arrows*) (see also Fig. 5.59).

occurs of the wall but not in the thrombus in the centre of the (posterior) part of the sagittal sinus that is perpendicularly imaged on an axial CT slice (Figs 5.59, 5.60 and 5.63). The name of this sign easily sticks in the mind but it is found in only a small number of patients.[392]

MR imaging

The way in which thrombus in dural sinuses appears on MR imaging depends very much on the interval from the time the thrombus began to form to scanning.[393,394] Three stages can be distinguished in its evolution:

- In the acute stage (days 1–5) it appears strongly hypointense on T2-weighted images and isointense on T1-weighted images (rather as for arterial thrombi (Fig. 5.61).
- In the subacute stage (up to day 15) the thrombus signal is strongly hyperintense, initially on T1-weighted images and subsequently also on T2-weighted images.
- The third stage begins 3–4 weeks after symptom onset: the thrombus signal becomes isointense on T1-weighted images but on T2-weighted images it remains hyperintense, although often non-homogeneous. Recanalization may occur over months in up to one-third of patients, but persistent abnormalities are

common and do not signify recurrent thrombosis.[393,395] In the brain parenchyma, early changes of venous congestion can be demonstrated on T2-weighted images or with fluid attenuated inversion recovery (FLAIR) techniques, while diffusion-weighted images show only subtle changes, unlike ischaemia from arterial occlusion.[396,397]

> Persistent abnormalities in the sinus at the site of the original thrombosis are not uncommon and do not signify recurrent thrombosis.

Transcranial Doppler ultrasound

Transcranial Doppler with colour coding and contrast enhancement may show decreased, increased or reversed venous flow parallel to the major intracranial sinuses,[398] abnormal flow velocities in the transverse sinus or in the deep venous system,[399–401] but a normal test far from excludes the diagnosis. It is unlikely that many clinicians will rely on ultrasound techniques alone for making the diagnosis of intracranial venous thrombosis.

References

1 Sudlow CLM, Warlow CP. Comparable studies of the incidence of stroke and its pathological types: results from an international collaboration. *Stroke* 1997; **28**:491–9.

2 Feigin VL, Lawes CM, Bennett DA, Anderson CS. Stroke epidemiology: a review of population-based studies of incidence, prevalence, and case-fatality in the late 20th century. *Lancet Neurol* 2003; **2**:43–53.

3 Keir S, Wardlaw JM, Warlow CP. Have epidemiological studies of stroke incidence underestimated the frequency of primary intracerebral haemorrhage? *Cerebrovasc Dis* 2000; **10**:50.

4 Johansson B, Norrving B, Lindgren A. Increased stroke incidence in Lund-Orup, Sweden, between 1983 to 1985 and 1993 to 1995. *Stroke* 2000; **31**:481–6.

5 Hamad I, Ayman H, Sokrab S, Momani S, Mesraoua B, Ahmed AR. Incidence of stroke in Qatar. *J Stroke Cerebrovasc Dis* 2000; **9**:83–4.

6 Ueda K, Kiyohara Y, Fujishima M. Epidemiology: stroke risk factors in general population: the Hisayama study. *J Stroke Cerebrovasc Dis* 2000; **9**:27–8.

7 Thrift AG, Dewey HM, Macdonell RAL, McNeil JJ, Donnan GA. Incidence of the major stroke subtypes: initial findings from the North East Melbourne Stroke Incidence Study (NEMESIS). *Stroke* 2001; **32**:1732–8.

8 Tanizaki Y, Kiyohara Y, Kato I, Iwamoto H, Nakayama K, Shinohara N *et al*. Incidence and risk factors for subtypes of cerebral infarction in a general population; The Hisayama Study. *Stroke* 2001; **31**:2616–22.

9 Wardlaw JM, Keir SL, Dennis MS. The impact of delays in computed tomography of the brain on the accuracy of diagnosis and subsequent management in patients with minor stroke. *J Neurol Neurosurg Psychiatry* 2003; **74**:77–81.

10 Rowe CC, Donnan GA, Bladin PF. Intracerebral haemorrhage: incidence and use of computed tomography. *Br Med J* 1988; **297**:1177–8.

11 Hayward R. VOMIT (victims of modern imaging technology): an acronym for our times. *Br Med J* 2003; **326**:1273.

12 Cameron EW. Transient ischaemic attacks due to meningioma: report of 4 cases. *Clin Radiol* 1994; **49**:416–18.

13 Allen CM. Clinical diagnosis of the acute stroke syndrome. *Q J Med* 1983; **52**:515–23.

14 Poungvarin N, Viriyavejakul A, Komontri C. Siriraj stroke score and validation study to distinguish supratentorial intracerebral haemorrhage from infarction. *Br Med J* 1991; **302**:1565–7.

15 Besson G, Robert C, Hommel M, Perret J. Is it clinically possible to distinguish nonhemorrhagic infarct from hemorrhagic stroke? *Stroke* 1995; **26**:1205–9.

16 Lindley R, Sandercock PAG, Wardlaw JM, Sellar R. Can antithrombotic therapy be started in acute stroke patients without CT scanning. In: *Book of Abstracts from the Proceedings of the Second International Conference on Stroke, The World Federation of Neurology*, Geneva, 12–15 May 1993, p. 20.

17 Celani MG, Ceravolo MG, Duca E, Minciotti P, Caputo N, Orlandini M. Was it infarction or haemorrhage? A clinical diagnosis by means of the Allen score. *J Neurol* 1992; **239**:411–13.

18 Weir CJ, Murray GD, Adams FG, Muir KW, Grosset DG, Lees KR. Poor accuracy of stroke scoring systems for differential clinical diagnosis of intracranial haemorrhage and infarction. *Lancet* 1994; **344**:999–1002.

19 Hawkins GC, Bonita R, Broad JB, Anderson NE. Inadequacy of clinical scoring systems to differentiate stroke subtypes in population-based studies. *Stroke* 1995; **26**:1338–42.

20 Sohn YH, Kim SM, Kim JS, Kim DI. Benign brainstem haemorrhage simulating transient ischaemic attack. *Yonsei Med J* 1991; **32**:91–3.

21 Aparicio A, Sobrino J, Arboix A, Torres M. Hematoma intraparenquimatoso que simula un accidente isquemico transitorio. *Medicina Clinica* 1995; **104**:478–9.

22 Gunathilake SB. Rapid resolution of symptoms and signs of intracerebral haemorrhage: case reports. *Br Med J* 1998; **316**:1495–6.

23 Ivo L. CT scanning can differentiate between ischaemic attack and haemorrhage. *Lancet* 1999; **319**:1197–8.

24 Evyapan D, Kumral E. Cerebral hemorrhage with transient signs. *Cerebrovasc Dis* 2000; **10**:483–4.

25 Chen WH, Liu JS, Wu SC, Chang YY. Transient global amnesia and thalamic hemorrhage. *Clin Neurol Neurosurg* 1996; **98**:309–11.

26 Scott WR, Miller BR. Intracerebral haemorrhage with rapid recovery. *Arch Neurol* 1985; **42**:133–6.

27 Fishman RA. Cerebrospinal fluid in cerebrovascular disorders. In: Barnett HJM, Mohr JP, Stein BM, Yatsu FM, eds. *Stroke: Pathophysiology, Diagnosis and Management.* New York: Churchill Livingstone, 1992, pp. 103–10.

28 Marchi N, Rasmussen P, Kapural M, Fazio V, Kight K, Mayberg MR *et al.* Peripheral markers of brain damage and blood–brain barrier dysfunction. *Restor. Neurol Neurosci* 2003; **21**:109–21.

29 Barber M, Langhorne P, Rumley A, Lowe GDO, Stott DJ. Hemostatic function and progressing ischemic stroke: D-dimer predicts early clinical progression. *Stroke* 2004; **35**:1421–5.

30 Montaner J, Fernandez-Cadenas I, Molina CA, Ribo M, Huertas R, Rosell A *et al.* Post-stroke C-reactive protein is a powerful prognostic tool among candidates for thrombolysis. *Stroke* 2006; **37**:1205–10.

31 Montaner J, Molina CA, Monasterio J, Abilleira S, Arenillas JF, Ribo M *et al.* Matrix metalloproteinase-9 pretreatment level predicts intracranial hemorrhagic complications after thrombolysis in human stroke. *Circulation* 2003; **107**:598–603.

32 Montaner J, Ribo M, Delgado P, Purroy F, Quintana M, Penalba A *et al.* Biochemical diagnosis of acute stroke using a panel of plasma biomarkers. *Cerebrovasc Dis* 2005; **19**(S2):47.

33 Ambrose J. Computerised transverse axial scanning (tomography): part 2: clinical application. *Br J Radiol* 1973; **46**:1023–47.

34 Paxton R, Ambrose J. EMI scanner: brief review of first 650 patients. *Br J Radiol* 1974; **47**:530–65.

35 Kistler JP, Hochberg FH, Brooks BR, Richardson EP, Jr., New PF, Schnur J. Computerized axial tomography: clinicopathologic correlation. *Neurology* 1975; **25**:201–9.

36 Kinkel WR, Jacobs L. Computerized axial transverse tomography in cerebrovascular disease. *Neurology* 1976; **26**:924–30.

37 Royal College of Radiologists. *Making the Best Use of a Department of Clinical Radiology*, 5th edn. London: Royal College of Radiologists, 2003.

38 Wardlaw JM, Keir SL, Seymour J, Lewis S, Sandercock PA, Dennis MS, Cairns J. What is the best imaging strategy for acute stroke? *Health Technol Assess* 2004; **8**(1):1–180.

39 International Stroke Trial Collaborative Group. The International Stroke Trial (IST): a randomised trial of aspirin, subcutaneous heparin, both, or neither among 19435 patients with acute ischaemic stroke. *Lancet* 1996; **349**:1569–81.

40 Wardlaw JM, Seymour J, Cairns J, Keir S, Lewis S, Sandercock P. Immediate computed tomography scanning of acute stroke is cost-effective and improves quality of life. *Stroke* 2004; **35**:2477–83.

41 Masson M, Prier S, Desbleds MT, Colombani JM, Juliard JM. Transformation d'un infarctus cerebral en hemorragie au cours d'un examen tomodensitometrique, chez un patient sous traitement anticoagulant. *Rev Neurol* (Paris) 1984; **140**(8–9):502–6.

42 Franke FL, Ramos LMP, van Gijn J. Development of multifocal haemorrhage in a cerebral infarct during computed tomography. *J Neurol Neurosurg Psychiatry* 1990; **53**:531–2.

43 Dennis MS, Bamford JM, Molyneux AJ, Warlow CP. Rapid resolution of signs of primary intracerebral haemorrhage in computed tomograms of the brain. *Br Med J* 1987; **295**:379–81.

44 Franke CL, van Swieten JC, van Gijn J. Residual lesions on computed tomography after intracerebral hemorrhage. *Stroke* 1991; **22**:1530–3.

45 Sung CY, Chu NS. Late CT manifestations in spontaneous putaminal haemorrhage. *Neuroradiology* 1992; **34**:200–4.

46 Bradley WG, Jr. Hemorrhage and hemorrhagic infections in the brain. *Neuroimaging Clin N Am* 1994; **4**:707–32.

47 Pierce JN, Taber KH, Hayman LA. Acute intracranial hemorrhage secondary to thrombocytopenia: CT appearances unaffected by absence of clot retraction. *Am J Neuroradiol* 1997; **15**:213–15.

48 Packard AS, Kase CS, Aly AS, Barest GD. 'Computed tomography-negative' intracerebral hemorrhage. *Arch Neurol* 2003; **60**:1156–9.

49 Schriger DL, Kalafut M, Starkman S, Krueger M, Saver JL. Cranial computed tomography interpretation in acute stroke: physician accuracy in determining eligibility for thrombolytic therapy. *J Am Med Assoc* 1998; **279**:1293–7.

50 Pfleger MJ, Hardee EP, Contant CF, Jr., Hayman LA. Sensitivity and specificity of fluid-blood levels for coagulopathy in acute intracerebral hematomas. *Am J Neuroradiol* 1994; **15**:217–23.

51 Miller JH, Wardlaw JM, Lammie GA. Intracerebral haemorrhage and cerebral amyloid angiopathy: CT features with pathological correlation. *Clin Radiol* 1999; **54**:422–9.

52 Bakac G, Wardlaw JM. Problems in the diagnosis of intracranial venous infarction. *Neuroradiology* 1997; **39**:566–70.

53 Inoue Y, Takemoto K, Miyamoto T, Yoshikawa N, Taniguchi S, Saiwai S. Sequential computed tomography scans in acute cerebral infarction. *Radiology* 1980; **135**:655–62.

54 Wall SD, Brant-Zawadzki M, Jeffrey RB, Barnes B. High frequency CT findings within 24 hours after cerebral infarction. *Am J Roentgenol* 1982; **138**:307–11.

55 Tomura N, Uemura K, Inugami A, Fujita H, Higano S, Shishido F. Early CT finding in cerebral infarction: obscuration of the lentiform nucleus. *Radiology* 1988; **168**:463–7.

56 Truwit CL, Barkovich AJ, Gean-Marton A, Hibri N, Norman D. Loss of the insuar ribbon: another early CT

sign of acute middle cerebral artery infarction. *Radiology* 1990; **176**:801–6.

57 Grond M, von Kummer R, Sobesky J, Schmulling S, Heiss WD. Early computed-tomography abnormalities in acute stroke. *Lancet* 1997; **350**:1595–6.

58 Von Kummer R, Allen KL, Holle R, Bozzao L, Bastianello S, Manelfe C *et al*. Acute stroke: usefulness of early CT findings before thrombolytic therapy. *Radiology* 1997; **205**:327–33.

59 Wardlaw JM, Mielke O. Early signs of brain infarction at CT: observer reliability and outcome after thrombolytic treatment: systematic review. *Radiology* 2005; **235**:444–53.

60 Von Kummer R, Holle R, Gizyska U, Hofmann E, Jansen O, Petersen D *et al*. Interobserver agreement in assessing early CT signs of middle cerebral artery infarction. *Am J Neuroradiol* 1996; **17**:1743–8.

61 Barber PA, Demchuk AM, Zhang J, Buchan AM. Validity and reliability of a quantitative computed tomography score in predicting outcome of hyperacute stroke before thrombolytic therapy. ASPECTS Study Group. Alberta Stroke Programme Early CT Score. *Lancet* 2000; **355**:1670–4.

62 Wardlaw JM, Sellar RJ. A simple practical classification of cerebral infarcts on CT and its interobserver reliability. *Am J Neuroradiol* 1994; **15**:1933–9.

63 Silver B, Demaerschalk B, Merino JG, Wong E, Tamayo A, Devasenapathy A *et al*. Improved outcomes in stroke thrombolysis with pre-specified imaging criteria. *Can J Neurol Sci* 2001; **28**:113–19.

64 Dzialowski I, Weber J, Doerfler A, Forsting M, von Kummer R. Brain tissue water uptake after middle cerebral artery occlusion assessed with CT. *J Neuroimaging* 2004; **14**:42–8.

65 Gibbs J, Wise R, Leenders K, Jones T. The relationship of regional cerebral blood flow, blood volume, and oxygen metabolism in patients with carotid occlusion: evaluation of perfusion reserve. *J Cereb Blood Flow Metab* 1983; **3**:S590–1.

66 Astrup J, Siesjo BK, Symon L. Thresholds in cerebral ischemia: the ischemic penumbra. *Stroke* 1981; **12**:723–5.

67 Gacs G, Merei FT, Bodosi M. Balloon catheter as a model of cerebral emboli in humans. *Stroke* 1982; **13**:39–42.

68 Leys D, Pruvo JP, Godefroy O, Rondepierre P, Leclerc X. Prevalence and significance of hyperdense middle cerebral artery in acute stroke. *Stroke* 1992; **23**:317–24.

69 Barber PA, Demchuk AM, Hudon ME, Pexman JH, Hill MD, Buchan AM. Hyperdense sylvian fissure MCA 'dot' sign: A CT marker of acute ischemia. *Stroke* 2001; **32**:84–8.

70 Bastianello S, Pierallini A, Colonnese C, Brughitta G, Angeloni U, Antonelli M *et al*. Hyperdense middle cerebral artery CT sign. Comparison with angiography in the acute phase of ischemic supratentorial infarction. *Neuroradiology* 1991; **33**:207–11.

71 Hankey GJ, Khangure MS, Stewart-Wynne EG. Detection of basilar artery thrombosis by computed tomography. *Clin Radiol* 1988; **39**:140–3.

72 Bettle N, Lyden PD. Thrombosis of the posterior cerebral artery (PCA) visualized on computed tomography. The dense PCA sign. *Arch Neurol* 2004; **61**:1960–1.

73 Ehsan T, Hayat G, Malkoff MD, Selhorst JB, Martin D, Manepalli A. Hyperdense basilar artery. An early computed tomography sign of thrombosis. *J Neuroimaging* 1994; **4**:200–5.

74 Koo CK, Teasdale E, Muir KW. What constitutes a true hyperdense middle cerebral artery sign? *Cerebrovasc Dis* 2000; **10**:419–23.

75 Maramattom BV, Wijdicks EFM. A misleading hyperdence MCA sign. *Neurology* 2004; **63**:586.

76 Rauch RA, Bazan C, III, Larsson EM, Jinkins JR. Hyperdense middle cerebral arteries identified on CT as a false sign of vascular occlusion. *Am J Neuroradiol* 1993; **14**:669–73.

77 Furlan A, Higashida R, Wechsler L, Gent M, Rowley H, Kase C *et al*. Intra-arterial prourokinase for acute ischemic stroke. The PROACT II study: a randomized controlled trial. Prolyse in Acute Cerebral Thromboembolism. *J Am Med Assoc* 1999; **282**:2003–11.

78 Manelfe C, Larrue V, von Kummer R, Bozzao L, Ringleb P, Bastianello S *et al*. Association of hyperdense middle cerebral artery sign with clinical outcome in patients treated with tissue plasminogen activator. *Stroke* 1999; **30**:769–72.

79 Yang SS, Ryu SJ, Wu CL. Early CT diagnosis of cerebral ischaemia. *Stroke* 1990; **2**:1–121.

80 Hakim AM, Ryder-Cooke MD, Melanson D. Sequential computerized tomographic appearance of strokes. *Stroke* 1983; **14**:893–7.

81 Skriver EB, Olsen JS, McNair P. Mass effect and atrophy after stroke. *Acta Radiologica* 1990; **31**:431–8.

82 Wardlaw JM, Dennis MS, Lindley RI, Warlow CP, Sandercock PAG, Sellar R. Does early reperfusion of a cerebral infarct influence cerebral infarct swelling in the acute stage or the final clinical outcome? *Cerebrovasc Dis* 1993; **3**:86–93.

83 Wardlaw JM, Sellar R. In: *Book of Abstracts from the Proceedings of the Second International Conference on Stroke, The World Federation of Neurology*, Geneva, 12–15 May 1993, p. 23.

84 Berrouschot J, Barthel H, Hesse S, Knapp WH, Schneider D, von Kummer R. Reperfusion and metabolic recovery of brain tissue and clinical outcome after ischemic stroke and thrombolytic therapy. *Stroke* 2000; **31**:1545–51.

85 Skriver EB, Olsen TS. Transient disappearance of cerebral infarcts on CT scan, the so-called fogging effect. *Neuroradiology* 1981; **22**:61–5.

86 Becker H, Desch H, Hacker H, Pencz A. CT fogging effect with ischemic cerebral infarcts. *Neuroradiology* 1979; **18**:185–92.

87 Wing SD, Norman D, Pollock JA, Newton TH. Contrast enhancement of cerebral infarcts in computed tomography. *Radiology* 1976; **121**:89–92.

88 Davis KR, Ackerman RH, Kistler JP, Mojr JP. Computed tomography of cerebral infarction: hemorrhagic, contrast enhancement, and time of appearance. *Comput Tomogr* 1977; **1**:71–86.

89 Pullicino P, Kendall BE. Contrast enhancement in ischaemic lesions. I. Relationship to prognosis. *Neuroradiology* 1980; **19**:235–9.

90 Sage MR. Blood–brain barrier: phenomenon of increasing importance to the imaging clinician. *Am J Roentgenol* 1982; **138**:887–98.

91 Kendall BE, Pullicino P. Intravascular contrast injection in ischaemic lesions. II. Effect on prognosis. *Neuroradiology* 1980; **19**:241–3.

92 Morcos SK, Thomsen HS, Exley CM. Contrast media: interactions with other drugs and clinical tests. *Eur Radiol* 2005; **15**:1463–8.

93 Pislaru S, Pislaru C, Szilard M, Arnout J, Van de WF. In vivo effects of contrast media on coronary thrombolysis. *J Am Coll Cardiol*. 1998; **32**:1102–8.

94 Dehmer GJ, Gresalfi N, Daly D, Oberhardt B, Tate DA. Impairment of fibrinolysis by streptokinase, urokinase and recombinant tissue-type plasminogen activator in the presence of radiographic contrast agents. *J Am Coll Cardiol*. 1995; **25**:1069–75.

95 Wardlaw JM, Lewis SC, Dennis MS, Counsell C, McDowall M. Is visible infarction on computed tomography associated with an adverse prognosis in acute ischemic stroke? *Stroke* 1998; **29**:1315–19.

96 Wardlaw JM, West TM, Sandercock PA, Lewis SC, Mielke O. Visible infarction on computed tomography is an independent predictor of poor functional outcome after stroke, and not of haemorrhagic transformation. *J Neurol Neurosurg Psychiatry* 2003; **74**:452–8.

97 Donnan GA, Tress BM, Bladin PF. A prospective study of lacunar infarction using computerized tomography. *Neurology* 1982; **32**:49–56.

98 Bamford J, Sandercock P, Jones L, Warlow C. The natural history of lacunar infarction: the Oxfordshire Community Stroke Project. *Stroke* 1987; **18**:545–51.

99 Lindgren A, Norrving B, Rudling O, Johansson BB. Comparison of clinical and neuroradiological findings in first-ever stroke: a population-based study. *Stroke* 1994; **25**:1371–7.

100 Bonke B, Koudstaal PJ, Dijkstra G, van Hilligersberg R, van Knippenberg FC, Duivenvoorden HJ, Kappelle LJ. Detection of lacunar infarction in brain CT-scans: no evidence of bias from accompanying patient information. *Neuroradiology* 1989; **31**:170–3.

101 Anderson CS, Taylor BV, Hankey GJ, Stewart-Wynne EG, Jamrozik KD. Validation of a clinical classification for subtypes of acute cerebral infarction. *J Neurol Neurosurg Psychiatry* 1994; **57**:1173–9.

102 Mead GE, O'Neill PA, Murray H, Farrell A, McCollum CN. Does the Oxfordshire Community Stroke Project classification predict the site of cerebral infarction. *Cerebrovasc Dis* 1996; **6**:32–178.

103 Wardlaw JM, Dennis MS, Lindley RI, Sellar RJ, Warlow CP. The validity of a simple clinical classification of acute ischaemic stroke. *J Neurol* 1996; **243**:274–9.

104 Al-Buhairi AR, phillips SJ, Llwellyn G, Jan MSJ. Prediction of infarct topography using the Oxfordshire Community

Stroke Project classification of stroke subtypes. *J Stroke Cerebrovasc Dis* 1998; **7**:339–43.

105 Savoiardo M. *CT Scanning*. New York: Churchill Livingstone, 1986, pp. 189–219.

106 Bamford J, Sandercock P, Dennis M, Burn J, Warlow C. Classification and natural history of clinically identifiable subtypes of cerebral infarction. *Lancet* 1991; **337**:1521–6.

107 Mead GE, Lewis S, Wardlaw JM, Dennis MS, Warlow CP. Should computed tomography appearance of lacunar stroke influence patient management? *J Neurol Neurosurg Psychiatry* 1999; **67**:682–4.

108 Lindgren A, Staaf G, Geijer B, Brockstedt S, Stahlberg F, Holtas S, Norrving B. Clinical lacunar syndromes as predictors of lacunar infarcts: a comparison of acute clinical lacunar syndromes and findings on diffusion-weighted MRI. *Acta Neurol Scand* 2000; **101**:128–34.

109 Toni D, Del Duca R, Fiorelli M, Sacchetti ML, Bastianello S, Giubilei F *et al*. Pure motor hemiparesis and sensorimotor stroke: accuracy of very early clinical diagnosis of lacunar strokes. *Stroke* 1994; **25**:92–6.

110 Toni D, Iweins F, von Kummer R, Busse O, Bogousslavsky J, Falcou A *et al*. Identification of lacunar infarcts before thrombolysis in the ECASS I study. *Neurology* 2000; **54**:684–8.

111 Wardlaw JM. What causes lacunar stroke? *J Neurol Neurosurg Psychiatry* 2005; **76**:617–19.

112 Bamford J. Clinical examination in diagnosis and subclassification of stroke. *Lancet* 1992; **339**:400–2.

113 Kittner SJ, Sharkness CM, Price TR, Plotnick GD, Dambrosia JM, Wolf PA *et al*. Infarcts with a cardiac source of embolism in the NINCDS Stroke Data Bank: historical features. *Neurology* 1990; **40**:281–4.

114 Adams HP, Jr., Bendixen BH, Kappelle LJ, Biller J, Love BB, Gordon DL, Marsh EE, III. Classification of subtype of acute ischemic stroke. Definitions for use in a multicenter clinical trial. TOAST. Trial of Org 10172 in Acute Stroke Treatment. *Stroke* 1993; **24**:35–41.

115 Sacco RL, Ellenberg JH, Mohr JP, Tatemichi TK, Hier DB, Price TR, Wolf PA. Infarcts of undetermined cause: the NINCDS Stroke Data Bank. *Ann Neurol* 1989; **25**:382–90.

116 Jackson C, Sudlow C. Are lacunar strokes really different? A systematic review of differences in risk factor profiles between lacunar and non-lacunar infarcts. *Stroke* 2005; **36**:891–904.

117 Hill MD, Buchan AM, for the Canadian Alteplase for Stroke Effectiveness Study (CASES) Investigators. Thrombolysis for acute ischemic stroke: results of the Canadian Alteplase for Stroke Effectiveness Study. *Can Med Assoc J* 2005; **172**:1307–12.

118 Patel SC, Levine SR, Tilley BC, Grotta JC, Lu M, Frankel M *et al*. for the National Institute of Neurological Disorders and Stroke rt-PA Stroke Study Group. Lack of clinical significance of early ischemic changes on computed tomography in acute stroke. *J Am Med Assoc* 2001; **286**:2830–8.

119 Cornu C, Boutitie F, Candelise L, Boissel JP, Donnan GA, Hommel M *et al*. Streptokinase in acute ischemic stroke: an

individual patient data meta-analysis : The Thrombolysis in Acute Stroke Pooling Project. *Stroke* 2000; **31**:1555–60.

120 Hill MD, Rowley HA, Adler F, Eliasziw M, Furlan A, Higashida RT *et al.* for the PROACT-II Investigators. Selection of acute ischemic stroke patients for intra-arterial thrombolysis with pro-urokinase by using ASPECTS. *Stroke* 2003; **34**:1925–31.

121 Demchuk AM, Hill MD, Barber PA, Silver B, Patel SC, Levine SR. Importance of early ischemic computed tomography changes using ASPECTS in NINDS rt-PA Stroke Study. *Stroke* 2005; **36**:2110–15.

122 Hill MD, Barber PA, Demchuk AM, Buchan AM, Warwick JH, Hu W *et al.* Validation of the ASPECT score as a pedictor of outcome: analysis of the ATLANTIS-B Study. *Stroke* 2002; **33**(1):381.

123 Dzialowski I, Hill MD, Coutts SB, Demchuk AM, Kent DM, Wunderlich O, von Kummer R. Extent of early ischemic changes on computed tomography (CT) before thrombolysis: prognostic value of the Alberta Stroke Program Early CT Score in ECASS II. *Stroke* 2006; **37**:973–8.

124 Finocchi C, Gandolfo C, Gasparetto B, Del Sette M, Croce R, Loeb C. Value of early variables as predictors of short-term outcome in patients with acute focal cerebral ischemia. *Ital J Neurol Sci* 1996; **17**:341–6.

125 Heinsius T, Bogousslavsky J, Van Melle G. Large infarcts in the middle cerebral artery territory. Etiology and outcome patterns. *Neurology* 1998; **50**:341–50.

126 Candelise L, Pinardi G, Morabito A, the Italian Acute Stroke Study Group. Mortality in acute stroke with atrial fibrillation. *Stroke* 1991; **22**:169–74.

127 Coutts SB, Demchuk AM, Barber PA, Hu WY, Simon JE, Buchan AM, Hill MD, for the VISION Study Group. Interobserver variation of ASPECTS in real time. *Stroke* 2004; **35**:e103–e105.

128 Lee D, Fox A, Vinuela F, Pelz D, Lau C, Donald A, Merskey H. Interobserver variation in computed tomography of the brain. *Arch Neurol* 1987; **44**:30–1.

129 Shinar D, Gross CR, Hier DB, Caplan LR, Mohr JP, Price TR *et al.* Interobserver reliability in the interpretation of computed tomographic scans of stroke patients. *Arch Neurol* 1987; **44**:149–55.

130 Damasio H. A computed tomographic guide to the identification of cerebral vascular territories. *Arch Neurol* 1983; **40**:138–42.

131 Torvik A. The pathogenesis of watershed infarcts in the brain. *Stroke* 1984; **15**:221–3.

132 Graeber MC, Jordan JE, Mishra SK, Nadeau SE. Watershed infarction on computed tomographic scan. An unreliable sign of hemodynamic stroke. *Arch Neurol* 1992; **49**:311–13.

133 Van der Zwan A, Hillen B, Tulleken CAF, Dujovny M, Dragovic L. Variability of the territories of the major cerebral arteries. *J Neurosurg* 1992; **77**:927–40.

134 Lang EW, Daffertshofer M, Daffertshofer A, Wirth SB, Chesnut RM, Hennerici M. Variability of vascular territory in stroke. Pitfalls and failure of stroke pattern interpretation. *Stroke* 1995; **26**:942–5.

135 Weiller C, Ringelstein EB, Reiche W, Thron A, Buell U. The large striatocapsular infarct. A clinical and pathophysiological entity. *Arch Neurol* 1990; **47**:1085–91.

136 Angeloni U, Bozzao L, Fantozzi L, Bastianello S, Kushner M, Fieschi C. Internal borderzone infarction following acute middle cerebral artery occlusion. *Neurology* 1990; **40**:1196–8.

137 Donnan GA, Bladin PF, Berkovic SF, Longley WA, Saling MM. The stroke syndrome of striatocapsular infarction. *Brain* 1991; **114** (Pt 1A):51–70.

138 Wardlaw JM, Lewis SC, Dennis MS, Warlow CP. Is it reasonable to assume a particular embolic source from the type of stroke? *Cerebrovasc Dis* 1999; **9**:14.

139 Wintermark M, Sesay M, Barbier E, Borbely K, Dillon WP, Eastwood JD *et al.* Comparative overview of brain perfusion imaging techniques. *Stroke* 2005; **36**:2032–2034.

140 Meuli RA. Imaging viable brain tissue with CT scan during acute stroke. *Cerebrovasc Dis* 2004; **17**:28–34.

141 Parsons MW, Pepper EM, Chan V, Siddique S, Rajaratnam S, Bateman GA, Levi CR. Perfusion computed tomography: prediction of final infarct extent and stroke outcome. *Ann Neurol* 2005; **58**:672–9.

142 Murphy BD, Fox AJ, Lee DH, Sahlas DJ, Black SE, Hogan MJ *et al.* Identification of penumbra and infarct in acute ischemic stroke using computed tomography perfusion-derived blood flow and blood volume measurements. *Stroke* 2006; **37**:1771–7.

143 Wintermark M, Flanders AE, Velthuis B, Meuli R, van Leeuwen M, Goldsher D *et al.* Perfusion-CT assessment of infarct core and penumbra. Receiver operating characteristic curve analysis in 130 patients suspected of acute hemispheric stroke. *Stroke* 2006; **37**:979–85.

144 Bandera E, Botteri M, Minelli C, Sutton A, Abrams KR, Latronico N. Cerebral blood flow threshold of ischemic penumbra and infarct core in acute ischemic stroke. A systematic review. *Stroke* 2006; **37**:1334–9.

145 Warach S. Stroke neuroimaging. *Stroke* 2003; **34**:345–7.

146 Ritter MA, Poeplau T, Schaefer A, Kloska SP, Dziewas R, Ringelstein EB *et al.* CT angiography in acute stroke: does it provide additional information on occurence of infarction and functional outcome after 3 months? *Cerebrovasc Dis* 2006; **22**:362–7.

147 Fischer U, Arnold M, Nedeltchev K, Brekenfeld C, Ballinari P, Remonda L *et al.* NIHSS score and arteriographic findings in acute ischemic stroke. *Stroke* 2005; **36**:2121–5.

148 King-Im JM, Trivedi RA, Graves MJ, Harkness K, Eales H, Joubert I *et al.* Utility of an ultrafast magnetic resonance imaging protocol in recent and semi-recent strokes. *J Neurol Neurosurg Psychiatry* 2005; **76**:1002–5.

149 Singer OC, Sitzer M, du Mesnil de Rochemont R, Neumann-Haefelin T. Practical limitations of acute stroke MRI due to patient-related problems. *Neurology* 2004; **62**:1848–9.

150 Hand PJ, Wardlaw JM, Rowat AM, Haisma JA, Lindley RI, Dennis MS. Magnetic resonance brain imaging in patients with acute stroke: feasibility and patient-related difficulties. *J Neurol Neurosurg Psychiatry* 2005; **76**:1525–7.

151 Barber PA, Hill MD, Eliasziw M, Demchuk AM, Pexman JH, Hudon ME et al, for the ASPECTS Study Group. Imaging of the brain in acute ischaemic stroke: comparison of computed tomography and magnetic resonance diffusion-weighted imaging. *J Neurol Neurosurg Psychiatry* 2005; **76**:1528–33.

152 Rowat AM, Wardlaw JM, Dennis MS, Warlow CP. Patient positioning influences oxygen saturation in the acute phase of stroke. *Cerebrovasc Dis* 2001; **12**:66–72.

153 Wardlaw JM, Keir SL, Dennis MS. The impact of delays in CT brain imaging on the accuracy of diagnosis and subsequent management in patients with minor stroke. *J Neurol Neurosurg Psychiatry* 2003; **74**:77–81.

154 Koroshetz WJ, Gonzales RG. Imaging stroke in progress: magnetic resonance advances but computed tomography is poised for counterattack. *Ann Neurol* 1999; **46**:556–8.

155 Lev MH. CT versus MR for acute stroke imaging: is the 'obvious' choice necessarily the correct one? *Am J Neuroradiol* 2003; **24**:1930–1.

156 Powers WJ, Zivin J. Magnetic resonance imaging in acute stroke: not ready for prime time. *Neurology* 1998; **50**:842–3.

157 Ringelstein EB. Ultrafast magnetic resonance imaging protocols in stroke. *J Neurol Neurosurg Psychiatry* 2005; **76**:905.

158 Dimigen M, Keir S, Dennis M, Wardlaw J. Long-term visibility of primary intracerebral haemorrhage on MRI. *J Stroke Cerebrovasc Dis* 2004; **13**:104–8.

159 Schellinger PD, Jansen O, Fiebach JB, Hacke W, Sartor K. A standardized MRI stroke protocol: comparison with CT in hyperacute intracerebral hemorrhage. *Stroke* 1999; **30**:765–8.

160 Melhem ER, Patel RT, Whitehead RE, Bhatia RG, Rockwell DT, Jara H. MR imaging of hemorrhagic brain lesions: a comparison of dual-echo gradient- and spin-echo and fast spin-echo techniques. *Am J Neuroradiol* 1998; **3**:797–802.

161 Linfante I, Llinas RH, Caplan LR, Warach S. MRI features of intracerebral hemorrhage within 2 hours from symptom onset. *Stroke* 1999; **30**:2263–7.

162 Fiebach JB, Schellinger PD, Gass A, Kucinski T, Siebler M, Villringer A et al, for the Kompetenznetzwerk Schlaganfall B5. Stroke magnetic resonance imaging is accurate in hyperacute intracerebral hemorrhage. A multicenter study on the validity of stroke imaging. *Stroke* 2004; **35**:502–7.

163 Alemany RM, Stenborg A, Sonninen P, Terent A, Raininko R. Detection and appearance of intraparenchymal haematomas of the brain at 1.5 T with spin-echo, FLAIR and GE sequences: poor relationship to the age of the haematoma. *Neuroradiology* 2004; **46**:435–43.

164 Liang L, Korogi Y, Sugahara T, Shigematsu Y, Okuda T, Ikushima I, Takahashi M. Detection of intracranial hemorrhage with susceptibility-weighted MR sequences. *Am J Neuroradiol* 1999; **20**:1527–34.

165 Haacke EM, Cheng NY, House MJ, Liu Q, Neelavalli J, Ogg RJ et al. Imaging iron stores in the brain using magnetic resonance imaging. *Magn Reson Imaging* 2005; **23**:1–25.

166 Patel MR, Edelman RR, Warach S. Detection of hyperacute primary intraparenchymal hemorrhage by magnetic resonance imaging. *Stroke* 1996; **27**:2321–4.

167 Garcia JH, Ho K-L, Caccamo DV. Intracerebral hemorrhage: pathology of selected topics. In: Kase CS, Caplan LR, eds. *Intracerebral Hemorrhage*. Newton MA: Butterworth-Heinemann, 1994, pp. 48–50.

168 Wardlaw JM, Statham PF. How often is haemosiderin not visible on routine MRI following traumatic intracerebral haemorrhage? *Neuroradiology* 2000; **42**:81–4.

169 Viswanathan A, Chabriat H. Cerebral microhemorrhage. *Stroke* 2006; **37**:549–54.

170 Koennecke HC. Cerebral microbleeds on MRI: prevalence, associations, and potential clinical implications. *Neurology* 2006; **66**:165–71.

171 Cordonnier C, Al-Shahi R, and Wardlaw JM. Brain microbleeds: systematic review, subgroup analyses and standards for study design and reporting. *Brain* 2007; doi: 10.1093/brain/aw1387

172 Offenbacher H, Fazekas F, Schmidt R, Koch M, Fazekas G, Kapeller P. MR of cerebral abnormalities concomitant with primary intracerebral haematomas. *Am J Neuroradiol* 1996; **17**:573–8.

173 Scharf J, Braunherr E, Forsting M, Sartor K. Significance of haemorrhagic lacunes on MRI in patients with hypertensive cerebrovascular disease and intracerebral haemorrhage. *Neuroradiology* 1994; **36**:504–8.

174 Tanaka A, Ueno Y, Nakayama Y, Takano K. Small chronic haemorrhages and ischaemic lesions in association with spontaneous intracerebral haematomas. *Stroke* 1999; **30**:1637–42.

175 Roob G, Schmidt R, Kapeller P, Lechner A, Hartung HP, Fazekas F. MRI evidence of past cerebral microbleeds in a healthy elderly population. *Neurology* 1999; **52**:991.

176 Jeerakathil T, Wolf PA, Beiser A, Hald JK, Au R, Kase CS, Massaro JM, DeCarli C. Cerebral microbleeds: prevalence and associations with cardiovascular risk factors in the Framingham Study. *Stroke* 2004; **35**:1831–5.

177 Lee SH, Kwon SJ, Kim KS, Yoon BW, Roh JK. Cerebral microbleeds in patients with hypertensive stroke. Topographical distribution in the supratentorial area. *J Neurol* 2004; **251**:1183–9.

178 Lee S-H, Bae H-J, Ko S-B, Kim H, Yoon B-W, Roh J-K. Comparative analysis of the spatial distribution and severity of cerebral microbleeds and old lacunes. *J Neurol Neurosurg Psychiatry* 2004; **75**:423–7.

179 Fazekas F, Kleinert R, Roob G, Kleinert G, Kapeller P, Schmidt R, Hartung HP. Histopathologic analysis of foci of signal loss on gradient-echo T2*-weighted MR images in patients with spontaneous intracerebral hemorrhage: evidence of microangiopathy-related microbleeds. *Am J Neuroradiol* 1999; **20**:637–42.

180 Kwa VIH, Franke CL, Verbeeten B Jr., Stam J. Silent intracerebral microhemorrhages in patients with ischaemic stroke. *Ann Neurol* 1998; **44**:372–7.

181 Smith EE, Gurol ME, Eng JA, Engel CR, Nguyen TN, Rosand J, Greenberg SM. White matter lesions, cognition,

and recurrent hemorrhage in lobar intracerebral hemorrhage. *Neurology* 2004; **63**:1606–12.

182 Roob G, Lechner A, Schmidt R, Flooh E, Hartung HP, Fazekas F. Frequency and location of microbleeds in patients with primary intracerebral hemorrhage. *Stroke* 2000; **31**:2665–9.

183 Lee SH, Bae HJ, Kwon SJ, Kim H, Kim YH, Yoon BW, Roh JK. Cerebral microbleeds are regionally associated with intracerebral hemorrhage. *Neurology* 2004; **62**:72–6.

184 Wardlaw JM, Lewis SC, Keir SL, Dennis MS, Shenkin S. Cerebral microbleeds are associated with lacunar stroke defined clinically and radiologically, indepently of white matter lesions. *Stroke* 2006; **37**:2633–6.

185 Werring DJ, Frazer DW, Coward LJ, Losseff NA, Watt H, Cipolotti L et al. Cognitive dysfunction in patients with cerebral microbleeds on T2*-weighted gradient-echo MRI. *Brain* 2004; **127**:2265–75.

186 Hiroki M, Miyashita K, Oe H, Takaya S, Hirai S, Fukuyama H. Link between linear hyperintensity objects in cerebral white matter and hypertensive intracerebral hemorrhage. *Cerebrovasc Dis* 2004; **18**:166–73.

187 Fan YH, Zhang L, Lam WWM, Mok VCT, Wong KS. Cerebral microbleeds as a risk factor for subsequent intracerebral hemorrhages among patients with acute ischemic stroke. *Stroke* 2003; **34**:2462.

188 Imaizumi T, Horita Y, Chiba M, Hashimoto Y, Honma T, Niwa J. Dot-like hemosiderin spots on gradient echo T2*-weighted magnetic resonance imaging are associated with past history of small vessel disease in patients with intracerebral hemorrhage. *J Neuroimaging* 2004; **14**:251–7.

189 Nighoghossian N, Hermier M, Adeleine P, Blanc-Lasserre K, Derex L, Honnorat J et al. Old microbleeds are a potential risk factor for cerebral bleeding after ischemic stroke. A gradient-echo T2*-weighted brain MRI study. *Stroke* 2002; **33**:735–42.

190 Kidwell CS, Saver JL, Villablanca JP, Duckwiler G, Fredieu A, Gough K et al. Magnetic resonance imaging detection of microbleeds before thrombolysis: an emerging application. *Stroke* 2002; **33**:95–8.

191 Wong KS, Chan YL, Liu JY, Gao S, Lam WW. Asymptomatic microbleeds as a risk factor for aspirin-associated intracerebral hemorrhages. *Neurology* 2003; **60**:511–13.

192 Chalela JA, Kang D-W, Warach S. Multiple cerebral microbleeds: MRI marker of a diffuse hemorrhage-prone state. *J Neuroimaging* 2004; **14**:54–7.

193 Derex L, Hermier M, Adeleine P, Honnorat J, Berthezene Y, Froment JC et al. Usefulness of T2-weighted MRI sequences before intravenous tPA for acute ischemic stroke. In: *Proceedings of the 7th International Symposium on Thrombolysis and Acute Stroke Therapy*, Lyon, France, 2002, p. 83.

194 Walker DA, Broderick DF, Kotsenas AL, Rubino FA. Routine use of gradient-echo MRI to screen for cerebral amyloid angiopathy in elderly patients. *Am J Roentgenol* 2004; **182**:1547–50.

195 Rosand J. Hypertension and the brain: stroke is just the tip of the iceberg. *Neurology* 2004; **63**:6–7.

196 Dichgans M, Holtmannspotter M, Herzog J, Peters N, Bergmann M, Yousry TA. Cerebral microbleeds in CADASIL: a gradient-echo magnetic resonance imaging and autopsy study. *Stroke* 2002; **33**:67–71.

197 Fisher M, Albers GW. Applications of diffusion-perfusion magnetic resonance imaging in acute ischemic stroke. *Neurology* 1999; **52**:1750–6.

198 Latchaw RE. The roles of diffusion and perfusion MR imaging in acute stroke management. *Am J Neuroradiol* 1999; **20**:957–9.

199 Prichard JW, Grossman RI. New reasons for early use of MRI in stroke. *Neurology* 1999; **52**:1733–6.

200 Mead GE, Wardlaw JM. Detection of intraluminal thrombus in acute stroke by proton density MR imaging. *Cerebrovasc Dis* 1998; **8**:133–4.

201 Flacke S, Urbach H, Keller E, Traber F, Hartmann A, Textor J et al. Middle cerebral artery (MCA) susceptibility sign at susceptibility-based perfusion MR imaging: clinical importance and comparison with hyperdense MCA sign at CT. *Radiology* 2000; **215**:476–82.

202 Assouline E, Benziane K, Reizine D, Guichard JP, Pico F, Merland JJ, Bousser MG, Chabriat H. Intra-arterial thrombus visualized on T2* gradient echo imaging in acute ischemic stroke. *Cerebrovasc Dis* 2005; **20**:6–11.

203 Fisher M, Sotak CH, Minematsu K, Li L. New magnetic resonance techniques for evaluating cerebrovascular disease. *Ann Neurol* 1995; **32**:122.

204 Yoneda Y, Tokui K, Hanihara T, Kitagaki H, Tabuchi M, Mori E. Diffusion-weighted magnetic resonance imaging: detection of ischemic injury 39 minutes after onset in a stroke patient. *Ann Neurol* 1999; **45**:794–7.

205 Kidwell CS, Saver JL, Mattiello J, Starkman S, Vinuela F, Duckwiler G et al. Thrombolytic reversal of acute human cerebral ischemic injury shown by diffusion/perfusion magnetic resonance imaging. *Ann Neurol* 2000; **47**:462–9.

206 Guadagno JV, Warburton EA, Aigbirhio FI, Smielewski P, Fryer TD, Harding S et al. Does the acute diffusion-weighted imaging lesion represent penumbra as well as core? A combined quantitative PET/MRI voxel-based study. *J Cereb Blood Flow Metab* 2004; **24**:1249–54.

207 Rivers CS, Wardlaw JM. What has diffusion imaging in animals told us about diffusion imaging in patients with ischaemic stroke? *Cerebrovasc Dis* 2005; **19**:328–36.

208 Ay H, Oliveira-Filho J, Buonanno FS, Schaefer PW, Furie KL, Chang YC et al. 'Footprints' of transient ischemic attacks: a diffusion-weighted MRI study. *Cerebrovas Dis* 2002; **14**:177–86.

209 Ay H, Buonanno FS, Rordorf G, Schaefer PW, Schwamm LH, Wu O et al. Normal diffusion-weighted MRI during stroke-like deficits. *Neurology* 1999; **52**:1784–92.

210 Hasso AN, Stringer WA, Brown KD. Cerebral ischaemia and infarction. *Neuroimaging Clinics of North America* 1994; **4**:733–52.

211 Ida M, Mizunuma K, Hata Y, Tada S. Subcortical low intensity in early cortical ischemia. *Am J Neuroradiol* 1994; **15**:1387–93.

212 Brant-Zawadzki M, Atkinson DJ, Detrick M, Bradley WG, Scidmore G. fluid-attenuated inversion recovery (FLAIR)

for assessment of cerebral infarction. Initial cllinical experience in 50 patients. *Stroke* 1996; **27**:1187–91.

213 Noguchi K, Ogawa T, Inugami A, Fujita H, Hatazawa J, Shimosegawa E *et al*. MRI of acute cerebral infarction: a comparison of FLAIR and T2-weighted fast spin-echo imaging. *Neuroradiology* 1997; **39**:406–10.

214 Cosnard G, Duprez T, Grandin C, Smith AM, Munier T, Peeters A. Fast FLAIR sequence for detecting major vascular abnormalities during the hyperacute phase of stroke: a comparison with MR angiography. *Neuroradiology* 1999; **41**:342–6.

215 Burdette JH, Elster AD, Ricci PE. Acute cerebral infarction: quantification of spin-density and T2 shine-through phenomena on diffusion-weighted MR images. *Radiology* 1999; **212**:333–9.

216 Schlaug G, Siewert B, Benfield A, Edelman RR, Warach S. Time course of the apparent diffusion coefficient (ADC) abnormality in human stroke. *Neurology* 1997; **49**:113–19.

217 Burdette JH, Ricci PE, Petitti N, Elster AD. Cerebral infarction: time course of signal intensity changes on diffusion-weighted MR images. *Am J Roentgenol* 1998; **171**:791–5.

218 Warach S, Gaa J, Siewert B, Wielopolski P, Edelman RR. Acute human stroke studied by whole brain echo planar diffusion-weighted magnetic resonance imaging. *Ann Neurol* 1995; **37**:231–41.

219 Eastwood JD, Engelter ST, MacFall JF, DeLong DM, Provenzale JM. Quantitative assessment of the time course of infarct signal intensity on diffusion-weighted images. *Am J Neuroradiol* 2003; **24**:680–7.

220 Lansberg MG, Thijs VN, O'Brien MW, Ali JO, de Crespigny AJ *et al*. Evolution of apparent diffusion coefficient diffusion-weighted, and T2-weighted signal intensity of acute stroke. *Am J Neuroradiol* 2001; **22**:637–44.

221 Muñoz Maniega S, Bastin ME, Armitage PA, Farrall AJ, Carpenter TK, Hand PJ *et al*. Temporal evolution of water diffusion parameters is different in grey and white matter in human ischaemic stroke. *J Neurol Neurosurg Psychiatry* 2004; **75**:1714–18.

222 Rivers CS, Wardlaw JM, Armitage PA, Bastin M, Carpenter T, Cvoro V *et al*. Persistent infarct hyperintensity on diffusion-weighted imaging late after stroke indicates heterogeneous, delayed, infarct evolution. *Stroke* 2006; **14**:18–23.

223 Schlaug G, Baird AE, Picone M, Edelman RR, Wararch S. Early normalization of the apparent diffusion coefficient (ADC) after reperfusion. 23rd International Joint Conference on Stroke and Cerebral Circulation Florida, USA 1998. *Stroke* 1998; **29**(1):280.

224 Del Zoppo GJ, Schmid-Schonbein GW, Mori E, Copeland BR, Chang CM. Polymorphonuclear leukocytes occlude capillaries following middle cerebral artery occlusion and reperfusion in baboons. *Stroke* 1991; **22**:1276–83.

225 Geijer B, Lindgren A, Brockstedt S, Stahlberg F, Holtas S. Persistent high signal on diffusional-weighted MRI in the late stages of small cortical and lacunar ischaemic lesions. *Neuroradiology* 2001; **43**:115–22.

226 Schulz UGR, Briley D, Meagher T, Molyneux A, Rothwell PM. Abnormalities on diffusion weighted magnetic resonance imaging performed several weeks after a minor stroke or transient ischaemic attack. *J Neurol Neurosurg Psychiatry* 2003; **74**:734–8.

227 Wardlaw JM, Armitage P, Dennis MS, Lewis S, Marshall I, Sellar R. The use of diffusion-weighted magnetic resonance imaging to identify infarctions in patients with minor strokes. *J Stroke Cerebrovasc Dis* 2000; **9**:70–5.

228 Falcao AL, Reutens DC, Markus R, Koga M, Read SJ, Tochon-Danguy H *et al*. The resistance to ischemia of white and gray matter after stroke. *Ann Neurol* 2004; **56**:695–701.

229 Sorensen GA, Buonanno FS, Gonzalez RG, Schwamm LH, Lev MH, Huang-Hellinger FR. Hyperacute stroke: evaluation with combined multisection diffusion-weighted and hemodynamically weighted echo-planar MR imaging. *Radiology* 1996; **199**:391–401.

230 Baird AE, Benfield A, Schlaug G, Siewert B, Lovblad KO, Edelman RR. Enlargement of human cerebral ischemic lesion volumes measured by diffusion-weighted magnetic resonance imaging. *Ann Neurol* 1997; **41**:581–9.

231 Brant-Zawadzki M, Weinstein P, Bartkowski H, Moseley M. MR imaging and spectroscopy in clinical and experimental cerebral ischemia: a review. *Am J Roentgenol* 1987; **148**:579–88.

232 DeWitt LD, Kistler JP, Miller DC, Richardson EP Jr., Buonanno FS. NMR – neuropathologic correlation in stroke. *Stroke* 1987; **18**:342–51.

233 Pereira AC, Doyle VL, Griffiths JR, Brown MM. Disappearing cerebral infarcts: a longitudinal MRI study of 16 patients. *Cerebrovasc Dis* 1997; **7**:30.

234 Torigoe R, Harad K, Matsuo H. Assessment of cerebral infarction by MRI – particularly fogging effect. *No-To-Shinkei* 1990; **42**:547–52.

235 O'Brien P, Sellar RJ, Wardlaw JM. Fogging on T2-weighted MR after acute ischaemic stroke: how often might this occur and what are the implications? *Neuroradiology* 2004; **46**:635–41.

236 Bryan RN, Levy LM, Whitlow WD, Killian JM, Preziosi TJ, Rosario JA. Diagnosis of acute cerebral infarction: comparison of CT and MR imaging. *Am J Neuroradiol* 1991; **12**:611–20.

237 Merten CL, Knitelius HO, Assheuer J, Bergmann-Kurz B, Hedde JP, Bewermeyer H. MRI of acute cerebral infarcts: increased contrast enhancement with continuous infusion of gadolinium. *Neuroradiology* 1999; **41**:242–8.

238 Elster AD. MR contrast enhancement in brainstem and deep cerebral infarction. *Am J Neuroradiol* 1991; **12**:1127–32.

239 Samuelson M, Lindell D, Norrving B. Gadolinium-enhanced magnetic resonance imaging in patients with presumed lacunar infarcts. *Cerebrovasc Dis* 1994; **4**:12–19.

240 Simmons Z, Biller J, Adams HP, Jr., Dunn V, Jacoby CG. Cerebellar infarction: comparison of computed tomography and magnetic resonance imaging. *Ann Neurol* 1986; **19**:291–3.

241 Keir S, Wardlaw JM, Bastin ME, Dennis MS. In which patients is diffusion-weighted magnetic resonance imaging most useful in routine stroke care? *J Neuroimaging* 2004; **14**:118–22.

242 Noguchi K, Nagayoshi T, Watanabe N, Kanazawa T, Toyoshima S, Morijiri M *et al*. Diffusion-weighted echo-planar MRI of lacunar infarcts. *Neuroradiology* 1998; **40**:448–51.

243 Ohta K, Obara K, and Suzuki N. Diagnostic usefulness of echo planner diffusion-weighted magnetic resonance image in acute phase of lacunar stroke. *Cerebrovasc Dis* 1999; **9**(S1):69.

244 Wardlaw JM, Armitage P, Dennis MS, Lewis S, Marshall I, Sellar R. The use of diffusion-weighted magnetic resonance imaging to identify infarctions in patients with minor strokes. *J Stroke Cerebrovasc Dis* 2000; **9**:70–5.

245 Gass A, Ay H, Szabo K, Koroshetz WJ. Diffusion-weighted MRI for the 'small stuff': the details of acute cerebral ischaemia. *Lancet Neurol* 2004; **3**:39–45.

246 Marks MP, de Crespigny A, Lentz D, Enzmann DR, Albers GW, Moseley ME. Acute and chronic stroke: navigated spin-echo diffusion-weighted MR imaging. *Radiology* 1996; **199**:403–8.

247 Altieri M, Metz R, Muller C, Maeder P, Meuli R, Bogousslavsky J. Differentiation of acute versus chronic infarcts by diffusion weighted MRI in patients with multiple ischemic lesions. *Cerebrovasc Dis* 1997; **7**(4):6.

248 Lindgren A, Geijer B, Brockstedt S, Staaf G, Stahlberg F. The use of diffusion-MRI to differentiate acute cerebral infarcts from chronic lesions. *Cerebrovasc Dis* 1997; **7**:60.

249 Fitzek C, Tintera J, Muller-Forell W, Urban P, Thomke F, Fitzek S *et al*. Differentiation of recent and old cerebral infarcts by diffusion-weighted MRI. *Neuroradiology* 1998; **40**:778–82.

250 Bartylla K, Hagen T, Globel H, Jost V, Schneider G. Diffusion-weighted magnetic resonance imaging for demonstration of cerebral infarcts. *Radiologe* 1997; **37**:859–64.

251 Wang AM, Shetty AN, Woo H, Rao SK, Manzione JV, Moore JR. Diffusion weighted MR imaging in evaluation of CNS disease. *Rivista di Neuroradiologia* 1998; **11**:109–12.

252 Warach S, Kidwell CS. The redefinition of TIA: the uses and limitations of DWI in acute ischemic cerebrovascular syndromes. *Neurology* 2004; **62**:359–60.

253 Kidwell CS, Alger JR, Di Salle F, Starkman S, Villablanca P, Bentson J, Saver JL. Diffusion MRI in patients with transient ischemic attacks. *Stroke* 1999; **30**:1174–80.

254 Crisostomo RA, Garcia MM, Tong DC. Detection of diffusion-weighted MRI abnormalities in patients with transient ischemic attack: correlation with clinical characteristics. *Stroke* 2003; **34**:932–7.

255 Ay H, Koroshetz WJ, Benner T, Vangel MG, Wu O, Schwamm LH, Sorensen AG. Transient ischemic attack with infarction: a unique syndrome? *Ann Neurol* 2005; **57**:679–86.

256 Purroy F, Montaner J, Rovira A, Delgado P, Quintana M, Alvarez-Sabin J. Higher risk of further vascular events among transient ischemic attack patients with diffusion-weighted imaging acute ischemic lesions. *Stroke* 2004; **35**:2313–19.

257 Coutts SB, Simon JE, Eliasziw M, Sohn CH, Hill MD, Barber PA *et al*. Triaging transient ischemic attack and minor stroke patients using acute magnetic resonance imaging. *Ann Neurol* 2005; **57**:848–54.

258 Douglas VC, Johnston CM, Elkins J, Sidney S, Gress DR, Johnston SC. Head computed tomography findings predict short-term stroke risk after transient ischemic attack. *Stroke* 2003; **34**:2894–8.

259 Yuh WTC, Crain MR, Loes DJ, Greene GM, Ryals TJ, Sato Y. MR imaging of cerebral ischaemia: findings in the first 24 hours. *Am J Neuroradiol* 1991; **12**:621–9.

260 Hommel M, Grand S, Devoulon P, Le Bas J-F. New directions in magnetic resonance in acute cerebral ischemia. *Cerebrovasc Dis* 1994; **4**:3–11.

261 Mohr JP, Biller J, Hilal SK, Yuh WTC, Tatemichi TK, Hedges S *et al*. Magnetic resonance versus computed tomographic imaging in acute stroke. *Stroke* 1995; **26**:807–12.

262 Sato A, Takahashi S, Soma Y, Ishii K, Kikuchi Y, Watanabe T, Sakamoto K. Cerebral infarction: early detection by means of contrast-enhanced cerebral arteries at MR imaging. *Radiology* 1991; **178**:433–9.

263 Alberts MJ, Faulstich ME, Gray L. Stroke with negative brain magnetic resonance imaging. *Stroke* 1992; **23**:663–7.

264 Lovblad KO, Weber J, Heid O, Mattle HP, Schroth G. Clinical and radiological patterns of human stroke as defined by echo-planar diffusion-weighted MR imaging. *Rivista di Neuroradiologia* 1998; **11**:227–30.

265 Lecouvet FE, Duprez TP, Raymackers JM, Peeters A, Cosnard G. Resolution of early diffusion-weighted and FLAIR MRI abnormalities in a patient with TIA. *Neurology* 1999; **52**:1085–7.

266 Lefkowitz D, LaBenz M, Nudo SR, Steg RE, Bertoni JM. Hyperacute ischaemic stroke missed by diffusion-weighted imaging. *Am J Neuroradiol* 2000; **20**:1871–5.

267 Wang PY, Barker PB, Wityk RJ, Ulug AM. Diffusion-negative stroke: a report of two cases. *Am J Neuroradiol* 1999; **20**:1876–80.

268 Kertesz A, Black SE, Nicholson L, Carr T. The sensitivity and specificity of MRI in stroke. *Neurology* 1987; **37**:1580–5.

269 Ueda T, Yuh WTC, Maley JE, Quets JP, Hahn PY, Magnotta VA. Outcome of acute lesions evaluated by diffusion and perfusion MR imaging. *Am J Neuroradiol* 1999; **20**:983–9.

270 Kohno K, Hoehn-Berlage M, Mies G, Back T, Hossmann KA. Relationship between diffusion-weighted MR images, cerebral blood flow, and energy state in experimental brain infarction. *Magn Reson Imaging* 1995; **13**:73–80.

271 Beaulieu C, de Crespigny A, Tong DC, Moseley ME, Albers GW, Marks MP. Longitudinal magnetic resonance imaging study of perfusion and diffusion in stroke: evolution of lesion volume and correlation with clinical outcome. *Ann Neurol* 1999; **46**:568–78.

272 Kidwell C, Mattiello J, Alger J, Duckwiler G, Starkman S, Liebeskind D, Saver, J, for the UCLA MRI Thrombolysis

Investigators. MRI ADC thresholds indicating increased risk of hemorrhagic transformation and of ischemic infarction with intra-arterial thrombolysis. *Stroke* 2000; **31**:9(067).

273 Neumann-Haefelin T, Wittsack H-J, Wenserski F, Siebler M, Seitz RJ. Diffusion- and perfusion-weighted MRI. The DWI/PWI mismatch region in acute stroke. *Stroke* 1999; **30**:1591–7.

274 Schlaug G, Benfield A, Baird AE, Siewert B, Lovblad KO, Parker RA, Edelman RR, Warach S. The ischemic penumbra: operationally defined by diffusion and perfusion MRI. *Neurology* 1999; **53**:1528–37.

275 Thijs VN, Adami A, Neumann-Haefelin T, Moseley ME, Marks MP, Albers GW. Relationship between severity of MR perfusion deficit and DWI lesion evolution. *Neurology* 2001; **57**:1205–11.

276 Fiehler J, Foth M, Kucinski T, Knab R, von Bezold M, Weiller C *et al*. Severe ADC decreases do not predict irreversible tissue damage in humans. *Stroke* 2002; **33**:79–86.

277 Bykowski JL, Latour LL, Warach S. More accurate identification of reversible ischemic injury in human stroke by cerebrospinal fluid suppressed diffusion-weighted imaging. *Stroke* 2004; **35**:1100–6.

278 Desmond PM, Lovell AC, Rawlinson AA, Parsons MW, Barber PA, Yang Q *et al*. The value of apparent diffusion coefficient maps in early cerebral ischemia. *Am J Neuroradiol* 2001; **22**:1260–7.

279 Lee TY, Murphy BD, Aviv RI, Fox AJ, Black SE, Sahlas DJ, *et al*. Cerebral blood flow threshold of ischemic penumbra and infarct core in acute ischemic stroke: a systematic review. *Stroke* 2006; **37**:2201.

280 Wardlaw JM, Keir SL, Bastin ME, Armitage PA, Rana AK. Is diffusion imaging appearance an independent predictor of outcome after ischaemic stroke? *Neurology* 2002; **59**:1381–7.

281 Hand PJ, Wardlaw JM, Rivers CS, Armitage PA, Bastin ME, Lindley RI, Dennis MS. MR diffusion-weighted imaging and outcome prediction after ischemic stroke. *Neurology* 2006; **66**:1159–63.

282 Warach S, Pettigrew LC, Dashe JF, Pullicino P, Lefkowitz DM, Sabounjian L *et al*. Effect of citicoline on ischemic lesions as measured by diffusion-weighted magnetic resonance imaging. Citicoline 010 Investigators. *Ann Neurol* 2000; **48**:713–22.

283 Phan TG, Donnan GA, Davis SM, Byrnes G. Proof-of-Principle Phase II MRI studies in stroke. Sample size estimates from dichotomous and continuous data. *Stroke* 2006; **37**:2521–5.

284 Warach S, Dashe JF, Edelman RR. Clinical outcome in ischaemic stroke predicted by early diffusion-weighted and perfusion magnetic resonance imaging: a preliminary analysis. *J Cereb Blood Flow Metab* 1996; **16**:53–9.

285 Lovblad KO, Baird AE, Schlaug G, Benfield A, Siewert B, Voetsch B *et al*. Ischemic lesion volumes in acute stroke by diffusion-weighted magnetic resonance imaging correlate with clinical outcome. *Ann Neurol* 1997; **42**:164–70.

286 Barber PA, Darby DG, Desmond PM, Yang Q, Gerraty RP, Jolley D. Prediction of stroke outcome with echoplanar perfusion- and diffusion-weighted MRI. *Neurology* 1998; **51**:418–26.

287 Van Everdingen KJ, van der Grond J, Kappelle LJ, Ramos LM, Mali WP. Diffusion-weighted magnetic resonance imaging in acute stroke. *Stroke* 1998; **29**:1783–90.

288 Thijs VN, Lansberg MG, Beaulieu C, Marks MP, Moseley ME, Albers GW. Is early ischemic lesion volume on diffusion-weighted imaging an independent predictor of stroke outcome? A multivariable analysis. *Stroke* 2000; **31**:2597–602.

289 Baird AE, Dambrosia J, Janket S, Eichbaum Q, Chaves C, Silver B *et al*. A three-item scale for the early prediction of stroke recovery. *Lancet* 2001; **357**:2095–9.

290 Schellinger PD, Fiebach JB, Jansen O, Ringleb PA, Mohr A, Steiner T *et al*. Stroke magnetic resonance imaging within 6 hours after onset of hyperacute cerebral ischemia. *Ann Neurol* 2001; **49**:460–9.

291 Fiehler J. ADC and metabolites in stroke: even more confusion about diffusion? *Stroke* 2003; **34**:7.

292 Engelter ST, Provenzale JM, Petrella JR, DeLong DM, Alberts MJ. Infarct volume on apparent diffusion coefficient maps correlates with length of stay and outcome after middle cerebral artery stroke. *Cerebrovasc Dis* 2003; **15**:188–91.

293 Engelter ST, Wetzel SG, Radue EW, Rausch M, Steck AJ, Lyrer PA. The clinical significance of diffusion-weighted MR imaging in infratentorial strokes. *Neurology* 2004; **62**:574–80.

294 Wyatt JC, Altman DG. Prognostic models: clinically useful or quickly forgotten? *Br Med J* 1995; **311**:1539–41.

295 Counsell C, Dennis M. Systematic review of prognostic models in patients with acute stroke. *Cerebrovasc Dis* 2001; **12**:159–70.

296 Counsell C, Dennis M, McDowall M, Warlow C. Predicting outcome after acute and subacute stroke. Development and validation of new prognostic models. *Stroke* 2002; **33**:1041–7.

297 Augustin M, Bammer R, Simbrunner J, Stollberger R, Hartung HP, Fazekas F. Diffusion-weighted imaging of patients with subacute cerebral ischemia: comparison with conventional and contrast-enhanced MR imaging. *Am J Neuroradiol* 2000; **21**:1596–602.

298 Singer MB, Chong J, Lu D, Schonewille WJ, Tuhrim S, Atlas SW. Diffusion-weighted MRI in acute subcortical infarction. *Stroke* 1998; **29**:133–6.

299 Roh JK, Kang DW, Lee SH, Yoon BW, Chang KH. Significance of acute multiple brain infarction on diffusion-weighted imaging. *Stroke* 2000; **31**:688–94.

300 Ay H, Oliveira-Filho J, Buonanno FS, Ezzeddine M, Schaefer PW, Rordorf G *et al*. Diffusion-weighted imaging identifies a subset of lacunar infarction associated with embolic source. *Stroke* 1999; **30**:2644–50.

301 Oliveira-Filho J, Ay H, Schaefer PW, Buonanno FS, Chang Y, Gonzalez RG, Koroshetz WJ. Diffusion-weighted magnetic resonance imaging identifies the 'clinically

relevant' small-penetrator infarcts. *Arch Neurol* 2000; **57**:1009–14.

302 Schonewille WJ, Tuhrim S, Singer MB, Atlas SW. Diffusion-weighted MRI in acute lacunar syndromes: a clinical-radiological correlation study. *Stroke* 1999; **30**:2066–9.

303 Yonemura K, Kimura K, Minematsu K, Uchino M, Yamaguci T. Small centrum ovale infarcts on diffusion-weighted magnetic resonance imaging. *Stroke* 2002; **33**:1541–4.

304 Albers GW, Caplan LR, Easton JD, Fayad PB, Mohr JP, Saver JL, Sherman DG. Transient ischemic attack: proposal for a new definition. *N Engl J Med* 2002; **347**:1713–16.

305 Goldstein LB, Simel DL. Is this patient having a stroke? *J Am Med Assoc* 2005; **293**:2391–402.

306 Latchaw RE, Yonas H, Hunter GJ, Yuh WT, Ueda T, Sorensen AG *et al*. Guidelines and recommendations for perfusion imaging in cerebral ischemia: a scientific statement for healthcare professionals by the writing group on perfusion imaging, from the Council on Cardiovascular Radiology of the American Heart Association. *Stroke* 2003; **34**:1084–104.

307 Chalela JA, Alsop DC, Gonzalez-Atavales JB, Maldjian JA, Kasner SE, Detre JA. Magnetic resonance perfusion imaging in acute ischemic stroke using continuous arterial spin labeling. *Stroke* 2000; **31**:680–7.

308 Calamante F, Gadian DG, Connelly A. Quantification of perfusion using bolus tracking magnetic resonance imaging in stroke: assumptions, limitations, and potential implications for clinical use. *Stroke* 2002; **33**:1146–51.

309 Carpenter T, Armitage PA, Bastin ME, Wardlaw JM. DSC perfusion MRI: quantification and reduction of systematic errors arising in areas of reduced cerebral blood flow. *Magn Reson Med* 2006; **55**:1342–9.

310 Kane I, Sandercock P, Wardlaw J. Magnetic resonance perfusion diffusion mismatch in acute ischaemic stroke: systematic review of methods used, influence on prognosis and impact on response to thrombolytic therapy. *J Neurol Neurosurg Psychiatry* 2007; **78**:485–491.

311 Rivers CS, Wardlaw JM, Armitage P, Bastin ME, Carpenter TK, Cvoro V *et al*. Do acute diffusion- and perfusion-weighted MRI lesions identify final infarct volume in ischemic stroke? *Stroke* 2006; **37**:98–104.

312 Ostergaard L, Weisskoff RM, Chesler D, Gyldensted C, Rosen BR. High resolution measurement of cerebral blood flow using intravascular tracer bolus passages. Part I: mathematical approach and statistical analysis. *Magn Reson Med* 1996; **36**:715–25.

313 Ostergaard L, Sorensen AG, Kwong KK, Weisskoff RM, Gyldensted C, Rosen BR. High resolution measurement of cerebral blood flow using intravascular tracer bolus passages. Part II: experimental comparison and preliminary results. *Magn Reson Med* 1996; **36**:726–36.

314 Teng MM, Cheng HC, Kao YH, Hsu LC, Yeh TC, Hung CS *et al*. MR perfusion studies of brain for patients with unilateral carotid stenosis or occlusion: evaluation of maps of 'time to peak' and 'percentage of baseline at peak'. *J Comput Assist Tomogr* 2001; **25**:121–5.

315 Zierler KL. Equations for measuring blood flow by external monitoring of radioisotopes. *Circ Res* 1965; **XVI**:309–21.

316 Rohl L, Ostergaard L, Simonsen CZ, Vestergaard-Poulsen P, Andersen G, Sakoh M *et al*. Viability thresholds of ischemic penumbra of hyperacute stroke defined by perfusion-weighted MRI and apparent diffusion coefficient. *Stroke* 2001; **32**:1140–6.

317 Parsons MW, Yang Q, Barber PA, Darby DG, Desmond PM, Gerraty RP *et al*. Perfusion magnetic resonance imaging maps in hyperacute stroke: relative cerebral blood flow most accurately identifies tissue destined to infarct. *Stroke* 2001; **32**:1581–7.

318 Rose SE, Janke AL, Griffin M, Finnigan S, Chalk JB. Improved prediction of final infarct volume using bolus delay-corrected perfusion-weighted MRI: implications for the ischemic penumbra. *Stroke* 2004; **35**:2466–71.

319 Baird AE, Lovblad KO, Dashe JF, Connor A, Burzynski C, Schlaug GS, Straroselskaya I, Edelman RR, Warach S. Clinical correlations of diffusion and perfusion lesion volumes in acute ischemic stroke. *Cerebrovasc Dis* 2000; **10**:441–8.

320 Barber PA, Parsons MW, Desmond PM, Bennett DA, Donnan GA, Tress BM, Davis SM. The use of PWI and DWI measures in the design of 'proof-of-concept' stroke trials. *J Neuroimaging* 2004; **14**:123–32.

321 Butcher K, Parsons M, Baird T, Barber A, Donnan G, Desmond P *et al*. Perfusion thresholds in acute stroke thrombolysis. *Stroke* 2003; **34**:2159–64.

322 Rohl L, Geday J, Ostergaard L, Simonsen CZ, Vestergaard-Poulsen P *et al*. Correlation between diffusion- and perfusion-weighted MRI and neurological deficit measured by the Scandinavian Stroke Scale and Barthel Index in hyperacute subcortical stroke (< or = 6 hours). *Cerebrovasc Dis* 2001; **12**:203–13.

323 Rose SE, Chalk JB, Griffin MP, Janke AL, Chen F, McLachan GJ *et al*. MRI based diffusion and perfusion predictive model to estimate stroke evolution. *Magn Reson Imaging* 2001; **19**:1043–53.

324 Simonsen CZ, Rohl L, Vestergaard-Poulsen P, Gyldensted C, Anderson G, Ostergaard L. Final infarct size after acute stroke: prediction with flow heterogeneity. *Neuroradiology* 2002; **225**:269–75.

325 Hjort N, Butcher K, Davis SM, Kidwell CS, Koroshetz WJ, Rother J *et al*. Magnetic resonance imaging criteria for thrombolysis in acute cerebral infarct. *Stroke* 2005; **36**:388–97.

326 Hacke W, Albers G, Al Rawi Y, Bogousslavsky J, Davalos A, Eliasziw M *et al*. The Desmoteplase in Acute Ischemic Stroke Trial (DIAS): a phase II MRI-based 9-hour window acute stroke thrombolysis trial with intravenous desmoteplase. *Stroke* 2005; **36**:66–73.

327 Butcher KS, Parsons M, MacGregor L, Barber PA, Chalk J, Bladin C *et al*, for the EPITHET Investigators. Refining the perfusion-diffusion mismatch hypothesis. *Stroke* 2005; **36**:1153–9.

328 Markus R, Reutens DC, Kazui S, Read S, Wright P, Pearce DC *et al*. Hypoxic tissue in ischaemic stroke: persistence

and clinical consequences of spontaneous survival. *Brain* 2004; **127**:1427–36.

329 Baker LL, Kucharczyk J, Sevick RJ, Mintorovitch J, Moseley ME. Recent advances in MR imaging/spectroscopy of cerebral ischemia. *Am J Roentgenol* 1991; **156**:1133–43.

330 Fisher M, Prichard JW, Warach S. New magnetic resonance techniques for acute ischemic stroke. *J Am Med Assoc* 1995; **274**:908–11.

331 Warach S, Li W, Ronthal M, Edelman RR. Acute cerebral ischaemia: evaluation with dynamic contrast-enhanced MR imaging and MR angiography. *Radiology* 1992; **182**:41–7.

332 Wardlaw JM, Chappell FM, Best JJK, Wartolowska K, Berry E, on behalf of the NHS Research & Development Health Technology Assessment Carotid Stenosis Imaging Group. Non-invasive imaging compared with intra-arterial angiography in the diagnosis of symptomatic carotid stenosis: a meta-analysis. *Lancet* 2006; **367**:1503–12.

333 Bottomley PA. Human in vivo NMR spectroscopy in diagnostic medicine: clinical tool or research probe? *Radiology* 1989; **170**:1–15.

334 Howe FA, Maxwell RJ, Saunders DE, Brown MM, Griffiths JR. Proton spectroscopy in vivo. *Magn Reson Q* 1993; **9**:31–59.

335 Ross B, Michaelis T. Clinical applications of magnetic resonance spectroscopy. *Magn Reson Q* 1994; **10**:191–247.

336 Saunders DE, Clifton AG, Brown MM. Measurement of infarct size using MRI predicts prognosis in middle cerebral artery infarction. *Stroke* 1995; **26**:2272–6.

337 Wardlaw JM, Marshall I, Wild J, Dennis MS, Cannon J, Lewis SC. Studies of acute ischemic stroke with proton magnetic resonance spectroscopy: relation between time from onset, neurological deficit, metabolite abnormalities in the infarct, blood flow, and clinical outcome. *Stroke* 1998; **29**:1618–24.

338 Wild JM, Wardlaw JM, Marshall I, Warlow CP. N-acetyl aspartate distribution in proton spectroscopic images of ischemic stroke: relationship to infarct appearance on T2-weighted magnetic resonance imaging. *Stroke* 2000; **31**:3008–14.

339 Baron JC, Cohen LG, Cramer SC, Dobkin BH, Johansen-Berg H, Loubinoux I *et al*. Neuroimaging in stroke recovery: a position paper from the First International Workshop on Neuroimaging and Stroke Recovery. *Cerebrovasc Dis* 2004; **18**:260–7.

340 Kidwell CS, Chalela JA, Saver JL, Starkman S, Hill MD, Demchuk AM *et al*. Comparison of MRI and CT for detection of acute intracerebral hemorrhage. *J Am Med Assoc* 2004; **292**:1823–30.

341 Fiebach JB, Schellinger PD, Jansen O, Meyer M, Wilde P, Bender J *et al*. CT and diffusion-weighted MR imaging in randomized order: diffusion-weighted imaging results in higher accuracy and lower interrater variability in the diagnosis of hyperacute ischemic stroke. *Stroke* 2002; **33**:2206–10.

342 Urbach H, Flacke S, Keller E, Textor J, Berlis A, Hartmann A *et al*. Detectability and detection rate of acute cerebral

hemisphere infarcts on CT and diffusion-weighted MRI. *Neuroradiology* 2000; **42**:722–7.

343 Fiebach J, Jansen O, Schellinger P, Knauth M, Hartmann M, Heiland S *et al*. Comparison of CT with diffusion-weighted MRI in patients with hyperacute stroke. *Neuroradiology* 2001; **43**:628–32.

344 Barber PA, Darby DG, Desmond PM, Gerraty RP, Yang Q, Li T *et al*. Identification of major ischemic change: diffusion-weighted imaging versus computed tomography. *Stroke* 1999; **30**:2059–65.

345 Lansberg MG, Albers GW, Beaulieu C, Marks MP. Comparison of diffusion-weighted MRI and CT in acute stroke. *Neurology* 2000; **54**:1557–61.

346 Witt J-P, Holl K, Heissler HE, Dietz H. Stable xenon CT CBF: effects of blood flow alterations on CBF calculations during inhalation of 33% stable xenon. *Am J Neuroradiol* 1991; **12**:973–5.

347 Merrick MV. Cerebral perfusion studies. *Eur J Nucl Med* 1990; **17**:98.

348 De Bruine JF, Limburg M, van Royen EA, Hijdra A, Hill TC, and Van Der Schoot JB. SPET brain imaging with 201 diethyldithiocarbamate in acute ischaemic stroke. *Eur J Nucl Med* 1990; **17**(5):248–51.

349 Hayman LA, Taber KH, Jhingran SG, Killian JM, and Carroll RG. Cerebral infarction: diagnosis and assessment of prognosis by using IMP-SPECT and CT. *Am J Neuroradiol* 1989; **10**(3):557–62.

350 Limburg M, van Royen EA, Hijdra A, de Bruine JF, Verbeeten BW, Jr. Single-photon emission computed tomography and early death in acute ischemic stroke. *Stroke* 1990; **21**:1150–5.

351 Alexandrov AV, Masdeu JC, Devous MD, Sr., Black SE, Grotta JC. Brain single-photon emission CT with HMPAO and safety of thrombolytic therapy in acute ischemic stroke. Proceedings of the meeting of the SPECT Safe Thrombolysis Study Collaborators and the members of the Brain Imaging Council of the Society of Nuclear Medicine. *Stroke* 1997; **28**:1830–4.

352 Baird AE, Austin MC, McKay WJ, Donnan GA. Changes in cerebral tissue perfusion during the first 48 hours of ischaemic stroke: relation to clinical outcome. *J Neurol Neurosurg Psychiatry* 1996; **61**:26–9.

353 Barber PA, Davis SM, Infeld B, Baird AE, Donnan GA, Jolley D, Lichtenstein M. Spontaneous reperfusion after ischemic stroke is associated with improved outcome. *Stroke* 1998; **29**:2522–8.

354 Baird AE, Donnan GA, Austin MC, Fitt GJ, Davis SM, McKay WJ. Reperfusion after thrombolytic therapy in ischemic stroke measured by single-photon emission computed tomography. *Stroke* 1994; **25**:79–85.

355 Ueda T, Sakaki S, Yuh WTC, Nochide I, Ohta S. Outcome in acute stroke with successful intra-arterial thrombolysis and predictive value of initial single-photon emission-computed tomography. *J Cereb Blood Flow Metab* 1999; **19**(1):99–108.

356 Moretti J-L, Defer G, Cinotti L, Cesaro P, Degos JD, Vigneron N *et al*. 'Luxury perfusion' with ^{99m}Tc-HMPAO

and ^{123}I-IMP SPECT imaging during the subacute phase of stroke. *Eur J Nucl Med* 1990; **16**:17–22.

357 Raynaud C, Rancurel G, Tzourio N, Soucy JP, Baron JC, Pappata S *et al*. SPECT analysis of recent cerebral infarction. *Stroke* 1989; **20**:192–204.

358 Bowler JV, Wade JP, Jones BE, Nijran K, Jewkes RF, Cuming R, Steiner TJ. Contribution of diaschisis to the clinical deficit in human cerebral infarction. *Stroke* 1995; **26**:1000–6.

359 Andrews RJ. Transhemispheric diaschisis. A review and comment. *Stroke* 1991; **22**:943–9.

360 Yasata M, Read SJ, O'Keefe GJ, Egan GF, Pointas O, McKay WJ, Donnan GA. Positron emission tomography in ischemic stroke: cerebral perfusion and metabolism after stroke onset. *J Clin Neurosci* 1998; **5**:413–416.

361 Baron JC. Mapping the ischaemic penumbra with PET: implications for acute stroke treatment. *Cerebrovasc Dis* 1999; **9**:193–201.

362 Baron JC. How healthy is the acutely reperfused ischemic penumbra? *Cerebrovasc Dis* 2005; **20**(S2):25–31.

363 Dobkin JA, Mintun MA. Clinical PET: Aesop's tortoise? *Radiology* 1993; **186**:13–15.

364 Davis SM, Donnan GA. Advances in penumbra imaging with MR. *Cerebrovasc Dis* 2004; **17**(S3):23–7.

365 Heiss W-D. Experimental evidence of ischemic thresholds and functional recovery. *Stroke* 1992; **23**:1668–72.

366 Heiss WD, Huber M, Fink GR, Herholz K, Pietrzyk U, Wagner R, Wienhard K. Progressive derangement of periinfarct viable tissue in ischemic stroke. *J Cereb Blood Flow Metab* 1992; **12**:193–203.

367 Baron JC, von Kummer R, del Zoppo GJ. Treatment of acute stroke. Challenging the concept of a rigid and universal time window. *Stroke* 1995; **26**:2219–21.

368 Read SJ, Hirano T, Abbott DF, Sachinidis VI, Tochon-Danguy HJ, Chan JG, *et al*. Identifying hypoxic tissue after acute ischemic stroke using PET and 18F-fluoromisonidazole. *Neurology* 1998; **51**:1617–1621.

369 Marchal G, Beaudouin V, Rioux P, de la Sayette V, Le Doze F, Viader F *et al*. Prolonged persistence of substantial volumes of potentially viable brain tissue after stroke: a correlative PET-CT study with voxel-based data analysis. *Stroke* 1996; **27**(4):599–606.

370 Heiss W-D, Grond M, Thiel A, von Stockhausen H-M, Rudolf J. Ischaemic brain tissue salvaged from infarction with alteplase. *Lancet* 1997; **349**:1600.

371 Marchal G, Benali K, Iglesias S, Viader F, Derlon JM, Baron JC. Voxel-based mapping of irreversible ischaemic damage with PET in acute stroke. *Brain* 1999; **123**:2387–400.

372 Sobesky J, Zaro WO, Lehnhardt FG, Hesselmann V, Neveling M, Jacobs A, Heiss WD. Does the mismatch match the penumbra? Magnetic resonance imaging and positron emission tomography in early ischemic stroke. *Stroke* 2005; **36**:980–5.

373 Bogousslavsky J, Regli F, Uske A, Maeder P. Early spontaneous hematoma in cerebral infarct: is primary cerebral hemorrhage overdiagnosed? *Neurology* 1991; **41**:837–40.

374 Lindley RI, Wardlaw JM, Sandercock PAG, Rimdusid P, Lewis SC, Signorini DF, Ricci S. Frequency and risk factors for spontaneous hemorrhagic transformation of cerebral infarction. *J Stroke Cerebrovasc Dis* 2004; **13**:235–46.

375 Motto C, Aritzu E, Boccardi E, De Grandi C, Piana A, Candelise L. Reliability of hemorrhagic transformation diagnosis in acute ischemic stroke. *Stroke* 1997; **28**:302–6.

376 Tanne D, Kasner SE, Demchuk AM, Koren-Morag N, Hanson S, Grond M, Levine SR, and the Multicentre rt-PA Stroke Survey Group. Markers of increased risk of intracerebral hemorrhage after intravenous recombinant tissue plasminogen activator therapy for acute ischemic stroke in clinical practice. The Multicentre rt-PA Acute Stroke Survey. *Circulation* 2002; **105**:1679–85.

377 Rimdusid P, Wardlaw J, Lindley RI, Sandercock P on behalf of the International Stroke Trial Collaboration Group. Haemorrhagic infarction in acute ischaemic stroke patients. *Cerebrovasc Dis* 1995; **5**:264.

378 Kent DM, Hinchey J, Price LL, Levine SR, Selker HP. In acute ischemic stroke, are asymptomatic intracranial hemorrhages clinically innocuous? *Stroke* 2004; **35**:1141–6.

379 Fisher M, Adams RD. Observations on brain embolism with special reference to the mechanism of haemorrhagic infarction. *J Neuropathol Exp Neurol* 1951; **10**:92–4.

380 Pessin MS, Teal PA, Caplan LR. Hemorrhagic infarction: guilt by association? *Am J Neuroradiol* 1992; **12**:1123–6.

381 Globus JH, Epstein JA. Massive cerebral haemorrhage: spontaneous and experimentally induced. *J Neuropathol Exp Neurol* 1953; **12**:107–31.

382 Ogata J, Yutani C, Imakita M, Ishibashi-Ueda H, Saku Y, Minematsu K *et al*. Hemorrhagic infarct of the brain without a reopening of the occluded arteries in cardioembolic stroke. *Stroke* 1989; **20**:876–83.

383 Bozzao L, Angeloni U, Bastianello S, Fantozzi LM, Pierallini A, Fieschi C. Early angiographic and CT findings in patients with hemorrhagic infarction in the distribution of the middle cerebral artery. *Am J Neuroradiol* 1992; **158**:1115–21.

384 Mori E, Tabuchi M, Ohsumi Y. Intra-arterial urokinase infusion therapy in acute thromboembolic stroke. *Stroke* 1990; **21**:1–74.

385 Wardlaw JM, Lammie GA, Whittle IR. A brain haemorrhage? *Lancet* 1998; **351**:1028.

386 Bousser MG. Cerebral venous thrombosis: diagnosis and management. *J Neurol* 2000; **247**:252–8.

387 Perkin GD. Cerebral venous thrombosis: development in imaging and treatment. *J Neurol Neurosurg Psychiatry* 1995; **59**:1–3.

388 Lafitte F, Boukobza M, Guichard JP, Hoeffel C, Reizine D, Ille O *et al*. MRI and MRA for diagnosis and follow-up of cerebral venous thrombosis (CVT). *Clin Radiol* 1997; **52**:672–9.

389 Virapongse C, Cazenave C, Quisling R, Sarwar M, Hunter S. The empty delta sign: frequency and significance in 76 cases of dural sinus thrombosis. *Radiology* 1987; **162**:779–85.

390 Duncan IC, Fourie PA. Imaging of cerebral isolated cortical vein thrombosis. *Am J Roentgenol* 2005; **184**:1317–19.

391 Buonanno E, Moody DM, Ball MR, Laster DW. Computed cranial tomographic findings in cerebral sino-venous occlusion. *J Comput Assist Tomography* 1978; **2**:281–90.

392 Bousser MG, Chiras J, Bories J, Castaigne P. Cerebral venous thrombosis: a review of 38 cases. *Stroke* 1985; **16**:199–213.

393 Dormont D, Anxionnat R, Evrard S, Louaille C, Chiras J, Marsault C. MRI in cerebral venous thrombosis. *J Neuroradiol* 1994; **21**(2):81–99.

394 Isensee Ch, Reul J, Thron A. Magnetic resonance imaging of thrombosed dural sinuses. *Stroke* 1994; **25**:29–34.

395 Mas J-L, Meder J-F, Meary E. Dural sinus thrombosis: long-term follow up by magnetic resonance imaging. *Cerebrovasc Dis* 1992; **2**:137–44.

396 Keller E, Flacke S, Urbach H, Schild HH. Diffusion- and perfusion-weighted magnetic resonance imaging in deep cerebral venous thrombosis. *Stroke* 1999; **30**:1144–6.

397 Corvol JC, Oppenheim C, Manai R, Logak M, Dormont D, Samson Y *et al.* Diffusion-weighted magnetic resonance imaging in a case of cerebral venous thrombosis. *Stroke* 1998; **29**:2649–52.

398 Wardlaw JM, Vaughan GT, Steers AJW, Sellar RJ. Transcranial Doppler ultrasound findings in cerebral venous sinus thrombosis. *J Neurosurg* 1994; **80**:332–5.

399 Stolz E, Kaps M, Dorndorf W. Assessment of intracranial venous hemodynamics in normal individuals and patients with cerebral venous thrombosis. *Stroke* 1999; **30**:70–5.

400 Ries S, Steinke W, Neff KW, Hennerici M. Echocontrast-enhanced transcranial color-coded sonography for the diagnosis of transverse sinus venous thrombosis. *Stroke* 1997; **28**:696–700.

401 Valdueza JM, Hoffmann O, Weih M, Mehraein S, Einhaupl KM. Monitoring of venous hemodynamics in patients with cerebral venous thrombosis by transcranial Doppler ultrasound. *Arch Neurol* 1999; **56**:229–34.

6

What caused this transient or persisting ischaemic event?

6.1 Introduction

Having decided that a patient has had a stroke or transient ischaemic attack (TIA) (Chapter 3), where the brain lesion is (Chapter 3) and its relationship to the vascular supply (Chapter 4), and that the cause is ischaemic rather than haemorrhagic (Chapter 5), the next step is to define the cause of the ischaemia. What caused *this* ischaemic event? If, for whatever reason, it has been impossible to distinguish an ischaemic stroke from non-traumatic intracerebral haemorrhage (ICH), then the causes of the latter (Chapter 8) must be considered as well. Naturally, how far one pursues 'the cause' must depend on how much this will influence the subsequent management and outcome of an individual patient, how far an individual patient or their family might want to pursue matters, or even – in some healthcare systems – how much they can afford.

So often physicians regard stroke as though it is a single disease. But a stroke is a clinical syndrome with many causes and the particular cause in an individual may determine the immediate outcome (section 10.2), have a substantial impact on the risk of recurrence

Stroke: practical management, 3rd edition. C. Warlow, J. van Gijn, M. Dennis, J. Wardlaw, J. Bamford, G. Hankey, P. Sandercock, G. Rinkel, P. Langhorne, C. Sudlow and P. Rothwell. Published 2008 Blackwell Publishing. ISBN 978-1-4051-2766-0.

(section 16.2) and influence the choice of both immediate (Chapters 12 and 13) and long-term treatment (Chapter 16). Moreover, identification of the cause may have unanticipated later relevance; for example, ischaemic stroke caused by carotid dissection as a consequence of a car accident (rather than caused by atherothrombosis) may lead to substantial compensation from an insurance company. Finding the likely cause is therefore important and may not be very difficult. The first clue is the clinical syndrome (where and how big is the area of brain ischaemia or infarction, section 6.7), then the general examination – which may provide more information about the cause than neurological examination (e.g. atrial fibrillation) – and a few well-targeted investigations should complete the picture (section 6.8). Sometimes, of course, a patient may have several competing causes, making it impossible to know which one is *the* cause.

A 70-year-old man suddenly developed weakness of the left arm and leg, which recovered after a few days. When he went to his doctor 3 days after the onset, there was a left hemiparesis but no visual field defect, nor any obvious sensory inattention or neglect. He was known to be hypertensive, discovered to be in atrial fibrillation and his ECG showed an unsuspected but probably old anterior myocardial infarction. There was a loud right carotid bruit. Brain CT was normal but MRI showed multiple presumed lacunar infarcts of indeterminate age in the periventricular white matter of both cerebral hemispheres. Therefore, this stroke might have been caused by any one of the following:

- *embolism from the heart (either from thrombus in the fibrillating left atrium or from thrombus in the left ventricle as a result of the myocardial infarction) causing a cortical infarct invisible even on MRI (any cortical signs having disappeared by the time the patient went to the doctor);*
- *embolism from atherothrombotic carotid stenosis to cause a cortical infarct invisible even on MRI;*
- *low flow distal to severe atherothrombotic carotid stenosis or occlusion;*
- *intracranial small vessel disease causing lacunar infarction; or*
- *something unusual, such as thrombocythaemia.*

6.2 What to expect

There is no *qualitative* difference between an ischaemic stroke and a transient ischaemic attack (TIA); anything which causes an ischaemic stroke may, if less severe or less prolonged, cause a TIA, while anything which causes a TIA may, if more severe or more prolonged, cause an ischaemic stroke. The *quantitative* difference is arbitrary and enshrined in the temporal boundary of symptoms lasting more or less than 24 h. This is, of course, irrelevant if a patient is seen within 24 h and is still symptomatic, where the concept of 'brain attack' is more appropriate (section 3.2.3). It is therefore not surprising that imaging evidence of relevant infarction is more likely the longer the duration of the symptoms (Fig. 3.2),[1–5] that all types of ischaemic stroke are about equally likely to be preceded by TIAs[6] (Table 6.1) and that the risk factor profiles

of ischaemic stroke and TIA are so similar.[7,8] Therefore, there is no great difference between searching for the cause of an ischaemic stroke and searching for the cause of a TIA.[9]

> Anything which causes an ischaemic stroke may, if less severe or less prolonged, cause a transient ischaemic attack, while anything which causes a transient ischaemic attack may, if more severe or more prolonged, cause an ischaemic stroke.

In population-based studies in white people, about one-half of cerebral ischaemic events, whether permanent or transient, are probably caused by the thrombotic and embolic complications of atheroma, which is a disorder of large and medium-sized arteries, about one-quarter to intracranial small vessel disease causing lacunar infarction, about one-fifth to embolism from the heart, and the rest to rarities[10–12] (Fig. 6.1) (Table 6.2). Not surprisingly, where admission rates are low, hospital-referred stroke patients are rather less likely to have lacunar strokes (because they are conscious without any cognitive defect and therefore easier to look after at home) and more likely to have something unusual, particularly if the hospital has a special interest in stroke or one of its causes – so-called hospital referral bias[12,13] (section 10.2.6). Age will colour expectations too: a 21-year-old female is unlikely to have atheroma, while an 81-year-old male is relatively unlikely to have a rare cause of cerebral ischaemia, such as a patent foramen ovale, and even if he has it is less likely to be relevant than in a 20-year-old male.

Table 6.1 The frequency of transient ischaemic attacks before various types of ischaemic stroke. (Unpublished data collected by Dr Claudio Sacks from the Oxfordshire Community Stroke Project.)

Stroke type	Percentage with preceding transient ischaemic attacks
All ischaemic strokes	14
Total anterior circulation infarction	16
Partial anterior circulation infarction	15
Lacunar infarction	12
Posterior circulation infarction	12
Presumed cardioembolic ischaemic stroke	16

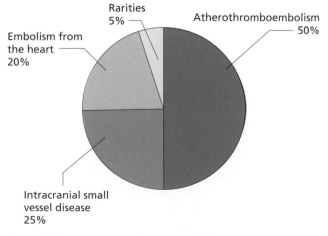

Fig. 6.1 The approximate frequency of the main causes of ischaemic stroke and transient ischaemic attacks in white populations.

Table 6.2 The causes of ischaemia affecting the arterial circulation of the brain and eye, largely disorders of the vessel wall (see Chapter 7 for unusual causes); haematological causes of ischaemic stroke are listed in Table 7.3 and the cardiac causes in Table 6.4.

Atherothromboembolism (section 6.3)
Embolism (section 6.3.2)
Occlusive thrombosis (section 6.3.2–6.3.5)
Low blood flow without acute occlusion (section 6.7.5)
Dolichoectasia (section 6.3.6)
Intracranial small vessel disease
'Complex' small vessel disease (section 6.4)
Hyaline arteriosclerosis or 'simple' small vessel disease (section 6.4)
Mural, junctional and microatheroma (section 6.4)
Cerebral amyloid angiopathy (section 8.2.2)
CADASIL (section 7.20.1)
Connective tissue, inflammatory vascular disorders (and other obscure vasculopathies)
Giant-cell arteritis* (section 7.3.1)
Takayasu's arteritis (section 7.3.2)
Systemic lupus erythematosus (section 7.3.3)
Antiphospholipid syndrome* (section 7.3.4)
Sneddon syndrome (section 7.3.5)
Primary systemic vasculitis (section 7.3.6)
   classic polyarteritis nodosa
   microscopic polyangiitis
   Churg–Strauss syndrome
   Wegener's granulomatosis
Kawasaki disease (section 7.3.7)
Henoch–Schönlein purpura (section 7.3.8)
Rheumatoid disease (section 7.3.9)
Sjögren syndrome (section 7.3.10)
Behçet's disease (section 7.3.11)
Relapsing polychondritis (section 7.3.12)
Progressive systemic sclerosis (scleroderma) (section 7.3.13)
Essential cryoglobulinaemia (section 7.3.14)
Malignant atrophic papulosis (Kohlmeier–Degos disease) (section 7.3.15)
Sarcoidosis (section 7.3.16)
Primary angiitis of the central nervous system (section 7.3.17)
Idiopathic reversible cerebral 'vasoconstriction' (section 7.3.18)
Buerger's disease (thromboangiitis obliterans) (section 7.3.19)
Paraneoplastic vasculitis (section 7.3.20)
Therapeutic drugs (section 7.3.21)
Acute posterior multifocal placoid pigment epitheliopathy (section 7.3.22)
Susac syndrome (section 7.3.23)
Eales disease (section 7.3.24)
Cogan syndrome (section 7.3.25)
Secondary inflammatory vascular disordesr
Infections (section 7.11)
Drugs* (section 7.15)
Irradiation (section 7.12)
Inflammatory bowel disease (section 7.17)
Coeliac disease (section 7.17)
Congenital
Fibromuscular dysplasia (section 7.4.1)
Hypoplastic carotid and vertebral arteries (7.4.2)
Internal carotid artery loops (7.4.3)
*Arterial dissection**
Trauma (section 7.1)
Cystic medial necrosis (section 7.2.1)
Fibromuscular dysplasia (section 7.4.1)

Marfan syndrome (section 7.20.7)
Ehlers–Danlos syndrome type 4 (section 7.20.7)
Inflammatory arterial disease (section 7.3)
Infective arterial disease (e.g. syphilis) (section 7.11)
Alpha – 1 antitrypsin deficiency (section 7.2.1)
Autosomal dominant polycystic kidney disease (section 7.2.1)
Osteogenesis imperfecta (section 7.2.1)
Trauma
Penetrating neck injury (section 7.1.1)
   neck laceration/surgery
   missile wounds
   oral trauma
   tonsillectomy
   cerebral catheter angiography
   attempted jugular vein catheterization
Non-penetrating (blunt) neck injury (section 7.1.2, 3 and 5)
   carotid compression
   cervical manipulation
   blow to the neck
   cervical flexion–extension 'whiplash' injury
   minor head movements?
   cervical rib
   fractured clavicle
   bronchoscopy
   endotracheal intubation
   head-banging
   labour
   epileptic seizures
   yoga
   attempted strangulation
   atlanto-occipital instability
   atlanto-axial dislocation
   fractured base of skull
   faulty posture of neck during general anaesthesia, or even a prolonged telephone conversation or vomiting
Head injury (section 7.1.4)
Single gene disorders
CADASIL (section 7.20.1)
Homocystinuria (section 7.20.2)
Fabry's disease (section 7.20.3)
Tuberous sclerosis (section 7.20.4)
Neurofibromatosis (section 7.20.5)
Oxalosis (section 7.20.6)
Inherited disorders of connective and elastic tissue (section 7.20.7)
Metabolic disorders (section 7.16)
Miscellaneous
Fibrocartilaginous embolism (section 7.1.6)
Air embolism (section 7.1.7)
Fat embolism (section 7.1.8)
Arterial aneurysms (section 7.6)
Cholesterol embolization syndrome (7.7)
Migraine (section 7.8)
Cancer (section 7.12)
Irradiation (section 7.12)
Oral contraceptives/oestrogens (section 7.13)
Pregnancy and the puerperium (section 7.14)
Perioperative (section 7.18)
Mitochodrial diseases (section 7.19)

*The most common 'rare' causes of arterial disease, in total, well under 5% of all patients with ischaemic stroke/transient ischaemic attack.
CADASIL, cerebral autosomal dominant arteriopathy with subcortical infarcts and leukoencephalopathy;
MELAS, mitochondrial encephalopathy, lactic acidosis and stroke-like episodes.

About 95% of ischaemic strokes and transient ischaemic attacks are caused by the embolic, thrombotic or low-flow consequences of atheroma affecting large and medium-sized arteries, intracranial small vessel disease or embolism from the heart.

This chapter will consider the nature of the three main causes of cerebral ischaemia: atherothromboembolism (section 6.3), intracranial small vessel disease (section 6.4) and embolism from the heart (section 6.5). The more unusual causes will be described in Chapter 7.

6.3 Atheroma and large vessel disease

Atheroma is by far the most frequent, but certainly not the only, arterial disorder. It is almost universal in the elderly, at least in developed countries. When complicated by thrombosis and embolism, and sometimes by low flow distal to a severely stenosed or occluded artery, it is the most common cause of cerebral ischaemia and infarction. Although very difficult to prove, atheroma itself – uncomplicated by thrombosis and embolism – may *not* have become more prevalent during the first half of the 20th century, despite the rising mortality attributed to stroke and coronary events at the time, nor less prevalent more recently as vascular disease mortality has declined (section 18.2.1).[14–16] The clinically important consequences of atheroma – ischaemic stroke, myocardial infarction and peripheral vascular disease – are probably more to do with the thrombotic complications of atheroma than the atheroma itself. It is, after all, remarkable how widespread atheroma can be at postmortem in patients with no clinically obvious events. Also, both ischaemic stroke and myocardial infarction can occur even when atheroma is relatively restricted; is this bad atheroma, bad clotting or just bad luck?

The current view is that atheroma is initiated by some sort of endothelial injury and, perhaps in genetically susceptible individuals, is then amplified by lifestyle and environmental factors, and it is already apparent even in children and young adults.[17–19] Evidence comes from animal models of atheroma, postmortem examination of human arteries, and epidemiological studies of 'risk factors', although these may be as much risk factors for the complicating thrombosis as for the underlying atheroma itself, if, indeed, the two processes can be separated.[20]

6.3.1 The distribution of atheroma

Atheroma affects mainly large and medium-sized arteries, particularly at points of arterial branching, curvature and confluence[18,19,21–26] (Fig. 6.2). The most common extracranial sites for atheroma are the aortic arch, the proximal subclavian arteries, the carotid bifurcation and the vertebral artery origins. Plaques in the subclavian arteries frequently extend into the origin of the vertebral arteries and plaques may occasionally occur at the origin of the innominate arteries. Frequently, the second portion of the vertebral artery as it passes through the transverse foramen is also affected but the atheroma, which tends to form a ladder-like arrangement opposite cervical discs and osteophytes, does not normally restrict the lumen size significantly.[27]

Intracranial arteries are morphologically different from extracranial arteries, having no external elastic lamina, fewer elastic fibres in the media and adventitia and a thinner intimal layer (Fig. 4.2). The carotid siphon, the proximal middle cerebral artery and the anterior cerebral artery around the anterior communicating artery origin are the most common sites for intracranial atheroma formation in the anterior circulation. In the posterior circulation, the intracranial vertebral arteries are often affected just after they penetrate the dura and distally near the basilar artery origin. Plaques are also found in the proximal basilar artery and also before the origin of the posterior cerebral arteries. The mid-basilar segment may be affected around the origins of the cerebellar arteries. Occlusion of a branch artery at its origin by disease in the parent vessel seems to occur more commonly in the posterior circulation (e.g. 'basilar branch occlusion') than in the anterior circulation where occlusion of the small perforating arteries is usually caused by intrinsic small vessel disease (section 6.4).

It is remarkable how free of atheroma some arterial sites can be; for example, the internal carotid artery (ICA) between just distal to its origin in the neck (the carotid sinus) and the carotid siphon in the head, and the main cerebral arteries distal to the circle of Willis. Occlusion of the middle cerebral artery (MCA) can sometimes be caused by *in situ* thrombosis complicating an unstable atheromatous plaque, but is much more likely to be caused by embolism from the heart or from a proximal arterial site.[28–30] Indeed, even occlusion of the carotid siphon is seldom caused by *in situ* atherothrombosis, but more likely by embolism or a non-atheromatous arterial disorder.[31] Another unexplained oddity is how the upper limb arteries are far less affected by atheroma than the lower limb arteries.

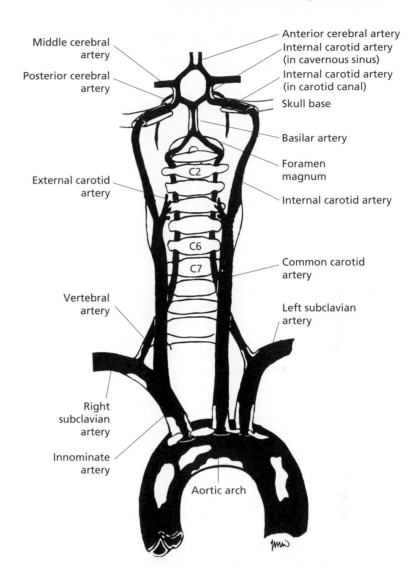

Middle cerebral artery
Posterior cerebral artery
Anterior cerebral artery
Internal carotid artery (in cavernous sinus)
Internal carotid artery (in carotid canal)
Skull base
Basilar artery
Foramen magnum
External carotid artery
C2
Internal carotid artery
C6
C7
Common carotid artery
Vertebral artery
Left subclavian artery
Right subclavian artery
Innominate artery
Aortic arch

Fig. 6.2 The distribution of atheroma (white indentations of the arterial lumen) in the arteries supplying the brain and eye in white populations. Intracranial atheroma is relatively more severe in Japanese, Chinese and black populations.

> Atheroma affects large and medium-sized arteries, particularly at places of branching, tortuosity and confluence. It is a multifocal rather than a diffuse disease.

Possible explanations for this multifocal distribution of atheroma are:
- high haemodynamic shear stress and so endothelial trauma, a notion now largely discredited;
- low haemodynamic shear stress, boundary-zone flow separation, directional and stagnation changes in the blood, all leading to intimal proliferation and the accumulation of platelets; and
- turbulence, leading to endothelial damage;

all of which might promote thrombosis, which itself is clearly involved in the progression, if not the very beginnings, of atheroma.[32,33] Interestingly, there can be very severe atherothrombotic stenosis at a particular site on one side of the body, but none at all at the mirror-image site on the other side, perhaps reflecting intra-individual geometric differences in arterial anatomy.[34,35] Alternatively, perhaps once an atheromatous plaque is established, its growth becomes self-promoting as a result of a positive feedback loop, either biochemical or haemodynamic. This asymmetry clearly cannot be because of asymmetric exposure to vascular risk factors, such as smoking. On the whole, however, individuals with atheroma affecting one artery tend to have it affecting many others, subclinically if not clinically. Therefore, patients with cerebral ischaemia or carotid disease often already have (Table 6.3) or develop (section 16.2) angina, myocardial infarction and peripheral vascular disease.[36-41] Presumably, genetic predisposition determines *who* is likely to develop atheroma, or to have particularly

Table 6.3 The prevalence of vascular risk factors and diseases in 244 patients with a first-ever-in-a-lifetime ischaemic stroke. Data from the Oxfordshire Community Stroke Project (Sandercock *et al.* 1989).[10]

Risk factor	Number	Percentage
Hypertension (blood pressure > 160/90 mmHg, at least twice pre-stroke)	126	52
Angina and/or past myocardial infarction	92	38
Current smoker	66	27
Claudication and/or absent foot pulses	60	25
Major cardiac embolic source	50	20
Transient ischaemic attack	35	14
Cervical arterial bruit	33	14
Diabetes mellitus	24	10
Any of the above	196	80

extensive or severe atheroma when exposed to causal risk factors, such as hypertension, while the arterial anatomy determines *where* the atheroma occurs.

There appear to be important racial differences in the distribution of atheroma, and race is an independent predictor of lesion location.[42] White males tend to develop atheroma in the extracranial cerebral vessels, the aorta and coronary arteries while intracranial large vessel disease appears to be relatively more common in black, Hispanic and Asian populations[43–45] and tends to affect younger patients[43,45] and those with type 1 diabetes mellitus.[43] Some sources report that women have more intracranial disease compared to men but this is disputed by others.[44] However, carotid bifurcation stenosis does appear to be becoming more frequent in Oriental populations either because the pattern of atheroma is evolving as a result of lifestyle changes, or because previous studies were confounded by selection and other biases.[44,46,47] There are very few data on the aetiology of stroke in Africa, but reports from stroke registers in South Africa show that atheroma is a less common cause of stroke in blacks than in whites.[48]

> Individuals with atheroma affecting one artery almost always have atheroma affecting many other arteries, with or without clinical manifestations.

6.3.2 The nature, progression and clinical consequences of atheroma

Atheroma begins as intimal fatty streaks in children, it is thought in response to endothelial injury[18,19] (Fig. 6.3).

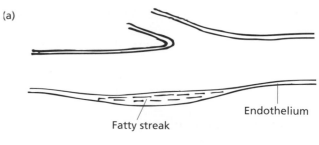

(a)

Endothelium

Fatty streak

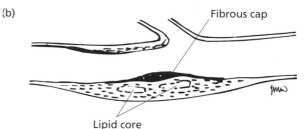

(b)

Fibrous cap

Lipid core

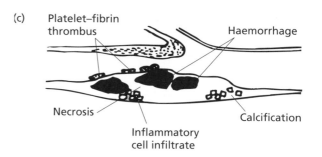

(c)

Platelet–fibrin thrombus

Haemorrhage

Necrosis

Calcification

Inflammatory cell infiltrate

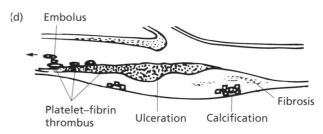

(d)

Embolus

Platelet–fibrin thrombus

Ulceration

Calcification

Fibrosis

Fig. 6.3 The growth, progression and complications of atheromatous plaques: (a) early deposition of lipid in the artery wall as a fatty streak; (b) further build-up of fibrous and lipid material; (c) necrosis, inflammatory cell infiltrate, calcification and new vessel formation, leading to (d) plaque instability, ulceration and platelet–fibrin thrombus formation on the plaque surface.

Over many years, circulating monocyte-derived macrophages adhere to and invade the arterial wall. As a result, there is an inflammatory response with cytokine production and T-lymphocyte activation. Intra- and later extracellular cholesterol and other lipids are deposited, particularly in macrophages, which are then described as foam cells. Arterial smooth-muscle cells migrate into the lesion and proliferate, fibrosis occurs and so fibrolipid plaques are formed. These plaques, with their lipid core and fibrous cap, encroach upon the media and spread around and along the arterial wall. Some become necrotic, ulcerated and calcified with neovascularization and haemorrhage – so-called complicated plaques. The arterial wall thickens, the vessel dilates or the lumen narrows and the artery becomes stiffer and tortuous.

Atherosclerotic lesions may cause ischaemic stroke through acute vessel occlusion, or by reducing vessel diameter and thus regional cerebral blood flow. Whether acute occlusion of a cerebral vessel, or reduction in cerebral blood flow, leads to infarction depends on not only for how long the blood flow is impaired, but also the availability and functional capability of the collateral circulation[49–53] (section 4.2).

Arterial occlusion secondary to atheroma occurs by three mechanisms. First, thrombi may form on lesions and cause local occlusion. Second, embolization of plaque debris or thrombus may block a more distal vessel; emboli are usually the cause of obstruction of the anterior circulation intracranial vessels[29,30] at least in white males in whom intracranial atheroma is relatively rare. Third, small vessel origins may be occluded by growth of plaque in the parent vessel. This is seen particularly in the basilar artery and the subclavian artery around the vertebral origin. Low regional cerebral blood flow secondary to atheroma occurs when plaque growth causes severe reduction in the diameter of the vessel lumen and hypoperfusion of distal brain regions, particularly in the border zones where blood supply is poorest. This may lead to 'borderzone infarction' (section 6.7.5) of these regions following severe hypotension or hypoxia. The mechanisms of atherosclerosis-related stroke are discussed further below.

6.3.3 Atheromatous plaques complicated by thrombosis: atherothrombosis

From an early stage, or perhaps even from the very first stage, atheromatous plaques promote platelet adhesion, activation and aggregation, which initiates blood coagulation and thus mural thrombosis.[54–56] At first, any thrombus may be lysed by fibrinolytic mechanisms in the vessel wall, or incorporated into the plaque, which re-endothelializes and so 'heals'. Gradually, the athero- and then atherothrombotic plaque grows, in part because of repeated episodes of mural thrombosis layering one on top of the other, and eventually the lumen may become obstructed. Such occlusive intraluminal thrombus may then propagate proximally or distally in the column of stagnant blood, but usually no further than the next arterial branching point.

Thrombosis is opposed by the release of prostacyclin and nitric oxide, both vasodilators, from the vascular endothelium and by endothelium-derived plasminogen activator. The balance of these pro- and antithrombotic factors may determine whether a thrombus complicating an atheromatous plaque or an occlusive embolus grows, is lysed or becomes incorporated into the arterial wall and so contributes to the gradually enlarging atherothrombotic plaque.

Symptomatic *in situ* acute atherothrombotic occlusion – rather than artery-to-artery embolism – does not appear to be a very common cause for ischaemic stroke or transient ischaemic attacks (TIAs) in the carotid territory. Perhaps this is because atheroma affects the larger arteries (e.g. internal carotid artery (ICA) rather than middle cerebral artery) and it takes a very large plaque to occlude them, or because the potential for collateral blood flow is better distal to larger arteries.[29,57] Indeed, once the ICA has occluded, the risk of ipsilateral ischaemic stroke appears to be less than for severe stenosis.[58–60] On the other hand, symptomatic *in situ* atherothrombotic occlusion may be more common in the posterior circulation (e.g. of the basilar artery) but even here artery-to-artery embolism is well described.[61–65]

6.3.4 Embolism from atherothrombotic plaques: atherothromboembolism

Atheroma and/or thrombus may embolize – in whole or in part – to obstruct a smaller distal artery, usually at a branching point – the same one or different ones on several occasions. Emboli consist of any combination of cholesterol crystals and other debris from the plaque, platelet aggregates, and fibrin which may be recently formed and relatively friable or old and well organized. Depending on their size, composition, consistency and age – and presumably the blood flow conditions at the site of impaction – emboli may be lysed, fragment and then be swept on into the microcirculation. Alternatively, they may permanently occlude the distal artery and promote local antero- and retrograde thrombosis, which is further encouraged by the release of thromboxane A2 from platelets, which is also a vasoconstrictor.

Emboli are transmitted to the brain or eye via their normal arterial supply, which itself varies somewhat in distribution between individuals (section 4.2). An embolus from an atherosclerotic carotid bifurcation – usually a plaque at the origin of the internal carotid artery (ICA) but sometimes the distal common or proximal external carotid arteries – normally goes to the eye or the anterior two-thirds of the cerebral hemisphere. But, on occasion, it may go to the occipital cortex if blood is flowing from the ICA via the posterior communicating artery to the posterior cerebral artery, or if there is a fetal origin (section 4.2.3) of the posterior cerebral artery from the distal ICA (5–10% of individuals). However, if an artery is already occluded, then an embolus may travel via the collateral circulation and impact in an unexpected place. For example, with severe vertebral arterial disease, and therefore poor flow distally into the basilar artery, an embolus from the ICA origin may reach the basilar artery via the circle of Willis.

With ICA occlusion, it is still possible to have an ipsilateral middle cerebral artery (MCA) distribution cerebral infarct as a result of:

• an embolus travelling from the *contralateral* ICA origin via the anterior communicating artery;
• an embolus from any blind stump of the occluded ICA, or from disease of the ipsilateral external carotid artery (ECA), via the ECA and orbital collaterals to the MCA;
• an embolus from the tail of thrombus in the ICA distal to the occlusion; or
• low flow distal to the ICA occlusion, perhaps within a boundary zone (section 6.7.5), particularly if the collateral blood supply is poor, cerebrovascular reactivity is impaired and the oxygen extraction ratio high.[652,66–69]

Curiously, emboli from the neck arteries (or from the heart) seldom seem to enter the small perforating arteries of the brain to cause lacunar infarction (section 6.4) perhaps as a consequence of the fact that the perforating vessels arise at a 90° angle from the parent vessel.

6.3.5 Atherothrombosis/embolism as an acute-on-chronic disorder: plaque instability

Like the coronary arteries, atheromatous plaques in the cerebral circulation – particularly at the carotid bifurcation – become 'active' or 'unstable' from time to time with fissuring, cracking or rupture of the fibrous cap, or ulceration. The histological features of plaque instability are a thin fibrous cap, large lipid core, reduced smooth muscle content and high macrophage density[31,70–72] (Fig. 6.4a). If the thrombogenic centre of the plaque is exposed to flowing blood, then complicating thrombosis occurs. Plaque instability may even be a 'systemic' tendency because irregularity on catheter angiography – and so presumed instability and ulceration – of symptomatic carotid stenosis is associated with irregularity of the asymptomatic contralateral carotid artery, and with coronary events assumed to be caused by plaque rupture.[73] At other times the plaque is quiescent with a thick fibrous cap, or slowly growing, without causing any clinical symptoms[30,31,74–77] (Fig. 6.4b). In other words, atherothromboembolism is an 'acute-on-chronic disorder'. It is no surprise therefore that the clinical complications of atheroma reflect this:

• transient ischaemic attacks (TIA) tend to cluster in time[78] (section 3.2.1);
• stroke tends to occur early after a TIA and affect the same arterial territory[79] (section 16.2.1);

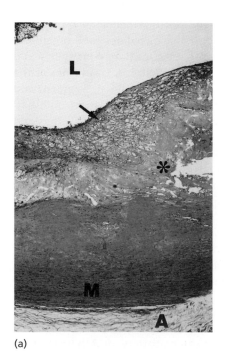

(a)

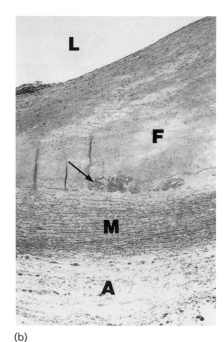

(b)

Fig. 6.4 Photomicrographs of transverse sections of the carotid sinus illustrating the pathological features of atherosclerotic plaque stability. (a) An unstable plaque characterized by a large necrotic core (✱), and a thin fibrous cap heavily infiltrated by macrophages (*arrow*). Elsewhere the plaque is ulcerated and the lumen occluded by thrombus, part of which had embolized to the ipsilateral middle cerebral artery causing a fatal ischaemic stroke. (b) A comparable stenotic but stable plaque, comprising largely fibrous tissue (F) with focal calcification (*arrow*). There is no significant necrotic core or inflammatory cell infiltrate. L lumen; A tunica adventitia; M tunica media. (Provided by Dr Alistair Lammie.)

- the risk of ischaemic stroke ipsilateral to severe carotid stenosis is highest soon after symptomatic presentation and then declines,[73,80] even though the stenosis itself seldom regresses (Fig. 16.38);
- presumed artery-to-artery embolic strokes tend to recur particularly early[81] (section 16.2.3);
- emboli are more often detected with transcranial Doppler sonography if carotid stenosis is severe or recently symptomatic;[82–87] and
- the rate of Doppler-detected emboli in the middle cerebral artery tends to decline with time after stroke.[88]

Increasing severity of symptomatic atherothrombotic stenosis, at least at the origin of the internal carotid artery, is undoubtedly a powerful predictor and cause of ischaemic stroke ipsilateral to the lesion.[89] However, this cannot be the whole explanation because:

- the risk of stroke distal to an asymptomatic stenosis is far less than distal to a recently symptomatic stenosis of the same severity (section 16.12.5);
- by no means all patients with severe stenosis have a stroke (section 16.11.5); and
- relatively mildly stenosed plaques can be complicated by acute carotid occlusion.[31]

Curiously, there is not such an obvious relationship between increasing coronary artery stenosis and coronary events. This may be because the coronary arteries are harder to image repeatedly and are more anatomically complicated, because coronary events are more often 'silent', or because the coronary arteries are smaller and more likely to be blocked if even a small plaque ruptures.[90]

Independently of the severity of stenosis, plaque irregularity on catheter angiography is associated with increased stroke risk, probably because irregularity represents plaque ulceration and instability with thrombosis and so likely complicating embolism[71,85,91] (section 16.11.8).

> Atherothromboembolism is an acute-on-chronic disorder, both in its pathology and in its clinical manifestations. Although the formation of atherothrombotic plaques must be a long and gradual process over many years, the clinical manifestations usually occur acutely (e.g. an ischaemic stroke) and tend to cluster in time. For example, stroke tends to occur sooner rather than later after a transient ischaemic attack, perhaps as a result of the breakdown and 'instability' of an atherothrombotic plaque which later 'heals'.

Exactly why one plaque becomes unstable (and then perhaps ulcerates with complicating thrombosis) and another does not, is unknown. Histological comparisons of recently symptomatic with asymptomatic carotid plaques – matched for stenosis severity – are not easy to perform. However, it seems as though intraplaque haemorrhage, calcification and the lipid core are similar in both but, crucially, the thickness of the fibrous cap has not generally been assessed.[92–94] Similar problems arise with attempts to compare inflammatory processes and the expression of adhesion molecules,[95,96] metalloproteinase expression,[97] differences in plaque tissue factor[98] and in plaque geometry and motion and so potential stresses on the fibrous cap.[99,100] Whether infection causes plaque instability is very unclear (section 6.6.17). In all these cross-sectional studies there is always the possibility of reverse causality – that by becoming symptomatic a plaque is changed in its anatomy, motion, biochemistry, and so on.

6.3.6 Dolichoectasia

This somewhat unusual pattern of arterial disease tends to affect the medium-sized arteries at the base of the brain, particularly the basilar artery, mostly in the elderly but occasionally in children[101–105] (section 4.2.3). The arteries are widened, tortuous, elongated and are often enlarged enough to be seen as characteristic flow voids on MRI, and as tortuous channels – even without enhancement – or by virtue of calcification in their walls on brain CT[106] (Fig. 6.5). When found in an individual, this arterial abnormality is not necessarily the cause of any ischaemic stroke (and very rarely of intracranial haemorrhage, despite the aneurysmal dilatation). However, these enlarged vessels can contain thrombus which embolizes, or occludes the origin of small branch arteries of the ectatic vessel, or even occludes the ectatic vessel itself. Cranial nerve and brainstem dysfunction due to direct compression or small vessel ischaemia, or hydrocephalus caused by cerebrospinal fluid pathway compression, are other occasional complications of basilar (or vertebral) ectasia.[104,105,107–109] Atheroma is the most common cause.[110] Other causes include various types of congenital defect in the vessel wall, Marfan syndrome, pseudoxanthoma elasticum and Fabry's disease[111] – both in homozygotic males and heterozygotic females.

6.4 Intracranial small vessel disease

There are a number of pathologies which affect the small (40–400 µm diameter) arteries, arterioles and veins

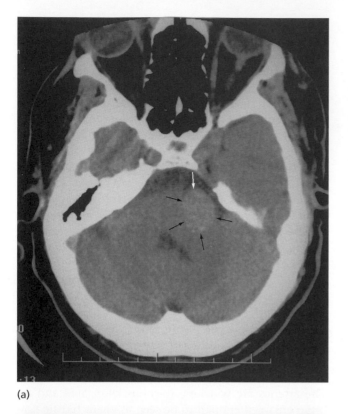

(a)

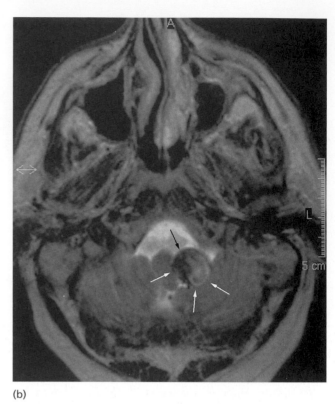

(b)

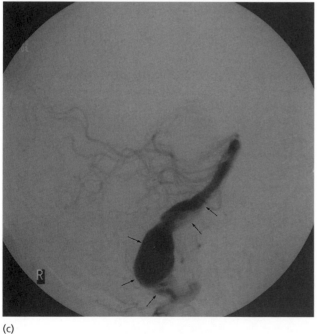

(c)

Fig. 6.5 Vertibrobasilar dolichoectasia. (a) On the brain CT scan there is a 1.5–2 cm rounded mass (*arrows*) which is of slightly higher density than adjacent brain and sits in the left cerebellopontine angle. The mass is indenting the brainstem. On adjacent sections the mass was obviously longitudinal and contiguous with the vertebral and top end of the basilar arteries. (b) MR examination of the same patient shows the mixed signal mass (*arrows*). The presence of increased signal indicates either very slowly flowing or partially clotted blood. (c) Catheter angiography shows a lateral projection of the vertebrobasilar circulation. Although the main area of expansion of the arterial system is in the lower basilar artery (*arrows*), the dolichoectasia actually extends from the upper right vertebral artery almost to the very tip of the basilar artery.

of the meninges and brain – for example, cerebral amyloid angiopathy (section 8.2.2); vasculitis (section 7.3); atheroma near the origin of the small perforating arteries (see below); and the angiopathy underlying cerebral autosomal dominant arteriopathy with subcortical infarcts and leucoenceophalopathy (CADASIL)

(section 7.20.1). Much more common, however, is what has been termed hyaline arteriosclerosis. This is an almost universal change in the small arteries and arterioles of the aged brain, particularly it is said in the presence of hypertension or diabetes, but sometimes in quite young patients without any of the classical

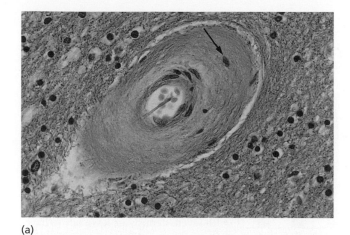

(a)

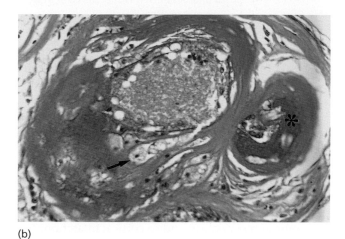

(b)

Fig. 6.6 Photomicrograph of perforating lenticulostriate artery branches in the putamen, illustrating two distinctive patterns of vessel pathology. (a) Concentric hyaline wall thickening with a few remaining vascular smooth-muscle cell nuclei (*arrow*). The lumen remains patent. Such 'simple' small vessel disease is an almost invariable feature of elderly brains, most prominent in hypertensive and diabetic patients. (b) A complex, disorganized vessel segment showing an asymmetrical destructive process with focal fibrinoid material (*) and mural foam cells (*arrow*). The lumen is visible cut in two planes of section. In this case the vascular lesion was adjacent to and, presumably, the cause of a right striatocapsular lacunar infarct. This 'complex' vessel lesion corresponds with what Miller Fisher termed 'lipohyalinosis'. (Provided by Dr Alistair Lammie.)

vascular risk factors[112] (Fig. 6.6). Important factors in its development appear to include not only hypertension and diabetes, but also breakdown of the blood–brain barrier with incorporation of plasma proteins into the vessel wall, possibly due to endothelial dysfunction.[113] The smooth muscle cells in the wall are eventually replaced by collagen, which reduces vascular distensibility, and presumably reactivity, but not necessarily the size of the lumen.

Unfortunately, over the years, the pathological nomenclature for small vessel disease has been very confusing and, as a result, the 'simple' small vessel disease (SVD) described above has frequently been confused with a more aggressive-looking disorder of small arteries with disorganization of their walls and foam cell infiltration. It is this 'complex' SVD that Fisher first called 'segmental arterial disorganization' and then 'lipohyalinosis'. The term fibrinoid vessel wall necrosis refers to a different, characteristic, but more acute change in the vessel wall seen, for example, as a consequence of accelerated hypertension and as a reactive phenomenon around acute intracerebral haematomas, spontaneous or traumatic. When healed, this probably takes on the appearance of 'complex' SVD[114,115] (Fig. 6.6). However, it is by no means certain that 'complex' SVD and acute fibrinoid necrosis are more advanced forms of 'simple' SVD, and there is no evidence that 'simple' SVD is the 'healed' version of complex SVD. Nonetheless, both 'simple' and 'complex' SVD tend to affect the lenticulostriate perforating branches of the middle cerebral artery, the thalamoperforating branches of the proximal posterior cerebral artery, the perforating branches of the basilar artery to the brainstem, and the vessels in the periventricular white matter.[116]

Most of what is known about small vessel disease and lacunar stroke comes from a very small number of very careful clinicoanatomical observations by Fisher. He did not describe 'simple' SVD as the underlying vascular pathology of lacunes, but what we prefer to call 'complex' SVD in some cases, and atheroma affecting the origins of the small vessels where they come off the circle of Willis and major cerebral arteries in others.[117–119] In theory, one can think of 'mural atheroma' affecting the parent arteries, 'junctional atheroma' affecting the origin of the small perforating arteries where they leave the parent artery, and 'microatheroma' affecting the proximal parts of these small arteries. In practice, these distinctions are more or less impossible to make at postmortem and the contribution of intracranial atheroma to lacunar infarction has still to be established.

The current view is that both 'complex' SVD and atheroma at or near the origin of the small perforating vessels arising from the major cerebral arteries cause most, but not all, of the small deep infarcts responsible for lacunar ischaemic strokes (and, by implication, lacunar transient ischaemic attacks) which make up about one-quarter of symptomatic cerebral ischaemic events[9,12,58,120–124] (sections 4.3.2 and 6.7.3). However, this hypothesis is not universally accepted[125,126] since there is remarkably little *direct* postmortem evidence of occlusion of these vessels leading to lacunar infarcts,

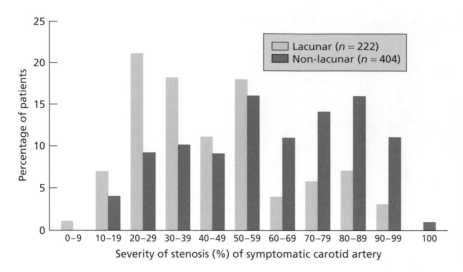

Fig. 6.7 The relationship between the severity of symptomatic carotid stenosis and the likelihood of finding a non-lacunar (territorial) or lacunar infarct on the baseline brain CT in 626 patients in the European Carotid Surgery Trial. Those with severe stenosis are less likely to have lacunar infarcts. (With permission from Boiten *et al.* 1996.[150])

largely because the case fatality of lacunar stroke is so low and pathological material so scanty.

The main supporting evidence for a specific small vessel lesion leading to lacunar infarction is indirect:

- The relative *lack* of large vessel atheroma or embolic sources in the heart in the vast majority of lacunar patients, compared to those with cortical infarcts[12,127–136] (Fig. 6.7).

- Emboli are rarely if ever detected in the middle cerebral or common carotid artery by Doppler ultrasound in most studies of patients with lacunar infarction. However, it is not clear at what stage after the onset of stroke it is best to look – too early and an occluded middle cerebral artery might prevent the passage of emboli, too late and any proximal embolic source may have 'healed'.[88,137–140]

- The low risk of early recurrence also argues against the concept of an active embolic source, either in the heart or an unstable atheromatous plaque.[11,81,135,136]

- The 'capsular warning syndrome' might suggest that a single perforating vessel is intermittently on the verge of occluding before it finally does so (section 6.7.3).

- The impaired cerebrovascular reactivity in lacunar patients might suggest a specific problem, if not pathology, of the small intracerebral resistance vessels,[141] such as endothelial dysfunction.[113]

It is conceivable that 'complex' SVD causes vessel rupture, leading to intracerebral haemorrhage as well as arterial occlusion, maybe at sites of so-called Charcot–Bouchard microaneurysms, although these may be artifacts of the pathological specimens. In fact, whether they are real or not is semantic, because what matters is not if the vessel wall bulges, but what weakens it in the first place[122,142–146] (section 8.2.1). On the other hand, leukoaraiosis appears to be more associated with 'simple'

SVD, and indeed this may be one underlying vascular cause, although it is clearly insufficient on its own, being so common in elderly brains.

Interestingly, 'cortical' (presumed atherothrombotic) and 'lacunar' ischaemic stroke patients probably have a similar vascular risk factor profile (section 6.6), including hypertension.[6,12,135,136,147–151] It is conceivable therefore that the same type of individual (i.e. hypertensive, diabetic, etc.) develops *either* small vessel disease (complex or atheroma) and so lacunar infarcts, *or* large vessel atherothromboembolism and so cortical infarction. The difference in the type of 'degenerative' vascular disease that occurs may perhaps reflect differing genetic susceptibilities. But, on the other hand, many individual patients have these different ischaemic stroke types at different times.[144,152] On balance, we believe it likely that the lacunar hypothesis is correct and so, whatever the exact nature of the underlying small vessel lesion, lacunar infarction is seldom the result of embolization from proximal sites.

> About one-quarter of all ischaemic strokes and transient ischaemic attacks are 'lacunar' and many, if not most, lacunar infarcts are caused by disease of the small intracranial perforating arteries, either 'complex' small vessel disease, or atheroma affecting their proximal parts as they arise from their parent cerebral arteries.

One question that has never been answered is whether there is a similar small vessel disease that affects the blood supply to the optic nerve and retina: are there 'lacunar' ocular syndromes equivalent to lacunar cerebral syndromes? What is clear, however, is that a high proportion of patients with ischaemic amaurosis fugax, retinal infarction and anterior ischaemic optic neuropathy do not have any detectable and likely proximal source of embolism (or evidence of low flow) in the arterial supply to the eye or the heart. Perhaps it is these patients who have small vessel disease like patients with ischaemic lacunar strokes.[58,153,154]

6.5 Embolism from the heart

That embolic material can pass from the heart to the brain, and from the venous system through the heart to the brain (paradoxical embolism), as well as to other organs, is undisputed. However, not all cardiac sources of embolism pose equal threats. For example, a mechanical prosthetic valve is much more likely to cause thromboembolism than mitral leaflet prolapse. In developed countries, embolism from the heart probably causes about one-fifth of ischaemic stroke and transient ischaemic attacks (TIAs), although a *potential* embolic source may be present in nearer one-third[155–160]. However, there are two very real and tiresome problems. As technology advances, more and more *potential* cardiac sources of embolism are being identified (Table 6.4), and patients may have two or more competing causes of cerebral ischaemia, such as carotid stenosis and atrial fibrillation. Therefore, it may well be unclear whether embolism from the heart is *the* cause in an individual patient, especially when the cardiac lesion is common in normal people.[57,58,154,161–163]

Not all emboli are of the same size, of the same age, or made of the same thing (fibrin, platelets, calcium, infected vegetations, tumour, etc.). Some are large and impact permanently in the mainstem of the middle cerebral artery to cause total anterior circulation infarction, others impact in a more distal branch of a cerebral artery to cause a partial anterior circulation infarct, others merely cause a transient ischaemic attack, and still others are asymptomatic.[164–167] Emboli may also occlude the basilar artery and its branches, and even the internal carotid artery in the neck.[61,165]

> Embolism from the heart causes about one-fifth of ischaemic strokes and transient ischaemic attacks. The most substantial embolic threats are non-rheumatic and rheumatic atrial fibrillation, infective endocarditis, prosthetic heart valve, recent myocardial infarction, dilated cardiomyopathy, intracardiac tumours and rheumatic mitral stenosis.

Table 6.4 Cardiac sources of embolism in anatomical sequence.

Right-to-left shunt (paradoxical embolism from the venous system or right-atrial thrombus) (section 6.5.12)
Patent foramen ovale
Atrial septal defect
Ventriculoseptal defect
Pulmonary arteriovenous fistula
Left atrium
Thrombus
   atrial fibrillation* (section 6.5.1)
   sinoatrial disease (sick sinus syndrome) (section 6.5.14)
   atrial septal aneurysm (section 6.5.12)
Myxoma and other cardiac tumours* (section 6.5.13)
Mitral valve
Rheumatic endocarditis (stenosis* or regurgitation) (section 6.5.4)
Infective endocarditis* (section 6.5.9)
Mitral annulus calcification (section 6.5.6)
Non-bacterial thrombotic (marantic) endocarditis (section 6.5.10)
Systemic lupus erythematosus/antiphospholipid syndrome (section 7.3.3 and 4)
Prosthetic heart valve* (section 6.5.3)
Papillary fibroelastoma (section 6.5.13)
Mitral leaflet prolapse (uncertain) (section 6.5.7)
Mitral valve strands (uncertain) (section 6.5.8)
Left ventricle
Mural thrombus
   acute myocardial infarction (previous few weeks)* (section 7.10)
   left-ventricular aneurysm or akinetic segment (section 7.10)
   dilated or restrictive cardiomyopathy* (section 6.5.11)
   mechanical 'artificial' heart*
   blunt chest injury (myocardial contusion)
Myxoma and other cardiac tumours* (section 6.5.13)
Hydatid cyst
Primary oxalosis (uncertain, section 7.20.6)
Aortic valve
Rheumatic endocarditis (stenosis or regurgitation) (section 6.5.4)
Infective endocarditis* (section 6.5.9)
Syphilis
Non-bacterial thrombotic (marantic) endocarditis (section 6.5.10)
Systemic lupus erythematosus/antiphospholipid syndrome (section 7.3.3 and 4)
Prosthetic heart valve* (section 6.5.3)
Calcific stenosis/sclerosis/calcification (section 6.5.6)
Aneurysm of the sinus of Valsalva
Congenital heart disease (particularly with right-to-left shunt)
Cardiac manipulation/surgery/catheterization/ valvuloplasty/angioplasty* (section 7.18.1)

*Substantial risk of embolism.

Table 6.5 Prevalence of potential cardiac sources of embolism in 244 patients with a first-ever-in-a-lifetime ischaemic stroke in the Oxfordshire Community Stroke Project (Sandercock *et al.* 1989).[10]

Source	Number	Percentage
Any atrial fibrillation	31	13
without rheumatic heart disease	28	11
with rheumatic heart disease	3	1
Mitral regurgitation	15	6
Recent (<6 weeks) myocardial infarction	12	5
Prosthetic heart valve	3	1
Mitral stenosis	2	1
Paradoxical embolism	1	1
Any of the above	50	20
Other sources of uncertain significance (aortic stenosis/ sclerosis, mitral annulus calcification, mitral leaflet prolapse, etc.)	28	11

6.5.1 Atrial fibrillation

Non-rheumatic atrial fibrillation (AF), with clot formed in the left atrium and then embolizing to the brain, is by far the most common cause of cardioembolic stroke in developed countries (Table 6.5). However, it is unlikely to cause more than about one-sixth of all strokes at most, because it is present in less than this proportion of ischaemic stroke patients,[8,12,168] although this proportion increases if paroxysmal AF identified on Holter monitoring is taken into account.[169] AF may also be responsible for a greater proportion of ischaemic strokes in the very elderly, where its frequency in the population is highest.[170] The average absolute risk of stroke in un-anticoagulated non-rheumatic AF patients without prior stroke is about 4% per year, six times greater than in those in sinus rhythm[171–174] (section 16.6.2).

> Non-rheumatic atrial fibrillation is the most common cause of embolism from the heart to the brain in developed countries.

In fibrillating stroke patients, the AF cannot always be causal because:
- some patients have had an intracerebral haemorrhage (ICH), although it is conceivable that ICH has been confused with haemorrhagic transformation of an infarct on computed tomography (section 5.7);
- the AF may have been caused by the stroke;
- perhaps 20% of the fibrillating ischaemic stroke patients have other possible causes, such as carotid stenosis or

aortic arch atheroma[175] and coagulation abnormalities have also been described;[176]
- and yet others have lacunar (presumed non-embolic) ischaemic strokes;[163,168,177–180]
- also, AF is often caused by either coronary or hypertensive heart disease, both of which may be associated with stroke by mechanisms other than embolism from the left atrium, such as carotid stenosis or intracerebral haemorrhage;[181,182]
- furthermore, 'only' about 13% or less of non-rheumatic atrial fibrillation patients have detectable thrombus in the left atrium by transoesophageal echocardiography (although some thrombi may have completely embolized or be too small to be detected). It is not known whether these patients definitely have a higher stroke risk than those without detectable thrombus.[183,184]

Nonetheless, AF is clearly the cause of ischaemic stroke in many patients, as supported by:
- postmortem evidence[185–189]
- case–control studies[190]
- most, but not all, cohort studies[191–194] and
- the lower prevalence of AF in lacunar ischaemic stroke probably caused by small vessel disease.[135,136,168]

The effective prevention of stroke by anticoagulating fibrillating patients (section 16.6.2) is not necessarily a good supporting argument, because it is conceivable that anticoagulation may prevent artery-to-artery as well as heart-to-artery embolic events although existing trial evidence (section 16.6.1) does not suggest that anticoagulation is superior to antiplatelet drugs for prevention of non-cardioembolic strokes.[195]

Within the fibrillating population, there must be some individuals at particularly high risk and others at particularly low risk of embolization. For example, those with no other detectable cardiac disease (so-called lone AF) have a low absolute risk of stroke, while those with rheumatic mitral valve disease have a much higher risk.[191,196–198] Other risk factors include a previous embolic event, increasing age, hypertension, diabetes and – as defined by echocardiography – left ventricular dysfunction and enlarged left atrium.[176,199–203] Spontaneous echo contrast in the left atrium, probably a consequence of blood stasis, left atrial thrombi, left atrial appendage size and dysfunction, and various haemostatic variables may perhaps be additional risk factors.[184,204–206]

What is really needed, however, is not just a list of risk factors predicting stroke, with slightly different weightings depending on the study, but validated statistical models to predict the probability of stroke in individual fibrillating patients (as is available for symptomatic carotid stenosis, section 16.11.8). The absolute risk of stroke varies 20-fold among atrial fibrillation patients, depending on age and associated risk factors. Estimating the individual's stroke risk is the initial step in decisions regarding antithrombotic prophylaxis (section 16.6.2).

At least ten similar stroke risk stratification schemes have been published.[176,207] The best validated of these, the CHADS2 score, awards 1 point each for congestive heart failure, hypertension, age ≥ 75 years and diabetes mellitus and 2 points for prior stroke or transient ischaemic attack. The score has been validated in hospital clinic cohorts[208,209] and in randomized trial cohorts.[210] Patients with a CHADS2 score of 0 have a low risk of stroke averaging 0.5% per year, while those with a CHADS2 score of 1 have a stroke risk of 1.5% per year.[209] If echocardiographic data are available, the Stroke Prevention in Atrial Fibrillation (SPAF) III risk stratification scheme has also been validated in several, albeit smaller, cohorts.[211] Patient preference, availability of anticoagulation monitoring, and estimated bleeding risk are all key issues in deciding on antithrombotic prophylaxis and several patient decision aids have been developed.[212,213] It should be pointed out, however, that the risk prediction systems described above refer mainly to the primary prevention situation. Although it is generally considered that warfarin is indicated in the secondary prevention setting, provided there are no contraindications, there is probably still a need for tools to predict the balance of risk and benefit.

Paroxysmal AF carries the same stroke risk as persistent AF[214,215] and should thus be treated similarly. There is no evidence that conversion to sinus rhythm followed by pharmacotherapy to try and maintain such rhythm is superior to rate control in terms of mortality and stroke risk (section 16.10.1).[211,216,217]

6.5.2 Coronary heart disease

Embolism from left ventricular mural thrombus complicating acute myocardial infarction, or a chronic left ventricular aneurysm long after myocardial infarction, is considered in section 7.10, and the complications of cardiac surgery in section 7.18.1.

6.5.3 Prosthetic heart valves

Prosthetic heart valves, particularly mechanical rather than tissue ones, have long been known to be complicated by thrombosis, followed sometimes by embolism. Furthermore, infective endocarditis is a potential risk for any type of prosthetic valve. Asymptomatic emboli, at least as detected by transcranial Doppler, are surprisingly frequent, but are probably gaseous cavitation bubbles

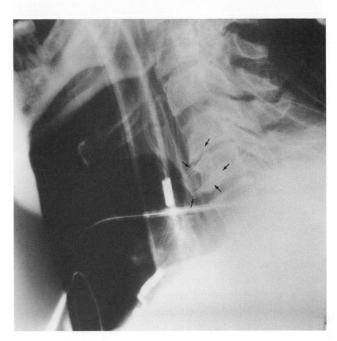

Fig. 6.8 Lateral neck X-ray of a patient whose mechanical heart valve had disintegrated. Part of the valve (*arrows*) has impacted in the carotid artery.

of no clinical consequence and not solid fragments of thrombus.[218,219] There is little discernible difference in stroke risk between the different types of mechanical valve, but those in the mitral position are more prone to thrombosis than those in the aortic position. For all valves, the overall risk of embolism is about 2% per year, provided patients with mechanical valves are on anticoagulants.[220] Some Bjork–Shiley convexoconcave valves (no longer in use) have disintegrated with not only serious cardiac consequences but also embolization of their components to the cerebral circulation[221] (Fig. 6.8). There are some reports of possible embolization of minute metal fragments from apparently normally functioning valves.[222]

Bioprostheses provide an excellent alternative to mechanical prostheses for heart valve replacement in patients unable to comply with systemic anticoagulations and in the elderly. Tissue valves available include the Carpentier-Edwards and Hancock porcine heterograft valves and the Carpentier-Edwards pericardial valve; the overall results are similar to mechanical valves, being about equal at the end of 10 years.[223,224]

The characteristics of each type of valve substitute dictate the selection of one prosthesis in preference to others for a particular patient. Mechanical prostheses are recommended for patients without contraindications to anticoagulants. Tissue valves are reserved for patients over 65 years of age, for patients in whom anticoagulation is contraindicated, for patients whose ejection fraction is less than 40%, or whose life expectancy is less than 10 years.[223,224] Current bioprostheses have significantly better durability than earlier bioprostheses.[224] Some disagreement remains about the need for systemic anticoagulation during the first few months after insertion of a bioprosthesis, when the embolic stroke risk is highest.[225]

6.5.4 Rheumatic valvular disease

Rheumatic valvular disease, particularly mitral, is a well-recognized cause of embolism to the brain, particularly when the patient is in atrial fibrillation and has thrombosis in the left atrium. But even when the patient is in sinus rhythm and there is no thrombus in the left atrium, degenerate and sometimes calcific fragments of valve can be discharged into the circulation. Infective endocarditis (see below) and intracerebral haemorrhage caused by anticoagulation (section 8.4.1) are among the many other causes of stroke in these patients.[226–228]

6.5.6 Non-rheumatic sclerosis and calcification of the aortic and mitral valves

Non-rheumatic sclerosis, and particularly calcification, of the aortic and mitral valves can occasionally be a source of embolism of thrombotic or calcific material. However, these valvular abnormalities are so common in elderly people that a cause-and-effect relationship is difficult to establish in an individual unless, very unusually, calcific emboli are seen in the retina, on brain CT or at postmortem. Any associated atrial fibrillation, coronary disease or carotid stenosis compounds the diagnostic problem.[229–235]

6.5.7 Mitral leaflet (or valve) prolapse

Mitral leaflet prolapse (MLP) can be familial,[236] and is a common clinical and echocardiographic finding in healthy people, but the diagnostic criteria are so variable, and many studies so flawed by referral bias, that there is a wide range of reported prevalence. Almost certainly, MLP has been over-diagnosed in the past.[237–239] Therefore, it is all but impossible to pin down MLP as the cause of an ischaemic stroke or transient ischaemic attack (TIA) in an individual unless there is complicating infective endocarditis, atrial fibrillation, gross mitral regurgitation or thrombus in the left atrium. MLP is often associated with myxomatous degeneration of the valve leaflets, which can occasionally be complicated by rupture.[240]

> Uncomplicated mitral leaflet prolapse should no longer be considered a cause of embolism from the heart to the brain; there must be something additional, such as gross mitral regurgitation, atrial fibrillation or infective endocarditis.

Although MLP may be more common than expected in young TIA patients,[241] it was always odd, if the relationship is causal, that thrombus on the valve cusps is so rare in uncomplicated MLP and that embolism to anywhere other than the brain or eye has never been described.[242,243] Furthermore, MLP does not appear to be more frequent than expected in ischaemic stroke[244–246] and there is no definite excess risk of first-ever stroke or recurrent stroke in patients with uncomplicated MLP.[247–249] Therefore, in an individual patient, we would not regard uncomplicated MLP as a *definite* cause of ischaemic stroke/TIA, even if no other cause can be found. It is much more likely to be an innocent bystander.

6.5.8 Mitral valve strands

Strands are mobile, thread-like filaments attached to cardiac valves that can be seen on transoesophageal echocardiography. Although suggested as sources of embolism, or perhaps as increasing the risk of embolism in patients whose valves are abnormal for whatever reason, the evidence so far is not persuasive.[250,251]

6.5.9 Infective endocarditis

About one-fifth of patients with acute or subacute infective endocarditis have an ischaemic stroke or transient ischaemic attack as a result of embolism of valvular vegetations. Cerebrovascular symptoms can be the presenting feature, but they more often occur in someone who is clearly unwell, perhaps already in hospital, but before the infection has been controlled.[252–254] Haemorrhagic transformation of an infarct occurs in 20–40% and may be excacerbated or precipitated by unwise anticoagulation. Primarily haemorrhagic strokes – intracerebral or, rarely, subarachnoid or mixed intracerebral and subdural[255] – are as or more commonly caused by a pyogenic vasculitis and vessel wall necrosis than by the more well-known mycotic aneurysms which can be single or multiple and most often affect the distal branches of the middle cerebral artery[256,257] (section 8.2.11) (Fig. 6.9). These aneurysms do not always rupture and they tend to resolve with time so that, on balance, cerebral angiography to detect unruptured aneurysms with a view to surgery is unnecessary, and so is surgical repair of any asymptomatic aneurysm.[258]

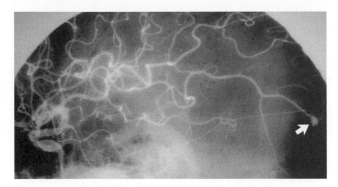

Fig. 6.9 Selective catheter carotid angiogram (lateral skull view) showing a mycotic cerebral aneurysm on a distal branch of the middle cerebral artery (*arrow*).

Early institution of the correct antibiotic therapy is the most effective way to prevent thromboembolism in infective endocarditis, the risks of which are highest in the first 24–48 h after diagnosis. Anticoagulation should not be given to patients with native valve or bioprosthetic valve endocarditis because of the risk of intracerebral haemorrhage from mycotic aneurysms and arteritis, and the reduction in embolism risk with antibiotic therapy. For patients with mechanical valves who are on long-term anticoagulation at the time of developing infective endocarditis, the correct management is unclear. Some advocate withholding anticoagulation in all such patients because warfarin has not been shown to be associated with a reduction in systemic embolization, and the risk of haemorrhagic complications has been up to 40% in some studies. Others continue anticoagulation unless embolic stroke or haemorrhage occur. Some authors have stated that large ischaemic stroke, haemorrhage on CT, presence of mycotic aneurysm, uncontrolled infection and infection with *Staphylococcus aureus* are all contraindications to anticoagulants in mechanical valve endocarditis.

There is no direct evidence that antiplatelet drugs are effective in ischaemic stroke secondary to infective endocarditis although animal studies suggest that they may reduce vegetation size and systemic embolization. On balance, given the risks of warfarin described above, antiplatelet drugs are probably the best option in most cases.

Other neurological complications of infective endocarditis include: meningitis; a diffuse encephalopathy, perhaps as a result of showers of small emboli; acute mononeuropathy; rarely, cerebral abscess; discitis; and headache.[252,259]

It is important to realize that fever, a cardiac murmur and vegetations seen on echocardiography are not invariably present in patients with infective endocarditis.

Therefore, in an otherwise unexplained ischaemic or haemorrhagic stroke, blood cultures are indicated, particularly if the erythrocyte sedimentation rate is raised, with a mild anaemia, neutrophil leucocytosis and disturbed liver function, or if the patient is an intravenous drug user.

> In infective endocarditis the blood cultures can occasionally be negative and the echocardiogram may not show any valvular vegetations. A high index of diagnostic suspicion is required in any unexplained stroke, particularly if there is a cardiac murmur.

6.5.10 Non-bacterial thrombotic (marantic) endocarditis

Small sterile vegetations, consisting of fibrin and platelets, appear on the cardiac valves in cachectic and debilitated patients as a result of cancer (usually adenocarcinomas) and sometimes of disseminated intravascular coagulation, burns and septicaemia, usually but not only in elderly people (Fig. 6.10). Similar vegetations are found in systemic lupus erythematosus and the antiphospholipid syndrome (sections 7.3.3 and 7.3.4), and possibly protein C deficiency (section 7.9.11). These vegetations are friable and may embolize to cause ischaemic stroke (and sometimes global encephalopathy because of multiple emboli), ischaemia in other organs, and pulmonary embolism. The vegetations are so small that they are all but impossible to diagnose during life, although the larger ones can be seen on transoesophageal echocardiography. The diagnosis should be suspected in an ischaemic stroke/transient ischaemic attack patient who is cachectic and who may have additional evidence of systemic embolization without any other cause being found, or if there are antiphospholipid

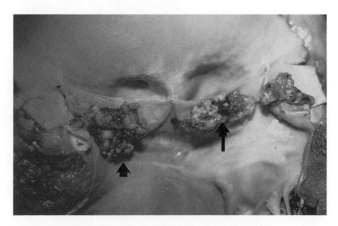

Fig. 6.10 A close-up view of non-infective marantic vegetations (*arrows*) on the cusps of the aortic valve.

antibodies.[260–263] Sometimes however, the patient, even with cancer, can appear remarkably well.[264]

6.5.11 Non-ischaemic 'primary' cardiomyopathies

Non-ischaemic 'primary' cardiomyopathies are well known to be complicated by intracardiac thrombus and so embolism, particularly if they are of the dilated or restrictive type and there is severe ventricular dysfunction, atrial fibrillation, infective endocarditis or intracardiac thrombus on echocardiography.[265] Hypertrophic cardiomyopathies are most unlikely to be complicated by embolism.

6.5.12 Paradoxical embolism, patent foramen ovale and atrial septal aneurysm

A number of convincing postmortem examples (Fig. 6.11) have established that paradoxical embolism can occur from thrombi in the venous system of the legs (or pelvis) through the right to the left side of the heart – and exceptionally from thrombus in the right atrium as a result of cardiac disease or possibly an indwelling venous line – and on to the brain. The right-to-left cardiac conduits for emboli are a patent foramen ovale (PFO) which, depending as always on the diagnostic criteria, is found in about one-quarter of unselected postmortems and a similar proportion of healthy people by using transoesophageal echocardiography; an atrial septal defect; and, rarely, a ventriculoseptal defect.[244,266,267] However, although

bubbles can frequently be shown to move from the right to the left side of the heart, and appear in the cerebral circulation detected by transcranial Doppler, it is very rare for thrombus to do so, unless the right atrial pressure is raised (section 6.9.3).

There is an increased prevalence of PFO in patients with cryptogenic stroke[268,269] but the risk of recurrent stroke in patients with a PFO is low and far more information is required from ongoing randomized trials before embarking on routine endovascular closure.[270–276] Reports of a continuing risk of stroke after closure of PFO[277] highlight the need for reliable data from large trials.

Atrial septal aneurysm, a bulging of the inter-atrial septum into the right or left atrium or both, is an echocardiographic finding in some normal people who seldom have any cardiac signs. The diagnostic criteria are variable which makes it difficult to compare studies and to generalize their results. Perhaps such aneurysms can be complicated by thrombus, embolism and so cerebral ischaemia, perhaps also by atrial fibrillation, but very often they are associated with a patent foramen ovale and so the potential for paradoxical embolism from the venous system.[244,278–281] There is evidence that the combination of atrial septal aneurysm and PFO carries a higher stroke risk than PFO alone,[268,269] with a risk of recurrent stroke of maybe 2% per annum, albeit based on small numbers of cases. However, a 3-year prospective Spanish multicentre cohort study recently reported that right-to-left shunting was not

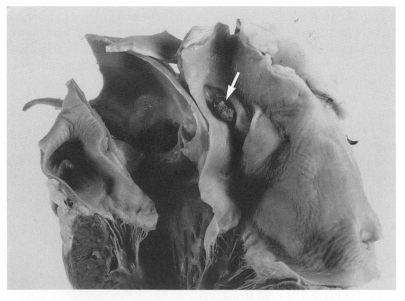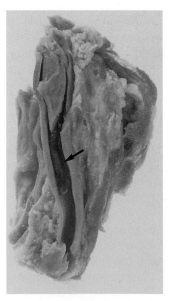

Fig. 6.11 Paradoxical embolism. A postmortem specimen showing: (a) a venous thrombus (arrow) protruding through a patent foramen ovale into the left atrium; and (b) part of the same thrombus (*arrow*) in the right common carotid artery. (c) See colour plate section for a colour reproduction of paradoxical embolism. (Courtesy of Dr John Webb.)

associated with an increased risk of recurrent stroke.[282] Neither large shunts nor a shunt and an atrial septal aneurysm in combination predicted recurrent stroke in 500 patients of all ages, or in 168 patients less than 55 years old.

Consequently, it is uncertain whether closure of PFO is indicated in these patients. At present there are no reliable data from randomized controlled trials to guide management. If closure of a PFO is being considered it is important to first make sure that all other causes of stroke in a young person are excluded. It is also important to determine whether any aspects of the clinical history increase the likelihood of a causal association between the PFO and the stroke, including a recent venous thrombosis, recent prolonged travel, or straining at onset of stroke.

Interestingly, there appears to be an association between PFO and migraine, particularly migraine with aura, stronger where there is a coexistent atrial septal aneurysm. Following anecdotal reports of improvement in migraine symptoms following PFO closure,[283,284] several observational studies have suggested that PFO closure is associated with a reduction in migraine frequency.[285] Randomized trials of shunt closure have been started but only one completed, the MIST trial (Migraine Intervention with STARFLEX Technology) which showed a significant reduction of migraine with aura after closure compared with control, but the benefit was more modest than expected from the observational studies.[285]

Another, but very unusual, route for emboli to reach the brain via the venous system is through or from a pulmonary arteriovenous fistula, either isolated or in patients with hereditary haemorrhagic telangiectasia. Diagnostic clues are finger-clubbing, cyanosis, haemoptysis, bruit over the chest and a 'coin lesion' on the chest X-ray[286] (Fig. 6.12).

> Although a patent foramen ovale is common in healthy individuals, it is unusual for cerebral ischaemia to be caused by paradoxical embolism from the right to the left side of the heart, and so to the brain. There is no good evidence that closing the heart defect reduces the risk of stroke (or of migraine).

6.5.13 Intracardiac tumours

Myxomas, found in the left atrium much more often than in any other cardiac chamber, are the most common intracardiac tumour but are still extremely rare. Some are familial.[287–289] Tumour or complicating thrombus may embolize to the brain, eye and elsewhere. Myxomatous emboli cause not only focal cerebral ischaemia but also fusiform and irregular aneurysmal dilatations at sites of earlier symptomatic or even asymptomatic embolic occlusions, and these can rupture to cause intracerebral or subarachnoid haemorrhage[290] (Fig. 6.13). Brain metastases have also been described.[291] Like other cardiac tumours, myxomas can also cause intracardiac obstruction with shortness of breath, palpitations and syncope. Often but not always they cause constitutional problems, such as malaise, fatigue, weight loss, fever, rash, arthralgia, myalgia, anaemia, raised erythrocyte sedimentation rate and hypergammaglobulinaemia. Recurrent neurological problems after resection of the cardiac tumour are very unusual.[292,293]

Other, even rarer, primary and secondary cardiac tumours may embolize, such as valvular fibroelastoma.[294–296]

6.5.14 Sinoatrial disease (sick sinus syndrome)

Sinoatrial disease can be associated with intracardiac thrombus and embolism, particularly if bradycardia

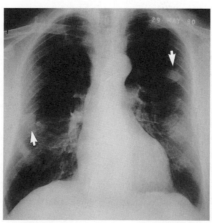 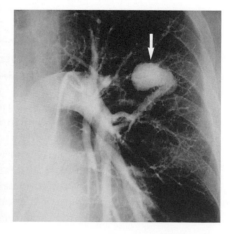

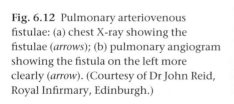

Fig. 6.12 Pulmonary arteriovenous fistulae: (a) chest X-ray showing the fistulae (*arrows*); (b) pulmonary angiogram showing the fistula on the left more clearly (*arrow*). (Courtesy of Dr John Reid, Royal Infirmary, Edinburgh.)

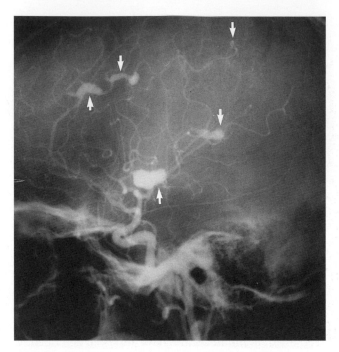

Fig. 6.13 Catheter carotid angiogram showing multiple aneurysmal dilatations of cerebral arteries (*arrows*) as a result of embolism from a cardiac myxoma. (Courtesy of Professor Alastair Compston.)

Table 6.6 Factors associated with an increased risk of occlusive vascular disorders (i.e. ischaemic stroke, myocardial infarction, claudication, etc.).

Increasing age (section 6.6.1)
Male sex (section 6.6.2)
Increasing blood pressure (section 6.6.3)
Cigarette-smoking (section 6.6.4)
Diabetes mellitus (section 6.6.5)
Blood lipids (section 6.6.6)
Increasing plasma fibrinogen (section 6.6.7)
Raised haematocrit (section 6.6.7)
High plasma factor VII coagulant activity (section 6.6.7)
Raised von Willebrand factor antigen (section 6.6.7)
Low blood fibrinolytic activity (section 6.6.7)
Raised tissue plasminogen activator antigen (section 6.6.7)
Hyperhomocystinaemia (section 6.6.8)
Physical inactivity (section 6.6.9)
Obesity (section 6.6.10)
The metabolic syndrome (section 6.6.11)
Diet (salt, antioxidants, etc.) (section 6.6.12)
Alcohol (none, or heavy drinking) (section 6.6.13)
Ethnicity (section 6.6.14)
Genotype (section 6.6.15)
Social deprivation (section 6.6.16)
Infection (section 6.6.17)
'Stress' (section 6.6.18)

alternates with tachycardia or the patient is in atrial fibrillation. It can be familial.[297–299]

6.5.15 Other unusual causes of embolism from the heart to the brain

Myocardial *hydatid cysts*, thrombus in an *aneurysm of the sinus of Valsalva* and intracardiac calcification caused by *primary oxalosis* are extremely rare causes of embolism to the brain.[300–303] *Myocardial contusion* as a result of blunt chest injury can be associated with left ventricular thrombus and embolism.[304]

6.6 Risk factors for ischaemic stroke

Since large vessel disease (atheroma) causes around 50% of ischaemic stroke in white populations, it is not surprising that many of the risk factors for stroke are also risk factors for atheroma. Moreover, atheroma affects the coronary as well as the cerebral circulation resulting in cardioembolic stroke, and intracranial small vessel disease seems to share many of the same risk factors as atheroma, so the risk factors and causes of ischaemic

stroke and other vascular diseases overlap to a considerable extent.

Whatever the exact mechanisms of the development of atherosclerosis, it is quite clear that certain individual and population characteristics (risk factors) are associated with the *clinical* consequences of atheroma (i.e. ischaemic stroke, myocardial infarction, peripheral vascular disease and so on) (Table 6.6). As it turns out, there is much more information about risk factors for coronary events than for ischaemic stroke,[305] in part because heart patients have tended to be more intensively investigated, but also because heart disease receives much higher levels of research funding.[306,307] The tendency for epidemiologists to lump all types of stroke together (haemorrhage with infarct, lacunar infarct with cortical infarct, etc.) might, in part, explain the curious *quantitative* differences between stroke and coronary heart disease (CHD) risk factors, although *qualitatively* they are the same. Why are smoking, raised plasma cholesterol and male sex far stronger risk factors for myocardial infarction, while hypertension is a far stronger risk factor for stroke? Could it be that some types of stroke are not to do with cholesterol, smokers and male sex? If these stroke types could be identified and removed from the analysis, together with strokes caused by embolism from the heart, would the remaining ischaemic strokes have a more similar risk factor profile to CHD which, it seems, is less heterogeneous than stroke and mostly caused by atherothrombosis? Furthermore, why is it that some populations, like the Japanese and black Africans, seem to be afflicted far more by stroke than coronary events? For black Africans this appears to be due to the fact that African countries are generally earlier in epidemiological transition than developed countries, at which stage hypertension and cardioembolic stroke due to rheumatic heart disease are common but atherothrombosis is still relatively rare.[48]

> It is curious that some risk factors are so much stronger for ischaemic stroke (e.g. increasing blood pressure) and yet others are so much stronger for coronary heart disease (e.g. increasing plasma cholesterol) if the underlying vascular pathology (atheroma) is much the same.

It is important to be clear that a risk factor merely indicates an association between that factor and the disease of interest (Table 6.7). This association may be causal, coincidental or a reflection of reverse causality (i.e. the disease itself changes the risk factor level or prevalence). In some but by no means all instances there is a plausible biological explanation for the causal associations, through atherothrombotic arterial disease to the clinical syndrome. A causal rather than a coincidental relationship is suggested by a number of rather circumstantial pieces of evidence that on their own may not be very convincing:[308]

- a strong association between the risk factor and the disease (i.e. a high relative risk or relative odds);
- consistency of association across several types of studies at different times in different places;
- a dose–response relationship (i.e. the greater the exposure to the risk factor, the greater the risk of the disease);
- independence from confounding variables, particularly age (Fig. 6.14);
- a clear temporal sequence of exposure to the risk factor *before* disease onset, remembering that the onset of atheroma is years before the onset of its clinical manifestations;
- biological and epidemiological plausibility, although there is no end to human ingenuity in constructing plausible hypotheses to explain the natural world; and
- most convincing of all but not always feasible, demonstration that attenuation of the risk factor leads to a fall in disease incidence, preferably by means of a randomized controlled trial. However, a trial can be negative if the intervention is too little (i.e. not enough blood-pressure lowering for long enough), too late (the arterial damage is already done and the clinical consequences are inevitable) or the trial is too small (type II error).

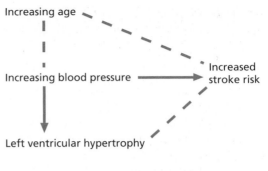

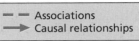

Fig. 6.14 'Confounding' in observational studies which relate a risk factor to a disease such as stroke. In this example, increasing age is associated with both increasing blood pressure and increasing risk of stroke. In fact, age and blood pressure are independent of the confounding effect of one on the other. In other words, for a population of the same age, there is an increasing risk of stroke with increasing blood pressure, and for a population with the same blood pressure, there is an increasing risk of stroke with increasing age. Therefore, irrespective of age, increasing blood pressure is strongly associated with stroke risk. Also, increasing age is associated with increasing stroke risk, not because age and blood pressure are associated, which they are, but because of something else (perhaps increasing prevalence of atrial fibrillation with age, etc.). On the other hand, although left ventricular hypertrophy is associated with increasing stroke risk, this association more or less disappears if blood pressure is controlled for because, presumably, increasing blood pressure causes *both* stroke and left ventricular hypertrophy. So hypertension is a confounding factor and explains the left ventricular hypertrophy–stroke relationship. It is not possible to adjust for confounding factors if they are not measured or even suspected and, even when they are, statistical adjustment is not always easy or possible, so that some associations said to be unconfounded may not be.

It is most important to realize that even if a risk factor is associated with a high relative risk of stroke and the relationship is causal, the factor may still contribute very little to the incidence of stroke if it is rarely present in the population (e.g. rheumatic atrial fibrillation) or if there is a low baseline risk of stroke in the population where the risk factor is acting (e.g. oral contraceptives in young women). In other words, the impact of a risk factor is low if the proportion of stroke cases attributable to that risk factor is low (low population-attributable risk). On the other hand, a causal risk factor with a rather modest relative risk may be of major importance in contributing to stroke incidence if it is very prevalent (e.g. moderate hypertension) and/or the background risk of stroke in the population is high (e.g. in elderly people). The population-attributable risk is then high.

Cohort studies

A longitudinal study of a cohort of individuals, some of whom have a risk factor for stroke $(a+b)$, and some of whom develop a stroke during follow-up $(a+c)$

Stroke during follow-up

		Yes	No
Risk factor at baseline	Yes	a	b
	No	c	d

The risk of stroke in those with the risk factor $(R+)$ is $\dfrac{a}{a+b}$

The risk of stroke in those without the risk factor $(R-)$ is $\dfrac{c}{c+d}$

Therefore: the relative risk (or risk ratio) $=\dfrac{R+}{R-}$, i.e. $\dfrac{a}{a+b}\times\dfrac{c+d}{c}=\dfrac{ac+ad}{ac+bc}$

and the absolute risk difference $=(R+)-(R-)$

The odds of stroke in those with the risk factor $(O+)$ is $\dfrac{a}{b}$

The odds of stroke in those without the risk factor $(O-)$ is $\dfrac{c}{d}$

Therefore: the relative odds (or odds ratio) $=\dfrac{O+}{O-}$, i.e. $\dfrac{ad}{bc}$

Note: when stroke is rare (i.e. a and c are small compared with b and d), then the relative risk and relative odds are about the same

Case–control studies

Patients with stroke $(a+c)$ and controls without a stroke $(b+d)$ from the same population are identified and the previous exposure to the risk factor compared using the odds ratio

Stroke, and non-stroke
control patients identified
at one point in time

		Yes	No
Risk factor present	Yes	a	b
	No	c	d

The odds of a stroke patient having the risk factor are $\dfrac{a}{c}$

The odds of a control patient having the risk factor are $\dfrac{b}{d}$

Therefore: the relative odds (or the odds ratio) $=\dfrac{a}{c}\div\dfrac{b}{d}=\dfrac{ad}{bc}$

Table 6.7 The association between a risk factor and disease; calculating relative risk and relative odds in cohort and case–control studies.

> It is important to be clear that a risk factor merely indicates an association between that factor and the disease of interest. This association may be causal, coincidental or a reflection of reverse causality (i.e. the disease itself changes the risk factor level or prevalence).

This epidemiological approach to defining risk factors and possible causation has tended to lump all strokes together, more so in prospective cohort than in case–control studies. Therefore, the heterogeneous nature of the pathology and causes of stroke may obscure any relationship between a particular risk factor and, for example, a particular type of stroke, such as haemorrhagic rather than ischaemic, or a lacunar infarct rather than a cardioembolic infarct. Furthermore, stroke itself may:

• change some risk factors, e.g. blood glucose increases temporarily after acute stroke (section 11.18.3) while plasma cholesterol falls (section 6.8.1);

- make information of past activities impossible to obtain because of the patient's confusion or aphasia;
- lead to bias in recording risk factors in case–control studies because it is impossible to blind assessors to stroke or control patient status; or
- require treatment which modifies risk factors (e.g. stopping smoking or lowering blood pressure).

Therefore, quick and relatively easy case–control studies based on stroke survivors are fraught with surprising difficulty, especially hospital-based studies which tend to exclude mild cases and those that die before admission.[12] Using transient ischaemic attack (TIA) patients as a surrogate for ischaemic stroke, and extracting information from medical records written *before* the TIA, could avoid some of these problems. Studies relating stroke mortality to various risk factors are problematic if the factor itself increases case fatality (such as diabetes mellitus), and also if haemorrhagic and ischaemic strokes are lumped together because haemorrhagic strokes are more likely to cause death. The most unbiased information comes from large prospective community-based cohort studies where all strokes are counted. However, these take many years to complete and if a baseline variable has not been collected – or even thought of at the time – it clearly cannot be related to later stroke risk, unless it involves analysis of a baseline stored blood sample, for DNA for example.

Studying easily accessible arteries directly with ultrasound, such as the carotid bifurcation, is a relatively recent approach. This gets closer to risk factors for very early changes in the vessel wall (increasing intima-media thickness, IMT) and also for atherothrombotic plaque, although ultrasound cannot always reliably distinguish plaque constituents.[309–312] Increased IMT is now widely used as a measure of the early development of arterial disease,[313,314] although it is still not completely clear exactly how increased IMT is related to the development of early atherosclerosis. With improvements in ultrasound imaging, direct measurement of the total burden of early plaque formation around the carotid bifurcation is now possible,[315] and plaque area might be a better surrogate measure of future vascular risk than IMT.

This 'arterial' rather than 'patient' approach is still prone to the familiar problems of observational epidemiology: inadequate sample size, the numerous potential biases in case–control studies, confounding, chance effects in small samples, lack of blinding to case or control status and inappropriate subgroup analyses. Also, in prospective cohort studies, it is not easy to quantify progression or regression of arterial wall thickness or plaques over time. Alterations in a plaque may be as much to do with the difficulty in imaging exactly the same plaque at the same angle, and changes in any

complicating thrombus (such as lysis), as with growth or resolution of atheroma in the vessel wall, or as a result of temporary changes in the plaque, such as haemorrhage. In practice, looking at arteries rather than people has not yet led to any new aetiological insights, perhaps because the sample sizes have been too small and other methodological problems.

As can be seen in Table 6.3, the vast majority of ischaemic stroke patients, necessarily taken as a group in most epidemiological studies and therefore including those resulting from small vessel disease and embolism from the heart as well as atheroma, have one or more of the definite vascular risk factors, which will be discussed below.

6.6.1 Age

Increasing age is the strongest risk factor for TIAs and ischaemic stroke, and almost certainly for the various subcategories of ischaemic stroke (Fig. 6.15). For example, an 80-year-old has about 30 times the risk of ischaemic stroke as a 50-year-old.[316]

6.6.2 Sex

There is much less of an excess of ischaemic strokes and TIAs in men than in women (Fig. 6.16) compared with coronary events and peripheral arterial disease.[316] Notwithstanding popular dogma, the equalization of vascular risk in elderly males and females is probably not

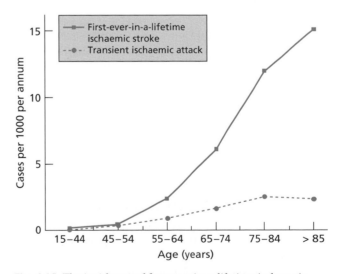

Fig. 6.15 The incidence of first-ever-in-a-lifetime ischaemic stroke and transient ischaemic attack (TIA) in the Oxfordshire Community Stroke Project. The flattening of TIA and, to some extent, stroke incidence in old age may be because cases did not come to medical attention or, when they did, they were not correctly diagnosed in the elderly.

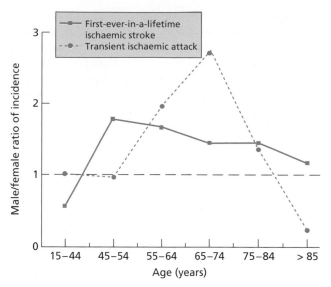

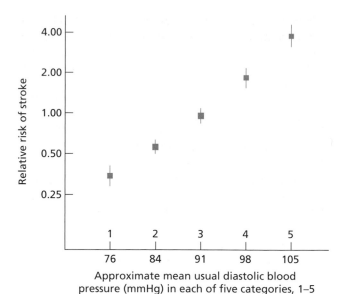

Fig. 6.16 The ratio of male : female incidence of first-ever-in-a-lifetime ischaemic stroke and transient ischaemic attack in the Oxfordshire Community Stroke Project.

Fig. 6.17 The risk of stroke related to the usual diastolic blood pressure in five categories, defined by usual baseline blood pressure, from a pooled analysis of seven prospective observational studies. Solid squares represent stroke risks relative to risk in the whole study population; their size is proportional to the number of strokes in each blood pressure category. The vertical lines represent 95% confidence intervals. Note the doubling scale of the y-axis. (With permission from MacMahon *et al.* 1990.[325])

explained by the natural menopause, although bilateral oophorectomy without oestrogen replacement about doubles the risk of vascular events.[317,318] Use of hormone replacement therapy in women after the menopause does not confer a benefit in terms of reduced cardiovascular morbidity, in fact there is evidence that such treatment is associated with an *increased* risk of acute coronary syndrome, stroke and venous thromboembolism[319–321] (section 7.13.2).

6.6.3 Blood pressure

In healthy populations of both sexes and independently of age, increasing blood pressure is strongly associated with overall stroke risk, and of all the main pathological types, including ischaemic stroke.[322–324] The relationship between usual diastolic blood pressure and subsequent stroke is log–linear with no threshold below which stroke risk becomes stable, at least not within the 'normal' range of 70–110 mmHg (Fig. 6.17). The proportional increase in stroke risk associated with a given increase in blood pressure is similar at all levels of blood pressure. This risk almost doubles with each 7.5 mmHg increase in usual diastolic blood pressure in Western populations, and with each 5.0 mmHg in Japanese and Chinese populations.[325–327] Because moderately raised blood pressure is so common in the middle-aged and elderly in developed countries, high blood pressure probably accounts for more ischaemic strokes than any other risk factor.

The strength of the association between blood pressure and stroke is attenuated with increasing age, although

the absolute risk of stroke in the elderly is far higher than in the young.[327] Nevertheless, hypertension is still a risk factor in the very elderly, although it is weaker because stroke may be associated with low blood pressure secondary to cardiac failure and other comorbid conditions.[328] Moreover, in patients with bilateral severe carotid stenosis, stroke risk is higher at low blood pressures suggesting that aggressive blood-pressure lowering may be harmful in this group (section 16.3.1).[329]

The relationship between stroke and systolic blood pressure is possibly stronger than with diastolic pressure, and even 'isolated' systolic hypertension with a 'normal' diastolic blood pressure is associated with increased stroke risk.[327,330–333]

There is no doubt, as confirmed by the results of randomized controlled trials, that the relationship between increasing blood pressure and stroke risk is causal (section 16.3). However, it is not clear whether all types of stroke are prevented by reducing blood pressure, largely because in the clinical trials they have all been lumped together, haemorrhagic with ischaemic strokes of various types[182,334–337] (section 16.3.2). Progression of carotid stenosis, at least as assessed by ultrasound, is slowed by treating hypertension.[338]

Hypertension seems to increase the risk of ischaemic stroke by increasing the extent and severity of atheroma (section 6.3) as well as the prevalence of 'simple' and 'complex' intracranial small vessel disease[339–344] (section 6.4).

6.6.4 Smoking

Cigarette-smoking is associated with approximately double the risk of ischaemic stroke in males and females, but less obviously in the elderly, and there is a dose–response relationship.[345–350] There are not as many data on passive smoking and stroke as there are for coronary events where the association is surprisingly strong.[351–354] As one would expect, most of the ultrasound and angiogram studies link carotid disease with smoking.[344,355–357] Although cigar-smoking increases the risk of coronary events by about one-quarter, there are insufficient data to link either pipe- or cigar-smoking with stroke, perhaps because there are fewer people who still indulge in these habits.[358] The risk of stroke gradually declines after stopping smoking so supporting a causal relationship, but a satisfactory randomized controlled trial proved impossible.[345,350,359–361]

6.6.5 Diabetes mellitus

Any studies linking diabetes with fatal stroke will exaggerate the association, because diabetics who have a stroke are more likely to die of it than non-diabetics[362] (sections 10.2.7 and 11.18.3). Indeed, the the risk of fatal stroke is higher in those with a higher HbA1C at diagnosis[363] In fact, diabetes about doubles the risk of ischaemic stroke over and above confounding with hypertension and other risk factors.[364–370] Diabetics also have thicker carotid arterial walls but the relationship with carotid stenosis is less clear, probably because of lack of patient

numbers.[311,344,371] So far, randomized trials have not shown that diabetic treatment definitely reduces the risk of stroke[372] (section 16.9), although improved glycaemic control does lead to a reduction in overall rates of vascular complications of diabetes and a reduction in premature death. In the UKPDS study, overweight patients with type 2 diabetes who were treated with metformin had a 32% reduction in diabetes-related adverse outcomes and a 42% reduction in diabetes-related deaths.[372]

6.6.6 Blood lipids

Increasing plasma total cholesterol, increasing low-density lipoprotein-cholesterol and decreasing levels of high-density lipoprotein-cholesterol are all strong risk factors for coronary heart disease, whereas triglyceride levels are not. A long-term reduction of plasma cholesterol by 1 mmol/L should and does reduce the relative risk of coronary events by at least one-third,[373] and also reduces coronary risk in the elderly.[374–379] On the other hand, the relationship with ischaemic stroke is less clear. Very large systematic reviews of cohort studies have not revealed any association between all stroke types combined and increasing plasma total cholesterol at baseline, except perhaps under the age of 45 years[326,380] (Fig. 6.18). Case–control studies provide less reliable measures of association because of their biases, particularly the changes in plasma lipids following stroke[381] (section 6.8.1). Relating carotid intima-media thickness or stenosis with blood lipids is perhaps too far from the clinical consequences of atheroma to be relevant, or the studies have been too small to be reliable.[310,312,342,344,382,383]

Surprisingly therefore, the Heart Protection Study of cholesterol lowering in patients with known vascular disease or diabetes showed that simvastatin definitely reduced the risk of stroke on follow-up, although it did

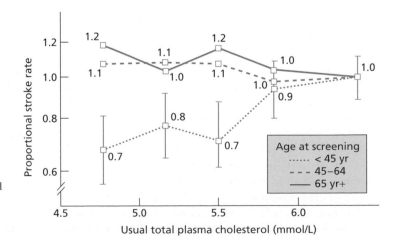

Fig. 6.18 Adjusted proportional risk of stroke (with 95% confidence intervals) by age and usual plasma cholesterol from a systematic review of 45 prospective observational studies. (With permission from the Prospective Studies Collaboration 1995.[380])

not reduce the risk of recurrent stroke[384,385] (section 16.4.2). This may have been because incident strokes occurred on average 4.6 years before the study onset and hence, at the time of the study, patients would have been at low risk of recurrent stroke but at high risk of coronary vascular disease. More recently, the Stroke Prevention by Aggressive Reduction in Cholesterol Levels (SPARCL) trial showed that atorvastatin in patients who had had a stroke or TIA within 1–6 months before study entry did reduce stroke risk.[386] However, statin treatment was associated with a small but significant increase in risk of haemorrhagic stroke. Interestingly, the same trend had been found in the Heart Protection Study (HPS) in the 3280 patients with previous stroke or TIA,[384] in whom simvastatin 40 mg *increased* the risk of haemorrhagic stroke. Thus, the randomized evidence does suggest that there is a causal association between plasma LDL cholesterol and risk of ischaemic stroke – but more work is required to determine whether the increase in risk of haemorrhagic stroke is genuine.

The marked contrast between coronary disease and ischaemic stroke in their association with plasma cholesterol is even more curious now it is clear that cholesterol lowering reduces the risk of myocardial infarction *and* stroke.[384,386,387] It appears that the observational epidemiology has missed an ischaemic stroke–lipid connection, possibly because:

- the seemingly negative association between increasing plasma cholesterol and intracranial haemorrhage has obscured a positive association with ischaemic stroke in studies where the pathological type of stroke was not accounted for (Fig. 6.19), which would tie in with the possibility that reducing plasma cholesterol with statins increases the risk of haemorrhagic stroke;
- the over-representation of fatal, and therefore more likely to be haemorrhagic, strokes in some studies;
- the narrow range of cholesterol levels examined in many studies;
- the loss of stroke-susceptible individuals from the study population by prior death from coronary disease;
- uncertainties about the effect of stroke itself on lipid levels in case–control studies; and
- not differentiating ischaemic strokes likely to be caused by intracranial small vessel disease from those caused by large vessel atherothrombosis.

Alternatively, the lack of a strong plasma cholesterol association with ischaemic stroke may be correct and perhaps the statins reduce stroke risk by some mechanism other than by cholesterol lowering.[388,389] Both acute plaque-stabilizing effects of statins[390] and neuroprotective effects[391,392] have been postulated. Some support for potentially non-lipid effects comes from the

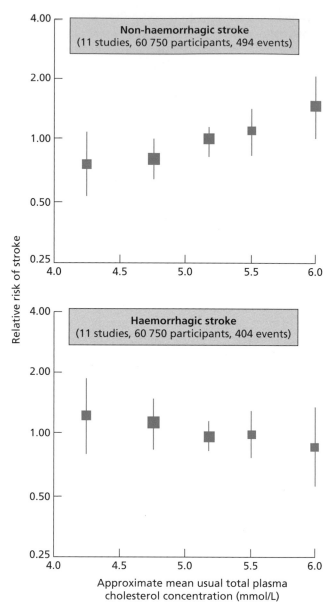

Fig. 6.19 Overall adjusted relative risk (95% confidence intervals) of non-haemorrhagic and haemorrhagic stroke by usual plasma cholesterol from a systematic review of prospective observational studies in China and Japan. The size of the solid squares is proportional to the number of strokes in each cholesterol category. Note the doubling scale of the y-axis. (With permission from the Eastern Stroke & Coronary Heart Disease Collaborative Research Group, 1998.[326])

apparent short-term effect of statins on risk of stroke after acute coronary syndromes.[393] The inconsistency between the association between total or LDL cholesterol and ischaemic stroke and the effectiveness of statins in preventing ischaemic stroke also raises the possibility that other lipid subfractions that are affected by statins might be better predictors of ischaemic stroke.[394]

Any association between plasma lipoprotein (a) and apolipoprotein E genotype with ischaemic stroke is still rather uncertain,[395–397] but apolipoproteins (apo A1 and apo B), which make up the protein moiety of lipoproteins, do appear to be predictive of ischaemic stroke.[398,399] Apo A1 is mainly found in HDL and apo B in LDL. Differences in prognostic value of apolipoproteins and LDL cholesterol are possible for several reasons. First, measurement of LDL cholesterol is an estimate of the mass of cholesterol in the LDL fraction of plasma, whereas measurements of apo B and apo A1 provide information on the total number of atherogenic (apo B) or anti-atherogenic (apo A1) particles. Second, the ratio of apo B : apo A1 best reflects the status of cholesterol transport to and from peripheral tissues. Third, unlike the relationships between total and LDL cholesterol and CHD, which weaken with age, apo B retains its predictive power in the elderly.[400]

Apo B is an established risk factor for coronary vascular events,[400,401] and statin-mediated coronary event risk reduction has been attributed to apo B reduction.[402] Data on apolipoproteins and ischaemic stroke risk are somewhat limited and conflicting, although there appears to be a relationship between raised apo B and an increased risk of ischaemic stroke, and an inverse correlation with apo A1 levels.[398,399]

6.6.7 Haemostatic variables

Despite much effort, very few consistent associations have been found between coagulation parameters, fibrinolytic activity, platelet behaviour and vascular disease.[403,404] Often these variables are altered by acute stroke so that most case–control studies are invalid, and it has not been practical to carry out very many long-term cohort studies.

Plasma fibrinogen has a strong and consistent positive association with stroke and coronary events, including recurrent stroke.[405,406] Cigarette-smoking is a confounding variable so the effect of cigarette-smoking on stroke may be mediated, at least in part, by increasing the fibrinogen level, thus accelerating thrombosis. Less important but still confusing confounding factors include age, hypertension, diabetes, hyperlipidaemia, lack of exercise, social class, social activity, season of the year, alcohol consumption and stress. It is not yet certain therefore whether increasing plasma fibrinogen really is a causal factor and, if so, whether it acts by increasing plasma viscosity or through promoting thrombosis. The confusion is compounded because there is no standard method for measuring plasma fibrinogen, it tends to rise after acute events including infections, it is not easy to lower plasma fibrinogen, and no satisfactory randomized controlled trials have been reported.[344,381,405–412]

Raised haematocrit is an uncertain risk factor for stroke and other acute vascular events, although it does seem to be associated with an increased case fatality in ischaemic stroke.[413] The association is confounded by the fact that cigarette-smoking, blood pressure and plasma fibrinogen are all positively associated with haematocrit.[414–416] Both raised haematocrit and raised plasma fibrinogen increase *whole blood viscosity*, another potentially causal risk factor.[411] No randomized trials are available of lowering haematocrit, viscosity or fibrinogen.

Raised plasma factor VII coagulant activity may be a risk factor for coronary events, and also polymorphisms of the factor VII gene, but there are very few data for stroke.[417–419]

Raised von Willebrand factor antigen is another possible risk factor for ischaemic stroke.[417,420]

Low blood fibrinolytic activity and *high plasma plasminogen-activator type I* are coronary risk factors and *raised tissue plasminogen activator antigen* may be associated with both coronary and stroke risk, perhaps because it is a marker of endogenous fibrinolytic activity.[417,421–426]

Abnormal platelet behaviour has not been convincingly linked with subsequent stroke in cohort studies, and any case–control studies after stroke have great potential for bias as stroke alters platelet function.[427] Polymorphisms of platelet membrane glycoprotein IIIa were at first associated with stroke but, as seems to happen so often with genetic studies, then rejected on the basis of larger and more methodologically sound work.[428]

6.6.8 Plasma homocysteine

Because the rare inborn recessive condition of homocystinuria is complicated by arterial and venous thrombosis (section 7.20.2), it is natural to imagine that mildly raised levels of plasma homocysteine could be a risk factor for or even a cause of vascular disease in general. Raised plasma homocysteine is positively associated with increasing age, abnormal lipids, smoking, diabetes, chronic renal failure and hypertension, and it is also raised in nutritional deficiencies and probably after stroke and myocardial infarction. The observational data linking coronary events, stroke, venous thromboembolism and carotid intima-media thickness and stenosis with increasing plasma homocysteine (hyperhomocysteinaemia) are now fairly robust.[429–435]

In view of the strength of the epidemiological association between homocysteine and risk of stroke, several trials of homocysteine-lowering with folic acid and pyridoxine are being performed, some of which have now been reported, but so far the results are not promising and hyperhomocystinaemia cannot yet be regarded as a causal risk factor (section 16.8.1).

6.6.9 Physical exercise

Physical exercise somewhat reduces blood pressure, weight, plasma cholesterol, plasma fibrinogen and the risk of non-insulin-dependent diabetes mellitus and is associated with less cigarette-smoking.[436,437] Therefore, not surprisingly, lack of exercise is associated with coronary events and there is also strong evidence of a similar association with stroke.[438–443] So far there is insufficient evidence from randomized trials to be sure that deliberately increasing exercise levels, in sporting activities or as part of a generally healthy lifestyle, reduces the risk of vascular events in the general population[444] (section 16.7.4). However, there is evidence (see below) that exercise can prevent progression to diabetes in patients with the metabolic syndrome as part of an overall lifestyle modification programme.[445,446]

6.6.10 Obesity

Any relationship between obesity and stroke is likely to be confounded by the positive association of obesity with hypertension, diabetes, hypercholesterolaemia and lack of exercise, and the negative association with smoking and concurrent illness. Nevertheless, stroke is more common in the obese and so is overall mortality. How to measure obesity is itself somewhat controversial; a raised waist : hip ratio as a measure of central obesity, and perhaps change in body weight, may be stronger risk factors than the traditional measure of weight compared with height (see below).[447–451]

6.6.11 The metabolic syndrome

Obesity, specifically visceral obesity, plays a key role in the development of the metabolic syndrome and type 2 diabetes. Visceral adipocytes are insulin-resistant and highly metabolically active and promote dyslipidaemia, hypertension and reduced systemic thrombolysis, as well as leading to a relatively pro-inflammatory state.[452] The constellation of metabolic abnormalities including central obesity, decreased HDL, raised triglycerides and blood pressure, and hyperglycaemia is known as the metabolic syndrome, and this is associated with a threefold increased risk of type 2 diabetes and a twofold increase in cardiovascular risk, including stroke.[453,454] It is thought to be the main driver for the modern-day epidemic of diabetes and vascular disease. As well as the prevention of acute vascular events in patients with the metabolic syndrome, primary prevention of which is mostly the same as for other groups,[453,454] one additional aim should be to prevent progression to frank diabetes. Two strategies have been shown to be effective in this regard – lifestyle modification with diet and

exercise;[445,446] and angiotensin-converting enzyme (ACE) inhibitors or A2 blockers (ARB).[455–457]

6.6.12 Diet

It is technically difficult to measure what people eat and how they cook it, relate any particular diet to events such as stroke that occur years later, and to be sure that any association is not better explained by a confounding variable.[458] For example, people who eat a lot of fruit tend to have a generally 'healthy' lifestyle, not to smoke, and they may use less salt.[459] Salt, by increasing systemic blood pressure, is probably associated with increased stroke risk but this issue is still controversial.[460–463] In observational studies, diets low in the following may be associated with a raised risk of coronary disease and stroke:[464]

- potassium[465–467]
- calcium[466,468]
- fresh fruit and vegetables[469,470]
- fish[469–473]
- antioxidants such as vitamin E,[474–476] vitamin C,[477–479] beta-carotene[480–482] and flavonols.[483,484]

On the whole, randomized trials of dietary interventions and vitamin supplementation have been disappointing (section 16.7.3). Either the theory is wrong, or the interventions were too little, too late, for insufficient time or the trials were too small.[385,455,485–489] The effect of a vegetarian diet is unclear.[490]

Despite earlier enthusiasm, it now appears that there is no association between coffee consumption and vascular disease.[491–494]

6.6.13 Alcohol

The relationship between alcohol, ischaemic stroke and carotid atheroma is complex and may be U-shaped.[495] While heavy alcohol consumption may be an independent and perhaps causal risk factor, it seems that modest consumers are protected to some extent compared with abstainers.[496–504] Whether 'binge' drinking is associated with stroke is uncertain[505,506] but it is possible that irregular drinking carries a higher risk.[507] Much of the confusion in relating alcohol consumption with stroke is because:[508]

- people are not always truthful about their alcohol consumption;
- it is difficult to measure alcohol consumption accurately, particularly over time;
- there are varied ways of expressing alcohol consumption (per day, per week, grams, units, number of drinks, regular, binge, etc.);
- different types of alcoholic drinks may have different effects;

- pattern of drinking behaviour may change over time;
- combining ex-drinkers, some of whom may have given up drinking because of symptoms of vascular or other diseases, with lifetime non-drinkers in the analyses;
- the biases inherent in case–control studies;
- publication bias;
- small numbers and so imprecise estimates;
- confounding with cigarette-smoking, hypertension and deprivation which are positively related, and with exercise which is negatively related with alcohol consumption;
- confounding with unknown or unmeasurable factors which might link no drinking or heavy drinking with an excess risk of vascular disease (e.g. healthy vs risky lifestyle);
- lumping ischaemic and haemorrhagic strokes together.

It is difficult to think of the same biological reason for ischaemic stroke in non-drinkers and heavy drinkers. Possible causal explanations, at least in heavy drinkers, are that alcohol almost certainly increases the blood pressure; traumatic arterial dissection in the neck during an alcohol-related injury; dehydration, hyperviscosity and platelet activation perhaps; sleep apnoea and hypoxia; and that alcohol can cause both atrial fibrillation and cardiomyopathy with embolism to the brain.[509–512]

Perhaps it would be more productive to ask why modest drinking is protective, if it really is. Increased plasma high-density lipoprotein-cholesterol and lower fibrinogen levels are possibilities.[513] It is most unlikely that a randomized trial of modest alcohol consumption, in the hope of reducing the risk of vascular disorders without increasing the risk of other disorders, will ever be feasible. Therefore, we are left trying to interpret, with difficulty, the available observational data (section 16.7.2).

6.6.14 Ethnicity

There are no good population-based data on stroke incidence in developing countries, with yawning gaps particularly in South and South-East Asia and sub-Saharan Africa[48,514,515] (section 18.2.2). Nonetheless, and notwithstanding the difficulty in defining ethnicity, stroke incidence does seem greater in black than white people living in Western countries, probably both ischaemic stroke and intracerebral haemorrhage.[516–520] The high prevalence of hypertension, diabetes, sickle cell trait and social deprivation in black people may be part of the explanation.[521–523] South Asian populations in the UK have a high stroke mortality as well as a high prevalence of coronary disease, central obesity, insulin resistance, diabetes mellitus and other risk factors.[524,525] This is in part because they are genetically more at risk than white populations by virtue of higher serum lipoprotein (a) concentrations.[526–529] Also, Maori and Pacific people living in New Zealand have a higher stroke risk than white New Zealanders.[530] Moreover, the fall in stroke incidence that has occurred in white New Zealanders has not been mirrored by any similar fall in the Maori and Pacific population.[531]

6.6.15 Specific genes for common types of ischaemic stroke

Based on the assumption that at least some of the risk for stroke is genetic, large numbers of studies have now been done or are being done in an attempt to identify the genes involved.[532] However, on the whole, methodological rigour – and so the reliability of the results of these studies – has been limited. It seems likely that the genetic component of stroke risk is modest and that many (probably hundreds) of genes are involved, each one contributing only a small increased risk. But, studies so far have generally not been large enough to detect reliably the sort of relative risks (i.e. the risk ratio comparing one genotype with another at a particular genetic locus) that might realistically be expected (probably about 1.2 to 1.5). Other methodological limitations include: poor choice of controls in case–control studies and/or failure to use methods designed to detect and control for selection bias; inadequate distinction between the different pathological types and subtypes of stroke for which genetic influences may differ; failure to replicate positive results in an independent and adequately sized study; and testing of multiple genetic or subgroup hypotheses with no adjustment of p-values for declaring statistical significance.[533,534]

Candidate gene studies

Most genetic studies so far have been candidate gene studies, in which the frequency of different genotypes at a specific locus or loci within a gene or genes thought likely to be in some way connected with stroke risk are compared between stroke cases and stroke-free controls. Candidate genes have generally been selected on the basis of their known or presumed involvement in the control of factors or pathways likely to influence stroke risk: blood pressure, lipid metabolism, inflammation, coagulation, homocysteine metabolism and so on.[535,536] Rigorous meta-analyses of candidate gene studies, both in stroke and other vascular diseases such as coronary heart disease, have highlighted the various methodological issues discussed above. In particular, they have drawn attention to the problems of small study size (most studies have included a few hundred or less, rather than the required 1000 or more cases and controls), leading to the potential for publication bias (i.e. small positive studies are far more likely to be published and available for inclusion in meta-analyses than small negative ones), with very large studies tending to detect either much smaller relative risks or no evidence of altered risk at all.[534,537,538] Large numbers of candidate gene studies have together identified a handful of genes (those encoding factor V Leiden, methylenetetrahydrofolate reductase, prothrombin and angiotensin-converting enzyme) which, on the basis of results from meta-analyses, seem likely to influence risk of ischaemic stroke modestly.[536] However, since none of the contributing studies was large enough to be independently reliable, occult publication bias might still account for the apparent effects of these few genes, and confirmation in further very large studies is needed.

Linkage studies

As yet there have been far fewer stroke genetics studies that use more traditional genetic study designs, based on collecting information and DNA from related individuals with and without the disease of interest. This is at least partly because family members of stroke patients (who of course tend to be elderly) are often no longer still alive, and so obtaining information and samples for DNA extraction from large enough numbers of relatives is challenging.[539] There are some exceptions, though. For example, the Icelandic population has excellent genealogical records allowing the construction of complex pedigrees, along with stored DNA and medical histories on large numbers of people in the population. Family or pedigree-based genetic study designs allow for linkage analysis, which has the attraction of not being driven by hypotheses about specific candidates, but instead sets out to identify which regions of the genome may influence disease risk, through analysing the degree of sharing of genetic information (at markers across the whole genome) between related individuals with and without disease. The Icelandic deCODE group has carried out a number of linkage studies to identify regions of the genome likely to influence risk of various common diseases, including stroke (see http://www.decode.com/Population-Approach.php). Through this process, two candidate genes for ischaemic stroke, encoding the enzymes phosphodiesterase-4D and arachidonate 5-lipoxygenase-activating protein ALOX5AP, have been identified.[540] There is still some debate, however, about their influence in non-Icelandic populations, since their effect on ischaemic stroke risk has been confirmed in some, but not all, subsequent studies, and the confirmatory studies have not been free of the methodological problems discussed above.[541,542]

Whole genome association studies

The combination of technological developments allowing rapid throughput genotyping at multiple loci, the attraction of non-hypothesis-driven genetic studies, and the recognized limitations of traditional linkage approaches have together led to a new wave of genome-wide association studies, where multiple (up to 500 000 or more) polymorphisms across the genome are genotyped and compared in cases and controls, looking for loci where significant differences may suggest genetic influences on disease risk. The statistical considerations required for such studies are considerable, since huge numbers of potential genetic risk factors, albeit not completely independent of each other (because segments of the genome tend to be transmitted together during meiosis – linkage dysequilibrium), are tested simultaneously.[543,544] Thus, there is great potential for missing real genetic effects or for finding spurious ones. Nonetheless, this approach has had a few (perhaps lucky) successes in common diseases; one small, preliminary study in stroke has now been published, and no doubt others will follow.[545]

Genetic studies of other vascular diseases, known vascular risk factors and intermediate phenotypes

The results of genetic studies of other vascular diseases (in particular coronary heart disease) may also prove useful in identifying likely genetic candidates for ischaemic stroke. In addition, since much of the genetic risk of stroke seems likely to be mediated through already-known risk factors such as cholesterol and blood pressure (sections 6.6.3 and 6.6.6), studies of these may also provide useful information about likely stroke risk genes. Finally, genetic studies have started to emerge of so-called 'intermediate phenotypes', markers of predisposition to stroke (or other vascular diseases), which can be measured in large numbers of subjects both with and without vascular risk factors or disease. These intermediate phenotypes include carotid intima media thickness and leukoaraiosis (measured or graded on CT or MR brain scans), and both linkage and candidate gene approaches have been used.[533,546] As with studies of clinically manifest disease, methodological rigour and adequate study size are crucial, and so systematic review and meta-analysis approaches will be helpful in interpreting the large numbers of studies and quantities of data emerging.[547]

We are still far from being able to quantify the genetic influences on stroke, or to identify reliably the genes involved. One serious challenge is that the available laboratory technology is currently outstripping our ability to properly analyse and interpret the results. In the future, only careful integration of information from all of the different approaches described above, together with the results of laboratory studies of gene expression and function, from the molecular to the animal model level, will shed useful light on the genetic influences on stroke, hopefully allowing us to understand better the way in which already-known risk factors influence stroke, and reliably to identify new ones.

6.6.16 Social deprivation

Social deprivation, low socioeconomic status and un-employment are all inextricably linked and associated with increased stroke risk.[548,549] This association is partly caused by a higher prevalence of vascular risk factors, stress and adverse health behaviours, such as smoking, poor diet and lack of exercise in deprived populations.[550] For example, these factors appear to account for most of the north–south gradient in stroke mortality in the UK.[551] Also, it has been suggested that poor health and nutrition *in utero* or infancy are associated with the development of vascular risk factors such as hyperten-sion and adult vascular disease, including stroke.[552–555] It is extremely difficult to disentangle early from later life influences on health and so, not surprisingly, the 'early life' or 'Barker' hypothesis has been refuted by some.[556–559] The possibility of reducing stroke risk by tackling social deprivation is yet another reason to add to the many others to support what has to be political rather than medical action.

6.6.17 Infection

There has been interest in the notion that infection contributes to the development of atheroma, the pro-gression of the atherothrombotic plaque, and perhaps plaque instability. However, the evidence from observa-tional epidemiological studies of infections in general,[560] and of chronic dental infection,[561] together with serological evidence of specific infectious agents, such as *Chlamydia pneumoniae*, *Helicobacter pylori* and cyto-megalovirus, is not very convincing, even for coronary disease where there are – as usual – more data than for stroke.[562–569] The generalized inflammatory response in patients with coronary artery disease may be too non-specific to be convincing evidence of infection, and there may well be the familiar problems of confounding and publication bias.[412,563,564,570] Nonetheless, the fact that evidence of chlamydial infection can be found in atherosclerotic plaques is certainly interesting although reverse causality is a possibility, i.e. atheroma *becomes* infected more often than normal arterial wall.[571] An early randomized trial to eliminate chlamydia was far too small to be reliable despite being published in a high-impact journal.[572] Further antibiotic intervention trials are ongoing.[573,574]

6.6.18 'Stress'

It is part of folklore that stress causes strokes: 'I was so upset, I nearly had a stroke'. Indeed, there are some striking anecdotes.

This 82-year-old lady was admitted for investigation of anaemia and hepatomegaly. She was found to have multiple liver metastases. When she was told the news, she stopped speaking and never spoke again. It took a day or so before the medical staff realized that her mute state was not 'psychological' but that she was aphasic. A brain CT scan showed a left cortical infarct. She died some days later from her malignancy.

However, showing that long-term psychological stressors are associated with stroke, or that shorter-term ones precipitate stroke, is not easy. There is some evid-ence that severely threatening life events,[575,576] anxiety and depression,[577] high levels of anger expression[578,579] and psychological stress[577,580,581] may trigger the onset of stroke, perhaps in people already at risk of stroke.

6.6.19 Non-stroke vascular disease

Because atheroma in one artery is likely to be accompanied by atheroma in others (section 6.3.1), and because embolism from the heart is a common cause of ischaemic stroke (section 6.5), non-stroke vascular disorders are associated with (i.e. are risk factors for) ischaemic stroke and transient ischaemic attack (Table 6.8).

Coronary heart disease (e.g. angina or myocardial infarc-tion) has been repeatedly associated with an increased risk of stroke in postmortem,[582,583] twin,[584] case–control[190,585–587] and cohort studies.[170,194,330] Therefore, it is not surprising that electrocardiogram abnormalities and cardiac failure are also associated with increased risk of stroke because they both so often reflect coronary

Table 6.8 Degenerative vascular disorders outside the head associated with an increased risk of ischaemic stroke and transient ischaemic attack.

Myocardial infarction/angina
Cardiac failure
Left ventricular hypertrophy
Atrial fibrillation
Cervical arterial bruit/stenosis
Peripheral arterial disease

disease and hypertension, as is left ventricular hypertrophy.[330,588–592] Atrial fibrillation is considered in section 6.5.1.

Cervical bruits (carotid or supraclavicular) are generally caused by stenosis of the underlying arteries (section 6.7.7), mostly as a result of atheroma, and so become more common with age; about 5% of asymptomatic people over the age of 75 years have bruits.[593–595] Carotid bruits are clearly a risk factor for ischaemic stroke, but not necessarily in the same arterial territory as the bruit, and also for coronary events, because atheroma of one artery is likely to be accompanied by atheroma of other arteries in the same predisposed individual.[596,597] The risk of these various vascular events increases with carotid stenosis severity (section 16.11.5).

Atheroma affecting the leg arteries is associated with cerebrovascular and coronary disease in the same individuals so often that it is not surprising that claudicants have an increased risk of stroke and other serious vascular events.[194,598–602]

Little seems to be known about the prevalence of *abdominal aortic aneurysms* in ischaemic stroke/TIA patients. It is said to be quite high, about 10–20%, depending on the selection of patients and the size criterion for what constitutes an aneurysm.[602–605] The incidence of aneurysm rupture in the general population is 5–10 times higher in men than in women,[316] and so there might be an argument for screening men presenting with transient ischaemic attack or stroke, particularly perhaps if the cause is thought to be atherothromboembolism and bearing in mind the advantages of screening even in 'normal' elderly men from the Multicentre Aneurysm Screening Study (MASS).[606]

6.6.20 Other risk factors

Innumerable other risk factors for coronary heart disease, and/or ischaemic stroke, have been suggested and supported by varying degrees of evidence. However, it may take many years, even decades, before a particular risk factor is accepted as causal, as has been the case for hypertension and smoking. So often initial discoveries of 'new' risk factors are found subsequently to be spurious.[607] Even by 1981, 246 risk factors had been counted and by now there must be many more.[608] Some may or may not be important in the causal pathway to stroke but, even if not, they may still conceivably be helpful in predicting future stroke in individuals and populations. This distinction is important: for example, claudication is clearly not on the causal pathway to stroke but is so strongly associated with stroke risk that it is included in many statistical models which predict later stroke (section 16.2).

6.7 From symptoms, signs and clinical syndrome to cause

Once the diagnosis of ischaemic stroke or transient ischaemic attack (TIA) has been made, the cause of the ischaemic event needs to be established since this has implications for treatment, prognosis and risk of recurrence. Four clinical syndromes, based on the history and examination, can be identified: total anterior circulation infarction, partial anterior circulation infarction, lacunar infarction and posterior circulation infarction. The clinical syndrome reasonably predicts the site and size of the brain lesion, which takes one a long way towards the likely cause of the ischaemic event (Fig. 6.20). Clinical localization is easier if the patient has had an established stroke with stable physical signs rather than being in the very early stages when the signs are still evolving (brain attack), or has had a TIA and any signs have disappeared.

However, stroke localization based on the history and examination is by no means infallible: in about one-quarter of cases where a recent lesion is visible on brain imaging, it is not in the expected place to explain the clinical syndrome.[133] For example, although most pure motor strokes are caused by a lacunar infarct as a result of small vessel disease, in a few cases the CT or MR scan shows striatocapsular infarction which is likely to be caused by middle cerebral artery occlusion with good cortical collaterals (sections 4.2.2 and 6.7.2; fig. 6.20e). And in a recent study of 150 patients with minor stroke and a single acute lesion on DWI, agreement on localization to anterior or posterior vascular territory between DWI and the clinical judgements of three independent neurologists was only moderate (kappa = 0.5).[609] Thus, brain imaging, in particular new techniques such as MR DWI, can and if possible should be used to refine lesion localization and thus aid in the search for the cause of the ischaemic stroke/TIA in an individual patient.

In acute stroke, computed tomography or magnetic resonance imaging should be neither the first nor only way to classify patients on the basis of the size and site of any ischaemic brain lesion. Imaging is used to confirm and refine where the symptoms and neurological signs – in other words, the clinical syndrome – suggest the lesion is. From there, it is possible to narrow down the potential causes of the infarct.

6.7.1 Total anterior circulation infarction

The acute ischaemic stroke clinical syndrome of a total anterior circulation infarction (TACI) comprises a hemiparesis, with or without hemisensory loss, homonymous hemianopia, and a new cortical deficit such as aphasia or neglect. It is a good predictor of infarction of most of the middle cerebral artery (MCA) territory on brain CT, as a consequence of occlusion of either the MCA mainstem (or proximal large branch) or the internal carotid artery (ICA) in the neck (section 4.3.4) (Fig. 6.20c). Occasionally, a TACI can be caused by occlusion of the posterior cerebral artery, but the hemiparesis is usually rather mild. The *cause* of the arterial occlusion therefore is usually in the heart (e.g. embolism as a consequence of atrial fibrillation, recent myocardial infarction, etc.), or it is atherothrombosis complicated by embolism or occasionally propagating thrombosis of the ICA, or embolism from the aortic arch. Therefore, if the heart is clinically normal (history, examination, chest X-ray and electrocardiogram) and if there is no evidence of arterial disease in the neck (bruits, palpation perhaps, but mainly duplex sonography), then it is important to consider rarities, for example, infective endocarditis (echocardiogram, blood cultures) and carotid dissection (MR angiogram, and certainly recheck for past history of neck trauma, or associated neck or face pain). Although transcranial Doppler may confirm an MCA mainstem occlusion (but not if it has already recanalized), it will not help much in the search for a cause.[134] A catheter angiogram *might* be diagnostically helpful if it could be justified on the basis of changing the patient's management (e.g. traumatic carotid dissection could lead to later litigation, fibromuscular dysplasia could stop the search for other explanations, a giant aneurysm with contained thrombus might be surgically treatable, and so on). MRI and MR angiography, and CT angiography, are now widely and more appropriately used to show lesions, such as dissection and aneurysms, but they are still not always easily available in patients in the acute stage of stroke (sections 6.8.3 and 6.8.4).

6.7.2 Partial anterior circulation infarction

Partial anterior circulation infarction (PACI) is a more restricted clinical syndrome with only two out of the three components of a TACI; or a new isolated cortical deficit, such as aphasia; or a predominantly proprioceptive deficit in one limb; or a motor/sensory deficit restricted to one body area or part of one body area (e.g. one leg, one hand, etc.) (section 4.3.5). This syndrome is reasonably predictive of a restricted cortical infarct caused by occlusion of a branch of the middle cerebral artery (MCA) or, much less commonly, of the anterior cerebral artery, as a result of embolism from the heart or from proximal sites of atherothrombosis (usually the

carotid bifurcation), or to any other cause of a TACI (Fig. 6.20b).

Investigation is therefore similar to that for the patient with a TACI, except it is usually easier because the patient is fully conscious and less neurologically impaired. However, investigation must be quicker because of the higher risk of early recurrence (section 16.2.3)[79,80] and because the patient has more to lose from a recurrence which might, next time, be a TACI. The potential for secondary prevention must be considered, particularly eligibility for carotid endarterectomy, and this requires early duplex sonography to find any severe carotid stenosis (section 6.8.5), and eligibility for anticoagulation if the patient is in atrial fibrillation. Transcranial Doppler (TCD) is unlikely to demonstrate the blocked cerebral artery because this is almost always distal to the MCA mainstem, at a point where TCD is not particularly sensitive.[134] Occasionally, however, patients with a large PACI, but falling short of the full definition of a TACI, do have MCA mainstem occlusion, presumably because good collateral flow to the margins of the central infarcted area of brain restricts the clinical syndrome. This is particularly likely with striatocapsular infarction, which usually presents as a PACI (Figs 4.14, 6.20e). Some other PACI syndromes are caused by infarction in the centrum semiovale (section 4.2.2) and in boundary zones (section 6.7.5). Anterior choroidal artery infarcts may also present as a PACI (or a lacunar) syndrome and they seem to be caused by either embolism from proximal sites or intracranial small vessel disease (section 4.2.2).

> Total and partial anterior circulation infarction/transient ischaemic attacks are usually caused by occlusion of the mainstem or a branch of the middle cerebral artery, by occlusion of the anterior cerebral artery, or by occlusion of the internal carotid artery. Such occlusions are usually caused by embolism from the heart, embolism from proximal arterial sites of atherothombosis (the internal carotid artery origin, the aortic arch, etc.), and sometimes by thrombotic occlusion of severe internal carotid artery stenosis.

6.7.3 Lacunar infarction

Lacunar syndromes, the vast majority of which are ischaemic rather than due to intracerebral haemorrhage, are almost always caused by small, deep, infarcts more likely to be seen on MRI than brain CT (section 4.3.2) (Fig. 6.20d). These small, deep, infarcts are mostly caused by a vasculopathy affecting the small perforating arteries of the brain, and not by embolism from proximal

(a)

(b)

(c)

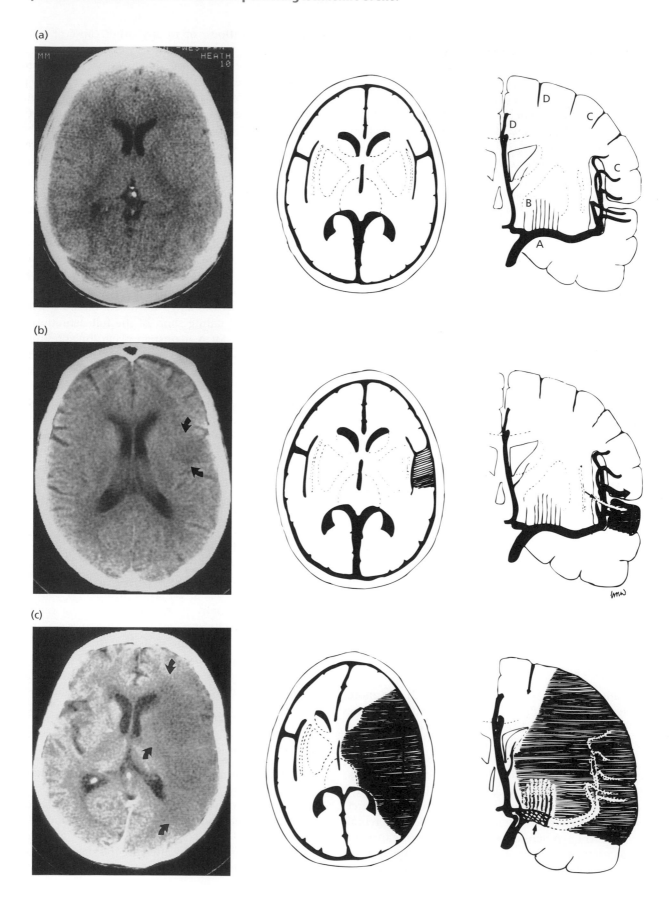

(d)

(e)

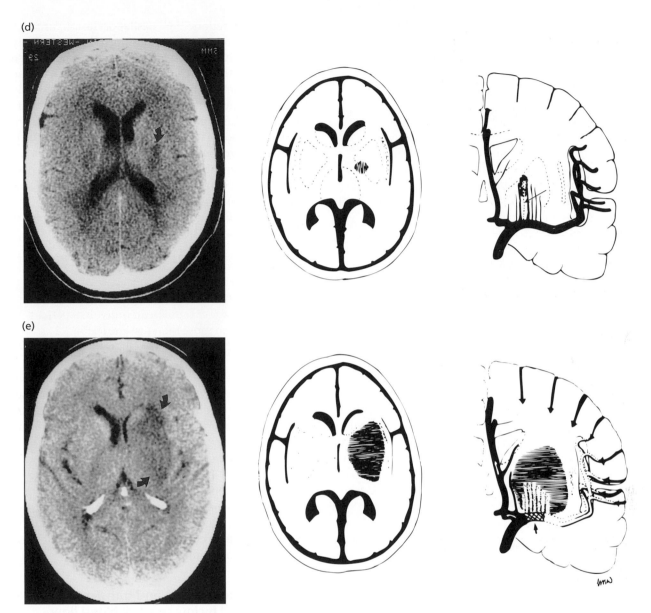

Fig. 6.20 (*opposite & above*) Various patterns of arterial occlusion cause different types of ischaemic stroke. *Left-hand columns*: axial CT brain scan at the level of the basal ganglia; middle columns, diagram to correspond with the CT brain scan with the area of infarction shaded; *right-hand columns*: diagram of the middle cerebral artery (MCA) and anterior cerebral arteries on a coronal brain section with the area of infarction shaded. A, main trunk of MCA; B, lenticulostriate perforating branches of the MCA; C, cortical branches of the MCA; D, cortical branches of the anterior cerebral arteries. (a) Normal arterial anatomy and CT scan. (b) Occlusion – usually embolic (*straight arrow*) from heart, aorta or internal carotid artery – of a cortical branch of the MCA and restricted cortical infarct on CT (*curved arrows*); partial anterior circulation infarction (PACI). (c) Occlusion – usually embolic (*straight arrow*) as in (b) above – of MCA mainstem to cause infarction of entire MCA territory (*curved arrows*); total anterior circulation infarction (TACI). (d) Occlusion of one lenticulostriate artery (*straight arrow*) to cause a lacunar infarct (*curved arrow*); lacunar infarction (LACI). Note that the patient has an old lacunar infarct in the opposite hemisphere. (e) Occlusion of the MCA mainstem (*straight arrow*) but with good cortical collaterals from the anterior and posterior cerebral arteries to cause a striatocapsular infarct (*curved arrows*).

arterial sources or the heart (section 6.4) and thus have a low risk of early recurrence[71] There is not therefore the same urgency to rule out a cardiac source of embolism or severe carotid stenosis as there is for a partial anterior circulation infarction (PACI) (section 6.7.2).

> The vast majority of lacunar stroke syndromes are caused by ischaemia rather than haemorrhage. Most ischaemic lacunar strokes are the result of a small, deep, not a cortical, infarct. These small, deep infarcts are usually within the distribution of a small, perforating artery. The underlying vascular pathology is probably 'complex' small vessel disease, which differs from atheroma, but sometimes atheroma of the parent artery may occlude the mouth of the perforating artery. Lacunar infarcts are seldom caused by embolism from the heart or from proximal arterial sources.

The *capsular warning syndrome* has a rather characteristic pattern. Over hours or days, there is cluster of transient ischaemic attacks (TIAs), consisting typically of weakness down the whole of one side of the body without any cognitive or language deficit (i.e. pure motor lacunar TIAs). These may be followed within hours or days by a lacunar infarct in the internal capsule. This syndrome is presumably caused by intermittent closure of a single lenticulostriate or other perforating artery, followed by complete occlusion, and one is unlikely to find a proximal arterial or cardiac cause, as in any other type of lacunar ischaemic stroke.[346]

6.7.4 Posterior circulation infarction

Ischaemia and infarction in the brainstem and/or occipital region is aetiologically more heterogeneous than in the other three main clinical syndromes[61,62] (section 4.3.3). Emboli from the heart may reach a small artery supplying the brainstem (e.g. superior cerebellar artery) to cause a fairly restricted deficit, block the basilar artery to produce a major brainstem stroke, travel on to block one or both posterior cerebral arteries to cause a homonymous hemianopia or cortical blindness, or any combination of these deficits. Similarly, embolism from the vertebral artery (as a result of atherothrombosis usually, but sometimes another disorder such as dissection) or from atherothrombosis of the basilar artery, aortic arch or innominate or subclavian arteries produces exactly the same neurological features as embolism from the heart.[63,165,610] Even embolism from the carotid territory can, in some individuals with a dominant posterior communicating artery or a persistent trigeminal artery, cause occlusion of the posterior cerebral artery and even

brainstem infarction.[611,612] Basilar occlusion, usually as a result of severe atherothrombotic stenosis, is likely to produce massive brainstem infarction. Obstruction, usually by atherothrombosis, of the origin of the small arteries arising from the basilar artery, can produce restricted brainstem syndromes, as can 'complex' small vessel disease within the brainstem; certainly some patients with a lacunar syndrome have a small infarct in the brainstem. A posterior circulation infarction (POCI) does not therefore provide much of a clue to the cause of the ischaemic event. An exception is the patient with simultaneous brainstem signs and a homonymous hemianopia, where embolism from the heart or a proximal artery must be the likely cause and not small vessel disease.

> Posterior circulation infarction/transient ischaemic attack can be due to almost any cause of cerebral ischaemia, which makes it very difficult to be certain of the exact cause in an individual patient if one knows no more than just the lesion localization.

Cerebellar ischaemic strokes (section 4.2.3) are mostly caused by embolism from the heart, vertebral and basilar arteries, or by atherothrombotic occlusion at the origin of the cerebellar arteries; some are said to result from low blood flow alone.[613–616]

Thalamic infarcts (section 4.2.3) can be caused by: 'complex' small vessel disease affecting one of the small perforating arteries; atheromatous occlusion of these same arteries where they arise from the posterior cerebral and other medium-sized arteries; and occlusion of these latter arteries by embolism from the heart, basilar, vertebral and other proximal arterial sites.[617–619]

6.7.5 Ischaemic strokes and transient ischaemic attacks caused by low cerebral blood flow

The pressure gradient across, and blood flow through, large arteries is not affected until their diameter is reduced by more than 50%, often not until by much more.[620–622] Not surprisingly, therefore, even if there is severe disease of the carotid or vertebral arteries, cerebral perfusion pressure is usually normal. However, in some patients, as the stenosis becomes more severe, flow does fall, and eventually cerebral vasodilatation (autoregulation) cannot compensate for the low cerebral perfusion pressure. Regional cerebral blood flow (CBF) then falls, particularly if the collateral circulation is compromised because the circle of Willis, for example, is incomplete or diseased[53,66,623–625] (section 4.2.2). At this stage of exhausted cerebral perfusion reserve, the ratio of cerebral blood flow : cerebral blood volume falls below about 6.0, oxygen extraction fraction starts to rise and stroke risk probably also rises[53,626–629] (section 12.1.2).

Using transcranial Doppler (TCD) to demonstrate impaired cerebrovascular reactivity to a chemical rather than perfusion challenge is an indirect but more practical alternative to positron emission tomography (PET), but the correlation is not perfect[624] (section 6.8.9). Isotopic measurement of the mean cerebral transit time,[630] gradient echo and perfusion-weighted MRI,[625,631] MR angiography,[632] CT perfusion[633,634] and near-infrared spectroscopy[635] are other possibilities.

Therefore, although the notion that ischaemic strokes may be caused by 'hypotension' goes back many years, low regional CBF alone is not particularly common and cannot easily explain more than a small fraction of strokes. Severe arterial stenosis or occlusion, or good evidence of a fall in systemic blood pressure just before onset, are simply not present in most ischaemic stroke cases.[636] Most ischaemic strokes and transient ischaemic attacks (TIAs) must be caused, we believe, by embolic or *in situ* acute (usually thrombotic) occlusion of an artery to the brain causing blood flow to be suddenly cut off, so causing ischaemia in its territory of supply.

Naturally, at times, focal ischaemia *could* also be caused just by low flow without *acute* vessel occlusion but usually only distal to a severely stenosed or occluded internal carotid (ICA) or other artery. This is where the vascular bed is likely to be maximally dilated and therefore where the brain is particularly vulnerable to any fall in perfusion pressure (even more so if arteries carrying collateral blood flow are also diseased). Under these circumstances, a small drop in systemic blood pressure might cause transient or permanent focal ischaemia without any acute occlusive event. Under *normal* circumstances quite a large fall in blood pressure does not cause cerebral symptoms, provided it is transient. This is because of autoregulation of CBF (section 12.1.2). If it does, the symptoms are much more likely to be non-focal (faintness, bilateral blurring of vision, etc.) than focal[637] (sections 3.2.1 and 3.4.12).

Boundary-zone ischaemia and infarction

Sometimes, ischaemia occurs not *within* but *between* major arterial territories in their boundary zones (section 4.2.4). Because this is where perfusion pressure is likely to be most attenuated, it is conceivable that 'low flow' as a result of low perfusion pressure, as well as the more common acute arterial occlusion caused by embolism, can cause ischaemia in these areas.[638] The alternative term of watershed infarction is a misnomer based on geographical ignorance. A watershed is the line separating the water flowing *into* different river basins (i.e. the

high ground *between* two drainage areas), which is quite different from the pattern of arterial supply where flow is from larger to smaller vessels.

The evidence that at least some boundary-zone infarcts are caused by low flow rather than acute arterial occlusion is that sudden, profound and relatively prolonged hypotension (e.g. as a result of cardiac arrest or cardiac surgery) sometimes causes infarction bilaterally in the posterior boundary zones, between the supply territories of the middle cerebral artery (MCA) and the posterior cerebral artery in the parieto-occipital region. The clinical features include cortical blindness, visual disorientation and agnosia, and amnesia. Unilateral posterior boundary-zone infarction causes contralateral hemianopia, cortical sensory loss and, if in the dominant hemisphere, aphasia. Also, distal to severe carotid stenosis or occlusion, unilateral infarction is well recognized in the anterior boundary zone between the supply territories of the MCA and anterior cerebral artery in the frontoparasagittal region, but this does not necessarily mean that the cause was low flow rather than embolism. The clinical features are contralateral weakness of the leg more than the arm and sparing the face, some impaired sensation in the same distribution, and aphasia if in the dominant hemisphere[57,162,639] There is an internal or subcortical boundary zone in the corona radiata and centrum semiovale, lateral and/or above the lateral ventricle. This lies between the supply of the lenticulostriate perforating branches from the MCA trunk, and the medullary perforating arteries which arise from the cortical branches of the MCA and the anterior and, perhaps, posterior cerebral arteries. Infarction can occur within this internal boundary zone, usually causing a lacunar or partial anterior circulation syndrome, in association with severe carotid disease and sometimes an obvious haemodynamic precipitating cause.[640]

The diagnosis of 'low flow' as the cause of ischaemic strokes and TIAs

It would be simplistic to presume that all ischaemic strokes are caused by acute arterial occlusion. However, the definitive separation of stroke resulting from 'low flow' from acute arterial occlusion is far from easy. It is probably best inferred from the circumstances surrounding the onset of the symptoms, and to some extent by their nature, and not very much from either the neurological signs or the site of any visible infarct on brain imaging. Unfortunately, any clinical guideance to 'low flow' ischaemic episodes cannot be validated against a 'gold standard' because at present there is none.

Most ischaemic strokes and TIAs occur 'out of the blue' with no precipitating activity. However, on the basis of a number of convincing case reports, a fall in cerebral perfusion pressure as the cause – mostly resulting from a fall in systemic blood pressure – should be suspected if the symptoms start under certain circumstances:

- on standing or sitting up quickly, even if postural hypotension cannot be demonstrated in the clinic;
- immediately after a heavy meal;
- in very hot weather;
- after a hot bath or warming the face;
- with exercise, coughing or hyperventilation;
- during a Valsalva manoeuvre, but paradoxical embolism is another possibility;
- during a clinically obvious episode of cardiac dysrhythmia (chest pain, palpitations, etc.), but embolism from the heart is also possible;
- during operative hypotension (section 7.18); or
- if the patient has recently been started on or increased the dose of any drug likely to cause hypotension, such as calcium blockers or vasodilators.

In addition, there is usually very obvious evidence of severe arterial disease in the neck, i.e. bruits and/or absent pulsations.[641–653]

Transient ischaemic attacks (TIAs) caused by low flow may be atypical 'limb shaking TIAs' and tend to develop over minutes rather than seconds. These consist of stereotyped jerking and shaking of one arm and/or leg contralateral to the cerebral ischaemia and so are easily confused with focal motor seizures (section 3.3.4), or there is monocular or binocular visual blurring, dimming, fragmentation or bleaching, often only in bright light (section 3.3.6). Movement disorders including chorea have also been reported but involvement of the face is thought not to occur, perhaps because the blood flow to the facial motor cortex is not significantly compromised. 'Limb shaking TIAs' typically occur on standing up and may be abolished by a reduction in any hypertensive therapy, or carotid surgery, since they are frequently associated with severe occlusive carotid disease. There may be additional non-focal features, such as faintness, mental vagueness or even loss of consciousness.[654–659] Low-flow ischaemic oculopathy is discussed in section 3.3.6.

It is very important to note that boundary-zone infarction on brain imaging (or at postmortem) is *not* necessarily caused by low cerebral blood flow (without acute arterial occlusion) but this assumption has bedevilled much of the literature. The brain CT/MRI-defined site and size of any visible recent infarction is *not* an accurate way to diagnose a low-flow ischaemic stroke. This is, first, because some boundary-zone infarcts result from embolism.[638,660,661] Second, there is much variation between individuals in *where* the boundary zones are, and they may even change with time in the same individual in response to changes in peripheral vascular resistance (Fig. 6.21). Third, however boundary-zone infarcts are defined on imaging, there is little difference between them and territorial presumed-embolic infarcts in patient demographic characteristics, vascular risk

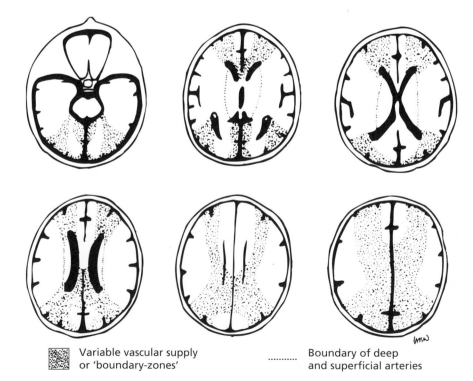

| | Variable vascular supply or 'boundary-zones' | .... | Boundary of deep and superficial arteries |

Fig. 6.21 The anterior and posterior boundary zones between the territories of the middle, anterior and posterior cerebral arteries. The maximum extent of these variable zones is shown on CT templates (see also Figs 4.11, 4.17, 4.23 and 4.25).

factors and even in the prevalence of arterial disease in the neck severe enough to cause low flow, which is far more often assumed than measured.[662–665] However, there have not been many comparative studies, definitions of boundary zones vary and the numbers of patients have been small.

On balance, although some boundary-zone infarcts may have a haemodynamic (i.e. low flow) cause, many others could be caused by embolism or acute occlusive thrombosis. After all, any arterial territory has a terminal zone which forms a boundary with adjacent arterial territories and which is probably particularly vulnerable to ischaemia. There is no reason to suppose that this zone is more susceptible to ischaemia caused by low flow without *acute* arterial occlusion, than as a result of acute arterial occlusion. Another possibility is that boundary-zone infarcts are caused by a *combination* of embolization to the margins of the territorial supply of a cerebral artery, as well as insufficient perfusion pressure to clear the emboli because of severe arterial disease in the neck, or operative hypotension.[661] Clearly, in view of the diagnostic difficulties, it is quite conceivable that low flow is a more frequent cause of cerebral ischaemia, or less frequent, than currently believed.

> The exact sites of the boundary zones between the territories of supply of the major cerebral arteries are so variable between, and even within, individuals that the diagnosis of infarction in a boundary zone based on CT/MRI alone is all but impossible. Boundary-zone infarction can be caused by acute arterial obstruction, while low blood flow does not necessarily cause infarction only within boundary zones.

Implications for treatment

Being certain that an ischaemic episode is caused either by low flow alone, or by acute arterial obstruction, seldom really matters. It makes very little difference if ischaemic stroke or TIA caused by low flow is recognized as such because unless the precipitating factor(s) can be avoided or reversed (particularly over-treatment of hypertension), the management is exactly the same as for presumed embolic causes of ischaemia, i.e. antithrombotic drugs, statins, careful blood pressure lowering, management of any other causal vascular risk factors and surgical relief of any obstruction to blood flow if it is practical and safe to do so (Chapter 16). However, there is certainly a case for less aggressive treatment of hypertension if there is good evidence of low flow symptoms. And one must acknowledge that in a patient with or without known severe arterial disease in the neck, an ischaemic episode may *occasionally* be caused by low

flow rather than embolism or some other cause of acute arterial obstruction, and even that different episodes at different times in the same patient can be caused by different mechanisms.

6.7.6 Clues from the history

The vast majority of transient ischaemic attacks (TIAs) and ischaemic strokes start suddenly, without any obvious provocation, and there are few if any symptoms other than those of a focal neurological or ocular deficit. Sometimes there can be clues to the cause in the history (Table 6.9), as well as to whether the patient has had a stroke or TIA in the first place (Chapter 3). These clues may require some tenacity to recognize, or perhaps just an ability to take a history instead of rushing to order lots of tests.

> There will be no clues from the history if no one bothers to take a history in the rush to organize a brain scan.

Gradual onset

Gradual onset of ischaemic stroke or TIA over hours or days, rather than seconds or minutes, is unusual but is becoming more recognized now that strokes are being seen much earlier (section 3.3.8). If the onset is gradual, and ischaemic stroke or TIA is not likely to be caused by low flow (section 6.7.5) or migraine (section 7.8), then the diagnosis should be considered particularly carefully and a structural intracranial (or ocular) lesion looked for again, or for the first time if brain imaging has not already been carried out (e.g. intracranial tumour, chronic subdural haematoma, cerebral abscess, section 3.4.4). Under the age of 50 years, multiple sclerosis should also be considered (section 3.4.10). However, *a priori*, focal neurological deficits which develop over hours, and even over 1 or 2 days, in *elderly* patients are still more likely to have a vascular than a non-vascular cause because in them vascular causes are so much more common than conditions such as brain tumours. It is only when progression occurs over a longer period that the likelihood of a non-vascular cause (such as chronic subdural haematoma) starts to rise.

Precipitating factors

The exact activity and time of onset may both be important (section 3.3.9). Anything to suggest a drop in cerebral perfusion or blood pressure may be relevant (section 6.7.5), as is any operative procedure (section 7.18).

Table 6.9 Important clues from the history which may suggest the cause of an ischaemic stroke or transient ischaemic attack, or that the diagnosis of cerebrovascular disease should be reconsidered.

Gradual onset	*Non-stroke vascular disease or vascular risk factors*
Low cerebral blood flow without acute occlusion (section 6.7.5)	Heart disease (section 6.6.19)
Migraine (section 7.8)	Claudication (section 6.6.19)
Structural intracranial lesion (section 3.4.4)	Hypertension (section 6.6.3)
Multiple sclerosis (section 3.4.10)	Smoking (section 6.6.4)
Precipitating factors	*Drugs*
Suspected systemic hypotension or low cerebral perfusion pressure (standing up or sitting up quickly, heavy meal, hot weather, hot bath, warming the face, exercise, coughing, hyperventilation, chest pain or palpitations, starting or changing blood pressure-lowering drugs) (section 6.7.5)	Oral contraceptives (section 7.13.1)
	Oestrogens in men (section 7.13)
	Blood pressure-lowering/vasodilators (section 6.7.5)
	Hypoglycaemic drugs (section 7.16)
	Cocaine (section 7.15.1)
	Amphetamines (section 7.15.1)
Pregnancy/puerperium (section 7.14)	Ephedrine (section 7.15.1)
Surgery (section 7.18)	Phenylpropanolamine (section 7.15.1)
Head-turning (section 7.1.5)	'Ecstasy' (section 7.15.1)
Hypoglycaemia (section 7.16)	Anti-inflammatory drugs (section 7.15.2)
Valsalva manoeuvre (paradoxical embolism, section 6.5.12; or low flow, section 6.7.5)	Antipsychotic drugs (section 7.15.3)
	Deoxycoformycin (section 7.3.21)
	Allopurinol (section 7.3.21)
Recent headache	L-asparaginase (section 7.12)
Carotid/vertebral dissection (section 7.2.1)	*Injury*
Migrainous stroke/transient ischaemic attack (section 7.8.1)	Chronic subdural haematoma (section 3.4.4)
	Vertebral/carotid artery dissection (section 7.2.1)
Intracranial venous thrombosis (section 7.21.2)	Cerebral air embolism (section 7.1.7)
Giant-cell arteritis (or other inflammatory vascular disorders) (section 7.3.1)	Fat embolism (section 7.1.8)
	Self-audible bruits
Structural intracranial lesion (section 3.4.4)	Internal carotid artery stenosis (distal) (section 6.7.6)
Epileptic seizures	Dural arteriovenous fistula (section 8.2.8)
Intracranial venous thrombosis (section 7.21.2)	Glomus tumour
Mitochondrial diseases (section 7.19)	Caroticocavernous fistula (section 8.2.14)
Non-vascular intracranial lesion (section 3.4.4)	Raised intracranial pressure
Malaise	Intracranial venous thrombosis (section 7.21.2)
Inflammatory arterial disorders (section 7.3)	*Past medical history*
Infective endocarditis (section 6.5.9)	Inflammatory bowel disease (section 7.17)
Cardiac myxoma (section 6.5.13)	Coeliac disease (section 7.17)
Cancer (section 7.12)	Homocystinuria (section 7.20.2)
Thrombotic thrombocytopenic purpura (section 7.9.3)	Cancer (section 7.12)
Sarcoidosis (section 7.3.16)	Irradiation of the head or neck (section 7.12)
Chest pain	Recurrent deep venous thrombosis (sections 7.3.4 and 7.9.11)
Myocardial infarction (section 7.10)	Recurrent miscarriages (section 7.3.4)
Aortic dissection (section 7.2.3)	Recent surgery/long distance travel (section 6.5.12)
Paradoxical embolism (sections 6.5.12)	Family history (Table 6.10)

Head-turning is an occasional cause (section 7.1.5). Recurrent attacks first thing in the morning or during exercise suggest hypoglycaemia, which is easy to think of in a diabetic patient on hypoglycaemic drugs but more difficult if there is a less obvious cause of hypoglycaemia, such as the very rare insulinoma or drugs such as pentamidine (sections 3.4.5 and 7.16). Onset during a Valsalva manoeuvre (e.g. lifting a heavy object) suggests a low flow ischaemic stroke (section 6.7.5) or paradoxical embolism (section 6.5.12), and so sets off a search for

deep venous thrombosis if there is evidence on echocardiography of a patent foramen ovale (section 6.9.3).

Headache

Headache at around the onset of ischaemic stroke or TIA occurs in about 25% of patients, is usually mild and, if localized at all, tends to be related to the position of the brain/eye lesion (sections 3.3.10 and 11.9). It is more common with vertebrobasilar than carotid

Table 6.10 Causes of familial stroke (including intracranial haemorrhage) and transient ischaemic attack.

Connective tissue disorders
Ehlers–Danlos syndrome (section 7.20.7)
Pseudoxanthoma elasticum (section 7.20.7)
Marfan syndrome (section 7.20.7)
Fibromuscular dysplasia (section 7.4.1)
Familial mitral leaflet prolapse (section 6.5.7)
Haematological disorders
Sickle cell disease/trait (section 7.9.8)
Antithrombin III deficiency (section 7.9.11)
Protein C deficiency (section 7.9.11)
Protein S deficiency (section 7.9.11)
Plasminogen abnormality/deficiency (section 7.9.11)
Haemophilia and other inherited coagulation factor
  deficiencies (section 8.4.4)
Others
Familial hypercholesterolaemia
Neurofibromatosis (section 7.20.5)
Homocystinuria (section 7.20.2)
Fabry's disease (section 7.20.3)
Tuberous sclerosis (section 7.20.4)
Dutch and Icelandic cerebral amyloid angiopathy
  (section 8.2.2)
Migraine (section 7.8)
Familial cardiac myxoma (section 6.5.13)
Familial cardiomyopathies (section 6.5.11)
Mitochondrial diseases (section 7.19)
CADASIL (section 7.20.1)
Sneddon syndrome (section 7.3.5)
Arteriovenous malformations (section 8.2.4)
Cavernous malformations (section 8.2.5)
Intracranial saccular aneurysms (section 8.2.3)

CADASIL, cerebral autosomal dominant arteriopathy with subcortical infarcts and leukoencephalopathy.

distribution ischaemia, and less common with lacunar ischaemia.[666–671] Severe pain unilaterally in the head, face, neck or eye at around or before the time of stroke onset is highly suggestive of carotid dissection, while vertebral dissection tends to cause unilateral or sometimes bilateral occipital pain (section 7.2.1). Migrainous stroke may be accompanied by headache (section 7.8.1) and patients with cerebral autosomal dominant arteriopathy with subcortical infarcts and leucoencephalo-pathy (CADASIL) usually have a history of migraine (section 7.20.1). In the context of the differential diagnosis of TIAs, migraine should be fairly obvious, unless there is no headache (section 3.4.1). It is important to note that vertebrobasilar ischaemia may cause similar symptoms to migraine with headache, gradual onset of focal neurological symptoms and visual disturbance.

Although intracranial venous thrombosis usually causes either intracranial hypertension alone or a subacute encephalopathy, a focal onset does occur and headache (occurring in around 75% of patients) can be a clue (section 7.21.2). Stroke or TIA in the context of a patient who has had a headache for days or weeks previously must raise the possibility of giant-cell arteritis and other inflammatory vascular disorders (section 7.3.1). Pain in the jaw muscles with chewing, which resolves with rest, strongly suggests claudication, which is caused by external carotid artery disease as a result of giant-cell arteritis far more often than atherothrombosis.

Epileptic seizures

Epileptic seizures, partial or generalized, within hours of stroke onset are distinctly unusual in adults (about 5%) and should lead to a reconsideration of non-stroke brain pathologies (section 3.4.4). They are rather more common in childhood stroke. They are more likely with haemorrhagic than ischaemic strokes and if the infarct is extensive and involves the cerebral cortex (section 11.8).[672–676] They are also likely with venous infarction (up to 40%) (section 7.21.12) and mitochondrial disorders (section 7.19). Partial motor seizures can be confused with limb-shaking TIAs, but the former are more clonic and the jerking spreads in a typical Jacksonian way from one body part to another and the latter are supposed never to involve the face (sections 3.3.4 and 6.7.5). Very rarely, transient focal ischaemia seems to cause just partial epileptic seizures, but proving a causal relationship is seldom possible.[677] Interestingly, onset of idiopathic seizures late in life is a powerful independent predictor of subsequent stroke.[678]

Because the diagnosis of stroke may be wrong if a tumour on CT is misinterpreted as an infarct (contrast enhancement can look very similar in both, section 5.4.2), partial seizures after a 'stroke' should always be an indication to re-examine the diagnosis and reassess the imaging. Also, seizures in the presence of a history of a few days of malaise, headache and fever should suggest encephalitis and the need for an electroencephalogram to show bilateral diffuse rather than unilateral focal slow waves, and cerebrospinal fluid examination (raised white cell count, but this can also occur in stroke, section 6.8.11).

Malaise

Stroke in the context of a patient who has been generally unwell for days, weeks or months suggests an inflammatory arterial disorder, particularly giant-cell arteritis (section 7.3.1), infective endocarditis (section 6.5.9), cardiac myxoma (section 6.5.13), cancer (section 7.12), thrombotic thrombocytopenic purpura (section 7.9.3) or even sarcoidosis (section 7.3.16).

Chest pain

Chest pain may suggest a recent myocardial infarction with complicating stroke (section 7.10); aortic dissection, particularly if the pain is also interscapular (section 7.2.3); and pleuritic pain suggests pulmonary embolism and the possibility of paradoxical embolism (section 6.5.12).

Vascular risk factors

Vascular risk factors (section 6.6) and diseases should be sought. It is most unusual for an ischaemic stroke or TIA to occur in someone with *no* vascular risk factors, unless they are very old, or are young with some unusual cause of stroke (Table 6.3). Heart disease of any sort may be relevant (source of embolism to the brain, dysrhythmias causing low-flow ischaemia, etc.) and cardiac symptoms should be specifically elicited in the history: angina, shortness of breath, palpitations, and so on.

Drugs and drug users

Drugs may well be relevant: oral contraceptives and hormone replacement therapy in women and oestrogens in men (section 7.13); anything which lowers the blood pressure (section 6.7.5); hypoglycaemic agents (section 7.16); and illicit drugs (section 7.15.1).

Injury

Any injury in the days and weeks before ischaemic stroke or TIA onset is crucial information. A head injury might have caused a chronic subdural haematoma (highly unlikely if more than 3 months previously) although this should have been considered earlier at the stroke vs non-stroke stage (section 3.4.4). Of possible relevance is an injury to the neck in the hours, days or even few weeks before onset, because this may cause carotid or vertebral dissection (section 7.2.1). After long bone fracture, fat embolism may cause a generalized encephalopathy, but occasionally there are additional focal features (section 7.1.8).[679–682] It is therefore essential to ask about any injury, strangulation, car crash, unusual yoga exercises, neck manipulation and so forth, in any unexplained stroke (Table 6.2).

Self-audible bruits

Pulsatile self-audible bruits are rare. They can be differentiated from tinnitus because they are in time with the pulse. They may be audible to the examiner on auscultation of the neck, orbit or cranium. They are unlikely to be caused by carotid bifurcation atherothrombosis because the source of the sound is too far from the ear. They are much more likely to indicate *distal* internal carotid artery stenosis (due to dissection or, rarely, atherothrombosis), dural arteriovenous fistula near the petrous temporal bone, glomus tumour, caroticocavernous fistula, intracranial venous thrombosis, symptomatic and idiopathic intracranial hypertension, a loop in the internal carotid artery, or just heightened awareness of one's own pulse.[683,684]

Past medical history

Past medical history of inflammatory bowel disease (section 7.17), coeliac disease (section 7.17), irradiation of the head and neck (section 7.12), cancer (section 7.12) or even homocystinuria (section 7.20.2) may be important. Recurrent deep venous thrombosis (DVT) suggests thrombophilia (section 7.9.11), particularly if there is a family history, or the antiphospholipid syndrome (section 7.3.4). Recurrent miscarriage is another feature of the antiphospholipid syndrome. *Any* reason for a recent DVT (e.g. a long cramped journey, admission to hospital for an acute medical disorder, or surgery) should raise the question of paradoxical embolism (sections 6.5.12 and 6.9.3).

> If a patient has, or has had, deep venous thrombosis in the legs, then consider paradoxical embolism to the brain, a familial clotting factor problem or the antiphospholipid syndrome.

Previous strokes and/or transient ischaemic attacks

Previous strokes and/or TIAs in *different* vascular territories are more likely with a proximal embolic source in the heart, or arch of the aorta, than with a single arterial lesion in the neck or head. Attacks going back months or more make some causes unlikely (e.g. infective endocarditis, arterial dissection).

Family history

There are several rare familial conditions that may be complicated by ischaemic stroke and TIAs (Table 6.10). There is also increasing interest in complex genetic disorders thought to be caused by multiple gene interactions, presumably influenced by environmental factors (section 6.6.15).[535,685–687] However, family history of stroke is only a modest risk factor for ischaemic stroke.[687] Moreover, much of the association appears to be secondary to hereditability of risk factors for stroke such as hypertension and diabetes.[687,688] On the other hand, these same risk factors are clearly influenced by the environment (for example, diets rich in fat and in salt tend to raise the plasma cholesterol and blood pressure, respectively). Just how easy it will be to separate out shared genes from shared environment in a disease as common as stroke remains to be seen. Disentangling the interactions and working out the pathway from genotype to phenotype will be a monumental task (section 6.6.15). Whatever the mechanism(s), one can at least reassure patients with TIA or stroke that a family history of stroke is associated with little or no increase in the risk of a future stroke.[689,690]

6.7.7 Clues from the examination

Neurological examination

Neurological examination is primarily to localize the brain lesion; of course, in patients with transient ischaemic attacks (TIAs), or those seen some days after a minor stroke, there will probably be no signs at all (section 3.3.1). Occasionally, however, there may be a clue to the cause. A Horner syndrome ipsilateral to a carotid distribution infarct (i.e. not as the result of a brainstem stroke, where it might be expected) suggests dissection of the internal carotid artery (ICA) or sometimes acute atherothrombotic carotid occlusion (section 7.2.1). Lower cranial nerve lesions ipsilateral to a hemispheric cerebral infarct can also occur in carotid dissection and, like Horner syndrome, are caused by stretching and bulging of the arterial wall in relation to the affected nerves, or ischaemia. Ocular ischaemia, as well as third, fourth and sixth cranial nerve palsies – sometimes with orbital pain – has been described ipsilateral to acute ICA occlusion and stenosis, presumably caused by ischaemia of the nerve trunks.[691,692]

In a total anterior circulation infarct or brainstem stroke some drowsiness is expected, but with more restricted infarcts, consciousness is normal. Therefore if consciousness is impaired and yet the 'stroke' itself seems mild, it is important to:

- reconsider the differential diagnosis (particularly chronic subdural haematoma) (section 3.4.4);
- consider the diffuse encephalopathic disorders which have focal features and which may masquerade as stroke, e.g. cerebral vasculitis of some sort (section 7.3), endocarditis (sections 6.5.9 and 6.5.10), intracranial venous thrombosis (section 7.21), mitochondrial disorders (section 7.19), thrombotic thrombocytopenic purpura (section 7.9.3), familial hemiplegic migraine[693] and Hashimoto's encephalitis;[694]

- remember that comorbidity, such as pneumonia, sedative drugs, infection and hypoglycaemia, may all make the neurological deficit seem worse than it really is (section 11.4).

> If the neurological deficit is mild and yet the patient is drowsy, then consider chronic subdural haematoma, cerebral vasculitis, non-bacterial thrombotic endocarditis, intracranial venous thrombosis, mitochondrial disorders, thrombotic thrombocytopenic purpura, sedative drugs, hypoglycaemia, familial hemiplegic migraine and comorbidity, such as pneumonia or other infections.

Eyes

The eyes may provide general clues to the cause of a stroke (e.g. diabetic or hypertensive retinopathy), or may reveal papilloedema which would make the diagnosis of ischaemic stroke, or even intracerebral haemorrhage, most unlikely. In addition, it is worth searching thoroughly for evidence of emboli which are very often completely asymptomatic[695,696] (section 3.3.6):

- Fibrin–platelet emboli are dull greyish-white amorphous plugs but are rarely observed, perhaps because they move through the retinal circulation and disperse; they suggest embolism from the heart or proximal sources of atherothrombosis.
- Cholesterol emboli quite often stick at arteriolar branching points, usually without obstructing the blood flow, and appear as glittering orange or yellow bodies reflecting the ophthalmoscope light; obviously these strongly suggest embolization from proximal atheromatous plaques, but they are often asymptomatic.
- 'Calcific' retinal emboli appear as solid, white and non-reflective bodies and tend to lodge near the edge of the optic disc; they suggest embolism from aortic or mitral valve calcification.

Localized areas of periarteriolar sheathing, seen as opaque white obliteration of segments of the retinal arterioles, suggest embolism, usually cholesterol, in the past. Roth spots in the retina are very suggestive of infective endocarditis (section 6.5.9). Dislocated lenses should suggest Marfan syndrome (section 7.20.7) or homocystinuria (section 7.20.2); angioid streaks in the retina suggest pseudoxanthoma elasticum (section 7.20.7); and in hyperviscosity syndromes there is a characteristic retinopathy (section 7.9.10).

Dilated episcleral vessels are a clue to abnormal anastomoses between branches of the external carotid artery (ECA) and orbital branches of the internal carotid artery (ICA), distal to severe ICA disease.[697] With very severe ICA disease, usually accompanied by severe disease of the ipsilateral ECA, the eye may occasionally become so ischaemic that *venous stasis retinopathy* develops, although arterial disease does not invariably underlie this condition[698] (section 3.3.6). Haemorrhages are scattered around the retina with microaneurysms, and the retinal veins are dilated and irregular. The retinal blood flow is extremely impaired, as demonstrated by lightly compressing the eye with one finger while observing the fundus and noting collapse of the central retinal artery. With more extreme ischaemia, *ischaemic oculopathy* may develop with impaired visual acuity, eye pain, rubeosis of the iris (dilated blood vessels), fixed dilated pupil, 'low pressure' glaucoma, cataract and corneal oedema.[699,700] Pre-existing raised intraocular pressure, i.e. glaucoma, makes the eye more susceptible to low blood flow and ischaemia as a result.

Arterial pulses

It is always worth feeling *both* radial pulses simultaneously. Any inequality in timing or volume suggests subclavian or innominate stenosis or occlusion, and this is further supported if there is an ipsilateral supraclavicular bruit or lower blood pressure in the arm with the weak or delayed pulse.

An elderly patient presented with a sudden left-sided hemiparesis and no other symptoms. She had right carotid and supraclavicular bruits. Brain CT was normal. Three days later the duplex examination showed narrowing of the right common carotid artery which appeared to be caused by dissection of the aortic arch. Only then did she admit to some mild chest pain before the stroke. Unequal pulses and blood pressures were found in her upper limbs, and chest CT confirmed the aortic dissection. The lessons are that any pain in or around the chest may be relevant and should have been more thoroughly sought, and in all stroke patients both radial pulses must be felt routinely before, not after, arterial imaging.

Normally, the *internal* carotid artery pulse is too deep and rostral to be felt in the neck. Therefore, any loss of the 'carotid' pulsation reflects common carotid artery (CCA) or innominate occlusion or severe stenosis, both rather rare situations or, perhaps more likely, the artery is too deep to be felt or the neck too thick.

> The arterial pulse felt in the neck comes from the common, not the internal, carotid artery.

The superficial temporal pulses should be easily felt and symmetrical. If there is unilateral absence or delay,

this suggests external carotid artery (ECA) or CCA disease. Tenderness of any of the branches of the ECA (occipital, facial, superficial temporal) points towards giant-cell arteritis. Tenderness of the carotid artery in the neck (i.e. the CCA) can occur in acute carotid occlusion but is more likely to be a sign of dissection, or possibly arteritis.

Absence of several neck and arm pulses in a young person suggests Takayasu's arteritis (section 7.3.2). Other causes of widespread disease of the aortic arch are atheroma, giant-cell arteritis, syphilis, subintimal fibrosis, arterial dissection and trauma.[264,701,702]

Delayed or absent leg pulses suggest coarctation of the aorta or, much more commonly, peripheral vascular disease (PVD) which is very common in patients with TIA and ischaemic stroke (Table 6.3) and may need treating in its own right. Furthermore, PVD is an important predictor of future serious vascular events (Table 16.4). The state of the femoral artery is important to assess before cerebral angiography via the femoral route (section 6.8.5) and, if after angiography the leg pulses disappear, then it was a complication of the angiography. Obviously, any evidence of systemic embolism would direct the search towards a source of emboli in the heart (section 6.5).

Finally, while the hand is on the abdomen, aortic aneurysm should be considered while searching for any masses or hepatosplenomegaly. Although the prevalence of aortic aneurysm in these stroke/TIA patients is unknown, it could well be quite high, particularly in men and if the patient has carotid stenosis (section 6.6.19). Diagnosis is important because of the benefits of surgery in patients with larger aneurysms.[606]

Cervical bruits

Listening to the neck is a favourite occupation for inquisitive physicians, and acquisitive surgeons, and can lead to some useful information (Fig. 6.22). A localized bruit, occasionally palpable, over the carotid bifurcation (i.e. high up under the jaw) is predictive of some degree of carotid stenosis, but very tight stenosis (or occlusion) may not cause a bruit at all (Fig. 6.23) (Table 6.11). External carotid stenosis can also cause a bruit in the same place. An innocent carotid bruit is more common in women,[703] probably due to sex differences in carotid bifurcation anatomy.[704]

Bruits transmitted from the heart become attenuated as one listens further up the neck towards the angle of the jaw, thyroid bruits are bilateral and more obviously over the gland, a hyperdynamic circulation tends to cause a diffuse bruit, and venous hums are more continuous and roaring, and are obliterated by light pressure over

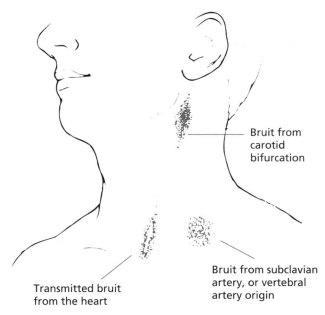

Fig. 6.22 The sites of various cervical bruits. Note that a bruit arising from the carotid bifurcation is high up under the angle of the jaw. Localized supraclavicular bruits are caused either by subclavian or vertebral origin artery stenosis.

Table 6.11 The source of neck bruits.

Carotid bifurcation arterial bruit
Internal carotid artery origin stenosis
External carotid artery origin stenosis
Supraclavicular arterial bruit
Subclavian artery stenosis
Vertebral artery origin stenosis
Can be normal in young adults
Diffuse neck bruit
Thyrotoxicosis
Hyperdynamic circulation (pregnancy, anaemia, fever, haemodialysis)
Transmitted bruit from the heart and great vessels
Aortic stenosis/regurgitation
Mitral regurgitation
Patent ductus arteriosus
Coarctation of the aorta
Venous hum

> Carotid bruits are neither sufficiently specific nor sensitive to diagnose carotid stenosis severe enough to consider surgery. Arterial imaging is needed. Physicians and surgeons desperate to use their stethoscopes would do better to measure the blood pressure and listen to the heart.

Cardiac examination

Cardiac examination is important, particularly to look for any cardiac source of embolism (section 6.5). If physicians feel under-confident about their cardiological abilities, then they should get properly trained or a cardiologist will have to be consulted. Atrial fibrillation (AF) will already have been suspected from the radial pulse; left ventricular hypertrophy suggests hypertension or aortic stenosis, and most *major* cardiac sources of embolism are fairly obvious clinically (e.g. AF, mitral stenosis, prosthetic heart valve).

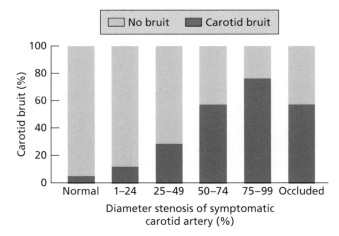

Fig. 6.23 The percentage of patients with a localized bruit over the symptomatic carotid bifurcation for various degrees of stenosis as estimated (using the European Carotid Surgery Trial method) from 298 carotid angiograms. (Adapted with permission from Hankey and Warlow, 1990.[790])

Fever

Fever is distinctly unusual in the first few hours after stroke onset. Any raised temperature at this time must therefore be taken seriously and endocarditis or other infections, inflammatory vascular disorders, deep venous thrombosis or cardiac myxoma considered. Later on, fever is quite common and usually reflects some complication of the stroke (section 11.12).

Skin and nails

the ipsilateral jugular vein.[593] An arterial bruit in the supraclavicular fossa suggests either subclavian or proximal vertebral arterial disease, but a transmitted bruit from aortic stenosis must also be considered. Normal young adults quite often have a short supraclavicular bruit; the reason is unknown.

The skin and nails occasionally provide clues to the cause of ischaemic stroke or transient ischaemic attack (Table 6.12).

Finger-clubbing	Right-to-left intracardiac shunt (section 6.5.12)
	Cancer (section 7.12)
	Pulmonary arteriovenous malformation (section 6.5.12)
	Infective endocarditis (section 6.5.9)
	Inflammatory bowel disease (section 7.17)
Splinter haemorrhages	Infective endocarditis (section 6.5.9)
	Cholesterol embolization syndrome (section 7.7)
	Vasculitis (section 7.3)
Scleroderma	Systemic sclerosis (section 7.3.13)
Livedo reticularis	Sneddon syndrome (section 7.3.5)
	Systemic lupus erythematosus (section 7.3.4)
	Polyarteritis nodosa (section 7.3.6)
	Cholesterol embolization syndrome (section 7.7)
Lax skin	Ehlers–Danlos syndrome (section 7.20.7)
	Pseudoxanthoma elasticum (section 7.20.7)
Skin colour	Anaemia (section 7.9.7)
	Polycythaemia (section 7.9.1)
	Cyanosis (right-to-left intracardiac shunt, pulmonary arteriovenous malformation) (section 6.5.12)
Porcelain-white papules/scars	Kohlmeier–Degos disease (section 7.3.15)
Skin scars	Ehlers–Danlos syndrome (section 7.20.7)
Petechiae/purpura/bruising	Thrombotic thrombocytopenic purpura (section 7.9.3)
	Fat embolism (section 7.1.8)
	Cholesterol embolization syndrome (section 7.7)
	Ehlers–Danlos syndrome (section 7.20.7)
Orogenital ulceration	Behçet's disease (section 7.3.11)
Rash	Fabry's disease (section 7.20.3)
	Systemic lupus erythematosus (section 7.3.3)
	Tuberous sclerosis (section 7.20.4)
Epidermal naevi	Epidermal naevus syndrome
Café-au-lait patches	Neurofibromatosis (section 7.20.5)
Thrombosed superficial veins, needle marks	Intravenous drug users (section 7.15.1)

Table 6.12 Clues to the cause of ischaemic stroke/transient ischaemic attack from examination of the skin and nails.

> Getting to the bottom of the cause of an ischaemic stroke or transient ischaemic attack requires much more than just neurological skills. Stroke medicine, like neurology, is part of general internal medicine. It is important therefore that doctors looking after stroke patients have a good general internal medical training.

6.8 Investigation

Investigations are mainly to help unravel the pathological type of stroke (ischaemic stroke vs intracerebral haemorrhage vs subarachnoid haemorrhage, as discussed in Chapter 5) and then to determine the cause of the cerebral ischaemia (or intracranial haemorrhage; Chapters 8 and 9), particularly a cause that will influence immediate treatment or long-term management. Investigation may also provide important prognostic information, e.g. severe carotid stenosis on ultrasound (section 16.11.8). In addition, the many patients who also have angina or other cardiac symptoms, claudication or suspected aortic aneurysm may well need specific investigations directed at these problems with a view to appropriate treatment.

> Ideally, any investigation should be practical, feasible, accurate, safe, non-invasive, inexpensive and, most importantly, informative in the sense that the result (positive or negative, high or low, etc.) will influence patient management and outcome. Idle curiosity or financial gain are not good reasons to order any test.

6.8.1 Routine investigations

Although there are no absolute rules, all ischaemic stroke/transient ischaemic attack (TIA) patients, unless they are already heavily dependent or institutionalized, or have already been recently investigated for a previous event or some other problem, should have basic non-invasive first-line investigations within a few hours of presentation. None of these necessarily require hospital admission, although brain imaging does require attendance at hospital (Table 6.13). The chance of picking up a relevant abnormality (yield) may be very low for some tests – e.g. full blood count and erythrocyte sedimentation rate (ESR) – but these are cheap and the consequences of missing a treatable disorder, such as giant-cell arteritis, are serious. There is a higher chance of picking up a treatable abnormality with the blood glucose, urine analysis and electrocardiogram (ECG). Depending on the definition, many or even most patients are hypercholesterolaemic, and how this should be acted on is discussed in section 16.4; immediately after stroke, but probably not TIA, there is a transient fall in plasma cholesterol, which will underestimate the usual level.[705,706] Brain imaging is discussed in sections 5.4, 5.5 and 6.8.3. If patients have the basic tests and if the results are read, written in the records and acted upon,

this may well do more good than the inappropriate ordering of a huge range of further tests while missing some crucial clue from one of the routine investigations (such as an ESR of 100 mm in the first hour).

> All patients should have a full blood count, erythrocyte sedimentation rate, plasma glucose, urea, electrolytes and cholesterol, urine analysis, and electrocardiogram. Most should also have a CT and/or MR brain scan.

6.8.2 Second-line investigations for selected patients

Second-line investigations (Table 6.14) are usually more costly, invasive and/or dangerous, so they must be targeted on patients most likely to gain from a useful change in management as a consequence of the test result. The likelihood of a relevant result depends on the selection of patients for the investigation – a balance must be struck between over-investigation (inconvenience, high cost, possibly high-risk, low yield, false-positive results

Table 6.13 First-line investigations for ischaemic stroke/transient ischaemic attack.

Investigation	Disorders suggested	Yield* (%)
Full blood count	Anaemia, polycythaemia, leukaemia, thrombocythaemia, heparin-induced thrombocytopenia with thrombosis, infections	1
Erythrocyte sedimentation rate	Vasculitis, infections, cardiac myxoma, hyperviscosity, cholesterol embolization syndrome, non-bacterial thrombotic endocarditis	2
Plasma glucose	Diabetes mellitus, hypoglycaemia	5
Urea and electrolytes	Diuretic-induced hypokalaemia, renal failure, hyponatraemia	3
Plasma cholesterol	Hypercholesterolaemia	45
Syphilis serology	Syphilis, anticardiolipin syndrome	<1†
Urinalysis	Diabetes, renal disease, infective endocarditis, vasculitis, Fabry's disease	5
ECG	Dysrhythmia, left-ventricular hypertrophy, silent myocardial infarction	17
Unenhanced CT brain scan	Intracerebral haemorrhage, non-vascular intracranial mimic of stroke-syndrome	20

*The yield represents the proportion of patients in whom a positive test result may lead to a useful change in management (e.g. the diagnosis of diabetes in a previously undiagnosed case). The figures assume that *all* ischaemic stroke/transient ischaemic attack patients have the investigations. Data have been taken from various more or less reliable sources but should not be regarded as precise statements of some universal truth.

†In the Oxfordshire Community Stroke Project, eight of 675 first-ever-in-a-lifetime strokes had positive syphilis serology, of which only one turned out to have previously undiagnosed secondary syphilis. It may be therefore that this investigation should not be routine but only performed in young or middle-aged patients, those likely to have been exposed to infection, and in high-risk populations.

Table 6.14 Second-line investigations for selected ischaemic stroke/transient ischaemic attack patients.

Investigation	Indications	Possible disorders
Blood		
Liver function	Fever, malaise, raised ESR, suspected malignancy	Giant-cell arteritis and other inflammatory vascular disorders, infective endocarditis, non-bacterial thrombotic endocarditis
Calcium	Recurrent focal neurological symptoms very rarely caused by hypercalcaemia	Hypercalcaemia
Thyroid function tests	Atrial fibrillation	Thyrotoxicosis
Activated partial thromboplastin time, dilute Russell's viper time, antinuclear and other autoantibodies	Young (<50 years) and no other cause found, past or family history of venous thrombosis, especially if unusual sites (cerebral, mesenteric, hepatic veins), recurrent miscarriage, thrombocytopenia, cardiac valve vegetations, livedo reticularis, raised ESR, malaise, positive syphilis serology	Antiphospholipid syndrome, vasculitis, systemic lupus erythematosus
Serum proteins, serum protein electrophoresis, plasma viscosity	Raised ESR	Paraproteinaemias, nephrotic syndrome, cardiac myxoma
Haemoglobin electrophoresis	Black patients	Sickle cell trait or disease and other haemoglobinopathies
Protein C and S, antithrombin III, activated protein C resistance, thrombin time*	Personal or family history of thrombosis (usually venous, particularly in unusual sites, such as hepatic vein) at unusually young age	Thrombophilias
Blood cultures	Fever, cardiac murmur, haematuria, deranged liver function, raised ESR, malaise, unexplained stroke	Infective endocarditis
HIV serology	Young (<40 years), drug addict, homosexual, blood products/transfusion, systemically unwell, lymphadenopathy, pneumonia, cytomegalovirus retinitis, etc.	HIV infection
Lipoprotein fractionation	Raised plasma cholesterol or strong family history	Hyperlipoproteinaemia
Serum homocystine	Marfanoid habitus, high myopia, dislocated lenses, osteoporosis, mental retardation, young patient	Homocystinuria
Leucocyte α-galactosidase A	Corneal opacities, cutaneous angiokeratomas, paraesthesias and pain, renal failure	Fabry's disease
Blood/CSF lactate	Young patient, basal ganglia calcification, epilepsy, parieto-occipital ischaemia	Mitochondrial diseases
Serum fluorescent treponemal antibody absorption test	Positive screening serology tests	Syphilis
Cardiac enzymes	History or ECG evidence of recent myocardial infarction	Myocardial infarction
Drug screen	Young patient, no other obvious cause	Cocaine/amphetamine, etc.-induced ischaemic stroke
Genetic analysis	Familial stroke with periventricular changes on CT/MRI	CADASIL
Urine		
Amino acids	Marfanoid habitus, high myopia, dislocated lenses, osteoporosis, mental retardation, young patient	Homocystinuria
Drug screen	Young patient, no other obvious cause	Cocaine/amphetamine, etc.-induced ischaemic stroke
Imaging		
Chest X-ray	Hypertension, finger-clubbing, cardiac murmur or abnormal ECG, young patient, ill patient	Enlarged heart, pulmonary arteriovenous malformation, calcified heart valves, baseline in ill patients
MRI	Suggestion of arterial dissection, uncertain diagnosis of stroke	Arterial dissection, multiple sclerosis
Carotid ultrasound with a view to carotid surgery	Carotid TIA or mild ischaemic stroke	Extracranial carotid stenosis
Catheter angiography (now less used with improved MR and CT angiography)	Carotid ultrasound suggests severe stenosis of recently symptomatic internal carotid artery and patient fit and willing for surgery, suspected arterial dissection, arteriovenous malformation or aneurysm	Arterial dissection, arteriovenous malformation, carotid stenosis
Arch aortography (MR angiography)	Symptoms of subclavian steal and unequal brachial pulses and blood pressures	Subclavian or innominate stenosis

Table 6.14 (*continued*)

Investigation	Indications	Possible disorders
Cardiac		
Echocardiography (transthoracic, transoesophageal)	Young (<50 years), or clinical, ECG or chest X-ray evidence of heart disease, likely to cause embolism, aortic arch dissection	Cardiac source of embolism, aortic arch atheroma or dissection
24-h ECG	Palpitations or loss of consciousness during a suspected TIA, suspicious resting ECG	Intermittent atrial fibrillation or heart block
Others		
Electroencephalogram	Doubt about diagnosis of TIA or stroke: ?epilepsy, ?generalized encephalopathy	Seizure disorder, structural brain lesion, encephalitis, diffuse encephalopathy caused by inflammatory vascular disorders, Creutzfeldt–Jakob disease
CSF	Positive syphilis serology, young patient, ?infective endocarditis, possibility of multiple sclerosis	Vasculitis, syphilis, multiple sclerosis, infective endocarditis
Red cell mass	Raised haematocrit	Primary polycythaemia
Temporal artery biopsy	Older (>60 years), jaw claudication, headache, polymyalgia, malaise, anaemia, raised ESR	Giant-cell arteritis
Skin biopsy	Familial stroke with periventricular changes on CT/MRI	CADASIL

*Repeat to ensure persistently raised. Transient falls occur after stroke so any low level must be repeated and family members investigated.
CADASIL, cerebral autosomal dominant arteriopathy with subcortical infarcts and leukoencephalopathy; CSF, cerebrospinal fluid; CT, computerized tomography; ECG, electrocardiogram; ESR, erythrocyte sedimentation rate; MRI, magnetic resonance imaging; TIA, transient ischaemic attack.

leading to even more over-investigation) and under-investigation (low cost, low-risk, high yield, but occasional missed diagnosis). This balance depends on the consequences of overlooking a particular diagnosis. For example, missing severe carotid stenosis would be harmful, because carotid endarterectomy reduces the risk of stroke, whereas missing the lupus anticoagulant whose relevance is unknown, and where the effect of any treatment is uncertain, may be of little consequence. Also, the balance will be affected by a reasonable tendency to search particularly hard for a cause in an unusual case without any evidence of atherothromboembolism (section 6.9.1), small vessel disease (section 6.9.2) or embolism from the heart (section 6.9.3).

The main indications for the second-line investigations and the disorders likely to be detected are listed in Table 6.14. These are discussed in further detail in other sections of this chapter and in Chapter 7, although at this stage it will be helpful to discuss imaging the brain, cerebral and coronary circulation, lumbar puncture and the electroencephalogram.

6.8.3 Imaging the brain

The development of brain and cerebral vessel imaging has advanced the management of acute stroke by providing information regarding the diagnosis and underlying cause of the stroke thus enabling treatment to be targeted to a specific individual patient.

Computed tomography

Unenhanced computed tomography (CT) scanning of the brain should be a routine investigation for stroke although some centres now use MRI. It is the key to distinguishing ischaemic stroke from intracerebral haemorrhage (section 5.4). This fundamental distinction determines the strategy for looking for the cause of a stroke; it is crucial in decisions about continuing, stopping or starting antithrombotic and inevitably anti-haemostatic treatments, such as anticoagulants, aspirin or thrombolysis; and it is also crucial in any later decision that may have to be made about carotid endarterectomy. The limited, but important, role for CT in excluding intracranial structural lesions that can occasionally present as a transient ischaemic attack (TIA) or stroke has already been discussed in section 3.4.4. Some would argue that CT is unnecessary in patients with a *single* suspected TIA because it cannot possibly confirm the clinical diagnosis but only rule out intracerebral haemorrhage which has hardly ever been reported to cause focal symptoms lasting less than 24 h[707] although the sensitivity of CT for microbleeds is poor. Microbleeds are more likely to occur in hypertensive patients and are shown on gradient echo MRI (see below) and it is possible that increased use of this technique will show microbleeds as a cause of TIA (whether that will change their management remains to be seen). A structural brain lesion in a TIA patient, such as a subdural haematoma, is very unlikely unless the symptoms recur. But, as always, these arguments must be seen in the context of the availability, convenience, risk and cost of the investigation under debate. All agree that transient monocular blindness is certainly one type of TIA where brain CT is not necessary because examining the eye clinically will exclude any structural cause of the symptoms.

It cannot be overemphasized that very early CT brain scanning is *not* to demonstrate infarcts, but to exclude haemorrhage. Within the first few hours of stroke onset, the main thrust of management – and indeed research into acute treatment – is to *prevent* the appearance of infarction on CT and so, one hopes, to reduce case fatality and disability. There is therefore usually no need to delay CT in the hope that any infarct will become visible. If the CT shows no infarct and the localization of the stroke is unclear (for example, transient hemiparesis in a patient who does not attempt to speak *could* be caused by a cortical, internal capsule or pontine lesion) MRI, and DWI in particular, are much more sensitive than CT and should if possible be performed in preference to a repeat CT scan. MRI/MR venography will help where there is a possibility of venous rather than arterial infarction.

On the whole, a *clinically* definite stroke with a normal CT can be assumed to be caused by an infarct. The clinical syndrome is usually predictive enough of the site and size of the brain lesion (sections 4.3.2– 4.3.6), and so its likely cause (sections 6.7.1–6.7.4), for routine management. Infarct localization in patients with periventricular low density (leukoaraiosis) may be very difficult using CT (or conventional MRI) since there are so many small and often asymptomatic infarcts, or so much cortical atrophy, that a small *recently* symptomatic infarct simply cannot be distinguished (section 5.4.2) but DWI may show the acute lesion in these patients. DWI is particularly useful in patients presenting with TIA or minor stroke, especially in patients presenting late after a minor stroke, to exclude haemorrhage.[688,708]

The problem of reliably detecting boundary-zone infarction has been discussed earlier, and it is looking increasingly likely that many so-called boundary-zone infarcts on CT (or MRI) may not result from low flow but acute arterial occlusion (section 6.7.5).

Occasionally, on an unenhanced CT scan within hours of stroke onset, the middle cerebral or basilar artery is hyperdense, particularly if thin slices are obtained

(section 5.4.2) (Fig. 6.24). This is caused by an acute embolus or *in situ* thrombosis in the arterial lumen. Although fairly specific for arterial occlusion, it is not sensitive enough to exclude it. If it is really necessary to know the pattern of intracranial arterial occlusion, then catheter angiography is needed, or possibly MR angiography, CT angiography or transcranial Doppler sonography will do instead (sections 6.8.4–6.8.5 and 6.8.9). Therefore, in routine practice, the dense artery sign has little impact on determining the cause of cerebral ischaemia, the clinical syndrome being as good or a better predictor of the likely site and size of any infarct, and so of which arterial territory is involved, and of prognosis.

> Very early CT brain scanning of stroke patients is mainly to exclude intracerebral haemorrhage and the occasional structural lesion mimicking stroke, it is not to demonstrate infarcts although early ischaemic change may be used to guide decisions regarding suitability for thrombolysis.

In general, therefore, brain CT has little role in determining the cause of an ischaemic event, because if one needs to know within hours of the onset, the scan will probably be normal anyway (section 5.4.2). Later on the scan can still be normal and any infarct already reasonably well predicted, both in site and size, on the basis of the neurological symptoms and signs (section 4.3). If there is an anatomically relevant and recent infarct in a slightly inappropriate place for the clinical syndrome, it is probably best to follow the scan rather than the syndrome (section 4.3.7) (i.e. the infarct is in the correct general area of the brain, such as an internal capsule lacunar infarct on CT/MRI in a patient with a partial anterior circulation clinical syndrome).[133] It follows that repeat CT scanning, with or without intravenous contrast enhancement, is seldom necessary in the search for the cause of an ischaemic event, but it may be needed if there is uncertainty that the patient has had a stroke at all, or even a TIA in some circumstances (but MRI is much more sensitive), or if the patient deteriorates (section 11.5).

> The demonstration of the site and size of an infarct on brain imaging helps in determining the underlying cause of an ischaemic stroke. DWI has greater sensitivity than CT or conventional MRI in acute stroke.

Magnetic resonance imaging

Magnetic resonance imaging (MRI) of the brain is more sensitive than CT[709] (section 5.5.4). It displays smaller infarcts, especially in the brainstem and cerebellum, and

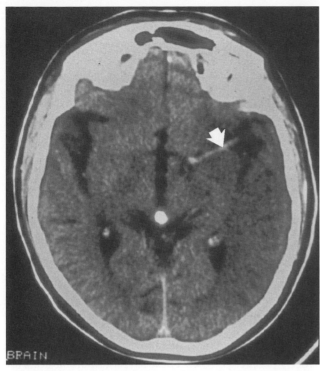

(a)

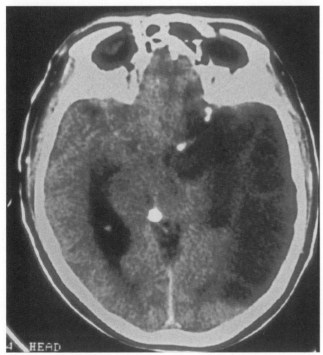

(b)

Fig. 6.24 (a) Hyperdense middle cerebral artery (*arrow*) on an unenhanced CT brain scan within hours of the onset of a total anterior circulation infarct. At this point the infarct is hardly visible. However, the next day (b) the large left hemisphere infarct is clearly visible and the hyperdense sign has vanished.

is even more sensitive after gadolinium enhancement, which may indicate which of several lesions on an unenhanced scan is the recently symptomatic one, even lacunar infarcts sometimes, and more sensitive again with diffusion-weighted MR imaging (DWI). Gradient echo MRI is also better than CT at demonstrating small amounts of blood, e.g. petechial haemorrhages at the borders of an infarct (section 5.5.1), although it is unclear whether this has any practical impact on stroke management (MRI may simply be demonstrating what is already suspected from postmortem studies). Unfortunately, MRI is less practical than CT in acutely ill, confused stroke patients, particularly those requiring some form of monitoring, so it is likely that CT will remain the first-line brain imaging investigation for acute stroke for the foreseeable future, reserving MRI for more complicated cases.

Despite the superior sensitivity of MRI over CT, it is still possible to have the clinical syndrome of a stroke, and certainly of a TIA, and yet no relevant and visible brain lesion, even with DWI, or at least any relevant lesion that can be differentiated from diffuse or multiple periventricular high-signal areas[2,124,185,688,710–712] (section 5.5.2).

Conventional MRI is poor at distinguishing acute from chronic infarction, particularly in patients with multiple infarcts and in the elderly, in whom multiple T2-weighted abnormalities in the corona radiata, basal ganglia and brainstem are common and in whom focal neurological symptoms may appear with intercurrent illness on a background of previous stroke. However, conventional MRI can certainly help in some important ways:

- loss of flow void in a major cerebral vessel may provide direct information about exactly which artery (or vein) is blocked, and where;
- it may be possible to visualize the widening of the arterial wall and mural haematoma in cervical artery dissection, but only if the neck as well as the brain is imaged, so making invasive catheter angiography unnecessary (section 7.2.1);
- it may demonstrate arterial ectasia (section 6.3.6);
- it may demonstate the typical periventricular changes of cerebral autosomal dominant arteriopathy with sub-cortical infarcts and leucoencephalopathy (CADASIL) (section 7.20.1); and
- it may come up with surprises which cannot normally be seen on CT, such as the features of multiple sclerosis (section 3.4.10) which can be clinically confused with stroke in young adults, and small focal infarcts in the cerebellum in some patients with 'isolated vertigo' who in previous times would have been diagnosed as 'acute labyrinthitis', because the less sensitive CT was normal (sections 3.3.7 and 3.4.7).

Diffusion-weighted MR imaging (DWI) is becoming increasingly important in the assessment of stroke since it is highly sensitive in acute stroke and is able to distinguish between acute and chronic infarction, unlike CT and other MRI sequences,[185,712] although it should be noted that other conditions such as seizure, encephalitis and multiple sclerosis can all cause DWI changes. Thus, DWI can confirm that a new ischaemic cerebrovascular event has occurred in a confused elderly patient with previous strokes, or in patients with non-specific symptoms such as confusion or dizziness. Inter-observer agreement is better for DWI than with conventional MRI[713,714] but there appears to be a lower sensitivity for DWI in posterior circulation acute stroke (19–31% false negative), particularly where lesions are small and within the first 24 h after symptom onset.[715]

Identification of ischaemic stroke subtype cannot reliably be made on the basis of clinical criteria and early CT alone[716] and DWI shows localization in a different vascular territory from that initially suspected on the basis of clinical features and conventional MRI in around 18% of patients.[688,717] The presence of bilateral multiple acute infarcts on DWI suggests cardioembolism prompting further cardiac investigation, whereas one acute infarct with several old infarcts in the same vascular territory is more suggestive of a thromboembolic event in one arterial territory. Multiple recent infarcts in the anterior circulation of the same hemisphere suggest either critical carotid stenosis[718] or proximal middle cerebral artery stenosis.[719] Demonstration of posterior circulation infarction may prompt further assessment of the vertebrobasilar vessels. The presence of an acute DWI lesion in the anterior circulation in the absence of extracranial internal carotid stenosis may warrant imaging of the distal carotid and intracranial vessels.

DWI is also valuable in the assessment of TIA patients, around 50% of whom have a focal abnormality if scanned within 24 h, and many of whom do not have a lesion correlate on T2-weighted MRI.[711,720] Thus DWI can alter the attending physician's opinion regarding anatomical and so vascular localization and probable TIA mechanism in a significant number of patients.[688,717,718]

Many patients with TIA or minor stroke delay seeking medical attention, and often there is a further delay before they are seen by specialist stroke services. In these patients, a clear history may be more difficult to obtain, clinical signs may have resolved, and it may be difficult to make a definite diagnosis of a cerebral ischaemic event or to be certain of the vascular territory or territories involved. DWI is of particular use in this situation[688,708] because it detects clinically appropriate ischaemic lesions in a high proportion of minor stroke patients when scanned 2 weeks or more after their event.[688] Inter-observer agreement for identifying recent ischaemic lesions in this patient group is much higher for DWI than for T2-weighted scans and DWI provides useful information over and above T2-imaging in about one-third of patients, most commonly by increasing diagnostic certainty and by indicating the vascular territory involved.

The presence of presumed recent infarct on CT in patients with TIA is associated with an increased likelihood of recurrent stroke.[721] Similarly, preliminary studies using DWI suggest that the presence, absence and pattern of DWI lesions in patients with TIA and minor stroke provide prognostic information.[722–724]

'Silent – or unrecognized – cerebral infarction'

Focal low-density areas are often seen on CT (or MRI) in patients with transient ischaemic attack or stroke in areas of the brain that are clearly irrelevant to the presenting or any past clinical event; distal to asymptomatic carotid stenosis; in patients with coronary heart disease or atrial fibrillation; and even in apparently normal elderly people.[669,725–732] These asymptomatic lesions are usually small and deep, rather than large and cortical, and are often now termed 'white matter hyperintensities' on MRI.[731] The assumption is usually made, but without pathology verification, that the lesions are a result of previous subclinical infarction, or perhaps intracerebral haemorrhage, or that the patient had not recognized or had simply forgotten a previous symptomatic event. The reported frequency of 'silent infarcts' varies enormously, depending on the precise definition of the radiological abnormality, the imaging technique used, how the patients were selected, how certain one can really be about the lack of previous neurological symptoms, whether the observer was blind to any presenting clinical syndrome, and the demographic characteristics of the patients. Also, it is not always easy to differentiate small infarcts from dilatated perivascular spaces on MRI.[733] However, the presence of widespread white matter hyperintensities is associated with impaired cognitive abilities[187,734–736] and with an increased risk of stroke.[737,738] Also, a very obvious and large cortical infarct, even without previous symptoms, might at least make one reconsider proximal sources of embolism to the brain.

6.8.4 Imaging the cerebral circulation

It would obviously be of interest to image the cerebral circulation repeatedly in everyone with an ischaemic stroke or transient ischaemic attack (TIA) to display which artery is blocked, how quickly recanalization occurs, and where any embolus may have originated.

However, at present this information does not often influence clinical management and therefore should not be sought *routinely* because of the risk, inconvenience and cost. Indeed, sometimes it simply cannot be sought at all because the technology is either not available (e.g. MRA) or it is difficult to use accurately (e.g. ultrasound). In practice, imaging the cerebral circulation must always be carefully directed to answer a relevant clinical question and any answer must be likely to influence the patient's management.[739,740]

The main indications for imaging the cerebral circulation are if the patient is a potential candidate for carotid surgery (sections 6.9.1 and 16.11), the possibility of arterial dissection (section 7.2.1), acute ischaemic stroke patients (e.g. to demonstrate vessel occlusion and thus consideration of thrombolysis; section 12.5), intracranial venous thrombosis (section 7.21), frequent vertebrobasilar TIAs, particularly with subclavian steal (sections 6.8.6 and 16.16), to demonstrate the site of large vessel stenosis with a view to possible endovascular intervention, and research.

6.8.5 Carotid imaging

The risks and benefits of carotid endarterectomy are sometimes quite finely balanced and so it is essential that imaging the carotid bifurcation to help select patients for surgery is more or less completely risk-free and accurate (section 16.11). The critical imaging question is 'how severe is any stenosis at the origin of the internal carotid artery (ICA) ipsilateral to the cerebral or ocular ischaemia?' The 'gold standard' is intra-arterial selective catheter angiography. However, even this is not a perfect test without any inter-observer variation, but it is reasonably reliable at the severe end of the stenosis spectrum where surgical decisions have to be made.[741,742] It is still the gold standard because it was the first way the whole of the anatomy of the cerebral circulation could be displayed; it has intuitive face validity; and, most importantly, it was the only accurate imaging technique available when the large randomized trials of surgery were recruiting patients. Therefore, any criterion for making the surgery vs no-surgery decision based on the severity of the stenosis, and then applying the inferences from those trials to routine clinical practice, is implicitly based on catheter angiography. If this decision is now to be based on non-invasive measurement of carotid stenosis, then it must be very certain that what is measured non-invasively can be 'translated' to what would have been measured if catheter angiography had been performed.[743]

Performing intra-arterial catheter angiography in everyone with a mild carotid ischaemic event is clearly unacceptable because there is a risk, as well as a cost (see below). Furthermore, less than 20% of these patients actually have severe carotid stenosis; even if only those with 'cortical' rather than 'lacunar' events are selected, the proportion is still less than 30%.[129,744,745] The rest presumably have an unsuspected source of embolism in the heart; or an arterial embolic source which is not imaged, such as in the aortic arch and common carotid arteries; or intracranial small vessel disease; or less severe carotid bifurcation disease which may still have been the source of embolism but is perhaps unlikely to be so again in the near future; or ischaemia in the vertebrobasilar distribution. Confining angiography to patients with a carotid bifurcation bruit will miss some patients with severe stenosis and still subject too many with mild or moderate stenosis to the risks, but with nothing to gain from carotid surgery (Fig. 6.23). Nor will a combination of a cervical bruit with various clinical features do much better.[745]

Catheter angiography

Catheter angiography is inconvenient, invasive, uncomfortable, costly, carries a risk and normally requires hospital admission which may introduce unnecessary delay before carotid endarterectomy and so risk an avoidable stroke in the meantime. About 4% of patients have a transient ischaemic attack (TIA) or stroke – one-quarter of them permanent – as a result of catheter angiography, probably more if the patient has *severe* carotid disease. TIAs and strokes complicating angiography occur because, first, the catheter tip dislodges atheromatous plaque or dissects the arterial wall during insertion, injection or flushing; second, thrombus may form at the catheter tip or in blood contaminating the contrast-containing syringe; and, finally, exceptionally, as a result of the almost inevitable injection of some air.[746] In addition, there are systemic and allergic adverse effects of the contrast material, particularly during intravenous digital subtraction angiography where large quantities are used. Some patients develop a haematoma, aneurysm or nerve injury at the site of arterial puncture (which is usually into the femoral artery in the groin), and the occasional patient develops *de novo* or has worsened symptoms of peripheral vascular disease in the leg distal to the puncture site, sometimes even leading to amputation. The cholesterol embolization syndrome is very rare, but it can be fatal (section 7.7).

Compared with cut-film selective intra-arterial catheter angiography recorded directly onto X-ray film, intra-arterial digital subtraction angiography is quicker, the images are easier to manipulate and store, contrast resolution is better although spatial resolution is less, but

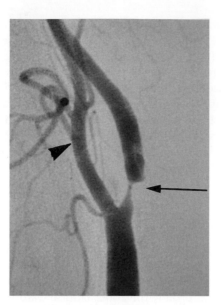

Fig. 6.25 Anteroposterior view of a selective intra-arterial digital subtraction catheter carotid angiogram showing stenosis (*arrow*) at the origin of the internal carotid artery which can be differentiated easily from the external carotid artery (*arrowhead*) because the former has no branches in the neck.

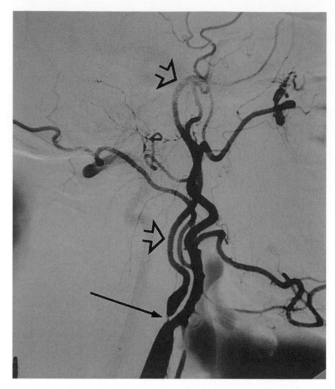

Fig. 6.26 Lateral view of selective catheter carotid angiogram showing almost complete occlusion of the internal carotid artery (*arrow*) with poor flow distal to the lesion (*open arrows*) and delayed filling of the carotid siphon. Normally the carotid siphon fills well before the branches of the external carotid artery.

there is no evidence that less contrast is used or that it is much safer[747] (Fig. 6.25). Neither *intravenous* digital subtraction angiography (IVDSA) nor arch aortography is a satisfactory alternative to selective intra-arterial angiography. So often the images are poor and stenoses impossible to measure (particularly with IVDSA), vessels may overlap, there is no accurate information about intracranial vessels and the techniques are not necessarily safer.[748,749] All of these factors combine to reduce the prognostic value of the degree of stenosis measured by non-selective angiography.[89] Even with selective angiography, there can be difficulty in distinguishing occlusion from extreme internal carotid artery stenosis, and then late views are needed to see contrast eventually passing up into the head (Fig. 6.26).

Biplanar, but preferably triplanar,[750] views of the carotid bifurcation are required to measure the degree of carotid stenosis accurately, i.e. to visualize the residual lumen without overlap of other vessels, to measure at the narrowest point, and to compare with a suitable denominator to derive the percentage diameter stenosis. This is the measurement on which decisions concerning carotid endarterectomy have to be made because this is what the randomized controlled trials used (section 16.11). The residual lumen *alone* is unsatisfactory, because normal arteries vary in size between individuals and are larger in men than women, and there is also variation in the X-ray magnification factor between different

centres. Area stenosis is impossible to measure on catheter angiograms.

> The severity of any carotid stenosis must be measured as accurately as possible; guesswork is unacceptable.

There are three possible methods of measuring carotid stenosis on catheter angiograms (Fig. 6.27): that used in the North American Symptomatic Carotid Endarterectomy Trial (NASCET), that used in the European Carotid Surgery Trial (ECST) and the common carotid method.[741] It is, however, quite possible for two observers to differ in their assessment of moderate/severe stenosis by 20%.[751] Increasing stenosis measured by all three methods predicts equally well the risk of ipsilateral ischaemic stroke and they are therefore all valid in this sense.[741] Fortunately, it is easy to convert the measurement by one method to either of the other two because they are all linearly related, at least within the moderate and severe stenosis range.[751] The ECST and common carotid method give essentially identical results and 30%, 50% and 70% by these methods equates to about 50%, 70% and 85% stenosis respectively by the NASCET method of measurement.

It might be imagined that irregularity of an athero-thrombotic plaque on an angiogram suggests plaque ulceration, instability, complicating thrombosis and embolism, and therefore predicts what really matters, i.e. ipsilateral ischaemic stroke. However, angiography tends to underestimate the ulceration observed by vascular surgeons and pathologists. In fact, it is not clear what the 'gold standard' of ulceration is supposed to be, either at postmortem or by imaging,[72] and there is only moderate inter-observer agreement in the angiographic diagnosis of 'ulceration'[749,752] as well as lack of data regarding the reproducibility of the classification of histological abnormalities.[72] However, angiographic irregularity of a stenotic plaque does predict a higher risk of stroke than if the plaque is smooth, given the same degree of stenosis[91,753] and there is good correlation between catheter angiographic plaque morphology and histology when the latter is rigorously evaluated.[71] What effect the angiographic demonstration of a 'floating thrombus' has on the risk of stroke is unknown.[754]

At present therefore the main *angiographic* criteria for the prediction of ipsilateral ischaemic stroke are, despite some inter-observer variability, percentage diameter stenosis, together with plaque irregularity/ulceration.

Duplex sonography

This technique combines real-time ultrasound imaging to display the arterial anatomy combined with pulsed Doppler flow analysis at any point of interest in the vessel lumen (Fig. 6.28). Its accuracy is enhanced and it is technically easier to carry out if the Doppler signals are colour coded to show the direction of blood flow and its velocity. Power Doppler and intravenous echo-contrast may also help.[755–759] The degree of carotid luminal stenosis is calculated not only from the real-time ultrasound image, which can be inaccurate when the lesion is echolucent or calcification scatters the ultrasound beam, but also from the blood flow velocities derived from the Doppler signal. If colour Doppler is not available, but only grey-scale duplex, it is usually helpful to first insonate the supraorbital artery with a simple continuous-wave Doppler probe, because *inward* flow of blood strongly suggests severe internal carotid artery (ICA) stenosis or occlusion, although not necessarily at the origin.

Although duplex sonography is non-invasive and widely available, there are some difficulties that any ultrasound service must acknowledge and deal with.

- It is very operator dependent and so requires skill, training and considerable experience to be sure of

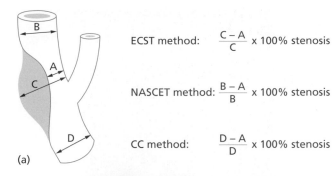

ECST method: $\dfrac{C-A}{C} \times 100\%$ stenosis

NASCET method: $\dfrac{B-A}{B} \times 100\%$ stenosis

CC method: $\dfrac{D-A}{D} \times 100\%$ stenosis

(a)

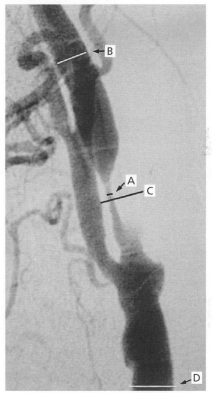

(b)

Fig. 6.27 (a) Three methods of measuring percentage diameter stenosis at the origin of the internal carotid artery (ICA) in the neck. All use as the numerator the minimum residual lumen where the stenosis is most severe (A). However, the denominator differs. In the European Carotid Surgery Trial (ECST) method, it is an *estimate* (C) of the normal lumen diameter at the site of the stenosis (whether this is at the bifurcation, more distal in the ICA or in the distal common carotid artery). In the North American Symptomatic Carotid Endarterectomy Trial (NASCET) method, it is the diameter of the ICA lumen when it becomes normal and free of disease, usually well beyond the bulb (B), and in the cases of near occlusion of the ICA an arbitrary 95% stenosis is assigned. In the common carotid method, it is the diameter of the common carotid artery proximal to the bifurcation, where it is free of disease and the diameter is fairly constant (D). (b) An illustrative example from a carotid angiogram in which (A)–(D) correspond with the measurements described in (a) above. The stenosis measures 89% by the ECST method, 88% by the common carotid method and 85% by the NASCET method.

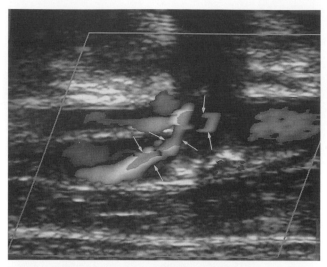

(a)

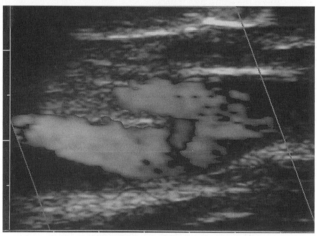

(b)

Fig. 6.28 (a) Duplex sonography examination of the carotid bifurcation to show a stenotic plaque (*arrows*) at the origin of the internal carotid artery. (b) Normal artery for comparison. In both, the head is to the left of the picture, the heart to the right.

accurate measurements of stenosis and the avoidance of pitfalls, such as confusing the external with the internal carotid artery.

- It may be difficult to interpret, particularly if there is plaque or periarterial calcification.
- It is not completely reliable in distinguishing very severe (>90%) stenosis (which is operable) from occlusion (which is not), unless used and interpreted with very great care.[760]
- It is not completely sensitive and specific for severe (70–99%) ICA stenosis.
- Different machines vary in their accuracy in measuring carotid stenosis.[761]

- It provides little information about the proximal arterial anatomy, although this is seldom affected by disease or relevant to the surgeon, or about distal anatomy. Just how often the latter is a really important problem is not at all clear (e.g. the position of the upper limit of the stenotic lesion, intracranial stenosis and asymptomatic intracranial aneurysms).[762]

As staff change and machines are updated, constant audit of the results against any subsequent catheter angiography is essential, but this is becoming more and more impractical as fewer catheter angiograms are being performed.[763] Another problem is that the technique is still evolving and any conclusions about accuracy in measuring the severity and character of carotid lesions can become dated, and must be applied in the context of the institution.[764,765] Unfortunately, the literature comparing the accuracy of ultrasound vs the 'gold standard' of catheter angiography is bedevilled by poor epidemiological and statistical methods and seldom conforms to standard guidelines for evaluating this kind of diagnostic test[766,767] (Table 6.15). Nonetheless, with stringent quality control and confirmation of stenosis by an independent observer (see below), duplex sonography is now the most common way that carotid stenosis severe enough to warrant surgery is diagnosed.[768]

There are no standard and commonly used definitions for the ultrasound appearance of plaques (soft, hard, calcified, etc.) and there is also considerable variation in reporting between and even within the same observers at different times.[769] Therefore, although unstable and ulcerated plaques are more likely to be symptomatic than stable plaques with fibrous caps (section 6.3.5), the

Table 6.15 Methodological criteria for comparing a test for measuring carotid stenosis against the 'gold-standard' of intra-arterial catheter angiography.

Prospective study design
Consecutive series of patients, or random sample
Adequate description of the study population
A spectrum of stenosis severity over the clinically relevant range
No exclusion of patients with poor images
Adequate details of the imaging techniques
Images assessed by one technique 'blind' to the images of the other
Adequate detail of exactly how the stenosis is measured by both techniques
Proper statistical methodology for comparing continuous and discontinuous variables
Reproducibility of measurements reported (inter- and intra-observer reliability)
Appropriate sample size for adequate power

ultrasound inaccuracy compromises any study of the relationship between plaque characteristics on duplex sonography and the risk of later stroke, and so the selection for carotid surgery.[770] Indeed, the appropriate natural history studies have never been carried out, and now probably never can be, at least not in *symptomatic* patients who mostly require endarterectomy if they have severe ICA stenosis, irrespective of what the plaque looks like on ultrasound. In *asymptomatic* stenosis, there is some evidence that a hypoechoic plaque predicts stroke risk,[771] but this was not confirmed in the Asymptomatic Carotid Surgery Trial.[772] Until it becomes possible to translate carotid plaque irregularity as seen on catheter angiography, which does add to the risk of stroke over and above the degree of stenosis (section 16.11.8), into what is seen on duplex sonography, it will remain tantalizingly difficult to use anything other than stenosis to predict stroke risk if only duplex is being used.

Despite all these limitations, duplex sonography is a remarkably quick and simple investigation in experienced hands, and it is neither unpleasant nor risky. Very rarely, the pressure of the Doppler probe on the carotid bifurcation can dislodge thrombus, or cause enough carotid sinus stimulation to lead to bradycardia or hypotension.[773,774] The same conceivably applies to the various arterial compression manoeuvres that may be carried out during transcranial Doppler or extracranial Doppler sonography, and any such compression should be avoided in patients who may have carotid bifurcation disease.[775,776]

> Reliable duplex sonography in a laboratory with stringent quality control, with any carotid stenosis confirmed by an independent observer, is now generally the best way to diagnose stenosis that is severe enough for carotid endarterectomy to be worthwhile.

CT angiography

This is now a widely used method for imaging the carotid arteries and cerebral circulation (section 5.4.3).[777–779] It requires a large dose of intravenous contrast to outline the arterial lumen, there is X-ray exposure, it gives only a limited view of a short segment of the neck arteries usually with no intracranial information, the images obtained depend on the proficiency of the operator in their selection, and it tends to underestimate stenosis. However, it does provide multiple viewing angles, three-dimensional reconstruction, and imaging of calcium deposits separately from the vessel lumen outlined by the contrast[780–782] (Fig. 6.29). Furthermore,

the technology is constantly improving so that views of the entire cerebral circulation, from the arch of the aorta to the cerebral arteries, are now possible.

Magnetic resonance angiography

Although non-invasive and safe, magnetic resonance angiography (MRA) alone, particularly non-enhanced imaging (or 'time of flight' imaging) is unlikely to be accurate enough in estimating carotid stenosis, at least at the present stage of development.[768,783,784] The pictures are not always adequate to allow measurement of the carotid stenosis (movement and swallowing artifacts are particular problems); the severity of the stenosis tends to be overestimated; there may be a flow gap distal to a stenosis of as little as 60%, making precise stenosis measurement impossible, and even in the posterior part of the carotid bulb, in both cases probably because of loss of laminar flow and increased residence times of the blood; irregularity/ulceration are not well seen; and severe stenosis can be confused with occlusion[785–787] (Fig. 6.30). However, image quality and reproducibility of measurement of stenosis are significantly improved with contrast-enhanced MRA.[784,788] So far, there have not been enough methodologically sound comparisons (Table 6.15) of MRA with catheter angiography.[768,789] The comparative studies that have been carried out have frequently been overtaken by changes in MR technology. Despite the limitations of MRA, its use is increasing as the role of MRI brain imaging in stroke expands (section 5.5.2).

Imaging of the internal carotid artery: advantages and disadvantages of non-invasive and invasive methods

The main advantage of non-invasive methods over catheter angiography is there is no serious procedural risk, and they can usually be done very quickly. In fact the procedural risk may have been overestimated in the past. Although an early systematic review of prospective studies of the risks of catheter angiography in patients with cerebrovascular disease reported a 0.1% risk of death and a 1.0% risk of permanent neurological sequelae,[790] more recent studies have reported lower risks in both academic centres and community hospitals.[791] Also it should be noted that most studies counted all strokes that occurred within 24 h of angiography as procedural complications. Given that the risk of stroke shortly after presentation with symptomatic carotid stenosis and prior to endarterectomy is about 0.5% per day, the excess risk of permanent neurological sequelae due to angiography in recently symptomatic patients may be less than 1.0%.[792]

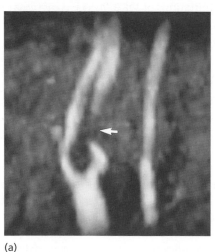

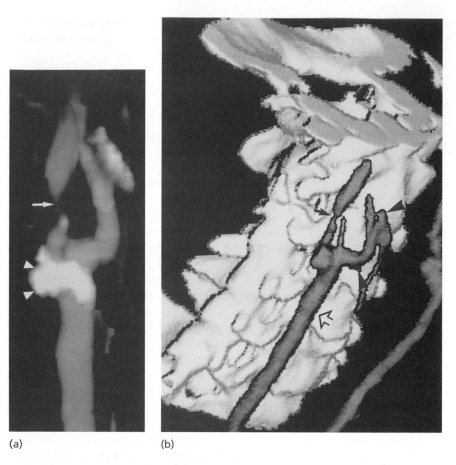

(a)   (b)

Fig. 6.29 CT angiogram of the carotid bifurcation. (a) Two-dimensional reconstruction to show severe stenosis at the origin of the internal carotid artery (*arrow*) as well as areas of calcification of the distal common carotid artery (*arrowheads*). (b) Three-dimensional reconstruction of the same artery to show the relationship with the cervical vertebrae. Common (*open arrow*), internal carotid stenosis (*arrow*) and external carotid arteries and branches (*arrowheads*).

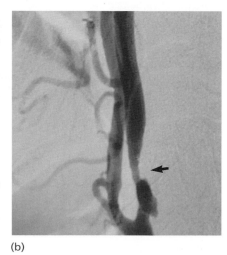

(a)   (b)

Fig. 6.30 (a) MR angiogram (three-dimensional time of flight) showing severe internal carotid stenosis. While the stenosis is clearly 'severe', it is not possible to measure its exact extent because of the 'flow gap' (*arrow*) distal to the lesion. (b) On the other hand, catheter angiography shows the lesion clearly (*arrow*) so that a stenosis of 82% (by the European Carotid Surgery Trial or common carotid artery method) or 71% (by the North American Symptomatic Carotid Endarterectomy Trial method) can be measured. The marked irregularity of the surface of the stenosis is also clearly visible, whereas this feature was lost on the MRA.

In contrast to pharmaceutical products, new diagnostic or imaging strategies are not subject to stringent regulatory control, and no standards are set for validation. Given that the available techniques of carotid imaging use completely different source data to estimate stenosis, that there is major variation in carotid bifurcation anatomy between individuals, and between the sexes, translation of measurements of stenosis from one technique to another is not at all straightforward. Although several hundred studies of carotid imaging have been published over the last two decades, most are undermined by poor design, inadequate sample size and inappropriate analysis and presentation of data.[767] A meta-analysis of the methodologically sound studies of non-invasive carotid imaging published prior to 1995 concluded that non-invasive methods could not substitute for catheter angiography as the sole pre-endarterectomy imaging technique because of the frequency with which the degree of stenosis was misclassified.[766] More recent studies have confirmed this.[768,791,793,794]

Because benefit from endarterectomy is highly dependent on the degree of symptomatic carotid stenosis as measured on catheter angiography, misclassification of stenosis with non-invasive methods will lead to some patients being operated unnecessarily, and others being denied appropriate surgery. This harm must be balanced against the small excess risk of stroke associated with catheter angiography, perhaps as low as one additional stroke per 200 patients. For example, given the 33% reduction in the 8-year absolute risk of stroke with endarterectomy in patients with 90–99% symptomatic stenosis,[795] for every three patients who are not operated on, possibly because a complete occlusion is misdiagnosed with Doppler ultrasound, one stroke will go unprevented. A risk of misclassification of 90–99% stenosis as complete occlusion of only few per cent would therefore be sufficient to offset the risk of catheter angiography. In practice, misclassification rates can be much higher. In a recent comparison of catheter angiography with Doppler ultrasound in 569 consecutive patients in 'accredited' laboratories with experienced radiologists, 28% of decisions about endarterectomy based on Doppler ultrasound alone were inappropriate.[791] Misclassification in non-accredited laboratories is likely to be even greater.

Given the major shortcomings of a Doppler ultrasound alone in selection of patients for endarterectomy, the combination of Doppler ultrasound with other non-invasive methods of imaging, usually MRA, has been studied. Inappropriate decisions in comparison with catheter angiography were reduced to less than 10% in patients in whom the results of Doppler ultrasound and MRA were concordant.[791] Catheter angiography is still required in the patients in whom Doppler ultrasound and MRA do not produce concordant results.

Present policy

At present, in all recently symptomatic 'carotid' patients who are fit for and willing to consider carotid endarterectomy, we first perform duplex sonography, if possible blinded to which carotid artery is symptomatic to avoid observer bias. If the first duplex shows stenosis above about 60%, or occlusion, another observer is asked (blinded to the results of the first duplex) to repeat the duplex (either CT or MR angiography are acceptable non-invasive alternatives if more convenient). If *both* observers agree that the patient has severe stenosis, within about 10 percentage points of each other, then the

option of surgery is considered further (section 16.11.8). Similar approaches based on two different methods of non-invasive imaging have been shown by other groups to be effective in routine clinical practice.[791,796,797] If the observers/techniques disagree, then catheter angiography is recommended, but usually only of the symptomatic artery to keep any risk to a minimum.

6.8.6 Vertebrobasilar transient ischaemic attacks

Vertebrobasilar transient ischaemic attacks (TIAs) were thought for many years to be associated with a lower risk of stroke than carotid territory TIAs.[798–800] However, recent work has shown that the risk of stroke is at least as high, and possibly higher in the first few weeks after the event.[801,802] It is not clear that vascular surgery has much to offer other than in the rather special situation of subclavian steal (section 16.16). However, there are an increasing number of reports of angioplasty and stenting of atherothrombotic stenoses of the vertebral or proximal basilar arteries. MR or CT angiography are the most useful non-invasive methods of imaging the posterior circulation, although catheter angiography is often still necessary to confirm or exclude significant stenosis.

Although asymptomatic subclavian steal is quite common (reversed vertebral artery flow detected by ultrasound or vertebral angiography), *symptomatic* subclavian steal is rare, presumably because collateral blood flow to the brainstem is enough to compensate for the reversed vertebral artery blood flow distal to ipsilateral subclavian stenosis or occlusion (section 4.2.3). The clinical syndrome is quite easily recognized by unequal blood pressures between the two arms, a supraclavicular bruit and vertebrobasilar TIAs which may or may not be brought on by exercise of the arm ipsilateral to the subclavian stenosis or occlusion, so increasing blood flow *down* the vertebral artery from the brainstem to the arm muscles.[803–806] It is only this sort of symptomatic patient who may require surgery and therefore who has to accept the risk of any preceding angiography. *Innominate artery steal* is even rarer, with retrograde vertebral artery flow distal to innominate rather than subclavian artery occlusion.[807,808]

6.8.7 The diagnosis of cervical arterial dissection

Although arterial dissection tends to heal without any treatment, and many physicians do not use anticoagulants or any other specific treatment (section 7.2.1), it is still often necessary to make a definitive diagnosis because this aborts unnecessary further investigation to look for the cause of an ischaemic stroke or transient ischaemic attack; there may be medicolegal issues, such as litigation against some assailant or other person responsible for any trauma; the patient (and their life insurance company, employers, and so on) can be reassured that the risk of recurrence is low; and long-term antithrombotic drugs and other conventional secondary prevention treatments are not needed. The 'gold standard' imaging used to be catheter angiography because ultrasound and other non-invasive methods were neither specific nor sensitive enough to rely on. However, there is now a widespread consensus that cross-sectional MRI, to show haematoma within the widened arterial wall, combined with magnetic resonance angiography, is the safer and best option (Fig. 7.2).

6.8.8 Vascular imaging in acute ischaemic stroke

Patients with ischaemic stroke may have symptomatic atheromatous stenosis of their extracranial carotid artery and be candidates for carotid endarterectomy. Severe internal carotid artery origin stenosis can be excluded by duplex sonography once there is enough recovery to make surgery an option. The role of imaging in therapeutic decision-making in acute stroke is dealt with in section 12.5. Other potential indications for angiography include suspicion of any of the following.

- Cervical arterial dissection (section 7.2.1).
- An aneurysm of the extra- or intracranial circulation large enough to contain thrombus which might embolize to the brain or eye. This is very rare, but surgery may be required to clip or remove an aneurysm, or anticoagulation might be indicated (section 7.6).
- Fibromuscular dysplasia – although whether and how it should be treated is not at all clear (section 7.4.1).
- Cerebral vasculitis, which can be associated with beading and narrowing of cerebral arteries, although this is neither a specific nor sensitive feature. This diagnosis is better made by serological tests, extracranial tissue biopsy (renal, skin, etc.) or by meningeal/cortical biopsy, if clinically justifiable (section 7.3).
- Moyamoya syndrome is exceedingly rare and any treatment possibilities are severely limited (section 7.5).

6.8.9 Transcranial Doppler sonography

Transcranial Doppler (TCD) sonography provides information on the velocity of blood flow and its direction in relation to the ultrasound probe, in the major intracranial arteries at the base of the brain, and so whether they are occluded or stenosed (Fig. 6.31). It is non-invasive, repeatable on demand, can be performed at the bedside, is not expensive and not too difficult to perform

accurately. It is very safe, although during tests involving compression of the carotid artery it is conceivable that emboli can be released from an underlying atheromatous plaque, and bradycardia can occur. However, the patient has to keep reasonably still; the examination can take as long as an hour; the skull is impervious to ultrasound in 5–10% of cases, more with increasing age and in females, but less if intravenous echocontrast is used; exact vessel identification may be difficult, but colour-flow real-time imaging makes this easier; spatial resolution is poor; diagnostic criteria vary; and the technique is not always accurate in comparison with cerebral catheter angiography.[809–815]

Despite the fact that TCD, like positron emission tomography (PET), has increased our knowledge of the cerebral circulation in health and disease, and even though it is inexpensive and quite widely available and repeatable on demand (very unlike PET), it still has rather a minor role in *routine* clinical management. As well as monitoring during carotid endarterectomy (section 16.11.2), the diagnosis of patent foramen ovale (section 6.5.12), sickle cell disease (section 7.9.8), and perhaps in helping define stroke risk[85–87,816] there are four other possible indications: display of intracranial arterial occlusion and stenosis; emboli detection; assessment of cerebrovascular reactivity; and acceleration of clot lysis following treatment with a thrombolytic agent in acute ischaemic stroke (section 12.6.3).[817,818]

Display of intracranial arterial occlusion and stenosis

Stenosis can be difficult to distinguish from hyperaemia because both increase flow velocity, but TCD can display occlusion of the MCA mainstem if not the branches, the anterior cerebral artery and, less easily, of the basilar and posterior cerebral arteries. It cannot demonstrate occlusion of smaller arteries which cannot be seen. However, at present, this information is of limited clinical relevance although it may aid in selection of patients for thrombolysis (section 12.5).

Emboli detection

What may become of more clinical relevance is the detection of emboli as high-intensity transient signals on the sonogram, so-called microembolic signals (MES) (Fig. 6.32). Although the vast majority of MES appear to be asymptomatic, their detection may help in distinguishing cardiac and aortic arch from carotid emboli, because with the first two, emboli should be detected in several arterial distributions, whereas with the last in only the one arterial distribution distal to the supposed embolic source.[87,819,820] However, the frequency of

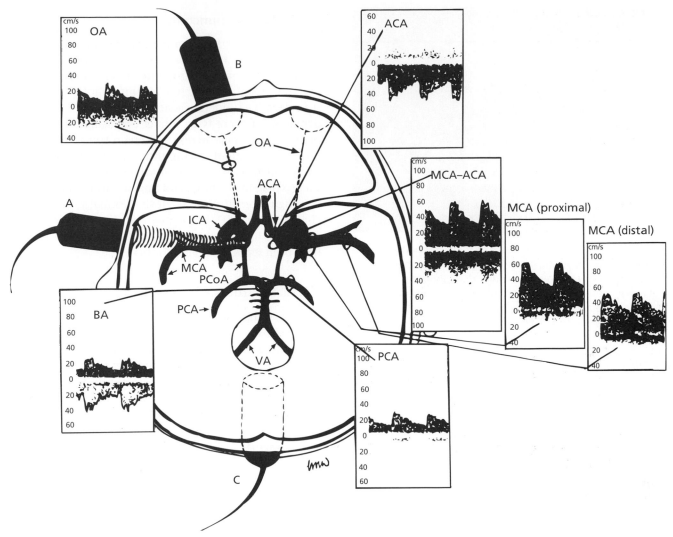

Fig. 6.31 Transcranial Doppler sonography. The base of the skull looked at from above (eyes at the top of the diagram) to illustrate the cranial sonographic windows (A temporal; B orbital; C foramen magnum) and typical waveforms obtained from the major intracranial arteries. Note that the power output of the transducer must be reduced to 10% of the maximum for the transorbital approach to avoid damage to the eyes. ACA anterior cerebral artery; BA basilar artery; ICA internal carotid artery; MCA middle cerebral artery; OA ophthalmic artery; PCA posterior cerebral artery; PCoA posterior communicating artery; VA vertebral artery.

MES can be so frustratingly low and variable that their detection requires prolonged monitoring and automation.[86,87,815] Conceivably, MES detection might help distinguish organic from hysterical events, be used to monitor acute ischaemic stroke treatment, surgical or medical, and as a surrogate outcome in trials of secondary prevention of stroke.[86,87]

Assessment of cerebrovascular reactivity

Transcranial Doppler sonography can also be used to assess cerebrovascular reactivity, i.e. the capacity for intracranial vasodilatation in response to acetazolamide, carbon dioxide inhalation or breath-holding, although these three methods do not always produce concordant results[53,821–823] (section 12.1.2). However, there is still debate about exactly how to standardize this test (what exactly is 'abnormal'?) and it is not routinely used. It may even be important to recognize normal variation during the day.[824] Interestingly, impaired reactivity may have some prognostic significance for identifying individual patients at particularly high risk of stroke from among those with carotid stenosis (section 16.11.5) and internal carotid artery occlusion, although the

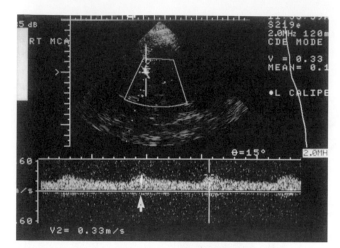

Fig. 6.32 Transcranial Doppler signals from the middle cerebral artery. Arrow shows the high intensity microembolic signal (MES) of an embolus. Note that the embolic signal does not extend beyond the Doppler trace and is of higher intensity (brightness) than the rest of the Doppler signal.

numbers studied have been small and the situation is not yet clear-cut.[53,66,624] With time, and presumably increasing collateralization, any impairment of reactivity can return to normal.[825–828]

6.8.10 Imaging the coronary circulation

Symptomatic coronary heart disease (CHD) is very common in transient ischaemic attack (TIA) and ischaemic stroke patients; about one-third have angina or have had a myocardial infarction (Table 6.3). It clearly requires the usual cardiological investigation and treatment. In addition, a substantial proportion of patients *without* symptomatic CHD have evidence of subclinical coronary artery lesions, the exact figure depending on how intensively the patients are investigated (section 6.3.1). Therefore, it is hardly surprising that the future risk of serious coronary events is high (section 16.2.3). However, the detection of *asymptomatic* coronary artery disease does not at present influence the long-term management of ischaemic stroke/TIA patients because vascular risk factors will be treated and antithrombotic drugs and statins used anyway, and it is unknown whether coronary artery surgery/stenting has any impact on the long-term prognosis in this category of patient. There is no indication therefore for exercise ECG testing, thallium-201 dipyridamole scintigraphy or coronary angiography, unless the patient has cardiac symptoms or other reasons, such as an abnormal resting ECG, to suggest coronary artery disease requiring surgical or endovascular treatment.

6.8.11 Lumbar puncture

Lumbar puncture is certainly not a routine investigation in acute stroke. It is of no use in differentiating intracerebral haemorrhage from ischaemic stroke (section 5.3.2) although it still has an important place in CT scan-negative sudden headache (section 3.7.3). It can be dangerous if there is an infarct or haematoma causing brain shift or obstruction to cerebrospinal fluid (CSF) flow, and in patients taking anticoagulant drugs it can be complicated by spinal haemorrhage. It is only useful if there is diagnostic doubt and a possibility of encephalitis, meningitis or multiple sclerosis. Normally, there is no change in the CSF after acute ischaemic stroke but there can be up to 100 white blood cells/mm³, more if there have been septic emboli to the brain.[829]

6.8.12 Electroencephalogram

Infarcts, or haemorrhages, involving the cerebral cortex are likely to cause ipsilateral slowing of the electroencephalogram (EEG), but there are better clinical and imaging ways of distinguishing them from deep lesions such as lacunar infarcts. If the diagnosis of stroke is unclear and encephalitis or some other generalized encephalopathy are possibilities, or even Creutzfeldt–Jakob disease, then a bilaterally abnormal EEG would weigh against stroke. Also, when there is confusion between stroke and epilepsy masquerading as stroke, or epilepsy making an old stroke seem worse (sections 11.4 and 11.8), focal seizure activity on the EEG is informative.[830] An EEG may also help distinguish a transient ischaemic attack from focal epilepsy (section 3.4.2) but a *routine* EEG is not necessary.

6.8.13 Cost-effectiveness

Wherever there is uncertainty, as there certainly is in how far to investigate stroke patients, there is always considerable variation in practice between and within countries – and doctors. Not everyone will agree with our views on the investigation of ischaemic stroke/transient ischaemic attack patients. However, we must emphasize that the criteria for *any* investigation have nothing to do with scientific curiosity or financial profit, which can both so easily distort recommendations. We are only interested if the result of an investigation is likely to influence the patient's management in a useful way, without unacceptable risk, and potentially improve their outcome. What is meant by 'unacceptable' must depend on the *balance* of the risk of investigation and the risk of *not* doing the investigation and so prejudicing a patient's outcome; this balance will surely change as new and safer investigations are developed, and treatments improve. Thus, we are 'minimalist' and should, as a result, be cost-effective. On the other hand, those who are more aggressive in their treatments (in our view, very often relying on theory rather than evidence from randomized trials and meta-analysis), would clearly regard our minimalist investigation strategy as sloppy and seriously lacking in detail, perhaps even negligent.

> How far a patient is investigated for the cause of their stroke or transient ischaemic attack depends on how the results of any investigation will influence treatment decisions, and these treatment decisions will depend on how far one is driven by theory rather than evidence based on randomized trials and systematic reviews.

The debate about cost-effectiveness should ideally concentrate on where the real money is (such as MR angiography) and not on inexpensive investigations (such as the erythrocyte sedimentation rate) which even if performed in extremely large numbers will have a negligible impact on the overall investigation budget. Moreover, the cost of investigation must be seen within the context of the total hospital costs of stroke. Even in a specialist neuroscience unit, the investigation cost is only about 12% of the budget, while in general internal medical and geriatric units, where the vast majority of strokes are managed in the UK, the proportion is less than 2% (section 17.16).

6.9 Identifying the three most common causes of ischaemic stroke and transient ischaemic attack

About 95% of ischaemic strokes and transient ischaemic attacks (TIAs) are caused by atherothromboembolism, small vessel disease, or embolism from the heart (Fig. 6.1). The 5% comprising the rarities may or may not be reasonably obvious from the clinical history, examination and routine first-line investigations and should be looked for particularly assiduously, with further appropriate investigations, where they are most likely to be present, i.e. in young and middle-aged patients, or if there is no good evidence for one of three main causes of cerebral ischaemia or any of the main stroke risk factors (hypertension, smoking, diabetes mellitus, atrial fibrillation (AF), carotid bruit, and evidence of coronary or peripheral vascular disease). If there is the problem of

two, three or even four competing causes for cerebral ischaemia in an individual patient then one must concentrate on the treatable. In the region of 10% of ischaemic stroke patients have evidence of both atherothrombosis and a cardiac source of embolism,[161,831] while about two-thirds of patients with an identifiable rare cause of cerebral ischaemia also have one or more of the common vascular risk factors (Table 6.16). Naturally, if a transient ischaemic attack (TIA) patient definitely has giant-cell arteritis then that should be treated, whether or not the patient also has hypertension and AF. As the giant-cell arteritis comes under control, one should consider lowering the blood pressure, giving a statin and using anticoagulants or antiplatelet drugs as one might for primary prevention in people who have never had a stroke (Chapter 16).

In the first minutes of medical contact after a stroke, all that is available diagnostically is the clinical syndrome but this can take one a long way towards establishing the cause, and then a CT brain scan is usually required to rule out cerebral haemorrhage (section 5.4.1). In the next few hours and days, during which further investigations can be carried out, a more precise idea of the cause may be formed which, although too late to influence any acute treatment, may modify

Table 6.16 Non-atheromatous, non-cardioembolic conditions causing or predisposing to ischaemic stroke amongst 244 cases of first-ever-in-a-lifetime ischaemic stroke in the Oxfordshire Community Stroke Project. (Adapted from Sandercock *et al.* 1989.[10])

	Total number	Percentage
Arteritis	9	4
Migraine	7	3
Major operation	3	1
Inflammatory bowel disease	3	1
Neck trauma	2	1
Carcinoma of the thyroid	1	<1
Autoimmune disease*	1	<1
Leukaemia	1	<1
Oral contraceptive use (in the past)	1	<1
Total	28†	12

*One patient with rheumatoid arthritis, glomerulonephritis and myasthenia gravis.
†Eighteen of these 28 patients also had one or more vascular risk factors (hypertension, heart disease, peripheral vascular disease, cervical bruit, diabetes mellitus, etc.), making the exact cause of their ischaemic stroke uncertain. Non-atheromatous, non-embolic conditions were the *only* predisposing factors in 10 of the 244 patients (4%).

further management. The stroke clinical syndrome is not very helpful in deciding between more than one competing cause in an individual patient, although a lacunar event is unlikely to be caused by embolism from the heart, aorta or carotid bifurcation, even if one or more of these embolic sources are present. Nonetheless, many physicians feel that severe carotid stenosis should be operated on (section 16.11.9), and patients with non-rheumatic AF should be prescribed anticoagulants (section 16.6.2), even if the patient has had a recent lacunar ischaemic stroke since there is evidence of benefit.

Our guidelines to distinguish the three main causes of ischaemic stroke/TIA are based on common sense and the scientific literature, as far as it goes, but have not and cannot be thoroughly validated, because there is no 'gold standard' to define the cause in *every* case (Table 6.17). Even for those who die, the postmortem can still leave uncertainties. Therefore, uncertainty must be accepted and, given the difficulty in defining a precise cause in an individual patient, it is not surprising that in many cases – depending on the diagnostic criteria and how far investigation is taken – no certain cause is found. However, in clinical practice, the exact cause is less important than deciding what to do next, if anything,

i.e. would the result of a particular investigation, and knowing the cause of the stroke, influence the choice of treatment for this particular case? For example, one would not prescribe anticoagulants for a fibrillating stroke patient who was an elderly alcoholic given to falling over, but aspirin instead. If a patient has a patent foramen ovale (PFO) and no other cause of cerebral ischaemia, then paradoxical embolism might have been responsible, but because it is unclear what the risk of recurrence is, or whether antithrombotic drugs or closure of the defect influences this risk, then in a sense the PFO is of no *clinical* relevance (section 6.5.12). However, it would be of great *scientific* interest if a large number of similar patients were followed up to study the risk of recurrence so that future clinical practice could be improved, particularly if they were invited to participate in randomized controlled trials.

> It is very difficult, and usually impossible, to be sure of the actual cause of an ischaemic stroke or transient ischaemic attack if several potential causes are present in the same individual, and sometimes even if only one is present.

Table 6.17 The strength of the evidence for the three main causes of ischaemic stroke and transient ischaemic attack in an individual patient based on a number of clinical variables and investigations.

Variable	Atherothromboembolism	Small vessel disease	Embolism from the heart
Age	>50	>50	Any
Total/partial anterior circulation ischaemia (clinical syndrome ± brain imaging)	+++	–	+++
Lacunar ischaemia (clinical syndrome ± brain imaging)	+	+++	+
Boundary-zone ischaemia (brain imaging)	+++	–	–
Posterior cerebral artery ischaemia (clinical syndrome ± brain imaging)	+++	+	+++
Brainstem ischaemia (clinical syndrome ± brain imaging)	++	++	++
Cerebellar ischaemia (clinical syndrome ± brain imaging)	++	+	++
Cholesterol retinal emboli	+++	–	–
Calcific retinal emboli	–	–	++
Recent ischaemic episodes in more than one arterial territory, particularly in more than one organ	+	–	+++
Arterial bruits (neck, legs), absent/unequal pulses (neck, arms, legs)	+++	+	–
Duplex sonography/angiogram evidence of severe stenosis/occlusion	+++	+	–
Major cardiac source of embolism	+	–	++
Clinical evidence of atherothrombosis elsewhere (angina, myocardial infarction, claudication)	++	+	+
Vascular risk factors (hypertension, diabetes, etc.)	++	++	–
Clear evidence of an alternative cause, such as dissection, vasculitis, etc.	–	–	–

+++, Strong supportive evidence; ++, reasonable supportive evidence; +, weak evidence; –, evidence against.
Note: neither the speed of onset of symptoms nor a past history of transient ischaemic attack are helpful.

6.9.1 Atherothromboembolism

Although atherothromboembolism is the most common cause of ischaemic stroke/transient ischaemic attack (TIA), about 50% of patients have other causes and so it must not be assumed that every stroke is caused by this admittedly common vascular disorder (section 6.3). More positive evidence, if possible, is required (Table 6.17). It is not realistic to be precise in every individual, but there are some criteria that make atherothromboembolism more likely:

- a total or partial anterior circulation syndrome without any cardiac embolic source (sections 4.3.4, 4.3.5, 6.7.1 and 6.7.2);
- the presence of vascular risk factors, such as smoking, hyperlipidaemia and hypertension;
- absent or diminished pulses or vascular bruits, particularly over the symptomatic artery, together with duplex or angiogram-confirmed stenosis;
- cholesterol emboli in the retina;
- boundary-zone infarction on brain imaging;
- MR-DWI showing multiple acute infarcts in the anterior circulation territory of one hemisphere.

This problem is more difficult when dealing with vertebrobasilar rather than carotid ischaemia, because there are more causal possibilities and because it is still difficult to image the vertebral circulation non-invasively. However, a large infarct in the cerebellum or in the territory of the posterior cerebral artery is likely to be atherothromboembolic if there is no cardiac source of embolism.

If possible, it is worth making a positive diagnosis of atherothromboembolism because this stops the fruitless search for alternatives; it directs attention to defining the degree of any symptomatic carotid stenosis and therefore the need for carotid endarterectomy (section 16.11); it also emphasizes the control of vascular risk factors (sections 16.3 and 16.4) and the use of antiplatelet drugs (section 16.5). It is impossible to be absolutely precise about whether an event was caused by acute arterial occlusion or low flow, or either mechanism at different times but, fortunately, this difficulty seldom affects clinical management (section 6.7.5).

6.9.2 Intracranial small vessel disease

That an ischaemic stroke or transient ischaemic attack (TIA) was caused by intracranial small vessel disease is highly likely if the clinical syndrome is lacunar – easier in stroke than TIA patients to be sure – and particularly if there is no cardiac source of embolism clinically, no clinical or ultrasound evidence of arterial disease in the neck, and no reasonably obvious rare cause of stroke clinically or on the routine investigations (sections 4.3.2 and 6.7.3) (Table 6.17). It is very likely that there will be stroke risk factors but, apart from recent myocardial infarction and atrial fibrillation (AF), these are about as likely as in atherothromboembolic ischaemic stroke (section 6.4). From the management point of view, a positive diagnosis of small vessel disease reduces the urgency for the detection of severe carotid stenosis which, if found, is difficult to interpret. Is it really caused by embolism or low flow (in which case carotid endarterectomy may be indicated) or is it 'asymptomatic', in which case it perhaps should be left alone? Our view is that, even if the syndrome is lacunar, carotid endarterectomy might well be recommended, but only if the patient has severe carotid stenosis on the symptomatic side and other factors in favour of surgery, as perhaps for primary stroke prevention (section 16.11.9). We would be more likely to prescribe anticoagulants for a lacunar patient in AF, even though the AF *might* not be relevant. At least we could reassure ourselves that worthwhile *primary* stroke prevention is definitely achieved by anticoagulation in patients who are able to handle the treatment (section 16.6.2).

6.9.3 Embolism from the heart

The diagnosis of ischaemic stroke or transient ischaemic attack (TIA) caused by embolism from the heart should only be considered at all if there is an identifiable cardioembolic source, which is the case in about 20–30% of ischaemic stroke/TIA patients (section 6.5) (Table 6.4), a higher proportion in recent studies using transoesophageal echocardiography. However, in perhaps one-third the cardiac source is of uncertain relevance, because there is another, maybe more likely, cause of cerebral ischaemia, such as carotid stenosis.

Other than lacunar syndromes (which are seldom caused by cardiac embolism), the neurological and conventional brain CT/MRI features of any cerebral ischaemic event do not reliably distinguish a cardioembolic from some other cause of ischaemic stroke.[157,158,832] However, DWI may demonstrate several acute lesions in multiple arterial territories suggesting a cardioembolic source (but also an aortic arch source). In fact, most cardiac lesions with a substantial embolic threat can be suspected, and even definitively diagnosed, by competent clinical examination, an electrocardiogram (ECG) and a chest X-ray. In addition, *transthoracic* echocardiography may be indicated to refine the clinical diagnosis and guide the management of any suspected lesions (e.g. mitral stenosis, atrial myxoma). *Transoesophageal* echocardiography, with intravenous echo contrast, is somewhat invasive, uncomfortable, occasionally risky (bronchospasm, hypoxia, angina, cardiac dysrhythmias, vocal

Transthoracic echcocardiography preferred	Transoesophageal echocardiography preferred
Left-ventricular thrombus*	Left atrial thrombus*
Left-ventricular dyskinesis	Left atrial appendage thrombus*
Mitral stenosis	Spontaneous echo contrast
Mitral annulus calcification	Intracardiac tumours
Aortic stenosis	Atrial septal defect†
	Atrial septal aneurysm
	Patent foramen ovale†
	Mitral and aortic valve vegetations
	Prosthetic heart valve malfunction
	Aortic arch atherothrombosis/dissection
	Mitral leaflet prolapse

Table 6.18 Comparison of transthoracic vs transoesophageal echocardiography for detecting potential cardiac sources of embolism.

*The detection of intracardiac thrombus is not *necessarily* relevant, because not all thrombi embolize and the lack of intracardiac thrombus may not be relevant, either because it is too small to be detected or it has all embolized already.
†A less invasive alternative is to inject air bubbles or other echocontrast material intravenously and, if there is a patent foramen ovale, they can be detected by transcranial Doppler sonography of the middle cerebral artery, particularly with a provocative Valsalva manoeuvre. There is considerable variation in the methods and this influences the diagnostic sensitivity and specificity. It is also uncertain what size of shunt is 'clinically relevant', and some bubbles may pass to the brain through pulmonary rather than cardiac shunts (Droste *et al.* 1999[84]).

cord paresis, bacteraemia, pharyngeal bleeding, oesophageal laceration or perforation, and endocarditis) and perhaps difficult to perform in acute stroke.[833,834] However, it undoubtedly provides more information (e.g. patent foramen ovale, valvular vegetations, thrombus in the left atrium) and displays atheromatous plaques in at least part of the aortic arch[835–839] (Table 6.18). None the less, *routine* transthoracic, and certainly *routine* transoesophageal echocardiography without preceding transthoracic echocardiography, is not justifiable because the yield in unselected patients is extremely low, particularly in the crucial sense of changing management rather than collecting anatomical information for no very obvious purpose other than research. Putting patients to inconvenience and risk in the search for a diagnosis that does not then lead on to a change – preferably evidence-based – in their management cannot be justified.[840–844] Transthoracic and then – if necessary – transoesophageal echocardiography may well help if a cardiac source of embolism is suspected on the basis of the history (past rheumatic fever, ischaemic events in more than one vascular territory, etc.), cardiac examination (murmurs, etc.), ECG (atrial fibrillation, recent myocardial infarction), *particularly* if there is no reasonable alternative cause (such as severe carotid stenosis, giant-cell arteritis, etc.). Moreover, in young patients with no obvious cause of cerebral ischaemia, it is justifiable to examine the heart in considerable detail, even as far as transoesophageal echocardiography, because degenerative arterial disease is so rare in them.[845,846]

> The presence of intracardiac thrombus on echocardiography does not necessarily mean that embolism has occurred, while the absence of intracardiac thrombus does not necessarily mean that embolism has not occurred. In either case, embolism may recur sooner or later.

The decision whether an identified potential embolic source in the heart was the cause of the ischaemic stroke or TIA can be quite easy if most of the criteria in Table 6.17 are fulfilled; for example, if the patient is aged 30 years, has a mechanical prosthetic heart valve and no vascular disorder or risk factors. Also, some cardiac lesions are much more threatening causes of embolism than others (Table 6.4). On the other hand, it can be clinically impossible; for example, if the patient is a 70-year-old and has both atrial fibrillation and severe carotid stenosis ipsilateral to a single cortical infarct confined on DWI, when one might be tempted (correctly perhaps) to recommend anticoagulation as well as carotid endarterectomy. Some cardiac lesions are so common in the normal stroke-free population (e.g. patent foramen ovale, mitral annulus calcification) that their relevance in an individual ischaemic stroke patient is unassessable without additional evidence of embolism. One comes back to treating what is treatable (to prevent stroke recurrence), provided the risks are not thought to outweigh the potential benefits and the patient is prepared to accept the risk of treatment, as well as the benefit. Whether emboli detection with transcranial Doppler becomes helpful in sorting out the origin of emboli remains to be seen, it is certainly not a routinely available investigation as yet (section 6.8.9).

Long-term monitoring of the electrocardiogram

The frequency of cardiac dysrhythmias in transient ischaemic attack (TIA) patients is similar to the frequency in the normal population of the same age.[161] Therefore, unless a dysrhythmia can be shown to *coincide* with a cerebral ischaemic event (which is unlikely unless the events are occurring, if not daily, at least several times a week), its relevance (in the sense of causing hypotension and so focal cerebral ischaemia) to any neurological symptoms is uncertain. Hypotensive *focal* cerebral ischaemic events are very uncommon (section 6.7.5). We only monitor the ECG if the ischaemic events are occurring frequently enough to be captured on tape, and particularly if no embolic cause is likely, and the focal neurological symptoms are accompanied by faintness, chest pain, shortness of breath or palpitations. Treatment of the dysrhythmia might then reduce the risk of recurrent symptoms.

Other indications for ECG monitoring are a patient in sinus rhythm, who *might* have paroxysmal atrial fibrillation (AF) (history of palpitations or possibly irregular pulse, etc.) and so require anticoagulation[847] (section 16.6), or to check that any treatment to return a fibrillating patient to sinus rhythm has been effective. In a recent study of 465 consecutive patients admitted with a diagnosis of new ischaemic stroke, 210 underwent 24-h ECG recording.[169] Previously undiscovered AF was identified in five cases (2.4%). In three cases, the Holter test was negative despite AF documented on an admission ECG. The authors postulated that the standard 24-h duration of monitoring might have underestimated the real prevalence of paroxysmal AF in their population.

Venography

Ultrasound to detect deep venous thrombosis (DVT) of the legs may be required in the rare case where paradoxical embolism is suspected.[848] If negative, X-ray venography of the legs or MR venography of the pelvic veins is more sensitive[849] (section 11.13). Criteria to suspect paradoxical embolism include:[850–852]

- an ischaemic event occurring in the context of a Valsalva manoeuvre (lifting, straining, coughing, trumpet playing, etc.), or anything else likely to increase right atrial pressure and so encourage blood flow from the right to left atrium;
- a patent foramen ovale or other septal defect identified with contrast echocardiography or transcranial Doppler sonography;
- echocardiographically visible clot in the right atrium or across the inter-atrial septum;
- a reason for DVT or pelvic venous thrombosis (e.g. recent surgery or lengthy travel); and
- no other more likely cause.

However, these clues are far from specific and sensitive for the reliable diagnosis of paradoxical embolism in an individual patient.[853] Furthermore, any venography must be performed early (within 48 h at most) because DVT is so common as a *consequence* of stroke, particularly in a paralysed leg[854,855] (section 11.13).

References

1 Koudstaal PJ, van Gijn J, Frenken CW, Hijdra A, Lodder J, Vermeulen M *et al*. TIA, RIND, minor stroke: a continuum, or different subgroups? Dutch TIA Study Group. *J Neurol Neurosurg Psychiatry* 1992; **55**:95–7.

2 Engelter ST, Provenzale JM, Petrella JR, Alberts MJ. Diffusion MR imaging and transient ischemic attacks. *Stroke* 1999; **30**:2762–3.

3 Kimura K, Minematsu K, Yasaka M, Wada K, Yamaguchi T. The duration of symptoms in transient ischaemic attack. *Neurology* 1999; **52**:976–80.

4 Crisostomo RA, Garcia MM, Tong DC. Detection of diffusion-weighted MRI abnormalities in patients with transient ischemic attack: correlation with clinical characteristics. *Stroke* 2003; **34**:932–7.

5 Coutts SB, Simon JE, Eliasziw M, Sohn CH, Hill MD, Barber PA *et al*. Triaging transient ischemic attack and minor stroke patients using acute magnetic resonance imaging. *Ann Neurol* 2005; **57**:848–54.

6 Petty GW, Brown RD, Jr, Whisnant JP, Sicks JD, O'Fallon WM, Wiebers DO. Ischemic stroke subtypes: a population-based study of incidence and risk factors. *Stroke* 1999; **30**:2513–16.

7 Whisnant JP, Brown RD, Petty GW, O'Fallon WM, Sicks JD, Wiebers DO. Comparison of population-based models of risk factors for TIA and ischemic stroke. *Neurology* 1999; **53**:532–6.

8 Rothwell PM, Coull AJ, Giles MF, Howard SC, Silver LE, Bull LM *et al*. Change in stroke incidence, mortality, case-fatality, severity, and risk factors in Oxfordshire, UK

from 1981 to 2004 (Oxford Vascular Study). *Lancet* 2004; **363**:1925–33.

9 Sempere AP, Duarte J, Cabezas C, Claveria LE. Etiopathogenesis of transient ischemic attacks and minor ischemic strokes: a community-based study in Segovia, Spain. *Stroke* 1998; **29**:40–5.

10 Sandercock PA, Warlow CP, Jones LN, Starkey IR. Predisposing factors for cerebral infarction: the Oxfordshire community stroke project. *Br Med J* 1989; **298**:75–80.

11 Bamford J, Sandercock P, Dennis M, Burn J, Warlow C. Classification and natural history of clinically identifiable subtypes of cerebral infarction. *Lancet* 1991; **337**:1521–6.

12 Schulz UG, Rothwell PM. Differences in vascular risk factors between etiological subtypes of ischemic stroke: importance of population-based studies. *Stroke* 2003; **34**:2050–9.

13 Giroud M, Lemesle M, Quantin C, Vourch M, Becker F, Milan C *et al*. A hospital-based and a population-based stroke registry yield different results: the experience in Dijon, France. *Neuroepidemiology* 1997; **16**:15–21.

14 Morris JN. Recent history of coronary disease. *Lancet* 1951; **1**:69–73.

15 Joseph A, Ackerman D, Talley JD, Johnstone J, Kupersmith J. Manifestations of coronary atherosclerosis in young trauma victims: an autopsy study. *J Am Coll Cardiol* 1993; **22**:459–67.

16 Enriquez-Sarano M, Klodas E, Garratt KN, Bailey KR, Tajik AJ, Holmes DR, Jr. Secular trends in coronary atherosclerosis: analysis in patients with valvular regurgitation. *N Engl J Med* 1996; **335**:316–22.

17 Berenson GS, Srinvasan SR, Bao W *et al*. Association between multiple cardiovascular risk factors and atherosclerosis in children and young adults. *N Engl J Med* 1998; **338**: 1650–6.

18 Goldschmidt-Clermont PJ, Creager MA, Losordo DW, Lam GK, Wassef M, Dzau VJ. Atherosclerosis 2005: recent discoveries and novel hypotheses. *Circulation* 2005; **112**:3348–53.

19 Gotto AM, Jr. Evolving concepts of dyslipidemia, atherosclerosis, and cardiovascular disease: the Louis F. Bishop Lecture. *J Am Coll Cardiol* 2005; **46**:1219–24.

20 Ebrahim S, Harwood R. *Stroke: Epidemiology, Evidence and Clinical Practice*. Oxford: Oxford University Press, 1999.

21 Fisher CM. Occlusion of the internal carotid artery. *Arch Neurol Psychiatry* 1951; **65**:346–77.

22 Fisher CM. Occlusion of the carotid arteries. *Arch Neurol Psychiatry* 1954; **72**:187–204.

23 Hutchinson EC, Yates PO. Carotico-vertebral stenosis. *Lancet* 1957; **272**:2–8.

24 Schwartz CJ, Mitchell JR. Atheroma of the carotid and vertebral arterial systems. *Br Med J* 1961; **5259**:1057–63.

25 Cornhill JF, Akins D, Hutson M, Chandler AB. Localization of atherosclerotic lesions in the human basilar artery. *Atherosclerosis* 1980; **35**:77–86.

26 Heinzlef O, Cohen A, Amarenco P. An update on aortic causes of ischemic stroke. *Curr Opin Neurol* 1997; **10**:64–72.

27 Moosy J. Morphology, sites and epidemiology of cerebral atherosclerosis in research publications. *Assoc Res Nerv Ment Dis* 2002; **51**:1–22.

28 Constantinides P. Pathogenesis of cerebral artery thrombosis in man. *Arch Pathol* 1967; **83**:422–8.

29 Lhermitte F, Gautier JC, Derouesne C. Nature of occlusions of the middle cerebral artery. *Neurology* 1970; **20**:82–8.

30 Ogata J, Masuda J, Yutani C, Yamaguchi T. Mechanisms of cerebral artery thrombosis: a histopathological analysis on eight necropsy cases. *J Neurol Neurosurg Psychiatry* 1994; **57**:17–21.

31 Lammie GA, Sandercock PA, Dennis MS. Recently occluded intracranial and extracranial carotid arteries: relevance of the unstable atherosclerotic plaque. *Stroke* 1999; **30**:1319–25.

32 Nicholls SC, Phillips DJ, Primozich JF, Lawrence RL, Kohler TR, Rudd TG *et al*. Diagnostic significance of flow separation in the carotid bulb. *Stroke* 1989; **20**:175–82.

33 Malek AM, Alper SL, Izumo S. Hemodynamic shear stress and its role in atherosclerosis. *J Am Med Assoc* 1999; **282**:2035–42.

34 Gnasso A, Irace C, Carallo C, De Franceschi MS, Motti C, Mattioli PL *et al*. In vivo association between low wall shear stress and plaque in subjects with asymmetrical carotid atherosclerosis. *Stroke* 1997; **28**:993–8.

35 Schulz UG, Rothwell PM. Major variation in carotid bifurcation anatomy: a possible risk factor for plaque development? *Stroke* 2001; **32**:2522–9.

36 Mitchell JR, Schwartz CJ. Relationship between arterial disease in different sites. A study of the aorta and coronary, carotid, and iliac arteries. *Br Med J* 1962; **5288**:1293–301.

37 Hertzer NR, Young JR, Beven EG, Graor RA, O'Hara PJ, Ruschhaupt WF, III *et al*. Coronary angiography in 506 patients with extracranial cerebrovascular disease. *Arch Intern Med* 1985; **145**:849–52.

38 Craven TE, Ryu JE, Espeland MA, Kahl FR, McKinney WM, Toole JF *et al*. Evaluation of the associations between carotid artery atherosclerosis and coronary artery stenosis: a case–control study. *Circulation* 1990; **82**:1230–42.

39 Chimowitz MI, Poole RM, Starling MR, Schwaiger M, Gross MD. Frequency and severity of asymptomatic coronary disease in patients with different causes of stroke. *Stroke* 1997; **28**:941–5.

40 O'Leary DH, Polak JF, Kronmal RA, Manolio TA, Burke GL, Wolfson SK, Jr. Carotid-artery intima and media thickness as a risk factor for myocardial infarction and stroke in older adults. Cardiovascular Health Study Collaborative Research Group. *N Engl J Med* 1999; **340**:14–22.

41 Clark TG, Murphy MF, Rothwell PM. Long term risks of stroke, myocardial infarction, and vascular death in 'low risk' patients with a non-recent transient ischaemic attack. *J Neurol Neurosurg Psychiatry* 2003; **74**:577–80.

42 Inzitari D, Hachinski VC, Taylor DW, Barnett HJ. Racial differences in the anterior circulation in cerebrovascular disease: how much can be explained by risk factors? *Arch Neurol* 1990; **47**:1080–4.

43 Sacco RL, Kargman DE, Gu Q, Zamanillo MC. Race-ethnicity and determinants of intracranial

atherosclerotic cerebral infarction. The Northern Manhattan Stroke Study. *Stroke* 1995; **26**:14–20.

44 Wityk RJ, Lehman D, Klag M, Coresh J, Ahn H, Litt B. Race and sex differences in the distribution of cerebral atherosclerosis. *Stroke* 1996; **27**:1974–80.

45 Gorelick PB. Distribution of atherosclerotic cerebrovascular lesions: effects of age, race, and sex. *Stroke* 1993; **24**:I16–I19.

46 Leung SY, Ng TH, Yuen ST, Lauder IJ, Ho FC. Pattern of cerebral atherosclerosis in Hong Kong Chinese: severity in intracranial and extracranial vessels. *Stroke* 1993; **24**:779–86.

47 Chen WH, Ho DS, Ho SL, Cheung RT, Cheng SW. Prevalence of extracranial carotid and vertebral artery disease in Chinese patients with coronary artery disease. *Stroke* 1998; **29**:631–4.

48 Connor MD, Walker R, Modi G, Warlow CP. Burden of stroke in black populations in sub-Saharan Africa. *Lancet Neurol* 2007; **6**:269–78.

49 Norris JW, Bornstein NM. Progression and regression of carotid stenosis. *Stroke* 1986; **17**:755–7.

50 Vane JR, Anggard EE, Botting RM. Regulatory functions of the vascular endothelium. *N Engl J Med* 1990; **323**:27–36.

51 Caplan LR, Hennerici M. Impaired clearance of emboli (washout) is an important link between hypoperfusion, embolism, and ischemic stroke. *Arch Neurol* 1998; **55**:1475–82.

52 Derdeyn CP, Grubb RL, Jr, Powers WJ. Re: Stages and thresholds of hemodynamic failure. *Stroke* 2003; **34**:589.

53 Derdeyn CP, Grubb RL, Jr, Powers WJ. Indications for cerebral revascularization for patients with atherosclerotic carotid occlusion. *Skull Base* 2005; **15**:7–14.

54 Ware JA, Heistad DD. Seminars in medicine of the Beth Israel Hospital, Boston: platelet-endothelium interactions. *N Engl J Med* 1993; **328**:628–35.

55 Libby P. Atheroma: more than mush. *Lancet* 1996; **348**(Suppl 1):s4–s7.

56 Viles-Gonzalez JF, Fuster V, Badimon JJ. Atherothrombosis: a widespread disease with unpredictable and life-threatening consequences. *Eur Heart J* 2004; **25**:1197–207.

57 Bogousslavsky J, Regli F. Unilateral watershed cerebral infarcts. *Neurology* 1986; **36**:373–7.

58 Hankey GJ, Warlow CP. Prognosis of sympomatic carotid artery occlusion: an overview. *Cerebrovasc Dis* 1991; **1**:245–56.

59 European Carotid Surgery Trialists Collaborative Group. Risk of stroke in the distribution of an asymptomatic carotid artery. *Lancet* 1995; **345**:209–12.

60 Klijn CJ, Kappelle LJ, Tulleken CA, van Gijn J. Symptomatic carotid artery occlusion: a reappraisal of hemodynamic factors. *Stroke* 1997; **28**:2084–93.

61 Castaigne P, Lhermitte F, Gautier JC, Escourelle R, Derousené C, Der Agopian P *et al*. Arterial occlusions in the vertebro-basilar system: a study of 44 patients with post-mortem data. *Brain* 1973; **96**:133–54.

62 Caplan LR, Tettenborn B. Vertebrobasilar occlusive disease: review of selected aspects. 2. Posterior circulation embolism. *Cerebrovasc Dis* 1992; **2**:320–6.

63 Koennecke HC, Mast H, Trocio SS, Jr, Sacco RL, Thompson JL, Mohr JP. Microemboli in patients with vertebrobasilar ischemia: association with vertebrobasilar and cardiac lesions. *Stroke* 1997; **28**:593–6.

64 Schwarz S, Egelhof T, Schwab S, Hacke W. Basilar artery embolism: clinical syndrome and neuroradiologic patterns in patients without permanent occlusion of the basilar artery. *Neurology* 1997; **49**:1346–52.

65 Martin PJ, Chang HM, Wityk R, Caplan LR. Midbrain infarction: associations and aetiologies in the New England Medical Center Posterior Circulation Registry. *J Neurol Neurosurg Psychiatry* 1998; **64**:392–5.

66 Vernieri F, Pasqualetti P, Matteis M, Passarelli F, Troisi E, Rossini PM *et al*. Effect of collateral blood flow and cerebral vasomotor reactivity on the outcome of carotid artery occlusion. *Stroke* 2001; **32**:1552–8.

67 Markus H, Cullinane M. Severely impaired cerebrovascular reactivity predicts stroke and TIA risk in patients with carotid artery stenosis and occlusion. *Brain* 2001; **124**:457–67.

68 Silvestrini M, Vernieri F, Pasqualetti P, Matteis M, Passarelli F, Troisi E *et al*. Impaired cerebral vasoreactivity and risk of stroke in patients with asymptomatic carotid artery stenosis. *J Am Med Assoc* 2000; **283**:2122–7.

69 Rutgers DR, Klijn CJ, Kappelle LJ, van der Grond J. Recurrent stroke in patients with symptomatic carotid artery occlusion is associated with high-volume flow to the brain and increased collateral circulation. *Stroke* 2004; **35**:1345–9.

70 Fuster V, Fayad ZA, Badimon JJ. Acute coronary syndromes: biology. *Lancet* 1999; **353**(Suppl 2):SII5–SII9.

71 Lovett JK, Gallagher PJ, Hands LJ, Walton J, Rothwell PM. Histological correlates of carotid plaque surface morphology on lumen contrast imaging. *Circulation* 2004; **110**:2190–7.

72 Redgrave JN, Lovett JK, Gallagher PJ, Rothwell PM. Histological assessment of 526 symptomatic carotid plaques in relation to the nature and timing of ischemic symptoms: the Oxford plaque study. *Circulation* 2006; **113**:2320–8.

73 Rothwell PM, Villagra R, Gibson R, Donders RC, Warlow CP. Evidence of a chronic systemic cause of instability of atherosclerotic plaques. *Lancet* 2000; **355**:19–24.

74 Torvik A, Svindland A, Lindboe CF. Pathogenesis of carotid thrombosis. *Stroke* 1989; **20**:1477–83.

75 Ogata J, Masuda J, Yutani C, Yamaguchi T. Rupture of atheromatous plaque as a cause of thrombotic occlusion of stenotic internal carotid artery. *Stroke* 1990; **21**:1740–5.

76 Davies MJ. The composition of coronary-artery plaques. *N Engl J Med* 1997; **336**:1312–14.

77 Lovett JK, Redgrave JN, Rothwell PM. A critical appraisal of the performance, reporting, and interpretation of studies comparing carotid plaque imaging with histology. *Stroke* 2005; **36**:1091–7.

78 Rothwell PM, Warlow CP. Timing of TIAs preceding stroke: time window for prevention is very short. *Neurology* 2005; **64**:817–20.

79 Coull AJ, Lovett JK, Rothwell PM. Population based study of early risk of stroke after transient ischaemic attack or minor stroke: implications for public education and organisation of services. *Br Med J* 2004; **328**:326.

80 Fairhead JF, Mehta Z, Rothwell PM. Population-based study of delays in carotid imaging and surgery and the risk of recurrent stroke. *Neurology* 2005; **65**:371–5.

81 Lovett JK, Coull AJ, Rothwell PM. Early risk of recurrence by subtype of ischemic stroke in population-based incidence studies. *Neurology* 2004; **62**:569–73.

82 Molloy J, Khan N, Markus HS. Temporal variability of asymptomatic embolization in carotid artery stenosis and optimal recording protocols. *Stroke* 1998; **29**:1129–32.

83 Wijman CA, Babikian VL, Matjucha IC, Koleini B, Hyde C, Winter MR *et al.* Cerebral microembolism in patients with retinal ischemia. *Stroke* 1998; **29**:1139–43.

84 Droste DW, Dittrich R, Kemeny V, Schulte-Altedorneburg G, Ringelstein EB. Prevalence and frequency of microembolic signals in 105 patients with extracranial carotid artery occlusive disease. *J Neurol Neurosurg Psychiatry* 1999; **67**:525–8.

85 Molloy J, Markus HS. Asymptomatic embolization predicts stroke and TIA risk in patients with carotid artery stenosis. *Stroke* 1999; **30**:1440–3.

86 Dittrich R, Ritter MA, Kaps M, Siebler M, Lees K, Larrue V *et al.* The use of embolic signal detection in multicenter trials to evaluate antiplatelet efficacy: signal analysis and quality control mechanisms in the CARESS (Clopidogrel and Aspirin for Reduction of Emboli in Symptomatic carotid Stenosis) trial. *Stroke* 2006; **37**:1065–9.

87 Markus HS. Can miroemboli on transcranial Doppler identify patients at increased stroke risk? *Nature Clin Pract Cardiovasc Med* 2006; **3**:246–7.

88 Kaposzta Z, Young E, Bath PM, Markus HS. Clinical application of asymptomatic embolic signal detection in acute stroke: a prospective study. *Stroke* 1999; **30**:1814–18.

89 Cuffe RL, Rothwell PM. Effect of nonoptimal imaging on the relationship between the measured degree of symptomatic carotid stenosis and risk of ischemic stroke. *Stroke* 2006; **37**:1785–91.

90 Fuster V, Badimon L, Badimon JJ, Chesebro JH. The pathogenesis of coronary artery disease and the acute coronary syndromes (1). *N Engl J Med* 1992; **326**:242–50.

91 Rothwell PM, Gibson R, Warlow CP. Interrelation between plaque surface morphology and degree of stenosis on carotid angiograms and the risk of ischemic stroke in patients with symptomatic carotid stenosis. On behalf of the European Carotid Surgery Trialists' Collaborative Group. *Stroke* 2000; **31**:615–21.

92 Hatsukami TS, Ferguson MS, Beach KW, Gordon D, Detmer P, Burns D *et al.* Carotid plaque morphology and clinical events. *Stroke* 1997; **28**:95–100.

93 Golledge J, Greenhalgh RM, Davies AH. The symptomatic carotid plaque. *Stroke* 2000; **31**:774–81.

94 Fisher M, Paganini-Hill A, Martin A, Cosgrove M, Toole JF, Barnett HJ *et al.* Carotid plaque pathology: thrombosis, ulceration, and stroke pathogenesis. *Stroke* 2005; **36**:253–7.

95 DeGraba TJ, Siren AL, Penix L, McCarron RM, Hargraves R, Sood S *et al.* Increased endothelial expression of intercellular adhesion molecule-1 in symptomatic versus asymptomatic human carotid atherosclerotic plaque. *Stroke* 1998; **29**:1405–10.

96 Jander S, Sitzer M, Schumann R, Schroeter M, Siebler M, Steinmetz H *et al.* Inflammation in high-grade carotid stenosis: a possible role for macrophages and T cells in plaque destabilization. *Stroke* 1998; **29**:1625–30.

97 Loftus IM, Naylor AR, Goodall S, Crowther M, Jones L, Bell PR *et al.* Increased matrix metalloproteinase-9 activity in unstable carotid plaques. A potential role in acute plaque disruption. *Stroke* 2000; **31**:40–7.

98 Ardissino D, Merlini PA, Ariens R, Coppola R, Bramucci E, Mannucci PM. Tissue-factor antigen and activity in human coronary atherosclerotic plaques. *Lancet* 1997; **349**:769–71.

99 Richardson PD, Davies MJ, Born GV. Influence of plaque configuration and stress distribution on fissuring of coronary atherosclerotic plaques. *Lancet* 1989; **2**:941–4.

100 Meairs S, Hennerici M. Four-dimensional ultrasonographic characterization of plaque surface motion in patients with symptomatic and asymptomatic carotid artery stenosis. *Stroke* 1999; **30**:1807–13.

101 Little JR, St Louis P, Weinstein M, Dohn DF. Giant fusiform aneurysm of the cerebral arteries. *Stroke* 1981; **12**:183–8.

102 Nishizaki T, Tamaki N, Takeda N, Shirakuni T, Kondoh T, Matsumoto S. Dolichoectatic basilar artery: a review of 23 cases. *Stroke* 1986; **17**:1277–81.

103 Ince B, Petty GW, Brown RD, Jr, Chu CP, Sicks JD, Whisnant JP. Dolichoectasia of the intracranial arteries in patients with first ischemic stroke: a population-based study. *Neurology* 1998; **50**:1694–8.

104 Idbaih A, Pico F, Guichard JP, Bousser MG, Chabriat H. Clinical course and MRI changes of basilar artery dolichoectasia: three case reports. *Cerebrovasc Dis* 2004; **17**:262–4.

105 Savitz SI, Ronthal M, Caplan LR. Vertebral artery compression of the medulla. *Arch Neurol* 2006; **63**:234–41.

106 Aichner TT, Flever SR, Birbamer GG, Posch A. Magnetic resonance imaging and magnetic resonance angiography of vertebrobasilar dolichoectasia. *Cerebrovasc Dis* 1993; **3**:280–4.

107 Pessin MS, Chimowitz MI, Levine SR, Kwan ES, Adelman LS, Earnest MP *et al.* Stroke in patients with fusiform vertebrobasilar aneurysms. *Neurology* 1989; **39**:16–21.

108 Schwartz A, Rautenberg W, Hennerici M. Dolichoectatic intracranial arteries: review of selected aspects. *Cerebrovasc Dis* 1993; **3**:273–9.

109 Passero S, Filosomi G. Posterior circulation infarcts in patients with vertebrobasilar dolichoectasia. *Stroke* 1998; **29**:653–9.

110 Hegedus K. Ectasia of the basilar artery with special reference to possible pathogenesis. *Surg Neurol* 1985; **24**:463–9.

111 Rolfs A, Bottcher T, Zschiesche M, Morris P, Winchester B, Bauer P *et al.* Prevalence of Fabry disease in patients with cryptogenic stroke: a prospective study. *Lancet* 2005; **366**:1794–6.

112 Lammie GA, Brannan F, Slattery J, Warlow C. Nonhypertensive cerebral small-vessel disease: an autopsy study. *Stroke* 1997; **28**:2222–9.

113 Hassan A, Hunt BJ, O'Sullivan M, Parmar K, Bamford JM, Briley D *et al*. Markers of endothelial dysfunction in lacunar infarction and ischaemic leukoaraiosis. *Brain* 2003; **126**:424–32.

114 Lammie GA. Pathology of small vessel stroke. *Br Med Bull* 2000; **56**:296–306.

115 Lammie GA. Hypertensive cerebral small vessel disease and stroke. *Brain Pathol* 2002; **12**:358–70.

116 Lammie GA, Wardlaw JM. Small centrum ovale infarcts: a pathological study. *Cerebrovasc Dis* 1999; **9**:82–90.

117 Fisher CM. The arterial lesions underlying lacunes. *Acta Neuropathol (Berl)* 1968; **12**:1–15.

118 Fisher CM. Capsular infarcts: the underlying vascular lesions. *Arch Neurol* 1979; **36**:65–73.

119 Fisher CM. Lacunar infarcts: a review. *Cerebrovasc Dis* 1991; **1**:311–20.

120 Bamford J, Sandercock P, Jones L, Warlow C. The natural history of lacunar infarction: the Oxfordshire Community Stroke Project. *Stroke* 1987; **18**:545–51.

121 Bamford JM, Warlow CP. Evolution and testing of the lacunar hypothesis. *Stroke* 1988; **19**:1074–82.

122 Besson G, Hommel M, Perret J. Historical aspects of the lacunar concept. *Cerebrovasc Dis* 1991; **1**:306–10.

123 Donnan GA, Norrving B, Bamford J, Bogousslavsky J. *Lacunar and Other Subcortical Infarctions*. Oxford: Oxford University Press, 1995.

124 Ay H, Oliveira-Filho J, Buonanno FS, Ezzeddine M, Schaefer PW, Rordorf G *et al*. Diffusion-weighted imaging identifies a subset of lacunar infarction associated with embolic source. *Stroke* 1999; **30**:2644–50.

125 Millikan C, Futrell N. The fallacy of the lacune hypothesis. *Stroke* 1990; **21**:1251–7.

126 Horowitz DR, Tuhrim S, Weinberger JM, Rudolph SH. Mechanisms in lacunar infarction. *Stroke* 1992; **23**:325–7.

127 Olsen TS, Skriver EB, Herning M. Cause of cerebral infarction in the carotid territory: its relation to the size and the location of the infarct and to the underlying vascular lesion. *Stroke* 1985; **16**:459–66.

128 Lodder J, Bamford JM, Sandercock PA, Jones LN, Warlow CP. Are hypertension or cardiac embolism likely causes of lacunar infarction? *Stroke* 1990; **21**:375–81.

129 Hankey GJ, Warlow CP. Lacunar transient ischaemic attacks: a clinically useful concept? *Lancet* 1991; **337**:335–8.

130 Landi G, Motto C, Cella E, Musicco M, Lipari S, Boccardi E *et al*. Pathogenetic and prognostic features of lacunar transient ischaemic attack syndromes. *J Neurol Neurosurg Psychiatry* 1993; **56**:1265–70.

131 Mast H, Thompson JL, Voller H, Mohr JP, Marx P. Cardiac sources of embolism in patients with pial artery infarcts and lacunar lesions. *Stroke* 1994; **25**:776–81.

132 Gan R, Sacco RL, Kargman DE, Roberts JK, Boden-Albala B, Gu Q. Testing the validity of the lacunar hypothesis: the Northern Manhattan Stroke Study experience. *Neurology* 1997; **48**:1204–11.

133 Mead GE, Lewis SC, Wardlaw JM, Dennis MS, Warlow CP. Should computed tomography appearance of lacunar stroke influence patient management? *J Neurol Neurosurg Psychiatry* 1999; **67**:682–4.

134 Mead GE, Wardlaw JM, Dennis MS, Lewis SC, Warlow CP. Relationship between pattern of intracranial artery abnormalities on transcranial doppler and Oxfordshire Community Stroke Project clinical classification of ischemic stroke. *Stroke* 2000; **31**:714–19.

135 Jackson C, Sudlow C. Comparing risks of death and recurrent vascular events between lacunar and non-lacunar infarction. *Brain* 2005; **128**:2507–17.

136 Jackson C, Sudlow C. Are lacunar strokes really different? a systematic review of differences in risk factor profiles between lacunar and nonlacunar infarcts. *Stroke* 2005; **36**:891–901.

137 Tegeler CH, Knappertz VA, Nagaraja D, Mooney M, Dalley GM. Relationship of common carotid artery high intensity transient signals in patients with ischaemic stroke to white matter versus territorial infarct pattern on brain CT scan. *Cerebrovasc Dis* 1995; **5**:128–32.

138 Daffertshofer M, Ries S, Schminke U, Hennerici M. High-intensity transient signals in patients with cerebral ischemia. *Stroke* 1996; **27**:1844–9.

139 Koennecke HC, Mast H, Trocio SH, Jr, Sacco RL, Ma W, Mohr JP *et al*. Frequency and determinants of microembolic signals on transcranial Doppler in unselected patients with acute carotid territory ischemia: a prospective study. *Cerebrovasc Dis* 1998; **8**:107–12.

140 Serena J, Segura T, Castellanos M, Davalos A. Microembolic signal monitoring in hemispheric acute ischaemic stroke: a prospective study. *Cerebrovasc Dis* 2000; **10**:278–82.

141 Molina C, Sabin JA, Montaner J, Rovira A, Abilleira S, Codina A. Impaired cerebrovascular reactivity as a risk marker for first-ever lacunar infarction: a case–control study. *Stroke* 1999; **30**:2296–301.

142 Fisher CM. Cerebral miliary aneurysms in hypertension. *Am J Pathol* 1972; **66**:313–30.

143 Challa VR, Moody DM, Bell MA. The Charcot-Bouchard aneurysm controversy: impact of a new histologic technique. *J Neuropathol Exp Neurol* 1992; **51**:264–71.

144 Samuelsson M, Lindell D, Norrving B. Presumed pathogenic mechanisms of recurrent stroke after lacunar infarction. *Cerebrovasc Dis* 1996; **6**:128–36.

145 Kwa VI, Franke CL, Verbeeten B, Jr, Stam J. Silent intracerebral microhemorrhages in patients with ischemic stroke. Amsterdam Vascular Medicine Group. *Ann Neurol* 1998; **44**:372–7.

146 Roob G, Schmidt R, Kapeller P, Lechner A, Hartung HP, Fazekas F. MRI evidence of past cerebral microbleeds in a healthy elderly population. *Neurology* 1999; **52**:991–4.

147 Sacco SE, Whisnant JP, Broderick JP, Phillips SJ, O'Fallon WM. Epidemiological characteristics of lacunar infarcts in a population. *Stroke* 1991; **22**:1236–41.

148 Boiten J, Lodder J. Prognosis for survival, handicap and recurrence of stroke in lacunar and superficial infarction. *Cerebrovasc Dis* 1993; **3**:221–6.

149 van Zagten M, Lodder J, Franke C, Heuts-van Raak L, Claassens C, Kessels F. Different vascular risk factor profiles in primary intracerebral haemorrhage and small deep infarcts do not suggest similar types of underlying small vessel disease. *Cerebrovasc Dis* 1994; **4**:121–4.

150 Boiten J, Rothwell PM, Slattery J, Warlow C. for the European Carotid Surgery Trialists' Collaborative Group. Ischaemic lacunar stroke in the European Carotid Surgery Trial: risk factors, distribution of carotid stenosis, effect of surgery and type of recurrent stroke. *Cerebrovasc Dis* 1996; **6**:281–7.

151 Schmal M, Marini C, Carolei A, Di Napoli M, Kessels F, Lodder J. Different vascular risk factor profiles among cortical infarcts, small deep infarcts, and primary intracerebral haemorrhage point to different types of underlying vasculopathy. A study from the L'Aquila Stroke Registry. *Cerebrovasc Dis* 1998; **8**:14–19.

152 Kappelle LJ, van Latum JC, van Swieten JC, Algra A, Koudstaal PJ, van Gijn J. Recurrent stroke after transient ischaemic attack or minor ischaemic stroke: does the distinction between small and large vessel disease remain true to type? Dutch TIA Trial Study Group. *J Neurol Neurosurg Psychiatry* 1995; **59**:127–31.

153 Bogousslavsky J, Regli F, Despland PA, Zografos L. Optic nerve head infarction: small artery disease, large artery disease and cardioembolism. *Cerebrovasc Dis* 1991; **1**:341–4.

154 Fry CL, Carter JE, Kanter MC, Tegeler CH, Tuley MR. Anterior ischemic optic neuropathy is not associated with carotid artery atherosclerosis. *Stroke* 1993; **24**:539–42.

155 Nishide M, Irino T, Gotoh M, Naka M, Tsuji K. Cardiac abnormalities in ischemic cerebrovascular disease studied by two-dimensional echocardiography. *Stroke* 1983; **14**:541–5.

156 Cerebral Embolism Task Force. Cardiogenic brain embolism: the second report of the cerebral embolism task force. *Arch Neurol* 1989; **46**:727–43.

157 Kittner SJ, Sharkness CM, Price TR, Plotnick GD, Dambrosia JM, Wolf PA *et al*. Infarcts with a cardiac source of embolism in the NINCDS Stroke Data Bank: historical features. *Neurology* 1990; **40**:281–4.

158 Kittner SJ, Sharkness CM, Sloan MA, Price TR, Dambrosia JM, Tuhrim S *et al*. Features on initial computed tomography scan of infarcts with a cardiac source of embolism in the NINDS Stroke Data Bank. *Stroke* 1992; **23**:1748–51.

159 Hart RG. Cardiogenic embolism to the brain. *Lancet* 1992; **339**:589–94.

160 Oppenheimer SM, Lima J. Neurology and the heart. *J Neurol Neurosurg Psychiatry* 1998; **64**:289–97.

161 De Bono DP, Warlow CP. Potential sources of emboli in patients with presumed transient cerebral or retinal ischaemia. *Lancet* 1981; **1**:343–6.

162 Bogousslavsky J, Regli F. Borderzone infarctions distal to internal carotid artery occlusion: prognostic implications. *Ann Neurol* 1986; **20**:346–50.

163 Bogousslavsky J, Van Melle G, Regli F, Kappenberger L. Pathogenesis of anterior circulation stroke in patients with nonvalvular atrial fibrillation: the Lausanne Stroke Registry. *Neurology* 1990; **40**:1046–50.

164 Kempster PA, Gerraty RP, Gates PC. Asymptomatic cerebral infarction in patients with chronic atrial fibrillation. *Stroke* 1988; **19**:955–7.

165 Caplan LR. Brain embolism, revisited. *Neurology* 1993; **43**:1281–7.

166 Cullinane M, Wainwright R, Brown A, Monaghan M, Markus HS. Asymptomatic embolization in subjects with atrial fibrillation not taking anticoagulants: a prospective study. *Stroke* 1998; **29**:1810–15.

167 Nabavi DG, Arato S, Droste DW, Schulte-Altedorneburg G, Kemeny V, Reinecke H *et al*. Microembolic load in asymptomatic patients with cardiac aneurysm, severe ventricular dysfunction, and atrial fibrillation: clinical and hemorheological correlates. *Cerebrovasc Dis* 1998; **8**:214–21.

168 Sandercock P, Bamford J, Dennis M, Burn J, Slattery J, Jones L *et al*. Atrial fibrillation and stroke: prevalence in different types of stroke and influence on early and long-term prognosis (Oxfordshire Community Stroke Project). *Br Med J* 1992; **305**:1460–5.

169 Shafqat S, Kelly PJ, Furie KL. Holter monitoring in the diagnosis of stroke mechanism. *Intern Med J* 2004; **34**:305–9.

170 Wolf PA, Abbott RD, Kannel WB. Atrial fibrillation as an independent risk factor for stroke: the Framingham Study. *Stroke* 1991; **22**:983–8.

171 Narayan SM, Cain ME, Smith JM. Atrial fibrillation. *Lancet* 1997; **350**:943–50.

172 Anderson DC, Koller RL, Asinger RW, Bundlie SR, Pearce LA. Atrial fibrillation and stroke: epidemiology, pathophysiology and management. *Neurologist* 1998; **4**:235–58.

173 Hart RG, Benavente O, McBride R, Pearce LA. Antithrombotic therapy to prevent stroke in patients with atrial fibrillation: a meta-analysis. *Ann Intern Med* 1999; **131**:492–501.

174 Lip GY. Atrial fibrillation (recent onset). *Clin Evid* 2005; **14**:71–89.

175 Chang YJ, Ryu SJ, Lin SK. Carotid artery stenosis in ischemic stroke patients with nonvalvular atrial fibrillation. *Cerebrovasc Dis* 2002; **13**:16–20.

176 Lip GY, Boos CJ. Antithrombotic treatment in atrial fibrillation. *Heart* 2006; **92**:155–61.

177 Weinberger J, Rothlauf E, Materese E, Halperin J. Noninvasive evaluation of the extracranial carotid arteries in patients with cerebrovascular events and atrial fibrillations. *Arch Intern Med* 1988; **148**:1785–8.

178 Vingerhoets F, Bogousslavsky J, Regli F, Van Melle G. Atrial fibrillation after acute stroke. *Stroke* 1993; **24**:26–30.

179 Kanter MC, Tegeler CH, Pearce LA, Weinberger J, Feinberg WM, Anderson DC *et al*. Carotid stenosis in patients with atrial fibrillation: prevalence, risk factors, and relationship to stroke in the Stroke Prevention in Atrial Fibrillation Study. *Arch Intern Med* 1994; **154**:1372–7.

180 Blackshear JL, Pearce LA, Hart RG, Zabalgoitia M, Labovitz A, Asinger RW *et al*. Aortic plaque in atrial fibrillation:

prevalence, predictors, and thromboembolic implications. *Stroke* 1999; **30**:834–40.

181 Davies MJ, Pomerance A. Pathology of atrial fibrillation in man. *Br Heart J* 1972; **34**:520–5.

182 MacMahon S, Rodgers A. The effects of blood pressure reduction in older patients: an overview of five randomized controlled trials in elderly hypertensives. *Clin Exp Hypertens* 1993; **15**:967–78.

183 Daniel WG. Should transesophageal echocardiography be used to guide cardioversion? *N Engl J Med* 1993; **328**:803–4.

184 Stollberger C, Chnupa P, Kronik G, Brainin M, Finsterer J, Schneider B *et al*. Transesophageal echocardiography to assess embolic risk in patients with atrial fibrillation. ELAT Study Group. Embolism in Left Atrial Thrombi. *Ann Intern Med* 1998; **128**:630–8.

185 Sitburana O, Koroshetz WJ. Magnetic resonance imaging: implication in acute ischemic stroke management. *Curr Atheroscler Rep* 2005; **7**:305–12.

186 Aberg H. Atrial fibrillation. I. A study of atrial thrombosis and systemic embolism in a necropsy material. *Acta Med Scand* 1969; **185**:373–9.

187 EAFT Study Group. Silent brain infarction in non-rheumatic atrial fibrillation. *Neurology* 2007; **46**:159–65.

188 Britton M, Gustafsson C. Non-rheumatic atrial fibrillation as a risk factor for stroke. *Stroke* 1985; **16**:182–8.

189 Yamanouchi H, Nagura H, Mizutani T, Matsushita S, Esaki Y. Embolic brain infarction in nonrheumatic atrial fibrillation: a clinicopathologic study in the elderly. *Neurology* 1997; **48**:1593–7.

190 Friedman GD, Loveland DB, Ehrlich SP, Jr. Relationship of stroke to other cardiovascular disease. *Circulation* 1968; **38**:533–41.

191 Wolf PA, Dawber TR, Thomas HE, Jr, Kannel WB. Epidemiologic assessment of chronic atrial fibrillation and risk of stroke: the Framingham study. *Neurology* 1978; **28**:973–7.

192 Davis PH, Dambrosia JM, Schoenberg BS, Schoenberg DG, Pritchard DA, Lilienfeld AM *et al*. Risk factors for ischemic stroke: a prospective study in Rochester, Minnesota. *Ann Neurol* 1987; **22**:319–27.

193 Flegel KM, Shipley MJ, Rose G. Risk of stroke in non-rheumatic atrial fibrillation. *Lancet* 1987; **1**:526–9.

194 Harmsen P, Rosengren A, Tsipogianni A, Wilhelmsen L. Risk factors for stroke in middle-aged men in Goteborg, Sweden. *Stroke* 1990; **21**:223–9.

195 Hart RG, Pearce LA, Miller VT, Anderson DC, Rothrock JF, Albers GW *et al*. Cardioembolic vs. noncardioembolic strokes in atrial fibrillation: frequency and effect of antithrombotic agents in the stroke prevention in atrial fibrillation studies. *Cerebrovasc Dis* 2000; **10**:39–43.

196 Close JB, Evans DW, Bailey SM. Persistent lone atrial fibrillation: its prognosis after clinical diagnosis. *J R Coll Gen Pract* 1979; **29**:547–9.

197 Brand FN, Abbott RD, Kannel WB, Wolf PA. Characteristics and prognosis of lone atrial fibrillation: 30-year follow-up in the Framingham Study. *J Am Med Assoc* 1985; **254**:3449–53.

198 Kopecky SL, Gersh BJ, McGoon MD, Whisnant JP, Holmes DR, Jr, Ilstrup DM *et al*. The natural history of lone atrial fibrillation: a population-based study over three decades. *N Engl J Med* 1987; **317**:669–74.

199 Atrial Fibrillation Investigators. Risk factors for stroke and efficacy of antithrombotic therapy in atrial fibrillation: analysis of pooled data from five randomised controlled trials. *Arch Intern Med* 1994; **154**:1449–57.

200 Atrial Fibrillation Investigators. Echocardiographic predictors of stroke in patients with atrial fibrillation: a prospective study of 1066 patients from 3 clinical trials. *Arch Intern Med* 1998; **158**:1316–20.

201 Benjamin EJ, D'Agostino RB, Belanger AJ, Wolf PA, Levy D. Left atrial size and the risk of stroke and death. The Framingham Heart Study. *Circulation* 1995; **92**: 835–41.

202 Van Latum JC, Koudstaal PJ, Venables GS, van Gijn J, Kappelle LJ, Algra A. Predictors of major vascular events in patients with a transient ischemic attack or minor ischemic stroke and with nonrheumatic atrial fibrillation. European Atrial Fibrillation Trial (EAFT) Study Group. *Stroke* 1995; **26**:801–6.

203 Hart RG, Pearce LA, McBride R, Rothbart RM, Asinger RW. Factors associated with ischemic stroke during aspirin therapy in atrial fibrillation: analysis of 2012 participants in the SPAF I-III clinical trials. The Stroke Prevention in Atrial Fibrillation (SPAF) Investigators. *Stroke* 1999; **30**:1223–9.

204 Chimowitz MI, DeGeorgia MA, Poole RM, Hepner A, Armstrong WM. Left atrial spontaneous echo contrast is highly associated with previous stroke in patients with atrial fibrillation or mitral stenosis. *Stroke* 1993; **24**:1015–19.

205 Lip GY. Does atrial fibrillation confer a hypercoagulable state? *Lancet* 1995; **346**:1313–14.

206 The Stroke Prevention in Atrial Fibrillation Investigators Committee on Echocardiography. Transesophageal echocardiographic correlates of thromboembolism in high-risk patients with nonvalvular atrial fibrillation. *Ann Intern Med* 1998; **128**:639–47.

207 Nattel S, Opie LH. Controversies in atrial fibrillation. *Lancet* 2006; **367**:262–72.

208 Gage BF, Waterman AD, Shannon W, Boechler M, Rich MW, Radford MJ. Validation of clinical classification schemes for predicting stroke: results from the National Registry of Atrial Fibrillation. *J Am Med Assoc* 2001; **285**:2864–70.

209 Go AS, Hylek EM, Chang Y, Phillips KA, Henault LE, Capra AM *et al*. Anticoagulation therapy for stroke prevention in atrial fibrillation: how well do randomized trials translate into clinical practice? *J Am Med Assoc* 2003; **290**:2685–92.

210 Gage BF, van Walraven C, Pearce L, Hart RG, Koudstaal PJ, Boode BS *et al*. Selecting patients with atrial fibrillation for anticoagulation: stroke risk stratification in patients taking aspirin. *Circulation* 2004; **110**:2287–92.

211 Hart RG, Halperin JL, Pearce LA, Anderson DC, Kronmal RA, McBride R *et al*. Lessons from the Stroke Prevention in Atrial Fibrillation trials. *Ann Intern Med* 2003; **138**:831–8.

212 Man-Son-Hing M, Laupacis A, O'Connor AM, Hart RG, Feldman G, Blackshear JL *et al.* Development of a decision aid for atrial fibrillation who are considering antithrombotic therapy. *J Gen Intern Med* 2000; **15**:723–30.

213 McAlister FA, Man-Son-Hing M, Straus SE, Ghali WA, Anderson D, Majumdar SR *et al.* Impact of a patient decision aid on care among patients with nonvalvular atrial fibrillation: a cluster randomized trial. *Can Med Assoc J* 2005; **173**:496–501.

214 Lip GY, Hee FL. Paroxysmal atrial fibrillation. *QJM* 2001; **94**:665–78.

215 Saxonhouse SJ, Curtis AB. Risks and benefits of rate control versus maintenance of sinus rhythm. *Am J Cardiol* 2003; **91**:27D–32D.

216 Segal JB, McNamara RL, Miller MR, Powe NR, Goodman SN, Robinson KA *et al.* Anticoagulants or antiplatelet therapy for non-rheumatic atrial fibrillation and flutter. *Cochrane Database Syst Rev* 2001; CD001938.

217 Blackshear JL, Safford RE. AFFIRM and RACE trials: implications for the management of atrial fibrillation. *Card Electrophysiol Rev* 2003; **7**:366–9.

218 Sliwka U, Georgiadis D. Clinical correlations of Doppler microembolic signals in patients with prosthetic cardiac valves: analysis of 580 cases. *Stroke* 1998; **29**:140–3.

219 Georgiadis D, Baumgartner RW, Uhlmann F, Lindner A, Zerkowski HR, Zierz S. Venous microemboli in patients with artificial heart valves. *Cerebrovasc Dis* 1999; **9**:238–41.

220 Vongpatanasin W, Hillis LD, Lange RA. Prosthetic heart valves. *N Engl J Med* 1996; **335**:407–16.

221 O'Neill WW, Chandler JG, Gordon RE, Bakalyar DM, Abolfathi AH, Castellani MD *et al.* Radiographic detection of strut separations in Bjork-Shiley convexo-concave mitral valves. *N Engl J Med* 1995; **333**:414–19.

222 Naumann M, Hofmann E, Toyka KV. Multifocal brain MRI hypointensities secondary to embolic metal fragments from a mechanical heart valve prosthesis: a possible source of epileptic seizures. *Neurology* 1998; **51**:1766–7.

223 Peterseim DS, Cen YY, Cheruvu S, Landolfo K, Bashore TM, Lowe JE *et al.* Long-term outcome after biologic versus mechanical aortic valve replacement in 841 patients. *J Thorac Cardiovasc Surg* 1999; **117**:890–7.

224 Ruel M, Kulik A, Rubens FD, Bedard P, Masters RG, Pipe AL *et al.* Late incidence and determinants of reoperation in patients with prosthetic heart valves. *Eur J Cardiothorac Surg* 2004; **25**:364–70.

225 Orszulak TA, Schaff HV, Mullany CJ, Anderson BJ, Ilstrup DM, Puga FJ *et al.* Risk of thromboembolism with the aortic Carpentier-Edwards bioprosthesis. *Ann Thorac Surg* 1995; **59**:462–8.

226 Daley R, Mattingly TW, Holt CL, Bland EF, White PD. Systemic arterial embolism in rheumatic heart disease. *Am Heart J* 1951; **42**:566–81.

227 Coulshed N, Epstein EJ, McKendrick CS, Galloway RW, Walker E. Systemic embolism in mitral valve disease. *Br Heart J* 1970; **32**:26–34.

228 Swash M, Earl CJ. Transient visual obscurations in chronic rheumatic heart-disease. *Lancet* 1970; **2**:323–6.

229 Holley KE, Bahn RC, McGoon DC, Mankin HT. Spontaneous calcific embolisation associated with calcific aortic stenosis. *Circulation* 1963; **27**:197–202.

230 Penner R, Font RL. Retinal embolism from calcified vegetations of aortic valve: spontaneous complication of rheumatic heart disease. *Arch Ophthalmol* 1969; **81**:565–8.

231 De Bono DP, Warlow CP. Mitral-annulus calcification and cerebral or retinal ischaemia. *Lancet* 1979; **2**:383–5.

232 Boon A, Lodder J, Cheriex E, Kessels F. Risk of stroke in a cohort of 815 patients with calcification of the aortic valve with or without stenosis. *Stroke* 1996; **27**:847–51.

233 Mouton P, Biousse V, Crassard I, Bousson V, Bousser MG. Ischemic stroke due to calcific emboli from mitral valve annulus calcification. *Stroke* 1997; **28**:2325–6.

234 Shanmugam V, Chhablani R, Gorelick PB. Spontaneous calcific cerebral embolus. *Neurology* 1997; **48**:538–9.

235 Adler Y, Koren A, Fink N, Tanne D, Fusman R, Assali A *et al.* Association between mitral annulus calcification and carotid atherosclerotic disease. *Stroke* 1998; **29**:1833–7.

236 Devereux RB, Brown WT, Kramer-Fox R, Sachs I. Inheritance of mitral leaflet prolapse: effect of age and sex on gene expression. *Ann Intern Med* 1982; **97**:826–32.

237 Devereux RB, Kramer-Fox R, Shear MK, Kligfield P, Pini R, Savage DD. Diagnosis and classification of severity of mitral leaflet prolapse: methodologic, biologic, and prognostic considerations. *Am Heart J* 1987; **113**:1265–80.

238 Freed LA, Levy D, Levine RA, Larson MG, Evans JC, Fuller DL *et al.* Prevalence and clinical outcome of mitral-valve prolapse. *N Engl J Med* 1999; **341**:1–7.

239 Theal M, Sleik K, Anand S, Yi Q, Yusuf S, Lonn E. Prevalence of mitral leaflet prolapse in ethnic groups. *Can J Cardiol* 2004; **20**:511–15.

240 Leong SW, Soor GS, Butany J, Henry J, Thangaroopan M, Leask RL. Morphological findings in 192 surgically excised native mitral valves. *Can J Cardiol* 2006; **22**:1055–61.

241 Barnett HJ, Boughner DR, Taylor DW, Cooper PE, Kostuk WJ, Nichol PM. Further evidence relating mitral-valve prolapse to cerebral ischemic events. *N Engl J Med* 1980; **302**:139–44.

242 Geyer SJ, Franzini DA. Myxomatous degeneration of the mitral valve complicated by nonbacterial thrombotic endocarditis with systemic embolization. *Am J Clin Pathol* 1979; **72**:489–92.

243 Chesler E, King RA, Edwards JE. The myxomatous mitral valve and sudden death. *Circulation* 1983; **67**:632–9.

244 Cabanes L, Mas JL, Cohen A, Amarenco P, Cabanes PA, Oubary P *et al.* Atrial septal aneurysm and patent foramen ovale as risk factors for cryptogenic stroke in patients less than 55 years of age: a study using transesophageal echocardiography. *Stroke* 1993; **24**:1865–73.

245 Marini C, Carolei A, Roberts RS, Prencipe M, Gandolfo C, Inzitari D *et al.* Focal cerebral ischemia in young adults: a collaborative case–control study. The National Research Council Study Group. *Neuroepidemiology* 1993; **12**:70–81.

246 Gilon D, Buonanno FS, Joffe MM, Leavitt M, Marshall JE, Kistler JP *et al.* Lack of evidence of an association between mitral-valve prolapse and stroke in young patients. *N Engl J Med* 1999; **341**:8–13.

247 Orencia AJ, Petty GW, Khandheria BK, Annegers JF, Ballard DJ, Sicks JD et al. Risk of stroke with mitral leaflet prolapse in population-based cohort study. *Stroke* 1995; **26**:7–13.

248 Orencia AJ, Petty GW, Khandheria BK, O'Fallon WM, Whisnant JP. Mitral leaflet prolapse and the risk of stroke after initial cerebral ischemia. *Neurology* 1995; **45**:1083–6.

249 Avierinos JF, Brown RD, Foley DA, Nkomo V, Petty GW, Scott C et al. Cerebral ischemic events after diagnosis of mitral leaflet prolapse: a community-based study of incidence and predictive factors. *Stroke* 2003; **34**:1339–44.

250 Cohen A, Tzourio C, Chauvel C, Bertrand B, Crassard I, Bernard Y et al. Mitral valve strands and the risk of ischemic stroke in elderly patients. The French Study of Aortic Plaques in Stroke (FAPS) Investigators. *Stroke* 1997; **28**:1574–8.

251 Homma S, Di Tullio MR, Sciacca RR, Sacco RL, Mohr JP. Effect of aspirin and warfarin therapy in stroke patients with valvular strands. *Stroke* 2004; **35**:1436–42.

252 Jones HR, Jr, Siekert RG. Neurological manifestations of infective endocarditis: review of clinical and therapeutic challenges. *Brain* 1989; **112**:1295–315.

253 Hart RG, Foster JW, Luther MF, Kanter MC. Stroke in infective endocarditis. *Stroke* 1990; **21**:695–700.

254 Salgado AV. Central nervous system complications of infective endocarditis. *Stroke* 1991; **22**:1461–3.

255 Bamford J, Hodges J, Warlow C. Late rupture of a mycotic aneurysm after 'cure' of bacterial endocarditis. *J Neurol* 1986; **233**:51–3.

256 Masuda J, Yutani C, Waki R, Ogata J, Kuriyama Y, Yamaguchi T. Histopathological analysis of the mechanisms of intracranial hemorrhage complicating infective endocarditis. *Stroke* 1992; **23**:843–50.

257 Krapf H, Skalej M, Voigt K. Subarachnoid hemorrhage due to septic embolic infarction in infective endocarditis. *Cerebrovasc Dis* 1999; **9**:182–4.

258 Van der Meulen JH, Weststrate W, van Gijn J, Habbema JD. Is cerebral angiography indicated in infective endocarditis? *Stroke* 1992; **23**:1662–7.

259 Kanter MC, Hart RG. Neurologic complications of infective endocarditis. *Neurology* 1991; **41**:1015–20.

260 Graus P, Rogers LR, Posner JB. Cerebrovascular complications in patients with cancer. *Medicine* 1985; **64**:16–35.

261 Lopez JA, Ross RS, Fishbein MC, Siegel RJ. Nonbacterial thrombotic endocarditis: a review. *Am Heart J* 1987; **113**:773–84.

262 Walz ET, Slivka AP, Tice FD, Gray PC, Orsinelli DA, Pearson AC. Non-infective mitral valve vegetations identified by transoesophageal echocardiography as a cause of stroke. *J Stroke Cerebrovasc Dis* 1998; **7**:310–14.

263 Levine SR, Brey RL, Tilley BC, Thompson JL, Sacco RL, Sciacca RR et al. Antiphospholipid antibodies and subsequent thrombo-occlusive events in patients with ischemic stroke. *J Am Med Assoc* 2004; **291**:576–84.

264 Wickremaratchi M, Hughes T, Warlow C, Hourihan M, Lammie L. Three strokes and a heart attack in a fit and relatively young woman. *Pract Neurol* 2004; **4**:228–37.

265 Kozdag G, Ciftci E, Vural A, Selekler M, Sahin T, Ural D et al. Silent cerebral infarction in patients with dilated cardiomyopathy: echocardiographic correlates. *Int J Cardiol* 2006; **107**:376–81.

266 Gautier JC, Durr A, Koussa S, Lascault G, Grosgogeat Y. Paradoxical cerebral embolism with a patent foramen ovale: a report of 29 patients. *Cerebrovasc Dis* 1991; **1**:193–202.

267 Jeanrenaud X, Kappenberger L. Patent foramen ovale and stroke of unknown origin. *Cerebrovasc Dis* 1991; **1**:184–92.

268 Mas JL, Arquizan C, Lamy C, Zuber M, Cabanes L, Derumeaux G et al. Recurrent cerebrovascular events associated with patent foramen ovale, atrial septal aneurysm, or both. *N Engl J Med* 2001; **345**:1740–6.

269 Lamy C, Giannesini C, Zuber M, Arquizan C, Meder JF, Trystram D et al. Clinical and imaging findings in cryptogenic stroke patients with and without patent foramen ovale: the PFO-ASA Study. Atrial Septal Aneurysm. *Stroke* 2002; **33**:706–11.

270 Bogousslavsky J, Garazi S, Jeanrenaud X, Aebischer N, Van Melle G. Stroke recurrence in patients with patent foramen ovale: the Lausanne Study. Lausanne Stroke with Paradoxal Embolism Study Group. *Neurology* 1996; **46**:1301–5.

271 Homma S, Di Tullio MR, Sacco RL, Sciacca RR, Smith C, Mohr JP. Surgical closure of patent foramen ovale in cryptogenic stroke patients. *Stroke* 1997; **28**:2376–81.

272 Mas JL. Specifics of patent foramen ovale. *Adv Neurol* 2003; **92**:197–202.

273 Kizer JR, Devereux RB. Clinical practice: patent foramen ovale in young adults with unexplained stroke. *N Engl J Med* 2005; **353**:2361–72.

274 Homma S, Sacco RL. Patent foramen ovale and stroke. *Circulation* 2005; **112**:1063–72.

275 Amarenco P. Patent foramen ovale and the risk of stroke: smoking gun guilty by association? *Heart* 2005; **91**:441–3.

276 Messe SR, Cucchiara B, Luciano J, Kasner SE. PFO management: neurologists vs cardiologists. *Neurology* 2005; **65**:172–3.

277 Wahl A, Meier B, Haxel B, Nedeltchev K, Arnold M, Eicher E et al. Prognosis after percutaneous closure of patent foramen ovale for paradoxical embolism. *Neurology* 2001; **57**:1330–2.

278 Silver MD, Dorsey JS. Aneurysms of the septum primum in adults. *Arch Pathol Lab Med* 1978; **102**:62–5.

279 Nater B, Bogousslavsky J, Regli F, Stauffer J. Stroke patterns with atrial septal aneurysm. *Cerebrovasc Dis* 1992; **2**:342–6.

280 Agmon Y, Khandheria BK, Meissner I, Gentile F, Whisnant JP, Sicks JD et al. Frequency of atrial septal aneurysms in patients with cerebral ischemic events. *Circulation* 1999; **99**:1942–4.

281 Berthet K, Lavergne T, Cohen A, Guize L, Bousser MG, Le Heuzey JY et al. Significant association of atrial vulnerability with atrial septal abnormalities in young patients with ischemic stroke of unknown cause. *Stroke* 2000; **31**:398–403.

282 CODICE Study Group. Recurrent stroke is not associated with massive right-to-left shunt: preliminary results from

the 3-year prospective Spanish Multicentre Centre (CODICE study). *Cerebrovasc Dis* 2006; **21**:1.

283 Holmes DR, Jr. Strokes and holes and headaches: are they a package deal? *Lancet* 2004; **364**:1840–2.

284 Diener HC, Weimar C, Katsarava Z. Patent foramen ovale: paradoxical connection to migraine and stroke. *Curr Opin Neurol* 2005; **18**:299–304.

285 Schwerzmann M, Nedeltchev K, Meier B. Patent foramen ovale closure: a new therapy for migraine. *Catheter Cardiovasc Interv* 2007; **69**:277–84.

286 Dennis MS. Neurological complications of pulmonary arteriovenous malformations. *Br Med J (Clin Res)* 1985; **290**:1392–3.

287 Markel ML, Waller BF, Armstrong WF. Cardiac myxoma: a review. *Medicine (Baltimore)* 1987; **66**:114–25.

288 Burke AP, Virmani R. Cardiac myxoma: a clinicopathologic study. *Am J Clin Pathol* 1993; **100**:671–80.

289 Reynen K. Cardiac myxomas. *N Engl J Med* 1995; **333**:1610–17.

290 Suzuki T, Nagai R, Yamazaki T, Shiojima I, Maemura K, Yamaoki K *et al*. Rapid growth of intracranial aneurysms secondary to cardiac myxoma. *Neurology* 1994; **44**:570–1.

291 Ng HK, Poon WS. Cardiac myxoma metastasizing to the brain: case report. *J Neurosurg* 1990; **72**:295–8.

292 Roeltgen DP, Weimer GR, Patterson LF. Delayed neurologic complications of left atrial myxoma. *Neurology* 1981; **31**:8–13.

293 Mattle HP, Maurer D, Sturzenegger M, Ozdoba C, Baumgartner RW, Schroth G. Cardiac myxomas: a long-term study. *J Neurol* 1995; **242**:689–94.

294 Joynt RJ, Zimmerman G, Khalifeh R. Cerebral emboli from cardiac tumours. *Arch Neurol* 1965; **12**:84–91.

295 Chalmers N, Campbell IW. Left atrial metastasis presenting as recurrent embolic strokes. *Br Heart J* 1987; **58**:170–2.

296 Giannesini C, Kubis N, N'Guyen A, Wassef M, Mikol J, Woimant F. Cardiac papillary fibroelastoma: a rare cause of ischemic stroke in the young. *Cerebrovasc Dis* 1999; **9**:45–9.

297 Bathen J, Sparr S, Rokseth R. Embolism in sinoatrial disease. *Acta Med Scand* 1978; **203**:7–11.

298 Fisher M, Kase CS, Stelle B, Mills RM, Jr. Ischemic stroke after cardiac pacemaker implantation in sick sinus syndrome. *Stroke* 1988; **19**:712–15.

299 Pierre P, Bogousslavsky J, Menetrey R, Regli F, Kappenberger L. Familial sick sinus disease: another Mendelian aetiology of stroke. *Cerebrovasc Dis* 1993; **3**:120–2.

300 Shields DA. Multiple emboli in hydatid disease. *Br Med J* 1990; **301**:213–14.

301 Benomar A, Yahyaoui M, Birouk N, Vidailhet M, Chkili T. Middle cerebral artery occlusion due to hydatid cysts of myocardial and intraventricular cavity cardiac origin: two cases. *Stroke* 1994; **25**:886–8.

302 Stollberger C, Seitelberger R, Fenninger C, Prainer C, Slany J. Aneurysm of the left sinus of Valsalva: an unusual source of cerebral embolism. *Stroke* 1996; **27**:1424–6.

303 Lammie GA, Wardlaw J, Dennis M. Thrombo-embolic stroke, moya-moya phenomenon and primary oxalosis. *Cerebrovasc Dis* 1998; **8**:45–50.

304 Dugani BV, Higginson LA, Beanlands DS, Akyurekli Y. Recurrent systemic emboli following myocardial contusion. *Am Heart J* 1984; **108**:1354–7.

305 Bhatia M, Rothwell PM. A systematic comparison of the quality and volume of published data available on novel risk factors for stroke versus coronary heart disease. *Cerebrovasc Dis* 2005; **20**:180–6.

306 Rothwell PM. The high cost of not funding stroke research: a comparison with heart disease and cancer. *Lancet* 2001; **357**:1612–16.

307 Pendlebury ST, Rothwell PM, Algra A, Ariesen MJ, Bakac G, Czlonkowska A *et al*. Underfunding of stroke research: a Europe-wide problem. *Stroke* 2004; **35**:2368–71.

308 Glynn JR. A question of attribution. *Lancet* 1993; **342**:530–2.

309 Bonithon-Kopp C, Touboul PJ, Berr C, Magne C, Ducimetiere P. Factors of carotid arterial enlargement in a population aged 59 to 71 years: the EVA study. *Stroke* 1996; **27**:654–60.

310 Crouse JR, Goldbourt U, Evans G, Pinsky J, Sharrett AR, Sorlie P *et al*. Risk factors and segment-specific carotid arterial enlargement in the Atherosclerosis Risk in Communities (ARIC) cohort. *Stroke* 1996; **27**:69–75.

311 O'Leary DH, Polak JF, Kronmal RA, Savage PJ, Borhani NO, Kittner SJ *et al*. Thickening of the carotid wall: a marker for atherosclerosis in the elderly? Cardiovascular Health Study Collaborative Research Group. *Stroke* 1996; **27**:224–31.

312 Wilson PW, Hoeg JM, D'Agostino RB, Silbershatz H, Belanger AM, Poehlmann H *et al*. Cumulative effects of high cholesterol levels, high blood pressure, and cigarette smoking on carotid stenosis. *N Engl J Med* 1997; **337**:516–22.

313 Lorenz MW, Markus HS, Bots ML, Rosvall M, Sitzer M. Prediction of clinical cardiovascular events with carotid intima-media thickness: a systematic review and meta-analysis. *Circulation* 2007; **115**:459–67.

314 Pruissen DM, Gerritsen SA, Prinsen TJ, Dijk JM, Kappelle LJ, Algra A. Carotid intima-media thickness is different in large- and small-vessel ischemic stroke: the SMART study. *Stroke* 2007; **38**:1371–3.

315 Spence JD. Technology insight: ultrasound measurement of carotid plaque: patient management, genetic research, and therapy evaluation. *Nat Clin Pract Neurol* 2006; **2**:611–19.

316 Rothwell PM, Coull AJ, Silver LE, Fairhead JF, Giles MF, Lovelock CE *et al*. Population-based study of event-rate, incidence, case fatality, and mortality for all acute vascular events in all arterial territories (Oxford Vascular Study). *Lancet* 2005; **366**:1773–83.

317 Van der Schouw YT, van der Graaf Y, Steyerberg EW, Eijkemans JC, Banga JD. Age at menopause as a risk factor for cardiovascular mortality. *Lancet* 1996; **347**:714–18.

318 Hu FB, Grodstein F, Hennekens CH, Colditz GA, Johnson M, Manson JE *et al*. Age at natural menopause and risk of cardiovascular disease. *Arch Intern Med* 1999; **159**:1061–6.

319 Cho L, Mukherjee D. Hormone replacement therapy and secondary cardiovascular prevention: a meta-analysis of randomized trials. *Cardiology* 2005; **104**:143–7.

320 Farquhar CM, Marjoribanks J, Lethaby A, Lamberts Q, Suckling JA. Long term hormone therapy for perimenopausal and postmenopausal women. *Cochrane Database Syst Rev* 2005; CD004143.

321 Gabriel SR, Carmona L, Roque M, Sanchez GL, Bonfill X. Hormone replacement therapy for preventing cardiovascular disease in post-menopausal women. *Cochrane Database Syst Rev* 2005; CD002229.

322 Whelton PK. Epidemiology of hypertension. *Lancet* 1994; **344**:101–6.

323 Gil-Nunez AC, Vivancos-Mora J. Blood pressure as a risk factor for stroke and the impact of antihypertensive treatment. *Cerebrovasc Dis* 2005; **20**(Suppl 2):40–52.

324 Goldstein LB, Hankey GJ. Advances in primary stroke prevention. *Stroke* 2006; **37**:317–19.

325 MacMahon S, Peto R, Cutler J, Collins R, Sorlie P, Neaton J *et al*. Blood pressure, stroke, and coronary heart disease. Part 1, Prolonged differences in blood pressure: prospective observational studies corrected for the regression dilution bias. *Lancet* 1990; **335**:765–74.

326 Eastern Stroke and Coronary Heart Disease Collaborative Research Group. Blood pressure, cholesterol and stroke in eastern Asia. *Lancet* 1998; **352**:1801–7.

327 Lewington S, Clarke R, Qizilbash N, Peto R, Collins R. Age-specific relevance of usual blood pressure to vascular mortality: a meta-analysis of individual data for one million adults in 61 prospective studies. *Lancet* 2002; **360**:1903–13.

328 Birns J, Markus H, Kalra L. Blood pressure reduction for vascular risk: is there a price to be paid? *Stroke* 2005; **36**:1308–13.

329 Rothwell PM, Howard SC, Spence JD. Relationship between blood pressure and stroke risk in patients with symptomatic carotid occlusive disease. *Stroke* 2003; **34**:2583–90.

330 Shaper AG, Phillips AN, Pocock SJ, Walker M, Macfarlane PW. Risk factors for stroke in middle-aged British men. *Br Med J* 1991; **302**:1111–15.

331 Keli S, Bloemberg B, Kromhout D. Predictive value of repeated systolic blood pressure measurements for stroke risk. The Zutphen Study. *Stroke* 1992; **23**:347–51.

332 Sagie A, Larson MG, Levy D. The natural history of borderline isolated systolic hypertension. *N Engl J Med* 1993; **329**:1912–17.

333 Petrovitch H, Curb D, Bloom-Marcus E. Isolated systolic hypertension and risk of stroke in Japanese-American men. *Stroke* 1995; **26**:25–9.

334 MacMahon S, Rodgers A. Antihypertensive agents and stroke prevention. *Cerebrovasc Dis* 1994; **4**(suppl.1):11–15.

335 Collins R, MacMahon S. Blood pressure, antihypertensive drug treatment and the risks of stroke and of coronary heart disease. *Br Med Bull* 1994; **50**:272–98.

336 Mulrow CD, Cornell JA, Herrera CR, Kadri A, Farnett L, Aguilar C. Hypertension in the elderly: implications and generalizability of randomized trials. *J Am Med Assoc* 1994; **272**:1932–8.

337 Turnbull F. Effects of different blood-pressure-lowering regimens on major cardiovascular events: results of prospectively-designed overviews of randomised trials. *Lancet* 2003; **362**:1527–35.

338 Sutton-Tyrrell K, Wolfson SK, Jr, Kuller LH. Blood pressure treatment slows the progression of carotid stenosis in patients with isolated systolic hypertension. *Stroke* 1994; **25**:44–50.

339 Ross Russell RW. How does blood pressure-cause stroke? *Lancet* 1975; **2**:1283–5.

340 Chobanian AV. The influence of hypertension and other hemodynamic factors in atherogenesis. *Prog Cardiovasc Dis* 1983; **26**:177–96.

341 Lusiani L, Visona A, Castellani V, Ronsisvalle G, Scaldalai E, Carraro L *et al*. Prevalence of atherosclerotic involvement of the internal carotid artery in hypertensive patients. *Int J Cardiol* 1987; **17**:51–6.

342 Reed DM, Resch JA, Hayashi T, MacLean C, Yano K. A prospective study of cerebral artery atherosclerosis. *Stroke* 1988; **19**:820–5.

343 Sutton-Tyrrell K, Alcorn HG, Wolfson SK, Jr, Kelsey SF, Kuller LH. Predictors of carotid stenosis in older adults with and without isolated systolic hypertension. *Stroke* 1993; **24**:355–61.

344 Fine-Edelstein JS, Wolf PA, O'Leary DH, Poehlman H, Belanger AJ, Kase CS *et al*. Precursors of extracranial carotid atherosclerosis in the Framingham Study. *Neurology* 1994; **44**:1046–50.

345 Shinton R, Beevers G. Meta-analysis of relation between cigarette smoking and stroke. *Br Med J* 1989; **298**:789–94.

346 Donnan GA, O'Malley HM, Quang L, Hurley S, Bladin PF. The capsular warning syndrome: pathogenesis and clinical features. *Neurology* 1993; **43**:957–62.

347 Doll R, Peto R, Wheatley K, Gray R, Sutherland I. Mortality in relation to smoking: 40 years' observations on male British doctors. *Br Med J* 1994; **309**:901–11.

348 Robbins AS, Manson JE, Lee IM, Satterfield S, Hennekens CH. Cigarette smoking and stroke in a cohort of US male physicians. *Ann Intern Med* 1994; **120**:458–62.

349 Haheim LL, Holme I, Hjermann I, Leren P. Smoking habits and risk of fatal stroke: 18 years follow-up of the Oslo Study. *J Epidemiol Commun Health* 1996; **50**:621–4.

350 Bonita R, Duncan J, Truelsen T, Jackson RT, Beaglehole R. Passive smoking as well as active smoking increases the risk of acute stroke. *Tob Control* 1999; **8**:156–60.

351 Law MR, Morris JK, Wald NJ. Environmental tobacco smoke exposure and ischaemic heart disease: an evaluation of the evidence. *Br Med J* 1997; **315**:973–80.

352 Jamrozik K, Dobson A. Please put out that cigarette, grandpa. *Tob Control* 1999; **8**:125–6.

353 He J, Vupputuri S, Allen K, Prerost MR, Hughes J, Whelton PK. Passive smoking and the risk of coronary heart disease: a meta-analysis of epidemiologic studies. *N Engl J Med* 1999; **340**:920–6.

354 You RX, Thrift AG, McNeil JJ, Davis SM, Donnan GA. Ischemic stroke risk and passive exposure to spouses' cigarette smoking. Melbourne Stroke Risk Factor Study (MERFS) Group. *Am J Public Health* 1999; **89**:572–5.

355 Haapanen A, Koskenvou M, Kaprio J, Kesaniemi YA, Heikkila K. Carotid arteriosclerosis in identical twins

discordant for cigarette smoking. *Circulation* 1989; **80**:10–16.

356 O'Leary DH, Polak JF, Kronmal RA, Kittner SJ, Bond MG, Wolfson SK, Jr. *et al.* Distribution and correlates of sonographically detected carotid artery disease in the Cardiovascular Health Study. The CHS Collaborative Research Group. *Stroke* 1992; **23**:1752–60.

357 Howard G, Wagenknecht LE, Burke GL, Diez-Roux A, Evans GW, McGovern P *et al.* Cigarette smoking and progression of atherosclerosis: The Atherosclerosis Risk in Communities (ARIC) Study. *J Am Med Assoc* 1998; **279**:119–24.

358 Iribarren C, Tekawa IS, Sidney S, Friedman GD. Effect of cigar smoking on the risk of cardiovascular disease, chronic obstructive pulmonary disease, and cancer in men. *N Engl J Med* 1999; **340**:1773–80.

359 Donnan GA, McNeil JJ, Adena MA, Doyle AE, O'Malley HM, Neill GC. Smoking as a risk factor for cerebral ischaemia. *Lancet* 1989; **2**:643–7.

360 Rose G, Colwell L. Randomised controlled trial of anti-smoking advice: final (20 year) results. *J Epidemiol Commun Health* 1992; **46**:75–7.

361 Kawachi I, Colditz GA, Stampfer MJ, Willett WC, Manson JE, Rosner B *et al.* Smoking cessation and decreased risk of stroke in women. *J Am Med Assoc* 1993; **269**:232–6.

362 Jorgensen H, Nakayama H, Raaschou HO, Olsen TS. Stroke in patients with diabetes. The Copenhagen Stroke Study. *Stroke* 1994; **25**:1977–84.

363 Stevens RJ, Coleman RL, Adler AI, Stratton IM, Matthews DR, Holman RR. Risk factors for myocardial infarction case fatality and stroke case fatality in type 2 diabetes: UKPDS 66. *Diabetes Care* 2004; **27**:201–7.

364 Rosengren A, Welin L, Tsipogianni A, Wilhelmsen L. Impact of cardiovascular risk factors on coronary heart disease and mortality among middle-aged diabetic men: a general population study. *Br Med J* 1989; **299**: 1127–31.

365 Manson JE, Colditz GA, Stampfer MJ, Willett WC, Krolewski AS, Rosner B *et al.* A prospective study of maturity-onset diabetes mellitus and risk of coronary heart disease and stroke in women. *Arch Intern Med* 1991; **151**:1141–7.

366 Burchfield CM, Curb JD, Rodriguez BL, Abbott RD, Chiu D, Yano K. Glucose intolerance and 22-year stroke incidence. The Honolulu Heart Program. *Stroke* 1994; **25**:951–7.

367 Qureshi AI, Giles WH, Croft JB. Impaired glucose tolerance and the likelihood of nonfatal stroke and myocardial infarction: the Third National Health and Nutrition Examination Survey. *Stroke* 1998; **29**:1329–32.

368 Tuomilehto J, Rastenyte D. Diabetes and glucose intolerance as risk factors for stroke. *J Cardiovasc Risk* 1999; **6**:241–9.

369 Wannamethee SG, Perry IJ, Shaper AG. Nonfasting serum glucose and insulin concentrations and the risk of stroke. *Stroke* 1999; **30**:1780–6.

370 Rothwell PM. Prevention of stroke in patients with diabetes mellitus and the metabolic syndrome. *Cerebrovasc Dis* 2005; **20** (Suppl 1):24–34.

371 Niskanen L, Rauramaa R, Miettinen H, Haffner SM, Mercuri M, Uusitupa M. Carotid artery intima-media thickness in elderly patients with NIDDM and in nondiabetic subjects. *Stroke* 1996; **27**:1986–92.

372 UK Prospective Diabetes Study (UKPDS) Group. Intensive blood-glucose control with sulphonylureas or insulin compared with conventional treatment and risk of complications in patients with type 2 diabetes (UKPDS 33). *Lancet* 1998; **352**:837–53.

373 Lewington S, Clarke R. Combined effects of systolic blood pressure and total cholesterol on cardiovascular disease risk. *Circulation* 2005; **112**:3373–4.

374 Law MR, Wald NJ, Thompson SG. By how much and how quickly does reduction in serum cholesterol concentration lower risk of ischaemic heart disease? *Br Med J* 1994; **308**:367–72.

375 Hokanson JE, Austin MA. Plasma triglyceride level is a risk factor for cardiovascular disease independent of high-density lipoprotein cholesterol level: a meta-analysis of population-based prospective studies. *J Cardiovasc Risk* 1996; **3**:213–19.

376 Downs JR, Clearfield M, Weis S, Whitney E, Shapiro DR, Beere PA *et al.* Primary prevention of acute coronary events with lovastatin in men and women with average cholesterol levels: results of AFCAPS/TexCAPS. Air Force/Texas Coronary Atherosclerosis Prevention Study. *J Am Med Assoc* 1998; **279**:1615–22.

377 Huxley R, Lewington S, Clarke R. Cholesterol, coronary heart disease and stroke: a review of published evidence from observational studies and randomized controlled trials. *Semin Vasc Med* 2002; **2**:315–23.

378 Clarke R, Lewington S, Youngman L, Sherliker P, Peto R, Collins R. Underestimation of the importance of blood pressure and cholesterol for coronary heart disease mortality in old age. *Eur Heart J* 2002; **23**:286–93.

379 Baigent C, Keech A, Kearney PM, Blackwell L, Buck G, Pollicino C *et al.* Efficacy and safety of cholesterol-lowering treatment: prospective meta-analysis of data from 90,056 participants in 14 randomised trials of statins. *Lancet* 2005; **366**:1267–78.

380 Cholesterol, diastolic blood pressure, and stroke: 13,000 strokes in 450,000 people in 45 prospective cohorts. Prospective studies collaboration. *Lancet* 1995; **346**:1647–53.

381 Qizilbash N, Jones L, Warlow C, Mann J. Fibrinogen and lipid concentrations as risk factors for transient ischaemic attacks and minor ischaemic strokes. *Br Med J* 1991; **303**:605–9.

382 Homer D, Ingall TJ, Baker HL, Jr, O'Fallon WM, Kottke BA, Whisnant JP. Serum lipids and lipoproteins are less powerful predictors of extracranial carotid artery atherosclerosis than are cigarette smoking and hypertension. *Mayo Clin Proc* 1991; **66**:259–67.

383 Willeit J, Kiechl S, Santer P, Oberhollenzer F, Egger G, Jarosch E *et al.* Lipoprotein(a) and asymptomatic carotid artery disease. Evidence of a prominent role in the evolution of advanced carotid plaques: the Bruneck Study. *Stroke* 1995; **26**:1582–7.

384 Collins R, Armitage J, Parish S, Sleight P, Peto R. Effects of cholesterol-lowering with simvastatin on stroke and other major vascular events in 20,536 people with cerebrovascular disease or other high-risk conditions. *Lancet* 2004; **363**:757–67.

385 Heart Protection Study Collaborative Group. MRC/BHF Heat Protection Study of cholesterol lowering with simvastatin in 20,536 high-risk individuals: a randomised placebo-controlled trial. *Lancet* 2002; **360**:7–22.

386 Amarenco P, Bogousslavsky J, Callahan A, III, Goldstein LB, Hennerici M, Rudolph AE *et al*. High-dose atorvastatin after stroke or transient ischemic attack. *N Engl J Med* 2006; **355**:549–59.

387 Di Mascio R, Marchioli R, Tognoni G. Cholesterol reduction and stroke occurrence: an overview of randomized clinical trials. *Cerebrovasc Dis* 2000; **10**:85–92.

388 Ovbiagele B, Kidwell CS, Saver JL. Expanding indications for statins in cerebral ischemia: a quantitative study. *Arch Neurol* 2005; **62**:67–72.

389 Amarenco P. Effect of statins in stroke prevention. *Curr Opin Lipidol* 2005; **16**:614–18.

390 Akdim F, van Leuven SI, Kastelein JJ, Stroes ES. Pleiotropic effects of statins: stabilization of the vulnerable atherosclerotic plaque? *Curr Pharm Des* 2007; **13**:1003–12.

391 Cimino M, Balduini W, Carloni S, Gelosa P, Guerrini U, Tremoli E *et al*. Neuroprotective effect of simvastatin in stroke: a comparison between adult and neonatal rat models of cerebral ischemia. *Neurotoxicology* 2005; **26**:929–33.

392 Switzer JA, Hess DC. Statins in stroke: prevention, protection and recovery. *Expert Rev Neurother* 2006; **6**:195–202.

393 Schwartz GG, Olsson AG, Ezekowitz MD, Ganz P, Oliver MF, Waters D *et al*. Effects of atorvastatin on early recurrent ischemic events in acute coronary syndromes: the MIRACL study: a randomized controlled trial. *J Am Med Assoc* 2001; **285**:1711–18.

394 Sniderman AD, Furberg CD, Keech A, Roeters van Lennep JE, Frohlich J, Jungner I *et al*. Apolipoproteins versus lipids as indices of coronary risk and as targets for statin treatment. *Lancet* 2003; **361**:777–80.

395 Van Kooten F, van Krimpen J, Dippel DW, Hoogerbrugge N, Koudstaal PJ. Lipoprotein(a) in patients with acute cerebral ischemia. *Stroke* 1996; **27**:1231–5.

396 Margaglione M, Seripa D, Gravina C, Grandone E, Vecchione G, Cappucci G *et al*. Prevalence of apolipoprotein E alleles in healthy subjects and survivors of ischemic stroke: an Italian case-control study. *Stroke* 1998; **29**:399–403.

397 Peng DQ, Zhao SP, Wang JL. Lipoprotein (a) and apolipoprotein E epsilon 4 as independent risk factors for ischemic stroke. *J Cardiovasc Risk* 1999; **6**:1–6.

398 Simons LA, Simons J, Friedlander Y, McCallum J. Cholesterol and other lipids predict coronary heart disease and ischaemic stroke in the elderly, but only in those below 70 years. *Atherosclerosis* 2001; **159**:201–8.

399 Bhatia M, Howard SC, Clark TG, Neale R, Qizilbash N, Murphy MF *et al*. Apolipoproteins as predictors of ischaemic stroke in patients with a previous transient ischaemic attack. *Cerebrovasc Dis* 2006; **21**:323–8.

400 Walldius G, Jungner I, Holme I, Aastveit AH, Kolar W, Steiner E. High apolipoprotein B, low apolipoprotein A-I, and improvement in the prediction of fatal myocardial infarction (AMORIS study): a prospective study. *Lancet* 2001; **358**:2026–33.

401 Talmud PJ, Hawe E, Miller GJ, Humphries SE. Nonfasting apolipoprotein B and triglyceride levels as a useful predictor of coronary heart disease risk in middle-aged UK men. *Arterioscler Thromb Vasc Biol* 2002; **22**:1918–23.

402 Simes RJ, Marschner IC, Hunt D, Colquhoun D, Sullivan D, Stewart RA *et al*. Relationship between lipid levels and clinical outcomes in the Long-term Intervention with Pravastatin in Ischemic Disease (LIPID) Trial: to what extent is the reduction in coronary events with pravastatin explained by on-study lipid levels? *Circulation* 2002; **105**:1162–9.

403 Markus HS, Hambley H. Neurology and the blood: haematological abnormalities in ischaemic stroke. *J Neurol Neurosurg Psychiatry* 1998; **64**:150–9.

404 Sacco RL. Newer risk factors for stroke. *Neurology* 2001; **57**:S31–S34.

405 Rothwell PM, Howard SC, Power DA, Gutnikov SA, Algra A, van Gijn J *et al*. Fibrinogen concentration and risk of ischemic stroke and acute coronary events in 5113 patients with transient ischemic attack and minor ischemic stroke. *Stroke* 2004; **35**:2300–5.

406 Danesh J, Lewington S, Thompson SG, Lowe GD, Collins R, Kostis JB *et al*. Plasma fibrinogen level and the risk of major cardiovascular diseases and nonvascular mortality: an individual participant meta-analysis. *J Am Med Assoc* 2005; **294**:1799–809.

407 Cook NS, Ubben D. Fibrinogen as a major risk factor in cardiovascular disease. *Trends Pharmacol Sci* 1990; **11**:444–51.

408 Rosengren A, Wilhelmsen L, Welin L, Tsipogianni A, Teger-Nilsson AC, Wedel H. Social influences and cardiovascular risk factors as determinants of plasma fibrinogen concentration in a general population sample of middle-aged men. *Br Med J* 1990; **300**:634–8.

409 Ernst E, Resch KL. Fibrinogen as a cardiovascular risk factor: a meta-analysis and review of the literature. *Ann Intern Med* 1993; **118**:956–63.

410 Brunner E, Davey SG, Marmot M, Canner R, Beksinska M, O'Brien J. Childhood social circumstances and psychosocial and behavioural factors as determinants of plasma fibrinogen. *Lancet* 1996; **347**:1008–13.

411 Lowe GD, Lee AJ, Rumley A, Price JF, Fowkes FG. Blood viscosity and risk of cardiovascular events: the Edinburgh Artery Study. *Br J Haematol* 1997; **96**:168–73.

412 Danesh J, Collins R, Appleby P, Peto R. Association of fibrinogen, C-reactive protein, albumin, or leukocyte count with coronary heart disease: meta-analyses of prospective studies. *J Am Med Assoc* 1998; **279**:1477–82.

413 Allport LE, Parsons MW, Butcher KS, MacGregor L, Desmond PM, Tress BM *et al*. Elevated hematocrit is

associated with reduced reperfusion and tissue survival in acute stroke. *Neurology* 2005; **65**:1382–7.

414 Welin L, Svardsudd K, Wilhelmsen L, Larsson B, Tibblin G. Analysis of risk factors for stroke in a cohort of men born in 1913. *N Engl J Med* 1987; **317**:521–6.

415 Gagnon DR, Zhang TJ, Brand FN, Kannel WB. Hematocrit and the risk of cardiovascular disease – the Framingham study: a 34-year follow-up. *Am Heart J* 1994; **127**:674–82.

416 Wannamethee G, Perry IJ, Shaper AG. Haematocrit, hypertension and risk of stroke. *J Intern Med* 1994; **235**:163–8.

417 Qizilbash N, Duffy S, Prentice CR, Boothby M, Warlow C. Von Willebrand factor and risk of ischemic stroke. *Neurology* 1997; **49**:1552–6.

418 Lacoviello L, Di Castelnuovo A, De Kniff P, Diorazio *et al*. Polymorphisms in the coagulation factor VII gene and the risk of myocardial infarction. *N Engl J Med* 1998; **338**: 79–85.

419 Funk M, Endler G, Lalouschek W, Hsieh K, Schillinger M, Lang W *et al*. Factor VII gene haplotypes and risk of ischemic stroke. *Clin Chem* 2006; **52**:1190–2.

420 Smith A, Patterson C, Yarnell J, Rumley A, Ben Shlomo Y, Lowe G. Which hemostatic markers add to the predictive value of conventional risk factors for coronary heart disease and ischemic stroke? The Caerphilly Study. *Circulation* 2005; **112**:3080–7.

421 Meade TW, Ruddock V, Stirling Y, Chakrabarti R, Miller GJ. Fibrinolytic activity, clotting factors, and long-term incidence of ischaemic heart disease in the Northwick Park Heart Study. *Lancet* 1993; **342**:1076–9.

422 Ridker PM, Hennekens CH, Stampfer MJ, Manson JE, Vaughan DE. Prospective study of endogenous tissue plasminogen activator and risk of stroke. *Lancet* 1994; **343**:940–3.

423 Macko RF, Kittner SJ, Epstein A, Cox DK, Wozniak MA, Wityk RJ *et al*. Elevated tissue plasminogen activator antigen and stroke risk: The Stroke Prevention In Young Women Study. *Stroke* 1999; **30**:7–11.

424 Johansson L, Jansson JH, Boman K, Nilsson TK, Stegmayr B, Hallmans G. Tissue plasminogen activator, plasminogen activator inhibitor-1, and tissue plasminogen activator/plasminogen activator inhibitor-1 complex as risk factors for the development of a first stroke. *Stroke* 2000; **31**:26–32.

425 Kohler HP, Grant PJ. Plasminogen-activator inhibitor type 1 and coronary artery disease. *N Engl J Med* 2000; **342**:1792–801.

426 Van Goor ML, Garcia EG, Leebeek F, Brouwers GJ, Koudstaal P, Dippel D. The plasminogen activator inhibitor (PAI-1) 4G/5G promoter polymorphism and PAI-1 levels in ischemic stroke: a case-control study. *Thromb Haemost* 2005; **93**:92–6.

427 Van Kooten F, Ciabattoni G, Koudstaal PJ, Dippel DW, Patrono C. Increased platelet activation in the chronic phase after cerebral ischemia and intracerebral hemorrhage. *Stroke* 1999; **30**:546–9.

428 Kekomaki S, Hamalainen L, Kauppinen-Makelin R, Palomaki H, Kaste M, Kontula K. Genetic polymorphism of platelet glycoprotein IIIa in patients with acute myocardial

infarction and acute ischaemic stroke. *J Cardiovasc Risk* 1999; **6**:13–17.

429 Clarke R, Collins R. Can dietary supplements with folic acid or vitamin B6 reduce cardiovascular risk? Design of clinical trials to test the homocysteine hypothesis of vascular disease. *J Cardiovasc Risk* 1998; **5**:249–55.

430 Danesh J, Lewington S. Plasma homocysteine and coronary heart disease: systematic review of published epidemiological studies. *J Cardiovasc Risk* 1998; **5**:229–32.

431 Refsum H, Ueland PM, Nygard O, Vollset SE. Homocysteine and cardiovascular disease. *Annu Rev Med* 1998; **49**:31–62.

432 Welch GN, Loscalzo J. Homocysteine and atherothrombosis. *N Engl J Med* 1998; **338**:1042–50.

433 Kittner SJ, Giles WH, Macko RF, Hebel JR, Wozniak MA, Wityk RJ *et al*. Homocyst(e)ine and risk of cerebral infarction in a biracial population : the stroke prevention in young women study. *Stroke* 1999; **30**:1554–60.

434 Hankey GJ. Is homocysteine a causal and treatable risk factor for vascular diseases of the brain (cognitive impairment and stroke)? *Ann Neurol* 2002; **51**:279–81.

435 Hankey GJ, Eikelboom JW. Homocysteine and stroke. *Lancet* 2005; **365**:194–6.

436 Connelly JB, Cooper JA, Meade TW. Strenuous exercise, plasma fibrinogen, and factor VII activity. *Br Heart J* 1992; **67**:351–4.

437 Arroll B, Beaglehole R. Exercise for hypertension. *Lancet* 1993; **341**:1248–9.

438 Berlin JA, Colditz GA. A meta-analysis of physical activity in the prevention of coronary heart disease. *Am J Epidemiol* 1990; **132**:612–28.

439 Evenson KR, Rosamond WD, Cai J, Toole JF, Hutchinson RG, Shahar E *et al*. Physical activity and ischemic stroke risk. The atherosclerosis risk in communities study. *Stroke* 1999; **30**:1333–9.

440 Lee IM, Hennekens CH, Berger K, Buring JE, Manson JE. Exercise and risk of stroke in male physicians. *Stroke* 1999; **30**:1–6.

441 Wannamethee SG, Shaper AG. Physical activity and the prevention of stroke. *J Cardiovasc Risk* 1999; **6**:213–16.

442 Ellekjaer H, Holmen J, Ellekjaer E, Vatten L. Physical activity and stroke mortality in women. Ten-year follow-up of the Nord-Trondelag health survey, 1984–1986. *Stroke* 2000; **31**:14–18.

443 Hu FB, Stampfer MJ, Colditz GA, Ascherio A, Rexrode KM, Willett WC *et al*. Physical activity and risk of stroke in women. *J Am Med Assoc* 2000; **283**:2961–7.

444 O'Connor GT, Buring JE, Yusuf S, Goldhaber SZ, Olmstead EM, Paffenbarger RS, Jr. *et al*. An overview of randomized trials of rehabilitation with exercise after myocardial infarction. *Circulation* 1989; **80**:234–44.

445 Tuomilehto J, Lindstrom J, Eriksson JG, Valle TT, Hamalainen H, Ilanne-Parikka P *et al*. Prevention of type 2 diabetes mellitus by changes in lifestyle among subjects with impaired glucose tolerance. *N Engl J Med* 2001; **344**:1343–50.

446 Diabetes Prevention Program Research Group. Reduction in the incidence of Type 2 diabetes with lifestyle

intervention or Metformin. *N Engl J Med* 2002; **346**:393–403.

447 Walker SP, Rimm EB, Ascherio A, Kawachi I, Stampfer MJ, Willett WC. Body size and fat distribution as predictors of stroke among US men. *Am J Epidemiol* 1996; **144**:1143–50.

448 Rexrode KM, Hennekens CH, Willett WC, Colditz GA, Stampfer MJ, Rich-Edwards JW *et al*. A prospective study of body mass index, weight change, and risk of stroke in women. *J Am Med Assoc* 1997; **277**:1539–45.

449 Shaper AG, Wannamethee SG, Walker M. Body weight: implications for the prevention of coronary heart disease, stroke, and diabetes mellitus in a cohort study of middle-aged men. *Br Med J* 1997; **314**:1311–17.

450 Calle EE, Thun MJ, Petrelli JM, Rodriguez C, Heath CW, Jr. Body-mass index and mortality in a prospective cohort of US adults. *N Engl J Med* 1999; **341**:1097–105.

451 Yusuf S, Hawken S, Ounpuu S, Bautista L, Franzosi MG, Commerford P *et al*. Obesity and the risk of myocardial infarction in 27,000 participants from 52 countries: a case–control study. *Lancet* 2005; **366**:1640–9.

452 Shirai K. Obesity as the core of the metabolic syndrome and the management of coronary heart disease. *Curr Med Res Opin* 2004; **20**:295–304.

453 Eckel RH, Grundy SM, Zimmet PZ. The metabolic syndrome. *Lancet* 2005; **365**:1415–28.

454 Grundy SM, Cleeman JI, Daniels SR, Donato KA, Eckel RH, Franklin BA *et al*. Diagnosis and management of the metabolic syndrome: an American Heart Association/National Heart, Lung, and Blood Institute Scientific Statement. *Circulation* 2005; **112**:2735–52.

455 Yusuf S, Sleight P, Pogue J, Bosch J, Davies R, Dagenais G. Effects of an angiotensin-converting-enzyme inhibitor, ramipril, on cardiovascular events in high-risk patients. The Heart Outcomes Prevention Evaluation Study Investigators. *N Engl J Med* 2000; **342**:145–53.

456 Dahlof B, Devereux RB, Kjeldsen SE, Julius S, Beevers G, de Faire U *et al*. Cardiovascular morbidity and mortality in the Losartan Intervention For Endpoint reduction in hypertension study (LIFE): a randomised trial against atenolol. *Lancet* 2002; **359**:995–1003.

457 Julius S, Kjeldsen SE, Weber M, Brunner HR, Ekman S, Hansson L *et al*. Outcomes in hypertensive patients at high cardiovascular risk treated with regimens based on valsartan or amlodipine: the VALUE randomised trial. *Lancet* 2004; **363**:2022–31.

458 Ding EL, Mozaffarian D. Optimal dietary habits for the prevention of stroke. *Semin Neurol* 2006; **26**:11–23.

459 Ness AR, Powles JW. The role of diet, fruit and vegetables and antioxidants in the aetiology of stroke. *J Cardiovasc Risk* 1999; **6**:229–34.

460 Frost CD, Law MR, Wald NJ. By how much does dietary salt reduction lower blood pressure? II. Analysis of observational data within populations. *Br Med J* 1991; **302**:815–18.

461 Law MR, Frost CD, Wald NJ. By how much does dietary salt reduction lower blood pressure? I. Analysis of observational data among populations. *Br Med J* 1991; **302**:811–15.

462 Law MR, Frost CD, Wald NJ. By how much does dietary salt reduction lower blood pressure? III. Analysis of data from trials of salt reduction. *Br Med J* 1991; **302**:819–24.

463 He J, Ogden LG, Vupputuri S, Bazzano LA, Loria C, Whelton PK. Dietary sodium intake and subsequent risk of cardiovascular disease in overweight adults. *J Am Med Assoc* 1999; **282**:2027–34.

464 Diaz MN, Frei B, Vita JA, Keaney JF, Jr. Antioxidants and atherosclerotic heart disease. *N Engl J Med* 1997; **337**:408–16.

465 Khaw KT, Barrett-Connor E. Dietary potassium and stroke-associated mortality: a 12-year prospective population study. *N Engl J Med* 1987; **316**:235–40.

466 Iso H, Stampfer MJ, Manson JE, Rexrode K, Hennekens CH, Colditz GA *et al*. Prospective study of calcium, potassium, and magnesium intake and risk of stroke in women. *Stroke* 1999; **30**:1772–9.

467 Di Legge S, Spence JD, Tamayo A, Hachinski V. Serum potassium level and dietary potassium intake as risk factors for stroke. *Neurology* 2003; **60**:1870.

468 Umesawa M, Iso H, Date C, Yamamoto A, Toyoshima H, Watanabe Y *et al*. Dietary intake of calcium in relation to mortality from cardiovascular disease: the JACC Study. *Stroke* 2006; **37**:20–6.

469 Orencia AJ, Daviglus ML, Dyer AR, Shekelle RB, Stamler J. Fish consumption and stroke in men: 30-year findings of the Chicago Western Electric Study. *Stroke* 1996; **27**:204–9.

470 He FJ, Nowson CA, MacGregor GA. Fruit and vegetable consumption and stroke: meta-analysis of cohort studies. *Lancet* 2006; **367**:320–6.

471 Albert CM, Hennekens CH, O'Donnell CJ, Ajani UA, Carey VJ, Willett WC *et al*. Fish consumption and risk of sudden cardiac death. *J Am Med Assoc* 1998; **279**:23–8.

472 Bouzan C, Cohen JT, Connor WE, Kris-Etherton PM, Gray GM, Konig A *et al*. A quantitative analysis of fish consumption and stroke risk. *Am J Prev Med* 2005; **29**:347–52.

473 Brouwer IA, Heeringa J, Geleijnse JM, Zock PL, Witteman JC. Intake of very long-chain n-3 fatty acids from fish and incidence of atrial fibrillation. The Rotterdam Study. *Am Heart J* 2006; **151**:857–62.

474 Steinberg D. Antioxidant vitamins and coronary heart disease. *N Engl J Med* 1993; **328**:1487–9.

475 Hennekens CH, Buring JE, Peto R. Antioxidant vitamins: benefits not yet proved. *N Engl J Med* 1994; **330**:1080–1.

476 Gaziano JM. Vitamin E and cardiovascular disease: observational studies. *Ann N Y Acad Sci* 2004; **1031**:280–91.

477 Bulpitt CJ. Vitamin C and vascular disease. *Br Med J* 1995; **310**:1548–9.

478 Nyyssonen K, Parviainen MT, Salonen R, Tuomilehto J, Salonen JT. Vitamin C deficiency and risk of myocardial infarction: prospective population study of men from eastern Finland. *Br Med J* 1997; **314**:634–8.

479 Voko Z, Hollander M, Hofman A, Koudstaal PJ, Breteler MM. Dietary antioxidants and the risk of ischemic stroke: the Rotterdam Study. *Neurology* 2003; **61**:1273–5.

480 Greenberg ER, Baron JA, Karagas MR, Stukel TA, Nierenberg DW, Stevens MM *et al*. Mortality associated with low plasma concentration of beta carotene and the effect of oral supplementation. *J Am Med Assoc* 1996; **275**:699–703.

481 Tornwall ME, Virtamo J, Korhonen PA, Virtanen MJ, Albanes D, Huttunen JK. Postintervention effect of alpha tocopherol and beta carotene on different strokes: a 6-year follow-up of the Alpha Tocopherol, Beta Carotene Cancer Prevention Study. *Stroke* 2004; **35**:1908–13.

482 Hak AE, Ma J, Powell CB, Campos H, Gaziano JM, Willett WC *et al*. Prospective study of plasma carotenoids and tocopherols in relation to risk of ischemic stroke. *Stroke* 2004; **35**:1584–8.

483 Hertog MG, Feskens EJ, Kromhout D. Antioxidant flavonols and coronary heart disease risk. *Lancet* 1997; **349**:699.

484 Arts IC, Hollman PC. Polyphenols and disease risk in epidemiologic studies. *Am J Clin Nutr* 2005; **81**:317S–25S.

485 Steinberg D. Clinical trials of antioxidants in atherosclerosis: are we doing the right thing? *Lancet* 1995; **346**:36–8.

486 Stephens N. Anti-oxidant therapy for ischaemic heart disease: where do we stand? *Lancet* 1997; **349**:1710–11.

487 GISSI-Prevenzione Investigators. Dietary supplementation with n-3 polyunsaturated fatty acids and vitamin E after myocardial infarction: results of the GISSI-Prevenzione trial. *Lancet* 1999; **354**:447–55.

488 Hooper L, Capps N, Clements G *et al*. Foods or supplements in omega-3 fatty acids for preventing cardiovascular disease in patients with ischaemic heart disease (protocol for a Cochrance Review). *The Cochrane Library* 2000. Update Software: Oxford.

489 Leppala JM, Virtamo J, Fogelholm R, Huttunen JK, Albanes D, Taylor PR *et al*. Controlled trial of alpha-tocopherol and beta-carotene supplements on stroke incidence and mortality in male smokers. *Arterioscler Thromb Vasc Biol* 2000; **20**:230–5.

490 Key TJ, Appleby PN, Rosell MS. Health effects of vegetarian and vegan diets. *Proc Nutr Soc* 2006; **65**:35–41.

491 Kawachi I, Colditz GA, Stone CB. Does coffee drinking increase the risk of coronary heart disease? results from a meta-analysis. *Br Heart J* 1994; **72**:269–75.

492 Stensvold I, Tverdal A, Jacobsen BK. Cohort study of coffee intake and death from coronary heart disease over 12 years. *Br Med J* 1996; **312**:544–5.

493 Willett WC, Stampfer MJ, Manson JE, Colditz GA, Rosner BA, Speizer FE *et al*. Coffee consumption and coronary heart disease in women: a ten-year follow-up. *J Am Med Assoc* 1996; **275**:458–62.

494 Lopez-Garcia E, van Dam RM, Willett WC, Rimm EB, Manson JE, Stampfer MJ *et al*. Coffee consumption and coronary heart disease in men and women: a prospective cohort study. *Circulation* 2006; **113**:2045–53.

495 Van Gijn J, Stampfer MJ, Wolfe CD, Algra A. The association between alcohol and stroke. In: Vershuren PM, ed. *Health Issues Related to Alcohol Consumption*. Washington: ILSI Press, 1993, p. 44.

496 Camargo CA, Jr. Moderate alcohol consumption and stroke: the epidemiologic evidence. *Stroke* 1989; **20**:1611–26.

497 Marmot M, Brunner E. Alcohol and cardiovascular disease: the status of the U shaped curve. *Br Med J* 1991; **303**:565–8.

498 Wannamethee SG, Shaper AG. Patterns of alcohol intake and risk of stroke in middle-aged British men. *Stroke* 1996; **27**:1033–9.

499 Doll R. One for the heart. *Br Med J* 1997; **315**:1664–8.

500 Kiechl S, Willeit J, Rungger G, Egger G, Oberhollenzer F, Bonora E. Alcohol consumption and atherosclerosis: what is the relation? Prospective results from the Bruneck Study. *Stroke* 1998; **29**:900–7.

501 Berger K, Ajani UA, Kase CS, Gaziano JM, Buring JE, Glynn RJ *et al*. Light-to-moderate alcohol consumption and risk of stroke among US male physicians. *N Engl J Med* 1999; **341**:1557–64.

502 Hart CL, Davey Smith G, Hole DJ, Hawthorne VM. Alcohol consumption and mortality from all causes, coronary heart disease and stroke: results from a prospective cohort study of Scottish men with 21 years of follow up. *Br Med J* 1999; **318**:1725–9.

503 Sacco RL, Elkind M, Boden-Albala B, Lin IF, Kargman DE, Hauser WA *et al*. The protective effect of moderate alcohol consumption on ischemic stroke. *J Am Med Assoc* 1999; **281**:53–60.

504 Elkind MS, Sciacca R, Boden-Albala B, Rundek T, Paik MC, Sacco RL. Moderate alcohol consumption reduces risk of ischemic stroke: the Northern Manhattan Study. *Stroke* 2006; **37**:13–19.

505 Gorelick PB. Alcohol and stroke. *Stroke* 1987; **18**:268–71.

506 Hillbom M, Numminen H, Juvela S. Recent heavy drinking of alcohol and embolic stroke. *Stroke* 1999; **30**:2307–12.

507 Mazzaglia G, Britton AR, Altmann DR, Chenet L. Exploring the relationship between alcohol consumption and non-fatal or fatal stroke: a systematic review. *Addiction* 2001; **96**:1743–56.

508 Ben Shlomo Y, Markowe H, Shipley M, Marmot MG. Stroke risk from alcohol consumption using different control groups. *Stroke* 1992; **23**:1093–8.

509 MacMahon SW, Norton RN. Alcohol and hypertension: implications for prevention and treatment. *Ann Intern Med* 1986; **105**:124–6.

510 Puddey IB, Beilin LJ, Vandongen R. Regular alcohol use raises blood pressure in treated hypertensive subjects: a randomised controlled trial. *Lancet* 1987; **1**:647–51.

511 Marmot MG, Elliott P, Shipley MJ, Dyer AR, Ueshima H, Beevers DG *et al*. Alcohol and blood pressure: the INTERSALT study. *Br Med J* 1994; **308**:1263–7.

512 Kaplan NM. Alcohol and hypertension. *Lancet* 1995; **345**:1588–9.

513 Rimm EB, Williams P, Fosher K, Criqui M, Stampfer MJ. Moderate alcohol intake and lower risk of coronary heart disease: meta-analysis of effects on lipids and haemostatic factors. *Br Med J* 1999; **319**:1523–8.

514 Sudlow CL, Warlow CP. Comparable studies of the incidence of stroke and its pathological types: results from

an international collaboration. International Stroke Incidence Collaboration. *Stroke* 1997; **28**:491–9.

515 Feigin VL, Lawes CM, Bennett DA, Anderson CS. Stroke epidemiology: a review of population-based studies of incidence, prevalence, and case-fatality in the late 20th century. *Lancet Neurol* 2003; **2**:43–53.

516 Broderick J, Brott T, Kothari R, Miller R, Khoury J, Pancioli A *et al*. The Greater Cincinnati/Northern Kentucky Stroke Study: preliminary first-ever and total incidence rates of stroke among blacks. *Stroke* 1998; **29**:415–21.

517 Sacco RL, Boden-Albala B, Gan R, Chen X, Kargman DE, Shea S *et al*. Stroke incidence among white, black, and Hispanic residents of an urban community: the Northern Manhattan Stroke Study. *Am J Epidemiol* 1998; **147**:259–68.

518 Stewart JA, Dundas R, Howard RS, Rudd AG, Wolfe CD. Ethnic differences in incidence of stroke: prospective study with stroke register. *Br Med J* 1999; **318**:967–71.

519 Wolfe CD, Rudd AG, Howard R, Coshall C, Stewart J, Lawrence E *et al*. Incidence and case fatality rates of stroke subtypes in a multiethnic population: the South London Stroke Register. *J Neurol Neurosurg Psychiatry* 2002; **72**:211–16.

520 Wolfe CD, Smeeton NC, Coshall C, Tilling K, Rudd AG. Survival differences after stroke in a multiethnic population: follow-up study with the South London stroke register. *Br Med J* 2005; **331**:431.

521 Giles WH, Kittner SJ, Hebel JR, Losonczy KG, Sherwin RW. Determinants of black-white differences in the risk of cerebral infarction. The National Health and Nutrition Examination Survey Epidemiologic Follow-up Study. *Arch Intern Med* 1995; **155**:1319–24.

522 Davey SG, Neaton JD, Wentworth D, Stamler R, Stamler J. Mortality differences between black and white men in the USA: contribution of income and other risk factors among men screened for the MRFIT. MRFIT Research Group. Multiple Risk Factor Intervention Trial. *Lancet* 1998; **351**:934–9.

523 Gorelick PB. Cerebrovascular disease in African Americans. *Stroke* 1998; **29**:2656–64.

524 Balarajan R. Ethnic differences in mortality from ischaemic heart disease and cerebrovascular disease in England and Wales. *Br Med J* 1991; **302**:560–4.

525 Bhopal R, Rahemtulla T, Sheikh A. Persistent high stroke mortality in Bangladeshi populations. *Br Med J* 2005; **331**:1096–7.

526 McKeigue PM, Shah B, Marmot MG. Relation of central obesity and insulin resistance with high diabetes prevalence and cardiovascular risk in South Asians. *Lancet* 1991; **337**:382–6.

527 Bhatnagar D, Anand IS, Durrington PN, Patel DJ, Wander GS, Mackness MI *et al*. Coronary risk factors in people from the Indian subcontinent living in west London and their siblings in India. *Lancet* 1995; **345**:405–9.

528 Winkleby MA, Kraemer HC, Ahn DK, Varady AN. Ethnic and socioeconomic differences in cardiovascular disease risk factors: findings for women from the Third National Health and Nutrition Examination Survey, 1988–1994. *J Am Med Assoc* 1998; **280**:356–62.

529 Bhopal R, Unwin N, White M, Yallop J, Walker L, Alberti KG *et al*. Heterogeneity of coronary heart disease risk factors in Indian, Pakistani, Bangladeshi, and European origin populations: cross sectional study. *Br Med J* 1999; **319**:215–20.

530 Bonita R, Broad JB, Beaglehole R. Ethnic differences in stroke incidence and case fatality in Auckland, New Zealand. *Stroke* 1997; **28**:758–61.

531 Anderson CS, Carter KN, Hackett ML, Feigin V, Barber PA, Broad JB *et al*. Trends in stroke incidence in Auckland, New Zealand, during 1981 to 2003. *Stroke* 2005; **36**:2087–93.

532 Dichgans M. Genetics of ischaemic stroke. *Lancet Neurol* 2007; **6**:149–61.

533 Dichgans M, Markus HS. Genetic association studies in stroke: methodological issues and proposed standard criteria. *Stroke* 2005; **36**:2027–31.

534 Sudlow C, Martinez Gonzalez NA, Kim J, Clark C. Does apolipoprotein E genotype influence the risk of ischemic stroke, intracerebral hemorrhage, or subarachnoid hemorrhage? Systematic review and meta-analyses of 31 studies among 5961 cases and 17,965 controls. *Stroke* 2006; **37**:364–70.

535 Hassan A, Markus HS. Genetics and ischaemic stroke. *Brain* 2000; **123**(9):1784–812.

536 Casas JP, Hingorani AD, Bautista LE, Sharma P. Meta-analysis of genetic studies in ischemic stroke: thirty-two genes involving approximately 18,000 cases and 58,000 controls. *Arch Neurol* 2004; **61**:1652–61.

537 Keavney B, McKenzie C, Parish S, Palmer A, Clark S, Youngman L *et al*. Large-scale test of hypothesised associations between the angiotensin-converting-enzyme insertion/deletion polymorphism and myocardial infarction in about 5000 cases and 6000 controls. International Studies of Infarct Survival (ISIS) Collaborators. *Lancet* 2000; **355**:434–42.

538 Wheeler JG, Keavney BD, Watkins H, Collins R, Danesh J. Four paraoxonase gene polymorphisms in 11212 cases of coronary heart disease and 12786 controls: meta-analysis of 43 studies. *Lancet* 2004; **363**:689–95.

539 Hassan A, Sham PC, Markus HS. Planning genetic studies in human stroke: sample size estimates based on family history data. *Neurology* 2002; **58**:1483–8.

540 Gulcher JR, Gretarsdottir S, Helgadottir A, Stefansson K. Genes contributing to risk for common forms of stroke. *Trends Mol Med* 2005; **11**:217–24.

541 Rosand J, Bayley N, Rost N, de Bakker PI. Many hypotheses but no replication for the association between PDE4D and stroke. *Nat Genet* 2006; **38**:1091–2.

542 Gulcher JR, Kong A, Gretarsdottir S, Thorleifsson G, Stefansson K. Reply to 'Many hypotheses but no replication for the association between PDE4D and stroke'. *Nat Genet* 2006; **38**:1092–3.

543 Wang WY, Barratt BJ, Clayton DG, Todd JA. Genome-wide association studies: theoretical and practical concerns. *Nat Rev Genet* 2005; **6**:109–18.

544 Hirschhorn JN, Daly MJ. Genome-wide association studies for common diseases and complex traits. *Nat Rev Genet* 2005; **6**:95–108.

545 Matarin M, Brown WM, Scholz S, Simon-Sanchez J, Fung HC, Hernandez D *et al*. A genome-wide genotyping study in patients with ischaemic stroke: initial analysis and data release. *Lancet Neurol* 2007; **6**:414–20.

546 Humphries SE, Morgan L. Genetic risk factors for stroke and carotid atherosclerosis: insights into pathophysiology from candidate gene approaches. *Lancet Neurol* 2004; **3**:227–35.

547 Paternoster L, Martinez-Gonzalez N, Lewis S, Sudlow C. Association between apolipoprotein E genotype and carotid intima media thickness may suggest a specific effect on large artery atherothrombotic stroke. *Stroke* 2007; in press.

548 Kunst AE, del Rios M, Groenhof F, Mackenbach JP. Socioeconomic inequalities in stroke mortality among middle-aged men: an international overview. European Union Working Group on Socioeconomic Inequalities in Health. *Stroke* 1998; **29**:2285–91.

549 Van Rossum CT, van de Mheen H, Breteler MM, Grobbee DE, Mackenbach JP. Socioeconomic differences in stroke among Dutch elderly women: the Rotterdam Study. *Stroke* 1999; **30**:357–62.

550 Davey Smith, G. Down at heart: the meaning and implications of social inequalities in cardiovascular disease. *J R Coll Phys Lond* 1997; **31**:414–24.

551 Morris RW, Whincup PH, Emberson JR, Lampe FC, Walker M, Shaper AG. North-south gradients in Britain for stroke and CHD: are they explained by the same factors? *Stroke* 2003; **34**:2604–9.

552 Barker DJP. *Mothers, Babies, and Disease in Later Life*. London: BMJ Publishing, 1994.

553 Martyn CN, Barker DJ, Osmond C. Mothers' pelvic size, fetal growth, and death from stroke and coronary heart disease in men in the UK. *Lancet* 1996; **348**:1264–8.

554 Rich-Edwards JW, Stampfer MJ, Manson JE, Rosner B, Hankinson SE, Colditz GA *et al*. Birth weight and risk of cardiovascular disease in a cohort of women followed up since 1976. *Br Med J* 1997; **315**:396–400.

555 Forsen T, Eriksson JG, Tuomilehto J, Osmond C, Barker DJ. Growth in utero and during childhood among women who develop coronary heart disease: longitudinal study. *Br Med J* 1999; **319**:1403–7.

556 Lynch JW, Kaplan GA, Cohen RD, Kauhanen J, Wilson TW, Smith NL *et al*. Childhood and adult socioeconomic status as predictors of mortality in Finland. *Lancet* 1994; **343**:524–7.

557 Paneth N, Susser M. Early origin of coronary heart disease (the 'Barker hypothesis'). *Br Med J* 1995; **310**:411–12.

558 Lucas A, Fewtrell MS, Cole TJ. Fetal origins of adult disease: the hypothesis revisited. *Br Med J* 1999; **319**:245–9.

559 Huxley R, Neil A, Collins R. Unravelling the fetal origins hypothesis: is there really an inverse association between birthweight and subsequent blood pressure? *Lancet* 2002; **360**:659–65.

560 Grau AJ, Buggle F, Becher H, Zimmermann E, Spiel M, Fent T *et al*. Recent bacterial and viral infection is a risk factor for cerebrovascular ischemia: clinical and biochemical studies. *Neurology* 1998; **50**:196–203.

561 Beck J, Garcia R, Heiss G, Vokonas PS, Offenbacher S. Periodontal disease and cardiovascular disease. *J Periodontol* 1996; **67**:1123–37.

562 Markus HS, Mendall MA. *Helicobacter pylori* infection: a risk factor for ischaemic cerebrovascular disease and carotid atheroma. *J Neurol Neurosurg Psychiatry* 1998; **64**:104–7.

563 Danesh J, Youngman L, Clark S, Parish S, Peto R, Collins R. *Helicobacter pylori* infection and early onset myocardial infarction: case–control and sibling pairs study. *Br Med J* 1999; **319**:1157–62.

564 Danesh J, Whincup P, Walker M, Lennon L, Thomson A, Appleby P *et al*. *Chlamydia pneumoniae* IgG titres and coronary heart disease: prospective study and meta-analysis. *Br Med J* 2000; **321**:208–13.

565 Fagerberg B, Gnarpe J, Gnarpe H, Agewall S, Wikstrand J. *Chlamydia pneumoniae* but not cytomegalovirus antibodies are associated with future risk of stroke and cardiovascular disease: a prospective study in middle-aged to elderly men with treated hypertension. *Stroke* 1999; **30**:299–305.

566 Glader CA, Stegmayr B, Boman J, Stenlund H, Weinehall L, Hallmans G *et al*. *Chlamydia pneumoniae* antibodies and high lipoprotein(a) levels do not predict ischemic cerebral infarctions: results from a nested case-control study in Northern Sweden. *Stroke* 1999; **30**:2013–18.

567 Strachan DP, Carrington D, Mendall MA, Ballam L, Morris J, Butland BK *et al*. Relation of *Chlamydia pneumoniae* serology to mortality and incidence of ischaemic heart disease over 13 years in the Caerphilly prospective heart disease study. *Br Med J* 1999; **318**:1035–9.

568 Ngeh J, Gupta S, Goodbourn C, Panayiotou B, McElligott G. *Chlamydia pneumoniae* in elderly patients with stroke (C-PEPS): a case–control study on the seroprevalence of *Chlamydia pneumoniae* in elderly patients with acute cerebrovascular disease. *Cerebrovasc Dis* 2003; **15**:11–16.

569 Danesh J, Whincup P, Walker M. *Chlamydia pneumoniae* IgA titres and coronary heart disease: prospective study and meta-analysis. *Eur Heart J* 2003; **24**:881.

570 Ridker PM, Hennekens CH, Buring JE, Rifai N. C-reactive protein and other markers of inflammation in the prediction of cardiovascular disease in women. *N Engl J Med* 2000; **342**:836–43.

571 Yamashita K, Ouchi K, Shirai M, Gondo T, Nakazawa T, Ito H. Distribution of *Chlamydia pneumoniae* infection in the atherosclerotic carotid artery. *Stroke* 1998; **29**:773–8.

572 Gurfinkel E, Bozovich G, Daroca A, Beck E, Mautner B. Randomised trial of roxithromycin in non-Q-wave coronary syndromes: ROXIS Pilot Study. ROXIS Study Group. *Lancet* 1997; **350**:404–7.

573 Danesh J. Antibiotics in the prevention of heart attacks. *Lancet* 2005; **365**:365–7.

574 Jespersen CM, Als-Nielsen B, Damgaard M, Hansen JF, Hansen S, Helo OH *et al*. Randomised placebo-controlled multicentre trial to assess short-term clarithromycin for patients with stable coronary heart disease: CLARICOR trial. *Br Med J* 2006; **332**:22–7.

575 House A, Dennis M, Mogridge L, Hawton K, Warlow C. Life events and difficulties preceding stroke. *J Neurol Neurosurg Psychiatry* 1990; **53**:1024–8.

576 Rosengren A, Orth-Gomer K, Wedel H, Wilhelmsen L. Stressful life events, social support, and mortality in men born in 1933. *Br Med J* 1993; **307**:1102–5.

577 Hemingway H, Marmot M. Psychological factors in the aetiology and prognosis of coronary heart disease: systematic review of prospective cohort studies. *Br Med J* 1999; **318**:1460–7.

578 Everson SA, Kaplan GA, Goldberg DE, Lakka TA, Sivenius J, Salonen JT. Anger expression and incident stroke: prospective evidence from the Kuopio ischemic heart disease study. *Stroke* 1999; **30**:523–8.

579 Koton S, Tanne D, Bornstein NM, Green MS. Triggering risk factors for ischemic stroke: a case-crossover study. *Neurology* 2004; **63**:2006–10.

580 May M, McCarron P, Stansfeld S, Ben Shlomo Y, Gallacher J, Yarnell J *et al*. Does psychological distress predict the risk of ischemic stroke and transient ischemic attack? The Caerphilly Study. *Stroke* 2002; **33**:7–12.

581 Truelsen T, Nielsen N, Boysen G, Gronbaek M. Self-reported stress and risk of stroke: the Copenhagen City Heart Study. *Stroke* 2003; **34**:856–62.

582 Kagan AR. Atherosclerosis and myocardial lesions in subjects dying from fresh cerebrovascular disease. *Bull World Health Organ* 1976; **53**:597–600.

583 Stemmermann GN, Hayashi T, Resch JA, Chung CS, Reed DM, Rhoads GG. Risk factors related to ischemic and hemorrhagic cerebrovascular disease at autopsy: the Honolulu Heart Study. *Stroke* 1984; **15**:23–8.

584 Brass LM, Hartigan PM, Page WF, Concato J. Importance of cerebrovascular disease in studies of myocardial infarction. *Stroke* 1996; **27**:1173–6.

585 Herman B, Schmitz PI, Leyten AC, Van Luijk JH, Frenken CW, Op De Coul AA *et al*. Multivariate logistic analysis of risk factors for stroke in Tilburg, The Netherlands. *Am J Epidemiol* 1983; **118**:514–25.

586 Woo J, Lau E, Lam CW, Kay R, Teoh R, Wong HY *et al*. Hypertension, lipoprotein(a), and apolipoprotein A-I as risk factors for stroke in the Chinese. *Stroke* 1991; **22**:203–8.

587 Feigin VL, Wiebers DO, Nikitin YP, O'Fallon WM, Whisnant JP. Risk factors for ischemic stroke in a Russian community: a population-based case–control study. *Stroke* 1998; **29**:34–9.

588 Kagan A, Popper JS, Rhoads GG. Factors related to stroke incidence in Hawaii Japanese men. The Honolulu Heart Study. *Stroke* 1980; **11**:14–21.

589 Kannel WB, Wolf PA, Verter J. Manifestations of coronary disease predisposing to stroke. The Framingham study. *J Am Med Assoc* 1983; **250**:2942–6.

590 Knutsen R, Knutsen SF, Curb JD, Reed DM, Kautz JA, Yano K. Predictive value of resting electrocardiograms for 12-year incidence of stroke in the Honolulu Heart Program. *Stroke* 1988; **19**:555–9.

591 Pullicino PM, Halperin JL, Thompson JL. Stroke in patients with heart failure and reduced left ventricular ejection fraction. *Neurology* 2000; **54**:288–94.

592 Hueb JC, Zanati SG, Okoshi K, Raffin CN, Silveira LV, Matsubara BB. Association between atherosclerotic aortic plaques and left ventricular hypertrophy in patients with cerebrovascular events. *Stroke* 2006; **37**:958–62.

593 Sandok BA, Whisnant JP, Furlan AJ, Mickell JL. Carotid artery bruits: prevalence survey and differential diagnosis. *Mayo Clin.Proc.* 1982; **57**:227–30.

594 Mathiesen EB, Joakimsen O, Bonaa KH. Prevalence of and risk factors associated with carotid artery stenosis: the Tromso Study. *Cerebrovasc Dis* 2001; **12**:44–51.

595 Heeringa J, van der Kuip DA, Hofman A, Kors JA, van Rooij FJ, Lip GY *et al*. Subclinical atherosclerosis and risk of atrial fibrillation: the Rotterdam Study. *Arch Intern Med* 2007; **167**:382–7.

596 Wiebers DO, Whisnant JP, Sandok BA, O'Fallon WM. Prospective comparison of a cohort with asymptomatic carotid bruit and a population-based cohort without carotid bruit. *Stroke* 1990; **21**:984–8.

597 Touze E, Warlow CP, Rothwell PM. Risk of coronary and other nonstroke vascular death in relation to the presence and extent of atherosclerotic disease at the carotid bifurcation. *Stroke* 2006; **37**:2904–9.

598 Davey Smith G, Shipley MJ, Rose G. Intermittent claudication, heart disease risk factors and mortality. The Whitehall Study. *Circulation* 1990; **82**: 1925–31.

599 Leng GC, Fowkes FG, Lee AJ, Dunbar J, Housley E, Ruckley CV. Use of ankle brachial pressure index to predict cardiovascular events and death: a cohort study. *Br Med J* 1996; **313**:1440–4.

600 Allan PL, Mowbray PI, Lee AJ, Fowkes FG. Relationship between carotid intima-media thickness and symptomatic and asymptomatic peripheral arterial disease. The Edinburgh Artery Study. *Stroke* 1997; **28**:348–53.

601 Hankey GJ, Norman PE, Eikelboom JW. Medical treatment of peripheral arterial disease. *J Am Med Assoc* 2006; **295**:547–53.

602 Leys D, Woimant F, Ferrieres J, Bauters C, Touboul PJ, Guerillot M *et al*. Detection and management of associated atherothrombotic locations in patients with a recent atherothrombotic ischemic stroke: results of the DETECT survey. *Cerebrovasc Dis* 2006; **21**:60–6.

603 Carty GA, Nachtigal T, Magyar R, Herzler G, Bays R. Abdominal duplex ultrasound screening for occult aortic aneurysm during carotid arterial evaluation. *J Vasc Surg* 1993; **17**:696–702.

604 Karanjia PN, Madden KP, Lobner S. Coexistence of abdominal aortic aneurysm in patients with carotid stenosis. *Stroke* 1994; **25**:627–30.

605 Hollander M, Hak AE, Koudstaal PJ, Bots ML, Grobbee DE, Hofman A *et al*. Comparison between measures of atherosclerosis and risk of stroke: the Rotterdam Study. *Stroke* 2003; **34**:2367–72.

606 Ashton HA, Buxton MJ, Day NE, Kim LG, Marteau TM, Scott RA *et al*. The Multicentre Aneurysm Screening Study (MASS) into the effect of abdominal aortic aneurysm screening on mortality in men: a randomised controlled trial. *Lancet* 2002; **360**:1531–9.

607 Hankey GJ. Potential new risk factors for ischemic stroke: what is their potential? *Stroke* 2006; **37**: 2181–8.

608 Hopkins PN, Williams RR. A survey of 246 suggested coronary risk factors. *Atherosclerosis* 1981; **40**:1–52.

609 Flossmann E, Redgrave JN, Schulz UG, Briley D, Rothwell PM. Reliability of clinical diagnosis of the symptomatic vascular territory in patients with recent TIA or minor stroke. *Cerebrovasc Dis* 2006; **21**:18.

610 Yamamoto Y, Georgiadis AL, Chang HM, Caplan LR. Posterior cerebral artery territory infarcts in the New England Medical Center Posterior Circulation Registry. *Arch Neurol* 1999; **56**:824–32.

611 Zeman A, Anslow P, Greenhall R. Persistent trigeminal artery and brain stem stroke. *Cerebrovasc Dis* 1993; **3**:236–40.

612 Gasecki AP, Fox AJ, Lebrun LH, Daneault N. Bilateral occipital infarctions associated with carotid stenosis in a patient with persistent trigeminal artery. The Collaborators of the North American Carotid Endarterectomy Trial (NASCET). *Stroke* 1994; **25**:1520–3.

613 Tohgi H, Takahashi S, Chiba K, Hirata Y. Cerebellar infarction: clinical and neuroimaging analysis in 293 patients. The Tohoku Cerebellar Infarction Study Group. *Stroke* 1993; **24**:1697–701.

614 Chaves CJ, Caplan LR, Chung CS, Tapia J, Amarenco P, Teal P *et al*. Cerebellar infarcts in the New England Medical Center Posterior Circulation Stroke Registry. *Neurology* 1994; **44**:1385–90.

615 Min WK, Kim YS, Kim JY, Park SP, Suh CK. Atherothrombotic cerebellar infarction: vascular lesion-MRI correlation of 31 cases. *Stroke* 1999; **30**:2376–81.

616 Savitz SI, Caplan LR. Vertebrobasilar disease. *N Engl J Med* 2005; **352**:2618–26.

617 Castaigne P, Lhermitte F, Buge A, Escourolle R, Hauw JJ, Lyon-Caen O. Paramedian thalamic and midbrain infarct: clinical and neuropathological study. *Ann Neurol* 1981; **10**:127–48.

618 Bogousslavsky J, Caplan LR. Vertebrobasilar occlusive disease: review of selected aspects. 3. Thalamic infarcts. *Cerebrovasc Dis* 1993; **3**:193–205.

619 Voetsch B, DeWitt LD, Pessin MS, Caplan LR. Basilar artery occlusive disease in the New England Medical Center Posterior Circulation Registry. *Arch Neurol* 2004; **61**:496–504.

620 Brice JG, Dowsett DJ, Lowe RD. Haemodynamic effects of carotid artery stenosis. *Br Med J* 1964; **5421**:1363–6.

621 Deweese JA, May AG, Lipchik EO, Rob CG. Anatomic and hemodynamic correlations in carotid artery stenosis. *Stroke* 1970; **1**:149–57.

622 Archie JP, Jr, Feldtman RW. Critical stenosis of the internal carotid artery. *Surgery* 1981; **89**:67–72.

623 Derlon JM, Bouvard G, Viader F, Petit MC, Dupuy B, Khoury S *et al*. Impaired cerebral hemodynamics in internal carotid occlusion. *Cerebrovasc Dis* 1992; **2**:72–81.

624 Derdeyn CP, Grubb RL, Jr, Powers WJ. Cerebral hemodynamic impairment: methods of measurement and association with stroke risk. *Neurology* 1999; **53**:251–9.

625 Kluytmans M, van der GJ, van Everdingen KJ, Klijn CJ, Kappelle LJ, Viergever MA. Cerebral hemodynamics in relation to patterns of collateral flow. *Stroke* 1999; **30**:1432–9.

626 Gibbs JM, Wise RJ, Leenders KL, Jones T. Evaluation of cerebral perfusion reserve in patients with carotid-artery occlusion. *Lancet* 1984; **1**:310–14.

627 Powers WJ, Press GA, Grubb RL, Jr, Gado M, Raichle ME. The effect of hemodynamically significant carotid artery disease on the hemodynamic status of the cerebral circulation. *Ann Intern Med* 1987; **106**:27–34.

628 Schumann P, Touzani O, Young AR, Morello R, Baron JC, MacKenzie ET. Evaluation of the ratio of cerebral blood flow to cerebral blood volume as an index of local cerebral perfusion pressure. *Brain* 1998; **121**(7):1369–79.

629 Grubb RL, Jr, Derdeyn CP, Fritsch SM, Carpenter DA, Yundt KD, Videen TO *et al*. Importance of hemodynamic factors in the prognosis of symptomatic carotid occlusion. *J Am Med Assoc* 1998; **280**:1055–60.

630 Naylor AR, Merrick MV, Gillespie I, Sandercock PA, Warlow CP, Cull RE *et al*. Prevalence of impaired cerebrovascular reserve in patients with symptomatic carotid artery disease. *Br J Surg* 1994; **81**:45–8.

631 Kleinschmidt A, Steinmetz H, Sitzer M, Merboldt KD, Frahm J. Magnetic resonance imaging of regional cerebral blood oxygenation changes under acetazolamide in carotid occlusive disease. *Stroke* 1995; **26**:106–10.

632 Mandai K, Sueyoshi K, Fukunaga R, Nukada M, Tsukaguchi I, Matsumoto M *et al*. Evaluation of cerebral vasoreactivity by three-dimensional time-of-flight magnetic resonance angiography. *Stroke* 1994; **25**:1807–11.

633 Binaghi S, Colleoni ML, Maeder P, Uske A, Regli L, Dehdashti AR *et al*. CT angiography and perfusion CT in cerebral vasospasm after subarachnoid hemorrhage. *Am J Neuroradiol* 2007; **28**:750–8.

634 Parsons MW, Pepper EM, Bateman GA, Wang Y, Levi CR. Identification of the penumbra and infarct core on hyperacute noncontrast and perfusion CT. *Neurology* 2007; **68**:730–6.

635 Smielewski P, Czosnyka M, Pickard JD, Kirkpatrick P. Clinical evaluation of near-infrared spectroscopy for testing cerebrovascular reactivity in patients with carotid artery disease. *Stroke* 1997; **28**:331–8.

636 Bladin CF, Chambers BR. Frequency and pathogenesis of hemodynamic stroke. *Stroke* 1994; **25**:2179–82.

637 Kendell RE, Marshall J. Role of hypotension in the genesis of transient focal cerebral ischaemic attacks. *Br Med J* 1963; **2**(5353):344–8.

638 Torvik A. The pathogenesis of watershed infarcts in the brain. *Stroke* 1984; **15**:221–3.

639 Yanagihara T, Sundt TM, Jr, Piepgras DG. Weakness of the lower extremity in carotid occlusive disease. *Arch Neurol* 1988; **45**:297–301.

640 Bladin CF, Chambers BR. Clinical features, pathogenesis, and computed tomographic characteristics of internal watershed infarction. *Stroke* 1993; **24**:1925–32.

641 Caplan LR, Sergay S. Positional cerebral ischaemia. *J Neurol Neurosurg Psychiatry* 1976; **39**:385–91.

642 Pantin CF, Young RA. Postprandial blindness. *Br Med J* 1980; **281**:1686.

643 Raymond LA, Sacks JG, Choromokos E, Khodadad G. Short posterior ciliary artery insufficiency with hyperthermia (Uhthoff's symptom). *Am J Ophthalmol* 1980; **90**:619–23.

644 Purvin VA, Dunn DW. Nitrate-induced transient ischemic attacks. *South Med J* 1981; **74**:1130–1.

645 Nobile-Orazio E, Sterzi R. Cerebral ischaemia after nifedipine treatment. *Br Med J (Clin Res)* 1981; **283**:948.

646 Stark RJ, Wodak J. Primary orthostatic cerebral ischaemia. *J Neurol Neurosurg Psychiatry* 1983; **46**:883–91.

647 Milder DG, Lance JW. Intermittent claudication of one cerebral hemisphere. *Neurology* 1984; **34**:692–4.

648 Hankey GJ, Gubbay SS. Focal cerebral ischaemia and infarction due to antihypertensive therapy. *Med J Aust* 1987; **146**:412–14.

649 Ross Russell RW. Cause and treatment of insufficiency in the cerebral circulation. *Clin Neurol Neurosurg* 1988; **90**:19–24.

650 Kamata T, Yokata T, Furukawa T, Tsukagoshi H. Cerebral ischaemic attack caused by postprandial hypotension. *Stroke* 1994; **25**:511–13.

651 Gironelli A, Rey A, Marti-Vilalta JL. Positional cerebral ischaemia. *Cerebrovasc Dis* 1995; **5**:313–14.

652 Schlingemann RO, Smit AA, Lunel HF, Hijdra A. Amaurosis fugax on standing and angle-closure glaucoma with clomipramine. *Lancet* 1996; **347**:465.

653 Leira EC, Ajax T, Adams HP, Jr. Limb-shaking carotid transient ischemic attacks successfully treated with modification of the antihypertensive regimen. *Arch Neurol* 1997; **54**:904–5.

654 Furlan AJ, Whisnant JP, Kearns TP. Unilateral visual loss in bright light: an unusual symptom of carotid artery occlusive disease. *Arch Neurol* 1979; **36**:675–6.

655 Ross Russell RW, Page NGR. Critical perfusion of brain and retina. *Brain* 1983; **106**:419–34.

656 Yanagihara T, Piepgras DG, Klass DW. Repetitive involuntary movement associated with episodic cerebral ischemia. *Ann Neurol* 1985; **18**:244–50.

657 Wiebers DO, Swanson JW, Cascino TL, Whisnant JP. Bilateral loss of vision in bright light. *Stroke* 1989; **20**:554–8.

658 Baumgartner RW, Baumgartner I. Vasomotor reactivity is exhausted in transient ischaemic attacks with limb shaking. *J Neurol Neurosurg Psychiatry* 1998; **65**:561–4.

659 Schulz UG, Rothwell PM. Transient ischaemic attacks mimicking focal motor seizures. *Postgrad Med J* 2002; **78**:246–7.

660 Angeloni U, Bozzao L, Fantozzi L, Bastianello S, Kushner M, Fieschi C. Internal borderzone infarction following acute middle cerebral artery occlusion. *Neurology* 1990; **40**:1196–8.

661 Belden JR, Caplan LR, Pessin MS, Kwan E. Mechanisms and clinical features of posterior border-zone infarcts. *Neurology* 1999; **53**:1312–18.

662 Hupperts RM, Lodder J, Heuts-van Raak EPM, Wilmink JT, Kessels AGH. Borderzone brain infarcts on CT taking into account the variability in vascular supply areas. *Cerebrovasc Dis* 1996; **6**:294–300.

663 Hupperts RM, Warlow CP, Slattery J, Rothwell PM. Severe stenosis of the internal carotid artery is not associated with borderzone infarcts in patients randomised in the European Carotid Surgery Trial. *J Neurol* 1997; **244**: 45–50.

664 Hupperts RM, Lodder, J, Heuts-van Raak L, Kessels F. Border-zone small deep infarcts: vascular risk factors and relationship with signs of small and large-vessel disease. *Cerebrovasc Dis* 1997; **7**:280–3.

665 Gandolfo C, Del Sette M, Finocchi C, Calautti C, Loeb C. Internal borderzone infarction in patients with ischemic stroke. *Cerebrovasc Dis* 1998; **8**:255–8.

666 Nichols FT, III, Mawad M, Mohr JP, Stein B, Hilal S, Michelsen WJ. Focal headache during balloon inflation in the internal carotid and middle cerebral arteries. *Stroke* 1990; **21**:555–9.

667 Koudstaal PJ, van Gijn J, Kappelle LJ. Headache in transient or permanent cerebral ischemia. Dutch TIA Study Group. *Stroke* 1991; **22**:754–9.

668 Vestergaard K, Andersen G, Nielsen MI, Jensen TS. Headache in stroke. *Stroke* 1993; **24**:1621–4.

669 Jorgensen HS, Jespersen HF, Nakayama H, Raaschou HO, Olsen TS. Headache in stroke: the Copenhagen Stroke Study. *Neurology* 1994; **44**:1793–7.

670 Kumral E, Bogousslavsky J, Van Melle G, Regli F, Pierre P. Headache at stroke onset: the Lausanne Stroke Registry. *J Neurol Neurosurg Psychiatry* 1995; **58**:490–2.

671 Mitsias PD, Ramadan NM, Levine SR, Schultz L, Welch KM. Factors determining headache at onset of acute ischemic stroke. *Cephalalgia* 2006; **26**:150–7.

672 Pohlmann-Eden B, Hoch DB, Cochius JI, Hennerici MG. Stroke and epilepsy: critical review of the literature. I. Epidemiology and risk factors. *Cerebrovasc Dis* 1996; **6**:332–8.

673 Pohlmann-Eden B, Cochius JI, Hoch DB, Hennerici MG. Stroke and epilepsy: critical review of the literature. II. Risk factors, pathophysiology and overlap syndrome. *Cerebrovasc Dis* 1997; **7**:2–9.

674 Arboix A, Garcia-Eroles L, Massons JB, Oliveres M, Comes E. Predictive factors of early seizures after acute cerebrovascular disease. *Stroke* 1997; **28**:1590–4.

675 Burn J, Dennis M, Bamford J, Sandercock P, Wade D, Warlow C. Epileptic seizures after a first stroke: the Oxfordshire Community Stroke Project. *Br Med J* 1997; **315**:1582–7.

676 Arboix A, Comes E, Garcia-Eroles L, Massons JB, Oliveres M, Balcells M. Prognostic value of very early seizures for in-hospital mortality in atherothrombotic infarction. *Eur Neurol* 2003; **50**:78–84.

677 Kaplan PW. Focal seizures resembling transient ischaemic attacks due to subclinical ischaemia. *Cerebrovasc Dis* 1993; **3**:241–3.

678 Cleary P, Shorvon S, Tallis R. Late-onset seizures as a predictor of subsequent stroke. *Lancet* 2004; **363**:1184–6.

679 Jacobson DM, Terrence CF, Reinmuth OM. The neurologic manifestations of fat embolism. *Neurology* 1986; **36**:847–51.

680 Fabian TC. Unravelling the fat embolism syndrome. *N Engl J Med* 1993; **329**:961–3.

681 Van Oostenbrugge RJ, Freling G, Lodder J, Lalisang R, Twijnstra A. Fatal stroke due to paradoxical fat embolism. *Cerebrovasc Dis* 1996; **6**:313–14.

682 Forteza AM, Koch S, Romano JG, Zych G, Bustillo IC, Duncan RC *et al*. Transcranial Doppler detection of fat emboli. *Stroke* 1999; **30**:2687–91.

683 Biousse V, Newman NJ, Lessell S. Audible pulsatile tinnitus in idiopathic intracranial hypertension. *Neurology* 1998; **50**:1185–6.

684 Waldvogel D, Mattle HP, Sturzenegger M, Schroth G. Pulsatile tinnitus: a review of 84 patients. *J Neurol* 1998; **245**:137–42.

685 Rastenyte D, Tuomilehto J, Sarti C. Genetics of stroke: a review. *J Neurol Sci* 1998; **153**:132–45.

686 Alberts MJ. *Genetics of Cerebrovascular Disease*. New York: Futura Publishing Company, 1999.

687 Flossmann E, Rothwell PM. Systematic review of methods and results of studies of the genetic epidemiology of ischaemic stroke. *Stroke* 2004; **35**:212–27.

688 Schulz UG, Briley D, Meagher T, Molyneux A, Rothwell PM. Diffusion-weighted MRI in 300 patients presenting late with subacute transient ischemic attack or minor stroke. *Stroke* 2004; **35**:2459–65.

689 Flossmann E, Rothwell PM. Family history of stroke in patients with TIA in relation to hypertension and other intermediate phenotypes. *Stroke* 2005; **36**:830–5.

690 Flossmann E, Rothwell PM. Family history of stroke does not predict risk of stroke after transient ischaemic attack. *Stroke* 2006; **37**:544–6.

691 Kapoor R, Kendall BE, Harrison MJ. Permanent oculomotor palsy with occlusion of the internal carotid artery. *J Neurol Neurosurg Psychiatry* 1991; **54**:745–6.

692 Hollinger P, Sturzenegger M. Painful oculomotor nerve palsy: a presenting sign of internal carotid artery stenosis. *Cerebrovasc Dis* 1999; **9**:178–81.

693 Pietrobon D. Familial hemiplegic migraine. *Neurotherapeutics* 2007; **4**:274–84.

694 Ferracci F, Bertiato G, Moretto G. Hashimoto's encephalopathy: epidemiologic data and pathogenetic considerations. *J Neurol Sci* 2004; **217**:165–8.

695 Arruga J, Sanders MD. Ophthalmologic findings in 70 patients with evidence of retinal embolism. *Ophthalmology* 1982; **89**:1336–47.

696 Mitchell P, Wang JJ, Li W, Leeder SR, Smith W. Prevalence of asymptomatic retinal emboli in an Australian urban community. *Stroke* 1997; **28**:63–6.

697 Countee RW, Gnanadev A, Chavis P. Dilated episcleral arteries: a significant physical finding in assessment of patients with cerebrovascular insufficiency. *Stroke* 1978; **9**:42–5.

698 Kersemakers P, Beintema M, Lodder J. Venous stasis retinopathy unlikely results from internal carotid artery obstruction alone. *Cerebrovasc Dis* 1992; **2**:305–7.

699 Sturrock GD, Mueller HR. Chronic ocular ischaemia. *Br J Ophthalmol* 1984; **68**:716–23.

700 Ross Russell RW, Ikeda H. Clinical and electrophysiological observations in patients with low pressure retinopathy. *Br J Ophthalmol* 1986; **70**:651–6.

701 Ross RS, McKusick VA. Aortic arch syndromes: diminished or absent pulses in arteries arising from arch of aorta. *AMA Arch Intern Med* 1953; **92**:701–40.

702 Dalal PM, Deshpande CK, Daftary SG. Aortic arch syndrome. *Neurol India* 1971; **19**:155–71.

703 Ford CS, Howard VJ, Howard G, Frye JL, Toole JF, McKinney WM. The sex difference in manifestations of carotid bifurcation disease. *Stroke* 1986; **17**:877–81.

704 Schulz UG, Rothwell PM. Sex differences in carotid bifurcation anatomy and the distribution of atherosclerotic plaque. *Stroke* 2001; **32**:1525–31.

705 Mendez I, Hachinski V, Wolfe B. Serum lipids after stroke. *Neurology* 1987; **37**:507–11.

706 Woo J, Lam CW, Kay R, Wong HY, Teoh R, Nicholls MG. Acute and long-term changes in serum lipids after acute stroke. *Stroke* 1990; **21**:1407–11.

707 Gunatilake SB. Rapid resolution of symptoms and signs of intracerebral haemorrhage: case reports. *Br Med J* 1998; **316**:1495–6.

708 Schulz UG, Briley D, Meagher T, Molyneux A, Rothwell PM. Abnormalities on diffusion weighted magnetic resonance imaging performed several weeks after a minor stroke or transient ischaemic attack. *J Neurol Neurosurg Psychiatry* 2003; **74**:734–8.

709 Chalela JA, Kidwell CS, Nentwich LM, Luby M, Butman JA, Demchuk AM *et al*. Magnetic resonance imaging and computed tomography in emergency assessment of patients with suspected acute stroke: a prospective comparison. *Lancet* 2007; **369**:293–8.

710 Bhadelia RA, Anderson M, Polak JF, Manolio TA, Beauchamp N, Knepper L *et al*. Prevalence and associations of MRI-demonstrated brain infarcts in elderly subjects with a history of transient ischemic attack. The Cardiovascular Health Study. *Stroke* 1999; **30**:383–8.

711 Kidwell CS, Alger JR, Di Salle F, Starkman S, Villablanca P, Bentson J *et al*. Diffusion MRI in patients with transient ischemic attacks. *Stroke* 1999; **30**:1174–80.

712 Schaefer PW, Copen WA, Lev MH, Gonzalez RG. Diffusion-weighted imaging in acute stroke. *Neuroimaging Clin N Am* 2005; **15**:503–30, ix–x.

713 Lutsep HL, Albers GW, DeCrespigny A, Kamat GN, Marks MP, Moseley ME. Clinical utility of diffusion-weighted magnetic resonance imaging in the assessment of ischemic stroke. *Ann Neurol* 1997; **41**:574–80.

714 Lansberg MG, Norbash AM, Marks MP, Tong DC, Moseley ME, Albers GW. Advantages of adding diffusion-weighted magnetic resonance imaging to conventional magnetic resonance imaging for evaluating acute stroke. *Arch Neurol* 2000; **57**:1311–16.

715 Oppenheim C, Stanescu R, Dormont D, Crozier S, Marro B, Samson Y *et al*. False-negative diffusion-weighted MR findings in acute ischemic stroke. *Am J Neuroradiol* 2000; **21**:1434–40.

716 Madden KP, Karanjia PN, Adams HP, Jr, Clarke WR. Accuracy of initial stroke subtype diagnosis in the TOAST

study. Trial of ORG 10172 in Acute Stroke Treatment. *Neurology* 1995; **45**:1975–9.

717 Albers GW, Lansberg MG, Norbash AM, Tong DC, O'Brien MW, Woolfenden AR *et al*. Yield of diffusion-weighted MRI for detection of potentially relevant findings in stroke patients. *Neurology* 2000; **54**: 1562–7.

718 Gass A, Ay H, Szabo K, Koroshetz WJ. Diffusion-weighted MRI for the 'small stuff': the details of acute cerebral ischaemia. *Lancet Neurol* 2004; **3**:39–45.

719 Lee DK, Kim JS, Kwon SU, Yoo SH, Kang DW. Lesion patterns and stroke mechanism in atherosclerotic middle cerebral artery disease: early diffusion-weighted imaging study. *Stroke* 2005; **36**:2583–8.

720 Ay H, Oliveira-Filho J, Buonanno FS, Schaefer PW, Furie KL, Chang YC *et al*. 'Footprints' of transient ischemic attacks: a diffusion-weighted MRI study. *Cerebrovasc Dis* 2002; **14**:177–86.

721 Douglas VC, Johnston CM, Elkins J, Sidney S, Gress DR, Johnston SC. Head computed tomography findings predict short-term stroke risk after transient ischemic attack. *Stroke* 2003; **34**:2894–8.

722 Wen HM, Lam WW, Rainer T, Fan YH, Leung TW, Chan YL *et al*. Multiple acute cerebral infarcts on diffusion-weighted imaging and risk of recurrent stroke. *Neurology* 2004; **63**:1317–19.

723 Purroy F, Montaner J, Rovira A, Delgado P, Quintana M, Alvarez-Sabin J. Higher risk of further vascular events among transient ischemic attack patients with diffusion-weighted imaging acute ischemic lesions. *Stroke* 2004; **35**:2313–19.

724 Bang OY, Lee PH, Heo KG, Joo US, Yoon SR, Kim SY. Specific DWI lesion patterns predict prognosis after acute ischaemic stroke within the MCA territory. *J Neurol Neurosurg Psychiatry* 2005; **76**:1222–8.

725 Dennis M, Bamford J, Sandercock P, Molyneux A, Warlow C. Computed tomography in patients with transient ischaemic attacks: when is a transient ischaemic attack not a transient ischaemic attack but a stroke? *J Neurol* 1990; **237**:257–61.

726 Herderschee D, Hijdra A, Algra A, Koudstaal PJ, Kappelle LJ, van Gijn J. Silent stroke in patients with transient ischemic attack or minor ischemic stroke. The Dutch TIA Trial Study Group. *Stroke* 1992; **23**:1220–4.

727 Tanaka H, Sueyoshi K, Nishino M, Ishida M, Fukunaga R, Abe H. Silent brain infarction and coronary artery disease in Japanese patients. *Arch Neurol* 1993; **50**:706–9.

728 Boon A, Lodder J, Heuts-van Raak L, Kessels F. Silent brain infarcts in 755 consecutive patients with a first-ever supratentorial ischemic stroke: relationship with index-stroke subtype, vascular risk factors, and mortality. *Stroke* 1994; **25**:2384–90.

729 Brott T, Tomsick T, Feinberg W, Johnson C, Biller J, Broderick J *et al*. Baseline silent cerebral infarction in the Asymptomatic Carotid Atherosclerosis Study. *Stroke* 1994; **25**:1122–9.

730 Caplan LR. Silent brain infarcts. *Cerebrovasc Dis* 1994; **4**(Suppl. 1):32–9.

731 Wardlaw JM, Ferguson KJ, Graham C. White matter hyperintensities and rating scales–observer reliability varies with lesion load. *J Neurol* 2004; **251**:584–90.

732 Naka H, Nomura E, Takahashi T, Wakabayashi S, Mimori Y, Kajikawa H *et al*. Combinations of the presence or absence of cerebral microbleeds and advanced white matter hyperintensity as predictors of subsequent stroke types. *Am J Neuroradiol* 2006; **27**:830–5.

733 Takao M, Koto A, Tanahashi N, Fukuuchi Y, Takagi M, Morinaga S. Pathologic findings of silent, small hyperintense foci in the basal ganglia and thalamus on MRI. *Neurology* 1999; **52**:666–8.

734 Price TR, Manolio TA, Kronmal RA, Kittner SJ, Yue NC, Robbins J *et al*. Silent brain infarction on magnetic resonance imaging and neurological abnormalities in community-dwelling older adults. The Cardiovascular Health Study. CHS Collaborative Research Group. *Stroke* 1997; **28**:1158–64.

735 Au R, Massaro JM, Wolf PA, Young ME, Beiser A, Seshadri S *et al*. Association of white matter hyperintensity volume with decreased cognitive functioning: the Framingham Heart Study. *Arch Neurol* 2006; **63**:246–50.

736 Van den Heuvel DM, ten Dam VH, de Craen AJ, Admiraal-Behloul F, Olofsen H, Bollen EL *et al*. Increase in periventricular white matter hyperintensities parallels decline in mental processing speed in a non-demented elderly population. *J Neurol Neurosurg Psychiatry* 2006; **77**:149–53.

737 Jeerakathil T, Wolf PA, Beiser A, Massaro J, Seshadri S, D'Agostino RB *et al*. Stroke risk profile predicts white matter hyperintensity volume: the Framingham Study. *Stroke* 2004; **35**:1857–61.

738 Dufouil C, Chalmers J, Coskun O, Besancon V, Bousser MG, Guillon P *et al*. Effects of blood pressure lowering on cerebral white matter hyperintensities in patients with stroke: the PROGRESS (Perindopril Protection Against Recurrent Stroke Study) Magnetic Resonance Imaging Substudy. *Circulation* 2005; **112**:1644–50.

739 Hankey GJ, Warlow CP. Cost-effective investigation of patients with suspected transient ischaemic attacks. *J Neurol Neurosurg Psychiatry* 1992; **55**:171–6.

740 Sellar RJ. Imaging blood vessels of the head and neck. *J Neurol Neurosurg Psychiatry* 1995; **59**:225–37.

741 Rothwell PM, Gibson RJ, Slattery J, Warlow CP. Prognostic value and reproducibility of measurements of carotid stenosis: a comparison of three methods on 1001 angiograms. European Carotid Surgery Trialists' Collaborative Group. *Stroke* 1994; **25**:2440–4.

742 Dippel DW, van Kooten F, Bakker SL, Koudstaal PJ. Interobserver agreement for 10% categories of angiographic carotid stenosis. *Stroke* 1997; **28**:2483–5.

743 Rothwell PM, Warlow CP. Making sense of the measurement of carotid stenosis. *Cerebrovasc Dis* 1996; **6**:54–8.

744 Hankey GJ, Slattery JM, Warlow CP. The prognosis of hospital-referred transient ischaemic attacks. *J Neurol Neurosurg Psychiatry* 1991; **54**:793–802.

745 Mead GE, Wardlaw JM, Lewis SC, McDowall M, Dennis MS. Can simple clinical features be used to identify patients with severe carotid stenosis on Doppler ultrasound? *J Neurol Neurosurg Psychiatry* 1999; **66**:16–19.

746 Gerraty RP, Bowser DN, Infeld B, Mitchell PJ, Davis SM. Microemboli during carotid angiography: association with stroke risk factors or subsequent magnetic resonance imaging changes? *Stroke* 1996; **27**:1543–7.

747 Warnock NG, Gandhi MR, Bergvall U, Powell T. Complications of intraarterial digital subtraction angiography in patients investigated for cerebral vascular disease. *Br J Radiol* 1993; **66**:855–8.

748 Pelz DM, Fox AJ, Vinuela F. Digital subtraction angiography: current clinical applications. *Stroke* 1985; **16**:528–36.

749 Rothwell PM, Gibson RJ, Villagra R, Sellar R, Warlow CP. The effect of angiographic technique and image quality on the reproducibility of measurement of carotid stenosis and assessment of plaque surface morphology. *Clin Radiol* 1998; **53**:439–43.

750 Jeans WD, Mackenzie S, Baird RN. Angiography in transient cerebral ischaemia using three views of the carotid bifurcation. *Br J Radiol* 1986; **59**:135–42.

751 Rothwell PM, Gibson RJ, Slattery J, Sellar RJ, Warlow CP. Equivalence of measurements of carotid stenosis: a comparison of three methods on 1001 angiograms. European Carotid Surgery Trialists' Collaborative Group. *Stroke* 1994; **25**:2435–9.

752 Streifler JY, Eliaziw M, Fox AJ *et al*. for the North American Symptomatic Carotid Endarterectomy Trial. Angiographic detection of carotid plaque ulceration: comparison with surgical observations in a multicentre study. *Stroke* 1994; **25**:1130–2.

753 Eliasziw M, Streifler JY, Fox AJ, Hachinski VC, Ferguson GG, Barnett HJ. Significance of plaque ulceration in symptomatic patients with high-grade carotid stenosis. North American Symptomatic Carotid Endarterectomy Trial. *Stroke* 1994; **25**:304–8.

754 Martin R, Bogousslavsky J, Miklossy J *et al*. Floating thrombus in the innominate artery as a cause of cerebral infarction in young adults. *Cerebrovasc Dis* 1992; **2**:177–81.

755 Furst H, Hartl WH, Jansen I, Liepsch D, Lauterjung L, Schildberg FW. Color-flow Doppler sonography in the identification of ulcerative plaques in patients with high-grade carotid artery stenosis. *Am J Neuroradiol* 1992; **13**:1581–7.

756 Griewing B, Morgenstern C, Driesner F, Kallwellis G, Walker ML, Kessler C. Cerebrovascular disease assessed by color-flow and power Doppler ultrasonography: comparison with digital subtraction angiography in internal carotid artery stenosis. *Stroke* 1996; **27**:95–100.

757 Droste DW, Jurgens R, Nabavi DG, Schuierer G, Weber S, Ringelstein EB. Echocontrast-enhanced ultrasound of extracranial internal carotid artery high-grade stenosis and occlusion. *Stroke* 1999; **30**:2302–6.

758 Wardlaw JM, Lewis S. Carotid stenosis measurement on colour Doppler ultrasound: agreement of ECST, NASCET and CCA methods applied to ultrasound with intra-arterial angiographic stenosis measurement. *Eur J Radiol* 2005; **56**:205–11.

759 Gaitini D, Soudack M. Diagnosing carotid stenosis by Doppler sonography: state of the art. *J Ultrasound Med* 2005; **24**:1127–36.

760 Furst G, Saleh A, Wenserski F, Malms J, Cohnen M, Aulich A *et al*. Reliability and validity of noninvasive imaging of internal carotid artery pseudo-occlusion. *Stroke* 1999; **30**:1444–9.

761 Howard G, Baker WH, Chambless LE, Howard VJ, Jones AM, Toole JF. An approach for the use of Doppler ultrasound as a screening tool for hemodynamically significant stenosis (despite heterogeneity of Doppler performance): a multicenter experience. Asymptomatic Carotid Atherosclerosis Study Investigators. *Stroke* 1996; **27**:1951–7.

762 Griffiths PD, Worthy S, Gholkar A. Incidental intracranial vascular pathology in patients investigated for carotid stenosis. *Neuroradiology* 1996; **38**:25–30.

763 Elgersma OE, van Leersum M, Buijs PC, van Leeuwen MS, van de Schouw YT, Eikelboom BC *et al*. Changes over time in optimal duplex threshold for the identification of patients eligible for carotid endarterectomy. *Stroke* 1998; **29**:2352–6.

764 Ringelstein EB. Skepticism toward carotid ultrasonography: a virtue, an attitude, or fanaticism? *Stroke* 1995; **26**:1743–6.

765 Carpenter JP, Lexa FJ, Davis JT. Determination of duplex Doppler ultrasound criteria appropriate to the North American Symptomatic Carotid Endarterectomy Trial. *Stroke* 1996; **27**:695–9.

766 Blakeley DD, Oddone EZ, Hasselblad V, Simel DL, Matchar DB. Noninvasive carotid artery testing: a meta-analytic review. *Ann Intern Med* 1995; **122**:360–7.

767 Rothwell PM, Pendlebury ST, Wardlaw J, Warlow CP. Critical appraisal of the design and reporting of studies of imaging and measurement of carotid stenosis. *Stroke* 2000; **31**:1444–50.

768 Wardlaw JM, Chappell FM, Best JJK, Wartowska K, Berry E on behalf of the NHS Research and Development Health Technology Assessment Carotid Stenosis Imaging Group. Non-invasive imaging compared with intra-arterial angiography in the diagnosis of symptomatic carotid stenosis: a meta-analysis. *Lancet* 2006; **376**:1503–12.

769 Arnold JA, Modaresi KB, Thomas N, Taylor PR, Padayachee TS. Carotid plaque characterization by duplex scanning: observer error may undermine current clinical trials. *Stroke* 1999; **30**:61–5.

770 Gronholdt ML. Ultrasound and lipoproteins as predictors of lipid-rich, rupture-prone plaques in the carotid artery. *Arterioscler Thromb Vasc Biol* 1999; **19**:2–13.

771 Polak JF, Shemanski L, O'Leary DH, Lefkowitz D, Price TR, Savage PJ *et al*. Hypoechoic plaque at US of the carotid artery: an independent risk factor for incident stroke in adults aged 65 years or older. Cardiovascular Health Study. *Radiology* 1998; **208**:649–54.

772 Halliday A, Mansfield A, Marro J, Peto C, Peto R, Potter J *et al.* Prevention of disabling and fatal strokes by successful carotid endarterectomy in patients without recent neurological symptoms: randomised controlled trial. *Lancet* 2004; **363**:1491–502.

773 Rosario JA, Hachinski VC, Lee DH, Fox AJ. Adverse reactions to duplex scanning. *Lancet* 1987; **2**:1023.

774 Friedman SG. Transient ischemic attacks resulting from carotid duplex imaging. *Surgery* 1990; **107**:153–5.

775 Khaffaf N, Karnik R, Winkler WB, Valentin A, Slany J. Embolic stroke by compression maneuver during transcranial Doppler sonography. *Stroke* 1994; **25**:1056–7.

776 Karnik R, Winkler WB, Valentin A, Khaffaf N, Slany J. Carotid sinus massage and the risk of cerebral embolization. *Stroke* 1995; **26**:1124–5.

777 Brink JA, McFarland EG, Heiken JP. Helical/spiral computed body tomography. *Clin Radiol* 1997; **52**:489–503.

778 Bartlett ES, Symons SP, Fox AJ. Correlation of carotid stenosis diameter and cross-sectional areas with CT angiography. *Am J Neuroradiol* 2006; **27**:638–42.

779 Bartlett ES, Walters TD, Symons SP, Fox AJ. Quantification of carotid stenosis on CT angiography. *Am J Neuroradiol* 2006; **27**:13–19.

780 Heiken JP, Brink JA, Vannier MW. Spiral (helical) CT. *Radiology* 1993; **189**:647–56.

781 Leclerc X, Godefroy O, Pruvo JP, Leys D. Computed tomographic angiography for the evaluation of carotid artery stenosis. *Stroke* 1995; **26**:1577–81.

782 Nandalur KR, Baskurt E, Hagspiel KD, Finch M, Phillips CD, Bollampally SR *et al.* Carotid artery calcification on CT may independently predict stroke risk. *Am J Roentgenol* 2006; **186**:547–52.

783 Graves MJ. Magnetic resonance angiography. *Br J Radiol* 1997; **70**:6–28.

784 DeMarco JK, Huston J, III, Nash AK. Extracranial carotid MR imaging at 3T. *Magn Reson Imaging Clin N Am* 2006; **14**:109–21.

785 Siewart B, Patel MR, Warach S. Magnetic resonance angiography. *Neurologist* 1995; **1**:167–84.

786 Levi CR, Mitchell A, Fitt G, Donnan GA. The accuracy of magnetic resonance angiography in the assessment of extracranial carotid artery occlusive disease. *Cerebrovasc Dis* 1996; **6**:231–6.

787 Fox AJ, Eliasziw M, Rothwell PM, Schmidt MH, Warlow CP, Barnett HJ. Identification, prognosis, and management of patients with carotid artery near occlusion. *Am J Neuroradiol* 2005; **26**:2086–94.

788 Mitra D, Connolly D, Jenkins S, English P, Birchall D, Mandel C *et al.* Comparison of image quality, diagnostic confidence and interobserver variability in contrast enhanced MR angiography and 2D time of flight angiography in evaluation of carotid stenosis. *Br J Radiol* 2006; **79**:201–7.

789 King-Im JM, Hollingworth W, Trivedi RA, Cross JJ, Higgins NJ, Graves MJ *et al.* Cost-effectiveness of diagnostic strategies prior to carotid endarterectomy. *Ann Neurol* 2005; **58**:506–15.

790 Hankey GJ, Warlow CP. Symptomatic carotid ischaemic events: safest and most cost-effective way of selecting patients for angiography, before carotid endarterectomy. *Br Med J* 1990; **300**:1485–91.

791 Johnston DC, Goldstein LB. Clinical carotid endarterectomy decision making: noninvasive vascular imaging versus angiography. *Neurology* 2001; **56**:1009–15.

792 Norris JW, Rothwell PM. Noninvasive carotid imaging to select patients for endarterectomy: is it really safer than conventional angiography? *Neurology* 2001; **56**:990–1.

793 Norris JW, Morriello F, Rowed DW, Maggisano R. Vascular imaging before carotid endarterectomy. *Stroke* 2003; **34**:e16.

794 Norris JW, Halliday A. Is ultrasound sufficient for vascular imaging prior to carotid endarterectomy? *Stroke* 2004; **35**:370–1.

795 Rothwell PM, Eliasziw M, Gutnikov SA, Fox AJ, Taylor DW, Mayberg MR *et al.* Analysis of pooled data from the randomised controlled trials of endarterectomy for symptomatic carotid stenosis. *Lancet* 2003; **361**:107–16.

796 Johnston DC, Eastwood JD, Nguyen T, Goldstein LB. Contrast-enhanced magnetic resonance angiography of carotid arteries: utility in routine clinical practice. *Stroke* 2002; **33**:2834–8.

797 Barth A, Arnold M, Mattle HP, Schroth G, Remonda L. Contrast-enhanced 3-D MRA in decision making for carotid endarterectomy: a 6-year experience. *Cerebrovasc Dis* 2006; **21**:393–400.

798 Sivenius J, Riekkinen PJ, Smets P, Laakso M, Lowenthal A. The European Stroke Prevention Study (ESPS): results by arterial distribution. *Ann Neurol* 1991; **29**:596–600.

799 Mohr JP, Gautier JC, Pessin MS. Internal carotid artery disease. In Barnett HJ, Mohr JP, Stein B, Yatsu FM, eds. *Stroke.* New York: Churchill Livingstone, 1992, p. 311.

800 Caplan LR. *Posterior Circulation Disease: Clinical Findings, Diagnosis and Management.* Cambridge, MA; Oxford, UK: Blackwell Science, 1996.

801 Flossmann E, Rothwell PM. Prognosis of vertebrobasilar transient ischaemic attack and minor ischaemic stroke. *Brain* 2003; **126**:1940–54.

802 Flossmann E, Touze E, Giles MF, Lovelock CE, Rothwell PM. The early risk of stroke after vertebrobasilar TIA is higher than after carotid TIA. *Cerebrovasc Dis* 2006; **21**(suppl 4):6.

803 Fields WS, Lemak NA. Joint Study of extracranial arterial occlusion. VII. Subclavian steal: a review of 168 cases. *J Am Med Assoc* 1972; **222**:1139–43.

804 Bohmfalk GL, Story JL, Brown WE, Marlin AE. Subclavian steal syndrome. Part 1: Proximal vertebral to common carotid artery transposition in three patients, and historical review. *J Neurosurg* 1979; **51**:628–40.

805 Bornstein NM, Norris JW. Subclavian steal: a harmless haemodynamic phenomenon? *Lancet* 1986; **2**:303–5.

806 Hennerici M, Klemm C, Rautenberg W. The subclavian steal phenomenon: a common vascular disorder with rare neurologic deficits. *Neurology* 1988; **38**:669–73.

807 Kempczinski R, Hermann G. The innominate steal syndrome. *J Cardiovasc Surg (Torino)* 1979; **20**:481–6.

808 Grosveld WJ, Lawson JA, Eikelboom BC, vander Windt JM, Ackerstaff RG. Clinical and hemodynamic significance of innominate artery lesions evaluated by ultrasonography and digital angiography. *Stroke* 1988; **19**:958–62.

809 Ley-Pozo J, Ringelstein EB. Noninvasive detection of occlusive disease of the carotid siphon and middle cerebral artery. *Ann Neurol* 1990; **28**:640–7.

810 Petty GW, Wiebers WO, Meissner I. Transcranial Doppler ultrasonography: clinical applications in cerebrovascular disease. *Mayo Clin Proc* 1990; **65**:1350–64.

811 Bornstein NM, Norris JW. Transcranial Doppler sonography is at present of limited clinical value. *Arch Neurol* 1994; **51**:1057–9.

812 Baumgartner RW, Mattle HP, Aaslid R, Kapps M. Transcranial colour-coded duplex sonography in arterial cerebrovascular disease. *Cerebrovasc Dis* 1997; **7**:57–63.

813 Baumgartner RW. Transcranial color-coded duplex sonography. *J Neurol* 1999; **246**:637–47.

814 Gerriets T, Seidel G, Fiss I, Modrau B, Kaps M. Contrast-enhanced transcranial color-coded duplex sonography: efficiency and validity. *Neurology* 1999; **52**:1133–7.

815 Markus H, Cullinane M, Reid G. Improved automated detection of embolic signals using a novel frequency filtering approach. *Stroke* 1999; **30**:1610–15.

816 Babikian VL, Wijman CA, Hyde C, Cantelmo NL, Winter MR, Baker E *et al.* Cerebral microembolism and early recurrent cerebral or retinal ischemic events. *Stroke* 1997; **28**:1314–18.

817 Alexandrov AV, Molina CA, Grotta JC, Garami Z, Ford SR, Alvarez-Sabin J *et al.* Ultrasound-enhanced systemic thrombolysis for acute ischemic stroke. *N Engl J Med* 2004; **351**:2170–8.

818 Kim YS, Garami Z, Mikulik R, Molina CA, Alexandrov AV. Early recanalization rates and clinical outcomes in patients with tandem internal carotid artery/middle cerebral artery occlusion and isolated middle cerebral artery occlusion. *Stroke* 2005; **36**:869–71.

819 Markus HS, Droste DW, Brown MM. Detection of asymptomatic cerebral embolic signals with Doppler ultrasound. *Lancet* 1994; **343**:1011–12.

820 Sliwka U, Lingnau A, Stohlmann WD, Schmidt P, Mull M, Diehl RR *et al.* Prevalence and time course of microembolic signals in patients with acute stroke: a prospective study. *Stroke* 1997; **28**:358–63.

821 Bishop CC, Powell S, Insall M, Rutt D, Browse NL. Effect of internal carotid artery occlusion on middle cerebral artery blood flow at rest and in response to hypercapnia. *Lancet* 1986; **1**:710–12.

822 Markus HS, Harrison MJ. Estimation of cerebrovascular reactivity using transcranial Doppler, including the use of breath-holding as the vasodilatory stimulus. *Stroke* 1992; **23**:668–73.

823 Dahl A, Russell D, Rootwelt K, Nyberg-Hansen R, Kerty E. Cerebral vasoreactivity assessed with transcranial Doppler and regional cerebral blood flow measurements: dose, serum concentration, and time course of the response to acetazolamide. *Stroke* 1995; **26**:2302–6.

824 Ameriso SF, Mohler JG, Suarez M, Fisher M. Morning reduction of cerebral vasomotor reactivity. *Neurology* 1994; **44**:1907–9.

825 Kleiser B, Widder B. Course of carotid artery occlusions with impaired cerebrovascular reactivity. *Stroke* 1992; **23**:171–4.

826 Widder B, Kleiser B, Krapf H. Course of cerebrovascular reactivity in patients with carotid artery occlusions. *Stroke* 1994; **25**:1963–7.

827 Gur AY, Bova I, Bornstein NM. Is impaired cerebral vasomotor reactivity a predictive factor of stroke in asymptomatic patients? *Stroke* 1996; **27**:2188–90.

828 Vernieri F, Pasqualetti P, Passarelli F, Rossini PM, Silvestrini M. Outcome of carotid artery occlusion is predicted by cerebrovascular reactivity. *Stroke* 1999; **30**:593–8.

829 Powers WJ. Should lumbar puncture be part of the routine evaluation of patients with cerebral ischemia? *Stroke* 1986; **17**:332–3.

830 Faught E. Current role of electroencephalography in cerebral ischemia. *Stroke* 1993; **24**:609–13.

831 Bogousslavsky J, Hachinski VC, Boughner DR, Fox AJ, Vinuela F, Barnett HJ. Cardiac and arterial lesions in carotid transient ischemic attacks. *Arch Neurol* 1986; **43**:223–8.

832 Bogousslavsky J, Hachinski VC, Boughner DR, Fox AJ, Vinuela F, Barnett HJ. Clinical predictors of cardiac and arterial lesions in carotid transient ischemic attacks. *Arch Neurol* 1986; **43**:229–33.

833 Daniel WG, Erbel R, Kasper W, Visser CA, Engberding R, Sutherland GR *et al.* Safety of transesophageal echocardiography: a multicenter survey of 10,419 examinations. *Circulation* 1991; **83**:817–21.

834 Daniel WG, Mugge A. Transesophageal echocardiography. *N Engl J Med* 1995; **332**:1268–79.

835 Tegeler CH, Downes TR. Cardiac imaging in stroke. *Stroke* 1991; **22**:1206–11.

836 Adams HP, Love BB. Transesophageal echocardiography in the evaluation of young adults with ischemic stroke: promises and concerns. *Cerebrovasc Dis* 1995; **5**:323–7.

837 Donnan GA, Jones EF. Aortic arch atheroma and stroke. *Cerebrovasc Dis* 1995; **5**:10–13.

838 Stollberger C, Brainin M, Abzieher F, Slany J. Embolic stroke and transoesophageal echocardiography: can clinical parameters predict the diagnostic yield? *J Neurol* 1995; **242**:437–42.

839 Macleod MR, Amarenco P, Davis SM, Donnan GA. Atheroma of the aortic arch: an important and poorly recognised factor in the aetiology of stroke. *Lancet Neurol* 2004; **3**:408–14.

840 Burnett PJ, Milne JR, Greenwood R, Giles MR, Camm J. The role of echocardiography in the investigation of focal cerebral ischaemia. *Postgrad Med J* 1984; **60**:116–19.

841 Good DC, Frank S, Verhulst S, Sharma B. Cardiac abnormalities in stroke patients with negative arteriograms. *Stroke* 1986; **17**:6–11.

842 Leung DY, Black IW, Cranney GB, Walsh WF, Grimm RA, Stewart WJ *et al.* Selection of patients for transesophageal echocardiography after stroke and systemic embolic

events: role of transthoracic echocardiography. *Stroke* 1995; **26**:1820–4.

843 Rauh G, Fischereder M, Spengel FA. Transoesophageal echocardiography in patients with focal cerebral ischaemia of unknown cause. *Stroke* 1996; **27**:691–4.

844 Censori B, Colombo F, Valsecchi MG, Clivati L, Zonca A, Camerlingo M *et al*. Early transoesophageal echocardiography in cryptogenic and lacunar stroke and transient ischaemic attack. *J Neurol Neurosurg Psychiatry* 1998; **64**:624–7.

845 Biller J, Johnson MR, Adams HP, Jr, Kerber RE, Toffol GJ, Butler MJ. Echocardiographic evaluation of young adults with nonhemorrhagic cerebral infarction. *Stroke* 1986; **17**:608–12.

846 DeRook FA, Comess KA, Albers GW, Popp RL. Transesophageal echocardiography in the evaluation of stroke. *Ann Intern Med* 1992; **117**:922–32.

847 Van Walraven C, Hart RG, Singer DE, Laupacis A, Connolly S, Petersen P *et al*. Oral anticoagulants vs aspirin in nonvalvular atrial fibrillation: an individual patient meta-analysis. *J Am Med Assoc* 2002; **288**:2441–8.

848 Kearon C, Julian JA, Newman TE, Ginsberg JS. Noninvasive diagnosis of deep venous thrombosis. McMaster Diagnostic Imaging Practice Guidelines Initiative. *Ann Intern Med* 1998; **128**:663–77.

849 Cramer SC, Rordorf G, Kaufman JA, Buonanno F, Koroshetz WJ, Schwamm L. Clinically occult pelvic-vein thrombosis in cryptogenic stroke. *Lancet* 1998; **351**:1927–8.

850 Mas JL. Patent foramen ovale, stroke and paradoxical embolism. *Cerebrovasc Dis* 1991; **1**:181–3.

851 Ranoux D, Cohen A, Cabanes L, Amarenco P, Bousser MG, Mas JL. Patent foramen ovale: is stroke due to paradoxical embolism? *Stroke* 1993; **24**:31–4.

852 Brogno D, Lancaster G, Rosenbaum M. Embolism interruptus. *N Engl J Med* 1994; **330**:1761–2.

853 Petty GW, Khandheria BK, Chu CP, Sicks JD, Whisnant JP. Patent foramen ovale in patients with cerebral infarction: a transesophageal echocardiographic study. *Arch Neurol* 1997; **54**:819–22.

854 Warlow C. Venous thromboembolism after stroke. *Am Heart J* 1978; **96**:283–5.

855 Landi G, D'Angelo A, Boccardi E, Candelise L, Mannucci PM, Morabito A *et al*. Venous thromboembolism in acute stroke: prognostic importance of hypercoagulability. *Arch Neurol* 1992; **49**:279–83.

7 Unusual causes of ischaemic stroke and transient ischaemic attack

Neither atherothromboembolism (section 6.3) nor 'complex' small vessel disease (section 6.4) are likely causes of ischaemic stroke or transient ischaemic attacks under the age of 40 years. However, over the age of 60 these pathologies become overwhelmingly more likely than anything else, other than embolism from the heart – mostly due to atrial fibrillation in this age group (section 6.5). Naturally, young patients tend to get more intensively investigated, which is not unreasonable because the *proportion* with an unusual (and sometimes treatable) cause is undoubtedly higher than in the elderly. However, the *range* of causes of ischaemic stroke is similar in older people compared with young adults – for example, just because an old person is a hypertensive smoker does not mean that a stroke was not due to carotid dissection; every case must be considered carefully on its merits and investigated appropriately.

> The usual causes of ischaemic stroke in older people are degenerative arterial disorders and atrial fibrillation, but older people may occasionally have unusual causes (such as arterial dissection) although these are proportionally far less likely than in young adults.

There have many series of 'young stroke patients' meaning anything from age under 30 to age under 50 years, and a few series in children. The mix of causes and the proportion with 'no cause' depend on referral bias, investigation intensity, differences in diagnostic criteria,

---

Stroke: practical management, 3rd edition. C. Warlow, J. van Gijn, M. Dennis, J. Wardlaw, J. Bamford, G. Hankey, P. Sandercock, G. Rinkel, P. Langhorne, C. Sudlow and P. Rothwell. Published 2008 Blackwell Publishing. ISBN 978-1-4051-2766-0.

what is deemed *the* cause of the stroke rather than merely an innocent bystander, and fashion, which changes as more new causes are discovered and later often rejected (e.g. uncomplicated mitral leaflet prolapse in the first edition of this book). In practice, the main causes in young adults are arterial dissection, embolism from the heart, inflammatory vascular disorders and migrainous stroke – and about one-quarter remain stubbornly unexplained.

Many books devote 95% of the section on the causes of ischaemic stroke to the 5% or so which turn out to have a rare or unusual cause. Although we will not be nearly so extreme, it is not unreasonable to discuss rare disorders in some detail, even at the risk of being encyclopaedic, particularly if their diagnosis leads to specific treatment for the acute episode, prevention of recurrence, or genetic counselling. Also, many specific and unusual causes are confusing and require explanation (the treatment of some will be described in this chapter, while the management of the common causes is described in Chapters 12 and 16).

7.1 Trauma

Increasingly, ischaemic strokes and transient ischaemic attacks (TIAs), particularly in young and middle-aged patients, are recognized as being caused by arterial trauma, perhaps because physicians are now more attuned to asking the right questions about antecedent trauma, as well as because of improved diagnostic technology.

7.1.1 Penetrating neck injury

Penetrating neck injury is more likely to damage the carotid than the better-protected vertebral arteries (Table 6.2).[1,2] This type of arterial injury causes laceration, dissection (section 7.2.1), intimal tears and occasionally an arteriovenous fistula, all of which may be complicated by thrombosis occluding the artery, and by embolism of mural thrombus to the brain or eye hours, days or even weeks after the injury. A traumatic aneurysm can gradually develop, perhaps over several years, and any contained thrombus may embolize to the brain or eye (section 7.6).

7.1.2 Non-penetrating (blunt) neck injury

Non-penetrating (blunt) neck injury (Table 6.2) is a more subtle cause of ischaemic stroke and transient ischaemic attack. The injury may have seemed rather trivial at the time, or any cerebrovascular symptoms may have been overshadowed by more obvious injuries such as fractures, and stroke can occur hours, days or even weeks later.[3–6] The internal carotid artery and, very rarely, the common carotid artery are more vulnerable to a direct blow to the neck or to compression, and the vertebral arteries are more vulnerable to rotational and hyperextension injuries at the level of the atlas and axis.[7–12] Blunt, like penetrating trauma, can also cause intimal tearing or dissection with complicating thrombosis and embolism. Traumatic rupture of an atheromatous plaque, vasospasm, and delayed aneurysm formation are probably all exceptionally rare.[1]

7.1.3 Subclavian artery injury

The subclavian artery can be damaged distal to the vertebral artery origin by a fractured clavicle or cervical rib, or by clumsy central venous line insertion. This may cause mural thrombosis and, as a result of the normal reversal of subclavian blood flow in diastole, embolization up the vertebral artery on either side, or even up the carotid system on the right.[13,14] Presumably, this same flow reversal might also cause spontaneous embolism of atherothrombotic material from the distal subclavian arteries, and even from the descending aortic arch, to the brain.

> Subclavian artery trauma can lead to a posterior and even sometimes to an anterior circulation ischaemic stroke.

7.1.4 Head injury

In rare instances, ischaemic stroke occurs soon after a head injury but with no obvious neck trauma. However, any associated sudden movement of the neck may still have caused extracranial arterial dissection (section 7.1.2). Other rarer possibilities are:
- intracranial arterial dissection (section 7.2.2);
- compression of the distal internal carotid or middle cerebral artery against the bony structures at the base of the skull, causing intimal damage and thrombosis;[15]
- fracture of the skull base involving the carotid canal;
- fractured vertebra damaging the vertebral artery;
- and perhaps vasospasm.[16]

Transient focal neurological episodes have been described minutes after minor head injury in children.[17]

7.1.5 Head turning (rotational vertebral artery occlusion)

Turning the head can certainly sometimes occlude one of the vertebral arteries against a spondylotic spur of a vertebra. But, bearing in mind that the basilar artery usually receives blood from both vertebral arteries and from the carotid arteries via the circle of Willis, it is hardly surprising that unilateral vertebral occlusion has seldom been convincingly demonstrated to have caused a brainstem ischaemic stroke or transient ischaemic attack; there must be stenosis or hypoplasia of the contralateral non-compressed vertebral artery in addition[18-24] (section 4.2.3). Of course, non-specific 'dizziness' or 'light-headedness' during neck extension or head turning is common in the elderly, but the exact cause is very uncertain and may lie in the peripheral vestibular apparatus, as in benign positional vertigo (section 3.4.7). Symptomatic positional occlusion of the carotid artery has hardly ever been reported.[25]

Unusual or forced neck turning very rarely causes arterial dissection, for example after vigorous neck manipulation.[26,27]

7.1.6 Fibrocartilaginous embolism

Fibrocartilaginous embolism is extraordinarily rare in humans (but curiously not in dogs). Embolic material from a disrupted intervertebral disc, perhaps as a result of trauma, somehow reaches the arterial or venous circulation of the spinal cord, rarely of the brain, to cause infarction. This is all but impossible to diagnose during life although there are presumed non-fatal cases.[28-30]

7.1.7 Cerebral air embolism

Air sometimes enters the cerebral circulation to cause sudden focal, but more often global, ischaemic deficits as the result of arterial or cardiac catheterization, cardiac surgery, carotid surgery, intracranial surgery in the sitting position, lung surgery and biopsy, haemodialysis, central venous catheterization generally with air passing through a patent foramen ovale, tension pneumothorax and scuba diving accidents. Early brain CT may show the gas bubbles and MR diffusion-weighted imaging the ischaemic regions.[31,32] Hyperbaric oxygen is said to be effective but no randomized trials are available.[33]

7.1.8 Fat embolism

Fat embolism, most commonly occurring 12 h to a few days after long bone injury or surgery, generally causes a rather acute global encephalopathy (along with respiratory distress and skin petechiae); additional focal features are unusual, and stroke-like features without coma must be very rare indeed.[34]

7.2 Arterial dissection in the neck, head and thorax

7.2.1 Cervical arterial dissection

Cervical arterial dissection is generally the result of trauma (section 7.1) or coincides with an apparently trivial neck movement.[35,36] Sometimes it seems truly spontaneous, perhaps because the patients have cystic medial necrosis, fibromuscular dysplasia, Marfan syndrome, Ehlers-Danlos syndrome type 4, alpha-1-antitrypsin deficiency, autosomal dominant polycystic kidney disease, osteogenesis imperfecta, or other less well-characterized, familial, connective tissue disorders. There is some not very good evidence that recent infection as well as various non-specific transient and more permanent arteriopathies may play a part.[37,38]

Blood splits the arterial wall to form an intramural haematoma of variable length, and this may extend with time. There are usually one or more intimal tears so the false and true lumen are in communication (Fig. 7.1). Aneurysms sometimes form but seldom become symptomatic. Dissection can occur anywhere in the extracranial internal carotid artery (ICA) as far distal as the skull base, but is unusual at the carotid bifurcation (the most common site for atheroma). In the vertebral artery it tends to affect the portion in relation to the first and second cervical vertebrae, occasionally extending intracranially. Sometimes cervical dissection is an extension from dissection more proximally in the aorta (section 7.2.3). Usually only one artery is affected, but sometimes two or more arteries in the neck and even elsewhere appear to be affected more or less simultaneously, perhaps because whatever caused the problem in one artery affected others at the same time (e.g. neck trauma, aortic arch dissection or even infection perhaps).

The incidence of diagnosed *carotid* dissection is about 3 per 100 000 per annum, but may now be higher with improved awareness and diagnostic imaging, both in stroke patients and in those at particular risk, such as after head and neck trauma.[35] Although fairly common in young adults, where it is often thought of and investigated, dissection can still occur in older people.

Ischaemic stroke, transient ischaemic attack, retinal infarction, ischaemic oculopathy – and even spinal cord infarction in the case of vertebral dissection – are caused by occlusion of the true arterial lumen by the expanded vessel wall with distal hypoperfusion; occlusive and propagating thrombosis within the true lumen; and – probably most often although it is difficult to be sure just from patterns of infarction on brain imaging – by embolism from thrombus within the true lumen.[39-41]

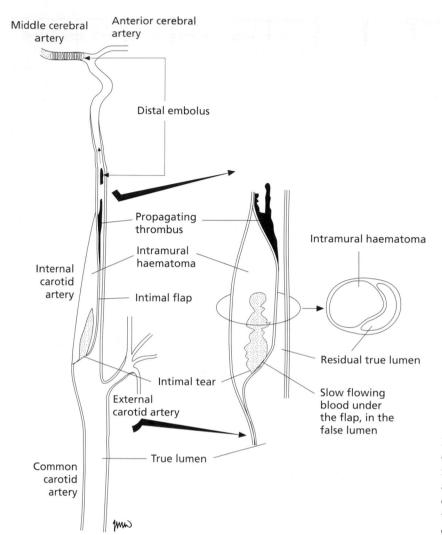

Fig. 7.1 Arterial dissection at the origin of the internal carotid artery showing: intramural haematoma which thromboses and becomes organized; intimal tear; complicating non-occlusive thrombosis in the true lumen with embolism causing distal occlusion of the middle cerebral artery.

Diagnostic clues, which may be present singly or in combination, are:

- pain in the face, around the eye, in the neck or side of the head ipsilateral to ICA dissection, or pain in the back of the head and neck – usually unilaterally – for vertebral dissection; sometimes the pain is distant from the site of the dissection; the pain of dissection may start suddenly or gradually, and be continuous or intermittent;
- Horner syndrome as a result of damage to the sympathetic nerve fibres around the dissected ICA;
- self-audible bruit because carotid dissection tends to spread distally to the base of the skull, or is only present distally;
- occasionally, ipsilateral palsies of one or more lower cranial nerves, particularly the hypoglossal, as a result of pressure from the expanded ICA wall at the base of the skull, or of nerve ischaemia, causing false localizing signs suggesting a brainstem stroke; ocular

motor palsies ipsilateral to an ICA dissection are very rare;

- cervical nerve root lesions have recently been described in vertebral dissection, either caused by ischaemia or pressure from the bulging arterial wall.

One or more of these features may occur, even just headache alone, without any stroke at all, but very often they precede, as well as accompany, the onset of cerebral ischaemia by hours or days but, in some cases, none of these features are present.[42–46]

Although ICA (but less often vertebral) dissection can be suspected on duplex sonography, often because of the damping of flow due to distal occlusion rather than direct visualization of the dissection, the definitive investigation is a combination of axial magnetic resonance imaging (MRI) through the lesion to show the intramural haematoma, combined with MR angiography (MRA) to display the length and distribution of the arterial pathology with irregular narrowing of the

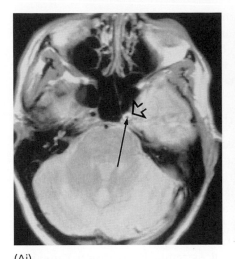
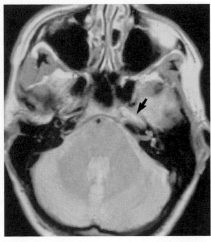
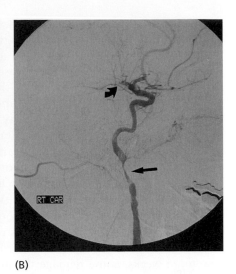

(Ai)   (Aii)   (B)

Fig. 7.2 (A) Carotid dissection on MRI. Expansion of the arterial wall by blood clot is more or less diagnostic but is not seen in every case because the lesion may be too small; the MRI cuts are not through the affected part of the artery; there is intraluminal thrombus which cannot be differentiated from intramural haematoma; or perhaps the clot is so fresh that there is not enough methaemoglobin to enhance the signal on T1-weighted images. It is also conceivable that haemorrhage within an atheromatous plaque could be confused with dissection, but atheroma is usually in a different part of the artery. The true lumen is seen as an eccentric signal void on T1- and T2-weighted axial images and is surrounded by semilunar hyperintensity, corresponding with the intramural haematoma, but the signal intensity does depend on the age of the haematoma and the pulse sequence selected. In the example shown (proton density-weighted axial MRI), the dissected distal internal carotid artery is seen passing through the skull base in the carotid canal. (Ai) The high signal of the intramural haematoma (*open arrow*) and central flow void (*thin arrow*) are clearly seen, rather like a shooting target. (Aii) Slice immediately rostral of (Ai) showing the high signal of the occluded internal carotid artery (*arrow*). (B) Carotid dissection on catheter angiography. The diagnostic features include an elongated and tapering stenosis (*arrow*), often irregular and possibly with complete occlusion of the lumen. Sometimes there is aneurysmal bulging of the adventitial wall, an intimal flap, a floating thrombus or an obviously double lumen. Unlike carotid atheroma, dissection is usually well distal to the internal carotid origin and also it seldom reaches beyond the base of the skull. The middle cerebral artery is occluded, presumably as a result of embolism (*curved arrow*).

vessel lumen, sometimes with aneurysm formation or occlusion.[47,48] If there is any doubt, catheter angiography is necessary, particularly when a correct diagnosis is vital, for example in potential medicolegal cases (Fig. 7.2). CT angiography is a possible alternative to MRA; it can show high attenuation thrombus in the arterial wall.

Although any imaging modality may demonstrate complete arterial occlusion, this in itself is non-specific and does not imply dissection unless there is the typical long tapering 'rat's tail' appearance, a double-lumen, an intimal flap, or a haematoma in the arterial wall. Imaging must be performed within days of symptom onset because dissections usually resolve spontaneously, sometimes within days. Because ocasionally several arteries may be involved at the same time (e.g. both carotids or one carotid and both vertebrals) it is important to examine the other neck arteries carefully and also to document the proximal and distal extent of the dissection.

> Cervical arterial dissection is diagnosed by first asking the right question: 'In the last few days or weeks have you injured or damaged your neck, has anyone grabbed or manipulated your neck, have you had a car crash or a recent operation, have you recently been through labour, or done anything to twist your neck?' The correct investigations should then be performed before the dissection heals: magnetic resonance imaging and angiography and, if there is still uncertainty, selective catheter angiography.

Recurrence of dissection, in the same or a different artery, is distinctly unusual; around 1% per annum, except in familial cases where it is more common.[35,49] This argues against an underlying but as yet unrecognized abnormality of the arterial wall in most patients, and favours a 'one off' event such as trauma, although a combination of both is possible.

The treatment of cervical arterial dissection is controversial, largely because there are no randomized trials[50,51] and so we must rely on our – as always – incomplete understanding of the pathophysiology. Acutely, intra-venous thrombolysis has been used and is said to be safe in a small number of reported cases.[52] Longer-term antithrombotic drugs may reduce the tendency for thrombus to form in the true lumen and so perhaps prevent distal embolization, but they may also increase the risk of further bleeding in the false lumen. The options are to do nothing, give aspirin as an antithrombotic drug (section 16.5.3) for some weeks on the assumption that unless there is a persisting cause for the dissection it will have healed by then and the risk of recurrence is very low (which is our practice), or formal anticoagula-tion with heparin and then warfarin for a matter of weeks (section 16.6), perhaps followed by aspirin for a few more weeks. Some reimage the artery and do not stop antithrombotics until the wall is normal. It might be reasonable to anticoagulate if the patient worsens on aspirin, or has a recurrent ischaemic event which if it is going to occur tends to occur early,[53] and if the cause appears to be due to thromboembolism. Best of all, we would join a well-founded randomized trial of anti-thrombotic treatment, both in the short and longer term.

Presumably it is wise to avoid any further activities of the sort that caused the dissection, if possible, although not to the extent of inducing phobias by insisting on ludicrous restrictions like never looking over one's shoulder when reversing the car.

7.2.2 Intracranial arterial dissection

Intracranial dissection may be caused by a blow on the head, as well as by the other causes of dissection listed in Table 6.2, but most often no cause is found. It seems to be much rarer than extracranial dissection and more often affects the vertebral and basilar arteries than the internal carotid artery and its branches. It is more likely to present with subarachnoid haemorrhage than with cere-bral ischaemia (it is therefore a cause of non-aneurysmal subarachnoid haemorrhage, section 9.1.3).[42,54–58] haem-orrhage is the result of rupture of the bulging arterial adventitia, given the lack of external elastic lamina in the intradural section of the arteries, or dissection in the adventitial rather than medial layer of the arterial wall (section 9.1.3).[59] Basilar dissection may also compress the brainstem and lower cranial nerves.

The diagnosis of unruptured dissections can be sus-pected by the young age of the patient, and often severe headache immediately before the focal neurological fea-tures (not dissimilar to intracranial venous thrombosis). On cerebral angiography (MRA or, more reliably, by catheter) the findings include a focal area of constric-tion or dilatation although this appearance can also be caused by a clearing embolus; a long tapered occlusion; an intimal flap; an aneurysm; and – probably the only pathognomonic feature – a double lumen which is actually seldom seen (Fig. 9.6). MRI may demonstrate intramural haematoma.

7.2.3 Aortic arch dissection

Aortic arch dissection generally causes global cerebral ischaemia, syncope and coma.[60–65] However, it can cause *focal* cerebral ischaemia (i.e. ischaemic stroke or transi-ent ischaemic attack) if the dissection extends up one of the major neck arteries to cause occlusion, or mural thrombosis and embolism. More often, any cerebral ischaemia is generalized, perhaps causing low-flow infarc-tion, as a result of systemic hypotension caused by cardiac tamponade, acute aortic regurgitation or myo-cardial infarction. Clues to the diagnosis are:

- sudden and severe anterior chest pain and/or inter-scapular pain which may move as the dissection extends (sometimes there is no pain at all) (section 6.7.6);
- syncope;
- hypotension;
- diminished, unequal or absent arterial pulses and blood pressures in the arms, neck and sometimes legs (often not looked for by neurologists and others);
- acute aortic regurgitation and cardiac failure;
- cardiac tamponade;
- simultaneous or sequential ischaemia in carotid, subclavian, vertebral, spinal, coronary and other aortic branches if the dissection extends over several centimetres;
- mediastinal widening and left pleural effusion on the chest X-ray.

The electrocardiogram is generally normal unless there is complicating acute myocardial infarction, cardiac tamponade or acute left ventricular strain. Intra-arterial aortography is diagnostic and allows full evaluation of the extent of the lesion. However, transoesophageal echocardiography and contrast CT or MRI of the aortic arch are safer and perhaps quicker, but give less informa-tion about coronary patency. The management lies in the hands of cardiologists and cardiothoracic surgeons.

7.3 Inflammatory vasculopathies and connective tissue diseases

Most of the autoimmune or collagen vascular and related disorders (Table 6.2) can be complicated by, or occasionally present with, various peripheral and central neurological syndromes, including stroke and transient ischaemic attack.[66–72]

> Vasculitic disorders affecting the central nervous system may cause not only thrombosis within arteries and veins, but also rupture of affected vessels with subarachnoid or intracerebral haemorrhage.

Usually in these conditions – but not always – there is an acute, subacute or chronic inflammatory reaction in the arterial and/or venous wall, with or without granuloma formation, i.e. vasculitis which in the literature, and in clinical practice, is often assumed rather than demonstrated histopathologically (Fig. 7.3). This mural cellular proliferation, necrosis and subsequent fibrosis may be sufficient to occlude the vessel lumen; precipitate thrombosis, which may be complicated by embolism; and promote aneurysm formation, dissection or even wall rupture. Therefore, these vessel changes may cause not only focal and generalized cerebral ischaemia, either by arterial or venous occlusion, but also intracranial haemorrhage. In addition, non-neurological complications (e.g. hypertension caused by renal involvement in a systemic vasculitic disorder) and adverse effects of treatment (e.g. opportunistic meningeal and cerebral infections resulting from immunosuppression) may lead to cerebral ischaemia or haemorrhage.

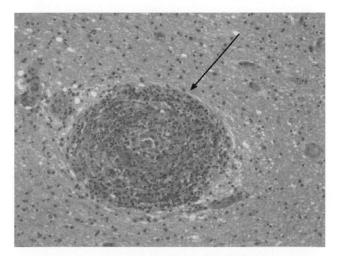

Fig. 7.3 Cerebral vasculitis: there is lymphocytic infiltration and destruction of a small blood vessel in the brain parenchyma (*arrow*). The vessel is completely occluded by the thickened vessel wall. Stain H&E, × 40 magnification. (Also reproduced in colour in the plate section.) Courtesy of Dr Colin Smith, Edinburgh.

> In all cases it is crucial not just to assume that a known inflammatory vascular disorder is the cause of the stroke or transient ischaemic attack, but always to consider the possibility of the adverse effects of immunosuppression or an opportunistic infection.

Among patients presenting with stroke or transient ischaemic attack there are very few who are already known to have, or who are discovered to have, an auto-immune or inflammatory vascular disorder. In fact, patients with cerebral involvement due to a collagen vascular disorder are generally more likely to have a generalized encephalopathy or aseptic chronic meningitis, with or without focal features, which does not really fit with the 'typical stroke patient'. Nonetheless, these disorders are well worth looking out for, even in stroke and TIA patients, because their presence will require a detailed general evaluation of the patient in terms of renal function, joint problems, etc., and they will certainly change the way the patient is managed. On the other hand, one should not over-react to a moderately raised erythrocyte sedimentation rate (ESR) in a stroke patient who is otherwise well with no clinical features of a systemic disorder. An inflammatory vascular disorder – or even paraproteinaemia – should certainly be considered, but as often as not the raised ESR reflects some intercurrent infection before or possibly complicating the stroke. The same caution should be applied to an antinuclear factor antibody titre of only 1 : 40.

Clues to the diagnosis of an autoimmune or inflammatory vascular disorder, unless it is already known, are:
- preceding or accompanying systemic features such as weight loss, headache, malaise, skin rash, livedo reticularis, arthropathy, renal failure and fever;
- the lack of any other obvious or more common cause of stroke;
- younger patient in most cases (an exception being giant-cell arteritis);
- a raised ESR and C-reactive protein (the latter is usually normal in systemic lupus erythematosus);
- anaemia and leucocytosis in the routine blood screening tests; and
- when diagnostic suspicion is aroused, specific immunological tests, such as raised serum antiphospholipid, double-stranded DNA and antineutrophil cytoplasmic antibodies (ANCA) (a positive antinuclear factor antibody is far too non-specific to be useful on its own, even in relatively high titre).

Unless obvious, the diagnosis must usually be confirmed by biopsy of the superficial temporal artery, meninges, cerebral cortex, skin, kidney, etc., as appropriate to the clinical syndrome. However, false-negative

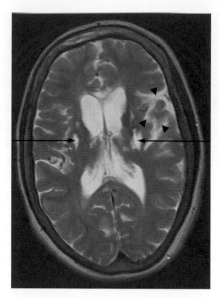

Fig. 7.4 MRI (T2-weighted) of cerebral vasculitis. Note the lesions (infarcts) affect grey (*arrowheads*) as well as white matter (*arrows*), unlike in multiple sclerosis, where only white matter is affected.

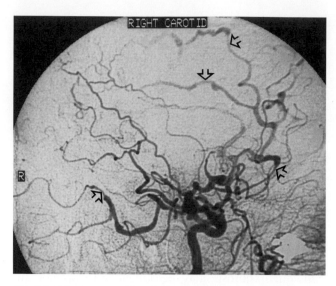

Fig. 7.5 Selective carotid catheter angiogram to show focal dilatations and constrictions of branches of the middle and anterior cerebral arteries (*arrows*). Brain and meningeal biopsies were negative but many years later the patient presented with an acute abdomen and histologically proven vasculitis of the gastrointestinal tract.

biopsies can occur because the vascular lesions can and do heal and they are anyway often very patchy in distribution. Any abnormalities in the cerebrospinal fluid (CSF) are usually non-specific: a lymphocyte, or occasionally neutrophil, inflammatory reaction; raised protein; and oligoclonal bands confined to the CSF, all of which can also occur in multiple sclerosis for example[73] (matching CSF and serum oligoclonal bands are, however, less likely in multiple sclerosis). Brain CT and the more sensitive MRI may both show areas of presumed infarction, and sometimes haemorrhage, in both grey and white matter, sometimes with diffuse meningeal and subependymal involvement (Fig. 7.4) (cf. multiple sclerosis where the lesions are confined to the periventricular white matter and corpus callosum, but the distinction from vasculitis is impossible in many cases).[73] There are no *specific* angiographic criteria for cerebral vasculitis; focal narrowing, dilatation and beading of medium-sized and small cerebral arteries, sometimes with aneurysm formation, are seen in many other situations (Table 7.1) (Fig. 7.5). Moreover, angiography is often normal even in biopsy-proven vasculitis, particularly if MR or CT rather than catheter angiography – the most reliable method to show the subtle features of vasculitis – is relied on. The electro-encephalogram may help in the sense that bilateral diffuse slowing in a patient who clinically seems to have only a unilateral hemispheric lesion suggests a diffuse encephalopathic process of some sort, which may be vasculitic.

Table 7.1 Some causes of segmental narrowing, dilatation and beading of the cerebral arteries seen on angiography.

> Cerebral vasculitis (section 7.3)
> Tumour emboli (section 7.12)
> Irradiation (section 7.12)
> Malignant meningitis
> Chronic meningeal infections (section 7.11)
> Drug misuse (cocaine, amphetamines, etc.) (section 7.15)
> Multiple emboli
> Idiopathic reversible cerebral vasoconstriction (puerperal angiopathy) (sections 7.3.18 and 7.14)
> Arterial dissection (section 7.2.2)
> Intravascular lymphoma (section 7.9.5)
> Malignant hypertension (section 3.4.5)
> Fabry's disease (section 7.20.3)
> Phaeochromocytoma (section 3.7.2)

> 'Beading' of intracranial arteries on cerebral angiography is neither a specific nor sensitive sign of cerebral vasculitis, which cannot be diagnosed reliably without meningeal or cerebral histopathology if there is no safer tissue to biopsy, or if there are no definitely diagnostic serum autoantibodies.

The treatment of these various conditions, largely dependent on corticosteroids with or without immuno-suppresion, is largely based on experience, and occasional randomized trials in the far more common patients with non-neurological problems. Obviously, the numerous adverse effects of treatment have to be carefully monitored (e.g. osteoporosis and diabetes with corticosteroids, marrow suppression and bladder cancer with cyclophosphamide). It makes sense for neurologists and stroke physicians to collaborate with rheumatologists or other specialists with particular experience in managing patients with inflammatory connective tissue disorders.

7.3.1 Giant-cell arteritis

Giant-cell (temporal) arteritis is the most common 'vasculitic' cause of ischaemic stroke. It *should* be easily suspected because of the almost invariable presence of one or more accompanying systemic features such as malaise, polymyalgia, headache, weight loss, low-grade fever, depression and – usually but not always – an ESR over 50 and often over 100 mm in the first hour, and even more often a raised C-reactive protein (raised plasma viscosity is probably as informative as a raised ESR).[74] The patients are seldom under the age of 60 and almost never under the age of 50 years. There is frequently a mild normochromic normocytic anaemia, a raised platelet count and slightly disturbed liver function. Alternative diagnostic possibilities include other inflammatory vascular disorders, infective endocarditis, malignancy and paraproteinaemias.

Any medium or large artery may be affected (carotid, vertebral, coronary, subclavian, femoral, aorta, etc.), most commonly:

- branches of the external carotid artery (superficial temporal, occipital, facial) which causes headache and facial pain, scalp tenderness and sometimes jaw claudication;
- the ophthalmic, posterior ciliary and central retinal arteries which causes infarction of the optic nerve (ischaemic optic neuropathy, section 3.5.2 and Fig. 3.45) more often than of the retina;
- the extradural vertebral arteries more often than the internal carotid arteries which causes ischaemic stroke or transient ischaemic attacks.[75,76] Curiously, the anterior, middle and posterior cerebral and basilar arteries and their branches are less often affected (Fig. 7.6).

Arterial biopsy is the definitive investigation to show giant cells and other evidence of chronic inflammation in the vessel wall with destruction of the internal elastic lamina[77] (Fig. 7.7). A clinical diagnosis *alone* is seldom enough to commit elderly patients to months or years of the risks of corticosteroids; if steroid complications occur some months after the start of treatment, the knowledge that a biopsy was positive is immensely reassuring. To maximize the chance of a positive biopsy, it is best to examine an extracranial artery that is *tender*, if possible.

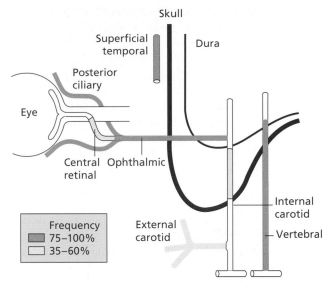

Fig. 7.6 The typical distribution of giant cell arteritis affecting the arteries of the head and neck. The most frequently affected arteries are the ophthalmic, posterior ciliary, superficial temporal and vertebral. Less often affected are the central retinal, distal internal carotid and other external carotid artery branches. (With permission from Wilkinson & Ross Russell, 1972.)[625]

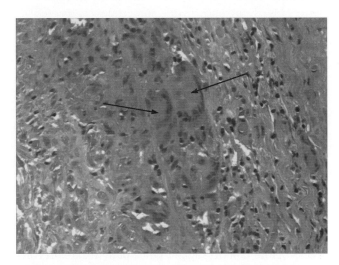

Fig. 7.7 Giant cell arteritis: superficial temporal artery biopsy showing multinucleated giant cells (*arrows*) lying in relation to the damaged internal elastic lamina of the vessel wall. Stain H&E, ×60 magnification. (Also reproduced in colour in the plate section.) Courtesy of Dr Colin Smith, Edinburgh.

Otherwise, at least 2 cm of the superficial temporal artery should be taken and, if negative and the case is still a puzzle, many physicians biopsy another scalp artery, such as the contralateral superficial temporal artery. Unfortunately, a negative biopsy does not rule out the diagnosis because the arterial lesions can be patchy and so a short segment of artery may miss them, particularly if multiple sections have not been examined. Therefore, the clinical diagnosis has sometimes to be accepted, backed up by the complete resolution of the systemic symptoms (polymyalgia, headache, etc.) within 24–48 h of starting high-dose corticosteroids and a normal ESR within about 1 month. The temporal artery biopsy should be performed as soon as the diagnosis is suspected but, if this is impractical, corticosteroids must be started at once in case of impending eye or brain ischaemia; it seems that corticosteroids will not interfere with the histological appearance if the biopsy is performed within a few days, but presumably the sooner the biopsy is done the better.[78] If there is still diagnostic doubt, corticosteroids should be slowly withdrawn and, if symptoms recur or the ESR rises, the diagnostic process must be repeated.

> If a patient presents with cerebral or ocular ischaemia and is aged over 50 years, and there is a recent history of malaise and headache not likely to be caused by infective endocarditis or other infection, then an erythrocyte sedimentation rate must be performed urgently. If it is raised, high doses of corticosteroids should be started before the results of any temporal artery biopsy are known, and sometimes even before the biopsy is performed (which must be within a few days).

Treatment starts with high-dose oral prednisolone (60 mg daily), tapered over a few weeks to about 20 mg daily, and then more slowly to 10–15 mg daily. Every 6 months or so cautious attempts should be made to withdraw the steroids, reducing every month by perhaps 1–2 mg. Eventually, in a matter of months to years, the patient will be in remission and the steroids can be stopped. A close watch must be kept for recurrent symptoms and a rising ESR unexplained by, for example, intercurrent infection – either or both should lead to an immediate increase in the steroid dose for a few weeks before tapering again. Once patients are on corticosteroids they are unlikely to have any serious vascular events such as stroke or ischaemic optic neuropathy, but this is not guaranteed.[79] For patients who are running into adverse effects, there is some evidence that methotrexate can be used as a steroid sparing agent, but a meta-analysis of the available, not very large, trials is needed.[80,81]

7.3.2 Takayasu's arteritis

Takayasu's arteritis is histologically identical to giant-cell arteritis but preferentially affects the aorta and the large

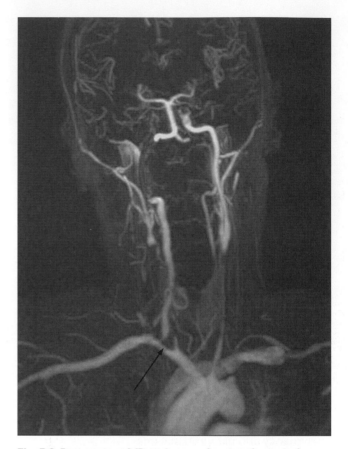

Fig. 7.8 Post-contrast MR angiogram showing the typical features of Takayasu's arteritis with smooth short and long stenoses and occlusions of the major arteries in the neck. *Long arrow*: stenosis of the right subclavian artery and origin of the right vertebral artery. *Arrowheads*: smooth long stenosis of the left common carotid artery. Blood reaches the internal carotid arteries via collaterals in the neck.

arteries arising from it, mainly but not exclusively in young Asian women.[82–86] There are multiple regions of smooth stenosis, irregularity, occlusion and aneurysmal bulging which, with catheter angiography or non-invasive vascular imaging, in the correct clinical context, gives the diagnosis (Fig. 7.8). Curiously, the distribution of the arterial pathology differs in various parts of the world. As with giant-cell arteritis, but not so frequently, there can be systemic features such as malaise, fever, weight loss, anaemia and a raised ESR, at least in the early stages of the illness.

The neurological features are thought to reflect the gradually increasing ischaemia of the tissues as their supplying arteries become stenosed and occluded: claudication of jaw muscles; headache; ischaemic oculopathy (section 3.5.2; Fig. 3.45); syncope, particularly on sitting or standing up; epileptic seizures; confusion; and low-flow cerebral ischaemia with, sometimes, focal ischaemic strokes and transient ischaemic attacks. There is some evidence for embolism as another potential cause of ischaemia.[87] There may also be ischaemic necrosis of the lips, nasal septum and palate. The arms and hands, and sometimes also the legs, may become ischaemic with unequal or absent pulses and blood pressures, as may the kidneys to cause hypertension (which can be difficult to diagnose if the upper limb arteries are also affected). Aortic regurgitation and coronary artery occlusion are further complications.

The treatment is as for giant-cell arteritis although, given the fact that the arterial occlusions may stabilize and the ESR is not necessarily raised, and the relative rarity of the condition, there is not a lot of experience to draw on and no randomized trials.[88] Not surprisingly various surgical revascularization procedures have been attempted, and now of course stenting (of the renal as well as the arteries to the brain), which makes sense in the more chronic phase of the disease when the arteries become fibrotic rather than inflamed.

7.3.3 Systemic lupus erythematosus

This is a chronic autoimmune multisystem disease affecting mainly young women.[89–91] It much more often causes a generalized subacute or chronic encephalopathy than focal ischaemic or haemorrhagic cerebral episodes.[92–95] Scattered cerebral infarcts and haemorrhages, of varying size, are found in some but not all 'encephalopathic' cases at postmortem. If any *vascular* lesion is found, it is seldom a florid vasculitis but rather bland intimal proliferation involving small vessels, although this may possibly represent healed vasculitis. Why the occasional patient has large artery occlusion is unknown, but embolism from heart valves affected by systemic lupus erythematosus (SLE) is obviously one possibility. Indeed, embolism from non-infective cardiac valvular vegetations to cerebral arteries is probably quite common.[96,97] Finally, it appears that, for some reason, SLE patients have a higher prevalence of coronary artery and carotid lesions, i.e. presumed atheroma, on the basis of CT[98] and ultrasound respectively.[99]

Most patients have circulating antinuclear antibodies of various sorts, as well as non-neurological features of SLE, such as arthropathy. A raised antinuclear factor is a highly sensitive but not at all specific finding in SLE. Double-stranded DNA and anti-Sm antibodies are much more specific but are found in less than half of cases. A high proportion also have antiphospholipid antibodies (section 7.3.4) which seem to be particularly associated with cardiac valvular vegetations and arterial thrombosis.[100]

The treatment should generally be in collaboration with rheumatologists, or other specialists who have more experience of the condition than most neurologists and stroke physicians. Despite the very small number of randomized trials, the general view is that corticosteroids, often with cyclophosphamide or methotrexate, are effective, or chloroquine for milder cases.[101,102] For those with high levels of antiphospholipid antibodies, there is an argument for antithrombotic drugs (section 7.3.4), and if premature atherosclerosis is likely then the usual secondary prevention strategies (Chapter 16).

7.3.4 Antiphospholipid syndrome

A number of ischaemic stroke/transient ischaemic attack patients, generally young women, have raised circulating IgG or, probably less relevant, IgM, anticardiolipin antibodies and/or the lupus anticoagulant detected by the activated partial thromboplastin time or the dilute Russell's viper venom time. The exact proportion depends on selection of patients as ever, timing of the blood sample after symptom onset, laboratory methods used which are not yet standardized, and what level is deemed 'abnormal', bearing in mind the spontaneous fluctuations in titre in individuals. However, very few patients have some or all of the constellation of features of the antiphospholipid syndrome (APS): recurrent miscarriage, venous and less often arterial thrombosis in any sized vessel (but not vasculitis) and, variably, livedo reticularis, heart valve vegetations, migraine-like headaches, thrombocytopenia, haemolytic anaemia, circulating lupus anticoagulant and false-positive non-specific serological tests for syphilis.[103,104] If a patient has the typical syndrome but no antibodies, then the test should be repeated after a few weeks because the titres may fall during the acute episode.[105] Raised antibodies in a stroke patient without the APS should probably be ignored as having no bearing on prognosis or management.

Antiphospholipid antibodies are not specific to the APS, particularly if they are not present in high titres on *repeated* testing. They can be found in some normal individuals, and also in SLE and other collagen vascular disorders, malignancy, lymphoma, paraproteinaemias, human immunodeficiency virus (HIV) and other infections, patients with multiple vascular risk factors, in the elderly, on haemodialysis, and as a result of a variety of drugs such as phenothiazines, hydralazine, phenytoin, valproate, procainamide and quinidine.[106]

The cause of thrombosis, the prognosis for recurrent stroke and the nature of the relationship and overlap with SLE are all uncertain.[107]

The antiphospholipid syndrome cannot be diagnosed on the basis of a single raised titre of antibody in the serum. The titre must be substantially raised on several occasions and associated not only with cerebral ischaemia but also with some combination of deep venous thrombosis, recurrent miscarriage, livedo reticularis, cardiac valvular vegetations, thrombocytopenia and migraine.

Because thrombosis appears to be more of an issue in the APS than in SLE, long-term warfarin has become the most commonly used treatment, with a target INR of about 3.0 (notwithstanding the serious lack of randomized trials of any size in patients with arterial rather than venous thrombosis where the evidence is better). Presumably aspirin would provide some protection in those unable or unwilling to take warfarin for the rest of their lives, or if prescribed by physicians who are unconvinced by the weak evidence supporting warfarin.[108,109]

It is unclear whether ischaemic stroke patients with the antiphospholipid syndrome gain more protection from recurrent ischaemic events when given long-term warfarin rather than aspirin, and whether the risks of haemorrhage are less than any benefits.

7.3.5 Sneddon syndrome

Sneddon syndrome – most commonly seen in young women – is the rare combination of widespread and prominent livedo reticularis (Fig. 7.9) which is a rather non-specific skin appearance[110] (Table 7.2), ischaemic stroke/transient ischaemic attacks but rarely intracerebral haemorrhage, and sometimes autoantibodies associated with SLE (particularly antiphospholipid antibodies and the lupus anticoagulant), if not the full-blown syndrome (sections 7.3.3 and 7.3.4).[111–113] It might be one variety of the antiphospholipid syndrome, itself part of the spectrum of SLE.[114,115] It is unclear whether it should be treated more like SLE with immunosuppression, or the antiphospholipid syndrome with an antithrombotic drug, or with both.

7.3.6 Primary systemic vasculitis

This is a group of related multisystem disorders which are defined rather variably: classic polyarteritis nodosa, Wegener's granulomatosis, the Churg–Strauss syndrome and microscopic polyangiitis.[116,117] While involvement of the kidneys, lungs, peripheral and cranial nerves, and skin is quite common, cerebrovascular complications

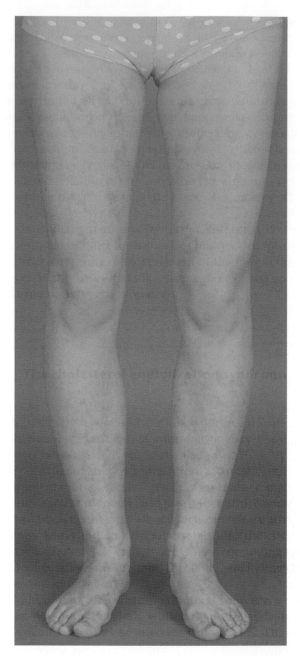

Fig. 7.9 The typical appearance of livedo reticularis affecting the legs. Also reproduced in colour in the plate section.

are rare. But ischaemia and haemorrhage can affect the brain and eye, with clinical features rather like SLE.[118–123] However, in contrast to SLE, the vascular lesion is generally but not always a vasculitis affecting small and medium-sized arteries, arterioles, venules and capillaries. The serum antibodies characteristic of SLE are seldom present while eosinophilia, raised serum ANCA and haematuria are all more likely.

Table 7.2 The causes of livedo reticularis.

Vessel wall disease
Vasculitis (section 7.3)
Atherosclerosis
Intravascular obstruction
Hypercoagulability (section 7.9.11)
Paraproteinaemia (section 7.9.10)
Mixed essential cryoglobulinaemia (section 7.3.14)
Cholesterol embolization syndrome (section 7.7)
Disseminated intravascular coagulation (section 7.9.12)
Decompression sickness
Infections
Tuberculosis
Meningococcal septicaemia
Endocarditis
Syphilis
Typhus fever
Drugs
Amantadine
Quinine
Catecholamines
Metabolic/endocrine
Cushing's disease
Hypothyroidism
Pellagra
Miscellaneous
Cardiac failure
Lymphoma
Oxalosis
Acute pancreatitis

Depending on the clinical severity, treatment is generally with a combination of prednisolone (60 mg per day, oral) perhaps preceded by high-dose iv methyl-prednisolone (1 g daily for 3 days), and cysclo-phophamide (2–3 mg per kg per day, oral) and then, once the disease is under control, tapering prednisolone over several months and substituting the rather safer azathioprine (2 mg/kg/day, oral) for the cyclopho-sphamide. Normally rheumatologists rather than neurologists take the lead in treatment because they are more familiar with these disorders and the use of cyclophosphamide.

7.3.7 Kawasaki disease

This is another systemic vasculitis, but more or less confined to infants and children.[124] The illness is self-limiting and acute, with fever, conjunctival injection, fissuring of the lips, cervical lymphadenopathy, rash and reddening of the palms of the hands and soles of the feet. While coronary arteritis with aneurysm formation is the most common serious complication, occasionally there are neurological features: aseptic meningitis, facial palsy, epileptic seizures and encephalopathy.[69]

7.3.8 Henoch–Schönlein purpura

This small-vessel vasculitis, mainly occurring in children, typically involves the skin, gut and kidneys and is associated with arthritis. Subacute encephalopathy, perhaps with focal features, and peripheral nerve involvement are both rare.[125,126] Meningoccocal meningitis is an important differential diagnosis.

7.3.9 Rheumatoid disease

Rheumatoid disease is very rarely complicated by cerebral vasculitis.[127–129] Atlanto-occipital dislocation can cause symptomatic vertebral artery compression with posterior circulation ischaemia.[130]

7.3.10 Sjögren syndrome

Dry eyes and dry mouth as a result of inflammation and destruction of the lacrimal and salivary glands are the defining features of Sjögren syndrome – a systemic autoimmune disorder.[131] Characteristically, antinuclear and antibodies to SS-A/Ro or SS-B/La, as well sometimes as rheumatoid factor, are present. Peripheral neuropathy is the most frequent neurological complication. Rarely, there is a systemic and cerebral vasculitis, the latter causing transient or permanent focal neurological deficits, aseptic meningitis and global encephalopathy.[132–136]

7.3.11 Behçet's disease

This is an inflammatory relapsing and remitting syndrome of orogenital ulceration and uveitis, often along with skin, joint and gut involvement and recurrent venous thrombosis. Both a large- and small-vessel vasculitis is well described, but florid necrotizing vasculitis appears to be distinctly unusual.

Behçet's disease can be complicated by chronic aseptic meningitis which affects cerebral arteries, perhaps more commonly those supplying the brainstem, to cause ischaemic stroke/transient ischaemic attack and intracerebral and sometimes subarachnoid haemorrhage.[137–140] A more global subacute and relapsing encephalopathy is well recognized, as often with low-grade inflammation within the brain as in the vessels, while intracranial venous thrombosis (section 7.21) is probably the most commonly encountered neurological complication of the disease – presenting with intracranial hypertension without other neurological features, as well as with intracerebral haemorrhagic infarction. The neurological symptoms tend to start a few years after the onset of the disease and coincide with flare-ups of the mucocutaneo-ocular symptoms, but can antedate them.

There are no specific circulating autoantibodies and the diagnosis is usually made by the clinical manifestations and sometimes a positive pathergy test (cutaneous needle prick causes an erythematous nodule 48 h later).

Thalidomide, colchicine, corticosteroids, azathioprine and ciclosporin are all recommended as treatments but, although there are randomized trials, none have been in patients with neuro-Behçet's disease.[139]

7.3.12 Relapsing polychondritis

Relapsing polychondritis is a very rare condition characterized by febrile episodes of inflammation affecting the cartilage of the ears, nose, larynx, trachea and ribs. It affects men and women in middle age. There is often an arthropathy, inflammation in the eyes and optic nerve, deafness and vertigo, anaemia and a high ESR.[141] It is sometimes complicated by a systemic and cerebral vasculitis with subacute aseptic meningitis, cranial nerve palsies, global encephalopathy, epileptic seizures, stroke/transient ischaemic attack, aortic arch syndromes and peripheral neuropathy.[142–145] There are no specific diagnostic tests.

7.3.13 Progressive systemic sclerosis

Progressive systemic sclerosis is characterized by widespread and slowly progressive fibrous sclerosis affecting the skin, lungs, kidneys, gut and heart. It is hardly ever complicated by stroke, but a carotid and cerebral arteritis has been described as well as nondescript intracerebral small-vessel disease.[146,147] Linear scleroderma has also been associated with an inflammatory vascular disorder of the brain.[148]

7.3.14 Mixed essential cryglobulinaemia

Peripheral neuropathy is the most common neurological complication of this chronic disease manifested by purpura, Raynaud's phenomenon, arthralgia, hepatic dysfunction and progressive renal failure. Plasma cryoglobulins are present without any evidence of other causes of cryoglobulinaemia such as malignancy, infections or circulating monoclonal and/or polyclonal immunoglobulins.[149,150] There can be a widespread systemic vasculitis and there have been occasional reports of cerebral vasculitis, although in some cases the vessel wall itself was histologically normal while the lumen was plugged with immunoglobulin-rich deposits.[151]

7.3.15 Malignant atrophic papulosis (Kohlmeier–Degos disease)

Malignant atrophic papulosis is another very rare vasculopathy. Crops of painless but occasionally itchy, umbilicated, pinkish papules appear mainly on the trunk, which heal to form distinctive, circular, porcelain-white scars. Intimal endothelial proliferation and thrombosis in small arteries can cause ischaemia and haemorrhage in the brain, spinal cord, gut and other organs.[152,153] Muscle and nerve are sometimes affected.

7.3.16 Sarcoid vasculitis

Sarcoidosis is a systemic, multiorgan, non-caseating, granulomatous disorder which mostly affects the lungs, lymph nodes, eyes and skin.[154–156] The illness tends to be subacute and self-limiting, but it may recur, and it is occasionally chronic.

As well as intracerebral granulomatous mass lesions, aseptic meningitis and cranial nerve palsies, typically with marked CT or MR contrast enhancement of the leptomeninges, sarcoid can cause a vasculitis of the small arteries and veins of the meninges and brain. This may lead to a subacute global encephalopathy. Focal cerebral ischaemia and haemorrhage causing stroke is much rarer. Because involvement of the nervous system without any systemic features at all is so unusual, the diagnosis should be reasonably obvious from the almost invariable non-neurological features, such as hilar lymphadenopathy, uveitis, etc. A raised serum (or CSF) angiotensin-converting enzyme level is neither sensitive nor specific so, as usual with suspected vasculitis, a tissue biopsy may be necessary for diagnosis, either of a lymph node or very occasionally of brain and meninges.[157–159]

There are no randomized trials specifically in neuro-sarcoidosis and so the usual treatment for pulmonary sarcoidosis is generally used; corticosteroids are the first choice and, if necessary for steroid sparing, antimalarials or cytotoxics.[155,156] Recently some success has been reported with infliximab, a TNF alpha inhibitor.[160]

7.3.17 Primary angiitis of the central nervous system

Primary – or isolated – angiitis of the central nervous system is a rare disorder affecting mainly young adults and the middle-aged (about 1–2 cases per million per year). Occasionally a similar vasculitis is associated with herpes zoster infection, lymphoma and cerebral amyloid angiopathy.[161–163]

A focal and segmental vasculitis affects the small leptomeningeal, cortical and spinal cord blood vessels to cause a subacute global encephalopathy with headache and seizures, with or without stroke-like episodes caused by ischaemia or occasionally haemorrhage, and sometimes a myelopathy or even radiculopathy.[164,165] Systemic symptoms are uncommon, but sometimes there is fever, raised ESR and a raised CSF protein with lymphocytosis. A definite diagnosis can only be made from meningeal/cortical biopsy of non-dominant frontal lobe, or an affected area shown on brain imaging. Although biopsy is somewhat risky, a positive result is helpful so that treatment can be confidently given, and sometimes a completely unexpected and yet treatable disorder is discovered (e.g. encephalitis, lymphoma, sarcoidosis, TB).[166,167]

So-called benign cases have been described (section 7.3.18). However, unless there is confirmatory histopathology, any diagnosis of vasculitis is speculative, even if based on cerebral angiography because it is so non-specific[168] (Table 7.1).

Although there are no randomized trials, high-dose corticosteroids have become the standard treatment and usually some improvement can be expected. It is however extremely difficult to monitor the dose, and to know when to withdraw treatment, because there are no markers for disease activity (e.g. ESR). Some add cyclophosphamide, either from the start or only if the patient does not improve with steroids. Despite this, many patients deteriorate and die.

7.3.18 Idiopathic reversible cerebral 'vasoconstriction'

This is a curious and rather poorly characterized syndrome in which apparently healthy adolescents or young adults suffer severe headaches which may start suddenly, nausea and vomiting, fluctuating and sometimes bilateral focal neurological deficits and seizures.[169,170] On cerebral angiography there is segmental narrowing and dilatation of cerebral arteries which is assumed to be caused by vasoconstriction, notwithstanding the numerous other causes of this appearance (Table 7.1). This syndrome may be a relatively benign form of primary angiitis of the central nervous system (section 7.3.17), but without any histology to demonstrate the vascular pathology one cannot be sure – in fact, in a few biopsied cases there has been no evidence of vasculitis.

The arterial changes, if not the neurological impairments, seem to resolve, usually completely, over a matter of weeks, and it is unclear if corticosteroids affect the natural history. A similar syndrome has been described with the use of triptans and in the puerperium (section 7.14), and in some drug users (section 7.15.1).

7.3.19 Buerger's disease (thromboangiitis obliterans)

Buerger's disease is a rare, but seemingly distinct, inflammatory disorder of mainly distal small and medium arteries and veins, in the lower and upper limbs of young adults, causing digital gangrene. It is much more common in men than women, and almost all are smokers.[171] It is often associated with superficial thrombophlebitis and Raynaud's phenomenon but not with the systemic or laboratory disturbances so often seen in other forms of vasculitis. Cerebrovascular complications have very occasionally been described, but without a standardized definition of the vasculopathy it is difficult to know if the cases reported have all been of the same condition.[172–175]

7.3.20 Paraneoplastic vasculitis

Cutaneous and systemic vasculitis of various types, sometimes affecting the brain, is recognized as being very rarely associated with some malignant tumours, particularly lymphoproliferative disorders.[176,177]

7.3.21 Therapeutic drugs

Various therapeutic drugs have been implicated, with varying levels of evidence, in hypersensitivity reactions which may include cerebral vasculitis, e.g. allopurinol and deoxycoformycin.[178] Non-therapeutic drugs of abuse are discussed in section 7.15.1.

7.3.22 Acute posterior multifocal placoid pigment epitheliopathy

This is a well-defined but rare sporadic chorioretinal disorder with bilateral, rapidly deteriorating, central vision which usually recovers spontaneously in weeks or months. It is occasionally complicated by a systemic, including cerebral, vasculitis with stroke/transient ischaemic attack, aseptic meningitis and global encephalopathy.[179]

7.3.23 Susac syndrome

The combination of a microangiopathy of the brain and retina, with bilateral sensorineural hearing loss, is known as Susac syndrome. Microinfarcts in the brain lead to personality change, subacute encephalopathy and stroke/transient ischaemic attack-like episodes which tend to relapse and remit and then become self-limiting. It is much more common in young women than men.[180,181]

7.3.24 Eales disease

This rare sporadic disorder predominantly affects young men who develop retinal 'perivasculitis' causing recurrent, bilateral, retinal and vitreous haemorrhage. Stroke and transient ischaemic attack have been described as the result of cerebral and leptomeningeal vasculitis, but myelopathy is more common.[182,183]

7.3.25 Cogan syndrome

This is another rare, sporadic, subacute syndrome seen in children and adults.[184] It is characterized by non-syphilitic interstitial keratitis together with vertigo, tinnitus and deafness mimicking Meniere syndrome. There are systemic symptoms along with a vasculitis which can affect the aorta, medium and small vessels, sometimes involving the brain.[185,186]

7.4 Congenital arterial anomalies

There are several rather unusual arterial abnormalities which are probably congenital, and which may be an occasional cause of cerebral and ocular ischaemia.

7.4.1 Fibromuscular dysplasia

Fibromuscular dysplasia (FMD) is an uncommon, sometimes familial, segmental disorder of medium-sized arteries presenting at any age, more commonly in females than males, and usually affecting more than one artery in an individual.[187–189] The renal arteries are the most commonly involved, causing renovascular hypertension. In the neck, the mid to high cervical portion of the internal carotid artery (ICA) and the vertebral artery at the level of the first two cervical vertebrae are the most common sites, i.e. well away from the usual sites of atheroma.

The pathology is neither atheromatous nor inflammatory: the arterial wall is fibrosed and thickened in one or more segments, so the typical angiographic appearance is of a 'string of beads', or tubular segmental or longer areas of stenosis (Fig. 7.10). Sometimes there is enlargement, and a fibrous 'web' obstructing the proximal ICA, which looks more smooth and regular than typical atherothrombotic stenosis.[190] FMD is occasionally associated with intracranial aneurysms and vascular malformations, and can itself be complicated by aneurysm formation and dissection. It is unknown how often

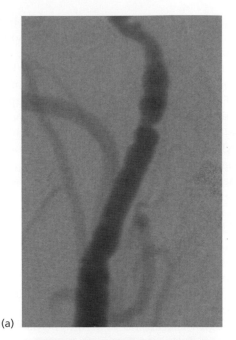

(a)

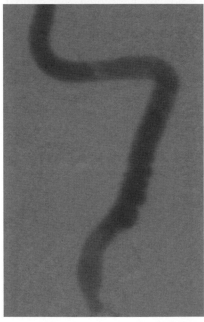

(b)

Fig. 7.10 Selective catheter angiogram showing fibromuscular dysplasia of the internal carotid artery. Note the irregular 'beaded' appearance of (a) the right and (b) the left carotid arteries.

uncomplicated FMD causes thrombosis and embolism. Therefore, when FMD is found on an angiogram (much less often with duplex ultrasound), it is not necessarily relevant to any neurological symptoms.

It is uncertain whether either antithrombotic drugs or angioplasty/stenting are sensible treatments, particularly as the natural history is not really known. The blood pressure should be carefully monitored for life, with a low threshold for investigation for renal artery stenosis.

7.4.2 Hypoplastic carotid and vertebral arteries

Hypoplastic, or even absent, carotid arteries have been described.[191] Presumably the brain is then more likely to become ischaemic, especially when atheroma develops in the other extracranial arteries, and intracranial haemorrhage from fine collaterals can occur. This anomaly is usually an incidental finding when angiography is performed for some unrelated reason, or absent carotid canals are noticed on CT of the skull base.[192] A hypoplastic, or absent, vertebral artery is much more common, and usually the other vertebral artery is enlarged to compensate; there is some recent evidence that vertebral artery hypoplasia makes a posterior circulation stroke more likely, but it is unclear whether the associated strokes are more severe.[193] It is important not to confuse these anomalies with the appearances of dissection on imaging.

7.4.3 Internal carotid artery loops

Internal carotid artery loops are probably congenital and of no consequence unless complicated by aneurysmal swelling (section 7.6), hypoglossal nerve palsy or, possibly, pulsatile tinnitus.[194,195] Focal ischaemia on head movement must be extraordinarily rare. An association with carotid dissection has been suggested.[196] Some degree of kinking, buckling and tortuosity of the carotid artery is quite common, becomes more common with increasing age, and is likely to be caused by atheroma or fibromuscular dysplasia, but it can be congenital.[197] Although various surgical procedures to 'normalize' the anatomy have been described, there is no good evidence they reduce the risk of stroke.

7.5 Moyamoya syndrome

Moyamoya is as rare as the name is memorable. It is not a specific vascular pathology, but a *radiologically* defined pattern of severe stenosis or occlusion of one, or more often both, *distal* internal carotid arteries (ICA), frequently with additional involvement of parts of the circle of Willis and sometimes of the proximal cerebral and basilar arteries.[198,199] It may progress after diagnosis.[200] Numerous tiny collaterals develop from the lenticulostriate,

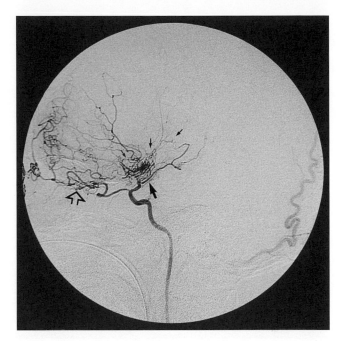

Fig. 7.11 Lateral view of a selective carotid catheter angiogram from a patient with moyamoya syndrome. The internal carotid artery ends in numerous small dilated lenticulostriate arteries (*thin arrows*) and meningeal and ophthalmic artery collaterals (*fat arrow* and *open arrow*, respectively). Courtesy of Professor Takenori Yamaguchi, National Cardiovascular Centre, Osaka, Japan.

thalamoperforating and pial arteries at the base of the brain; orbital and ethmoidal branches of the external carotid artery (ECA); leptomeningeal collaterals from the posterior cerebral artery; and transdural vessels from branches of the ECA. This pattern of collaterals looks like a puff of smoke (moyamoya in Japanese) in the basal ganglia region on the cerebral angiogram (Fig. 7.11). There can be associated intracranial aneurysms.[201]

> The moyamoya syndrome is a radiologically defined pattern of arterial occlusion at the base of the brain displayed by cerebral angiography. There are several causes but often there is no explanation.

This pattern of arterial obstruction is found mostly, but not entirely, in Japanese and other East Asians. It can be familial[202,203] or congenital, and various acquired disorders can cause arterial occlusion including basal meningeal or nasopharyngeal infection; vasculitis (section 7.3); irradiation (section 7.12); trauma; fibromuscular dysplasia (section 7.4.1); a generalized fibrous disorder of arteries;[204,205] sickle cell disease (section 7.9.8); Down syndrome;[206] neurofibromatosis (section 7.20.5); and primary oxalosis (section 7.20.6). Atheroma

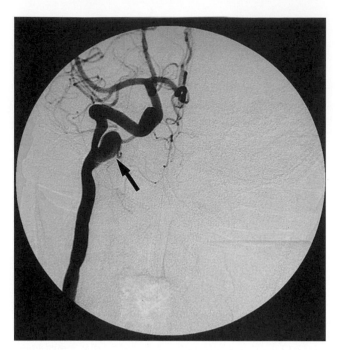

Fig. 7.12 Selective carotid catheter angiogram showing a traumatic extracranial aneurysm of the internal carotid artery (*arrow*). Courtesy of Dr Evelyn Teasdale, Institute of Neurological Sciences, Glasgow, UK.

is very rarely responsible, perhaps because it is not usually distributed so distally in the ICA. In most cases, however, no cause is found.

Children with the syndrome present with recurrent focal cerebral ischaemia and infarction, cognitive impairment, headache, seizures and, occasionally, involuntary movements, all presumably the consequences of low cerebral blood flow. Adults can present in the same way, but also with subarachnoid, intracerebral or intraventricular haemorrhage caused by rupture of the collaterals, or of any associated aneurysms[207,208] (section 8.2.12).

Not surprisingly, surgical revascularization of brain distal to occluded arteries has been attempted, and success claimed, but it is impossible to know whether the natural history is changed for the better.[209]

7.6 Embolism from arterial aneurysms

Aneurysms may contain thrombus which can embolize distally, although it is difficult to be certain if this is the cause of cerebral ischaemia unless there is no other more likely cause, and no possibility of vasospasm complicating rupture of an intracranial aneurysm. This course of events has occasionally been described with intracranial saccular and fusiform aneurysms.[210,211] It also occurs with extracranial carotid or vertebral aneurysms caused by blunt or penetrating trauma, infection, carotid surgery, irradiation, atheroma, fibromuscular dysplasia or inherited disorders of connective tissue such as Marfan syndrome and Ehlers–Danlos syndrome type IV.[212–215] The diagnosis of the aneurysm, and demonstration of any contained thrombus, is made by catheter, CT or magnetic resonance angiography (Fig. 7.12).

Extracranial aneurysms should be suspected if there is a pulsatile swelling in the neck or pharynx, dysphagia, a Horner syndrome or compression of the lower cranial nerves at the base of skull; compression of the spinal cord and roots is exceptional.[216]

7.7 The cholesterol embolization syndrome

This is a rarely recognized clinical syndrome in patients with widespread atheroma, although it may be much more common than is currently diagnosed.[217–219] It can be spontaneous, but is more often a complication of instrumentation or surgical repair of large atheromatous arteries, such as the aorta, and possibly of anticoagulants or thrombolytic therapy, all of which can release atheromatous debris and cholesterol crystals into the circulation.[220] Cholesterol emboli are found occluding the microcirculation throughout the body, including the brain and spinal cord.

Hours or days after instrumentation or surgery, a subacute syndrome develops with rather similar features to systemic vasculitis or infective endocarditis. There is malaise, fever, proteinuria, haematuria, renal failure, abdominal pain, gastrointestinal bleeding, drowsiness and confusion, skin petechiae, splinter haemorrhages, livedo reticularis, cyanosis of fingers and toes, peripheral gangrene, raised erythrocyte sedimentation rate, anaemia, thrombocytopenia, neutrophil leucocytosis, eosinophilia and hypocomplementaemia.[221–224]

The diagnosis is made by demonstrating cholesterol debris in the microcirculation of biopsy material from kidney, skin or muscle. However, the specificity of this finding is uncertain because similar debris can be found in people without the syndrome, albeit rarely.

Iloprost, a prostacyclin analogue, may be an effective treatment.[225]

7.8 Migraine

A 'normal' stroke (caused, say, by embolism from severe carotid stenosis) can start during the course of a typical migrainous episode for that particular individual and so appear to have been provoked by the migraine – but both conditions are common and may coincide by chance. Sometimes a 'normal' stroke, or just asymptomatic low cerebral blood flow, can provoke migrainous episodes with an aura previously experienced by that particular patient. And sometimes a 'normal' stroke can be followed by typical migraine with aura which has never been previously experienced. In practice, it is not always easy to sort out the exact chronological, let alone the exact aetiological, relationship between migraine and stroke in a particular case.[226] However, strokes in migraineurs should be investigated in the same way as in non-migraineurs bearing in mind that, with a careful history, it may be possible to recognize 'migrainous' strokes (section 7.8.1).

7.8.1 Migrainous stroke

A *migrainous* stroke should never be a diagnosis of desperation when no other cause for ischaemic stroke can be found, but a *positive* statement to describe a characteristic clinical syndrome in the absence of no more likely cause of stroke (section 3.4.1). The occasional patient, from thousands, who has previously had migrainous auras (with or without headache), may one day, for no known reason, experience their typical aura, which then persists as a focal neurological deficit. Brain imaging may or may not show a relevant lesion, presumed infarction. To make the diagnosis, there must not be any reason to suspect that the stroke was caused by anything else after full investigation, particularly anything which can be associated or confused with migraine, such as arterial dissection (section 7.2), the antiphospholipid syndrome (section 7.3.4), CADASIL (section 7.20.1), mitochondrial cytopathy (section 7.19) or even an arteriovenous malformation (section 8.2.4).[227,228]

A migrainous stroke most often results in a homonymous hemianopia (reflecting the common visual disturbance in migrainous auras), seldom seems to cause persisting and severe disability, and perhaps does not recur very often, although data are sparse. Arterial occlusion has very rarely been demonstrated and it is not clear why it occurs. 'Vasospasm' is often postulated and is said to have been observed in the retinal circulation during transient monocular blindness in a few patients.[229]

Recurrent spontaneous extracranial internal carotid artery (ICA) 'vasospasm' has been described, but not in a migraneur or with clearly the phenotype of migrainous stroke[230] and also in the extracranial ICA.[231] Migraine has very rarely been blamed for intracerebral haemorrhage (section 8.3.2).

Migrainous auras lasting the usual 20–30 min can be confused with transient ischaemic attacks, a problem which has been discussed earlier (section 3.4.1).

> A migrainous stroke is a well-defined clinical syndrome. It is not a diagnosis of exclusion or desperation.

7.8.2 Migraine as a risk factor for stroke

Migraine with, and possibly even without, aura may be associated with about a doubling of the risk of ischaemic stroke, possibly more in women on oral contraceptives (section 7.13.1), although this estimate is based mainly on case–control rather than more reliable cohort studies where the association is less obvious.[232–234] Any relationship with myocardial infarction is less certain, but recently has become rather more compelling.[234,235] If the association with stroke is causal, the explanation cannot be 'migrainous stroke' because this is too rare, and in any event this would not explain the association with myocardial infarction. Possibilities include:

- some factor associated with migraine also causing stroke and other vascular disorders, perhaps vasospasm, platelet hyperaggregability, patent foramen ovale,[236] or treatments for migraine such as ergotamine, triptans etc.;
- both migraine and stroke sharing some causal factor – possibly genetic;
- or that migraineurs simply have a worse vascular risk profile and that observational epidemiological studies have not been able to fully adjust for this as a confounder.[237]

7.9 Haematological disorders

Occasionally, ischaemic strokes, intracranial venous thrombosis and transient ischaemic attacks complicate an underlying haematological disorder, which itself may be quite common (such as sickle cell disease in Afro-Caribbeans) or extremely rare (such as protein S deficiency)[238,239] (Table 7.3). The diagnosis is not usually

Quantitative abnormalities of formed blood elements
Polycythaemia rubra vera (section 7.9.1)
Relative polycythaemia (section 7.9.1)
Secondary polycythaemia (section 7.9.1)
Essential thrombocythaemia (section 7.9.2)
Thrombotic thrombocytopenic purpura and haemolytic–uraemic syndrome
   (section 7.9.3)
Iron-deficiency anaemia (section 7.9.7)
Qualitative abnormalities of formed blood elements
Haemoglobinopathies (e.g. sickle cell disease, thalassaemia) (section 7.9.8)
Paroxysmal nocturnal haemoglobinuria (section 7.9.9)
Leukaemia (section 7.9.4)
Intravascular lymphoma (section 7.9.5)
Abnormalities of platelet secretion, adhesion, aggregation? (section 7.9.11)
Hyperviscosity
Polycythaemia (section 7.9.1)
Waldenström's macroglobulinaemia (section 7.9.10)
Multiple myeloma (section 7.9.10)
Coagulation disorders (thrombophilias) (section 7.9.11)
Antithrombin III deficiency
Protein S deficiency
Protein C deficiency
Activated protein C resistance most commonly caused by a mutation of factor V
   protein (factor V Leiden)
Prothrombin (factor II) mutation
Factor VII deficiency
Elevated factor VIII
Plasminogen abnormality or deficiency
Elevated concentrations of factors II, VII, VIII
Antifibrinolytic drugs
Activated factor VIIa
Prothrombotic states of uncertain cause
Cancer (section 7.12)
Disseminated intravascular coagulation (section 7.9.12)
Pregnancy and the puerperium (section 7.14)
Oral contraceptives (section 7.13.1)
Heparin-associated thrombocytopenia with thrombosis (section 7.9.11)
Antiphospholipid syndrome (section 7.3.4)
L-asparaginase (section 7.12)
Nephrotic syndrome (section 7.9.11)
Desmopressin (section 7.9.11)
Intravenous immunoglobulin (section 7.9.11)
Androgens (section 7.9.11)
Hypereosinophilic syndrome (section 7.9.11)
Snake bite/scorpion bite/wasp sting (section 7.9.11)

Table 7.3 Haematological disorders that may cause or predispose to cerebral and ocular ischaemia.

difficult because the routine first-line investigations will pick up most of the disorders (full blood count, platelet count and ESR) and, if there is no obvious other cause, fairly standard haematological tests will pick up the rest (Table 6.14). But, as with cardiac embolism, it can be difficult to know if a diagnosed haematological disorder is *the* cause of an ischaemic stroke when there is also a competing cause, or whether a haematological disorder has merely increased the risk or severity of stroke caused by – for example – coexistent atherothromboembolism. Exactly what the risk of vascular events is, including stroke, in these conditions has not been at all studied but presumably it is higher in those who have already had an event than in those who are still event-free. However, because the haematological disorder often needs treating in its own right (of course in collaboration with haematologists), management decisions are usually fairly straightforward.

7.9.1 Polycythaemia

Polycythaemia is conventionally defined as a haematocrit above 0.50 in males and 0.47 in females, provided the patient is rested and normally hydrated and the blood taken without venous occlusion. Above this level, the exact diagnosis should be refined by measuring the red cell mass.

Polycythaemia rubra vera (primary proliferative polycythaemia) may be complicated by transient ischaemic attacks, ischaemic stroke or intracranial venous thrombosis. The exact risk is unknown because the disease is rare, and no reliable prospective studies are available.[240,241] In patients selected for a trial, the risk of stroke, myocardial infarction or vascular death was about 5% in the placebo group and 2% in the aspirin group over about 3 years, but this estimate must be imprecise being based on only 18 events.[242] The presumed thrombotic tendency is not just a result of the increased whole-blood viscosity; the platelet count is often raised, and platelet activity and endothelial cell function may be altered as well. Curiously, there can also be a haemostatic defect which is the result of defective platelet function, so causing intracranial haemorrhage. The 'hyperviscosity syndrome' is another complication (section 7.9.10).

Relative polycythaemia is caused by reduced plasma volume (diuretics, alcohol, dehydration, hypertension, obesity) and *secondary polycythaemia* to a raised red cell mass (chronic hypoxia, smoking, cerebellar haemangioblastoma, renal tumour). Whether the raised haematocrit of relative and secondary polycythaemia is a risk factor for stroke is unclear; a direct causal relationship is rather unlikely (section 6.6.7). It is conceivable that increased whole-blood viscosity might have a particularly adverse effect in the microcirculation of a cerebral infarct caused by something else, e.g. embolism from the heart, so affecting recovery.

7.9.2 Essential thrombocythaemia

Essential thrombocythaemia (idiopathic primary thrombocytosis) defined by a sustained platelet count $> 600 \times 10^9$/L can be associated with both arterial and venous thrombosis.[243,244] Occasionally, paradoxically, there is a bleeding tendency because platelet function is defective. Headache, transient focal and non-focal disturbances are the most common neurological symptoms.[245–248] Before making the diagnosis, other causes of thrombocytosis should be excluded: malignancy, splenectomy or hyposplenism, surgery and other trauma, haemorrhage, iron deficiency, infection, polycythaemia rubra vera, myelofibrosis and leukaemia.

7.9.3 Thrombotic thrombocytopenic purpura

Although rare, thrombotic thrombocytopenic purpura (TTP) is a treatable acute or subacute disease, rather similar to and overlapping with the *haemolytic–uraemic syndrome* in children.[249–252] Platelet microthrombi cause infarcts in many organs, including the brain, leading to a fluctuating encephalopathic illness, with confusion and epileptic seizures, with or without focal features, rather than a simple stroke syndrome.[253–256] Brain CT and MRI may be normal or show infarcts and posterior cerebral oedema; occasionally intracerebral haemorrhage occurs, possibly caused or exacerbated by therapeutic heparinization or acute hypertension rather than the TTP itself.[257] The patient is ill, with malaise, fever, skin purpura, renal failure, proteinuria and haematuria. The blood film shows thrombocytopenia, microangiopathic haemolytic anaemia and fragmented red cells, and the plasma lactate dehydrogenase levels are very high.

7.9.4 Leukaemia

Leukaemia more often causes intracranial haemorrhage (section 8.4.5) or the 'hyperviscosity syndrome' (section 7.9.10) than cerebral arterial or venous occlusion. Vascular occlusion when it does occur may be the result of increased whole-blood viscosity, opportunistic infections, or non-bacterial thrombotic endocarditis.[258]

7.9.5 Intravascular lymphoma (intravascular lymphomatosis)

Patients with this rare form of B-cell lymphoma, in which neoplastic lymphocytes proliferate within the lumen of small vessels in almost every organ, can present with multifocal stroke and transient ischaemic attack-like episodes, typically in late middle age.[259–262] But, more often, the cerebral features are diffuse with subacute progressive global dementia. Spinal cord, roots and peripheral nerves can also be involved. Characteristically, there are skin nodules and plaques, malaise and a raised plasma lactate dehydrogenase. Brain imaging is non-specific with infarct-like and mass lesions, and sometimes meningeal enhancement (Fig. 7.13). The diagnosis can only be made by biopsy, typically of skin or brain. The course is relentlessly progressive to death within a few months.

7.9.6 Lymphomatoid granulomatosis

Lymphomatoid granulomatosis is a rare disorder, possibly lymphomatous. It affects mostly the lungs with diffuse infiltration and nodules, but also the skin and the central and peripheral nervous systems with vascular

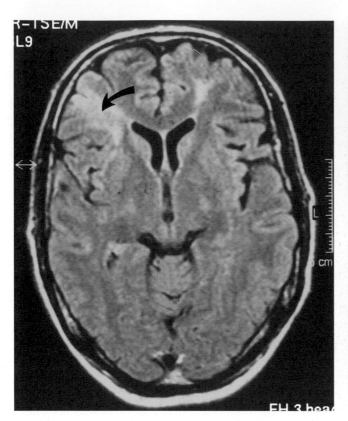

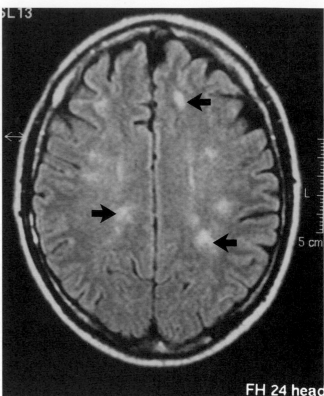

Fig. 7.13 Fluid-attenuated inversion recovery (FLAIR) MRI axial views in a patient with histologically proven intravascular lymphoma. Areas of infarction are seen in grey (*curved arrow*) and white matter (*straight arrows*).

infiltration by abnormal lymphocytes and plasmacytoid cells, and a necrotizing vasculitis. The neurological syndrome is of a subacute encephalopathy, cranial neuropathies, seizures and stroke.[263–265]

7.9.7 Anaemia

Iron-deficiency anaemia (and presumably other types of anaemia as well), if severe, may it seems provoke transient ischaemic attacks, particularly if there is already severe cerebral arterial disease.[266,267] Anaemia has also been associated with intracranial venous thrombosis[268] and with ischaemic arterial stroke, perhaps because of the associated thrombocythaemia.[269,270] In practice, anaemia is much more likely to cause non-specific neurological symptoms such as generalized weakness, fatigue, poor concentration and faintness. Of course, the anaemia may be symptomatic of some other cause of stroke, such as non-bacterial thrombotic endocarditis in a patient with cancer.

7.9.8 Sickle cell disease

Homozygous children, and less often adults, very often develop ischaemic stroke and, sometimes, intracranial haemorrhage due to fragile collaterals and aneurysms –

the overall stroke risk is about 1% per annum – and also 'silent' cerebral infarction and cognitive decline.[271–275] Stroke is very much rarer in heterozygotes except perhaps in the context of a hypoxia-provoked sickle cell crisis.[276,277]

Small and large arteries and veins are occluded by thrombi not just as a result of the rigid red blood cells but also by their complex interactions with the endothelium, platelets, the coagulation system and leucocytes.[278] There is also fibrous proliferation of the intima which causes arterial stenosis and ectasia of the main cerebral arteries which can be seen on catheter and MR angiography, and inferred from transcranial Doppler of the middle cerebral artery.[279,280]

Stroke prevention at present depends on prophylactic red cell transfusion in children at high risk, but there is a serious problem of iron overload.[281]

Stroke may complicate *haemoglobin SC disease*[282] and has also been associated with *thalassaemia*, perhaps as a result of the associated thrombocythaemia, atrial fibrillation, cardiomyopathy, cardiac failure or pseudoxanthoma elasticum.[283]

7.9.9 Paroxysmal nocturnal haemoglobinuria

Paroxysmal nocturnal haemoglobinuria is a very rare acquired disorder in which haemopoietic stem cells become peculiarly sensitive to complement-mediated lysis. Venous, and exceptionally arterial, thrombosis occurs in the brain and elsewhere. The patients are almost always anaemic at neurological presentation and there may be a history of abdominal pain, recurrent deep venous thrombosis, dark urine, haemolysis and a low platelet and granulocyte count.[284,285]

7.9.10 The paraproteinaemias

Waldenström's macroglobulinaemia, multiple myeloma and the POEMS syndrome can all sometimes be complicated by arterial or venous cerebral infarction as a result of occlusion of vessels with acidophilic material, thought to be a precipitant of the abnormal plasma proteins.[238,286–289] Intracranial haemorrhage also occurs because of the reduced number and impaired reactivity of platelets, perhaps as a result of uraemia. However, patients seldom present with strokes or transient ischaemic attacks but more often have the 'hyperviscosity syndrome' of rather uncertain pathology and varying severity: headache, ataxia, diplopia, dysarthria, lethargy, poor concentration, confusion, drowsiness, coma, visual blurring and deafness; the retina shows dilatation and tortuosity of the veins, venous occlusions, papilloedema and haemorrhages.[290] Similar symptoms may also be caused by uraemia, hypercalcaemia or lymphoma complicating the paraproteinaemia.

7.9.11 Thrombophilias and other causes of 'hypercoagulability'

The thrombophilias are a number of rare, usually familial, conditions in which spontaneous and recurrent venous thrombosis occurs (usually in the legs but sometimes in the head). Arterial thrombosis is very seldom a presenting or complicating feature.[291–293] There may be additional causes, or at least precipitants, of stroke in the very small number of cases with thrombophilia described (such as oral contraceptives, pregnancy, etc.). Furthermore, although familial deficiencies of antithrombin III, protein C and protein S can undoubtedly cause venous thrombosis, as can activated protein C resistance with factor V Leiden mutation and the prothrombin G20210A mutation, the patients are asymptomatic for most of their lives; these abnormalities may, therefore, be better regarded as risk factors rather than causes of thrombotic events, including possibly stroke. The role of protein Z is very uncertain.[294]

In patients discovered to have these coagulation abnormalities, it is very possible that the cause of any arterial ischaemic stroke is something quite different (e.g. arterial dissection), so they must be thoroughly investigated and not just assumed to have a thrombophilic stroke. Paradoxical embolism from the venous system is another possible cause, or even that a venous cerebral infarct has been misdiagnosed as an arterial stroke (Table 5.4). Another problem is that acute stroke (and pregnancy) may reduce the level of some of these coagulation factors, so the tests must be repeated on several later occasions (with due allowance if the patient is anticoagulated). To make the diagnosis of familial deficiency, the family members must be tested too. The risks of recurrence and what if any treatment should be are quite unknown, although many haematologists favour lifelong anticoagulation, at least for venous if not arterial thrombosis.

Therefore, it is very uncertain how relevant these coagulation abnormalities really are in 'stroke' patients, and whether they should be looked for at all, but there is more of an argument in favour for venous compared with arterial stroke.[295]

> If a coagulation abnormality (thrombophilia) is found in a patient with an arterial or venous stroke, then the abnormality must be confirmed weeks or months after the acute event before any persisting and definite 'thrombophilia' can be reliably diagnosed. Even then, the cause of the stroke might be something else and the thrombophilia is either an additional cause, or totally unrelated.

Despite many attempts to relate quantitative abnormalities of platelet behaviour, impaired fibrinolysis and an increase in coagulation factors to ischaemic stroke and transient ischaemic attack in general, no definite cause-and-effect relationship has been demonstrated (section 6.6.7). In most cases, any changes in these haematological variables are a consequence rather than the cause of the cerebral ischaemic event.

A hypercoagulable state may occur with the following conditions, but whether the arterial and venous strokes reported are due to this or something else, or are merely coincidental, is often difficult to say:

- nephrotic syndrome can be complicated by ischaemic arterial stroke and intracranial venous thrombosis, perhaps as a result of 'hypercoagulability';[296,297]
- antiphospholipid syndrome (section 7.3.4);
- widespread malignancy (section 7.12);
- immune-mediated heparin-induced thrombocytopenia is associated with an increased risk of thrombosis in cerebral arteries and veins;[298–300]
- desmopressin;[301]
- intravenous immunoglobulin carries a small risk of stroke and probably should be avoided in patients with known vascular disease or multiple vascular risk factors;[302–304]

- androgens;[305]
- hypereosinophilic syndrome;[306,307]
- antifibrinolytic drugs have been reported to cause both cerebral venous and arterial thrombosis;[308]
- recombinant human erythropoietin (epoetin) by increasing the haematocrit may induce a hypercoagulable state and so perhaps venous if not arterial ischaemic stroke in dialysis patients and sportsmen;[309,310]
- snake or scorpion bite are more likely to cause defibrination, acute hypertension and bleeding than ischaemic stroke although this has been described,[311–314] as it has after wasp stings.[315]

7.9.12 Disseminated intravascular coagulation

Here there are widespread haemorrhagic cerebral infarcts and intracranial haemorrhages which cause an acute or subacute global encephalopathy rather than stroke-like episodes.[316–318] Because patients are so often critically ill as a result of their primary disease – obstetric disasters, septicaemia, trauma, etc. – it can be very difficult to disentangle any *added* effect of disseminated intravascular coagulation (DIC) on the brain. The diagnosis is supported by a low platelet count, prolonged prothrombin and activated partial thromboplastin times, low plasma fibrinogen, raised fibrin degradation products in plasma, and raised D-dimers.

7.10 Stroke in association with acute myocardial infarction

Cerebral and coronary arterial atheroma are so often present in the same patient that it is hardly surprising that there is a past history of myocardial infarction or current angina in about one-third of ischaemic stroke and TIA patients (Table 6.3), and that myocardial infarction occurs not infrequently during their long-term follow-up (section 16.2.3). However, if a stroke (or transient ischaemic attack) occurs within hours or days of an acute myocardial infarction, it is tempting, and often correct, to suspect a cause-and-effect relationship rather than a coincidence (Table 7.4).

Left ventricular mural thrombus, diagnosed by echocardiography, occurs within days of an acute myocardial infarction in about 20% of patients, mostly in those with large anterior infarcts, although this frequency is probably declining with more frequent use of antithrombotic drugs.[319] Such thrombi may embolize, but most seem to do little harm because *clinically* evident systemic

Table 7.4 Causes of stroke and transient ischaemic attacks within hours or days of acute myocardial infarction.

Ischaemic stroke/transient ischaemic attack
Embolism from left-ventricular mural thrombus (section 7.10)
Instrumentation of the aorta/coronary arteries (section 7.18.1)
Low-flow infarcts caused by hypotension/cardiac arrest (section 6.7.5)
Atrial fibrillation and embolism from the left atrium (section 6.5.1)
Paradoxical embolism (section 6.5.12)
Intracerebral haemorrhage
Anticoagulants (section 8.4.1)
Antiplatelet drugs (section 8.4.2)
Thrombolytic drugs (section 8.4.3)
Both myocardial infarction and ischaemic stroke caused by the same disorder
Giant cell arteritis (section 7.3.1)
Infective endocarditis (section 6.5.9)
Aortic arch dissection (section 7.2.3)
Embolism from the heart to both cerebral and coronary arteries (e.g. from atrial myxoma, valvular vegetations)

embolism to the brain and elsewhere complicates less than 5% of all acute myocardial infarctions.[320–322] Furthermore, most patients with emboli detected with transcranial Doppler do not have a stroke.[323] Of course, ischaemic stroke after an acute myocardial infarction can have other causes: emboli as a result of cardiac catheterization,[324] angioplasty or surgery (section 7.18.1), or atrial fibrillation (section 6.5.1); low-flow infarction caused by systemic hypotension or cardiac arrest (section 6.7.5); or paradoxical embolism caused by deep venous thrombosis and a patent foramen ovale (section 6.5.12). Rarely, some non-atheromatous pathological mechanism may cause more or less simultaneous brain and heart ischaemia (Table 7.4). Naturally it must never be assumed that any stroke is ischaemic unless brain imaging has excluded intracerebral haemorrhage, which is more likely in the present age of thrombolytic treatment than it was as a consequence of anticoagulants or aspirin.

The overall low stroke risk after acute myocardial infarction still seems much the same as ever it was before the thrombolytic era although if it does occur the case fatality is unsurprisingly high.[325–327] The risk of stroke is even lower in patients with acute coronary syndromes without ST-segment elevation on the electrocardiogram (ECG).[328]

Stroke complicating acute myocardial infarction is
not necessarily caused by embolism from the heart,
or hypotension. It may be caused by intracerebral
haemorrhage, often secondary to thrombolytic
treatment. Brain imaging is always required, as in
other stroke patients.

Occasionally, acute myocardial infarction can be
clinically 'silent'. The diagnostic clues are raised cardiac
enzymes if measured in an ischaemic stroke patient (but
these may be unreliable because an increase can occur
solely as a result of the stroke) and, more tellingly, an
ECG showing recent ischaemic changes, such as ST
elevation, particularly if the changes evolve typically
over time.[329,330]

After the acute period, the risk of stroke is much lower,
about 8% within 5 years, but still higher than the background stroke risk in the population.[322,331–333] Not all
these strokes are caused by embolism from the heart.
Many of the patients have atherothrombosis of their
extra- and intracranial arteries as well as other non-
cardiac causes of stroke.[334] Whether a left ventricular
aneurysm adds to the risk of embolic stroke is unclear.

7.11 Infections

Ischaemic stroke has long been known to complicate
chronic meningeal infections which cause inflammation
and so secondary thrombosis – and rarely rupture – of
arteries and veins on the surface of the brain.[335] Therefore, focal or multifocal ischaemic events in patients
with *tuberculous*,[336] *fungal*, or *syphilitic meningitis*[337–339]
are not unexpected (Table 7.5). Occasionally, acute *bacterial meningitis* can be similarly complicated by cerebral
infarction.[340–342]

Herpes zoster can cause intracranial periarterial
inflammation and thrombosis. As a result, stenosis and
occlusion of arteries at the base of the brain and of the
main cerebral arteries – and very rarely, intracerebral
haemorrhage – can occur a few weeks after ophthalmic
zoster and occasionally in other areas of the skin,[66,343–346]
and sometimes after chickenpox.[347] A more widespread
encephalopathy caused by varicella zoster results from
multiple infarcts and haemorrhages secondary to a small
artery vasculopathy.[348]

HIV infection can be complicated by ischaemic or
haemorrhagic stroke in a variety of *indirect* ways such
as infectious or non-infectious endocarditis, non-HIV
viral vasculitis, meningovascular syphilis, TB and fungal

Table 7.5 Infections causing ischaemic stroke and transient
ischaemic attacks.

Chronic meningitis
Tuberculosis
Fungal (cryptococcus, candida, aspergillus, mucormycosis)
Syphilis
Acute bacterial meningitis
Meningococcal
Pneumococcal
Haemophilus
Borrelia
Leptospirosis
Viral
Herpes zoster
Human immunodeficiency virus (HIV) (Table 7.6)
Cytomegalovirus
Hepatitis C
Mycoplasma
Worms
Neurotrichinosis
Cysticercosis
Hydatid disease
Cat-scratch disease
Carotid inflammation
Pharyngitis
Tonsillitis
Lymphadenitis
Infective endocarditis (section 6.5.9)

Table 7.6 Potential causes of stroke in HIV/AIDS.

Intracranial haemorrhage
Disseminated intravascular coagulation (section 7.9.12)
Thrombocytopenia (section 8.4.5)
Ischaemic stroke/TIA
Chronic tuberculous, syphilitic and fungal meningitis
 (section 7.11)
Herpes zoster vasculopathy (section 7.11)
Cytomegalovirus vasculopathy (section 7.11)
Infective endocarditis (section 6.5.9)
Non-bacterial thrombotic (marantic) endocarditis
 (section 6.5.10)
Irradiation (section 7.12)
Aneurysms/ectasia

meningitis, thrombocytopenia and drug use[349–352]
(Table 7.6). The HIV-associated small vessel vasculopthy
with hyaline change is probably not a *direct* cause of
stroke[353] and stroke patients who are HIV positive are
very similar to those who are HIV negative.[354] At present,
therefore, it does not seem that HIV is a *direct* cause of
stroke – a positive HIV blood test is clearly not a reason to
stop looking for the cause of a stroke, either an indirect
cause as above or some other cause unrelated to HIV.

Various other infections have occasionally been implicated with ischaemic or haemorrhagic stroke, or both

– with varying proposed mechanisms (vasculitis, endocarditis, hypercoagulability, etc.) and degrees of evidence:

- borrelia;[355–358]
- leptospirosis;[359]
- chlamydia;[360]
- mycoplasma;[361,362]
- hepatitis C virus related to essential cryoglobulinaemia;[363,364]
- cytomegalovirus;[365]
- neurotrichinosis;[366]
- cysticercosis;[367–371]
- cat-scratch disease;[372]
- hydatid cysts.[373–375]

Inflammation of the carotid artery in the neck, with secondary thrombosis, can very occasionally complicate pharyngitis, tonsillitis and lymphadenitis, particularly in children.[376]

7.12 Cancer and its treatment

Stroke and cancer are both so common that their association in an individual may be no more than coincidence, rather than cause and effect. Any difficulty in sorting out causal relationship is compounded by the fact that stroke in cancer patients may not be fully investigated because of their poor prognosis, and so the exact cause of any stroke may be unclear, and because neurological problems can also be caused by radiotherapy or chemotherapy.[377] In fact, there seem to be several ways that cancer patients may develop a stroke (Table 7.7) but knowing the exact cause in an individual makes little if any difference to the stroke outcome, the risk of recurrence, or the overall prognosis – at least in most cases.[258,378–380]

Table 7.7 Possible causes of stroke in patients with cancer.

Non-bacterial thrombotic (marantic) endocarditis with embolism to the brain (section 6.5.10)

Tumour embolism, sometimes with intracranial aneurysm formation and rupture to cause intracranial haemorrhage

Opportunistic meningeal infections (herpes zoster, fungi) (section 7.11)

Haemorrhage into primary tumours (section 8.5.1)
    malignant astrocytoma
    oligodendroglioma
    medulloblastoma
    haemangioblastoma

Haemorrhage into metastases (section 8.5.1)
    melanoma
    bronchus
    germ cell tumours
    hypernephroma
    choriocarcinoma

Subdural/extradural haemorrhage due to tumour invasion of dura/skull

Carotid artery rupture complicating surgery or radiotherapy for neck cancer (section 7.12)

Coagulopathy/thrombocytopenia and intracranial haemorrhage

Thrombocythaemia (section 7.9.2)

Hyperviscosity syndrome (section 7.9.10)

'Hypercoagulability' (section 7.9.11)

Disseminated intravascular coagulation (section 7.9.12)

Paraneoplastic vasculitis (section 7.3.20)

Neoplastic compression/invasion of extra- or intracranial vessels

Irradiation damage to extra- or intracranial arteries (section 7.12)

Intracranial venous thrombosis caused by tumour infiltration or compression, hypercoagulability, etc. (section 7.21)

Drugs (section 7.12)
    ciclosporin
    carboplatin
    L-asparaginase
    methotrexate
    + any causing haemostatic defect

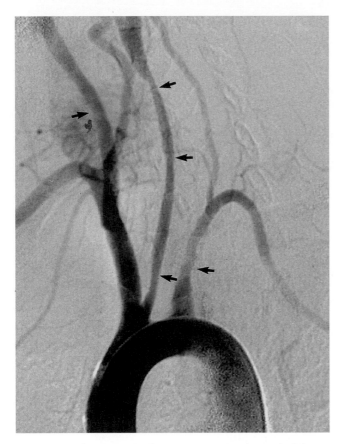

Fig. 7.14 Arch aortogram showing narrowing (*arrows*) of the large arteries in the neck 20 years after irradiation of cervical lymph nodes affected by Hodgkin's disease.

Irradiation of the head or neck can cause damage not only to the microvasculature but also to intra- and extra-cranial large and medium-sized arteries (Fig. 7.14).[377,381–384] Months or more often years after irradiation, a localized, stenotic and accelerated atheromatous lesion in the radiation field may become symptomatic, to cause ischaemic stroke or transient ischaemic attack. Fibrosis of the arterial wall and aneurysm formation with rupture have also been described, as well as the moyamoya syndrome (section 7.5).[385,386] Ascribing any stroke to irradiation in an individual can be difficult unless:

- the vascular lesion is in an unusual place for atheroma (e.g. terminal carotid artery) or for an aneurysm (e.g. well away from the circle of Willis);
- the lesion is directly within the radiation field;
- and there is no other more likely cause.

Chemotherapy has been associated with stroke:

- *Ciclosporin*, usually in transplant recipients, can cause headache, nausea, vomiting, cortical blindness, seizures, confusion and coma as the result of a subacute and reversible posterior leucoencephalopathy, perhaps in part because of a vasculopathy and hypertension. This

syndrome may start suddenly enough to be mistaken for a posterior circulation stroke[387–389] (section 3.4.5).

- *Cisplatin* and *carboplatin* cause similar problems[390] while cisplatin, mostly in association with other anti-cancer drugs, has been implicated in ischaemic stroke.[391]
- *L-asparaginase* treatment for leukaemia can cause both cerebral ischaemia and haemorrhage.[392]
- High doses of systemic *methotrexate* can be followed a few days later by various transient focal neurological symptoms, rather like a stroke, and merging into a more global encephalopathy with behavioural abnormalities and seizures.[393]
- *Tamoxifen* approximately doubles the risk of ischaemic stroke.[394]

Finally, a cerebral vasculitis has been reported after bone marrow transplantation for leukaemia.[395]

7.13 Exogenous female sex hormones

High-dose *exogenous oestrogen* given to men increases their risk of vascular death, and presumably also of stroke and other non-fatal vascular events.[396–398] Also ovarian induction therapy for *in vitro* fertilization has been reported to cause both arterial and venous ischaemic strokes in the midst of the ovarian hyperstimulation syndrome.[399]

7.13.1 Oral contraceptives

Women on oral contraceptives have about triple the risk of ischaemic stroke, but a smaller or perhaps no increased risk of haemorrhagic stroke; this excess risk declines rapidly on stopping oral contraceptives.[400–404] However, these excess risks are only derived from observational studies since no randomized trials have ever been done, and the exact mechanisms to explain any association are unknown (does the pill cause a specific coagulopathy or vasculopathy, or does is it merely facilitate some other cause of stroke?). Modern oral contraceptives with a low oestrogen content may have much the same or a negligible risk compared with earlier preparations, but this is difficult to quantify, in part perhaps because women perceived as being at higher risk of stroke may be preferentially prescribed the lowest dose pills.[405] The role of any progestogen component is also difficult to assess, mainly because of small sample sizes in the studies.[406] On the whole, probably the lower the oestrogen dose the better, while it is not clear whether progestogen-only pills are safer.

Increasing the very low risk of stroke in young women by prescribing the pill by even three times makes little difference unless their background risk is raised as a result of smoking, hypertension, by being over the age of about 35 years, and perhaps by having migraine, although it is very unclear whether this applies only to migraine with aura or to any migraine (section 7.8.2). The blanket recommendation that young women with migraine with aura should avoid oestrogen-containing oral contraceptives seems over-cautious[407] and still lingers in the British National Formulary. However, it is commonsense to stop oral contraception if a woman's migraines – with or without aura – become more frequent or severe while on the pill, or perhaps if she develops migraine with aura for the first time.[408] Fortunately, where any stroke risk is deemed unacceptable, there are several alternative contraceptive strategies. Clearly, when giving advice to women on contraception, any small excess risk of stroke and other vascular disorders must be set in the context of the risks of pregnancy, both unplanned and planned, and the reduced risk of ovarian cancer.[409,410] In fact, oral contraceptives only account for 2–8 strokes per 100 000 women years.

In an individual case, whether the pill is the cause of a stroke, a contributory cause in the presence of some other cause such as a patent foramen ovale perhaps, or an innocent bystander is difficult if not impossible to say. Nonetheless, if a woman has a stroke, either arterial or venous, while on the pill, it seems very reasonable to stop oral contraceptives indefinitely, even if a plausible alternative cause of stroke emerges. If, despite thorough investigation, no cause is found then it is often assumed – without much proof – that the oral contraceptive was responsible for the stroke although, even in non-pill-takers, strokes of unknown cause quite frequently occur.

> If a woman on any type of oral contraceptive has a stroke, do not jump to cause-and-effect conclusions too easily. It is important to investigate for all potential causes of stroke in young women. Whether or not a cause is found, it is wise for the woman to avoid oral contraception thereafter.

There seems to be an especially high risk of intracranial *venous* thrombosis in women who are both taking oral contraceptives and carrying mutations for factor V Leiden and prothrombin 20210A.[411]

7.13.2 Hormone replacement therapy

There have been endless arguments about the balance of risks and benefits of postmenopausal oestrogen replacement, along with considerable commercial pressure to prescribe. In the last edition we pointed out that this argument would never be properly resolved until appropriate randomized trials had been carried out. They now have been and despite the fact that oestrogen replacement, with or without progestogen:

- is associated with a favourable lipid profile;[412–414]
- has a better haemostatic profile;[412,415]
- and in observational studies there did not appear to be any increased risk of stroke;[416,417] and perhaps even a reduced risk of myocardial infarction,[418]

the randomized trials have shown, not a protective effect for vascular disease, but about a one-third increase in the risk of ischaemic stroke, probably without any excess risk of haemorrhagic stroke.[419] Quite what the mechanism is to explain this excess risk is unclear. Clearly the observational studies were biased, particularly by hormone replacement therapy (HRT) being more likely to be given to women without vascular risk factors, and requested by women more likely to look after their health.[420] Of course the excess stroke risk has to be set against the advantages of HRT (less post-menopausal symptoms, less osteoporosis, possibly less colon cancer) and other disadvantages (more breast cancer, coronary events and venous thromboembolism).[421] It would surely be unwise for a woman to take HRT if she is at high risk of stroke, or already has had an ischaemic stroke or transient ischaemic attack.

> If a woman on hormone replacement therapy has a stroke, this is a very good reason to stop it.

7.14 Pregnancy and the puerperium

Stroke complicating pregnancy and the puerperium is so rare – about 1 per 10 000 deliveries in developed countries – that it is impossible to estimate the exact risk, and even the size of any excess risk over and above what is expected in non-pregnant females of childbearing age. It tends to occur more in the third trimester and puerperium.[422–425] Among the usual causes of strokes in non-pregnant young women, there are some which may be particularly associated with pregnancy:

- intracranial venous thrombosis is probably more likely in women with thrombophilia, much more often in the puerperium than during pregnancy, but with a low risk of recurrence in later pregnancies, it seems;[426]
- acute middle cerebral or other large artery occlusion, perhaps caused by paradoxical embolism from the legs or pelvic veins;
- cervical arterial dissection during labour;[427]

- low-flow infarction or disseminated intravascular coagulation complicating obstetric disasters;
- ergot-type, bromocriptine and other vasoconstricting drugs have been associated with so-called postpartum cerebral segmental vasoconstriction or puerperal cerebral angiopathy[428,429] although this also occurs without any drug exposure and may be due to vasculitis rather than 'vasospasm'.[430–432] This subacute syndrome of headache, seizures, focal infarcts and even intracranial haemorrhage may be related to or is the same as idiopathic reversible cerebral 'vasoconstriction' (section 7.3.18). Exactly how this syndrome differs from postpartum eclampsia seems rather uncertain;[433,434]
- infective endocarditis (section 6.5.9);
- peripartum dilating cardiomyopathy and embolism;[435]
- sickle cell crisis (section 7.9.8);
- intracranial haemorrhage caused by anticoagulants, disseminated intravascular coagulation, or rupture of an aneurysm or vascular malformation.

Eclampsia causes a global encephalopathic syndrome with seizures, headache, cortical blindness and impaired consciousness. It is due to increasing blood pressure, cerebral oedema, and sometimes vasospasm and haemorrhage, complicated by disseminated intravascular coagulation.[436–438] Typically, there are bilateral hypodensities on CT and increased signal on T2-weighted MRI, particularly in the occipital and parietal lobes. It should be distinguished from focal cerebral infarction or haemorrhage due to other causes, intracranial venous thrombosis and postpartum cerebral segmental vasoconstriction (if indeed it is a different entity to the last).

Haemorrhagic choriocarcinoma metastases can look very like multiple intracerebral haemorrhages on CT, the diagnostic test being a raised serum human chorionic gonadotrophin level (sections 3.4.4 and 8.5.1). There is a curious tendency for migraine auras without headache to occur in pregnancy, and these should be differentiated from transient ischaemic attacks (section 3.4.1).

In general therefore, stroke in pregnancy or the puerperium should be investigated in the same way as any other stroke in a young, otherwise healthy female, bearing in mind fetal exposure to any diagnostic irradiation – MR appears to be safe (section 5.5). The risk of arterial stroke recurrence in any future pregnancy is surprisingly low, suggesting that most pregnancy-associated strokes must be due to 'one off' events rather than any persisting abnormality such as thrombophilia;[439] the risk of future oral contraception is also unknown, but this is perhaps best avoided as there are several alternatives.

7.15 Drugs, including drugs of misuse

7.15.1 Drugs of misuse

Cocaine – snorted, smoked or injected – is the most commonly implicated drug of misuse causing stroke[440,441] (sections 8.5.4 and 9.1.4). Within hours of administration, it can cause ischaemic stroke, transient ischaemic attack, intracerebral, intraventricular and subarachnoid haemorrhage, or paraplegia.[442–445] A vasculitis has been rarely described on brain biopsy but inferred much more commonly – probably wrongly – by non-specific beading on cerebral angiography.[446,447] More likely explanations for stroke are an acute rise of systemic blood pressure causing rupture of an unsuspected arteriovenous malformation or aneurysm; cerebral vasoconstriction with complicating thrombosis and ischaemia; and possibly cardiac dysrhythmias, myocardial infarction or cardiomyopathy and so cerebral embolism.[448–453] Moyamoya has also been described.[454]

Amphetamines seem occasionally to cause a small-vessel vasculopathy (in at least one case due to vasculitis) leading to intracranial haemorrhage, but acute hypertension is another possible factor; ischaemic stroke is much less common[455–458] (section 8.5.3).

Other sympathomimetic drugs (often found in nasal decongestants and appetite suppressants) may cause stroke in similar ways to amphetamines:
- ephedrine and pseudoephedrine;[459]
- ephedra alkaloids (ma huang);[460]
- phenylpropanolamine;[461–463]
- oxymetazoline;
- diethylproprion;
- phentermine;
- fenfluramine;
- methylene dioxymethylamphetamine ('ecstasy').[464–466]

Cannabis has been associated with ischaemic stroke in a handful of case reports but whether this is a causal relationship, and if so what the mechanism is, is unknown.[467]

Additional causes of stroke, or stroke-like syndromes, likely in drug-users, should not be forgotten:
- infective endocarditis (section 6.5.9);
- head or neck trauma (section 7.1);
- embolization of intravenously injected particulate foreign matter;
- alcohol abuse (sections 6.6.13 and 8.5.2);
- complications of human immunodeficiency virus infection (section 7.11);
- syphilis (section 7.11);
- hepatitis C (section 7.11).

7.15.2 Anti-inflammatory drugs

Rofecoxib (Vioxx), a selective cyclo-oxygenase (COX)-2 inhibitor non-steroidal anti-inflammatory drug which has now been withdrawn, is associated with a small increased risk of myocardial infarction and possibly (although the numbers are small) of stroke too, a problem which has become enveloped in political, scientific and corporate recriminations – plus a lot of confusion.[468,469] Similar concerns have been expressed over related drugs – valdecoxib, celecoxib, etoricoxib and lumiracoxib – presumably reflecting a class effect, most likely by inhibition of the production of prostacyclin in the vascular endothelium.[470-472] It is, therefore, prudent for ischaemic stroke survivors to avoid a COX-2 inhibitor if possible, and if anti-inflammatory analgesia is really necessary they should probably use a traditional non-steroidal anti-inflammatory (more COX-1 and less COX-2 inhibition) about which there is somewhat less concern, at least in moderate dosage – naproxen or ibuprofen perhaps being the safest.[471,473] And if they develop indigestion then adding a proton pump inhibitor may be preferable to switching to a COX-2 inhibitor.

7.15.3 Atypical antipsychotic drugs

In elderly patients with dementia, there have been concerns that both risperidone and olanzapine are associated with a modest increased risk of stroke, the mechanism for any causal association being unknown. This association is however rather uncertain at present.[474] And now concerns are emerging about conventional antipsychotics.[475]

7.15.4 Sildenafil

Although one might expect sildenafil (Viagra) to cause ischaemic stroke by acutely lowering the blood pressure, there are remarkably few case reports of this complication.[476]

7.15.5 Tibolone

There is as yet incompletely published evidence that tibolone – a drug to reduce osteoporosis – is associated with an increased risk of stroke.[477]

7.16 Hypoglycaemia and other metabolic causes of stroke-like syndromes

Hypoglycaemia, almost always caused by hypoglycaemic drugs rather than an insulinoma, is the most common 'metabolic' cause of focal cerebral episodes.[478] Curiously, consciousness is usually normal and there are seldom any of the usual systemic manifestations of hypoglycaemia, such as sweating and tachycardia. The episodes tend to occur soon after waking or after exercise. By the time the patient is seen, the blood glucose may well have returned to normal.[479-485] The episodes may last hours or sometimes a day or so – focal changes on MR DWI have been reported[486] (section 3.4.5).

Hypo- and hypercalcaemia,[487-489] non-ketotic hyperglycaemia[478,490-492] and hyponatraemia[478,493,494] have all occasionally been reported to cause transient ischaemic attack and stroke-like episodes, but some may some may actually have been partial epileptic seizures (section 3.4.5).

7.17 Gastrointestinal disorders

There are a number of case reports of ischaemic stroke, transient ischaemic attack and intracranial venous thrombosis complicating *ulcerative* and *Crohn's colitis*.[495-500] The bowel disease is not necessarily active at the time and may even present *after* the stroke. Causal possibilities include thrombocytosis, hypercoagulability, immobility and paradoxical embolism from the legs, vasculitis and dehydration. Curiously, these colitic patients, even without neurological symptoms, are apparently more likely than controls to have what *may* be 'vasculitic' lesions on brain MRI.[501]

Cerebral vasculitis has been described with *coeliac disease* but coeliac patients present neurologically more often with an encephalopathy than with a focal stroke-like syndrome.[502]

Food embolism to the brain through an oesophageal–atrial fistula as a complication of oesophageal cancer is a curiosity.[503]

7.18 Perioperative stroke

7.18.1 Cardiac surgery

During surgery, or within the next few days, about 3% of coronary artery bypass procedures are complicated by stroke, somewhat more often with valve surgery, and even more often after cardiac transplantation.[504–506] Much more common are what seem to be clinically silent brain lesions on imaging[507] and, perhaps of more consequence, a diffuse neurological syndrome with postoperative confusion, soft neurological signs, poor memory and other neuropsychological impairments.[508–510] This syndrome, which must be distinguished from depression, mostly resolves in days or weeks, perhaps coinciding with the resolution of the brain swelling which has been demonstrated immediately postoperatively.[511] Progressive long-term cognitive decline has been reported in some patients, perhaps due to comorbid cerebrovascular disease rather than the surgery itself.[509]

There are many possible explanations for these complications, the most common probably being embolism from the heart or aortic arch (Table 7.8). They are more likely with increasing age, previous stroke, other vascular disorders and risk factors, intraoperative hypotension, the use of aprotinin to reduce intraoperative bleeding, severe aortic arch atheroma and lengthy extracorporeal circulation.[508,512–514] A risk index has been suggested but not yet externally validated.[510] It is now becoming increasingly clear from several randomized trials that off-pump beating heart surgery is associated with fewer strokes and perhaps less clinically relevant cognitive decline than conventional coronary surgery under cardiopulmonary bypass.[515–517]

Whether asymptomatic carotid stenosis or occlusion is causally associated with perioperative stroke is much discussed. Certainly the extent of any association is uncertain because:

- the number of strokes in any one study is far too small for precise estimates of *relative* risk even though the *absolute* risk can appear quite high;
- often patients who might have had a stroke have been excluded from a series by having an elective carotid endarterectomy before cardiac surgery;
- the proportion of all operative strokes caused by severe carotid disease, presumably in association with a fall in systemic blood pressure, is probably rather small;
- most studies have been retrospective;
- and by no means all patients in the studies have had imaging to assess the severity of any carotid stenosis.

Table 7.8 Possible causes of stroke and cognitive decline complicating cardiac surgery.

Embolization to the brain during surgery of:
    platelet aggregates
    fibrin
    calcific valvular debris
    intracardiac thrombus
    atheromatous debris from the aorta
    fat, air and silicone or particulate matter from the pump–oxygenator system
    vegetations complicating infective endocarditis
Embolism after surgery from:
    thrombus on suture lines or on prosthetic material
    left ventricular thrombus complicating myocardial infarction
    atrial fibrillation
    infective endocarditis
Global hypoperfusion and ischaemia resulting from perioperative hypotension (section 6.7.5)
Haemodilution during surgery
Simultaneous carotid endarterectomy under the same anaesthetic (section 16.14)
Cholesterol embolization syndrome (section 7.7)
Thrombosis associated with heparin-induced thrombocytopenia (section 7.9.11)
The systemic inflammatory response
Non-specific effect of general anaesthesia
Intracranial haemorrhage caused by:
    thrombocytopenia
    disseminated intravascular coagulation
    uncontrolled hypertension
    antithrombotic drugs
Paradoxical embolism from postoperative deep venous thrombosis (section 6.5.12)

With recently symptomatic carotid stenosis the stroke risk may be higher.[518] Pending a large, prospective and methodologically sound study to clarify this issue, a systematic review of all the available studies is much needed.

Instrumentation of the coronary arteries and aorta may dislodge valvular, intracardiac or atheromatous aortic and other large-artery thrombus and debris to cause cerebral ischaemia. Although under 1% of procedures are complicated by stroke of any consequence, minor events including subtle neurocognitive abnormalities may well have passed unnoticed or been under-reported, while apparently asymptomatic changes on MR DWI are fairly common.[324,507,519,520] Thrombus may also form on the intra-arterial catheter tip, a fragment of catheter may break off and embolize, there may be systemic hypotension, cerebral air embolism is a possibility, and the cholesterol embolization syndrome is a rare complication (section 7.7). Large doses of intravenous contrast

Table 7.9 Possible causes of stroke during or soon after general surgery.

Intra- or postoperative hypotension causing low-flow infarction, particularly if there are stenotic or occluded arteries supplying the brain (section 6.7.5)

Haemostatic defect resulting from antithrombotic drugs, or disseminated intravascular coagulation, causing intracranial haemorrhage

Occlusion or dissection of neck arteries caused by faulty handling and positioning during general anaesthesia (section 7.2.1)

Paradoxical embolism from postoperative deep venous thrombosis (section 6.5.12)

Withdrawal of long-term warfarin therapy for stroke prevention

Penetrating trauma of a neck artery during attempted venous catheterization or neck surgery (section 7.1.1)

Perioperative myocardial infarction or atrial fibrillation

Infective endocarditis (section 6.5.9)

Fat embolism after long bone surgery (section 7.1.8)

Air embolism (section 7.1.7)

The rather nebulous concept of postoperative 'hypercoagulability'

may cause temporary cortical blindness, and even normal doses can cause migrainous aura.[521,522]

7.18.2 General surgery

General surgery is less frequently complicated by stroke than cardiac surgery – less than 1% of operations depending on age – most often in patients with a past history of stroke, widespread vascular disease or chronic obstructive airways disease.[523,524] As after cardiac surgery, there is some evidence of early and perhaps longer-term postoperative cognitive decline, but the studies are bedevilled with methodological problems.[525] There are many possible causes of perioperative stroke but so often the stroke is not recognized very quickly in sick postoperative patients, and investigation is generally less than optimal in surgical wards (Table 7.9). Sometimes the stroke is coincidental, particularly in elderly people with multiple vascular risk factors who increasingly are having surgery as anaesthesia becomes safer.

7.19 Mitochondrial diseases

This large group of rare multisystem disorders is associated with structural abnormalities of mitochondria, together with biochemical defects in the respiratory chain.[526–530] Many are now known to be caused by various deletions and point mutations in mitochondrial DNA, where inheritance of point mutations is usually through the maternal line, and also sometimes by defects in nuclear DNA.[529,531] There are a number of rather characteristic, but often overlapping, clinical phenotypes, one of which can present as 'stroke': mitochondrial encephalopathy, lactic acidosis and stroke-like episodes (MELAS).

MELAS usually presents in children, adolescents or middle-aged adults with recurrent focal cerebral episodes, usually first affecting the occipital lobes, and caused by lesions which were originally regarded as infarcts but not corresponding with the territories of the main cerebral arteries.[532,533] These episodes tend to be complicated in the acute stage, or later, by partial and secondary generalized epileptic seizures. Eventually the patient becomes demented and usually cortically blind. The cause of the brain lesions is uncertain; perhaps a defect in brain oxidative metabolism, or the structural changes that can be seen in small cerebral blood vessels rather than overt vessel occlusion,[534,535] the former possibility being supported by MR DWI studies.[536] MELAS patients are often rather short, with sensorineural deafness, migraine, episodic vomiting, diabetes mellitus and some learning disability. There may be additional features more characteristic of other mitochondrial syndromes, such as proximal muscle weakness, myoclonus, ataxia, exercise intolerance, cardiomyopathy, progressive external ophthalmoplegia, pigmentary retinopathy and ovarian and testicular failure.

The diagnosis of MELAS should be suspected in any young patient with an ischaemic stroke, particularly if it is in the occipital lobe and complicated by epilepsy, and if there is no other fairly obvious cause.[537] CT frequently shows basal ganglia calcification and also areas of low density in the grey and white matter of the cerebral hemispheres, and these may show mass effect and enhancement in the acute stage, and then disappear, eventually to be followed by atrophy, more obvious on MRI[538] (Fig. 7.15).

The fasting plasma and, particularly, cerebrospinal fluid (CSF) lactate is raised, usually at rest. However, CSF lactate may also be raised for some days after epileptic seizures, subarachnoid haemorrhage, meningitis and stroke and is anyway not diagnostically helpful because either an abnormal or normal test result must be followed up if there is diagnostic suspicion in the first place – biochemical or molecular confirmation is ultimately always required.[539] In many but not all patients, muscle biopsy shows ragged red fibres on Gomori's trichrome staining and, with electron microscopy, large numbers

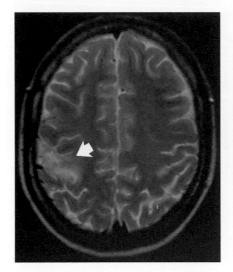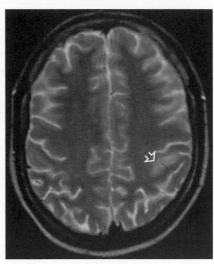

Fig. 7.15 Mitochondrial encephalomyopathy, lactic acidosis and stroke-like episodes (MELAS): T2-weighted MR scan. The first scan (*left-hand panel*) shows an infarct-like hyperintensity in the parieto-occipital cortex (*white arrow*). The second scan (*right-hand panel*) was obtained 2 weeks later and shows a new lesion in the left parieto-occipital cortex (*open white arrow*); the earlier lesion has vanished.

of abnormal mitochondria. The point mutation in mitochondrial DNA (usually at base pair 3243 but occasionally at one of several other sites) can be demonstrated in white blood cells, but sometimes only in muscle. However, not all MELAS patients have known mutations, and sometimes the known mutations can be found in other mitochondrial clinical syndromes, in relatives of MELAS patients who may or may not be symptomatic, and in some normal people.[540–542] At present, there is no specific treatment.

Children with autosomal recessive cytochrome oxidase deficiency and lactic acidosis have been reported to have stroke-like episodes.[543]

7.20 Single gene disorders

7.20.1 Cerebral autosomal dominant arteriopathy with subcortical infarcts and leucoencephalopathy

Cerebral autosomal dominant arteriopathy with subcortical infarcts and leucoencephalopathy (CADASIL) is an increasingly recognized but rare autosomal dominant – and occasionally sporadic – disorder of small blood vessels caused by various mutations of the Notch 3 gene on chromosome 19.[544–546]

Migraine with aura (which can be prolonged, complicated and easily confused with strokes and transient ischaemic attacks) tends to develop in patients in their 20s, recurrent – mainly lacunar ischaemic – strokes and transient ischaemic attacks in their 40s, progressive subcortical dementia in their 50s, and the patients die in

their 60s; early on, depressive symptoms and other mood disorders are common.[547–550] However, affected individuals vary in the frequency and severity of the various manifestations and age of onset, sometimes within the same family, the phenotype is constantly being expanded, and cognitive decline may even be present very early on.[551]

On CT, and more obviously on MRI, there are very characteristic focal, diffuse and confluent lesions in the periventricular and subcortical cerebral white matter, also sometimes in the brainstem, looking very similar to ischaemic leukoaraiosis and even multiple sclerosis, but typically there are also changes in the temporal poles which is not the case with either of these differential diagnoses; the MR changes very often start before the patients are symptomatic, and progress with time[187,552,553] (Fig. 7.16). Multifocal microhaemorrhages on gradient echo MRI – and at autopsy – are another common feature, perhaps in part a consequence of antiplatelet drug treatment, hypertension or diabetes, although clinically apparent haemorrhagic stroke is unusual.[554–556] Catheter angiography should be avoided because of the apparent excess risk of neurological complications.[557] The CSF may show a mildly raised protein level, and very occasionally unmatched oligoclonal bands.

The changes in the vessel wall are distinctive with deposits of eosinophilic periodic-acid-Schiff positive material within the leptomeningeal and perforating arteries of the brain.[558] The basal lamina of the affected vessels is thickened by granular osmiophilic material which is dense under electron microscopy. Despite the lack of any obvious clinical consequences, similar changes can be found in the small vessels of skin, muscle, nerve and other viscera which occasionally allows histological, and particularly electron microscopy, confirmation of

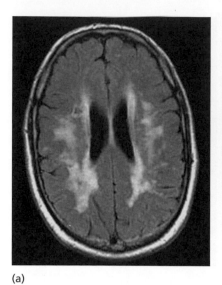
(a)

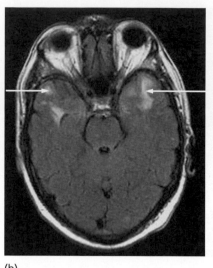
(b)

Fig. 7.16 Cerebral autosomal dominant arteriopathy with subcortical infarcts and leukoencephalopathy (CADASIL): FLAIR MR brain scan showing (a) numerous abnormal high signal areas in the cerebral white matter bilaterally and, typically, (b) in the anterior temporal lobes (*arrows*) which would be most unusual in multiple sclerosis, for example.

the diagnosis from skin or muscle biopsy, although this may not always be reliable;[559–561] the utility can however be improved with immunostaining with a Notch 3 monoclonal antibody.[562] Genetic testing will generally detect known mutations but these vary in different populations, it is therefore time-consuming because there are so many mutations, and it may be negative.[563]

It is clear therefore that the diagnosis of CADASIL is not as straightforward as it once seemed. The clinical phenotype varies and obviously overlaps with migraine, stroke and dementia – particularly in the early stages when only one manifestation may be present, such as migraine; the MR scan is almost always abnormal but shares many features with multiple sclerosis in young adults and ischaemic leukoaraiosis in older people; there is not always a family history; the skin biopsy is not always positive; and Notch 3 mutations are not always found, perhaps because not enough have been tested for in an individual patient or there are more to be discovered.

Other than paying attention to any vascular risk factors in the normal way (Chapter 16), and perhaps adding aspirin as an antithrombotic drug, there is no specific treatment. Genetic counselling is of course important, with all the problems inherent in a long-term but ultimately fatal condition which can be predicted from a blood test, and which so often becomes manifest after those affected have themselves had children.

Other even rarer familial small-vessel disorders have also been described including cerebral autosomal recessive arteriopathy with subcortical infarcts and leucoencephalopathy (CARASIL), hereditary endotheliopathy with retinopathy, nephropathy and stroke syndrome (HERNS), cerebroretinal vasculopathy, familial amyloid angiopathy, and others as yet unnamed.[564]

7.20.2 Homocystinuria

This rare autosomal recessive inborn error of metabolism, usually caused by cystathione synthase deficiency, is complicated by cerebral arterial and intracranial venous thrombosis, usually in children and young adults, for reasons that are unclear.[565] The underlying vascular pathology has rarely been studied but seems to be atheromatous-like in some cases but not others.[566–569] The diagnosis should be suspected if there are epileptic seizures, learning disability, marfanoid habitus, osteoporosis, high myopia and dislocated lenses but these are not invariably very obvious or even present.[568,570–572] Hyperhomocysteinaemia, insufficiently severe to cause the clinical syndrome of homocystinuria, may be a risk factor for degenerative vascular disease (section 6.6.8).

7.20.3 Fabry's disease

This rare, X-linked, recessive lysosomal storage disorder in which there is a deficiency of alpha-galactosidase A results in the accumulation of glycolipids in vascular endothelial and other cells.[573,574]

The patients are young males (and increasingly recognized heterozygous females) who are affected by skin angiokeratomas in the bathing-trunks area, hypohidrosis, and burning pain and paraesthesia in the hands and feet (but seldom any signs) caused by a small fibre neuropathy. Additional complications include corneal dystrophy, cataract, renal failure and secondary hypertension, cardiomyopathy, myocardial ischaemia and conduction abnormalities. Death generally occurs in middle age.

Clinically evident as well as 'silent' strokes, both cortical and subcortical, are caused by: occlusion of small blood vessels; larger vessel ectasia; embolism from the heart; and rarely intracranial haemorrhage.[575] Fabry's disease is worth looking for in young stroke patients with no obvious cause, particularly males, occurring in maybe 1% or so.[576]

7.20.4 Tuberous sclerosis

This multisystem, autosomal dominant disorder may be complicated by cerebral emboli from a cardiac rhabdomyosarcoma.[577] It has also been uncertainly associated with intracranial aneurysms and the moyamoya syndrome (section 7.5).

7.20.5 Neurofibromatosis

This is another multisystem, autosomal dominant disorder. It may be complicated by: distal carotid stenosis or occlusion, sometimes but not always the result of irradiation for optic nerve glioma, and this in turn may cause the moyamoya syndrome (section 7.5); ectasia and occlusion of cerebral arteries; intracranial and extracranial aneurysms perhaps; and tumour compression of intracranial arteries.[578–580]

7.20.6 Primary oxalosis

This rare autosomal recessive disorder is complicated by renal stones and failure. It may rarely be complicated by ischaemic stroke due to embolism from the heart, or the moyamoya syndrome.[581]

7.20.7 Inherited disorders of connective and elastic tissue

Ehlers–Danlos syndrome type IV (section 9.1.1), pseudoxanthoma elasticum, Marfan's syndrome and osteogenesis imperfecta are all rare disorders which can affect arteries and so occasionally be complicated by, or present with, arterial dissection, local aneurysm formation or even rupture, intracranial aneurysm formation, caroticocavernous fistula and embolism from cardiac lesions.[582–587]

7.21 Intracranial venous thrombosis

The advent of non-invasive brain imaging in the 1980s resulted in greatly increased recognition of intracranial venous thrombosis (ICVT), although it is still far less frequent than arterial ischaemic stroke.[588–590] Before then, only physicians with a high index of suspicion considered the diagnosis in patients with otherwise unexplained headache, focal deficits, seizures, impaired consciousness, or combinations of these features; all too often the diagnosis was made at postmortem – as it was in the first recorded case by Thomas Willis.[591] Not surprisingly it used to be regarded as a rare disease that was commonly fatal, whereas now it is seen as a relatively common disease which is rarely fatal.

7.21.1 Predisposing factors

Unlike arterial thrombosis, damage to the vessel wall – due to infection, infiltration, or trauma to cortical veins or dural sinuses – is a causal factor in only about 10% of patients with ICVT.[592] More important are disorders of coagulation[592] (Table 7.10). The most common inherited coagulation defect is factor V Leiden mutation, which is found in some 20% of patients without other obvious predisposing causes.[593–595] The third component of Virchow's triad of causes of thrombosis – stagnant flow – contributes no more than a few per cent (associated with dehydration or with dural puncture, sometimes in combination with hyperosmolar contrast agents).[596] In about 20% of patients no contributing factors can be identified and the cause remains shrouded in mystery. Perhaps as yet undiscovered prothrombotic mutations are responsible to some extent.

Often there is no single cause but a combination of contributing factors, for example the postpartum period *and* protein S deficiency,[597] pregnancy *and* Behçet's disease,[598] oral contraceptives *and* the factor V Leiden mutation,[599,600] or the same combinations with dural puncture as a third factor.[601]

In neonates, ICVT is usually associated with acute systemic problems such as perinatal complications or dehydration; in older children the most frequent underlying conditions are local infection (the leading cause until the antibiotic era), coagulopathy[602,603] and – more in Mediterranean countries – Behçet's disease.[604]

7.21.2 Clinical features

Unlike arterial ischaemic stroke, ICVT relatively more commonly affects neonates, infants, children and young adults than older people, but no age is exempt. The clinical features consist essentially of headache, focal neurological deficits, epileptic seizures and impairment of consciousness, in different combinations and degrees of severity. The symptoms and signs depend to some extent on which vein or venous sinus is affected, and to an important extent on whether the thrombotic process is limited to the dural sinuses or extends to the cortical veins.[592]

Prothrombotic states
Pregnancy and puerperium, particularly in developing countries (section 7.14)
Ovarian hyperstimulation syndrome (section 7.13)
Hereditary coagulopathies
Protein C or S deficiency (section 7.9.11)
Antithrombin III deficiency (section 7.9.11)
Factor II (prothrombin) gene mutations (section 7.9.11)
Factor V Leiden mutations (section 7.9.11)
von Willebrand's disease
5,10 methylene tetrahydrofolate reductase mutation
Homocystinuria (section 7.20.2) and hyperhomocysteinaemia
Coagulopathies secondary to blood diseases
Thrombocythaemia (section 7.9.2)
Primary polycythaemia (section 7.9.1)
Leukaemia (section 7.9.4)
Paroxysmal nocturnal haemoglobinuria (section 7.9.9)
Iron deficiency anaemia (section 7.9.7)
Sickle cell disease (section 7.9.8)
Disseminated intravascular coagulation (section 7.9.12)
After bone marrow transplantation
Secondary to systemic disease
Behçet's disease (section 7.3.11)
Systemic lupus erythematosus/antiphospholipid syndrome (sections 7.3.3 and
    7.3.4)
Systemic vasculitis (section 7.3.6)
Carcinoma (breast, prostate, etc.) (section 7.12)
Lymphoma
Hyperviscosity syndromes (section 7.9.10)
Nephrotic syndrome (section 7.9.11)
Ulcerative colitis or Crohn's disease (section 7.17)
Dehydration
Sarcoidosis (section 7.3.16)
Systemic infectious disease (bacterial, fungal)
Drugs
Oral contraceptives (section 7.13.1)
Corticosteroids
Dihydroergotamine
Asparaginase (section 7.12)
Androgens
Ecstasy (section 7.15.1)
Recombinant human erythropoietin
Antifibrinolytic drugs
Thalidomide?
Local infection or infiltration
Otitis, mastoiditis, sinusitis
Dental abscess
Tonsillitis
Meningitis (acute or chronic, bacterial, fungal)
Subdural empyema
Obstruction of dural sinus by tumour
Malignant meningitis
Thrombosis of vein draining venous malformation
Dural puncture
Epidural anaesthesia
Metrizamide myelography
Diagnostic tap
Trauma
Head injury, open or closed, with or without fracture
Jugular vein, including catheterization
Neurosurgical procedures

Table 7.10 Predisposing factors for intracranial venous thrombosis.

Dural sinus thrombosis causes raised intracranial pressure with headache and papilloedema (without hydrocephalus). In the past, patients with so-called 'benign intracranial hypertension' may well have had unrecognized sinus thrombosis; although they are more often non-obese males, they can be clinically indistinguishable from patients with what should now be called idiopathic intracranial hypertension.[605] Papilloedema can cause transient visual obscurations and sometimes irreversible constriction of the visual fields, beginning in the inferonasal quadrants.[606] The increased pressure of the cerebrospinal fluid may give rise to sixth nerve palsies, and sometimes to other cranial nerve deficits. The onset of the headache is usually gradual over some days, but in up to 15% of patients it is sudden, which may initially suggest the diagnosis of a ruptured aneurysm intracranial.[607] Very few patients seem to go on to develop problems with cortical venous infarction, although a few do.

Involvement of cortical veins causes one or more areas of venous infarction, which are usually highly oedematous, with or without haemorrhagic transformation. If the affected veins drain into the sagittal sinus, the venous infarcts are typically located near the midline in the parasagittal and parieto-occipital regions, often on both sides. In the case of the lateral sinus, the venous infarct is usually located in the posterior temporal area. If the thrombotic process extends to the petrosal sinus, the fifth or sixth cranial nerves may be affected, and with jugular vein thrombosis the ninth to eleventh cranial nerves;[592] sometimes the lower cranial nerve palsies are isolated with no other clinical signs.[608]

Clinically, the infarcts present typically with headache and focal epileptic seizures with or without secondary generalization, and with focal deficits such as hemiparesis or aphasia (transient or more permanent). If unilateral weakness develops (with thrombosis originating in the superior sagittal sinus), it tends to predominate in the leg, in keeping with the parasagittal location of most venous infarcts. Obstruction of cortical veins draining into the posterior part of the superior sagittal sinus, or into the lateral sinus, will relatively often lead to hemianopia, aphasia or a confusional state. A generalized encephalopathy with impairment of consciousness may result from multiple infarcts in the cerebral hemispheres, or from transtentorial herniation and compression of the brainstem. Either epilepsy or a focal deficit is a presenting feature in 10–15% of patients;[609] during the course of the illness seizures occur in 10–60%, and focal deficits in 30–80%.[609-612] Occasionally the presentation can be with headache alone, mimicking subarachnoid haemorrhage.

Involvement of the cortical veins, without sinus thrombosis and its associated signs of increased CSF pressure, is rare but can present as 'stroke' and so may be under-recognized, particularly when the clinical features are rather mild and there is no haemorrhagic transformation of any infarct, or any infarct at all, on imaging.[609,610,613] One wonders if ICVT is responsible for many transient ischaemic attacks; presumably it must be, but is unrecognized.

Thrombosis of the deep venous system, including the great vein of Galen, may lead to bilateral haemorrhagic infarction of the corpus striatum, thalamus, hypothalamus, the ventral corpus callosum, the medial occipital lobes and the upper part of the cerebellum.[614] The clinical picture is dominated by coma, disordered eye movements and pupillary reflexes, with a high case fatality. However, there are partial syndromes which can be survived, sometimes with surprisingly few sequelae.[610,615,616]

Thrombosis of cerebellar veins leads to clinical features resembling those of arterial territory infarcts in the cerebellum (dominated by headache, vertigo, vomiting and ataxia, sometimes followed by impaired consciousness), but with a more gradual onset.[606,617,618]

7.21.3 Diagnosis and investigations

The main trick is to think of the diagnosis in a patient who appears to have idiopathic intracranial hypertension, an encephalopathy with multiple cerebral 'haemorrhages', sudden headache not due to subarachnoid haemorrhage, or a 'stroke' (either ischaemic or haemorrhagic) with epileptic seizures and headache in a young patient – particularly if the patient is or has recently been pregnant, has a past history of venous thrombosis elsewhere, or systemic risk factors for venous thrombosis. However, these days the first suggestion often comes from CT or MR imaging (section 5.8). Once the radiological diagnosis is made, then clearly the cause has to be searched for along the lines outlined in Table 7.10. But even if one 'cause' is found, others must also be considered because so often one or more act synergistically to cause ICVT, perhaps in half the cases. However, in about 20% of cases no cause is found. D-dimer assay is neither specific nor sensitive enough to be useful.[590]

7.21.4 Prognosis and treatment

Dural sinus thrombosis alone generally has a very good prognosis without any treatment, and even patients with widespread haemorrhagic venous infarcts have made surprising recoveries – venous infarcts are clearly different from arterial infarcts in this respect. However,

ICVT can still be a very serious disorder and a few patients die, usually of transtentorial herniation.[619] In the acute phase of an encephalopathy, raised intracranial pressure may have to be treated with mannitol, large haemorrhagic infarcts removed surgically, and even decompressive hemicraniectomy may be required for major cerebral swelling (despite the lack of formal evidence of benefit). It is uncertain whether corticosteroids are helpful.

The treatment of patients with just raised intracranial pressure should probably be along the same lines as for idiopathic intracranial hypertension (acetazolamide, repeat lumbar punctures, CSF diversion), notwithstanding the very poor evidence on which this is based.[620]

Some patients are left with residual neurological disability, epilepsy and – exceptionally – a dural or pial arteriovenous fistula.[621,622]

For years the logical treatment for thrombosis within veins – anticoagulation – was avoided because of the fear of causing haemorrhagic transformation of venous infarcts. However, as people became aware that this was seldom a problem, and that even if haemorrhagic transformation was actually present patients still seemed to do well on anticoagulants, three randomized trials were organized; in aggregate they showed a non-significant trend in favour of treatment: 54% relative reduction in death and disability (95% confidence interval 84–31% increase)[589,623] (Fig. 7.17). Under the circumstances, most physicians are now prepared to heparinize patients, even in the presence of haemorrhagic infarcts, and then to switch after a few days to warfarin with a target INR of 2–3. Presumably, if there is a definite contraindication to anticoagulation, aspirin or another antiplatelet drug would have some useful antithrombotic effect. Endovascular thrombolysis, with or without mechanical clot disruption, has been attempted but there is no good evidence that it is effective; it should be reserved for randomized trials or patients who are doing badly even with anticoagulation. Naturally any underlying cause should be treated (infections, vasculitis, etc.) and, if this is successful, anticoagulation can be withdrawn in a matter of months. More difficult is whether anticoagulation should be continued indefinitely in patients with an inherited or aquired coagulopathy, or indeed in patients with no obvious 'cause'; maybe it should be, particularly if recurrent venous thromboses have occurred, although the risk of recurrence of ICVT appears to be very small, even in any subsequent pregnancy.[426]

Pulmonary embolism may be more frequent than one might anticipate for the severity of any leg paralysis or length of bed rest, perhaps it is due to propagation of thrombus from the intracranial sinuses to the pulmonary veins, or because of an underlying thrombophilia.[624]

7.22 The ischaemic stroke or transient ischaemic attack case with no cause – what to do?

Even over 50–60 years of age, ischaemic strokes should not carelessly be put down to 'degenerative arterial

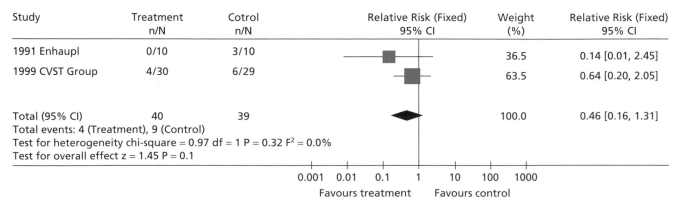

Fig. 7.17 The Cochrane Review of anticoagulation treatment for intracranial venous thrombosis.[623] The outcome is death and dependency. Each of the two trials is represented by a box describing the relative reduction in risk of a poor outcome with the horizontal line representing the 95% confidence interval (fixed effects method). The diamond represents the overall reduction in risk with its 95% confidence interval (copyright Cochrane Collaboration, reproduced with permission).

disease' unless there are clear-cut risk factors (hypertension, smoking, etc.) and/or clear-cut evidence of arterial disease elsewhere (bruits, claudication, angina) *and* no more obvious cause, such as giant-cell arteritis. Nor should ischaemic strokes be ascribed to embolism from the heart unless there is a major and threatening cardiac source (e.g. atrial fibrillation, prosthetic heart valve, etc.). Of course, there are many other, admittedly rare, possibilities to be considered from Fabry's disease to CADASIL. But, after taking an exhaustive history, examining the patient obsessionally and undertaking appropriate investigations, there are still some patients where no reasonable explanation for their stroke can be found or in whom any putative cause is marginal (e.g. uncomplicated mitral leaflet prolapse, patent foramen ovale, oral contraceptives with no prothrombotic or other abnormality, an uncertain diagnosis of migrainous stroke); the stroke is then deemed 'cryptogenic'. Naturally, the intensity of the search for a cause must depend on the previous level of dependency and the age of the patient, the severity of the stroke (aggressive investigation is reasonable in milder strokes where there is more to lose from a disabling recurrence), and the consequences of missing the diagnosis. For example, at any age, it is vital to diagnose infective endocarditis as without treatment it can be fatal, whereas traumatic arterial dissection with no medicolegal consequences is perhaps less important because – as yet – there is no generally accepted treatment, and recurrence is unlikely. Nonetheless, the diagnosis of dissection or a migrainous stroke would at least stop the patient having to take the full range of vascular risk-reducing drugs (Chapter 16) for the rest of their lives, and also improve their chances of getting life insurance.

In a puzzling case, it is important to go over the history and examination again, re-read all the medical records and to check not only that the appropriate investigations have been carried out but also that the results have been discussed by the medical team and are available in the medical records. It may turn out that the diagnosis of stroke or transient ischaemic attack has to be revised, particularly if a 'stroke' patient deteriorates or fails to improve in a typical way after the acute stage, taking one back to the 'stroke' vs 'not-stroke' issues discussed in Chapter 3. It is surprising how often, in young people, multiple sclerosis can be confused with stroke, in elderly patients how the pseudobulbar palsy of motor neurone disease can be called a stroke, and at any age how migraine aura without headache can be confused with transient ischaemic attacks. A 'psychogenic' disorder is also easily confused with stroke. So 'no cause for a stroke' may simply mean that the patient has not had a stroke in the first place – double check.

> If there is no obvious cause for a stroke or transient ischaemic attack, it is important to retake the history, re-examine the patient and check not only that all the relevant investigations have been carried out but that the results have been seen and discussed by the medical team. If there is still no cause, then follow-up, or a recurrence, may provide the crucial clue.

If the ischaemic stroke or transient ischaemic attack diagnosis is secure, all the relevant investigations are negative, the heart is normal, and there are no vascular risk factors or evidence of vascular disease outside the head, then there is little to be done except recommend aspirin as an antithrombotic drug along perhaps with a statin (at least for a while), await events and hope that any recurrence does not bring to light a diagnosis which should have led to an effective treatment at the time of the first stroke. In general, the problem is seldom the lack of a key investigation but more often the lack of a good clinical history. Therefore, other than checking out all the possible investigations in Tables 6.13 and 6.14, it is best to retake the history, re-examine the patient and follow up the patient carefully, at least for a while. Fortunately, as far as one call tell, strokes with truly no discernable cause seldom seem to recur.

References

1 Davis JM, Zimmerman RA. Injury of the carotid and vertebral arteries. *Neuroradiology* 1983;**25**(2):55–69.

2 Inamasu J, Guiot BH. Iatrogenic vertebral artery injury. *Acta Neurol Scand* 2005; **112**(6):349–57.

3 Auer RN, Krcek J, Butt JC. Delayed symptoms and death after minor head trauma with occult vertebral artery injury. *J Neurol Neurosurg Psychiatry* 1994; **57**(4):500–2.

4 Viktrup L, Knudsen GM, Hansen SH. Delayed onset of fatal basilar thrombotic embolus after whiplash injury. *Stroke* 1995; **26**(11):2194–6.

5 Martin PJ, Humphrey PR. Disabling stroke arising five months after internal carotid artery dissection. *J Neurol Neurosurg Psychiatry* 1998; **65**(1):136–7.

6 Nazir FS, Muir KW. Prolonged interval between vertebral artery dissection and ischemic stroke. *Neurology* 2004; **62**(9):1646–7.

7 Hughes JT, Brownell B. Traumatic thrombosis of the internal carotid artery in the neck. *J Neurol Neurosurg Psychiatry* 1968; **31**(4):307–14.

8 Hilton-Jones D, Warlow CP. Non-penetrating arterial trauma and cerebral infarction in the young. *Lancet* 1985; 1(8443):1435–8.

9 Pozzati E, Giuliani G, Poppi M, Faenza A. Blunt traumatic carotid dissection with delayed symptoms. *Stroke* 1989; 20(3):412–16.

10 Frisoni GB, Anzola GP. Vertebrobasilar ischemia after neck motion. *Stroke* 1991; 22(11):1452–60.

11 Thie A, Hellner D, Lachenmayer L, Janzen RW, Kunze K. Bilateral blunt traumatic dissections of the extracranial internal carotid artery: report of eleven cases and reivew of the literature. *Cerebrovasc Dis* 1993; 3:295–303.

12 Tulyapronchote R, Selhorst JB, Malkoff MD, Gomez CR. Delayed sequelae of vertebral artery dissection and occult cervical fractures. *Neurology* 1994; 44(8):1397–9.

13 English R, Macaulay M. Subclavian artery thrombosis with contralateral hemiplegia. *Br Med J* 1977; 2(6102):1583.

14 Prior AL, Wilson LA, Gosling RG, Yates AK, Ross Russell RW. Retrograde cerebral embolism. *Lancet* 1979; 2(8151):1044–7.

15 Sawauchi S, Terao T, Tani S, Ogawa T, Abe T. Traumatic middle cerebral artry occlusion from boxing. *J Clin Neurosci* 1999; 6:63–7.

16 Zubkov AY, Pilkington AS, Bernanke DH, Parent AD, Zhang J. Posttraumatic cerebral vasospasm: clinical and morphological presentations. *J Neurotrauma* 1999; 16(9):763–70.

17 Haas DC, Pineda GS, Lourie H. Juvenile head trauma syndromes and their relationship to migraine. *Arch Neurol* 1975; 32(11):727–30.

18 Sakai F, Ishii K, Igarashi H, Suzuki S, Kitai N, Kanda T, Tazaki Y. Regional cerebral blood flow during an attack of vertebrobasilar insufficiency. *Stroke* 1988; 19(11):1426–30.

19 Rosengart A, Hedges TR, III, Teal PA, DeWitt LD, Wu JK, Wolpert S, Caplan LR. Intermittent downbeat nystagmus due to vertebral artery compression. *Neurology* 1993; 43(1):216–18.

20 Sturzenegger M, Newell DW, Douville C, Byrd S, Schoonover K. Dynamic transcranial Doppler assessment of positional vertebrobasilar ischemia. *Stroke* 1994; 25(9):1776–83.

21 Kawaguchi T, Fujita S, Hosoda K, Shibata Y, Iwakura M, Tamaki N. Rotational occlusion of the vertebral artery caused by transverse process hyperrotation and unilateral apophyseal joint subluxation: case report. *J Neurosurg* 1997; 86(6):1031–5.

22 Kuether TA, Nesbit GM, Clark WM, Barnwell SL. Rotational vertebral artery occlusion: a mechanism of vertebrobasilar insufficiency. *Neurosurgery* 1997; 41(2):427–32.

23 Strupp M, Planck JH, Arbusow V, Steiger HJ, Bruckmann H, Brandt T. Rotational vertebral artery occlusion syndrome with vertigo due to 'labyrinthine excitation'. *Neurology* 2000; 54(6):1376–9.

24 Choi KD, Shin HY, Kim JS, Kim SH, Kwon OK, Koo JW *et al.* Rotational vertebral artery syndrome: oculographic analysis of nystagmus. *Neurology* 2005; 65(8):1287–90.

25 Nehls DG, Marano SR, Spetzler RF. Positional intermittent occlusion of the internal carotid artery: case report. *J Neurosurg* 1985; 62(3):435–7.

26 Rothwell DM, Bondy SJ, Williams JI. Chiropractic manipulation and stroke: a population-based case-control study. *Stroke* 2001; 32(5):1054–60.

27 Haldeman S, Kohlbeck FJ, McGregor M. Stroke, cerebral artery dissection, and cervical spine manipulation therapy. *J Neurol* 2002; 249(8):1098–104.

28 Toro-Gonzalez G, Navarro-Roman L, Roman GC, Cantillo J, Serrano B, Herrera M, Vergara I. Acute ischemic stroke from fibrocartilaginous embolism to the middle cerebral artery. *Stroke* 1993; 24(5):738–40.

29 Tosi L, Rigoli G, Beltramello A. Fibrocartilaginous embolism of the spinal cord: a clinical and pathogenetic reconsideration. *J Neurol Neurosurg Psychiatry* 1996; 60(1):55–60.

30 Beer S, Kesselring J. Fibrocartilaginous embolisation of the spinal cord in a 7-year-old girl. *J Neurol* 2002; 249(7):936–7.

31 Brouns R, De SD, Neetens I, De Deyn PP. Fatal venous cerebral air embolism secondary to a disconnected central venous catheter. *Cerebrovasc Dis* 2006; 21(3):212–14.

32 Caulfield AF, Lansberg MG, Marks MP, Albers GW, Wijman CA. MRI characteristics of cerebral air embolism from a venous source. *Neurology* 2006; 66(6):945–6.

33 Murphy BP, Harford FJ, Cramer FS. Cerebral air embolism resulting from invasive medical procedures: treatment with hyperbaric oxygen. *Ann Surg* 1985; 201(2):242–5.

34 Jacobson DM, Terrence CF, Reinmuth OM. The neurologic manifestations of fat embolism. *Neurology* 1986; 36(6):847–51.

35 Schievink WI. Spontaneous dissection of the carotid and vertebral arteries. *N Engl J Med* 2001; 344(12):898–906.

36 Arnold M, Bousser MG. Carotid and vertebral artery dissection. *Pract Neurol* 2005; 5(2):100–9.

37 Rubinstein SM, Peerdeman SM, van Tulder MW, Riphagen I, Haldeman S. A systematic review of the risk factors for cervical artery dissection. *Stroke* 2005; 36(7):1575–80.

38 Volker W, Besselmann M, Dittrich R, Nabavi D, Konrad C, Dziewas R *et al.* Generalized arteriopathy in patients with cervical artery dissection. *Neurology* 2005; 64(9):1508–13.

39 O'Connell BK, Towfighi J, Brennan RW, Tyler W, Mathews M, Weidner WA, Saul RF. Dissecting aneurysms of head and neck. *Neurology* 1985; 35(7):993–7.

40 Koch S, Rabinstein AA, Romano JG, Forteza A. Diffusion-weighted magnetic resonance imaging in internal carotid artery dissection. *Arch Neurol* 2004; 61(4):510–12.

41 Benninger DH, Georgiadis D, Kremer C, Studer A, Nedeltchev K, Baumgartner RW. Mechanism of ischemic infarct in spontaneous carotid dissection. *Stroke* 2004; 35(2):482–5.

42 Caplan L, Tettenborn B. Vertebrobasilar occlusive disease: review of selected aspects. I. Spontaneous dissection of extracranial and intracranial posterior circulation arteries. *Cerebrovasc Dis* 1992; 2:256–65.

43 Hetzel A, Berger W, Schumacher M, Lucking CH. Dissection of the vertebral artery with cervical nerve root lesions. *J Neurol* 1996; 243(2):121–5.

44 De Bray JM, Penisson-Besnier I, Dubas F, Emile J. Extracranial and intracranial vertebrobasilar dissections:

diagnosis and prognosis. *J Neurol Neurosurg Psychiatry* 1997; **63**(1):46–51.

45 Laufs H, Weidauer S, Heller C, Lorenz M, Neumann-Haefelin T. Hemi-spinal cord infarction due to vertebral artery dissection in congenital afibrinogenemia. *Neurology* 2004; **63**(8):1522–3.

46 Arnold M, Cumurciuc R, Stapf C, Favrole P, Berthet K, Bousser MG. Pain as the only symptom of cervical artery dissection. *J Neurol Neurosurg Psychiatry* 2006; **77**(9):1021–4.

47 Mullges W, Ringelstein EB, Leibold M. Non-invasive diagnosis of internal carotid artery dissections. *J Neurol Neurosurg Psychiatry* 1992; **55**(2):98–104.

48 Auer A, Felber S, Schmidauer C, Waldenberger P, Aichner F. Magnetic resonance angiographic and clinical features of extracranial vertebral artery dissection. *J Neurol Neurosurg Psychiatry* 1998; **64**(4):474–81.

49 Touze E, Gauvrit JY, Moulin T, Meder JF, Bracard S, Mas JL. Risk of stroke and recurrent dissection after a cervical artery dissection: a multicenter study. *Neurology* 2003; **61**(10):1347–51.

50 Norris JW. Extracranial arterial dissection: anticoagulation is the treatment of choice: for. *Stroke* 2005; **36**(9):2041–2.

51 Lyrer PA. Extracranial arterial dissection: anticoagulation is the treatment of choice: against. *Stroke* 2005; **36**(9):2042–3.

52 Georgiadis D, Lanczik O, Schwab S, Engelter S, Sztajzel R, Arnold M *et al*. IV thrombolysis in patients with acute stroke due to spontaneous carotid dissection. *Neurology* 2005; **64**(9):1612–14.

53 Beletsky V, Nadareishvili Z, Lynch J, Shuaib A, Woolfenden A, Norris JW. Cervical arterial dissection: time for a therapeutic trial? *Stroke* 2003; **34**(12):2856–60.

54 Yoshimoto Y, Wakai S. Unruptured intracranial vertebral artery dissection: clinical course and serial radiographic imagings. *Stroke* 1997; **28**(2):370–4.

55 Mori K, Nakayama T, Cho K, Hirano A, Maeda M. Dissecting aneurysms limited to the basilar artery: report of two cases and review of the literature. *J Stroke Cerebrovasc Dis* 1998; **7**:213–21.

56 Chaves C, Estol C, Esnaola MM, Gorson K, O'Donoghue M, De Witt LD, Caplan LR. Spontaneous intracranial internal carotid artery dissection: report of 10 patients. *Arch Neurol* 2002; **59**(6):977–81.

57 Marushima A, Yanaka K, Okazaki M, Kojima H, Nose T. Repeated vertebral artery dissections: an autopsy case report. *Cerebrovasc Dis* 2005; **20**(1):61–5.

58 Kneyber MCJ, Rinkel GJE, Ramos LMP, Tulleken CAF, Braun KPJ. Early posttraumatic subarachnoid hemorrhage due to dissecting aneurysms in three children. *Neurology* 2005; **65**(10):1663–5.

59 Farrell MA, Gilbert JJ, Kaufmann JC. Fatal intracranial arterial dissection: clinical pathological correlation. *J Neurol Neurosurg Psychiatry* 1985; **48**(2):111–21.

60 Gerber O, Heyer EJ, Vieux U. Painless dissections of the aorta presenting as acute neurologic syndromes. *Stroke* 1986; **17**(4):644–7.

61 DeSanctis RW, Doroghazi RM, Austen WG, Buckley MJ. Aortic dissection. *N Engl J Med* 1987; **317**(17):1060–7.

62 Carrel T, Laske A, Jenny R, von Segesser L, Turina M. Neurological complications associated with acute aortic dissection: is there a place for a surgical approach? *Cerebrovasc Dis* 1991; **1**:296–301.

63 Pretre R, Von Segesser LK. Aortic dissection. *Lancet* 1997; **349**(9063):1461–4.

64 Hagan PG, Nienaber CA, Isselbacher EM, Bruckman D, Karavite DJ, Russman PL *et al*. The International Registry of Acute Aortic Dissection (IRAD): new insights into an old disease. *J Am Med Assoc* 2000; **283**(7):897–903.

65 Gaul C, Dietrich W, Friedrich I, Sirch J, Erbguth FJ. Neurological symptoms in type A aortic dissections. *Stroke* 2007; **38**(2):292–7.

66 Sigal LH. The neurologic presentation of vasculitic and rheumatologic syndromes: a review. *Medicine (Baltimore)* 1987; **66**(3):157–80.

67 Ferro JM. Vasculitis of the central nervous system. *J Neurol* 1998; **245**(12):766–76.

68 Moore PM, Richardson B. Neurology of the vasculitides and connective tissue diseases. *J Neurol Neurosurg Psychiatry* 1998; **65**(1):10–22.

69 Jennekens FGI, Kater L. *Neurology of the Inflammatory Connective Tissue Diseases*. London: Saunders, 1999.

70 Scolding NJ. *Immunological and Inflammatory Disorders of the Central Nervous System*. Oxford: Butterworth Heinemann, 1999.

71 Joseph FG, Scolding NJ. Cerebral vasculitis: a practical approach. *Pract Neurol* 2002; **2**(2):80–93.

72 Sofat N, Malik O, Higgens CS. Neurological involvement in patients with rheumatic disease. *Q J Med* 2006; **99**(2):69–79.

73 McLean BN, Miller D, Thompson EJ. Oligoclonal banding of IgG in CSF, blood–brain barrier function, and MRI findings in patients with sarcoidosis, systemic lupus erythematosus, and Behcet's disease involving the nervous system. *J Neurol Neurosurg Psychiatry* 1995; **58**(5):548–54.

74 Salvarini C, Cantini F, Boiardi L, Hunder GG. Polymyalgia rheumatica and giant cell arteritis. *N Engl J Med* 2002; **347**:261–71.

75 Caselli RJ, Hunder GG, Whisnant JP. Neurologic disease in biopsy-proven giant cell (temporal) arteritis. *Neurology* 1988; **38**(3):352–9.

76 Hayreh SS. Steroid therapy for visual loss in patients with giant-cell arteritis. *Lancet* 2000; **355**(9215):1572–3.

77 Smetana GW, Shmerling RH. Does this patient have temporal arteritis? *J Am Med Assoc* 2002; **287**(1):92–101.

78 Achkar AA, Lie JT, Hunder GG, O'Fallon WM, Gabriel SE. How does previous corticosteroid treatment affect the biopsy findings in giant cell (temporal) arteritis? *Ann Intern Med* 1994; **120**(12):987–92.

79 Staunton H, Stafford F, Leader M, O'Riordain D. Deterioration of giant cell arteritis with corticosteroid therapy. *Arch Neurol* 2000; **57**(4):581–4.

80 Jover JA, Hernandez-Garcia C, Morado IC, Vargas E, Banares A, Fernandez-Gutierrez B. Combined treatment of giant-cell arteritis with methotrexate and prednisone. a

randomized, double-blind, placebo-controlled trial. *Ann Intern Med* 2001; **134**(2):106–14.

81 Hoffman GS, Cid MC, Hellmann DB, Guillevin L, Stone JH, Schousboe J *et al.* A multicenter, randomized, double-blind, placebo-controlled trial of adjuvant methotrexate treatment for giant cell arteritis. *Arthritis Rheum* 2002; **46**(5):1309–18.

82 Lupi-Herrera E, Sanchez-Torres G, Marcushamer J, Mispireta J, Horwitz S, Vela JE. Takayasu's arteritis: clinical study of 107 cases. *Am Heart J* 1977; **93**(1):94–103.

83 Hall S, Barr W, Lie JT, Stanson AW, Kazmier FJ, Hunder GG. Takayasu arteritis: a study of 32 North American patients. *Medicine (Baltimore)* 1985; **64**(2):89–99.

84 Numano F, Kobayashi Y. Takayasu arteritis: beyond pulselessness. *Intern Med* 1999; **38**(3):226–32.

85 Numano F, Okawara M, Inomata H, Kobayashi Y. Takayasu's arteritis. *Lancet* 2000; **356**(9234):1023–5.

86 Mwipatayi BP, Jeffrey PC, Beningfield SJ, Matley PJ, Naidoo NG, Kalla AA, Del Kahn. Takayasu arteritis: clinical features and management: report of 272 cases. *ANZ J Surg* 2005; **75**:110–17.

87 Kumral E, Evyapan D, Aksu K, Keser G, Kabasakal Y, Balkir K. Microembolus detection in patients with Takayasu's arteritis. *Stroke* 2002; **33**(3):712–16.

88 Kerr GS, Hallahan CW, Giordano J, Leavitt RY, Fauci AS, Rottem M, Hoffman GS. Takayasu arteritis. *Ann Intern Med* 1994; **120**(11):919–29.

89 Mills JA. Systemic lupus erythematosus. *N Engl J Med* 1994; **330**(26):1871–9.

90 Hama N, Boumpas DT. Cerebral lupus erythematosus: diagnosis and rational drup treatment. *CNS Drugs* 1995; 3:416–26.

91 D'Cruz DP, Khamashta MA, Hughes GR. Systemic lupus erythematosus. *Lancet* 2007; **369**(9561):587–96.

92 Haas LF. Stroke as an early manifestation of systemic lupus erythematosus. *J Neurol Neurosurg Psychiatry* 1982; **45**(6):554–6.

93 Devinsky O, Petito CK, Alonso DR. Clinical and neuropathological findings in systemic lupus erythematosus: the role of vasculitis, heart emboli, and thrombotic thrombocytopenic purpura. *Ann Neurol* 1988; **23**(4):380–4.

94 Kitagawa Y, Gotoh F, Koto A, Okayasu H. Stroke in systemic lupus erythematosus. *Stroke* 1990; **21**(11):1533–9.

95 Mitsias P, Levine SR. Large cerebral vessel occlusive disease in systemic lupus erythematosus. *Neurology* 1994; **44**(3 Pt 1):385–93.

96 Roldan CA, Shively BK, Crawford MH. An echocardiographic study of valvular heart disease associated with systemic lupus erythematosus. *N Engl J Med* 1996; **335**(19):1424–30.

97 Dahl A, Omdal R, Waterloo K, Joakimsen O, Jacobsen EA, Koldingsnes W, Mellgren SI. Detection of cerebral embolic signals in patients with systemic lupus erythematosus. *J Neurol Neurosurg Psychiatry* 2006; **77**(6):774–9.

98 Asanuma Y, Oeser A, Shintani AK, Turner E, Olsen N, Fazio S *et al.* Premature coronary-artery atherosclerosis in systemic lupus erythematosus. *N Engl J Med* 2003; **349**(25):2407–15.

99 Roman MJ, Shanker BA, Davis A, Lockshin MD, Sammaritano L, Simantov R *et al.* Prevalence and correlates of accelerated atherosclerosis in systemic lupus erythematosus. *N Engl J Med* 2003; **349**(25):2399–406.

100 Khamashta MA, Cervera R, Asherson RA, Font J, Gil A, Coltart DJ *et al.* Association of antibodies against phospholipids with heart valve disease in systemic lupus erythematosus. *Lancet* 1990; **335**(8705):1541–4.

101 Ruiz-Irastorza G, Khamashta MA, Castellino G, Hughes GR. Systemic lupus erythematosus. *Lancet* 2001; **357**(9261):1027–32.

102 Flanc RS, Roberts MA, Strippoli GF, Chadban SJ, Kerr PG, Atkins RC. Treatment for lupus nephritis. *Cochrane Database Syst Rev* 2004; (1):CD002922.

103 Greaves M. Antiphospholipid antibodies and thrombosis. *Lancet* 1999; **353**(9161):1348–53.

104 Levine JS, Branch DW, Rauch J. The antiphospholipid syndrome. *N Engl J Med* 2002; **346**(10):752–63.

105 Drenkard C, Sanchez-Guerrero J, Alarcon-Segovia D. Fall in antiphospholipid antibody at time of thromboocclusive episodes in systemic lupus erythematosus. *J Rheumatol* 1989; **16**(5):614–17.

106 Tanne D, D'Olhaberriague L, Schultz LR, Salowich-Palm L, Sawaya KL, Levine SR. Anticardiolipin antibodies and their associations with cerebrovascular risk factors. *Neurology* 1999; **52**(7):1368–73.

107 Verro P, Levine SR, Tietjen GE. Cerebrovascular ischemic events with high positive anticardiolipin antibodies. *Stroke* 1998; **29**(11):2245–53.

108 Lockshin MD, Erkan D. Treatment of the antiphospholipid syndrome. *N Engl J Med* 2003; **349**(12):1177–9.

109 Lim W, Crowther MA, Eikelboom JW. Management of antiphospholipid antibody syndrome: a systematic review. *J Am Med Assoc* 2006; **295**(9):1050–7.

110 Burton JL. Livedo reticularis, porcelain-white scars, and cerebral thromboses. *Lancet* 1988; **1**(8597):1263–5.

111 Stockhammer G, Felber SR, Zelger B, Sepp N, Birbamer GG, Fritsch PO, Aichner FT. Sneddon's syndrome: diagnosis by skin biopsy and MRI in 17 patients. *Stroke* 1993; **24**(5):685–90.

112 Boortz-Marx RL, Clark HB, Taylor S, Wesa KM, Anderson DC. Sneddon's syndrome with granulomatous leptomeningeal infiltration. *Stroke* 1995; **26**(3):492–5.

113 Aquino Gondim FA, Leacock RO, Subrammanian TA, Cruz-Flores S. Intracerebral hemorrhage associated with Sneddon's syndrome: is ischemia-related angiogenesis the cause? Case report and review of the literature. *Neuroradiology* 2003; **45**(6):368–72.

114 Kalashnikova LA, Nasonov EL, Stoyanovich LZ, Kovalyov VU, Kocheleva NM, Reshetnyak TM. Sneddon's syndrome and the primary antiphospholipid syndrome. *Cerebrovasc Dis* 1994; **4**:76–82.

115 Geschwind DH, FitzPatrick M, Mischel PS, Cummings JL. Sneddon's syndrome is a thrombotic vasculopathy:

neuropathologic and neuroradiologic evidence. *Neurology* 1995; **45**(3 Pt 1):557–60.

116 Jennette JC, Falk RJ. Small-vessel vasculitis. *N Engl J Med* 1997; **337**(21):1512–23.

117 Bosch X, Guilabert A, Font J. Antineutrophil cytoplasmic antibodies. *Lancet* 2006; **368**(9533):404–18.

118 Nishino H, Rubino FA, Parisi JE. The spectrum of neurologic involvement in Wegener's granulomatosis. *Neurology* 1993; **43**(7):1334–7.

119 Sehgal M, Swanson JW, DeRemee RA, Colby TV. Neurologic manifestations of Churg-Strauss syndrome. *Mayo Clin Proc* 1995; **70**(4):337–41.

120 Reichart MD, Bogousslavsky J, Janzer RC. Early lacunar strokes complicating polyarteritis nodosa: thrombotic microangiopathy. *Neurology*; **54**(4):883–9.

121 De Groot K, Schmidt DK, Arlt AC, Gross WL, Reinhold-Keller E. Standardized neurologic evaluations of 128 patients with Wegener granulomatosis. *Arch Neurol* 2001; **58**(8):1215–21.

122 Nardone R, Lochner P, Tezzon F. Wegener's granulomatosis presenting with intracerebral hemorrhages. *Cerebrovasc Dis* 2004; **17**(1):81–2.

123 Maramattom BV, Giannini C, Manno EM, Wijdicks EF. Wegener's granulomatosis and vertebro-basilar thrombosis. *Cerebrovasc Dis* 2005; **20**(1):65–8.

124 Burns JC, Glode MP. Kawasaki syndrome. *Lancet* 2004; **364**(9433):533–44.

125 Belman AL, Leicher CR, Moshe SL, Mezey AP. Neurologic manifestations of Schoenlein-Henoch purpura: report of three cases and review of the literature. *Pediatrics* 1985; **75**(4):687–92.

126 Sokol DK, McIntyre JA, Short RA, Gutt J, Wagenknecht DR, Biller J, Garg B. Henoch-Schonlein purpura and stroke: antiphosphatidylethanolamine antibody in CSF and serum. *Neurology* 2000; **55**(9):1379–81.

127 Watson P, Fekete J, Deck J. Central nervous system vasculitis in rheumatoid arthritis. *Can J Neurol Sci* 1977; **4**(4):269–72.

128 Beck DO, Corbett JJ. Seizures due to central nervous system rheumatoid meningovasculitis. *Neurology* 1983; **33**(8):1058–61.

129 Neamtu L, Belmont M, Miller DC, Leroux P, Weinberg H, Zagzag D. Rheumatoid disease of the CNS with meningeal vasculitis presenting with a seizure. *Neurology* 2001; **56**(6):814–15.

130 Howell SJ, Molyneux AJ. Vertebrobasilar insufficiency in rheumatoid atlanto-axial subluxation: a case report with angiographic demonstration of left vertebral artery occlusion. *J Neurol* 1988; **235**(3):189–90.

131 Fox RI. Sjogren's syndrome. *Lancet* 2005; **366**(9482):321–31.

132 De la Monte SM, Hutchins GM, Gupta PK. Polymorphous meningitis with atypical mononuclear cells in Sjogren's syndrome. *Ann Neurol* 1983; **14**(4):455–61.

133 Bragoni M, Di P, V, Priori R, Valesini G, Lenzi GL. Sjogren's syndrome presenting as ischemic stroke. *Stroke* 1994; **25**(11):2276–9.

134 Li JY, Lai PH, Lam HC, Lu LY, Cheng HH, Lee JK, Lo YK. Hypertrophic cranial pachymeningitis and lymphocytic

hypophysitis in Sjogren's syndrome. *Neurology* 1999; **52**(2):420–3.

135 Lafitte C, Amoura Z, Cacoub P, Pradat-Diehl P, Picq C, Salachas F *et al.* Neurological complications of primary Sjogren's syndrome. *J Neurol* 2001; **248**(7):577–84.

136 Delalande S, de Seze J, Fauchais AL, Hachulla E, Stojkovic T, Ferriby D *et al.* Neurologic manifestations in primary Sjogren syndrome: a study of 82 patients. *Medicine (Baltimore)* 2004; **83**(5):280–91.

137 Farah S, Al-Shubaili A, Montaser A, Hussein JM, Malaviya AN, Mukhtar M *et al.* Behcet's syndrome: a report of 41 patients with emphasis on neurological manifestations. *J Neurol Neurosurg Psychiatry* 1998; **64**(3):382–4.

138 Serdaroglu P. Behcet's disease and the nervous system. *J Neurol* 1998; **245**(4):197–205.

139 Akman-Demir G, Serdaroglu P. Neuro-Behcet's disease: a practical approach to diagnosis and treatment. *Pract Neurol* 2002; **2**(6):340–7.

140 Al-Araji A, Sharquie K, Al-Rawi Z. Prevalence and patterns of neurological involvement in Behcet's disease: a prospective study from Iraq. *J Neurol Neurosurg Psychiatry* 2003; **74**(5):608–13.

141 Isaak BL, Liesegang TJ, Michet CJ, Jr. Ocular and systemic findings in relapsing polychondritis. *Ophthalmology* 1986; **93**(5):681–9.

142 Stewart SS, Ashizawa T, Dudley AW, Jr., Goldberg JW, Lidsky MD. Cerebral vasculitis in relapsing polychondritis. *Neurology* 1988; **38**(1):150–2.

143 Ragnaud JM, Tahbaz A, Morlat P, Sire S, Gin H, Aubertin J. Recurrent aseptic purulent meningitis in a patient with relapsing polychondritis. *Clin Infect Dis* 1996; **22**(2):374–5.

144 Kothare SV, Chu CC, VanLandingham K, Richards KC, Hosford DA, Radtke RA. Migratory leptomeningeal inflammation with relapsing polychondritis. *Neurology* 1998; **51**(2):614–17.

145 Irani SR, Soni A, Beynon H, Athwal BS. Relapsing 'encephalo' polychondritis. *Pract Neurol* 2006; **6**(6):372–5.

146 Hietaharju A, Jaaskelainen S, Hietarinta M, Frey H. Central nervous system involvement and psychiatric manifestations in systemic sclerosis (scleroderma): clinical and neurophysiological evaluation. *Acta Neurol Scand* 1993; **87**(5):382–7.

147 Heron E, Fornes P, Rance A, Emmerich J, Bayle O, Fiessinger JN. Brain involvement in scleroderma: two autopsy cases. *Stroke* 1998; **29**(3):719–21.

148 Stone J, Franks AJ, Guthrie JA, Johnson MH. Scleroderma 'en coup de sabre': pathological evidence of intracerebral inflammation. *J Neurol Neurosurg Psychiatry* 2001; **70**(3):382–5.

149 Gorevic PD, Kassab HJ, Levo Y, Kohn R, Meltzer M, Prose P, Franklin EC. Mixed cryoglobulinemia: clinical aspects and long-term follow-up of 40 patients. *Am J Med* 1980; **69**(2):287–308.

150 Monti G, Galli M, Invernizzi F, Pioltelli P, Saccardo F, Monteverde A *et al.* Cryoglobulinaemias: a multi-centre study of the early clinical and laboratory manifestations of primary and secondary disease. GISC. Italian Group

for the Study of Cryoglobulinaemias. *Q J Med* 1995; **88**(2):115–26.

151 Ince PG, Duffey P, Cochrane HR, Lowe J, Shaw PJ. Relapsing ischemic encephaloenteropathy and cryoglobulinemia. *Neurology* 2000; 55(10):1579–81.

152 Subbiah P, Wijdicks E, Muenter M, Carter J, Connolly S. Skin lesion with a fatal neurologic outcome (Degos' disease). *Neurology* 1996; **46**(3):636–40.

153 Amato C, Ferri R, Elia M, Cosentino F, Schepis C, Siragusa M, Moschini M. Nervous system involvement in Degos disease. *Am J Neuroradiol* 2005; **26**(3):646–9.

154 Nowak DA, Widenka DC. Neurosarcoidosis: a review of its intracranial manifestation. *J Neurol* 2001; **248**(5):363–72.

155 Baughman RP, Lower EE, du Bois RM. Sarcoidosis. *Lancet* 2003; **361**(9363):1111–18.

156 Hoitsma E, Faber CG, Drent M, Sharma OP. Neurosarcoidosis: a clinical dilemma. *Lancet Neurol* 2004; **3**(7):397–407.

157 Sethi KD, el Gammal T, Patel BR, Swift TR. Dural sarcoidosis presenting with transient neurologic symptoms. *Arch Neurol* 1986; **43**(6):595–7.

158 Zadra M, Brambilla A, Erli LC, Grandi R, Finazzi G. Neurosarcoidosis, stroke and antiphospholipid antibodies: a case report. *Eur J Neurol* 1996; **3**:146–8.

159 Libman RB, Sharfstein S, Harrington W, Lerner P. Recurrent intracerebral haemorrhage from sarcoid angiitis. *J Stroke Cerebrovasc Dis* 1997: **6**:373–5.

160 Kobylecki C, Shaunak S. A difficult case: refractory neurosarcoidosis responding to infliximab. *Pract Neurol* 2007; **7**(2):112–15.

161 Hankey GJ. Isolated angiitis/angiopathy of the central nervous system. *Cerebrovasc Dis* 1991; **1**:2–15.

162 Delobel P, Brassat D, Danjoux M, Lotterie JA, Irsutti-Fjortoft M, Clanet M, Laurent G. Granulomatous angiitis of the central nervous system revealing Hodgkin's disease. *J Neurol* 2004; **251**(5):611–12.

163 Scolding NJ, Joseph F, Kirby PA, Mazanti I, Gray F, Mikol J *et al.* Abeta-related angiitis: primary angiitis of the central nervous system associated with cerebral amyloid angiopathy. *Brain* 2005; **128**(Pt 3):500–15.

164 Vollmer TL, Guarnaccia J, Harrington W, Pacia SV, Petroff OA. Idiopathic granulomatous angiitis of the central nervous system: diagnostic challenges. *Arch Neurol* 1993; 5B0(9):925–30.

165 Lanthier S, Lortie A, Michaud J, Laxer R, Jay V, deVeber G. Isolated angiitis of the CNS in children. *Neurology* 2001; **56**(7):837–42.

166 Hunn M, Robinson S, Wakefield L, Mossman S, Abernethy D. Granulomatous angiitis of the CNS causing spontaneous intracerebral haemorrhage: the importance of leptomeningeal biopsy. *J Neurol Neurosurg Psychiatry* 1998; **65**(6):956–7.

167 Alrawi A, Trobe JD, Blaivas M, Musch DC. Brain biopsy in primary angiitis of the central nervous system. *Neurology* 1999; **53**(4):858–60.

168 Woolfenden AR, Tong DC, Marks MP, Ali AO, Albers GW. Angiographically defined primary angiitis of the CNS: is it really benign? *Neurology* 1998; **51**(1):183–8.

169 Call GK, Fleming MC, Scalfon S, Levine H, Kistler JP, Fisher CM. Reversible cerebral segmental vasoconstriction. *Stroke* 1988; **19**(9):1159–70.

170 Miteff F, Anderson N, Snow B. Idiopathic reversible segmental cerebral vasoconstriction. *Pract Neurol* 2006; **6**(6):382–3.

171 Olin JW. Thromboangiitis obliterans (Buerger's disease). *N Engl J Med* 2000; **343**(12):864–9.

172 Biller J, Asconape J, Challa VR, Toole JF, McLean WT. A case for cerebral thromboangiitis obliterans. *Stroke* 1981; **12**(5):686–9.

173 Drake ME, Jr. Winiwarter-Buerger disease ('thromboangiitis obliterans') with cerebral involvement. *J Am Med Assoc* 1982; **248**(15):1870–2.

174 Bischof F, Kuntz R, Melms A, Fetter M. Cerebral vein thrombosis in a case with thromboangiitis obliterans. *Cerebrovasc Dis* 1999; **9**(5):295–7.

175 Larner AJ, Kidd D, Elkington P, Rudge P, Scaravilli F. Spatz-Lindenberg disease: a rare cause of vascular dementia. *Stroke* 1999; **30**(3):687–9.

176 Wooten MD, Jasin HE. Vasculitis and lymphoproliferative diseases. *Semin Arthritis Rheum* 1996; **26**(2):564–74.

177 Fortin PR. Vasculitides associated with malignancy. *Curr Opin Rheumatol* 1996; **8**(1):30–3.

178 Steinmetz JC, DeConti R, Ginsburg R. Hypersensitivity vasculitis associated with 2-deoxycoformycin and allopurinol therapy. *Am J Med* 1989; **86**(4):498–9.

179 Al KA, Wang DZ, Kishore K, Kattah JC. A case of ischemic cerebral infarction associated with acute posterior multifocal placoid pigment epitheliopathy, CNS vasculitis, vitamin B(12) deficiency and homocysteinemia. *Cerebrovasc Dis* 2004; **18**(4):338–9.

180 Fialho D, Holmes P, Riordan-Eva P, Silber E. A blinding headache falling on deaf ears (Susac's syndrome). *Pract Neurol* 2002; **2**(6):358–61.

181 Gross M, Eliashar R. Update on Susac's syndrome. *Curr Opin Neurol* 2005; **18**(3):311–14.

182 Herson RN, Squier M. Retinal perivasculitis with neurological involvement: a case report with pathological findings. *J Neurol Sci* 1978; **36**(1):111–17.

183 Gordon MF, Coyle PK, Golub B. Eales' disease presenting as stroke in the young adult. *Ann Neurol* 1988; **24**(2):264–6.

184 Lunardi C, Bason C, Leandri M, Navone R, Lestani M, Millo E *et al.* Autoantibodies to inner ear and endothelial antigens in Cogan's syndrome. *Lancet* 2002; **360**(9337):915–21.

185 Vollertsen RS, McDonald TJ, Younge BR, Banks PM, Stanson AW, Ilstrup DM. Cogan's syndrome: 18 cases and a review of the literature. *Mayo Clin Proc* 1986; **61**(5):344–61.

186 Grasland A, Pouchot J, Hachulla E, Bletry O, Papo T, Vinceneux P. Typical and atypical Cogan's syndrome: 32 cases and review of the literature. *Rheumatology (Oxford)* 2004; **43**(8):1007–15.

187 Chabriat H, Tournier-Lasserve E, Bousser MG. Vasculopathies. In: Alberts MJ, ed. *Genetics of Cerebrovascular Disease*. New York: Futura, 1999, pp. 195–208.

188 Leary MC, Finley A, Caplan LR. Cerebrovascular complications of fibromuscular dysplasia. *Curr Treat Options Cardiovasc Med* 2004; **6**(3):237–48.

189 Slovut DP, Olin JW. Fibromuscular dysplasia. *N Engl J Med* 2004; **350**(18):1862–71.

190 Kubis N, Von Langsdorff D, Petitjean C, Brouland JP, Guichard JP, Chapot R *et al.* Thrombotic carotid megabulb: fibromuscular dysplasia, septae, and ischemic stroke. *Neurology* 1999; **52**(4):883–6.

191 Schlenska GK. Absence of both internal carotid arteries. *J Neurol* 1986; **233**(5):263–6.

192 Kubis N, Zuber M, Meder JF, Mas JL. CT scan of the skull base in internal carotid artery hypoplasia. *Cerebrovasc Dis* 1996; **6**:40–4.

193 Perren F, Poglia D, Landis T, Sztajzel R. Vertebral artery hypoplasia: a predisposing factor for posterior circulation stroke? *Neurology* 2007; **68**(1):65–7.

194 Sarkari NBS, Macdonald Holmes J, Bickerstaff ER. Neurological manifestations associated with internal carotid loops and kinks in children. *J Neurol Neurosurg Psychiatry* 1970; **33**:194–200.

195 Desai B, Toole JF. Kinks, coils, and carotids: a review. *Stroke* 1975; **6**(6):649–53.

196 Barbour PJ, Castaldo JE, Rae-Grant AD, Gee W, Reed JF, III, Jenny D, Longennecker J. Internal carotid artery redundancy is significantly associated with dissection. *Stroke* 1994; **25**(6):1201–6.

197 Metz H, Murray-Leslie RM, Bannister RG, Bull JW, Marshall J. Kinking of the internal carotid artery. *Lancet* 1961; **1**:424–6.

198 Bruno A, Adams HP, Jr., Biller J, Rezai K, Cornell S, Aschenbrener CA. Cerebral infarction due to moyamoya disease in young adults. *Stroke* 1988; **19**(7):826–33.

199 Chen ST, Liu YH, Hsu CY, Hogan EL, Ryu SJ. Moyamoya disease in Taiwan. *Stroke* 1988; **19**(1):53–9.

200 Kuroda S, Ishikawa T, Houkin K, Nanba R, Hokari M, Iwasaki Y. Incidence and clinical features of disease progression in adult moyamoya disease. *Stroke* 2005; **36**(10):2148–53.

201 Herreman F, Nathal E, Yasui N, Yonekawa Y. Intracranial aneurysms in Moyamoya disease: report of ten cases and review of the literature. *Cerebrovasc Dis* 1994; **4**:329–36.

202 Kitahara T, Ariga N, Yamaura A, Makino H, Maki Y. Familial occurrence of moya-moya disease: report of three Japanese families. *J Neurol Neurosurg Psychiatry* 1979; **42**(3):208–14.

203 Mineharu Y, Takenaka K, Yamakawa H, Inoue K, Ikeda H, Kikuta KI *et al.* Inheritance pattern of familial moyamoya disease: autosomal dominant mode and genomic imprinting. *J Neurol Neurosurg Psychiatry* 2006; **77**(9):1025–9.

204 Ikeda E. Systemic vascular changes in spontaneous occlusion of the circle of Willis. *Stroke* 1991; **22**(11):1358–62.

205 Aoyagi M, Fukai N, Yamamoto M, Nakagawa K, Matsushima Y, Yamamoto K. Early development of intimal thickening in superficial temporal arteries in patients with moyamoya disease. *Stroke* 1996; **27**(10):1750–4.

206 Cramer SC, Robertson RL, Dooling EC, Scott RM. Moyamoya and Down syndrome: clinical and radiological features. *Stroke* 1996; **27**(11):2131–5.

207 Iwama T, Hashimoto N, Murai BN, Tsukahara T, Yonekawa Y. Intracranial rebleeding in moyamoya disease. *J Clin Neurosci* 1997; **4**(2):169–72.

208 Chiu D, Shedden P, Bratina P, Grotta JC. Clinical features of moyamoya disease in the United States. *Stroke* 1998; **29**(7):1347–51.

209 Yilmaz EY, Pritz MB, Bruno A, Lopez-Yunez A, Biller J. Moyamoya: Indiana University Medical Center experience. *Arch Neurol* 2001; **58**(8):1274–8.

210 Steinberger A, Ganti SR, McMurtry JG, III, Hilal SK. Transient neurological deficits secondary to saccular vertebrobasilar aneurysms: report of two cases. *J Neurosurg* 1984; **60**(2):410–3.

211 Brownlee RD, Tranmer BI, Sevick RJ, Karmy G, Curry BJ. Spontaneous thrombosis of an unruptured anterior communicating artery aneurysm: an unusual cause of ischemic stroke. *Stroke* 1995; **26**(10):1945–9.

213 Nesbit RR, Jr., Neistadt A, May AG. Bilateral internal carotid artery aneurysms. *Arch Surg* 1979; **114**(3):293–5.

214 Mokri B, Piepgras DG. Cervical internal carotid artery aneurysm with calcific embolism to the retina. *Neurology* 1981; **31**(2):211–14.

215 Catala M, Rancurel G, Koskas F, Martin-Dealassalle E, Kiefer E. Ischaemic stroke due to spontaneous extracranial vertebral giant aneurysm. *Cerebrovasc Dis* 1993; **3**:322–6.

216 Dubard T, Pouchot J, Lamy C, Hier DB, Caplan L, Mas JL. Upper limb peripheral motor deficits due to extracranial vertebral artery dissection. *Cerebrovasc Dis* 1994; **4**:88–91.

217 Fine MJ, Kapoor W, Falanga V. Cholesterol crystal embolization: a review of 221 cases in the English literature. *Angiology* 1987; **38**(10):769–84.

218 Orr WP, Banning AP. Aortic atherosclerotic debris detected by trans-oesophageal echocardiography: a risk factor for cholesterol embolization. *Q J Med* 1999; **92**(6):341–6.

219 Cuddy E, Robertson S, Cross S, Isles C. Risks of coronary angiography. *Lancet* 2005; **366**(9499):1825.

220 Blankenship JC, Butler M, Garbes A. Prospective assessment of cholesterol embolization in patients with acute myocardial infarction treated with thrombolytic vs conservative therapy. *Chest* 1995; **107**(3):662–8.

221 Coppeto JR, Lessell S, Lessell IM, Greco TP, Eisenberg MS. Diffuse disseminated atheroembolism: three cases with neuro-ophthalmic manifestation. *Arch Ophthalmol* 1984; **102**(2):225–8.

222 Cosio FG, Zager RA, Sharma HM. Atheroembolic renal disease causes hypocomplementaemia. *Lancet* 1985; **2**(8447):118–21.

223 Cross SS. How common is cholesterol embolism? *J Clin Pathol* 1991; **44**(10):859–61.

224 Rhodes JM. Cholesterol crystal embolism: an important 'new' diagnosis for the general physician. *Lancet* 1996; **347**(9016):1641.

225 Elinav E, Chajek-Shaul T, Stern M. Improvement in cholesterol emboli syndrome after iloprost therapy. *Br Med J* 2002; **324**(7332):268–9.

226 Olesen J, Friberg L, Olsen TS, Andersen AR, Lassen NA, Hansen PE, Karle A. Ischaemia-induced (symptomatic) migraine attacks may be more frequent than migraine-induced ischaemic insults. *Brain* 1993; **116**(Pt 1):187–202.

227 Shuaib A. Stroke from other etiologies masquerading as migraine-stroke. *Stroke* 1991; **22**(8):1068–74.

228 Bousser MG, Welch KM. Relation between migraine and stroke. *Lancet Neurol* 2005; **4**(9):533–42.

229 Winterkorn JM, Kupersmith MJ, Wirtschafter JD, Forman S. Brief report: treatment of vasospastic amaurosis fugax with calcium-channel blockers. *N Engl J Med* 1993; **329**(6):396–8.

230 Yokoyama H, Yoneda M, Abe M, Sakai T, Sagoh T, Adachi Y, Kondo T. Internal carotid artery vasospasm syndrome: demonstration by neuroimaging. *J Neurol Neurosurg Psychiatry* 2006; **77**(7):888–9.

231 Janzarik WG, Ringleb PA, Reinhard M, Rauer S. Recurrent extracranial carotid artery vasospasms: report of 2 cases. *Stroke* 2006; **37**(8):2170–3.

232 Etminan M, Takkouche B, Isorna FC, Samii A. Risk of ischaemic stroke in people with migraine: systematic review and meta-analysis of observational studies. *Br Med J* 2005; **330**(7482):63.

233 Kurth T, Slomke MA, Kase CS, Cook NR, Lee IM, Gaziano JM *et al*. Migraine, headache, and the risk of stroke in women: a prospective study. *Neurology* 2005; **64**(6):1020–6.

234 Kurth T, Gaziano JM, Cook NR, Logroscino G, Diener HC, Buring JE. Migraine and risk of cardiovascular disease in women. *J Am Med Assoc* 2006; **296**(3):283–91.

235 Sternfeld B, Stang P, Sidney S. Relationship of migraine headaches to experience of chest pain and subsequent risk for myocardial infarction. *Neurology* 1995; **45**(12):2135–42.

236 Anzola GP, Morandi E, Casilli F, Onorato E. Different degrees of right-to-left shunting predict migraine and stroke: data from 420 patients. *Neurology* 2006; **66**(5):765–7.

237 Scher AI, Terwindt GM, Picavet HS, Verschuren WM, Ferrari MD, Launer LJ. Cardiovascular risk factors and migraine: the GEM population-based study. *Neurology* 2005; **64**(4):614–20.

238 Davies-Jones GAB. Neurological manifestations of haematological disorders. In: Aminoff MJ, ed. *Neurology and General Medicine*. New York: Churchill Livingstone, 1995; 219.

239 Markus HS, Hambley H. Neurology and the blood: haematological abnormalities in ischaemic stroke. *J Neurol Neurosurg Psychiatry* 1998; **64**(2):150–9.

240 Silverstein A, Gilbert H, Wasserman LR. Neurologic complications of polycythemia. *Ann Intern Med* 1962; **57**:909–16.

241 Wetherley-Mein G, Pearson TC, Burney PG, Morris RW. Polycythaemia study. A project of the Royal College of Physicians Research Unit. 1. Objectives, background and design. *J R Coll Physicians Lond* 1987; **21**(1):7–16.

242 Landolfi R, Marchioli R, Kutti J, Gisslinger H, Tognoni G, Patrono C, Barbui T. Efficacy and safety of low-dose aspirin in polycythemia vera. *N Engl J Med* 2004; **350**(2):114–24.

243 Harrison CN, Linch DC, Machin SJ. Desirability and problems of early diagnosis of essential thrombocythaemia. *Lancet* 1998; **351**(9106):846–7.

244 Bazzan M, Tamponi G, Schinco P, Vaccarino A, Foli C, Gallone G, Pileri A. Thrombosis-free survival and life expectancy in 187 consecutive patients with essential thrombocythemia. *Ann Hematol* 1999; **78**(12):539–43.

245 Preston FE, Martin JF, Stewart RM, Davies-Jones GA. Thrombocytosis, circulating platelet aggregates, and neurological dysfunction. *Br Med J* 1979; **2**(6204):1561–3.

246 Murphy MF, Clarke CR, Brearley RL. Superior sagittal sinus thrombosis and essential thrombocythaemia. *Br Med J (Clin Res Ed)* 1983; **287**(6402):1344.

247 Michiels JJ, Koudstaal PJ, Mulder AH, van Vliet HH. Transient neurologic and ocular manifestations in primary thrombocythemia. *Neurology* 1993; **43**(6):1107–10.

248 Arboix A, Besses C, Acin P, Massons JB, Florensa L, Oliveres M, Sans-Sabrafen J. Ischemic stroke as first manifestation of essential thrombocythemia: report of six cases. *Stroke* 1995; **26**(8):1463–6.

249 Sheth KJ, Swick HM, Haworth N. Neurological involvement in hemolytic-uremic syndrome. *Ann Neurol* 1986; **19**(1):90–3.

250 Moake JL. Thrombotic microangiopathies. *N Engl J Med* 2002; **347**(8):589–600.

251 Franchini M, Zaffanello M, Veneri D. Advances in the pathogenesis, diagnosis and treatment of thrombotic thrombocytopenic purpura and hemolytic uremic syndrome. *Thromb Res* 2006; **118**(2):177–84.

252 George JN. Clinical practice: thrombotic thrombocytopenic purpura. *N Engl J Med* 2006; **354**(18):1927–35.

253 Kelly PJ, McDonald CT, Neill GO, Thomas C, Niles J, Rordorf G. Middle cerebral artery main stem thrombosis in two siblings with familial thrombotic thrombocytopenic purpura. *Neurology* 1998; **50**(4):1157–60.

254 Oberlander DA, Biller J, McCarthy LJ. Thrombotic thrombocytopenic purpura: a neurological perspective. *J Stroke Cerebrovasc Dis* 1995; **5**:175–9.

255 Garrett WT, Chang CW, Bleck TP. Altered mental status in thrombotic thrombocytopenic purpura is secondary to nonconvulsive status epilepticus. *Ann Neurol* 1996; **40**(2):245–6.

256 Scheid R, Hegenbart U, Ballaschke O, Von Cramon DY. Major stroke in thrombotic-thrombocytopenic purpura (Moschcowitz syndrome). *Cerebrovasc Dis* 2004; **18**(1):83–5.

257 Bakshi R, Shaikh ZA, Bates VE, Kinkel PR. Thrombotic thrombocytopenic purpura: brain CT and MRI findings in 12 patients. *Neurology* 1999; **52**(6):1285–8.

258 Graus F, Rogers LR, Posner JB. Cerebrovascular complications in patients with cancer. *Medicine (Baltimore)* 1985; **64**(1):16–35.

259 Glass J, Hochberg FH, Miller DC. Intravascular lymphomatosis. A systemic disease with neurologic manifestations. *Cancer* 1993; **71**(10):3156–64.

260 Chapin JE, Davis LE, Kornfeld M, Mandler RN. Neurologic manifestations of intravascular lymphomatosis. *Acta Neurol Scand* 1995; **91**(6):494–9.

261 Al-Shahi R, Warlow CP, Jansen GH, Frijns CJ, van Gijn J. A 59-year-old man with progressive spinal cord and peripheral nerve dysfunction culminating in encephalopathy: Edinburgh advanced clinical neurology course, 1999. *J Neurol Neurosurg Psychiatry* 2001; **71**(5):696–703.

262 Beristain X, Azzarelli B. The neurological masquerade of intravascular lymphomatosis. *Arch Neurol* 2002; **59**(3):439–43.

263 Liebow AA. The J. Burns Amberson lecture: pulmonary angiitis and granulomatosis. *Am Rev Respir Dis* 1973; **108**(1):1–18.

264 Patton WF, Lynch JP, III. Lymphomatoid granulomatosis: clinicopathologic study of four cases and literature review. *Medicine (Baltimore)* 1982; **61**(1):1–12.

265 Schmidt BJ, Meagher-Villemure K, Del CJ. Lymphomatoid granulomatosis with isolated involvement of the brain. *Ann Neurol* 1984; **15**(5):478–81.

266 Siekert RG, Whisnant JP, Millikan CH. Anaemia and intermittent focal cerebral arterial insufficiency. *Archives of Neurology* 1960; **3**:386–90.

267 Shahar A, Sadeh M. Severe anemia associated with transient neurological deficits. *Stroke* 1991; **22**(9):1201–2.

268 Belman AL, Roque CT, Ancona R, Anand AK, Davis RP. Cerebral venous thrombosis in a child with iron deficiency anemia and thrombocytosis. *Stroke* 1990; **21**(3):488–93.

269 Saxena VK, Brands C, Crols R, Moens E, Marien P, De Deyn PP. Multiple cerebral infarctions in a young patient with secondary thrombocythemia due to iron deficiency anemia. *Acta Neurol (Napoli)* 1993; **15**(4):297–302.

270 Akins PT, Glenn S, Nemeth PM, Derdeyn CP. Carotid artery thrombus associated with severe iron-deficiency anemia and thrombocytosis. *Stroke* 1996; **27**(5):1002–5.

271 Adams RJ, Nichols FT, McKie V, McKie K, Milner P, Gammal TE. Cerebral infarction in sickle cell anemia: mechanism based on CT and MRI. *Neurology* 1988; **38**(7):1012–17.

272 DeBaun MR, Schatz J, Siegel MJ, Koby M, Craft S, Resar L *et al.* Cognitive screening examinations for silent cerebral infarcts in sickle cell disease. *Neurology* 1998; **50**(6):1678–82.

273 Prengler M, Pavlakis SG, Prohovnik I, Adams RJ. Sickle cell disease: the neurological complications. *Ann Neurol* 2002; **51**(5):543–52.

274 Steen RG, Xiong X, Langston JW, Helton KJ. Brain injury in children with sickle cell disease: prevalence and etiology. *Ann Neurol* 2003; **54**(5):564–72.

275 Switzer JA, Hess DC, Nichols FT, Adams RJ. Pathophysiology and treatment of stroke in sickle-cell disease: present and future. *Lancet Neurol* 2006; **5**(6):501–12.

276 Greenberg J, Massey EW. Cerebral infarction in sickle cell trait. *Ann Neurol* 1985; **18**(3):354–5.

277 Feldenzer JA, Bueche MJ, Venes JL, Gebarski SS. Superior sagittal sinus thrombosis with infarction in sickle cell trait. *Stroke* 1987; **18**(3):656–60.

278 Stuart MJ, Nagel RL. Sickle-cell disease. *Lancet* 2004; **364**(9442):1343–60.

279 Rothman SM, Fulling KH, Nelson JS. Sickle cell anemia and central nervous system infarction: a neuropathological study. *Ann Neurol* 1986; **20**(6):684–90.

280 Adams RJ, McKie VC, Carl EM, Nichols FT, Perry R, Brock K *et al.* Long-term stroke risk in children with sickle cell disease screened with transcranial Doppler. *Ann Neurol* 1997; **42**(5):699–704.

281 Adams RJ, Brambilla D. Discontinuing prophylactic transfusions used to prevent stroke in sickle cell disease. *N Engl J Med* 2005; **353**(26):2769–78.

282 Fabian RH, Peters BH. Neurological complications of hemoglobin SC disease. *Arch Neurol* 1984; **41**(3):289–92.

283 Singh R, Venketasubramanian N. Recurrent cerebral infarction in beta thalassaemia major. *Cerebrovasc Dis* 2004; **17**(4):344–5.

284 Al-Hakim M, Katirji B, Osorio I, Weisman R. Cerebral venous thrombosis in paroxysmal nocturnal hemoglobinuria: report of two cases. *Neurology* 1993; **43**(4):742–6.

285 Socie G, Mary JY, de Gramont A, Rio B, Leporrier M, Rose C *et al.* Paroxysmal nocturnal haemoglobinuria: long-term follow-up and prognostic factors. French Society of Haematology. *Lancet* 1996; **348**(9027):573–7.

286 Scheithauer BW, Rubinstein LJ, Herman MM. Leukoencephalopathy in Waldenstrom's macroglobulinemia. Immunohistochemical and electron microscopic observations. *J Neuropathol Exp Neurol* 1984; **43**(4):408–25.

287 Steck AJ. Neurological manifestations of malignant and non-malignant dysglobulinaemias. *J Neurol* 1998; **245**(10):634–9.

288 Kang K, Chu K, Kim DE, Jeong SW, Lee JW, Roh JK. POEMS syndrome associated with ischemic stroke. *Arch Neurol* 2003; **60**(5):745–9.

289 Caswell R, Warner T, Mehta A, Ginsberg L. POEMS syndrome. *Pract Neurol* 2006; **6**(2):111–16.

290 Preston FE, Cooke KB, Foster ME, Winfield DA, Lee D. Myelomatosis and the hyperviscosity syndrome. *Br J Haematol* 1978; **38**(4):517–30.

291 Munts AG, van Genderen PJ, Dippel DW, van Kooten F, Koudstaal PJ. Coagulation disorders in young adults with acute cerebral ischaemia. *J Neurol* 1998; **245**(1):21–5.

292 Ortel TL. Genetics of coagulation disorders. In: Alberts MJ, ed. *Genetics of Cerebrovascular Disease*. New York: Futura, 1999; 129–56.

293 Grieves M. Thrombophilia. *Pract Neurol* 2002; **3**:161–7.

294 McQuillan AM, Eikelboom JW, Hankey GJ, Baker R, Thom J, Staton J *et al.* Protein Z in ischemic stroke and its etiologic subtypes. *Stroke* 2003; **34**(10):2415–19.

295 Hankey GJ, Eikelboom JW, van Bockxmeer FM, Lofthouse E, Staples N, Baker RI. Inherited thrombophilia in ischemic stroke and its pathogenic subtypes. *Stroke* 2001; **32**(8):1793–9.

296 Lau SO, Bock GH, Edson JR, Michael AF. Sagittal sinus thrombosis in the nephrotic syndrome. *J Pediatr* 1980; **97**(6):948–50.

297 Chaturvedi S. Fulminant cerebral infarctions with membranous nephropathy. *Stroke* 1993; **24**(3):473–5.

298 Pohl C, Harbrecht U, Greinacher A, Theuerkauf I, Biniek R, Hanfland P, Klockgether T. Neurologic complications in immune-mediated heparin-induced thrombocytopenia. *Neurology* 2000; **54**(6):1240–5.

299 Pohl C, Klockgether T, Greinacher A, Hanfland P, Harbrecht U. Neurological complications in heparin-induced thrombocytopenia. *Lancet* 1999; **353**(9165):1678–9.

300 Chong BH. Heparin-induced thrombocytopenia. *J Thromb Haemost* 2003; **1**(7):1471–8.

301 Grunwald Z, Sather SD. Intraoperative cerebral infarction after desmopressin administration in infant with end-stage renal disease. *Lancet* 1995; **345**(8961):1364–5.

302 Reinhart WH, Berchtold PE. Effect of high-dose intravenous immunoglobulin therapy on blood rheology. *Lancet* 1992; **339**(8794):662–4.

303 Velioglu SK, Ozmenoglu M, Boz C. Cerebral infarction following intravenous immunoglobulin therapy for Guillain-Barre syndrome. *J Stroke Cerebrovasc Dis* 2001; **10**:290–2.

304 Paran D, Herishanu Y, Elkayam O, Shopin L, Ben-Ami R. Venous and arterial thrombosis following administration of intravenous immunoglobulins. *Blood Coagul Fibrinolysis* 2005; **16**(5):313–18.

305 Jaillard AS, Hommel M, Mallaret M. Venous sinus thrombosis associated with androgens in a healthy young man. *Stroke* 1994; **25**(1):212–13.

306 Weaver DF, Heffernan LP, Purdy RA, Ing VW. Eosinophil-induced neurotoxicity: axonal neuropathy, cerebral infarction, and dementia. *Neurology* 1988; **38**(1):144–6.

307 Kwon SU, Kim JC, Kim JS. Sequential magnetic resonance imaging findings in hypereosinophilia-induced encephalopathy. *J Neurol* 2001; **248**(4):279–84.

308 Achiron A, Gornish M, Melamed E. Cerebral sinus thrombosis as a potential hazard of antifibrinolytic treatment in menorrhagia. *Stroke* 1990; **21**(5):817–19.

309 Finelli PF, Carley MD. Cerebral venous thrombosis associated with epoetin alfa therapy. *Arch Neurol* 2000; **57**(2):260–2.

310 Lage JM, Panizo C, Masdeu J, Rocha E. Cyclist's doping associated with cerebral sinus thrombosis. *Neurology* 2002; **58**(4):665.

311 Bashir R, Jinkins J. Cerebral infarction in a young female following snake bite. *Stroke* 1985; **16**(2):328–30.

312 Rai M, Shukla RC, Varma DN, Bajpai HS, Gupta SK. Intracerebral hemorrhage following scorpion bite. *Neurology* 1990; **40**(11):1801.

313 Polo JM, varez de AA, Cid C, Berciano J. Aphasia in a farmer following viper bite. *Lancet* 2002; **359**(9324):2164.

314 Bartholdi D, Selic C, Meier J, Jung HH. Viper snakebite causing symptomatic intracerebral haemorrhage. *J Neurol* 2004; **251**(7):889–91.

315 Crawley F, Schon F, Brown MM. Cerebral infarction: a rare complication of wasp sting. *J Neurol Neurosurg Psychiatry* 1999; **66**(4):550–1.

316 Schwartzman RJ, Hill JB. Neurologic complications of disseminated intravascular coagulation. *Neurology* 1982; **32**(8):791–7.

317 Levi M, Ten CH. Disseminated intravascular coagulation. *N Engl J Med* 1999; **341**(8):586–92.

318 Toh CH, Dennis M. Disseminated intravascular coagulation: old disease, new hope. *Br Med J* 2003; **327**(7421):974–7.

319 Dutta M, Hanna E, Das P, Steinhubl SR. Incidence and prevention of ischemic stroke following myocardial infarction: review of current literature. *Cerebrovasc Dis* 2006; **22**(5–6):331–9.

320 Sloan MA, Gore JM. Ischemic stroke and intracranial hemorrhage following thrombolytic therapy for acute myocardial infarction: a risk–benefit analysis. *Am J Cardiol* 1992; **69**(2):21A–38A.

321 Vaitkus PT, Barnathan ES. Embolic potential, prevention and management of mural thrombus complicating anterior myocardial infarction: a meta-analysis. *J Am Coll Cardiol* 1993; **22**(4):1004–9.

322 Witt BJ, Brown RD, Jr., Jacobsen SJ, Weston SA, Yawn BP, Roger VL. A community-based study of stroke incidence after myocardial infarction. *Ann Intern Med* 2005; **143**(11):785–92.

323 Nadareishvili ZG, Choudary Z, Joyner C, Brodie D, Norris JW. Cerebral microembolism in acute myocardial infarction. *Stroke* 1999; **30**(12):2679–82.

324 Khatri P, Kasner SE. Ischemic strokes after cardiac catheterization: opportune thrombolysis candidates? *Arch Neurol* 2006; **63**(6):817–21.

325 Fibrinolytic Therapy Trialists' (FTT) Collaborative Group. Indications for fibrinolytic therapy in suspected acute myocardial infarction: collaborative overview of early mortality and major morbidity results from all randomised trials of more than 1000 patients. *Lancet* 1994; **343**(8893):311–22.

326 Mooe T, Eriksson P, Stegmayr B. Ischemic stroke after acute myocardial infarction. A population-based study. *Stroke* 1997; **28**(4):762–7.

327 Sloan MA, Price TR, Terrin ML, Forman S, Gore JM, Chaitman BR *et al*. Ischemic cerebral infarction after rt-PA and heparin therapy for acute myocardial infarction. The TIMI-II pilot and randomized clinical trial combined experience. *Stroke* 1997; **28**(6):1107–14.

328 Cronin L, Mehta SR, Zhao F, Pogue J, Budaj A, Hunt D, Yusuf S. Stroke in relation to cardiac procedures in patients with non-ST-elevation acute coronary syndrome: a study involving >18 000 patients. *Circulation* 2001; **104**(3):269–74.

329 Chin PL, Kaminski J, Rout M. Myocardial infarction coincident with cerebrovascular accidents in the elderly. *Age Ageing* 1977; **6**(1):29–37.

330 Von Arbin M, Britton M, de Faire U, Helmers C, Miah K, Murray V. Myocardial infarction in patients with acute cerebrovascular disease. *Eur Heart J* 1982; **3**(2):136–41.

331 Tanne D, Goldbourt U, Zion M, Reicher-Reiss H, Kaplinsky E, Behar S. Frequency and prognosis of stroke/TIA among 4808 survivors of acute myocardial infarction. The SPRINT Study Group. *Stroke* 1993; **24**(10):1490–5.

332 Bodenheimer MM, Sauer D, Shareef B, Brown MW, Fleiss JL, Moss AJ. Relation between myocardial infarct location and stroke. *J Am Coll Cardiol* 1994; **24**(1):61–6.

333 Loh E, Sutton MS, Wun CC, Rouleau JL, Flaker GC, Gottlieb SS *et al*. Ventricular dysfunction and the risk of stroke after myocardial infarction. *N Engl J Med* 1997; **336**(4):251–7.

334 Martin R, Bogousslavsky J. Mechanism of late stroke after myocardial infarct: the Lausanne Stroke Registry. *J Neurol Neurosurg Psychiatry* 1993; **56**(7):760–4.

335 Dalal PM, Dalal KP. Cerebrovascular manifestations of infectious disease. In: Vinken PJ, Bruyn GW, Klawans HL, eds. *Handbook of Clinical Neurology*. New York: Elsevier Science, 1989; 411.

336 Chan KH, Cheung RT, Lee R, Mak W, Ho SL. Cerebral infarcts complicating tuberculous meningitis. *Cerebrovasc Dis* 2005; **19**(6):391–5.

337 Landi G, Villani F, Anzalone N. Variable angiographic findings in patients with stroke and neurosyphilis. *Stroke* 1990; **21**(2):333–8.

338 Del Mar Saez de Ocariz M, Nader JA, Del Brutto OH, Santos Zambrano JA. Cerebrovascular complications of neurosyphilis: the return of an old problem. *Cerebrovasc Dis* 1996; **6**:195–201.

339 Flint AC, Liberato BB, Anziska Y, Schantz-Dunn J, Wright CB. Meningovascular syphilis as a cause of basilar artery stenosis. *Neurology* 2005; **64**(2):391–2.

340 Igarashi M, Gilmartin RC, Gerald B, Wilburn F, Jabbour JT. Cerebral arteritis and bacterial meningitis. *Arch Neurol* 1984; **41**(5):531–5.

341 Perry JR, Bilbao JM, Gray T. Fatal basilar vasculopathy complicating bacterial meningitis. *Stroke* 1992; **23**(8):1175–8.

342 Chang CJ, Chang WN, Huang LT, Chang YC, Huang SC, Hung PL *et al*. Cerebral infarction in perinatal and childhood bacterial meningitis. *Q J Med* 2003; **96**(10):755–62.

343 Eidelberg D, Sotrel A, Horoupian DS, Neumann PE, Pumarola-Sune T, Price RW. Thrombotic cerebral vasculopathy associated with herpes zoster. *Ann Neurol* 1986; **19**(1):7–14.

344 Fukumoto S, Kinjo M, Hokamura K, Tanaka K. Subarachnoid hemorrhage and granulomatous angiitis of the basilar artery: demonstration of the varicella-zoster-virus in the basilar artery lesions. *Stroke* 1986; **17**(5):1024–8.

345 Gilden DH, Lipton HL, Wolf JS, Akenbrandt W, Smith JE, Mahalingam R, Forghani B. Two patients with unusual forms of varicella-zoster virus vasculopathy. *N Engl J Med* 2002; **347**(19):1500–3.

346 Lanthier S, Armstrong D, Domi T, deVeber G. Post-varicella arteriopathy of childhood: natural history of vascular stenosis. *Neurology* 2005; **64**(4):660–3.

347 Leopold NA. Chickenpox stroke in an adult. *Neurology* 1993; **43**(9):1852–3.

348 Gilden DH, Kleinschmidt-DeMasters BK, LaGuardia JJ, Mahalingam R, Cohrs RJ. Neurologic complications of the reactivation of varicella-zoster virus. *N Engl J Med* 2000; **342**(9):635–45.

349 Park YD, Belman AL, Kim TS, Kure K, Llena JF, Lantos G *et al*. Stroke in pediatric acquired immunodeficiency syndrome. *Ann Neurol* 1990; **28**(3):303–11.

350 Kieburtz KD, Eskin TA, Ketonen L, Tuite MJ. Opportunistic cerebral vasculopathy and stroke in patients with the acquired immunodeficiency syndrome. *Arch Neurol* 1993; **50**(4):430–2.

351 Dubrovsky T, Curless R, Scott G, Chaneles M, Post MJ, Altman N *et al*. Cerebral aneurysmal arteriopathy in childhood AIDS. *Neurology* 1998; **51**(2):560–5.

352 Evers S, Nabavi D, Rahman NU, Heese C, Reichart MD, Husstedt I-W. Ischaemic cerebrovascular events in HIV infection. *Cerebrovasc Dis* 2003; **15**:199–205.

353 Connor MD, Lammie GA, Bell JE, Warlow CP, Simmonds P, Brettle RD. Cerebral infarction in adult AIDS patients: observations from the Edinburgh HIV Autopsy Cohort. *Stroke* 2000; **31**(9):2117–26.

354 Patel VB, Sacoor Z, Francis P, Bill PL, Bhigjee AI, Connolly C. Ischemic stroke in young HIV-positive patients in Kwazulu-Natal, South Africa. *Neurology* 2005; **65**(5):759–61.

355 Uldry PA, Regli F, Bogousslavsky J. Cerebral angiopathy and recurrent strokes following *Borrelia burgdorferi* infection. *J Neurol Neurosurg Psychiatry* 1987; **50**(12):1703–4.

356 Reik L, Jr. Stroke due to Lyme disease. *Neurology* 1993; **43**(12):2705–7.

357 Oksi J, Kalimo H, Marttila RJ, Marjamaki M, Sonninen P, Nikoskelainen J, Viljanen MK. Intracranial aneurysms in three patients with disseminated Lyme borreliosis: cause or chance association? *J Neurol Neurosurg Psychiatry* 1998; **64**(5):636–42.

358 Schmiedel J, Gahn G, von KR, Reichmann H. Cerebral vasculitis with multiple infarcts caused by lyme disease. *Cerebrovasc Dis* 2004; **17**(1):79–81.

359 Forwell MA, Redding PJ, Brodie MJ, Gentleman DD. Leptospirosis complicated by fatal intracerebral haemorrhage. *Br Med J (Clin Res Ed)* 1984; **289**(6458):1583.

360 Minnerop M, Bos M, Harbrecht U, Maass M, Urbach H, Klockgether T, Schroder R. CNS infection with *Chlamydia pneumoniae* complicated by multiple strokes. *J Neurol* 2002; **249**(9):1329–31.

361 Mulder LJ, Spierings EL. Stroke due to intravascular coagulation in Mycoplasma pneumoniae infection. *Lancet* 1987; **2**(8568):1152–3.

362 Antachopoulos C, Liakopoulou T, Palamidou F, Papathanassiou D, Youroukos S. Posterior cerebral artery occlusion associated with Mycoplasma pneumoniae infection. *J Child Neurol* 2002; **17**(1):55–7.

363 Tembl JI, Ferrer JM, Sevilla MT, Lago A, Mayordomo F, Vilchez JJ. Neurologic complications associated with hepatitis C virus infection. *Neurology* 1999; **53**(4):861–4.

364 Marchioni E, Ceroni M, Erbetta A, Alfonsi E, Bottanelli M, Imbesi F, Ricevuti G. Severe acute cerebrovascular disease revealing hepatitis C virus infection: effectiveness of alpha-interferon. *J Neurol* 2002; **249**(8):1111–13.

365 Koeppen AH, Lansing LS, Peng SK, Smith RS. Central nervous system vasculitis in cytomegalovirus infection. *J Neurol Sci* 1981; **51**(3):395–410.

366 Fourestie V, Douceron H, Brugieres P, Ancelle T, Lejonc JL, Gherardi RK. Neurotrichinosis. A cerebrovascular disease associated with myocardial injury and hypereosinophilia. *Brain* 1993; **116**(Pt 3):603–16.

367 Del Brutto OH. Cysticercosis and cerebrovascular disease: a review. *J Neurol Neurosurg Psychiatry* 1992; **55**(4):252–4.

368 Bang OY, Heo JH, Choi SA, Kim DI. Large cerebral infarction during praziquantel therapy in neurocysticercosis. *Stroke* 1997; **28**(1):211–13.

369 Jha S, Kumar V. Neurocysticercosis presenting as stroke. *Neurol India* 2000; **48**(4):391–4.

370 Aditya GS, Mahadevan A, Santosh V, Chickabasaviah YT, Ashwathnarayanarao CB, Krishna SS. Cysticercal chronic basal arachnoiditis with infarcts, mimicking tuberculous pathology in endemic areas. *Neuropathology* 2004; **24**(4):320–5.

371 Garcia HH, Gonzalez AE, Tsang VCW, for the Cysticerocosis Working Group in Peru. Neurocysticercosis: some of the essentials. *Pract Neurol* 2006; **6**:288–97.

372 Selby G, Walker GL. Cerebral arteritis in cat-scratch disease. *Neurology* 1979; **29**(10):1413–18.

373 Shields DA. Multiple emboli in hydatid disease. *Br Med J* 1990; **301**(6745):213–14.

374 Benomar A, Yahyaoui M, Birouk N, Vidailhet M, Chkili T. Middle cerebral artery occlusion due to hydatid cysts of myocardial and intraventricular cavity cardiac origin: two cases. *Stroke* 1994; **25**(4):886–8.

375 Singh NP, Arora SK, Gupta A, Anuradha S, Sridhara G, Agarwal SK, Gulati P. Stroke: a rare presentation of cardiac hydatidosis. *Neurol India* 2003; **51**(1):120–1.

376 Bickerstaff ER. Aetiology of acute hemiplegia in childhood. *Br Med J* 1964; **2**(5401):82–7.

377 Keime-Guibert F, Napolitano M, Delattre JY. Neurological complications of radiotherapy and chemotherapy. *J Neurol* 1998; **245**(11):695–708.

378 Hickey WF, Garnick MB, Henderson IC, Dawson DM. Primary cerebral venous thrombosis in patients with cancer: a rarely diagnosed paraneoplastic syndrome. Report of three cases and review of the literature. *Am J Med* 1982; **73**(5):740–50.

379 Bick RL. Cancer-associated thrombosis. *N Engl J Med* 2003; **349**(2):109–11.

380 Rogers LR. Cerebrovascular complications in cancer patients. *Neurol Clin* 2003; **21**(1):167–92.

381 Murros KE, Toole JF. The effect of radiation on carotid arteries. A review article. *Arch Neurol* 1989; **46**(4):449–55.

382 Griewing B, Guo Y, Doherty C, Feyerabend M, Wessel K, Kessler C. Radiation-induced injury to the carotid artery: a longitudinal study. *Eur J Neurol* 1995; **2**:379–83.

383 Grill J, Couanet D, Cappelli C, Habrand JL, Rodriguez D, Sainte-Rose C, Kalifa C. Radiation-induced cerebral vasculopathy in children with neurofibromatosis and optic pathway glioma. *Ann Neurol* 1999; **45**(3):393–6.

384 Lam WW, Liu KH, Leung SF, Wong KS, So NM, Yuen HY, Metreweli C. Sonographic characterisation of radiation-induced carotid artery stenosis. *Cerebrovasc Dis* 2002; **13**(3):168–73.

385 Scodary DJ, Tew JM, Jr., Thomas GM, Tomsick T, Liwnicz BH. Radiation-induced cerebral aneurysms. *Acta Neurochir (Wien)* 1990; **102**(3–4):141–4.

386 Bitzer M, Topka H. Progressive cerebral occlusive disease after radiation therapy. *Stroke* 1995; **26**(1):131–6.

387 Reece DE, Frei-Lahr DA, Shepherd JD, Dorovini-Zis K, Gascoyne RD, Graeb DA *et al.* Neurologic complications in allogeneic bone marrow transplant patients receiving cyclosporin. *Bone Marrow Transplant* 1991; **8**(5):393–401.

388 Hinchey J, Chaves C, Appignani B, Breen J, Pao L, Wang A *et al.* A reversible posterior leukoencephalopathy syndrome. *N Engl J Med* 1996; **334**(8):494–500.

389 Gijtenbeek JM, van den Bent MJ, Vecht CJ. Cyclosporine neurotoxicity: a review. *J Neurol* 1999; **246**(5):339–46.

390 O'Brien ME, Tonge K, Blake P, Moskovic E, Wiltshaw E. Blindness associated with high-dose carboplatin. *Lancet* 1992; **339**(8792):558.

391 El AM, Heinzlef O, Debroucker T, Roullet E, Bousser MG, Amarenco P. Brain infarction following 5-fluorouracil and cisplatin therapy. *Neurology* 1998; **51**(3):899–901.

392 Feinberg WM, Swenson MR. Cerebrovascular complications of L-asparaginase therapy. *Neurology* 1988; **38**(1):127–33.

393 Walker RW, Allen JC, Rosen G, Caparros B. Transient cerebral dysfunction secondary to high-dose methotrexate. *J Clin Oncol* 1986; **4**(12):1845–50.

394 Bushnell CD, Goldstein LB. Risk of ischemic stroke with tamoxifen treatment for breast cancer: a meta-analysis. *Neurology* 2004; **63**(7):1230–3.

395 Padovan CS, Bise K, Hahn J, Sostak P, Holler E, Kolb HJ, Straube A. Angiitis of the central nervous system after allogeneic bone marrow transplantation? *Stroke* 1999; **30**(8):1651–6.

396 The Coronary Drug Project. Initial findings leading to modifications of its research protocol. *J Am Med Assoc* 1970; **214**(7):1303–13.

397 Henriksson P, Edhag O. Orchidectomy versus oestrogen for prostatic cancer: cardiovascular effects. *Br Med J (Clin Res Ed)* 1986; **293**(6544):413–15.

398 Byar DP, Corle DK. Hormone therapy for prostate cancer: results of the Veterans Administration Cooperative Urological Research Group studies. *NCI Monogr* 1988; (7):165–70.

399 Worrell GA, Wijdicks EF, Eggers SD, Phan T, Damario MA, Mullany CJ. Ovarian hyperstimulation syndrome with ischemic stroke due to an intracardiac thrombus. *Neurology*; **57**(7):1342–4.

400 Stampfer MJ, Willett WC, Colditz GA, Speizer FE, Hennekens CH. Past use of oral contraceptives and cardiovascular disease: a meta-analysis in the context of the Nurses' Health Study. *Am J Obstet Gynecol* 1990; **163**(1 Pt 2):285–91.

401 WHO Collaborative Study of Cardiovascular Disease and Steroid Hormone Contraception. Ischaemic stroke and combined oral contraceptives: results of an international, multicentre, case-control study. *Lancet* 1996; **348**(9026):498–505.

402 WHO Collaborative Study of Cardiovascular Disease and Steroid Hormone Contraception. Haemorrhagic stroke, overall stroke risk, and combined oral contraceptives: results of an international, multicentre, case-control study. *Lancet* 1996; **348**(9026):505–10.

403 Beral V, Hermon C, Kay C, Hannaford P, Darby S, Reeves G. Mortality associated with oral contraceptive use: 25 year follow-up of cohort of 46 000 women from Royal College of General Practitioners' oral contraception study. *Br Med J* 1999; **318**(7176):96–100.

404 Gillum LA, Johnston SC. Oral contraceptives and stroke risk: the debate continues. *Lancet Neurol* 2004; **3**(8):453–4.

405 Rosendaal FR, Van H, V, Tanis BC, Helmerhorst FM. Estrogens, progestogens and thrombosis. *J Thromb Haemost* 2003; **1**(7):1371–80.

406 Poulter NR, Chang CL, Farley TM, Marmot MG, Meirik O. WHO Collaborative Study of Cardiovascular Disease and Steroid Hormone Contraception. Effect on stroke of different progestagens in low oestrogen dose oral contraceptives. *Lancet* 1999; **354**(9175):301–2.

407 MacGregor EA, Guillebaud J. Recommendations for clinical practice: combined oral contraceptives, migraine and ischaemic stroke. *Br J Fam Planning* 1998; **24**:53–60.

408 Becker WJ. Use of oral contraceptives in patients with migraine. *Neurology* 1999; **53**(4 Suppl 1):S19–S25.

409 Skegg DC. Oral contraception and health. *Br Med J* 1999; **318**(7176):69–70.

410 Vessey M, Painter R, Yeates D. Mortality in relation to oral contraceptive use and cigarette smoking. *Lancet* 2003; **362**(9379):185–91.

411 Vandenbroucke JP. Cerebral sinus thrombosis and oral contraceptives: there are limits to predictability. *Br Med J* 1998; **317**(7157):483–4.

412 Nabulsi AA, Folsom AR, White A, Patsch W, Heiss G, Wu KK, Szklo M. Association of hormone-replacement therapy with various cardiovascular risk factors in postmenopausal women. The Atherosclerosis Risk in Communities Study Investigators. *N Engl J Med* 1993; **328**(15):1069–75.

413 Belchetz PE. Hormonal treatment of postmenopausal women. *N Engl J Med* 1994; **330**(15):1062–71.

414 Effects of estrogen or estrogen/progestin regimens on heart disease risk factors in postmenopausal women. The Postmenopausal Estrogen/Progestin Interventions (PEPI) Trial. The Writing Group for the PEPI Trial. *J Am Med Assoc* 1995; **273**(3):199–208.

415 Koh KK, Mincemoyer R, Bui MN, Csako G, Pucino F, Guetta V *et al*. Effects of hormone-replacement therapy on fibrinolysis in postmenopausal women. *N Engl J Med* 1997; **336**(10):683–90.

416 Pedersen AT, Lidegaard O, Kreiner S, Ottesen B. Hormone replacement therapy and risk of non-fatal stroke. *Lancet* 1997; **350**(9087):1277–83.

417 Petitti DB, Sidney S, Quesenberry CP, Jr., Bernstein A. Ischemic stroke and use of estrogen and estrogen/progestogen as hormone replacement therapy. *Stroke* 1998; **29**(1):23–8.

418 Grady D, Rubin SM, Petitti DB, Fox CS, Black D, Ettinger B *et al*. Hormone therapy to prevent disease and prolong life in postmenopausal women. *Ann Intern Med* 1992; **117**(12):1016–37.

419 Bath PM, Gray LJ. Association between hormone replacement therapy and subsequent stroke: a meta-analysis. *Br Med J* 2005; **330**(7487):342.

420 Rodstrom K, Bengtsson C, Lissner L, Bjorkelund C. Pre-existing risk factor profiles in users and non-users of hormone replacement therapy: prospective cohort study in Gothenburg, Sweden. *Br Med J* 1999; **319**(7214):890–3.

421 Grady D. Postmenopausal hormones: therapy for symptoms only. *N Engl J Med* 2003; **348**(19):1835–7.

422 Grosset DG, Ebrahim S, Bone I, Warlow C. Stroke in pregnancy and the puerperium: what magnitude of risk? *J Neurol Neurosurg Psychiatry* 1995; **58**(2):129–31.

423 Jaigobin C, Silver FL. Stroke and pregnancy. *Stroke* 2000; **31**(12):2948–51.

424 Skidmore FM, Williams LS, Fradkin KD, Alonso RJ, Biller J. Presentation, aetiology, and outcome of stroke in pregnancy and puerperium. *J Stroke Cerebrovasc Dis* 2001; **10**:1–10.

425 Jeng J-S, Tang S-C, Yip P-K. Incidence and aetiologies of stroke during pregnancy and puerperium as evidenced in Taiwanese women. *Cerebrovasc Dis* 2004; **18**:290–5.

426 Mehraein S, Ortwein H, Busch M, Weih M, Einhaupl K, Masuhr F. Risk of recurrence of cerebral venous and sinus thrombosis during subsequent pregnancy and puerperium. *J Neurol Neurosurg Psychiatry* 2003; **74**(6):814–16.

427 Gasecki AP, Kwiecinski H, Lyrer PA, Lynch TG, Baxter T. Dissections after childbirth. *J Neurol* 1999; **246**(8):712–15.

428 Janssens E, Hommel M, Mounier-Vehier F, Leclerc X, Guerin du MB, Leys D. Postpartum cerebral angiopathy possibly due to bromocriptine therapy. *Stroke* 1995; **26**(1):128–30.

429 Comabella M, Alvarez-Sabin J, Rovira A, Codina A. Bromocriptine and postpartum cerebral angiopathy: a causal relationship? *Neurology* 1996; **46**(6):1754–6.

430 Ursell MR, Marras CL, Farb R, Rowed DW, Black SE, Perry JR. Recurrent intracranial hemorrhage due to postpartum cerebral angiopathy: implications for management. *Stroke* 1998; **29**(9):1995–8.

431 Calado S, Vale-Santos J, Lima C, Viana-Baptista M. Postpartum cerebral angiopathy: vasospasm, vasculitis or both? *Cerebrovasc Dis* 2004; **18**(4):340–1.

432 Singhal AB. Postpartum angiopathy with reversible posterior leukoencephalopathy. *Arch Neurol* 2004; **61**(3):411–16.

433 Dziewas R, Stogbauer F, Freund M, Ludemann P, Imai T, Holzapfel C, Ringelstein PB. Late onset postpartum eclampsia: a rare and difficult diagnosis. *J Neurol* 2002; **249**(9):1287–91.

434 Munjuluri N, Lipman M, Valentine A, Hardiman P, Maclean AB. Postpartum eclampsia of late onset. *Br Med J* 2005; **331**(7524):1070–1.

435 Dyken ME, Biller J. Peripartum cardiomyopathy and stroke. *Cerebrovasc Dis* 1994; **4**:325–8.

436 Drislane FW, Wang AM. Multifocal cerebral hemorrhage in eclampsia and severe pre-eclampsia. *J Neurol* 1997; **244**(3):194–8.

437 Sawle GV, Ramsay MM. The neurology of pregnancy. *J Neurol Neurosurg Psychiatry* 1998; **64**(6):711–25.

438 Walker JJ. Pre-eclampsia. *Lancet* 2000; **356**(9237):1260–5.

439 Lamy C, Hamon JB, Coste J, Mas JL. Ischemic stroke in young women: risk of recurrence during subsequent pregnancies. French Study Group on Stroke in Pregnancy. *Neurology* 2000; **55**(2):269–74.

440 Caplan LR, Hier DB, Banks G. Current concepts of cerebrovascular disease–stroke: stroke and drug abuse. *Stroke* 1982; **13**(6):869–72.

441 Sloan MA, Kittner SJ, Feeser BR, Gardner J, Epstein A, Wozniak MA *et al.* Illicit drug-associated ischemic stroke in the Baltimore-Washington Young Stroke Study. *Neurology* 1998; **50**(6):1688–93.

442 Cregler LL, Mark H. Medical complications of cocaine abuse. *N Engl J Med* 1986; **315**(23):1495–500.

443 Levine SR, Brust JC, Futrell N, Brass LM, Blake D, Fayad P *et al.* A comparative study of the cerebrovascular complications of cocaine: alkaloidal versus hydrochloride: a review. *Neurology* 1991; **41**(8):1173–7.

444 Aggarwal SK, Williams V, Levine SR, Cassin BJ, Garcia JH. Cocaine-associated intracranial hemorrhage: absence of vasculitis in 14 cases. *Neurology* 1996; **46**(6):1741–3.

445 Nolte KB, Brass LM, Fletterick CF. Intracranial hemorrhage associated with cocaine abuse: a prospective autopsy study. *Neurology* 1996; **46**(5):1291–6.

446 Krendel DA, Ditter SM, Frankel MR, Ross WK. Biopsy-proven cerebral vasculitis associated with cocaine abuse. *Neurology* 1990; **40**(7):1092–4.

447 Fredericks RK, Lefkowitz DS, Challa VR, Troost BT. Cerebral vasculitis associated with cocaine abuse. *Stroke* 1991; **22**(11):1437–9.

448 Daras M, Tuchman AJ, Marks S. Central nervous system infarction related to cocaine abuse. *Stroke* 1991; **22**(10):1320–5.

449 Daras M, Tuchman AJ, Koppel BS, Samkoff LM, Weitzner I, Marc J. Neurovascular complications of cocaine. *Acta Neurol Scand* 1994; **90**(2):124–9.

450 Sauer CM. Recurrent embolic stroke and cocaine-related cardiomyopathy. *Stroke* 1991; **22**(9):1203–5.

451 Libman RB, Masters SR, de Paola A, Mohr JP. Transient monocular blindness associated with cocaine abuse. *Neurology* 1993; **43**(1):228–9.

452 Konzen JP, Levine SR, Garcia JH. Vasospasm and thrombus formation as possible mechanisms of stroke related to alkaloidal cocaine. *Stroke* 1995; **26**(6):1114–18.

453 Kaufman MJ, Levin JM, Ross MH, Lange N, Rose SL, Kukes TJ *et al.* Cocaine-induced cerebral vasoconstriction detected in humans with magnetic resonance angiography. *J Am Med Assoc* 1998; **279**(5):376–80.

454 Storen EC, Wijdicks EF, Crum BA, Schultz G. Moyamoya-like vasculopathy from cocaine dependency. *Am J Neuroradiol* 2000; **21**(6):1008–10.

455 Harrington H, Heller HA, Dawson D, Caplan L, Rumbaugh C. Intracerebral hemorrhage and oral amphetamine. *Arch Neurol* 1983; **40**(8):503–7.

456 Rothrock JF, Rubenstein R, Lyden PD. Ischemic stroke associated with methamphetamine inhalation. *Neurology* 1988; **38**(4):589–92.

457 Heye N, Hankey GJ. Amphetamine-associated stroke. *Cerebrovasc Dis* 1996; **6**:149–55.

458 Buxton N, McConachie NS. Amphetamine abuse and intracranial haemorrhage. *J R Soc Med* 2000; **93**(9):472–7.

459 Bruno A, Nolte KB, Chapin J. Stroke associated with ephedrine use. *Neurology* 1993; **43**(7):1313–16.

460 Haller CA, Benowitz NL. Adverse cardiovascular and central nervous system events associated with dietary supplements containing ephedra alkaloids. *N Engl J Med* 2000; **343**(25):1833–8.

461 Arauz A, Velasquez L, Cantu C, Nader J, Lopez M, Murillo L, Aburto Y. Phenylpropanolamine and intracranial hemorrhage risk in a Mexican population. *Cerebrovasc Dis* 2003; **15**(3):210–14.

462 Cantu C, Arauz A, Murillo-Bonilla LM, Lopez M, Barinagarrementeria F. Stroke associated with sympathomimetics contained in over-the-counter cough and cold drugs. *Stroke* 2003; **34**(7):1667–72.

463 Worrall BB, Phillips CD, Henderson KK. Herbal energy drinks, phenylpropanoid compounds, and cerebral vasculopathy. *Neurology* 2005; **65**(7):1137–8.

464 Harries DP, De SR. 'Ecstasy' and intracerebral haemorrhage. *Scott Med J* 1992; **37**(5):150–2.

465 Henry JA, Jeffreys KJ, Dawling S. Toxicity and deaths from 3,4-methylenedioxymethamphetamine ('ecstasy'). *Lancet* 1992; **340**(8816):384–7.

466 Rothwell PM, Grant R. Cerebral venous sinus thrombosis induced by 'ecstasy'. *J Neurol Neurosurg Psychiatry* 1993; **56**(9):1035.

467 Mateo I, Pinedo A, Gomez-Beldarrain M, Basterretxea JM, Garcia-Monco JC. Recurrent stroke associated with cannabis use. *J Neurol Neurosurg Psychiatry* 2005; **76**(3):435–7.

468 Juni P, Nartey L, Reichenbach S, Sterchi R, Dieppe PA, Egger M. Risk of cardiovascular events and rofecoxib: cumulative meta-analysis. *Lancet* 2004; **364**(9450):2021–9.

469 Waxman HA. The lessons of Vioxx: drug safety and sales. *N Engl J Med* 2005; **352**(25):2576–8.

470 Drazen JM. COX-2 inhibitors: a lesson in unexpected problems. *N Engl J Med* 2005; **352**(11):1131–2.

471 Kearney PM, Baigent C, Godwin J, Halls H, Emberson JR, Patrono C. Do selective cyclo-oxygenase-2 inhibitors and traditional non-steroidal anti-inflammatory drugs increase the risk of atherothrombosis? Meta-analysis of randomised trials. *Br Med J* 2006; **332**(7553):1302–8.

472 Vonkeman HE, Brouwers JR, van de Laar MA. Understanding the NSAID related risk of vascular events. *Br Med J* 2006; **332**(7546):895–8.

473 Rodriguez LA, Patrignani P. The ever growing story of cyclo-oxygenase inhibition. *Lancet* 2006; **368**(9549):1745–7.

474 Herrmann N, Lanctot KL. Do atypical antipsychotics cause stroke? *CNS Drugs* 2005; **19**:91–103.

475 Wang PS, Schneeweiss S, Avorn J, Fischer MA, Mogun H, Solomon DH, Brookhart MA. Risk of death in elderly users of conventional vs. atypical antipsychotic medications. *N Engl J Med* 2005; **353**(22):2335–41.

476 Morgan JC, Alhatou M, Oberlies J, Johnston KC. Transient ischemic attack and stroke associated with sildenafil (Viagra) use. *Neurology* 2001; **57**(9):1730–1.

477 Cummings SR. LIFT study is discontinued. *Br Med J* 2006; **332**(7542):667.

478 Berkovic SF, Bladin PF, Darby DG. Metabolic disorders presenting as stroke. *Med J Aust* 1984; **140**(7):421–4.

479 Illangasekera VL. Insulinoma masquerading as carotid transient ischaemic attacks. *Postgrad Med J* 1981; **57**(666):232–4.

480 Wallis WE, Donaldson I, Scott RS, Wilson J. Hypoglycemia masquerading as cerebrovascular disease (hypoglycemic hemiplegia). *Ann Neurol* 1985; **18**(4):510–12.

481 Pell AC, Frier BM. Restoration of perception of hypoglycaemia after hemiparesis in an insulin dependent diabetic patient. *Br Med J* 1990; **300**(6721):369–70.

482 Rother J, Schreiner A, Wentz KU, Hennerici M. Hypoglycemia presenting as basilar artery thrombosis. *Stroke* 1992; **23**(1):112–13.

483 Shintani S, Tsuruoka S, Shiigai T. Hypoglycaemic hemiplegia: a repeat SPECT study. *J Neurol Neurosurg Psychiatry* 1993; **56**(6):700–1.

484 Service FJ. Hypoglycemic disorders. *N Engl J Med* 1995; **332**(17):1144–52.

485 Shanmugam V, Zimnowodski S, Curtin J, Gorelick PB. Hypoglycaemic hemiplegia: insulinoma masquerading as stroke. *J Stroke Cerebrovasc Dis* 1997; **6**:368–9.

486 Cordonnier C, Oppenheim C, Lamy C, Meder JF, Mas JL. Serial diffusion and perfusion-weighted MR in transient hypoglycemia. *Neurology* 2005; **65**(1):175.

487 Longo DL, Witherspoon JM. Focal neurologic symptoms in hypercalcemia. *Neurology* 1980; **30**(2):200–1.

488 Walker GL, Williamson PM, Ravich RB, Roche J. Hypercalcaemia associated with cerebral vasospasm causing infarction. *J Neurol Neurosurg Psychiatry* 1980; **43**(5):464–7.

489 Ayuk J, Matthews T, Tayebjee M, Gittoes NJ. A blind panic. *Lancet* 2001; **357**(9264):1262.

490 Maccario M. Neurological dysfunction associated with nonketotic hyperglycemia. *Arch Neurol* 1968; **19**(5):525–34.

491 Carril JM, Guijarro C, Portocarrero JS, Solache I, Jimenez A, Valera de SE. Speech arrest as manifestation of seizures in non-ketotic hyperglycaemia. *Lancet* 1992; **340**(8829):1227.

492 Lavin PJ. Hyperglycemic hemianopia: a reversible complication of non-ketotic hyperglycemia. *Neurology* 2005; **65**(4):616–19.

493 Ruby RJ, Burton JR. Acute reversible hemiparesis and hyponatraemia. *Lancet* 1977; **1**(8023):1212.

494 Daggett P, Deanfield J, Moss F. Neurological aspects of hyponatraemia. *Postgrad Med J* 1982; **58**(686):737–40.

495 Johns DR. Cerebrovascular complications of inflammatory bowel disease. *Am J Gastroenterol* 1991; **86**(3):367–70.

496 Jorens PG, Delvigne CR, Hermans CR, Haber I, Holvoet J, De Deyn PP. Cerebral arterial thrombosis preceding ulcerative colitis. *Stroke* 1991; **22**(9):1212.

497 Jackson M, Lennox G, Jaspan T, Lowe J. Cerebral venous and systemic thrombosis in resolving ulcerative colitis. *Cerebrovasc Dis* 1993; **3**:178–9.

498 Lossos A, River Y, Eliakim A, Steiner I. Neurologic aspects of inflammatory bowel disease. *Neurology* 1995; **45**(3 Pt 1):416–21.

499 Wills A, Hovell CJ. Neurological complications of enteric disease. *Gut* 1996; **39**(4):501–4.

500 Jackson LM, O'Gorman PJ, O'Connell J, Cronin CC, Cotter KP, Shanahan F. Thrombosis in inflammatory bowel disease: clinical setting, procoagulant profile and factor V Leiden. *Q J Med* 1997; **90**(3):183–8.

501 Geissler A, Andus T, Roth M, Kullmann F, Caesar I, Held P *et al*. Focal white-matter lesions in brain of patients with inflammatory bowel disease. *Lancet* 1995; **345**(8954):897–8.

502 Mumford CJ, Fletcher NA, Ironside JW, Warlow CP. Progressive ataxia, focal seizures, and malabsorption syndrome in a 41 year old woman. *J Neurol Neurosurg Psychiatry* 1996; **60**(2):225–30.

503 Reynolds P, Walker FO, Eades J, Smith JD, Lantz PE. Food embolus. *J Neurol Sci* 1997; **149**(2):185–90.

504 Roach GW, Kanchuger M, Mangano CM, Newman M, Nussmeier N, Wolman R *et al*. Adverse cerebral outcomes after coronary bypass surgery. Multicenter Study of Perioperative Ischemia Research Group and the Ischemia Research and Education Foundation Investigators. *N Engl J Med* 1996; **335**(25):1857–63.

505 Likosky DS, Marrin CA, Caplan LR, Baribeau YR, Morton JR, Weintraub RM *et al*. Determination of etiologic mechanisms of strokes secondary to coronary artery bypass graft surgery. *Stroke* 2003; **34**(12):2830–4.

506 Belvis R, Marti-Fabregas J, Cocho D, Garcia-Bargo MD, Franquet E, Agudo R *et al*. Cerebrovascular disease as a complication of cardiac transplantation. *Cerebrovasc Dis* 2005; **19**(4):267–71.

507 Bendszus M, Stoll G. Silent cerebral ischaemia: hidden fingerprints of invasive medical procedures. *Lancet Neurol* 2006; **5**(4):364–72.

508 Newman SP, Harrison MJ. Coronary-artery bypass surgery and the brain: persisting concerns. *Lancet Neurol* 2002; **1**(2):119–25.

509 Selnes OA, McKhann GM. Neurocognitive complications after coronary artery bypass surgery. *Ann Neurol* 2005; **57**(5):615–21.

510 Newman MF, Mathew JP, Grocott HP, Mackensen GB, Monk T, Welsh-Bohmer KA *et al*. Central nervous system

injury associated with cardiac surgery. *Lancet* 2006; **368**(9536):694–703.

511 Harris DN, Bailey SM, Smith PL, Taylor KM, Oatridge A, Bydder GM. Brain swelling in first hour after coronary artery bypass surgery. *Lancet* 1993; **342**(8871):586–7.

512 Hogue CW, Jr., Murphy SF, Schechtman KB, Davila-Roman VG. Risk factors for early or delayed stroke after cardiac surgery. *Circulation* 1999; **100**(6):642–7.

513 Stamou SC, Hill PC, Dangas G, Pfister AJ, Boyce SW, Dullum MK *et al*. Stroke after coronary artery bypass: incidence, predictors, and clinical outcome. *Stroke* 2001; **32**(7):1508–13.

514 Mangano DT, Tudor IC, Dietzel C. The risk associated with aprotinin in cardiac surgery. *N Engl J Med* 2006; **354**(4):353–65.

515 Taggart D. About impaired minds and closed hearts. *Br Med J* 2002; **325**(7375):1255–6.

516 Al-Ruzzeh S, George S, Bustami M, Wray J, Ilsley C, Athanasiou T, Amrani M. Effect of off-pump coronary artery bypass surgery on clinical, angiographic, neurocognitive, and quality of life outcomes: randomised controlled trial. *Br Med J* 2006; **332**(7554):1365.

517 Sedrakyan A, Wu AW, Parashar A, Bass EB, Treasure T. Off-pump surgery is associated with reduced occurrence of stroke and other morbidity as compared with traditional coronary artery bypass grafting: a meta-analysis of systematically reviewed trials. *Stroke* 2006; **37**(11):2759–69.

518 Dashe JF, Pessin MS, Murphy RE, Payne DD. Carotid occlusive disease and stroke risk in coronary artery bypass graft surgery. *Neurology* 1997; **49**(3):678–86.

519 Ayas N, Wijdicks. Cardiac catheterization complicated by stroke: 14 patients. *Cerebrovasc Dis* 1995; **5**:304–7.

520 Leker RR, Pollak A, Abramsky O, Ben-Hur T. Abundance of left hemispheric embolic strokes complicating coronary angiography and PTCA. *J Neurol Neurosurg Psychiatry* 1999; **66**(1):116–17.

521 Sticherling C, Berkefeld J, Auch-Schwelk W, Lanfermann H. Transient bilateral cortical blindness after coronary angiography. *Lancet* 1998; **351**(9102):570.

522 Hankey GJ. Recurrent migraine aura triggered by coronary angiography. *Pract Neurol* 2004; **4**(5):308–9.

523 Hart R, Hindman B. Mechanisms of perioperative cerebral infarction. *Stroke* 1982; **13**(6):766–73.

524 Limburg M, Wijdicks EF, Li H. Ischemic stroke after surgical procedures: clinical features, neuroimaging, and risk factors. *Neurology* 1998; **50**(4):895–901.

525 Selwood A, Orrell M. Long term cognitive dysfunction in older people after non-cardiac surgery. *Br Med J* 2004; **328**(7432):120–1.

526 Jackson MJ, Schaefer JA, Johnson MA, Morris AA, Turnbull DM, Bindoff LA. Presentation and clinical investigation of mitochondrial respiratory chain disease: a study of 51 patients. *Brain* 1995; **118**(Pt 2):339–57.

527 Chinnery PF, Turnbull DM. Mitochondrial medicine. *Q J Med* 1997; **90**(11):657–67.

528 Chinnery PF, Turnbull DM. Mitochondrial DNA and disease. *Neth J Med* 1998; **53**(1):4–6.

529 Chinnery PF. The mitochondrion and its disorders. *Pract Neurol* 2003; **3**(2):100–5.

530 Schapira AH. Mitochondrial disease. *Lancet* 2006; **368**(9529):70–82.

531 McFarland R, Taylor RW, Turnbull DM. The neurology of mitochondrial DNA disease. *Lancet Neurol* 2002; **1**(6):343–51.

532 Ciafaloni E, Ricci E, Shanske S, Moraes CT, Silvestri G, Hirano M *et al*. MELAS: clinical features, biochemistry, and molecular genetics. *Ann Neurol* 1992; **31**(4):391–8.

533 Majamaa K, Turkka J, Karppa M, Winqvist S, Hassinen IE. The common MELAS mutation A3243G in mitochondrial DNA among young patients with an occipital brain infarct. *Neurology* 1997; **49**(5):1331–4.

534 Clark JM, Marks MP, Adalsteinsson E, Spielman DM, Shuster D, Horoupian D, Albers GW. MELAS: Clinical and pathologic correlations with MRI, xenon/CT, and MR spectroscopy. *Neurology* 1996; **46**(1):223–7.

535 Gilchrist JM, Sikirica M, Stopa E, Shanske S. Adult-onset MELAS. Evidence for involvement of neurons as well as cerebral vasculature in strokelike episodes. *Stroke* 1996; **27**(8):1420–3.

536 Oppenheim C, Galanaud D, Samson Y, Sahel M, Dormont D, Wechsler B, Marsault C. Can diffusion weighted magnetic resonance imaging help differentiate stroke from stroke-like events in MELAS? *J Neurol Neurosurg Psychiatry* 2000; **69**(2):248–50.

537 Chinnery PF, Turnbull DM. Clinical features, investigation, and management of patients with defects of mitochondrial DNA. *J Neurol Neurosurg Psychiatry* 1997; **63**(5):559–63.

538 Sue CM, Crimmins DS, Soo YS, Pamphlett R, Presgrave CM, Kotsimbos N *et al*. Neuroradiological features of six kindreds with MELAS tRNA(Leu) A2343G point mutation: implications for pathogenesis. *J Neurol Neurosurg Psychiatry* 1998; **65**(2):233–40.

539 Chinnery PF. Could it be mitochondrial? When and how to investigate. *Pract Neurol* 2006; **6**(2):90–101.

540 Koo B, Becker LE, Chuang S, Merante F, Robinson BH, MacGregor D *et al*. Mitochondrial encephalomyopathy, lactic acidosis, stroke-like episodes (MELAS): clinical, radiological, pathological, and genetic observations. *Ann Neurol* 1993; **34**(1):25–32.

541 Taylor RW, Chinnery PF, Haldane F, Morris AA, Bindoff LA, Wilson J, Turnbull DM. MELAS associated with a mutation in the valine transfer RNA gene of mitochondrial DNA. *Ann Neurol* 1996; **40**(3):459–62.

542 Chinnery PF, Howell N, Lightowlers RN, Turnbull DM. Molecular pathology of MELAS and MERRF: the relationship between mutation load and clinical phenotypes. *Brain* 1997; **120**(Pt 10):1713–21.

543 Morin C, Dube J, Robinson BH, Lacroix J, Michaud J, De Braekeleer M *et al*. Stroke-like episodes in autosomal recessive cytochrome oxidase deficiency. *Ann Neurol* 1999; **45**(3):389–92.

544 Joutel A, Dodick DD, Parisi JE, Cecillon M, Tournier-Lasserve E, Bousser MG. De novo mutation in the Notch3 gene causing CADASIL. *Ann Neurol* 2000; **47**(3):388–91.

545 Razvi SS, Muir KW. Cerebral autosomal dominant arteriopathy with subcortical infarcts and leukoencephalopathy (CADASIL). *Pract Neurol* 2004; **4**(1):50–5.

546 Miao Q, Paloneva T, Tuisku S, Roine S, Poyhonen M, Viitanen M, Kalimo H. Arterioles of the lenticular nucleus in CADASIL. *Stroke* 2006; **37**(9):2242–7.

547 Chabriat H, Vahedi K, Iba-Zizen MT, Joutel A, Nibbio A, Nagy TG *et al*. Clinical spectrum of CADASIL: a study of 7 families: cerebral autosomal dominant arteriopathy with subcortical infarcts and leukoencephalopathy. *Lancet* 1995; **346**(8980):934–9.

548 Hutchinson M, O'Riordan J, Javed M, Quin E, Macerlaine D, Wilcox T *et al*. Familial hemiplegic migraine and autosomal dominant arteriopathy with leukoencephalopathy (CADASIL). *Ann Neurol* 1995; **38**(5):817–24.

549 Desmond DW, Moroney JT, Lynch T, Chan S, Chin SS, Mohr JP. The natural history of CADASIL: a pooled analysis of previously published cases. *Stroke* 1999; **30**(6):1230–3.

550 Vahedi K, Chabriat H, Levy C, Joutel A, Tournier-Lasserve E, Bousser MG. Migraine with aura and brain magnetic resonance imaging abnormalities in patients with CADASIL. *Arch Neurol* 2004; **61**(8):1237–40.

551 Amberla K, Waljas M, Tuominen S, Almkvist O, Poyhonen M, Tuisku S *et al*. Insidious cognitive decline in CADASIL. *Stroke* 2004; **35**(7):1598–602.

552 Chabriat H, Mrissa R, Levy C, Vahedi K, Taillia H, Iba-Zizen MT *et al*. Brain stem MRI signal abnormalities in CADASIL. *Stroke* 1999; **30**(2):457–9.

553 O'Sullivan M, Jarosz JM, Martin RJ, Deasy N, Powell JF, Markus HS. MRI hyperintensities of the temporal lobe and external capsule in patients with CADASIL. *Neurology* 2001; **56**(5):628–34.

554 Dichgans M, Holtmannspotter M, Herzog J, Peters N, Bergmann M, Yousry TA. Cerebral microbleeds in CADASIL: a gradient-echo magnetic resonance imaging and autopsy study. *Stroke* 2002; **33**(1):67–71.

555 Viswanathan A, Guichard JP, Gschwendtner A, Buffon F, Cumurcuic R, Boutron C *et al*. Blood pressure and haemoglobin A1c are associated with microhaemorrhage in CADASIL: a two-centre cohort study. *Brain* 2006; **129**(Pt 9):2375–83.

556 Choi JC, Kang SY, Kang JH, Park JK. Intracerebral hemorrhages in CADASIL. *Neurology* 2006; **67**(11):2042–4.

557 Dichgans M, Petersen D. Angiographic complications in CADASIL. *Lancet* 1997; **349**(9054):776–7.

558 Jung HH, Bassetti C, Tournier-Lasserve E, Vahedi K, Arnaboldi M, Arifi VB, Burgunder JM. Cerebral autosomal dominant arteriopathy with subcortical infarcts and leukoencephalopathy: a clinicopathological and genetic study of a Swiss family. *J Neurol Neurosurg Psychiatry* 1995; **59**(2):138–43.

559 Furby A, Vahedi K, Force M, Larrouy S, Ruchoux MM, Joutel A, Tournier-Lasserve E. Differential diagnosis of a vascular leukoencephalopathy within a CADASIL family: use of skin biopsy electron microscopy study

and direct genotypic screening. *J Neurol* 1998; **245**(11):734–40.

560 Ruchoux MM, Maurage CA. Endothelial changes in muscle and skin biopsies in patients with CADASIL. *Neuropathol Appl Neurobiol* 1998; **24**(1):60–5.

561 Mayer M, Straube A, Bruening R, Uttner I, Pongratz D, Gasser T *et al*. Muscle and skin biopsies are a sensitive diagnostic tool in the diagnosis of CADASIL. *J Neurol* 1999; **246**(7):526–32.

562 Joutel A, Favrole P, Labauge P, Chabriat H, Lescoat C, Andreux F *et al*. Skin biopsy immunostaining with a Notch3 monoclonal antibody for CADASIL diagnosis. *Lancet* 2001; **358**(9298):2049–51.

563 Dotti MT, Federico A, Mazzei R, Bianchi S, Scali O, Conforti FL *et al*. The spectrum of Notch3 mutations in 28 Italian CADASIL families. *J Neurol Neurosurg Psychiatry* 2005; **76**(5):736–8.

564 Verreault S, Joutel A, Riant F, Neves G, Rui SM, Maciazek J *et al*. A novel hereditary small vessel disease of the brain. *Ann Neurol* 2006; **59**(2):353–7.

565 Yap S. Classical homocystinuria: vascular risk and its prevention. *J Inherit Metab Dis* 2003; **26**(2–3):259–65.

566 Gibson JB, Carson NA, Neill DW. Pathological findings in homocystinuria. *J Clin Pathol* 1964; **17**:427–37.

567 McCully KS. Vascular pathology of homocysteinemia: implications for the pathogenesis of arteriosclerosis. *Am J Pathol* 1969; **56**(1):111–28.

568 Schimke RN, McKusick VA, Huang T, Pollack AD. Homocystinuria: studies of 20 families with 38 affected members. *J Am Med Assoc* 1965; **193**:711–19.

569 Rubba P, Mercuri M, Faccenda F, Iannuzzi A, Irace C, Strisciuglio P *et al*. Premature carotid atherosclerosis: does it occur in both familial hypercholesterolemia and homocystinuria? Ultrasound assessment of arterial intima-media thickness and blood flow velocity. *Stroke* 1994; **25**(5):943–50.

570 Mudd SH, Skovby F, Levy HL, Pettigrew KD, Wilcken B, Pyeritz RE *et al*. The natural history of homocystinuria due to cystathionine beta-synthase deficiency. *Am J Hum Genet* 1985; **37**(1):1–31.

571 Visy JM, Le Coz P, Chadefaux B, Fressinaud C, Woimant F, Marquet J *et al*. Homocystinuria due to 5,10-methylenetetrahydrofolate reductase deficiency revealed by stroke in adult siblings. *Neurology* 1991; **41**(8):1313–15.

572 Cardo E, Campistol J, Caritg J, Ruiz S, Vilaseca MA, Kirkham F, Blom HJ. Fatal haemorrhagic infarct in an infant with homocystinuria. *Dev Med Child Neurol* 1999; **41**(2):132–5.

573 Ginsberg L, Valentine A, Mehta A. Fabry disease. *Pract Neurol* 2005; **5**(2):110–13.

574 Fellgiebel A, Muller MJ, Ginsberg L. CNS manifestations of Fabry's disease. *Lancet Neurol* 2006; **5**(9):791–5.

575 Garzuly F, Marodi L, Erdos M, Grubits J, Varga Z, Gelpi E *et al*. Megadolichobasilar anomaly with thrombosis in a family with Fabry's disease and a novel mutation in the alpha-galactosidase A gene. *Brain* 2005; **128**(Pt 9):2078–83.

576 Rolfs A, Bottcher T, Zschiesche M, Morris P, Winchester B, Bauer P *et al*. Prevalence of Fabry disease in patients with

cryptogenic stroke: a prospective study. *Lancet* 2005; 366(9499):1794–6.

577 Kandt RS, Gebarski SS, Goetting MG. Tuberous sclerosis with cardiogenic cerebral embolism: magnetic resonance imaging. *Neurology* 1985; 35(8):1223–5.

578 Rizzo JF, III, Lessell S. Cerebrovascular abnormalities in neurofibromatosis type 1. *Neurology* 1994; 44(6):1000–2.

579 Rosser TL, Vezina G, Packer RJ. Cerebrovascular abnormalities in a population of children with neurofibromatosis type 1. *Neurology* 2005; 64(3):553–5.

580 Ryan AM, Hurley M, Brennan P, Moroney JT. Vascular dysplasia in neurofibromatosis type 2. *Neurology* 2005; 65(1):163–4.

581 Lammie GA, Wardlaw J, Dennis M. Thrombo-embolic stroke, moya-moya phenomenon and primary oxalosis. *Cerebrovasc Dis* 1998; 8(1):45–50.

582 Schievink WI, Michels VV, Piepgras DG. Neurovascular manifestations of heritable connective tissue disorders: a review. *Stroke* 1994; 25(4):889–903.

583 North KN, Whiteman DA, Pepin MG, Byers PH. Cerebrovascular complications in Ehlers-Danlos syndrome type IV. *Ann Neurol* 1995; 38(6):960–4.

584 Van den Berg JS, Hennekam RC, Cruysberg JR, Steijlen PM, Swart J, Tijmes N, Limburg M. Prevalence of symptomatic intracranial aneurysm and ischaemic stroke in pseudoxanthoma elasticum. *Cerebrovasc Dis* 2000; 10(4):315–19.

585 Pepin M, Schwarze U, Superti-Furga A, Byers PH. Clinical and genetic features of Ehlers-Danlos syndrome type IV, the vascular type. *N Engl J Med* 2000; 342(10):673–80.

586 Wityk RJ, Zanferrari C, Oppenheimer S. Neurovascular complications of marfan syndrome: a retrospective, hospital-based study. *Stroke* 2002; 33(3):680–4.

587 Judge DP, Dietz HC. Marfan's syndrome. *Lancet* 2005; 366(9501):1965–76.

588 Ferro JM, Canhao P. Cerebral venous and dural sinus thrombosis. *Pract Neurol* 2003; 3(4):214–19.

589 Stam J. Thrombosis of the cerebral veins and sinuses. *N Engl J Med* 2005; 352(17):1791–8.

590 Bousser MG, Ferro JM. Cerebral venous thrombosis: an update. *Lancet Neurol* 2007; 6(2):162–70.

591 Williams AN. Cerebral venous thrombosis: the first reported case of adolescent stroke? *J R Soc Med* 2000; 93(10):552–3.

592 Bousser MG, Ross Russell RW. *Cerebral Venous Thrombosis*. London: W B Saunders, 1997.

593 Martinelli I, Landi G, Merati G, Cella R, Tosetto A, Mannucci PM. Factor V gene mutation is a risk factor for cerebral venous thrombosis. *Thromb Haemost* 1996; 75(3):393–4.

594 Zuber M, Toulon P, Marnet L, Mas JL. Factor V Leiden mutation in cerebral venous thrombosis. *Stroke* 1996; 27(10):1721–3.

595 Ludemann P, Nabavi DG, Junker R, Wolff E, Papke K, Buchner H *et al.* Factor V Leiden mutation is a risk factor for cerebral venous thrombosis: a case–control study of 55 patients. *Stroke* 1998; 29(12):2507–10.

596 Canhao P, Batista P, Falcao F. Lumbar puncture and dural sinus thrombosis: a causal or casual association? *Cerebrovasc Dis* 2005; 19(1):53–6.

597 Galan HL, McDowell AB, Johnson PR, Kuehl TJ, Knight AB. Puerperal cerebral venous thrombosis associated with decreased free protein S: a case report. *J Reprod Med* 1995; 40(12):859–62.

598 Wechsler B, Genereau T, Biousse V, Vauthier-Brouzes D, Seebacher J, Dormont D, Godeau P. Pregnancy complicated by cerebral venous thrombosis in Behcet's disease. *Am J Obstet Gynecol* 1995; 173(5):1627–9.

599 Dulli DA, Luzzio CC, Williams EC, Schutta HS. Cerebral venous thrombosis and activated protein C resistance. *Stroke* 1996; 27(10):1731–3.

600 De Bruijn SF, Stam J, Koopman MM, Vandenbroucke JP. Case–control study of risk of cerebral sinus thrombosis in oral contraceptive users and in [correction of who are] carriers of hereditary prothrombotic conditions. The Cerebral Venous Sinus Thrombosis Study Group. *Br Med J* 1998; 316(7131):589–92.

601 Wilder-Smith E, Kothbauer-Margreiter I, Lammle B, Sturzenegger M, Ozdoba C, Hauser SP. Dural puncture and activated protein C resistance: risk factors for cerebral venous sinus thrombosis. *J Neurol Neurosurg Psychiatry* 1997; 63(3):351–6.

602 Lancon JA, Killough KR, Tibbs RE, Lewis AI, Parent AD. Spontaneous dural sinus thrombosis in children. *Pediatr Neurosurg* 1999; 30(1):23–9.

603 DeVeber G, Andrew M, Adams C, Bjornson B, Booth F, Buckley DJ, Camfield CS *et al*. Cerebral sinovenous thrombosis in children. *N Engl J Med* 2001; 345(6):417–23.

604 Saatci I, Arslan S, Topcu M, Eldem B, Karagoz T, Saatci U. Case of the month. *Eur J Pediatr* 1996; 155(1):63–4.

605 Biousse V, Ameri A, Bousser MG. Isolated intracranial hypertension as the only sign of cerebral venous thrombosis. *Neurology* 1999; 53(7):1537–42.

606 Bousser MG, Chiras J, Bories J, Castaigne P. Cerebral venous thrombosis: a review of 38 cases. *Stroke* 1985; 16(2):199–213.

607 De Bruijn SF, Stam J, Kappelle LJ. Thunderclap headache as first symptom of cerebral venous sinus thrombosis. CVST Study Group. *Lancet* 1996; 348(9042):1623–5.

608 Kuehnen J, Schwartz A, Neff W, Hennerici M. Cranial nerve syndrome in thrombosis of the transverse/sigmoid sinuses. *Brain* 1998; 121(Pt 2):381–8.

609 Cantu C, Barinagarrementeria F. Cerebral venous thrombosis associated with pregnancy and puerperium: review of 67 cases. *Stroke* 1993; 24(12):1880–4.

610 Ameri A, Bousser MG. Cerebral venous thrombosis. *Neurol Clin* 1992; 10(1):87–111.

611 Daif A, Awada A, Al-Rajeh S, Abduljabbar M, Al Tahan AR, Obeid T, Malibary T. Cerebral venous thrombosis in adults: a study of 40 cases from Saudi Arabia. *Stroke* 1995; 26(7):1193–5.

612 Tsai FY, Wang AM, Matovich VB, Lavin M, Berberian B, Simonson TM, Yuh WT. MR staging of acute dural sinus thrombosis: correlation with venous pressure

measurements and implications for treatment and prognosis. *Am J Neuroradiol* 1995; **16**(5):1021–9.

613 Park DC, Sohn YH, Lee PH. Neurologic deficits with isolated cortical venous congestion. *Neurology* 1999; **52**(3):671–2.

614 Rahman NU, al-Tahan AR. Computed tomographic evidence of an extensive thrombosis and infarction of the deep venous system. *Stroke* 1993; **24**(5):744–6.

615 Baumgartner RW, Landis T. Venous thalamic infarction. *Cerebrovasc Dis* 1992; **2**:353–8.

616 Van den Bergh WM, van der Schaaf I, van Gijn J. The spectrum of presentations of venous infarction caused by deep cerebral vein thrombosis. *Neurology* 2005; **65**(2):192–6.

617 Eng LJ, Longstreth WT, Jr., Shaw CM, Eskridge JM, Bahls FH. Cerebellar venous infarction: case report with clinicopathologic correlation. *Neurology* 1990; **40**(5):837–8.

618 Nayak AK, Karnad D, Mahajan MV, Shah A, Meisheri YV. Cerebellar venous infarction in chronic suppurative otitis media: a case report with review of four other cases. *Stroke* 1994; **25**(5):1058–60.

619 Canhao P, Ferro JM, Lindgren AG, Bousser MG, Stam J, Barinagarrementeria F. Causes and predictors of death in cerebral venous thrombosis. *Stroke* 2005; **36**(8):1720–5.

620 Lueck CJ, McIlwaine GG. Idiopathic intracranial hypertension. *Pract Neurol* 2002; **2**:262–71.

621 Ozawa T, Miyasaka Y, Tanaka R, Kurata A, Fujii K. Dural-pial arteriovenous malformation after sinus thrombosis. *Stroke* 1998; **29**(8):1721–4.

622 Ferro JM, Correia M, Pontes C, Baptista MV, Pita F. Cerebral vein and dural sinus thrombosis in Portugal: 1980–1998. *Cerebrovasc Dis* 2001; **11**:177–82.

623 Stam J, de Bruijn SF, deVeber G. Anticoagulation for cerebral sinus thrombosis. *Cochrane Database Syst Rev* 2002; (4):CD002005.

624 Cakmak S, Nighoghossian N, Desestret V, Hermier M, Cartalat-Carel S, Derex L *et al.* Pulmonary embolism: an unusual complication of cerebral venous thrombosis. *Neurology* 2005; **65**(7):1136–7.

625 Wilkinson IM, Ross Rossini RW. Arteries of the head and neck in giant cell arteritis: a pathological study to show the pattern of arterial involvement. *Arch Neurol* 1972; **27**(5):378–91.

8 What caused this intracerebral haemorrhage?

8.1 Introduction

The separation of all the causes for non-traumatic intracerebral haemorrhage (ICH) listed in Table 8.1 is slightly simplistic. As a rule, there is no single cause for non-traumatic intracerebral haemorrhage, but an interaction of several factors, some of which are interrelated. Take the classical example of a so-called hypertensive haemorrhage: a haematoma developing in the region of the basal ganglia, in an elderly patient on anticoagulants for chronic atrial fibrillation and for an even longer period on antihypertensive drugs. Should chronic hypertension or anticoagulants be considered *the* cause of the intracerebral haemorrhage? Both are major risk factors.[1,2] The relative weight of each of these two factors depends on the degree of structural damage to the small arteries in the brain as a result of previously raised blood pressure (unknown), on the actual blood pressure immediately before the onset of the haemorrhage (also unknown) and on the intensity of anticoagulation. But even a combination of recognized 'causes', such as hypertension and anticoagulants, does not invariably lead to intracerebral haemorrhage. Apparently, the presence or absence of

other factors, of minor importance by themselves, can be decisive. Examples of such additional factors are age, sex, alcohol consumption, and plasma cholesterol,[1] and even genetic make-up associated with skin colour.[3] Not uncommonly, a combination of minor factors may lead to ICH, because some patients do not seem to have even one of the major 'causes'. In general, therefore, we are dealing with multiple rather than with single causes, and even for major factors the relationship with intracerebral haemorrhage is neither sufficient nor necessary. For example: why do some arteriovenous malformations of the brain bleed and others not?

With these qualifications, the known causal factors can be broadly grouped into three major categories (Table 8.1): structural factors (lesions or malformations of the vasculature in the brain), haemodynamic factors (blood pressure) and haemostatic factors (to do with platelet function or with the coagulation system). Lesions of the vascular system account for the vast majority of haemorrhages. The type of underlying abnormality varies with age: below the age of 40 years arteriovenous malformations and cavernous malformations are the most common single cause of ICH, whereas between 40 and 70 years the most frequent cause is deep haemorrhage from rupture of small perforating arteries, and in the elderly one also finds haemorrhages in the white matter ('lobar' haemorrhages), commonly attributed to amyloid angiopathy. The exact proportions depend on the age distribution and the control of risk factors within a given population. These relative probabilities

Stroke: practical management, 3rd edition. C. Warlow, J. van Gijn, M. Dennis, J. Wardlaw, J. Bamford, G. Hankey, P. Sandercock, G. Rinkel, P. Langhorne, C. Sudlow and P. Rothwell. Published 2008 Blackwell Publishing. ISBN 978-1-4051-2766-0.

Structural factors: lesions or malformations of the cerebral blood vessels
Changes in perforating arteries associated with chronic hypertension (section 8.2.1)
Amyloid angiopathy (section 8.2.2)
Saccular aneurysms (section 8.2.3)
Cerebral arteriovenous malformations (section 8.2.4)
Cavernous malformations (section 8.2.5)
Venous malformations (section 8.2.6)
Teleangiectasias (section 8.2.7)
Dural arteriovenous fistulae (section 8.2.8)
Haemorrhagic transformation of arterial infarction (section 8.2.9)
Intracranial venous thrombosis (section 8.2.10 and 7.21)
Septic arteritis and mycotic aneurysms (section 8.2.11)
Moyamoya syndrome (sections 8.2.12 and 7.5)
Arterial dissection (sections 8.2.13 and 7.2)
Caroticocavernous fistula (section 8.2.14)
Haemodynamic factors
Arterial hypertension, chronic or acute (sections 8.3.1 and 6.3.3)
Migraine (sections 8.3.2 and 7.8)
Haemostatic factors
Anticoagulants (section 8.4.1)
Antiplatelet drugs (section 8.4.2)
Thrombolytic treatment (section 8.4.3)
Clotting factor deficiency (section 8.4.4)
Leukaemia and thrombocytopenia (sections 8.4.5 and 7.9)
Other factors
Cerebral tumours (section 8.5.1)
Alcohol (sections 8.5.2 and 6.6.13)
Amphetamines (sections 8.5.3 and 7.1.1)
Cocaine and other drugs (sections 8.5.4 and 7.1.1)
Vasculitis (sections 8.5.5 and 7.3)
Trauma ('spät-Apoplexie'; section 8.5.6)

Table 8.1 Causes of non-traumatic intracerebral haemorrhage.

are discussed in more detail in section 8.6, in relation to the site of the haemorrhage.

8.2 Structural factors

8.2.1 Changes in perforating arteries associated with chronic hypertension

Chronically raised blood pressure is – with age – by far the most powerful risk factor for stroke in general, whether ischaemic or haemorrhagic (section 6.6.3). In many cases, it is chronic hypertension that underlies the degenerative change in small perforating arteries, which ultimately leads to their rupture in the basal ganglia, cerebellum or brainstem, or less often in the subcortical white matter. Few prospective studies have assessed the risk of increasing blood pressure for haemorrhagic stroke separately from ischaemic stroke. Those

that did found that the risk of haemorrhagic and ischaemic stroke increased to a similar degree with blood pressure, in Australia,[4] as well as in China and Japan, the stroke rate doubling for each 5 mmHg increase of diastolic pressure.[5]

Nevertheless, as pointed out in the introduction to this chapter, hypertension is neither a sufficient nor a necessary cause of ICH. The problem is compounded by questions of definition, blood pressure being not only a continuous but also an inconstant variable, dependent on technical equipment to boot. In hospital series of ICH patients, the proportion with hypertension (as determined by history and from the chest X-ray, ECG or heart weight) ranges mostly between 45% and 60%.[6] The population-attributable risk of hypertension has been estimated at 52% for deep brain haemorrhages,[7] and for intracerebral haemorrhage in general between 42% (Asians) and 34% (whites).[7] A systematic review of studies comparing blood pressure in deep compared with lobar haemorrhages found that in population-based studies of first strokes with a pre-stroke definition of hypertension the excess of hypertension was rather modest; OR 1.50 (95% CI 1.09–2.07); in other words, 'hypertension' is not all that much more common in deep compared with lobar haemorrhages.[8] All these pieces of evidence from different sources suggest that the term 'hypertensive intracerebral haemorrhage' is a misnomer. Furthermore, the 'normotensive' patients in these series may have had mild degrees of hypertension, without cardiac hypertrophy or other overt organ damage. After all, as in any disorder, 'high-risk' patients make up only a small proportion of the entire group of patients with the disorder in question; the majority are patients at only moderate risk – the prevention paradox (section 18.5.1).

> Factors other than hypertension must contribute to the rupture of small perforating vessels, because this occurs in some, but not all, people with hypertension, and sometimes even without hypertension.

Microaneurysms

In the 1860s Charcot and Bouchard examined the brains of patients who had died from ICH by immersing them in running water to remove not only unclotted blood but also most of the brain tissue. In this way they found multiple, minute outpouchings of small blood vessels, which they called miliary aneurysms.[9] These lesions, now called Charcot-Bouchard aneurysms (*très étonnés de se trouver ensemble*; section 2.7) were mostly found in the thalamus and corpus striatum, and to a somewhat lesser extent in the pons, cerebellum and cerebral white matter (Fig. 8.1). The view that these microaneurysms were commonly the source of bleeding held sway until the beginning of the 20th century, when at least some of these outpouchings were attributed to nothing more than perivascular collections of blood clot,[10,11] a finding that has been confirmed by later histological studies.[12] Other explanations for intracerebral haemorrhage gained ascendancy, particularly an older theory that haemorrhages were in fact secondary to previous brain infarction (sections 2.7 and 5.7).

In 1963 Ross Russell not only rediscovered the existence of microaneurysms, but also established a close relationship between these abnormalities and hypertension.[13] He performed postmortem studies of the brains of hypertensive and normotensive elderly people, by injecting barium sulphate into the basal arteries of the brain and then examining brain slices after fixation. Microaneurysms were found in 15 of 16 brains from hypertensive patients but in just 10 of 38 brains from normotensives; only previously hypertensive patients had more than 10 microaneurysms, with one dubious

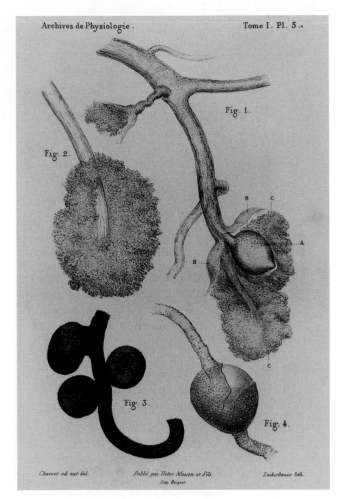

Fig. 8.1 'Miliary aneurysms' (Charcot & Bouchard, 1868).[9] (Fig. 1) a microaneurysm within a clot; (Fig. 2) a clot only; (Fig. 3) and (Fig. 4) microaneurysms without surrounding clot.

exception in the control group. The microaneurysms measured 300–900 μm in diameter and were found on small arteries 100–300 μm in diameter, commonly branches of the lateral lenticulostriate arteries in the region of the basal ganglia (Fig. 8.2). The relation between microaneurysms and hypertension was confirmed and expanded in a larger study by Cole and Yates of the brains of 100 normotensive patients, seven of whom had microaneurysms, and of 100 hypertensive patients, with microaneurysms in 46 patients, mostly above the age of 50.[14] The distribution of microaneurysms through the brain paralleled that of small perforating vessels, most often in the deep regions of the brain (Fig. 8.3). Accordingly, haemorrhages unexplained by detectable vascular lesions most often occur in these same regions: basal ganglia (Figs 8.4, 8.27a), internal capsule (Fig. 8.27b) and thalamus (Fig. 8.28); less often in the cerebellum (Fig. 8.29), midbrain (Fig. 8.30), pons (Fig. 8.31) and medulla oblongata (Fig. 8.32).

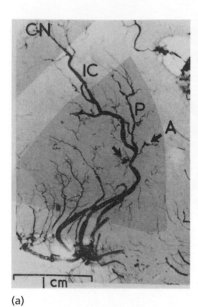

(a)

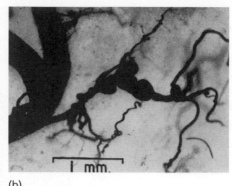

(b)

Fig. 8.2 Microaneurysms. (a) X-ray of striate arteries in coronal section of basal ganglia from elderly hypertensive subject; barium sulphate had been injected into the arterial tree before formalin fixation of the brain. Irregularity of main trunks, attenuation of small arteries and a number of microaneurysms (*arrows*). (b) Enlarged view of an area showing multiple aneurysms. (From Ross Russell, 1963;[13] by kind permission of the author and *Brain*.)

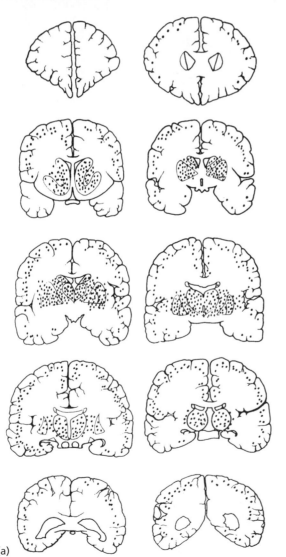

(a)

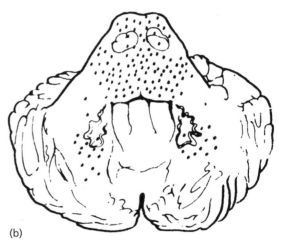

(b)

Fig. 8.3 (a) Sites of all microaneurysms discovered in the cerebral hemispheres of 53 patients (46/100 with hypertension and 7/100 normotensives). Successive front-to-back sections, from left to right and top to bottom. (b) Sites of microaneurysms in the hindbrains of the 53 patients, represented in a single section. (From Cole & Yates, 1967;[14] by kind permission of the authors and the *Journal of Pathology and Bacteriology*.)

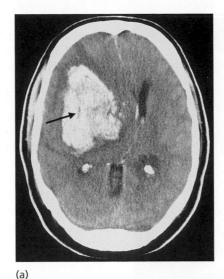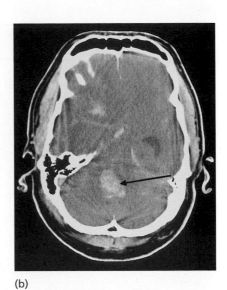

Fig. 8.4 Massive and rapidly fatal haemorrhage shown on CT brain scans in basal ganglia of right hemisphere (*arrow*) (a), with secondary haemorrhage in brainstem (*arrow*) as a result of transtentorial herniation (b).

(a)   (b)

Nevertheless, the role of microaneurysms in the pathogenesis of ICH remains controversial. About their existence there should be little doubt, despite the retrospective critique that Charcot and Bouchard may have misinterpreted not only clots in perivascular spaces but also twists and coils in perforating arteries.[15] The problem remains that just a few observations have directly traced an intracerebral haemorrhage to a specific microaneurysm. Cole and Yates found this in only a single patient of the 21 they studied after death from massive ICH. A Japanese study of surgical specimens demonstrated microaneurysms in 7 of 14 patients with deep brain haemorrhages and normal angiograms, but that they were the actual source of bleeding was no more than probable.[16] Ironically, the best documented patient in recent times was a normotensive 44-year-old woman with a relatively large 'microaneurysm' of 2 mm, visible on an angiogram.[17]

Probably perforating arterioles can rupture as a consequence of lesions other than microaneurysms. Fisher microscopically examined the border region of the haematoma in two patients with putaminal haemorrhage and in one patient with a pontine haemorrhage. In all three he found not single but multiple points of bleeding, in the form of 'fibrin globes' consisting of a plug of platelets occluding the lumen of a small artery (Fig. 8.5).[18] He found degenerative changes in the walls of the small perforating vessels, consisting of a segmental process of fatty changes ('lipohyalinosis') and fibrinoid necrosis. These changes were associated with local thinning, in other words places which might well be vulnerable to microtrauma in the form of an adjacent haemorrhage. Others have also found fibrinoid necrosis of the walls of these perforating arterioles as an almost

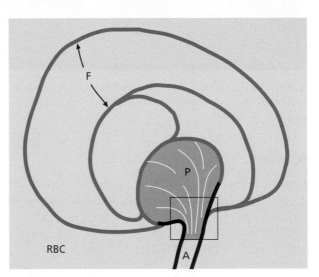

Fig. 8.5 Schematic representation of an occlusive thrombus at the site of rupture in a small perforating artery. A, ruptured artery; F, fibrin; P, platelets; RBC, red blood cells. (Redrawn after Fisher, 1971;[18] by kind permission of the author and Charles C. Thomas, publisher.)

invariable phenomenon in patients with deep ICH,[19] or atrophy and fragmentation of smooth muscle cells, with the site of rupture most commonly at distal bifurcations of lenticulostriate arteries.[20] Finally, penetrating arteries studied after surgical evacuation of deep haematomas showed evidence of dissection as often as degenerative changes.[21]

Not surprisingly, small deep infarcts are relatively common in patients presenting with deep haemorrhages. After all, small vessel disease commonly underlies both occlusion (section 6.4) and rupture.

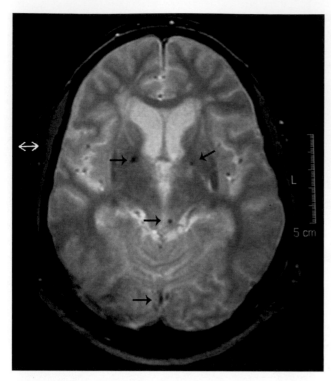

Fig. 8.6 Gradient-echo T2*-weighted MRI sequence showing microbleeds as black 'holes' (*arrows*) in different regions of the brain

Microbleeds

Magnetic resonance imaging of the brain with T2*-weighted gradient echo sequences has allowed the identification of traces of haemosiderin, suggesting small, 'silent' haemorrhages in the past, especially in patients with intracerebral haemorrhage (section 5.5.1; Fig. 8.6).[22,23] Histological study in postmortem specimens has confirmed the presence of haemosiderin in about two-thirds (21/34) of these lesions.[24] It should be recalled, though, that such 'microbleeds', as they are now commonly called, had already been identified in the 1960s by Cole and Yates, in the white matter, basal ganglia and internal capsule of 13 of the 46 brains of hypertensive patients with microaneurysms.[25]

In the general population such microbleeds are found especially among elderly males, while associations with hypertension, white matter changes and small, deep infarcts are less consistent.[26,27] Among stroke patients in general, they are relatively common in patients with intracerebral haemorrhage.[28,29] Haemorrhages tend to be larger if microbleeds are present.[30] Their preferential location is in the deep regions of the brain or in the border zone between cortex and white matter.[31] In patients with ischaemic stroke their presence has been found to predict haemorrhagic transformation.[32] It is uncertain

whether microbleeds predict the occurrence of ICH in general,[33] but if they are associated with evidence of presumed amyloid angiopathy on MRI (i.e. cortical border zone ICH) the risk is probably increased.[34] In patients with transient cerebral ischaemia or ischaemic stroke the presence of microbleeds heralds an increased risk of future stroke in general – of any type.[35]

One might speculate that microbleeds represent small leaks from perforating aneurysms damaged by chronic hypertension, or, in the case of microbleeds at the border of cortex and white matter, as a result of amyloid angiopathy (section 8.2.2). These minute haemorrhages are associated with moderate cognitive deficits,[36] while focal symptoms may appear as soon as they are a few mm in size.

The dynamics of extensive haemorrhage from deep arterioles

Fisher proposed that rupture of a single small artery might lead to subsequent rupture of other fragile arterioles, thus causing an 'avalanche' of secondary haemorrhages.[18] Another postmortem study confirmed multiple sites of rupture in single perforating arteries, 2 to 11 in number.[20] Indirect support for the 'avalanche' theory is provided by imaging *in vivo*. A systematic study of 103 patients with deep ICH in whom the first computed tomography (CT) scan was performed within 3 h of the first symptoms and who underwent a second CT scan 1 h later, found in one-quarter of these patients an increase in size of the haematoma.[37] A further 15–20% showed expansion 3–24 h after the onset.[37,38] Clinical deterioration in this group of patients is common, depending on the degree of enlargement.[39] The process of early haematoma expansion correlates with evidence of extravasation on CT angiography or magnetic resonance imaging,[40,41] and also with molecular markers of vascular injury and inflammation.[42] Already taking antiplatelet drugs probably increases the risk of haematoma expansion, even after correction for confounding factors.[43] Blood pressure and heart rate have no influence.[44] Expansion by rebleeding is rarely documented after 24 h.[38] All this evidence implicates a dynamic process, with a stable phase being reached in a matter of hours. Clinical deterioration later than 2 days after deep ICH is not caused by continued extravasation, but by perifocal oedema.[45]

> 'Hypertensive' intracerebral haemorrhage results from degenerative changes in small perforating vessels, most of which are found in deep regions: basal ganglia, thalamus, cerebellum and brainstem. Microaneurysms occur on these vessels but are not necessarily the site of rupture.

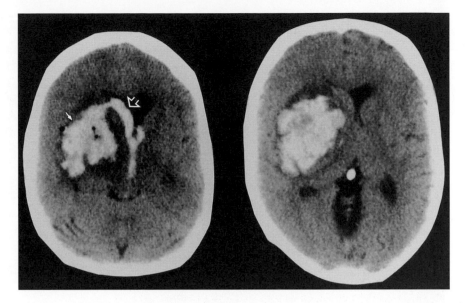

Fig. 8.7 Rebleeding in a 40-year-old woman with 'hypertensive' intracerebral haemorrhage (CT brain scans). *Left*: large haematoma in the right basal ganglia (*small arrow*), with rupture into the frontal horn of the right lateral ventricle (*open arrow*); the haematoma was surgically removed on the same day, because of progressive deterioration of consciousness. *Right*: fresh haemorrhage, indicated by sudden deterioration, 8 months after the initial episode; angiography was normal.

Recurrence of deep intracerebral haemorrhage

Deep brain haemorrhages are not necessarily a one-off event (Fig. 8.7).[46] In a systematic review of ten prospective studies with a minimum follow-up period of 3 months, the aggregate rebleeding rate was 2.3% per annum, which exceeded the rate of subsequent ischaemic stroke (1.1%).[47] Recurrences of deep haemorrhages were less common (2.1% per annum) than with haemorrhages at the border between white and grey matter (4.4% per annum), presumably caused by amyloid angiopathy (section 8.2.2). The site of the second haemorrhage is only rarely the same as the first one.[48]

8.2.2 Cerebral amyloid angiopathy

It is only in the last few decades that this disorder has been recognized as a cause of ICH, particularly of superficial ('lobar') haemorrhages (Fig. 8.8).[49,50] In patients with deep haemorrhages amyloid angiopathy is no more common than in controls aged over 65, i.e. less than 10%.[51]

Case reports of 'congophilic angiopathy' (or other descriptive terms) started to appear at the beginning of the 20th century,[52] but the first series of patients were not reported until the 1970s.[53,54] Haemorrhages associated with amyloid angiopathy typically occur at the border of the grey and white matter of the cerebral hemispheres and are irregular (Fig. 8.9);[55] also they may rupture towards the surface and spread through the subarachnoid space.[56] Cerebellar haemorrhages associated with amyloid angiopathy are less common.[57,58] The amyloid-laden vessels may be so brittle that even mild head trauma precipitates a haemorrhage.[59] One of our

own patients was an old lady who bled in both cerebral hemispheres when she tripped getting off a bus, without any direct head injury. In the same way, intracranial haemorrhage distant from the site of a neurosurgical intervention may well have to be attributed to amyloid angiopathy.[60] Thrombolytic therapy for myocardial infarction can be another precipitating factor (section 8.4.3).

Recurrence of haemorrhage associated with amyloid angiopathy is much more common than with 'hypertensive' small vessel disease (section 8.2.1);[47] case histories with 4–8 episodes are on record.[61–63] Recurrent haemorrhages often appear in the same region of the brain.[64] Serial MR scanning with gradient echo sequences may uncover asymptomatic new haemorrhages,[65] including small, punctate haemorrhages for which gradient echo MRI is most sensitive.[66] These microbleeds also occur with 'hypertensive' small vessel disease (section 8.2.1), but if they are associated with lobar haemorrhage the risk of recurrent major bleeding is proportional to their number.[67]

Manifestations other than lobar haemorrhage

Three non-haemorrhagic manifestations of cerebral amyloid angiopathy merit attention. The most frequent is intellectual deterioration associated with diffuse demyelination of the subcortical white matter. This is often found not only in patients with proven amyloid angiopathy,[66,68] but also with lobar haemorrhage in general.[69] On the other hand, white matter changes may also result from atherosclerotic changes in the long perforators from the cerebral convexity to the white matter, which is much more common in the general population (leukoaraiosis). A distinguishing feature is that with amyloid angiopathy the white matter is most affected in

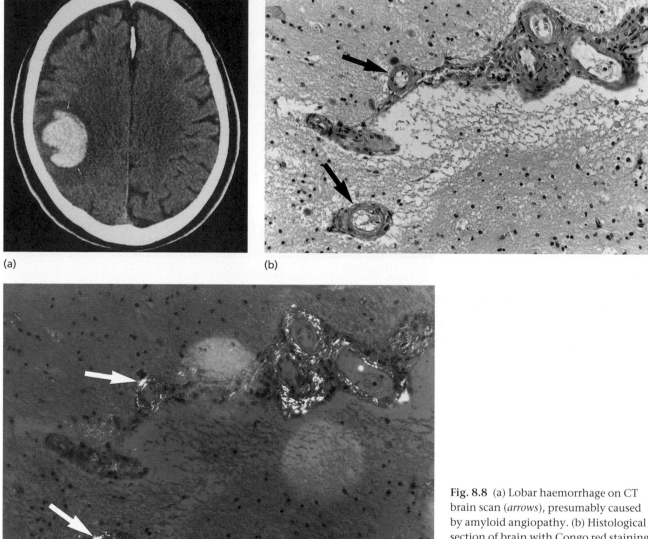

(a)

(b)

(c)

Fig. 8.8 (a) Lobar haemorrhage on CT brain scan (*arrows*), presumably caused by amyloid angiopathy. (b) Histological section of brain with Congo red staining, showing amyloid angiopathy in walls of arterioles (*arrows*) (magnification 200×). (c) As in (b), showing birefringence under polarized light (*arrows*).

the temporal region and in the splenium.[70] Occasionally amyloid angiopathy causes full-blown dementia without preceding haemorrhage.[71,72]

A much rarer problem is recurrent, transient episodes of focal weakness, paraesthesiae, numbness with spread and, less often, visual distortion. These attacks may be caused by transient ischaemia or by small haemorrhages with a focal seizure.[73–76] Often the diagnosis of amyloid angiopathy can be made only in retrospect, when a large lobar haemorrhage supervenes, but MRI may suggest amyloid angiopathy as the cause of stereo-typed 'TIAs' if T2*-weighted imaging reveals an area of signal loss consistent with bleeding within cortical

subarachnoid spaces, while conventional T2 imaging shows leukoaraiosis.[77]

A recently recognized complication of amyloid angiopathy other than haemorrhage is perivascular inflammation,[78] which clinically manifests as a combination of headaches, seizures, cognitive decline and focal deficits.[78–80] The white matter abnormalities on neuroimaging and the pleocytosis with raised protein level in the CSF are indistinguishable from the idiopathic variant of primary angiitis of the central nervous system (section 7.3.17); only brain biopsy or post-mortem allows the diagnosis to be made. Occasionally the inflammatory reaction gives rise to a local, reversible

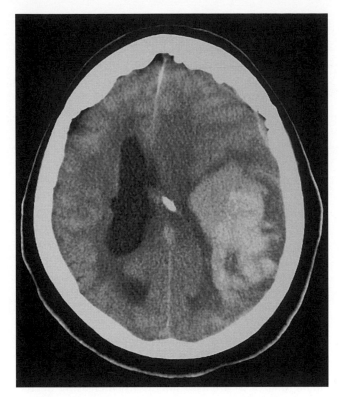

Fig. 8.9 CT brain scan showing non-homogeneous lobar haemorrhage in an 89-year-old woman, probably caused by amyloid angiopathy.

leukoencephalopathy,[81] or to local granuloma presenting as a space-occupying lesion.[82]

Diagnosis

A diagnosis of amyloid angiopathy in an elderly patient with lobar haemorrhage may be suspected but definitive proof is difficult. Fortunately, the distinction from deep haemorrhages is reliable between trained radiologists.[83] The occurrence of multiple 'lobar' haemorrhages, either at the same time or separated only by days, is a fairly typical, although not unique, characteristic of haemorrhages associated with amyloid angiopathy (Fig. 8.10).[84] Other causes of multiple intracerebral haemorrhages are listed in Table 8.2 and range from unsuspected head injury to sepsis and diffuse intravascular coagulation. Multifocal haemorrhages are distinctly rare in deep locations.

In the case of a single lobar haemorrhage, which makes up approximately 30–40% of all ICHs in community studies,[85,86] 30% overall are attributable to amyloid angiopathy.[58] The set of criteria proposed by the Boston Cerebral Amyloid Angiopathy Group proved valid on postmortem examination in all 13 cases with a diagnosis of 'probable cerebral amyloid angiopathy' on clinical

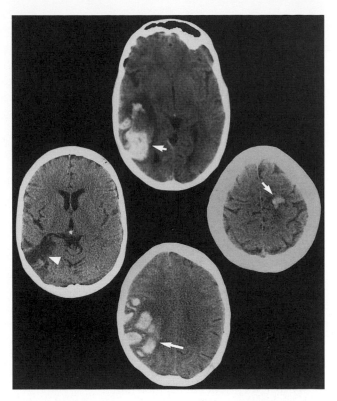

Fig. 8.10 Multiple haemorrhages from familial amyloid angiopathy in a single patient (CT scans). *Top*: haemorrhage in right temporal lobe (*arrow*), at age 51 years. *Left and right*: small haemorrhage (*arrow*) at the convexity of the left hemisphere, at age 54 years; the previous haemorrhage has left a hypodense scar (*arrowhead*). *Bottom*: haemorrhage in right parietal lobe (*arrow*), at age 55 years. The patient died after a fourth episode at the age of 56 years.

Table 8.2 Causes of multiple haemorrhages in the brain.

Intracranial venous thrombosis (sections 5.8, 7.21 and 8.2.10)
Thrombolytic treatment (section 8.4.3)
Metastases, especially melanoma, bronchial carcinoma, renal carcinoma, choriocarcinoma (section 8.5.1)
Cerebral vasculitis (section 7.3 and 8.5.5)
Diffuse intravascular coagulation (section 7.9.12)
Haemostatic disorder (sections 8.4.3 and 8.4.4)
Leukaemia (section 8.4.5)
Eclampsia (section 8.3.1 and 7.14)
Unsuspected head injury

grounds, but recurrent lobar haemorrhage was required for inclusion in this category.[87] On the other hand, with single lobar haemorrhages (category 'possible') the same study from Boston as well as another study from Kiel with histological verification found misclassification in 25–50% of lobar haemorrhages initially regarded as amyloid-related on the basis of CT scanning.[87,88]

Misclassification involves not only 'hypertensive' haemorrhages but also rare causes of lobar haemorrhage such as CADASIL (section 7.20.1).[89]

So other factors than a superficial location need to be taken into account to make a diagnosis of amyloid angiopathy. Magnetic resonance imaging (MRI) may give support to the diagnosis by showing evidence of previous punctate haemorrhages,[34,65,67] although these 'microbleeds' are also found in patients with 'hypertensive' haemorrhages (section 8.2.1). Radiological features in patients with lobar haemorrhage, confirmed at postmortem as due to amyloid angiopathy, are: an non-homogeneous, rather variable hyperattenuation of the haematoma on CT (compared with haematomas caused by rupture of an AVM or saccular aneurysm); a tendency to sedimentation of blood in the posterior regions of the haematoma; and rupture to the cerebral surface or the ventricular system.[55] However, the specificity of these characteristics has not been tested by comparison with lobar haemorrhages from other causes. A cortical biopsy is very sensitive and also specific if fibrinoid necrosis is found in amyloid-laden vessels,[90] but this is rarely indicated and may even be dangerous because it may provoke new episodes of haemorrhage.

There is a need for new diagnostic criteria, in which clinical factors (age, cognitive deterioration) and radiological characteristics (non-homogeneous density, evidence of small previous haemorrhages on gradient echo MRI) can be entered into the equation for an estimate of the probability of amyloid angiopathy in a patient with a single lobar haematoma. Unfortunately histological studies are indispensable for the validation of any set of criteria, but nowadays postmortem examination is – unfortunately – becoming the exception rather than the rule.

Origin and genetics of intravascular amyloid in sporadic cases

Cerebral amyloid angiopathy has no relation to systemic amyloidosis. The condition is not limited to humans, as it has been found in an aged woodpecker.[91] The amyloid deposits are patchy and are located in the muscle layer of small and medium-sized cortical arteries (Fig. 8.8). Several variants of amyloid protein occur.[92] The Aβ amyloid protein is found in sporadic cases, which is by far the most common form.

The general view, supported by a transgenic mouse model, is that the abnormal protein is derived from precursor proteins synthesized *in situ* by smooth muscle cells.[93,94] Others assume a relationship with peri-arterial interstitial fluid drainage pathways,[95] in that peptides such as Aβ would be eliminated along these perivascular spaces and so become entrapped in the walls of cerebral arteries.[96]

Some degree of accumulation of Aβ amyloid is found in cortical vessels of asymptomatic individuals, the proportion increasing with age, from 5–10% in those aged between 60 and 69 years, approximately 25% between ages 70 and 79 years, 40% between 80 and 89 years, to more than 50% for those over 90 years.[57,97–100] Arteries in the occipital, parietal and frontal lobes are most often involved. Affected arteries are found mostly in the cortex but also in the leptomeninges and in subcortical areas.

The difference between amyloid angiopathy with or without haemorrhages is twofold. First, amyloid deposition is more extensive in those with haemorrhages, not so much reflected by the proportion of affected cortical vessels but rather by the degree of involvement per vessel.[101,102] Second, cortical arteries of patients with amyloid-associated haemorrhages relatively often show evidence of dilatation, disruption and fibrinoid necrosis.[101,103]

The genetic background in sporadic cases is largely unknown. The only traces of knowledge so far relate to the apolipoprotein E gene. Increasing doses of the ε4 allele (0, 1 or 2) are associated with increasing degrees of amyloid deposition,[102] whereas the ε2 allele predisposes to amyloid-associated damage to the vessel wall, especially fibrinoid necrosis,[104,105] and also to actual haemorrhages.[106,107] Some suggest that not only the risk of haemorrhage but also the anatomical distribution differs according to the apolipoprotein genotype, in that meningeal vessels are affected in ε2-associated amyloid angiopathy (the 'haemorrhagic type') but not in ε4-associeted vasculopathy, whereas for cortical capillaries it is the other way around.[108]

> Haemorrhages into the white matter ('lobar' haemorrhages) are most often caused by the same type of 'hypertensive' arteriolar disease that is associated with deep haemorrhages, but in those aged over 70 years cerebral amyloid angiopathy is also a common underlying condition, in approximately 30%. Amyloid angiopathy can be more specifically suspected with multiple or recurrent haemorrhages, preceding episodes of transient deficits or, very rarely, a family history of intracerebral haemorrhage.

Amyloid angiopathy and Alzheimer's disease

There is a complex relationship between amyloid angiopathy and Alzheimer's disease.[109] Both are associated with accumulation of Aβ amyloid, in the case of Alzheimer's disease in the brain parenchyma, and both are associated with the apolipoprotein ε4 genotype. But perhaps that is where the similarity ends, because it is well established that amyloid angiopathy leading to lobar haemorrhage may occur without clinical evidence of dementia and also without amyloid plaques or any of the other hallmarks of Alzheimer's disease in the brain parenchyma,[110] and vice versa.[111] A possible synthesis is offered by observations that if amyloid angiopathy is associated with Alzheimer's disease there is a distinct profile of the type and distribution of Aβ, with deposits predominantly in cortical capillaries and consisting of a peptide of 42 or 43 amino acids, similar to amyloid in senile plaques of the same patient.[112,113] In contrast, amyloid angiopathy proper, in cortical and leptomeningeal arteries, the type commonly associated with haemorrhages, consists mainly of a shorter Aβ peptide, of 40 amino acids.[113] The relationship with the apolipoprotein genotypes mentioned above is striking (ε4 for capillary amyloid associated with Alzheimer's disease vs ε2 for arterial and meningeal amyloid associated with haemorrhages).

> Sporadic amyloid angiopathy associated with lobar haemorrhages is concentrated in cortical and meningeal arteries, is associated with the apolipoprotein ε2 genotype and consists mainly of Aβ peptides with 40 amino acids. In contrast, amyloid angiopathy associated with Alzheimer's disease is found mainly in cortical capillaries, is associated with the apolipoprotein ε2 genotype and consists mainly of Aβ peptides with 42 or 43 amino acids.

Familial forms of amyloid angiopathy

Specific mutations have been identified in autosomal dominant forms of amyloid angiopathy with cerebral haemorrhage. In the Icelandic type, with a median age of onset of 30 years,[114] the amyloid protein consists of a mutant cystatin C.[115,116] All other heritable forms of cerebral amyloid angiopathy are associated with mutations in the beta-amyloid precursor protein, so far at four sites, all situated within the beta-amyloid peptide sequence itself.[117]

For the Dutch type, in which all three pedigrees could be traced back to two nearby villages on the North Sea coast, the median age at the time of a first haemorrhage is 50 years, often with preceding cognitive decline.[118,119] The Dutch type is caused by a point mutation in the gene for the amyloid precursor protein (APP),[120] resulting in accumulation in cerebral vessels of mostly Aβ42 peptides with a single amino acid substitution at residue 22 of Aβ (codon 693 of APP). Variants with early-onset dementia in addition to haemorrhages are caused by a different mutation in the same codon (Arctic variant),[121] and by a mutation in the adjoining codon 692 of the APP gene.[122] The 'Iowa mutation' at codon 694 causes cerebral haemorrhages in one kindred,[123] but leukoencephalopathy with dementia in another.[124] An Italian kindred with recurrent haemorrhages from an amino acid substitution at residue 34 of Aβ (corresponding with a mutation in codon 705 of the APP gene) showed amyloid only in cerebral arteries and not at all in the parenchyma.[125] Other mutations of the Aβ sequence outside residues 21–23 (or codons 692–694 of the APP gene) are associated with pure dementia, including rarer forms of familial Alzheimer's disease.[92,126]

8.2.3 Saccular aneurysms

In large hospital series, one-quarter to one-third of the patients with subarachnoid haemorrhage (SAH) from a ruptured aneurysm (section 9.1.1) have an associated intracerebral haemorrhage (ICH).[127,128] Patients with large ICHs often die early, so highly specialized referral centres will see a smaller proportion of haematomas associated with aneurysmal haemorrhages. No prospective studies have addressed the relative frequency of ICH from ruptured saccular aneurysms. However, an educated guess can be made from the overall annual incidence (per 100 000 in a current white population): for first-ever in a lifetime strokes the rate critically depends on age distribution (Table 17.15) but overall it is approximately 200,[129,130] some 12% or 24 per 100 000 consisting of ICHs, and some 3% or six per 100 000 of SAH.[131] Given that two out of six patients with SAH have an ICH, this corresponds with two out of every 26 patients with ICH. In other words, about one in 13 ICHs is secondary to rupture of a saccular aneurysm. However, this is the ratio for all ages combined. Below the age of 65, SAH and deep ICH are about equally common,[132] in which case the proportion of ICHs from aneurysmal haemorrhage will be around one in six.

> About one in 13 of all intracerebral haemorrhages are due to a ruptured saccular aneurysm, but more like two in 13 under the age of 65 years.

Intracerebral haemorrhage from aneurysmal haemorrhage can be fairly reliably diagnosed on the basis of at least one of two characteristics: the association with blood in the basal cisterns and a fairly typical location (section 9.4.1).[133] It is important to distinguish between an intracerebral haematoma secondary to a ruptured aneurysm and intracerebral haemorrhage originating in the parenchyma, whether deep or lobar, because a patient with a ruptured aneurysm requires

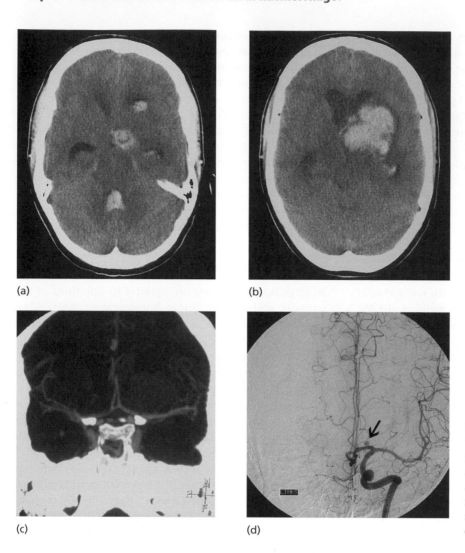

(a)

(b)

(c)

(d)

Fig. 8.11 CT brain scans showing 'hypertensive' intracerebral haemorrhage in a 45-year-old woman (a,b). A CT angiogram – of less than optimal quality according to present standards – was normal (c), but a later catheter angiogram showed an aneurysm of the anterior cerebral artery (d, *arrow*).

urgent treatment to occlude the site of bleeding, apart from problems caused by the ICH (Fig. 8.11); section 14.4). It should be kept in mind that demonstration of an aneurysm in the vicinity of the ICH does not exclude other causes, such as rupture of a cavernous malformation.[134]

> If the location of an intracerebral haemorrhage is compatible with a ruptured aneurysm, the patient should be urgently transferred to a neurosurgical facility for evacuation to at least be considered, especially if the patient's clinical condition is poor.

8.2.4 Cerebral arteriovenous malformations

Haemorrhage is the initial *clinical* manifestation in about half of patients known to have arteriovenous malformations (AVMs).[135] The next most common manifestation is epilepsy (about one-quarter), while many are asymptomatic at the time of detection.[136] Demonstrable

AVMs are the most common single cause of ICH in the young, but they account for no more than about one-third of those cases. The annual detection rate of AVMs is approximately 1 per 100 000 per year.[135,137]

AVMs are tangles of dilated arteries and veins, without a capillary network between them; the intervening brain tissue is usually normal. On angiography, they are recognizable by the large feeding arteries and the rapid shunting of blood to veins that are enlarged and tortuous, often with a central nidus of dilated vessels, between the arteries and veins. Multiple AVMs are exceptional, but their frequency is probably underestimated because a second AVM is often very small; about half the patients with multiple AVMs have hereditary haemorrhagic telangiectasia (Rendu-Osler-Weber syndrome).[138] Familial occurrence of AVMs is even more exceptional.[139,140]

There are saccular aneurysms on the feeding arteries or within the nidus itself in about 20% of AVMs, the aneurysms being likely sources of bleeding.[141] Also AVMs in which one or more aneurysms have formed are

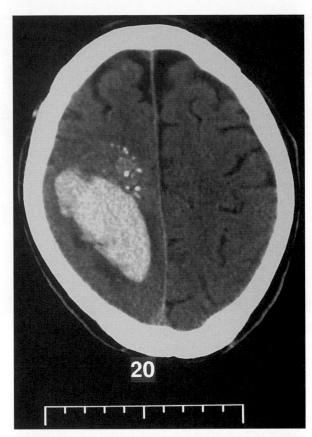

(a)

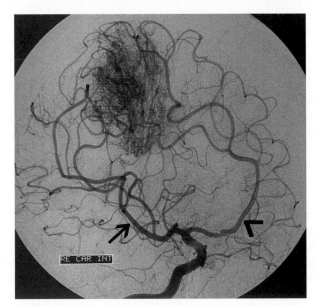

(b)

Fig. 8.12 CT brain scan showing intracerebral haemorrhage in the right parietal lobe, in a 27-year-old man (a). The adjacent calcifications suggest the presence of an arteriovenous malformation. The catheter angiogram (b) shows the malformation is fed by branches of the middle cerebral artery (*arrow*) as well as of the anterior cerebral artery (*arrowhead*).

more likely to (re)rupture: the annual risk of bleeding is as high as 7%, against the usual rate of 2–3%/year for AVMs without associated aneurysm (section 15.3.2).

Haemorrhages from AVMs are mostly in the white matter ('lobar'; Fig. 8.12), but they also occur in the deep nuclei of the cerebral hemisphere. Subarachnoid haemorrhage results if the haematoma reaches the surface of the brain, but of all haemorrhages secondary to a ruptured AVM only 4% are purely subarachnoid, without a parenchymal component.[142] If there is no associated aneurysm on the arterial side, the site of rupture is usually on the venous side of the malformation. Rupture of a vein might perhaps explain the often slower onset and better recovery of the clinical deficits as the result of haemorrhages from AVMs compared with ICHs from rupture of perforating arteries, or saccular aneurysms.[143,144]

> Rupture of arteriovenous malformations almost invariably results in an intracerebral haemorrhage, and only exceptionally (4%) in a purely subarachnoid haemorrhage.

Very small vascular malformations may not be seen on angiography. In a series of 72 patients under 45 years with ICH, the proportion of unexplained haemorrhages was as high as 25%, perhaps in part because not every AVM could be seen on conventional (catheter) angiography.[145] Before modern neuroimaging techniques, specifically MRI, became widely available, angiographically occult lesions were categorized as 'microangiomas' but in retrospect these were probably cavernous malformations.[146,147]

8.2.5 Cavernous malformations

Cerebral cavernous malformations are small (1 mm to several cm in diameter), thin-walled vascular structures, consisting of a mulberry-like conglomerate lined by endothelium without muscular or elastic layers and with no intervening brain tissue; they are single or multiple, and occasionally calcified.[148] Cavernous malformations may also occur in the skin, orbit and almost any internal organ. In the brain they are often asymptomatic – even if complicated by haemorrhage, which is mostly minute.

Cavernous malformations are encountered in 0.5% of routine postmortems.[149] It was only after the advent of CT, and especially MRI (Fig. 8.13), that these lesions became regularly recognized during life. A review of more than 14 000 consecutive MR scans in the late 1980s discovered them in again 0.5%.[150] On T2-weighted MRI, cavernous malformations are characterized by a combination of a reticulated core of mixed signal intensity with a

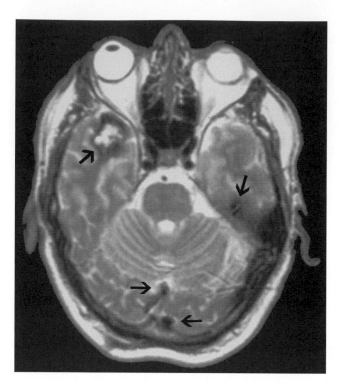

Fig. 8.13 Multiple cavernous malformations (*arrows*) detected by MRI scanning (T2 weighted, axial view) through the brainstem, cerebellum and temporal poles.

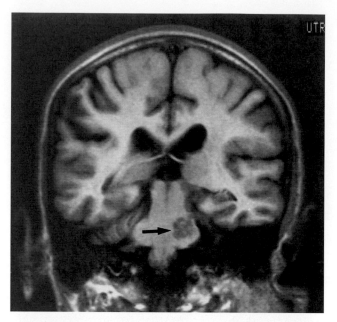

Fig. 8.14 Probable cavernous malformation of the brainstem. MR scan (T1-weighted in the coronal plane) of a 48-year-old woman who had experienced an attack, lasting several hours, of vertigo, tinnitus, a burning feeling around the nose, and pins and needles of the right half of her body below the face. The marginated but rather sharply demarcated border of the abnormality in the left half of the pons and middle cerebellar peduncle in the absence of space-occupying effect suggests a cavernous malformation (*arrow*). Left vertebral catheter angiography was normal. Three years later, the lesion had not changed.

surrounding rim of decreased signal intensity, corresponding to haemosiderin (Fig. 8.14). Smaller lesions appear as areas of decreased signal intensity (black dots) and are picked up even better by T2-weighted gradient echo MRI.[151,152] The lesions are not static but often grow or shrink,[153] and can even appear *de novo* in sporadic cases.[154] Brain radiation in children is a probable risk factor.[155–157]

Cavernous malformations are located in the hemispheric white matter or cortex in about one-half of all cases, in the posterior fossa (most often the brainstem) in one-third, and in the basal ganglia or thalamus in one-sixth.[158–160] Exceptional locations include the ventricular system, where cavernous malformations may become extremely large,[161] the pineal region,[162] the cavernous sinus,[163] the optic chiasm or other cranial nerves,[164] and the spinal cord.[165] Coexistence of spinal and cerebral cavernous malformations is not uncommon.[166]

If a cavernous malformation is symptomatic, epileptic seizures are at least as common a manifestation as haemorrhage, despite the bias that the studies have tended to originate from neurosurgical services.[167] The third main clinical syndrome is that of a transient or permanent focal deficit corresponding to a brain region or a cranial nerve, sometimes associated with an expanding cavernous malformation. Not unexpectedly this occurs relatively often with lesions in the brainstem. The deficits

usually develop in a gradual fashion but may remit, mimicking multiple sclerosis,[168] or they may cause myoclonus of the face or palate.[169]

Estimates of the risk of haemorrhage in patients in whom a cavernous malformation has been detected vary widely, between 0.25% and 6% per annum.[148] This is because of differences in study design with varying degrees of referral bias according to clinical presentation (no symptoms, epilepsy, haemorrhage or focal deficits; familial or sporadic occurrence), retrospective case finding, and variation in the definition of what constitutes a haemorrhage on imaging. Factors possibly predisposing to a relatively high risk of haemorrhage are a previous haemorrhage,[158] deep location of the cavernous malformation (brainstem, cerebellum, basal ganglia or thalamus),[160] age below 35 on first presentation,[170] and – not surprisingly – the presence of multiple lesions, which mostly occur in familial forms (see below).[171] On the other hand, haemorrhages from a cavernous malformation are usually limited (Fig. 8.15) and rarely fatal. Despite this, many neurosurgeons favour resection of symptomatic cavernous malformations in the brainstem

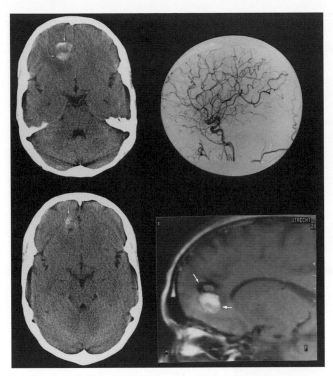

Fig. 8.15 Suspected cavernous malformation in a 25-year-old woman. *Top, left*: CT brain scan showing a parasagittal haemorrhage (*arrow*) in the right frontal lobe (clinically manifested by sudden headache, followed by a seizure). *Top, right*: normal right carotid catheter angiogram (the left carotid angiogram was also normal). *Bottom, left*: CT scan, 3 months after the event; residual lesion with calcification (*arrow*) and a region of hypodensity. *Bottom, right*: sagittal MR scan (T1-weighted), 4 months after the event; sharply demarcated, hypodense lesion (*thin arrow*), with residual, hyperintense region (haemosiderin) at its ventral border (*thick arrow*).

or spinal cord, where even a small bleed can cause considerable deficits (section 13.3.8).

A familial form of the disorder was first detected in Mexican-American families, and accounts for some half of all cases in people of Mexican origin.[172] Subsequently, familial forms have also been detected in several European countries, where sporadic forms are in the large majority, estimated at 80–90%,[173] and in Asia.[174] In contrast to sporadic cases with a single cavernous malformation most familial cases have multiple cavernous malformations, the number increasing with advancing age; conversely, in a given patient with multiple cavernous malformations there is a 75% chance that first-degree relatives are affected as well.[175]

Loci for the genes in question have been mapped on chromosomes 7q (CCM1; 40% of familial cases), 7p (CCM2; 20%) and 3q (CCM3; 20%) For CCM1 the gene has been identified; it encodes *Krit1*, a 736-amino acid protein; at the time of writing some 75 different

mutations have been found in this gene, all of which led to premature stop codons.[173] Clinical as well as radiological penetrance is incomplete: in a study of 138 relatives (of 64 probands) who were mutation carriers, half were asymptomatic and one in ten had no lesions on gradient echo MR imaging.[173] In Spanish families, the CCM1 mutations are different from those in Mexican-Americans,[176] in whom the mutation is highly stereotyped and probably inherited from a single founder.[177] The CCM2 gene has only recently been identified.[178] The expression patterns of the three CCM genes is similar in a variety of tissues; given the identical aspect of the malformations, this suggests the three gene products have similar actions.[179,180]

8.2.6 Venous malformations

Venous malformations consist of several dilated veins, without an abnormal input on the arterial side, converging into a single abnormal vein, which in turn drains into the venous system on the surface of the brain or, less commonly, into the deep venous system. The radial orientation of the peripheral veins creates the impression of a caput medusae (Fig. 8.16). The annual rate of symptomatic haemorrhage in patients with unruptured venous malformations is very low, between 0.15 and 0.34%.[181,182] If such lesions bleed at all, one should search for an associated abnormality, such as a cavernous malformation,[182] or an arteriovenous malformation.[183] Venous malformations are the most common vascular anomaly incidentally encountered at postmortem: in a series of over 4000 consecutive postmortems, 4% of all brains harboured one or more vascular malformations, 63% of which were venous malformations.[184] Most occur in the frontal lobes, followed by the parietal lobes and the cerebellum.[181,185] Their appearance on MR scans is that of a tubular area of decreased signal intensity in the white matter of the brain (Fig. 8.17).

As with cavernous malformations, common manifestations of venous malformations are not only haemorrhagic episodes, but also seizures, transient focal deficits or tinnitus.[181,185,186] Headache is also mentioned in these series, but probably this symptom represents the reason for ordering a head scan rather than being a true consequence of the lesion.[181,182,185,187]

These days there is increasing awareness that in the majority the 'lesion' is a variant of venous drainage rather than a pathological malformation, which is why some have proposed the term 'developmental venous anomaly' over 'venous malformation'.[187,188] The enlarged vein, which is the pathognomonic feature of venous malformations, is an indispensable conduit for the

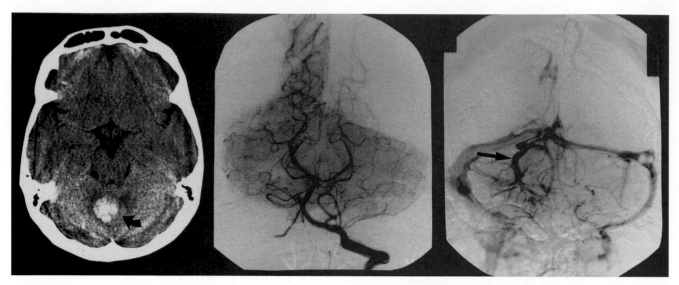

Fig. 8.16 Venous malformation in a 44-year-old man. *Left*: CT scan, showing intracerebral haemorrhage in the vermis of the cerebellum (*arrow*). *Middle*: left vertebral catheter angiogram, showing normal arterial phase. *Right*: left vertebral angiogram in the venous phase showing the venous malformation, with abnormal venous structures converging towards a single draining vein (caput medusae, *arrow*).

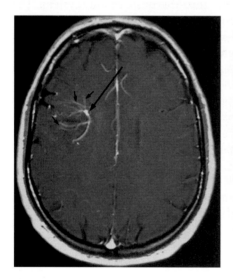

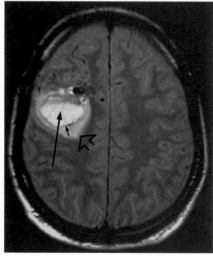

Fig. 8.17 Appearance of ruptured venous malformation on MR scanning, in a 31-year-old man. *Left*: gadolinium-enhanced T1-weighted MR scan shows the radial orientation of the contributing veins (*small arrows*), towards a central draining vein (*large arrow*). *Right* (early T2-weighted image): haematoma in the right centrum semiovale, represented by a hyperintense core of methaemoglobin (*long arrow*), surrounded by a hypointense rim of intracellular deoxyhaemoglobin (*short arrow*) and a hyperintense zone of oedema (*open arrow*). The central draining vein is represented by a tubular area of hypointensity ('signal void'), caused by the flow of blood.

drainage of blood from the brain, as the usual drainage pathways are inadequate or absent. Operative intervention aimed at resection or collapse of such large veins can therefore be disastrous.[189] We personally know of a case history with fatal brain swelling a few days after resection of a venous malformation in the frontal lobe. Even spontaneous thrombosis of the central draining vein can result in venous swelling and infarction.[190] Operative treatment is therefore not warranted.

8.2.7 Telangiectasias

Telangiectasias are small lesions in which the vessels resemble capillaries but have a larger lumen (20–500 μm),

separated by normal brain tissue. They occur most often in the pons. They have a very low potential for bleeding unless they are multiple, in the context of hereditary haemorrhagic teleangiectasia (Rendu-Osler-Weber disease), a condition in which other organs are more often affected, notably lungs, mucous membranes, gut and liver.[191] The vascular abnormalities in hereditary haemorrhagic teleangiectasia consist not only of telangiectasias but also of arteriovenous malformations, especially in the lung; in fact two-thirds of the neurological complications (mostly brain abscesses) of Rendu-Osler-Weber disease are secondary to pulmonary AVMs.[192] The risk of brain haemorrhage from telangiectasias in patients is low and even then the outcome is good.[193]

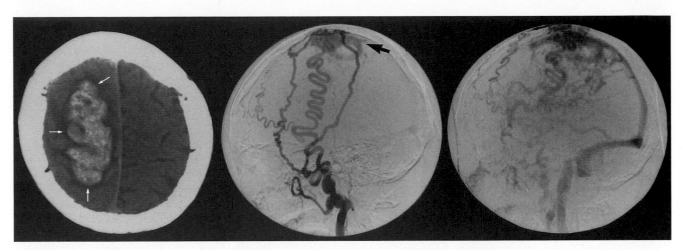

Fig. 8.18 Dural fistula with intracerebral haemorrhage. *Left*: CT scan showing a marginated haemorrhage at the convexity of the right hemisphere (*arrows*); the clinical deficit, a left hemiparesis, had developed gradually, over about 1 h. *Middle*: right external carotid catheter angiogram (arterial phase), showing abnormally large meningeal branches, converging towards the dural fistula (*arrow*). *Right*: right external carotid angiogram (venous phase) showing filling of abnormal, dilated intracranial veins.

Occasionally telangiectasias give rise to brainstem deficits without haemorrhage.[194]

8.2.8 Dural arteriovenous fistulae

Dural arteriovenous fistulae are fed by meningeal vessels, most often branches of the middle meningeal or occipital branches of the external carotid artery, more rarely from the internal carotid or vertebral artery. As a rule, drainage is directly into dural sinuses, most often the transverse or sigmoid sinus, less commonly the superior sagittal or cavernous sinus (Fig. 8.18). In a minority the anomaly communicates retrogradely with superficial veins of the cerebral convexity or the cerebellum, or with perimesencephalic or perimedullary veins.[195] If drainage occurs via spinal veins the clinical features may result from venous congestion rather than haemorrhage.[196] In adults the lesions are acquired, mostly (40%) through thrombotic or neoplastic occlusion of a major venous sinus, the venous hypertension resulting in abnormal anastomoses between dural arteries and veins.[197,198] Previous head injury accounts for less than 10% of arteriovenous fistulae,[199] presumably through thrombosis of the dural sinus in question;[200] rarely a fracture of the anterior skull base underlies the development of a dural fistula.[201]

Haemorrhage is the presenting event in only 15% of patients with a dural arteriovenous fistula.[202] The danger of haemorrhage is relatively high with multiple lesions and if drainage occurs through cortical veins;[203,204] in those cases rebleeding is not infrequent.[205] The bleeding may be confined to the subarachnoid space (section 9.1.4). It should not be forgotten that cerebellar haemorrhage can also be secondary to arteriovenous fistulae.[206] In contrast, the risk of haemorrhage from arteriovenous fistulae without cortical drainage is rather low.[207]

The most common manifestations of dural fistulae are pulsatile tinnitus (if the fistula is near the temporal bone),[208] or headache and visual symptoms from papilloedema.[209] The papilloedema reflects increased pressure of cerebrospinal fluid, through increased pressure in the superior sagittal sinus; it presents with visual obscurations, inferior nasal field defects or concentric field constriction, and eventually impaired visual acuity. A distinctly rare presentation is progressive dementia.[210]

8.2.9 Haemorrhagic transformation of an arterial infarct

A popular theory at the beginning of this century had it that cerebral infarction preceded *all* instances of non-traumatic intracerebral haemorrhage (section 2.7), a view that is clearly wrong. Haemorrhagic transformation occurs in *some* patients with cerebral infarction (15–45%, depending on patient selection and radiological criteria (section 5.7).[211,212] What concerns us here is that in some patients with haemorrhagic transformation of an infarct, the haemorrhage is so dense that it would have been regarded as a primary intracerebral haemorrhage, had not an earlier CT scan soon after symptom onset shown no haemorrhage.[213] One possible but very uncommon cause of this is *in situ* dissection of the wall of the middle cerebral artery following embolic occlusion.[214]

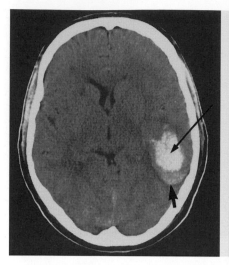
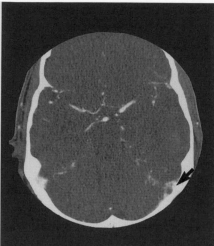
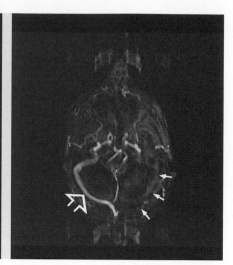

Fig. 8.19 Intracerebral haemorrhage caused by intracranial venous thrombosis in a 55-year-old man. *Left*: CT scan showing a haemorrhagic lesion in the left temporal lobe; the hyperdense core (*long arrow*) is surrounded by a rim of slight hyperintensity (*short arrow*), consistent with haemorrhagic transformation of an infarct. *Middle*: CT angiogram showing a filling defect in the left sigmoid sinus (*arrow*). *Right*: MR venogram, with non-filling of the left tranverse and sigmoid sinus (*short arrows*). Note the normal right transverse and sigmoid sinus (*open arrow*).

Dense intracerebral haemorrhage secondary to infarction is relatively frequent in patients with ischaemic stroke treated with thrombolytic agents. This risk is highest with increasing age, severe clinical deficits, early changes of ischaemia on CT scanning and evidence of microbleeds on MRI (sections 5.7 and 8.4.3).[32,215,216]

8.2.10 Intracranial venous thrombosis

There are many causes of intracranial venous thrombosis (section 7.21). Extensive haemorrhages occur in only a minority of patients, although the precise proportion depends on referral patterns and also on the assiduousness with which the diagnosis is pursued in patients with a diagnosis of idiopathic intracranial hypertension where ICH is exceptional.[217] Haemorrhages are most often the result of engorgement caused by obstruction of cortical veins ('venous infarction'; Fig. 8.19). Therefore, the haemorrhage is usually preceded by an ischaemic phase, manifested by focal deficits, seizures or a global encephalopathy, without radiological evidence of extravasation of blood, the interval being hours or days. Occasionally an ICH may be the presenting feature of intracranial venous thrombosis. The diagnosis can be suspected from a location that is unusual for the more common causes: parasagittal and often bilateral with thrombosis or the superior sagittal sinus (Fig. 5.59), at the cerebral convexity with rupture of a thrombosed cortical vein,[218] or in the temporal lobe with thrombosis of the lateral sinus (Fig. 8.19);[219] in which case the cerebellum may be involved as well[220] (section 5.8).

> Intracranial venous thrombosis is an underdiagnosed condition. Apart from other presentations (headache, visual symptoms secondary to papilloedema, ischaemic neurological deficits), it should be included in the differential diagnosis of intracerebral haemorrhage. The diagnosis should be strongly suspected if the patient is a young woman, if the haemorrhage has been preceded by some of the other manifestations of intracranial venous thrombosis, and if the haemorrhage is multiple, in the parasagittal or temporal regions.

8.2.11 Septic arteritis and 'mycotic' aneurysms

Infective endocarditis (section 6.5.9) is complicated by intracerebral haemorrhage (ICH) in about 5% of cases.[221] It most commonly results not from rupture of 'mycotic' aneurysms – actually bacteria as well as fungi may be involved – but as a result of acute, pyogenic necrosis of the arterial wall early in the disease, caused by virulent organisms such as *Staphylococcus aureus*.[222] Mycotic aneurysms may develop and rupture later, during antimicrobial therapy or with less virulent bacteria, such as *Streptococcus viridans*, *Strep. sanguis*, *Staph. epidermidis* or *Salmonella* species.[223,224]

In general, lobar haemorrhage is an exceptional first sign of endocarditis, i.e. in a patient without any history of heart disease, recent cerebral ischaemia, recent malaise, fever or loss of weight (Fig. 8.20). The combined case fatality of ICH and the underlying endocarditis is in the

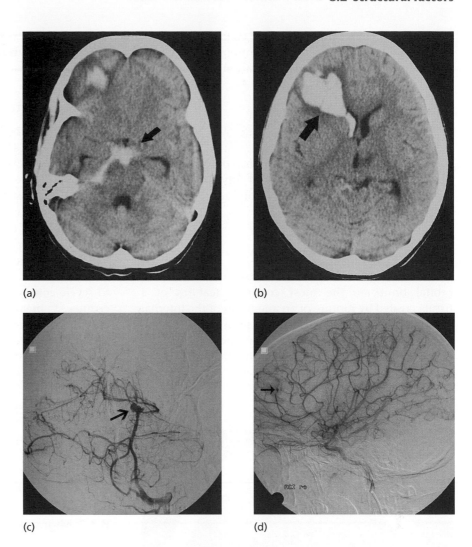

Fig. 8.20 Haemorrhages from a septic arteritis in a 16-year-old girl, refugee from another continent. CT scanning shows subarachnoid haemorrhage in the basal cisterns (a; *arrow*), and also a right frontal haematoma (b; *arrow*). Catheter angiography demonstrated an irregular aneurysm at the top of the basilar artery (c; *arrow*), and another aneurysm on a distal branch of the middle cerebral artery (d; *arrow*). Echocardiography showed mitral vegetations and regurgitation.

order of 25–50%, higher than that of ICH alone in the corresponding age group.[225–227] Valve replacement is urgent in cases of heart failure, but otherwise it is best deferred until at least 4 weeks after the haemorrhage.[228]

In patients with AIDS, toxoplasmosis or tuberculoma of the brain may lead to ICH, presumably through arteritis.[229] In tropical countries, parasitic infections of the brain such as sparganosis can be associated with ICH.[230]

8.2.12 Moyamoya syndrome

Moyamoya syndrome is a chronic condition characterized by stenosis or occlusion of the terminal portions of the internal carotid arteries or proximal middle cerebral arteries, with an abnormal collateral network in the vicinity of the arterial occlusion (section 7.5). The network which gives the condition its name represents only the sequel, while the actual disease process consists of arterial narrowing, most often by an idiopathic proliferative process in the endothelium,[231] rarely by an identifiable cause such as atherosclerosis or chronic cocaine use.[232] A positive family history is obtained in one out of ten cases;[233] genetic factors are likely to operate in many sporadic cases as well.

In Asia, intracerebral haemorrhage, subarachnoid haemorrhage or, occasionally, intraventricular haemorrhage is the most common manifestation of the moyamoya syndrome in adults, whereas in children it is more often encountered as a cause of ischaemic stroke.[234] In contrast, adult patients of European descent also most often present with infarction.[235] The bleeding is caused by rupture of one of the widened perforating vessels acting as collaterals, or sometimes of an associated aneurysm. Therefore, most haemorrhages occur in the basal ganglia. Without the angiographic diagnosis of the primarily occlusive disorder, these cannot be distinguished from the much more common 'hypertensive' haemorrhages, as a result of small vessel disease. Several case reports document an association with pregnancy,[236] not only in Asian women but also in African-Americans and whites.[237,238]

The risk of rebleeding from dilated collateral pathways has been estimated at 4–7% per annum.[239,240] A controlled trial of revascularization operation to prevent this from occurring is under way.[241]

8.2.13 Arterial dissection

(See also section 7.2.)

Haemorrhage is an uncommon complication of intracranial arterial dissection, and any extravasation that occurs is almost invariably confined to the subarachnoid space (section 9.1.3).

8.2.14 Caroticocavernous fistula

Pulsating exophthalmos, conjunctival injection and orbital bruit are the most common features of a fistula created by rupture of an aneurysm of the internal carotid artery within the cavernous sinus, or by trauma. Exceptionally, rupture of one of the dilated and congested veins that drain into the cavernous sinus occurs, resulting in an intracerebral haemorrhage (Fig. 8.21).[242–244]

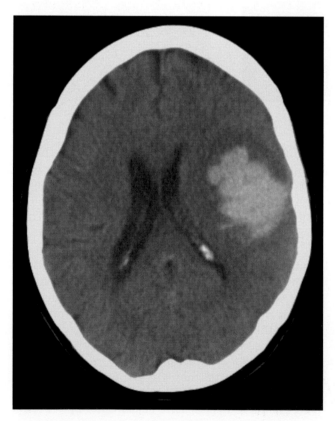

Fig. 8.21 Haemorrhage in the left temporal lobe due to venous engorgement in a patient with a caroticocavernous fistula.

8.3 Haemodynamic factors

8.3.1 Acute arterial hypertension

Acutely raised blood pressure can precipitate intracerebral haemorrhage (ICH), particularly in previously normotensive individuals whose autoregulation has not been reset towards a higher range (section 12.1.2).[245] The rapid increase in pressure is transmitted to the wall of small arterioles, which are not relatively protected by previous hypertrophy as occurs in long-standing hypertension. Case reports document intracerebral haemorrhage in a variety of situations associated with high blood pressure, such as phaeochromocytoma,[246] eclampsia,[247] exposure to severe cold weather,[248] pain induced by dental procedures,[249] break dancing,[250] unconventional medical treatments such as 'coining',[251] emotional upset,[252] and sildenafil-assisted sexual intercourse.[253] ICH associated with use of amphetamines and cocaine where no structural lesion is found is also attributed to acute hypertension (sections 8.5.3 and 8.5.4).

After carotid endarterectomy for severe stenosis, there may be relative hypertension in a previously underperfused hemisphere, in some cases resulting in intracerebral haemorrhage in the previously ischaemic region (section 16.11.3),[254] or – exceptionally – as a classical 'hypertensive' haemorrhage in the deep parts of the brain.[255]

8.3.2 Migraine

Migraine may be indirectly associated with intracerebral haemorrhage, through the presence of an arteriovenous malformation if any such association is real,[256,257] but also directly. Medication with sumutriptan has been implicated as an additional factor, though rather unconvincingly.[258] Lobar haemorrhages after an unusually severe attack of migraine have been reported in three women with a long history of migrainous attacks, with tenderness of the carotid artery in the neck and on angiography evidence of extensive vasospasm in the ipsilateral internal carotid or intracranial arteries; the density and compactness of the haemorrhages on brain CT argued against the possibility that the haemorrhages were secondary to infarction.[259] Surgical specimens in two of these patients had evidence of necrosis in the walls of intracranial vessels, probably as a result of ischaemia, with secondary inflammatory changes. Curiously enough these observations came from a single centre and they have not been confirmed, apart from an isolated report of a woman with bilateral deep haemorrhages during a migraine attack.[260]

8.4 Haemostatic factors

8.4.1 Anticoagulants

Intracerebral haemorrhage (ICH) associated with anticoagulants is mostly in the deep regions of the brain, reflecting the distribution of degenerative changes in small arteries (section 8.2.1).[261] But lobar haemorrhages also occur, especially with advancing age, perhaps therefore reflecting pre-existing amyloid angiopathy (section 8.2.2);[262] because of the age factor lobar haemorrhages associated with anticoagulants may be underrepresented in hospital series. During treatment with oral anticoagulants, the risk of ICH, compared with age-matched controls not on anticoagulants, is increased by between seven and ten times and amounts to an absolute risk of about 1% per year (section 16.6.4).[2] Part of this excess risk should of course be attributed to the underlying arteriolar degeneration associated with the vascular condition for which the treatment may have been given (i.e. confounding by indication).

Not surprisingly, the risk of ICH increases with the intensity of anticoagulation;[2] this gradient applies in equal measure to patients in whom the indication is non-neurological[263–265] and to patients with cerebral ischaemia, whether of cardiac or arterial origin.[261,266] Nevertheless, in most patients with ICH during treatment with oral anticoagulants the intensity of anticoagulation is within the therapeutic range. This is another illustration of the paradox that the absolute number of disease events is greater among patients at medium risk (representing a small proportion of a very large group) than among patients at highest risk (a large proportion of a small group) (section 18.5.1).

Risk factors, other than the intensity of the international normalized ratio, for ICH in patients taking anticoagulants are advanced age, especially in the first few months of treatment,[267–269] and also previous ischaemic stroke, especially those with leukoaraiosis.[261,270] The evidence for insulin-dependent diabetes as a risk factor is somewhat less strong.[271]

> The risk of intracerebral haemorrhage in patients on oral anticoagulants increases with the intensity of anticoagulation, but in most patients with intracerebral haemorrhage while on anticoagulants the international normalized ratio values are within appropriate limits.

A remarkable feature of ICH precipitated by anticoagulants is the gradual progression of the clinical deficits.[272]

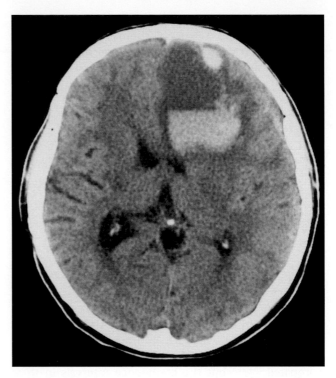

Fig. 8.22 CT brain scan showing an intracerebral haemorrhage in the left frontal lobe, with a horizontal border representing the interface between sedimented red blood cells and supernatant plasma, indicating impaired coagulation. There is also distortion of the ventricle and loss of sulci, indicating mass effect.

Accordingly, the average volume of the haemorrhage is larger than in ICH not associated with anticoagulants,[273,274] the shape is more often irregular,[275] and the rate of subsequent expansion is greater.[276] A fluid-blood level within the haematoma (Fig. 8.22), i.e. a horizontal interface between unclotted serum (hypodense) and sedimentated red cells (hyperdense), occurs in 60% of anticoagulant-related ICHs, which is more often than in other situations (section 5.4.1).[57,277]

8.4.2 Antiplatelet drugs

In a complete overview, up to 1997, of all randomized trials of antiplatelet drugs (mostly aspirin and involving almost 90 000 patients), for any indication, in which haemorrhagic and ischaemic strokes had been distinguished as an outcome event, the relative increase of (fatal or non-fatal) intracerebral haemorrhage (ICH) in treated patients was 22%, but this was outweighed by a relative decrease in fatal or non-fatal ischaemic stroke of 30%[278] (section 16.5.1). In absolute terms and with temporary disregard for the net benefits of treatment, one haemorrhagic stroke will occur for every 1000 patients treated with aspirin for a period of 3–5 years, depending on the baseline risk.[279] In patients with a history of cerebral ischaemia, the risk of haemorrhagic stroke on aspirin is similar for patients with a cardiac or an arterial source of thromboembolism.[280] If antiplatelet drugs are prescribed in survivors of ICH, the risk of recurrent haemorrhage does not appear to be high.[281]

The combination of clopidogrel and aspirin is associated with a small but statistically significant increase of ICH, in comparison with clopidogrel alone.[282] Compared with aspirin alone this combination also resulted in an increased risk of haemorrhage, but not in the brain.[283]

> Antiplatelet drugs are probably only a relatively minor contributory factor in the pathogenesis of intracerebral haemorrhage against a background of much more powerful determinants, most often small vessel disease.

The dose of aspirin is not an important factor with regard to the risk of ICH, at least not according to the few studies in which different doses were directly compared,[284,285] but the confidence intervals in these comparisons are wide.

Intracerebral haemorrhage in aspirin users is more often lobar and more often associated with microbleeds than in non-aspirin users.[29,286] This is probably explained by the characteristics of aspirin users that predispose to amyloid angiopathy (section 8.2.2), especially advanced age. A single study reported a relatively high case fatality of ICH in current aspirin users,[287] but the question remains whether this association is causal or indirect.

8.4.3 Thrombolytic treatment for non-neurological indications

Intracerebral haemorrhage (ICH) is a serious and potentially fatal complication of thrombolytic therapy for acute myocardial infarction, occurring in about 1% of patients, usually within 24 h (section 7.10).[288,289] Factors associated with a relatively high risk are advanced age, female sex, low body weight (in other words, a relatively high dose of thrombolytic drug), previous stroke, hypertension left untreated on admission to hospital, treatment with tissue plasminogen activator rather than another agent, and bolus injection rather than infusion.[288-291] Two clues incriminate amyloid angiopathy as the most frequent anatomical abnormality underlying this complication.[292] First, a disproportionate number of ICHs after thrombolysis occur in the white matter instead of in the deep regions of the brain, and multiple ICHs occur in about one-third.[293] Second, in the few patients in whom brain tissue could be examined after operation or postmortem, blood vessels showed amyloid changes.[292] Amyloid angiopathy is also the obvious explanation for lobar haemorrhage occurring after thrombolysis for ischaemic stroke, at a site that is remote from the initial lesion.[294]

A state of systemically enhanced thrombolysis from these drugs adversely affects the process of haemostasis in the brain, as reflected by fluid levels in lobar haematomas (Fig. 8.22),[294] by relatively little perilesional oedema,[295] and by a high case fatality, about 50–60%.[288,296]

> Intracerebral haemorrhage after thrombolytic treatment for myocardial infarction is mostly of the lobar type, related to amyloid angiopathy in elderly patients; this complication is fatal in at least half the patients.

8.4.4 Clotting factor deficiency

Spontaneous intracranial bleeding may occur in haemophilia, with severe deficiency of factors VIII, IX, or rarely XIII; most patients are children.[297] Head injury may provoke brain haemorrhage in patients with mild or subclinical degrees of haemophilia or von Willebrand's disease.[298] The case fatality is high. Acquired immune deficiency syndrome (AIDS) is sometimes a contributory factor, because factor replacement therapy may be delayed by a patient's impaired judgement.[299]

Rare clotting disorders associated with spontaneous ICH are congenital afibrinogenaemia,[300] type 1 cryoglobulinaemia (section 7.3.14),[301] terminal liver cirrhosis (Fig. 8.23),[302] factor X deficiency[303] and antibodies against factor XIIIa associated with lupus erythematosus (section 7.3.3).[304] A few studies have claimed an association between polymorphisms for certain clotting factors and ICH,[305,306] but such associations may just be a chance finding.[307]

8.4.5 Leukaemia and thrombocytopenia

(See also section 7.9.4.)

Myeloid leukaemia is complicated by intracerebral haemorrhage (ICH) in around 20% of cases,[308] occasionally as a first manifestation,[309] whereas ICH is exceptional in lymphatic leukaemia or in hairy cell leukaemia. There are many intermediate causes. Most often the direct cause is the formation of aggregates of tumour cells, which obstruct arterioles or capillaries in the cortex or subcortical white matter. This is followed by local proliferation of white blood cells, with erosion of the vessel wall. Other causes are disseminated intravascular

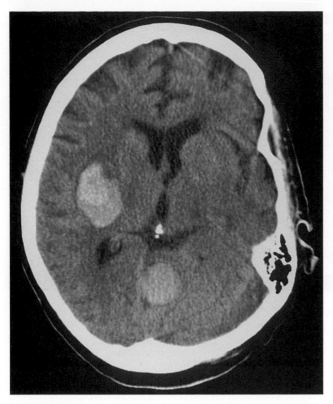

Fig. 8.23 Multifocal intracerebral haemorrhages in a 59-year-old woman with liver cirrhosis.

coagulation and consumption coagulopathy, or thrombocytopenia by infiltration of the bone marrow, with or without transplantation.[310] However, thrombocytopenia should not be accepted as a cause of ICH if the platelet count is above 20×10^9/L, because above this value the bleeding time is normal (provided platelet function is intact). Apart from leukaemia, thrombocytopenia may be associated with myelofibrosis, aplastic anaemia, diffuse intravascular coagulation,[311] leptospirosis,[312] idiopathic thrombocytopenic purpura (Werlhof's disease)[313,314] and, in children, with immune-mediated thrombocytopenic purpura.[315]

8.5 Other factors

8.5.1 Cerebral tumours

Haemorrhage into a cerebral tumour accounts for approximately 5% of all intracerebral haemorrhage (ICH).[316] To suspect such a connection is not too difficult if the patient is already known to have an intracerebral tumour, and it should also come readily to mind with a known extracranial malignant tumour.

On brain scanning, several features suggest an underlying tumour (section 5.4.1) including:

- an irregular, mottled appearance of the haematoma, especially a low-density area in the centre of the haemorrhage, suggesting necrosis (Fig. 8.24);
- multiple haemorrhages (a feature shared with some other types of haemorrhage; Table 8.2);
- a disproportionate degree of surrounding oedema or mass effect;
- nodular enhancement of surrounding tissue after intravenous contrast, other than the ring enhancement that represents the inflammatory response to the haemorrhage (Fig. 8.25; section 5.4.1);
- multiple tumours on brain imaging suggest metastases.

The issue can often generally be resolved by a search for the primary tumour, or by repeating the scan after an interval of several weeks or months (Fig. 8.24).

Glioblastomas, metastases and meningiomas are the most frequent tumours that cause ICH.[316] Metastases include melanoma, bronchial carcinoma (Fig. 8.25), renal carcinoma and choriocarcinoma.

8.5.2 Alcohol

Definitions of heavy drinking depend on nationality and gender, but increasing doses of alcohol per day are consistently associated with an increased risk of intracerebral haemorrhage (ICH).[1] Compared with those who report moderate drinking (less than 36 g per day), the odds ratio is around 2 for daily quantities between 36 and 56 g of alcohol per day and around 4 for an intake above 56 g (for readers who wish to convert this into millilitres: the density of alcohol being 0.79, the multiplication factor is 1.27; or, a standard 125-mL glass of wine with an alcohol content of 12% contains 12 grams of alcohol). This effect may be partly related to a mild inhibitory action of alcohol on platelets and clotting factors.[317] Whether brief spells of excessive drinking ('binge drinking') can precipitate ICH, subarachnoid haemorrhage or even stroke in general is controversial;[318] obviously there are several confounding factors such as trauma and associated lifestyle factors (section 6.6.13). Massive ICH may occur in alcoholics with liver damage associated with a low platelet count and abnormalities of the clotting system.

8.5.3 Amphetamines

(See also section 7.15.1.)

There are several case reports of intracerebral haemorrhage (ICH) after ingestion of amphetamine,

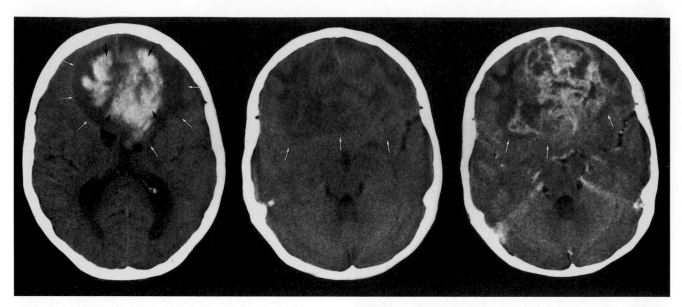

Fig. 8.24 Haemorrhage caused by primary brain tumour in a 71-year-old woman. *Left*: CT scan 1 day after sudden loss of consciousness, showing a bifrontal intracerebral haemorrhage (*black arrows*) with irregular shape and disproportionate oedema (hypodense margin around the haematoma; *white arrows*). *Middle*: CT scan 3 months later, after a gradual recovery had been followed by secondary deterioration; diffuse oedema in both frontal lobes with considerable mass effect (*arrows*). *Right*: after injection of intravenous contrast a grossly irregular tumour emerges (glioblastoma).

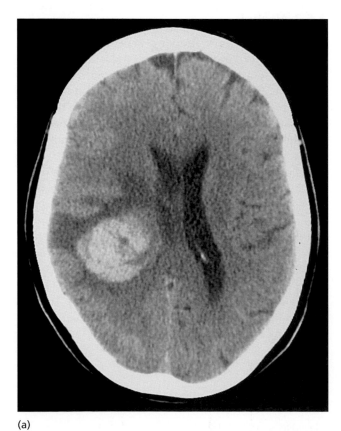

(a)

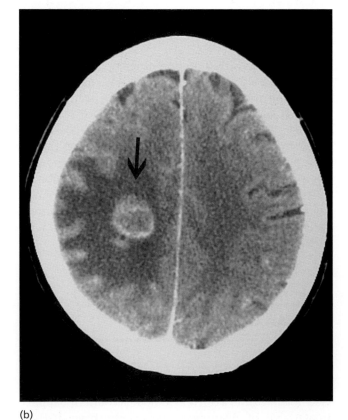

(b)

Fig. 8.25 Haemorrhage in the right parietal lobe on CT scanning in a 55-year-old woman with non-small cell bronchial carcinoma (a). A higher slice shows a metastasis after injection of contrast (b; *arrow*).

methamphetamine or ring-substituted amphetamine (MDMA or 'ecstasy'), less often of dextroamphetamine, with any route of administration and after relatively low doses. The interval between ingestion and haemorrhage can be as short as a few minutes, never longer than a few hours.

Frequently there is an underlying anatomical abnormality such as an arteriovenous malformation or saccular aneurysm.[319] In other patients angiography may show scattered segments of narrowing and dilatation ('beading') or occlusion.[320] At postmortem, these lesions correspond with areas of fibrinoid necrosis in small and medium-sized vessels in the brain, as well as in other organs.[321] Nevertheless, in some fatal cases the cerebral vasculature is completely intact;[322] a sudden rise in blood pressure may have been the precipitating factor (section 8.3.1).

8.5.4 Cocaine and other drugs

(See also section 7.15.1.)

As with amphetamines, cocaine-associated brain haemorrhage may occur after oral ingestion, intravenous injection or inhalation, but relatively more often after inhalation of 'crack' cocaine, a mixture of cocaine hydrochloride and ammonia or baking soda.[323] African-Americans are more susceptible than whites.[324] These haemorrhages occur mostly in the white matter of the cerebral hemispheres and are often multiple.[325] As with amphetamines, there is a high likelihood of an underlying vascular abnormality such as an aneurysm, in the order of 50%, at least in patients with adequate angiographic or postmortem studies.[326] In the remaining group, postmortem mostly fails to show vasculopathic changes;[327,328] the normal blood vessels suggest haemodynamic rather than structural factors, an explanation supported by a higher frequency of pre-existing hypertension than in patients with aneurysms.[329] Evidence of vasculitis is exceptional.[330]

Intracerebral haemorrhage (ICH) has also been reported in association with the use of ephedrine or epinephrine.[331,332] Ergot alkaloids such as bromocriptine and lisuride may cause ICH through vasoconstriction and probably vessel necrosis, especially in the postpartum period (section 7.14).[333,334]

8.5.5 Vasculitis

Primary angiitis of the central nervous system is by definition not associated with any systemic involvement (section 7.3.17). The cause is obscure and it is uncertain whether the condition is a nosological entity.[335,336] Presenting features include subacute headache, mental deterioration, seizures and focal ischaemia. Occasionally, intracerebral haemorrhage (ICH) may be the first clinical manifestation.[337,338] Clinically silent haemorrhages can be detected by gradient echo MRI.[339] The haemorrhages may recur;[340] in these cases they may be associated with aneurysmal dilatations at changing arterial sites.[341] Other vasculitic disorders affecting the brain can sometimes present with, or be complicated by, ICH (section 7.3) including bacterial meningitis,[342] Wegener's granulomatosis,[343–345] HLTV-1 associated myelopathy[346] and herpes zoster, in isolation or as a complication of AIDS.[347]

8.5.6 Trauma ('spät-Apoplexie')

The antiquity of this notion can be surmised from its exotic name.[348,349] There is of course no doubt that even minor head trauma may result in rupture of vulnerable arteries, specifically in patients with amyloid angiopathy (section 8.2.2). Also there is abundant evidence from serial CT scans after head trauma that a superficial brain contusion may change its aspect within hours or days, from a slightly hypodense, mottled, or even normal appearance to an extensive, space-occupying lesion.[350] Patients on anticoagulants are at increased risk.[351] In all these cases the initial lesion immediately follows the trauma, and it is usually accompanied by neurological deficits, focal or general.

Just by chance there must be a few patients with an intracerebral haemorrhage (ICH) who had sustained a head injury in the preceding period,[352] but to assume a cause-and-effect relationship without other evidence is a violation of the rules of causality. It must be regarded as a medico-legal myth that minor head trauma can contribute to the development of deep ICH after an interval of days or even weeks, certainly if initial investigations have not shown a brain lesion.

8.6 Relative frequency of causes of intracerebral haemorrhage, according to age and location

We pointed out in the introduction to this chapter that age is an important factor in determining the a priori probability of a particular cause of an intracerebral haemorrhage (ICH) in an individual patient. Arteriovenous malformations and cavernous malformations are the leading cause in the young, and degenerative intracranial small vessel disease in the middle-aged and the aged, while amyloid angiopathy is another important cause to consider in the aged. Some refinements of this rule of thumb are possible, not only by listing causes less common than these three, but also by considering factors other than age, particularly the location of the haematoma. Table 8.3 lists the frequency of the different causes of ICH, according to age group by location. This ranking is based partly on hospital series of young adults (under 45 years) with ICH,[353,354] partly on a surgical series of lobar haemorrhages with negative angiography and with thorough histological study of the specimens,[355] and finally – where nothing else is available – on guesswork. The relative importance of causes also depends to some extent on social factors, for instance in the case of drug use or endocarditis. The order given here reflects the relative frequencies in Europe and should be adjusted where necessary for any cultural and geographical differences.

> Arteriovenous malformations are the most common cause of intracerebral haemorrhage in the young, degenerative small vessel disease in middle and old age, and amyloid angiopathy in old age.

8.7 Clues from the history

The cause of intracerebral haemorrhage (ICH) may occasionally be identified from the history:

- A *past history of ICH in the same location* may suggest a structural lesion such as an arteriovenous malformation not detected on the earlier occasion; if the recurrent haemorrhage is distant from the earlier lesion the underlying condition may be cerebral amyloid angiopathy (section 8.2.2), especially when there is evidence of associated leukoaraiosis.
- A *family history* of ICH at a relatively young age may suggest cavernous malformations, hereditary haemorrhagic teleangiectasia, or a familial variant of amyloid angiopathy.
- Previous *epileptic seizures* should raise suspicions about the presence of an arteriovenous or cavernous malformation, a tumour or, if focal and of recent onset, cerebral amyloid angiopathy.[75,356]
- Cerebral amyloid angiopathy should also come to mind with a history of *transient ischaemic attacks, intellectual deterioration*, or both.[66,75]
- Long-standing *hypertension* suggests small vessel diseases as the most probable underlying condition in a patient with an ICH in the basal ganglia or in the

posterior fossa; on the other hand, hypertension is so common that it may coexist with other conditions.

- If the patient is known to have had *cancer*, especially melanoma, bronchial carcinoma or renal carcinoma, or if the patient is a woman with a recent pregnancy, haemorrhage into a brain metastasis should be reckoned with.
- *Valvular heart disease* must raise the suspicion of septic embolism, although this is not the cause even in the majority of those cases, because infective endocarditis is a rare disease, much rarer than many other causes of ICH such as cerebral amyloid angiopathy.
- If *haemorrhages at other sites*, such as in the skin, have preceded the haemorrhagic stroke, a disorder of haemostasis is almost too obvious to be missed. In any patient with *haemophilia*, a 'stroke', unexplained sudden coma or severe headache signifies intracranial bleeding until proved otherwise.
- The use of *oral anticoagulants* is a vital piece of information, because, in consultation with the cardiologist and haematologist, their action should probably be neutralized as soon as possible by intravenous prothrombin complex concentrate and vitamin K (section 12.4.7).
- It is equally important to know about the use of *recreational drugs*, particularly cocaine and amphetamines; this information may be withheld for weeks.[357]
- Finally, the circumstances preceding ICH may contribute to identifying its cause: an earlier phase of the illness with a dense neurological deficit (*haemorrhagic transformation of an infarct*), *puerperium* (intracranial venous thrombosis, choriocarcinoma), or *severe neck trauma* (dissection of the vertebral or carotid artery).

In general, headache as a new symptom may be the only clue to the diagnosis of ICH, especially if the onset is within seconds or minutes.

8.8 Clues from the examination

8.8.1 General examination

Inspection provides rather few clues to the cause of an intracerebral haemorrhage (ICH), with the exception of *petechiae* or *bruising*, indicating a generalized haemostatic disorder, *telangiectasias* in the skin and mucous membranes, or signs of malignant disease such as *cutaneous melanoma*.

Finding *hypertension* on admission is the rule, but only in about 50% of patients is this a contributing factor (section 8.2.1), in the others it is merely a reactive phenomenon (section 11.7.1). *Hypertensive vascular changes in the retina* or *left ventricular hypertrophy* support the idea that hypertension is a contributing factor, but their absence does not exclude it. A *collapsed lung* or *enlargement of the liver or spleen* may point towards underlying cancer. *Heart murmurs* may be coincidental but should at least raise the possibility of infective endocarditis as a cause of ICH, as should finding needle marks in possible drug addicts.

8.8.2 Neurological examination

The clinical manifestations of intracerebral haemorrhage (ICH) almost always include focal deficits, with or without a decreased level of consciousness. Coma or a lesser degree of obtundation in general is a non-localizing feature, except with haemorrhage in the posterior fossa.

Auscultating the skull for detecting arteriovenous malformations is useful for impressing naive readers of textbooks as well as medical students and patients, but is not very rewarding (we are still offering a free copy of this book to anyone who had no other clues and only by auscultation diagnosed an arteriovenous malformation of the brain in an adult). *Subhyaloid haemorrhages* on fundoscopy indicate intracranial acute bleeding in general, most often subarachnoid haemorrhage.[358]

A *decreased level of consciousness* is one of the classical features of ICH as taught to medical students, but it is absent in a sizeable proportion of patients (section 5.3.1). Given that infarcts are four times as common as haemorrhages in white populations, and on the assumption that half the patients with ICH have a normal level of consciousness, it follows that if the distinction is based only on the level of consciousness, one out of nine times an infarct is diagnosed it will in fact be an ICH. A decrease in consciousness after admission, which occurs in about one-third of all patients with ICH, may result from:

- enlargement of the ICH;[37,38]
- formation of oedema around an already large ICH (especially if the deterioration occurs after 48 h);[45]
- obstructive hydrocephalus with posterior fossa ICH;[359]
- a medical complication such as hyponatraemia or neurogenic pulmonary oedema (sections 11.18 and 14.2.5).

The *focal deficits* in ICH are of course determined by the site and size of the haemorrhage. The pace at which these symptoms and signs develop is usually a matter of seconds or minutes, rarely of hours. Rapid resolution of deficits as a rule suggests ischaemia rather than haemorrhage, but not invariably (Fig. 8.26).[360,361]

Some general comments are appropriate:

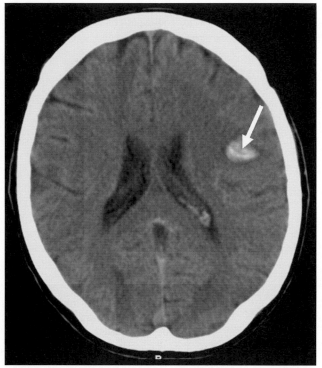

(a)

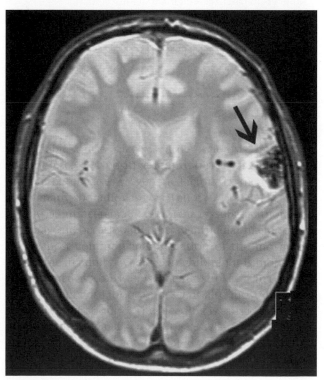

(b)

Fig. 8.26 Intracerebral haemorrhage on a CT brain scan (a; *arrow*) in a 46-year-old man with a 'TIA' (disturbance of spoken language, for several hours). The cause was a small arteriovenous malformation, evident on early T2-weighted MRI (b; *arrow*).

Table 8.3 A priori probabilities in rank order for structural causes of intracerebral haemorrhage (coagulopathies and haemodynamic factors excluded), according to the patient's age and the location of the haematoma.

Age (years)	Basal ganglia/thalamus	Lobar	Cerebellum/brainstem
Below 45	1 AVM or cavernous malformation 2 Small vessel disease 3 Moyamoya syndrome (4) Amphetamines/cocaine	1 AVM or cavernous malformation 2 Saccular aneurysm* 3 Tumour 4 Intracranial venous thrombosis† (5) Amphetamines/cocaine 6 Infective endocarditis‡	1 AVM or cavernous malformation 2 Small vessel disease 3 Tumour
45–69	1 Small vessel disease 2 AVM or cavernous malformation 3 Atherosclerotic moyamoya syndrome (4) Tumour (5) Amyloid angiopathy 6 Intracranial venous thrombosis† 7 Infective endocarditis‡	1 Small vessel disease 2 AVM or cavernous malformation 3 Saccular aneurysm* (4) Amyloid angiopathy	1 Small vessel disease 2 AVM or cavernous malformation (3) Tumour
70 and over	1 Small vessel disease (2) Tumour (3) AVM or cavernous malformation (4) Intracranial venous thrombosis 5 Infective endocarditis‡	1 Small vessel disease 2 Amyloid angiopathy 3 Saccular aneurysm* 4 AVM or cavernous malformation	1 Small vessel disease 2 Amyloid angiopathy 3 Tumour

AVM arteriovenous malformation; * haematomas in specific locations (see text); † haematoma usually in parasagittal area;
‡ with history of valvular heart disease.
Numbers in parentheses: rank order not certain.

- With *thalamic haemorrhage*, the nature of the deficits critically depends on the location within the thalamus,[362] as this conglomerate of nuclei has connections with almost every part of the cerebral cortex. A fairly characteristic feature with posterolateral thalamic lesions, especially haemorrhages, is distortion of the vertical orientation of the body, with a tendency to push away from the non-paralysed side.[363]
- *Caudate haemorrhage* may produce few focal deficits but a predominance of general symptoms (headache, vomiting and a decrease in the level of consciousness, or only cognitive impairment) by rapid extension of the bleed into the ventricular system; these features may mimic subarachnoid haemorrhage.[364]
- All *haemorrhages in the posterior fossa* may be complicated by obstructive hydrocephalus, whether in the cerebellum,[359] midbrain, or pons.[365]
- The prognosis of *haemorrhages in the pons* is not always as bleak as was believed before the CT scan era, when the diagnosis was made only in fatal cases; in prospective series from primary referral centres, survival is around 40%.[365,366]
- In fact, small haemorrhages in the pons, midbrain, thalamus and internal capsule may cause a wide variety of 'lacunar syndromes' (section 4.3.2), in these cases the result of small deep haemorrhages rather than small deep infarcts; an entire monograph could

Table 8.4 Approximate frequency of the different locations of primary intracerebral haemorrhage (regardless of age).

Location	Frequency (%)
Putamen or internal capsule	30
Lobar[85]	30
Thalamus	15
Cerebellum	10
Entire basal ganglia region	5
Caudate nucleus[400]	5
Pons or midbrain	5

be filled with an inventory of such case reports, but in truth these merely serve to confirm the established facts of neurological semiology.

The relative probabilities of intracerebral haemorrhage occurring in the locations shown in Table 8.3 are estimated in Table 8.4. The proportions in this table are only an approximation of the truth, for three reasons:
- First, most estimates are based on hospital series[367,368] which suffer from bias in that referral is less often considered for moribund patients or, at the other extreme, for patients with only mild deficits.
- Second, population studies are unbiased but they contain such a small proportion of haemorrhages that any subdivisions are subject to chance effects.

- Finally, many series date back to the 1980s; it is odd but true that more recent observations of the subdivisions of haemorrhages according to location are no longer newsworthy.

8.9 Investigations

8.9.1 Laboratory studies

Routine laboratory investigations (section 6.8.1) should not be forgotten from the point of view of general medical management, but they seldom uncover the cause of intracerebral haemorrhage (ICH) (e.g. massive liver damage).

Abnormalities of haemostasis may have contributed to the development of ICH, although we should reiterate that identified and possible causes are not necessarily the only or even the true cause. Nonetheless, haemostatic factors should be considered in every patient with ICH. Sometimes the relationship is obvious, e.g. if the patient is on anticoagulants. But, in other instances the relationship may be more indirect, such as the haemostatic defect in renal failure. If ICH is caused by a disorder of haemostasis, this is usually because of impaired clotting, that is, the secondary phase of haemostasis, which depends on adequate levels of coagulation factors. Abnormalities of primary haemostasis have to do with defects of platelet function or with thrombocytopenia; most commonly these result in haemorrhages in the skin and mucous membranes, much more rarely in haemorrhages in organs such as the brain. The overview of the Antithrombotic Trialists' Collaboration, discussed earlier in section 8.4.2, found a slightly increased risk of ICH in patients on antiplatelet drugs, but in absolute terms the excess risk is very small.[278]

The most important screening test of primary haemostatic function is the platelet count. But thrombocytopenia precipitates ICH only with values less than 20×10^9/L. A normal platelet count is reassuring, but only if platelet function is normal; if this is uncertain, for example with renal failure or in the presence of antiplatelet antibodies, determination of the bleeding time may be helpful, despite its broad normal range.

The clotting system (coagulation factors) can be assessed with the partial thromboplastin time (PTT), the prothrombin time (PT), the thrombin time (TT) or, preferably, the international normalized ratio (INR). Circulating antibodies (usually of the IgG class) may impair the activity of specific coagulation factors (inhibitor syndromes); they develop especially in patients with factor VIII or factor IX deficiency who have received multiple plasma infusions, but also with autoimmune diseases or in patients being treated with penicillin or streptomycin. Appropriate tests can uncover these specific autoantibodies.

If infective endocarditis is suspected, the diagnosis may be supported by a high erythrocyte sedimentation rate or C-reactive protein, and of course if there is any suspicion blood cultures should be taken. Peripheral blood leucocytosis up to 12.500×10^9/L may result from the ICH itself, especially if it is large.[369]

8.9.2 CT brain scanning

This is the most important single investigation in patients with suspected ICH (section 5.4.1). Because of its sensitivity in the recognition of intracerebral blood, CT has led to an increased awareness of the diagnosis of ICH. Whether a small brain haemorrhage on CT in the acute stage can be missed is controversial.[370] After months or years have passed, it is difficult if not impossible to attribute brain lesions to either haemorrhage or infarction, but there are some clues (section 5.4.1).

The location of the haematoma may to some extent point to the underlying cause (Figs 8.27–8.32; Table 8.3). *Intraventricular extension* of the haemorrhage occurs relatively often with deep haemorrhages associated with rupture of damaged perforating arteries (section 8.2.1), but also with aneurysms. It carries a relatively poor prognosis, depending not only on the volume of intraventricular blood but also on the underlying cause.[371,372] A *fluid-blood level* is seen with an underlying coagulopathy,[277] but also without; a horizontal border may falsely suggest a disorder of coagulation, a question that can be resolved by repositioning the patient because the position of a true fluid level will then change accordingly. An *irregular and indistinct margin* of a lobar haemorrhage suggests cerebral amyloid angiopathy, as does *inhomogeneous density*, extension through the cortex with *rupture into the subarachnoid space* and coexistence of *microhaemorrhages* in the cortical or subcortical region.[55] If *multiple or recurrent haemorrhages in the white matter* are identified on CT (Table 8.2), this should also raise the possibility of amyloid angiopathy, at least in an elderly patient (Figs 8.8, 8.9, 8.10); of intracranial venous thrombosis if the irregular shape and parasagittal location suggest infarction as a result of venous congestion, with haemorrhagic transformation (Fig. 8.19); or of metastases if there is a history of malignant disease. *Calcifications* adjacent to the haematoma should bring to mind that an arteriovenous malformation might be the underlying cause (Fig. 8.12).

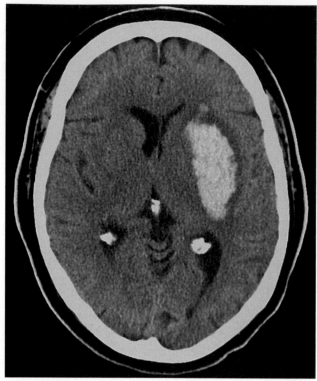

(a)

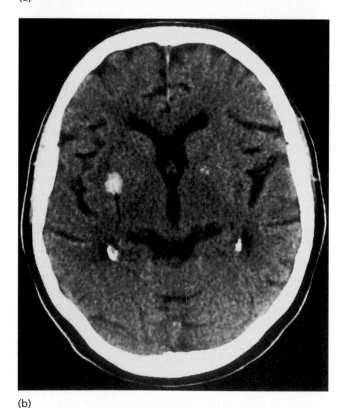

(b)

Fig. 8.27 CT brain scan showing a haemorrhage in the putaminal region of the basal ganglia; (a) large haemorrhage in the left basal ganglia. (b) CT scan showing a small haemorrhage in the right internal capsule (*arrow*).

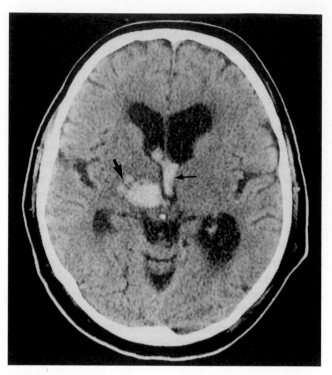

Fig. 8.28 CT brain scan showing a haemorrhage in the right thalamus (*thick arrow*), with rupture into the third ventricle (*thin arrow*), resulting in obstructive hydrocephalus.

Repeat brain CT before and after injection of contrast may be required for picking up underlying vascular lesions such as tumours and arteriovenous malformations. These can be most easily identified at a stage, weeks or months later, when the lesion is no longer obscured by mass effects and the haemorrhage has resolved, at least partially. CT angiography is mostly used for picking up ruptured aneurysms (section 9.4.4) but arteriovenous malformations can also be identified.[373]

8.9.3 Magnetic resonance imaging of the brain

Intraparenchymal haemorrhages can be detected by magnetic resonance imaging (MRI) even a few hours after onset, but special echo sequences and expertise are necessary for an unequivocal diagnosis (section 5.5.1).[374,375] It is especially for the demonstration of associated vascular anomalies that MR scanning is useful in patients with ICH. As flowing blood is not susceptible in the same way as brain tissue to the changes induced by strong magnetic fields, vascular channels appear as strongly hypointense, 'empty' regions ('signal voids'), representing flowing blood (Figs 8.17, 8.33). MR scanning may in this way identify arteriovenous malformations and sometimes even saccular aneurysms. Cavernous malformations are best detected

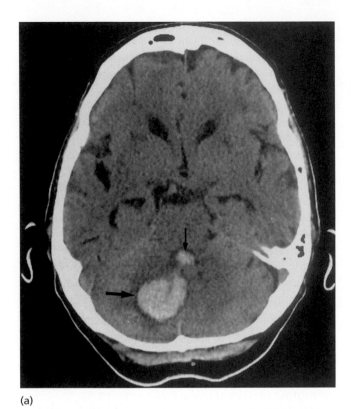

(a)

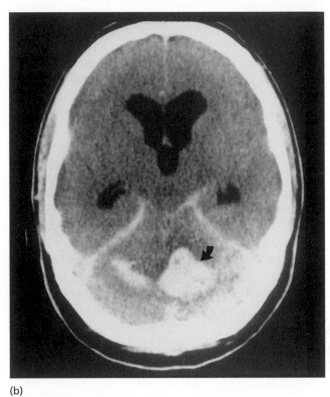

(b)

Fig. 8.29 (a) CT brain scan showing a haemorrhage in the right cerebellar hemisphere (*thick arrow*), with rupture into the fourth ventricle (*thin arrow*). (b) CT brain scan showing a large haemorrhage in the left cerebellar hemisphere (*arrow*) and vermis (and smaller haemorrhage in right cerebellar hemisphere), with compression of the fourth ventricle and obstructive hydrocephalus.

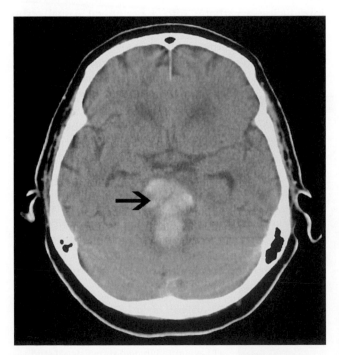

Fig. 8.30 CT scan of 'hypertensive' haemorrhage in the midbrain, extending into the pons and cerebellum (*arrow*).

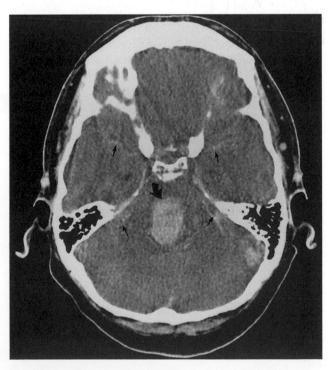

Fig. 8.31 CT brain scan showing a haemorrhage in the pons (*thick arrow*), with some blood being visible in the subarachnoid space (*thin arrows*) through rupture into the fourth ventricle (not visible).

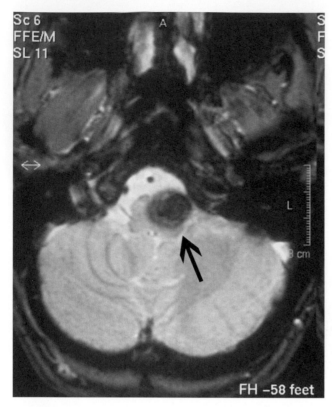

Fig. 8.32 MR brain scan (T2-weighted image) of 'hypertensive' haemorrhage in the medulla oblongata (hypointense or dark area; *arrow*).

with a gradient echo technique.[151,152] Signs of congestion of pial vessels suggest a dural fistula draining into cortical veins (section 8.2.8). Dedicated techniques for demonstrating moving blood (MR angiography, MRA)

are even more sensitive for the detection of vascular lesions than MR techniques used for cross-sectional brain imaging (section 5.5.2; for aneurysms, see section 9.4.5) The developments of this technique are so rapid that it is well on its way to replace catheter angiography.

If intracranial *venous thrombosis* is suspected as a cause of ICH, MRI is useful in showing the two complementary features that are necessary for the diagnosis: filling defects and thrombus (section 7.21). Filling defects alone may represent hypoplasia and are not sufficient for the diagnosis; they can be seen on standard MRI sequences and even better on contrast-enhanced whole-brain venography.[376] Demonstrating *thrombi within dural sinuses* is more complicated, since the abnormalities are time-dependent.[377–379] In the acute stage (days 1–5), the thrombus appears isointense on T1-weighted images and strongly hypointense on T2-weighted images (especially with the T2*-susceptibility-weighted technique), in the subacute stage (up to day 15) the thrombus signal is strongly hyperintense on T1 as well as on T2-weighted images, and after the third week the thrombus signal is decreased in all sequences, until the restitution of normal blood flow (section 5.8).

MR digital subtraction angiography can be used to detect arteriovenous malformations and fistulae.[380,381]

8.9.4 Catheter angiography

Introducing a catheter into a peripheral (usually the femoral) artery and guiding it through the aorta to the extracranial and then intracranial vessels and then injecting radio-opaque fluid is not without risk, at least

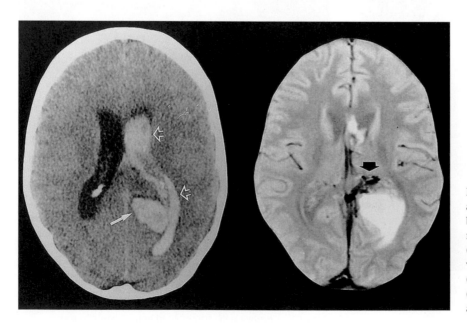

Fig. 8.33 Intracerebral haemorrhage from an arteriovenous malformation. *Left*: CT brain scan showing a haematoma in the medial part of the left occipital lobe (*arrow*), with rupture into the lateral ventricle (*open arrows*). *Right*: MR scan (T1-weighted image) shows signal void (black, *arrow*) from malformation, and large draining vein.

not in patients with ischaemic cerebrovascular disease (section 6.8.5).[382,383] Arterial dissection and contrast hypersensitivity are among the greatest dangers. Nonetheless, in patients with ICH, catheter angiography is still often indicated to detect underlying vascular lesions that are amenable to specific treatment, particularly arteriovenous malformations and saccular aneurysms. This applies essentially to all patients under 50 years of age with ICH, provided they are fit for operation or neuroradiological intervention (the probability of finding a treatable lesion is in the order of 50–80% in normotensive patients under 45 with lobar haemorrhage.[384,385] Angiography may be especially indicated if the pattern of haemorrhage is compatible with a saccular aneurysm but it should preferably be preceded by CT angiography, which may avoid the need for a catheter angiogram (section 9.4.4).[386] Catheter angiography is definitely indicated if MR scanning shows 'flow voids' consistent with an arteriovenous malformation.

Unless an aneurysm is anticipated with its high early risk of rebleeding, it is wise to defer angiography until the space-occupying effect of the haematoma has resolved, because in the acute stage the vascular lesion may be too compressed to be seen.[387,388]

> In any patient with intracerebral haemorrhage who is fit for surgery, one should at least consider catheter angiography, with a view to detecting surgically or radiologically treatable lesions, particularly saccular aneurysms and arteriovenous malformations. The indication is strongest if the patient is under the age of about 50 years, if the haemorrhage is lobar rather than in the deep regions of the brain, and if the patient is not hypertensive.

Given the increasing sensitivity of CT and MR angiography, catheter angiography is rarely indicated in patients over 65 years old, and in hypertensive patients with haemorrhage in the basal ganglia or the posterior fossa. How often this invasive procedure provides extra information that influences management to the benefit of patients in this age group is not precisely known, but probably any such gains are offset by the risks.

8.10 Subdural haematoma

Although subdural haematomas are outside the brain, they are still included in this chapter because most of their many possible causes overlap with those of intracerebral

Table 8.5 Causes of spontaneous subdural haematomas without associated intracerebral or subarachnoid haemorrhage.

Acute, of arterial origin
- Rupture of a small pial artery, spontaneous,[395,397] or in association with cocaine (section 8.5.4)[401]
- Saccular aneurysm of major intracerebral artery (section 9.1.1)[402,403]
- Arteriovenous malformation (section 8.2.4)[404]
- Intracavernous aneurysm of the carotid artery[405]
- Aneurysm of middle meningeal artery[406]
- Moyamoya syndrome (sections 8.2.12 and 7.5)[407]

Chronic, by rupture of a (bridging) vein
- Anticoagulant treatment (section 8.4.1)[394]
- Thrombolytic treatment (section 8.4.3)[408]
- Coagulation defects, genetically determined or acquired (section 8.4.4)[409]
- Low cerebrospinal fluid pressure, secondary to spontaneous leak from a spinal root sleeve,[410] lumbar puncture,[411] or with unknown cause[392,412]
- Tension pneumocephalus[413]
- Rupture of an arachnoid cyst[414]
- Dural arteriovenous fistula (section 8.2.8)[415]
- Dural metastasis[416]
- Autosomal dominant polycystic kidney disease[417,418]

haemorrhage (Table 8.5). Subdural haematomas without attendant haemorrhage in the subarachnoid space or in the brain parenchyma mostly arise from rupture of a bridging vein and are traditionally associated with head trauma in the elderly, but they can also occur 'spontaneously' (or, one might speculate, after trauma that was too trivial to be remembered). Anticoagulants are the most common precipitant (Fig. 8.34) in urbanized areas of Western Europe, accounting for approximately 20% of all chronic forms of subdural haematomas.[389] In young patients, other coagulation disorders may precipitate bleeding in the subdural space.[390] In such cases rapid correction of the coagulation status is mandatory (section 12.4.7), often followed by craniotomy. With most subdural haematomas of venous origin the evolution of symptoms is gradual and by the time they present they may have evolved into fluid collections that appear hypodense on CT scans ('hygromas').

Low cerebrospinal fluid pressure is increasingly recognized as a cause of chronic subdural haematomas, thanks to the characteristic appearances on MRI scanning: diffuse enhancement of the dura and sometimes descent of the brain mimicking a Chiari malformation.[391,392] The leak may be iatrogenic (by lumbar puncture or operation) but also spontaneous, most often from a dural root sleeve.[393]

Arterial sources of bleeding are less common causes of spontaneous bleeding in the subdural space than

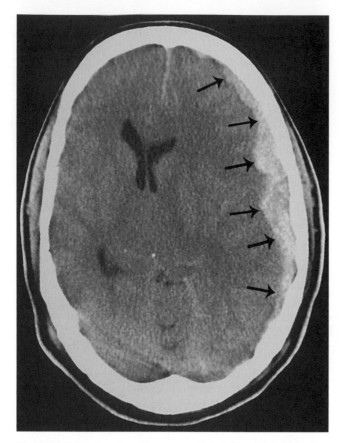

Fig. 8.34 CT brain scan of an acute subdural haematoma in a 54-year-old man treated with oral anticoagulants (*arrows*).

coagulopathies.[394] They include rupture of a small pial artery,[395] most often in the region of the sylvian fissure;[396] angiography may show a small peripheral aneurysm or extravasation from a small artery at the surface of the brain into the subdural space.[397] Subdural haematomas may also be caused by aneurysm rupture; as a rule there is a tell-tale extravasation of blood in the subarachnoid space as well but occasionally the subdural haematoma is the only manifestation (section 9.4.1).

Most spontaneous subdural haematomas occur over the convexity of the cerebral hemisphere, but they may also be found in the posterior interhemispheric fissure, as a rule from a ruptured aneurysm,[398] and in the posterior fossa.[399]

References

1 Ariesen MJ, Claus SP, Rinkel GJE, Algra A. Risk factors for intracerebral hemorrhage in the general population: a systematic review. *Stroke* 2003; **34**:2060–5.

2 Hart RG, Boop BS, Anderson DC. Oral anticoagulants and intracranial hemorrhage: Facts and hypotheses. *Stroke* 1995; **26**:1471–7.

3 Labovitz DL, Halim A, Boden-Albala B, Hauser WA, Sacco RL. The incidence of deep and lobar intracerebral hemorrhage in whites, blacks, and Hispanics. *Neurology* 2005; **65**:518–22.

4 Jamrozik K, Broadhurst RJ, Anderson CS, Stewart Wynne EG. The role of lifestyle factors in the etiology of stroke. A population-based case-control study in Perth, Western Australia. *Stroke* 1994; **25**:51–9.

5 Rodgers A, MacMahon S, Yee T *et al*. Blood pressure, cholesterol, and stroke in eastern Asia. *Lancet* 1998; **352**:1801–7.

6 Woo D, Sauerbeck LR, Kissela BM *et al*. Genetic and environmental risk factors for intracerebral hemorrhage: preliminary results of a population-based study. *Stroke* 2002; **33**:1190–5.

7 Zhang XF, Attia J, D'Este C, Yu XH. Prevalence and magnitude of classical risk factors for stroke in a cohort of 5092 Chinese steelworkers over 13.5 years of follow-up. *Stroke* 2004; **35**:1052–6.

8 Jackson CA, Sudlow CL. Is hypertension a more frequent risk factor for deep than for lobar supratentorial intracerebral haemorrhage? *J Neurol Neurosurg Psychiatry* 2006; **77**(11):1244–52.

9 Charcot JM, Bouchard C. Nouvelles recherches sur la pathogénie de l'hémorrhagie cérébrale. *Arch Physiol norm pathol* 1868; **1**:110–27, 643–65, 725–34.

10 Ellis AG. The pathogenesis of spontaneous intracerebral hemorrhage. *Proc Pathol Soc Philadelphia* 1909; **12**:197–235.

11 Adams RD, vander Eecken HM. Vascular diseases of the brain. *Ann Rev Med* 1953; **4**:213–52.

12 Cole FM, Yates PO. Pseudo-aneurysms in relation to massive cerebral haemorrhage. *J Neurol Neurosurg Psychiatry* 1967; **30**:61–6.

13 Ross Russell RW. Observations on intracerebral aneurysms. *Brain* 1963; **86**:425–42.

14 Cole FM, Yates PO. The occurrence and significance of intracerebral micro-aneurysms. *J Pathol Bacteriol* 1967; **93**:393–411.

15 Challa VL, Moody DM, Bell MA. The Charcot-Bouchard aneurysm controversy: impact of a new histologic technique. *J Neuropathol Exp Neurol* 1992; **51**:264–71.

16 Wakai S, Nagai M. Histological verification of microaneurysms as a cause of cerebral haemorrhage in surgical specimens. *J Neurol Neurosurg Psychiatry* 1989; **52**:595–9.

17 Horn EM, Zabramski JM, Feiz-Erfan I, Lanzino G, McDougall CG. Distal lenticulostriate artery aneurysm rupture presenting as intraparenchymal hemorrhage: case report. *Neurosurgery* 2004; **55**:E708–E712.

18 Fisher CM. Pathological observations in hypertensive cerebral hemorrhage. *J Neuropathol Exp Neurol* 1971; **30**:536–50.

19 Ooneda G, Yoshida Y, Suzuki K, Sekiguchi T. Morphogenesis of plasmatic arterionecrosis as the cause

of hypertensive intracerebral hemorrhage. *Virchows Arch A Pathol Anat* 1973; **361**:31–8.

20 Takebayashi S, Kaneko M. Electron microscopic studies of ruptured arteries in hypertensive intracerebral hemorrhage. *Stroke* 1983; **14**:28–36.

21 Mizutani T, Kojima H, Miki Y. Arterial dissections of penetrating cerebral arteries causing hypertension-induced cerebral hemorrhage. *J Neurosurg* 2000; **93**:859–62.

22 Offenbacher H, Fazekas F, Schmidt R, Koch M, Fazekas G, Kapeller P. MR of cerebral abnormalities concomitant with primary intracerebral hematomas. *Am J Neuroradiol* 1996; **17**:573–8.

23 Kwa VIH, Franke CL, Verbeeten B, Jr., Stam J, Amsterdam Vascular Medicine Group. Silent intracerebral microhemorrhages in patients with ischemic stroke. *Ann Neurol* 1998; **44**:372–7.

24 Fazekas F, Kleinert R, Roob G *et al.* Histopathologic analysis of foci of signal loss on gradient-echo T2*-weighted MR images in patients with spontaneous intracerebral hemorrhage: evidence of microangiopathy-related microbleeds. *Am J Neuroradiol* 1999; **20**:637–42.

25 Cole FM, Yates P. Intracerebral microaneurysms and small cerebrovascular lesions. *Brain* 1967; **90**:759–68.

26 Roob G, Schmidt R, Kapeller P, Lechner A, Hartung HP, Fazekas F. MRI evidence of past cerebral microbleeds in a healthy elderly population. *Neurology* 1999; **52**:991–4.

27 Jeerakathil T, Wolf PA, Beiser A *et al.* Cerebral microbleeds: prevalence and associations with cardiovascular risk factors in the Framingham Study. *Stroke* 2004; **35**:1831–5.

28 Kato H, Izumiyama M, Izumiyama K, Takahashi A, Itoyama Y. Silent cerebral microbleeds on T2*-weighted MRI: correlation with stroke subtype, stroke recurrence, and leukoaraiosis. *Stroke* 2002; **33**:1536–40.

29 Wong KS, Chan YL, Liu JY, Gao S, Lam WWM. Asymptomatic microbleeds as a risk factor for aspirin-associated intracerebral hemorrhages. *Neurology* 2003; **60**:511–13.

30 Lee SH, Kim BJ, Roh JK. Silent microbleeds are associated with volume of primary intracerebral hemorrhage. *Neurology* 2006; **66**:430–2.

31 Roob G, Lechner A, Schmidt R, Flooh E, Hartung HP, Fazekas F. Frequency and location of microbleeds in patients with primary intracerebral hemorrhage. *Stroke* 2000; **31**:2665–9.

32 Nighoghossian N, Hermier M, Adeleine P *et al.* Old microbleeds are a potential risk factor for cerebral bleeding after ischemic stroke: a gradient-echo T2*-weighted brain MRI study. *Stroke* 2002; **33**:735–42.

33 Koennecke HC. Cerebral microbleeds on MRI: prevalence, associations, and potential clinical implications. *Neurology* 2006; **66**:165–71.

34 Viswanathan A, Chabriat H. Cerebral microhemorrhage. *Stroke* 2006; **37**:550–5.

35 Boulanger JM, Coutts SB, Eliasziw M *et al.* Cerebral microhemorrhages predict new disabling or fatal strokes in patients with acute ischemic stroke or transient ischemic attack. *Stroke* 2006; **37**:911–14.

36 Werring DJ, Frazer DW, Coward LJ *et al.* Cognitive dysfunction in patients with cerebral microbleeds on T2*-weighted gradient-echo MRI. *Brain* 2004; **127**:2265–75.

37 Brott T, Broderick J, Kothari R *et al.* Early hemorrhage growth in patients with intracerebral hemorrhage. *Stroke* 1997; **28**:1–5.

38 Kazui S, Naritomi H, Yamamoto H, Sawada T, Yamaguchi T. Enlargement of spontaneous intracerebral hemorrhage: incidence and time course. *Stroke* 1996; **27**:1783–7.

39 Davis SM, Broderick J, Hennerici M *et al.* Hematoma growth is a determinant of mortality and poor outcome after intracerebral hemorrhage. *Neurology* 2006; **66**:1175–81.

40 Murai Y, Ikeda Y, Teramoto A, Tsuji Y. Magnetic resonance imaging-documented extravasation as an indicator of acute hypertensive intracerebral hemorrhage. *J Neurosurg* 1998; **88**:650–5.

41 Murai Y, Takagi R, Ikeda Y, Yamamoto Y, Teramoto A. Three-dimensional computerized tomography angiography in patients with hyperacute intracerebral hemorrhage. *J Neurosurg* 1999; **91**:424–31.

42 Silva Y, Leira R, Tejada J, Lainez JM, Castillo J, Davalos A. Molecular signatures of vascular injury are associated with early growth of intracerebral hemorrhage. *Stroke* 2005; **36**:86–91.

43 Toyoda K, Okada Y, Minematsu K *et al.* Antiplatelet therapy contributes to acute deterioration of intracerebral hemorrhage. *Neurology* 2005; **65**:1000–4.

44 Jauch EC, Lindsell CJ, Adeoye O *et al.* Lack of evidence for an association between hemodynamic variables and hematoma growth in spontaneous intracerebral hemorrhage. *Stroke* 2006; **37**:2061–5.

45 Zazulia AR, Diringer MN, Derdeyn CP, Powers WJ. Progression of mass effect after intracerebral hemorrhage. *Stroke* 1999; **30**:1167–73.

46 Gonzalez-Duarte A, Cantu C, Ruíz-Sandoval JL, Barinagarrementeria F. Recurrent primary cerebral hemorrhage: frequency, mechanisms, and prognosis. *Stroke* 1998; **29**:1802–5.

47 Bailey RD, Hart RG, Benavente O, Pearce LA. Recurrent brain hemorrhage is more frequent than ischemic stroke after intracranial hemorrhage. *Neurology* 2001; **56**:773–7.

48 Bae HG, Jeong DS, Doh JW, Lee KS, Yun IG, Byun BJ. Recurrence of bleeding in patients with hypertensive intracerebral hemorrhage. *Cerebrovasc Dis* 1999; **9**:102–8.

49 Vinters HV. Cerebral amyloid angiopathy. A critical review. *Stroke* 1987; **18**:311–24.

50 Smith EE, Eichler F. Cerebral amyloid angiopathy and lobar intracerebral hemorrhage. *Arch Neurol* 2006; **63**:148–51.

51 Ritter MA, Droste DW, Hegedus K *et al.* Role of cerebral amyloid angiopathy in intracerebral hemorrhage in hypertensive patients. *Neurology* 2005; **64**:1233–7.

52 Fischer O. Die presbyophrene Demenz, deren anatomische Grundlage und klinische Abgrenzung. *Z gesamte Neurol Psychiatr* 1910; **3**:371–471.

53 Torack RM. Congophilic angiopathy complicated by surgery and massive hemorrhage. A light and electron microscopic study. *Am J Pathol* 1975; **81**:349–65.

54 Jellinger K. Cerebrovascular amyloidosis with cerebral hemorrhage. *J Neurol* 1977; **214**:195–206.

55 Miller JH, Wardlaw JM, Lammie GA. Intracerebral haemorrhage and cerebral amyloid angiopathy: CT features with pathological correlation. *Clin Radiol* 1999; **54**:422–9.

56 Yamada M, Itoh Y, Otomo E, Hayakawa M, Miyatake T. Subarachnoid haemorrhage in the elderly: a necropsy study of the association with cerebral amyloid angiopathy. *J Neurol Neurosurg Psychiatry* 1993; **56**:543–7.

57 Masuda J, Tanaka K, Ueda K, Omae T. Autopsy study of incidence and distribution of cerebral amyloid angiopathy in Hisayama, Japan. *Stroke* 1988; **19**:205–10.

58 Itoh Y, Yamada M, Hayakawa M, Otomo E, Miyatake T. Cerebral amyloid angiopathy: a significant cause of cerebellar as well as lobar cerebral hemorrhage in the elderly. *J Neurol Sci* 1993; **116**:135–41.

59 McCarron MO, Nicoll JAR, Ironside JW, Love S, Alberts MJ, Bone I. Cerebral amyloid angiopathy-related hemorrhage interaction of APOE ε2 with putative clinical risk factors. *Stroke* 1999; **30**:1643–6.

60 Brisman MH, Bederson JB, Sen CN, Germano IM, Moore F, Post KD. Intracerebral hemorrhage occurring remote from the craniotomy site. *Neurosurgery* 1996; **39**:1114–21.

61 Finelli PF, Kessimian N, Bernstein PW. Cerebral amyloid angiopathy manifesting as recurrent intracerebral hemorrhage. *Arch Neurol* 1984; **41**:330–3.

62 Neau JP, Ingrand P, Couderq C *et al.* Recurrent intracerebral hemorrhage. *Neurology* 1997; **49**:106–13.

63 Weir NU, van Gijn J, Lammie GA, Wardlaw JM, Warlow CP. Recurrent cerebral haemorrhage in a 65-year-old man: advanced clinical neurology course, Edinburgh, 1997. *J Neurol Neurosurg Psychiatry* 1999; **66**:104–10.

64 Rosand J, Muzikansky A, Kumar A *et al.* Spatial clustering of hemorrhages in probable cerebral amyloid angiopathy. *Ann Neurol* 2005; **58**:459–62.

65 Greenberg SM, O'Donnell HC, Schaefer PW, Kraft E. MRI detection of new hemorrhages: Potential marker of progression in cerebral amyloid angiopathy. *Neurology* 1999; **53**:1135–8.

66 Greenberg SM, Gurol ME, Rosand J, Smith EE. Amyloid angiopathy-related vascular cognitive impairment. *Stroke* 2004; **35**:2616–9.

67 Greenberg SM, Eng JA, Ning M, Smith EE, Rosand J. Hemorrhage burden predicts recurrent intracerebral hemorrhage after lobar hemorrhage. *Stroke* 2004; **35**:1415–20.

68 Gray F, Dubas F, Roullet E, Escourolle R. Leukoencephalopathy in diffuse hemorrhagic cerebral amyloid angiopathy. *Ann Neurol* 1985; **18**:54–9.

69 Smith EE, Gurol ME, Eng JA *et al.* White matter lesions, cognition, and recurrent hemorrhage in lobar intracerebral hemorrhage. *Neurology* 2004; **63**:1606–12.

70 Salat DH, Smith EE, Tuch DS *et al.* White matter alterations in cerebral amyloid angiopathy measured by diffusion tensor imaging. *Stroke* 2006; **37**:1759–64.

71 Hendricks HT, Franke CL, Theunissen PH. Cerebral amyloid angiopathy: diagnosis by MRI and brain biopsy. *Neurology* 1990; **40**:1308–10.

72 Caulo M, Tampieri D, Brassard R, Christine GM, Melanson D. Cerebral amyloid angiopathy presenting as nonhemorrhagic diffuse encephalopathy: neuropathologic and neuroradiologic manifestations in one case. *Am J Neuroradiol* 2001; **22**:1072–6.

73 Smith DB, Hitchcock M, Philpott PJ. Cerebral amyloid angiopathy presenting as transient ischemic attacks. Case report. *J Neurosurg* 1985; **63**:963–4.

74 Gras P, Grosmaire N, Fayolle H, Vion P, Giroud M, Dumas R. [Transient neurologic deficit preceding intracerebral hemorrhage. Physiopathological hypotheses] Déficits neurologiques transitoires précédant les hémorragies intraparenchymateuses. Hypotheses physiopathologiques. *Rev Neurol (Paris)* 1993; **149**:224–6.

75 Greenberg SM, Vonsattel JP, Stakes JW, Gruber M, Finklestein SP. The clinical spectrum of cerebral amyloid angiopathy: presentations without lobar hemorrhage. *Neurology* 1993; **43**:2073–9.

76 Peysson S, Nighoghossian N, Derex L, Jouvet A, Hermier M, Trouillas P. Angiopathie amyloide cérébrale revelée par des accidents neurologiques transitoires. Interêts diagnostiques et physiopathologiques de l'IRM [Cerebral amyloid angiopathy revealed by transient ischemic events: contribution of MRI to diagnosis and pathophysiology study]. *Rev Neurol (Paris)* 2003; **159**:203–5.

77 Roch JA, Nighoghossian N, Hermier M *et al.* Transient neurologic symptoms related to cerebral amyloid angiopathy: usefulness of T2*-weighted imaging. *Cerebrovasc Dis* 2005; **20**:412–14.

78 Wong SH, Robbins PD, Knuckey NW, Kermode AG. Cerebral amyloid angiopathy presenting with vasculitic pathology. *J Clin Neurosci* 2006; **13**:291–4.

79 Eng JA, Frosch MP, Choi K, Rebeck GW, Greenberg SM. Clinical manifestations of cerebral amyloid angiopathy-related inflammation. *Ann Neurol* 2004; **55**:250–6.

80 Scolding NJ, Joseph F, Kirby PA *et al.* Abeta-related angiitis: primary angiitis of the central nervous system associated with cerebral amyloid angiopathy. *Brain* 2005; **128**:500–15.

81 Oh U, Gupta R, Krakauer JW, Khandji AG, Chin SS, Elkind MS. Reversible leukoencephalopathy associated with cerebral amyloid angiopathy. *Neurology* 2004; **62**:494–7.

82 Polivka M, Vallat AV, Woimant F *et al.* Cerebral amyloid angiopathy (CAA) with presentation as a brain inflammatory pseudo-tumour. *Clin Exp Pathol* 1999; **47**:303–10.

83 Wermer MJH, Rinkel GJE, Van Rooij WJ, Witkamp TD, Ziedses Des Plantes BG, Algra A. Interobserver agreement in the assessment of lobar versus deep location of intracerebral haematomas on CT. *J Neuroradiol* 2002; **29**:271–4.

84 Gilles C, Brucher JM, Khoubesserian P, Vanderhaeghen JJ. Cerebral amyloid angiopathy as a cause of multiple intracerebral hemorrhages. *Neurology* 1984; **34**:730–5.

85 Broderick J, Brott T, Tomsick T, Leach A. Lobar hemorrhage in the elderly. The undiminishing importance of hypertension. *Stroke* 1993; **24**:49–51.

86 Anderson CS, Chakera TM, Stewart Wynne EG, Jamrozik KD. Spectrum of primary intracerebral haemorrhage in Perth, Western Australia, 1989–90: incidence and outcome. *J Neurol Neurosurg Psychiatry* 1994; **57**:936–40.

87 Knudsen KA, Rosand J, Karluk D, Greenberg SM. Clinical diagnosis of cerebral amyloid angiopathy: Validation of the Boston Criteria. *Neurology* 2001; **56**:537–9.

88 Lang EW, Ya ZR, Preul C *et al*. Stroke pattern interpretation: The variability of hypertensive versus amyloid angiopathy hemorrhage. *Cerebrovasc Dis* 2001; **12**:121–30.

89 Maclean AV, Woods R, Alderson LM *et al*. Spontaneous lobar haemorrhage in CADASIL. *J Neurol Neurosurg Psychiatry* 2005; **76**:456–7.

90 Greenberg SM, Vonsattel JP. Diagnosis of cerebral amyloid angiopathy: sensitivity and specificity of cortical biopsy. *Stroke* 1997; **28**:1418–22.

91 Nakayama H, Katayama KI, Ikawa A *et al*. Cerebral amyloid angiopathy in an aged great spotted woodpecker (*Picoides major*). *Neurobiol Aging* 1999; **20**:53–6.

92 Revesz T, Ghiso J, Lashley T *et al*. Cerebral amyloid angiopathies: a pathologic, biochemical, and genetic view. *J Neuropathol Exp Neurol* 2003; **62**:885–98.

93 Coria F, Rubio I. Cerebral amyloid angiopathies. *Neuropathol Appl Neurobiol* 1996; **22**:216–27.

94 Christie R, Yamada M, Moskowitz M, Hyman B. Structural and functional disruption of vascular smooth muscle cells in a transgenic mouse model of amyloid angiopathy. *Am J Pathol* 2001; **158**:1065–71.

95 Abbott NJ. Evidence for bulk flow of brain interstitial fluid: significance for physiology and pathology. *Neurochem Int* 2004; **45**:545–52.

96 Weller RO, Nicoll JA. Cerebral amyloid angiopathy: pathogenesis and effects on the ageing and Alzheimer brain. *Neurol Res* 2003; **25**:611–16.

97 Tomonaga M. Cerebral amyloid angiopathy in the elderly. *J Am Geriatr Soc* 1981; **29**:151–7.

98 Vinters HV, Gilbert JJ. Cerebral amyloid angiopathy: incidence and complications in the aging brain. II. The distribution of amyloid vascular changes. *Stroke* 1983; **14**:924–8.

99 Mastaglia FL, Byrnes ML, Johnsen RD, Kakulas BA. Prevalence of cerebral vascular amyloid-beta deposition and stroke in an aging Australian population: a postmortem study. *J Clin Neurosci* 2003; **10**:186–9.

100 Love S, Nicoll JA, Hughes A, Wilcock GK. APOE and cerebral amyloid angiopathy in the elderly. *Neuroreport* 2003; **14**:1535–6.

101 Vonsattel JP, Myers RH, Hedley-Whyte ET, Ropper AH, Bird ED, Richardson EP, Jr. Cerebral amyloid angiopathy without and with cerebral hemorrhages: a comparative histological study. *Ann Neurol* 1991; **30**:637–49.

102 Alonzo NC, Hyman BT, Rebeck GW, Greenberg SM. Progression of cerebral amyloid angiopathy: Accumulation of amyloid-β40 in affected vessels. *J Neuropathol Exp Neurol* 1998; **57**:353–9.

103 Maeda A, Yamada M, Itoh Y, Otomo E, Hayakawa M, Miyatake T. Computer-assisted three-dimensional image analysis of cerebral amyloid angiopathy. *Stroke* 1993; **24**:1857–64.

104 Greenberg SM, Vonsattel JPG, Segal AZ *et al*. Association of apolipoprotein E ε2 and vasculopathy in cerebral amyloid angiopathy. *Neurology* 1998; **50**:961–5.

105 McCarron MO, Nicoll JAR, Stewart J *et al*. The apolipoprotein E ε2 allele and the pathological features in cerebral amyloid angiopathy-related hemorrhage. *J Neuropathol Exp Neurol* 1999; **58**:711–18.

106 McCarron MO, Nicoll JAR. Apolipoprotein E genotype and cerebral amyloid angiopathy-related hemorrhage. *Ann NY Acad Sci* 2000; **903**:176–9.

107 Sudlow C, Martinez Gonzalez NA, Kim J, Clark C. Does apolipoprotein E genotype influence the risk of ischemic stroke, intracerebral hemorrhage, or subarachnoid hemorrhage? Systematic review and meta-analyses of 31 studies among 5961 cases and 17,965 controls. *Stroke* 2006; **37**:364–70.

108 Thal DR, Ghebremedhin E, Rüb U, Yamaguchi H, Del Tredici K, Braak H. Two types of sporadic cerebral amyloid angiopathy. *J Neuropathol Exp Neurol* 2002; **61**:282–93.

109 Love S. Contribution of cerebral amyloid angiopathy to Alzheimer's disease. *J Neurol Neurosurg Psychiatry* 2004; **75**:1–4.

110 Kalyan Raman UP, Kalyan Raman K. Cerebral amyloid angiopathy causing intracranial hemorrhage. *Ann Neurol* 1984; **16**:321–9.

111 Tian J, Shi J, Bailey K, Mann DM. Negative association between amyloid plaques and cerebral amyloid angiopathy in Alzheimer's disease. *Neurosci Lett* 2003; **352**:137–40.

112 Gravina SA, Ho L, Eckman CB *et al*. Amyloid beta protein (A beta) in Alzheimer's disease brain. Biochemical and immunocytochemical analysis with antibodies specific for forms ending at A beta 40 or A beta 42(43). *J Biol Chem* 1995; **270**:7013–16.

113 Attems J, Lintner F, Jellinger KA. Amyloid beta peptide 1-42 highly correlates with capillary cerebral amyloid angiopathy and Alzheimer disease pathology. *Acta Neuropathol (Berl)* 2004; **107**:283–91.

114 Gudmundsson G, Hallgrímsson J, Jónasson TÁ, Bjarnason Ó. Hereditary cerebral haemorrhage with amyloidosis. *Brain* 1972; **95**:387–404.

115 Calero M, Pawlik M, Soto C *et al*. Distinct properties of wild-type and the amyloidogenic human cystatin C variant of hereditary cerebral hemorrhage with amyloidosis, Icelandic type. *J Neurochem* 2001; **77**:628–37.

116 Palsdottir A, Snorradottir AO, Thorsteinsson L. Hereditary cystatin C amyloid angiopathy: genetic, clinical, and pathological aspects. *Brain Pathol* 2006; **16**:55–9.

117 Zhang-Nunes SX, Maat-Schieman ML, van Duinen SG, Roos RA, Frosch MP, Greenberg SM. The cerebral beta-amyloid angiopathies: hereditary and sporadic. *Brain Pathol* 2006; **16**:30–9.

118 Luyendijk W, Bots GTAM, Vegter-van der Vlis M, Went LN, Frangione B. Hereditary cerebral haemorrhage caused by cortical amyloid angiopathy. *J Neurol Sci* 1988; **85**:267–80.

119 Wattendorff AR, Frangione B, Luyendijk W, Bots GTAM. Hereditary cerebral haemorrhage with amyloidosis, Dutch type (HCHWA-D): Clinicopathological studies. *J Neurol Neurosurg Psychiatry* 1995; **58**:699–705.

120 Bakker E, van Broeckhoven C, Haan J et al. DNA diagnosis for hereditary cerebral hemorrhage with amyloidosis (Dutch type). *Am J Hum Genet* 1991; **49**:518–21.

121 Nilsberth C, Westlind-Danielsson A, Eckman CB et al. The 'Arctic' APP mutation (E693G) causes Alzheimer's disease by enhanced Abeta protofibril formation. *Nat Neurosci* 2001; **4**:887–93.

122 Hendriks L, Van Duijn CM, Cras P et al. Presenile dementia and cerebral haemorrhage linked to a mutation at codon 692 of the beta-amyloid precursor protein gene. *Nat Genet* 1992; **1**:218–21.

123 Greenberg SM, Shin Y, Grabowski TJ et al. Hemorrhagic stroke associated with the Iowa amyloid precursor protein mutation. *Neurology* 2003; **60**:1020–2.

124 Grabowski TJ, Cho HS, Vonsattel JPG, Rebeck GW, Greenberg SM. Novel amyloid precursor protein mutation in an Iowa family with dementia and severe cerebral amyloid angiopathy. *Ann Neurol* 2001; **49**:697–705.

125 Obici L, Demarchi A, de Rosa G et al. A novel AbetaPP mutation exclusively associated with cerebral amyloid angiopathy. *Ann Neurol* 2005; **58**:639–44.

126 Sleegers K, Brouwers N, Gijselinck I et al. APP duplication is sufficient to cause early onset Alzheimer's dementia with cerebral amyloid angiopathy. *Brain* 2006; **129**(Pt 11):2977–83.

127 Van Gijn J, van Dongen KJ. The time course of aneurysmal haemorrhage on computed tomograms. *Neuroradiology* 1982; **23**:153–6.

128 Abbed KM, Ogilvy CS. Intracerebral hematoma from aneurysm rupture. *Neurosurg Focus* 2003; **15**(4):1–5.

129 Bamford J, Sandercock P, Dennis M et al. A prospective study of acute cerebrovascular disease in the community: the Oxfordshire Community Stroke Project 1981–86. 1. Methodology, demography and incident cases of first-ever stroke. *J Neurol Neurosurg Psychiatry* 1988; **51**:1373–80.

130 Thrift AG, Dewey HM, Macdonell RA, McNeil JJ, Donnan GA. Stroke incidence on the east coast of Australia: the North East Melbourne Stroke Incidence Study (NEMESIS). *Stroke* 2000; **31**:2087–92.

131 Linn FHH, Rinkel GJE, Algra A, van Gijn J. Incidence of subarachnoid hemorrhage: role of region, year, and rate of computed tomography: A meta-analysis. *Stroke* 1996; **27**:625–9.

132 Broderick JP, Brott T, Tomsick T, Miller R, Huster G. Intracerebral hemorrhage more than twice as common as subarachnoid hemorrhage. *J Neurosurg* 1993; **78**:188–91.

133 Laissy JP, Normand G, Monroc M, Duchateau C, Alibert F, Thiebot J. Spontaneous intracerebral hematomas from vascular causes. Predictive value of CT compared with angiography. *Neuroradiology* 1991; **33**:291–5.

134 Krings T, Mayfrank L, Thron A. Bleeding from a cavernous angioma mimicking rupture of a middle cerebral artery aneurysm. *Neuroradiology* 2001; **43**:985–9.

135 Al-Shahi R, Bhattacharya JJ, Currie DG et al. Prospective, population-based detection of intracranial vascular malformations in adults: the Scottish Intracranial Vascular Malformation Study (SIVMS). *Stroke* 2003; **34**:1163–9.

136 Al Shahi R, Warlow C. A systematic review of the frequency and prognosis of arteriovenous malformations of the brain in adults. *Brain* 2001; **124**:1900–26.

137 Stapf C, Mast H, Sciacca RR et al. The New York Islands AVM Study: design, study progress, and initial results. *Stroke* 2003; **34**:e29–e33.

138 Willinsky RA, Lasjaunias P, Terbrugge K, Burrows P. Multiple cerebral arteriovenous malformations (AVMs). Review of our experience from 203 patients with cerebral vascular lesions. *Neuroradiology* 1990; **32**:207–10.

139 Yokoyama K, Asano Y, Murakawa T et al. Familial occurrence of arteriovenous malformation of the brain. *J Neurosurg* 1991; **74**:585–9.

140 Larsen PD, Hellbusch LC, Lefkowitz DM, Schaefer GB. Cerebral arteriovenous malformation in three successive generations. *Pediatr Neurol* 1997; **17**:74–6.

141 Stapf C, Mohr JP, Pile-Spellman J et al. Concurrent arterial aneurysms in brain arteriovenous malformations with haemorrhagic presentation. *J Neurol Neurosurg Psychiatry* 2002; **73**:294–8.

142 Aoki N. Do intracranial arteriovenous malformations cause subarachnoid haemorrhage? Review of computed tomography features of ruptured arteriovenous malformations in the acute stage. *Acta Neurochir (Wien)* 1991; **112**:92–5.

143 Hartmann A, Mast H, Mohr JP et al. Morbidity of intracranial hemorrhage in patients with cerebral arteriovenous malformation. *Stroke* 1998; **29**:931–4.

144 Choi JH, Mast H, Sciacca RR et al. Clinical outcome after first and recurrent hemorrhage in patients with untreated brain arteriovenous malformation. *Stroke* 2006; **37**:1243–7.

145 Toffol GJ, Biller J, Adams HP, Jr. Nontraumatic intracerebral hemorrhage in young adults. *Arch Neurol* 1987; **44**:483–5.

146 Robinson JR, Jr., Awad IA, Masaryk TJ, Estes ML. Pathological heterogeneity of angiographically occult vascular malformations of the brain. *Neurosurgery* 1993; **33**:547–54.

147 Tomlinson FH, Houser OW, Scheithauer BW, Sundt TM, Jr., Okazaki H, Parisi JE. Angiographically occult vascular malformations: a correlative study of features on magnetic resonance imaging and histological examination. *Neurosurgery* 1994; **34**:792–9.

148 Raychaudhuri R, Batjer HH, Awad IA. Intracranial cavernous angioma: a practical review of clinical and biological aspects. *Surg Neurol* 2005; **63**:319–28.

149 Otten P, Pizzolato GP, Rilliet B, Berney J. [131 cases of cavernous angioma (cavernomas) of the CNS, discovered by retrospective analysis of 24,535 autopsies] A propos de 131 cas d'angiomes caverneux (cavernomes) du s.n.c.,

répérés par l'analyse rétrospective de 24 535 autopsies. *Neurochirurgie* 1989; **35**:82–3,128–31.

150 Robinson JR, Awad IA, Little JR. Natural history of the cavernous angioma. *J Neurosurg* 1991; **75**:709–14.

151 Duchene M, Caldas JG, Benoudiba F, Cerri GG, Doyon D. Séquences de résonance magnétique dans la détection de cavernomes [MRI sequences in the detection of cavernous angiomas]. *J Radiol* 2002; **83**:1843–6.

152 Lehnhardt FG, von Smekal U, Rückriem B *et al*. Value of gradient-echo magnetic resonance imaging in the diagnosis of familial cerebral cavernous malformation. *Arch Neurol* 2005; **62**:653–8.

153 Clatterbuck RE, Moriarity JL, Elmaci I, Lee RR, Breiter SN, Rigamonti D. Dynamic nature of cavernous malformations: a prospective magnetic resonance imaging study with volumetric analysis. *J Neurosurg* 2000; **93**:981–6.

154 Labauge P, Brunereau L, Coubes P *et al*. Appearance of new lesions in two nonfamilial cerebral cavernoma patients. *Eur Neurol* 2001; **45**:83–8.

155 Larson JJ, Ball WS, Bove KE, Crone KR, Tew JM, Jr. Formation of intracerebral cavernous malformations after radiation treatment for central nervous system neoplasia in children. *J Neurosurg* 1998; **88**:51–6.

156 Duhem R, Vinchon M, Leblond P, Soto-Ares G, Dhellemmes P. Cavernous malformations after cerebral irradiation during childhood: report of nine cases. *Childs Nerv Syst* 2005; **21**(10):922–5.

157 Lew SM, Morgan JN, Psaty E, Lefton DR, Allen JC, Abbott R. Cumulative incidence of radiation-induced cavernomas in long-term survivors of medulloblastoma. *J Neurosurg* 2006; **104**:103–7.

158 Kondziolka D, Lunsford LD, Kestle JR. The natural history of cerebral cavernous malformations. *J Neurosurg* 1995; **83**:820–4.

159 Bertalanffy H, Benes L, Miyazawa T, Alberti O, Siegel AM, Sure U. Cerebral cavernomas in the adult. Review of the literature and analysis of 72 surgically treated patients. *Neurosurg Rev* 2002; **25**:1–53.

160 Porter PJ, Willinsky RA, Harper W, Wallace MC. Cerebral cavernous malformations: natural history and prognosis after clinical deterioration with or without hemorrhage. *J Neurosurg* 1997; **87**:190–7.

161 Nieto J, Hinojosa J, Munoz MJ, Esparza J, Ricoy R. Intraventricular cavernoma in pediatric age. *Childs Nerv Syst* 2003; **19**:60–2.

162 Vishteh AG, Nadkarni T, Spetzler RF. Cavernous malformation of the pineal region: short report and review of the literature. *Br J Neurosurg* 2000; **14**:147–51.

163 Sohn CH, Kim SP, Kim IM, Lee JH, Lee HK. Characteristic MR imaging findings of cavernous hemangiomas in the cavernous sinus. *Am J Neuroradiol* 2003; **24**:1148–51.

164 Deshmukh VR, Albuquerque FC, Zabramski JM, Spetzler RF. Surgical management of cavernous malformations involving the cranial nerves. *Neurosurgery* 2003; **53**:352–7.

165 Santoro A, Piccirilli M, Frati A *et al*. Intramedullary spinal cord cavernous malformations: report of ten new cases. *Neurosurg Rev* 2004; **27**:93–8.

166 Cohen-Gadol AA, Jacob JT, Edwards DA, Krauss WE. Coexistence of intracranial and spinal cavernous malformations: a study of prevalence and natural history. *J Neurosurg* 2006; **104**:376–81.

167 Stefan H, Hammen T. Cavernous haemangiomas, epilepsy and treatment strategies. *Acta Neurol Scand* 2004; **110**:393–7.

168 Cader MZ, Winer JB. Lesson of the week: cavernous haemangioma mimicking multiple sclerosis. *Br Med J* 1999; **318**:1604–5.

169 Kumral E, Özdemirkiran T, Bayülkem G. Facio-oculo-palatal myoclonus due to pontine cavernous angioma. *Cerebrovasc Dis* 2002; **13**:217–18.

170 Kupersmith MJ, Kalish H, Epstein F *et al*. Natural history of brainstem cavernous malformations. *Neurosurgery* 2001; **48**:47–53.

171 Zabramski JM, Wascher TM, Spetzler RF *et al*. The natural history of familial cavernous malformations: results of an ongoing study. *J Neurosurg* 1994; **80**:422–32.

172 Rigamonti D, Hadley MN, Drayer BP *et al*. Cerebral cavernous malformations. Incidence and familial occurrence. *N Engl J Med* 1988; **319**:343–7.

173 Denier C, Labauge P, Brunereau L *et al*. Clinical features of cerebral cavernous malformations patients with KRIT1 mutations. *Ann Neurol* 2004; **55**:213–20.

174 Chen DH, Lipe HP, Qin Z, Bird TD. Cerebral cavernous malformation: novel mutation in a Chinese family and evidence for heterogeneity. *J Neurol Sci* 2002; **196**:91–6.

175 Labauge P, Laberge S, Brunereau L, Levy C, Tournier-Lasserve E, Soc FN. Hereditary cerebral cavernous angiomas: clinical and genetic features in 57 French families. *Lancet* 1998; **352**:1892–7.

176 Lucas M, Solano F, Zayas MD *et al*. Spanish families with cerebral cavernous angioma do not bear 742C—>T Hispanic American mutation of the *KRIT1* gene. *Ann Neurol* 2000; **47**:836.

177 Gunel M, Awad IA, Finberg K *et al*. A founder mutation as a cause of cerebral cavernous malformation in Hispanic Americans. *N Engl J Med* 1996; **334**:946–51.

178 Denier C, Goutagny S, Labauge P *et al*. Mutations within the MGC4607 gene cause cerebral cavernous malformations. *Am J Hum Genet* 2004; **74**:326–37.

179 Seker A, Pricola KL, Guclu B, Ozturk AK, Louvi A, Gunel M. CCM2 expression parallels that of CCM1. *Stroke* 2006; **37**:518–23.

180 Petit N, Blecon A, Denier C, Tournier-Lasserve E. Patterns of expression of the three cerebral cavernous malformation (CCM) genes during embryonic and postnatal brain development. *Gene Expr Patterns* 2006; **6**:495–503.

181 Sarwar M, McCormick WF. Intracerebral venous angioma. Case report and review. *Arch Neurol* 1978; **35**:323–5.

182 Garner TB, Del Curling O, Jr., Kelly DL, Jr., Laster DW. The natural history of intracranial venous angiomas. *J Neurosurg* 1991; **75**:715–22.

183 Naff NJ, Wemmer J, Hoenig-Rigamonti K, Rigamonti DR. A longitudinal study of patients with venous malformations: documentation of a negligible hemorrhage risk and benign natural history. *Neurology* 1998; **50**:1709–14.

184 Malinvaud D, Lecanu JB, Halimi P, Avan P, Bonfils P. Tinnitus and cerebellar developmental venous anomaly. *Arch Otolaryngol Head Neck Surg* 2006; **132**:550–3.

185 McLaughlin MR, Kondziolka D, Flickinger JC, Lunsford S, Lunsford LD. The prospective natural history of cerebral venous malformations. *Neurosurgery* 1998; **43**:195–200.

186 Töpper R, Jürgens E, Reul J, Thron A. Clinical significance of intracranial developmental venous anomalies. *J Neurol Neurosurg Psychiatry* 1999; **67**:234–8.

187 Mullan S, Mojtahedi S, Johnson DL, Macdonald RL. Cerebral venous malformation arteriovenous malformation transition forms. *J Neurosurg* 1996; **85**:9–13.

188 Lasjaunias P, Burrows P, Planet C. Developmental venous anomalies (DVA): the so-called venous angioma. *Neurosurg Rev* 1986; **9**:233–42.

189 Abe M, Hagihara N, Tabuchi K, Uchino A, Miyasaka Y. Histologically classified venous angiomas of the brain: a controversy. *Neurol Med Chir (Tokyo)* 2003; **43**:1–10.

190 Masson C, Godefroy O, Leclerc X, Colombani JM, Leys D. Cerebral venous infarction following thrombosis of the draining vein of a venous angioma (developmental abnormality). *Cerebrovasc Dis* 2000; **10**:235–8.

191 Letteboer TG, Mager JJ, Snijder RJ *et al.* Genotype-phenotype relationship in hereditary haemorrhagic telangiectasia. *J Med Genet* 2006; **43**:371–7.

192 Guttmacher AE, Marchuk DA, White RI, Jr. Hereditary hemorrhagic telangiectasia. *N Engl J Med* 1995; **333**:918–24.

193 Maher CO, Piepgras DG, Brown RD, Jr., Friedman JA, Pollock BE. Cerebrovascular manifestations in 321 cases of hereditary hemorrhagic telangiectasia. *Stroke* 2001; **32**:877–82.

194 Scaglione C, Salvi F, Riguzzi P, Vergelli M, Tassinari CA, Mascalchi M. Symptomatic unruptured capillary telangiectasia of the brain stem: report of three cases and review of the literature. *J Neurol Neurosurg Psychiatry* 2001; **71**:390–3.

195 Sarma D, ter Brugge K. Management of intracranial dural arteriovenous shunts in adults. *Eur J Radiol* 2003; **46**:206–20.

196 Renner C, Helm J, Roth H, Meixensberger J. Intracranial dural arteriovenous fistula associated with progressive cervical myelopathy and normal venous drainage of the thoracolumbar cord: case report and review of the literature. *Surg Neurol* 2006; **65**:506–10.

197 Tsai LK, Jeng JS, Liu HM, Wang HJ, Yip PK. Intracranial dural arteriovenous fistulas with or without cerebral sinus thrombosis: analysis of 69 patients. *J Neurol Neurosurg Psychiatry* 2004; **75**:1639–41.

198 Vilela P, Willinsky R, Terbrugge K. Dural arteriovenous fistula associated with neoplastic dural sinus thrombosis: two cases. *Neuroradiology* 2001; **43**:816–20.

199 Obrador S, Soto M, Silvela J. Clinical syndromes of arteriovenous malformations of the transverse-sigmoid sinus. *J Neurol Neurosurg Psychiatry* 1975; **38**:436–51.

200 Chaudhary MY, Sachdev VP, Cho SH, Weitzner I, Jr., Puljic S, Huang YP. Dural arteriovenous malformation of the major venous sinuses: an acquired lesion. *Am J Neuroradiol* 1982; **3**:13–9.

201 Ishikawa T, Houkin K, Tokuda K, Kawaguchi S, Kashiwaba T. Development of anterior cranial fossa dural arteriovenous malformation following head trauma: case report. *J Neurosurg* 1997; **86**:291–3.

202 Davies MA, Terbrugge K, Willinsky R, Coyne T, Saleh J, Wallace MC. The validity of classification for the clinical presentation of intracranial dural arteriovenous fistulas. *J Neurosurg* 1996; **85**:830–7.

203 Van Dijk JMC, TerBrugge KG, Willinsky RA, Wallace MC. Multiplicity of dural arteriovenous fistulas. *J Neurosurg* 2002; **96**:76–8.

204 Van Dijk JMC, TerBrugge KG, Willinsky RA, Wallace MC. Clinical course of cranial dural arteriovenous fistulas with long-term persistent cortical venous reflux. *Stroke* 2002; **33**:1233–6.

205 Duffau H, Lopes M, Janosevic V *et al.* Early rebleeding from intracranial dural arteriovenous fistulas: report of 20 cases and review of the literature. *J Neurosurg* 1999; **90**:78–84.

206 Satoh K, Satomi J, Nakajima N, Matsubara S, Nagahiro S. Cerebellar hemorrhage caused by dural arteriovenous fistula: a review of five cases. *J Neurosurg* 2001; **94**:422–6.

207 Satomi J, Van Dijk JMC, TerBrugge KG, Willinsky RA, Wallace C. Benign cranial dural arteriovenous fistulas: outcome of conservative management based on the natural history of the lesion. *J Neurosurg* 2002; **97**:767–70.

208 Shah SB, Lalwani AK, Dowd CF. Transverse/sigmoid sinus dural arteriovenous fistulas presenting as pulsatile tinnitus. *Laryngoscope* 1999; **109**:54–8.

209 Cognard C, Casasco A, Toevi M, Houdart E, Chiras J, Merland JJ. Dural arteriovenous fistulas as a cause of intracranial hypertension due to impairment of cranial venous outflow. *J Neurol Neurosurg Psychiatry* 1998; **65**:308–16.

210 Bernstein R, Dowd CF, Gress DR. Rapidly reversible dementia. *Lancet* 2003; **361**:392.

211 Motto C, Aritzu E, Boccardi E, De Grandi C, Piana A, Candelise L. Reliability of hemorrhagic transformation diagnosis in acute ischemic stroke. *Stroke* 1997; **28**:302–6.

212 Lindley RI, Wardlaw JM, Sandercock PAG *et al.* Frequency and risk factors for spontaneous hemorrhagic transformation of cerebral infarction. *J Stroke Cerebrovasc Dis* 2004; **18**:235–46.

213 Bogousslavsky J, Regli F, Uske A, Maeder P. Early spontaneous hematoma in cerebral infarct: is primary cerebral hemorrhage overdiagnosed? *Neurology* 1991; **41**:837–40.

214 De Freitas GR, Carruzzo A, Tsiskaridze A, Lobrinus JA, Bogousslavsky J. Massive haemorrhagic transformation in cardioembolic stroke: the role of arterial wall trauma and dissection. *J Neurol Neurosurg Psychiatry* 2001; **70**:672–4.

215 Larrue V, Von Kummer R, del Zoppo G, Bluhmki E. Hemorrhagic transformation in acute ischemic stroke: potential contributing factors in the European Cooperative Acute Stroke Study. *Stroke* 1997; **28**:957–60.

216 Berger C, Fiorelli M, Steiner T et al. Hemorrhagic transformation of ischemic brain tissue: Asymptomatic or symptomatic? *Stroke* 2001; **32**:1330–5.

217 Tehindrazanarivelo A, Evrard S, Schaison M, Mas J-L, Dormont D, Bousser M-G. Prospective study of cerebral sinus venous thrombosis in patients presenting with benign intracranial hypertension. *Cerebrovasc Dis* 1992; **2**:22–7.

218 Tang OS, Ng EHY, Cheng PW, Ho PC. Cortical vein thrombosis misinterpreted as intracranial haemorrhage in severe ovarian hyperstimulation syndrome. *Hum Reprod* 2000; **15**:1913–16.

219 Thaler DE, Lev MH, Frosch MP, Buonanno FS. A 41-year-old woman with global headache and an intracranial mass: cerebral venous thrombosis, resulting in hemorrhagic infarction of the posterior left temporal lobe. *N Engl J Med* 2002; **346**:1651–8.

220 Wardlaw JM, Lammie GA, Whittle IR. A brain haemorrhage? *Lancet* 1998; **351**:1028.

221 Kanter MC, Hart RG. Neurologic complications of infective endocarditis. *Neurology* 1991; **41**:1015–20.

222 Masuda J, Yutani C, Waki R, Ogata J, Kuriyama Y, Yamaguchi T. Histopathological analysis of the mechanisms of intracranial hemorrhage complicating infective endocarditis. *Stroke* 1992; **23**:843–50.

223 Gomez-Moreno J, Moar C, Roman F, Perez-Maestu R, Lopez de Letona JM. Salmonella endocarditis presenting as cerebral hemorrhage. *Eur J Intern Med* 2000; **11**:96–7.

224 Voermans NC, Hart W, van Engelen BG. Klinisch denken en beslissen in de praktijk. Een 23-jarige vrouw met malaise, anorexie en gedragsveranderingen [Clinical reasoning and decision making in practice. A 23 year old woman with malaise, anorexia, fever and behavior changes]. *Ned Tijdschr Geneeskd* 2004; **148**:1079–86.

225 Hart RG, Kagan Hallet K, Joerns SE. Mechanisms of intracranial hemorrhage in infective endocarditis. *Stroke* 1987; **18**:1048–56.

226 Monsuez JJ, Vittecoq D, Rosenbaum A et al. Prognosis of ruptured intracranial mycotic aneurysms: a review of 12 cases. *Eur Heart J* 1989; **10**:821–5.

227 Ruttmann E, Willeit J, Ulmer H et al. Neurological outcome of septic cardioembolic stroke after infective endocarditis. *Stroke* 2006; **37**:2094–9.

228 Angstwurm K, Borges AC, Halle E, Schielke E, Einhaupl KM, Weber JR. Timing the valve replacement in infective endocarditis involving the brain. *J Neurol* 2004; **251**:1220–6.

229 Roquer J, Palomeras E, Knobel H, Pou A. Intracerebral haemorrhage in AIDS. *Cerebrovasc Dis* 1998; **8**:222–7.

230 Jeong SC, Bae JC, Hwang SH, Kim HC, Lee BC. Cerebral sparganosis with intracerebral hemorrhage: A case report. *Neurology* 1998; **50**:503–6.

231 Fukui M, Kono S, Sueishi K, Ikezaki K. Moyamoya disease. *Neuropathology* 2000; **20** Suppl:S61–S64.

232 Storen EC, Wijdicks EFM, Crum BA, Schultz G. Moyamoya-like vasculopathy from cocaine dependency. *Am J Neuroradiol* 2000; **21**:1008–10.

233 Yamauchi T, Tada M, Houkin K et al. Linkage of familial moyamoya disease (spontaneous occlusion of the circle of Willis) to chromosome 17q25. *Stroke* 2000; **31**:930–5.

234 Suzuki J, Kodama N. Moyamoya disease: a review. *Stroke* 1983; **14**:104–9.

235 Hallemeier CL, Rich KM, Grubb RL, Jr. et al. Clinical features and outcome in North American adults with moyamoya phenomenon. *Stroke* 2006; **37**:1490–6.

236 Kim TS, Lee JH, Kim IY et al. Moyamoya disease with repeated intracranial haemorrhage in two consecutive pregnancies. *J Clin Neurosci* 2004; **11**:525–7.

237 Williams DL, Martin IL, Gully RM. Intracerebral hemorrhage and moyamoya disease in pregnancy. *Can J Anaesth* 2000; **47**:996–1000.

238 Tzeng DZ, Fein J, Boe N, Chan A. A pregnant woman with headaches, seizures, and hypertension. *Lancet* 2005; **365**:2150.

239 Yoshida Y, Yoshimoto T, Shirane R, Sakurai Y. Clinical course, surgical management, and long-term outcome of moyamoya patients with rebleeding after an episode of intracerebral hemorrhage: an extensive follow-up study. *Stroke* 1999; **30**:2272–6.

240 Kobayashi E, Saeki N, Oishi H, Hirai S, Yamaura A. Long-term natural history of hemorrhagic moyamoya disease in 42 patients. *J Neurosurg* 2000; **93**:976–80.

241 Miyamoto S. Study design for a prospective randomized trial of extracranial-intracranial bypass surgery for adults with moyamoya disease and hemorrhagic onset: the Japan Adult Moyamoya Trial Group. *Neurol Med Chir (Tokyo)* 2004; **44**:218–19.

242 D'Angelo VA, Monte V, Scialfa G, Fiumara E, Scotti G. Intracerebral venous hemorrhage in 'high-risk' carotid-cavernous fistula. *Surg Neurol* 1988; **30**:387–90.

243 Hiramatsu K, Utsumi S, Kyoi K et al. Intracerebral hemorrhage in carotid-cavernous fistula. *Neuroradiology* 1991; **33**:67–9.

244 Van Rooij WJ, Sluzewski M, Beute GN. Ruptured cavernous sinus aneurysms causing carotid cavernous fistula: incidence, clinical presentation, treatment, and outcome. *Am J Neuroradiol* 2006; **27**:185–9.

245 Caplan L. Intracerebral hemorrhage revisited. *Neurology* 1988; **38**:624–7.

246 Gelis A, Pelissier J, Blard JM, Pages M. Hémorragie intracranienne et pheochromocytome [Intracranial haemorrhage associated with phaeochromocytoma]. *Rev Neurol (Paris)* 2004; **160**:945–8.

247 Drislane FW, Wang AM. Multifocal cerebral hemorrhage in eclampsia and severe pre-eclampsia. *J Neurol* 1997; **244**:194–8.

248 Caplan LR, Neely S, Gorelick P. Cold-related intracerebral hemorrhage. *Arch Neurol* 1984; **41**:227.

249 Barbas N, Caplan L, Baquis G, Adelman L, Moskowitz M. Dental chair intracerebral hemorrhage. *Neurology* 1987; **37**:511–12.

250 Lee KC, Clough C. Intracerebral hemorrhage after break dancing [letter]. *N Engl J Med* 1990; **323**:615–16.

251 Ponder A, Lehman LB. 'Coining' and 'coning': an unusual complication of unconventional medicine. *Neurology* 1994; **44**:774–5.

252 Lammie GA, Lindley R, Keir S, Wiggam I. Stress-related primary intracerebral hemorrhage: autopsy clues to underlying mechanism. *Stroke* 2000; **31**:1426–8.

253 Marti I, Marti Masso JF. Hemiballism due to sildenafil use. *Neurology* 2004; **63**:534.

254 Russell DA, Gough MJ. Intracerebral haemorrhage following carotid endarterectomy. *Eur J Vasc Endovasc Surg* 2004; **28**:115–23.

255 Buhk JH, Cepek L, Knauth M. Hyperacute intracerebral hemorrhage complicating carotid stenting should be distinguished from hyperperfusion syndrome. *Am J Neuroradiol* 2006; **27**:1508–13.

256 Troost BT, Mark LE, Maroon JC. Resolution of classic migraine after removal of an occipital lobe AVM. *Ann Neurol* 1979; **5**:199–201.

257 Spierings ELH. Daily migraine with visual aura associated with an occipital arteriovenous malformation. *Headache* 2001; **41**:193–7.

258 Combremont PC, Marcus EM. Intracranial hemorrhages associated with sumatriptan. *Neurology* 2001; **56**:1243–4.

259 Cole AJ, Aubé M. Migraine with vasospasm and delayed intracerebral hemorrhage. *Arch Neurol* 1990; **47**:53–6.

260 Raabe A, Krug U. Migraine associated bilateral intracerebral haemorrhages. *Clin Neurol Neurosurg* 1999; **101**:193–5.

261 Gorter JW, Stroke Prevention in Reversible Ischemia Trial (SPIRIT) Group, European Atrial Fibrillation Trial (EAFT) Group. Major bleeding during anticoagulation after cerebral ischemia: patterns and risk factors. *Neurology* 1999; **53**:1319–27.

262 Rosand J, Hylek EM, O'Donnell HC, Greenberg SM. Warfarin-associated hemorrhage and cerebral amyloid angiopathy: a genetic and pathologic study. *Neurology* 2000; **55**:947–51.

263 Hylek EM, Singer DE. Risk factors for intracranial hemorrhage in outpatients taking warfarin. *Ann Intern Med* 1994; **120**:897–902.

264 Cannegieter SC, Rosendaal FR, Wintzen AR, Van der Meer FJM, Vandenbroucke JP, Briët E. Optimal oral anticoagulant therapy in patients with mechanical heart valves. *N Engl J Med* 1995; **333**:11–17.

265 Azar AJ, Koudstaal PJ, Wintzen AR, Van Bergen PF, Jonker JJ, Deckers JW. Risk of stroke during long-term anticoagulant therapy in patients after myocardial infarction. *Ann Neurol* 1996; **39**:301–7.

266 Chesebro JH, Wiebers DO, Holland AE *et al*. Bleeding during antithrombotic therapy in patients with atrial fibrillation. *Arch Intern Med* 1996; **156**:409–16.

267 Berwaerts J, Webster J. Analysis of risk factors involved in oral-anticoagulant-related intracranial haemorrhages. *Q J Med* 2000; **93**:513–21.

268 Torn M, Algra A, Rosendaal FR. Oral anticoagulation for cerebral ischemia of arterial origin: high initial bleeding risk. *Neurology* 2001; **57**:1993–9.

269 Hart RG, Tonarelli SB, Pearce LA. Avoiding central nervous system bleeding during antithrombotic therapy: recent data and ideas. *Stroke* 2005; **36**:1588–93.

270 Smith EE, Rosand J, Knudsen KA, Hylek EM, Greenberg SM. Leukoaraiosis is associated with warfarin-related hemorrhage following ischemic stroke. *Neurology* 2002; **59**:193–7.

271 Dawson I, van Bockel JH, Ferrari MD, van der Meer FJ, Brand R, Terpstra JL. Ischemic and hemorrhagic stroke in patients on oral anticoagulants after reconstruction for chronic lower limb ischemia. *Stroke* 1993; **24**:1655–63.

272 Sjöblom L, Hårdemark HG, Lindgren A *et al*. Management and prognostic features of intracerebral hemorrhage during anticoagulant therapy: a Swedisih multicenter study. *Stroke* 2001; **32**:2567–74.

273 Franke CL, de Jonge J, van Swieten JC, Op de Coul AAW, van Gijn J. Intracerebral hematomas during anticoagulant treatment. *Stroke* 1990; **21**:726–30.

274 Neau JP, Couderq C, Ingrand P, Blanchon P, Gil R, VGP Study Group. Intracranial hemorrhage and oral anticoagulant treatment. *Cerebrovasc Dis* 2001; **11**:195–200.

275 Huttner HB, Steiner T, Hartmann M *et al*. Comparison of ABC/2 estimation technique to computer-assisted planimetric analysis in warfarin-related intracerebral parenchymal hemorrhage. *Stroke* 2006; **37**:404–8.

276 Flibotte JJ, Hagan N, O'Donnell J, Greenberg SM, Rosand J. Warfarin, hematoma expansion, and outcome of intracerebral hemorrhage. *Neurology* 2004; **63**:1059–64.

277 Pfleger MJ, Hardee EP, Contant CF, Jr., Hayman LA. Sensitivity and specificity of fluid-blood levels for coagulopathy in acute intracerebral hematomas. *Am J Neuroradiol* 1994; **15**:217–23.

278 Baigent C, Sudlow C, Collins R, Peto R, for the Antithrombotic Trialists Collaboration. Collaborative meta-analysis of randomised trials of antiplatelet therapy for prevention of death, myocardial infarction, and stroke in high risk patients. *Br Med J* 2002; **324**:71–86.

279 Gorelick PB, Weisman SM. Risk of hemorrhagic stroke with aspirin use: an update. *Stroke* 2005; **36**:1801–7.

280 Ariesen MJ, Algra A, Koudstaal PJ, Rothwell PM, Van Walraven C. Risk of intracerebral hemorrhage in patients with arterial versus cardiac origin of cerebral ischemia on aspirin or placebo: analysis of individual patient data from 9 trials. *Stroke* 2004; **35**:710–14.

281 Viswanathan A, Rakich SM, Engel C *et al*. Antiplatelet use after intracerebral hemorrhage. *Neurology* 2006; **66**:206–9.

282 Diener HC, Bogousslavsky J, Brass LM *et al*. Aspirin and clopidogrel compared with clopidogrel alone after recent ischaemic stroke or transient ischaemic attack in high-risk patients (MATCH): randomised, double-blind, placebo-controlled trial. *Lancet* 2004; **364**:331–7.

283 Bhatt DL, Fox KA, Hacke W *et al*. Clopidogrel and aspirin versus aspirin alone for the prevention of atherothrombotic events. *N Engl J Med* 2006; **354**:1706–17.

284 UK-TIA Study Group. The United Kingdom transient ischaemic attack (UK-TIA) aspirin trial: final results. *J Neurol Neurosurg Psychiatry* 1991; **54**:1044–54.

285 The Dutch TIA Trial Study Group. A comparison of two doses of aspirin (30 mg vs. 283 mg a day) in patients after a transient ischemic attack or minor ischemic stroke. *N Engl J Med* 1991; **325**:1261–6.

286 Wong KS, Mok V, Lam WWM *et al.* Aspirin-associated intracerebral hemorrhage: clinical and radiologic features. *Neurology* 2000; **54**:2298–301.

287 Saloheimo P, Ahonen M, Juvela S, Pyhtinen J, Savolainen ER, Hillbom M. Regular aspirin-use preceding the onset of primary intracerebral hemorrhage is an independent predictor for death. *Stroke* 2006; **37**:129–33.

288 Brass LM, Lichtman JH, Wang Y, Gurwitz JH, Radford MJ, Krumholz HM. Intracranial hemorrhage associated with thrombolytic therapy for elderly patients with acute myocardial infarction: results from the cooperative cardiovascular project. *Stroke* 2000; **31**:1802–11.

289 Ruiz-Bailen M, Brea-Salvago JF, de Hoyos EA *et al.* Post-thrombolysis intracerebral hemorrhage: data from the Spanish Register ARIAM. *Crit Care Med* 2005; **33**:1829–38.

290 Mehta SR, Eikelboom JW, Yusuf S. Risk of intracranial haemorrhage with bolus versus infusion thrombolytic therapy: a meta-analysis. *Lancet* 2000; **356**:449–54.

291 Barron HV, Rundle AC, Gore JM, Gurwitz JH, Penney J, Natl RM. Intracranial hemorrhage rates and effect of immediate beta-blocker use in patients with acute myocardial infarction treated with tissue plasminogen activator. *Am J Cardiol* 2000; **85**:294–8.

292 McCarron MO, Nicoll JA. Cerebral amyloid angiopathy and thrombolysis-related intracerebral haemorrhage. *Lancet Neurol* 2004; **3**:484–92.

293 Gebel JM, Sila CA, Sloan MA *et al.* Thrombolysis-related intracranial hemorrhage: a radiographic analysis of 244 cases from the GUSTO-1 trial with clinical correlation. *Stroke* 1998; **29**:563–9.

294 Trouillas P, von Kummer R. Classification and pathogenesis of cerebral hemorrhages after thrombolysis in ischemic stroke. *Stroke* 2006; **37**:556–61.

295 Gebel JM, Brott TG, Sila CA *et al.* Decreased perihematomal edema in thrombolysis-related intracerebral hemorrhage compared with spontaneous intracerebral hemorrhage. *Stroke* 2000; **31**:596–600.

296 Mahaffey KW, Granger CB, Sloan MA *et al.* Neurosurgical evacuation of intracranial hemorrhage after thrombolytic therapy for acute myocardial infarction: Experience from the GUSTO-I Trial. *Am Heart J* 1999; **138**:493–9.

297 de Tezanos Pinto M., Fernandez J, Perez Bianco PR. Update of 156 episodes of central nervous system bleeding in hemophiliacs. *Haemostasis* 1992; **22**:259–67.

298 Johansson L, Jansson JH, Stegmayr B, Nilsson TK, Hallmans G, Boman K. Hemostatic factors as risk markers for intracerebral hemorrhage: a prospective incident case-referent study. *Stroke* 2004; **35**:826–30.

299 Andes WA, Wulff K. Intracranial hemorrhage in hemophiliacs with AIDS [letter]. *Thromb Haemost* 1990; **63**:326.

300 Henselmans JML, Meijer K, Haaxma R, Hew J, van der Meer J. Recurrent spontaneous intracerebral hemorrhage in a congenitally afibrinogenemic patient: diagnostic pitfalls and therapeutic options. *Stroke* 1999; **30**:2479–82.

301 Mazzola L, Antoine JC, Camdessanche JP, Barral FG, Reynaud J, Michel D. Brain hemorrhage as a complication of type I cryoglobulinemia vasculopathy. *J Neurol* 2003; **250**:1376–8.

302 Boudouresques G, Hauw JJ, Meininger V *et al.* Étude neuropathologique des hémorragies intra-craniennes de l'adulte. Données génerales a propos de 500 observations. [Neuropathological study of adult intracranial hemorrhage. General data in 500 cases]. *Rev Neurol (Paris)* 1979; **135**:197–210.

303 Thachil JV, Caswell M, Keenan R *et al.* Factor X deficiency presenting as a pseudotumor. Case report. *J Neurosurg* 2006; **104**:202–5.

304 Lorand L, Velasco PT, Hill JM, Hoffmeister KJ, Kaye FJ. Intracranial hemorrhage in systemic lupus erythematosus associated with an autoantibody against factor XIII. *Thromb Haemost* 2002; **88**:919–23.

305 Reiner AP, Schwartz SM, Frank MB *et al.* Polymorphisms of coagulation factor XIII subunit A and risk of nonfatal hemorrhagic stroke in young white women. *Stroke* 2001; **32**:2580–5.

306 Corral J, Iniesta JA, González-Conejero R, Villalón M, Vicente V. Polymorphisms of clotting factors modify the risk for primary intracranial hemorrhage. *Blood* 2001; **97**:2979–82.

307 Dichgans M, Markus HS. Genetic association studies in stroke: methodological issues and proposed standard criteria. *Stroke* 2005; **36**:2027–31.

308 Yamauchi K, Umeda Y. Symptomatic intracranial haemorrhage in acute nonlymphoblastic leukaemia: analysis of CT and autopsy findings. *J Neurol* 1997; **244**:94–100.

309 Arboix A, Oliveres M, Besses C. Sensorimotor stroke due to gangliocapsular hematoma as first manifestation of chronic myelocytic leukemia. *Cerebrovasc Dis* 2000; **10**:81–2.

310 Pomeranz S, Naparstek E, Ashkenazi E *et al.* Intracranial haematomas following bone marrow transplantation. *J Neurol* 1994; **241**:252–6.

311 Wijdicks EFM, Silbert PL, Jack CR, Parisi JE. Subcortical hemorrhage in disseminated intravascular coagulation associated with sepsis. *Am J Neuroradiol* 1994; **15**:763–5.

312 Theilen HJ, Lück C, Hanisch U, Ragaller M. Fatal intracerebral hemorrhage due to leptospirosis. *Infection* 2002; **30**:109–12.

313 Lee MS, Kim WC. Intracranial hemorrhage associated with idiopathic thrombocytopenic purpura: Report of seven patients and a meta-analysis. *Neurology* 1998; **50**:1160–3.

314 Cohen YC, Djulbegovic B, Shamai-Lubovitz O, Mozes B. The bleeding risk and natural history of idiopathic thrombocytopenic purpura in patients with persistent low platelet counts. *Arch Intern Med* 2000; **160**:1630–8.

315 Butros LJ, Bussel JB. Intracranial hemorrhage in immune thrombocytopenic purpura: a retrospective analysis. *J Pediatr Hematol Oncol* 2003; **25**:660–4.

316 Licata B, Turazzi S. Bleeding cerebral neoplasms with symptomatic hematoma. *J Neurosurg Sci* 2003; **47**:201–10.

317 Salem RO, Laposata M. Effects of alcohol on hemostasis. *Am J Clin Pathol* 2005; **123** Suppl:S96–105.

318 Puddey IB, Rakic V, Dimmitt SB, Beilin LJ. Influence of pattern of drinking on cardiovascular disease and cardiovascular risk factors: a review. *Addiction* 1999; **94**:649–63.

319 McEvoy AW, Kitchen ND, Thomas DG. Intracerebral haemorrhage and drug abuse in young adults. *Br J Neurosurg* 2000; **14**:449–54.

320 Brust JC. Vasculitis owing to substance abuse. *Neurol Clin* 1997; **15**:945–57.

321 Shibata S, Mori K, Sekine I, Suyama H. Subarachnoid and intracerebral hemorrhage associated with necrotizing angiitis due to methamphetamine abuse: an autopsy case. *Neurol Med Chir Tokyo* 1991; **31**:49–52.

322 McGee SM, McGee DN, McGee MB. Spontaneous intracerebral hemorrhage related to methamphetamine abuse: autopsy findings and clinical correlation. *Am J Forensic Med Pathol* 2004; **25**:334–7.

323 Levine SR, Brust JC, Futrell N *et al.* A comparative study of the cerebrovascular complications of cocaine: alkaloidal versus hydrochloride: a review. *Neurology* 1991; **41**:1173–7.

324 Qureshi AI, Mohammad Y, Suri MF *et al.* Cocaine use and hypertension are major risk factors for intracerebral hemorrhage in young African Americans. *Ethn Dis* 2001; **11**:311–19.

325 Green RM, Kelly KM, Gabrielsen T, Levine SR, Vanderzant C. Multiple intracerebral hemorrhages after smoking 'crack' cocaine. *Stroke* 1990; **21**:957–62.

326 Peterson PL, Roszler M, Jacobs I, Wilner HI. Neurovascular complications of cocaine abuse. *J Neuropsychiatry Clin Neurosci* 1991; **3**:143–9.

327 Aggarwal SK, Williams V, Levine SR, Cassin BJ, Garcia JH. Cocaine-associated intracranial hemorrhage: Absence of vasculitis in 14 cases. *Neurology* 1996; **46**:1741–3.

328 Nolte KB, Brass LM, Fletterick CF. Intracranial hemorrhage associated with cocaine abuse: A prospective autopsy study. *Neurology* 1996; **46**:1291–6.

329 Kibayashi K, Mastri AR, Hirsch CS. Cocaine induced intracerebral hemorrhage: Analysis of predisposing factors and mechanisms causing hemorrhagic strokes. *Hum Pathol* 1995; **26**:659–63.

330 Krendel DA, Ditter SM, Frankel MR, Ross WK. Biopsy-proven cerebral vasculitis associated with cocaine abuse. *Neurology* 1990; **40**:1092–4.

331 Bruno A, Nolte KB, Chapin J. Stroke associated with ephedrine use. *Neurology* 1993; **43**:1313–16.

332 Cartwright MS, Reynolds PS. Intracerebral hemorrhage associated with over-the-counter inhaled epinephrine. *Cerebrovasc Dis* 2005; **19**:415–16.

333 Comabella M, Alvarez-Sabin J, Rovira A, Codina A. Bromocriptine and postpartum cerebral angiopathy: a causal relationship? *Neurology* 1996; **46**:1754–6.

334 Rob JK, Park KS. Postpartum cerebral angiopathy with intracerebral hemorrhage in a patient receiving lisuride. *Neurology* 1998; **50**:1152–4.

335 Hankey GJ. Isolated angiitis/angiopathy of the central nervous sytem. *Cerebrovasc Dis* 1991; **1**:2–15.

336 MacLaren K, Gillespie J, Shrestha S, Neary D, Ballardie FW. Primary angiitis of the central nervous system: emerging variants. *QJM* 2005; **98**:643–54.

337 Biller J, Loftus CM, Moore SA, Schelper RL, Danks KR, Cornell SH. Isolated central nervous system angiitis first presenting as spontaneous intracranial hemorrhage. *Neurosurgery* 1987; **20**:310–15.

338 Hunn M, Robinson S, Wakefield L, Mossman S, Abernethy D. Granulomatous angiitis of the CNS causing spontaneous intracerebral haemorrhage: the importance of leptomeningeal biopsy. *J Neurol Neurosurg Psychiatry* 1998; **65**:956–7.

339 Ay H, Sahin G, Saatci I, Soylemezoglu F, Saribas O. Primary angiitis of the central nervous system and silent cortical hemorrhages. *Am J Neuroradiol* 2002; **23**:1561–3.

340 Clifford Jones RE, Love S, Gurusinghe N. Granulomatous angiitis of the central nervous system: a case with recurrent intracerebral haemorrhage. *J Neurol Neurosurg Psychiatry* 1985; **48**:1054–6.

341 Nishikawa M, Sakamoto H, Katsuyama J, Hakuba A, Nishimura S. Multiple appearing and vanishing aneurysms: primary angiitis of the central nervous system: case report. *J Neurosurg* 1998; **88**:133–7.

342 Kastenbauer S, Pfister HW. Pneumococcal meningitis in adults: spectrum of complications and prognostic factors in a series of 87 cases. *Brain* 2003; **126**:1015–25.

343 Nardone R, Lochner P, Tezzon F. Wegener's granulomatosis presenting with intracerebral hemorrhages. *Cerebrovasc Dis* 2004; **17**:81–2.

344 Memet B, Rudinskaya A, Krebs T, Oelberg D. Wegener granulomatosis with massive intracerebral hemorrhage: remission of disease in response to rituximab. *J Clin Rheumatol* 2005; **11**:314–18.

345 Granziera C, Michel P, Rossetti AO, Lurati F, Reymond S, Bogousslavsky J. Wegener granulomatosis presenting with haemorrhagic stroke in a young adult. *J Neurol* 2005; **252**:615–16.

346 Smith D, Lucas S, Jacewicz M. Multiple cerebral hemorrhages in HTLV-I-associated myelopathy. *Neurology* 1993; **43**:412–14.

347 Lipton SA, Schaefer PW, Adams RD, Ma MJ. A 37-year-old man with AIDS, neurologic deterioration, and multiple hemorrhagic cerebral lesions: Varicella-zoster leukoencephalitis with hemorrhage and large-vessel vasculopathy – acquired immunodeficiency syndrome. *N Engl J Med* 1996; **335**:1587–95.

348 DeJong RN. Delayed traumatic intracerebral hemorrhage. *Arch Neurol Psych* 1942; **48**:257–66.

349 Bollinger O. *Über traumatische Spät-Apoplexie: ein Beitrag zur Lehre von der Hirnerschütterung. Festschrift, Rudolf Virchow gewidmet zur Vollendung seines 70en Lebensjahres.* Berlin: A. Hirschwald, 1891, pp. 457–70.

350 Oertel M, Kelly DF, McArthur D *et al.* Progressive hemorrhage after head trauma: predictors and consequences of the evolving injury. *J Neurosurg* 2002; **96**:109–16.

351 Li J, Brown J, Levine M. Mild head injury, anticoagulants, and risk of intracranial injury. *Lancet* 2001; **357**:771–2.

352 Alvarez-Sabín J, Turon A, Lozano-Sánchez M, Vázquez J, Codina A. Delayed posttraumatic hemorrhage: 'Spät-apoplexie'. *Stroke* 1995; **26**:1531–5.

353 Ruíz-Sandoval JL, Cantu C, Barinagarrementeria F. Intracerebral hemorrhage in young people: analysis of risk factors, location, causes, and prognosis. *Stroke* 1999; **30**:537–41.

354 Gras P, Arveux P, Giroud M *et al.* [Spontaneous intracerebral hemorrhages in young patients. Study of 33 cases] Les hémorragies intracérébrales spontanées du sujet jeune. Étude de 33 cas. *Rev Neurol (Paris)* 1991; **147**:653–7.

355 Wakai S, Kumakura N, Nagai M. Lobar intracerebral hemorrhage. A clinical, radiographic, and pathological study of 29 consecutive operated cases with negative angiography. *J Neurosurg* 1992; **76**:231–8.

356 Passero S, Rocchi R, Rossi S, Ulivelli M, Vatti G. Seizures after spontaneous supratentorial intracerebral hemorrhage. *Epilepsia* 2002; **43**:1175–80.

357 Heye N, Hankey GJ. Amphetamine-associated stroke. *Cerebrovasc Dis* 1996; **6**:149–55.

358 McCarron MO, Alberts MJ, McCarron P. A systematic review of Terson's syndrome: frequency and prognosis after subarachnoid haemorrhage. *J Neurol Neurosurg Psychiatry* 2004; **75**:491–3.

359 Jensen MB, St Louis EK. Management of acute cerebellar stroke. *Arch Neurol* 2005; **62**:537–44.

360 Gunatilake SB. Rapid resolution of symptoms and signs of intracerebral haemorrhage. *Br Med J* 1998; **316**:1495–6.

361 Evyapan D, Kumral E. Cerebral hemorrhage with transient signs. *Cerebrovasc Dis* 2000; **10**:483–4.

362 Chung CS, Caplan LR, Han WC, Pessin MS, Lee KH, Kim JM. Thalamic haemorrhage. *Brain* 1996; **119**:1873–86.

363 Karnath HO, Johannsen L, Broetz D, Kuker W. Posterior thalamic hemorrhage induces 'pusher syndrome'. *Neurology* 2005; **64**:1014–19.

364 Liliang PC, Liang CL, Lu CH *et al.* Hypertensive caudate hemorrhage prognostic predictor, outcome, and role of external ventricular drainage. *Stroke* 2001; **32**:1195–200.

365 Murata Y, Yamaguchi S, Kajikawa H, Yamamura K, Sumioka S, Nakamura S. Relationship between the clinical manifestations, computed tomographic findings and the outcome in 80 patients with primary pontine hemorrhage. *J Neurol Sci* 1999; **167**:107–11.

366 Wijdicks EFM, St Louis E. Clinical profiles predictive of outcome in pontine hemorrhage. *Neurology* 1997; **49**:1342–6.

367 Schutz H, Bodeker RH, Damian M, Krack P, Dorndorf W. Age-related spontaneous intracerebral hematoma in a German community. *Stroke* 1990; **21**:1412–18.

368 Kase CS, Mohr JP, Caplan LR. Intracerebral hemorrhage. In: Barnett HJM, Mohr JP, Stein BM, Yatsu FM, eds. *Stroke: pathophysiology, diagnosis, and management.* New York: Churchill Livingstone, 1998, pp. 649–700.

369 Suzuki S, Kelley RE, Dandapani BK, Reyes Iglesias Y, Dietrich WD, Duncan RC. Acute leukocyte and temperature response in hypertensive intracerebral hemorrhage. *Stroke* 1995; **26**:1020–3.

370 Packard AS, Kase CS, Aly AS, Barest GD. 'Computed tomography-negative' intracerebral hemorrhage: case report and implications for management. *Arch Neurol* 2003; **60**:1156–9.

371 Roos YB, Hasan D, Vermeulen M. Outcome in patients with large intraventricular haemorrhages: A volumetric study. *J Neurol Neurosurg Psychiatry* 1995; **58**:622–4.

372 Tuhrim S, Horowitz DR, Sacher M, Godbold JH. Volume of ventricular blood is an important determinant of outcome in supratentorial intracerebral hemorrhage. *Crit Care Med* 1999; **27**:617–21.

373 Aoki S, Sasaki Y, Machida T *et al.* 3D-CT angiography of cerebral arteriovenous malformations. *Radiat Med* 1998; **16**:263–71.

374 Fiebach JB, Schellinger PD, Gass A *et al.* Stroke magnetic resonance imaging is accurate in hyperacute intracerebral hemorrhage: a multicenter study on the validity of stroke imaging. *Stroke* 2004; **35**:502–6.

375 Oppenheim C, Touze E, Hernalsteen D *et al.* Comparison of five MR sequences for the detection of acute intracranial hemorrhage. *Cerebrovasc Dis* 2005; **20**:388–94.

376 Lovblad KO, Schneider J, Bassetti C *et al.* Fast contrast-enhanced MR whole-brain venography. *Neuroradiology* 2002; **44**:681–8.

377 Isensee C, Reul J, Thron A. Magnetic resonance imaging of thrombosed dural sinuses. *Stroke* 1994; **25**:29–34.

378 Dormont D, Anxionnat R, Evrard S, Louaille C, Chiras J, Marsault C. MRI in cerebral venous thrombosis. *J Neuroradiol* 1994; **21**:81–99.

379 Idbaih A, Boukobza M, Crassard I, Porcher R, Bousser MG, Chabriat H. MRI of clot in cerebral venous thrombosis: high diagnostic value of susceptibility-weighted images. *Stroke* 2006; **37**:991–5.

380 Aoki S, Yoshikawa T, Hori M *et al.* MR digital subtraction angiography for the assessment of cranial arteriovenous malformations and fistulas. *Am J Roentgenol* 2000; **175**:451–3.

381 Griffiths PD, Hoggard N, Warren DJ, Wilkinson ID, Anderson B, Romanowski CA. Brain arteriovenous malformations: assessment with dynamic MR digital subtraction angiography. *Am J Neuroradiol* 2000; **21**:1892–9.

382 Hankey GJ, Warlow CP, Sellar RJ. Cerebral angiographic risk in mild cerebrovascular disease. *Stroke* 1990; **21**:209–22.

383 Cloft HJ, Joseph GJ, Dion JE. Risk of cerebral angiography in patients with subarachnoid hemorrhage, cerebral aneurysm, and arteriovenous malformation: a meta-analysis. *Stroke* 1999; **30**:317–20.

384 Halpin SF, Britton JA, Byrne JV, Clifton A, Hart G, Moore A. Prospective evaluation of cerebral angiography and computed tomography in cerebral haematoma. *J Neurol Neurosurg Psychiatry* 1994; **57**:1180–6.

385 Zhu XL, Chan MS, Poon WS. Spontaneous intracranial hemorrhage: Which patients need diagnostic cerebral

angiography? A prospective study of 206 cases and review of the literature. *Stroke* 1997; **28**:1406–9.

386 Velthuis BK, Rinkel GJE, Ramos LMP *et al.* Subarachnoid hemorrhage: Aneurysm detection and preoperative evaluation with CT angiography. *Radiology* 1998; **208**:423–30.

387 Willinsky RA, Fitzgerald M, Terbrugge K, Montanera W, Wallace M. Delayed angiography in the investigation of intracerebral hematomas caused by small arteriovenous malformations. *Neuroradiology* 1993; **35**:307–11.

388 Hino A, Fujimoto M, Yamaki T, Iwamoto Y, Katsumori T. Value of repeat angiography in patients with spontaneous subcortical hemorrhage. *Stroke* 1998; **29**:2517–21.

389 Gonugunta V, Buxton N. Warfarin and chronic subdural haematomas. *Br J Neurosurg* 2001; **15**:514–17.

390 Albanese A, Tuttolomondo A, Anile C *et al.* Spontaneous chronic subdural hematomas in young adults with a deficiency in coagulation factor XIII. Report of three cases. *J Neurosurg* 2005; **102**:1130–2.

391 Lin WC, Lirng JF, Fuh JL *et al.* MR findings of spontaneous intracranial hypotension. *Acta Radiol* 2002; **43**:249–55.

392 Whiteley W, Al-Shahi R, Myles L, Lueck CJ. Spontaneous intracranial hypotension causing confusion and coma: a headache for the neurologist and the neurosurgeon. *Br J Neurosurg* 2003; **17**:456–8.

393 Mizuno J, Mummaneni PV, Rodts GE, Barrow DL. Recurrent subdural hematoma caused by cerebrospinal fluid leakage. Case report. *J Neurosurg Spine* 2006; **4**:183–5.

394 Depreitere B, Van CF, van LJ. A clinical comparison of non-traumatic acute subdural haematomas either related to coagulopathy or of arterial origin without coagulopathy. *Acta Neurochir (Wien)* 2003; **145**:541–6.

395 Hori E, Ogiichi T, Hayashi N, Kuwayama N, Endo S. Case report: acute subdural hematoma due to angiographically unvisualized ruptured aneurysm. *Surg Neurol* 2005; **64**:144–6.

396 Matsuyama T, Shimomura T, Okumura Y, Sakaki T. Acute subdural hematomas due to rupture of cortical arteries: a study of the points of rupture in 19 cases. *Surg Neurol* 1997; **47**:423–7.

397 Yasui T, Komiyama M, Kishi H *et al.* Angiographic extravasation of contrast medium in acute 'spontaneous' subdural hematoma. *Surg Neurol* 1995; **43**:61–7.

398 Marinelli L, Parodi RC, Renzetti P, Bandini F. Interhemispheric subdural haematoma from ruptured aneurysm. A case report. *J Neurol* 2005; **252**:364–6.

399 Pal D, Gnanalingham K, Peterson D. A case of spontaneous acute subdural haematoma in the posterior fossa following anticoagulation. *Br J Neurosurg* 2004; **18**:68–9.

400 Stein RW, Kase CS, Hier DB *et al.* Caudate hemorrhage. *Neurology* 1984; **34**:1549–54.

401 Alves OL, Gomes O. Cocaine-related acute subdural hematoma: an emergent cause of cerebrovascular accident. *Acta Neurochir (Wien)* 2000; **142**:819–21.

402 Nonaka Y, Kusumoto M, Mori K, Maeda M. Pure acute subdural haematoma without subarachnoid haemorrhage caused by rupture of internal carotid artery aneurysm. *Acta Neurochir (Wien)* 2000; **142**:941–4.

403 Koerbel A, Ernemann U, Freudenstein D. Acute subdural haematoma without subarachnoid haemorrhage caused by rupture of an internal carotid artery bifurcation aneurysm: case report and review of literature. *Br J Radiol* 2005; **78**:646–50.

404 Oikawa A, Aoki N, Sakai T. Arteriovenous malformation presenting as acute subdural haematoma. *Neurol Res* 1993; **15**:353–5.

405 McLaughlin MR, Jho HD, Kwon Y. Acute subdural hematoma caused by a ruptured giant intracavernous aneurysm: Case report. *Neurosurgery* 1996; **38**:388–91.

406 Korosue K, Kondoh T, Ishikawa Y, Nagao T, Tamaki N, Matsumoto S. Acute subdural hematoma associated with nontraumatic middle meningeal artery aneurysm: case report. *Neurosurgery* 1988; **22**:411–13.

407 Oppenheim JS, Gennuso R, Sacher M, Hollis P. Acute atraumatic subdural hematoma associated with moyamoya disease in an African-American. *Neurosurgery* 1991; **28**:616–18.

408 Uglietta JP, O'Connor CM, Boyko OB, Aldrich H, Massey EW, Heinz ER. CT patterns of intracranial hemorrhage complicating thrombolytic therapy for acute myocardial infarction. *Radiology* 1991; **181**:555–9.

409 Bonnaud I, Saudeau D, de TB, Autret A. Recurrence of spontaneous subdural haematoma revealing acquired haemophilia. *Eur Neurol* 2003; **49**:253–4.

410 Fujimaki H, Saito N, Tosaka M, Tanaka Y, Horiguchi K, Sasaki T. Cerebrospinal fluid leak demonstrated by three-dimensional computed tomographic myelography in patients with spontaneous intracranial hypotension. *Surg Neurol* 2002; **58**:280–4.

411 Vos PE, de Boer WA, Wurzer JA, van Gijn J. Subdural hematoma after lumbar puncture: two case reports and review of the literature. *Clin Neurol Neurosurg* 1991; **93**:127–32.

412 De Noronha RJ, Sharrack B, Hadjivassiliou M, Romanowski CA. Subdural haematoma: a potentially serious consequence of spontaneous intracranial hypotension. *J Neurol Neurosurg Psychiatry* 2003; **74**:752–5.

413 Wessling H, de las Heras P. Spontaneous acute subdural haematoma caused by tension pneumocephalus. *Acta Neurochir (Wien)* 2005; **147**:89–92.

414 Donaldson JW, Edwards-Brown M, Luerssen TG. Arachnoid cyst rupture with concurrent subdural hygroma. *Pediatr Neurosurg* 2000; **32**:137–9.

415 Maiuri F, Iaconetta G, Sardo L, Briganti F. Dural arteriovenous malformation associated with recurrent subdural haematoma and intracranial hypertension. *Br J Neurosurg* 2001; **15**:273–6.

416 Caputi F, Lamaida E, Gazzeri R. Acute subdural hematoma and pachymeningitis carcinomatosa: case report. *Rev Neurol (Paris)* 1999; **155**:383–5.

417 Wijdicks EFM, Torres VE, Schievink WI. Chronic subdural hematoma in autosomal dominant polycystic kidney disease. *Am J Kidney Dis* 2000; **35**:40–3.

418 Holthouse D, Wong G. Chronic subdural hematoma in a 50-year-old man with polycystic kidney disease. *Am J Kidney Dis* 2001; **38**:E6.

9 What caused this subarachnoid haemorrhage?

9.1 Causes of spontaneous subarachnoid haemorrhage

Spontaneous (i.e. non-traumatic) subarachnoid haemorrhage (SAH) is a serious disorder that occurs in relatively young patients and has a poor prognosis. If the 15% of patients who die before reaching hospital are taken into account, the case fatality of aneurysmal SAH is around 50%, while another 20% remain dependent in activities of daily living.[1] SAH accounts for around 5% of all strokes. In most populations the incidence is around 9 per 100 000 per year, but in Finland and Japan the incidence is twice as high.[2] The incidence increases with age, but half the patients are younger than 55 years at the time of the SAH.[2] Because of the young age at which SAH occurs and the poor prognosis, the loss of productive life years from SAH in the population is as large as that from ischaemic stroke.[3] Although advances have been made in the treatment of patients with SAH (Chapter 14), the case fatality has only slightly decreased[1,4]. The main reason for this slow progress is that only a proportion of patients reach centres which specialize in treating SAH (Fig. 9.1).

Rupture of a saccular aneurysm at the base of the brain is not the cause in every patient with an SAH, but it is in approximately 85%. About 10% of patients have a so-called perimesencephalic haemorrhage, the cause of which is unknown (section 9.1.2). The rest are due to intracranial arterial dissections (section 9.1.3) or a variety

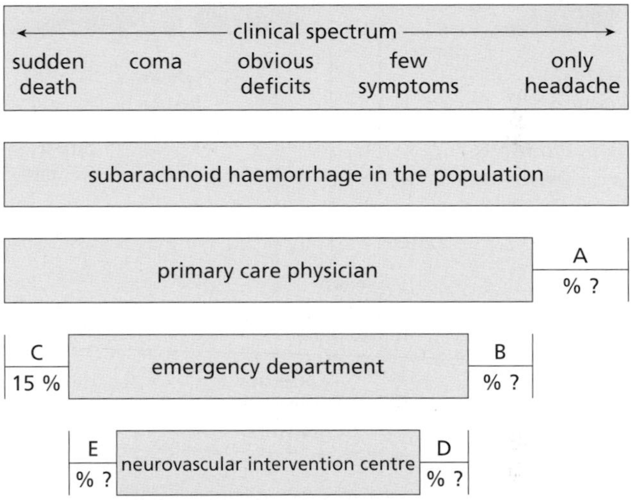

Fig. 9.1 Clinical spectrum of aneurysmal subarachnoid haemorrhage and reasons for failing to reach a neurovascular intervention centre where specialized treatment can be applied. A: some patients with only headache do not consult their primary care physician. B: in some patients the primary care physician does not recognize the cause of the headache or other symptoms. C: 15% of patients die suddenly or before reaching hospital. D: in some patients the emergency physician does not recognize the cause of the headache or other symptoms. E: some patients die before reaching the specialist centre.

of even rarer conditions (section 9.1.4). But, whatever the cause, in the vast majority of patients there is haemorrhage in the basal cisterns (Fig. 9.2).

> Subarachnoid haemorrhage is not synonymous with a ruptured aneurysm. About 85% of all spontaneous subarachnoid haemorrhages are caused by rupture of an intracranial saccular aneurysm, 10% by non-aneurysmal perimesencephalic haemorrhage, and 5% by rarities.

Stroke: practical management, 3rd edition. C. Warlow, J. van Gijn, M. Dennis, J. Wardlaw, J. Bamford, G. Hankey, P. Sandercock, G. Rinkel, P. Langhorne, C. Sudlow and P. Rothwell. Published 2008 Blackwell Publishing. ISBN 978-1-4051-2766-0.

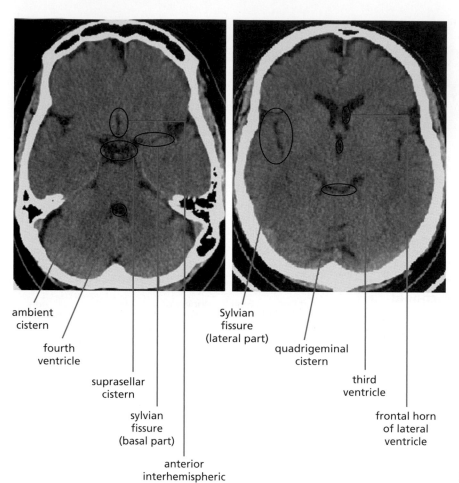

ambient
cistern

fourth
ventricle

suprasellar
cistern

sylvian
fissure
(basal part)

anterior
interhemispheric
fissure

Sylvian
fissure
(lateral part)

quadrigeminal
cistern

third
ventricle

frontal horn
of lateral
ventricle

Fig. 9.2 CT brain showing the basal
cisterns.

The presenting features of patients with all these different causes are usually indistinguishable: a severe headache of sudden onset, a depressed level of consciousness, or both; sometimes there are focal deficits or cranial nerve palsies (section 9.3.6). The exception is perimesencephalic non-aneurysmal haemorrhage, where explosive headache is usually the only symptom at onset. In the following sections on the pathological and pathophysiological background of all these causes, we will occasionally run ahead of the story by mentioning the findings on CT scanning, because this technique, as an early adjunct to the history and examination, provides an *in vivo* picture of the pathology.

9.1.1 Intracranial saccular aneurysms

Aneurysms of the cerebral vessels are not congenital but develop during the course of life, usually after the second decade.[5] In the exceptional case of childhood aneurysms, there is often an underlying cause such as trauma, infection or connective tissue disorder (Table 9.1).[6–10] The absolute frequencies of intracranial

aneurysms in adults to some degree depend on whether fatal cases of SAH have been included, on the definition of the minimal size for a lesion to be called an aneurysm, and finally on the diligence with which the search for unruptured aneurysms has been performed. In our systematic review of studies reporting the prevalence of all intracranial aneurysms in patients studied for reasons other than SAH, the best estimate of the frequency for an average adult without specific risk factors was 2.3% (95% confidence interval, 1.7–3.1%); this proportion tended to increase with age.[5]

> Intracranial aneurysms are not congenital but generally develop during life.

Saccular aneurysms arise at sites of arterial branching, usually at the base of the brain, either on the circle of Willis itself or at a nearby branching point (Fig. 9.3). The exact reason why aneurysms develop is unknown. In the search for answers attention has been paid to (ultra) structural abnormalities, familial intracranial aneurysms, conditions predisposing to intracranial aneurysms such

Table 9.1 Hereditary and congenital conditions associated with saccular aneurysms.

Disorders of connective tissue
- Ehlers-Danlos syndrome type IV[30,347]
- Autosomal dominant polycystic kidney disease*[5,11,27,28]
- (Infantile) fibromuscular dysplasia[348,349]

Disorders of angiogenesis
- Hereditary haemorrhagic telangiectasia (section 8.2.7)[350]
- Progressive hemifacial atrophy (Parry-Romberg syndrome)[351]

Associated hypertension
- Congenital heart disease[352]
- Coarctation of the aorta[353]
- Aortitis syndrome[354]

Local haemodynamic stress
- Anomalies of the circle of Willis;[355] these occur more often in women[356]
- Arteriovenous malformations (section 9.1.4)
- Moyamoya syndrome[357] (section 7.5)

*In polycystic kidney disease, hypertension may contribute to the formation of intracranial aneurysms, but aneurysms do occur in patients who have no hypertension.
Note: In the following conditions a relationship with cerebral aneurysms has been assumed in the past but subsequently questioned: neurofibromatosis type 1,[358] Marfan's syndrome,[359,360] and pseudoxanthoma elasticum.[361]

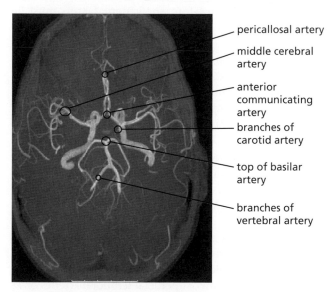

pericallosal artery

middle cerebral artery

anterior communicating artery

branches of carotid artery

top of basilar artery

branches of vertebral artery

Fig. 9.3 MR angiogram of the circle of Willis, showing the sites were aneurysms are usually found.

as autosomal dominant polycystic kidney disease and Ehlers-Danlos type IV, genetic abnormalities at the chromosomal or molecular level, the development of new aneurysms after a first episode of SAH, and finally to the important issue of acquired risk factors. In terms of attributable risk, the modifiable risk factors – alcohol, smoking and hypertension – account for about half of first SAH episodes, genetic factors for only about one-tenth.[11] In patients with multiple aneurysms a predominance of genetic factors is suggested by the fact that these patients are younger at the time of rupture than patients with SAH and a single aneurysm.[12] Other factors that have been linked with multiple aneurysms are female gender, smoking and hypertension.[13–15]

Structural abnormalities in the vessel wall

It is unknown why only some adults develop aneurysms at arterial bifurcations while most do not, except in specific, mostly genetically determined, conditions (Table 9.1). The once popular notion of a congenital gap in the muscle layer of the wall (tunica media), through which the inner layers of the arterial wall could bulge, has been largely dispelled. Defects in the muscle layer of intracranial arteries are equally common in patients with and without aneurysms, and are usually strengthened by densely packed collagen fibrils.[16–18]

Studies at the ultrastructural level have however shown definite abnormalities.[19] The proteins of the extracellular matrix that are decreased in the intracranial arterial wall of many ruptured aneurysms, in skin biopsies, and in intracranial and extracranial arteries of patients with aneurysms are collagen type III, collagen type IV and elastin fibres. Therefore, because the disruption of the extracellular matrix proteins has been found not only in aneurysms but also in skin and unaffected intracranial and extracranial arteries, intracranial aneurysms might not represent a localized disease but rather a more general disorder of the extracellular matrix. This decrease in extracellular matrix proteins might be explained by disrupted synthesis. On the other hand, there is constant degradation and synthesis of the constituents of the extracellular matrix regulated by a range of proteases (matrix metalloproteinases, neutrophil or leucocyte elastase) and their inhibitors (tissue inhibitor of matrix metalloproteinases and α1 antitrypsin), growth factors and cytokines. Accelerated protein degradation may, therefore, also be caused by an imbalance between these proteases and protease inhibitors.[19]

Familial occurrence of aneurysms

Around 10% of patients with SAH have one or more affected parents, siblings or children, i.e. first-degree relatives.[20,21] In familial SAH, aneurysms are more often large and multiple than in patients with sporadic SAH.[22] But, because familial SAH constitutes only 10% of all cases of SAH, in practice more large and multiple aneurysms are associated with sporadic rather than with familial SAH. Patients with familial SAH are in general younger than those with sporadic SAH, and in families with two generations affected the age at onset in the younger generation is earlier than in the older generation.[22,23]

Some degree of familial clustering also occurs in so-called sporadic SAH. The risk of SAH in first-degree relatives of index patients with SAH is approximately five times higher than in the general population.[20,24,25] Undoubtedly this familial clustering can to some extent be explained by shared classical (acquired) vascular risk factors, which are associated with ruptured aneurysms (see below). Nevertheless, classical risk factors such as hypertension explain only part of the familial aggregation.[24]

Autosomal dominant polycystic kidney disease

In patients with autosomal dominant polycystic kidney disease (ADPKD) intracranial aneurysms are found in approximately 10%.[5] But, although SAH frequently occurs in patients with ADPKD,[27] the relative rarity of ADPKD is the reason why the proportion of patients with ADPKD in series of patients with SAH is less than 1%.[11,27] Hypertension is not a necessary factor for the development of aneurysms in patients with ADPKD.[27] In 85% of the patients the gene responsible for the disease is on chromosome 16p (PKD1) and in the remaining 15% it is in most cases on chromosome 4q (PKD2). Most aneurysms are found in PKD1 patients and the position of the mutation predicts the development of intracranial aneurysms.[29]

Ehlers-Danlos disease type IV

Ehlers-Danlos disease is frequently mentioned as an important association with intracranial aneurysms, but given its rarity it too is a very infrequent cause of SAH. In our own database, which now includes over 2000 consecutive patients with SAH, we have only one patient on record who later proved to have Ehlers-Danlos disease. Ehlers-Danlos type IV is especially associated with arterial dissection and aneurysms of large and medium-sized arteries, including intracranial arteries. Intracranial aneurysms can be either saccular or fusiform. In a survey of 131 patients who had died from Ehlers-Danlos type IV, 7% did so from an SAH.[30] Patients with Ehlers-Danlos type IV have a defect in collagen type III. This association between a defect in collagen type III and aneurysms has prompted interest in the association between patients with aneurysms and collagen type III in general; however, in a consecutive series of patients only a minority showed reduced production of collagen type III, and there was no defect in the collagen type III gene.[31]

Genetic studies

CANDIDATE GENES

So far, in intracranial aneurysms, there have only been association studies of functional and positional candidate genes, those involved in maintaining the integrity of the extracellular matrix being proposed as the most likely candidates.[32] So far positive associations have been found for the genes of collagen type III-A1 (a single small study), collagen type I-A2, α1 antitrypsin and – more recently – for member 3 of clade A of serine proteinase inhibitors (SERPINA3, known previously as alpha-1-antichymotrypsin),[33] whereas results have been negative or conflicting for lysyl oxidase, fibrillin 2, different metalloproteinases, inhibitors of metalloproteinases, endoglin, angiotensin converting enzyme, NADPH oxidase, P22PHOX and phospholipase C.

LINKAGE STUDIES

Linkage studies can establish whether there is co-segregation of a disease phenotype with DNA markers of known location, dispersed throughout the genome, in families with the disease. This type of study mainly detects genetic factors with large effects. Fine mapping is not possible and, therefore, the genetic factors must lie in large regions of several hundreds of genes. Also, the mode of inheritance needs to be defined, except with affected sibling-pair analysis, but given the high case fatality in SAH that type of analysis is rarely possible. So far six linkage regions have been identified:[19] 7q11 (in more than one study; it includes the candidate gene for collagen type I-A2), 14q22, 19q13.3, 5q22–q31 (which region includes the candidate genes for lysyl oxidase and fibrillin 2), 2p13 and 1p34.3–p36.13 (possible candidate genes in this region include polycystic kidney disease-like 1, fibronectin type III domain-containing gene, and collagen type XVI-A2).

GENE EXPRESSION STUDIES

To date, the expression of a selection of genes has been analysed in samples of 24 ruptured and unruptured intracranial aneurysms, superficial temporal arteries of 43 intracranial aneurysm patients, and 19 control patients without intracranial aneurysms.[34] Concentrations of prostacyclin-stimulating factor and the protein RAI, both implicated in the process of tissue repair, were lower in those with ruptured intracranial aneurysms than in superficial temporal arteries of patients with intracranial aneurysms. Furthermore, there was a decrease of collagen-type-III expression.

New aneurysms after SAH

Because aneurysms develop during life, patients who have survived an SAH and in whom all aneurysms have been treated may still be at risk of developing new aneurysms and new episodes of SAH. Indeed, in the first 10 years after SAH the chance of finding a new aneurysm on screening is 16%.[35] Moreover, in the first 10 years after an SAH with successful clipping of the detected aneurysms, the risk of a recurrent SAH is 2–3%, about 20 times higher than expected in a population of comparable age and sex.[36,37] Besides this relatively high risk of recurrent SAH, patients who have survived an SAH may also be at increased risk of vascular diseases in general. In a Finnish study, those who had made a good recovery from an SAH had a twofold risk of dying from cerebrovascular or cardiovascular disorders compared with the general population.[37]

Acquired risk factors

A recent systematic review included much new information that has become available over the last few years.[37] The analysis included only studies in the English language that gave crude data (actual numbers of those exposed or non-exposed), and studies in which the diagnosis of SAH had been confirmed by CT angiography or postmortem in at least 70% of patients. Given these constraints, it contained 14 longitudinal and 23 case–control studies. Statistically significant risk factors were:
- current smoking (risk ratio [RR] 2.2 [95% CI 1.3–3.6]);
- hypertension (RR 2.5 [2.0–3.1]); and
- excessive alcohol intake (RR 2.1 [1.5–2.8]).

Non-white ethnicity was a less robust risk factor (RR 1.8 [0.8–4.2]). Oral contraceptives did not definitely affect the risk (RR 5.4 [0.7–43.5]). Lower risks were found for hormone replacement therapy (RR 0.6 [0.2–1.5]), hypercholesterolaemia (RR 0.8 [0.6–1.2]) and – surprisingly – diabetes (RR 0.3 [0–2.2]). Data were inconsistent for lean body mass index (RR 0.3 [0.2–0.4]) and rigorous exercise (RR 0.5 [0.3–1.0]).

Seasonal variation in the occurrence of SAH is found in some studies but not in most. There is clear variation, with lower rates of rupture during the night than during waking hours.[40,41] This variation suggests that activity is a risk factor for aneurysmal rupture, but does not prove it because only time of onset was recorded, not the activities preceding onset.

Some vascular malformations may predispose to the formation of aneurysms, especially arteriovenous malformations (AVMs) (section 9.1.4) and cerebellar haemangioblastoma,[42] but in these cases the aneurysm is seldom in one of the common locations at or near the circle of Willis, but rather on an artery closely related to the AVM or angioma.

Iatrogenic causes include:
- radiation therapy[43–46] (section 7.12);
- acrylate applied externally to an intracranial artery for microvascular decompression;[47]
- superficial temporal artery–middle cerebral artery bypass surgery, with the aneurysm forming at the site of the anastomosis.[48,49]

Triggers for aneurysm rupture

SAH from an aneurysm is the end result of the development and finally rupture of an aneurysm but little is known about what actually precipitates the rupture. A plausible factor is a sudden increase in arterial pressure. If this does play an important role, factors that increase it may be associated with the onset of SAH.

A few studies have collected data on the activities immediately preceding the onset of SAH:
- physical exertion preceding the haemorrhage was found in 2–20% of patients;[50–52]
- sexual intercourse in 0–11%;[48,50–52]
- activities with a Valsalva manoeuvre in 4–20%;[50,53,54]
- stress in 1–2%.[50,53]

Because none of these studies accounted for the usual frequency of these factors in everyday life, it is uncertain whether they actually increase the risk of aneurysm rupture or not.

In a case–control study, the risk of SAH was increased by smoking in the 3 h before the onset of SAH with never smokers as the reference group (OR 7.0; 95% CI 3.7–13.1) and by drinking more than 5 units of alcohol in the 24 h before the onset with teetotallers as reference (OR 4.3; 95% CI 1.5–12.3).[55] In a study where vigorous activity preceding the SAH occurred in 3% of patients, it increased the risk of SAH, in comparison with episodes without vigorous activity in the same patient (RR 15.0; 95% CI 4.3–52.2).[51] In another study with a case-crossover design, moderate to extreme exertion in the 2 h before SAH, which occurred in 19% of patients, also increased the risk, but to a lesser extent (RR 2.7; 95% CI 1.6–4.6).[52]

9.1.2 Non-aneurysmal perimesencephalic haemorrhage

In this radiologically distinct and strikingly harmless variety of SAH, the extravasated blood is confined to the cisterns around the midbrain.[56–58] This disease entity is entirely defined by the characteristic distribution of the

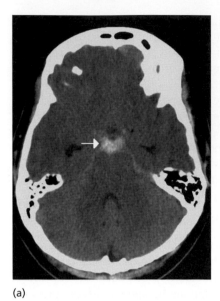

(a)

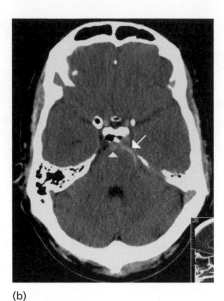

(b)

Fig. 9.4 (a) Typical example on CT scan of a perimesencephalic haemorrhage with blood adjacent to the brainstem in the suprasellar cistern (*arrow*). (b) Another example of a perimesencephalic haemorrhage on CT scan with blood in front of the pons (*arrowhead*) and in the left ambient cistern (*arrow*).

extravasated blood on brain CT, in combination with a normal angiographic study. The densest collection of extravasated blood is mostly immediately anterior to the midbrain, in the interpeduncular cistern (Fig. 9.4). In some patients, most or even the only evidence of blood is found in the quadrigeminal cistern,[59–61] or anterior to the pons.[62,63] There is no extension of the haemorrhage to the lateral sylvian fissures or to the anterior part of the interhemispheric fissure. Some sedimentation of blood in the posterior horns of the lateral ventricles may occur, but frank intraventricular haemorrhage or extension of the haemorrhage into the brain parenchyma rules out this particular condition.[56–58] However, the pattern of bleeding is not entirely specific: one in 20–40 patients with a perimesencephalic pattern of haemorrhage has a ruptured aneurysm of the basilar or vertebral artery.[57,64,65] Conversely, about 10–20% of all ruptured posterior fossa aneurysms have a perimesencephalic pattern of subarachnoid bleeding on CT.[66–68] To exclude an aneurysm, imaging of the cerebral vasculature is therefore indispensable, but repeated studies after a technically satisfactory initial study that is negative are not needed (section 9.4.1).

Perimesencephalic haemorrhage accounts for approximately 10% of all episodes of SAH and two-thirds of those with a normal angiogram.[64,69–71] It can occur at any age, including childhood,[10,72] but most patients are in their sixth decade, as with aneurysmal haemorrhage. In one-third of the patients, strenuous activities immediately precede the onset of symptoms, a proportion similar to that found in aneurysmal haemorrhage.[56]

There is a distinct and benign variety of subarachnoid haemorrhage, in which the distribution of extravasated blood on the brain CT scan is different from aneurysmal haemorrhage, in the cisterns around the midbrain or ventral to the pons. The cause of the bleeding is unknown but it is not a ruptured aneurysm. The long-term outcome is invariably excellent. This condition accounts for 10% of all subarachnoid haemorrhages and two-thirds of subarachnoid haemorrhages with a normal angiogram.

Clinically, there is little to distinguish this idiopathic perimesencephalic haemorrhage from aneurysmal haemorrhage. The headache onset is more often gradual (minutes rather than seconds) than with aneurysmal haemorrhage, but this has poor predictive value (section 9.2.1).[72] Loss of consciousness and focal symptoms are exceptional, and then only transient; a seizure at onset virtually rules out the diagnosis.[73] A memory gap of a few hours after the haemorrhage occurs in about one-third, and is associated with enlargement of the temporal horns on the initial CT scan.[74] On admission, all patients are in perfect clinical condition, apart from their headache.[56,75] Typically, the subsequent course is uneventful, rebleeding and delayed cerebral ischaemia simply do not occur. About 20% of patients have acute hydrocephalus on their admission brain CT scan (Fig. 9.5), associated with extravasation of blood in all the perimesencephalic cisterns, which probably causes obstruction of the cerebrospinal fluid circulation at the tentorial hiatus.[76] Only a small proportion have symptoms from this ventricular

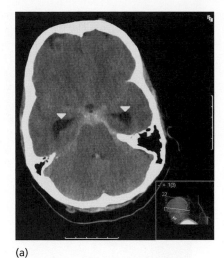
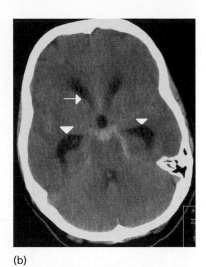

(a) (b)

Fig. 9.5 CT scans of a patient with perimesencephalic haemorrhage with blood in all perimesencephalic cisterns and hydrocephalus with dilatation of the temporal (*arrowheads*) and frontal horns (*arrow*).

dilatation, and even then an excellent outcome can be anticipated.[77,78] The period of convalescence is short, and almost invariably patients are able to resume their previous work and other activities.[78,79] Rebleeding after the hospital period has not been convincingly documented so far and life expectancy is not reduced compared to the general population.[80]

For the time being, the definition of this mild and idiopathic variant of SAH remains a purely descriptive one, based on a combination of radiological and clinical criteria. The cause of the bleeding is unknown, largely because postmortem studies have not been done, the very reason being that the outcome is so good. The mild clinical features, the limited extension of the extravasated blood on brain CT and the normal angiograms are all against bleeding from an aneurysm, or in fact from any other arterial source. Instead, rupture of a vein or a venous malformation in the prepontine or interpeduncular cistern seems a reasonable hypothesis. Indeed variants of venous drainage of the brainstem have been demonstrated in a proportion of these patients.[81,82] The hypothesis of a venous source of the haemorrhage is further supported by a single patient with a perimesencephalic pattern of haemorrhage caused by a spinal dural arteriovenous fistula.[83] In this patient the fistula was located at the C1 level and drained into a perimedullary vein connected to the venous system of the posterior cranial fossa.

We have already emphasized that a perimesencephalic pattern of haemorrhage may *occasionally* (in 2.5–5%) be caused by a ruptured posterior fossa aneurysm. By the same token, even rarer vascular abnormalities may also cause haemorrhage in the cisterns ventral to the lower brainstem: a (possible) capillary telangiectasia in the pons,[84] lacunar infarction in the vicinity of the haemorrhage, with the conjecture that a small perforating artery had occluded and subsequently ruptured,[85,86]

or small bulges of the basilar artery.[87] However, it is rather unlikely that any of these rare lesions cause *all* instances of idiopathic perimesencephalic haemorrhage.

9.1.3 Intracranial arterial dissection

Vertebral artery dissection

Dissection in general tends to be recognized more often in the carotid than in the vertebral artery (section 7.2.1), but SAH from arterial dissection most often occurs from the vertebral artery (Fig. 9.6), preferentially starting in the extracranial segment (section 7.2.2).[88,89] Blunt rotational or hyperextension trauma, even if slight, is a common cause of vertebral artery dissection,[90] in adults and also in children.[91] Iatrogenic causes include not only osteopathic manipulation but also surgery for glioma.[92] In middle-aged patients, dissection may occur more or less spontaneously. Sometimes there is an interval of days or even months between ischaemic symptoms and SAH from vertebral dissection.[93] What proportion of all SAHs arises from a dissected vertebral artery is not exactly known but all miscellaneous causes together (including dissection) account for only about 5%. In a postmortem study of fatal SAH, dissection was found in 5 of 110 patients.[94]

Neurological deficits may accompany SAH from vertebral artery dissection (section 4.2.3): ninth and tenth cranial nerve palsies, by subadventitial dissection, or Wallenberg syndrome, partial or complete, indicating subintimal dissection with impairment of blood flow in the territory of the posterior inferior cerebellar artery, resulting in ischaemia of the dorsolateral medulla. Rebleeding is common, between 30% and 70% in different series; the interval may be as short as a few hours or as long as a few weeks[95–98] and it may occur even after proximal clipping of the artery.[99] Recurrent bleeding

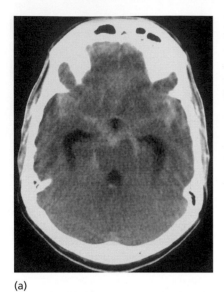

(a)

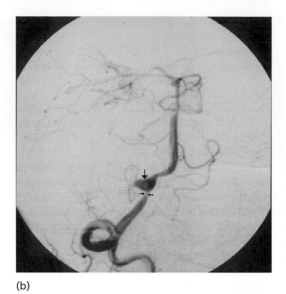

(b)

Fig. 9.6 CT scan (a) and CT angiogram (b) from a patient with subarachnoid haemorrhage from vertebral arterial dissection. The dissection shows as a narrowing (*small arrows*) followed by a dilatation (*large arrow*).

from a dissected vertebral artery is fatal in approximately half the patients.

Dissection of arteries in the anterior circulation

The intracranial portion of the internal carotid artery, or one of its branches, as the site of dissection is far less common than with the internal carotid artery in the neck, a condition encountered several times a year in most major neurology centres (section 7.2.1). It should especially be suspected if cerebral angiography is negative despite a pattern of haemorrhage on CT that suggests aneurysmal rupture in the anterior circulation.[100,101] Reported cases have affected the terminal portion of the internal carotid artery,[102–104] the middle cerebral artery[105–108] and the anterior cerebral artery[109–112] (Fig. 9.7).

Subarachnoid haemorrhage is not an invariable consequence of dissection in the anterior circulation; as with patients with vertebral artery dissection, the neurological symptoms may also result from ischaemia.[101,113] In patients with haemorrhage from a dissection, rebleeding has been reported in up to half the patients within the first 2 weeks after the initial haemorrhage, resulting in a poor outcome in most patients.[108]

9.1.4 Rare conditions causing subarachnoid haemorrhage

These are listed in Table 9.2 and some deserve comment.

Cerebral arteriovenous malformations

Cerebral AVMs were formerly believed to cause a substantial proportion of SAHs, but since the advent of CT it has become clear that haemorrhages from AVMs almost invariably involve the brain parenchyma (section 8.2.4). SAH may result if the haemorrhage reaches the surface of the brain, but of all haemorrhages secondary to a ruptured AVM only 4% are purely subarachnoid, without any parenchymal component.[114] Given that the annual incidence of haemorrhage from an AVM (per 100 000 in the general population) is of the order of 0.5,[115,116] against at least six for haemorrhage from ruptured aneurysms,[117] four of which are purely in the subarachnoid space,[118,119] at most only one in every 200 purely SAHs are caused by an AVM. It is therefore something of a mystery how in a small population-based study in Norway 9% (7/76) of SAH episodes were attributed to an AVM.[120]

Saccular aneurysms form on the feeding arteries of 10–20% of AVMs, presumably because of the greatly increased flow and the attendant strain on the arterial wall. If bleeding occurs in these cases, it is more often from the aneurysm than from the malformation itself, but the site of these aneurysms is different from the classical sites of saccular aneurysms on the circle of Willis, and again the haemorrhage is more often into the brain itself than into the subarachnoid space.[121–124]

> Very few arteriovenous malformations rupture only into the subarachnoid space. The vast majority form an intracerebral haematoma, with or without extension into the subarachnoid space. If there is an associated aneurysm this is generally the source of bleeding.

Cerebral fusiform aneurysms

A fusiform 'aneurysm' of an intracerebral artery is in fact an abnormal dilatation of a segment of the vessel.

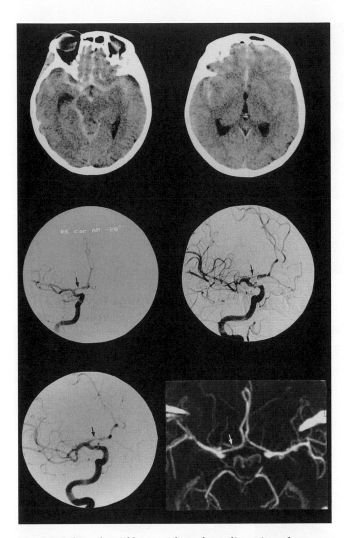

Fig. 9.7 Subarachnoid haemorrhage from dissection of an intracranial artery. *Top row*: CT brain scan within hours of the haemorrhage, showing diffuse extravasation of blood in the basal cisterns, predominantly on the right side. *Middle row, left*: right catheter carotid angiogram (antero-posterior view) after 1 day showing a narrowed segment in the proximal part of the anterior cerebral artery (*arrow*). *Middle row, right*: second angiogram (oblique view) after 11 days showing even more marked narrowing at the same site (*arrow*). *Lower row, left*: third angiogram (oblique view), 3 months after the haemorrhage; the affected segment has almost returned to a normal calibre (*arrow*). *Bottom row, right*: spiral CT scan after intravenous contrast, with maximal intensity projection, 9 months after the haemorrhage; the segment of the proximal right anterior cerebral artery is now completely normal (*arrow*).

Haemorrhages into the vessel wall are probably an important factor in their development (Fig. 9.8).[125] The presenting symptoms mostly result from ischaemia or local compression, but rupture may also occur (Fig. 9.9) when intraparenchymal extension of the haemorrhage is more common than purely subarachnoid haemorrhage (SAH).[126]

Table 9.2 Causes of subarachnoid haemorrhage, other than intracranial saccular aneurysms.

Idiopathic perimesencephalic haemorrhage (section 9.1.2)
Non-inflammatory lesions of intracerebral vessels
arterial dissection (sections 7.2.2 and 9.1.3)
cerebral arteriovenous malformations (section 9.1.4)
fusiform aneurysms (section 9.1.4)
cerebral dural arteriovenous fistulae (section 9.1.4)
intracerebral cavernous malformation[362] (section 8.2.5)
intracranial venous thrombosis (section 9.1.4)
cerebral amyloid angiopathy[363,364] (section 8.2.2)
blister-like bulges of the internal carotid artery[365,366]
rupture of circumferential artery in pontine cistern[367]
moyamoya syndrome[368] (section 7.5)
Vascular lesions in the spinal cord
saccular aneurysm of spinal artery (section 9.1.4)
spinal arteriovenous fistula or malformation (section 9.1.4)
cavernous malformation at spinal level[340,369]
Inflammatory lesions of cerebral arteries (section 7.3)
mycotic aneurysms (sections 6.5.9 and 9.1.4)
borreliosis[370] (section 7.11)
Behçet's disease[371] (section 7.3.11)
primary angiitis of the central nervous system
  (section 7.3.17)
polyarteritis nodosa[135,372,373] (section 7.3.6)
Churg-Strauss syndrome[374] (section 7.3.6)
Wegener's granulomatosis[375] (section 7.3.6)
Sickle cell disease (section 7.9.8 and 9.1.4)
Tumours
pituitary apoplexy (section 9.1.4)
cerebral metastases of cardiac myxoma (sections 6.5.13
  and 9.1.4)
malignant glioma[376]
acoustic neuroma[377]
cervical meningioma[378]
angiolipoma[379]
schwannoma of accessory nerve or spinal root[380–383]
spinal meningeal carcinomatosis[384]
melanoma of the cauda equina[385]
cervical spinal cord haemangioblastoma[386]
Drugs
cocaine use (sections 7.15.1 and 9.1.4)
anticoagulants (section 9.1.4)
Head trauma (section 9.1.4)
Superficial siderosis of the central nervous system
(section 9.1.4)

The abnormality most often occurs in the vertebro-basilar system, where dilatation is often accompanied by elongation and tortuosity, so-called dolichoectasia (section 6.3.6). The haemorrhage in patients with verte-brobasilar dolichoectasia may be the initial event,[127] but most often it follows other symptoms.[126,128,129] The risk of rupture is relatively high, according to analyses from a few patient series, if there is evidence of aneurysm

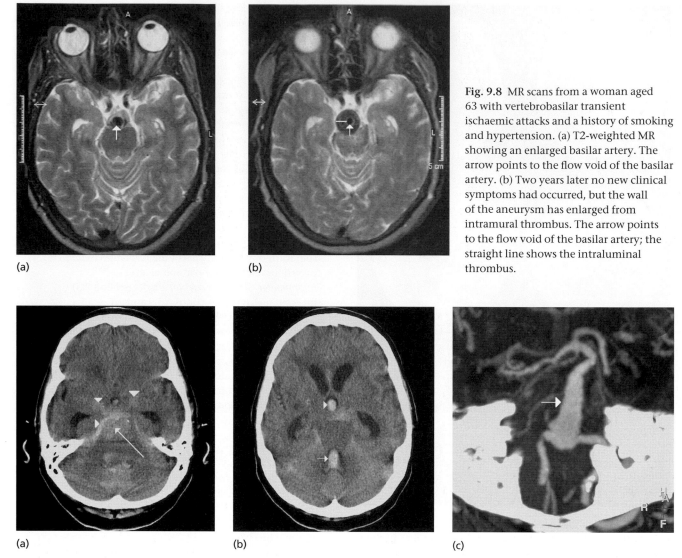

Fig. 9.8 MR scans from a woman aged 63 with vertebrobasilar transient ischaemic attacks and a history of smoking and hypertension. (a) T2-weighted MR showing an enlarged basilar artery. The arrow points to the flow void of the basilar artery. (b) Two years later no new clinical symptoms had occurred, but the wall of the aneurysm has enlarged from intramural thrombus. The arrow points to the flow void of the basilar artery; the straight line shows the intraluminal thrombus.

Fig. 9.9 Subarachnoid haemorrhage from a ruptured fusiform aneurysm of the basilar artery. (a) CT brain scan showing thrombus in the wall of the basilar artery (*arrow*) and blood in the basal cisterns (*arrowheads*). (b) CT brain scan showing subarachnoid blood as well as blood in the third (*arrowhead*) and fourth (*arrow*) ventricle. (c) CT angiogram showing the enlarged lumen of the basilar artery (*arrow*).

enlargement, if the aneurysm configuration is transitional between a fusiform and a dolichoectatic abnormality,[129] with extensive lateral displacement of the basilar artery, in the presence of hypertension, if the patient is taking antiplatelet drugs or anticoagulants, or if the patient is female.[126]

SAH may also occur from large fusiform aneurysms of the middle cerebral artery (Fig. 9.10); the dilatation may be secondary to dissection or to atherosclerosis.[130,131] Other locations are even rarer, such as the anterior cerebral artery,[132] the posterior cerebral artery,[133] the superior cerebellar artery,[134] the anterior inferior cerebellar artery (secondary to polyarteritis nodosa)[135] and the posterior inferior cerebellar artery.[136] If intracranial fusiform aneurysms are multiple, a cardiac myxoma should be suspected (section 6.5.13 and see below).[137]

Cerebral dural arteriovenous fistulae

Dural arteriovenous fistulae of the tentorium or the basal parts of the dura can give rise to a basal haemorrhage that is indistinguishable on CT from aneurysmal haemorrhage[138] (section 8.2.8); other patients present with intracerebral or subdural haemorrhage.[139] The anomaly is rare and can be found from adolescence to old age. Rebleeding may occur.[139,140]

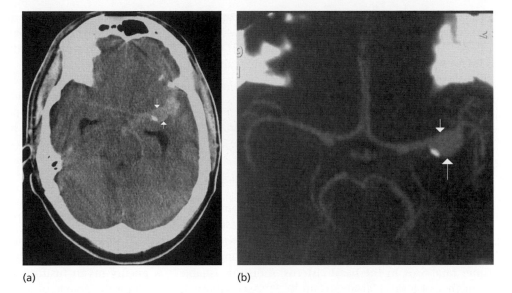

Fig. 9.10 Subarachnoid haemorrhage from a fusiform aneurysm of the left middle cerebral artery. (a) CT brain scan and (b) CT angiography showing the aneurysm (*arrows*).   (a)   (b)

Intracranial venous thrombosis

(See section 7.21)

Rarely, intracranial venous thrombosis presents with both the clinical and radiological features that initially suggest SAH from a ruptured aneurysm. In such cases, the diagnosis is largely based on neuroimaging. Recognition of intracranial venous thrombosis-induced SAH is important because in both conditions treatment should be initiated without delay, while the nature of the interventions is completely different: venous thrombosis-induced SAH should be treated with anticoagulants,[141] whereas these are obviously contraindicated in aneurysmal SAH until the the aneurysm has been occluded.

The clinical features of intracranial venous thrombosis may closely mimic SAH since the headache may be sudden in onset.[142] Also any extravasation of blood may be at the base of the brain if the venous congestion affects the basal parts of the temporal lobe as with thrombosis of the transverse, sigmoid or straight sinus.[143,144] The diagnosis is much easier if subarachnoid blood is located at the convexity, as may occur with thrombosis of the superior sagittal sinus or cortical veins,[145,146] which practically excludes a ruptured aneurysm.

Pituitary apoplexy

Pituitary apoplexy is a somewhat archaic term for arterial haemorrhage within a pituitary tumour, probably caused by tissue necrosis involving the wall of one or more hypophyseal arteries. There can also be diffuse haemorrhage in the basal cisterns, mimicking a ruptured aneurysm.[147–149] The pituitary tumour may have already been known about, or the haemorrhage may be the first

symptom. Potential precipitating factors are starting anticoagulation, general surgery, vaginal delivery, and discontinuation of dopamine agonists for prolactinoma.[150] The initial features are a sudden and severe headache, with or without nausea, vomiting, neck stiffness and depressed consciousness.[151–153] Circulatory shock is not uncommon.[154] Characteristics to distinguish pituitary apoplexy from other causes of SAH are an accompanying decrease in visual acuity or a disturbance of eye movements through compression of the oculomotor, trochlear and abducens nerves in the adjacent cavernous sinus.[155] Brain CT or MR scanning reveals the pituitary fossa as the source of the haemorrhage, and in most instances the adenoma itself is visible; associated radiological features may be extension of the haemorrhage into the frontal lobe,[156] or thickening of the mucosa of the sphenoid sinus.[157]

Cerebral mycotic aneurysms

Mycotic aneurysms underlying SAH are most frequently caused by infective endocarditis (section 6.5.9) or aspergillosis (section 7.11). Of course, in the context of infective endocarditis most strokes are (haemorrhagic) infarcts or intracerebral haemorrhages from pyogenic arteritis (section 8.2.11). Aneurysms associated with infective endocarditis are most often located on distal branches of the middle cerebral artery, because the septic emboli tend to lodge at the periphery of the arterial tree Fig. 6.9. Only about 10% of the aneurysms develop at more proximal sites.[158] Consequently, haemorrhages from mycotic aneurysms occur mostly in the cortex and in the underlying white matter, and only occasionally in the subarachnoid space, at the convexity of the brain or even at its base.[159] However, in SAH associated with infective endocarditis an aneurysm is not always identified,[160] presumably because pyogenic arteritis can also lead to rupture of the arterial wall without aneurysm formation.[161]

> Most mycotic aneurysms associated with infective endocarditis are located superficially in the cerebral hemisphere, in the cortex or underlying white matter; they rupture mostly into brain tissue, but sometimes into the subarachnoid space.

Aspergillosis is a dreaded complication in immunosuppressed patients. Mycotic aneurysms from aspergillosis are usually located on the proximal part of the basilar or carotid artery and rupture causes massive and sometimes fatal SAH in the basal cisterns, indistinguishable from that of a saccular aneurysm.[162–164] Aspergillosis is difficult to diagnose but should particularly be suspected in patients undergoing long-term treatment with antibiotics or immunosuppressive agents. Most patients with haematogenous dissemination have pulmonary lesions, but the chest X-ray may be normal early in the course.[165] Tests to detect metabolites produced by the fungus, or aspergillus-specific antibodies in serum, are now available, but their diagnostic properties have not yet been established.[166]

Other sources of microorganisms leading to the formation of mycotic aneurysms include the teeth (*Pseudomonas aeruginosa*).[167]

Cerebral metastases from cardiac myxoma

Cardiac myxoma is an extremely rare cause of aneurysm formation; the tumour can, after metastasizing to an intracranial artery, infiltrate the wall and thus cause an aneurysm to develop, sometimes more than 1 year after operation for the primary tumour[168] (section 6.5.13). These aneurysms have also been reported in children.[169] The aneurysms are often fusiform and may be multiple (Fig. 6.13).[137] On MR imaging, T1 sequences may show unusual foci of signal dropout surrounded by hyperintense rims around the aneurysms, similar in appearance to the artifacts produced by metallic aneurysm clips; these are probably caused by dense accumulation of iron and haemosiderin produced by recurrent intramural haemorrhages.

Spinal arteriovenous malformations and dural arteriovenous fistulas

Spinal arteriovenous malformations (AVMs) and dural arteriovenous fistulas (DAVFs) are an extremely rare

cause of (intracranial) subarachnoid haemorrhage. In our database of 2142 patients in the period 1985–2004, we have only one patient, while a review of the literature found 35 patients.[170] The arteriovenous shunt was located at the craniocervical junction in 14 patients, at the cervical level in 11 and at the thoracolumbar level in the remaining 11 patients. Intracranial SAH from a spinal arteriovenous shunt occurred at any age (4–72 years). Most patients (*n* = 26, 72%) had no disabling deficits at discharge or follow-up but rebleeding may occur, even repeatedly.[171]

Aneurysms of spinal arteries

SAH from aneurysms of spinal arteries is also extremely rare, with only about 20 patients on record.[172,173] These aneurysms are fusiform rather than saccular and develop along the course of an artery rather than at branching sites. A spinal aneurysm may form in the nidus of a spinal AVM,[174] or on a feeding artery of a spinal AVF.[175] As with AVMs of the spinal cord, the clinical features of spinal SAH may be accompanied by those of a transverse lesion of the cord, partial or complete.

Sickle cell disease

Sickle cell disease is commonly complicated by ischaemic stroke (section 7.9.8), but seldom by SAH.[176,177] Thirty per cent of patients with sickle cell disease and SAH are children; their CT scans show blood mostly in the superficial cortical sulci and angiograms reveal no aneurysms but often multiple distal branch occlusions and a leptomeningeal collateral circulation.[178,179] The outcome is poor. Young adults in whom sickle cell disease underlies SAH usually have one or more aneurysms at the base of the brain.

Cocaine use

Cocaine use is associated with haemorrhagic as well as with ischaemic stroke (sections 7.15.1 and 8.5.4). In patients with SAH, about half have a vascular anomaly, an aneurysm or arteriovenous malformation,[180] but the patients are younger and the aneurysms smaller than usual.[181] Rebleeding does occur, even in patients with a normal angiogram, and the outcome is often poor.[182,183] The source of the haemorrhage in patients without a vascular anomaly is unknown. Although biopsy-proven vasculitis has been found,[184] angiography seldom shows the changes suggestive of vasculitis but this is a very insensitive test.[180,185] Ingestion of *ephedrine* or 'ecstasy' may also precipitate aneurysmal SAH.[186,187]

Anticoagulation-related subarachnoid haemorrhage

If aneurysmal rupture occurs in patients on anti-coagulants the outcome is almost invariably poor.[188] Anticoagulants, however, are a rare cause for SAH in itself. In a series of 116 patients with intracranial, but extracerebral, haemorrhage while on anticoagulants, seven had only SAH, and in just three of these patients was there no cause for the haemorrhage other than anti-coagulation.[189] Severe coagulopathy, other than anti-coagulant-induced, for example congenital deficiency of factor VII, is also a rare cause of haemorrhage confined to the subarachnoid space.[190]

Head trauma

Trauma and spontaneous SAH are sometimes difficult to disentangle. Patients may be found alone after having been beaten up in a brawl or hit by a drunken driver who drove off. There may be no external wounds to indicate an accident, a decreased level of consciousness making it impossible to obtain a history, and neck stiffness causing the patient to be worked up for SAH (Fig. 9.11). Conversely, patients who rupture an aneurysm while riding a bicycle or driving a car may hit a tree or another vehicle, and the initial diagnosis will be 'traffic accident'.[191] The diagnostic conundrum becomes really difficult when patients after aneurysmal rupture fall, hit their head and sustain a skull fracture,[192] or when head trauma causes an aneurysm to burst.[193,194] Meticul-ous reconstruction of traffic or sports accidents may

therefore be rewarding, especially in patients with dis-proportionate headache or neck stiffness.

> Spontaneous subarachnoid haemorrhage may lead to head trauma, while head injury may cause superficial contusion of the brain, with accumulation of blood in the subarachnoid space. If there is any doubt, it is vital to disentangle the course of events as accurately as possible.

If trauma is the cause of SAH, CT scanning usually shows most of the blood in the superficial sulci at the convexity of the brain, adjacent to a fracture or to an intracerebral contusion.

Superficial siderosis of the central nervous system

This condition is characterized by iron overload of the pial membranes, through chronic oozing of blood from any source in the subarachnoid space. It has been included in this section on SAH only for the sake of completeness. The CSF contains blood or haemosiderin, but the clinical picture is completely different and does not include sudden headache.[195,196] The syndrome almost invariably includes subacute sensorineural deaf-ness (95% of patients), cerebellar ataxia (88%) and pyra-midal signs (76%). Less frequent features are cognitive impairment,[197] bladder disturbance and anosmia. Men are more often affected than women (3 : 1). A source of bleeding has been identified in a little more than half of the cases reported up to 1995.[196]

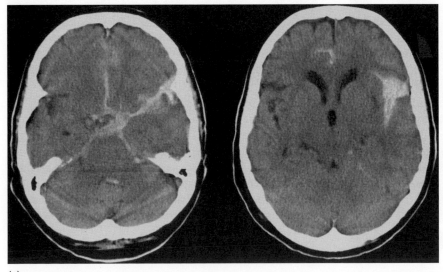

(a)

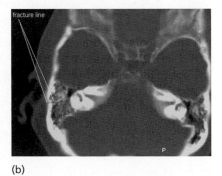

(b)

Fig. 9.11 CT brain scan of a 66-year-old woman with (a) a 'contre coup' subarachnoid haemorrhage and (b) a skull base fracture (indicated) after a fall on the floor. She had had repeated episodes of falling before; on admission after this traumatic subarachnoid haemorrhage, sick sinus syndrome was diagnosed.

Causes of chronic bleeding include:

- spinal pseudomeningoceles, spontaneous[198] or secondary to traumatic root avulsion;[199,200]
- vascular abnormalities of the dura surrounding the spinal cord or cervical roots;[201]
- a vascular tumour such as an ependymoma of the cauda equina; not really the first place to look if the problem is deafness;[202]
- as a late complication of neurosurgical interventions;[203,204]
- or any other vascular abnormality, including rarities such as familial transthyretin-related amyloidosis of meningeal vessels.[205,206]

Probably the remaining cases are also due to chronic haemorrhage, but it is not clear from where. The high iron content of the pial membranes cause a characteristic signal on MR scanning (Fig. 9.12).[199,207]

Idiopathic subarachnoid haemorrhage

In some patients no cause for a SAH is ever found, even after extensive and repeated radiological examinations of the head and spinal canal. Although non-aneurysmal types of SAH were distinguished more than 20 years ago,[56] a steady stream of publications in which SAH patients with a normal angiogram are still treated as a single group has continued to clutter up the scientific literature. That they contribute so little knowledge is to some extent the result of the invariably retrospective design, but the most serious flaw is that they contain a mixed bag of patients. The three most common subgroups are:

- patients whose 'SAH' is not real but in whom a misdiagnosis results from a traumatic lumbar puncture (section 3.7.3);
- patients with non-aneurysmal types of haemorrhage (section 9.1.2);
- patients with a pattern of haemorrhage that is entirely consistent with a ruptured aneurysm but who nevertheless have a normal angiogram. It is this last category of patient that we shall consider here. This group is getting smaller as the neuroradiological investigations become more sophisticated, but it is probably still heterogeneous, encompassing unidentified lesions of arteries, arterioles, capillaries and veins.

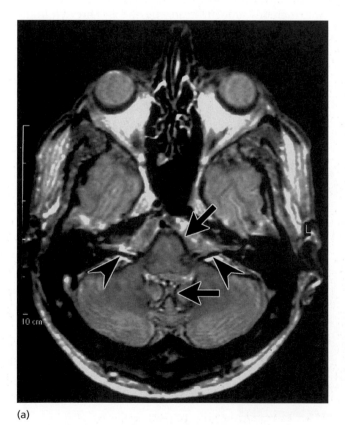

(a)

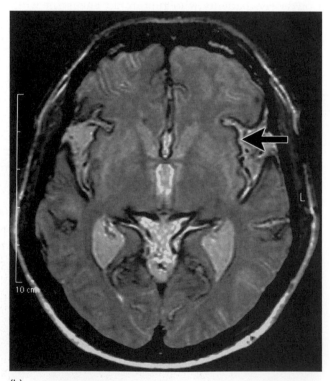

(b)

Fig. 9.12 Superficial siderosis of the nervous system. A T2-weighted magnetic resonance image of the brain in a 50-year-old man who presented with bilateral sensorineural hearing loss. The accumulation of ferric ions causes signal loss (black), due to a paramagnetic effect, over the entire pial surface (arrows), and in the acoustic nerves (arrowheads). (With permission from Padberg & Hoogenraad 2000.)

There are three studies of patients with an aneurysmal pattern of bleeding on CT who were separately distinguished among a larger group with SAH and one or more negative angiograms. After a single negative angiogram, saccular aneurysms still may become symptomatic in a minority of patients, by rebleeding, delayed cerebral ischaemia or compression of a cranial nerve.[69,208] After three negative angiograms, no episodes of aneurysmal rebleeding were documented, at least in a small series of 15 patients followed up for an average period of 5.5 years, but some patients had an ischaemic stroke or an intracerebral haemorrhage in the meantime.[209] The occurrence of all these complications is in stark contrast to patients with a non-aneurysmal perimesencephalic pattern of haemorrhage, in whom the subsequent course is almost invariably uneventful.

The substantial risk of rebleeding in patients with an aneurysmal pattern of haemorrhage and a single negative angiogram means that at least in some patients an aneurysm escapes radiological detection. Other than technical reasons, such as insufficient use of oblique projections or misreading the films,[210] this may be because of:

- Narrowing of blood vessels by 'vasospasm' which has been suggested in some cases.[211,212]
- Thrombosis of the neck of the aneurysm, or of the entire sac, is another possible reason.[212]
- Obliteration of the aneurysm by pressure of an adjacent haematoma may also prevent visualization, particularly with aneurysms of the anterior communicating artery.[213]

9.1.5 Spontaneous intraventricular haemorrhage

Intraventricular haemorrhage is usually caused by either a ruptured aneurysm (most often on the anterior communicating artery complex)[214] or by extension of an intracerebral haemorrhage. In both situations, the outcome is worse with intraventricular rupture than without, and an intraventricular clot of more than 20 mL is invariably fatal without surgical intervention.[215,216] In contrast, the outcome of 'primary' intraventricular haemorrhage, i.e. without detectable cause, is much better than if it is associated with subarachnoid or intracerebral haemorrhage; patients may survive even with intraventricular haemorrhages far exceeding 20 mL.[216,217] The advent of CT scanning proved that intraventricular haemorrhage is not the invariably lethal condition it was once thought to be when the diagnosis was made only in those who died.

'Primary' – or idiopathic – intraventricular haemorrhage is often speculatively attributed to occult vascular malformations in the ependymal wall. But only

Table 9.3 Causes of primary intraventricular haemorrhage.

Uncommon aneurysms
Posterior inferior cerebellar artery,[387,388] or its choroidal branch[389]
Anterior inferior cerebellar artery[390]
Arteriovenous malformations
In the ependymal lining[218–220]
Of the choroid plexus[391]
Dural fistula of a cerebral venous sinus[392,393]
Occlusive arterial disease
Moyamoya syndrome: idiopathic,[394] atherosclerotic[395] or with associated aneurysm[396] (section 7.5)
Lacunar infarction[397]
Clotting disorders
Haemophilia[398]
Tumours
Pituitary adenoma[399] or metastasis[400]
Ependymoma[401]
Meningioma[402]
Schwannoma[382]
Infectious diseases
Brain abscess[403]
Parasitic granuloma[404]
Drugs
Cocaine[180]
Amphetamine[405,406]
Wernicke's encephalopathy[407]

in exceptional cases have these actually been demonstrated.[218–220] Specific other causes range from tumours, which are immediately obvious on CT scanning, to small aneurysms at uncommon sites which only assiduous investigation can uncover (Table 9.3).

9.2 Clues from the history

The a priori probability of an aneurysm as the cause of subarachnoid haemorrhage (SAH) is so high (85%) that other conditions are very unlikely unless there are very strong clues in the history (head trauma, infective endocarditis, sickle cell disease, pituitary adenoma) or in any antecedent events (violent head movements, cocaine ingestion), or if the first pain was felt in the neck rather than in the head (arterial dissection, or spinal SAH).

9.2.1 Nature of the headache at onset

The key feature in diagnosing SAH is the sudden onset of an unusually severe headache. Classically it comes on in seconds ('a flash', 'just like that', 'a bolt from a blue sky', 'as if I was hit on the head'), or in a few minutes at most. However, the speed of onset of headache is of little help in distinguishing aneurysmal from perimesencephalic haemorrhage. Although headache develops more often in minutes rather than in a split second in patients with a perimesencephalic haemorrhage (35%) than in patients with aneurysmal haemorrhage (20%),[73] ruptured aneurysms are nine times as common as non-aneurysmal perimesencephalic haemorrhages.[89] Thus, only three of every 21 patients presenting with a more gradual onset of headache from SAH have a perimesencephalic haemorrhage, another example of the risk or prevention paradox (section 3.7.1). And nor does vomiting accompanying the headache discriminate between aneurysmal and perimesencephalic haemorrhage. In patients with perimesencephalic haemorrhage vomiting occurs in four out of every five patients,[73] which is no less than after aneurysmal rupture; it can even be the sole manifestation of the haemorrhage.[221]

Pain at onset in the lower part of the neck (upper neck pain is common with ruptured intracranial aneurysms), or a sudden and stabbing pain between the shoulder blades (*coup de poignard* or dagger thrust), with or without radiation to the arms, suggests a spinal arteriovenous malformation or fistula as the source of SAH (section 9.1.4).

> Sudden pain in the lower neck or between the shoulder blades is a pointer to spinal subarachnoid haemorrhage, particularly if the pain radiates to the shoulders or arms. Dissection of the thoracic aorta is another possibility.

9.2.2 Loss of consciousness

Loss of consciousness at onset occurs in over half the patients with aneurysmal SAH (section 3.7.1). Some patients complain of headache before they lose consciousness, and all patients have severe headache if they regain consciousness. Non-aneurysmal perimesencephalic SAH is typically associated with normal cognitive function; loss of consciousness or altered behaviour practically rules out this diagnosis, but amnesia may occur, mostly in association with an enlarged ventricular system.[74] Head trauma should always be considered in patients who are found unconscious (section 9.1.4).

9.2.3 Epileptic seizures

Epileptic seizures at the onset of aneurysmal SAH occur in about 10% of patients,[222–224] those with a large amount of cisternal blood on brain CT being relatively more often affected.[222] Almost every patient presenting

with de novo epilepsy over the age of 25 will have underlying conditions other than SAH, but the diagnosis should at least be suspected if any postictal headache is unusually severe or prolonged. Seizures have not been documented in patients with perimesencephalic SAH but they may well complicate haemorrhages from arterial sources other than aneurysms, such as dissection of the vertebral artery, or a vascular malformation.

9.2.4 Antecedent events

A previous episode of sudden headache hardly increases the likelihood of aneurysmal SAH despite a still widespread belief in the existence of so-called 'sentinel headaches', thought to be 'warning leaks' from the aneurysm that is eventually diagnosed. Indeed, on specific questioning, about one-third of patients recall a previous episode of headache that was unusually severe and lasted several hours.[225] Many neurosurgeons and neurologists are therefore convinced that important advances in the overall management of ruptured aneurysms can be expected from early recognition of minute episodes of subarachnoid haemorrhage, followed by emergency clipping or coiling of the aneurysm. A major difficulty with the notion of these 'warning leaks' is that almost all the studies have been hospital-based, most have been retrospective, and that even prospectively conducted studies are probably biased by hindsight (recall bias).

In a prospective study of 148 patients with sudden, severe headache identified in general practice, no neurological cause of headache was found in 93 and after 5 years of following them up there were no episodes of SAH. Only two of the 37 patients with SAH had had previous episodes of sudden headache on systematic questioning by the general practitioner at the time of presentation with the headache.[226] Also, in the 37 patients with SAH in this series, the amount and distribution of extravasated blood on brain CT, as well as the overall outcome, was similar to that in a previous hospital-based series of patients with SAH. In other words, first-ever episodes of SAH detected (or missed) in general practice are not 'small leaks', but the real thing and represent the same spectrum of severity as those seen in hospital.

A second approach to understanding the notion of 'warning leaks' is to study the clinical and radiological features in a prospective series of patients admitted to hospital with aneurysmal SAH and then to compare those with and without a history of preceding episodes of sudden severe headache. There is no difference between these two groups, whereas patients with documented rebleeding in hospital have more severe clinical deficits and more abnormalities on the CT scan.[227] In brief, the notion of frequent 'warning leaks' is not supported by epidemiological, clinical and radiological evidence. This does not mean that an episode of SAH cannot be missed by primary care physicians – or hospital doctors.

A history of even quite minor neck trauma or of sudden, unusual head movements before the onset of headache may provide a clue to the diagnosis of vertebral artery dissection as a cause of SAH. And head trauma and primary SAH may be confused as we have previously discussed (section 9.1.4). Trauma should always be suspected in patients found unconscious in the street, even if there is marked neck stiffness and no superficial wound. Conversely, a traffic accident may sometimes be the result rather than the cause of SAH, and invaluable information may be obtained from the police or ambulance workers. For example, in a patient known to have swerved from one side of the road to the other before crashing into someone else, the a priori *probabilities* are rather different (i.e. illness, falling asleep) from those in someone hit by a car that ignored a red traffic light.

9.2.5 Medical history

In patients with a distant history of head injury, and particularly if there was a skull fracture, a dural arteriovenous fistula should be suspected, since healing of the fracture may be accompanied by the development of such a lesion.[228]

Mycotic aneurysms may give rise to SAH even in patients not known to have a disorder of the heart valves, but this presentation of infective endocarditis is exceptional.[229] For practical purposes the possibility can be safely dismissed in a previously healthy patient in whom the haemorrhage is located at the base of the brain. A diagnosis of a ruptured mycotic aneurysm may well be entertained, however, if there is a history of malaise and a haemorrhage located at the convexity of the brain.

Usually it will not be hard for the physician to discover sickle cell disease, a history of cardiac myxoma, or the influence of coagulation disorders. The use of anticoagulants in itself should not be regarded as a sufficient explanation for SAH (section 9.1.4); the search for an underlying lesion ought to be just as vigorous as in other patients.

Pituitary apoplexy may be difficult to diagnose if an adenoma is not already known about, particularly if a decrease in the level of consciousness precludes a proper assessment of any visual and oculomotor deficits. Usually, the underlying adenoma has insidiously manifested itself before the dramatic occurrence of the haemorrhage, such as by a dull retro-orbital pain, fatigue, a gradual decrease of visual acuity, or constriction of the temporal fields, but often these symptoms lead to the diagnosis only in retrospect. On CT scanning the haemorrhage is usually confined within the tumour capsule, rarely extending throughout the basal cisterns as with ruptured aneurysms.

9.2.6 Family history

A family history of SAH can be a useful clue in patients with sudden headache, although of course that same fact may give rise to false alarms. There are some families in which numerous relatives suffer from ruptured aneurysms (section 9.1.1), but even in cases of so-called sporadic SAH, the risk in first-degree relatives is increased.[20,24,25] Families in which aneurysmal rupture has occurred in two or more first-degree relatives may have an underlying or associated disorder (Table 9.1), but these represent only a minority of familial aneurysms.

9.3 Clues from the examination

9.3.1 Level of consciousness

If the level of consciousness is depressed at the time of the initial examination, it is important to ascertain whether this was the situation from the onset, in which case it should probably be attributed to global perfusion failure caused by the high intracranial pressure at the time of rupture, or sometimes to an intracerebral or subdural haematoma. On the other hand, if the level of consciousness deteriorated later, other, often treatable causes should be suspected, such as acute hydrocephalus (section 14.2.4) or oedema formation around an intracerebral haemorrhage. If the level of consciousness was depressed from the outset, the bleeding is very likely to have been from an arterial source; patients with perimesencephalic haemorrhage have a normal level of consciousness at onset.[75] However, a depressed level of consciousness on arrival at the emergency department does not entirely rule out a perimesencephalic haemorrhage, because acute hydrocephalus leading to coma can occur within the first hours after the haemorrhage.[76]

A few patients with SAH (2–16%) enter a confused and agitated state (delirium).[230,231] Of course, in patients presenting with an acute confusional state to an emergency department, causes other than SAH are much more likely – SAH is the cause in only around 1% in this scenario.[232] However, more than once, such behaviour has been misinterpreted as psychological in origin. But on careful assessment most patients with SAH who do present with a confusional state have had an episode of loss of consciousness, severe headache or subtle signs on neurological examination which reveal the purely neurological cause of the behavioural disorder.[230]

9.3.2 Neck stiffness

Neck stiffness is a common sign in SAH of any cause but it takes hours to develop and therefore cannot be used to exclude the diagnosis if a patient is seen soon after the sudden-onset headache. Neck stiffness is also absent in deep coma. If present, the sign does not distinguish between the different causes of SAH, nor between SAH and meningitis (section 3.7.1).

9.3.3 Subhyaloid haemorrhages

Subhyaloid haemorrhages occur if a sudden increase in cerebrospinal fluid (CSF) pressure is transmitted to the CSF spaces surrounding the optic nerves and blocks the venous outflow from the retina, which in turn leads to rupture of retinal veins (section 3.7.1). Thus, subhyaloid haemorrhages point to an arterial source of the haemorrhage. Such intraocular haemorrhages occur in approximately 17% of patients with aneurysmal haemorrhage who survive the acute phase;[233,234] in half of them the blood remains confined to the space between the retina and the vitreous body, in the other half it ruptures into the vitreous body (Terson syndrome) (section 14.10.1).[235] Exceptionally, preretinal haemorrhages are the only sign of SAH.[236,237]

9.3.4 Pyrexia

In most patients the body temperature rises during the first 2–3 days after SAH, usually with no infection being found if the it does not exceed 38.5°C and the pulse rate has not increased. Patients with further or later increases in temperature should be carefully investigated for infection (section 14.3.3).

9.3.5 Blood pressure

In most patients with SAH, regardless of its cause, blood pressure is increased early after the onset of the haemorrhage. A low blood pressure in a patient with sudden headache should bring pituitary apoplexy to mind (section 9.1.4), or myocardial damage secondary to intracranial aneurysm rupture (section 14.9.3).

9.3.6 Focal neurological deficits

Classically, in the acute phase of aneurysmal SAH, there are no neurological signs other than those of meningeal irritation, but exceptions to this rule can provide useful information about the site or the extent of the haemorrhage (Table 9.4). Later, in the second or third week after rupture, focal deficits are not uncommon, most often as a consequence of secondary ischaemia (section 14.7.1).

In some patients, there may have been focal deficits or other symptoms before rupture, especially if the aneurysm is large. For example:

- cranial nerve palsies, especially of the olfactory, optic and oculomotor nerves;[238,239]
- deficits as a result of local compression of brain tissue;[240]
- ischaemic deficits through embolism (section 7.6);
- or focal epilepsy.[241]

But aneurysms smaller than 1 cm may occasionally cause such deficits without having ruptured.[242,243] An unruptured aneurysm may even cause intermittent ptosis ('pseudomyasthenia').[244]

Table 9.4 Focal neurological signs early after subarachnoid haemorrhage, and their explanation.

Sign	Most common explanation
Hemiparesis	Large subarachnoid haemorrhage in sylvian fissure (middle cerebral artery aneurysm)
Paraparesis	Aneurysm of anterior communicating artery; spinal arteriovenous malformation
Cerebellar ataxia, Wallenberg syndrome or both	Dissection of vertebral artery
IIIrd cranial nerve palsy	Aneurysm of internal carotid artery at the origin of posterior communicating artery; rarely aneurysm of basilar artery or superior cerebellar artery, or pituitary apoplexy
VIth cranial nerve palsy	Non-specific rise of intracranial pressure
IXth–XIIth cranial nerve palsy	Dissection of vertebral artery
Sustained downward gaze, and unreactive pupils	Acute hydrocephalus, with dilatation of the small proximal part of the sylvian aqueduct

Note: intracerebral haemorrhages may give rise to other deficits, depending on their site.

Visual field defects

Ruptured anterior communicating artery aneurysms may, in exceptional cases, compress the optic nerve or its blood supply and cause monocular blindness.[245,246] They may also penetrate one side of the optic chiasm, and with posterior lesions of the chiasm (optic tract) the visual field defect may be hemianopic.[247] However, involvement of the optic chiasm should always raise the possibility of haemorrhage into a pituitary tumour (section 9.1.4).

Third cranial nerve palsy

Complete or partial third nerve palsy is a well-recognized sign after rupture of aneurysms of the internal carotid artery at the origin of the posterior communicating artery.[248] It may also occasionally occur with aneurysms of the basilar tip, or of the superior cerebellar artery,[249] and has once been reported with non-aneurysmal peri-mesencephalic haemorrhage.[250] The pupil is most often dilated and unreactive but in some patients the pupil is spared.[251,252] Bilateral oculomotor palsies can result from pituitary apoplexy (section 9.1.4) and there may be an interval of several days between the oculomotor palsy and then the haemorrhage, presumably by expansion of the wall of the aneurysm first and later the rupture. Reactive CSF pleocytosis has been reported in aneurysmal third nerve palsies, which erroneously suggests a primary inflammatory process.[253]

Parinaud syndrome

After subarachnoid haemorrhage (SAH), small, unreactive pupils with impairment of vertical eye movements usually signify hydrocephalus rather than a direct impact of the haemorrhage on the midbrain. In a prospective study of 34 patients with acute hydrocephalus after SAH, 30 had an impaired level of consciousness, nine of these 30 had small, non-reactive pupils, and four of these nine also showed persistent downward deviation of the eyes, with otherwise intact brainstem reflexes.[254,255] The eye signs reflect dilatation of the proximal part of the aqueduct, which causes dysfunction of the pretectal area.[256] All nine patients with non-reactive pupils had a relative ventricular size of more than 1.2 and were in coma, i.e. they did not open their eyes, obey commands or utter words.

Sixth cranial nerve palsies

Sixth nerve palsies, often bilateral in the acute stage, usually result from the sustained rise of intracranial pressure, at the time of rupture or later. Therefore sixth nerve palsy has no localizing value, though occasionally aneurysms of the posterior circulation cause direct compression.[257]

Lower cranial nerve palsies

Transmural dissection of the vertebral artery may lead not only to SAH, but also to compression of the ninth or tenth nerve[258] and to ischaemia in the territory of the posterior inferior cerebellar artery.[95]

Hemiparesis

Hemiparesis at onset occurs in approximately 15% of patients with a ruptured aneurysm, usually of the middle cerebral artery.[259] As with other motor symptoms that are descibed below, the deficit may only be short-lived (for a period of a few minutes) but because these deficits may provide a clue to the cause of SAH, or the site of the aneurysm, they should not be disregarded. Aneurysms vastly outnumber all other potential causes of SAH, so the presence or absence of a hemiparesis does not contribute much to the diagnosis of rarer causes, in which hemiparesis may be relatively common, for example with ruptured mycotic aneurysms.

Cerebellar signs

Deficits indicating lesions of the cerebellum or brainstem, such as dysmetria, scanning speech, rotatory nystagmus or Horner syndrome, strongly suggest vertebral artery dissection (section 9.1.3).

Paraparesis

Early paraparesis may be a manifestation of a bifrontal haematoma complicating rupture of an anterior communicating artery complex aneurysm.[260] Later, if it develops after an interval of several days, it is more likely to reflect delayed ischaemia in the territory of both anterior cerebral arteries.[261]

Monoparesis

Weakness of one leg in the setting of SAH is most often caused by a ruptured aneurysm of the anterior communicating artery,[262] but occasionally and quite unexpectedly the aneurysm is of the posterior inferior cerebellar artery – explained by the close proximity of the aneurysm to the corticospinal tract to the contralateral leg.[263]

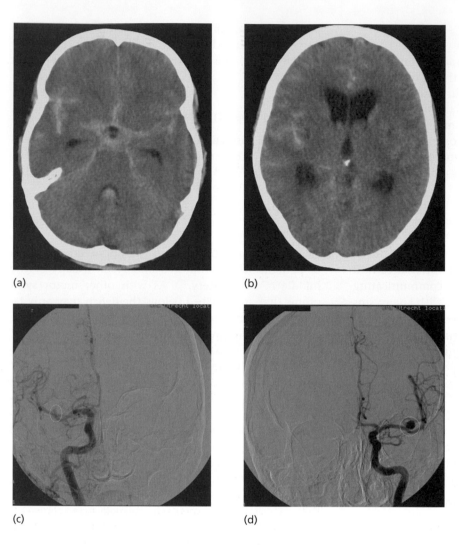

(a)

(b)

(c)

(d)

Fig. 9.13 A 47-year-old woman with a subarachnoid haemorrhage and two aneurysms. The pattern of haemorrhage points to the one that had ruptured. (a) CT scan showing diffuse haemorrhage in the basal cisterns. (b) CT scan showing more blood in the right than in the left sylvian fissure. (c) Catheter angiogram showing an aneurysm on the proximal part of the right middle cerebral artery (*circled*), it was this one which had ruptured. (d) Catheter angiogram showing a larger aneurysm on the proximal part of the left middle cerebral artery (*circled*).

9.4 Investigations

The following sections are devoted to the investigations aimed at detecting the underlying cause of SAH, with a view to treatment, but of course the other investigations needed to assess and monitor the patient's general medical condition remain essential: full blood count, glucose, urea, electrolytes, chest X-ray and an electrocardiogram.

9.4.1 CT scanning of the brain

CT brain scanning is still the first-line investigation if SAH is suspected because of the characteristic appearance of extravasated blood (section 3.7.3). On MR scanning, the abnormalities are much more subtle, at least in the acute stage. In this section, we will describe the patterns of bleeding in ruptured aneurysms, according to

their site, and also the radiological characteristics of non-aneurysmal sources of haemorrhage.

The distribution of extravasated blood on brain CT is an important though not infallible guide in determining the presence and site of the ruptured aneurysm. Identifying the source of haemorrhage from the scan is especially helpful if more than one aneurysm is found (Fig. 9.13) because there is a vast difference between the management of a ruptured aneurysm (urgent) (section 14.4) and an unruptured aneurysm (not urgent, if indicated at all) (section 15.2.4). This applies particularly to elderly patients, in whom surgical or endovascular repair of any additional unruptured aneurysms is not always indicated.

Intracerebral extension of the haemorrhage

Any intracerebral extension of the SAH is a good indicator of the site of the ruptured aneurysm, whether the

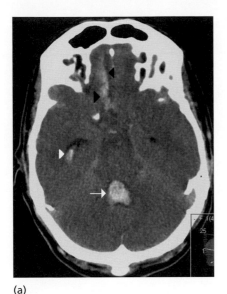

(a)

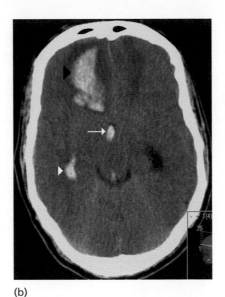

(b)

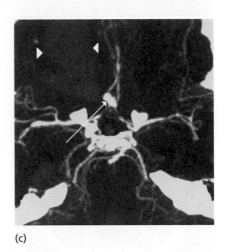

(c)

Fig. 9.14 CT brain scans after rupture of an aneurysm of the anterior communicating artery; the haemorrhage extends into the brain parenchyma and the ventricular system. (a) CT slice through the base of the brain shows a haematoma in the right gyrus rectus (*black arrowheads*), intraventricular blood in the temporal horn of the lateral ventricle (*white arrowhead*), and a large clot in the distended fourth ventricle (arrow). (b) A higher slice showing extension of the haematoma into the frontal lobe (*black arrowhead*), blood in the temporal horn of the lateral ventricle (*white arrowhead*), and the third ventricle (*arrow*). (c) CT angiogram shows the aneurysm (*arrow*) adjacent to the haematoma (*arrowheads*).

haematoma is truly intraparenchymal or only distends the subarachnoid space. The prediction of the site of the ruptured aneurysm is correct in at least 90% of haematomas.[264,265]

Haematomas from an aneurysm of the anterior communicating artery (Fig. 9.14) touch the midline with their deepest part; the extension into the frontal lobe may be paramedially, in the gyrus rectus on one or both sides,[266] or they may split the frontal lobe more laterally. A clot between the frontal horns, in the corpus callosum or the cavum septi pellucidi is a particularly reliable sign of a ruptured anterior communicating artery aneurysm.[267] A haematoma confined to the pericallosal cistern indicates that the aneurysm lies more distally on the anterior cerebral artery, usually at the origin of the pericallosal artery (Fig. 9.15).

Aneurysms arising from the internal carotid artery are most often at the origin of the posterior communicating artery, and any so intracerebral haematomas from rupture at this site are usually in the medial part of the temporal lobe (Fig. 9.16). Very large haematomas from such aneurysms, or from aneurysms at the top of the carotid artery, may also involve the frontal lobe (Fig. 9.17). Haematomas from an aneurysm at the origin of the ophthalmic artery tend to involve the frontal lobe on one side and do not reach the midline, which distinguishes them from intracerebral bleeding from an aneurysm of the anterior communicating artery.

Middle cerebral artery aneurysms are almost exclusively located close to the temporal bone, where the main stem of the artery divides and turns superiorly and posteriorly to enter the lateral part of the sylvian fissure. Haematomas from aneurysms of this type usually extend from this point posteriorly and superiorly, to follow the course of the lateral fissure. Less often, the haemorrhage is directed medially, in which case it can still be distinguished from a 'hypertensive' haemorrhage in the basal ganglia by its lateral extension to the inner table of the skull (Fig. 9.18).

Aneurysms arising from the posterior circulation rarely give rise to intracerebral extension of the haemorrhage.

However, it must be borne in mind that there will always be exceptional situations where physicians are wrong-footed by aneurysms at unusual locations. If doubt remains in a deteriorating patient, for whom rapid evacuation of the haematoma seems indicated, CT angiography may show – or to some extent exclude – an aneurysm (section 9.4.4).

Blood in the subarachnoid cisterns

The pattern of haemorrhage if the extravasated blood is confined to the subarachnoid cisterns is less specific for the site of the aneurysm, especially if the haemorrhage is diffuse rather than local.[268,269] Moreover, after an interval of 5 days, 50% of patients no longer show cisternal

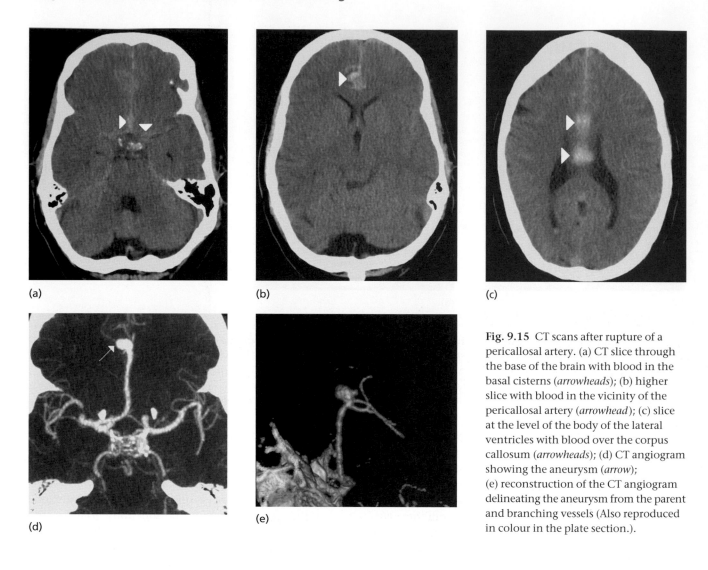

(a)

(b)

(c)

(d)

(e)

Fig. 9.15 CT scans after rupture of a pericallosal artery. (a) CT slice through the base of the brain with blood in the basal cisterns (*arrowheads*); (b) higher slice with blood in the vicinity of the pericallosal artery (*arrowhead*); (c) slice at the level of the body of the lateral ventricles with blood over the corpus callosum (*arrowheads*); (d) CT angiogram showing the aneurysm (*arrow*); (e) reconstruction of the CT angiogram delineating the aneurysm from the parent and branching vessels (Also reproduced in colour in the plate section.).

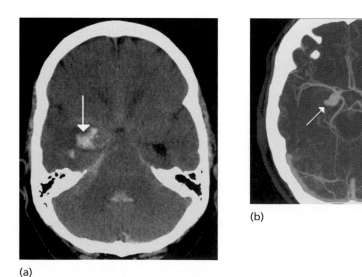

(a)

(b)

Fig. 9.16 Rupture of a posterior communicating artery aneurysm. (a) Brain CT showing a haematoma in the medial part of the right temporal lobe (*arrow*). (b) CT angiography showing a large aneurysm of the posterior communicating artery at its origin from the internal carotid artery (*arrow*).

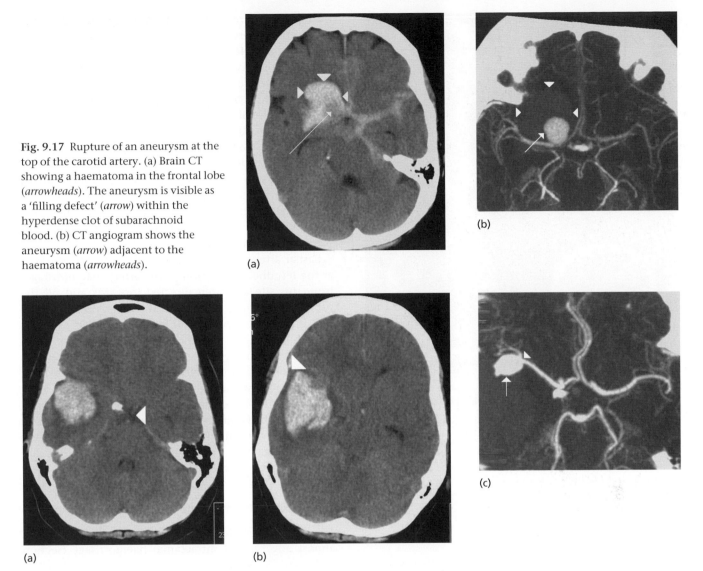

Fig. 9.17 Rupture of an aneurysm at the top of the carotid artery. (a) Brain CT showing a haematoma in the frontal lobe (*arrowheads*). The aneurysm is visible as a 'filling defect' (*arrow*) within the hyperdense clot of subarachnoid blood. (b) CT angiogram shows the aneurysm (*arrow*) adjacent to the haematoma (*arrowheads*).

(a)

(b)

(a)

(b)

(c)

Fig. 9.18 Haematoma from a ruptured aneurysm of the right middle cerebral artery. (a) Brain CT showing the haematoma extending medially from the sylvian fissure. Note the absence of blood in the suprasellar cistern (*arrowhead*). (b) The haematoma extends into the subinsular cortex and putamen, thereby partly mimicking a primary intracerebral haemorrhage from a ruptured perforating artery in the basal ganglia. The characteristic feature of aneurysmal bleeding is the extreme lateral extension of the haematoma, up to the inner table of the skull (*arrowhead*). (c) CT angiography to show the aneurysm (*arrow*) at the trifurcation of middle cerebral artery (*arrowhead*) that had caused the haemorrhage.

blood on CT,[118] and in exceptional cases the abnormalities have all but disappeared within a single day (Fig. 9.19). The source of SAH can be inferred if the haemorrhage remains confined to, or is most dense in a single cistern, near an arterial branching point site where aneurysms are known to arise (Fig. 9.3). Sometimes the hyperdensity is local but very subtle (Fig. 9.20), which may easily lead to a missed diagnosis of SAH in the middle of the night. It is helpful to specifically look for slight dilatation of the temporal horns of the lateral ventricles, and for fissures and sulci that should be present but are not visible, due to the presence of a small amount of blood that is isodense to the brain parenchyma.

The most common site for aneurysms is the anterior cerebral artery near the anterior communicating artery (Fig. 9.3) and these can be recognized from a region of hyperdensity in the deepest part of the frontal interhemispheric fissure (Fig. 9.21). Haemorrhage in the interhemispheric fissure at higher levels, particularly the supracallosal cistern (Fig. 9.15), suggests an aneurysm at the origin of the pericallosal artery, although occasionally

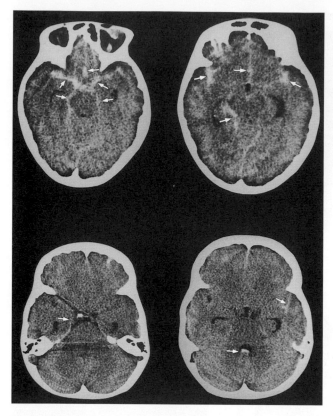

Fig. 9.19 Exceptionally rapid disappearance of subarachnoid blood. *Upper row*: CT brain scan 4 h after rupture of an aneurysm of the right posterior communicating artery, at its origin from the carotid artery. Abundant extravasation of blood, throughout the basal cisterns (*arrows*). *Lower row*: CT scan 24 h after symptom onset; only a small amount of blood remains (*arrows*). (From van der Wee *et al.*, 1995[408]; courtesy of the authors and the *Journal of Neurology, Neurosurgery and Psychiatry*.)

haemorrhages from an aneurysm of the anterior communicating artery complex may extend this far.[267]

An asymmetrical distribution of subarachnoid blood in the region of the suprasellar cisterns suggests an aneurysm of the internal carotid artery, usually at the origin of the posterior communicating artery; there may be some extension into the basal part of the sylvian fissure (Fig. 9.22). If the patient has an arachnoid cyst of the middle fossa, a posterior communicating artery aneurysm may bleed into the cyst.[270]

An aneurysm of the middle cerebral artery can be inferred from extravasation of blood at the junction of the basal and lateral parts of the sylvian fissure (Fig. 9.20). The haemorrhage may further extend into the lateral fissure.

Basilar artery aneurysms are almost invariably found at the terminal bifurcation of the artery; haemorrhages from this site are often directed forwards and fill the suprasellar, interhemispheric and (basal) sylvian cisterns (Fig. 9.23). The posterior inferior cerebellar artery is located near the base of the skull in the posterior fossa, a notoriously difficult region for CT; haemorrhages in this region can be detected only if the posterior fossa is adequately visualized[66] (Fig. 9.24). It is even more difficult if the aneurysm is on a loop of the posterior inferior cerebellar artery below the foramen magnum.[271] Fusiform aneurysms of the posterior circulation often bleed into the brain parenchyma as well as in the subarachnoid space (Fig. 9.9).

Intraventricular haemorrhage

The cerebral ventricles can fill with blood as a result of almost any type of intracranial haemorrhage (section

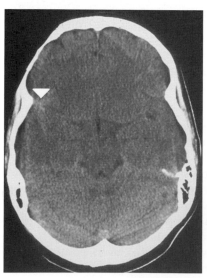

(a)

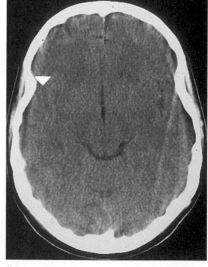

(b)

Fig. 9.20 Subtle sign of subarachnoid haemorrhage in a patient with a ruptured aneurysm of the right middle cerebral artery. (a) CT brain scan on the day of admission showing a small amount of blood in the right sylvian fissure (*arrowhead*). (b) Repeat CT scan 2 days after the initial scan showing disappearance of the blood (*arrowhead*).

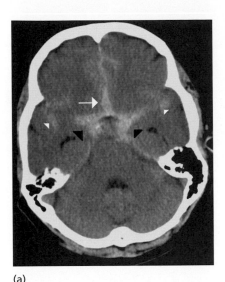
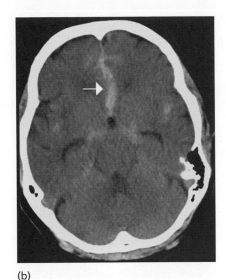
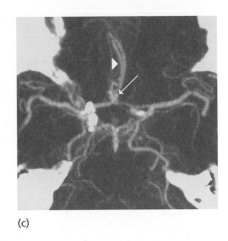

(a)   (b)   (c)

Fig. 9.21 Ruptured aneurysm of the anterior communicating artery. (a) CT brain scan slice through the base of the brain shows diffuse blood in the anterior interhemispheric fissure (*arrow*); blood is also present in the suprasellar cistern (*black arrowheads*) and sylvian fissures (*white arrowheads*). (b) On a higher slice the blood is most prominent in the anterior interhemispheric fissure (*arrow*). (c) CT angiogram showing the anterior communicating artery aneurysm (*arrow*); note the distortion of the anterior cerebral arteries (*arrowhead*) from the extravasated blood in the fissure.

Fig. 9.22 Ruptured aneurysm of the posterior communicating artery. (a) CT brain scan showing diffuse subarachnoid haemorrhage most dense in the left half of the suprasellar cistern extending into the basal part of the sylvian fissure (*arrowhead*). (b) CT angiogram shows the aneurysm of the posterior communicating artery, at its origin from the internal carotid artery (*arrow*).

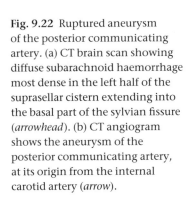
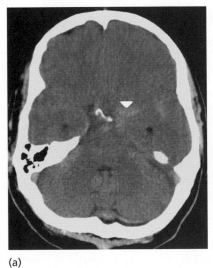
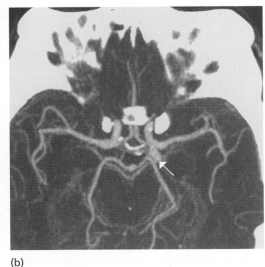

(a)   (b)

9.1.5). Transmission of pressure through the floor of the fourth ventricle can then cause acute failure of pontine and medullary functions, which accounts for 25–50% of early deaths after SAH.[272] Intraventricular haemorrhage occurs mostly with aneurysms of the anterior communicating artery, which bleed through the lamina terminalis to fill the third and lateral ventricles (Fig. 9.14).[214] Filling of the third, but not the lateral ventricles, suggests rupture of a basilar artery aneurysm, especially if the posterior part of the basal cisterns is filled as well. Similarly, rupture of an aneurysm of the posterior inferior cerebellar artery may preferentially fill the fourth ventricle (and sometimes also the third) from below (Fig. 9.24).

Subdural haematomas

Subdural haematomas develop in 2–3% of all cases of aneurysmal rupture,[273–275] more often after rebleeding than after a first episode.[227] They are most often associated with subarachnoid blood but can sometimes be the only manifestation of aneurysmal rupture.[276,277] The subdural collection is usually found at the convexity of

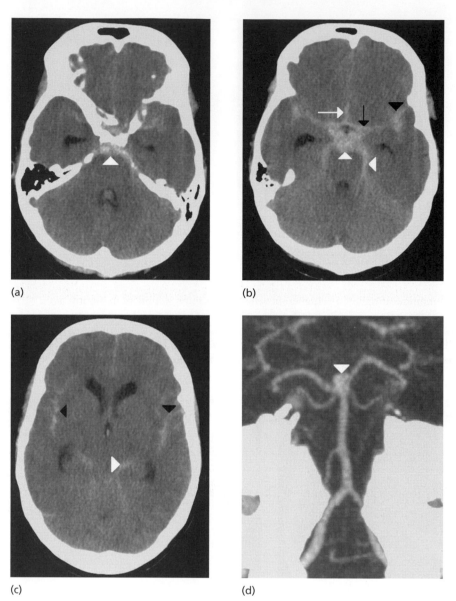

(a)

(b)

(c)

(d)

Fig. 9.23 Ruptured aneurysm at the top of the basilar artery. (a) CT brain scan shows blood in front of and alongside the pons (*arrowhead*); (b) higher slice showing blood in the basal part of the suprasellar cistern and in the ambient cistern (*white arrowheads*), extending into the frontal part of the suprasellar cistern (*black arrow*), the anterior interhemispheric fissure (*white arrow*) and the sylvian fissure (*black arrowhead*); (c) blood in the ambient cistern (*white arrowhead*) and in both sylvian fissures (*black arrowheads*); (d) CT angiogram showing the aneurysm at the top of the basilar artery (*arrowhead*).

the brain, seldom in the interhemispheric fissure. Subdural collections near the skull base are not well visualized on axial CT images. The ruptured aneurysm can be at any of the common sites, sometimes far removed from the subdural collection.[278] The most plausible explanation for the rupture through the arachnoid membrane is that the dome of the aneurysmal sac has become adherent to it, usually as a result of a previous rupture, recognized or unrecognized.[279] A more indirect pathogenesis is also conceivable, through traction on veins traversing the subdural space, but patients with subdural haematomas are no older than those without.[275] The distinction from subdural haematomas of traumatic origin can often be made on the basis of the associated extensive haemorrhage in the subarachnoid space, and also

because with trauma the haematoma is more often unilateral, hyperdense and crescentic in shape.[273]

Non-aneurysmal (perimesencephalic) patterns of haemorrhage

Fifteen per cent of patients with SAH do not have an aneurysm on angiographic studies, and two-thirds of these show basal haemorrhages of a distinct kind: mainly or only in the perimesencephalic cisterns, a pattern of haemorrhage that is seen only rarely in patients with a demonstrable aneurysm (Fig. 9.25) (section 9.1.2). A problem is that about one out of 20 patients with a perimesencephalic type of haemorrhage harbours an aneurysm after all, located on the posterior circulation

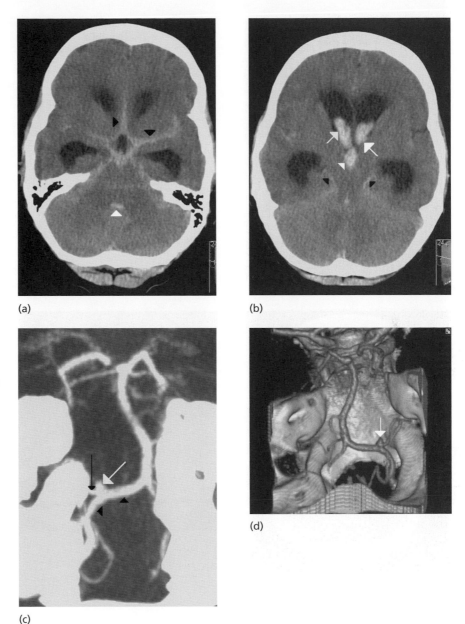

Fig. 9.24 Ruptured aneurysm of the posterior inferior cerebellar artery.
(a) Brain CT scan showing diffuse subarachnoid blood in the basal cisterns (*black arrowheads*) and blood in the fourth ventricle (*white arrowhead*); note also the enlarged lateral and third ventricles.
(b) A higher slice showing subarachnoid blood in both ambient cisterns (*black arrowheads*) and lateral (*white arrows*) and third ventricle (*white arrowhead*).
(c) CT angiogram showing the aneurysm (*white arrow*) at the origin of the posterior inferior cerebellar artery (*black arrow*) from the vertebral artery (*black arrowheads*). (d) Reconstruction of the CT angiogram showing better the relationship between the aneurysm (*arrow*) and parent and branching vessel. (Also reproduced in colour in the plate section.)

(a)

(b)

(c)

(d)

(Fig. 9.26).[57,64,68,280] An estimate of the balance of risks leads to the conclusion that withholding surgical or endovascular treatment in approximately 5% of patients with a perimesencephalic pattern of bleeding but an undetected basilar artery aneurysm is more unfavourable than the complications of 'unnecessary' angiographic imaging in the remaining 95%. However, there is no need to *repeat* a normal CT angiogram in a patient with a perimesencephalic pattern of haemorrhage,[281] or to proceed to catheter angiography after a normal CT angiogram.[282] A decision analysis indicates that a CT angiogram is sufficient to exclude a posterior fossa aneurysm,[283] provided the local radiological team has sufficient

experience with SAH patients and CT angiography.[284] In contrast, repeating a negative angiographic study is mandatory with aneurysmal patterns of haemorrhage on the CT scan (section 9.4.6).

> CT angiography (rather than catheter angiography) is still required in patients with a perimesencephalic subarachnoid pattern of subarachnoid haemorrhage, even though the chance of finding an aneurysm is extremely small. However, unlike with aneurysmal patterns of bleeding, there is no need to repeat the angiogram after a negative initial angiogram.

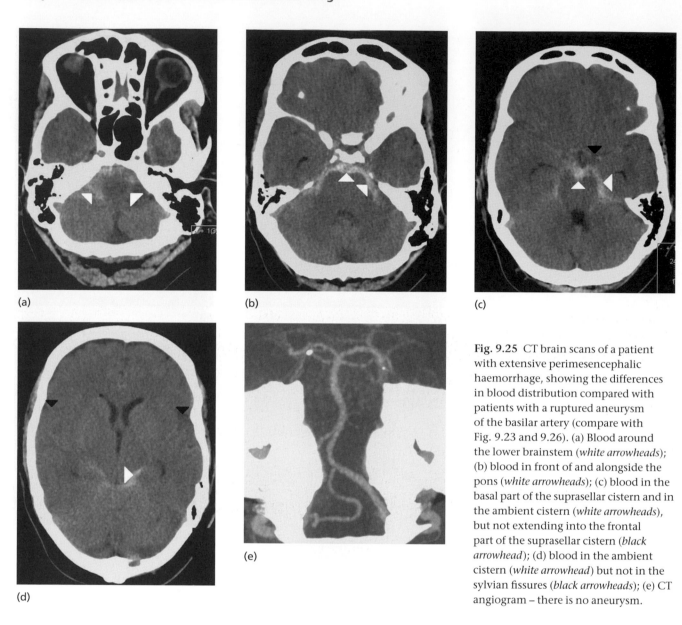

(a)

(b)

(c)

(d)

(e)

Fig. 9.25 CT brain scans of a patient with extensive perimesencephalic haemorrhage, showing the differences in blood distribution compared with patients with a ruptured aneurysm of the basilar artery (compare with Fig. 9.23 and 9.26). (a) Blood around the lower brainstem (*white arrowheads*); (b) blood in front of and alongside the pons (*white arrowheads*); (c) blood in the basal part of the suprasellar cistern and in the ambient cistern (*white arrowheads*), but not extending into the frontal part of the suprasellar cistern (*black arrowhead*); (d) blood in the ambient cistern (*white arrowhead*) but not in the sylvian fissures (*black arrowheads*); (e) CT angiogram – there is no aneurysm.

Other patterns and sources of haemorrhage

Basal haemorrhages, indistinguishable on CT scanning from those associated with a ruptured aneurysm, may result from vertebral artery dissection, a dural fistula of the tentorium, an arteriovenous malformation in the neck region, cocaine abuse without an associated aneurysm or a mycotic aneurysm with aspergillosis (section 9.1.4).

As already discussed (section 9.1.4), head trauma may result in SAH; if a patient is found unconscious or was seen to have caused an unexplained traffic accident, the question may arise whether the trauma or the SAH was the primary event. With traumatic brain injury, usually the brain CT shows an adjacent brain contusion at the convexity, different in shape and site from an aneurysmal haematoma. Nevertheless, some patients with basal-frontal contusions may show a pattern of haemorrhage resembling that of a ruptured anterior communicating artery aneurysm (Fig. 9.27), and in patients with blood confined to the sylvian fissure it may also be difficult to distinguish trauma from aneurysmal rupture by the pattern of haemorrhage alone. In some patients with shearing injury, pronounced accumulation of blood can be found in the posterior part of the ambient cistern at the level of the tentorial margin,[285,286] a site that makes a ruptured saccular aneurysm as source of the haemorrhage very unlikely. In patients with direct trauma to the neck, or with head injury associated with vigorous neck movement, the trauma can immediately be followed by

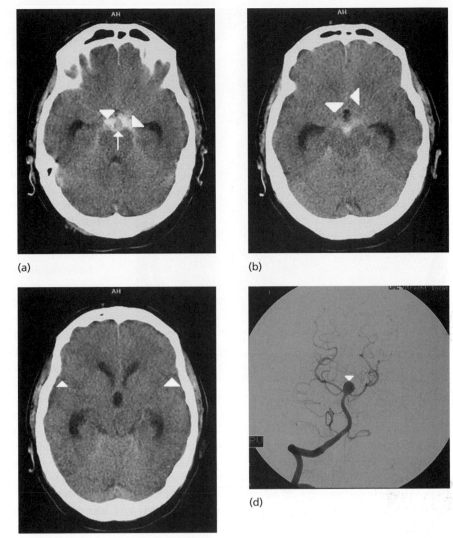

(a)

(b)

(c)

(d)

Fig. 9.26 A patient with a perimesencephalic pattern of haemorrhage but from a ruptured basilar artery aneurysm. (a) Brain CT scan showing subarachnoid blood in the basal part of the suprasellar cistern (*white arrowheads*); the aneurysm is already visible as a 'filling defect' (*arrow*) within the hyperdense clot of subarachnoid blood. (b) No apparent extension in the frontal part of the suprasellar cistern (*downward arrowhead*) or into the anterior interhemispheric fissure (*leftward arrowhead*). However, these subarachnoid spaces are not visible, which indicates that they contain blood. (c) No blood in the sylvian fissures (*arrowheads*). (d) Catheter angiogram confirming the aneurysm (*white arrowhead*).

massive basal haemorrhage resulting from a tear or even a complete rupture of one of the arteries of the posterior circulation, which tends to be rapidly fatal.[287]

9.4.2 Lumbar puncture

If there is no evidence of subarachnoid blood on brain CT in patients with clinical features suggesting SAH, examination of the CSF is extremely important for establishing or excluding the diagnosis (section 3.7.3). However, CSF analysis is of no use in establishing the cause of SAH.

9.4.3 Magnetic resonance imaging

In the acute stage of subarachnoid haemorrhage (SAH), particularly within the first 24 h, subarachnoid blood can be detected by MRI as a region of hyperintensity on spin echo T2-weighted images (Fig. 9.28),[288] and even better with gradient echo T2 sequences (on which the blood is hypointense),[289,290] fluid-attenuated inversion recovery (FLAIR),[291] fluid-attenuated turbo-inversion recovery (FLAT TIRE),[292] or proton density (PD) weighted images.[293,294] However FLAIR, fast spin echo T2 and PD sequences are in general relatively insensitive to blood regardless of where it is in the brain. Therefore, if bleeding is suspected or needs to be excluded, then a gradient echo sequence should always be done. Gadolinium enhancement may give a false impression of subarachnoid haemorrhage, especially on FLAIR images.

Some studies specifically emphasize the advantages of MRI with aneurysms of the posterior inferior cerebellar artery.[295] But there is undoubtedly some publication bias in that unfavourable performance with MRI in the acute

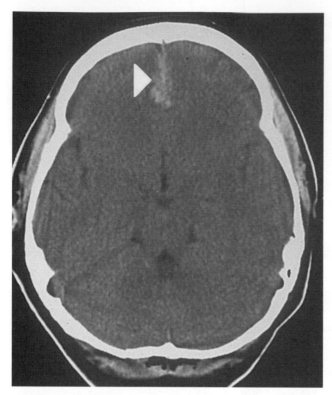

Fig. 9.27 CT brain scan showing extravasated blood in the frontal interhemispheric fissure (*arrowhead*) as a result of trauma (34-year-old woman who had fallen off her horse).

stage of SAH is less likely to have been reported, blinding of observers has been, at best, incomplete, and the number of patients no more 20–30 per study.

There is concern about the balance between sensitivity and specificity of MRI in the acute stage,[296] the facilities for MRI are much less readily available than CT scans, and when conscious level is impaired the relatively long scanning time increases the problem of movement artifacts and patient safety.

The hyperintensity of 'old' blood may last for at least 2 weeks on T1-weighted images[297] and even longer with FLAIR.[298] Therefore, for patients who are not seen until 1 or 2 weeks after onset when brain CT may no longer show any evidence of subarachnoid blood, MRI may identify the site of a ruptured aneurysm. However, in some patients it only shows traces of blood at the convexity of the brain,[299] which is not helpful in identifying the site of aneurysmal rupture although it does suggest that an SAH has occurred. For patients who are referred 1 or 2 weeks after the onset of the SAH, analysis of the CSF is more sensitive in detecting subarachnoid blood than MRI.[300]

In one study on 58 patients examined at least 3 months after proven aneurysmal rupture, T2-weighted images still revealed subarachnoid haemosiderin deposition in three of every four patients, whereas no deposition was seen in the healthy volunteers.[301] The haemosiderin was preferentially deposited in the subarachnoid space near the ruptured aneurysm. Thus, in patients presenting several weeks after the onset of headache MRI may be helpful in ruling in but not in ruling out SAH.

Aneurysms themselves can be identified by MRI as signal-void areas,[297] and special MR techniques that image moving blood have been developed for the detection of aneurysms, especially in asymptomatic subjects (section 9.4.5).

With arterial dissection, MRI (or CT) may detect a thrombus within the dissected wall of the artery[302–304] (section 7.2). In the case of chronic haemosiderosis (section 9.1.4), MR scanning shows diffuse deposition of

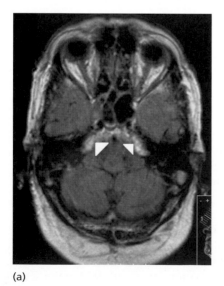

(a)

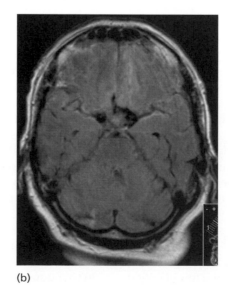

(b)

Fig. 9.28 MR brain scan of a patient who presented 5 days after the onset of headache from a ruptured aneurysm of the anterior communicating artery. (a) FLAIR sequence showing some remaining traces of blood as hyperintensities in front of the lower brainstem (*arrowheads*); (b) FLAIR at the level of the suprasellar cistern without any remaining blood.

haemosiderin in the subpial layers of the brain and spinal cord.

9.4.4 Computed tomographic angiography

Angiographic studies in general serve not only to identify one or more aneurysms as the potential cause of an SAH, but also to display the anatomical configuration of the aneurysm in relation to adjoining arteries which allows the optimal selection of treatment (coiling or clipping; Chapter 14).

CT angiography depends on the injection of iodinated contrast agent, just like conventional catheter angiography, but in this by the intravenous route. The technique of CT scanning has been considerably improved, first with spiral or helical scanning, which eliminates the problem of 'gaps' between imaged slices (improved spatial resolution), then with multislice techniques, which allow faster coverage (improved temporal resolution). And data processing techniques such as 'maximal intensity projection' compress three-dimensional information in a single plane, from many different angles (section 6.8.5) which can be used most effectively if the observer views the images on a computer screen, where it is possible to rotate the vessels in every possible direction. As a consequence, the sensitivity of CT angiography for detecting ruptured aneurysms, with conventional catheter angiography as the 'gold standard', is still improving, from about 90% in a review of eight methodologically sound studies up to 1998,[305] to 93% for 21 studies performed in 1995–2002.[306] In a recent report in which the multislice technique was used, the sensitivity was 95%,[307] while a study of helical CT in middle cerebral artery aneurysms (which are often difficult to detect) reported a sensitivity of 97%.[308] Not surprisingly, small aneurysms of 2–3 mm diameter may escape detection with CT angiography.[309,310] On the other hand, CT angiography may detect aneurysms that are missed by conventional catheter angiography[311] and often it provides the necessary information for choosing the best method for occluding the aneurysm.[312,313] Indeed, in many cases neurosurgeons are confident to base their operation on CT angiography alone[314,315] so that it will probably replace catheter angiography, except when coiling is the treatment of choice.

A great advantage of CT angiography over MR angiography and catheter angiography is the speed with which it can be performed, preferably immediately after the CT scan of the brain by which the diagnosis of aneurysmal haemorrhage is made, and while the patient is still in the machine.

For the purpose of detecting aneurysms in asymptomatic patients, CT scanning, however sophisticated, is less attractive than magnetic resonance angiography (section 9.4.5) because of the need for intravenous contrast and the small but inevitable risk of allergic reactions.

9.4.5 Magnetic resonance angiography

An important factor affecting the performance of magnetic resonance angiography (MRA) is the imaging protocol. For example, the sensitivity of time-of-flight MRA (for identification of at least one aneurysm per patient) is around 75% if the information is processed as maximal intensity projection (MIP) alone, but increases to 80–95% if axial base and spin echo images or a 3D-volume rendering algorithm are added (Fig. 15.4).[316–318] Aneurysm size is another important factor; for smaller than 3 mm, detection rates may be as low as 38%.[305]

To sum up, in patients with SAH, MRA is unlikely to replace contrast radiography in the near future. But, despite its limitations, and thanks to its non-invasive nature, MRA is being used to detect aneurysms in relatives of patients with SAH[319,320] and – perhaps appropriately – in patients who are followed up after coiling[301] for a ruptured aneurysm (section 14.4.2).

> Magnetic resonance angiography is almost without risk and is reasonably sensitive (90%) which makes it well suited for screening people at risk of intracranial aneurysms, but less suitable for patients with subarachnoid haemorrhage.

9.4.6 Cerebral catheter angiography

General consideration of risks and benefits

Catheter angiography is not innocuous. A systematic review of three prospective studies, in which patients with SAH were distinguished from other indications for catheter angiography, found a risk of transient or permanent neurological complications of 1.8%.[321] Also, the aneurysm may re-rupture during the procedure, in 1–2% overall,[322–324] and in the 6-h period after angiography the rupture risk has been estimated at 5%, which is higher than expected.[324] In certain parts of the world, the aim of making as accurate a diagnosis as possible overrides the balance of risks and benefits for the patient, and a catheter angiogram is felt to be justified in nearly every patient with SAH. By contrast, from a pragmatic point of view, we feel that catheter angiography should be omitted if clipping or coiling of an aneurysm is not a likely therapeutic option, for whatever reason.

> In general, catheter angiography in patients with subarachnoid haemorrhage should be performed only with a view to surgical or endovascular treatment or, in exceptional cases, to establish a more firm prognosis.

Timing and extent of angiography

In a patient with an aneurysmal pattern of haemorrhage on CT scanning, the timing of angiography is intricately linked with the timing of any proposed operation, or endovascular treatment. If operative occlusion is considered, many neurosurgeons advocate early clipping of the aneurysm, within 3 days of the initial bleed, but the evidence for such early intervention is weak (section 14.4.3). In any event, angiography with a view to clipping or coiling the aneurysm should be performed at the earliest opportunity if any intervention is planned within 3 days of SAH onset.

Exact information about the structure of the aneurysm and its relation to parent vessels is vital, but often CT angiography will supply this (section 9.4.4). If doubt remains, 3D rotational subtraction catheter angiography can help. This technique combines the high spatial resolution of digital subtraction angiography with acquisition of a three-dimensional data set. After Fourier transformation, this data set can be used in a volume rendering technique for reconstruction. These 3D images supply both the interventional neuroradiologist as well as the neurosurgeon with highly detailed information.

- With aneurysms of the anterior communicating artery, imaging of both carotid artery territories is necessary to identify the artery bearing the aneurysm and to determine from which side the distal parts of the anterior cerebral arteries are filled. But in practice this kind of information is usually already available from the CT angiogram, because in 90% of patients with aneurysms of the anterior communicating artery the A1 segments (the segment of the anterior cerebral artery between the carotid T-junction and the anterior communicating artery) are asymmetrical, which is reliably depicted on CT angiography.[325]
- With aneurysms of the carotid artery at the origin of the posterior communicating artery, it is often useful to know whether the posterior cerebral artery is sufficiently filled via the basilar artery, for example in the event that during operative treatment temporary clipping of the posterior communicating artery is required to control bleeding. Again, this feature is also often seen on CT angiography.[325]
- In contrast, with aneurysms of the middle cerebral artery it is not usually necessary to have information about any other arterial territory.

In a patient with a pattern of haemorrhage on CT scanning that is compatible with a posterior circulation aneurysm, an angiogram cannot be termed 'negative' until both vertebral arteries have been visualized, because aneurysms arising from the posterior inferior cerebellar artery or other proximal branches of the vertebral artery will be missed by imaging only one vertebral artery. Also 3D imaging of the region where the aneurysm is suspected may identify very small aneurysms (Fig. 9.29). Finally, if the patient's age and clinical condition warrant treatment of any unruptured as well as the ruptured aneurysm, that is good reason for displaying all the branches of both the carotid and vertebral arterial systems.

Suspicion of causes other than an aneurysm

In cases of suspected arterial dissection, the diagnosis rests on the angiographic demonstration of narrowing of the artery with signs of an intimal flap, a pseudoaneurysm or a double lumen (section 7.2.1). Catheter angiography may be warranted if CT angiography, MRI or MR angiography fails to confirm the clinical diagnosis of dissection, not with a view to treatment but for excluding other causes (sometimes with a medicolegal implication), and for giving a prognosis. Timing of imaging is difficult, because an early angiogram may be normal or show only non-specific arterial narrowing, while early abnormalities may have disappeared on a later angiogram.[326]

In patients in whom CT scanning suggests that the haemorrhage originates near the tentorium, angiography should be directed at the detection of a dural arteriovenous fistula. In that case, it is important to visualize the external carotid artery as well because its branches can be the main or only feeders.

Mycotic aneurysms were missed by angiography in 10% in older series, and even now they may be visible only on repeated studies. In patients with infective endocarditis but *no* intracranial haemorrhage, a policy of routine angiography to detect mycotic aneurysms is not justified by decision analysis.[327] However, in patients with endocarditis *and* intracranial haemorrhage, treatment of the ruptured aneurysm should be considered, and thus CT or catheter angiography should be performed.

Aneurysmal patterns of haemorrhage but negative initial angiography

In patients with an aneurysmal pattern of haemorrhage on CT and a negative initial CTA or catheter angiogram, repeat angiography is clearly indicated. The combined yield of a second catheter angiogram in 14 reported series

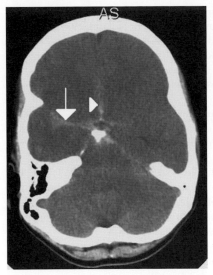

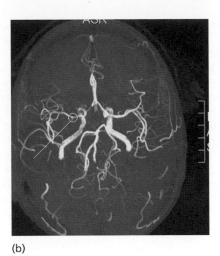

(b)

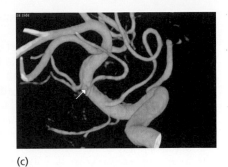

(c)

(a)

Fig. 9.29 A patient with a subarachnoid haemorrhage from a very small aneurysm on the proximal part of the middle cerebral artery. (a) CT brain scan showing diffuse blood in the basal part of the right sylvian fissure (*arrow*) and in the anterior interhemispheric fissure (*arrowhead*); (b) MR angiogram gives some suggestion of an aneurysm (*circle*); (c) Catheter three-dimensional angiogram confirms a very small aneurysm (*arrow*) which was clipped by the neurosurgeon.

was 58 aneurysms in 386 patients, or 15%.[212,213,328–338] If it is taken into account that patients with perimesencephalic non-aneurysmal haemorrhage were often not excluded from these series, the yield of repeat angiograms in patients with a diffuse or anteriorly located pattern of haemorrhage on CT scanning must be even higher. If a second angiogram again fails to demonstrate the suspected aneurysm, an aneurysm may still be demonstrated by exploratory craniotomy – or rebleeding.[69,339] If a first, as well as a second, angiogram is completely negative (not only both internal carotid arteries but also both vertebral arteries having been injected) despite an aneurysmal pattern of haemorrhage on the CT scan, the search for a vascular lesion should still be doggedly pursued. In a unique, consecutive series of 14 patients subjected to a third angiogram, a single aneurysm was found.[331] A reasonable approach is to perform a third investigation some 3 months after SAH onset, the choice (repeat catheter angiography, CT angiography, MRI/MRA) depending on the patient's clinical condition, age and personal wishes. CT angiography or MR angiography with three-dimensional projection will in due time probably replace catheter angiography in detecting 'occult' aneurysms.

9.4.7 Spinal imaging

In the case of subarachnoid haemorrhage from a spinal arteriovenous malformation, brain CT may show blood throughout the basal cisterns and ventricles, which makes it difficult to make the correct diagnosis.[340] Not only negative angiography of the cerebral circulation, but also clinical clues such as sudden backache, should suggest the need for spinal angiography. However, this procedure is not always diagnostic.[341,342] Also, angiography is impractical without localizing signs or symptoms because so many intercostal arteries have to be catheterized, while the procedure itself carries a risk of some 5% of a transient or even persisting neurological deficit.[343,344] In practice, if a vascular abnormality of the spinal cord is suspected, MRI, particularly in the sagittal plane, is the first-line investigation for detecting the characteristic serpiginous structures, usually on the dorsal aspect of the cord, indicating a dural arteriovenous fistula (section 9.1.4), or at least for detecting an associated extradural or subdural haematoma.[345,346] There are no systematic studies about the usefulness of spinal angiography after a negative MR scan of the spinal cord.

References

1 Hop JW, Rinkel GJE, Algra A, van Gijn J. Case-fatality rates and functional outcome after subarachnoid hemorrhage: a systematic review. *Stroke* 1997; **28**(3):660–4.
2 De Rooij NK, Linn FHH, van der Plas JAP, Algra A, Rinkel GJE. Incidence of Subarachnoid Haemorrhage: A systematic review with emphasis on region, age, gender

and time trends. *J Neurol Neurosurg Psychiatry*. 2007 May 2; [Epub ahead of print]

3 Johnston SC, Selvin S, Gress DR. The burden, trends, and demographics of mortality from subarachnoid hemorrhage. *Neurology* 1998; **50**:1413–18.

4 Koffijberg, H, Buskens E, Granath F, Adami J, Ekbom A, Rinkel G, Blomqvist P. Subarachnoid haemorrhage in Sweden 1987–2002: regional incidence and case fatality rates. *J Neurol Neurosurg Psychiatry* 2007; Jul 17; [Epub ahead of print].

5 Rinkel GJE, Djibuti M, Algra A, van Gijn J. Prevalence and risk of rupture of intracranial aneurysms: a systematic review. *Stroke* 1998; **29**:251–6.

6 Ferry PC, Kerber C, Peterson D, Gallo AA, Jr. Arteriectasis, subarachnoid hemorrhage in a three-month-old infant. *Neurology* 1974; **24**(5):494–500.

7 Stehbens WE. Intracranial berry aneurysms in infancy. *Surg Neurol* 1982; **18**(1):58–60.

8 Stehbens WE, Manz HJ, Uszinski R, Schellinger D. Atypical cerebral aneurysm in a young child. *Pediatr Neurosurg* 1995; **23**:97–100.

9 Proust F, Toussaint P, Garniéri J, Hannequin D, Legars D, Houtteville JP *et al*. Pediatric cerebral aneurysms. *J Neurosurg* 2001; **94**:733–9.

10 Anderson RC, Baskin J, Feldstein NA. Perimesencephalic nonaneurysmal subarachnoid hemorrhage in the pediatric population: case report and review of the literature. *Pediatr Neurosurg* 2002; **37**:258–61.

11 Ruigrok YM, Buskens E, Rinkel GJE. Attributable risk of common and rare determinants of subarachnoid hemorrhage. *Stroke* 2001; **32**:1173–5.

12 Pleizier CM, Ruigrok YM, Rinkel GJE. Relation between age and number of aneurysms in patients with subarachnoid haemorrhage. *Cerebrovasc Dis* 2002; **14**:51–3.

13 Ostergaard JR, Hog E. Incidence of multiple intracranial aneurysms. Influence of arterial hypertension and gender. *J Neurosurg* 1985; **63**:49–55.

14 Juvela S. Risk factors for multiple intracranial aneurysms. *Stroke* 2000; **31**:392–7.

15 Ellamushi HE, Grieve JP, Jäger HR, Kitchen ND. Risk factors for the formation of multiple intracranial aneurysms. *J Neurosurg* 2001; **94**:728–732.

16 Stehbens WE. Etiology of intracranial berry aneurysms. *J Neurosurg* 1989; **70**(6):823–31.

17 Fujimoto K. 'Medial defects' in the prenatal human cerebral arteries: an electron microscopic study. *Stroke* 1996; **27**:706–8.

18 Finlay HM, Whittaker P, Canham PB. Collagen organization in the branching region of human brain arteries. *Stroke* 1998; **29**:1595–601.

19 Ruigrok YM, Rinkel GJE, Wijmenga C. Genetics of intracranial aneurysms. *Lancet Neurol* 2005; **4**:179–89.

20 Bromberg JEC, Rinkel GJE, Algra A, Greebe P, van Duyn CM, Hasan D *et al*. Subarachnoid haemorrhage in first and second degree relatives of patients with subarachnoid haemorrhage. *Br Med J* 1995; **311**(1700):288–9.

21 Ronkainen A, Hernesniemi J, Ryynanen M. Familial subarachnoid hemorrhage in east Finland, 1977–1990. *Neurosurgery* 1993; **33**(5):787–96.

22 Ruigrok YM, Rinkel GJE, Algra A, Raaymakers TW, van Gijn J. Characteristics of intracranial aneurysms in patients with familial subarachnoid hemorrhage. *Neurology* 2004; **62**:891–4.

23 Bromberg JEC, Rinkel GJE, Algra A, van Duyn CM, Greebe P, Ramos LMP *et al*. Familial subarachnoid hemorrhage: distinctive features and patterns of inheritance. *Ann Neurol* 1995; **38**:929–34.

24 Gaist D, Vaeth M, Tsiropoulos I, Christensen K, Corder E, Olsen J *et al*. Risk of subarachnoid haemorrhage in first degree relatives of patients with subarachnoid haemorrhage: follow up study based on national registries in Denmark. *Br Med J* 2000; **320**:141–5.

25 Teasdale GM, Wardlaw JM, White PM, Murray G, Teasdale EM, Easton V. The familial risk of subarachnoid haemorrhage. *Brain* 2005; **128**:1677–85.

26 Bromberg JEC, Rinkel GJE, Algra A, Van den Berg UAC, Tjin-A-Ton MLR, van Gijn J. Hypertension, stroke, and coronary heart disease in relatives of patients with subarachnoid hemorrhage. *Stroke* 1996; **27**:7–9.

27 Belz MM, Hughes RL, Kaehny WD, Johnson AM, Fick-Brosnahan GM, Earnest MP *et al*. Familial clustering of ruptured intracranial aneurysms in autosomal dominant polycystic kidney disease. *Am J Kidney Dis* 2001; **38**:770–6.

28 Gieteling EW, Rinkel GJE. Characteristics of intracranial aneurysms and subarachnoid haemorrhage in patients with polycystic kidney disease. *J Neurol* 2003; **250**:418–23.

29 Rossetti S, Chauveau D, Kubly V, Slezak JM, Saggar-Malik AK, Pei Y *et al*. Association of mutation position in polycystic kidney disease 1 (PKD1) gene and development of a vascular phenotype. *Lancet* 2003; **361**:2196–201.

30 Pepin M, Schwarze U, Superti-Furga A, Byers PH. Clinical and genetic features of Ehlers-Danlos syndrome type IV, the vascular type [see comments]. *N Engl J Med* 2000; **342**:673–80.

31 Van den Berg JSP, Pals G, Arwert F, Hennekam RCM, Albrecht KW, Westerveld A *et al*. Type III collagen deficiency in saccular intracranial aneurysms: defect in gene regulation? *Stroke* 1999; **30**:1628–31.

32 Ruigrok YM, Rinkel GJ, Wijmenga C. Genetics of intracranial aneurysms. *Lancet Neurol* 2005; **4**:179–89.

33 Slowik A, Borratynska A, Turaj W, Pera J, Dziedzic T, Figlewicz DA *et al*. Alpha1-antichymotrypsin gene (SERPINA3) A/T polymorphism as a risk factor for aneurysmal subarachnoid hemorrhage. *Stroke* 2005; **36**:737–40.

34 Kassam AB, Horowitz M, Chang YF, Peters D. Altered arterial homeostasis and cerebral aneurysms: a molecular epidemiology study. *Neurosurgery* 2004; **54**:1450–60.

35 Wermer MJH, Van der Schaaf IC, Velthuis BK, Algra A, Buskens E, Rinkel GJE. Follow-up screening after subarachnoid haemorrhage: frequency and determinants of new aneurysms and enlargement of existing aneurysms. *Brain* 2005; **128**:2421–9.

36 Tsutsumi K, Ueki K, Usui M, Kwak S, Kirino T. Risk of recurrent subarachnoid hemorrhage after complete obliteration of cerebral aneurysms. *Stroke* 1998; **29**:2511–13.

37 Wermer MJH, Greebe P, Algra A, Rinkel GJE. Incidence of recurrent subarachnoid hemorrhage after clipping for ruptured intracranial aneurysms. *Stroke* 2005; **36**:2394–9.

38 Ronkainen A, Niskanen M, Rinne J, Koivisto T, Hernesniemi J, Vapalahti M. Evidence for excess long-term mortality after treated subarachnoid hemorrhage. *Stroke* 2001; **32**:2850–3.

39 Feigin VL, Rinkel GJ, Lawes CM, Algra A, Bennett DA, van Gijn J *et al.* Risk factors for subarachnoid hemorrhage: an updated systematic review of epidemiological studies. *Stroke* 2005; **36**:2773–80.

40 Vermeer SE, Rinkel GJE, Algra A. Circadian fluctuations in onset of subarachnoid hemorrhage: new data on aneurysmal and perimesencephalic hemorrhage and a systematic review. *Stroke* 1997; **28**(4):805–8.

41 Nyquist PA, Brown RD, Jr., Wiebers DO, Crowson CS, O'Fallon WM. Circadian and seasonal occurrence of subarachnoid and intracerebral hemorrhage. *Neurology* 2001; **56**:190–3.

42 Guzman R, Grady MS. An intracranial aneurysm on the feeding artery of a cerebellar hemangioblastoma: case report. *J Neurosurg* 1999; **91**:136–8.

43 Jensen FK, Wagner A. Intracranial aneurysm following radiation therapy for medulloblastoma: a case report and review of the literature. *Acta Radiol* 1997; **38**(1):37–42.

44 Pereira P, Cerejo A, Cruz J, Vaz R. Intracranial aneurysm and vasculopathy after surgery and radiation therapy for craniopharyngioma: case report. *Neurosurgery* 2002; **50**:885–7.

45 Sciubba DM, Gallia GL, Recinos P, Garonzik IM, Clatterbuck RE. Intracranial aneurysm following radiation therapy during childhood for a brain tumor: case report and review of the literature. *J Neurosurg* 2006; **105**:134–9.

46 Takao T, Fukuda, Kawaguchi T, Nishino K, Ito Y, Tanaka R *et al.* Ruptured intracranial aneurysm following gamma knife surgery for acoustic neuroma. *Acta Neurochir (Wien)* 2006; **148**:1317–18.

47 Tokuda Y, Inagawa T, Takechi A, Inokuchi F. Ruptured de novo aneurysm induced by ethyl 2-cyanoacrylate: case report. *Neurosurgery* 1998; **43**:626–8.

48 Sasaki T, Kodama N, Itokawa H. Aneurysm formation and rupture at the site of anastomosis following bypass surgery. *J Neurosurg* 1996; **85**:500–2.

49 Nishimoto T, Yuki K, Sasaki T, Murakami T, Kodama Y, Kurisu K. A ruptured middle cerebral artery aneurysm originating from the site of anastomosis 20 years after extracranial-intracranial bypass for moyamoya disease: case report. *Surg Neurol* 2005; **64**:261–5.

50 Ferro JM, Pinto AN. Sexual activity is a common precipitant of subarachnoid hemorrhage. *Cerebrovasc Dis* 1994; **4**:375.

51 Fann JR, Kukull WA, Katon WJ, Longstreth WT, Jr. Physical activity and subarachnoid haemorrhage: a population based case-control study. *J Neurol Neurosurg Psychiatry* 2000; **69**:768–72.

52 Anderson C, Ni MC, Scott D, Bennett D, Jamrozik K, Hankey G. Triggers of subarachnoid hemorrhage: role of physical exertion, smoking, and alcohol in the Australasian Cooperative Research on Subarachnoid Hemorrhage Study (ACROSS). *Stroke* 2003; **34**:1771–6.

53 Schievink WI, Karemaker JM, Hageman LM, van der Werf DJ. Circumstances surrounding aneurysmal subarachnoid hemorrhage. *Surg Neurol* 1989; **32**:266–72.

54 Matsuda M, Ohashi M, Shiino A, Matsumura K, Handa J. Circumstances precipitating aneurysmal subarachnoid hemorrhage. *Cerebrovasc Dis* 1993; **3**:285–8.

55 Longstreth WT, Jr., Nelson LM, Koepsell TD, van Belle G. Cigarette smoking, alcohol use, and subarachnoid hemorrhage. *Stroke* 1992; **23**(9):1242–9.

56 Van Gijn J, van Dongen KJ, Vermeulen M, Hijdra A. Perimesencephalic hemorrhage: a nonaneurysmal and benign form of subarachnoid hemorrhage. *Neurology* 1985; **35**(4):493–7.

57 Rinkel GJE, Wijdicks EFM, Vermeulen M, Ramos LMP, Tanghe HL, Hasan D *et al.* Nonaneurysmal perimesencephalic subarachnoid hemorrhage: CT and MR patterns that differ from aneurysmal rupture. *Am J Neuroradiol* 1991; **12**(5):829–34.

58 Schwartz TH, Solomon RA. Perimesencephalic nonaneurysmal subarachnoid hemorrhage: review of the literature. *Neurosurgery* 1996; **39**:433–40.

59 Rinkel GJE, van Gijn J. Perimesencephalic haemorrhage in the quadrigeminal cistern. *Cerebrovasc Dis* 1995; **5**:312–13.

60 Schwartz TH, Mayer SA. Quadrigeminal variant of perimesencephalic nonaneurysmal subarachnoid hemorrhage. *Neurosurgery* 2000; **46**:584–588.

61 Schwartz TH, Farkas J. Quadrigeminal non-aneurysmal subarachnoid hemorrhage: a true variant of perimesencephalic subarachnoid hemorrhage: case report. *Clin Neurol Neurosurg* 2003; **105**:95–8.

62 Zentner J, Solymosi L, Lorenz M. Subarachnoid hemorrhage of unknown etiology. *Neurol Res* 1996; **18**:220–6.

63 Schievink WI, Wijdicks EFM. Pretruncal subarachnoid hemorrhage: an anatomically correct description of the perimesencephalic subarachnoid hemorrhage. *Stroke* 1997; **28**:2572.

64 Pinto AN, Ferro JM, Canhao P, Campos J. How often is a perimesencephalic subarachnoid haemorrhage CT pattern caused by ruptured aneurysms? *Acta Neurochir (Wien)* 1993; **124**(2–4):79–81.

65 Van Calenbergh F, Plets C, Goffin J, Velghe L. Nonaneurysmal subarachnoid hemorrhage: prevalence of perimesencephalic hemorrhage in a consecutive series. *Surg Neurol* 1993; **39**(4):320–3.

66 Kayama T, Sugawara T, Sakurai Y, Ogawa A, Onuma T, Yoshimoto T. Early CT features of ruptured cerebral aneurysms of the posterior cranial fossa. *Acta Neurochir (Wien)* 1991; **108**(1–2):34–9.

67 Kallmes DF, Clark HP, Dix JE, Cloft HJ, Evans AJ, Dion JE *et al.* Ruptured vertebrobasilar aneurysms: frequency of

the nonaneurysmal perimesencephalic pattern of haemorrhage on CT scans. *Radiology* 1996; **201**:657–60.

68 Alen JF, Lagares A, Lobato RD, Gomez PA, Rivas JJ, Ramos A. Comparison between perimesencephalic nonaneurysmal subarachnoid hemorrhage and subarachnoid hemorrhage caused by posterior circulation aneurysms. *J Neurosurg* 2003; **98**:529–35.

69 Rinkel GJE, Wijdicks EFM, Hasan D, Kienstra GE, Franke CL, Hageman LM *et al.* Outcome in patients with subarachnoid haemorrhage and negative angiography according to pattern of haemorrhage on computed tomography. *Lancet* 1991; **338**(8773):964–8.

70 Farrés MT, Ferraz Leite H, Schindler E, Mühlbauer M. Spontaneous subarachnoid hemorrhage with negative angiography: CT findings. *J Comput Assist Tomogr* 1992; **16**(4):534–7.

71 Ferbert A, Hubo I, Biniek R. Non-traumatic subarachnoid hemorrhage with normal angiogram. Long-term follow-up and CT predictors of complications. *J Neurol Sci* 1992; **107**(1):14–18.

72 Sert A, Aydin K, Pirgon O, Emlik D, Ustun ME. Arterial spasm following perimesencephalic nonaneurysmal subarachnoid hemorrhage in a pediatric patient. *Pediatr Neurol* 2005; **32**:275–7.

73 Linn FHH, Rinkel GJE, Algra A, van Gijn J. Headache characteristics in subarachnoid haemorrhage and benign thunderclap headache. *J Neurol Neurosurg Psychiatry* 1998; **65**:791–3.

74 Hop JW, Brilstra EH, Rinkel GJE. Transient amnesia after perimesencephalic haemorrhage: the role of enlarged temporal horns. *J Neurol Neurosurg Psychiatry* 1998; **65**:590–3.

75 Rinkel GJE, Wijdicks EFM, Vermeulen M, Hasan D, Brouwers PJAM, van Gijn J. The clinical course of perimesencephalic nonaneurysmal subarachnoid hemorrhage. *Ann Neurol* 1991; **29**(5):463–4.

76 Rinkel GJE, Wijdicks EFM, Vermeulen M, Tans JTJ, Hasan D, van Gijn J. Acute hydrocephalus in nonaneurysmal perimesencephalic hemorrhage: evidence of CSF block at the tentorial hiatus. *Neurology* 1992; **42**(9):1805–7.

77 Rinkel GJE, Wijdicks EFM, Ramos LMP, van Gijn J. Progression of acute hydrocephalus in subarachnoid haemorrhage: a case report documented by serial CT scanning. *J Neurol Neurosurg Psychiatry* 1990; **53**(4):354–5.

78 Rinkel GJE, Wijdicks EFM, Vermeulen M, Hageman LM, Tans JT, van Gijn J. Outcome in perimesencephalic (nonaneurysmal) subarachnoid hemorrhage: a follow-up study in 37 patients. *Neurology* 1990; **40**(7):1130–2.

79 Brilstra EH, Hop JW, Rinkel GJE. Quality of life after perimesencephalic haemorrhage. *J Neurol Neurosurg Psychiatry* 1997; **63**:382–4.

80 Greebe P, Rinkel GJE. Life expectancy after perimesencephalic subarachnoid hemorrhage. *Stroke* 2007; **38**(4):1222–4.

81 Watanabe A, Hirano K, Kamada M, Imamura K, Ishii N, Sekihara Y *et al.* Perimesencephalic nonaneurysmal subarachnoid haemorrhage and variations in the veins. *Neuroradiology* 2002; **44**:319–25.

82 Van der Schaaf I, Velthuis BK, Gouw A, Rinkel GJE. Venous drainage in perimesencephalic hemorrhage. *Stroke* 2004; **35**:1614–18.

83 Hashimoto H, Iida J, Shin Y, Hironaka Y, Sakaki T. Spinal dural arteriovenous fistula with perimesencephalic subarachnoid haemorrhage. *J Clin Neurosci* 2000; **7**:64–6.

84 Wijdicks EFM, Schievink WI. Perimesencephalic nonaneurysmal subarachnoid hemorrhage: first hint of a cause? *Neurology* 1997; **49**:634–6.

85 Tatter SB, Buonanno FS, Ogilvy CS. Acute lacunar stroke in association with angiogram-negative subarachnoid hemorrhage: mechanistic implications of two cases. *Stroke* 1995; **26**:891–5.

86 Rogg JM, Smeaton S, Doberstein C, Goldstein JH, Tung GA, Haas RA. Assessment of the value of MR imaging for examining patients with angiographically negative subarachnoid hemorrhage. *Am J Roentgenol* 1999; **172**:201–6.

87 Matsumaru Y, Yanaka K, Muroi A, Sato H, Kamezaki T, Nose T. Significance of a small bulge on the basilar artery in patients with perimesencephalic nonaneurysmal subarachnoid hemorrhage: report of two cases. *J Neurosurg* 2003; **98**:426–9.

88 Kaplan SS, Ogilvy CS, Gonzalez R, Gress D, Pile Spellman J. Extracranial vertebral artery pseudoaneurysm presenting as subarachnoid hemorrhage. *Stroke* 1993; **24**(9):1397–9.

89 Rinkel GJE, van Gijn J, Wijdicks EFM. Subarachnoid hemorrhage without detectable aneurysm: a review of the causes. *Stroke* 1993; **24**(9):1403–9.

90 Chung YS, Han DH. Vertebrobasilar dissection: a possible role of whiplash injury in its pathogenesis. *Neurol Res* 2002; **24**:129–38.

91 Kneyber MC, Rinkel GJE, Ramos LMP, Tulleken CAF, Braun KPJ. Early posttraumatic subarachnoid hemorrhage due to dissecting aneurysms in three children. *Neurology* 2005; **65**:1663–5.

92 Nohjoh T, Houkin K, Takahashi A, Abe H. Ruptured dissecting vertebral artery aneurysm detected by repeated angiography: case report. *Neurosurgery* 1995; **36**(1):180–2.

93 Naito I, Iwai T, Sasaki T. Management of intracranial vertebral artery dissections initially presenting without subarachnoid hemorrhage. *Neurosurgery* 2002; **51**:930–7.

94 Sasaki O, Ogawa H, Koike T, Koizumi T, Tanaka R. A clinicopathological study of dissecting aneurysms of the intracranial vertebral artery. *J Neurosurg* 1991; **75**(6):874–82.

95 Caplan LR, Baquis GD, Pessin MS, D'Alton J, Adelman LS, DeWitt LD *et al.* Dissection of the intracranial vertebral artery. *Neurology* 1988; **38**(6):868–77.

96 Aoki N, Sakai T. Rebleeding from intracranial dissecting aneurysm in the vertebral artery. *Stroke* 1990; **21**(11):1628–31.

97 Yamaura A, Watanabe Y, Saeki N. Dissecting aneurysms of the intracranial vertebral artery. *J Neurosurg* 1990; **72**(2):183–8.

98 Mizutani T, Aruga T, Kirino T, Miki Y, Saito I, Tsuchida T. Recurrent subarachnoid hemorrhage from untreated

ruptured vertebrobasilar dissecting aneurysms. *Neurosurgery* 1995; **36**:905–13.

99 Kawamata T, Tanikawa T, Takeshita M, Onda H, Takakura K, Toyoda C. Rebleeding of intracranial dissecting aneurysm in the vertebral artery following proximal clipping. *Neurol Res* 1994; **16**(2):141–4.

100 Nakatomi H, Nagata K, Kawamoto S, Shiokawa Y. Ruptured dissecting aneurysm as a cause of subarachnoid hemorrhage of unverified etiology. *Stroke* 1997; **28**:1278–82.

101 Ohkuma H, Suzuki S, Ogane K. Dissecting aneurysms of intracranial carotid circulation. *Stroke* 2002; **33**:941–7.

102 Adams HP, Jr., Aschenbrener CA, Kassell NF, Ansbacher L, Cornell SH. Intracranial hemorrhage produced by spontaneous dissecting intracranial aneurysm. *Arch Neurol* 1982; **39**(12):773–6.

103 Massoud TF, Anslow P, Molyneux AJ. Subarachnoid hemorrhage following spontaneous intracranial carotid artery dissection. *Neuroradiology* 1992; **34**(1):33–5.

104 Ohkuma H, Nakano T, Manabe H, Suzuki S. Subarachnoid hemorrhage caused by a dissecting aneurysm of the internal carotid artery. *J Neurosurg* 2002; **97**:576–83.

105 Kunze S, Schiefer W. Angiographic demonstration of a dissecting aneurysm of the middle cerebral artery. *Neuroradiology* 1971; **2**(4):201–6.

106 Sasaki O, Koike T, Tanaka R, Ogawa H. Subarachnoid hemorrhage from a dissecting aneurysm of the middle cerebral artery: case report. *J Neurosurg* 1991; **74**(3):504–7.

107 Piepgras DG, McGrail KM, Tazelaar HD. Intracranial dissection of the distal middle cerebral artery as an uncommon cause of distal cerebral artery aneurysm: case report. *J Neurosurg* 1994; **80**(5):909–13.

108 Ohkuma H, Suzuki S, Shimamura N, Nakano T. Dissecting aneurysms of the middle cerebral artery: neuroradiological and clinical features. *Neuroradiology* 2003; **45**:143–8.

109 Guridi J, Gallego J, Monzon F, Aguilera F. Intracerebral hemorrhage caused by transmural dissection of the anterior cerebral artery. *Stroke* 1993; **24**(9):1400–2.

110 Koyama S, Kotani A, Sasaki J. Spontaneous dissecting aneurysm of the anterior cerebral artery: report of two cases. *Surg Neurol* 1996; **46**:55–61.

111 Mori K, Yamamoto T, Maeda M. Dissecting aneurysm confined to the anterior cerebral artery. *Br J Neurosurg* 2002; **16**:158–64.

112 Ohkuma H, Suzuki S, Kikkawa T, Shimamura N. Neuroradiologic and clinical features of arterial dissection of the anterior cerebral artery. *Am J Neuroradiol* 2003; **24**:691–9.

113 Kurino M, Yoshioka S, Ushio Y. Spontaneous dissecting aneurysms of anterior and middle cerebral artery associated with brain infarction: a case report and review of the literature. *Surg Neurol* 2002; **57**:428–36.

114 Aoki N. Do intracranial arteriovenous malformations cause subarachnoid haemorrhage? Review of computed tomography features of ruptured arteriovenous malformations in the acute stage. *Acta Neurochir (Wien)* 1991; **112**(3–4):92–5.

115 Al-Shahi R, Bhattacharya JJ, Currie DG, Papanastassiou V, Ritchie V, Roberts RC *et al*. Prospective, population-based detection of intracranial vascular malformations in adults: the Scottish Intracranial Vascular Malformation Study (SIVMS). *Stroke* 2003; **34**:1163–9.

116 Stapf C, Mast H, Sciacca RR, Berenstein A, Nelson PK, Gobin YP *et al*. The New York Islands AVM Study: design, study progress, and initial results. *Stroke* 2003; **34**:e29–e33.

117 Linn FHH, Rinkel GJE, Algra A, van Gijn J. Incidence of subarachnoid hemorrhage: Role of region, year, and rate of computed tomography: a meta-analysis. *Stroke* 1996; **27**:625–9.

118 Van Gijn J, van Dongen KJ. The time course of aneurysmal haemorrhage on computed tomograms. *Neuroradiology* 1982; **23**(3):153–6.

119 Abbed KM, Ogilvy CS. Intracerebral hematoma from aneurysm rupture. *Neurosurg Focus* 2003; **15**(4):1–5.

120 Kloster R. [Subarachnoid hemorrhage in Vestfold county. Occurrence and prognosis]. *Tidsskr Nor Laegeforen* 1997; **117**:1879–82.

121 Brown RD, Jr., Wiebers DO, Forbes GS. Unruptured intracranial aneurysms and arteriovenous malformations: frequency of intracranial hemorrhage and relationship of lesions. *J Neurosurg* 1990; **73**(6):859–63.

122 Marks MP, Lane B, Steinberg GK, Snipes GJ. Intranidal aneurysms in cerebral arteriovenous malformations: evaluation and endovascular treatment. *Radiology* 1992; **183**(2):355–60.

123 Stapf C, Mohr JP, Pile-Spellman J, Sciacca RR, Hartmann A, Schumacher HC *et al*. Concurrent arterial aneurysms in brain arteriovenous malformations with haemorrhagic presentation. *J Neurol Neurosurg Psychiatry* 2002; **73**:294–8.

124 Kim EJ, Halim AX, Dowd CF, Lawton MT, Singh V, Bennett J *et al*. The relationship of coexisting extranidal aneurysms to intracranial hemorrhage in patients harboring brain arteriovenous malformations. *Neurosurgery* 2004; **54**:1349–57.

125 Nakatomi H, Segawa H, Kurata A, Shiokawa Y, Nagata K, Kamiyama H *et al*. Clinicopathological study of intracranial fusiform and dolichoectatic aneurysms: insight on the mechanism of growth. *Stroke* 2000; **31**:896–900.

126 Passero SG, Calchetti B, Bartalini S. Intracranial bleeding in patients with vertebrobasilar dolichoectasia. *Stroke* 2005; **36**:1421–5.

127 Ricolfi F, Decq P, Brugieres P, Blustajn J, Melon E, Gaston A. Ruptured fusiform aneurysm of the superior third of the basilar artery associated with the absence of the midbasilar artery: case report. *J Neurosurg* 1996; **85**:961–5.

128 Flemming KD, Josephs K, Wijdicks EFM. Enlarging vertebrobasilar dolichoectasia with subarachnoid hemorrhage heralded by recurrent ischemia: case illustration. *J Neurosurg* 2000; **92**:504.

129 Flemming KD, Wiebers DO, Brown RD, Jr., Link MJ, Nakatomi H, Huston J, III *et al*. Prospective risk of hemorrhage in patients with vertebrobasilar nonsaccular intracranial aneurysm. *J Neurosurg* 2004; **101**:82–7.

130 Day AL, Gaposchkin CG, Yu CJ, Rivet DJ, Dacey RG, Jr. Spontaneous fusiform middle cerebral artery aneurysms: characteristics and a proposed mechanism of formation. *J Neurosurg* 2003; **99**:228–40.

131 Horie N, Takahashi N, Furuichi S, Mori K, Onizuka M, Tsutsumi K *et al*. Giant fusiform aneurysms in the middle cerebral artery presenting with hemorrhages of different origins: report of three cases and review of the literature. *J Neurosurg* 2003; **99**:391–6.

132 Fuentes S, Levrier O, Metellus P, Dufour H, Fuentes JM, Grisoli F. Giant fusiform intracranial A2 aneurysm: endovascular and surgical treatment. Case illustration. *J Neurosurg* 2004; **101**:704.

133 Selviaridis P, Spiliotopoulos A, Antoniadis C, Kontopoulos V, Foroglou G. Fusiform aneurysm of the posterior cerebral artery: report of two cases. *Acta Neurochir (Wien)* 2002; **144**:295–9.

134 Zicherman J, Roychowdhury S, Demarco JK, Shepard S, Schonfeld S, Keller I *et al*. Endovascular treatment of a ruptured giant serpentine aneurysm of the superior cerebellar artery in a patient with a Chiari II malformation. *Am J Neuroradiol* 2004; **25**:1077–9.

135 Sarkar A, Link MJ. Distal anterior inferior cerebellar artery aneurysm masquerading as a cerebellopontine angle tumor: case report and review of literature. *Skull Base* 2004; **14**:101–6.

136 Liew D, Ng PY, Ng I. Surgical management of ruptured and unruptured symptomatic posterior inferior cerebellar artery aneurysms. *Br J Neurosurg* 2004; **18**:608–12.

137 Josephson SA, Johnston SC. Multiple stable fusiform intracranial aneurysms following atrial myxoma. *Neurology* 2005; **64**:526.

138 Lasjaunias P, Chiu M, ter Brugge K, Tolia A, Hurth M, Bernstein M. Neurological manifestations of intracranial dural arteriovenous malformations. *J Neurosurg* 1986; **64**(5):724–30.

139 Duffau H, Lopes M, Janosevic V, Sichez JP, Faillot T, Capelle L *et al*. Early rebleeding from intracranial dural arteriovenous fistulas: report of 20 cases and review of the literature. *J Neurosurg* 1999; **90**:78–84.

140 Halbach VV, Higashida RT, Hieshima GB, Goto K, Norman D, Newton TH. Dural fistulas involving the transverse and sigmoid sinuses: results of treatment in 28 patients. *Radiology* 1987; **163**(2):443–7.

141 Ciccone A, Citterio A, Santilli I, Sterzi R. Subarachnoid haemorrhage treated with anticoagulants. *Lancet* 2000; **356**:1818.

142 De Bruijn SFTM, Stam J, Kappelle LJ. Thunderclap headache as first symptom of cerebral venous sinus thrombosis. *Lancet* 1996; **348**:1623–5.

143 Carviy Nievas M, Haas E, Hollerhage HG, Lorey T, Klein PJ. Cerebral vein thrombosis associated with aneurysmal subarachnoid bleeding: implications for treatment. *Surg Neurol* 2004; **61**:95–8.

144 Adaletli I, Sirikci A, Kara B, Kurugoglu S, Ozer H, Bayram M. Cerebral venous sinus thrombosis presenting with excessive subarachnoid hemorrhage in a 14-year-old boy. *Emerg Radiol* 2005; **12**:57–9.

145 Chang R, Friedman DP. Isolated cortical venous thrombosis presenting as subarachnoid hemorrhage: a report of three cases. *Am J Neuroradiol* 2004; **25**:1676–9.

146 Oppenheim C, Domigo V, Gauvrit JY, Lamy C, kowiak-Cordoliani MA, Pruvo JP *et al*. Subarachnoid hemorrhage as the initial presentation of dural sinus thrombosis. *Am J Neuroradiol* 2005; **26**:614–17.

147 Nakahara K, Oka H, Utsuki S, Lida H, Kurita M, Mochizuki T *et al*. Pituitary apoplexy manifesting as diffuse subarachnoid hemorrhage. *Neurol Med Chir (Tokyo)* 2006; **46**:594–7.

148 Satyarthee GD, Mahapatra AK. Pituitary apoplexy in a child presenting with massive subarachnoid and intraventricular hemorrhage. *Clin Neurosci* 2005; **12**:94–6.

149 Wohaibi MA, Russell NA, Ferayan AA, Awada A, Jumah MA, Omojola M. Pituitary apoplexy presenting as massive subarachnoid hemorrhage. *J Neurol Neurosurg Psychiatry* 2000; **69**:700–1.

150 Biousse V, Newman NJ, Oyesiku NM. Precipitating factors in pituitary apoplexy. *J Neurol Neurosurg Psychiatry* 2001; **71**:542–5.

151 Reid RL, Quigley ME, Yen SS. Pituitary apoplexy: a review. *Arch Neurol* 1985; **42**(7):712–19.

152 Dodick DW, Wijdicks EFM. Pituitary apoplexy presenting as a thunderclap headache. *Neurology* 1998; **50**:1510–11.

153 Al Wohaibi M, Russell NA, Al Ferayan A, Awada A, Al Jumah M, Omojola M. Pituitary apoplexy presenting as massive subarachnoid haemorrhage. *J Neurol Neurosurg Psychiatry* 2000; **69**:700–1.

154 Noordzij MJ, de Heide LJ, van den BG, Hoving EW. [Pituitary apoplexy: an endocrinologic emergency] Apoplexie van de hypofyse: een endocrinologisch spoedgeval. *Ned Tijdschr Geneeskd* 2005; **149**:2748–51.

155 McFadzean RM, Doyle D, Rampling R, Teasdale E, Teasdale G. Pituitary apoplexy and its effect on vision. *Neurosurgery* 1991; **29**(5):669–75.

156 Gazioglu N, Kadioglu P, Ocal E, Erman H, Akar Z, Oz B. An unusual presentation of Nelson's syndrome with apoplexy and subarachnoid hemorrhage. *Pituitary* 2002; **5**:267–74.

157 Arita K, Kurisu K, Tominaga A, Sugiyama K, Ikawa F, Yoshioka H *et al*. Thickening of sphenoid sinus mucosa during the acute stage of pituitary apoplexy: case report. *J Neurosurg* 2001; **95**:897–901.

158 Brust JC, Dickinson PC, Hughes JE, Holtzman RN. The diagnosis and treatment of cerebral mycotic aneurysms. *Ann Neurol* 1990; **27**(3):238–46.

159 Masuda J, Yutani C, Waki R, Ogata J, Kuriyama Y, Yamaguchi T. Histopathological analysis of the mechanisms of intracranial hemorrhage complicating infective endocarditis. *Stroke* 1992; **23**(6):843–50.

160 Chukwudelunzu FE, Brown RD, Jr., Wijdicks EF, Steckelberg JM. Subarachnoid haemorrhage associated with infectious endocarditis: case report and literature review. *Eur J Neurol* 2002; **9**:423–7.

161 Krapf H, Skalej M, Voigt K. Subarachnoid hemorrhage due to septic embolic infarction in infective endocarditis. *Cerebrovasc Dis* 1999; **9**:182–4.

162 Kowall NW, Sobel RA. Case records of the Massachusetts General Hospital. Weekly clinicopathological exercises. Case 7-1988. A 27-year-old man with acute myelomonocytic leukemia in remission and repeated intracranial hemorrhages. *N Engl J Med* 1988; **318**(7):427–40.

163 Lau AHC, Takeshita M, Ishii M. Mycotic (Aspergillus) arteriitis resulting in fatal subarachnoid hemorrhage: a case report. *Angiology* 1991; **42**:251–5.

164 Ho CL, Deruytter MJ. CNS aspergillosis with mycotic aneurysm, cerebral granuloma and infarction. *Acta Neurochir (Wien)* 2004; **146**:851–6.

165 Young RC, Bennett JE, Vogel CL, Carbone PP, DeVita VT. Aspergillosis. The spectrum of the disease in 98 patients. *Medicine (Baltimore)* 1970; **49**(2):147–73.

166 Hope WW, Walsh TJ, Denning DW. Laboratory diagnosis of invasive aspergillosis. *Lancet Infect Dis* 2005; **5**:609–22.

167 Knouse MC, Madeira RG, Celani VJ. *Pseudomonas aeruginosa* causing a right carotid artery mycotic aneurysm after a dental extraction procedure. *Mayo Clin Proc* 2002; **77**:1125–30.

168 Furuya K, Sasaki T, Yoshimoto Y, Okada Y, Fujimaki T, Kirino T. Histologically verified cerebral aneurysm formation secondary to embolism from cardiac myxoma: case report. *J Neurosurg* 1995; **83**:170–3.

169 Bobo H, Evans OB. Intracranial aneurysms in a child with recurrent atrial myxoma. *Pediatr Neurol* 1987; **3**:230–2.

170 Van Beijnum J, Straver DCG, Rinkel GJE, Klijn CJM. Spinal arteriovenous shunts presenting as intracranial subarachnoid haemorrhage. *J Neurol* 2007; [Epub ahead of print].

171 Aminoff MJ, Logue V. Clinical features of spinal vascular malformations. *Brain* 1974; **97**(1):197–210.

172 Rengachary SS, Duke DA, Tsai FY, Kragel PJ. Spinal arterial aneurysm: case report. *Neurosurgery* 1993; **33**:125–9.

173 Gonzalez LF, Zabramski JM, Tabrizi P, Wallace RC, Massand MG, Spetzler RF. Spontaneous spinal subarachnoid hemorrhage secondary to spinal aneurysms: diagnosis and treatment paradigm. *Neurosurgery* 2005; **57**:1127–31.

174 Sakamoto M, Watanabe T, Okamoto H. A case of ruptured aneurysm associated with spinal arteriovenous malformation presenting with hematomyelia: case report. *Surg Neurol* 2002; **57**:438–42.

175 Ohmori Y, Hamada J, Morioka M, Yoshida A. Spinal aneurysm arising from the feeding pedicle of a thoracic perimedullary arteriovenous fistula: case report. *Surg Neurol* 2005; **64**:468–70.

176 Anson JA, Koshy M, Ferguson L, Crowell RM. Subarachnoid hemorrhage in sickle-cell disease. *J Neurosurg* 1991; **75**(4):552–8.

177 Preul M, Cendes F, Just N, Mohr G. Intracranial aneurysms and sickle cell anemia: multiplicity and propensity for the vertebrobasilar territory. *Neurosurgery* 1998; **42**:971–7.

178 Carey J, Numaguchi Y, Nadell J. Subarachnoid hemorrhage in sickle cell disease. *Childs Nerv Syst* 1990; **6**(1):47–50.

179 Pegelow CH. Stroke in children with sickle cell anaemia: aetiology and treatment. *Paediatr Drugs* 2001; **3**:421–32.

180 Levine SR, Brust JC, Futrell N, Ho KL, Blake D, Millikan CH *et al.* Cerebrovascular complications of the use of the 'crack' form of alkaloidal cocaine. *N Engl J Med* 1990; **323**(11):699–704.

181 Nanda A, Vannemreddy PSSV, Polin RS, Willis BK. Intracranial aneurysms and cocaine abuse: analysis of prognostic indicators. *Neurosurgery* 2000; **46**:1063–7.

182 Simpson RK, Jr., Fischer DK, Narayan RK, Cech DA, Robertson CS. Intravenous cocaine abuse and subarachnoid haemorrhage: effect on outcome. *Br J Neurosurg* 1990; **4**(1):27–30.

183 Oyesiku NM, Colohan AR, Barrow DL, Reisner A. Cocaine-induced aneurysmal rupture: an emergent negative factor in the natural history of intracranial aneurysms? *Neurosurgery* 1993; **32**:518–25.

184 Krendel DA, Ditter SM, Frankel MR, Ross WK. Biopsy-proven cerebral vasculitis associated with cocaine abuse. *Neurology* 1990; **40**(7):1092–4.

185 Boco T, Macdonald RL. Absence of acute cerebral vasoconstriction after cocaine-associated subarachnoid hemorrhage. *Neurocrit Care* 2004; **1**:449–54.

186 Bruno A, Nolte KB, Chapin J. Stroke associated with ephedrine use. *Neurology* 1993; **43**(7):1313–16.

187 Auer J, Berent R, Weber T, Lassnig E, Eber B. Subarachnoid haemorrhage with 'ecstasy' abuse in a young adult. *Neurol Sci* 2002; **23**:199–201.

188 Rinkel GJE, Prins NEM, Algra A. Outcome of aneurysmal subarachnoid hemorrhage in patients on anticoagulant treatment. *Stroke* 1997; **28**:6–9.

189 Mattle H, Kohler S, Huber P, Rohner M, Steinsiepe KF. Anticoagulation-related intracranial extracerebral haemorrhage. *J Neurol Neurosurg Psychiatry* 1989; **52**(7):829–37.

190 Papa ML, Schisano G, Franco A, Nina P. Congenital deficiency of factor VII in subarachnoid hemorrhage. *Stroke* 1994; **25**(2):508–10.

191 Cummings TJ, Johnson RR, Diaz FG, Michael DB. The relationship of blunt head trauma, subarachnoid hemorrhage, and rupture of pre-existing intracranial saccular aneurysms. *Neurol Res* 2000; **22**:165–70.

192 Sakas DE, Dias LS, Beale D. Subarachnoid haemorrhage presenting as head injury. *Br Med J* 1995; **310**:1186–7.

193 Sahjpaul RL, Abdulhak MM, Drake CG, Hammond RR. Fatal traumatic vertebral artery aneurysm rupture: case report. *J Neurosurg* 1998; **89**:822–4.

194 Rosenow J, Das K, Weitzner I, Couldwell WT. Rupture of a large ophthalmic segment saccular aneurysm associated with closed head injury: case report. *Neurosurgery* 2000; **46**:1515–17.

195 Tomlinson BE, Walton JN. Superficial haemosiderosis of the central nervous system. *J Neurol Neurosurg Psychiatry* 1964; **27**:332–9.

196 Fearnley JM, Stevens JM, Rudge P. Superficial siderosis of the central nervous system. *Brain* 1995; **118**(4):1051–66.

197 Van Harskamp NJ, Rudge P, Cipolotti L. Cognitive and social impairments in patients with superficial siderosis. *Brain* 2005; **128**:1082–92.

198 Kumar N, Lindell EP, Wilden JA, Davis DH. Role of dynamic CT myelography in identifying the etiology of superficial siderosis. *Neurology* 2005; **65**:486–8.

199 Bonito V, Agostinis C, Ferraresi S, Defanti CA. Superficial siderosis of the central nervous system after brachial plexus injury: case report. *J Neurosurg* 1994; **80**(5):931–4.

200 Konitsiotis S, Argyropoulou MI, Kosta P, Giannopoulou M, Efremidis SC, Kyritsis AP. CNS siderosis after brachial plexus avulsion. *Neurology* 2002; **58**:505.

201 Li KW, Haroun RI, Clatterbuck RE, Murphy K, Rigamonti D. Superficial siderosis associated with multiple cavernous malformations: report of three cases. *Neurosurgery* 2001; **48**:1147–50.

202 Padberg M, Hoogenraad TU. Cerebral siderosis: deafness by a spinal tumour. *J Neurol* 2000; **247**:473.

203 Anderson NE, Sheffield S, Hope JKA. Superficial siderosis of the central nervous system: a late complication of cerebellar tumors. *Neurology* 1999; **52**:163–9.

204 McCarron MO, Flynn PA, Owens C, Wallace I, Mirakhur M, Gibson JM *et al.* Superficial siderosis of the central nervous system many years after neurosurgical procedures. *J Neurol Neurosurg Psychiatry* 2003; **74**:1326–8.

205 Mascalchi M, Salvi FP, Pirini MG, D'Errico A, Ferlini A, Lolli F *et al.* Transthyretin amyloidosis and superficial siderosis of the CNS. *Neurology* 1999; **53**:1498–503.

206 Jin K, Sato S, Takahashi T, Nakazaki H, Date Y, Nakazato M *et al.* Familial leptomeningeal amyloidosis with a transthyretin variant Asp18Gly representing repeated subarachnoid haemorrhages with superficial siderosis. *J Neurol Neurosurg Psychiatry* 2004; **75**:1463–6.

207 Uchino A, Aibe H, Itoh H, Aiko Y, Tanaka M. Superficial siderosis of the central nervous system: its MRI manifestations. *Clin Imaging* 1997; **21**:241–5.

208 Canhao P, Ferro JM, Pinto AM, Melo TP, Campos JG. Perimesencephalic and nonperimesencephalic subarachnoid haemorrhages with negative angiograms. *Acta Neurochir (Wien)* 1995; **132**:14–19.

209 Ruigrok YM, Rinkel GJE, van Gijn J. CT patterns and long-term outcome in patients with an aneurysmal type of subarachnoid hemorrhage and repeatedly negative angiograms. *Cerebrovasc Dis* 2002; **14**:221–7.

210 Du Mesnil de Rochemont R, Heindel W, Wesselmann C, Krüger K, Lanfermann H, Ernestus RI *et al.* Nontraumatic subarachnoid hemorrhage: value of repeat angiography. *Radiology* 1997; **202**(3):798–800.

211 Moritake K, Handa H, Ohtsuka S, Hashimoto N. Vanishing cerebral aneurysm in serial angiography. *Surg Neurol* 1981; **16**(1):36–40.

212 Kaim A, Proske M, Kirsch E, von Weymarn A, Radu EW, Steinbrich W. Value of repeat-angiography in cases of unexplained subarachnoid hemorrhage (SAH). *Acta Neurol Scand* 1996; **93**(5):366–73.

213 Iwanaga H, Wakai S, Ochiai C, Narita J, Inoh S, Nagai M. Ruptured cerebral aneurysms missed by initial angiographic study. *Neurosurgery* 1990; **27**(1):45–51.

214 Weisberg LA, Elliott D, Shamsnia M. Intraventricular hemorrhage in adults: clinical-computed tomographic

correlations. *Comput Med Imaging Graph* 1991; **15**(1):43–51.

215 Young WB, Lee KP, Pessin MS, Kwan ES, Rand WM, Caplan LR. Prognostic significance of ventricular blood in supratentorial hemorrhage: a volumetric study. *Neurology* 1990; **40**(4):616–19.

216 Roos YB, Hasan D, Vermeulen M. Outcome in patients with large intraventricular haemorrhages: a volumetric study. *J Neurol Neurosurg Psychiatry* 1995; **58**:622–4.

217 Verma A, Maheshwari MC, Bhargava S. Spontaneous intraventricular haemorrhage. *J Neurol* 1987; **234**(4):233–6.

218 Waga S, Shimosaka S, Kojima T. Arteriovenous malformations of the lateral ventricle. *J Neurosurg* 1985; **63**(2):185–92.

219 Darby DG, Donnan GA, Saling MA, Walsh KW, Bladin PF. Primary intraventricular hemorrhage: clinical and neuropsychological findings in a prospective stroke series. *Neurology* 1988; **38**(1):68–75.

220 Donnet A, Balzamo M, Royere ML, Grisoli F, Ali Cherif A. [Transient Korsakoff's syndrome after intraventricular hemorrhage] Syndrome de Korsakoff transitoire au décours d'une hémorragie intraventriculaire. *Neurochirurgie* 1992; **38**(2):102–4.

221 Caesar B, Middleton PM, Watkins LD. Sudden onset of vomiting as a presentation of perimesencephalic subarachnoid haemorrhage. *Eur J Emerg Med* 2005; **12**:185–7.

222 Hart RG, Byer JA, Slaughter JR, Hewett JE, Easton JD. Occurrence and implications of seizures in subarachnoid hemorrhage due to ruptured intracranial aneurysms. *Neurosurgery* 1981; **8**(4):417–21.

223 Pinto AN, Canhao P, Ferro JM. Seizures at the onset of subarachnoid haemorrhage. *J Neurol* 1996; **243**(2):161–64.

224 Claassen J, Peery S, Kreiter KT, Hirsch LJ, Du EY, Connolly ES *et al.* Predictors and clinical impact of epilepsy after subarachnoid hemorrhage. *Neurology* 2003; **60**:208–14.

225 Polmear A. Sentinel headaches in aneurysmal subarachnoid haemorrhage: what is the true incidence? A systematic review. *Cephalalgia* 2003; **23**:935–41.

226 Linn FHH, Wijdicks EFM, van der Graaf Y, Weerdesteyn-van Vliet FA, Bartelds AI, van Gijn J. Prospective study of sentinel headache in aneurysmal subarachnoid haemorrhage. *Lancet* 1994; **344**(8922):590–3.

227 Linn FHH, Rinkel GJE, Algra A, van Gijn J. The notion of 'warning leaks' in subarachnoid haemorrhage: are such patients in fact admitted with a rebleed? *J Neurol Neurosurg Psychiatry* 2000; **68**:332–6.

228 Chaudhary MY, Sachdev VP, Cho SH, Weitzner I, Jr., Puljic S, Huang YP. Dural arteriovenous malformation of the major venous sinuses: an acquired lesion. *Am J Neuroradiol* 1982; **3**(1):13–19.

229 Salgado AV, Furlan AJ, Keys TF. Mycotic aneurysm, subarachnoid hemorrhage, and indications for cerebral angiography in infective endocarditis. *Stroke* 1987; **18**(6):1057–60.

230 Reijneveld JC, Wermer MJH, Boonman Z, van Gijn J, Rinkel GJE. Acute confusional state as presenting feature

in aneurysmal subarachnoid hemorrhage: frequency and characteristics. *J Neurol* 2000; **247**:112–16.

231 Caeiro L, Menger C, Ferro JM, Albuquerque R, Figueira ML. Delirium in acute subarachnoid haemorrhage. *Cerebrovasc Dis* 2005; **19**:31–8.

232 Benbadis SR, Sila CA, Cristea RL. Mental status changes and stroke. *J Gen Intern Med* 1994; **9**:485–7.

233 Pfausler B, Belcl R, Metzler R, Mohsenipour I, Schmutzhard E. Terson's syndrome in spontaneous subarachnoid hemorrhage: a prospective study in 60 consecutive patients. *J Neurosurg* 1996; **85**:392–4.

234 Frizzell RT, Kuhn F, Morris R, Quinn C, Fisher WS, III. Screening for ocular hemorrhages in patients with ruptured cerebral aneurysms: a prospective study of 99 patients. *Neurosurgery* 1997; **41**:529–33.

235 Stiebel-Kalish H, Turtel LS, Kupersmith MJ. The natural history of nontraumatic subarachnoid hemorrhage-related intraocular hemorrhages. *Retina* 2004; **24**:36–40.

236 Kiriakopoulos ET, Gorn RA, Barton JJ. Small retinal hemorrhages as the only sign of an intracranial aneurysm. *Am J Ophthalmol* 1998; **125**:401–3.

237 Murthy S, Salas D, Hirekataur S, Ram R. Terson's syndrome presenting as an ophthalmic emergency. *Acta Ophthalmol Scand* 2002; **80**:665–6.

238 Manconi M, Paolino E, Casetta I, Granieri E. Anosmia in a giant anterior communicating artery aneurysm. *Arch Neurol* 2001; **58**:1474–5.

239 Haritoglou C, Müller-Schunk S, Weber C, Hoffmann U, Ulbig MW. Central retinal artery occlusion in association with an aneurysm of the internal carotid artery. *Am J Ophthalmol* 2001; **132**:270–1.

240 Kurita H, Kawamoto S, Ueki K, Kirino T. Dejerine syndrome caused by an aneurysmal compression. *Arch Neurol* 2000; **57**:1639–40.

241 Mizobuchi M, Ito N, Tanaka C, Sako K, Sumi Y, Sasaki T. Unidirectional olfactory hallucination associated with ipsilateral unruptured intracranial aneurysm. *Epilepsia* 1999; **40**:516–19.

242 Friedman JA, Piepgras DG, Pichelmann MA, Hansen KK, Brown RD, Jr., Wiebers DO. Small cerebral aneurysms presenting with symptoms other than rupture. *Neurology* 2001; **57**:1212–16.

243 Yanaka K, Matsumaru Y, Mashiko R, Hyodo A, Sugimoto K, Nose T. Small unruptured cerebral aneurysms presenting with oculomotor nerve palsy. *Neurosurgery* 2003; **52**:553–6.

244 Tummala RP, Harrison A, Madison MT, Nussbaum ES. Pseudomyasthenia resulting from a posterior carotid artery wall aneurysm: a novel presentation: case report. *Neurosurgery* 2001; **49**:1466–8.

245 Chan JW, Hoyt WF, Ellis WG, Gress D. Pathogenesis of acute monocular blindness from leaking anterior communicating artery aneurysms: report of six cases. *Neurology* 1997; **48**(3):680–3.

246 Hara N, Mukuno K, Ohtaka H, Shimizu K. Ischemic optic neuropathy associated with subarachnoid hemorrhage after rupture of anterior communicating artery aneurysm. *Ophthalmologica* 2003; **217**:79–84.

247 Date I, Akioka T, Ohmoto T. Penetration of the optic chiasm by a ruptured anterior communicating artery aneurysm: case report. *J Neurosurg* 1997; **87**:324–6.

248 Hyland HH, Barnett HJM. The pathogenesis of cranial nerve palsies associated with intracranial aneurysms. *Proc Roy Soc Med* 1954; **47**:141–6.

249 Vincent FM, Zimmerman JE. Superior cerebellar artery aneurysm presenting as an oculomotor nerve palsy in a child. *Neurosurgery* 1980; **6**(6):661–4.

250 Kamat AA, Tizzard S, Mathew B. Painful third nerve palsy in a patient with perimesencephalic subarachnoid haemorrhage. *Br J Neurosurg* 2005; **19**:247–50.

251 Nadeau SE, Trobe JD. Pupil sparing in oculomotor palsy: a brief review. *Ann Neurol* 1983; **13**(2):143–8.

252 Kissel JT, Burde RM, Klingele TG, Zeiger HE. Pupil-sparing oculomotor palsies with internal carotid-posterior communicating artery aneurysms. *Ann Neurol* 1983; **13**(2):149–54.

253 Keane JR. Aneurysmal third-nerve palsies presenting with pleocytosis. *Neurology* 1996; **46**:1176.

254 Van Gijn J, Hijdra A, Wijdicks EFM, Vermeulen M, van Crevel H. Acute hydrocephalus after aneurysmal subarachnoid hemorrhage. *J Neurosurg* 1985; **63**(3):355–62.

255 Maramattom BV, Wijdicks EFM. Dorsal mesencephalic syndrome and acute hydrocephalus after subarachnoid hemorrhage. *Neurocrit Care* 2005; **3**:57–8.

256 Swash M. Periaqueductal dysfunction (the Sylvian aqueduct syndrome): a sign of hydrocephalus? *J Neurol Neurosurg Psychiatry* 1974; **37**(1):21–6.

257 Fisher CM. Clinical syndromes in cerebral thrombosis, hypertensive hemorrhage, and ruptured saccular aneurysm. *Clin Neurosurg* 1975; **22**:117–47.

258 Senter HJ, Sarwar M. Nontraumatic dissecting aneurysm of the vertebral artery. *J Neurosurg* 1982; **56**:128–30.

259 Sarner M, Rose FC. Clinical presentation of ruptured intracranial aneurysm. *J Neurol Neurosurg Psychiatry* 1967; **30**:67–70.

260 Endo H, Shimizu H, Tominaga T. Paraparesis associated with ruptured anterior cerebral artery territory aneurysms. *Surg Neurol* 2005; **64**:135–9.

261 Greene KA, Marciano FF, Dickman CA, Coons SW, Johnson PC, Bailes JE *et al.* Anterior communicating artery aneurysm paraparesis syndrome: clinical manifestations and pathologic correlates. *Neurology* 1995; **45**(1):45–50.

262 Van de Warrenburg B, Vos P, Merx H, Kremer B. Paroxysmal leg weakness and hearing loss in a patient with subarachnoid hemorrhage. *Eur Neurol* 2000; **44**:186–7.

263 Ferrante L, Acqui M, Mastronardi L, Celli P, Lunardi P, Fortuna A. Posterior inferior cerebellar artery (PICA) aneurysm presenting with SAH and contralateral crural monoparesis: a case report. *Surg Neurol* 1992; **38**:43–45.

264 Laissy JP, Normand G, Monroc M, Duchateau C, Alibert F, Thiebot J. Spontaneous intracerebral hematomas from vascular causes. Predictive value of CT compared with angiography. *Neuroradiology* 1991; **33**(4):291–5.

265 Hillman J. Selective angiography for early aneurysm detection in acute subarachnoid haemorrhage. *Acta Neurochir (Wien)* 1993; **121**:20–5.

266 Kutluhan S, Oyar O, Ozmen S, Noyaner A, Guler K, Yesildag A. The unusually shaped bifrontal hematoma. *Stroke* 2002; **33**:876–7.

267 Jackson A, Fitzgerald JB, Hartley RW, Leonard A, Yates J. CT appearances of haematomas in the corpus callosum in patients with subarachnoid haemorrhage. *Neuroradiology* 1993; **35**(6):420–3.

268 Van der Jagt M, Hasan D, Bijvoet HWC, Pieterman H, Dippel DWJ, Vermeij FH *et al*. Validity of prediction of the site of ruptured intracranial aneurysms with CT. *Neurology* 1999; **52**:34–9.

269 Hino A, Fujimoto M, Iwamoto Y, Yamaki T, Katsumori T. False localization of rupture site in patients with multiple cerebral aneurysms and subarachnoid hemorrhage. *Neurosurgery* 2000; **46**:825–30.

270 Barker RA, Phillips RR, Moseley IF, Taylor WJ, Kitchen ND, Scadding JW. Posterior communicating artery aneurysm presenting with haemorrhage into an arachnoid cyst. *J Neurol Neurosurg Psychiatry* 1998; **64**:558–60.

271 Alliez B, Du Lac P, Trabulsi R. Anevrysme extra-cranien de l'artère cerebelleuse postéro- inférieure. Une observation. *Neurochirurgie* 1990; **36**(2):137–40.

272 Hijdra A, van Gijn J. Early death from rupture of an intracranial aneurysm. *J Neurosurg* 1982; **57**(6):765–8.

273 Weir B, Myles T, Kahn M, Maroun F, Malloy D, Benoit B *et al*. Management of acute subdural hematomas from aneurysmal rupture. *Can J Neurol Sci* 1984; **11**(3):371–6.

274 Kamiya K, Inagawa T, Yamamoto M, Monden S. Subdural hematoma due to ruptured intracranial aneurysm. *Neurol Med Chir Tokyo* 1991; **31**(2):82–6.

275 Ohkuma H, Shimamura N, Fujita S, Suzuki S. Acute subdural hematoma caused by aneurysmal rupture: incidence and clinical features. *Cerebrovasc Dis* 2003; **16**:171–3.

276 Inamasu J, Saito R, Nakamura Y, Ichikizaki K, Suga S, Kawase T *et al*. Acute subdural hematoma caused by ruptured cerebral aneurysms: diagnostic and therapeutic pitfalls. *Resuscitation* 2002; **52**:71–6.

277 Koerbel A, Ernemann U, Freudenstein D. Acute subdural haematoma without subarachnoid haemorrhage caused by rupture of an internal carotid artery bifurcation aneurysm: case report and review of literature. *Br J Radiol* 2005; **78**:646–50.

278 Pritz MB, Kaufman JK. Ruptured middle cerebral artery aneurysm and bilateral chronic subdural hematomas. *Surg Neurol* 2001; **55**:123–5.

279 Clarke E, Walton JN. Subdural haematoma complicating intracranial aneurysm and angioma. *Brain* 1953; **76**:378–404.

280 Schievink WI, Wijdicks EFM, Piepgras DG, Nichols DA, Ebersold MJ. Perimesencephalic subarachnoid hemorrhage. Additional perspectives from four cases. *Stroke* 1994; **25**(7):1507–11.

281 Huttner HB, Hartmann M, Kohrmann M, Neher M, Stippich C, Hahnel S *et al*. Repeated digital substraction angiography after perimesencephalic subarachnoid hemorrhage? *J Neuroradiol* 2006; **33**:87–9.

282 Kershenovich A, Rappaport ZH, Maimon S. Brain computed tomography angiographic scans as the sole diagnostic examination for excluding aneurysms in patients with perimesencephalic subarachnoid hemorrhage. *Neurosurgery* 2006; **59**:798–801.

283 Ruigrok YM, Rinkel GJE, Buskens E, Velthuis BK, van Gijn J. Perimesencephalic hemorrhage and CT angiography: a decision analysis. *Stroke* 2000; **31**:2976–83.

284 Velthuis BK, Rinkel GJE, Ramos LMP, Witkamp TD, Van Leeuwen MS. Perimesencephalic hemorrhage: exclusion of vertebrobasilar aneurysms with CT angiography. *Stroke* 1999; **30**:1103–9.

285 Lavin PJ, Troost BT. Traumatic fourth nerve palsy. Clinicoanatomic correlations with computed tomographic scan. *Arch Neurol* 1984; **41**(6):679–80.

286 Takenaka N, Mine T, Suga S, Tamura K, Sagou M, Hirose Y *et al*. Interpeduncular high-density spot in severe shearing injury. *Surg Neurol* 1990; **34**(1):30–8.

287 Dowling G, Curry B. Traumatic basal subarachnoid hemorrhage. Report of six cases and review of the literature. *Am J Forensic Med Pathol* 1988; **9**(1):23–31.

288 Jenkins A, Hadley DM, Teasdale GM, Condon B, Macpherson P, Patterson J. Magnetic resonance imaging of acute subarachnoid hemorrhage. *J Neurosurg* 1988; **68**(5):731–6.

289 Patel MR, Edelman RR, Warach S. Detection of hyperacute primary intraparenchymal hemorrhage by magnetic resonance imaging. *Stroke* 1996; **27**:2321–4.

290 Mitchell P, Wilkinson ID, Hoggard N, Paley MNJ, Jellinek DA, Powell T *et al*. Detection of subarachnoid haemorrhage with magnetic resonance imaging. *J Neurol Neurosurg Psychiatry* 2001; **70**:205–11.

291 Noguchi K, Ogawa T, Inugami A, Toyoshima H, Okudera T, Uemura K. MR of acute subarachnoid hemorrhage: a preliminary report of fluid-attenuated inversion-recovery pulse sequences. *Am J Neuroradiol* 1994; **15**(10):1940–3.

292 Chrysikopoulos H, Papanikolaou N, Pappas J, Papandreou A, Roussakis A, Vassilouthis J *et al*. Acute subarachnoid haemorrhage: detection with magnetic resonance imaging. *Br J Radiol* 1996; **69**:601–9.

293 Wiesmann M, Mayer TE, Yousry I, Medele R, Hamann GF, Brückmann HM. Detection of hyperacute subarachnoid hemorrhage of the brain by using magnetic resonance imaging. *J Neurosurg* 2002; **96**:684–9.

294 Fiebach JB, Schellinger PD, Geletneky K, Wilde P, Meyer M, Hacke W *et al*. MRI in acute subarachnoid haemorrhage; findings with a standardised stroke protocol. *Neuroradiology* 2004; **46**:44–8.

295 Stone JL, Crowell RM, Gandhi YN, Jafar JJ. Multiple intracranial aneurysms: magnetic resonance imaging for determination of the site of rupture. Report of a case. *Neurosurgery* 1988; **23**(1):97–100.

296 Atlas SW. MR imaging is highly sensitive for acute subarachnoid hemorrhage . . . not! *Radiology* 1993; **186**(2):319–22.

297 Matsumura K, Matsuda M, Handa J, Todo G. Magnetic resonance imaging with aneurysmal subarachnoid

hemorrhage: comparison with computed tomography scan. *Surg Neurol* 1990; **34**(2):71–8.

298 Noguchi K, Ogawa T, Seto H, Inugami A, Hadeishi H, Fujita H *et al*. Subacute and chronic subarachnoid hemorrhage: diagnosis with fluid-attenuated inversion-recovery MR imaging. *Radiology* 1997; **203**(1):257–62.

299 Dreier JP, Sakowitz OW, Harder A, Zimmer C, Dirnagl U, Valdueza JM *et al*. Focal laminar cortical MR signal abnormalities after subarachnoid hemorrhage. *Ann Neurol* 2002; **52**:825–9.

300 Mohamed M, Heasly DC, Yagmurlu B, Yousem DM. Fluid-attenuated inversion recovery MR imaging and subarachnoid hemorrhage: not a panacea. *Am J Neuroradiol* 2004; **25**:545–50.

301 Imaizumi T, Chiba M, Honma T, Niwa J. Detection of hemosiderin deposition by T2*-weighted MRI after subarachnoid hemorrhage. *Stroke* 2003; **34**:1693–8.

302 Quint DJ, Spickler EM. Magnetic resonance demonstration of vertebral artery dissection. Report of two cases. *J Neurosurg* 1990; **72**(6):964–7.

303 Schwaighofer BW, Klein MV, Lyden PD, Hesselink JR. MR imaging of vertebrobasilar vascular disease. *J Comput Assist Tomogr* 1990; **14**(6):895–904.

304 Woimant F, Spelle L. Spontaneous basilar artery dissection: contribution of magnetic resonance imaging to diagnosis. *J Neurol Neurosurg Psychiatry* 1995; **58**:540.

305 White PM, Wardlaw JM, Easton V. Can noninvasive imaging accurately depict intracranial aneurysms? A systematic review. *Radiology* 2000; **217**:361–70.

306 Chappell ET, Moure FC, Good MC. Comparison of computed tomographic angiography with digital subtraction angiography in the diagnosis of cerebral aneurysms: a meta-analysis. *Neurosurgery* 2003; **52**:624–30.

307 Wintermark M, Uske A, Chalaron M, Regli L, Maeder P, Meuli R *et al*. Multislice computerized tomography angiography in the evaluation of intracranial aneurysms: a comparison with intraarterial digital subtraction angiography. *J Neurosurg* 2003; **98**:828–36.

308 Villablanca JP, Hooshi P, Martin N, Jahan R, Duckwiler G, Lim S *et al*. Three-dimensional helical computerized tomography angiography in the diagnosis, characterization, and management of middle cerebral artery aneurysms: comparison with conventional angiography and intraoperative findings. *J Neurosurg* 2002; **97**:1322–32.

309 White PM, Teasdale E, Wardlaw JM, Easton V. What is the most sensitive non-invasive imaging strategy for the diagnosis of intracranial aneurysms? *J Neurol Neurosurg Psychiatry* 2001; **71**:322–8.

310 Van Gelder JM. Computed tomographic angiography for detecting cerebral aneurysms: implications of aneurysm size distribution for the sensitivity, specificity, and likelihood ratios. *Neurosurgery* 2003; **53**:597–605.

311 Hashimoto H, Iida J, Hironaka Y, Okada M, Sakaki T. Use of spiral computerized tomography angiography in patients with subarachnoid hemorrhage in whom subtraction angiography did not reveal cerebral aneurysms. *J Neurosurg* 2000; **92**:278–83.

312 Hirai T, Korogi Y, Ono K, Murata Y, Suginohara K, Omori T *et al*. Preoperative evaluation of intracranial aneurysms: usefulness of intraarterial 3D CT angiography and conventional angiography with a combined unit: initial experience. *Radiology* 2001; **220**:499–505.

313 Carvi y Nievas M, Haas E, Höllerhage HG, Drathen C. Complementary use of computed tomographic angiography in treatment planning for posterior fossa subarachnoid hemorrhage. *Neurosurgery* 2002; **50**:1283–8.

314 Velthuis BK, Van Leeuwen MS, Witkamp TD, Ramos LMP, Berkelbach van der Sprenkel JW, Rinkel GJE. Computerized tomography angiography in patients with subarachnoid hemorrhage: from aneurysm detection to treatment without conventional angiography. *J Neurosurg* 1999; **91**:761–7.

315 Matsumoto M, Sato M, Nakano M, Endo Y, Watanabe Y, Sasaki T *et al*. Three-dimensional computerized tomography angiography-guided surgery of acutely ruptured cerebral aneurysms. *J Neurosurg* 2001; **94**:718–27.

316 Ross JS, Masaryk TJ, Modic MT, Ruggieri PM, Haacke EM, Selman WR. Intracranial aneurysms: evaluation by MR angiography. *Am J Roentgenol* 1990; **155**(1):159–65.

317 Okahara M, Kiyosue H, Yamashita M, Nagatomi H, Hata H, Saginoya T *et al*. Diagnostic accuracy of magnetic resonance angiography for cerebral aneurysms in correlation with 3D-digital subtraction angiographic images – A study of 133 aneurysms. *Stroke* 2002; **33**:1803–8.

318 Mallouhi A, Felber S, Chemelli A, Dessl A, Auer A, Schocke M *et al*. Detection and characterization of intracranial aneurysms with MR angiography: comparison of volume-rendering and maximum-intensity-projection algorithms. *Am J Roentgenol* 2003; **180**:55–64.

319 Ronkainen A, Puranen MI, Hernesniemi JA, Vanninen RL, Partanen PL, Saari JT *et al*. Intracranial aneurysms: MR angiographic screening in 400 asymptomatic individuals with increased familial risk. *Radiology* 1995; **195**(1):35–40.

320 Raaymakers TWM, MARS Study Group. Aneurysms in relatives of patients with subarachnoid hemorrhage: frequency and risk factors. *Neurology* 1999; **53**:982–8.

321 Cloft HJ, Joseph GJ, Dion JE. Risk of cerebral angiography in patients with subarachnoid hemorrhage, cerebral aneurysm, and arteriovenous malformation: a meta-analysis. *Stroke* 1999; **30**:317–20.

322 Hayakawa I, Watanabe T, Tsuchida T, Sasaki A. Perangiographic rupture of intracranial aneurysms. *Neuroradiology* 1978; **16**:293–5.

323 Koenig GH, Marshall WH, Jr., Poole GJ, Kramer RA. Rupture of intracranial aneurysms during cerebral angiography: report of ten cases and review of the literature. *Neurosurgery* 1979; **5**(3):314–24.

324 Saitoh H, Hayakawa K, Nishimura K, Okuno Y, Teraura T, Yumitori K *et al*. Rerupture of cerebral aneurysms during angiography. *Am J Neuroradiol* 1995; **16**(3):539–42.

325 Velthuis BK, Van Leeuwen MS, Witkamp TD, Ramos LMP, Van der Sprenkel JWB, Rinkel GJE. Surgical anatomy of the cerebral arteries in patients with subarachnoid hemorrhage: comparison of computerized tomography

angiography and digital subtraction angiography. *J Neurosurg* 2001; **95**:206–12.

326 Friedman AH, Drake CG. Subarachnoid hemorrhage from intracranial dissecting aneurysm. *J Neurosurg* 1984; **60**(2):325–34.

327 Van der Meulen JHP, Weststrate W, van Gijn J, Habbema JD. Is cerebral angiography indicated in infective endocarditis? *Stroke* 1992; **23**(11):1662–7.

328 Ruelle A, Lasio G, Boccardo M, Gottlieb A, Severi P. Long-term prognosis of subarachnoid hemorrhages of unknown etiology. *J Neurol* 1985; **232**(5):277–9.

329 Spallone A, Ferrante L, Palatinsky E, Santoro A, Acqui M. Subarachnoid haemorrhage of unknown origin. *Acta Neurochir (Wien)* 1986; **80**(1–2):12–17.

330 Juul R, Fredriksen TA, Ringkjob R. Prognosis in subarachnoid hemorrhage of unknown etiology. *J Neurosurg* 1986; **64**(3):359–62.

331 Suzuki S, Kayama T, Sakurai Y, Ogawa A, Suzuki J. Subarachnoid hemorrhage of unknown cause. *Neurosurgery* 1987; **21**(3):310–13.

332 Giombini S, Bruzzone MG, Pluchino F. Subarachnoid hemorrhage of unexplained cause. *Neurosurgery* 1988; **22**(2):313–16.

333 Cioffi F, Pasqualin A, Cavazzani P, Da Pian R. Subarachnoid haemorrhage of unknown origin: clinical and tomographical aspects. *Acta Neurochir (Wien)* 1989; **97**(1–2):31–9.

334 du Mesnil de Rochemont R., Heindel W, Wesselmann C, Kruger K, Lanfermann H, Ernestus RI *et al.* Nontraumatic subarachnoid hemorrhage: value of repeat angiography. *Radiology* 1997; **202**:798–800.

335 Urbach H, Zentner J, Solymosi L. The need for repeat angiography in subarachnoid haemorrhage. *Neuroradiology* 1998; **40**:6–10.

336 Houben MP, Van Rooij WJ, Sluzewski M, Tijssen CC. [Subarachnoid hemorrhage without aneurysm on the angiogram: the value of repeat angiography]. *Ned Tijdschr Geneeskd* 2002; **146**:804–8.

337 Khan N, Schuknecht B, Yonekawa Y. Presentation and management of patients with initial negative 4-vessel cerebral angiography in subarachnoid hemorrhage. *Acta Neurochir Suppl* 2002; **82**:71–81.

338 Inamasu J, Nakamura Y, Saito R, Horiguchi T, Kuroshima Y, Mayanagi K *et al.* 'Occult' ruptured cerebral aneurysms revealed by repeat angiography: result from a large retrospective study. *Clin Neurol Neurosurg* 2003; **106**:33–7.

339 Di Lorenzo N, Guidetti G. Anterior communicating aneurysm missed at angiography: report of two cases treated surgically. *Neurosurgery* 1988; **23**(4):494–9.

340 Acciarri N, Padovani R, Pozzati E, Gaist G, Manetto V. Spinal cavernous angioma: a rare cause of subarachnoid hemorrhage. *Surg Neurol* 1992; **37**(6):453–6.

341 Kandel EI. Complete excision of arteriovenous malformations of the cervical cord. *Surg Neurol* 1980; **13**(2):135–9.

342 Swann KW, Ropper AH, New PF, Poletti CE. Spontaneous spinal subarachnoid hemorrhage and subdural hematoma. Report of two cases. *J Neurosurg* 1984; **61**(5):975–80.

343 Logue V. Angiomas of the spinal cord: review of the pathogenesis, clinical features, and results of surgery. *J Neurol Neurosurg Psychiatry* 1979; **42**(1):1–11.

344 Savader SJ, Williams GM, Trerotola SO, Perler BA, Wang MC, Venbrux AC *et al.* Preoperative spinal artery localization and its relationship to postoperative neurologic complications. *Radiology* 1993; **189**:27–8.

345 D'Angelo V, Bizzozero L, Talamonti G, Ferrara M, Colombo N. Value of magnetic resonance imaging in spontaneous extradural spinal hematoma due to vascular malformation: case report. *Surg Neurol* 1990; **34**(5):343–4.

346 Mohsenipour I, Ortler M, Twerdy K, Schmutzhard E, Attlmayr G, Aichner F. Isolated aneurysm of a spinal radicular artery presenting as spinal subarachnoid haemorrhage [letter]. *J Neurol Neurosurg Psychiatry* 1994; **57**(6):767–8.

347 Schievink WI, Limburg M, Oorthuys JW, Fleury P, Pope FM. Cerebrovascular disease in Ehlers-Danlos syndrome type IV. *Stroke* 1990; **21**(4):626–32.

348 Lee EK, Hecht ST, Lie JT. Multiple intracranial and systemic aneurysms associated with infantile-onset arterial fibromuscular dysplasia. *Neurology* 1998; **50**:828–9.

349 Cloft HJ, Kallmes DF, Kallmes MH, Goldstein JH, Jensen ME, Dion JE. Prevalence of cerebral aneurysms in patients with fibromuscular dysplasia: a reassessment. *J Neurosurg* 1998; **88**:436–40.

350 Román G, Fisher M, Perl DP, Poser CM. Neurological manifestations of hereditary hemorrhagic teleangiectasis (Rendu-Osler-Weber disease): report of two cases and review of the literature. *Ann Neurol* 1978; **4**:130–44.

351 Schievink WI, Mellinger JF, Atkinson JLD. Progressive intracranial aneurysmal disease in a child with progressive hemifacial atrophy (Parry-Romberg disease): case report. *Neurosurgery* 1996; **38**:1237–41.

352 Schievink WI, Mokri B, Piepgras DG, Gittenberger-de Groot AC. Intracranial aneurysms and cervicocephalic arterial dissections associated with congenital heart disease. *Neurosurgery* 1996; **39**:685–9.

353 Mercado R, López S, Cantú C, Sanchez A, Revuelta R, Gómez-Llata S *et al.* Intracranial aneurysms associated with unsuspected aortic coarctation – Report of three cases and review of the literature. *J Neurosurg* 2002; **97**:1221–5.

354 Asaoka K, Houkin K, Fujimoto S, Ishikawa T, Abe H. Intracranial aneurysms associated with aortitis syndrome: case report and review of the literature. *Neurosurgery* 1998; **42**:157–60.

355 Kayembe KN, Sasahara M, Hazama F. Cerebral aneurysms and variations in the circle of Willis. *Stroke* 1984; **15**(5):846–50.

356 Horikoshi T, Akiyama I, Yamagata Z, Sugita M, Nukui H. Magnetic resonance angiographic evidence of sex-linked variations in the circle of Willis and the occurrence of cerebral aneurysms. *J Neurosurg* 2002; **96**:697–703.

357 Nagamine Y, Takahashi S, Sonobe M. Multiple intracranial aneurysms associated with moyamoya disease: case report. *J Neurosurg* 1981; **54**(5):673–6.

358 Conway JE, Hutchins GM, Tamargo RJ. Lack of evidence for an association between neurofibromatosis type I and

intracranial aneurysms: autopsy study and review of the literature. *Stroke* 2001; **32**:2481–5.

359 Van den Berg JSP, Limburg M, Hennekam RCM. Is Marfan syndrome associated with symptomatic intracranial aneurysms. *Stroke* 1996; **27**:10–12.

360 Conway JE, Hutchins GM, Tamargo RJ. Marfan syndrome is not associated with intracranial aneurysms. *Stroke* 1999; **30**:1632–6.

361 Van den Berg JSP, Hennekam RCM, Cruysberg JRM, Steijlen PM, Swart J, Tijmes N *et al*. Prevalence of symptomatic intracranial aneurysm and ischaemic stroke in pseudoxanthoma elasticum. *Cerebrovasc Dis* 2000; **10**:315–19.

362 Escott EJ, Rubinstein D, Cajade-Law AG, Sze CI. Suprasellar cavernous malformation presenting with extensive subarachnoid hemorrhage. *Neuroradiology* 2001; **43**:313–16.

363 Ohshima T, Endo T, Nukui H, Ikeda S, Allsop D, Onaya T. Cerebral amyloid angiopathy as a cause of subarachnoid hemorrhage. *Stroke* 1990; **21**:480–3.

364 Takeda S, Yamazaki K, Miyakawa T, Onda K, Hinokuma K, Ikuta F *et al*. Subcortical hematoma caused by cerebral amyloid angiopathy: does the first evidence of hemorrhage occur in the subarachnoid space? *Neuropathology* 2003; **23**:254–61.

365 Ishikawa T, Nakamura N, Houkin K, Nomura M. Pathological consideration of a 'blister-like' aneurysm at the superior wall of the internal carotid artery: case report. *Neurosurgery* 1997; **40**:403–5.

366 Abe M, Tabuchi K, Yokoyama H, Uchino A. Blood blisterlike aneurysms of the internal carotid artery. *J Neurosurg* 1998; **89**:419–24.

367 Hochberg FH, Fisher CM, Roberson GH. Subarachnoid hemorrhage caused by rupture of a small superficial artery. *Neurology* 1974; **24**(4):319–21.

368 Marushima A, Yanaka K, Matsuki T, Kojima H, Nose T. Subarachnoid hemorrhage not due to ruptured aneurysm in moyamoya disease. *J Clin Neurosci* 2006; **13**:146–9.

369 Kim CH, Kim HJ. Cervical subarachnoid floating cavernous malformation presenting with recurrent subarachnoid haemorrhage. *J Neurol Neurosurg Psychiatry* 2002; **72**:668.

370 Chehrenama M, Zagardo MT, Koski CL. Subarachnoid hemorrhage in a patient with Lyme disease. *Neurology* 1997; **48**(2):520–3.

371 Nakasu S, Kaneko M, Matsuda M. Cerebral aneurysms associated with Behcet's disease: a case report. *J Neurol Neurosurg Psychiatry* 2001; **70**:682–4.

372 Munn EJ, Alloway JA, Diffin DC, Arroyo RA. Polyarteritis with symptomatic intracerebral aneurysms at initial presentation. *J Rheumatol* 1998; **25**:2022–5.

373 Takahashi JC, Sakai N, Iihara K, Sakai H, Higashi T, Kogure S *et al*. Subarachnoid hemorrhage from a ruptured anterior cerebral artery aneurysm caused by polyarteritis nodosa: case report. *J Neurosurg* 2002; **96**:132–4.

374 Calvo-Romero JM, del Carmen Bonilla-Gracia M, Bureo-Dacal P. Churg-Strauss syndrome presenting as spontaneous subarachnoid haemorrhage. *Clin Rheumatol* 2002; **21**:261–3.

375 Venning MC, Burn DJ, Bashir SH, Deopujari CE, Mendelow AD. Subarachnoid haemorrhage in Wegener's granulomatosis, with negative four vessel angiography. *Br J Neurosurg* 1991; **5**:195–8.

376 Hentschel S, Toyota B. Intracranial malignant glioma presenting as subarachnoid hemorrhage. *Can J Neurol Sci* 2003; **30**:63–6.

377 Yonemitsu T, Niizuma H, Kodama N, Fujiwara S, Suzuki J. Acoustic neurinoma presenting as subarachnoid hemorrhage. *Surg Neurol* 1983; **20**(2):125–30.

378 Scotti G, Filizzolo F, Scialfa G, Tampieri D, Versari P. Repeated subarachnoid hemorrhages from a cervical meningioma: case report. *J Neurosurg* 1987; **66**(5):779–81.

379 Vilela P, Saraiva P, Goulao A. Intracranial angiolipoma as cause of subarachnoid haemorrhage: case report and review of the literature. *Neuroradiology* 2005; **47**:91–6.

380 Corriero G, Iacopino DG, Valentini S, Lanza PL. Cervical neuroma presenting as a subarachnoid hemorrhage: case report. *Neurosurgery* 1996; **39**:1046–9.

381 Caputi F, De Sanctis S, Gazzeri G, Gazzeri R. Neuroma of the spinal accessory nerve disclosed by a subarachnoid hemorrhage: case report. *Neurosurgery* 1997; **41**:946–50.

382 Collignon FP, Friedman JA, Atkinson JLD. Recurrent intraventricular and subarachnoid hemorrhage due to an intracranial schwannoma: case illustration. *J Neurosurg* 2002; **96**:377.

383 Parmar H, Pang BC, Lim CC, Chng SM, Tan KK. Spinal schwannoma with acute subarachnoid hemorrhage: a diagnostic challenge. *Am J Neuroradiol* 2004; **25**:846–50.

384 Inci S, Bozkurt G, Gulsen S, Firat P, Ozgen T. Rare cause of subarachnoid hemorrhage: spinal meningeal carcinomatosis: case report. *J Neurosurg* Spine 2005; **2**:79–82.

385 Montinaro A, Cantisani P, Punzi F, D'Agostino A. Cauda equina melanoma presenting with subarachnoid hemorrhage: a case report. *J Neurosurg Sci* 2004; **48**:139–41.

386 Berlis A, Schumacher M, Spreer J, Neumann HP, van V, V. Subarachnoid haemorrhage due to cervical spinal cord haemangioblastomas in a patient with von Hippel-Lindau disease. *Acta Neurochir (Wien)* 2003; **145**:1009–13.

387 Kallmes DF, Lanzino G, Dix JE, Dion JE, Do H, Woodcock RJ *et al*. Patterns of hemorrhage with ruptured posterior inferior cerebellar artery aneurysms: CT findings in 44 cases. *Am J Roentgenol* 1997; **169**:1169–71.

388 Lewis SB, Chang DWJ, Peace DA, LaFrentz PJ, Day AL. Distal posterior inferior cerebellar artery aneurysms: clinical features and management. *J Neurosurg* 2002; **97**:756–66.

389 Horie N, Takahashi N, Furuichi S, Mori K, Onizuka M, Tsutsumi K *et al*. Ruptured aneurysm at the choroidal branch of the posterior inferior cerebellar artery: a case report and review of the literature. *Surg Neurol* 2003; **60**:540–4.

390 Oana K, Murakami T, Beppu T, Yamaura A, Kanaya H. Aneurysm of the distal anterior inferior cerebellar artery unrelated to the cerebellopontine angle: case report. *Neurosurgery* 1991; **28**(6):899–903.

391 van Rybroek JJ, Moore SA. Sudden death from choroid plexus vascular malformation hemorrhage: case report and review of the literature. *Clin Neuropathol* 1990; 9(1):39–45.

392 Kataoka K, Taneda M. Angiographic disappearance of multiple dural arteriovenous malformations: case report. *J Neurosurg* 1984; 60(6):1275–8.

393 Irie F, Fujimoto S, Uda K, Toyoda K, Hagiwara N, Inoue T *et al.* Primary intraventricular hemorrhage from dural arteriovenous fistula. *J Neurol Sci* 2003; 215:115–18.

394 Jabbour R, Taher A, Shamseddine A, Atweh SF. Moyamoya syndrome with intraventricular hemorrhage in an adult with factor V Leiden mutation. *Arch Neurol* 2005; 62:1144–6.

395 Masson C, Martin N, Masson M, Cambier J. Hémorragie intraventriculaire après endarteriectomie carotidienne. Role des suppléances de type moyamoya. *Rev Neurol (Paris)* 1986; 142(8–9):716–19.

396 Hamada J, Hashimoto N, Tsukahara T. Moyamoya disease with repeated intraventricular hemorrhage due to aneurysm rupture: report of two cases. *J Neurosurg* 1994; 80(2):328–31.

397 Gates PC, Barnett HJM, Vinters HV, Simonsen RL, Siu K. Primary intraventricular hemorrhage in adults. *Stroke* 1986; 17(5):872–7.

398 Stieltjes N, Calvez T, Demiguel V, Torchet MF, Briquel ME, Fressinaud E *et al.* Intracranial haemorrhages in French haemophilia patients (1991–2001): clinical presentation, management and prognosis factors for death. *Haemophilia* 2005; 11:452–8.

399 Tsubota A, Shishiba Y, Shimizu T, Ozawa Y, Sawano S, Yamada S. Masked Cushing's disease in an aged man associated with intraventricular hemorrhage and tuberculous peritonitis. *Jpn J Med* 1991; 30(3):233–7.

400 Pallud J, Nataf F, Roujeau T, Roux FX. Intraventricular haemorrhage from a renal cell carcinoma pituitary metastasis. *Acta Neurochir (Wien)* 2005; 147:1003–4.

401 Poon TP, Solis OG. Sudden death due to massive intraventricular hemorrhage into an unsuspected ependymoma. *Surg Neurol* 1985; 24(1):63–6.

402 Bosnjak R, Derham C, Popovic M, Ravnik J. Spontaneous intracranial meningioma bleeding: clinicopathological features and outcome. *J Neurosurg* 2005; 103:473–84.

403 Pascual J, Diez C, Carda JR, Vazquez Barquero A. Intraventricular haemorrhage complicating a brain abscess. *Postgrad Med J* 1987; 63(743):785–7.

404 Wong CW, Ho YS. Intraventricular haemorrhage and hydrocephalus caused by intraventricular parasitic granuloma suggesting cerebral sparganosis. *Acta Neurochir (Wien)* 1994; 129(3–4):205–8.

405 Imanse J, Vanneste JAL. Intraventricular hemorrhage following amphetamine abuse. *Neurology* 1990; 40(8):1318–19.

406 Moriya F, Hashimoto Y. A case of fatal hemorrhage in the cerebral ventricles following intravenous use of methamphetamine. *Forensic Sci Int* 2002; 129:104–9.

407 Pfister HW, Von Rosen F. Severe intraventricular haemorrhage shown by computed tomography as an unusual manifestation of Wernicke's encephalopathy. *J Neurol Neurosurg Psychiatry* 1995; 59:555–6.

408 Van der Wee N, Rinkel GJE, Hasan D, van Gijn J. Detection of subarachnoid haemorrhage on early CT scans: is lumbar puncture still indicated after a negative scan. *J Neurol Neurosurg Psychiatry* 1995; 58:357–359.

10 A practical approach to the management of stroke and transient ischaemic attack patients

This chapter introduces the general principles of managing patients with stroke. Because treatment is aimed at improving the patient's outcome, the chapter includes a section on the early prognosis of stroke and the factors that may help predict the progress of individual patients over the first year. It also introduces a model for treating patients that avoids the pitfalls of the traditional approach, which splits treatment artificially into acute care, rehabilitation and continuing care.

10.1 Aims of treatment

The aims of treatment can be summarized as optimizing the patient's chance of surviving and minimizing the impact of the stroke and any recurrent vascular events on the patient and carers. In minimizing the impact of the stroke, one has to think not just about the short-term effects of the stroke in causing the patient's neurological impairments, but also about its effect on the patient's function (i.e. disability) and role in society (i.e. handicap). Therefore, it is useful to consider the consequences of a stroke in terms of the original World Health Organization (WHO) International Classification of Impairments, Disabilities and Handicaps (ICIDH).[1]

Stroke: practical management, 3rd edition. C. Warlow, J. van Gijn, M. Dennis, J. Wardlaw, J. Bamford, G. Hankey, P. Sandercock, G. Rinkel, P. Langhorne, C. Sudlow and P. Rothwell. Published 2008 Blackwell Publishing. ISBN 978-1-4051-2766-0.

A revision of this original classification, the WHO International Classification of Functioning, Disabilities and Health substituted some new terms (Table 10.1) for old ones to emphasize positive aspects (i.e. activity, not disability; participation, not handicap) and to highlight the important 'contextual' factors – e.g. personal experiences, physical and social environment – that influence the impact of disease, at each level, on the individual.[2,3] However, we find the original version easier to relate to our patients' condition and therefore will refer to that version in the following sections.

Although not included in the WHO classifications, *quality of life* is obviously an important aspect of a patient's outcome. However, there is no generally accepted definition of quality of life, and it is therefore not surprising that it is difficult to measure (section 17.12.5).

> The consequences of a stroke must be considered at five levels: pathology, impairment, disability, handicap and quality of life.

The most obvious effects of a stroke are physical, but in many situations these may not be as important as the cognitive, psychological, social and even financial consequences. Thus, treatment that aims to minimize the impact of a stroke on patients and their carers must be directed at all of these various problems.

10.1.1 Aspects of treatment

Each patient has a unique blend of pathologies, impairments, disabilities and handicaps. Therefore it follows that treatment must be preceded by a comprehensive assessment and then tailored to that individual patient.

Table 10.1 Levels within the World Health Organization (WHO) International Classification of Impairments, Disabilities and Handicaps (with some new terms introduced in the WHO International Classification of Functioning, Disabilities and Health).

Pathology: the underlying pathological substrate of the stroke, e.g. ischaemic stroke due to embolic occlusion of a middle cerebral artery from thrombus in the left atrium, resulting from atrial fibrillation due to ischaemic heart disease. Specific medical and surgical treatments (e.g. thrombolytic or neuroprotective drugs) are directed at this level of the disease process (Chapters 12–15).

Impairment: any loss or abnormality of specific psychological, physiological, or anatomical structure or function caused by the stroke (e.g. muscle weakness or spasticity, loss of sensation, aphasia). Physical therapies, such as physiotherapy or electromyographic biofeedback, are directed at this level (section 11.21).

Disability (activity): any restriction or lack (resulting from an impairment) of ability to perform an activity in the manner or within the range considered normal for a human being (e.g. inability to walk, wash, feed, etc.) due to the stroke. Physical therapies are also used to try to reduce the disability related to impairments.

Handicap (participation): the disadvantage for a given individual, resulting from an impairment or disability, that limits or prevents the fulfilment of a role (depending on age, sex, social and cultural factors) for that individual – e.g. inability to continue the same job. Although more difficult to define and measure than the other levels of disease, handicap is probably the level that best reflects the patient's and carer's perspective. Many aspects of treatment will impact on handicap, but occupational therapy and social work are those most obviously aimed at influencing this level.

Traditionally, the discussion of the treatment of stroke is split into sections on: general treatment in the acute phase; acute medical and surgical treatments; secondary prevention; rehabilitation; and continuing care. However, this structure does not reflect the need for an integrated approach to the management of the patient, even though remnants of this structure remain in this book. For example, patients may develop acute problems (e.g. pneumonia, pulmonary embolism or urinary tract infection) or recurrent vascular events at any stage in their illness, quite often during what is commonly called rehabilitation.[4] Conversely, certain aspects of rehabilitation, such as teamwork and early mobilization, are just as important on the day of stroke onset as they are later on.

The term 'rehabilitation' means different things to different people. Unfortunately, to many physicians who are responsible for the care of stroke patients, the term is synonymous with physical therapy (e.g. physiotherapy, occupational therapy, and speech and language therapy).

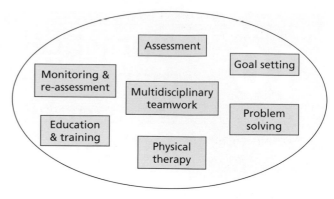

Fig. 10.1 The complex process called 'rehabilitation'.

Having referred the patient to one or more therapists, a physician then mistakenly believes that 'rehabilitation' has been organized. This is far too simplistic (Fig. 10.1). Although there is no universally accepted definition of rehabilitation, most people would view it as a 'goal-orientated' process aimed at minimizing the functional consequences of the stroke, minimizing the impact of the stroke on the lives of the patient and any carers, and maximizing their autonomy. If we include in our definition *all* those components of care that have these aims, it is apparent that rehabilitation must embrace most aspects of care, ranging from the acute medical treatment through to making alterations to the patient's home prior to hospital discharge and providing support later on. Achieving the best possible outcome for the patient requires a broad approach rather than one that just focuses on the primary lesion, or just on the resulting impairments.

Rehabilitation is not synonymous with physical therapies such as physiotherapy or occupational therapy – it is a far more complex process including assessment, goal-setting, physical therapies, reassessment and teamwork.

When the problem is thought of in this way, it becomes artificial – and perhaps even harmful – to separate stroke management into acute care, secondary prevention, rehabilitation and continuing care. All aspects are going on simultaneously. To compound the problem, these separate components of care may even be provided by different staff in different institutions, which leads to a breakdown in communication and lack of continuity of care. Often, in this modular system of care, one encounters a patient who is 'waiting for rehabilitation', i.e. the patient is in the department that normally deals with acute stroke patients but there is no immediate place in the rehabilitation facility and so the patient is not progressing. Conversely, one comes across patients in a 'rehabilitation setting' who have developed acute medical problems (e.g. epilepsy or chest pain) and who are

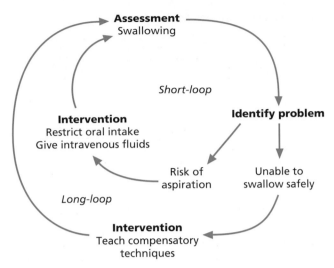

Fig. 10.2 'Short-loop' and 'long-loop' problems.

denied quick access to the necessary facilities or expertise to ensure optimum management of the problems.

> We should abandon the arbitrary division of treatment into acute and rehabilitation phases and adopt an integrated, problem- and goal-orientated approach.

10.1.2 An integrated, problem-orientated and goal-orientated approach

The patient's general management – as distinct from the specific treatment of the stroke pathology (Chapters 12–14) – is primarily aimed at anticipating and preventing potential problems, and solving existing ones that are identified at various stages of the illness. One can think of management in terms of many interwoven cycles or loops (Fig. 10.2). The assessment of a problem, or potential problem, includes not only detecting and perhaps measuring it, but also considering its likely cause and prognosis. This assessment may often have to include the patient's or carer's expectations or wishes (section 10.3.4). Furthermore, assessment is not just a 'once only' activity, but one that should be repeated throughout the illness so that management is tailored to the patient's needs as they change and evolve.

For some problems, this cycle can be completed in a few minutes (e.g. an obstructed airway is a short-loop problem), while for others, the cycle might take weeks to complete (e.g. depression is a long-loop problem). Quite often a problem such as dysphagia will demand both an immediate intervention – e.g. stopping oral intake and giving fluids and perhaps nutrition by an alternative route – and longer-term interventions, such as providing retraining to compensate for swallowing impairment (sections 11.17 and 11.19). Thus, in reality, the general management involves many such cycles layered on top

of each other and cycling at different rates, with each having some influence on the others. This model of management applies equally well to acute general care, rehabilitation and continuing care.

10.1.3 A guide to the following sections on management

We have tried to reflect our integrated approach in the structure of the following discussion on management, which is divided into several sections:

What is this patient's early prognosis? Section 10.2 deals with the prognosis of stroke over the first year or so, with respect to survival and function in groups of patients, and in individual patients.

Delivering an integrated management plan: Section 10.3 deals with general assessment of the patient, the role of the stroke team and its members, and problem-orientated and goal-orientated care.

Some difficult ethical dilemmas: In section 10.4, we discuss some of the ethical dilemmas that arise in treating stroke patients.

What are the patient's problems? A problem-orientated approach to management: Chapter 11 deals with the problems that may occur after stroke, their assessment, and interventions that may help to prevent or solve these problems.

Specific medical and surgical treatments in the acute phase: Chapters 12–14 deal with the pathophysiology of acute stroke and the drug and surgical treatments that aim to reduce the severity of brain injury.

Preventing recurrent stroke and other serious vascular events: Chapter 15 deals with specific interventions to prevent intracerebral haemorrhage while Chapter 16 completes the description of the prognosis of stroke by focusing on the early and later risks of further stroke and other serious vascular events, before moving on to describe various strategies to reduce these risks.

Organizing stroke services: Finally, Chapter 17 focuses on the organizational issues that are important when trying to deliver all these various aspects of treatment to large numbers of stroke patients as efficiently and equitably as possible.

10.2 What is this patient's prognosis?

10.2.1 Introduction

It is useful to try to predict the outcome of individual patients, because this may enable one to:

Table 10.2 Methodological features that are important in assessing a study of prognosis after stroke.[72]

Were the patients identified at an early and uniform point in the course of their disease, and were diagnostic criteria, disease severity, comorbidity and demographic details for inclusion clearly specified?

If they were, then this is called an 'inception cohort'. When applying data from a study of prognosis, it is important to consider whether the patients studied were similar to one's own patients.

Was the referral pattern described?

Did the study avoid the following:

– 'referral filter bias', which occurs when an inception cohort is assembled on selected cases that are not representative of all cases occurring in the population. This is a particular problem with specialist centres, which attract unusual cases (centripetal bias) or admit or track interesting cases (popularity bias).

– 'diagnostic access bias', which occurs if cases are defined by technology (e.g. intracerebral haemorrhage by CT scanning), but the patient's access to the technology is influenced by factors such as their wealth, which may affect their outcome.

Was consent bias avoided?

If inclusion in a cohort requires the patient to give explicit consent then those from whom consent could not be obtained will be excluded. This may include those who refuse consent or more often those in whom there were inadequate research resources to request consent. Patients from whom consent could not be obtained may differ systematically from those included and thus their exclusion may introduce bias in the assessment of prognosis.[73]

Was complete follow-up achieved?

Were all patients who were entered into the study accounted for, and was their clinical status known at the final follow-up? Patients who are lost to follow-up may be systematically different from those who are not. For example, patients with a good recovery may be more mobile or at work and therefore more difficult to follow up, whilst patients may not be followed up because they have died. Therefore, the effect of incomplete follow up on prognosis is difficult to predict.

Were objective outcome criteria developed and used, and were the criteria reproducible and accurate?

To make sense of prognostic data, it is important to know what the authors meant by terms such as 'recurrent stroke' or 'independent', so that one can apply the data to one's own patients. It is also important that the criteria were applied consistently.

Was outcome assessment blind?

In other words, were diagnostic suspicion bias and expectation bias avoided in the assessment of patient outcomes? If the observer has a preconceived view that a particular baseline factor is likely to be related to a particular outcome, knowledge of the presence or absence of that factor at the time of follow-up may bias that observer.

Was adjustment for extraneous prognostic factors carried out?

Where authors relate certain baseline factors to the likelihood of specific outcomes, it is important that they should allow for other baseline factors. The most common example of this is age, which partly explains the observed relationships between other factors, e.g. atrial fibrillation and early death. Before applying predictive equations to one's own patients, it is important for the equation to have been tested on an independent test cohort other than the one from which it was developed.

Was the study prospective or retrospective?

In general, prospective studies provide more reliable data than retrospective ones, because cases and events during the follow-up can be defined using strict criteria, complete data are more likely to be available, and these studies are less prone to bias.

CT, computerized tomography.

- have more informed discussions with the patient and/or their carers;
- set more appropriate short-term and long-term goals (section 10.3.3);
- weigh the potential risks and benefits of treatment options (e.g. one might reserve a particularly hazardous but nevertheless effective treatment for patients in whom the prognosis is poor);
- plan treatment and make early decisions about later discharge and long-term placement to optimize the efficiency of the service;
- make rationing decisions where resources are limited. Thus, if a particular patient is very unlikely to make a good recovery, one could divert resources from that patient to another with a better prognosis who may gain more from the interventions available. It is also

wasteful to use resources on patients who will make a good recovery without any intervention at all. Of course, by adopting this approach, one must avoid self-fulfilling prophecies – i.e. if one withdraws treatment from a patient, he or she may do badly because of the lack of input.

Before considering how to predict an *individual's* prognosis, we shall describe the prognosis of the 'average' patient, i.e. the outcome of an unselected cohort of stroke patients. Here, the prognosis with respect to survival and overall functional outcome is described, since this is relevant to all aspects of treatment. The prognosis for particular individual impairments, disabilities and handicaps is dealt with in the appropriate sections of Chapter 11, while that relating to the risk of late death, recurrent stroke and other vascular events is dealt with in Chapter 16. The prognosis of subarachnoid hae-morrhage is described in detail in Chapter 14.

10.2.2 Collecting reliable information about prognosis

If information about the prognosis of stroke is to be useful, it must have been collected using sound methods that minimize bias and maximize precision, accuracy and generalizability (Table 10.2).

Prognosis or natural history?

It is important to distinguish between these two terms. Natural history refers to the *untreated* course of an illness from its onset, while prognosis refers to the probability of a particular outcome occurring either in an individual or a group of patients over a defined period of time after the disease is first identified. The prognosis is likely to be influenced by any treatment given. Usually, but not always, the prognosis with treatment is better than the natural history, but it may be worse. This section describes the *prognosis* of stroke. No data on the natural history (strictly defined) are available, because in most parts of the world, patients with stroke are usually given some treatment, and in those places where minimal or no treatment is given, no studies of natural history have been reported. Even admission to a hospital, even without any medical or physical therapy, is an inter-vention and could be regarded as 'treatment' which may influence outcome.

Sources of prognostic data

No published study of prognosis after stroke completely fulfils all the criteria summarized in Table 10.2. We have mainly used data from two studies performed in Oxford-shire, UK, which used similar methods which at least partly met these criteria. The Oxfordshire Community Stroke Project collected data during the 1980s and the Oxford Vascular Study (OXVASC) over the last few years.[5,6] Other methodologically sound studies come to broadly similar conclusions, although to compare them directly is difficult because of their different methods, their varying styles of reporting, and because much of the variation in prognosis can be accounted for by differ-ences in case mix and by the play of chance as a result of relatively small sample sizes (section 17.12.6). Most studies have included predominantly white patients managed in quite well-organized healthcare systems – so one must be careful in extrapolating the results to other ethnic groups being cared for in different environments. There is some evidence that the prognosis of stroke may

be improving over time in some populations, although it is unclear whether this is due to improved health of the population, changing severity of stroke, improved treatment, or methodological factors such as improved detection of milder strokes[6-8] (section 18.2).

10.2.3 Prognosis for death

The risks of dying within the first 7 days or 30 days after a first-ever-in-a-lifetime stroke are about 10% and 20%, respectively (Table 10.3). The risk of dying in the years after a stroke remains higher than for stroke-free indi-viduals[9] (Fig. 10.3). Patients with haemorrhagic stroke, either intracerebral or subarachnoid, have a much higher early risk of dying than those with ischaemic stroke although this might be partly explained by studies missing small intracerebral haemorrhages due to delays in brain imaging (Figs 5.1 and 10.4). Patients with *major* ischaemic strokes, i.e. total anterior circulation infarc-tion (section 4.3.4), also have a very high early risk of death (Table 10.3).

Causes of death

Knowing the causes of these early deaths is import-ant if one is to prevent them (Fig. 10.5). In the first few days after stroke, most patients who die generally do so as a result of the direct effects of brain damage.[10] In brainstem strokes, the respiratory centre may be affected by the stroke itself, while in supratentorial ischaemic or haemorrhagic stroke, dysfunction of the

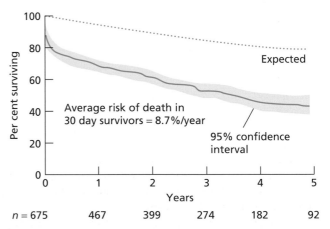

Fig. 10.3 A Kaplan–Meier plot, showing the proportion of patients surviving at increasing intervals after a first-ever-in-a-lifetime stroke compared with the expected survival of people of the same age and sex who have not had a stroke (data from the Oxfordshire Community Stroke Project). The expected survival was derived from all-cause mortality data for Oxfordshire (1985) (reproduced with permission from Dennis *et al.* 1993).[75]

(a) OCSP

Type of stroke	n	Case fatality (%)			
		7 days	30 days	6 months	1 year
All strokes	675	12	19	27	31
Subarachnoid haemorrhage	33	27	46	48	48
Intracerebral haemorrhage	66	40	50	58	62
All ischaemic stroke	545	5	10	18	23
Total anterior circulation infarct	92	17	39	57	60
Partial anterior circulation infarct	186	2	4	11	16
Lacunar infarct	138	2	2	7	11
Posterior circulation infarct	129	5	7	14	19

(b) OXVASC

Type of stroke	n	Case fatality (%)			
		7 days	30 days	6 months	1 year
All strokes	345	11	15	22	24
Subarachnoid haemorrhage	22	41	45	45	45
Intracerebral haemorrhage	33	42	52	58	61
All ischaemic stroke	290	5	9	16	18
Total anterior circulation infarct	22	41	50	64	64
Partial anterior circulation infarct	122	1	4	16	19
Lacunar infarct	80	0	0	1	3
Posterior circulation infarct	66	8	15	18	20

Table 10.3 Death after different pathological types, and ischaemic stroke subtypes, of first-ever-in-a-lifetime stroke. Data from (a) the Oxfordshire Community Stroke Project (OCSP) performed in the 1980s and (b) OXVASC performed in the same population since 2000.

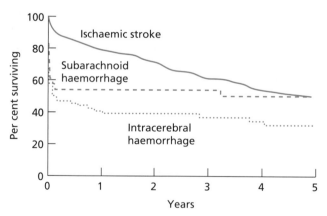

Fig. 10.4 A Kaplan–Meier plot, showing the proportion of patients surviving after a first-ever-in-a-lifetime ischaemic stroke (n = 545), intracerebral haemorrhage (n = 66) and subarachnoid haemorrhage (n = 33) (reproduced with permission from Dennis et al. 1993).[75]

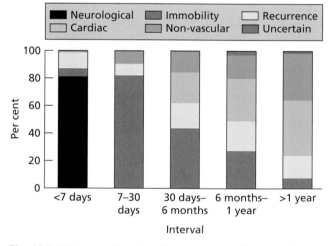

Fig. 10.5 Histogram showing the proportion of patients dying from different causes at increasing intervals after a first-ever-in-a-lifetime stroke (from Bamford et al.;[10] Dennis et al. 1993).[75]

brainstem results from displacement and herniation of oedematous supratentorial brain tissue (Figs 12.8 and 12.9). Deaths occurring within 1–2 h of onset are very unusual in ischaemic stroke, because it takes time for cerebral oedema to develop. Almost all such very early deaths after stroke result from intracranial hae-morrhage of some sort.[5] The very few sudden deaths

are probably due to coexisting cardiac pathology, or perhaps very rarely cardiac complications of the stroke (section 11.2.3).

> Death within a few hours of stroke onset can occur with intracerebral or subarachnoid haemorrhage, or rarely with massive brainstem infarction.

Having survived the first few days, patients may then develop various potentially fatal complications of immobility, the most common being pneumonia (section 11.12) and pulmonary embolism (section 11.13). In addition, pressure ulcers (section 11.16), dehydration (section 11.18.1) with renal failure, and urinary tract infection (section 11.12) may cause death where there is little if any basic care. Because some strokes occur in the context of other serious conditions, e.g. myocardial infarction (section 7.10), cardiac failure (section 6.5.11) and cancer (section 7.12), some early deaths can, at least in part, be attributed to these underlying problems. Also, because the risk of stroke recurrence is highest early after the first stroke – about 20% in the first year (section 16.2) – some patients will die from the direct or indirect effects of a recurrent stroke[11]. This is most likely in patients with aneurysmal subarachnoid haemorrhage (section 14.4.1), in whom the recurrence or rebleed rate is about 30% (without intervention), accounting for the majority of deaths (50% of the total) in the first 30 days.[12]

10.2.4 Prognosis for dependency in everyday activities

Stroke often leaves surviving patients with neurological impairments that prevent them from performing everyday activities and therefore dependent on others. Figures 10.6 and 10.7 show the proportions of survivors who are independent or dependent in everyday activities at various times after a first-ever-in-a-lifetime stroke and in strokes of different pathologies and subtypes. Other studies have produced similar data.[13] It is likely that a greater proportion of patients will become dependent after recurrent strokes. Details of the prognosis with respect to particular impairments, disabilities and handi-

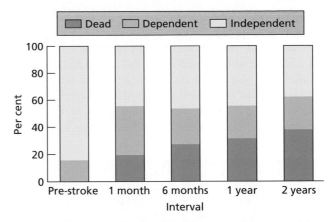

Fig. 10.6 Histogram showing the proportion of patients with different outcomes (i.e. dead, dependent (modified Rankin 3, 4 or 5) or independent (modified Rankin 0, 1 or 2) in activities of daily living) at increasing intervals after their first-ever-in-a-lifetime stroke (unpublished data from the Oxfordshire Community Stroke Project).

caps will be discussed in the specific sections dealing with their treatment (Chapter 11), but it is relevant here to discuss the general pattern of recovery after stroke.

10.2.5 Patterns of recovery

Patients who survive an acute stroke almost always improve to a greater or lesser extent. Improvement is reflected not just in a reduction in the neurological impairments but also in any resulting disability and handicap. The overall 'pattern of recovery' reflects several processes superimposed upon each other.[14] In the first few days after a stroke, ischaemic neurones that were not irreversibly damaged during the primary event (i.e

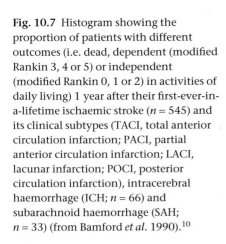

Fig. 10.7 Histogram showing the proportion of patients with different outcomes (i.e. dead, dependent (modified Rankin 3, 4 or 5) or independent (modified Rankin 0, 1 or 2) in activities of daily living) 1 year after their first-ever-in-a-lifetime ischaemic stroke (*n* = 545) and its clinical subtypes (TACI, total anterior circulation infarction; PACI, partial anterior circulation infarction; LACI, lacunar infarction; POCI, posterior circulation infarction), intracerebral haemorrhage (ICH; *n* = 66) and subarachnoid haemorrhage (SAH; *n* = 33) (from Bamford *et al.* 1990).[10]

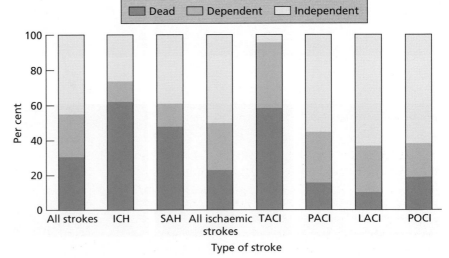

those in the ischaemic penumbra), may start to function because of improved blood supply, reversal of metabolic problems, or reduction of cerebral oedema (section 12.1.5). Resolution of diaschisis (section 5.6) is another explanation for early recovery, although this mechanism has not been well established. Neuroplasticity – the process by which other intact areas of the brain can take over some of the functions of those that have

been irreversibly damaged – might also explain some of the later improvement (Fig. 10.8). However, much of the later recovery with respect to disability and handicap is probably due to adaptive changes – i.e. patients learn techniques to compensate for their remaining impairments, and their environment is altered to maximize their autonomy. Although it is difficult to predict an individual patient's functional outcome, the

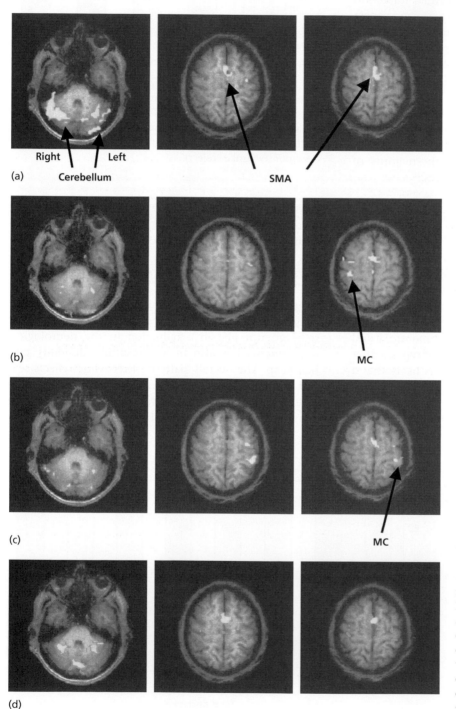

Fig. 10.8 Functional magnetic resonance imaging (fMRI) studies of dynamic changes in patterns of brain activation associated with hand movement accompanying recovery from an ischaemic stroke. The panels show the blood oxygenation level-dependent (*bold*) fMRI activations in the cerebral cortex and cerebellum accompanying flexion–extension of the digits of one hand at about 1.5 Hz. These activation volumes show local areas of increased blood flow with task-specific neuronal activation. The right hemisphere is represented on the left side of the images. Activation of the supplementary motor cortex (SMA), primary sensorimotor cortex (MC) and cerebellum are easily identified. (Also reproduced in colour in the plate section.) (Images courtesy of H. Johannsen-Berg, S. Pendlebury and P.M. Matthews, Centre for Functional Magnetic Resonance Imaging of the Brain, University of Oxford.)

From 2 weeks after the infarct (a) to 5 weeks after the infarct (b), there was functional improvement in the paretic left hand associated with increased activation of right hemisphere MC and decreased activation in SMA and the cerebellum. In contrast, movements of the unaffected right hand do not show clearly significant changes in the patterns of brain activation between the 2-week scan (c) and 5-week scan (d).

following general points can be made to patients and their relatives:

- the rate of recovery is usually fastest in the first few weeks after the initial stroke;
- functional improvement may continue, albeit at a slower rate, for many months and in some patients for 1–2 years;
- the speed and completeness of recovery varies from patient to patient and is relatively unpredictable, at least in the first few days and weeks after stroke onset.

> The pattern of recovery varies among patients and in individuals, and rarely follows that implied by grouped data. Only repeated assessments in individual patients can indicate their own pattern of recovery.

These generalizations are supported by our own experience and also by data from studies in which stroke patients' functional abilities have been repeatedly tested over a period of time.[15–17] Figure 10.9 shows grouped and individual patient data during recovery measured with the Barthel index. The chart shows grouped data which supports the idea that the 'pattern of recovery' follows an almost exponential trajectory. The individual patients within the cohort frequently have different patterns of recovery. Also, the apparent plateau in recovery after a few months may simply reflect the fact that the tools used to measure the function are often 'ordinal' rather than 'interval' scales (section 17.12.5), and also that there is a marked 'ceiling effect' – i.e. the measure is not sensitive to improvements at the upper end of the range of performance.[18] Therefore, the apparent differences in the patterns and duration of recovery for different impairments and disabilities may to some extent reflect the characteristics of the tools used to measure

them. For example, it is often said that language function continues to improve for a very long time after a stroke, while recovery in arm function does not. This different perception may simply be due to patients being acutely aware of even small differences in fluency, while they may only report an improvement in arm function if they can perform a new function with their hand. More research into the patterns of recovery after stroke that takes these points into account would be helpful.

It is unclear whether patterns of recovery differ among different pathological types of stroke (haemorrhagic vs ischaemic)[19–21] or subtypes of ischaemic stroke (lacunar vs cortical). Clinical experience suggests that recovery patterns do vary. For instance, we have seen late and dramatic improvements after intracerebral haemorrhage, but there are few reliable research data to confirm such observations. Although individual patients may continue to improve for a year or even two, the mean or median measure of function in a cohort of stroke patients peaks at about 6 months and then begins to slowly decline.[17] Any decline is presumably the result of a combination of subsequent ageing, recurrent strokes, progression of comorbidity, and perhaps withdrawal of physical therapy, other services and supports (section 11.6).

> The shape of so-called recovery curves may reflect the properties of the instrument used to measure function as much as the patient's rate of improvement.

10.2.6 Is this the prognosis of your patients?

The prognostic data presented in this section come mainly from two cohorts studies in Oxfordshire, UK performed about 20 years apart.[5–6] These prospectively registered

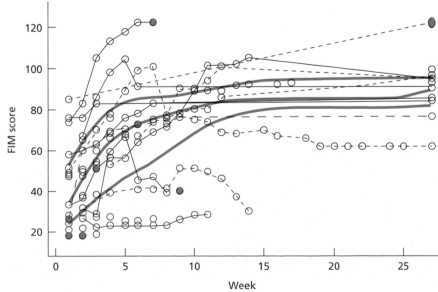

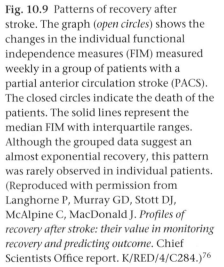

Fig. 10.9 Patterns of recovery after stroke. The graph (*open circles*) shows the changes in the individual functional independence measures (FIM) measured weekly in a group of patients with a partial anterior circulation stroke (PACS). The closed circles indicate the death of the patients. The solid lines represent the median FIM with interquartile ranges. Although the grouped data suggest an almost exponential recovery, this pattern was rarely observed in individual patients. (Reproduced with permission from Langhorne P, Murray GD, Stott DJ, McAlpine C, MacDonald J. *Profiles of recovery after stroke: their value in monitoring recovery and predicting outcome.* Chief Scientists Office report. K/RED/4/C284.)[76]

all patients from a well-defined population who had a first-ever-in-a-lifetime stroke. After assessment by a study neurologist, as soon after the stroke onset as possible, patients were prospectively followed up. Patients were included in the study whether referred to hospital or not, and so provided prognostic data on an unselected community-based cohort of patients with stroke. Studies of prognosis in other community-based series have provided broadly similar results, although higher case fatality has been reported in other populations, e.g. Belluno, Italy.[22] However, the prognosis of patients in one's own clinical practice may be different because of:

- *Different population characteristics*: The stroke population is different from that in Oxfordshire; patients may be younger or older, of different racial or ethnic background, have more or less severe strokes, more or less comorbidity, or a different pattern of stroke pathology. For example, a greater proportion of strokes are attributed to haemorrhage in Japan[23] (sections 5.2 and 18.2.2), and thus one might expect a higher early case fatality (Table 10.3).
- *Referral bias*: In any hospital, the prognosis of patients will be affected by referral bias (Table 10.2). In general, stroke patients referred to hospital can be expected to have a worse prognosis (i.e. a higher case fatality and worse functional outcome) because a greater proportion of milder cases are looked after by their family doctors at home. However, this is not always predictable, since in some places younger patients, who have on average a better prognosis (Fig. 10.10), may be referred to hospital more often than older patients. Furthermore, some patients with very severe strokes

that are likely to lead to death within a few hours, or who are already living in a nursing home, may not be admitted at all and therefore be underrepresented in a hospitalized cohort. Differences in outcome between hospitals are more likely to reflect the differences in the proportions of patients with severe stroke than any differences in treatment given (section 17.12.7).

- *Selection bias*: Hospital admission rates vary considerably from place to place, from country to country, and from time to time. For example, the admission rates in community-based studies have varied between 53% in Siberia, and at least 95% in Umea, Sweden.[24,25] These data have to be interpreted in the knowledge that definitions of hospital admission vary – e.g. did the patient actually spend a night in a hospital bed? And how were patients who had their stroke while in hospital, or who were admitted late after the stroke, handled in the analysis? The type of hospital (e.g. district general, university or tertiary referral hospital) and the specialties represented in it (e.g. neurosurgery, neurology, general medicine, care of the elderly, etc.), will have a major influence on case mix (section 17.12.7), so that clinicians working in different departments and institutions will form, from their own experience, widely differing views of the prognosis of stroke patients.[26]
- *Impact of time from onset*: If patients are seen very early after stroke onset (e.g. because the hospital is in a city, has an accident and emergency unit or provides a thrombolysis service), they are likely to have a worse prognosis than patients who are seen later (such as those referred to a distant tertiary referral centre), because they must survive long enough to be admitted (Table 10.2).
- *Follow-up method*: Unless patients are followed up using similar definitions of outcome and for the same time period as those in the published studies, their prognosis will be different (Table 10.2). Also, the reasons why patients are lost to follow-up may be related to their outcome. For example, if dead patients are lost to follow-up, this biases the prognostic data in a favourable direction, and if patients who have made a good recovery (and are mobile) are lost because they move away, this biases the prognostic data in the opposite direction (Table 10.2). Furthermore, if all patients are not followed up, the perceived prognosis is likely to be overly influenced by the outcome of the last few patients who are remembered most vividly (i.e. recall bias), or perhaps by the patients who had particularly good or particularly bad outcomes.
- *Random errors and small samples*: If the estimate of the outcome is based on the follow-up of too few patients,

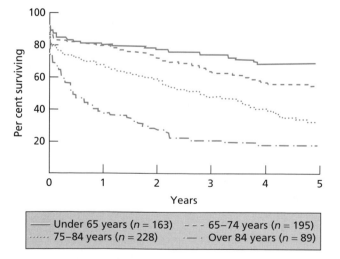

Fig. 10.10 A Kaplan–Meier plot showing the proportion of patients of different ages surviving after a first-ever-in-a-lifetime stroke (reproduced with permission from Dennis *et al.* 1993).[75]

it may differ from that in published studies simply by chance alone.

- *Differences in management*: Patients may be managed more or less effectively than those in Oxfordshire and other published studies, and thus the outcomes may be better or worse. However, the likely impact of differences in treatment between centres is likely to be swamped by other factors that have a much greater influence on outcome (e.g. case mix, section 17.12.7).

> The differences in outcome between your service and those of your colleagues in other hospitals are more likely to reflect differences in the patients you treat than any differences in the quality of care you provide.

10.2.7 Predicting outcome in individual patients

Unfortunately, it is difficult to predict an *individual* patient's outcome accurately enough for it to be of much value in clinical practice. It is also difficult to decide on the acceptable accuracy of any predictive tool, because this depends on the consequences, or cost, of getting it wrong. Taking an extreme example, if one was sure that a patient with an apparently severe stroke who was being supported on a ventilator was not going to have an acceptable long-term quality of life, then one might withdraw ventilatory support, particularly if the patient had left an appropriate advanced directive. However, in this situation one would have to be very confident of one's prediction.[27]

A large number of factors are associated with better than average or worse than average outcomes, including: clinical features shortly after stroke onset; the results of investigations; and the patient's progress over the initial post-stroke period (Table 10.4). Many are interrelated – e.g. conscious level and lesion size on brain computed tomography (CT) – so multiple regression statistical techniques are needed to identify the factors that *independently* predict outcome. Many studies have focused only on factors that are associated with an increased risk of death. However, a growing number also consider those factors that are related to a good or bad functional outcome, and in general, and not surprisingly, these factors are similar to those that predict death (Table 10.4). Unfortunately, methodological problems have so far limited the usefulness of these studies[28–30] (Table 10.5). Therefore, it is useful to have a list of criteria against which one can judge the quality of a study reporting the development of a predictive model to help decide whether it would be 'safe' to use in one's own practice (Table 10.6).

> At present, it is impossible to predict an individual's outcome early after stroke onset with enough accuracy for it to be of much value in clinical practice.

Predicting early death

Clinical features such as decreased conscious level, conjugate gaze palsy, severe bilateral weakness and abnormal breathing patterns which – alone or in combination – indicate severe brainstem dysfunction, due to direct damage or raised intracranial pressure, are highly predictive of early death. These clinical features in combination with radiological features such as massive intracerebral haemorrhage with mass effect can help guide management decisions.[27] However, many patients who die do not have these features, and occasionally patients with more than one of these features make an unexpectedly good recovery. Sometimes one sees patients with single predictive factors of a poor outcome, e.g. just periodic respiration (section 11.2.2) but, in isolation, these factors can be associated with a good recovery; it is the *combination* of prognostic factors that is the more powerful predictor.

Predicting longer-term outcomes

It is even more difficult to predict longer-term outcomes. Many of the factors that predict a high early risk of death also predict a high risk of long-term dependency if the patient survives. In general, the patient's age, pre-stroke health status and indicators of stroke severity (e.g. conscious level, motor impairment, disability, cognitive function) predict the likelihood of survival free of dependency. In predicting longer-term outcome, one also has the problem that further events – which may be related to the initial stroke (e.g. recurrent strokes and myocardial infarction) or may not (e.g. development of unrelated illness) – can occur and have a major and often quite unpredictable effect on outcome. It is even more difficult to estimate an individual's risk of further vascular events (section 16.2.1).

Methods of prediction

A variety of different approaches have been taken in predicting outcome after stroke.

THE SINGLE-FACTOR APPROACH

The simplest method is to identify a single factor, the presence or absence of which early after the stroke indicates the likelihood that the patient will have a good or bad outcome. The most widely used examples are age (Fig. 10.10), reduced level of consciousness (section 11.3)

	Poor survival	Poor survival or poor functional outcome
Demographic features		
Increasing age	+	+
Male sex	+	
Social factors		
Smoking	+	
Excess alcohol	+	+
Unmarried	+	
Living alone	+	
Past history		
Previous stroke/TIA	+	+
Ischaemic heart disease	+	
Peripheral vascular disease		+
Diabetes mellitus	+	
Cancer	+	
General clinical features		
Lost consciousness at onset	+	+
Post-stroke seizures	+	
Atrial fibrillation	+	+
Cardiac failure	+	
Fever	+	
Pneumonia	+	
Obstructive pulmonary disease	+	
Renal disease	+	
Tachycardia	+	
High systolic blood pressure	+	+
High diastolic blood pressure	+	
High pulse pressure		+
Urinary incontinence	+	+
Disability post-stroke	+	+
Neurological signs		
Reduced level of consciousness	+	+
Severe motor deficit	+	+
Bilateral extensor plantars	+	
Pupil abnormality	+	
Impaired proprioception		+
Visuospatial dysfunction		+
Cognitive impairment	+	+
Depression	+	
Poor balance/ataxia		+
Unable to walk	+	
Total anterior circulation syndrome	+	+
Early deterioration	+	
Simple laboratory tests		
High haematocrit	+	
High blood white cell count	+	
High erythrocyte sedimentation rate	+	
Hyperglycaemia	+	
High blood urea/creatinine	+	
High plasma cholesterol	+	
Low arterial Po_2		+
Abnormal electrocardiogram	+	+
Complex tests (CT or MR brain scan)		
Large stroke lesion (haematoma)	+	+
Site of brain lesion	+	+
Mass effect	+	+
Intraventricular blood (in haemorrhagic stroke)	+	+
Visible infarction		+

Table 10.4 Factors that have been shown to be statistically significant ($P < 0.05$) independent predictors of poor survival and/or poor functional outcome after stroke in at least one study including more than 100 patients.[74]

Note: many factors have been identified in just one or two studies, and many of these factors are probably interrelated (e.g. indicating common factors such as frailty, lesion size or stroke severity).

Table 10.5 Methodological problems in studies of prediction of outcome after stroke.

Failure to describe adequately the group of patients in whom the work was done

Use of unrepresentative cohorts of patients, e.g. highly selected patients in rehabilitation settings

Many studies are retrospective, which limits the range and perhaps the reliability of the baseline and outcome data

Failure to adequately define the baseline variables collected

Variation in the timing after stroke of the baseline patient assessments

Failure to measure outcome at a relevant and uniform point after the stroke, i.e. 6 months post-stroke rather than at hospital discharge

Failure to use reliable and valid measures of outcome

Inadequate sample size

Failure to use appropriate statistical techniques to adjust for the interactions between baseline variables

Failure to test the accuracy of any predictive model in an independent data set

---

and urinary incontinence, which have all been related to a poor survival and functional outcome.[30–32] Of course, if urinary catheterization, with all its risks, becomes the norm, urinary incontinence loses its predictive value (section 11.14). Measures of cognitive function at initial assessment (section 11.29) have also been related to poor functional outcomes.[30] Although such models are simple to use, and can guide clinical management, the user must be aware of their inaccuracy. They have a more obvious use in stratifying patients who are being randomized in clinical trials.

> Reduced conscious level and urinary incontinence in the first few days after stroke are both associated, in general, with a poor outcome. Unfortunately, this association is not reliable enough to be anything other than a very rough guide to prognosis in managing individual patients.

THE EXTENT OF BRAIN DAMAGE

In general, the greater the extent, the worse the clinical outcome, except for critically sited strokes, particularly in the brainstem, where even quite small lesions can be fatal. Many of the clinical indicators of poor prognosis relate quite closely to the size of the brain lesion. For example, the Oxfordshire Community Stroke Project classification (section 4.3.8) reflects the extent of brain damage, and so the prognosis of the different groups varies (Fig. 10.7). Imaging techniques, including CT, single-photon emission CT, and magnetic resonance imaging have so far added little to the accuracy of clinical predictors.[33–34] None of this is at all surprising,

---

Table 10.6 Criteria to judge the quality of a study reporting the development of a predictive model for stroke patients (adapted from Counsell 1998).[74]

Is the model externally valid? i.e. is it applicable to your patients?
  Was the model developed in a community-based cohort, i.e. unselected cases?
  Were patients with transient ischaemic attack and subarachnoid haemorrhage separated out?
  Were there any major exclusion criteria?
  Were the age and sex of the patients given?
  Were details of any treatment given?
Is the model internally valid?
  Was the delay between stroke onset and inclusion given, and was it short?
  Were less than 10% of the cohort excluded or lost?
  Were baseline and outcome data collected prospectively?
  Was outcome measured using valid and reliable instruments?
  Was outcome measured at a fixed point after the stroke?
  Was follow-up sufficiently long to provide useful data?
  Were important predictors included, e.g. stroke severity and age?
  Could the predictive variables be collected reliably?
Were statistical analyses appropriate?
  Was a stepwise analysis performed?
  Were the strengths of correlations between predictive variables assessed (i.e. collinearity). Strong correlations between predictive factors can cause multiple regression techniques to give spurious results.
  Was the outcome event per predictive factor ratio greater than 10?
  Was the ability of the model to discriminate between patients with a good and bad outcome tested? This is best done by establishing the sensitivity and specificity of the model over a full range of probabilities, plotting a receiver operating curve and establishing the area under that curve (Fig. 10.11).
  Was the model calibrated to establish any bias of predictions in grouped data? This can be done by plotting the proportions predicted to have a certain outcome against the proportion of patients who actually had that outcome in an independent test data set. Perfect calibration is indicated by the diagonal (Fig. 10.12).
Has the model been validated?
  Has the model been tested in the population from which it was derived?
  Has the model been tested in an independent population?
  Has the model been compared with other predictive systems, including informal clinical judgement?
  Has the model been evaluated in a randomized controlled trial, i.e. is its use associated with improved outcomes?
Is the model practical?
  Could the predictive variables be collected in practice?
  Was the actual model published?
  Were confidence intervals for the model given?

because the extent of the stroke lesion on brain imaging can so often be predicted from the clinical findings (section 4.3.7). Moreover, a substantial proportion of patients have a normal or near normal CT scan early after even a major ischaemic stroke, which weakens the early predictive utility of CT imaging (section 5.4.2). Other technologies, such as transcranial magnetic stimulation, have been shown to predict outcome though it is unclear how much they add to prediction based on simpler methods.[35]

> In general, the larger the stroke lesion, the worse the likely outcome, except for small, critically sited lesions, which may be associated with a poor outcome.

MATHEMATICAL MODELS

These are based on regression analyses and have been developed by several groups to predict both survival and functional outcome.[36–37] Although these are generally a little more accurate than models based on a single variable, any advantage may be offset by the practical difficulties in applying them.[38] Also, only a couple, a simple six-variable model (Table 10.7) and the Orpington Prognostic Score have been externally validated in independent cohorts of sufficient size[37,39,40] (Figs 10.11, 10.12). As one would predict, where they are externally validated they generally perform less well than in the cohort from which they were developed (internal validation).[31,37] If such models are to be used in routine clinical practice, they need to be further refined, tested prospectively in large independent cohorts of patients, and

made more reliable and 'user-friendly', so that they do not require the clinician to perform complex calculations.[41] Nonetheless, such models have been used to stratify groups of patients by predicted prognosis in large randomized trials, in which complex calculations are easily performed by computer during the randomization process.[42] Indeed, large randomized trials provide an excellent opportunity to test such predictive models prospectively.[43]

STROKE SCALES

These provide *scores* which, depending on the presence, absence, or severity of various neurological impairments, are frequently used to describe the severity of stroke in the acute phase and have also been used to predict outcome. However, because strokes scales such as the National Institutes of Health Stroke Scale (NIHSS) reflect stroke severity but not other predictive factors, such as age or pre-stroke function, the addition of these latter factors is bound to add to the scale's predictive accuracy for death or dependency.[44,45] Although the NIHSS has similar predictive accuracy to mathematical models (e.g. Guy's and Orpington prognostic scales), it contains items which add little to its performance (i.e. there is a lot of redundancy).[39,46,47]

PREDICTIONS BASED ON MEASURES OF FUNCTION EARLY AFTER A STROKE

Scales such as the Barthel index have been used to predict eventual functional outcome and may be particularly useful for those working in rehabilitation facilities.[30]

Variable†	Parameter coefficient, b (SE)	Odds ratio (95% CI)
Constant	15.586 (1.748)	
Age	–0.085 (0.014)	0.92‡ (0.89–0.94)
Living alone	0.384 (0.259)	0.68 (0.41–1.14)
Independent pre-stroke	–3.174 (0.639)	25.00 (6.67–100)
Normal Glasgow Coma Scale verbal	–2.177 (0.504)	9.09 (3.33–25)
Able to lift arms	–2.319 (0.513)	10.00 (3.70–25)
Able to walk	–1.154 (0.402)	3.12 (1.45–7.14)

† Dichotomous variables were coded 1 = yes, 2 = no.
‡ Per year of age.
Probability of outcome is calculated by: $P = e^Y/(1 + e^Y)$, where $Y = a + b_1X_1 + b_2X_2 + \ldots + b_iX_i$.
$Y = 15.586 – (0.085 \times age) + (0.384 \times living\ alone) – (3.174 \times independent\ pre$-stroke$) – (2.177 \times normal\ GCS\ verbal) – (2.319 \times able\ to\ lift\ arms) – (1.154 \times able\ to\ walk)$, where dichotomous variables have numeric values of 1 or 2 as described above.

Table 10.7 A mathematical model to predict the probability of survival free from dependency in activities of daily living 1 year after a stroke. This was derived from the Oxfordshire Community Stroke Project using logistic regression, and has been externally validated on two independent cohorts of stroke patients (Figs 10.11 and 10.12). Calculating the probability of an outcome is complex (see equation), but easily achieved using a programmable calculator or a nomogram. Health warning – this model should not be used to make firm predictions in individual patients!

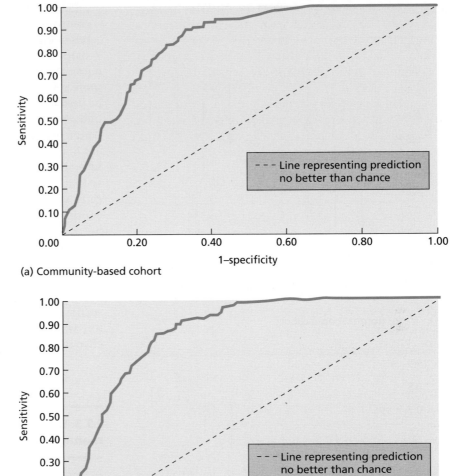

(a) Community-based cohort

(b) Hospital-based cohort

Fig. 10.11 Receiver operating characteristic (ROC) curves for a statistical model (Table 10.7) to predict the probability of survival free of dependency 1 year after stroke. The model was derived from the Oxfordshire Community Stroke Project, and has been tested on two independent cohorts of stroke patients: (a) a community-based cohort derived from the SEPIVAC and Perth Stroke Registries and (b) a hospital-based cohort, the Lothian Stroke Registry. The area under the curves indicates the accuracy of the model – i.e. the larger the area, the more discriminatory the model. The diagonal line indicates prediction no better than chance.

RATE OF CHANGE

Some repeated measure of the patient's condition during the early clinical course can be used to predict the likely longer-term outcome.[48,49] This might be likened to the growth curves used by paediatricians. Predictions for individuals would then depend on the pattern of recovery observed in large cohorts of patients.

INFORMAL JUDGEMENT

The most common method of prediction is the informal judgements we make about patients during our daily work. The accuracy seems to be similar to those of mathematical models, at least in predicting a simple dichotomous outcome (dependent or independent), but this is bound to depend on the experience of the clinician.[50]

In practice, the predictive systems developed so far are not sufficiently accurate to influence important clinical decisions in individuals. However, they may be useful as tools to:

- guide less experienced clinicians in what to say to patients and carers;
- choose who to randomize in trials of acute treatment;
- help decide which patient is likely to require an extended period of rehabilitation;
- assess the quality of care, for example by adjusting outcome data from different *groups* of patients for

(a) Community-based cohort

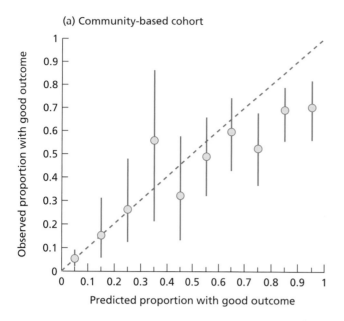

(b) Hospital-based cohort

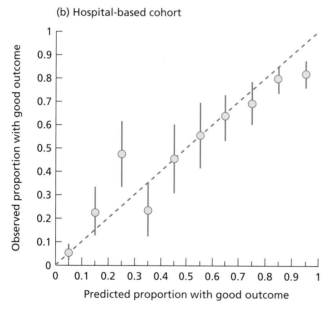

Fig. 10.12 Calibration of a statistical model (Table 10.7) to predict the probability of survival free of dependency 1 year after a stroke (i.e. good outcome). The model was derived from the Oxfordshire Community Stroke Project, and has been tested on two independent cohorts of stroke patients: (a) a community-based cohort derived from the SEPIVAC and Perth Stroke Registries and (b) a hospital based cohort, the Lothian Stroke Registry. The dotted line indicates perfect calibration. The vertical lines indicate the 95% confidence intervals, which depend on the number of patients in each at-risk group. The model calibrates better in the hospital-based than in the community-based cohort, and tends to be over-optimistic in those with the greatest probability of a good outcome (survival free of dependency).

differences in case mix at baseline, one can begin to compare the quality of care given by different hospitals or units (section 17.12.7).

In the future, we hope the fairly crude predictive models currently available will be replaced by more precise, more robust and better-validated models. These might be used to predict not only survival and basic functional outcome, but also the rate of recovery of individual impairments, disabilities and handicaps, which is so important in planning treatment. One might come to combine several approaches to predicting a patient's outcome, so that one relies on the mathematical modelling in the early stages, but as more data become available from continued observation of the patient, a patient's specific 'recovery curve' might be plotted.[48] One could imagine that these predictive systems could be presented in several forms for clinical use: wall charts; clinical slide rules; on pocket calculators; palm or desktop computers, or hospital-wide computer networks. Eventually, any such system will inevitably consume resources and therefore will have to be tested to show that it improves the effectiveness and efficiency of stroke services.

10.3 Delivering an integrated management plan

10.3.1 Introduction

The term 'stroke' embraces a very wide spectrum of clinical presentations ranging from neurological deficits lasting just one day to those leading rapidly to death or causing lifelong disability. These deficits are layered on a complex mix of pre-existing disease, personality, social and environmental factors. We have already seen the range of possible pathological types (Chapter 5) and causes (Chapters 6–9), but each patient requires a management plan tailored to his or her own individual needs. For a patient whose symptoms resolve completely within a few days, the emphasis should be on diagnosis and secondary prevention. In a patient with a major disabling stroke, the emphasis must be on treatment of the acute phase, prevention of complications and rehabilitation, although of course secondary prevention is still relevant. As ever, the essential first step in formulating a management plan is a full and detailed assessment. However, this will in practice often be staged so that one might perform a rapid, less detailed assessment very early to guide hyperacute treatment and follow this up with more detailed, time-consuming assessments later.

Stroke (Face Arm Speech Test)

Speech impairment	YES ☐	NO ☐	? ☐
Facial palsy	YES ☐	NO ☐	? ☐
Affected side	L ☐	R ☐	
Arm weakness	YES ☐	NO ☐	? ☐
Affected side	L ☐	R ☐	

Speech
 If the patient attempts a conversation
 − Look for NEW disturbance of speech
 − Check with companion
 − Look for slurred speech
 − Look for word-finding difficulties. This can be confirmed by asking the patient
   to name commonplace objects that may be nearby, such as a cup, chair, table,
   keys, pen
 − If there is a severe visual disturbance, place an object in the patient's hand
   and ask him/her to name it

Facial movements
 Ask patient to smile or show teeth
 − Look for NEW lack of symmetry − Tick the 'YES' box if there is an unequal smile
   or grimace, or obvious facial asymmetry
 − Note which side does not move well, and mark on the form whether it is the
   patient's right or left side

Arm movements
 − Lift the patient's arms together to 90° if sitting, 45° if supine and ask them to
   hold the position for 5 seconds then let go
 − Does one arm drift down or fall rapidly?
 − If one arm drifts down or falls, note whether it is the patient's left or right arm

Fig. 10.13 Face Arm Speech Test (FAST) to judge whether a stroke is likely. ?, uncertain.

10.3.2 Assessment

The assessment should aim to answer the following questions:

• is it a vascular event (transient ischaemic attack or stroke)? (Chapter 3);
• where is the lesion? (Chapters 3 and 4);
• what sort of stroke lesion is it (ischaemic or haemorrhagic)? (Chapter 5);
• what is the likely cause? (Chapters 6–9);
• what is this patient's prognosis? (sections 10.2 and 16.2);
• what are this patient's particular problems? (Chapter 11).

The answers to these questions will determine the management of the patient and which therapeutic interventions are appropriate. The first five questions have been discussed in previous sections, and before proceeding to discuss the assessment of specific problems to complete the diagnostic formulation (Chapter 11), some general principles and the organization of assessment must be considered.

In practice, the patient's first assessment is often carried out by either a general (family) practitioner in the patient's home, by a paramedic in the ambulance, or a triage nurse or a trainee hospital doctor in the emergency department. None may have had much training or experience in the assessment of patients with stroke. An average general practitioner with 2000 patients is likely to see only about four new cases of stroke each year. Simple assessment tools, such as the FAST[51,52] (Fig. 10.13) or ABCD[53,54] (Fig. 10.14), may enable non-experts to appropriately triage patients to the correct service in the appropriate time scale to allow effective treatment to be given. For example, the FAST test has been used to increase the proportion of patients treated with thrombolysis, and it has been suggested that the ABCD score could be used to triage transient ischaemic attack patients to ensure that those at highest risk of early stroke get earliest access to secondary prevention. Alternatively, assessments by a non-specialist are increasingly being augmented by a remote specialist via telemedicine links (section 17.5.6).

Guidelines, a protocol or, in hospital, a clerking or admission form may be useful tools to ensure that each patient has a thorough and relevant assessment. We, and others, have demonstrated a significant improvement

Factor		Score
Age	<60 years	0
	>60 years	1
Blood pressure	SBP <140 mmHg and DBP <90 mmHg	0
	SBP >140 mmHg and/or DBP >90 mmHg	1
Clinical features	No weakness or speech problem	0
	Dysarthria and/or dysphasia without weakness	1
	Definite weakness of face, arm or leg	2
Duration of longest TIA in last month	<10 mins	0
	10–59 mins	1
	≥60 min	2

Total score	Risk of stroke	Approx % risk in 7 days
≤1	Low	
2	Low	
3	Low	
4	Quite low	>1%
5	High	>10%
6	Very high	>20%

Fig. 10.14 ABCD scale to estimate the risk of stroke early after a transient ischaemic attack. DBP, diastolic blood pressure; SBP, systolic blood pressure.

in the completeness of the assessment of stroke patients following the introduction of a stroke clerking or admission form.[55,56] The use of the form also makes it much easier to access the information subsequently and to identify relevant items that are missing. However, one has to acknowledge the practical difficulties of introducing disease-specific assessment forms in situations – e.g. accident and emergency departments – where patients with a wide range of medical problems are being assessed. For example, it may not be clear until the end of the assessment what the most likely diagnosis is and therefore which form should have been used. One solution might be a 'core form' for all patients, with supplementary sheets for specific common conditions. There is reasonable evidence that patient-specific reminders (e.g. 'if ischaemic stroke, prescribe aspirin'), which can be included in such forms (perhaps as part of an integrated care pathway), improve adherence to management guidelines although randomized trials have not yet demonstrated improvements in patient outcomes.[57,58]

> A clerking or admission form will improve the completeness and relevance of the initial assessment and will facilitate communication and audit, but the introduction of diagnosis-specific forms is not without its problems.

Although a physician is often the first person to assess the patient, it is important to emphasize that assessment should often involve other members of the multidisciplinary team (section 10.3.5). It is often very valuable, even on the day of the stroke, to involve the nurse, the physiotherapist and a speech and language therapist. Advice on the patient's risk of pressure sores, lifting, handling and positioning and the patient's ability to

swallow safely are all relevant to their care from the moment of hospital admission, or indeed from the moment of assessment at home. The components of the initial assessment and their use are summarized in Table 10.8. It is important to emphasize again that assessment may well be staged; it is not a 'once only' process, but should continue throughout the course of the patient's recovery from stroke.

> Assessment is not a 'once only' process, but should continue throughout the course of the patient's recovery from stroke.

Health professionals involved in the initial assessment of stroke patients learn that, although the patient may be a useful source of information, other people often provide more information that is essential to planning treatment. This is particularly important when the patient, for a variety of reasons, cannot communicate. It is usually valuable to spend a little time interviewing the family, neighbours, general practitioner, ambulance technicians or nursing staff, using a telephone if necessary (Fig. 10.15).

> To complete an assessment it is usually valuable to talk to family, neighbours, or family doctor; essential information can often be collected by a telephone call to the appropriate person.

Social environment

The patient's social environment is a very important factor in determining the overall effect that a stroke will have on an individual and his or her family. Accurate knowledge of social networks is therefore critical when

Table 10.8 Information that should be collected during the initial assessment of a stroke patient, and the potential value.

Type of information	Diagnosis	Cause	Prognosis	Hyper-acute treatment	Problems	Secondary prevention
Demographics	+	+	+	+		+
History of onset	+	+	+	+		
Risk factors	+	+	+		+	+
Coexisting disease	+	+	+	+	+	+
Medication		+		+	+	+
Social details		+	+		+	+
Pre-stroke function			+		+	+
General examination	+	+	+	+	+	+
Neurological examination	+		+	+	+	
Investigations	+	+	+	+	+	+

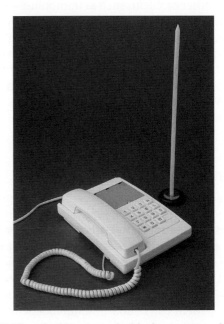

Fig. 10.15 The telephone is a valuable diagnostic tool.

setting longer-term goals for rehabilitation and in planning discharge from hospital. Moreover, this allows one to build up a picture of the patient as a person rather than as 'just another stroke' or 'that fibrillating hemiplegic in bed six'. It is often difficult to see the real person behind the facial weakness, severe aphasia, hemiplegia and incontinence. Finding out about the patient's pre-stroke life might encourage members of the team who are caring for the patient to treat him or her with more understanding and sympathy. Also, it is this background information that allows one to judge the likely effect that the individual's disabilities will have on their role in society, i.e. the likely handicap. This is important,

because one of the major aims of rehabilitation is to minimize handicap. For example, it may be more appropriate to put greater energy and resources into occupational therapy for a craftsman than for a schoolteacher, who might require relatively more speech therapy. The patient should, if possible, have a major role in deciding such priorities.

> It is so often difficult to see the real person behind the facial weakness, severe aphasia, hemiplegia and incontinence.

Although a lot of this background information can be collected over a longer period while the patient is recovering, it can be useful early on and may be more easily collected at the initial assessment. So often, the family – who may be the only source of this sort of information – disappear within a few hours of the admission and may then not reappear to be asked the relevant questions. It is therefore vital to seize the opportunity when a patient is first admitted, or at least during the next day or two, to obtain as much information from the family and friends as possible. Clearly, this may not be regarded as a medical priority, but professionals other than doctors, in particular the nursing staff, are often well placed to collect it. However, often this is not done very well. A complete picture of the patient's pre-stroke life will be useful when deciding how aggressively to manage a patient (e.g. neurosurgery for obstructive hydrocephalus). Because this background information is so important, but may not be available at the initial assessment, one needs to have some method of identifying which items of data are missing so they can be sought later on. The clerking or admission form, or a patient record that is shared by the different professions involved (the so-called 'combined' or 'single-patient' record), has the potential if properly used to fulfil this role. Many stroke units have introduced 'integrated care pathways', which usually include an admission form, multidisciplinary records and guidance on how to manage common problems (section 17.14).

> It is just as important to know the home and social circumstances of a stroke patient for early decision making (such as the desirability of emergency operation) as for later rehabilitation and discharge from hospital.

By the end of the initial assessment, which may be punctuated by giving a hyperacute treatment, one should have collected enough information to produce a diagnostic formulation, including certainty of stroke diagnosis, site and size of the brain lesion, and the likely causes. This leads on to choices about the amount of further investigation required (e.g. echocardiography or not?), and enables the physician to talk to the patient and/or the family about the likely diagnosis, prognosis and management. At this stage, it is valuable to consider, and even list, the particular problems the patient has, to ensure they have all been identified and addressed. It may also be useful to use a checklist of the most common ones that occur at this early stage (Table 10.9).

10.3.3 Identifying problems and setting goals

The patient's assessment, both initially and subsequently, should identify any major problems, and it is these that

Table 10.9 Important things to think about during the first day after a patient has had a severe stroke.

Maintenance of a clear airway
Treatment of co-existing or underlying disease
Need to review the patient's usual medication(s)
Investigation and avoidance of fever
Adequacy of oxygenation
Swallowing ability
Hydration
Nutritional status
Exclusion of urinary retention
Management of urinary incontinence
Exclusion of fractures if the patient may have fallen
Prevention of:
Deep venous thrombosis
Pressure ulcers
Aspiration
Trauma
Faecal impaction
Protection of a flaccid shoulder
Obtaining information from and giving information to the patient and family

determine the patient's management. Problems can occur at every level of the patient's illness – i.e. pathology, impairment, disability and handicap (section 10.1). For example, a problem at the pathology level might be 'diagnostic uncertainty' or 'raised erythrocyte sedimentation rate', which should lead on to further investigation if appropriate; while a problem at the level of handicap might be that the patient provides the only income for a large family, who now have no money to feed themselves. Having identified a problem, one can then formulate a plan to solve or at least alleviate that problem. Thus, a problem list can be turned into an action plan for the individual patient. Some problems can be dealt with very simply (e.g. antibiotics for a urinary tract infection). These are the 'short-loop problems' (section 10.1.2). The goal here is simply to remove the problem. Other problems such as immobility – which are more complex, respond more slowly to therapy and may require several different types of intervention – are the 'long-loop problems' (section 10.1.2); here it is useful to set a long-term goal of removing or alleviating the problem, but it is also helpful to set intermediate goals that allow one to judge whether progress is being made towards the long-term goal.

Why a goal-orientated approach has several advantages

Setting goals allows forward planning and provides a useful focus for multidisciplinary team meetings (section 10.3.7). Intermediate goals allow members of the team to coordinate their work, assuming that goals are achieved on time, and so improve efficiency. For example, if patients are to dress the lower half of their body, they must be able to stand. If the physiotherapist can estimate when the patient will be able to stand independently, the occupational therapist can plan when to start working on dressing the lower half. Setting longer-term goals can, for example, allow advanced planning of a pre-discharge home visit and final discharge to the community, which can reduce the patient's length of stay in hospital by the number of days or weeks needed to plan a home visit or to make any necessary adaptations to the patient's home before discharge (e.g. stair rails).

If realistic goals are set, they can then be used to help motivate patients, especially if they have been involved in choosing or setting the goal. Recovery from a stroke may be very slow, so slow that the patient and even the therapists are unable to discern any progress being made towards the long-term goal (e.g. to achieve independent mobility). If one sets and achieves intermediate goals (e.g. sitting balance), progress is more easily perceived and morale maintained. The management of patients

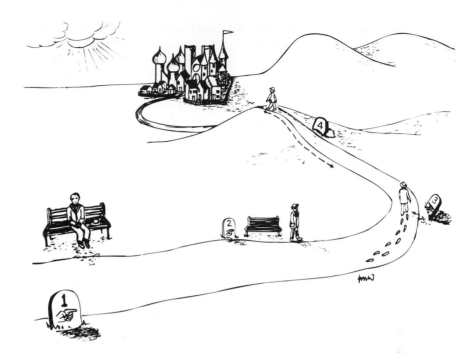

Fig. 10.16 The 'road' to recovery after a hemiplegic stroke, showing some mobility 'milestones': 1, sitting balance for 1 min; 2, standing for 10 s; 3, 10 steps unaided; 4, timed 10-m walk (Smith & Baer 1999).[59]

with stroke in hospital is often allowed to drift without direction or leadership. The clinician who is responsible for the patient waves to them on a weekly ward round, in the belief that the therapists are actively rehabilitating the patient. If the head of the multidisciplinary team maintains discipline, and encourages the setting of both intermediate and long-term goals, drift can be avoided. This discipline benefits the patients, the team members and the service as a whole. The greater efficiency reduces length of stay in hospital and allows a greater proportion of stroke patients to be treated in the stroke unit without the need for extra staff or beds.

Describing goals

Where the goal is simply the removal of a problem, such as a urinary tract infection, it is fairly easy to describe it and then measure progress, e.g. relief of symptoms and sterile urine on a repeat culture. Similarly, long-term goals are often easy to describe, but should take into account the patient's need for accommodation, physical and emotional support, how they might fill their time and what role they play in society. Judgements about whether these long-term goals have been achieved are relatively straightforward. For example, if the goal is to get a patient home to live with their family, or to return to work, one does not need any complex measures of outcome. In some areas, it is even fairly easy to set intermediate goals. For example, many patients with stroke

have problems with mobility, but usually the patient will achieve certain physical milestones on the road to recovery[59] (Fig. 10.16). Further improvement in mobility can be measured by recording the time it takes the patient to walk 10 m.[60] Thus, it is a fairly simple process to set an intermediate goal, which the patient or carer can understand, in terms of the level of function and the date by which it should be achieved.

If goals are to be reproducible, and therefore useful, a standard method for assessing attainment or not needs to be established and used. It is more complex to set goals for problems such as language or activities of daily living (ADL) than for mobility. For example, a goal for independent dressing a patient's top half would need to take account of important factors including the clothes worn, fasteners involved and the amount of prompting allowed (section 11.32.5). One could use a score on any one of the huge number of measures of language function or ADL as intermediate goals, but these scores are not easily understood by patients and carers, or even by the professionals using them. For example, it is unlikely to mean much to a patient, or even the team members, to aim for a Barthel index score of 12 (out of a maximum of 20) within the next 2 weeks. Despite these difficulties, the team should attempt to identify problems, specify intermediate and long-term goals, and introduce some meaningful measures to determine whether progress is being made towards achieving each of them.

> In every stroke patient, intermediate and long-term
> goals should be described so that progress towards
> them can be measured. Moreover, everyone will feel
> a sense of achievement when the goals are met.

10.3.4 Goal setting: a diagnostic tool

Goals may also be useful in identifying new or previously
unrecognized problems. If a patient is not achieving the
goals that have been set, it may be due to a number of
reasons, which can be divided into team factors, patient
factors and carer factors.

Team factors

If the goals are too ambitious because of inaccurate diagnosis, inadequate assessment or uncertainty about the
prognosis, then patients may fail to achieve them and
this will have a detrimental effect on the patient's and
the team's morale. If goals are too easy, then progress
may be slower than is, in fact, possible. Also, goal setting
must be realistic if one is to use it to coordinate care
(section 10.3.3). To set realistic goals in such a way that
they are more often achieved than not requires an
understanding of the prognosis and of the likely effectiveness of potential interventions. We have already seen
that accurate predictions of progress and outcome are
difficult in individual patients (section 10.2.7), but
informal judgements made by the team may be more
accurate, because they are based on past experience and
observation of the patient's progress over a period of
time. Another reason why a patient may not be achieving a goal might be lack of appropriate treatment. Thus,
progress may be hampered by too little therapy, or by the
wrong sort of therapy. However, since there is currently
so little information about the optimum amount or the
relative effectiveness of most interventions, it is difficult
to sort this out. Team members will much more often
have to modify their therapy based on their own experience rather than on evidence from properly conducted
randomized controlled trials.

> Goals should be meaningful and challenging, but
> achievable.

Patient and carer factors

New, unrecognized medical or psychological problems
(e.g. infection, recurrent stroke or depression) may not
present overtly – especially in their early stages – but may
develop in a less specific way, causing a patient's progress
to slow, stop, or even reverse. One can draw a parallel

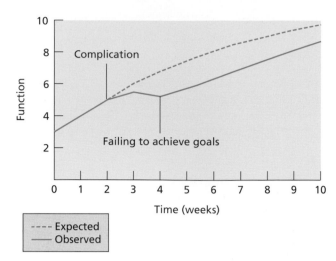

Fig. 10.17 'Failure to thrive' after a stroke. Deviation from
the expected recovery pattern might be due to any number of
factors, including recurrent stroke, infections, depression, etc.

with the concept of 'failure to thrive' in paediatric practice (Fig. 10.17). If a patient is failing to achieve his or her
goals (or milestones), then one needs to identify the
likely reason or reasons (Tables 11.5 and 11.7).

> When a patient is failing to achieve his or her goals (or
> milestones) then one must identify the reason, and if
> possible do something about it.

Sometimes the patient or the carer may have different
goals from those of the team looking after the patient.
This is 'goal mismatch'. For example, a patient who does
not want to live alone but would prefer to live with his
or her daughter may not achieve the level of independence expected. Therefore, when setting goals ideally one
should agree them with the patient and carers – although
they may be reticent about discussing such matters
openly. It is also important to involve the patient, and
perhaps the carer, in setting goals, to ensure that the
goals are really relevant to them. Most stroke patients
are retired, so that leisure activities may be particularly
important to their quality of life (section 11.33.3). The
patient may be less interested in a goal aiming at
achieving self-care in dressing than in being able to read
or do the gardening. In hospital practice, where activities
of daily living (ADL) abilities often determine the length
of stay, too much emphasis can be placed on ADL-related
goals because of the pressures on the team to make
beds available for new patients and to minimize costs
by discharging the patient as early as possible. There
are however important practical difficulties in involving patients in goal setting, including their cognitive,

communication and visuuospatial problems and the clinician's lack of experience or time.[61,62]

> Goal setting may sometimes involve just an individual professional, but ideally it should involve the rest of the team, the patient and sometimes the patient's family.

10.3.5 The stroke team

Although a physician usually has overall responsibility for the management of the patient, other members of the multidisciplinary team play an essential part. Stroke unit care reduces the case fatality, physical dependency and need for institutionalization compared with care on a general medical ward (section 17.6). The main difference between the two models of care is that stroke unit care is coordinated with a multidisciplinary team. Because stroke patients have such a broad range of problems, their care demands input from several professions. For coordination of the professionals' input, it is important that at least some of them should work as a core team, with regular meetings to discuss patients' progress and problems (Table 10.10). Other professionals (Table 10.11), who may not be regular members of the team, should be available for consultation about individual patients. Although well established in rehabilitation settings, the team has an important role in all phases of treatment, even on the day of the stroke. Of course, the type and intensity of input from different members of the team will vary at different stages of the patient's illness.

By working closely together and sharing information and skills, some blurring of the boundaries between the roles of the professions becomes possible, and this can provide greater flexibility and efficiency. For example, if the nursing staff are trained by the speech and language therapist to screen for dysphagia, this will provide every patient with early screening (even at weekends), enabling the speech and language therapist to focus on patients with definite swallowing or communication problems (sections 11.17 and 11.30). Some have suggested that we should develop a hybrid therapist who could take on several roles, but this interesting idea

Table 10.10 The core stroke team.

Physician
Nurse
Physiotherapist
Occupational therapist
Speech and language therapist
Social worker

Table 10.11 Other professionals who may be helpful in the management of particular stroke patients.

Others who may be consulted	Example of problem
Clinical psychologist	Antisocial behaviour
Psychiatrist	Severe depression
Neurosurgeon	Obstructive hydrocephalus
Vascular surgeon	Peripheral artery embolus
Radiologist	Unusual CT scan appearance
Rheumatologist	Painful shoulder
Orthopaedic surgeon	Fractured neck of femur
Optometrist	Refractive problems
Ophthalmologist	Persistent diplopia
Orthotist	Shortened leg, foot drop
Dietician	Weight loss
Pharmacist	Formulations for dysphagia
Dentist	Ill-fitting dentures

CT, computerized tomography.

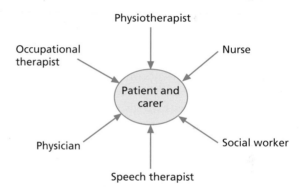

Fig. 10.18 The traditional model of care or rehabilitation, in which each member of the multidisciplinary team interacts independently with the patient and/or carer.

has, not surprisingly, met with considerable opposition from the existing professions. This concept may have particular merits in situations in which it is difficult to coordinate the activities of a multidisciplinary team, for example in a rural community rehabilitation setting.

Figures 10.18 and 10.19 illustrate two models of how members of the stroke team can provide input to patients and their carers. In the first, each professional predominantly works directly with the patient and/or carer, while in the second each professional has less direct patient contact, but influences the care given by a primary nurse. The two models represent the extremes, and it is likely that in the real world care is provided in an intermediate way. Although the model represented in Fig. 10.19 realistically means that patients must be treated in a stroke unit, it has other important advantages.

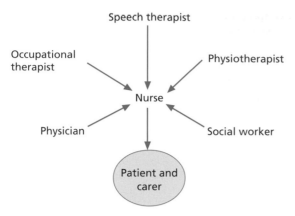

Fig. 10.19 The model of care or rehabilitation that can be adopted on a geographically defined stroke unit, in which each member of the multidisciplinary team influences the nursing input to the patients and carers, as well as having direct interaction with them.

Stroke patients, even on a stroke unit, are directly involved in therapeutic activity with therapists for only a small proportion of their time.[63] Training the nurses to practise with the patients the activities initiated by the therapists should encourage consistency and increase the total amount of therapy received by patients. After all, the nurses are caring for patients on a ward throughout the 24-h period. If, for example, the physiotherapists are teaching a patient how to transfer from bed to wheelchair, it is important that the patient should continue to do this in the same way *between* physiotherapy sessions. Otherwise, many of the skills the patient acquires during physiotherapy sessions may not be used during activities on the ward or, more importantly, at home. The same principles apply to input from other therapists. Whether therapy delivered by a non-specialist is as effective as therapy delivered by a highly trained specialist needs to be evaluated in randomized trials. One of the important functions of the team meeting is to harmonize the activity of the therapists and the nurses who provide much of the daily input to the patients. This may be at least one of the reasons why stroke units seem to achieve better outcomes (section 17.6).

10.3.6 The roles of the team members

This section outlines the main functions of the core members of the team. In practice, and certainly where a team is functioning well, there will be some blurring of the roles of the team members with each performing the less specialized functions of the others. The roles described and the professional labels used reflect those in our own clinical practice but they inevitably vary in different healthcare settings.

Physician

Few doctors really understand the important role that they can play in the care of stroke patients beyond making the initial diagnosis, searching for a treatable cause, giving acute medical therapies and initiating secondary preventive measures. The physician needs to be much more involved in the activities of the team for several reasons:

- *Team leader:* Usually, rightly or wrongly, political power in health services lies principally with doctors, and therefore if stroke patients are to have access to adequate facilities, the doctor must be involved.
- *Source of knowledge:* The physician should be knowledgeable about the disease processes – both stroke and non-stroke – that underlie the patients' functional problems, and should thus understand the prognosis and likely effect of interventions. This is essential for predicting outcome and setting appropriate goals.
- *Medical care underpinning rehabilitation:* Stroke patients commonly have coexisting and complicating medical problems (e.g. diabetes, heart failure, deep venous thrombosis), which need to be identified and treated.[4]
- *Ability to chair meetings effectively:* The physician will often have the broadest knowledge about stroke and is therefore in a good – although not necessarily unique – position to coordinate the team and to chair team meetings. This role is important, because team meetings can become very time-consuming and may lose direction without a strong chairperson (section 10.3.7). Overly long meetings are boring, demoralizing and inefficient.
- *Legal responsibility:* The legal responsibility for the patient is the doctor's, and therefore the doctor must be involved at all stages of the patient's care.

In the UK, to encourage specialist physician involvement in stroke care and management, there has been a move towards establishing stroke medicine as a subspecialty with its own training schemes (http://www.basp.ac.uk/2004specialtraining.pdf). Stroke physicians are trained to deal with the whole patient journey, from the hyperacute phase through to rehabilitation and long-term follow-up, and to manage most post-stroke problems (Chapter 11). In other countries these roles are often distributed among other specialists including neurologists, internal medicine specialists, rehabilitation specialists and geriatricians.

Nursing staff

The nursing staff probably have the broadest role in the management of patients with stroke, which includes at least four major components:

- A daily assessment of the patient's problems, both existing and new, and of their abilities and disabilities. Every week, our nurses assess the patients using the Barthel index, which focuses their attention on important functional issues. Based on this assessment, they evolve a care plan that aims to meet the individual's needs.
- Provision of all the basic needs of dependent patients after a stroke (e.g. feeding, washing, dressing, toileting, turning and transferring).
- Provision of skilled nursing to prevent the development of complications such as pressure ulcers (section 11.16), painful shoulders (section 11.24), other injuries (section 11.26) and aspiration pneumonia (sections 11.12 and 11.17). This involves correctly positioning and handling the immobile patient (section 11.11). If one adopts a model of teamworking approximating to that shown in Fig. 10.19, then the nurse's role will include many of the functions of other members of the team.
- Supporting the patient and family. With increasing emphasis by managers and politicians on improving easily measured clinical outcomes such as case fatality and disability, other aspects of caring for and about patients are easily forgotten. But these are very important to patients and close family members[64] – informing, reassuring, encouraging, advising, supporting and sympathizing. The nurses usually have greatest contact with the patients and family and therefore have an important role in this area.

In some healthcare systems trained nurses are not readily available, and much of the patient's day-to-day needs are met by relatives. In many countries specific training for stroke unit nurses is not yet available (http://www.nationalstrokenursingforum.com/). To fully realize the potential of stroke unit nurses requires considerable investment in specialist education and training.

Physiotherapist

The physiotherapist has several important roles in caring for stroke patients, depending on their individual needs and the stage of the illness (http://www.csp.org.uk/). Soon after a severe stroke, the physiotherapist may be involved in at least seven functions:

- Providing a detailed assessment of the motor and sensory problems of patients to help estimate their prognosis.
- Assessing and treating chest problems, including pneumonia and retention of secretions. Speech and language therapists often find it useful to have a physiotherapist present at swallowing assessments, to help position the patient and to deal promptly with any aspiration (section 11.17).

- Advising nurses and other carers on the best way to position patients to prevent unhelpful changes in muscle tone that may lead ultimately to contractures and further limitation of function (section 11.20).
- Teaching the nurses and informal carers the best way to handle the patient to avoid pain or injury to the patient or carer. This will often involve teaching proper methods of transferring, lifting, standing and walking the patient.
- Providing therapy to relieve the symptoms associated with painful shoulders or swollen limbs (sections 11.24 and 11.25).
- Providing therapy to improve the patient's mobility and arm function (section 11.21).
- Advising on walking aids and splints (section 11.32.1) that may sometimes improve a patient's function.

In some countries physiotherapists have a more limited role. They may not be so involved in assessment and formulation of treatment but simply deliver the interventions prescribed by a rehabilitation specialist.

Occupational therapist

Occupational therapists fulfil several roles in the management of stroke patients (http://www.cot.org.uk/specialist/nanot/forums/stroke.php). These are usually fairly limited in the very early period after a severe stroke, but become more important as the patient recovers and as self-care becomes more relevant. These roles include the following five components:

- An early assessment of patients to find out how each impairment is likely to restrict their function. This requires an assessment of what the patients were able to do before the stroke, what they can do now and what their home circumstances are, e.g. ease of access to the front door, bedroom, toilet, or bathroom; or the circumstances into which the patients will be discharged, e.g. a relative's home or nursing home.
- An assessment of the patient's visuospatial functioning. It is important to remember that many evaluations of the objective tests of visuospatial functioning use an occupational therapist's assessment as the 'gold standard'[65] (section 11.28).
- Training the patient and the carer to carry out everyday activities, despite the patient's impairments, is a crucial role (section 11.32). This involves finding the best way of achieving a particular activity for that individual patient. Most input is spent on the activities of daily living (Table 11.45), although in specialized units or those dealing with younger patients, therapy aimed at return to an occupation (section 11.33.2) or leisure activity (section 11.33.3) may be available.

- Provision of aids and adaptations to allow patients to function better. In the UK, this includes wheelchair provision, feeding and kitchen aids, and bathroom aids, among many others (section 11.32).
- Assessment of patients' ability to function in their own home, e.g. home visit which is often done before discharge with patients who have been admitted to hospital, and is an important element of discharge planning. It is important to identify problems that are specific to the patient's own home environment and which may have to be solved by further training or by provision of aids or adaptations.

Speech and language therapist

Speech and language therapists have several roles in the care of stroke patients (http://www.rcslt.org/). They include:

- Assessment of swallowing safety both initially and as the patients improve, so that their diet and fluid intake matches their swallowing abilities (section 11.17).
- Teaching the patient, nurses or family who are involved with feeding, techniques that help overcome a swallowing impairment and avoid aspiration.
- Teaching the patients exercises that *may* increase the rate of recovery of swallowing problems (section 11.17).
- Diagnosis and assessment of the patient's communication problems (section 11.30).
- Informing both formal and informal carers of the nature of the patient's communication problems. Patients, their families and even the professionals caring for the patient often have great difficulty in understanding what is wrong with a dysphasic patient. They may think the patient is 'confused', 'demented', or simply 'mad'. Because problems with communication so often lead to emotional distress, most speech and language therapists also take on a counselling role.
- Teaching patients, carers and even volunteers, strategies to allow the patients to communicate effectively using language (spoken or written), gesture, or communication aids where appropriate.
- Providing therapy that *may* enhance the recovery of communication difficulties (section 11.30).

Social worker

The role of the social worker is bound to vary in different societies. In the UK, Australia and the Netherlands (which are the countries where we have direct experience), the social worker is likely to:

- Provide patients and their families with practical advice and help at all stages of the patients' illness. For example, arranging subsidized transport for the family to visit the hospital, or extra home care for a dependent relative if the stroke patient was the main carer before admission. Social workers often help with any financial problems that have arisen because the main breadwinner has had a stroke, e.g. by applying for allowances or grants.
- Be involved helping to plan the patient's discharge from hospital, or change of accommodation. Social workers often spend a lot of time identifying the wishes and needs of the patient and family and then, with the rest of the team, trying to meet them. Where patients are unable to make decisions for themselves and have no close family, the social worker may need to act as the patient's advocate and make arrangements for financial affairs to be taken care of, perhaps even arranging any change of accommodation (e.g. transfer to a nursing home).
- Follow up patients and families after the patient's discharge from hospital, to identify their changing need for support and to make adjustments to any care package.
- Provide counselling that *may* be helpful in allowing patients and families to come to terms with the change in circumstances brought about by the stroke. Some organize groups of patients, carers, or both to help solve problems.

One function that should be shared by all members of the team is that of monitoring the patient's condition. Nurses and therapists, in particular, spend a lot of their time handling patients and observing the patient's performance, so they are often in an ideal position to notice the relatively minor changes that may be an early sign of a complication, which might benefit from early treatment.

> All members of the team should be alert to changes in the patient's condition that may indicate the development of a complication.

Are the interventions of the team members effective?

Although organized stroke care improves outcomes, some question the effectiveness of physiotherapy, occupational therapy, speech and language therapy and social work. They point to the lack of research evidence to support the effectiveness of these professionals (but interestingly, without questioning their own effectiveness), or they emphasize particular studies that appear to demonstrate the ineffectiveness of other professions. Unfortunately, these 'negative' studies have, in general, asked the wrong questions, measured the wrong outcomes, been too small, and have not evaluated the intervention in the context of a well-organized stroke team. This has possibly resulted in 'false-negative' studies,

MULTIDISCIPLINARY TEAM MEETINGS

WARD:

Addressograph

Date: / /

For CPR: Yes: No:

Week No: **Barthel:** **Milestones: None, Sit, Stand, Steps, 10m**

Falls Risk? YES/NO **Weight:**

Nursing: present/absent	**Medical**: Consultant present/absent
	Nutrition: Dietician present/absent
Physiotherapy: present/absent	**Speech & Language therapy**: present/absent
Occupational therapy: present/absent	**Social Work**: present/absent

Action Plan:
1.
2.
3.

Discharge within one week? Y/N

Signed: Designation:

Fig. 10.20 A proforma for recording the results of a multidisciplinary team meeting.

resulting in rejection of valuable team members. But, as everyone must realize, failure to demonstrate a definite effect cannot be taken as proof of a lack of effect.[66] There may be uncertainty about the effectiveness, optimum 'dose' and duration of some of the specific therapeutic manoeuvres that therapists use (in common with many medical practices) but, as we have shown, this type of input forms only a small part of their contribution to the care of stroke patients. In fact, there are an increasing number of well-conducted randomized trials that have established that interventions by therapists do improve patient outcome, as discussed in Chapter 11.[67–69]

10.3.7 Multidisciplinary team meetings

The team must meet regularly if it is to work effectively. All the stroke units included in the recent systematic review of the randomized controlled trials held at least weekly meetings of the multidisciplinary team, separate from conventional ward rounds.[70] These meetings have several important functions:

- The entire team can be introduced to new patients and their problems.
- Existing patients can be reviewed, and if individual team members have noted a change in their condition or a new problem, this can be communicated to the other members.
- After reviewing each patient's progress and any developing problems, realistic goals can be set jointly, and an appropriate course of action to meet those goals can be agreed (section 10.3.3).
- Verbal reports of individual therapists' assessments, and in particular the results of pre-discharge home visits, can be discussed and detailed plans for discharge can be made.
- Meetings have an educational role for the team members, students and visitors. For example, we often show the patient's brain CT and discuss the likely pathogenesis of the stroke and any rationale for treatment or therapy.

So that important details are not overlooked, it may be useful to agree a formal structure to the discussions which can be reinforced by using a standard form on which team discussions are recorded (Fig. 10.20). The structure we have adopted is discussed below. This is not rigidly adhered to, but provides a framework for discussions about individual patients.

Structure of team discussion

The medical details of any new patients are presented by the physician, including a brief account of the patient's symptoms and any relevant past history, including risk factors and the presumed cause of the stroke. The patient's social background is also presented briefly by the physician, but other members of the team are often able to contribute extra details. The patient's neurological impairments are discussed, and the therapists have often identified some that may not have been obvious to the physician. By the time of the meeting, the nursing staff can report on the functional consequences of these impairments (i.e. disability), and using the information about pre-stroke activities, some estimate of the stroke's

likely effect on the patient's life after the stroke can be made (i.e. predicted handicap).

At each subsequent meeting, we introduce the patient briefly with a résumé of the date of stroke, clinical type and presumed cause. We then summarize the problems, goals and actions that were agreed at the last meeting. Each member of the team is then invited to update the rest of the team on the patient's progress, what problems and goals have been solved or achieved, what new goals they plan to set, and how they plan to achieve them. Usually we do this in a set order that tends to reflect the way we think about patients, i.e. pathology, impairment, disability and handicap. The physician starts by updating the team on any changes in the patient's medical condition or the results of any important investigations that may be relevant to other team members. The nurses then give an overall report on the patient's progress, including current performance on the Barthel index. This usefully highlights many of the patient's functional problems, as well as giving an objective indication of progress. The therapists follow: first the physiotherapist, then the speech therapist and lastly the occupational therapist. The first two tend to focus more on impairments and the patient's basic functions such as mobility, swallowing and communication, while the occupational therapist usually focuses on the broader range of disabilities and how these are likely to affect the patient's everyday life. Lastly, the social worker reports on any problems which close contact with the family may have revealed and progress regarding discharge planning. This sequence also has the advantage that the occupational therapist and social worker can make use of the information from the others in formulating their own goals and actions.

The discussion is then opened up, and longer-term goals such as timing of home visits, discharges and case (family) conferences are set, and we decide who will do what by the next meeting including who will communicate with the patient and family to ensure that they are involved with the goal-setting process and that their views are being taken into account.

Multidisciplinary teams may lack effectiveness if each member is not given an equal chance to contribute. Inevitably, teams will include some more assertive individuals and other less outgoing members, the former tending to dominate discussions. It is important that the team leader – often the physician – ensures that individual members do not monopolize the discussions to the extent that others are not heard. The framework we have adopted lessens the likelihood of this arising, although of course not every member will necessarily have something useful to contribute in every case.

It is important that the person chairing the team meetings ensures that no individual member, including the chairperson, monopolizes the discussion to the extent that others are not heard.

We find it useful to have separate team meetings where patients are not discussed when we discuss general management issues, how the team is working, what the problems are, and any changes that might be made in the way we work.

Involving patients and carers in team meetings

Neither the patient nor the family have been mentioned yet as having a direct input into the team meetings, although their input is obviously crucial in setting goals and planning discharge from hospital. We do not invite them to attend each meeting, but we do seek their views on certain issues in advance of the meeting. We also try to ensure that the nature and conclusions of the discussion at the meeting are communicated back to the patient and/or family by the most appropriate team member, most often the nurse. Although it is sometimes vital to involve the patient and families in discussions, we feel that their attendance at each weekly meeting would inhibit the discussion and might be distressing for them. It would also make meetings longer and more unwieldy. We hold separate team meetings (case conferences or family meetings) to which the patient, family and any other people who are involved – such as the district (community) nurse and home care organizer – are invited. These meetings are useful in planning hospital discharge in complex cases and in resolving differences of opinion between the team members and the patient or family. The timing of these meetings is tailored to the individual patient.

Team building

It is useful to have separate team meetings at which patients are not discussed. On these occasions, we discuss general management issues, how the team is working, what the problems are, and any changes that might be made in the way we work. We discuss critical incidents to ensure that we learn from these. These sessions also allow individuals to tell the rest of the team about certain specialized aspects of their jobs. This, we believe, not only encourages some blurring of the distinctions between their functions but also aids team building. Each member can more fully appreciate the contribution made by other members. We also have weekly meetings, involving the consultants and trainees, to discuss patients entering our stroke register where we review their clinical and radiological details. These provide an additional opportunity for education, training, quality control and discussion of difficult cases with consultant colleagues.

Recording the work of the team

We have not yet found a totally satisfactory method of recording the work of the team. Traditionally, members have each kept their own records so that they may refer to them, but this inevitably leads to much unnecessary duplication. However, a unified record has disadvantages, the main one being that different members of the team require information of varying detail. Thus, the physiotherapist's record contains very detailed notes on the patient's motor functioning that are irrelevant to the social worker. Also, the records may be needed simultaneously by the physiotherapist in the gymnasium and by the pharmacist on the stroke unit. In our units, each profession has therefore kept its own records, but they do all make entries in a combined medical and nursing record. The nurses base their care plans on the discussions at the team meetings. This has been helped by their adoption of a problem-orientated approach, so that the nurses regularly record the patients' problems, the goals and actions aimed at attaining the goals. A compromise in which core details are collected once and shared, while more detailed records are kept by each team member, might provide the best and most efficient solution. We also increasingly use structured records in which the results of the most commonly used assessments (e.g. swallowing, continence) and actions taken require only a tick, date and signature. In the future, increased use of information technology may facilitate a combined patient record that avoids some of these problems but even now we do ensure that changes in the patient's condition, key decisions and proposed actions (by whom and by when) are recorded in the medical notes. This is important to avoid unnecessary and time-wasting repetition of discussions at future meetings and to ensure that decisions lead on to actions.

10.4 Some difficult ethical issues

When patients are judged unlikely to achieve a reasonable quality of life if they were to survive, many clinicians decide not to strive to ensure survival. However, this is an extremely difficult decision since, as we have already discussed, there are considerable difficulties in predicting outcome reliably at an early stage (section 10.2.7). Also the value that the patient would place on survival in a given state is impossible to judge. Patients who have had a major stroke are often not in a position to make decisions about their treatment because, due to a depressed conscious level, language or visuospatial problems, they are unable to understand or communicate. Under these circumstances, the family or potential carers should be included in the decision-making process. The family can often provide information allowing judgements to be made about what the patient's likely wishes are. However, some relatives may have their own interests and not just those of the patient to consider. Younger relatives may gain financially from the death of an older relative, and death removes the obligation to care for a severely disabled person. Patients may even have written down what they would like to happen in the event of a life-threatening illness (i.e. a living will). The legal status of these so-called 'living wills' varies from country to country, however. Also, it is not at all clear whether patients' judgements made while in good health about the value they might place on their life if they were in a dependent state remain true when they have become disabled. We have encountered many people who have become severely disabled and yet have accepted their disability and felt that their quality of life is acceptable or even very good.

> It is difficult to know how to react to patients' previously expressed view that they would never, ever want to live in a dependent state or go to a nursing home, when they then seem to cling to life after a major stroke.

One has to be particularly careful in assessing the likely prognosis of an individual patient with an apparently severe stroke. A relatively minor stroke that is complicated by another medical problem (e.g. pneumonia) may be impossible to differentiate from a severe stroke (section 11.4). If the complicating medical problem can be identified and treated then the patient may achieve a very satisfactory clinical outcome despite the apparently gloomy initial prognosis.

> It is not always easy to distinguish between a patient who has had a catastrophic stroke and one who has had a less severe stroke that is complicated and worsened by infection, epileptic seizures or metabolic problems. The prognosis is much worse for the former patient than the latter one.

Perhaps the most common dilemma is whether or not to give fluids or nutritional support to a patient with an 'apparently severe stroke' who is unable to swallow. Early nutritional support is likely to improve the proportion of patients surviving although not perhaps the functional status of survivors.[71] Few would argue against giving parenteral fluids to a conscious patient to prevent dehydration, thirst and discomfort. However, if the patient is unconscious and thus probably unaware of any discomfort, then there is more uncertainty about what to do for the best. Also, if the patient develops an infection very soon after the onset of the stroke, apart from the difficulties mentioned above in assessing the severity of stroke, the question arises as to how aggressively one should treat the patient. Are intravenous antibiotics, physiotherapy or even artificial ventilation and inotropic support appropriate in this situation?

There are some facts worth considering before making these difficult decisions. Most patients who are unconscious soon after a stroke die in the first few days from the direct neurological effects of the stroke on brainstem function, and not from dehydration or infection (section 10.2.3). Therefore, by simply giving fluids, it is unlikely that the lives of many patients will be greatly prolonged, but this may give more time to make an accurate assessment of prognosis. If one elects to give a patient fluids, antibiotics or even nutritional support via a feeding tube, this clearly does not have to be continued on a long-term basis. However, in some countries there are laws that prevent clinicians from withdrawing treatment of this kind, and many clinicians feel more uncomfortable about stopping a treatment that they have started than about not starting it in the first place. Apart from worrying about medicolegal issues, one has to consider the reaction of the family. However, in our experience, if the physician has spent enough time informing the family of the patient's state and likely prognosis, and has involved them in the decisions, then withdrawal of fluids, feeding or antibiotics is seldom a major problem. Unfortunately, in some countries there is a trend for such decisions – especially in severely brain-damaged children and patients in a persistent vegetative state – to be delegated to the legal profession. We cannot hope to have the answers to all these difficult problems, but perhaps it is worth suggesting a general approach that we have found practicable:

- First, collect accurate and unbiased information about the patient's life before the stroke. It is not good enough to base one's decisions on the severity of just the stroke, since this may be difficult to estimate accurately, and other factors will influence the prognosis (section 11.4). The patient's pre-stroke functional level and social activity are crucial in making these decisions. Unfortunately, this information is often not collected in sufficient detail during the acute phase, because its relevance to acute care is not recognized (section 10.3.2). One might be less aggressive in treating patient A, who was previously handicapped, miserable and in pain from severe arthritis and living in an institution, than patient B, who has an equally severe stroke but was previously living at home independently with his or her family. Usually, the patient's pre-stroke handicap sets the ceiling on the potential post-stroke outcome, so that these two patients have very different outlooks. It is still a difficult – some would say an impossible – judgement to say whether patient A's life is worth prolonging.

- Next, it is important to make a detailed assessment of the patient's condition in order to make the best possible judgement about the prognosis.
- Third, formulate the various alternative management plans that might be adopted. These should include those from the most aggressive to the most conservative.
- Finally, all options must be discussed with other members of the team and any close family members. The family needs to be given accurate information about the diagnosis, problems, likely outcomes and treatment possibilities. It is probably unfair to suggest that the decisions are all theirs, but any decision the clinician makes should ideally be compatible with their views. If one does not take the family's wishes into account one is inviting trouble, complaints – and nowadays litigation. It is worth making it clear to them that few decisions are irreversible (except perhaps turning off a ventilator), since circumstances change. One is often in a much better position to make an accurate prognosis having observed the patient's progress over a few days than on the day of the stroke, so what appeared to be an appropriate intervention on day 1 may appear less appropriate after a few days. It can also be useful to involve an independent and experienced clinician to provide a second opinion.

The development of better tools to help predict prognosis, and studies that give a better understanding of the effect of our supportive interventions, should make these difficult decisions somewhat easier in the future. Professional bodies often provide specific advice which is applicable to particular countries (e.g. http://www.gmc-uk.org/standards/default.htm).

Involve other members of the team and the patient's family in any decisions about how aggressively one should strive to keep a patient alive. Emphasize that most decisions can be reviewed – and reversed – in the light of the patient's progress.

References

1 WHO. *International Classification of Impairments, Disabilities and Handicaps*. Geneva: World Health Organization; 1980.
2 WHO. *International Classification of Functioning, Disability and Health (ICF)*. Geneva: World Health Organization; 2001.
3 Bornman J. The World Health Organization's terminology and classification: application to severe disability. *Disabil Rehabil* 2004; **26**(3):182–8.
4 Langhorne P, Stott DJ, Robertson L, MacDonald J, Jones L, McAlpine C *et al*. Medical complications after stroke: a multicenter study. *Stroke* 2000; **31**(6):1223–9.
5 Bamford J, Sandercock P, Dennis M, Burn J, Warlow C. A prospective study of acute cerebrovascular disease in the community: the Oxfordshire Community Stroke Project 1981–86. 2. Incidence, case fatality rates and overall outcome at one year of cerebral infarction, primary intracerebral and subarachnoid haemorrhage. *J Neurol Neurosurg Psychiatry* 1990; **53**(1):16–22.
6 Rothwell PM, Coull AJ, Giles MF, Howard SC, Silver LE, Bull LM *et al*. Change in stroke incidence, mortality, case-fatality, severity, and risk factors in Oxfordshire, UK from 1981 to 2004 (Oxford Vascular Study). *Lancet* 2004; **363**(9425):1925–33.
7 Bonita R, Broad JB, Beaglehole R. Changes in stroke incidence and case-fatality in Auckland, New Zealand, 1981–91. *Lancet* 1993; **342**(8885):1470–3.
8 Peltonnen M, Stegmayr B, Asplund K. Marked improvement since 1985 in short-term and long-term survival after stroke. *Cerebrovasc Dis* 1999; **9**(Suppl. 1): 62.
9 Gresham GE, Kelly-Hayes M, Wolf PA, Beiser AS, Kase CS, D'Agostino RB. Survival and functional status 20 or more years after first stroke: the Framingham Study. *Stroke* 1998; **29**(4):793–7.
10 Bamford J, Dennis M, Sandercock P, Burn J, Warlow C. The frequency, causes and timing of death within 30 days of a first stroke: the Oxfordshire Community Stroke Project. *J Neurol Neurosurg Psychiatry* 1990; **53**(10):824–9.
11 Burn J, Dennis M, Bamford J, Sandercock P, Wade D, Warlow C. Long-term risk of recurrent stroke after a first-ever stroke. The Oxfordshire Community Stroke Project. *Stroke* 1994; **25**(2):333–7.
12 Van GJ. Subarachnoid haemorrhage. *Lancet* 1992; **339**(8794):653–5.
13 Dombovy ML, Basford JR, Whisnant JP, Bergstralh EJ. Disability and use of rehabilitation services following stroke in Rochester, Minnesota, 1975–1979. *Stroke* 1987; **18**(5):830–6.
14 Kwakkel G, Kollen B, Lindeman E. Understanding the pattern of functional recovery after stroke: facts and theories. *Restor Neurol Neurosci* 2004; **22**(3–5):281–99.
15 Gray CS, French JM, Bates D, Cartlidge NE, James OF, Venables G. Motor recovery following acute stroke. *Age Ageing* 1990; **19**(3):179–84.

16 Duncan PW, Goldstein LB, Matchar D, Divine GW, Feussner J. Measurement of motor recovery after stroke. Outcome assessment and sample size requirements. *Stroke* 1992; **23**(8):1084–9.

17 Ashburn A. Physical recovery following stroke. *Physiotherapy* 1997; **83**:480–90.

18 Kwon S, Hartzema AG, Duncan PW, Min-Lai S. Disability measures in stroke: relationship among the Barthel Index, the Functional Independence Measure, and the Modified Rankin Scale. *Stroke* 2004; **35**(4):918–23.

19 Dennis MS. Outcome after brain haemorrhage. *Cerebrovasc Dis* 2003; **16** Suppl 1:9–13.

20 Barber M, Roditi G, Stott DJ, Langhorne P. Poor outcome in primary intracerebral haemorrhage: results of a matched comparison. *Postgrad Med J* 2004; **80**(940):89–92.

21 Lipson DM, Sangha H, Foley NC, Bhogal S, Pohani G, Teasell RW. Recovery from stroke: differences between subtypes. *Int J Rehabil Res* 2005; **28**(4):303–8.

22 Feigin VL, Lawes CM, Bennett DA, Anderson CS. Stroke epidemiology: a review of population-based studies of incidence, prevalence, and case-fatality in the late 20th century. *Lancet Neurol* 2003; **2**(1):43–53.

23 Tanaka H, Ueda Y, Date C, Baba T, Yamashita H, Hayashi M *et al*. Incidence of stroke in Shibata, Japan: 1976–1978. *Stroke* 1981; **12**(4):460–6.

24 Asplund K, Bonita R, Kuulasmaa K, Rajakangas AM, Schaedlich H, Suzuki K *et al*. Multinational comparisons of stroke epidemiology. Evaluation of case ascertainment in the WHO MONICA Stroke Study. World Health Organization Monitoring Trends and Determinants in Cardiovascular Disease. *Stroke* 1995; **26**(3):355–60.

25 Feigin VL, Nikitin I, Kholodov VA, Shishkin SV, Novokhatskaia MV, Belenko AI, Khatsenko VN. [The epidemiology of cerebral stroke in Siberia based on registry data]. *Zh Nevropatol Psikhiatr Im S S Korsakova* 1996; **96**(6):59–65.

26 Petty GW, Brown RD, Jr., Whisnant JP, Sicks JD, O'Fallon WM, Wiebers DO. Ischemic stroke: outcomes, patient mix, and practice variation for neurologists and generalists in a community. *Neurology* 1998; **50**(6):1669–78.

27 Wijdicks EF, Rabinstein AA. Absolutely no hope? Some ambiguity of futility of care in devastating acute stroke. *Crit Care Med* 2004; **32**(11):2332–42.

28 Counsell C, Dennis M. Systematic review of prognostic models in patients with acute stroke. *Cerebrovasc Dis* 2001; **12**(3):159–70.

29 Meijer R, Ihnenfeldt DS, van Limbeek J, Vermeulen M, de Haan RJ. Prognostic factors in the subacute phase after stroke for the future residence after six months to one year. A systematic review of the literature. *Clin Rehabil* 2003; **17**(5):512–20.

30 Meijer R, Ihnenfeldt DS, de Groot IJ, van Limbeek J, Vermeulen M, de Haan RJ. Prognostic factors for ambulation and activities of daily living in the subacute phase after stroke. A systematic review of the literature. *Clin Rehabil* 2003; **17**(2):119–29.

31 Gladman JR, Harwood DM, Barer DH. Predicting the outcome of acute stroke: prospective evaluation of five multivariate models and comparison with simple methods. *J Neurol Neurosurg Psychiatry* 1992; **55**(5):347–51.

32 Taub NA, Wolfe CD, Richardson E, Burney PG. Predicting the disability of first-time stroke sufferers at 1 year. 12-month follow-up of a population-based cohort in southeast England. *Stroke* 1994; **25**(2):352–7.

33 Wardlaw JM, Lewis SC, Dennis MS, Counsell C, McDowall M. Is visible infarction on computed tomography associated with an adverse prognosis in acute ischemic stroke? *Stroke* 1998; **29**(7):1315–9.

34 Nuutinen J, Liu Y, Laakso MP, Karonen JO, Roivainen R, Vanninen RL *et al*. Assessing the outcome of stroke: a comparison between MRI and clinical stroke scales. *Acta Neurol Scand* 2006; **113**(2):100–7.

35 Hendricks HT, Zwarts MJ, Plat EF, van Limbeek J. Systematic review for the early prediction of motor and functional outcome after stroke by using motor-evoked potentials. *Arch Phys Med Rehabil* 2002; **83**(9):1303–8.

36 Kwakkel G, Wagenaar RC, Kollen BJ, Lankhorst GJ. Predicting disability in stroke: a critical review of the literature. *Age Ageing* 1996; **25**(6):479–89.

37 Counsell C, Dennis M, McDowall M, Warlow C. Predicting outcome after acute and subacute stroke: development and validation of new prognostic models. *Stroke* 2002; **33**(4):1041–7.

38 Weingarten S, Bolus R, Riedinger MS, Maldonado L, Stein S, Ellrodt AG. The principle of parsimony: Glasgow Coma Scale score predicts mortality as well as the APACHE II score for stroke patients. *Stroke* 1990; **21**(9):1280–2.

39 Wright CJ, Swinton LC, Green TL, Hill MD. Predicting final disposition after stroke using the Orpington Prognostic Score. *Can J Neurol Sci* 2004; **31**(4):494–8.

40 Horgan NF, Cunningham CJ, Coakley D, Walsh JB, O'Neill D, O'Regan M *et al*. Validating the Orpington Prognostic Score in an Irish in-patient stroke population. *Ir Med J* 2005; **98**(6):172, 174–5.

41 Weir NU, Counsell CE, McDowall M, Gunkel A, Dennis MS. Reliability of the variables in a new set of models that predict outcome after stroke. *J Neurol Neurosurg Psychiatry* 2003; **74**(4):447–51.

42 Dennis MS, Lewis SC, Warlow C. Routine oral nutritional supplementation for stroke patients in hospital (FOOD): a multicentre randomised controlled trial. *Lancet* 2005; **365**(9461):755–63.

43 Counsell C, Dennis MS, Lewis S, Warlow C. Performance of a statistical model to predict stroke outcome in the context of a large, simple, randomized, controlled trial of feeding. *Stroke* 2003; **34**(1):127–33.

44 Frankel MR, Morgenstern LB, Kwiatkowski T, Lu M, Tilley BC, Broderick JP *et al*. Predicting prognosis after stroke: a placebo group analysis from the National Institute of Neurological Disorders and Stroke rt-PA Stroke Trial. *Neurology* 2000; **55**(7):952–9.

45 Weimar C, Konig IR, Kraywinkel K, Ziegler A, Diener HC. Age and National Institutes of Health Stroke Scale Score within 6 hours after onset are accurate predictors of outcome after cerebral ischemia: development and external validation of prognostic models. *Stroke* 2004; **35**(1):158–62.

46 Muir KW, Weir CJ, Murray GD, Povey C, Lees KR. Comparison of neurological scales and scoring systems for acute stroke prognosis. *Stroke* 1996; **27**(10):1817–20.

47 Lai SM, Duncan PW, Keighley J. Prediction of functional outcome after stroke: comparison of the Orpington Prognostic Scale and the NIH Stroke Scale. *Stroke* 1998; **29**(9):1838–42.

48 Tilling K, Sterne JA, Rudd AG, Glass TA, Wityk RJ, Wolfe CD. A new method for predicting recovery after stroke. *Stroke* 2001; **32**(12):2867–73.

49 Tilling K, Sterne JA, Wolfe CD. Multilevel growth curve models with covariate effects: application to recovery after stroke. *Stat Med* 2001; **20**(5):685–704.

50 Counsell C, Dennis M, McDowall M. Predicting functional outcome in acute stroke: comparison of a simple six variable model with other predictive systems and informal clinical prediction. *J Neurol Neurosurg Psychiatry* 2004; **75**(3):401–5.

51 Harbison J, Hossain O, Jenkinson D, Davis J, Louw SJ, Ford GA. Diagnostic accuracy of stroke referrals from primary care, emergency room physicians, and ambulance staff using the face arm speech test. *Stroke* 2003; **34**(1):71–6.

52 Nor AM, McAllister C, Louw SJ, Dyker AG, Davis M, Jenkinson D, Ford GA. Agreement between ambulance paramedic- and physician-recorded neurological signs with Face Arm Speech Test (FAST) in acute stroke patients. *Stroke* 2004; **35**(6):1355–9.

53 Rothwell PM, Giles MF, Flossmann E, Lovelock CE, Redgrave JN, Warlow CP, Mehta Z. A simple score (ABCD) to identify individuals at high early risk of stroke after transient ischaemic attack. *Lancet* 2005; **366**(9479):29–36.

54 Hill MD, Weir NU. Is the ABCD score truly useful? *Stroke* 2006; **37**(7):1636.

55 Davenport RJ, Dennis MS, Warlow CP. Improving the recording of the clinical assessment of stroke patients using a clerking pro forma. *Age Ageing* 1995; **24**(1):43–8.

56 Hancock RJ, Oddy M, Saweirs WM, Court B. The RCP stroke audit package in practice. *J R Coll Physicians Lond* 1997; **31**(1):74–8.

57 Bero LA, Grilli R, Grimshaw JM, Harvey E, Oxman AD, Thomson MA. Closing the gap between research and practice: an overview of systematic reviews of interventions to promote the implementation of research findings. The Cochrane Effective Practice and Organization of Care Review Group. *Br Med J* 1998; **317**(7156):465–8.

58 Kwan J, Sandercock P. In-hospital care pathways for stroke. [update of *Cochrane Database Syst Rev* 2002; (2):CD002924; PMID: 12076460]. *Cochrane Database Syst Rev* 2004; (4):CD002924.

59 Smith MT, Baer GD. Achievement of simple mobility milestones after stroke. *Arch Phys Med Rehabil* 1999; **80**(4):442–7.

60 Wade DT, Wood VA, Heller A, Maggs J, Langton HR. Walking after stroke. Measurement and recovery over the first 3 months. *Scand J Rehabil Med* 1987; **19**(1):25–30.

61 Parry RH. Communication during goal-setting in physiotherapy treatment sessions. *Clin Rehabil* 2004; **18**(6):668–82.

62 Wressle E, Eeg-Olofsson AM, Marcusson J, Henriksson C. Improved client participation in the rehabilitation process using a client-centred goal formulation structure. *J Rehabil Med* 2002; **34**(1):5–11.

63 Bernhardt J, Dewey H, Thrift A, Donnan G. Inactive and alone: physical activity within the first 14 days of acute stroke unit care. *Stroke* 2004; **35**(4):1005–9.

64 Pound P, Bury M, Gompertz P, Ebrahim S. Stroke patients' views on their admission to hospital. *Br Med J* 1995; **311**(6996):18–22.

65 Stone SP, Wilson B, Wroot A, Halligan PW, Lange LS, Marshall JC, Greenwood RJ. The assessment of visuo-spatial neglect after acute stroke. *J Neurol Neurosurg Psychiatry* 1991; **54**(4):345–50.

66 Altman DG, Bland JM. Absence of evidence is not evidence of absence. *Br Med J* 1995; **311**(7003):485.

67 Greener J, Enderby P, Whurr R. Speech and language therapy for aphasia following stroke. *Cochrane Database Syst Rev* 2000; (2):CD000425.

68 Walker MF, Leonardi-Bee J, Bath P, Langhorne P, Dewey M, Corr S *et al*. Individual patient data meta-analysis of randomized controlled trials of community occupational therapy for stroke patients. *Stroke* 2004; **35**(9):2226–32.

69 Steultjens EM, Dekker J, Bouter LM, Van de Nes JC, Cup EH, Van den Ende CH. Occupational therapy for stroke patients: a systematic review. *Stroke* 2003; **34**(3):676–87.

70 Langhorne P, Pollock A. What are the components of effective stroke unit care? *Age Ageing* 2002; **31**(5):365–71.

71 Dennis MS, Lewis SC, Warlow C. Effect of timing and method of enteral tube feeding for dysphagic stroke patients (FOOD): a multicentre randomised controlled trial. *Lancet* 2005; **365**(9461):764–72.

72 Sackett DL, Haynes RB, Guyatt GH, Tugwell MD. *Clinical Epidemiology: A Basic Science for Clinical Medicine*. 2nd ed. Boston: Little, Brown, 1991.

73 Al-Shahi R, Vousden C, Warlow C. Bias from requiring explicit consent from all participants in observational research: prospective, population based study. *Br Med J* 2005; **331**(7522):942.

74 Counsell C. *The Prediction of Outcome in Patients with Acute Stroke*. Cambridge: University of Cambridge; 1998.

75 Dennis MS, Burn JP, Sandercock PA, Bamford JM, Wade DT, Warlow CP. Long-term survival after first-ever stroke: the Oxfordshire Community Stroke Project. *Stroke* 1993; **24**(6):796–800.

76 Langhorne P, Murray GD, Stott DJ, McAlpine C, MacDonald J. *Profiles of Recovery after Stroke: Their Value in Monitoring Recovery and Predicting Outcome*. Chief Scientists Office report. K/RED/4/C284, in press.

11 What are this patient's problems?

A problem-based approach to the general management of stroke

Stroke: practical management, 3rd edition. C. Warlow, J. van Gijn,
M. Dennis, J. Wardlaw, J. Bamford, G. Hankey, P. Sandercock,
G. Rinkel, P. Langhorne, C. Sudlow and P. Rothwell. Published
2008 Blackwell Publishing. ISBN 978-1-4051-2766-0.

11.1 Introduction

The patient's general management, as distinct from the specific treatment of their stroke (Chapters 12–14), is primarily aimed at identifying and solving existing problems, as well as anticipating and preventing potential problems, at different stages of their illness. This chapter will cover the common problems which occur in patients who have had a stroke. Each section is loosely structured as follows:

- *General description of each problem* which includes a definition, its frequency, causes and clinical significance, and prognosis.
- *Assessment,* including methods of detection, simple clinical assessments and measures which may be appropriate for goal setting, audit or research.
- *Prevention and treatment,* including interventions which may reduce the risk of a problem developing or hasten recovery.

Post-stroke problems have seldom been systematically identified in community-based incidence studies (section 17.11.1) so their frequency in unselected populations is often unknown. Moreover, compared with other aspects of treatment there are few large randomized controlled trials (RCTs) or systematic reviews addressing these problems. This is partly because there are major methodological difficulties in performing RCTs and systematic reviews to evaluate non-pharmacological interventions (Table 11.1). However, the evidence base is improving. Existing trials are being systematically appraised (www.effectivestrokecare.org) and more trials are being performed. Where there is no high-quality evidence the content of this chapter reflects our own clinical experience. Many of the topics are not specific to stroke medicine but might be found in any textbook of internal medicine or surgery. Therefore, we have not attempted to provide comprehensive reviews, but instead have concentrated on those aspects of assessment and management which are particularly relevant to stroke patients.

11.2 Airway, breathing and circulation

Inadequate airway, breathing or circulation are life-threatening. Urgent resuscitative measures must be taken. Even if not an immediate threat to survival, it seems sensible to optimize the delivery of oxygen and glucose to the brain to minimize brain damage and so achieve the best possible outcome for the patient (section 12.1).

Table 11.1 Problems in performing randomized controlled trials and systematic reviews of physiotherapy interventions.

Lack of theoretical model or rationale founded on basic science for many interventions
Ethical problems of performing randomized controlled trials due to therapists' certainty about the effectiveness of their own therapy in individual patients
Difficulty in getting patients and therapists, to accept the possibility of 'no treatment'
Strong patient preferences based on their belief in the benefits and acceptability of therapy
Difficulty in blinding patients to treatment allocation
Difficulty in designing convincing placebo treatments, or establishing appropriate 'controls'
Difficulties in defining a therapy (in terms of type, dose, frequency, timing and duration) which has to be tailored to the individual patient; this leads to difficulties in applying the results in practice
Failure to identify key components or interactions between components of an intervention
Moderate treatment effects mean that large numbers of patients have to be randomized
The need to randomize large numbers of patients may necessitate multicentre trials but these raise difficulties in standardizing and monitoring treatment
Therapy is very labour-intensive and therefore expensive, so that bodies which fund research may not be willing to fund the therapy
Difficulties agreeing suitable measures of outcome which are sensitive to both what therapists expect to influence, and what is relevant to the patient and family
In unblinded trials, patient loyalty to a therapist may bias their responses to subjective outcome scales
Various different outcome measures which hinders systematic review of trials
Problems due to complex interactions with other therapies given simultaneously

11.2.1 Obstructed airway

Patients with a decreased level of consciousness, impaired bulbar function or who have aspirated may have an obstructed or partially obstructed airway. Central cyanosis, noisy airflow with grunting, snoring or gurgling, an irregular breathing pattern and indrawing of the suprasternal area and intercostal muscles may indicate an obstruction. Transient obstruction is common in the acute phase of stroke during sleep (section 11.2.2) and it is, therefore, important that apnoeic spells due to an obstructed airway are not mistakenly attributed to periodic respiration and so ignored (e.g. Cheyne–Stokes; section 11.2.2).

If an obstructed airway is suspected, the oropharynx should be cleared of any foreign matter with a sweep of a gloved finger, the patient's jaw pulled forward, and the neck extended to stop the tongue falling back to obstruct the airway (Fig. 11.1). Positioning the patient in the coma (i.e. recovery) position may be enough to keep the airway clear, although in some situations an oropharyngeal or nasopharyngeal airway, or even endotracheal intubation, may be required (Fig. 11.2).

Fig. 11.1 It is essential to maintain a patent airway in a patient with a decreased level of consciousness. (a) In comatose patients with their head in a resting or flexed position the tongue falls backwards to obstruct the hypopharynx (*arrow*) and the epiglottis obstructs the larynx. (b) Tilting the head back by lifting the chin stretches the anterior neck structures, which opens the airway.

(a)

(b)

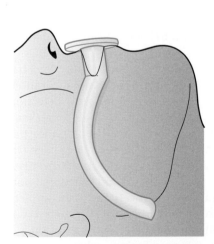

(a)

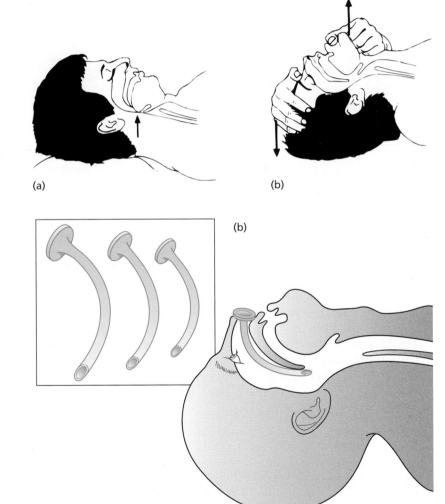

(b)

Fig. 11.2 Airways. (a) Oropharyngeal (Guedel) airway. To check that the airway is the correct size for the patient hold the airway across the cheek from corner of mouth to tip of ear lobe (the angle of the jaw bone may also be used). If this matches then the airway is the correct size. If too long or too short select another size. Incorrect sizing can result in the airway being blocked rather than kept open. Inserted upside down, they are moved along the roof of the mouth and rotated into position sitting behind the tongue and lifting it forward slightly. (b) Nasopharyngeal airway. To measure an appropriately sized nasopharyngeal airway, it is traditionally taught that the correct size is related to the patient's little finger or nostril. However these measures may not relate to the internal anatomy of their nose so it may more appropriate to size the airway by the patient's sex and height.[457,458]

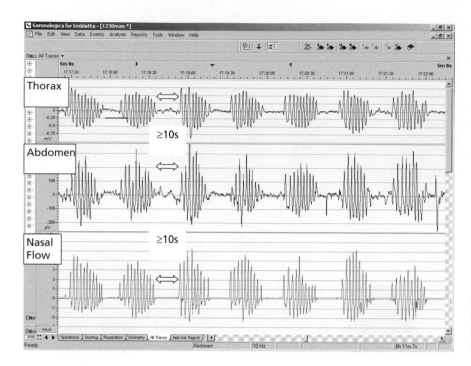

Fig. 11.3 Diagram showing Cheyne–Stokes breathing (courtesy of A Rowat); upper two traces show muscle activity, lower trace air flow.

Do not mistakenly attribute apnoeic spells due to intermittent airway obstruction to periodic or Cheyne–Stokes respiration.

11.2.2 Inadequate breathing

Strokes may weaken the intercostal muscles and the diaphragm, leading to reduced ventilation, poor cough and an increased risk of pneumonia.[1] Furthermore, the brain lesion itself may directly, or more often indirectly, impair the function of the respiratory centre in the medulla which results in various disordered patterns of breathing (Fig. 11.3) while the patient is awake, but much more commonly during sleep.[2]

Hypoxia

Hypoxic episodes (defined as saturations of < 90% for > 10% of monitoring period) have been described in about one-fifth of stroke patients within the first few hours of admission.[3] They occur more commonly during transfers between hospital departments and are associated with greater stroke severity and pre-existing cardiorespiratory disease. In patients with cardiorespiratory disease, hypoxia may be more marked in the supine position and reduced by sitting.[4] Hypoxia is associated with poorer survival but it is unclear whether this is an effect of hypoxia exacerbating the brain damage, or simply reflects co-existing severe cardiorespiratory disease occurring in severe strokes.[3]

Abnormal patterns of breathing

The abnormal patterns of breathing associated with stroke include obstructive and central sleep apnoea, periodic respiration (Cheyne–Stokes), hyperventilation ('forced respiration'), irregular (ataxic) breathing, apneustic (held in expiration) breathing and, ultimately, complete apnoea.[5]

Sleep apnoea is the commonest abnormality and has been identified in up to two-thirds of hospital-admitted patients, depending on the definitions and detection methods used. It is usually 'obstructive' although may occasionally be 'central'. Obstructive sleep apnoea has been associated with greater age, obesity, large neck circumference, and in some studies greater stroke severity.[2] It is associated with poorer survival and functional outcome but it is unclear whether this is due to incomplete adjustment for stroke severity, the associated hypoxia or fluctuations in blood pressure and cerebral perfusion.[6,7]

Periodic respiration (Cheyne–Stokes), where there are regular alternating phases of hyperventilation and hypoventilation, occurs in about a quarter of patients although it is seldom recognized by healthcare staff.[8] Other neurological functions, e.g. wakefulness, often vary in phase with breathing. The mechanisms of periodic respiration are still debated but it probably reflects a change in the sensitivity of the brainstem respiratory centre to the arterial pressure of carbon dioxide and/or slowed central circulation, with a resultant delay in the feedback loop controlling respiration.[9,10] Changes in oxygenation, pH and cerebral blood flow occur in periodic respiration but their importance is unclear. Periodic respiration is associated with greater stroke severity and poorer outcomes although it may be present in patients who are alert and who subsequently make a reasonable recovery.[8]

> Periodic respiration (Cheyne–Stokes) does not necessarily imply a hopeless prognosis.

Co-existing cardiopulmonary disease (e.g. chronic obstructive pulmonary disease, pneumonia) is probably a more frequent cause of inadequate ventilation than the abnormal breathing patterns due to the stroke itself. Its detection depends on a thorough initial assessment including an adequate history, physical examination and some simple investigations, e.g. chest X-ray and electrocardiogram (section 10.3.2).

Assessment

The adequacy of ventilation should be assessed clinically by checking for central cyanosis and examining the chest. We increasingly use pulse oximetry to assess and monitor our patients to detect hypoxaemia. Finger probes are more accurate than those on the ear, and it probably does not matter whether the probe is placed on the paretic or non-paretic hand.[11,12] Arterial blood gas analysis is useful in monitoring therapy in patients with type II respiratory failure, those requiring artificial ventilation and those with severe metabolic disturbances such as acidosis.

> It is easy to miss abnormalities in breathing pattern. Encourage all members of the team to observe the breathing pattern while they are assessing the patient.

Treatment

There are currently no data to support the *routine* administration of increased concentrations of oxygen to patients who are not hypoxic so do not automatically give oxygen to every admitted stroke patient.[13] However, if the patient has an oxygen saturation of < 95% in the first couple of days after stroke onset it seems sensible (although not supported by strong evidence) to increase incrementally the inspired oxygen concentration to achieve a saturation of > 95% and so reduce the the likelihood that any ischaemic but still viable brain tissue is

adversely affected. Patients prefer oxygen delivered via nasal prongs rather than with a face mask.[14] In patients with chronic lung disease and a tendency to hypercapnoea, 24% oxygen should be used initially with careful monitoring of the patient's respiration, neurological function (section 11.5) and arterial blood gases.

Although continuous positive airways pressure (CPAP) has been shown to reduce symptoms of obstructive sleep apnoea in general, in patients with recent stroke compliance with treatment tends to be very poor and there is no reliable evidence of benefit.[15–17] Treatment of any coexisting lung or cardiac disease should of course be given. Sitting the patient up may help to improve oxygenation.[4] If patients are sat out of bed, it is important that they are well supported in an upright position and not slumped in the chair, which worsens ventilation. Sitting may also reduce the intracranial pressure but may cause other problems (section 11.11). Sedative drugs, given to promote sleep, to facilitate imaging or to control seizures, may precipitate periodic respiration or respiratory failure and should generally be avoided if at all possible.

Tracheal intubation and mechanical ventilation may be used to maintain ventilation, or to reduce intracranial pressure (section 12.7.4). Indications vary between centres but generally include: deteriorating conscious level, severe hypoxia or hypercapnoea, and inability to maintain an airway. Depending on the indications and case mix, reported frequency of in-hospital case fatality among patients undergoing mechanical ventilation varies between 50 and 90%. Older age, evidence of brainstem dysfunction and comorbidities are predictably associated with worse outcomes; however, a small proportion of survivors make a reasonable recovery.[18–20] Often, such aggressive management is considered inappropriate because of the patient's low probability of regaining a good quality of life (section 10.4).

> If patients are nursed in a sitting position, it is best if they are well supported and upright in a chair rather than slumped in bed or a chair, which makes breathing more difficult.

11.2.3 Poor circulation

Both severe brainstem dysfunction and massive subarachnoid haemorrhage can cause major circulatory problems such as neurogenic pulmonary oedema, cardiac dysrhythmias and erratic blood pressure with severe hypertension or hypotension (section 14.9.3 and 14.9.4). More frequently, circulatory failure, with or without hypotension or hypoxia related to pulmonary oedema, is due to coexistent heart disease (e.g. congestive cardiac failure, myocardial infarction, atrial fibrillation), hypovolaemia (e.g. dehydration, bleeding) or severe infection.

Cardiac dysrhythmias

Cardiac dysrhythmias are quite common after an acute stroke, although they rarely cause major problems.[21] The most clinically important, in terms of frequency and effect on management, is atrial fibrillation which occurs in about one-fifth of patients with ischaemic stroke and one in ten of those with intracerebral haemorrhage.[22,23] In most cases, atrial fibrillation precedes the stroke and in some it is the most likely cause of the stroke (section 6.5.1). Of course, a small proportion of ischaemic strokes, perhaps 5%, occur in the context of a recent (within 6 weeks) myocardial infarction (section 7.10).[24]

Routine monitoring of the patient's cardiac rhythm, either at the bedside or preferably with ambulatory systems which do not inhibit early mobilization, will identify abnormalities, most commonly paroxysmal atrial fibrillation. The yield will depend on the duration of monitoring. A 24-h ECG monitor might detect previously undected atrial fibrillation in up to 5% and 7-day monitoring in a further 5% of hospitalized patients with ischaemic stroke.[25,26] The detection of atrial fibrillation will influence decisions about anticoagulation for secondary prevention (section 16.6). The feasibility and cost of routinely monitoring rhythm inevitably varies between centres and it is unclear what the yield is in terms of altering management, perhaps by starting anticoagulation and preventing recurrences. Certainly, as a minimum we would advise monitoring those with palpitations, syncope, unexplained breathlessness or recent myocardial infarction.

> Cardiac dysrhythmias, other than atrial fibrillation, are quite common after an acute stroke, but seldom seem to be a problem unless they are due not to the stroke itself but to a recent myocardial infarction.

Myocardial injury

It is important to identify the presence and likely cause of any circulatory failure, by clinical assessment of the cardiovascular system backed up with relevant investigations (e.g. cardiac enzymes, electrocardiogram (ECG) and echocardiography). Repolarization abnormalities and ischaemic-like changes on the ECG occur in about three-quarters of patients with subarachnoid haemorrhage but are far less common with other types of stroke.

In SAH the changes are most often secondary to the cerebral insult while in other stroke types they usually reflect associated cardiac disease.[27] The specificity of ECG changes for acute myocardial infarction in the context of an acute stroke is low.[28] Levels of plasma creatine kinase (CK) and of its more cardiac-specific isoenzyme CK muscle–brain (MB) are quite often raised but the interpretation may be difficult where the patient has fallen, been injured, lain on a hard floor or had a generalized seizure which may all increase the CK level. Indeed even when CK-MB is raised, troponins, which are more specific markers of myocardial injury, are often normal indicating that even CK-MB may not be of cardiac origin.[29] Raised troponins have been reported in up to a third of patients with stroke and may be markers of a concurrent myocardial infarction or small areas of myocardial necrosis, which have been identified at autopsy.[30] Raised troponins are associated with poorer survival even having adjusted for age and stroke severity.[27,31,32] Patients with circulatory failure, atrial fibrillation and recent myocardial infarction have a poor prognosis for survival and functional recovery after stroke.[22,33] Active treatment of these problems is likely to improve the outcome but a detailed account is beyond the scope of this book.

Gastrointestinal haemorrhage

About 3% of stroke patients have an upper gastrointestinal bleed in the first few weeks.[34] Bleeding most commonly occurs from petechiae, erosions and ulcers.[35] Bleeds are more common in the elderly, in more severe strokes and those with intracerebral haemorrhage; not surprisingly, therefore, gastrointestinal haemorrhage has been associated with high case fatality. Bleeding appears to be more common in patients fed via an enteral tube and may be more common with nasogastric, rather than percutaneous endoscopic, gastrostomy.[36] Clearly, resulting hypotension and anaemia might both exacerbate cerebral ischaemia and worsen the neurological outcome.

One should obviously be aware of this bleeding potential when prescribing antithrombotic and anti-inflammatory medication.[37] We try to avoid using nonsteroidal anti-inflammatory drugs (NSAIDs) unless there is a strong indication. Proton pump inhibitors (PPI), double dose H2 receptor antagonists and misoprostol have all been shown to reduce gastric and duodenal ulcers in patients (not stroke) taking NSAIDs chronically.[38] A meta-analysis of 20 trials with a total of 2624 mainly Chinese patients suggested an 80% odds reduction in stress-related gastrointestinal haemorrhage among stroke patients and even a reduction in mortality associated with PPI and H2 receptor antagonists.[39] However, the rate of bleeding in the control groups of

Table 11.2 The frequency of various clinical features among 675 patients with a first-ever-in-a-lifetime stroke at their initial assessment by a study neurologist (from the Oxfordshire Community Stroke Project, unpublished data).

Clinical feature	Number (%)	Not assessable (%)
Glasgow Coma Scale (motor < 6)	86 (13)	15 (2)
Glasgow Coma Scale (eyes < 4)	98 (15)	16 (2)
Glasgow Coma Scale (eyes + motor < 10)	111 (16)	16 (2)
High blood pressure (systolic > 160 mmHg)	311 (46)	19 (3)
Very high blood pressure (systolic > 200 mmHg)	90 (13)	19 (3)
High blood pressure (diastolic > 100 mmHg)	131 (19)	22 (3)
Very high blood pressure (diastolic > 120 mmHg)	23 (3)	22 (3)
Epileptic seizures within 24 h	14 (2)	0 (0)
Facial weakness	256 (38)	40 (6)
Arm or hand weakness	344 (51)	32 (5)
Leg weakness	307 (45)	34 (5)
Unilateral weakness of at least two of face, arm and leg	331 (49)	0 (0)
Sensory loss (proprioception)	101 (15)	168 (25)
Sensory loss (spinothalamic)	196 (29)	140 (21)
Homonymous visual field defect	113 (18)	134 (20)
Gaze palsy	50 (7)	36 (5)
Mental test score < 8/10[433]	85 (13)	135 (20)
Visuospatial dysfunction	81 (12)	179 (27)
Dysphasia	122 (19)	111 (16)
Dysarthria	135 (20)	127 (19)

these trials was far higher than that reported in observational studies in white populations. Management of active gastrointestinal haemorrhage is the same as in other situations.

11.3 Reduced level of consciousness

About 15% of stroke patients have a reduced level of consciousness during the first few days after the stroke (Table 11.2). The causes are not entirely clear (Table 11.3). It may arise from direct damage (haemorrhage or infarction) to the brainstem or more commonly indirect damage from supratentorial lesions associated with brain swelling and midline shift.[40,41] However, we not infrequently see patients with large ischaemic, apparently unilateral, hemispheric strokes who become drowsy within hours of onset, before one would expect enough oedema to have developed to raise intracranial pressure markedly, and with little or no apparent mass effect on brain imaging.[42] Indeed, in one study, only a minority of patients whose conscious level deteriorated after a large hemispheric ischaemic stroke had globally raised intracranial pressure on invasive monitoring.[43] It has

been argued that differences in pressure between brain compartments may be more important than the overall pressure. However, treatable complications of the stroke may also depress conscious level (Table 11.3).

Level of consciousness is an important indicator of the severity of the stroke and a valuable prognostic variable[44] (section 10.2.7).

Table 11.3 Remediable causes of a reduced level of consciousness after stroke.

Causes	Section
General	
Hypoxia	11.2.2
Hypotension	11.2.3
Severe infection	11.12
Electrolyte imbalance	11.18.1 and 11.18.2
Hypoglycaemia	11.18.4
Drugs: e.g. benzodiazepines, opiate analgesics	
Neurological	
Epileptic seizures	11.8
Raised intracranial pressure	12.7, 13.3.2
Obstructive hydrocephalus (e.g. due to cerebellar haematoma)	13.3.6, 14.8
Cerebral ischaemia after subarachnoid haemorrhage	14.5, 14.7

Assessment

The most commonly used measure of level of consciousness is the Glasgow Coma Scale (GCS) (Table 3.12), which reliably documents the patient's spontaneous actions as well as those in response to verbal and painful stimuli.[45] Although useful, the GCS, which was originally designed for patients with head injury, has a number of problems when applied to stroke. The most important is that many patients with stroke are aphasic and therefore have a reduced score on the verbal response scale. Thus, a patient may have a reduced total score on the GCS but a normal level of consciousness. Another problem is that inexperienced users may apply the motor scale to the affected arm in a patient with a hemiparesis and obtain a reduced motor response rather than the 'best' response. The GCS communicates most information if the component scores are recorded separately. Alternative measures include the reaction level scale and components of so-called 'stroke scales' (sections 10.2.7 and 17.12.5).[46]

Patients with a reduced level of consciousness are at greater risk of developing various complications (Table 11.4) so expert nursing care is needed to minimize these risks. Also, a falling level of consciousness may alert one to an important and potentially reversible condition (Table 11.3). Therefore, patients with severe strokes, in whom active treatment would be considered, should be monitored with the GCS for the first few days, especially where staff change frequently, to avoid delays in initiating investigation and treatment of any worsening in their condition. We usually reduce the frequency of monitoring, e.g. hourly, 2, 3 or 6-hourly, over the first few days after the stroke. The speed at which we do this will depend on the team's judgement about the likelihood of deterioration and the appropriateness and urgency of any intervention aimed at reversing the deterioration. Also, the availability of nursing staff to perform the measurements and the patient's need for

Table 11.4 Common complications in patients with a depressed level of consciousness after stroke.

Complication	Section
Airway obstruction	11.2.1
Aspiration	11.17
Fever and infection	11.12
Dehydration	11.18.1
Malnutrition	11.19
Urinary incontinence	11.14
Faecal incontinence or constipation	11.15
Pressure ulcers	11.16

unbroken sleep have to be taken into account. Therefore, one might monitor a patient's GCS hourly during the first 2 days after a cerebellar haematoma (in whom decompressive surgery would be considered) but only 6-hourly in a patient who is stable 2 days after a mild ischaemic stroke.

> The Glasgow Coma Scale is a useful tool for monitoring patients only if it is applied properly. Staff need to be trained in its proper use. Our patients are frequently said by medical and nursing staff to be confused or aphasic with a GCS of 15/15. Clearly this is nonsense!

The investigation and treatment of patients with a falling level of consciousness are similar to those with other indicators of worsening and are discussed in section 11.5. The specific treatment of patients with raised intracranial pressure is discussed in sections 12.7 and 13.3.2.

11.4 Severe stroke vs apparently severe stroke

It is important to be aware that severe concurrent illness, or stroke complications, may make a stroke appear much worse than it really is (Table 11.5). The clinical features which might indicate a severe stroke (e.g. reduced level of consciousness), and so a poor prognosis, may in fact be due to the complicating illness rather than the stroke itself. For example, a patient with a pure motor stroke (lacunar syndrome) (section 4.3.2) and a severe chest infection may be drowsy or confused. It is then difficult to distinguish this clinical picture from that due to a major middle cerebral artery territory infarction (section 4.3.4). Of course, an infection is more easily treated than a large volume of necrotic brain, so with appropriate therapy the prognosis of the two types of patient will be quite different.

A thorough general examination will identify signs such as fever, confusion, increased respiratory rate and reduced oxygen saturation, and usually reveals any relevant coexisting disorder. Simple investigations such as a white blood cell count, C-reactive protein, urea and electrolytes, urine microscopy and culture, chest X-ray, ECG and blood cultures are useful, not only to identify the cause of the stroke (sections 6.8.1 and 6.8.2), but also to alert one to serious coexisting non-stroke disease. Seizures that have occurred since stroke onset make the

Table 11.5 Causes of apparently severe strokes.

	Section
Non-neurological	
Infection	
Respiratory	11.12.1
Urinary	11.12.2
Septicaemia	
Metabolic	
Dehydration	11.18.1
Electrolyte disturbance	11.18.2, 11.18.3
Hypoglycaemia	11.18.4
Drugs	
Major and minor tranquillizers	11.29
Baclofen	11.20
Lithium toxicity	
Anti-epileptic drug toxicity	11.8
Anti-emetics	11.9
Hypoxia	
Pneumonia/chest infection	11.12.1
Pulmonary embolism	11.13
Chronic pulmonary disease	11.6
Pulmonary oedema	11.2.3
Hypercapnoea	
Chronic pulmonary disease	11.2.2
Limb or bowel ischaemia in patients with a cardiac or aortic arch source of embolism	
Neurological	
Obstructive hydrocephalus in patients with stroke in the posterior fossa, or subarachnoid haemorrhage	13.3.6, 12.7.3 and 14.8
Epileptic seizures, including complex partial seizures	11.8

assessment of stroke severity particularly difficult (section 11.8). It is also important not to overlook the possibility that any decreased conscious level is due to sedative drugs.

The treatment of apparently severe strokes will depend on the specific problem identified or suspected.

A 70-year-old man was found unconscious at home and admitted to hospital. In the receiving unit he had a partial seizure affecting his right side with secondary generalization. Subsequent neurological examination revealed a reduced conscious level, deviated gaze and a flaccid paralysis of the right side. Brain CT scan on the day of admission was normal. A diagnosis of a severe ischaemic stroke was made and the decision not to resuscitate was recorded in the notes. He was given intravenous fluids but no anti-epileptic drugs. He was later reviewed by the stroke physician who, having found occasional twitching movements of the right hand,

reversed the decision not to resuscitate and arranged an EEG which showed status epilepticus. Following intravenous phenytoin the patient improved and 4 days later was discharged from hospital without residual neurological deficits. Therefore, do not 'write off' people with apparently severe strokes and recent seizures.

11.5 Worsening after a stroke

Although stroke onset is usually abrupt, the patient's neurological condition may worsen hours, days or, rarely, weeks after the initial assessment (as well as improve). Patients may have a reducing level of consciousness, worsening of existing neurological deficits, or new deficits indicating dysfunction in another part of the brain. A large number of terms including 'stroke-in-evolution', 'stroke-in-progression', 'early neurological deterioration' and 'progressing stroke' have in the past been applied to this situation, which probably reflects the considerable level of interest in the problem and uncertainty as to its causes.[47] After all, here is a situation where one might be able to intervene to prevent a major stroke. One well-validated definition of 'progressing stroke' is based on a deterioration in the Scandinavian Stroke Scale[48] (Table 11.6) of at least two points on the conscious level, arm, leg or eye movement subscales and/or at least three points on the speech subscale between baseline and day 3.[49,50] The same change between consecutive measurements within the first 3 days was referred to as an 'early deterioration episode'.

Clearly, if we accept that the neurological deficit commonly increases over minutes or hours, then the earlier in the course of the stroke we first see the patient, the more likely we are to observe subsequent worsening. Indeed, it is likely that, as we attempt to introduce acute treatments for stroke, we will become much more aware of the 'normal' worsening over the first few hours after stroke onset. We will probably see patients earlier in the development of their stroke and monitor them more closely because they will be in clinical trials, or given a specific treatment for acute stroke. Not surprisingly therefore, estimates of the frequency of worsening in the first day or two have varied considerably but have been reported in up to 40% of hospital-admitted patients.[51]

Early worsening is more likely to be due to a neurological mechanism than a systemic complication of the stroke.[52] The factors underlying the progression of neurological deficits in the first day or two after stroke

Table 11.6 Scandinavian Stroke Scale.[48]

Consciousness:		☐
– fully conscious	6	
– somnolent, can be awaked to full consciousness	4	
– reacts to verbal command, but is not fully conscious	2	
– no reaction to verbal command	0	
Eye movement:		☐
– no gaze palsy	4	
– gaze palsy present	2	
– conjugate eye deviation	0	
Arm, motor power:*		☐
– raises arm with normal strength	6	
– raises arm with reduced strength	5	
– raises arm with flexion in elbow	4	
– can move, but not against gravity	2	
– paralysis	0	
Hand, motor power *:		☐
– normal strength	6	
– reduced strength in full range	4	
– some movement, fingertips do not reach palm	2	
– paralysis	0	
Leg, motor power *:		☐
– normal strength	6	
– raises straight leg with reduced strength	5	
– raises leg with flexion of knee	4	
– can move, but not against gravity	2	
– paralysis	0	
Orientation:		☐
– correct for time, place and person	6	
– two of these	4	
– one of these	2	
– completely disorientated	0	
Speech:		☐
– no aphasia	10	
– limited vocabulary or incoherent speech	6	
– more than yes/no, but not longer sentences	3	
– only yes/no or less	0	
Facial palsy:		☐
– none/dubious	2	
– present	0	
Gait:		☐
– walks 5 m without aids	12	
– walks with aids	9	
– walks with help of another person	6	
– sits without support	3	
– bedridden/wheelchair	0	
TOTAL		☐

*Motor power is assessed only on the affected side.

onset are unclear.[53] For example, what causes the progression of deficits in some patients with lacunar infarction?[54] Early worsening is likely to reflect complex interactions between biochemical and haemodynamic factors which are known to be important in the development of ischaemic stroke (sections 12.1.3 and 12.1.4). A history of diabetes or coronary heart disease, low and high arterial blood pressure, early computed tomography (CT) signs of infarction, evidence of siphon or middle cerebral artery occlusion, various biochemical (e.g. glucose and glutamate) and haematological (e.g. D-dimers) parameters have all been associated with a greater risk of early worsening.[47,55–57] Greater age, initial stroke severity and the presence of cerebral oedema on scanning have been associated with late deterioration.[47]

Worsening has a number of potential causes, some reversible, so it is important to detect and treat them early. The literature has tended to emphasize the neurological causes (Table 11.7) but it is important not to miss the non-neurological ones which tend to occur after the first couple of days and which are more treatable. There is, not surprisingly, considerable overlap with the causes of 'apparently severe stroke' (Table 11.5). The outcome of patients whose neurological condition worsens after initial presentation is predictably worse than that of patients who remain stable or improve rapidly.

Table 11.7 Causes of worsening after stroke.

	Section
Neurological	
Progression/completion of the stroke	
Extension/early recurrence	16.2
Haemorrhagic transformation of an infarct	5.7
Development of oedema around the infarct or haemorrhage*	12.1.5
Obstructive hydrocephalus in patients with stroke in the posterior fossa, or after subarachnoid haemorrhage*	13.2.6, 12.7.3 and 14.8
Epileptic seizures*	11.8
Delayed ischaemia* (in subarachnoid haemorrhage)	14.5, 14.7
Incorrect diagnosis	3.4
Intracranial tumour*	
Cerebral abscess*	
Encephalitis	
Chronic subdural haematoma*	
Subdural empyema*	
*Non-neurological**	
See Table 11.5	

*Remediable causes of worsening.

Table 11.8 Parameters to monitor and which can detect worsening.

	Section
Conscious level, i.e. Glasgow Coma Scale	3.3.2, 11.3
Pupillary responses	3.3.6
Eye movements	3.3.6
Limb movements	3.3.4
Stroke scale (e.g. Scandinavian Stroke Scale)	Table 11.6
Temperature	11.12
Pulse rate	11.2.3
Blood pressure	11.7
Respiratory rate	11.2.2, 11.12
Pulse oximetry	11.2.2
Fluid balance	11.18.1

Assessment

To ensure that clinical worsening is identified as early as possible, i.e. when the potential for therapeutic reversal is usually greatest, it is important to monitor the patient's condition. Regular measurements such as those in Table 11.8 will usually alert one to any problem. However, experienced nursing staff who have regular close contact with the patient may detect a problem at an early stage before it becomes obvious to other members of the team. Family members, who often spend long periods with ill patients, may also detect subtle but important changes in the patient's condition and they should be listened to. It is important that the physician caring for the patient encourages free communication so this sort of information is made known to those directing the patient's care.

Although there is a long list of potential causes of worsening, it is important to consider first those that are most readily reversible (Table 11.7). Most can be diagnosed by a clinical assessment supplemented by simple laboratory investigations. An urgent repeat CT brain scan is advisable in some situations, for example deterioration in conscious level in a patient with a cerebellar stroke or subarachnoid haemorrhage who may be developing obstructive hydrocephalus amenable to neurosurgical intervention. In a patient treated with thrombolytic drugs, an abrupt change in blood pressure, new onset of headache and/or vomiting or neurological deterioration should prompt an urgent CT scan to detect intracranial bleeding due to the treatment. The detection of haemorrhagic transformation of infarction in a patient receiving antithrombotic drugs may influence the decision to continue the medication or not, although there is no reliable evidence for the best policy

in this situation (sections 5.7, 12.4.2 and 12.5.7). A CT or MRI brain scan that shows that the deterioration was due to an early recurrent ischaemic stroke, especially one in a different arterial territory to the initial stroke, may encourage one to investigate further for a proximal arterial or cardiac source of embolism.

Treatment

Clearly, any treatment will depend on the reason for the worsening (see relevant sections) but it should be emphasized that at present there is little evidence from RCTs to support the use of treatments such as anticoagulants, thrombolysis, neuroprotection, haemodilution and manipulation of blood pressure for the treatment of worsening (Chapter 12). A small trial which randomized 98 patients to either routine care or intensive physiological monitoring showed that the more intensively monitored patients received more intensive treatment (e.g. supplementary oxygen) and deteriorated less frequently.[58] This preliminary finding, which needs to be confirmed in larger studies, could have important implications for the management of patients with acute stroke (section 17.6.2).

A 65-year-old woman had an acute ischaemic stroke affecting her cerebellum and brainstem. This occurred on a background of a previous occipital ischaemic stroke, impaired renal function and hypertension. After a stormy early course requiring drainage of obstructive hydrocephalus and ventilation on the intensive care unit, she made good progress. She could sit independently, help with washing herself and dressing, and could take a soft diet and fluids safely. She had diplopia, poor balance and complained of vertigo and vomiting which was exacerbated by movement. She was started on regular oral metoclopramide with some relief of these symptoms. She was transferred to a separate rehabilitation ward on a Friday afternoon. Over the weekend she deteriorated. Her speech became very unclear, her swallowing unsafe and she was unable to sit. Infection, metabolic abnormalities and recurrent hydrocephalus were excluded and a repeat MR scan showed no new stroke lesion although this seemed the most likely explanation for her deterioration. The family were advised that the prognosis was poor. The speech therapist, assessing the patient prior to insertion of a percutaneous endoscopic gastrostomy, remarked that the patient's tongue movements were like those of a patient with Parkinson's disease – the penny dropped! The drug chart was reviewed, the metoclopramide was withdrawn and the patient returned to her previous functional state over the next week. She was eventually discharged home, walking and requiring minimal help with everyday activities.

Table 11.9 Frequency of coexisting medical problems among 675 patients with a first-ever-in-a-lifetime stroke (from the Oxfordshire Community Stroke Project, unpublished data).

	n	(%)
Previous angina	106	(16)
Previous myocardial infarction	112	(17)
Cardiac failure	52	(8)
Intermittent claudication	112	(17)
Diabetes mellitus	63	(9)
Previous epileptic seizures	19	(3)
Previous malignancy	74	(11)
Dependent before stroke (Rankin > 2)	103	(15)

No data were available on respiratory or musculoskeletal problems.

11.6 Coexisting medical problems

Coexisting medical problems are common in stroke patients because they are usually elderly and have associated vascular disease (Table 11.9). Although we have already mentioned the importance of cardiorespiratory diseases in the immediate management of the patient (section 11.2), these and other conditions can be important for many other reasons, not least that they may require treatment in their own right. Severe non-stroke illness can make a mild stroke *appear* severe and thus lead to an inaccurate prognosis and possibly inappropriate treatment (section 11.4). Coexistent cardiorespiratory (e.g. angina, cardiac failure, chronic obstructive pulmonary disease), musculoskeletal (e.g. arthritis, back pain, amputation) and psychiatric conditions (e.g. depression, anxiety) often compound stroke-related disability. So, for example, after several months of rehabilitation, one might have taught a patient with a severe hemiparesis to walk again, but if he or she also has chronic obstructive pulmonary disease the added effort of walking with a hemiplegic gait may mean that the patient cannot walk any useful distance. It is important to be aware of the limitations on rehabilitation imposed by any pre-existing disease before spending months trying to make a patient walk. It may be more realistic to teach the patient to be independent in a wheelchair. Even if one cannot estimate the impact of non-stroke disease on recovery, knowledge of its existence may explain why patients are not achieving their rehabilitation goals (section 10.3.4).

Although most patients who survive a stroke improve over weeks or months, many of the coexisting problems, which contribute to disability, progress. Thus, a patient may reach their optimal functional recovery some months after a stroke and then deteriorate due to progression of a comorbid condition. If this kind of deterioration can be anticipated, it may allow for a more flexible package of care to cope with such fluctuations. There can be few things more dispiriting than to strive to discharge a patient into one form of accommodation and then hear that within a few months their condition has deteriorated to such an extent that the accommodation is no longer suitable. This can shatter the morale of the patient and their carer.

> Functional deterioration months after a stroke is unlikely to be due to the initial stroke and much more likely to be caused by a recurrent stroke or the progression of some comorbid condition such as angina, arthritis or intermittent claudication.

Assessment

A thorough history and examination at the time of admission, with reassessment when the patient is more active, should identify the main coexisting medical problems – the patient's medication will often provide a clue. An assessment of the patient's pre-stroke functional status (i.e. what could they do and not do?) is invaluable, not only in predicting outcome (section 10.2.7) but also for identifying comorbidities. Unfortunately, this is often not recorded in the medical records unless specifically prompted.[59,60] One approach might be to estimate routinely a pre-stroke Barthel Index (section 17.12.5) since this covers most of the important activities of daily living (ADL). This sort of ADL checklist is also useful in making a prognosis and in setting rehabilitation goals since, depending on the cause and duration, the pre-stroke functional impairment will determine the best achievable post-stroke functional status. If a patient has, as a result of arthritis, been immobile for 10 years before the stroke, it is ridiculous to try to get the patient to walk after the stroke. Unfortunately, this is often attempted simply because nobody has obtained an accurate picture of the patient's pre-stroke function. This is more likely to happen where the patient has difficulties with communication and no carer is available.

An assessment of the patient's pre-stroke function may also be very important in making decisions even within the first few hours after stroke. Although it may be impossible for anyone to judge a person's quality of life, other than that person themselves, one may deduce something from the patient's function. This may be important where, for example, one is considering antibiotics for a severe infection, or neurosurgery for acute obstructive hydrocephalus in a patient with a cerebellar stroke. It may be inappropriate to submit a previously very disabled or demented patient in a nursing home, who will almost certainly have a poor long-term outcome, to uncomfortable procedures (section 10.4).

Treatment

Clearly, one should aim to minimize the effect of any comorbidity by giving as effective treatments as possible. Where it is not possible to influence the disease directly, it is still important to take account of comorbidity in one's overall approach to the patient. One's intermediate and long-term goals also have to take this into account (section 10.3.3).

11.7 High and low blood pressure after stroke

11.7.1 High blood pressure

High blood pressure is often noted on admission to hospital after a stroke but it then usually falls spontaneously over the next few days. It is generally higher in patients with intracerebral haemorrhage than ischaemic stroke.[61,62] Although the raised blood pressure may, in part, reflect the physical and mental stress of hospital admission, or the 'white coat' effect, some of the rise seems to be due to the acute stroke itself. Raised blood pressure detected during the initial assessment may also indicate chronic hypertension since about half of stroke patients are hypertensive (i.e. at least two readings of > 160/90 mmHg) before the onset. They will tend to have higher blood pressures than those without previous hypertension and are more likely to have evidence of end-organ damage, e.g. hypertensive retinopathy, impaired renal function and left-ventricular hypertrophy. High blood pressure in the acute phase of both haemorrhagic and ischaemic strokes is associated with a poor outcome, an effect which appears to be independent of age and stroke severity (Fig. 11.4).[61,63–68]

Assessment

There is considerable variation in the methods used and the frequency of monitoring blood pressure after acute stroke. Traditionally, the blood pressure has been measured in the standard way with a sphygmomanometer and an appropriately sized cuff kept at the level of the

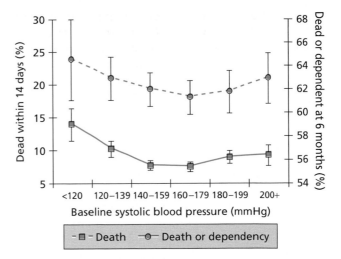

Fig. 11.4 Proportion of patients who died within 14 days (*solid lines*) or were dead or dependent at 6 months (*dashed lines*) by baseline systolic blood pressure. Squares and circles indicate the mean percentage of patients who had died within 14 days and patients who had died or were dependent at 6 months, respectively, within each blood pressure subgroup; 95% confidence intervals are represented by error bars. (From Leonardi-Bee *et al.*, 2002[66] with permission.)

patient's heart. However, increasingly, semi-automated non-invasive systems are used which allow more frequent monitoring (even when there are few nursing staff) and thus earlier intervention. These systems must be calibrated to avoid misleading readings.[69] The presence of atrial fibrillation reduces the reproducibility of both manual and semi-automated blood pressure recordings.[70,71] In the intensive care unit, intra-arterial monitoring is frequently used although this can very occasionally cause peripheral ischaemia. Perhaps not surprisingly, more intensive monitoring often leads to more manipulation of blood pressure, the value of which is currently unclear (see below).

> Semi-automatic blood pressure monitors should be properly calibrated to avoid misleading results. In patients with very low or high blood pressure, where the reading is likely to lead to a significant change in management, we would normally check the reading with a traditional sphygmomanometer.

There is no consistent difference between the blood pressure measured in the weak vs the unaffected arm, although there is often a difference between arms which is unrelated to the side of the stroke and probably reflects occlusive arterial disease affecting one arm.[72] Therefore, ideally the blood pressure should be checked in both arms on at least one occasion, and if the blood pressures are different, it should be monitored consistently in the arm giving the highest reading to avoid a spurious label of labile hypertension. If the blood pressure is raised on admission it should be monitored to establish whether or not it falls spontaneously and the patient examined to identify evidence of end-organ damage.

Treatment

There is considerable uncertainty about the risks and benefits of lowering the blood pressure in the acute phase of stroke. Treatment may theoretically reduce the likelihood of rebleeding in intracerebral and subarachnoid haemorrhage, and of brain oedema and haemorrhagic transformation in cerebral infarction. However, lowering the blood pressure may reduce cerebral perfusion where cerebral autoregulation is impaired and thus further increase ischaemic damage[73] (section 12.1.2). Intravenous calcium channel blockers which, apart from their potential neuroprotective action, also lower arterial blood pressure have been associated with worse outcomes in several randomized controlled trials (RCTs)[74] (section 12.8.3). Small trials have not established how blood pressure should be manipulated in the acute phase of stroke and larger trials are ongoing to determine how and when we should do so[61] (http://www.strokecenter.org/trials/).

Until RCTs are available, we offer the following advice:

- If the blood pressure remains raised (i.e. > 140/90 mmHg) for more than 1 week, or where there is evidence of end-organ damage, we would give the patient general advice (i.e. salt restriction, weight loss and moderation of alcohol intake) and start an antihypertensive drug, accepting that this timing is arbitrary. The issues of when to start antihypertensive treatment, the blood pressure level and the choice of agent, for the purposes of secondary prevention, are discussed in section 16.3.
- Our management is similar whatever the pathological type of stroke although we would be less inclined to lower blood pressure if the patient has severe stenoses or occlusions of the carotid and/or vertebral arteries.
- Where the patient is already on antihypertensive treatment, pending the results of ongoing RCTs, it seems reasonable to continue it as long as the patient can swallow the tablets safely and has not become hypovolaemic, which may increase the drug effect and lead to marked and potentially damaging hypotension.
- If the blood pressure is very high (i.e. > 220/ > 120 mmHg) there may be evidence of organ damage which would prompt earlier initiation of blood-pressure-lowering drugs (Table 11.10).

Table 11.10 Circumstances in which we would consider lowering the blood pressure immediately after an acute stroke.

Papilloedema or retinal haemorrhages and exudates
Marked renal failure with microscopic haematuria and proteinuria
Left ventricular failure diagnosed on clinical features and supported by evidence from the chest X-ray and/or echocardiogram
Features of hypertensive encephalopathy, e.g. seizures, reduced conscious level
Aortic dissection

Note: even these features may be misleading in acute stroke because left heart failure may frequently be due to coexistent ischaemic heart disease, and seizures and drowsiness may be due to the stroke itself.

- The aim of therapy should be a moderate reduction in blood pressure over a day or so, not minutes. An angiotensin-converting enzyme inhibitor (in the absence of contraindications) is a reasonable first choice. Thiazides probably have little effect in the acute phase although they remain a very reasonable choice later.[75,76] Transcutaneous glyceryl trinitrate is effective in lowering blood pressure, and the patches can easily be applied in dysphagic patients and withdrawn relatively quickly if blood pressure drops too far.[77] Intravenous labetalol, with very careful intra-arterial monitoring of blood pressure, may be useful in resistant cases.

> Do not lower the blood pressure in the first few days after a stroke unless there is evidence of accelerated hypertension or end-organ damage, or the patient is in of one of the ongoing multicentre randomized controlled trials (http://www.strokecenter.org/trials/).

11.7.2 Low blood pressure

It is difficult to define low blood pressure since, although one could set an arbitrary lower value for the systolic or mean blood pressure, clinically significant hypotension is that which leads to dysfunction of one or more organs. The level at which this occurs will depend on the patient's age, their usual blood pressure, the state of their arterial tree and whether cerebral autoregulation is intact or impaired. There is good evidence that autoregulation in the brain is impaired after stroke so that even if a patient has the same blood pressure after stroke as before, cerebral perfusion might still be reduced.

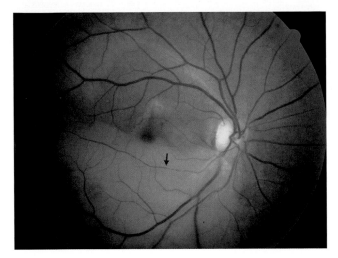

Plate 3.24 An ocular fundus photograph of a patient with inferior temporal branch retinal artery occlusion, showing pallor of the inferior half of the retina due to cloudy swelling of the retinal ganglion cells caused by retinal infarction. The inferior temporal branch arteriole is attenuated and contains embolic material (*arrow*).

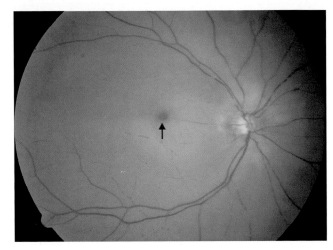

Plate 3.25 An ocular fundus photograph of a patient with central retinal artery occlusion, showing a cherry-red spot over the fovea (*arrow*). The cherry-red spot is the normal fovea (devoid of ganglion cells), which seems more obvious because the surrounding infarcted retina has lost its red colour and appears pale.

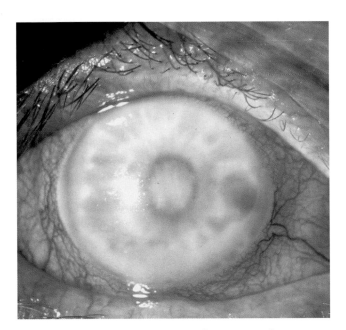

Plate 3.26 A photograph of the eye of a patient with acute glaucoma, showing congested sclera, cloudy cornea and oval pupil.

Plate 3.27 (a) and (b) Ischaemic oculopathy of the right eye; note episcleral vascular congestion, cloudy cornea, neovascularization of the iris (rubeosis of the iris) and mid-dilated pupil on external examination of the eye, which indicate chronic anterior segment ischaemia due to carotid occlusive disease (from Hankey & Warlow, 1994[2] by kind permission of the authors and W.B. Saunders Co. Ltd).

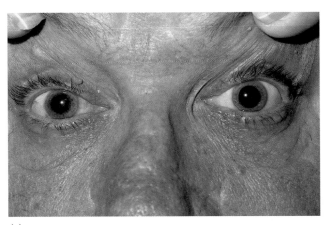

(a)

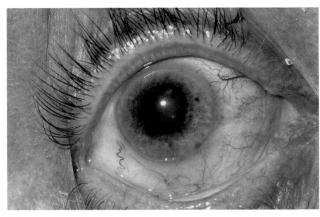

(b)

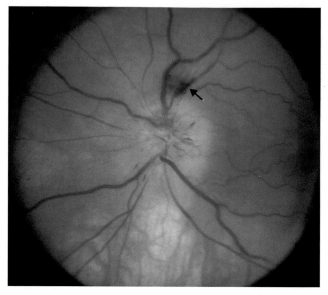

Plate 3.28 An ocular fundus photograph of a patient with anterior ischaemic optic neuropathy due to occlusion of the posterior ciliary artery as a result of giant cell arteritis. Note the oedema of the optic disc and flame-shaped haemorrhages (*arrow*).

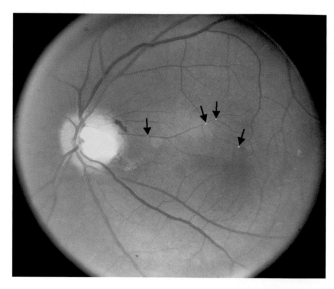

Plate 3.29 An ocular fundus photograph showing golden orange cholesterol crystals (Hollenshorst plaques) in the cilioretinal artery (*arrows*). The cilioretinal artery is present in only about one-third of the population. It originates from a branch of the short posterior ciliary artery and supplies the macula.

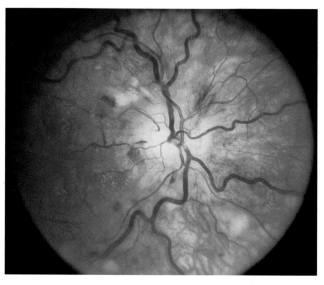

Plate 3.30 An ocular fundus photograph showing narrowing and tortuosity of retinal arterioles, arteriovenous nipping, retinal haemorrhages and papilloedema. These are the features of hypertensive retinopathy seen in malignant hypertension.

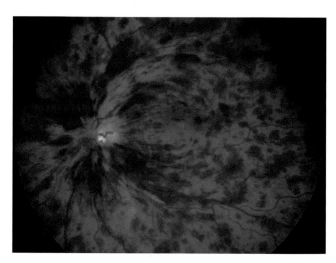

Plate 3.44 An ocular fundus photograph showing engorged retinal veins and multiple retinal haemorrhages due to central retinal vein thrombosis.

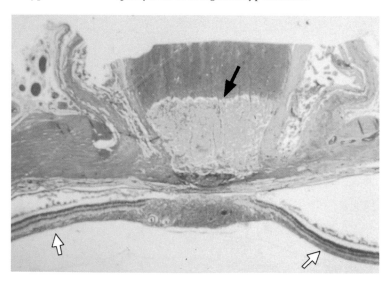

Plate 3.45 A photomicrograph of anterior ischaemic optic neuropathy caused by giant cell arteritis. The arrow indicates the infarcted optic nerve head and the open arrows the retina (courtesy of Dr J.F. Cullen, Western General Hospital, Edinburgh).

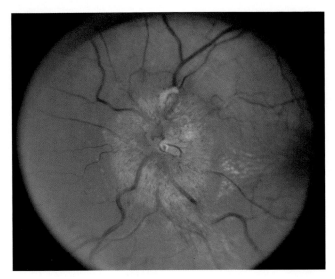

Plate 3.46 An ocular fundus photograph showing papilloedema. Note the congested, swollen disc, with loss of the physiological cup, a blurred disc margin and congested retinal veins.

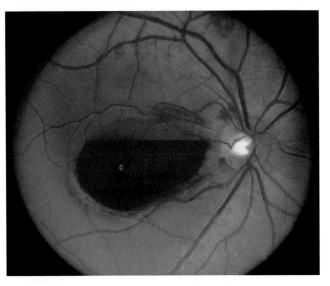

Plate 3.47 Ocular fundus of a patient with subhyaloid haemorrhage, appearing as sharply demarcated linear streaks of brick red-coloured blood or flame-shaped haemorrhage in the preretinal layer, adjacent to the optic disc and spreading out from the optic disc.

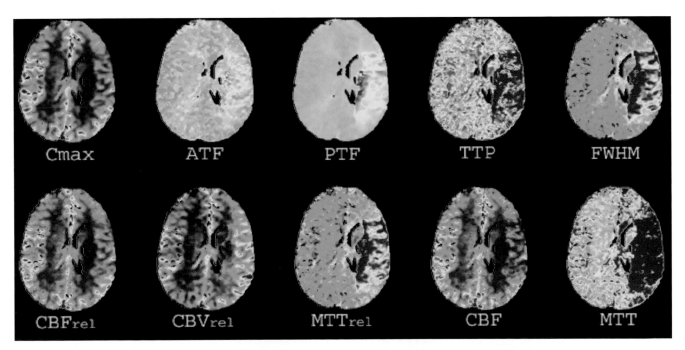

Plate 5.50 The different perfusion maps generated from the ten different perfusion processing methods (from curve in Fig. 5.49) applied to the same perfusion data acquisition from one patient (same slice shown for each of the 10 methods). See Fig. 5.49 for abbreviations. (Figure prepared by Dr Trevor Carpenter, Edinburgh.)

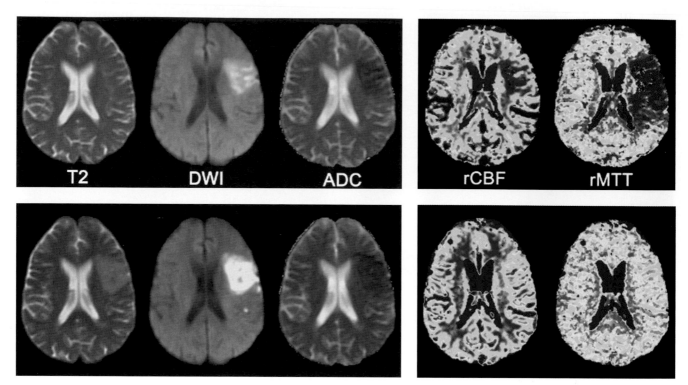

Plate 5.51 An example of MR diffusion-perfusion mismatch. *Top row*: 4 h after onset of right hemiparesis shows T2, diffusion, ADC, CBF and mean transit time (MTT) maps. There is early ischaemic change on diffusion and ADC but not on T2; a perfusion deficit is visible on CBF and MTT, largest on MTT, but larger than the diffusion lesion on both CBF and MTT. The 'DWI/CBF mismatch' would be smaller than the 'DWI/MTT mismatch'. *Bottom row*: 7 days after stroke, the infarct is now visible on T2, diffusion and ADC and there is no longer any lesion on CBF or MTT indicating reperfusion. The diffusion lesion does not seem to have grown particularly. This patient did not receive thrombolysis, so these perfusion changes were spontaneous.

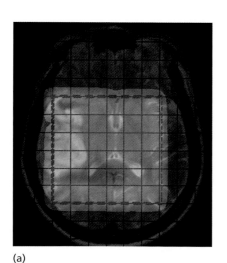

(a)

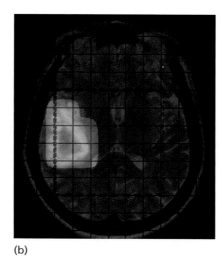

(b)

Plate 5.53 MR spectroscopic chemical shift imaging at 1 day after stroke in a patient with a right middle cerebral artery infarct. The T2-weighted image is in the background and the spectroscopic colour maps of the distribution of (a) the normal neuronal metabolite *N*-acetyl aspartate (NAA) and (b) the marker of anaerobic metabolism lactate, are superimposed. Red indicates large amounts and blues and greens small amounts of the metabolites. Note that the area of increased T2 signal of the infarct corresponds with the area of blue on the NAA map (in keeping with neuronal loss) and red on the lactate map (indicating anaerobic metabolism taking place in the infarct).

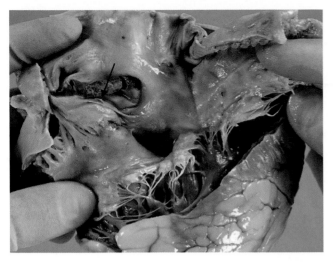

Plate 6.11 (c) Paradoxical embolus (*arrow*) straddling a patent foramen ovale.

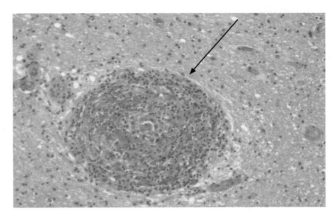

Plate 7.3 Cerebral vasculitis: there is lymphocytic infiltration and destruction of a small blood vessel in the brain parenchyma (*arrow*). The vessel is completely occluded by the thickened vessel wall which is infiltrated with lymphocytes. Stain H&E, × 40 magnification. Courtesy of Dr Colin Smith, Edinburgh.

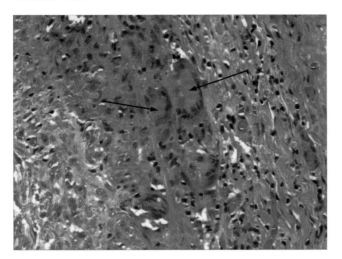

Plate 7.7 Giant cell arteritis: superficial temporal artery biopsy showing multinucleated giant cells (*arrows*) lying in relation to the damaged internal elastic lamina of the vessel wall. Stain H&E, × 60 magnification. Courtesy of Dr Colin Smith, Edinburgh.

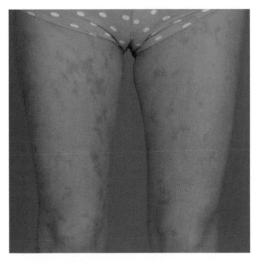

Plate 7.9 The typical appearance of livedo reticularis affecting the legs.

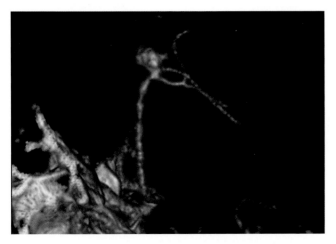

Plate 9.15 CT scan after rupture of a pericallosal artery; (e) reconstruction of the CT angiogram delineating the aneurysm from the parent and branching vessels.

Plate 9.24 (d) Reconstruction of the CT angiogram showing better the relationship between the aneurysm (*arrow*) and parent and branching vessel.

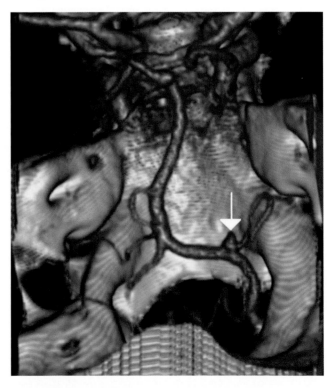

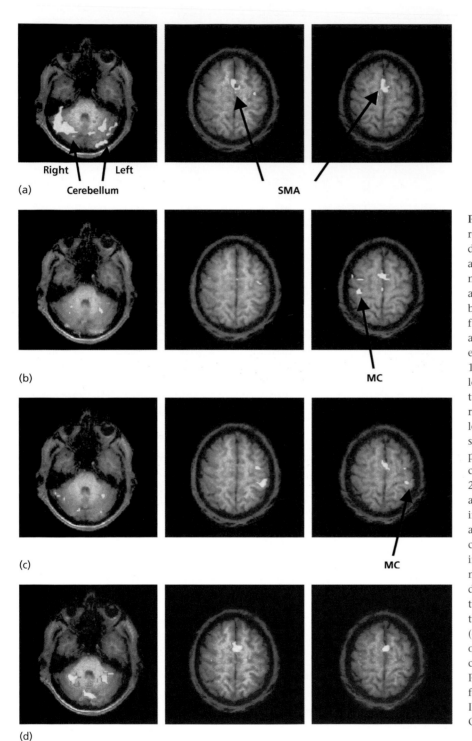

(a)

Right   Left

Cerebellum

SMA

(b)

MC

(c)

MC

(d)

Plate 10.8 Functional magnetic resonance imaging (fMRI) studies of dynamic changes in patterns of brain activation associated with hand movement accompanying recovery from an ischaemic stroke. The panels show the blood oxygenation level-dependent (*bold*) fMRI activations in the cerebral cortex and cerebellum accompanying flexion–extension of digits in one hand at about 1.5 Hz. These activation volumes show local areas of increased blood flow with task-specific neuronal activation. The right hemisphere is represented on the left side of the images. Activation of the supplementary motor cortex (SMA), primary sensorimotor cortex (MC) and cerebellum are easily identified. From 2 weeks after the infarct (a) to 5 weeks after the infarct (b), there was functional improvement in the paretic left hand associated with increased activation of contralateral MC and decreased activation in SMA and the cerebellum. In contrast, movements of the unaffected right hand do not show clearly significant changes in the patterns of brain activation between the 2-week scan (c) and 5-week scan (d). The right hemisphere is represented on the left side of the images. (Images courtesy of H. Johannsen-Berg, S. Pendlebury and P.M. Matthews, Centre for Functional Magnetic Resonance Imaging of the Brain, University of Oxford.)

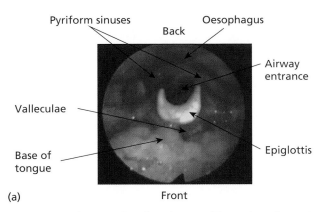

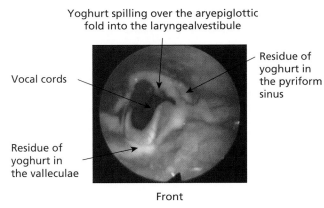

(a)

Plate 11.16 Photographs taken during a fibreoptic endoscopic evaluation of swallowing showing the main anatomic structures.

(b)

Pharyngeal residue after the swallow with risk of aspiration

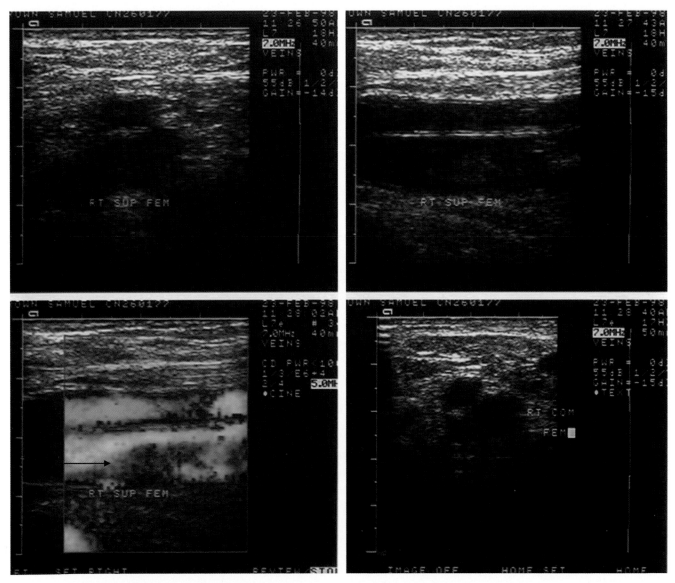

Plate 11.8 (b) A colour flow Doppler image of the femoral vein demonstrating thrombus within the lumen (*arrow*); this is usually associated with an inability to compress the vein and if the vein is occluded a loss of augmentation of flow with respiration or squeezing the calf.

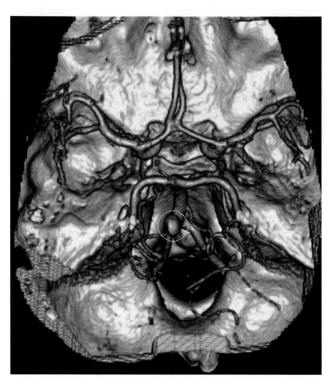

Plate 14.12 (b) Reconstruction of the CT angiogram showing an aneurysm (*circle*) at the origin of the posterior inferior cerebellar artery (which in this patient branches at the junction of the vertebral and basilar artery).

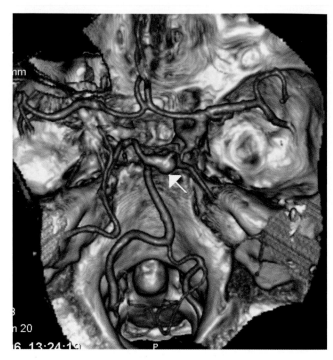

Plate 15.3 Follow-up CT angiogram in a patient with a ruptured posterior communicating artery aneurysm treated by neurosurgical clipping. (b) Reconstruction of the CT angiogram confirms the basilar artery tip aneurysm (*arrow*) and provides a better configuration of the anatomy. (Note that this reconstruction is a view from above, thus the right side of the patient is on the right.)

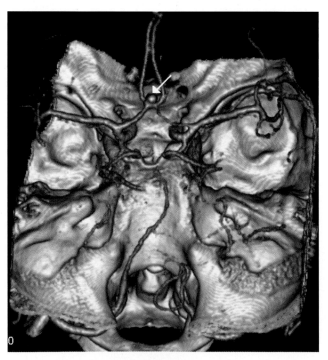

Plate 15.4 Follow-up after coiling of an anterior communicating artery aneurysm. (a) CT angiogram reconstruction showing an anterior communicating artery aneurysm (*arrow*).

Unfortunately, judgements about the optimal level of blood pressure after acute stroke are very difficult in routine practice since we have no easy and reliable techniques for assessing organ perfusion and more importantly function, other than the clinical state of the patient. Of course, when blood pressure is very low, patients may show signs of 'shock' (e.g. cold extremities, low urine output, worsening renal function, mental confusion, lactic acidosis) and actions to improve organ perfusion are required. In the International Stroke Trial, low blood pressure after acute stroke was associated with poor outcome, even after adjusting for stroke severity (Fig. 11.4).[66] However, the low blood pressure might not be the cause of the poor outcome but rather the consequence of important comorbidity (e.g. heart failure, atrial fibrillation) or complications (e.g. dehydration, pulmonary embolism).

Assessment

The monitoring of blood pressure after stroke has been discussed in section 11.7.1. The assessment of the clinical importance of hypotension should comprise a clinical examination and some simple investigations (e.g. blood urea, arterial blood gases) to identify the features of 'shock' mentioned already. Having established that the patient has low blood pressure which is associated with under-perfusion of tissues, it is then important to establish the cause. Is the patient hypovolaemic, due to dehydration (section 11.18.1) or blood loss (section 11.2.3)? Has the patient had a pulmonary embolus (section 11.13), or are they in heart failure (section 11.2.3) or septic (section 11.12)? Is the patient on drugs which could lower blood pressure excessively? These questions can normally be answered following a thorough clinical examination including assessment of the jugular venous pressure, review of the drug and fluid balance charts, and some simple investigations including haemoglobin and haematocrit, neutrophil count, C-reactive protein, urine and blood cultures, cardiac enzymes, an ECG and chest X-ray. Occasionally, further investigation with, for example, a CT pulmonary angiogram, an echocardiogram or measurement of right atrial or pulmonary wedge pressures is required to sort out the cause.

Treatment

This will obviously depend on the cause of the low blood pressure. In our experience, hypovolaemia is the most frequent problem and patients usually improve with intravenous fluids. Obviously, it is important to exclude cardiac failure before giving fluids in this way. There is little evidence on which to base a decision to increase the blood pressure in acute stroke.[78] Trials of sympathomimetics to raise blood pressure are in progress (http://www.strokecenter.org/trials/).

11.8 Epileptic seizures

11.8.1 Early seizures

About 5% of patients have an epileptic seizure within the first week or two of their stroke (so-called onset seizures), most occurring within 24 h. Inevitably, estimates of the frequency of onset seizures vary because of differences in case selection, diagnostic criteria, lack of witnesses and methods of follow-up. Most onset seizures are partial (focal) although often with secondary generalization (section 3.3.10) (Table 11.2). Onset seizures are more common in severe strokes, in haemorrhagic stroke and stroke involving the cerebral cortex.[79,80]

11.8.2 Later seizures

In population-based cohorts, which are relatively unaffected by hospital referral bias, the risk of having a first seizure, excluding onset seizures, is between 3% and 5% in the first year after a stroke and about 1–2% per year thereafter (Fig. 11.5). About 3% will have more than one seizure and could be regarded as having developed

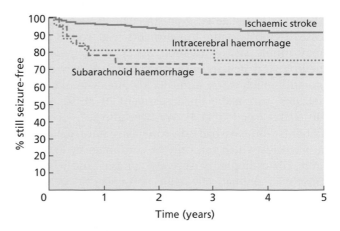

Fig. 11.5 A Kaplan–Meier plot showing the proportion of patients remaining seizure-free at increasing intervals after a first-ever-in-a-lifetime stroke in the Oxfordshire Community Stroke Project. Separate plots are shown for patients with ischaemic stroke ($n = 545$), non-truamatic intracerebral haemorrhage ($n = 66$) and subarachnoid haemorrhage ($n = 33$). Adapted from Burn et al., 1997.[80]

epilepsy following a stroke.[79] This represents a greatly increased relative risk of seizure (perhaps 20-fold) compared with stroke-free individuals of similar age. Patients with onset seizures, haemorrhagic strokes and infarcts involving the cerebral cortex have the highest overall risk of later seizures. Seizures may recur in about 50% of the patients, but are rarely troublesome if accurately diagnosed and appropriately treated. Patients who become functionally independent and who have not yet had a seizure are at very low risk of post-stroke seizures. The *theoretical* future risk of seizures is not great enough to prevent the patient driving an ordinary car in the UK where the acceptable risk of a seizure is < 20% per annum.

> The risk of having an epileptic seizure after a first-ever-in-a-lifetime stroke is, on average, about 5% in the first year and 1–2% per year thereafter. However, the risk is higher in patients with haemorrhagic stroke or with large ischaemic strokes involving the cortex, and lower in patients with lacunar and posterior circulation strokes.

Assessment

The diagnosis of seizures should, as usual, be based on a detailed description of the attack from the patient, and if possible a witness, and may very occasionally be confirmed by electroencephalography (EEG) during a seizure. Video-EEG monitoring is occasionally useful where patients are having frequent attacks of uncertain nature. If patients have seizures in the first few days after the stroke, and especially if they are partial (focal), they should be investigated. Non-stroke brain lesions complicated by post-seizure impairments (e.g. Todd's paresis) may mimic strokes (section 3.4.2). Also, because the neurological deficits and conscious level may be temporarily much worse immediately after a seizure, 'onset seizures' can make the assessment of stroke severity unreliable (section 11.4). We have also seen occasional patients who have had non-convulsive status epilepticus, a diagnosis which can only be confirmed by EEG, who may, for example, be severely aphasic, and who have improved dramatically with anti-epileptic treatment. Furthermore, seizures should not automatically be attributed to the stroke since many other causes may be present coincidentally, or as a consequence of the stroke (Table 11.11); appropriate investigations should be performed to exclude these. Finally, seizures may mimic recurrent stroke if associated with worsening of the original focal deficit; this is particularly confusing if any seizures have been unwitnessed and the patient presents with worsening of their earlier stroke (section 11.5).

Table 11.11 Causes of epileptic seizures after 'stroke'.

	Section
General	
Alcohol withdrawal	
Anti-epileptic drug withdrawal	
Hypoglycaemia	11.18.4
Hyperglycaemia, especially non-ketotic hyperglycaemia	11.18.3
Hyper/hyponatraemia	11.18.1 & 11.18.2
Hypocalcaemia or hypomagnesaemia	
Drugs:	
Baclofen given for spasticity	11.20
Antibiotics for infections, e.g. ciprofloxacin	11.12
Antidepressants given for emotionalism or depression	11.31
Phenothiazines given for agitation or hiccups	11.10 & 11.29.1
Anti-arrhythmics for associated atrial fibrillation	11.2.3
Neurological	
Due to the primary stroke lesion	
Haemorrhagic transformation of infarction	5.7
Underlying pathology:	
Arteriovenous malformation	8.2.4
Intracranial venous thrombosis	7.21
Mitochondrial cytopathy	7.19
Hypertensive encephalopathy	3.4.5
Wrong diagnosis	3.4
Herpes simplex encephalitis	
Cerebral abscess	
Intracranial tumour	
Subdural empyema	

Treatment

Any precipitating cause should be treated. Status epilepticus, although rare, should be managed in the normal way.[81] There is no evidence to support the routine use of prophylactic anti-epileptic drugs in stroke patients (including those with subarachnoid haemorrhage, section 14.3.3) who have not yet had a seizure but who are thought to be at high risk. Usually, an isolated seizure does not require treatment since the risk of further seizures is only about 50% over the next few years. However, if seizures recur, or if the patient wishes to minimize the risk of recurrence because of the implications for driving, employment or leisure activities, treatment after the first seizure may be warranted. We are not aware of any studies which have compared the efficacy of different anti-epileptic drugs in preventing seizures after stroke. Indeed, until recently there has been little evidence to suggest that any one of the most commonly used first-line drugs (i.e. phenytoin, sodium valproate, carbamazepine and lamotrigine) is more effective than any other in preventing partial (focal) or generalized seizures in adults.[82,83,461,462] The choice will depend on availability, efficacy the risk of adverse effects and cost. Recent evidence suggests that sodium valproate is the most effective agent in generalized seizures and lamotrigine in partial seizures.[461,462] Patients who have had a seizure should be advised not to drive (for a period which varies depending on national regulations), and to inform the necessary authorities (www.dvla.gov.uk/at_a_glance/ch1_neurological.htm, www.epilepsy.com/epilepsy/social_driving.html, http://www.ltsa.govt.nz/factsheets/17.html). However, many stroke patients who have seizures are too disabled to drive anyway (section 11.32.2).

> The risk of seizures after acute stroke, including subarachnoid haemorrhage, is not high enough to justify routine prophylactic anti-epileptic drugs. These may have significant adverse effects and are expensive.

11.9 Headache, nausea and vomiting

Headache is quite a common symptom at the time of stroke and may provide clues to the pathological type (e.g. haemorrhagic) and cause (e.g. giant-cell arteritis) (section 6.7.6). It is often associated with nausea or vomiting, most commonly in haemorrhagic and cerebellar strokes and less often in lacunar infarcts.[84–88] It is more common in those with prior migraine. Headache which occurs after the onset of stroke may be caused by treatment, for example due to intracranial bleeding secondary to thrombolysis or more commonly dipyridamole started for secondary prevention (section 16.5.5). Nausea or vomiting without headache is generally secondary to vertigo. These symptoms, which can be severe initially, usually improve within a few days. Having established that there is no important underlying cause (e.g. venous sinus thrombosis, giant-cell arteritis, arterial dissection) most patients simply require reassurance that the symptoms will improve, adequate analgesia and/or anti-emetics. However, these drugs may have adverse effects (see case history in section 11.5). Persistent vertigo which may be positional and associated with nausea or vomiting can be a particularly troublesome symptom, most commonly after

vertebrobasilar strokes. It may not respond to anti-emetics, indeed some believe that these may prevent tolerance developing. The place of so-called vestibular rehabilitation in such cases is unclear.

11.10 Hiccups

Hiccups are due to involuntary diaphragmatic contractions against a closed glottis. The precise cause is unclear. Although uncommon after stroke they may be persistent and troublesome in patients with strokes affecting the medulla.[89] If they persist, other causes should be considered (e.g. uraemia, diaphragmatic irritation). Numerous folk cures (e.g. sudden frights), acupuncture and drugs (Table 11.12) have been suggested as effective treatments.[90,91] It may be worth trying a short trial of each of the drugs in Table 11.12 when hiccups are persistent and distressing to the patient since any response is likely to be rapid and may not require ongoing drug treatment. Chlorpromazine, baclofen and gabapentin are probably the most frequently used. The choice should take into account the likely adverse effects.

11.11 Immobility and poor positioning

Immobility is a major consequence of impaired conscious level; severe motor deficits including weakness, ataxia and apraxia; and less commonly of sensory (i.e. proprioceptive) and visuospatial deficits. Immobility makes the patient vulnerable to a number of complications such as infections (section 11.12), deep venous

Table 11.12 Some of the drugs used to treat hiccups (most have important adverse effects).

Chlorpromazine
Haloperidol
Gabapentin
Baclofen
Metoclopramide
Sodium valproate
Phenytoin
Carbamazepine
Nifedipine
Amitriptyline

Table 11.13 Physiological factors to take into account when deciding in which position a patient should be nursed.

	Section
Maintenance of a clear airway	11.2.1
Cerebral perfusion	11.7.2
Cerebral oedema	11.3
Muscle tone	11.20
Swallowing	11.19
Limb oedema	11.25
Stimulation	11.31.3

thrombosis and pulmonary embolism (section 11.13), pressure ulcers (section 11.16), contractures (section 11.20) and falls and resulting injuries (section 11.26). Immobile patients are unable to position themselves to maintain comfort, to facilitate activities such as drinking and passing urine, and to relieve pressure over bony prominences. They are in the ignominious situation of always having to ask others to position them.

There has been little formal research of positioning after stroke.[92,93] For example, should the patient be nursed sitting or lying, and if lying, on which side? There is some evidence for the optimum positioning of mechanically ventilated patients: nursing semirecumbent is associated with a lower risk of pneumonia.[94] In the self-ventilating stroke patient the optimal position(s) are unclear but decisions should take into account the following physiological factors (Table 11.13):

- *Maintenance of a clear airway*: In unconscious patients correct positioning is vital to maintain a clear airway and so reduce the risk of aspiration (section 11.2.1).
- *Oxygenation*: Position may influence the patient's ability to breathe, ventilate their lungs and oxygenate their blood (section 11.2.2). Oxygenation is usually optimal in the sitting position.[92,95]
- *Cerebral perfusion*: Lying flat may increase cerebral perfusion.[96] Also, patients who are hypovolaemic may have reduced systemic blood pressure when sitting, which may reduce cerebral perfusion and possibly increase cerebral ischaemia.[92,97] However, if intracranial pressure falls further on sitting, cerebral perfusion pressure may increase.
- *Cerebral oedema*: Intracranial pressure is highly dependent on posture, being higher in supine patients and lower when sitting.[92,98] The relationships between oxygenation, cerebral perfusion, intracranial pressure and cerebral blood flow are so complex that it is difficult to predict the optimum position for nursing an individual patient (Fig. 11.6). Whether our own anecdotal observation that some patients with severe strokes are more alert when sitting up than when lying

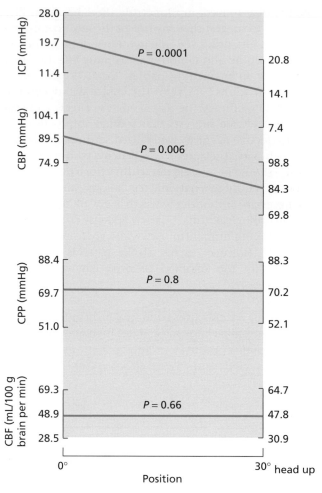

Fig. 11.6 Graph showing the interrelationships between intracranial pressure (ICP), carotid blood pressure (CBP), cerebral perfusion pressure (CPP) and cerebral blood flow (CBF) with changes in posture in patients with head injury. Data from Feldman *et al.*, 1992.[98]

is explained by reduced intracranial pressure, reduced cerebral oedema, improved oxygenation, and/or increased sensory or social stimulation is not at all clear.

- *Tone*: The position of a patient influences the tone in their trunk and limbs.[99] Positioning of the patient is used by physiotherapists and nurses to promote higher or lower tone, whichever seems most appropriate for that particular patient.[100] Spasticity and the tendency to develop contractures may be reduced by careful positioning to reduce tone (section 11.20), while patients who have low tone in their truncal muscles may benefit from positioning which promotes increased tone and leads to better truncal control. The positioning charts which are so often strategically placed by the patient's bed to guide nursing care give the impression that we know what we are doing (see Fig. 11.22). However, although there is some agreement about the optimum positioning of patients with hemiplegia (e.g. fingers extended, spine straight), there are many areas of uncertainty (e.g. optimum position of the head, foot and unaffected limbs).[100] There is clearly a need for further research into this area although this will be hampered by difficulties in prescribing specific positioning regimens, in ensuring compliance, and in reliably assessing outcomes (section 11.20).

- *Swallowing*: Swallowing is easier and safer if the patient is sitting up with their neck flexed (section 11.17).
- *Pressure area care*: For immobile patients who cannot shift their own weight, their position must be changed frequently enough to avoid developing ischaemia of the skin and subcutaneous tissues over bony prominences at weight-bearing points (section 11.16).
- *Limb oedema*: The ankles and the paralysed arm of immobile hemiparetic patients frequently become oedematous and painful. This may increase muscle tone and further reduce function (section 11.25).
- *Stimulation*: It is difficult for patients to see what is going on around them when lying flat. This lack of sensory and social stimulation and contact with daily events will encourage too much sleep during the day and may lead to boredom, reduced morale and sometimes confusion (section 11.31.3).

The team should assess (and regularly reassess) each patient and decide which of these potential problems are most important. For example, is the patient hypoxic or dysphagic or at particular risk of pressure ulcers? Depending on this assessment, a positioning regimen which sets out what are thought to be the best positions, and the frequency of repositioning, should be prescribed and re-evaluated. However, educational programmes for nursing staff are probably only moderately effective in increasing the proportion of time that patients are positioned according to the prescribed regime.[101] Equipment such as electrically operated multi-sectional profiling beds (Fig. 11.7) and specialist rehabilitation chairs

(Fig. 11.23) are, in our experience, valuable tools in positioning immobile stroke patients and they potentially allow some patients to reposition themselves to maintain comfort.

> Electrically operated multi-sectional profiling beds are helpful in positioning patients and may provide some immobile patients with the opportunity to reposition themselves. We also find them helpful for examining the jugular venous pressure and testing for postural hypotension, both essential to assessing patient fluid status.

11.12 Fever and infection

Fever is quite common after stroke although its frequency obviously depends on the population of stroke patients studied, the definitions used, and the method, timing and duration of monitoring. All published studies have been of hospital-referred patients, most have defined fever as an axillary or rectal temperature of > 37.5°C, and have monitored temperature for 2–7 days. Patients with fever during the first few days after stroke have a worse outcome than those without.[102,103] It is unclear whether this adverse prognosis is simply because fever is a marker of a severe stroke (i.e. due to loss of central temperature control or resorption of subarachnoid blood), an indicator of an infective complication (e.g. pneumonia or urinary infection), or increases cerebral damage. The last is an attractive, although unproven concept, since it is consistent with research in animal models which has shown that hyperthermia increases and hypothermia decreases ischaemic cerebral damage.[104] Table 11.14 lists some of the potential causes of fever after stroke, of which infection is probably the

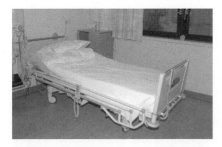
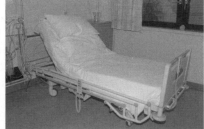
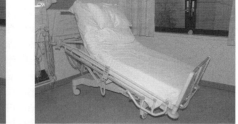

Fig. 11.7 A multi-sectional profiling bed – a useful tool for positioning stroke patients. It even helps assess patient hydration by facilitating examination of the jugular venous pressure, and testing for postural hypotension.

Table 11.14 Causes of fever after stroke.

Causes	Section
Infective/inflammatory complications of the stroke	
Urinary infection	11.14
Pneumonia	11.12.1
Deep venous thrombosis	11.13
Pulmonary embolism	11.13
Pressure ulcers	11.16
Infected intravenous access site	
Vascular problems, e.g. infarction of myocardium, bowel or limb	
Inflammatory causes of the stroke itself	
Infective endocarditis	6.5.9
Arteritis	7.3
Coincidental conditions	
Upper respiratory tract infection	
Drug allergy	

most common. Fever and infection may pre-date the stroke onset, and occasionally may actually cause or at least precipitate the stroke (sections 6.6.17 and 7.11).

Of course, immobile stroke patients are prone to infections, the most common sites being the chest and urinary tract.[105] There is some evidence that patients with stroke and other types of brain damage acquire an immune deficiency, mediated via the hypothalamic pituitary axis, which may contribute to their risk of infection.[106,107] However, the clinical relevance of these findings has yet to be established. Infections are (in general) associated with worse outcomes, even having adjusted for other important prognostic factors as far as it is possible to do so, and they cause many deaths, interrupt rehabilitation and slow recovery.[108]

11.12.1 Chest infections

Chest infections are much more common in the acute stage than later, occurring in about 20% of patients within the first month or two. Chest infections may be due to aspiration, failure to clear secretions, the patient's immobility, reduced chest wall or diaphragmatic movement on the hemiparetic side, or comorbidities including chronic airway disease.[109] However, there is no clear relationship between the side of any hemiparesis and side of pneumonia. Alterations in the bacterial flora in the mouth which have been observed after stroke[110] and in tube-fed individuals[111,112] may be associated with an increased risk of chest infection. Chest infections may be minimized by efforts to improve oral hygiene or alter the mouth flora[113] but further randomized trials are required to evaluate this approach. In the meantime careful positioning, physiotherapy and suction to avoid the

accumulation of secretions, and care to avoid aspiration seem sensible measures to take (section 11.17).

11.12.2 Urinary infections

About a quarter of hospitalized stroke patients develop a urinary infection within the first 2 months and this remains common over the subsequent months.[105] Urinary infections can be avoided by maintaining adequate hydration and thus urine output, and by avoiding unnecessary bladder catheterization (section 11.14). Given that incomplete bladder emptying is associated with an increased risk of infection it seems sensible to avoid constipation and drugs with anticholinergic effects if possible.[114] It is uncertain whether intermittent or continuous catheterization and/or prophylactic antibiotics are of benefit for patients with a persisting increased post-void residual volume.[115–117]

Assessment

The patient's temperature should be monitored at least 6-hourly during the first few days after the stroke and thereafter if there are any signs of infection or functional deterioration. However, fever may not accompany infection, especially in elderly and immunocompromised patients. Therefore, any functional deterioration or failure to attain a rehabilitation goal should prompt a search for occult infection, even if there is no fever. Obviously, the cause of fever should be identified using clinical assessment supplemented with appropriate investigations (e.g. blood neutrophil count, C-reactive protein, cultures of urine and blood, chest X-ray). Dipstick testing of a midstream urine to detect leucocytes and nitrates is insufficiently accurate to be relied on to exclude or confirm a urinary infection (section 11.14).[118]

Prevention and treatment

There is currently little evidence to support the use of prophylactic antipyretics to reduce fever after stroke (section 11.19). In fact, the routine use of paracetamol to lower body temperature and attempts to induce more profound hypothermia after stroke are being evaluated in ongoing RCTs[119] (http://www.strokecenter.org/trials/index.htm). A single-centre RCT of levofloxacin (a fluoroquinolone antibiotic) in acute stroke failed to demonstrate a reduction in infections but further trials will be required to establish whether alternative antibiotic regimes might be more effective.[120,121] The treatment of fever will depend on the cause (Table 11.14). We quite often start a broad-spectrum antibiotic, once specimens for microbiological testing have been taken,

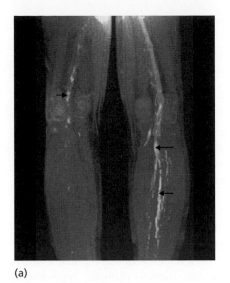

(a)

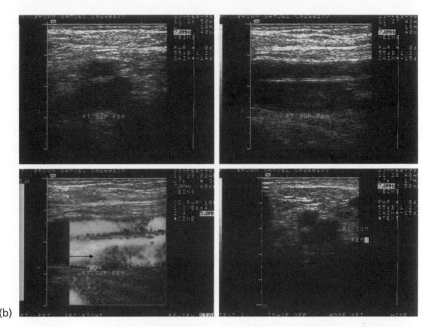

(b)

Fig. 11.8 (a) An MR scan of the legs using direct thrombus imaging to demonstrate extensive deep venous thrombosis (*arrows*). (b) A colour flow Doppler image of the femoral vein demonstrating thrombus within the lumen (*arrow*); this is usually associated with an inability to compress the vein and if the vein is occluded a loss of augmentation of flow with respiration or squeezing the calf. (Also reproduced in colour in the plate section.)

since delays in treating infections may impede patients' progress. However, with an increasing incidence of *Clostridium difficile* toxin-associated diarrhoea in many hospitals, the risks of early use of broad-spectrum antibiotics must be carefully weighed against the potential benefits.[122] Appropriate antibiotics and supportive treatment (e.g. physiotherapy, oxygen) should be given in established infection. Also, it seems reasonable, whatever the cause of the fever, to use a fan and prescribe paracetamol (acetaminophen) since fever may worsen outcome (see above). Even if such interventions appear to be without risk, one must remember that they take up a nurse's time which might be spent to greater effect in some other activity.

> Any functional deterioration or failure to attain a rehabilitation goal should prompt a search for occult infection.

11.13 Venous thromboembolism

Deep venous thrombosis (DVT) of the legs is common in patients with a recent stroke, particularly older patients with a severe hemiplegia who are immobile. Estimates of the frequency depend on the types of patients included, the use of preventive measures, and the timing and method of detection. The most sensitive techniques, such as MRI direct thrombus imaging, detect DVTs in about 40% of hospitalized patients treated with aspirin and graduated compression stockings and about half of these are above-knee[123] (Fig. 11.8a). Less sensitive, but more widely available, tests such as compression Doppler ultrasound (Fig. 11.8b) and plethysmography identify DVTs in about 20% of immobile hospitalized patients, above-knee in about half of these. Although DVT is said to be less common among Chinese a recent study has shown a similar incidence to that seen in white patients.[124] Clinically apparent DVT confirmed on investigation is less common, occurring in under 5%.

DVTs are most often asymptomatic, or unrecognized, but may still lead on to important complications.[123] Pulmonary embolism (PE) occurs in about 10% of hospitalized patients but like DVT is frequently not recognized.[123] It is an important cause of preventable death after stroke and is a frequent finding at autopsy.[125]

Assessment

DVT should be suspected if a patient's leg becomes swollen, hot or painful or if the patient develops a fever. Unfortunately, the clinical diagnosis can be difficult because many paretic legs become swollen, mostly because of the effects of gravity and lack of movement. If a paretic leg swells while a patient is still being nursed in bed, DVT is a likely cause, but where a patient is sitting out or mobilizing the clinical diagnosis is much less certain. Stroke patients who have communication difficulties, sensory loss or neglect may well not complain of discomfort or swelling, so that clinical detection will depend on the vigilance of members of the multidisciplinary team.

> Stroke patients who have communication difficulties, sensory loss or neglect may well not complain of discomfort or swelling associated with deep venous thrombosis, so that clinical detection will depend on the vigilance of members of the multidisciplinary team. If a patient develops a swollen leg on a stroke unit, deep venous thrombosis has to be actively excluded.

Where the patient develops clinical evidence of a DVT or pulmonary embolism, confirmatory investigations must be carried out if treatment with anticoagulants is being considered. We would normally use compression Doppler ultrasound in the first instance to confirm the diagnosis since this is non-invasive, widely available and reasonably sensitive (>90%) and specific (>90%) in detecting at least above-knee DVT in symptomatic patients.[126] However, it is operator dependent and if there is doubt about the result, or if one wishes to exclude thrombosis in the calf veins, contrast X-ray venography should be performed.

> The clinical diagnosis of deep venous thrombosis in stroke patients is particularly difficult because, on the one hand, a swollen leg may be due to paralysis and dependency while, on the other hand, a patient may not complain about pain and swelling because of language and perceptual problems.

The value of screening asymptomatic stroke patients for DVT has not been established. In considering such a policy one has to remember that the sensitivity and specificity of non-invasive tests, such as D-dimers and compression Doppler ultrasound, are lower in patients who do not have symptoms of DVT than in those with symptoms, and more 'positives' will be 'false-positives'.[127–129]

Given the high frequency of PE in hospitalized stroke patients, if a patient has clinical features compatible with PE – breathlessness and/or tachypnoea, with or without pleuritic chest pain and/or haemoptysis for which there is no other reasonable clinical explanation – the probability of PE is high. In such patients a CT pulmonary angiogram can be used to confirm or exclude a PE[130] because it is difficult to distinguish clinically between breathlessness due to pulmonary embolism and other causes without further investigation.

Prevention

Manoeuvres which may reduce the risk of DVT and pulmonary embolism include:

- *Early mobilization* of the patient and avoidance of prolonged bed rest, although the effectiveness of this regimen after stroke has never been tested in RCTs.
- *Hydration/fluids* may influence the risk of venous thromboembolism. A raised urea, probably indicating dehydration, is associated with a higher risk of DVT.[131] Also a systematic review of RCTs testing haemodilution in stroke indicated that this probably reduces the risk of DVT and PE (odds ratio 0.54, 95% confidence interval 0.30–0.99).[132] It is unclear whether this is a specific effect of haemodilution or a non-specific effect of improved hydration. We give intravenous saline to most of our patients with acute stroke and immobility, in part because they are often unable to take adequate fluids orally (sections 11.17 and 11.18.1).
- *Full-length graduated compression stockings.* Systematic reviews of RCTs in patients undergoing *surgery* have shown about a 60% reduction in the odds of developing DVT.[133,134] Most of these RCTs tested full-length stockings or did not specify the length. There is very little evidence that short (below-knee) stockings effectively prevent DVT.[134] But, in stroke, unlike surgery, stockings cannot be applied before the onset of the insult (i.e. the surgery itself), so DVTs may develop before stockings can be applied, and patients may be immobile for weeks and have prolonged leg paralysis. Moreover, compression stockings have potential hazards: they occasionally cause pressure ulcers (Fig. 11.9a) or acute limb ischaemia, the latter particularly in those with diabetes, peripheral neuropathy or peripheral vascular disease (Fig. 11.9b), they are uncomfortable and unpopular with patients and nurses; and considerable nursing resources are consumed in their application and monitoring. If used, stockings should be fitted in accordance with the manufacturer's instructions and removed daily to check for skin problems. The evidence for their effectiveness in stroke patients is inconclusive but a large randomized trial is in progress (www.clotstrial.com;[135] http://www.strokecenter.org/trials).
- *Aspirin,* started within 48 h of a presumed ischaemic stroke, reduces the relative risk of PE by about 30% and improves the patients' overall long-term outcome[136] (section 12.3). We start aspirin routinely (first dose

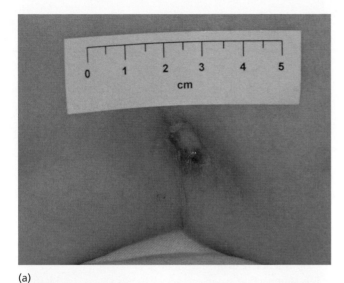

(a)

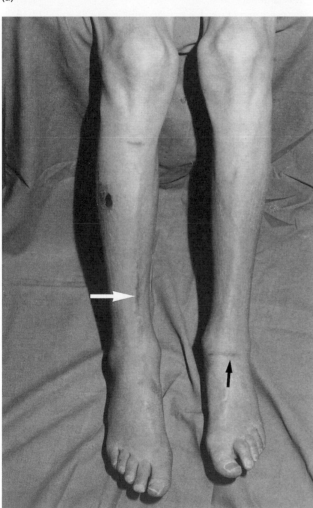

(b)

300 mg and 75 mg per day thereafter) as soon as we have excluded intracranial haemorrhage or other contraindications.

- *Heparin* has been shown to reduce the risk of DVT in patients with ischaemic stroke, but this benefit is offset by the risk of haemorrhagic complications so that routine use of heparin does not improve overall outcome[137] (section 12.4). We reserve unfractionated (5000 u twice per day) or low-molecular-weight heparin for patients we judge to be at particularly high risk of DVT and PE and low risk of haemorrhagic complications, accepting that these judgements are based on inadequate evidence. Such patients might include those with an ischaemic stroke with severe leg weakness and immobility, and cancer, thrombophilia or previous venous thromboembolism (section 12.4.3).
- *Other methods* of prophylaxis, e.g. external pneumatic compression and functional electrical stimulation, have been suggested but not evaluated adequately in stroke.[135,138]

Treatment

If a patient with a confirmed ischaemic stroke has a proven above-knee DVT or pulmonary embolism, we use subcutaneous low-molecular-weight heparin (LMWH) despite the lack of direct evidence that this is more effective than intravenous unfractionated heparin in stroke patients. We prefer LMWH because it is easier to use and does not need monitoring, and there is evidence in patients other than those with stroke that it is just as, or more, effective.[139–141] If patients are symptomatic we also usually treat DVT restricted to the calf veins although this depends on the presence of any relative contraindications to treatment.[142] In patients with DVT restricted to calf veins who have no symptoms we would also anticoagulate if a repeat Doppler ultrasound showed propagation of the thrombus in the popliteal or femoral veins. We normally continue heparin for a few days while starting oral anticoagulants which we continue for about 6 months, depending on our judgement of the patient's risk of recurrence, taking into account their

Fig. 11.9 (a) A pressure ulcer behind the knee due to graduated compression stockings and inadequate monitoring by nursing staff. (b) A patient with peripheral vascular disease and diabetes mellitus who was fitted with graduated compression stockings. Note the necrotic skin over the anterior border of the tibia (*white arrow*) and where the stockings were creased at the ankle (*black arrow*). There were also necrotic areas over both heels which failed to heal and led to a right above-knee amputation following an unsuccessful revascularization procedure.

immobility and risk of bleeding.[143] We do not believe that intracranial haemorrhage is an absolute contraindication to anticoagulation since, if a patient has had a life-threatening pulmonary embolus, the risk of anticoagulation may be worth taking. Alternatively one might consider insertion of a caval filter but there are no reliable studies which help us decide between these two treatments.[144] In a small number of patients, thrombolysis may need to be considered for massive PE or DVT but this has not been evaluated in stroke patients and would inevitably be associated with a risk of intracranial bleeding.

11.14 Urinary incontinence and retention

Between one- and two-thirds of acute stroke patients admitted to hospital are incontinent of urine in the first few days.[145,146] Urinary incontinence is more common in older patients, those with severe strokes, other disabling conditions and diabetes.[145,147] Urinary incontinence may be caused by the stroke itself, but perhaps one-fifth of patients have been incontinent before the stroke. Although detrusor instability is the most common single cause of urinary incontinence after the first 4 weeks, many other factors may contribute in the acute stage (Table 11.15). Urinary incontinence is an important cause of distress to patients and carers, increases the risk of pressure ulcers (section 11.16), often interferes with rehabilitation (e.g. by interrupting physiotherapy sessions or increasing spasticity; section 11.20) and influences the patient's requirements for ongoing nursing care.[147,148] Urinary incontinence may also cause patients to become dehydrated because patients tend to restrict their own fluid intake to limit urinary incontinence without telling the nurses or doctors.

> Urinary incontinence may cause patients to become dehydrated. This is because many patients restrict their own fluid intake to limit urinary incontinence – without telling the nurses or doctors.

Assessment

To identify patients with urinary incontinence one simply has to ask the carer or nursing staff. These are the people most aware of urinary problems since they have to deal with the consequences. It is important to ask, since many people consider incontinence an inevitable consequence of stroke and thus not worthy of mention.

Table 11.15 Factors which may contribute to urinary incontinence.

	Section
Reduced conscious level	11.3
Immobility (cannot get to the toilet in time)	11.11
Communication problems (cannot ask to go to the toilet)	11.30
Impaired upper limb function (cannot manipulate clothes or the urinal)	11.21
Dyspraxia	11.28
Loss of inhibition of bladder contraction (detrusor instability so cannot wait to go)	
Urinary infection (often without any other symptoms)	11.12.2
Urinary overflow due to outflow obstruction (e.g. prostatism)	
Faecal impaction	11.15
Excess urinary flow due to high fluid intake, diuretics and poorly controlled diabetes	11.18.3
Too few carers/nurses (cannot attend to patients in time)	
Importance of maintaining continence underestimated by carers/nurses	

Routine use of a measure such as the Barthel Index to monitor patient progress on the stroke unit should identify all patients with urinary incontinence. It is often useful, but frequently overlooked, to ask the patients themselves what they think is causing their incontinence. This may, for instance, help distinguish true incontinence from accidental spillage of urine from a urinal because of the patient's poor manual dexterity (Fig. 11.10). Many of our patients with severe stroke, often with some cognitive dysfunction, seem unaware of either voiding or being wet. They usually deny incontinence when asked. More detailed information, including urinary volumes, frequency and times of voiding, which can be collated with a micturition chart, may be useful in identifying the causes of incontinence (e.g. diuretics, communication difficulties) and in formulating a management plan.

> Many of our patients with severe stroke, often with some cognitive dysfunction, seem unaware of either voiding or being wet. They usually deny incontinence when asked. Although we exclude specific causes and try both behavioural and pharmacological interventions we usually resort to incontinence pads or an indwelling catheter.

Where the cause of urinary incontinence is unclear, and if it persists for more than a few days, the patient

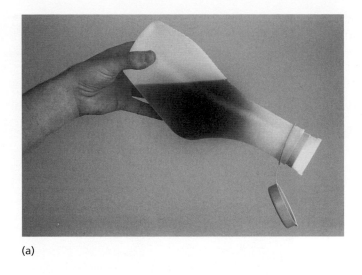

(a)

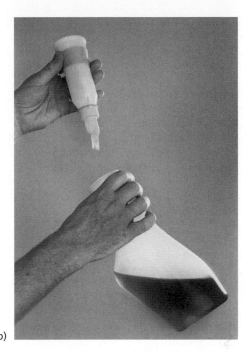

(b)

Fig. 11.10 Some patients have difficulty manipulating a urinal which leads to spills and, effectively, incontinence. (a) This urinal can be inverted without leaking; (b) a simple one-way valve inserted in the neck of the urinal prevents the contents spilling.

should be investigated. Urine dipstick testing for leucocytes and nitrates may help to exclude an infection but, given the high frequency of urinary infection in stroke patients (section 11.12.2), it is insufficiently accurate to be used as a single test; microscopy and culture should also be performed to exclude or confirm the diagnosis.[118] Measurement of postmicturition bladder volumes (by bladder ultrasound or catheterization) may be useful in assessing bladder sensation, contractility and outflow. We reserve formal urodynamic studies, which can better identify detrusor hyper- and hyporeflexia and bladder outflow problems, for the few patients with unexplained, troublesome incontinence which persists for weeks after the stroke and where the incontinence is out of proportion to the stroke severity.

A negative urine dipstick test for leucocytes and nitrates does not reliably exclude a urinary infection; a midstream urine collection should be obtained if possible and sent for microscopy and culture.

Prognosis

Urinary incontinence is an important predictor of poor survival and functional outcome after acute stroke (section 10.2.7): between 30% and 60% of incontinent patients die within the next few months.[145,149] However, among survivors, incontinence resolves in the majority, unless it pre-dated the stroke. Younger age, less severe stroke and lacunar stroke have all been associated with better rates of resolution.[147,149] Persisting urinary incontinence is associated with worse functional outcome and higher rates of institutionalization.[147,149,150]

Treatment

There is very little reliable evidence about the treatment of post-stroke incontinence.[151] If a patient is incontinent, but able to understand, then a careful explanation of the cause and likely prognosis should be given. Carers often benefit from such information too. Because urgency of micturition is such a common cause of incontinence in stroke patients, simple steps such as regular toileting, offering aphasic patients some means to alert the nurses to their needs, improving their mobility, or providing a commode by the bed, can all be effective. Provision of suitable clothing, such as trousers with a flap fastened with Velcro, may allow patients to use a urinal or commode independently and thus promote continence. Obviously, one should strive to treat the underlying cause (e.g. infection, outflow obstruction) and where possible remove exacerbating factors (e.g. excessive fluids, uncontrolled hyperglycaemia or diuretics). Having excluded easily treatable causes, we first employ 'bladder retraining' where patients are prompted to void

Table 11.16 Drugs used to inhibit bladder contractility, and their adverse effects.

Anticholinergic drugs
Flavoxate hydrochloride
Oxybutynin hydrochloride
Tolterodine tartrate
Propiverine hydrochloride
Propantheline bromide
Tricyclic antidepressants
Imipramine
Amitriptyline
Nortriptyline
Common adverse effects
Dry mouth
Blurred vision
Nausea/vomiting
Constipation/diarrhoea
Confusion in the elderly
Retention where there is bladder neck obstruction
Precipitation of acute glaucoma

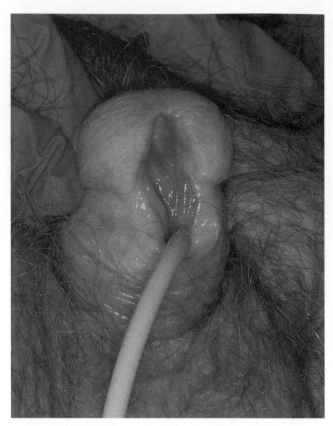

Fig 11.11 Traumatic hypospadias caused by an indwelling catheter. This is most likely to occur in a man with cognitive or communication problems who may not indicate he is uncomfortable, and who is being looked after by inadequately trained nursing staff.

regularly. If this does not achieve continence, we use a bedside ultrasound machine to exclude a postmicturition residual of 100 mL or more and then introduce an anticholinergic drug (e.g. oxybutinin or tolteridine) assuming there are no contraindications, e.g. closed angle glaucoma.[152] One must obviously be alert to the possible adverse effects of these drugs (Table 11.16). This approach achieves reasonable results with relatively few patients requiring formal urodynamic studies.[153]

An *indwelling catheter* should be avoided if at all possible because it makes resolution of urinary incontinence impossible to detect, and may lead to a number of complications (Fig. 11.11, Table 11.17). Intermittent catheterization facilitates detection of the resolution of incontinence and probably reduces the rate of bacturia but it is certainly more labour intensive and therefore may not be practical.[114] Other aids and appliances may be useful (Table 11.18) in avoiding unnecessary catheterization. However, when patients are at high risk of pressure ulcers (section 11.16), and other means have failed to keep them dry, or if accurate monitoring of fluid balance is required for some reason, an indwelling catheter is the best option. Catheterization may also be required to relieve urinary retention (see below) until any cause or precipitating factor can be removed, e.g. enlarged prostate, urinary infection, severe constipation, anticholinergic drugs. There is limited evidence that prophylactic antibiotics reduce the rate of bacturia in patients with indwelling catheters and this policy may increase bacterial resistance and rates of *Clostridium difficile*-associated diarrhoea.[112,114]

Occasionally, if urinary incontinence is a bar to discharge into the community, long-term catheterization with a silastic catheter may be the preferred option. This issue should be discussed with the patient and, where appropriate, their carer. Continence advisers, nurses with specialist training in the management of incontinence and access to information, aids and appliances, can often help other professionals, patients and their carers.[151] The choice of continence aids and catheters is huge but there are few rigorous studies to establish which are the most cost-effective, and most acceptable to patients and carers.[154,155] In many parts of the UK, laundry services run by health authorities or social services provide invaluable assistance to families having to cope with incontinence.

An indwelling catheter should be avoided if possible because this makes resolution of urinary incontinence impossible to detect and may lead to a number of complications.

Table 11.17 Problems (and solutions) of indwelling urinary catheters.[434]

Problem	Solution
Pain on insertion	Explain to the patient what is going to happen
	Use plenty of anaesthetic gel and allow time for it to work
Paraphimosis	Ensure foreskin is not left retracted after insertion
Traumatic hypospadius (Fig. 11.11)	Avoid traction and monitor carefully; if it occurs replace with suprapubic catheter
Poor self-esteem	Explain why catheter is needed, how it works and how long it will be in place
	Provide a discreet drainage bag
Immobility because of drainage bag	Use well-supported leg bag for mobile patients
Leakage	Use appropriate size of catheter
	Inhibit any involuntary bladder contraction which causes bypassing with an anticholinergic drug (Table 11.16)
	Change catheter if blocked
Blockage	Ensure adequate urine flow
	Remove encrusted catheter
Infection	Avoid unnecessary catheterization since no proven method of preventing infection
Catheter falls out due to urethral dilatation or pelvic floor laxity	Ensure balloon inflated to correct volume or use larger volume balloon
Catheter rejection due to bladder contraction	Avoid large volume balloon
	Inhibit with anticholinergic drug (Table 11.16)
Catheter pulled out by patient	Manage without a catheter to avoid further trauma
Pain on catheter removal	Avoid routine changes
	Explain procedure to patient
	Allow adequate time for balloon deflation
Failure of balloon deflation	Introduce ureteric catheter stylet along inflation channel

Table 11.18 Aids and appliances which may be useful in patients with urinary incontinence.[435]

Absorbent pads and pants
These vary in the volume of urine they can absorb, their shape, and the method of holding them in position.
Urinals
Useful for men who are immobile or have urgency which gives them insufficient time to reach the toilet. They can be fitted with a non-spill valve for patients who have poor manual dexterity (Fig. 11.10), or fluid absorbing granules, to reduce spillage.
Bedside commode
Useful where urgency is associated with poor mobility so the patient has insufficient time to get to the toilet (Fig. 11.33b).
Penile sheath
Often viewed as an alternative to an indwelling catheter in men without bladder outflow obstruction, but they easily fall off and are therefore unsuitable for agitated or confused patients. Other problems include skin erosions due to urinary stasis or the adhesive strip, and twisting of the sheath and penile retraction during voiding which causes leakage.

Urinary retention

Urinary retention, which may be acute or chronic, is common in stroke patients, more so in men. The main cause is pre-existing bladder outflow obstruction which may be exacerbated by constipation, immobility and drugs such as tricyclic antidepressants which have antimuscarinic effects.[156] Urinary retention may present with dribbling incontinence, agitation or confusion and is easily missed in patients with a reduced conscious level, communication difficulties or other cognitive problems. It is important to palpate the patient's abdomen or if in doubt perform a bladder ultrasound, on admission and later, if urinary problems or agitation develop, to exclude a distended bladder. Chronic retention with a postmicturition bladder volume of greater than 150 mL increases the risk of infection. A urethral catheter provides prompt relief. Removal of any exacerbating factors may avoid the need for a catheter or at least allow it to be removed quickly. In men with benign prostatic hypertrophy, alpha-blocking drugs (e.g. prazosin) or finasteride (which inhibits the metabolism of testosterone to dihydrotestosterone in the prostate) may enable one to remove the catheter without recurrence of retention. Surgeons and anaesthetists are often unwilling to consider transurethral resection of an enlarged prostate until several months have passed following a stroke. We are not aware of any evidence to indicate how long we should delay.

> It is important to palpate the patient's abdomen on admission and, later, if urinary problems or agitation develop, to exclude a distended bladder.

11.15 Faecal incontinence and constipation

Constipation is very common after stroke and may lead to abdominal discomfort, anxiety and faecal smearing or incontinence. Immobility, poor fluid and food intake, constipating analgesics and anticholinergic drugs are common causes. Faecal incontinence affects about one-third of patients after stroke and has been associated with increasing age, diabetes, other disabling conditions, stroke severity, immobility and size of brain lesion.[145,157]

Assessment

The frequency of bowel movements should be monitored. Simple monitoring will detect constipation and diarrhoea and may help establish the pattern of any faecal incontinence. Review of the drug chart will often identify possible causes. Abdominal and rectal examination will usually identify faecal impaction and indicate whether the constipated stool is hard or soft. Occasionally, if the patient has faecal incontinence associated with diarrhoea, it may be useful to culture the stool, and test for *Clostridium difficile* toxin to exclude infection or to X-ray the abdomen to exclude high faecal impaction. More detailed investigation is not required unless there are persistent unexplained problems.

Prognosis

Faecal incontinence early after stroke onset often resolves in survivors but may develop among those who were initially continent.[145,157] Later development of faecal incontinence is usually due to preventable causes such as drugs and inadequate staffing levels. Achieving continence can be a crucial step in discharging a patient home since faecal incontinence is so practically and socially difficult to cope with, and is invariably a considerable strain for the carer.

> Faecal incontinence which is not associated with severe cognitive problems is almost always remediable by dealing with constipation or diarrhoea. The rectum is often full of soft faeces which the patient cannot evacuate effectively.

Treatment

There is little reliable research to guide treatment.[158] Avoidance of constipation by ensuring an adequate intake of fluid and fibre is the best approach, but laxatives, suppositories and, occasionally, enemas are sometimes required. We find that stimulating laxatives (e.g. senna) are generally more effective than osmotic ones (e.g. lactulose) in elderly patients although the choice will be influenced by whether the stool is hard or soft. It is important to remember that laxatives may cause incontinence in immobile patients. Where patients are unable to toilet themselves, and a carer is not constantly available, it may be necessary to induce constipation, with for example codeine phosphate, and then relieve this with regular enemas to coincide with visits from a carer. Simple interventions including advice on diet, fluids and use of laxatives are helpful in reducing problems in the longer term.

11.16 Pressure ulcers

Pressure ulcers occur when local pressure on skin and subcutaneous tissues exceeds the capillary opening pressure for long enough to cause ischaemia. In addition, friction may cause blistering and tears in the skin. Pressure ulcers usually occur over weight-bearing bony prominences (Fig. 11.12). Ulcers occur in patients who are immobile and unable to redistribute their own weight when lying or sitting. The frequency of pressure ulcers in hospitalized stroke patients is bound to vary depending on the population studied, the prophylactic methods used and the diagnostic criteria. Pressure ulcers are more common in patients who are malnourished, infected, incontinent or have serious underlying disease.[159] They cause pain, increase spasticity, slow the recovery process, and may be fatal if complicated by severe sepsis. They prolong length of stay in hospital, often require intensive treatment and can therefore be extremely expensive to health services.[160] They can and should be prevented, although they may develop in the interval between the onset of the stroke and admission to hospital.

(a)

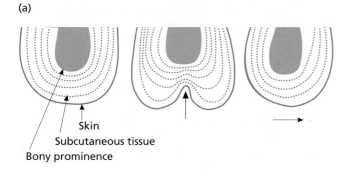

Skin
Subcutaneous tissue
Bony prominence

(b)

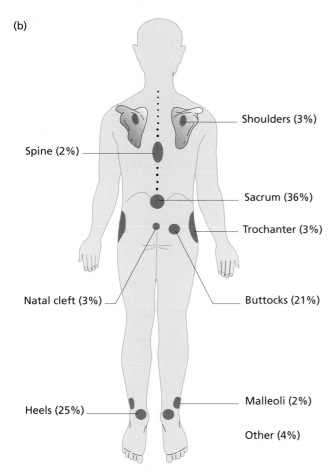

Shoulders (3%)

Spine (2%)

Sacrum (36%)

Trochanter (3%)

Natal cleft (3%)

Buttocks (21%)

Heels (25%)

Malleoli (2%)

Other (4%)

Fig. 11.12 (a) The distortions of tissues over a bony prominence due to compression or shear which may lead to pressure sores and (b) the anatomical distribution of established pressure sores based on data from a cross-sectional UK survey of pressure sores in patients being nursed on the Pegasus Airwave System. Although patients with cerebrovascular disease were the largest group in this sample, they made up only 14% of the whole group. (From St Clair, 1992.[459])

Assessment

Immobile patients should be examined regularly (sometimes several times in a day) to identify early signs of pressure damage, i.e. skin redness. It is important that patients who are at particular risk of developing pressure ulcers are identified as early as possible so that preventive measures can be taken. The Waterlow Scale (Table 11.19) is one of many clinical scoring systems developed to indicate an individual patient's risk. Most scales include some measure of mobility, continence, cognitive function and nutritional status and none, based on less than ideal evaluations, is clearly superior to the others.[161]

> Each patient's risk of pressure ulcers should be assessed and documented; actions, appropriate to the level of risk should be taken to prevent pressure ulcers developing. Pressure ulcers can be prevented by good nursing.

The clinician should be alert to behaviour which, in patients with communication and cognitive problems, may indicate a painful pressure area. Patients may repeatedly move themselves out of a desired position. For example, patients, colloquially known as 'thrusters', with a painful sacrum may force themselves out of a chair by extending their bodies at the waist. This may become a major problem for nursing staff. If patients develop pressure ulcers it is useful to have some objective measure of their severity so that healing or lack of healing can be monitored. Photographs incorporating a centimetre scale are a convenient and reliable method to demonstrate change, but where this facility is not available, tracing the limits of the ulcer or simply measuring it in several planes is useful.[162] Patients who are at risk, or who have established pressure ulcers, should be investigated to exclude malnutrition, hypoalbuminaemia, anaemia and infection (in the pressure ulcer or elsewhere), all of which can slow healing.[162]

Prevention

The most important way to prevent ulcers is to relieve the pressure on the tissues for long enough, and at frequent enough intervals, to allow the tissues to receive an adequate blood supply. This can usually be achieved by regular turning of patients (2- to 4-hourly depending on the assessment of risk) but this takes up a lot of skilled nursing resources. Although the introduction of a variety of special mattresses and cushions (Table 11.20) may reduce the need for regular turning, most patients do still need to be turned. Some beds are designed to turn the patient automatically (e.g. the net suspension bed).

Table 11.19 The Waterlow Scale.

Build/weight		Visual skin		Continence		Mobility		Sex/age		Appetite	
Average	0	Healthy	0	Complete	0	Fully mobile	0	Male	1	Average	0
Above average	2	Tissue paper	1	Occasionally incontinent	1	Restricted/difficult	1	Female	2	Poor	1
Below average	3	Dry	1	Catheter/incontinent of faeces	2	Restless/fidgety	2	14–49	1	Anorexic	2
		Oedematous	1	Doubly incontinent	3	Apathetic	3	50–64	2		
		Clammy	1			Inert/in traction	4	65–74	3		
		Discoloured	2					75–80	4		
		Broken	3					81+	5		

A total score of 10 indicates a patient is at risk of pressure ulcers, one of 15 indicates a high risk and a score of 20 a very high risk. In addition to the basic scale in which the scores for each of the six domains (i.e. weight, skin, continence, mobility, age/sex and appetite) are summed, additional points are added for special risk factors: poor nutrition (8 points); sensory deprivation including stroke (5 points); high-dose anti-inflammatory drugs, steroids (3 points); smoking > 10/day (1 point); orthopaedic surgery or fracture below waist (3 points).

Table 11.20 Specialized mattresses, cushions and beds.

Passive systems
Sheepskin fleeces and bootees which reduce skin shear and moisture; natural fleeces are better than man-made ones but they are rendered ineffective by poor cleaning and being covered by sheets.
Padded mattresses containing polyester fibres, e.g. Spenco.
Polystyrene bead system.
Foam mattresses (e.g. Vaperm) vary in their pressure-relieving properties.
Gel pads can be used under heels and sacrum.
Roho cushions are effective but very expensive (Fig. 11.13a).
Active systems
Ripple mattresses and airwave systems provide alternating pressure; the larger the cells the better but they tend to break down and leak.
Low air loss systems (e.g. Mediscus) providing constant low pressure; although effective, tend to be noisy, expensive and complex, needing regular maintenance and training (Fig. 11.13b).
Flotation beds and deep water beds are difficult to nurse patients on, are very heavy and some patients get motion sickness.
Dry flotation providing constant low pressure produced by glass microspheres blown by air. Air can be turned off when the patient needs to be repositioned. Effective but bulky and expensive.
Mechanical beds turn the patient, e.g. net suspension bed. Effectiveness uncertain, patients may not like being suspended (in full view of people around them). Useful for turning patients who are in pain.

Pressure-relieving mattresses and cushions (Fig. 11.13a) are divided into 'passive' and 'active' systems (Table 11.20). The 'passive' systems distribute the patient's weight through a larger area and make it easier for them to reposition themselves. High-specification foam mattresses are more effective than standard foam mattresses.[160] 'Active' systems (Fig. 11.13b) usually work by inflating and deflating air cells to relieve pressure on each point at regular intervals, and are more effective than the 'passive' systems in intensive care patients.[160] However, they are expensive and can make certain nursing tasks more difficult, e.g. positioning a patient to reduce the risk of contractures, to help breathing and to facilitate swallowing, because they offer a less firm base.

Other interventions such as staff education, nutritional support and local treatments (e.g. creams, lotions) applied to unbroken areas of skin may have a role in prevention but their effectiveness has not yet been demonstrated.[163,164]

The ultimate choice of preventive method will depend on an assessment of the individual patient's risk of pressure ulcer, the availability of nurses, the patient's other needs, e.g. positioning, and available resources. Further research is required to identify the most cost-effective strategy for preventing pressure ulcers.[160] Studies will have to take into account patients' absolute risk of developing ulcers, the reduction in risk with each intervention and the cost of the intervention, as well as the cost

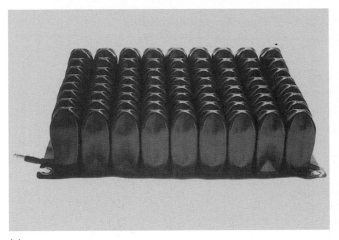

(a)

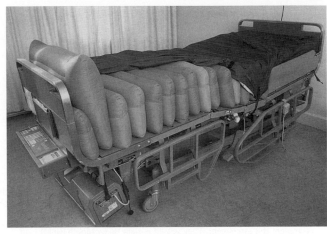

(b)

Fig. 11.13 Pressure-relieving cushion and bed: (a) Roho cushion; (b) low air-loss bed.

of treating any pressure ulcers which develop. However, we believe that, whatever technology is employed, adequate numbers of skilled nursing staff will still be essential if pressure ulcers are to be prevented.

Finally, it is important to recognize that certain management strategies (e.g. positioning in a chair, use of graduated compression stockings) may actually cause pressure ulcers unless they are properly applied and monitored (Fig. 11.9).

Treatment

For patients with established pressure ulcers, the relief of pressure probably remains the most important factor in promoting healing. 'Active' pressure-relieving systems are more effective than 'passive' ones.[165] In addition, it is important to optimize the patient's general condition by providing a good diet with adequate protein intake and by treating concurrent illness aggressively (e.g. infections, cardiac failure). This may need intensive nursing input in frail, elderly, anorexic patients who are drowsy or have swallowing problems. The pain associated with pressure ulcers may increase tone and lead to contractures (section 11.20) which may well hinder rehabilitation, while the discomfort may also affect the patient's morale and even further worsen their outcome. Adequate analgesia, with opiates if necessary, should be given to patients, especially before renewal of dressings. Antibiotics may be required if there is local or systemic infection (spreading cellulitis, osteomyelitis). Debridement to remove necrotic tissue, and skin grafting to achieve skin coverage, may sometimes be necessary.

A bewildering variety of local dressings and treatments (e.g. vitamin C, zinc, ultrasound, electrical stimulation, ultraviolet light) which aim to promote healing and reduce infection are available. Some small RCTs evaluating these interventions have been reported, but need to be systematically reviewed.[166,167]

11.17 Swallowing problems

Up to one-half of conscious patients admitted to hospital with an acute stroke cannot swallow safely on bedside testing.[168] However, estimates of the frequency of swallowing difficulties vary because of differences in definitions, timing and methods of detecting dysphagia and in selecting patients for study. Swallowing difficulties have been associated with a high case fatality and poor functional outcome and certainly put patients at risk of aspiration, pneumonia, dehydration and malnutrition.[168] However, much of the excess mortality and morbidity is probably due to the severity of the stroke itself rather than to swallowing difficulties.

11.17.1 Mechanisms of dysphagia

The following patterns of dysphagia after stroke have been identified with videofluoroscopy:[169,170]
- Poor oral control (oral preparatory phase) and delayed triggering of the swallow leads to aspiration before the swallow, i.e. liquid trickles over the back of the tongue before the swallow starts. In addition, patients with weakness or incoordination of the face or tongue often have difficulty keeping fluids in their mouth, and in chewing and manipulation of food to produce a well-formed food bolus.

- Failure of laryngeal adduction leads to aspiration during the swallow itself.
- Reduced pharyngeal 'peristalsis', or cricopharyngeal dysfunction, may allow food to collect in the pharynx and spill over, past the vocal cords and into the trachea. Thus, aspiration occurs after the swallow.

Poor oral control and delayed triggering of the swallow are the most common mechanisms causing dysphagia after stroke but more than one abnormality can usually be identified in any individual patient.

11.17.2 Detection of dysphagia

Despite their frequency, and the serious consequences of failing to detect them, swallowing problems are often not sought systematically in patients admitted to hospital with an acute stroke.[60] The current recommended approach is for a suitably trained nurse or other healthcare worker to perform a simple bedside swallow screen (Fig. 11.14), to distinguish patients able to take oral food and fluids safely from those who require a more detailed

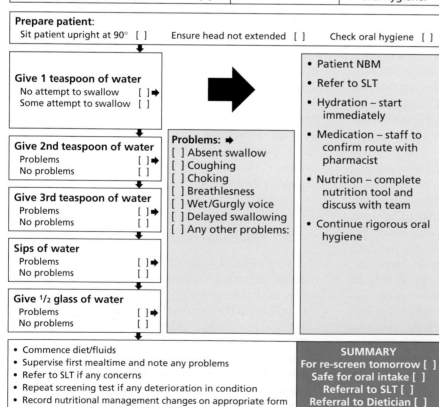

Fig. 11.14 Flow diagram for swallow screen and assessment from *Screening for Dysphagia* – an interactive training package developed by staff of NHS Lothian (http://www.elib.scot.nhs.uk/portal/stroke/dysphagia/index.asp). SLT, speech and language therapist.

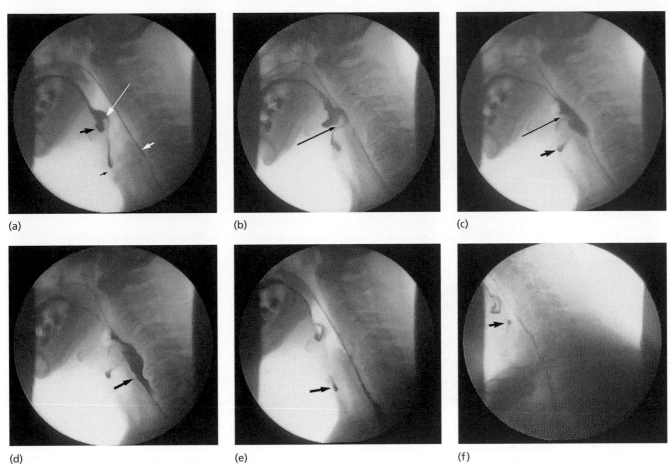

(a) (b) (c)

(d) (e) (f)

Fig. 11.15 A series of six frames taken from a videofluoroscopy examination in a stroke patient with swallowing difficulties. We have shown only the lateral views. (a) The food bolus containing radiodense material has been propelled into the pharynx by the tongue and has filled the vallecular space (*large black arrow*). Food is spilling over from the vallecular space, past the epiglottis (*long white arrow*) and is heading for the vocal cords (*small black arrow*). Note the nasogastric tube (*short white arrow*). The pharyngeal swallow has not yet been triggered. (b) The pharyngeal swallow has triggered (at last) with elevation and inversion of the epiglottis (*arrow*). (c) The epiglottis is fully inverted (*long arrow*). No further laryngeal penetration has occurred, indicating effective (but rather belated) laryngeal closure. However, some of the food bolus has passed the vocal cords (*short arrow*). (d) The food bolus is passing through the cricopharyngeal sphincter (*arrow*). (e) The swallow is complete but part of the food bolus remains below the vocal cords (*arrow*). The patient has not coughed, indicating that sensation is impaired, i.e. this patient has silent aspiration. (f) The patient has been asked to cough and this voluntary cough is effective in clearing the aspirated food back into the pharynx (*arrow*). (Videofluoroscopy provided by Diane Fraser.)

assessment.[171] In non-randomized studies a structured approach to swallow screening and appropriate feeding has been associated with fewer episodes of pneumonia.[172,173] Clinicians sometimes use the gag reflex to indicate swallowing safety but this is both inaccurate and unreliable.[174]

> The gag reflex is not a useful indicator of a stroke patient's swallowing ability.

The more detailed assessment of those patients who 'fail' their swallow screen usually comprises a detailed bedside assessment by a speech and language therapist, supplemented if necessary by an instrumental test such as videofluoroscopy (Fig. 11.15) or fibreoptic endoscopic evaluation of swallowing (FEES) (Fig. 11.16). Videofluoroscopy provides detailed information about the mechanism of dysphagia and can identify silent aspiration, which may be important since silent aspirators may be at greatest risk of complications.[175] It is regarded as the 'gold standard' method for assessing the swallow after stroke. The advantages and disadvantages of the main methods of assessment are summarized in Table 11.21. A clinical assessment might identify 40–90% of those with aspiration on videofluoroscopy.[176]

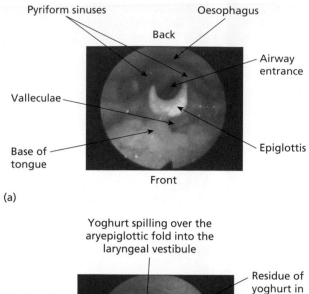

(a)

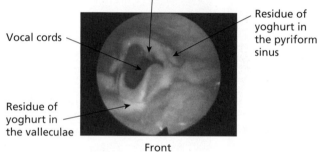

Pharyngeal residue after the swallow with
risk of aspiration

(b)

Fig. 11.16 Photographs taken during a fibreoptic endoscopic evaluation of swallowing showing the main anatomic structures. (Also reproduced in colour in the plate section.)

It is unclear whether dysphagia identified on a bedside swallowing assessment, or videofluoroscopy, is the better predictor of those who will develop complications such as pneumonia. Some workers have emphasized that the integrity of patients' laryngeal cough reflex may be a more important determinant of the risk of pneumonia than their ability to swallow.[177,178] The place of other techniques such as cervical auscultation, and pulse oximetry to detect oxygen desaturation during swallowing, is still unclear.[168] We suggest the following approach to screening for dysphagia:

- First, identify those patients who are *likely* to have problems swallowing, e.g. those with severe hemispheric, brainstem or bilateral strokes, or impaired consciousness. Table 11.22 lists those features which individually, or more particularly in combination, should alert one to a high risk of swallowing difficulty.
- Second, for patients without these features, or where access to a speech and language therapist with an

Table 11.21 Advantages and disadvantages of the available assessments of swallowing: bedside clinical, videofluoroscopy and fibreoptic endoscopic evaluation of swallowing.

Bedside clinical
Advantages
Performed at the bedside on the ward
Widely available, rapid and safe
No specialist equipment needed
Training in technique is readily available
Available in acute episode and easily repeated even on a daily basis
Wide range of foods, fluids and textures can be tried
Assesses effectiveness of therapeutic techniques
Disadvantages
Does not detect asymptomatic or silent aspiration
Limited predictive validity i.e. test result does not predict pneumonia or other patient outcomes
Little information about anatomy or actual mechanism of dysphagia
May not be available at weekends unless speech & language therapists offer this service

Videofluoroscopy
Advantages
Available in most hospitals, rapid and safe
Assessment of all anatomical stages of swallowing
Variety of foods can be tested
Allows the assessment of therapeutic manoeuvres
Considered the 'gold standard' method
Disadvantages
Radiation exposure and possibility of aspiration of barium
Rarely available in acute phase – usually needs to be pre-booked
Findings may not reflect ward behaviour
Density of barium means aspiration may not reflect risk with other foods
Training required for interpretation
Imperfect 'gold standard' – good 'face validity' but limited 'predictive validity' i.e. result does not predict pneumonia etc. better than alternatives

Fibreoptic endoscopic evaluation of swallowing
Advantages
Performed at the bedside with normal meals and variation in types, textures, etc.
Gives good anatomical data of the pharynx/larynx
Can be repeated regularly
Sensory testing can be undertaken
Disadvantages
Not widely available
Requires skilled operators
'White-out' often obscures the period of aspiration
No information is gathered on oral control
Limited data on validity so far

Table 11.22 Features that indicate a likelihood of swallowing problems, derived from several studies.[171,179,436,437]

Decreased level of consciousness (including confusion)
Poor sitting balance
Bilateral strokes
Older age
Abnormal tongue or palatal movement
Weak or absent voluntary cough
Moist or bubbling voice
Evidence of chest infection
Reduced pharyngeal sensation

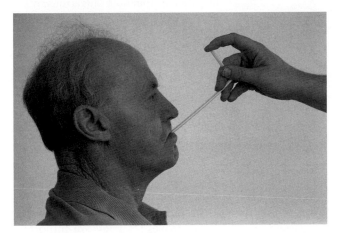

Fig. 11.17 One can control the volume of liquid a patient receives during a swallowing assessment with a drinking straw used as a pipette.

interest in swallowing difficulties is limited, a doctor or nurse can usefully assess swallowing. Ask the patient to swallow a total of perhaps 50 mL of water, initially in 5 mL aliquots, while sitting supported in the upright position, with neck flexed (which keeps the airway closed) and the head tilted to the unaffected side (which avoids the water slipping down the neglected side of the oropharynx). Suction equipment should be available. The volume and speed of delivery of the water can be controlled with a teaspoon, or using a drinking straw as a pipette (Fig. 11.17). Patients may, if simply handed a cup to drink from, attempt to drink it all and aspirate large volumes. After each swallow, wait for an involuntary cough and ask the patient to speak. A cough or a change in the patient's voice (i.e. wet voice) suggests aspiration. One should be particularly careful in assessing patients with existing respiratory disease who may be compromised by even minor degrees of aspiration.

- Finally, if swallowing difficulties are likely, or are demonstrated on simple bedside testing, put the patient on 'nil by mouth' and hydrate them via an alternative route until a more detailed assessment can be made (section 11.18.1). While the patient is 'nil by mouth' their mouth should be kept moist and clean with regular mouth care.

11.17.3 Prognosis and management

Prognosis

Most patients with swallowing difficulties immediately after their stroke either die, or improve, so dysphagia which persists in patients who survive for more than a week or two is relatively uncommon. Interestingly, many patients eating a normal diet have persisting abnormalities, including aspiration on videofluoroscopy, for several months after their stroke but the significance is unclear;[169] this raises questions about the validity of videofluoroscopy.

Treatment

An ongoing assessment of patients' swallowing abilities by a speech and language therapist is valuable in guiding their fluid and feeding regimen, so that patients are not unnecessarily deprived of nutrition or put at risk of aspiration (section 11.19). Speech and language therapists may not be any more accurate in detecting a swallowing problem than nurses or doctors, but they do provide a more detailed assessment and potential solutions. Their assessment includes feeding the patient: in various positions (e.g. leaning to one side or the other); with different food textures (e.g. liquid, thickened fluids, purée or solids); with increasing bolus size; with different methods of delivery; and with different verbal cues or instructions.[179] Videofluoroscopy and/or fibreoptic endoscopic evaluation of swallowing (FEES) can be useful in patients with persisting swallowing difficulties; if the cause of the dysphagia is uncertain; where percutaneous endoscopic gastrostomy (PEG) is being considered (section 11.19); or where silent aspiration is suspected in patients with repeated chest infections.

Based on their swallowing assessment, including videofluoroscopy and/or FEES or not, speech and language therapists can teach the patient and carer methods of compensating for their problems until recovery occurs.[171] Simple interventions which might allow a patient to swallow safely include:

- Ensure the patient is appropriately positioned, e.g. not slumped, semi-recumbent to their hemiplegic side.
- Teach the patient manoeuvres such as the 'chin tuck' or 'head turn' which make aspiration less likely.
- Tailor the consistency of fluids and food to the patient's swallowing abilities; for instance, thickened fluids are

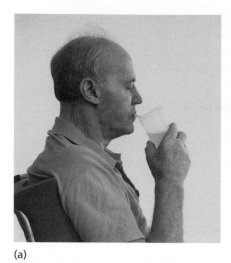
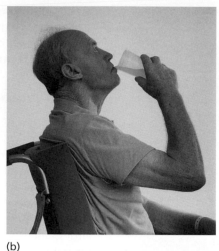

(a)   (b)

Fig. 11.18 Although beakers with a spout may prevent spills they have unfortunate associations with childhood which can make them unpopular with some patients. Also, they encourage patients to extend their neck when drinking which may lead to aspiration. This is the way *not* to do it: (a) bring the spout to the lips, (b) throw back the head, open the airway and inhale!

usually more easily swallowed than water because they move less rapidly through the oropharynx and so give more time for the initiation of the swallow. Ideally a range of diets of specified consistency should be available. It is important that those responsible for distributing meals and refreshments, including well-meaning relatives, are aware of patients' individual requirements.

- Choose an appropriate type of drinking vessel. If the patient does not have severe facial weakness and can suck, a drinking straw is often helpful. Beakers with spouts tend to encourage the patient to drink with an extended neck which opens the airway and encourages aspiration (Fig. 11.18).

These interventions, which involve swallowing food or fluids, are often termed compensatory or 'direct' strategies, while exercises which do not actually involve swallowing anything and which aim to improve motor control are referred to as 'indirect' strategies. One randomized single-centre trial has shown that a structured programme of assessment by a speech therapist, supplemented with videofluoroscopy when necessary, and both direct and indirect treatment strategies, achieved better recovery of swallowing than a less structured and formal approach.[180,181] Specific interventions such as oral stimulation have not yet been shown to improve swallowing performance.[182]

> All those involved in giving a patient food or fluids, including their relatives, must be made aware of the patient's swallowing difficulties and what the patient can, and can't, swallow safely. Staff training and effective communication are essential.

11.18 Metabolic disturbances

Metabolic disturbances, which may themselves occasionally mimic stroke (sections 3.4.5 and 7.16), are common in patients with severe strokes.[183] They are important because they may cause 'worsening' (section 11.5), but are often easily reversed.

11.18.1 Dehydration

Patients with stroke are vulnerable to dehydration because:

- swallowing difficulties are common after acute stroke (section 11.17);
- immobility means patients depend on others to provide them with drinks (section 11.11); they may even have been lying on the floor for several hours before being found;
- they may have communication problems (section 11.30) so cannot ask for drinks;
- they may have hemianopia or visual neglect (section 11.28) so may not see the jug of water beside them;
- they are often elderly and therefore may have reduced sensitivity to thirst;[184]
- they may have a fever, chest infection (section 11.12.1), hyperglycaemia (section 11.18.3) or be taking diuretics, all of which increase their fluid losses;[185]
- they may restrict their fluid intake to avoid embarrassing episodes of urinary incontinence (section 11.14).

Patients with dysphagia who require thickened fluids and those on diuretics are particularly vulnerable to

Table 11.23 Clinical indicators of dehydration.

> *General signs*
> Thirst
> Reduced skin turgor
> Dry mucous membranes
> Sunken eyes
> *Cardiovascular*
> Cool peripheries
> Collapsed peripheral veins
> Postural hypotension
> Low jugular venous pulse or central venous pressure
> Low urine output
> *Investigations*
> Rising urinary specific gravity
> Raised haemoglobin concentration
> Raised haematocrit
> Raised serum sodium (evidence of water depletion)
> Raised serum urea (out of proportion to the serum
>   creatinine)

dehydration.[185,186] Raised osmolality has been associated with worse survival at 3 months[187] and increased plasma urea with a greater frequency of venous thromboembolism[131] (section 11.13).

Assessment

Clinical signs (Table 11.23) are potentially helpful in identifying dehydration, but are difficult to assess reliably, especially in older patients.[188] Tachycardia, poor peripheral perfusion and low jugular venous pressure may be useful in severe cases. Modern electric profiling beds allow one to 'tilt' the patient to look for orthostatic hypotension even where standing would be impossible (Fig. 11.7). Investigations, including the measurement of urinary specific gravity or osmolality and plasma sodium, urea (and creatinine to allow the urea/creatinine ratio to be determined) and osmolality are probably more reliable than the bedside assessment.[189] Where a patient is very unwell with hypotension or renal failure, cannulation of a central vein to measure the right atrial pressure directly, and to monitor fluid replacement, may occasionally be valuable. In hospital, charting patients' fluid intake and output is also helpful but fluid charts are so often inaccurate, not least because it is difficult, although not impossible, if continence pads are weighed, to monitor output when patients are incontinent (section 11.14). Hypernatraemia is usually due to water depletion without concomitant sodium depletion and often occurs if patients do not drink adequate amounts. It can only be diagnosed by measuring the serum sodium since it is difficult to detect clinically. Very occasionally, hypernatraemia indicates a diabetic hyperosmolar state (section 11.18.3).

Prevention and treatment

Patients who are unable or unwilling to take adequate oral fluids to prevent or reverse dehydration should be given fluid replacement by another route, i.e. intravenously, subcutaneously or by nasogastric tube. Intravenous fluids are generally required where the patient is dehydrated while subcutaneous fluids are often sufficient to maintain hydration[190] (Table 11.24). There is a consensus that dextrose infusions should be avoided in the first day or two after acute stroke (section 11.18.3). Parenteral fluid replacement should be guided by regular monitoring of urea and electrolytes since patients' requirements for fluids are unpredictable (depending on urinary and insensible losses) and overhydration can occur.[191]

If patients are willing and able to take fluids orally they should be given adequate access to fluids (i.e. the cup and jug should be placed within their reach and not on the side of any neglect or hemianopia) and, importantly, regular encouragement to drink. Where the patient is hypernatraemic, adequate isotonic fluid replacement will usually normalize the serum sodium.

> Always ensure that patients who can swallow safely have ready access to fluids.

11.18.2 Hyponatraemia

Hyponatraemia is uncommon after ischaemic stroke and intracerebral haemorrhage, though it is more frequent after subarachnoid haemorrhage (section 14.9.1). It may be due to excess salt loss due to, for example, diuretics, or it may be dilutional (reflecting inappropriate secretion of antidiuretic hormone) in response to the brain injury, medication or medical complications.[191] Dilution is the conventional explanation for hyponatraemia after ischaemic stroke or intracerebral haemorrhage, but after subarachnoid haemorrhage, hyponatraemia has been attributed more often to excessive renal salt loss (section 14.9.1). It is unclear how often this so-called 'cerebral salt wasting' occurs in other types of stroke. Higher levels of antidiuretic hormone have been described in stroke patients than controls but in the absence of hyponatraemia.[192] Hyponatraemia may occasionally cause patients to deteriorate neurologically, so it is important to detect since it is usually reversible.

Table 11.24 Advantages and disadvantages of different methods of hydrating patients who are unable to swallow.

Intravenous:	*Advantages*
	Can give large volumes rapidly in hypovolaemia
	Can give intravenous drugs or irritative solutions via cannula
	Disadvantages
	Can overload patient if not properly supervised
	Requires skilled person to insert cannula (so administration may be interrupted if cannula needs replacing)
	Infection at cannula site can be serious
	Cannulae should be replaced regularly but they are expensive
Subcutaneous:	*Advantages*
	Can be started by relatively unskilled staff (which may reduce interruptions)
	Needle can be placed where patient cannot reach it and so lessen likelihood of removal
	Unlikely to administer large volumes rapidly and therefore fluid overload less likely
	Butterfly cannulae are relatively inexpensive
	Disadvantages
	May be associated with local oedema, redness or even abscess
	Absorption can be unpredictable
	Unable to give large volumes rapidly to reverse hypovolaemia and severe dehydration
	Cannot use cannulae for drug administration or irritative solutions
Nasogastric:	*Advantages*
	More 'physiological' and volume overload unlikely
	Can feed the patient via tube as well as just hydrating them
	Can give oral medications via tube
	Does not necessarily require expensive giving sets or sterile fluids
	Disadvantages
	May increase risk of aspiration
	Frequently pulled out by restless patients and thus fluid administration interrupted
	Probably less acceptable to patients and relatives
	Radiation exposure if X-rays used to check position

Table 11.25 Medications which have been associated with hyponatraemia and which are frequently used in stroke patients.

Medication	Likely indication	Section
Diuretics	High blood pressure/cardiac failure	11.7.1 and 16.3
Carbamazepine, oxcarbazepine	Seizures	11.8
Selective serotonin reuptake inhibitors (SSRI)	Depression/emotionalism	11.31.1 and 11.31.2
Angiotensin converting enzyme inhibitors (ACEI)	High blood pressure/cardiac failure	11.2.3 and 11.7.1

Assessment

We measure urea and electrolytes in all stroke patients as part of the baseline assessment, and we monitor them regularly where the baseline assessment indicates an abnormality, in patients with severe stroke, and those with swallowing problems. A low serum sodium should prompt a search for the cause including review of the medication (Table 11.25), a clinical assessment of hydration (Table 11.23) and fluid balance and, depending on the circumstances, some investigations, e.g. blood sugar, urea and creatinine, plasma and urine osmolality and urinary sodium concentration, plasma antidiuretic hormone level (where available) and perhaps a chest X-ray to identify an alternative cause of inappropriate secretion of antidiuretic hormone.

Treatment

The treatment of hyponatraemia obviously depends on the cause, e.g. stopping diuretics, fluid restriction in dilutional hyponatraemia and cautious administration of intravenous isotonic saline where salt wasting is confirmed (section 14.9.1). It is usually recommended that hyponatraemia is corrected slowly, over days rather than hours, to reduce the risk of central pontine myelinolysis.[193]

11.18.3 Hyperglycaemia

Hyperglycaemia (defined as a fasting glucose level of > 6.7 mmol/L, or 120 mg/dL) occurs in about one-third of non-diabetic acute stroke patients and two-thirds of those with diabetes.[194] About one-quarter of those with hyperglycaemia are known to have diabetes mellitus already and another quarter have a raised HbA1C which suggests that their blood glucose has been high for some time before the stroke, referred to as 'latent diabetes'.[195] Whether the hyperglycaemia in non-diabetics is due to release of catecholamines and corticosteroids as part of the stress response is controversial.[196]

Hyperglycaemia, after a stroke, at least in non-diabetic patients, is associated with increased case fatality and poor functional outcome.[194,197] This could be explained by more severe strokes producing a greater stress response and, thus, hyperglycaemia so that hyperglycaemia is simply a marker of severe stroke. However, some studies have demonstrated that hyperglycaemia is associated with a poor outcome having adjusted for stroke severity and other baseline prognostic factors.[194] This finding, along with some (but not all) animal work showing that hyperglycaemia can exacerbate ischaemic neuronal damage, has led many to believe there is a causal relationship between hyperglycaemia and poor outcome.[197,198]

Assessment

A random blood glucose should be measured in all patients with stroke. In those with hyperglycaemia, a fasting blood glucose and an HbA1C will help distinguish latent diabetes from hyperglycaemia due to the stroke itself. Blood sugar levels are likely to fall spontaneously in the first few days after stroke onset.[199] If necessary, a glucose tolerance test after the acute stage of the illness (i.e. when the patient is medically stable) may be helpful in sorting out which patients have diabetes or impaired glucose tolerance, and which simply have hyperglycaemia related to the acute stroke. Patients with established diabetes and latent diabetes should be assessed to exclude vascular (both micro and macro) and neurological complications.

Treatment

We currently aim to keep the blood sugar less than 11 mmol/L (200 mg/dL) in the first few days after an acute stroke. This will keep the patient free from thirst and avoid excessive diuresis which may cause dehydration (section 11.18.1). Whether more aggressive control of blood sugar, which has at least theoretical benefits for the ischaemic penumbra, is sensible will depend on any benefits, and the risks of hypoglycaemia, which will almost certainly depend on the intensity of monitoring available.[198] One small and one moderate sized, but underpowered RCT have shown that glucose-potassium-insulin (GKI) infusions can be used with reasonable safety to control hyperglycaemia in acute stroke but have not demonstrated any improvement in survival or functional outcomes.[199,200]

11.18.4 Hypoglycaemia

Hypoglycaemia may occasionally mimic stroke or transient ischaemic attack (sections 3.4.5 and 7.16). Ideally, it should be excluded on first contact with medical services (e.g. paramedics, primary care physician) by measuring the glucose on a capillary sample in all patients taking hypoglycaemic medication.[201] Hypoglycaemia also occurs after stroke because of efforts to normalize blood sugar in those with hyperglycaemia (section 11.18.3) and in diabetic patients receiving hypoglycaemic medication but a reduced food intake because of dysphagia (section 11.17) or other post-stroke problems (section 11.19.1). Since hypoglycaemia may, if severe or undetected, cause worsening of the neurological deficit, the blood sugar should be monitored particularly carefully in diabetic patients on hypoglycaemic medication.

11.19 Nutritional problems

11.19.1 Malnutrition

Malnutrition is a common and often unrecognized problem in patients admitted to hospital, especially the elderly.[202] Inevitably, the reported frequency of malnutrition after stroke has varied depending on patient selection, the definitions of malnutrition and the method and timing of assessments. Estimates vary from 8% to 34%.[203,204] It is not clear which factors are associated with malnutrition on admission, but the non-stroke literature suggests that malnutrition is more frequent in older patients, those living in institutions and poor social circumstances, and those with prior cognitive impairment, physical disability or gastrointestinal disease. In a proportion of stroke patients, nutritional status may worsen during hospital admission.[205,206]

Like any acute illness, stroke may cause a negative energy balance and greater nutritional demands but, at the same time, stroke patients may be less able to adapt to these.[207,208] They often have swallowing difficulties (section 11.17) and even those who can swallow may have a poor appetite because of lack of taste associated with the stroke itself[209] or medication, intercurrent illness, depression, or apathy; and they may eat slowly because of facial weakness, lack of dentures or poor arm function.

Poor nutrition has been associated with reduced muscle strength, reduced resistance to infection and impaired wound healing (although not specifically in stroke patients). Among patients with stroke, muscle weakness, infections and pressure ulcers are common and account for many deaths and much morbidity.[105] Malnutrition on admission is associated with increased case fatality and poorer functional outcomes even having adjusted for other factors, but it is unclear to what extent this association is causal.[210,211]

11.19.2 Obesity

Obesity is common among hospitalized stroke patients.[36,212] As well as being a risk factor for stroke (section 6.6.10), and presumably recurrent stroke obesity can also be a problem during recovery from stroke. Where patients have restricted mobility, especially where they rely on others for help with transfers, obesity can be a crucial factor in how long they remain in hospital and how much support they require. It is also a problem in the long term in achieving adequate control of vascular risk factors such as hypertension (section 16.7.3) and diabetes. Patients quite often gain weight after stroke, presumably because of decreased energy expenditure and excessive calorie intake.

11.19.3 Assessment

In routine clinical practice there are practical difficulties in assessing stroke patients' nutritional status. A dietary and weight history may not be available because of patients' communication problems and an alternative source of this information may not be available if, as is common, the patient lives alone. Simple assessments of weight and height to estimate the body mass index (BMI) pose problems in immobile stroke patients. Specialized equipment, of limited availability, such as weighing beds or hoists and scales which accommodate wheelchairs, may be required and height may have to be estimated from the patient's demi-span or heel–knee

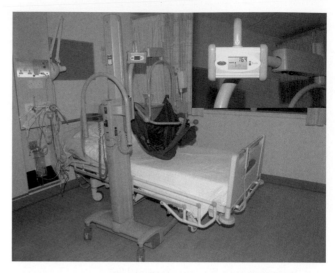

Fig. 11.19 A hoist which incorporates an electronic scale (inset) for weighing immobile stroke patients who are unable to stand or sit unaided.

length (Fig. 11.19). Laboratory parameters such as haemoglobin, serum protein, albumin and transferrin may not necessarily reflect nutritional status. More complex anthropometric measures, vitamin estimations, antigen skin testing and bioelectric impedance are all used in research but are not widely available.

Awareness of the possibility of malnutrition is a key factor in identifying malnourished patients. It is probably worthwhile using a standardized screening tool for nutritional problems in the stroke unit which can highlight those patients who would benefit from a dietician's input, but none have been adequately evaluated for stroke patients.[213,214] A simple and informal end-of-the-bed assessment (i.e. is the patient undernourished, normal or overweight?) is better than no assessment at all since it reliably identifies most stroke patients with a low BMI and abnormal anthropometry, as well as predicting outcome.[210,215] Estimation of the BMI, serial weights to identify weight loss, and monitoring of dietary intake should be used to screen patients on admission and monitor them while on the stroke unit. Simple laboratory tests including a serum albumin may be worth monitoring where there is clinical evidence of poor or worsening nutrition.

> All patients admitted to hospital with stroke should have an early assessment of their nutritional status. In the absence of a formal assessment tool the team's judgement of whether the patient is undernourished, normal or overweight is better than nothing. At least it focuses the team on this important aspect of care.

11.19.4 Prevention and treatment of malnutrition

General approach

It is useful to involve the speech and language therapist and dietician in the assessment and care of patients who have swallowing problems, or when nutritional intake may be inadequate for other reasons, e.g. confusion. Patients often eat very slowly after stroke and need supervision to ensure safe swallowing. Simple measures such as providing appetizing food of an appropriate consistency (section 11.17), placing the patient's meal in their intact visual field, and ensuring that the patient has well-fitting dentures should not be overlooked. Labelling a patient's dentures with their name while in hospital helps prevent losses and unfortunate mix-ups. Staff shortages may mean that patients receive insufficient food, which will eventually cause malnutrition, or have food forced into them hurriedly by unthinking staff, which is very demeaning and adversely affects morale. Where trained staff are unable to cope, the patient's family or even volunteers can be easily trained to help with feeding.

> Dentures are often lost during hospital admission. Labelling a patient's dentures with their name helps prevent losses and unfortunate mix-ups.

Most people do not like to be fed; they prefer to feed themselves. By providing patients with suitable feeding utensils or foods which they can pick up may allow them to feed themselves (section 11.32.6). If not, adequate staff or family members, who have been instructed in how to do it, need to be employed.

Oral nutritional supplements

Routine oral nutritional supplementation, which provide both proteins and calories, in hospitalized stroke patients is probably not worthwhile since they have not been shown to have a clinically useful impact on outcome. The FOOD trial randomly allocated 4023 patients with an acute stroke to routine oral nutritional supplements or not, for the duration of their hospital admission. There was no significant difference in survival or functional outcomes overall, but there were insufficient patients enrolled who were undernourished to determine if this subgroup might benefit.[212] Therefore, the results of the FOOD trial, taken along with a large number of much smaller single-centre RCTs of nutritional support in elderly patients, suggest that oral supplements are probably useful, but just in those who are identified as malnourished or who have inadequate food intake.[212]

Enteral tube feeding

Where swallowing is impaired, early introduction of nasogastric tube feeding probably reduces the risk of death although maybe at the expense of keeping more patients with severe disability alive (Fig. 11.20).[36] This also facilitates administration of important medications. Early tube feeding does not appear to influence the risk of chest infections but does seem to increase the risk of gastrointestinal haemorrhage (section 11.2.3) although it is unclear why this occurs and whether any preventive treatment such as a proton pump inhibitor would be effective (Table 11.26).

Inserting nasogastric tubes is often difficult and ensuring that they are in the stomach, rather than in the lungs, at the beginning of each feed is not straightforward.[216] Also, patients frequently find the nasogastric tube uncomfortable, and feeding is often interrupted by the patient repeatedly removing the tube. By restraining the patient (Fig. 11.21a,b) one can probably improve the continuity of nasogastric feeding but such restraints are not acceptable to some patients, their families and healthcare staff.

Although enteral feeding via a percutaneous endoscopic gastrostomy (PEG) is perceived as more comfortable and reliable in providing the prescribed feed, its routine early use is not associated with better survival or functional outcomes.[36] Indeed, the FOOD trial which included 321 patients allocated to initial tube feeding via nasogastric or PEG showed that patients allocated to PEG feeding tended to have worse outcomes (7.8% increased risk of death or severe disability (95% CI −0.08% to 15.5%). However, where a patient is likely to need prolonged tube feeding, or where nasogastric feeding is not practical, a PEG is usually the best option (Table 11.26). But one does have to take account of the associated complications. About one-fifth will develop aspiration pneumonia shortly after insertion, about 10% will develop a wound infection, and potentially life-threatening complications such as peritonitis and major bleeding occur in about 1%.[217-222] Patients, or more frequently their relatives, need to be counselled about these risks and the real possibility that their frail relative may die in the days following the procedure.

> The early introduction of PEG tube feeding, rather than persisting with a nasogastric tube, in dysphagic patients is unlikely to be associated with better outcomes. However, if nasogastric tube feeding becomes impractical there may be no alternative to PEG insertion.

Point estimate from FOOD trial
Feed 100 patients early
– prevent about six deaths

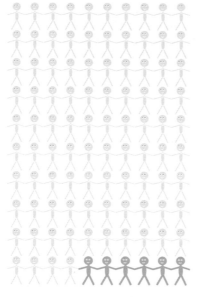

There was a 5.8% absolute (95% CI −0.8–12.5) reduction in the proportion of patients who had died at 6-months follow-up in the early enteral tube feeding group compared with the avoid early feed group. The reduction in death or dependency was only 1.2% (95% CI −4.2–6.6).

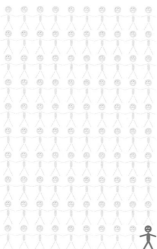

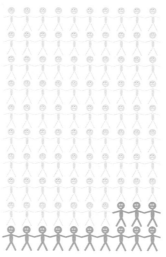

Lower 95% confidence interval: feed 100 patients early and cause about one additional death

Upper 95% confidence interval: feed 100 patients early and prevent about 13 deaths

Fig. 11.20 Results from the FOOD trial comparing outcomes (deaths by 6 months per 100 patients treated) following enteral tube feeding (mostly via nasogastric tube) started early after hospital admission versus avoiding enteral tube feeding for at least 1 week.

11.19.5 Treatment of obesity

Patients who are obese, in particular if this causes problems with mobility or control of diabetes or blood pressure, should be encouraged to lose weight and be offered dietary advice (section 16.7).

11.19.6 Other considerations

It is important to remember that eating plays an important role in our social lives and is a source of pleasure. Eating with other people during the recovery phase of stroke encourages communication and social

Table 11.26 Advantages and disadvantages of nasogastric and percutaneous endoscopic gastrostomy feeding.

	Advantages	Disadvantages
Nasogastric tube	Widely available Cheap	Easily inserted into lungs Often pulled out Unsightly Uncomfortable May lead to aspiration Nasal irritation/ulcer Gastric bleeding Interference with swallow
Percutaneous endoscopic gastrostomy	Tube rarely displaced Cosmetically acceptable Long-term use practical	Limited availability Expensive Aspiration when sedated for insertion Wound infection Bleeding Peritonitis

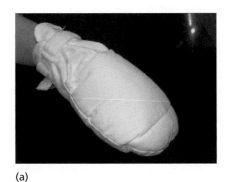

(a)

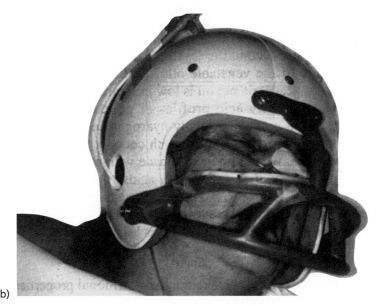

(b)

Fig. 11.21 (a) A mitten used to prevent a patient from removing a nasogastric tube. (b) An American football helmet to prevent a patient from pulling out a nasogastric tube. (Reproduced from Levine and Morris, 1995[460] with permission.)

interaction. Patients who are concerned by their appearance after a stroke (e.g. due to facial weakness) may gain confidence from this opportunity to socialize. On the other hand, dribbling or ending up with the food down their shirt, or on the table or floor, may distress patients and inhibit social interaction. Advice from the occupational therapist regarding equipment to allow the patient to eat independently should be sought to maximize the positive, and minimize the negative, aspects of eating in a communal setting (section 11.32.6).

11.20 Spasticity and contractures

Spasticity has been defined as a motor disorder characterized by velocity-dependent increase in muscle tone with exaggerated tendon reflexes. It develops in between one-fifth and one-third of hospital-admitted stroke patients over the first year and is more common in those with hemiparesis and after severe strokes, and is more common in the arm than the leg.[223,224] However, spasticity contributes to disability in only a minority of patients with hemiplegia.[224,225]

Spasticity is usually accompanied by muscle weakness and clumsiness and sometimes by flexor or extensor spasms. Immediately after a stroke the muscular tone in the limbs and trunk may be lower, the same as, or higher than normal. The reasons for this variation are unclear. Although tone may be lower than normal in the acute phase, in most patients who do not recover it tends to increase over the first few weeks. In patients with a hemiparesis, the tone in the arm is usually greater in the flexors than extensors, while in the leg it is greater in the extensors than the flexors. This explains the typical hemiplegic posture (i.e. elbow, wrist and fingers flexed and arm adducted and internally rotated with the leg extended at the hip and knee and the foot plantar flexed and inverted). Tone in the truncal muscles may also be abnormally high or low.

Tone may increase in any muscle group so much that it restricts the active movement which the residual muscle strength can produce. Imbalance in muscle tone can eventually result in shortening of muscles and permanent deformity and so restrict the full range of movement, i.e. contractures. Associated reactions are involuntary movements of the affected side (most typically flexion of the arm) elicited by a variety of stimuli including the use of unaffected limbs (e.g. self-propelling a wheelchair, yawning or coughing) and the upright posture.[99,226] Associated reactions become more obvious with increases in tone. Associated reactions may be misinterpreted as voluntary movements by family and ill-informed staff who should be educated about their significance to prevent them becoming unduly optimistic about the patient's motor recovery.

Spasticity and contractures may cause pain, deformity, disability and, if severe, secondary complications such as pressure ulcers at points of contact between soft tissues (e.g. on the inner aspect of the knees in a patient with contractures of the thigh adductors).

> Associated reactions may be misinterpreted as voluntary movements by family and ill-informed staff who should be educated about their significance to prevent them becoming unduly optimistic about the patient's motor recovery.

Assessment

Tone and spasticity: Physicians are trained to assess the tone in a limb by asking the patient to relax (which is almost guaranteed to have the opposite effect) and then moving the limb through its range of movement at each

Table 11.27 The modified Ashworth scale for the clinical assessment of muscle tone.[438]

0	No increase in muscle tone
1	Slight increase in muscle tone, manifested by a catch and release, or by a minimal resistance at the end of the range of motion when the affected part(s) is moved in flexion or extension
1+	Slight increase in muscle tone, manifested by a catch, followed by minimal resistance throughout the remainder (less than half) of the range of movement
2	More marked increase in muscle tone through most of the range of movement but affected parts easily moved
3	Considerable increase in muscle tone, passive movement difficult
4	Affected parts rigid in flexion or extension

joint at different speeds and noting any resistance to these movements. Unfortunately, many physicians do not appreciate how much tone is influenced by factors such as the patient's position, anxiety, fatigue, pain and medication. Tone may change from minute to minute. This makes it difficult to assess objectively with good inter-observer reliability. Physiotherapists, who spend far more time than physicians handling patients, are more aware of changes in tone and try to take advantage of them in their therapy.

Formal measurement of tone can be attempted using clinical scales (e.g. the modified Ashworth Scale, Table 11.27) or techniques such as electrogoniometry or quantitative neurophysiology. Unfortunately, the last two are not widely available or practical in routine clinical practice. The inter-observer reliability of the modified Ashworth Scale is generally good for assessing tone in the arm and around the knee but poor for assessing tone around the ankle.[227] When assessing the effectiveness of treatment in an individual patient, or in a group of patients in RCTs, it may be better to measure function (e.g. walking speed or dressing), or the achievement of a specific goal (to allow the palm of the hand to be accessed to maintain hygiene) than relying on measurement of tone itself. Indeed, the management of abnormal tone, like all other aspects of rehabilitation, should be directed at achieving realistic, relevant and measurable goals (section 10.3.3).

Contractures are easier to assess because, by definition, the deformity is fixed. Thus, one can objectively measure the range of movement around a joint and repeat the measure to determine whether or not an intervention has improved the range. However, occasionally an apparent contracture responds to injection of botulinum toxin (see below) indicating that the shortening is due to muscle contraction rather than permanent shortening of muscles or tendons.

Prevention and treatment

In rehabilitation our aim is to modulate changes in muscle tone to the patient's advantage. For instance, to increase tone in a flaccid leg and so provide the patient with a more secure base on which to walk, or reduce tone in the arm to facilitate more active movement. We use several complementary approaches to prevent the development of unwanted patterns of tone and to alleviate existing problems due to spasticity and contractures. Some are applicable to any patient while others are only required to deal with exceptional problems:

- *Avoidance of exacerbating factors*: Pain (section 11.23), urinary retention (section 11.14), severe constipation (section 11.15), skin irritation, pressure ulcers (section 11.16), anxiety (11.31.1) and any other unpleasant stimulus may cause an unwanted increase in tone. These factors must be avoided or alleviated.
- *Positioning and seating*: Poor positioning, especially in immobile patients, can lead to detrimental changes in tone. For example, long periods spent lying supine will increase extensor spasms, presumably by facilitation of basic reflexes. Regular positioning, such as external rotation of the shoulder, appears to reduce unwanted tonal changes.[228] Unfortunately, there seems to be quite a lot of uncertainty about the optimum positions for patients with hemiplegia and there are also practical difficulties in keeping them in the required position, i.e. patients tend to move.[229] The positioning charts which can be found on most stroke units (Fig. 11.22) can only be used as a general guide. Finding the optimum position for a patient is often a matter of trial and error and relies on the experience of the therapists and nurses. Appropriate seating which can be tailored to the individual patient is essential (Fig. 11.23). Ideally, patients should be seated in a balanced, symmetrical and stable position which they find comfortable and which enables them to function, e.g. eat, drink, etc.
- *Passive movements and physiotherapy*: It is important that muscles are not allowed to remain in a relaxed and shortened position for too long. For example, if the arm is left in a flexed posture at the elbow, or the foot plantar flexed in bed, this can lead to permanent shortening and contractures. Patients' limbs should be moved passively to stretch the muscles and maintain the range of movement, even in the very acute stages. However, it is important that carers are taught to do this without damaging vulnerable structures such as the shoulder (section 11.24). Also, handling methods, during transfers for example, can influence tone, at least in the short term.[230] Physiotherapists have an important role in teaching nurses and informal carers the correct positioning and handling techniques to minimize risk of injury (to patient and handler) and unwanted spasticity.

Patients with a hemiparesis often attempt to 'overuse' their sound side to achieve mobility but, as a consequence, the tone may increase in the affected side. Using the unaffected leg to self-propel a wheelchair is said to lead to increased spasticity in the affected arm and leg.[231] The impact of any changes in tone associated with such activities on functional recovery has not been established.[232]

The aim of many of the facilitation and inhibition techniques used by therapists is to use basic reflexes and postural changes in tone to promote function. However, these techniques, although widely accepted and practised, have not been evaluated adequately in RCTs (section 11.21). Various physical techniques including the application of cold, of heat, splinting and electrical stimulation can, at least for a short time, reduce spasticity.[230,233,234] This may relieve discomfort, allow improved hygiene, and plaster casts or splints to be applied. Whether these physical techniques have direct longer-term benefits is unclear:[233]

- *Splinting and casting*: Occasionally these may be necessary to prevent or treat contractures. Progressive splinting and application of casts can improve range of movement but the optimum duration and best methods are unclear. Also, badly fitted casts and splints can cause pain, pressure ulcers and tendon damage which may exacerbate rather than relieve spasticity and contractures.
- *Oral antispastic drugs*: Where spasticity is not adequately controlled by physical techniques, or where the patient is suffering from painful muscle spasms, certain drugs have been advocated: baclofen, dantrolene, tizanidine and diazepam which all reduce tone by altering neurotransmitter function or ion flux in the spinal cord, or in muscles. But there is little reliable evidence from RCTs to indicate that they usefully reduce spasticity or improve function in stroke patients.[235] Indeed, in our experience they rarely make much difference and they have a number of adverse effects (Table 11.28). Adverse effects are much more common in older patients but can be minimized by starting with low doses and increasing the dose slowly until the desired effect is achieved, or adverse effects necessitate withdrawal. We normally only use baclofen or tizanidine for a trial period in patients who our physiotherapists feel might benefit.
- *Local and regional treatments*: Injection of botulinum toxin directly into muscles can reduce troublesome spasticity. Small RCTs have confirmed that this does

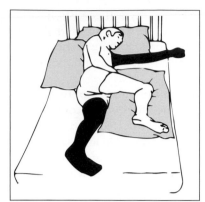

Lying on affected side
No backrest. One or two pillows for head.
Affected shoulder pulled well forward.
Place good leg forward on a pillow.
Pillow placed behind back.

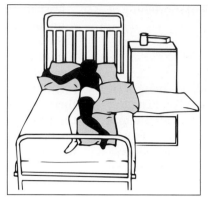

Lying on unaffected side
No backrest. One or two pillows for head.
Affected shoulder forward with arm
 on pillow.
Place affected leg backward on a pillow.
Pillow placed behind back.

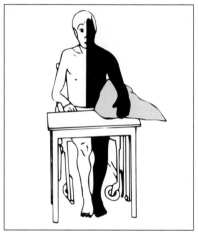

Sitting up
Sitting well back and in centre of chair.
Affected arm placed well forward on
 table or pillow.
Feet flat on floor.
Knees directly above the feet.

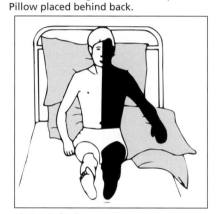

Sitting in bed
Sitting in bed is not desirable.
Affected arm placed on pillow.
Legs are straight.
Sitting upright and well supported.

Fig. 11.22 The typical chart used to guide
the positioning of stroke patients with
hemiplegia (shown in black) whilst in
bed.

indeed reduce tone, which may reduce clawing of the fingers and allow better skin hygiene.[236–238] This treatment appears to be safe, at least in the short term, but because its effects wear off over several months, repeated injections may be required and treatment costs can be very high. Sometimes, a single injection can allow simpler measures to be introduced which avoids the need for further injections. Further large trials are in progress to establish whether function really is improved (www.strokecentre.org).

Very occasionally, and usually where simple measures (see above) have been inadequate, spasticity can be so troublesome as to warrant more invasive procedures:

- local nerve blocks with ethanol or phenol although occasionally useful to solve specifc problems, can lead to unwanted muscle weakness and painful dysaesthesias;[239]
- intrathecal infusion of baclofen using implantable pumps;[240]
- surgical procedures such as anterior and posterior rhizotomy and more recently lesioning of the dorsal root entry zone (so-called drez-otomy);[233] and
- tendon lengthening and transfers which can, for example, help to reduce equinovarus deformity.[233]

Anecdotally, the prevalence of severe contractures appears to have declined dramatically over the last 30 years which is probably a result of improvements in the standards of general care. We now virtually never have to resort to the more invasive procedures described here.

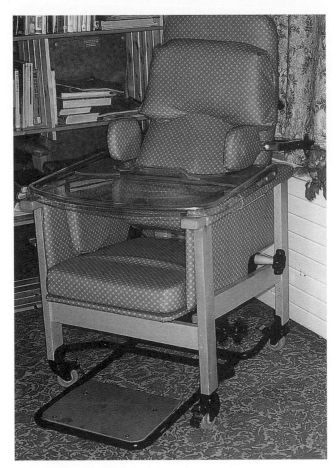

Fig. 11.23 A chair which can be tailored to the individual needs of the patient. This model can be raised, or lowered, the back rest and seat can be adjusted, arms can be altered and extra supports can be inserted.

11.21 Limb weakness, poor truncal control and unsteady gait

These three aspects of the patient's condition are impossible to separate and will therefore be discussed together. Weakness of an arm, leg or both, sometimes with unilateral facial weakness, is probably the most common and widely recognized impairment caused by stroke. However, there are often associated but less obvious problems with the axial muscles which impair truncal control and walking.

Facial weakness, which affects about 40% of patients (Table 11.2), apart from its cosmetic effects, may contribute to dysarthria (section 11.30.2) and cause problems with the oral preparatory phase of swallowing (section 11.17). Weakness of the upper limb, which affects about 50% of patients (Table 11.2), along with

changes in tone, is associated with the development of a painful shoulder (section 11.24) and swelling of the hand (section 11.25). Poor hand and arm function is a major cause of dependency in activities of daily living. Weakness of the leg, which affects about 45% of patients (Table 11.2), may be severe enough to immobilize the patient and thus predispose to the complications of immobility (section 11.11). Leg weakness, making it difficult to stand, transfer or walk independently, is one of the most important factors prolonging hospital stay in stroke patients. In patients with hemiparesis, which affects about 55% of patients, the arm is usually weaker than the leg (Table 11.2).

Assessment

In assessing function in a patient with stroke, unlike making the diagnosis, it is more useful to observe the range and control of voluntary movements of the limbs than assessing power in individual muscle groups. For instance, do the patients have only coarse control of movement around the hip or shoulder, or have they retained movement at the more distal joints? In stroke patients, distal movements are usually more severely impaired than proximal ones. The assessment of motor function and truncal control has already been described (section 3.3.4).

Recovery from a hemiplegic stroke has been likened to early infant development, in that the recovery of truncal control follows the same general pattern as that of a growing child. Head control returns first, followed by rolling over, sitting balance and then standing balance, and lastly the patient can walk with increasing steadiness and speed (Fig. 10.16). After a stroke it is useful to know where the patient is on this 'developmental ladder' when assessing prognosis and setting goals for rehabilitation.[241] It is also important to assess truncal control and gait since truncal ataxia can occur without limb incoordination in patients with midline cerebellar lesions. Indeed, it is not unknown for patients to undergo full gastrointestinal and metabolic investigation to elucidate the cause of vomiting before their truncal ataxia is noted and a cerebellar stroke diagnosed. It also seems absurd that, although immobility is the main reason for a stroke patient needing to stay in hospital for rehabilitation, mobility and balance are very often not assessed properly by doctors admitting stroke patients.[59]

Having stressed the importance of testing truncal control and gait, it is important that in doing so neither the patient nor the doctor are put at risk of injury. Poor handling and lifting technique may dislocate a patient's flaccid shoulder (section 11.24), result in a fracture from a fall (section 11.26) and may even injure the doctor's

Table 11.28 Adverse effects of antispasticity drugs.

Adverse effect	Baclofen	Diazepam	Dantrolene	Tizanidine
Sedation/central nervous system depression	++	+++	+	+
Confusion	+	+		
Hypotonia/weakness	+	+	++	+
Unsteadiness/ataxia	+	++	+	+
Exacerbation of epileptic seizures	++			
Psychosis/hallucinations	++		+	
Insomnia	+			+
Headache	+	+		
Urinary retention	+	+	+	
Dry mouth			++	
Hypotension	+	+		+
Nausea/vomiting	+	+		+
Diarrhoea/constipation	+	+	+	+
Abnormal liver function	+	+	+++	+
Hyperglycaemia	+			
Visual disturbance	+	+		
Skin rashes	+	+	+	
Pericarditis/pleural effusions			+	
Blood dyscrasia		+		
Withdrawal symptoms	+	++		
Drug interactions	++	+	+	

+ reported occasionally; ++ quite frequent; +++ potentially fatal.

back. Physiotherapists should ideally provide appropriate training to *all* staff, and informal carers, who are involved in handling patients.

The severity of weakness of individual muscle groups is often graded with the Medical Research Council (MRC) Scale[242] (Table 11.29). This was originally designed to assess motor weakness arising from injuries to single peripheral nerves, not stroke. Unfortunately, although the MRC Scale has good inter-observer reliability if applied rigorously,[227] it is often misused and the optional expansion to include extra grades (4 plus and 5 minus) makes it even less reliable in the routine recording of motor weakness. The motricity index, a modification of the MRC Scale (Table 11.29), for use in patients with stroke, allows the observer to grade the severity of the hemiparesis rather than each separate muscle group.[243] This can be useful in charting patients' progress for research purposes but is of limited value in routine clinical practice because it is difficult to remember the weights applied to individual movements and it requires a small block to assess grip strength. Several other tools are available for objectively measuring and recording motor function (Table 11.30).

Treatment

The amount of spontaneous recovery of motor function is highly variable. The more severe the initial impairment, the less likely is full recovery. One study suggested that motor and sensory function 5 days after stroke onset explained 74% of the variance in motor function at 6 months with the Fugl-Meyer Scale.[244] The pattern of recovery of motor function parallels that of other stroke-related deficits, with the most rapid recovery occurring in the first few weeks and then the pace of improvement slows over subsequent months (section 10.2.5). In patients with hemiparesis it is generally thought that motor function in the leg improves more than that in the arm, although this has been questioned.[245] Also, unless the patient has some return of grip within 1 month of the stroke, useful return of function is unlikely, although not impossible.[246]

Physiotherapy is the main therapeutic option in hemiparesis although techniques vary. The two broad approaches most commonly employed are the 'facilitation and inhibition' technique and the 'functional' approach.

Table 11.29 The MRC Scale of Weakness, and the motricity index which was developed from the MRC Scale for use in stroke patients.[242,243]

MRC Scale		
0	No contraction	
1	Flicker or trace of contraction	
2	Active movement with gravity eliminated	
3	Active movement against gravity	
4	Active movement against resistance	
5	Full strength	
The motricity index		
Arm	Pinch grip	—
	Elbow flexion (from 90°)	—
	Shoulder abduction (from chest)	—
	Total arm score	—
Leg	Ankle dorsiflexion (from plantar flexed)	—
	Knee extension (from 90°)	—
	Hip flexion	—
	Total leg score	—
Scoring system for pinch grip		
0	Pinch grip, no movement	
11	Beginnings of prehension	
19	Grips block (not against gravity)	
22	Grips block against gravity	
26	Against pull but weak	
33	Normal	
Scoring system for movements other than pinch grip		
0	No movement	
9	Palpable contraction only	
14	Movement but not against gravity/limited range	
19	Movement against gravity/full range	
25	Weaker than other side	
33	Normal	

Table 11.30 Measurements of motor function.[439]

Impairments	
MRC Scale (Table 11.29)	
Motricity index (Table 11.29)	
Trunk control test	
Motor club assessment	
Rivermead motor assessment	
Dynamometry	
Disability	
Arm	
Nine-hole peg test	
Frenchay arm test/battery	
Action research arm test	
Truncal control/mobility	
Standing balance	
Functional ambulation category	
Timed 10-m walk	
Truncal control	
Rivermead mobility index	
Subsection of Office of Population Censuses and Surveys (OPCS) scale[440]	

Table 11.31 Common features of facilitation/inhibition-based therapy.[249]

Recognition of the intimate relationship between sensation and movement
Recognition of the importance of basic reflex activity
Use of sensory input and different postures to facilitate or inhibit reflex activity and movement
Motor relearning based on repetition of activity and frequency of stimulation
Treatment of the body as an integrated unit rather than focusing on one part
Close personal interaction between the therapist and patient

- The facilitation and inhibition technique is based on the premise that posture and sensory stimuli can modify basic reflex patterns which emerge after cerebral damage. Several workers have developed different treatments based on this concept, the best-known being those of Bobath[247] and Brunnstrom.[248] Although these techniques differ, certain features are common to all[249] (Table 11.31): to achieve as normal a posture and pattern of movement on the affected side as possible.

- On the other hand, the functional approach simply aims, through training and strengthening of the unaffected side, to compensate for the impairment to achieve maximum function. For example, patients may be encouraged to transfer and walk as soon as possible after the stroke. Supporters of the facilitation and inhibition approach claim that, although the functional approach might achieve earlier independence, it results in more abnormal patterns of tone and movement which in the long term may lead to contractures and loss of function. Vigorous activity involving the unaffected side may increase the tone in the affected limbs during the activity. This does not seem to occur with all activities (e.g. pedalling) and any long-term effects on tone are unclear.[250]

We believe there is a place for both approaches in clinical practice. Quite often, where a patient has not achieved useful independent mobility despite a prolonged period of physiotherapy (with the facilitation and inhibition approach), we switch to a functional approach to maximize the patient's autonomy. For example, we will train patients to transfer independently and self-propel a wheelchair even though this may be associated with, at least in the short term, unwanted changes in tone.

There has been very little formal evaluation of the physiotherapy techniques. Although several small RCTs have been reported, no definite conclusions about their relative merits can be drawn.[251] In any case, comparisons of different techniques may have limited relevance to current clinical practice as many therapists adopt an eclectic approach, using selected aspects of each technique where appropriate for individual patients. There are, therefore, some important questions about physiotherapy after stroke which need to be answered in properly designed RCTs:

- When should physiotherapy start?
- How long should it continue?
- What is the optimum intensity of physiotherapy?[252]
- Which specific therapeutic interventions are the *most* effective?
- Is therapy provided by relatively unskilled therapists as effective as that provided by skilled therapists?
- Which patients gain most from physiotherapy and can we prospectively identify them?

The results of small RCTs support the hypothesis that physiotherapy, especially focused on achieving particular tasks, improves function even when started late after stroke.[253] The trials generally indicate that therapy has a greater impact on specific motor impairments than the resulting disability. This may be because the resulting disabilities are the consequence of sensory and cognitive as well as motor problems. The size of any treatment effect is probably influenced by the intensity of treatment.[252] However, many older, sicker patients may not be able to tolerate intensive regimes, which emphasizes the need for research to identify the optimum physiotherapy regime for particular subgroups of patients.[254] Given the methodological difficulties in systematically reviewing and performing RCTs of physiotherapy techniques (and those of other therapists), this is a daunting challenge (Table 11.1).

Other interventions

A large number of physical techniques have been developed with the aim of improving motor function or gait. Some have been evaluated in small RCTs which have included highly selected patients and focused more on impairment than disability as outcome measures. None are supported by enough evidence to recommend their routine use.[253] These techniques include:

- electromyographic, visual and auditory feedback;[255–257]
- functional electrical stimulation, which is effective as an orthosis; when applied it can reduce foot drop to facilitate gait, and probably increases muscle strength, but it is unclear whether it improves functional outcome and many patients find it uncomfortable;[253,258]
- acupuncture[259] and transcutaneous electrical nerve stimulation (TENS);[260]

- treadmill gait retraining with or without bodyweight support;[261]
- 'forced use' or 'constraint induced therapy' where the unaffected arm is immobilized for a major part of the day and during physiotherapy sessions;[262]
- drugs to enhance motor recovery.[263,264]

Other approaches

In this section we have dealt with interventions that aim to decrease disability by improving impairments. The complementary strategy of providing appropriate mobility aids, e.g. walking sticks, splints and wheelchairs is dealt with in section 11.32.1.

11.22 Sensory impairments

In about one-fifth of patients with acute stroke it is impossible to assess sensation adequately because of reduced conscious level, confusion or communication problems, but about one-third of the remainder have impairment of at least one sensory modality (Table 11.2). Sensory problems are more easily identified in patients with right rather than left hemisphere stroke, probably because they have fewer communication difficulties. Severe sensory loss may be as disabling as paralysis, especially when it affects proprioception. Furthermore, loss of pain and temperature sensation in a limb, or sensory loss with neglect, may put a patient at risk of injury from hot water, etc. And disordered sensation with numbness or paraesthesia, even without functional difficulties may, if persistent, be as distressing to some patients as central post-stroke pain (section 11.23). We have discussed some of the difficulties in assessing sensory function earlier (section 3.3.5).

> Patients often complain bitterly about what appears to the doctor to be a minor change in sensation. Do not underestimate the effect which facial numbness, or tingling in a hand, can have on the morale of a patient.

Little is known specifically about the recovery of sensation after stroke, although it probably follows a similar pattern seen in most other impairments (section 10.2.5). However, sensory symptoms may evolve and even become more distressing with time and they may worsen during intercurrent illness (e.g. infections) leading to concerns about recurrent stroke. Under these circumstances it is important to give appropriate explanation and reassurance to the patient and any carer.

Although patients may be given sensory stimulation as part of their therapy, the effect this or any other intervention has on sensation is unknown.[265] Where patients have lost temperature or pain sensation in a limb, especially if there is associated neglect, it is important to counsel them about commonsense strategies to avoid injury to the limb.

11.23 Pain (excluding headache)

Pain is a common complaint among stroke patients. Perhaps one-third require analgesia for pain (excluding shoulder pain) during hospital admission after an acute stroke and, although it becomes less of a problem with time, persisting severe pain may affect about one-fifth of patients.[105,266] There are many potential causes, some of which are coincidental and others which are in some way due to the stroke (Table 11.32). Usually, the cause becomes obvious after one has asked the patient about the distribution, nature and onset of the pain and has examined the relevant area. However, some pains (e.g. due to spasticity, axial arthritis and central post-stroke pain) may be difficult for patients to describe and localize. Diagnosis and assessment of analgesic requirements are particularly difficult in patients with communication and cognitive problems.

Table 11.32 Causes of pain after stroke.

	Section
Headache due to vascular pathology	3.7.1, 11.9
Painful shoulder	11.24
Deep venous thrombosis and pulmonary embolism	11.13
Pressure ulcers	11.16
Limb spasticity	11.20
Fractures	11.26
Arterial occlusion with ischaemia of limb, bowel or myocardium	
Coexisting arthritis exacerbated by immobility or therapy	
Instrumentation, e.g. catheter, intravenous cannulae, nasogastric tube	
Central *post-stroke* pain (thalamic pain/ Dejerine–Roussy syndrome)	11.23

The treatment of pain depends on the cause. Simple analgesics (e.g. paracetamol) along with some reassurance that the pain does not indicate any serious problem may be all that is needed. Other interventions such as local application of heat or cold, and transcutaneous electrical nerve stimulation (TENS) or acupuncture, may relieve symptoms with a low risk of adverse effects. Pain due to spasticity should initially be treated by alleviating exacerbating factors and by carefully positioning the patient (section 11.20). Antispasticity drugs are occasionally required, seldom work and have significant adverse effects (Table 11.28). Musculoskeletal pain can be treated with simple analgesics and, if these are ineffective and there are no contraindications, a non-steroidal anti-inflammatory drug. If a joint becomes acutely painful it may be necessary to rest it and investigate to exclude more serious causes, e.g. septic arthritis, fracture, or gout exacerbated by diuretics or aspirin. We find it useful to discuss the patient's pain at the multidisciplinary team meeting where one can establish the pattern, severity and control of pain in different settings, e.g. on the ward, at night, during therapy sessions. This provides important clues to its cause and the best approach to treatment.

Central post-stroke pain

This is variably described as a superficial burning, lacerating or pricking sensation often exacerbated by factors including touch, movement, cold and anxiety.[267] It usually affects one-half of the body but may be more localized, affecting a quadrant, one limb or just the face. It affects up to 10% of hospitalized patients surviving at 6 months in total, and 5% severely[268] though this estimate is certainly higher than we would expect in our clinical practice. A far less common, but related, problem is post-stroke pruritus.[269]

Central post-stroke pain is usually associated with some abnormality of pinprick or temperature sensation and may be accompanied by autonomic changes, for example sweating or cold.[270] It may start immediately after the stroke but more frequently after a delay of weeks or months.[267] Although the term 'thalamic pain' is commonly used synonymously with central post-stroke pain, this is misleading since the pain occurs in patients with stroke lesions affecting any part of the sensory pathways.[271]

Central post-stroke pain is often resistant to therapy. Avoidance of those factors which exacerbate the symptoms is an important first step. Tricyclic antidepressants (e.g. amitryptiline) may alleviate the symptoms and also lift any associated depression.[272] A small dose should be used initially, usually at bedtime, and be increased slowly until adequate symptom control is achieved or adverse effects become troublesome. If tricyclic anti-depressants are ineffective, addition of lamotrigine or gabapentin are reasonable second-line treatments. A range of alternative drugs including other anti-epileptics (e.g. carbamazepine, phenytoin, valproate, clonaze-pam), anti-arrhythmics (e.g. mexiletine), anaesthetics (e.g. ketamine), opiates and intrathecal baclofen have all been advocated but none adequately evaluated in placebo-controlled randomized trials.[272–274] Physical methods such as acupuncture and TENS are worth trying since they may occasionally provide relief and are at least fairly safe without any lasting adverse effects. Psychological interventions may help but have not been formally evaluated. More invasive and destructive tech-niques such as stereotactic mesencephalic tractotomy, or deep-brain stimulation, are occasionally used in severe cases which are resistant to other treatment modalities, but are not necessarily effective.

11.24 Painful shoulder

Shoulder pain is reported by at least one-fifth of patients in the first 6 months after stroke. Its frequency increases over the first few months. It is more common in those with severe sensorimotor deficits, and thus hospital-admitted patients, and usually affects the shoulder on the hemiparetic side.[275–277] Although many factors (Table 11.33) have been associated with painful shoulder, their role in its development is unclear.[277] A small proportion of patients who complain of a painful shoulder after a stroke have the other clinical features which comprise the syndrome of reflex sympathetic dystrophy or shoulder–hand syndrome (Table 11.34). It is unclear whether this represents a distinct entity or simply the severe end of a spectrum.

Our ignorance of the causes and prognosis of shoulder pain is in part due to major problems of definition and the lack of well-validated and reliable assessment tools.[278] But, although our understanding of the epi-demiology and causes of painful shoulder is incomplete, no one involved in stroke rehabilitation can doubt its importance. It causes patients great discomfort, it may seriously affect morale, and can inhibit recovery. In some patients it persists for months, even years.

Table 11.33 Factors associated with painful shoulder after stroke.

	Section
Associated features	
Shoulder pain before the stroke	
Low tone allowing glenohumeral subluxation/malalignment	Fig. 11.25
Spasticity	11.20
Severe weakness of the arm	11.21
Sensory loss	11.22
Neglect	11.28
Visual field deficits	11.27.1
Neurological mechanisms	
Reflex sympathetic dystrophy (shoulder–hand syndrome)	11.24
Central *post-stroke* pain	11.23
Brachial plexus injury	
Orthopaedic problems	
Adhesive capsulitis (frozen shoulder)	
Rotator cuff tears due to improper handling or positioning	
Acromioclavicular arthritis	
Glenohumeral arthritis	
Subdeltoid tendinitis	

Table 11.34 Features of reflex sympathetic dystrophy.

Pain and tenderness on abduction, flexion and external rotation of the arm at the shoulder
Pain and swelling over the carpal bones
Swelling of metacarpophalangeal and proximal interphalangeal joints
Changes in temperature, colour and dryness of the skin of the hand
Loss of dorsal hand skin creases, and nail changes
Osteoporosis

Note: there is probably considerable overlap between reflex sympathetic dystrophy and the cold arms described by Wanklyn[286,441] (section 11.25).

Prevention and treatment

Treatment of an established painful shoulder is often ineffective so that any measures to prevent its develop-ment are important. It is probably useful to introduce policies on the stroke unit which have been identified as being associated with a lower frequency of the problem in non-randomized studies (Table 11.35). It may also be useful to identify individuals who are at particularly high risk, based on the factors in Table 11.33, and make all staff aware of the potential problem. More specific

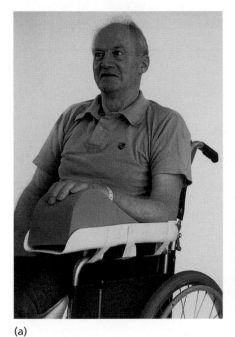
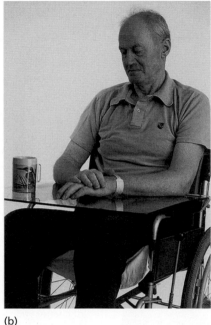
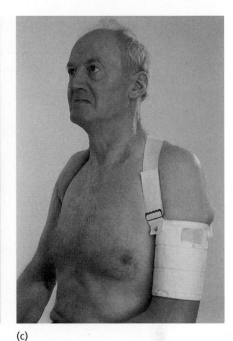

(a)   (b)   (c)

Fig. 11.24 By supporting the weight of the arm, glenohumeral subluxation can be reduced. This may be achieved when the patient is sitting using an arm support (a) which attaches to the chair or wheelchair or, alternatively, a perspex tray (b) which, because it is transparent, allows the patient to check on the position of their feet. Both are better than pillows which invariably end up on the floor. Several designs of sling (c) are available to reduce subluxation when patients are upright.

Table 11.35 General measures which may reduce the frequency of painful shoulder after stroke.

Instruct *all* staff and carers to:
Support the flaccid arm to reduce subluxation
Teach patients not to allow the affected arm to hang unsupported when sitting or standing. While sitting they might use one of several arm supports which attach to the chair or wheelchair. All are more effective than a pillow which spends most of the time on the floor. Shoulder/arm orthoses may, depending on their design, prevent subluxation but have not been shown to reduce the frequency of painful shoulder (Fig. 11.24c).
Avoid pulling on the affected arm when handling the patient
Staff and carers should be trained in methods of handling and lifting patients to avoid traction injuries.
Avoid any activity which causes shoulder discomfort
Therapy sessions sometimes do more harm than good.
Maintain range of passive shoulder movements

interventions including slings, cuffs and taping to support the flaccid arm (Fig. 11.24), and functional electrical stimulation may reduce subluxation but their effect on the frequency of painful shoulder and arm function is unproven.[279–281] Many therapists worry that the use of slings and cuffs will inhibit recovery of the arm because it is held in a position which promotes spasticity.

When a patient complains of shoulder pain it is important to exclude glenohumeral dislocation (Fig. 11.25), fracture or specific shoulder syndromes. For example, painful arc (supraspinatus tendinitis) may respond better to specific measures (e.g. local steroid injection) although even the evidence supporting treatments for these specific syndromes is poor.[282,283]

In established painful shoulder many treatments have been suggested, some have been evaluated in small RCTs, but further studies are needed to define the best treatments (Table 11.36). Some interventions are probably harmless (e.g. application of cold, heat, taping, TENS) and if they produce even short-term relief are worth trying. Others have potentially important adverse effects and costs (e.g. oral corticosteroids) and therefore need to be evaluated further before being adopted into routine clinical practice.[277]

Shoulder pain after stroke is common, ill understood, difficult to prevent and none of the suggested treatments are supported by reliable evidence.

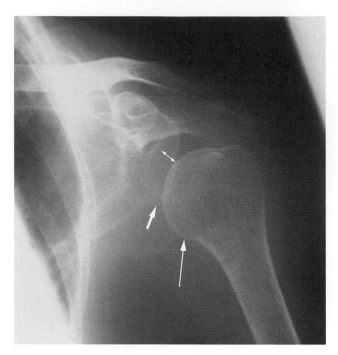

Fig. 11.25 X-ray of shoulder showing glenohumeral subluxation, a common finding in stroke patients, but does it matter? Note the widened joint space (*double-headed arrow*) and the increased distance between the lower border of the glenoid cavity (*short arrow*) and the lower border of the humeral head (*long arrow*). Photograph provided by Dr Allan Stephenson.

11.25 Swollen and cold limbs

Swelling with pitting oedema, and sometimes pain, quite often occurs in the paralysed or neglected hand, arm or leg, usually within the first few weeks.[284,285] The swelling may limit the movement of the affected part and the pain not only further restricts movement but also exacerbates spasticity and associated reactions (section 11.20). Some patients complain of coldness of the limb, more often of the arm than the leg.[286] Swelling more often occurs in the legs of patients who sit for prolonged periods (section 11.13). Gravity and lack of muscle contraction, which reduce venous and lymphatic return, presumably play a part but autonomic changes and control of regional blood flow may be relevant.[287] An isolated painful, swollen hand may be a mild form of the shoulder–hand syndrome. There are a number of other causes which need to be considered (Table 11.37). People with fractures or acute ischaemia of the limb usually complain of severe pain, but stroke patients with sensory loss, visuospatial dysfunction or communication

Table 11.36 Treatments used for painful shoulders.

Physiotherapy
Positioning and mobilization
Exercises
Heat or cold
Support
Strapping
Shoulder/arm orthoses (Fig. 11.24c)
Bobath sling
Rood shoulder support
Arm supports for bed or chairs
Lapboard (Fig. 11.24b)
Forearm support
Wheelchair outrigger (Fig. 11.24a)
Medication
Systemic
  Analgesics
  Non-steroidal anti-inflammatory drugs
  Corticosteroids[442]
  Antispastic drugs (Table 11.28)
  Phenoxybenzamine
  Antidepressants
Local
  Corticosteroid injection of shoulder
  Local anaesthetic
  Botulinum toxin to periarticular muscles
  Stellate ganglion block
Other physical
Ultrasound
Acupuncture
Biofeedback
Transcutaneous electrical nerve stimulation (TENS)
Surgery
Sympathectomy
Humeral head suspension
Relief of contractures

Table 11.37 Causes of swollen limb after stroke.

	Section
Gravity in a dependent limb	
Lack of muscle contraction	
Deep venous thrombosis	11.13
Compression of veins or lymphatics by tumour, etc.	
Cardiac failure	
Hypoalbuminaemia	11.19
Occult injury	11.26
Acute ischaemia	
Gout	
Reflex sympathetic dystrophy	11.24 (Table 11.34)

difficulties may not, which can lead to these diagnoses being overlooked.

Assessment

The other causes of a swollen limb should be excluded by clinical examination and appropriate investigation before attributing the swelling simply to immobility or dependency. Investigation is not usually necessary but Doppler ultrasound or venography to exclude deep venous thrombosis of the leg (section 11.13), a simple X-ray of a swollen wrist or ankle to exclude a fracture, and a serum albumin may be useful. One can monitor the effect of any intervention by simply measuring the circumference of the limb although plethysmography has been used in research studies.[288]

Treatment

The treatment obviously depends on the cause. Where the swelling appears to be due to immobility we try the following:

- elevation of the affected limb when at rest;
- encourage active movement (this may be impossible with severe weakness but is important if neglect is the main cause);
- graduated compression stocking on the leg (full length or below-knee depending on extent of swelling) or a bandage on the arm, although the latter may worsen swelling of the hand; and
- intermittent compression of the limb although this was shown to be ineffective in reducing arm swelling in a randomized trial.[289]

In addition, where the limb is painful, simple analgesia may ameliorate the secondary effects of pain on tone which leads to spasticity and contractures. Diuretics should be avoided unless there is evidence of heart failure, since immobile stroke patients have a tendency to become dehydrated (section 11.18.1) and incontinent (section 11.14).

11.26 Falls and fractures

Falls are common after stroke. About one-third of patients are expected to fall during their in-hospital care.[105,290–292] Falls are also frequent following discharge from hospital.[293,294] Many factors contribute to this tendency; some are listed in Table 11.38. Combinations of such factors are associated with higher risks, though

Table 11.38 Factors likely to contribute to falls after stroke.

	Section
The patient	
Muscle weakness (especially of quadriceps)	11.21
Sensory loss (especially visual impairments)	11.22 & 11.27
Impaired balance, righting reflexes and ataxia	11.21
Confusion	11.29
Visuospatial neglect, e.g. denial of hemiparesis	11.28
Deformity, e.g. plantarflexion causing toe catching	11.20
Epileptic seizures	11.8
Postural hypotension due to drugs or dehydration	11.2.3 & 11.18.1
The environment	
Inappropriate footwear, e.g. slippers	
Slippery floors, deep pile carpets and loose rugs	
Excess furniture	
Poorly positioned rails and inappropriate aids	
Lack of supervision	
Fire doors (these may close automatically and hit slow-moving stroke patients)	
Drugs:	
Sedatives and hypnotics	
Hypotensive drugs	
Antispastic drugs	Table 11.28
Anti-epileptic drugs	

patients with severe post-stroke impairments are often at lower risk because they are unable to mobilize at all.[294] Several 'falls risk scores' have been developed which incorporate these (and other) factors but none have yet been shown to be practical and sufficiently accurate to gain widespread use.[291,295,296]

A small proportion of falls occurring in hospital (<5%) or in the first few months at home (about 1%) result in serious injury, most often fracture of the hip, pelvis or wrist, but other injuries (e.g. head and soft tissue), fear and loss of confidence are very common consequences.[290,293,297] Also, falls are associated with an increased risk of intracranial haemorrhage associated with anticoagulation so that patients in atrial fibrillation often receive less than optimal secondary prevention.

The estimates of risk of any fracture, or specifically hip fractures, have varied from 22 to 36/1000 patient-years and 7 to 22/1000 patient-years respectively.[298] The risk of any fracture rises with age and is higher in women than men. The risk is highest in the first year after stroke (about 4%), higher than in stroke-free individuals.[298–302]

Most hip fractures affect the hemiparetic side, probably because patients tend to fall to that side, but the osteoporosis which develops on the side of the weakness may be a contributory factor.[303] Low vitamin D levels are common in stroke patients though their relevance is unclear.[304]

> Stroke patients with communication problems, sensory loss or neglect may not report injury or pain so it is important to look for signs of fracture, i.e. deformity, swelling, bruising, on admission and after any accident. One should have a low threshold for X-raying suspected fractures.

Prevention and treatment

One could avoid falls, and thus fractures, by keeping the patient in bed, clearly not a solution during rehabilitation. The risk of falls and injuries is minimized by the physiotherapist, nursing staff and carer all working closely together to ensure that patients are mobilizing with adequate supervision and support. It is also useful to identify patients who are at particular risk of falling (see above). Withdrawal of unnecessary diuretics and psychotropic drugs and avoidance of any relevant environmental causes should help reduce the risk of falls (Table 11.38). There is evidence, although not specifically in stroke patients, that a multidisciplinary approach which takes account of individuals' risk factors, environment and gives interventions tailored to that individual can reduce the risk of falls.[305,306]

There is currently insufficient evidence to recommend routine use of any interventions, including hip protectors, hormones, bisphosphonates, vitamins or oral supplements aimed at reducing injuries secondary to falls.[305,307] Large studies will be needed to demonstrate the effectiveness of bone protection, or any other method, in preventing fractures in stroke patients because their frequency is so low.[298,308]

Given the evidence in non-stroke patients it seems reasonable to recommend that stroke patients who have had an osteoporosis-related fracture are given bisphosphonates and possibly calcium and vitamin D to reduce the risk of recurrent fractures. Hormone replacement therapy should be avoided given the increased vascular events associated with its use[309] (section 7.13).

11.27 Visual problems

Stroke patients often have pre-existing visual problems due to refractive errors, cataracts, glaucoma, diabetic retinopathy and senile macular degeneration.[310] Although it is beyond the scope of this book to deal with their specific management, it is important that the clinician is aware of them, and their causes, because they may well have an important influence on the patient's function.

> Simple measures such as ensuring that a patient's glasses are clean, available and on their nose are obvious but easily overlooked.

11.27.1 Visual field defects

About one-fifth of stroke patients have a demonstrable field defect (Table 11.2). However, in an additional 20% vision is not assessable because of reduced conscious level or communication difficulties. The frequency of visual field loss in hospital patients will obviously depend on patient selection and the methods used to detect defects. Apart from their value in localizing the stroke lesion (section 3.3.6), visual field defects have some predictive value. For example, a homonymous visual field defect in association with motor and cognitive deficits is usually due to a large stroke lesion and is associated with a relatively poor prognosis (section 4.3.4).

Patients who are mobile and have field loss are at greater risk of falls and injury. Many patients with field defects find reading and watching television difficult, although some of their difficulty may be due to associated problems with cognition and concentration. Homonymous field defects (see Fig. 3.23) have important implications for patients who wish to drive (and sometimes for unfortunate pedestrians and cyclists) (section 11.32.2). Some of the difficulties in detecting field defects in stroke patients have already been discussed in section 3.3.6.

There have been very few studies of the recovery of visual field defects after stroke. One found that only about one-fifth of patients with complete homonymous hemianopia had normal visual fields 1 month after their stroke.[311] Most of any recovery occurred within the first 10 days. About 70% of patients with only an incomplete hemianopia initially recovered over the same period. This study supports our clinical impression that, although there are exceptions, visual field defects (especially hemianopia) that are still present at 7–10 days usually persist.

> Usually, although there are exceptions, visual field defects persist unless they resolve early.

No treatment is known to enhance the recovery of visual field defects. Therefore, interventions which aim to reduce the resulting disability and handicap are most important. It seems sensible to avoid putting patients with a homonymous field defect in a bed next to the wall so they cannot see anything going on around them. One can imagine that this 'sensory deprivation' might be bad for morale. It may be possible to teach the patient to compensate for a field defect by strategies such as scanning and head turning.[312] Hemianopia, even without associated neglect, makes reading difficult. Loss of the right visual field means that the patient has to track the words into a blind field, especially where they have no macular sparing. Loss of the left visual field makes it difficult to find the start of each line and patients lose their place easily. This can sometimes be helped by putting a ruler under each line and their hand or a bright coloured object at the left-hand margin, and to train them to look at this before starting a new line. Large print makes reading easier. Some patients with a right homonymous hemianopia find they can read more easily upside down because they can scan from right to left. The effects of bed orientation, computer assisted training and Fresnel's lenses, which shift images in the hemianopic field into the intact one, have been evaluated in small randomized trials but these have not demonstrated significant benefits[312–315] (http://www.effectivestrokecare.org/).

Patients with field defects often spend a lot of money on new glasses within a few months of their stroke because they mistakenly believe that the problem is with their eyes. It is therefore important that the nature of the problem is explained to the patient and any carer and that new glasses are only prescribed where there is an uncorrected refractive error.

> Patients often attribute their poor vision after a stroke to inadequate glasses. Explain to patients the nature and cause of their visual problems so they do not waste their money on inappropriate new glasses.

11.27.2 Disordered eye movements, diplopia and oscillopsia

Strokes may lead to conjugate gaze palsies so the patient is unable to look in a particular direction(s), or has diplopia due to dysconjugate eye movements (section 3.3.6). Diplopia occurs in about 5% and conjugate gaze palsies in about 8% of stroke patients in community-based studies[316] (Table 11.2). The pattern of abnormal eye movements after stroke helps localize the stroke lesion and the presence of a conjugate gaze palsy in a supratentorial stroke is associated with a poor outcome.

Conjugate gaze palsies rarely cause disability or handicap. Double vision, which may result from dysconjugate eye movements, and oscillopsia associated with nystagmus, are much more troublesome, sometimes exacerbating gait problems and making reading, watching television and driving difficult. The practical difficulties in assessing eye movements after stroke have been discussed earlier (section 3.3.6).

The most effective way of relieving patients of double vision in the early stages is a patch over one eye. We recommend patching the eye with the poorer acuity or movement although alternation is often recommended. Diplopia often resolves in a few weeks of the stroke but if it remains a problem it can be helped by glasses fitted with prism lenses. However, prisms are of no use where diplopia is associated with a variable degree of divergence. Of course, patients should be warned not to spend a lot of money on new glasses until they have reached a stable state. Oscillopsia occasionally persists and causes distress and difficulties with reading. Symptomatic improvement in individuals and small case series has been attributed to many drugs including gabapentin, memantine, clonazepam and baclofen.[317]

11.27.3 Visual hallucinations

Occasionally, patients report vivid visual hallucinations after strokes (section 3.3.6). However, more often they occur as part of an acute confusional state (section 11.29.1), associated with alcohol withdrawal or an adverse effect of medication and they resolve as the underlying cause is treated. If persistent it may be worth considering investigation to exclude epileptic seizures, particularly if the hallucinations are stereotyped and localized to a hemianopic field. Usually, patients simply require explanation and reassurance, although if hallucinations are associated with marked agitation sodium valproate or a major tranquillizer may be needed.

11.28 Visuospatial dysfunction

Visuospatial dysfunction includes visual and sensory neglect, visual and sensory inattention or extinction, constructional dyspraxia and agnosia. Unfortunately, the nomenclature is complex and confused by the use of different terms for the same phenomena (Table 3.17). The frequency of visuospatial dysfunction among stroke patients varies widely in the published literature because of patient selection, the timing of assessments and the use of different definitions and assessments.[318] Visual neglect has been reported in 33–85% of patients with right hemisphere strokes and 0–47% of those with left hemisphere strokes.[319] The frequency of visuospatial dysfunction in dominant hemisphere stroke may be underestimated because of the practical difficulties in

Table 11.39 Frequency of visuospatial problems among hospitalized patients within 3 days of a hemispheric first stroke.[319]

	% of assessable patients with phenomena		% not assessable	
	Right hemisphere (*n* = 69)	Left hemisphere (*n* = 102)	Right hemisphere	Left hemisphere
Visual neglect	82	65	11	27
Hemi-inattention	70	49	9	15
Tactile extinction	65	35	25	58
Allaesthesia	57	11	15	55
Visual extinction	23	2	13	21
Anosognosia	28	5	13	45
Anosodiaphoria	27	2	13	48
Non-belonging	36	29	20	53
Gaze paresis	29	25	0	3
Visual field defect	36	46	11	9

Note: The differences in frequency between left and right were statistically significant for all but non-belonging, gaze paresis and visual field defects. The relatively high frequency of these phenomena in this series (cf. Table 11.2) probably reflects the severity of the strokes in this hospital-referred series as well as the sensitivity of the test battery used.

Table 11.40 Components of the behavioural inattention test (from ref. 443, with permission).

Full version	Modified version
Line crossing	Pointing to objects in ward
Letter cancellation	Food on the plate
Star cancellation (Fig. 3.14)	Reading a menu
Figure and shape drawing	Reading a newspaper article
Line bisection	Star cancellation (Fig. 3.14)
Line cancellation	Picture scanning
Representational drawing	Coin selection
Telephone dialling	Figure copying
Menu reading	
Article reading	
Telling and setting time	
Coin sorting	
Address and sentence copying	
Map navigation	
Card sorting	

assessing patients with a paralysed dominant hand or problems with language (Table 11.39) (section 3.3.3).

Assessment

Test batteries which include assessments of a broad range of visuospatial problems (e.g. behavioural inattention test, BIT; Table 11.40) are inevitably more sensitive than simple screening tests used at the bedside (Table 3.16). The BIT contains tests to assess both sensory neglect (the patient's perception of incoming stimuli) and motor neglect (the patient's willingness to explore external space) but does not detect all neglect phenomena which may be noticed by the team[320] (Table 11.39). A variety of screening tests have been proposed including the wheelchair collision test.[321,322]

Prognosis

Visuospatial problems are major causes of disability and handicap, impede functional recovery and have been associated with a poor outcome[323,324] (Table 10.4). There have been few studies of the recovery of visuospatial function, but these suggest, as with most other stroke-related impairments, that recovery is most rapid in the first week or two and then slows[325] (section 10.2.5). If visual neglect is severe and associated with anosognosia it is less likely to resolve.[326]

Treatment

Visuospatial dysfunction has a major impact on rehabilitation. For instance, it is difficult to persuade patients with anosognosia or denial to become involved in therapy. There have been very few RCTs of interventions aimed at improving visuospatial function after stroke and they have all suffered from the difficulties outlined previously (Table 11.1). Several small RCTs have shown an effect of specific interventions for neglect on performance on test batteries but less impact on the more relevant activities of daily living.[327] In other words, any benefit of therapy appears to benefit performance on selected tasks but not usually on general visuospatial abilities.

Currently, therefore, we have to adopt strategies which do not necessarily influence the severity of the underlying impairment but may reduce the resulting disability and handicap, and help carers to cope. Carers are often bemused, frustrated or angered by the behavioural consequences of visuospatial dysfunction and so it is very important to spend time explaining the unusual nature of the deficit. If this is not done, then carers may wrongly conclude that the patient is dementing, wilfully obstructive or even deliberately ignoring them.

Patients with unilateral neglect are often positioned on the ward so they have their intact side facing a wall to encourage them to respond to stimuli on the affected side. However, since there is little evidence that this strategy influences outcome, we generally aim to position the patient in the middle of the ward so that he or she receives stimulation from both sides on the basis that their morale might suffer if they are not stimulated.[313]

In our experience, patients with unilateral neglect and hemiparesis can be taught to walk, but so often this is of limited functional use because they are so prone to fall. Unless supervised when walking, the patient's attention may become drawn to the unaffected side, which appears to inhibit activity on the affected side which leads to the fall. It can be difficult to persuade a patient who is unaware of their hemiparesis that they should only try to walk when supervised and that unsupervised walking carries a risk of falls and fractures (section 11.26). Patients with neglect are at risk in other situations, for example in the kitchen, because they are unaware of dangers to their affected side so that measures have to be taken to reduce this risk, for example using a microwave rather than a conventional cooker.

> Carers are often bemused, frustrated and angered by the behavioural consequences of visuospatial dysfunction so it is very important to spend time explaining the unusual nature of the deficit.

11.29 Cognitive dysfunction

Most patients with stroke are elderly and so pre-existing dementia is common. Its estimated frequency varies between 6% and 16% depending on the stroke population studied, the definitions and methods of ascertainment used.[328] In clinical practice, as well as formal studies, it is important to gather information from the family about the patient's pre-stroke cognitive state, especially where patients have communication problems: the Informant Questionnaire on Cognitive Decline in the Elderly (IQCODE) is a well-validated instrument which makes use of information from the patient and their family.[329] Without this information it is impossible to distinguish pre-stroke dementia from acute confusional states, and dementia secondary to the stroke itself. These possibilities will have different potentials for improvement.

11.29.1 Acute confusional states

In prospective hospital-based studies, the frequency of acute delirium in acute stroke, defined according to the criteria of the *Diagnostic and Statistical Manual of Mental Disorders* (DSM), version IIIR or IV, has varied between 10% and 48%. This is much higher than, for instance, those presenting with acute coronary syndromes.[330] Many risk factors have been identified but the most consistent are increasing age, pre-stroke dementia and greater stroke severity. The frequency of acute confusional states among unselected stroke patients (i.e. including those not admitted to hospital) is likely to be lower than in the published hospital-based series given the association with stroke severity.

Acute confusional states after stroke may be a direct consequence of the cerebral dysfunction or of non-cerebral complications (Table 11.41). Confusion with disorientation, poor memory and disruptive behaviour are distressing to other patients and carers and severely hamper rehabilitation.[331] Patients with acute confusional states are more likely to have longer hospital stays, are less likely to be discharged home and have worse physical and cognitive outcomes.[330]

Assessment

Cognitive impairments are often overlooked in elderly patients admitted to hospital.[332] Because non-structured assessments have poor inter-observer reliability (section 3.6), it is important to include one of the large number of assessment tools available, e.g. the ten-item Hodkinson Abbreviated Mental Test (Table 11.42) or the longer Mini Mental State Examination (MMSE) (Table 11.43), in the routine assessment of patients on admission to the stroke unit. However, both tend to be overly influenced by language difficulties (section 11.30.1). The Addenbrooke's Cognitive Assessment includes the MMSE but provides a more global assessment of cognition.[333,334] Having such a measure at baseline allows subsequent changes to be identified and the causes sought. Where patients are unable to communicate one usually

Table 11.41 Causes of cognitive dysfunction after stroke.

	Section
Coincidental (pre-existing)	
Alzheimer's disease and other dementing illnesses	
Directly caused by stroke	
Large hemisphere lesions	
Strategically located lesions, e.g. thalamus	3.3.3
Vascular dementia	
Amyloid angiopathy	8.2.2
Giant-cell arteritis*	7.3.1
Primary angiitis of the central nervous system*	7.3.17
Infective endocarditis*	6.5.9, 8.2.11
Complications of the stroke	
Infections*	11.12
Hypoxia, hypotension, etc.*	11.2
Metabolic abnormalities*	11.18
Depression*	11.31
Hydrocephalus*	14.2.4, 14.8
Epileptic seizures*	11.8
Urinary retention*	11.14
Alcohol and drug withdrawal*	
Drugs (e.g. neuroleptics, anticholinergic, antispastic, sedatives, antidepressants, diuretics)*	
Conditions mimicking stroke	3.4
Herpes encephalitis	3.4.6
Chronic subdural haematoma	3.4.4
Cerebral abscess or subdural empyema	3.4.6
Cerebral tumour	3.4.4
Creutzfeldt–Jakob disease	3.4.6

*Potentially reversible causes.

Table 11.42 Hodkinson Abbreviated Mental Test.[433]

Patient's age
Time (estimated to nearest hour)
Mr John Brown, 42 West Street, Gateshead (should be repeated to ensure that the patient has heard it correctly and then recalled at end of test)
Name of hospital/place
Current year
Recognition of two people (e.g. doctor, nurse)
Patient's date of birth
Dates of World War I*
Present monarch†
Count down from 20 to 1

Patient scores one point for each correct response.
*It may now be more appropriate to ask for dates of World War II.
†Clearly in some countries it is be more relevant to ask who the president is.

has to rely on the family, and the team's observation of the patient's behaviour and learning capacity.

Treatment

Treatment should focus on any potentially reversible underlying cause such as infection, electrolyte imbalance or hypoxia (Table 11.41). Confused patients require closer observation to reduce their risk of falling, and inappropriate removal of oxygen masks, intravenous cannulae, nasogastric tubes and urinary catheters. The balance of risk and benefit must be carefully weighed in each patient before one resorts to other measures such as mattresses on the floor (which may reduce injury but increase disorientation and make nursing more hazardous), physical restraints (which some regard as unethical and may cause injury) and psychotropic drugs (which have many adverse effects including confusion, hypotension, dehydration and involuntary movements).[335]

11.29.2 Post-stroke dementia

Perhaps 10–20% of patients who had no recognized cognitive problems before their stroke develop dementia which persists after the acute illness, or it develops over the following months.[336–339] Cognitive dysfunction, which may not be severe enough to be classified as dementia, is more common but often improves in the first few months after stroke.[337] Predictably, older age, low educational attainment and indicators of greater stroke severity are consistently associated with post-stroke dementia while other factors such as female sex, previous stroke, intracerebral haemorrhage and atrial fibrillation and other cardiovascular problems have been identified in individual studies. Post-stroke dementia is associated with a worse long-term survival and worse functional outcome.[340]

Assessment

It is important to reassess patients' cognitive function, even months or years after the stroke, especially where any deterioration in cognition or functional status has been noted by the patient or carer. Simple bedside assessments such as the Mini Mental State Examination (Table 11.43) and CAMCOG (the cognitive and self-contained part of the Cambridge Examination for Mental Disorders of the Elderly, CAMDEX)[341] are usually adequate for this purpose but one has to be aware that these tend to emphasize language dysfunction and are less sensitive in identifying, for example, visuospatial problems (section 11.28). More detailed neuropsychological assessments (e.g. Raven's Progressive Matrices[342] and the

Table 11.43 Mini Mental State Examination (adapted from ref. 444, with permission).

Section	Questions	Max. points	Patient score
1. Orientation	(a) Can you tell me today's (date)/(month)/(year)? Which (day of the week) is it today? Can you also tell me which (season) it is?	5	
	(b) What city/town are we in? What is the (county)/(country)? What (building) are we in and on what (floor)?	5	
2. Registration	I should like to test your memory (name three common objects, e.g. 'ball, car, man') Can you repeat the words I said? (*score one point for each word*) (repeat up to six trials until all three are remembered) (record number of trials needed here:)	3	
3. Attention and calculation	(a) From 100 keep subtracting 7 and give each answer: stop after five answers (93_86_79_72_65_) *Alternatively* (b) Spell the word 'WORLD' backwards (D_L_R_O_W)	5	
4. Recall	What were the three words I asked you to say earlier? (*skip this test if all three objects were not remembered during registration test*)	3	
5. Language	Name these objects (show a watch) (show a pencil)	2	
	Repeat the following: 'no ifs, ands or buts'	1	
6. Reading, writing	Show card or write 'CLOSE YOUR EYES': Read this sentence and do what it says	1	
	Now can you write a short sentence for me?	1	
7. Three stage command	Present paper: Take this paper in your left (or right) hand, fold it in half, and put it on the floor	3	
8. Construction	Will you copy this drawing please?	1	
Total score		**30**	

Addenbrooke's Cognitive Assessment) which depend less on intact language function may give a better indication of the patient's degree of cognitive deficit.

Prevention and treatment

Unfortunately, post-stroke dementia is rarely reversible but it may possibly be prevented and progression slowed by treating vascular risk factors and antithrombotic drugs. Many drugs are widely used in the treatment of vascular dementia (e.g. piracetam, oxypentifylline, naftidrofuryl oxalate, codergocrine mesylate) though there is little, if any, evidence of their benefit. Donepezil appears to improve cognitive function in patients with mild and moderate vascular dementia but it is unclear whether this translates into any usefully improved function.[343] Of course, one should seek to exclude anything which may cause acute confusion (section 11.29.1) and reversible causes of dementia (e.g. severe depression, hypothyroidism).[344] No specific therapy interventions

have been shown to improve cognitive deficits after stroke.[345,346]

In planning patients' rehabilitation, placement and longer-term care, it is important to know whether a patient's cognitive state will improve over months, is stable or worsening. Unfortunately, only regular reassessment over a prolonged period can do this. If patients are disorientated or have memory problems the 'carry over' between therapy sessions is often poor, leading to slow progress with rehabilitation.

Our current practice, which aims to make best use of scarce resources, is to try to identify patients with irreversible severe cognitive dysfunction as early as possible and, taking account of this, get on with planning long-term placement and a suitable package of care. Ideally, where cognitive dysfunction limits the patient's involvement in rehabilitation, one should be able to arrange suitable supportive care for a period, after which a further assessment of their ability to benefit from rehabilitation could be made. Alas, the inflexibility of most stroke services currently makes this approach difficult (section 17.9).

> Look systematically for pre- and post-stroke cognitive problems at an early stage in order to take account of them in the planning of rehabilitation, placement and long-term care.

11.30 Communication difficulties

The most common problems with communication after stroke are aphasia and dysarthria, which may occur separately but frequently coexist. Aphasia is almost invariably associated with dysgraphia and sometimes dyslexia (section 3.3.3). Patients occasionally talk very quietly after a stroke, which sometimes appears to be due to difficulties in coordinating speech and breathing. Other abnormalities include aprosody (loss of emotional content of speech) which occurs with non-dominant hemisphere lesions (section 3.3.3).

11.30.1 Aphasia

Estimates of the frequency of aphasia have inevitably depended on the population and screening methods used. In community-based studies about 20–30%[347] of assessable patients are aphasic at their first assessment (Table 11.2) while in the hospital-based Copenhagen Stroke Study about 40% of conscious patients were judged aphasic according to the Scandinavian Stroke Scale (Table 11.6).[348,349] About half the affected patients have fluent aphasia and half non-fluent in the acute stage.[348]

Assessment

A thorough assessment of patient communication abilities is not only important to localize and classify the stroke lesion (section 3.3.3) but also to:

- find a way for the patient to express his or her feelings, make their needs known to the carers and so avoid unnecessary distress caused by, for example, urinary incontinence (section 11.14);
- find out how much the patient is capable of understanding so that one can tailor information-giving to their level of understanding. Also, therapists need to find a way of asking the patient to follow quite complex instructions, and many therapists are masters of non-verbal communication;
- assess the patient's prognosis and set appropriate rehabilitation goals; and

- protect the patient from losing control of their affairs. We have seen lawyers, oblivious to patients' severe aphasia and dyslexia, explaining complex documents and asking for (and obtaining) patients' signatures. The hazards of such apparent 'comprehension and consent' are self-evident but often not considered by physicians. It is important that the family and lawyer are made aware of a patient's level of comprehension.

Although communication problems may be obvious, it is not always easy, as we have already discussed, to distinguish aphasia from dysarthria (section 3.3.3). Table 3.16 outlines a simple assessment of language function. It is important not to overlook pre-existing impairments such as deafness, ill-fitting dentures and poor vision which can all adversely affect a patient's ability to communicate. Before testing comprehension the patient must be wearing their hearing aid which should be turned on and functioning properly.

It is quite common for language function to vary with fatigue, anxiety and intercurrent illness. If patient communication deteriorates under these circumstances it is important to explain that this is not due to a recurrent stroke. Different members of the rehabilitation team may judge the severity of an individual patient's problems differently. In our experience, nurses often overestimate the patient's ability to understand language in part because, in dealing with the patient, they use a lot of non-verbal cueing which is of course of immense value.

More formal testing of language function with one of the standardized instruments (e.g. Western aphasia test, Aachen aphasia score, Porch index of communication ability, Boston diagnostic aphasia examination) is sometimes useful where there is doubt about the diagnosis, or in research projects, but these are usually administered by a speech and language therapist. The Frenchay aphasia screening test (FAST) has been developed for routine clinical practice by non-experts and has reasonable reliability and validity.[350,351]

> Having established that the patient has a communication problem, one should ensure that all the simple measures to optimize their ability to communicate are taken, e.g. correct false teeth, hearing aid and spectacles are being used. These simple things are easily overlooked but can make a great difference to the patient. The batteries of many hearing aids need replacing every week or two if used regularly.

Prognosis

Aphasia is a frequent cause of long-term disability and handicap. In general the severity decreases over time and the proportion classified as fluent aphasia increases.[348]

Those with mild aphasia and less severe stroke have a better outcome.[349]

Treatment

There is considerable controversy about the effectiveness of speech and language therapy in aphasia, mainly because of methodological weaknesses of trials to evaluate interventions, as outlined in Table 11.1.[352] One meta-analysis, of both randomized and non-randomized studies of the effectiveness of therapy on language, concluded that therapy, especially if intensive and started early, enhanced spontaneous recovery.[353] However, another systematic review, which included only randomized trials, concluded that there was insufficient evidence of benefit.[352] Both reviewers agree, however, that more methodologically robust RCTs are required to identify specific reproducible interventions which increase the rate of recovery of aphasia and decrease the residual impairment, disability and handicap.[352]

There is some evidence that drugs might improve language function or enhance the effects of language therapy.[354,355] The most intensively studied is piracetam although evidence of its ability to potentiate the effect of speech therapy comes from small RCTs or posthoc subgroup analyses of a larger one. We believe there is currently not enough evidence to recommend the routine use of piracetam or other drugs for enhancing the recovery of aphasia.

Even though there is doubt about the effect that speech therapy has on aphasia, few clinicians, patients or families doubt the value of involving a speech and language therapist in a patient's care. Therapists can assess the patient's communication problems, make a precise diagnosis and explain this to other members of the team and, most importantly, to the patient and carer. They also offer advice about the likely prognosis based on their findings and can devise strategies to allow the patient and the family to cope with the communication handicap, perhaps by achieving communication in other ways, e.g. gesture, word/picture charts. It may be appropriate to refer some patients to stroke clubs, which in the UK specialize in supporting aphasic patients and their families. Thus, therapists may or may not be able to influence recovery of language function measured by specific tests, but they can certainly help improve communication, in its broadest sense, and reduce the distress associated with communication difficulties after stroke.

11.30.2 Dysarthria

Dysarthria affects about 20% of assessable patients. It usually improves spontaneously and rarely causes major long-term problems. This is fortunate since, although speech and language therapists give patients exercises aimed at improving the clarity of speech, there has been little formal evaluation of these techniques.[356] In patients with dysarthria and intact language and cognitive functions, communication aids such as pen and paper, letter and picture charts, and electronic communicators may be helpful.

11.31 Psychological problems

11.31.1 Low mood and anxiety

Patients who have had a stroke have more psychological symptoms than age- and sex-matched controls.[357,358] Depressive symptoms, anxiety and non-specific psychological distress are particularly common.

Depression occurs in about one-third of patients in the first year after stroke although estimates of frequency vary due to differences in the definitions of depression, methods of detection, interval between stroke onset and assessment, and selection of patients.[359–361] Generalized anxiety disorders also occur in about one-quarter of patients.[362,363] Patients very often have symptoms of both anxiety and depression.

Previous depression, stroke severity, poor physical function and low social activity are the risk factors most consistently associated with depression after stroke.[364–366] Although the literature has been dominated by many small studies relating lesion location with post-stroke depression, systematic reviews have concluded that there is little or no evidence of such a relationship.[367–370] Of course, depression is a frequent consequence of other non-neurological diseases and therefore depression after stroke may be a non-specific reaction to illness rather than due to the brain lesion itself. The aetiology of mood disorders after stroke is bound to be multifactorial and 'post-stroke depression' is probably not a discrete disease entity.

Symptoms of anxiety are more common in women but less obviously associated with stroke severity and poor outcome than depression.[364,371] The high frequency of anxiety is not surprising since a stroke, even a minor one, is a considerable threat to most patients. Recently, researchers have found symptoms of post-traumatic stress syndrome among stroke survivors.[372] Patients are likely to be frightened of dying, being left disabled or having another stroke. Their role in the family and their livelihood may be threatened. Some of these threats are amplified by the patient's and their family's lack

Table 11.44 Self-report questionnaires which have been used to identify psychological problems after stroke (where data are available we have included estimates of sensitivity and specificity for diagnosing psychiatric disorder defined by psychiatric interview 'gold-standard').

Scale (and study)	Typical features	Response % (method of delivery)	Diagnosis	Sensitivity (%)	Specificity (%)
General Health Questionnaire	Several versions 12–60 item				
(445) *	30 item, cut-off 9/10	92% (interview)	DSM IV depression	85	64
(446) *	28 item, cut-off 5/6	—	DSM III depression	78	81
Beck Depression Inventory	21 item				
(447)	Cut-off 9/10	77–88% (self-report)	DSM III depression	92	75
Hospital Anxiety and Depression Questionnaire	14 item				
(446) *	Cut-off 5/6	—	DSM III depression	61	50
(445) *	Cut-off 6/7	76% (self-report)	DSM IV depression	80	79
Centre for Epidemiologic Studies depression scale	20 item				
(448)	Cut-off 15/16	—	DSM III depression	73	100
(449)	Cut-off 20	—	Informal clinical	56	91
Wakefield Depression Inventory	12 item	—	—		—
Geriatric depression scale	30 item				
(449)	Cut-off 10		Informal clinical	88	64
(446) *	Cut-off 10/11	—	DSM III depression	84	66
Zung depression scale	20 item				
(449)	Cut-off 45	—	Informal clinical	76	96
Patient Health Questionnaire PHQ	9 item				
(450)	Cut off ≥ 10		DSM IV depression	78	96
	2 item				
	Cut off ≥ 3			78	95
Visual analogue mood scale					
(447)	10-cm horizontal line	49%	—		—

*Some authors have published sensitivities and specificities for several cut-off points.
DSM, *Diagnostic and Statistical Manual of Mental Disorders*.

of knowledge concerning stroke, which adds to their uncertainty.

Depression after stroke is associated with worse survival, both short and longer term, and worse functional outcome.[373]

Assessment

Depressed mood, diminished interest or pleasure, fatigue or loss of energy, insomnia and psychomotor agitation/retardation may all indicate the presence of depression.[374] However, after a stroke it may be particularly difficult to diagnose depression, especially if the patient cannot communicate. A sad expression due to facial weakness, crying due to emotionalism (section 11.31.2) or frustration, apathy with right hemisphere lesions, and the loss of the normal modulation in tone when speaking (aprosody), may all lead to a mistaken impression of depression. And insomnia may be due to a noisy ward and loss of appetite to dysphagia or unappetizing hospital food, not depression. On the other hand, lack of progress with rehabilitation may indicate the onset of a depressive illness.

Single questions (e.g. do you often feel sad or depressed?') and questionnaires to detect depression and anxiety have been evaluated in stroke patients (Table 11.44).[375,376] The instruments are often quite sensitive, making them suitable for screening but their specificities are not high enough for them to be used as diagnostic tools. They are more useful in research, although a structured psychiatric interview, e.g. the Present State Examination (PSE), and Schedule for Affective Disorders and Schizophrenia (SADS), is recognized as the 'gold standard' for making an accurate psychiatric diagnosis.

Unfortunately, response rates in patients with communication and other cognitive difficulties are often low. Visual analogue scales and observer rating scales, for example, the stroke aphasia depression questionnaire (SADQ) and the aphasia depression rating scale (ADRS), have been developed to overcome this but inevitably validation has proved to be methodologically challenging and none can yet be recommended for routine use.[377,378]

Prognosis

While some patients recover spontaneously, up to one-third of patients have depression that persists during the first year or longer after the onset of stroke.[360] Patients with more severe symptoms at presentation appear less responsive to treatment and have a worse long-term prognosis.

Prevention

It may be possible to reduce psychological morbidity, in particular anxiety, by spending more time with the patient and carer explaining the nature, prognosis and consequences of stroke although the effectiveness of such information-giving on emotional outcome has not been established.[379] It is important that patients and carers are aware that although the symptoms of stroke come on quickly, improvement occurs over weeks or months; they should be neither surprised nor disappointed that their recovery does not also occur 'at a stroke' (section 10.2.5). Also, in our experience many patients have an overly pessimistic view of the risk of dying or of having a recurrent stroke. Some realistic information about the risks may provide reassurance (sections 10.2.3, 16.2 and 17.10.1). Patients are likely to need more than one opportunity to talk so that all the staff caring for the patient and their family should be able to address the issues in a consistent manner. Cognitive behavioural therapy, which aims to teach patients and their carers how to identify and solve problems, may improve mood but this approach needs further rigorous evaluation, particularly since the necessary resources are seldom available to deliver it.[380] No drug regime has been shown to prevent post-stroke mood abnormalities.[380]

> It is important that patients and carers are aware that although the symptoms of stroke come on quickly, improvement occurs over weeks or months; they should be neither surprised nor disappointed that their recovery does not also occur 'at a stroke'.

Treatment

In patients with a depressive illness after stroke, antidepressants appear to improve mood[381] although it is unclear whether this translates into better physical and social outcomes. It is wise to start with a small dose initially and then gradually increase to minimize adverse effects, but it is important not to use subtherapeutic doses in the mistaken belief that depression after a stroke is somehow more drug-sensitive than 'ordinary' depression. Improvements in mood attributable to antidepressants are usually delayed at least 2 weeks after treatment is started. There is no clear evidence that any one drug is more effective than another in this setting, although the frequency and type of adverse effects associated with each group of antidepressants generally determines the choice.[382,383] In elderly patients with a past history of depression who have previously relapsed when treatment has stopped, one should probably continue treatment indefinitely to prevent a relapse which could have serious functional consequences. Even where there is some doubt about the diagnosis of depression after stroke, perhaps because of communication difficulties, a trial of antidepressants may be worthwhile. Some drugs which are started after a stroke (e.g. beta-blockers to treat newly discovered hypertension) can themselves cause depression so it is important to review the drug chart before starting antidepressants.

Psychotherapy has not been shown to help mood after stroke in small RCTs and although electroconvulsive therapy may occasionally be required, and has been used without complications after stroke, it has not been formally evaluated.[384–386]

> Start with a small dose of antidepressant and gradually increase it to minimize adverse effects. It is important not to use subtherapeutic doses in the mistaken belief that depression after a stroke is particularly drug-sensitive.

11.31.2 Emotionalism

About one-quarter of patients have difficulty controlling the expression of emotion in the year following a stroke.[387] This problem has been described by a variety of overlapping terms including emotionalism, pathological emotionalism, emotional lability, emotional incontinence, pathological crying/laughing and pseudobulbar affect. The patient abruptly starts to weep, or less commonly to laugh uncontrollably, sometimes with no obvious precipitant. More often, episodes are triggered by a kind word (e.g. how are you feeling?) or a thought with emotional overtones (e.g. thinking of grandchildren), but the emotional response is out of all proportion to the degree of 'internal sadness' (or mirth). Usually, the episodes are short-lived but may occur frequently enough to disrupt completely a conversation, therapy session or social event. Such outbursts cause considerable distress to the patient and their carer and may be a major obstacle to rehabilitation and social integration. Although classically described as a characteristic of pseudobulbar palsy (e.g. with bilateral strokes), emotionalism often occurs after a single, unilateral stroke. It is most common early on although it may not be noticed in the first few days because of everything else that is going on. Usually, episodes of emotionalism become less severe and less frequent with time.[387] Patients with emotionalism have more severe strokes, more psychological symptoms, and tend to have worse cognitive function than unaffected patients so it is important not to overlook these additional sources of distress.[388]

Assessment

Emotionalism should be suspected if the patient is more tearful, or cries more easily, than before the stroke. Ask the patient, carer or staff whether the crying is of sudden onset and whether the patient can control it. Patients may describe similar problems controlling laughter, but this is much less common. Having established that crying is a problem, one needs to assess whether this is solely due to emotionalism or whether it reflects frustration or depression. Crying which always occurs when the patient is trying, with difficulty, to perform a task (e.g. an aphasic patient trying to speak) suggests that the emotional outburst is due to frustration, although this does not mean there are no other psychological problems as well. One needs to talk to the patient, the carers and staff to assess whether or not the patient is depressed (section 11.31.1). It can be useful to ask the patient to keep a diary to document the frequency and severity of emotional outbursts, especially if one is planning to start treatment.

Treatment

Patients and carers are often confused and distressed by emotionalism. Therefore, it is important to explain that the problem is due to the stroke, that it is relatively common, that it does not represent the degree of distress it suggests, and that it usually becomes less severe with time. Do not walk away when the patient bursts into tears, but take the opportunity to explain the nature of the problem to them. If it is a persistent problem, and is either causing major distress to the patient and family,

or disrupting therapy sessions, antidepressants appear to reduce the frequency of emotional outbursts, rather paradoxically because the problem is primarily one of psychomotor response rather than mood.[387] Symptoms are usually improved within the first few days of starting treatment, unlike the symptoms of depression which rarely respond in less than 2 weeks. Small doses are often effective. If the symptoms are not better in a week, increase the dose slowly until the patient responds or begins to have dose-related adverse effects. In patients with persisting problems and dose-related adverse effects it may be useful to switch to an alternative class of antidepressant.

> Emotionalism after stroke can occur with single or multiple lesions in more or less any part of the brain. It is usually triggered by some sort of emotion (such as seeing grandchildren), but the response is completely out of proportion to the stimulus.

11.31.3 Boredom

Patients who remain in hospital for a long period of rehabilitation often complain of boredom, not surprisingly because much of their time is spent doing nothing.[389,390] This is a particular problem during weekends and evenings when the patients are not receiving therapy, or at least not receiving it from the therapists. It may also be a problem for patients after discharge home if they are housebound, socially isolated and unable to resume their normal leisure or work activities. Boredom leads to reduced motivation, low morale and can ultimately affect recovery. The team should remain alert to the problem and ask patients about it. There are a number of ways to alleviate boredom in hospitalized patients, which include:

- be as flexible as possible about visiting hours to maximize social contact with family and friends;
- provide patients with a variety of leisure activities on the unit; some units even employ leisure activity coordinators;
- encourage families to take patients out of the hospital wherever this is practical, e.g. walks in the grounds, trips to the pub, trips home for a meal;
- introduce volunteers on the unit to work with patients and develop group activities at weekends;
- encourage patients to keep their own timetable so they can plan their free time; and
- provide individual televisions with remote controls and headphones, videos, DVD, and even computer games.

These interventions may be integrated with the rehabilitation programme and incorporated in goal setting, and so benefit the patient in other ways. Unfortunately, even in specialized stroke units, patients spend far too much of their time staring into space.[390,391] For patients at home there are often clubs, day centres and voluntary organizations which can help to get them out of the house, meet other people, and involved in leisure activities.

11.31.4 Fatigue

Between one- and two-thirds of patients with stroke complain of tiredness or fatigue – perhaps twice as many as those who are stroke-free.[392–394] This is often severe enough to limit involvement in rehabilitation and delay return to normal everyday activities. Although fatigue may be a symptom of depression, it often occurs in patients without other mood symptoms. Younger patients and particularly those with no residual neurological impairments seem to find the fatigue most troublesome, perhaps because their expectations of being able to function normally are greater. Fortunately in many patients fatigue spontaneously remits, but for others it persists for years.

Fatigue has been measured in stroke patients using the fatigue impact scale, a self-report questionnaire.[392] We normally look for obvious causes, such as depression or medications, e.g. beta-blockers, but in the majority we do not identify a cause. Nonetheless, simple acknowledgement by the stroke team that fatigue is a recognized problem after stroke, and that it usually resolves, may be helpful to patients.

11.32 Dependency in activities of daily living

In previous sections we have discussed many of the impairments which result from stroke. In this section we will concentrate on the resulting disabilities, and the measures which can be taken to limit them. Their frequency in stroke survivors is shown in Table 11.45. Interventions aimed at reducing physical, cognitive and emotional impairments may all improve activities of daily living (ADL) function. However, there is increasing evidence from RCTs that occupational therapy, including training and practice, the introduction of aids and appliances, and alterations to the patient's environment, can also reduce dependency in ADL, and handicap.[395] With a few exceptions, these trials have not reported the effects of therapy on individual items of ADL.[396]

Table 11.45 Frequency of dependency in activities of daily living (based on the Barthel Index) among 246 consecutive patients surviving 1 year after their first-ever-in-a-lifetime stroke in the Oxfordshire Community Stroke Project (unpublished data).

Function	Dependent (%)	Independent (%)
Bowel function	23 (9)	223 (91)
Grooming	26 (11)	220 (89)
Toileting	30 (12)	216 (88)
Transfers	33 (13)	213 (87)
Walking inside	36 (15)	210 (85)
Bladder function	41 (17)	205 (83)
Feeding	44 (18)	202 (82)
Dressing	53 (22)	193 (78)
Stairs	64 (26)	182 (74)
Walking outside	76 (31)	171 (69)
Bathing	80 (33)	166 (67)

It is notable that there is a hierachy with stairs, walking outside and bathing being the most difficult tasks, while continence of bowels, grooming and toileting are attained by most patients.

11.32.1 Mobility

Sections 11.11 and 11.21 described the immediate problems of immobility and the interventions aimed at preventing complications and reducing the impairment. This section will deal with the disability and handicap as a consequence of reduced mobility. Many patients have mobility problems 1 year after their stroke (Table 11.45). Although the neurological consequences of the stroke account for most of these problems, other pathologies, in particular arthritis and hip fractures, add to the burden of walking disability.[397]

Assessment

Simple history taking is surprisingly informative. Self-reported ability to turn over in bed, sit up, transfer (i.e. bed to chair, and sitting to standing), walk (and use walking aids, furniture) and climb stairs (up, down or both, with or without rails) gives a fairly clear picture of the patient's residual problems. It is useful to know whether the patient can (and does) walk outside, their range, and whether physical or verbal support from another person is needed. It is also important to establish the reason for any problem, i.e. is it due to painful joints or feet, breathlessness, angina, intermittent claudication, loss of confidence, lack of motivation due to depression, embarrassment, environmental factors such as high steps, lack of hand rails, or even the neighbour's aggressive

Table 11.46 Rivermead Mobility Index.[398]

1	*Turning over in bed*
	Do you turn over from your back to your side without help?
2	*Lying from sitting*
	From lying in bed, do you get up to sit on the edge of the bed on your own?
3	*Sitting balance*
	Do you sit on the edge of the bed without holding on for 10 s?
4	*Sitting to standing*
	Do you stand up (from any chair) in less than 15 s, and stand there for 15 s (using hands, and with an aid if necessary)?
5	*Standing unsupported*
	Observe standing for 10 s without any aid or support.
6	*Transfer*
	Do you manage to move, e.g. from bed to chair and back, without any help?
7	*Walking inside, with an aid if needed*
	Do you walk 10 m, with an aid or furniture if necessary, but with no stand-by help?
8	*Stairs*
	Do you manage a flight of stairs without help?
9	*Walking outside (even ground)*
	Do you walk around outside, on pavements without help?
10	*Walking inside (with no aid)*
	Do you walk 10 m inside with no caliper, splint, aid or use of furniture, and no stand-by help?
11	*Picking off floor*
	If you drop something on the floor, do you manage to walk 5 m, pick it up and then walk back?
12	*Walking outside (uneven ground)*
	Do you walk over uneven ground (grass, gravel, dirt, snow, ice, etc.) Without help?
13	*Bathing*
	Do you get in and out of a bath or shower unsupervised and wash yourself?
14	*Up and down four steps*
	Do you manage to go up and down four steps with no rail and without help, but using an aid if necessary?
15	*Running*
	Do you run 10 m without limping in 4 s (fast walk is acceptable)?

Note: only question 5 depends on direct observation. The index forms a hierarchy so that one does not have to ask all the questions. However, the authors point out that by asking all the questions, and finding out why patients cannot manage certain actions, useful information to guide management is obtained.

dog? It is useful to observe the patient and the carer carrying out the various manoeuvres in their own home since environmental factors so often determine the level of handicap associated with impaired mobility.

Several scales are available for measuring mobility, e.g. the Rivermead mobility index[398] (Table 11.46). The timed 10-m walk is particularly useful because it is simple, objective, requires no more equipment than a watch with a second hand, and age-related normative data are available, i.e. < 60 years 10 s; 60–69 years 12.5 s; > 70 years 16.6 s.[399]

Treatment

Where the patient has residual problems, a physiotherapist or occupational therapist can improve mobility.[400] Training aimed at improving cardiorespiratory function probably increases walking speed.[401] Patients' mobility quite often deteriorates, after a period of stability, in the months or years after a stroke. This may be attributed to further strokes, progression of coexisting pathology (e.g. arthritis) or attenuation of the benefits of regular physiotherapy. It is important that whoever is responsible for monitoring the patient's progress, most often the general (family) practitioner, is alert to this and refers the patient back to the physiotherapist. Although not backed up by RCTs, we have little doubt of the value of so-called 'top-up' physiotherapy in patients such as this, although its effectiveness will inevitably depend on the cause of any deterioration.

Therapy in the patient's own home may be more helpful than in a hospital outpatient department since the therapist can then deal with the real, everyday problems that the patient is experiencing. For example, patients can be taught to climb their *own* stairs and to overcome the particular problems associated with the layout

Table 11.47 Walking aids.[451]

Shoes

Should be comfortable, supportive and have non-slip soles

Occasionally, a smooth sole facilitates a smooth swing phase in patients with foot drop when walking on carpets

Walking sticks

May improve standing stability and walking speed but must be tailored to the patient (i.e. length, handle shape, weight and appearance)[452,453] but not evidence based;[454] a long stick can be used to encourage patients to put weight through their affected leg (Fig. 11.26d)

Replace worn rubber ferrule (i.e. rubber bit on end of stick)

Should be held in the unaffected hand in patients with hemiparesis but this means the patient's functioning hand is no longer available for other tasks

Other uses include extending the patient's reach, and 'self-defence'

Tripods and quadrapods

Provide a broader base of support than a walking stick

Their weight may cause associated reactions and may worsen the quality of gait[452]

Not useful on uneven ground

Walking frames (Fig. 11.26)

Available in many sizes and shapes with or without wheels

Useful where balance is poor, especially if the patient tends to lean backwards

Often give patients confidence

Needs good upper limb function and, of course, prevents patient from using hands or carrying things; many patients attach a basket or use a wheeled trolley to overcome this problem

Patients often try to pull up on their frame to rise from a chair, which can cause them to fall

Frames may trip up patients and be difficult to manoeuvre with lots of furniture and thick carpets

Cannot be used on stairs, therefore patients may require several frames, one on each level

Beware bent frames, protruding screws, loose hand-grips and worn ferrules

Other uses, drying underclothes

Ankle–foot orthosis or brace (Fig. 11.27)

Usually of thermoplastic construction and tailored to the individual

Occasionally useful in spastic foot drop to improve gait pattern,[455] but does not improve spasticity[456] and may actually exacerbate the problem

Beware in patients with oedema and tendency to leg ulcers

Knee brace

Occasionally required to prevent hyperextension of the knee

Functional electrical stimulation

An experimental treatment which has been used to correct foot drop after stroke (section 11.21)

Hand rails

Short grab-rails can be useful to provide support, especially at thresholds and doorways

Full-length rails on staircases are invaluable to those with poor balance, confidence or vision

Advice on positioning hand rails should be obtained from an occupational therapist; poorly placed hand rails can cause accidents or may not be used

---

of their *own* home. Two RCTs which compared the effectiveness of home vs hospital-based physiotherapy showed that improvement in ADL function was slightly greater in those treated at home, but other outcomes were no different.[402]

Although the therapist may be able to reduce the patient's degree of impairment, even when intervention starts very late after a stroke, the therapist's main tool at this point is the provision of mobility aids (Tables 11.47 and 11.48). When one prescribes an aid for patients, it is important to provide them and any carers with training in its use, and to ensure that it is maintained in good order (Figs 11.26–11.36). Many patients do not use the aids provided, which is both a waste of resources and an indication of the lack of value of that aid. It is important to follow up patients who have been given aids to ensure they fit the patient's needs and are actually being used, and to retrieve any unused equipment.

> If one prescribes an aid, one should teach the patient or carer how to use it, ensure that it solves the problem, check that it is maintained in good working order, and provide follow-up to ensure its continued use or appropriate removal.

Table 11.48 Other aids to mobility.

Chairs (Fig. 11.28)

Higher seats (but not so high as to cause the feet to dangle) without too much backward angle, and firm arm rests (of the correct height, shape and length) facilitate transfers

It is easier to stand from a chair if the patient can place his/her heels under it when preparing to stand

Chairs should be tailored to the individual's requirements, but existing chairs may be raised or lowered

Chairs on castors can be dangerous

Ejector chairs (Fig. 11.29)

The seat or chair may be sprung to provide an initial lift to allow the patient to rise

These must be tailored to the individual's weight to avoid the patient being catapulted across the room

Electric chairs which slowly bring the patient to a semi-erect position are occasionally useful but are expensive, bulky and require training to use properly

Beds

A firm mattress at the correct height will facilitate transfers from a bed

Blocks or leg extensions can be used to modify an existing bed

A grab-rail attached to the bed frame or floor can facilitate independent transfers (Fig. 11.30a)

It may be impossible to attach aids to a divan-style bed

Mechanical devices which help the patient to sit in bed can occasionally be helpful (Fig. 11.30b)

Wheelchairs

An invaluable means to improve mobility

Many hundreds of designs including self-propelled, carer-propelled and electric chairs

Need to be tailored to individual's requirements

Must be kept in good working order (Fig. 11.31)

Ramps

Useful to those in wheelchairs and their carers

Many designs available for different situations

Lifts

Many types, including:

    Domestic stair-lifts (Fig. 11.32) for those who cannot manage stairs

    Through-the-floor lifts for accessing upper floors in wheelchairs

    Short-rise lifts for accessing vehicles in wheelchairs or where there is insufficient space for a ramp

Lifts are expensive and may require structural alterations to accommodate them

Patients who are unable to walk outside, or who can walk only short distances, or who have difficulty using their own or public transport, may be helped by putting them in contact with any local transport schemes. For example, in the UK special financial allowances are available to help with the added cost of being immobile, specially adapted taxis can be provided and some shopping centres provide electric wheelchairs. In the last few years there has been a major campaign to improve access to public places for patients with disabilities.

11.32.2 Driving

Many people who have had a stroke never return to driving.[403,404] There are several reasons: severe residual motor, sensory, visual or cognitive impairments are the most common. In many countries the authorities place restrictions on driving after stroke, and particularly if the stroke is complicated by epileptic seizures (section 11.8). The variation in regulations probably reflects the dearth of relevant research in this area. Special, and usually more stringent, regulations apply to those who drive commercial vehicles, taxis and heavy goods vehicles. The main issue for driving authorities is not so much risk of recurrence – well under the 20% per annum for normal drivers in the UK – but physical disability and cognitive difficulties which can be so difficult to judge.

Patients are often not asked by their doctors whether they drive, thus many continue to drive and put lives at risk in contravention of their local regulations.[404–406] It is the doctor's responsibility to ask patients whether or not they drive so they can be given relevant information. Failure to do so might have serious consequences, although it is unclear whether patients who have had a stroke and return to driving are at increased risk of road traffic accidents.[407]

There appears to be little agreement about the optimal method of assessing a disabled patient's fitness to drive. Informal judgements are often made by patients or their family doctors.[404] Bedside testing of neurological

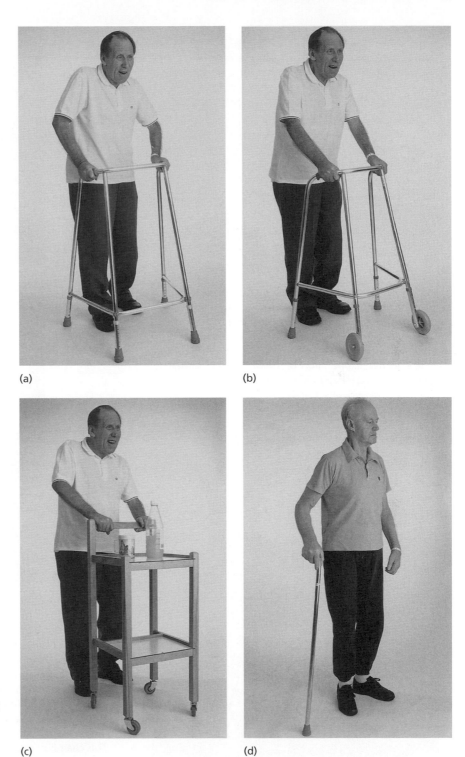

Fig. 11.26 Walking aids. (a) A typical light-weight walking frame of adjustable height which may be useful if a patient has poor balance but reasonable arm and hand function. (b) A walking frame with wheels which may be better than (a) in patients who tend to fall backwards or who have Parkinson's disease. (c) A tea trolley which will provide patients with support as well as allow them to take things from place to place. (d) A long walking stick held in the unaffected hand can be used to encourage the patient to put more of their weight through their affected leg.

impairments including cognitive function, assessments in driving simulators and road tests have all been advocated.[408] One might start with a bedside assessment to demonstrate any physical, and probably more importantly visual, visuospatial and cognitive impairments, which would make safe driving very unlikely.[409,410]

Patients who pass on the bedside testing could then be assessed on a driving simulator or an 'off-road' test which would identify those who are clearly unsafe to drive.[411] The remainder could then be given an on-road test in a dual-control car with an appropriately trained instructor,[412,413] which can be performed with good inter-rater

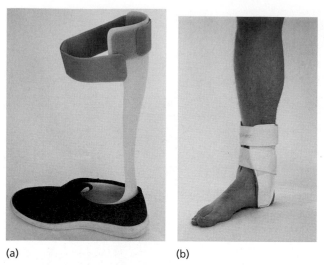

(a)   (b)

Fig. 11.27 Ankle supports. (a) A thermoplastic ankle–foot orthosis: the famous AFO splint. Although this is very useful in patients with foot drop secondary to lower motor neurone lesions, in stroke patients it can sometimes increase the tendency to plantarflexion by stimulating the sole of the foot. (b) A lateral ankle support may be useful in patients who have a tendency to invert their foot when walking.

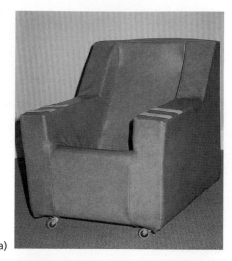

(a)

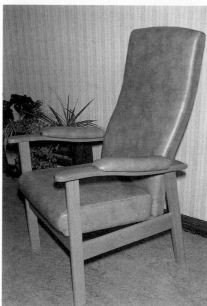

(b)

Fig. 11.28 Choosing an appropriate chair for a stroke patient who has difficulties getting from sitting to standing. (a) A bad chair to ensure the user never escapes! The seat is too low and slopes backwards, the arms are soft and offer little resistance to allow the person to push up on them, the base is solid so the patient cannot tuck their feet under them, and this chair is on castors so that if the patient eventually manages to stand the chair slides away and causes them to fall backwards. Note the Velcro pads on the arms to allow a tray to be fixed across the user's escape route. (b) A good chair to facilitate easy transfers. This chair is of reasonable height, is upright, has firm but padded arms and allows the user to tuck their feet underneath them which makes it easier to get their weight over their feet. This chair does not have wings, which may provide support for the user's head when sleeping but can stop interaction with other people sitting to either side.

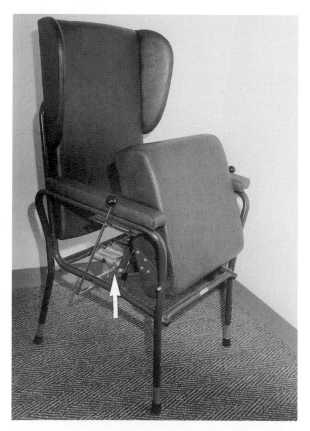

Fig. 11.29 An ejector chair. The number of springs (*arrow*) can be altered depending on the weight of the user. Some patients find that this type of chair pushes them off balance.

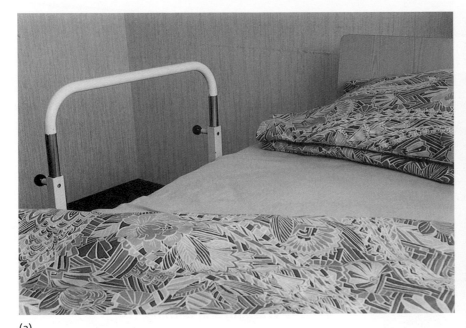

(a)

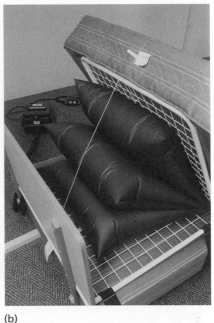

(b)

Fig. 11.30 Aids to getting out of bed. Although many people can get out of a bed independently during a therapy session when they are 'warmed up', they may need aids to get out in the middle of the night or first thing in the morning. (a) A grab-rail attached to the bed can facilitate transfers from lying to standing and may therefore prevent incontinence at night. The height of this model can be adjusted to suit the individual. (b) A pneumatic mattress elevator can be helpful in getting patients from lying to sitting.

Fig. 11.31 (*opposite*) Things to look for when examining a wheelchair. This wheelchair has many hazardous and uncomfortable features. Note the white sticky tape covering the name of the hospital on the side of this wheelchair, which wished, very reasonably, to remain anonymous. 1: Check that the tyres are properly inflated (*arrow*). Flat tyres make the wheelchair hard work to propel and the brakes inoperative. 2: Check the brakes work (*arrow*). 3: Check that the sides and arms (*arrow*) are removable to facilitate transfers onto toilets, into cars, etc. 4: Check that the foot plates are not fixed (*arrow*) or flapping about. Either problem may cause injury. The foot plates should fold neatly and securely out of the way when not in use. 5: Check that the arms (*arrow*) are properly padded to avoid discomfort and compression neuropathy of the ulnar nerve. 6: Check that the back (*arrow*) and seat (*arrow*) are not sagging and that the appropriate cushion is being used to reduce the risk of pressure ulcers. 7: Check that the grips on the handles are in good order (*arrow*).

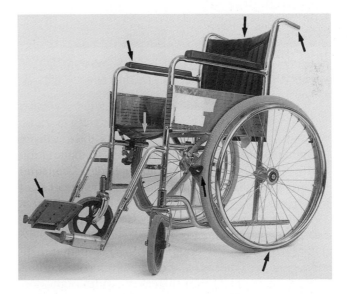

reliability. This stepwise approach should minimize the risk of injury to the patient, instructor and other road users. Many countries provide specialist centres for the assessment of disabled drivers. These centres not only assess driving skills, but also provide advice on vehicle adaptations which allow patients with severe physical disability to drive. Training on a driving simulator has been evaluated in a small RCT, and while definite conclusions are limited by methodological issues, this approach is promising.[414]

11.32.3 Toileting

The problems of urinary and faecal incontinence have been discussed in sections 11.14 and 11.15, respectively. About 10% of surviving patients are still dependent in

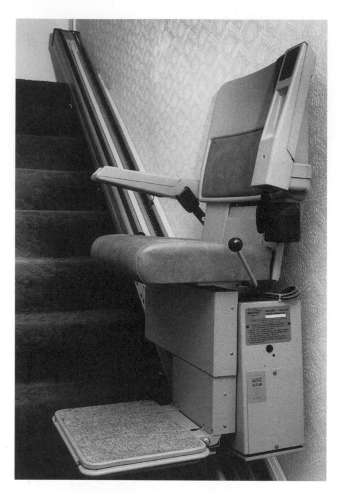

Fig. 11.32 A typical stair-lift for domestic use. The arm-rests fold out of the way to facilitate transfers. The foot-rest and seat fold up when not in use. The controls are on the arm-rests.

toileting 1 year after their first stroke due to inability to transfer independently, walk, or dress and undress (Table 11.45). For the cognitively intact patient, this is an embarrassing disability which severely damages their self-esteem.

An assessment by an occupation therapist should define the severity and cause of the problem. The patient's ability to toilet themselves is very dependent on the environment so that a home assessment may be particularly useful. Simple factors such as the width of the door to the toilet or bathroom, the position and height of the toilet, and the position of the toilet roll holder can make a crucial difference to whether or not the patient can use the toilet independently.

Therapy aimed at improving performance in mobility, transfers and dressing will all facilitate independence in toileting. Table 11.49 lists some common problems and simple solutions, and Fig. 11.33 shows some simple toilet aids.

Table 11.49 Toileting problems and solutions.

Cannot get to toilet because of mobility or access problems
Solutions: Urinal (Fig. 11.10)
Commode, many designs to suit individual needs (Fig. 11.33)
Chemical toilet, useful where regular emptying of a commode is not possible
Cannot transfer on and off the toilet, or poor balance making manipulation of clothes difficult
Solutions: Grab-rails
Toilet frame (Fig. 11.33)
Raised or adjustable toilet seat (Fig. 11.33)
Cannot clean myself
Solutions: Toilet paper holder on the unaffected side which can be used with one hand
Large aperture toilet seat
Self-cleaning toilet, like a bidet and toilet in one

11.32.4 Washing and bathing

About 10% and 30% are dependent in washing and bathing respectively 1 year after a first-ever-in-a-lifetime stroke (Table 11.45). Motor, sensory, visuospatial and cognitive impairments all contribute to these disabilities. Although poor arm function makes washing and grooming more difficult, most patients can perform these tasks with their unaffected arm, but those with visuospatial and cognitive deficits, even when arm function seems quite good, may still be unable to wash and groom themselves independently. Independence in bathing obviously requires some independence in mobility and transfers. Other disabling conditions in the elderly (e.g. painful arthritis) often contribute. A skilled assessment by an occupational therapist, preferably in the patient's own home, will delineate the problems. This assessment ensures there is adequate access to the bathroom (e.g. for a wheelchair). The size and layout of the bathroom will determine which aids can be used.

Therapy aimed at improving those impairments, especially motor impairments, which are contributing to the disability in bathing and washing may be of some help but, again, at this stage the provision of the wide range of available aids to allow the patient to compensate for their impairments is more effective (Fig. 11.34 and Table 11.50). Specific training in the use of bathing aids, both in hospital and in the patient's home, does appear to increase use of the bath.[415] Of course, in many countries patients prefer to take showers rather than a bath, which generally reduces the difficulty. One general point is that a patient who has trouble bathing should ensure that somebody else is in the house and that the bathroom door is left unlocked, so that if they fall or are unable to get out of the bath somebody can easily reach them.

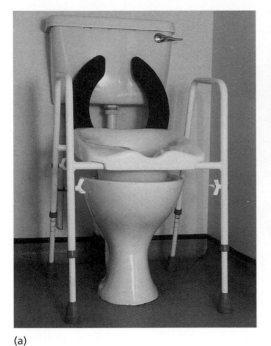

(a)

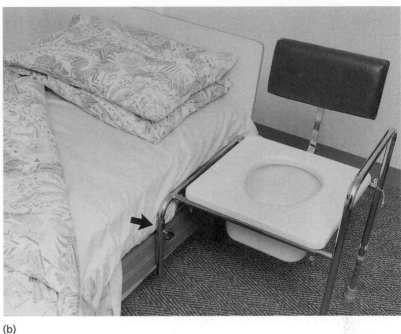

(b)

Fig. 11.33 Simple toilet aids. (a) A raised toilet seat with a frame. (b) A commode; this one attaches securely to the bed (*arrow*) for use at night.

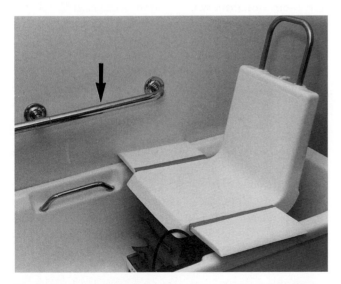

Fig. 11.34 A pneumatic bath aid to lower patients into and to lift them out of a bath. However, the humble bath rail (*arrow*) with some other simple aids is very commonly all that is needed to allow the person to use a bath independently.

> Patients who have difficulties bathing independently should not be left in their house alone while bathing. Some form of alarm or even a cordless or mobile telephone will increase safety.

Table 11.50 Problems with grooming or bathing/showering and solutions.

> *Cannot brush dentures with one hand*
> Solutions: Half fill sink with water, attach brush with a suction pad to the sink and brush dentures with functioning hand
> *Cannot get into, and even more important, out of the bath*
> Solutions: Grab-rails appropriately mounted around bath
> Non-slip bath mat
> Bath stool
> Bath board
> Inflatable or hydraulic bath seats which can lower patients into or raise them out of the bath (Fig. 11.34)
> Hoists
> Replace bath with shower

Some bathroom adaptations are expensive and cause considerable disruption to the patient's home. It is important that a proper assessment is done to avoid unnecessary building work and to ensure that any modifications really are likely to help the patient and/or carer. For some patients who live alone, or where aids and adaptations are not appropriate, it may be necessary to recommend either a simple strip wash or to introduce a nurse, care assistant or family member to help with bathing and so allow the patient to remain in their own home.

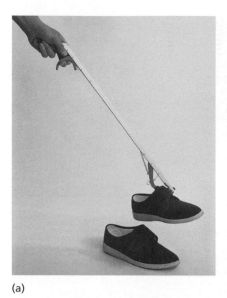

(a)

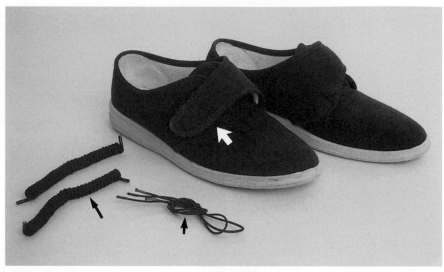

(b)

Fig. 11.35 Simple dressing aids. (a) A reaching aid. (b) Elastic laces (*short black arrow*), spiral laces which one simply pulls tight (*long black arrow*) and Velcro fasteners (*white arrow*) are invaluable dressing aids for those with only one functioning hand or poor manual dexterity.

Table 11.51 Problems with dressing and solutions (Fig. 11.35).

Cannot manage zips or buttons
Solutions: Button hook or toggle button hook allows patient to fasten buttons with one hand
Replace round buttons with oval ones
Hook to pull up zip
Replace zips and buttons with Velcro
Cannot get shoes on or tie shoe laces
Solutions: Long-handled shoe horn
Replace shoe laces with elastic ones or Velcro straps
Shoe ties
Cannot reach or pull up clothes
Solutions: Dressing hook or even a walking stick
Reaching aid

11.32.5 Dressing

About 20% of surviving patients need help from another person to dress 1 year after their first-ever-in-a-lifetime stroke (Table 11.45). Dependency in dressing is usually due to a combination of arm weakness or incoordination, inability to stand independently to pull up lower garments, and cognitive and visuospatial problems.[416] A painful shoulder makes dressing even more difficult (section 11.24). A detailed assessment by an occupational therapist should elucidate the causes and define the degree of disability.

Occupational therapists spend a considerable proportion of their time training patients to dress themselves. If the disability is due simply to a motor deficit, then 'dressing practice', where the patient is taught to compensate for their impairments, is often successful.[416] If the patient has cognitive or visuospatial problems or other non-stroke problems (e.g. arthritis), the benefit of this type of therapy is less obvious. There has been little formal evaluation of dressing practice.

Advice on the best type of clothes can allow patients to become independent, i.e. avoidance of tight clothes with small buttons or zips, and of shoes with laces. Oval buttons are easier to manipulate than round ones.[417] Velcro fastenings have revolutionized dressing for patients with only one functioning hand, being easier to use and preferred by patients than other fasteners.[417] Some of the common problems and possible solutions are shown in Table 11.51 and Fig. 11.35. If patients still cannot dress themselves, then care assistants or a member of the family will be needed to help.

11.32.6 Feeding

One year after a first-ever-in-a-lifetime stroke, about 20% of surviving patients need some help from another person to feed (Table 11.45).[418] Dependency in feeding is one of the most demeaning problems because of its associations with infancy. Impaired function of the arm and hand is the most common cause, although problems with sitting balance, facial weakness and visuospatial and sensory function may all be important as well. A small number of patients may have residual problems swallowing (section 11.17). Most problems can be

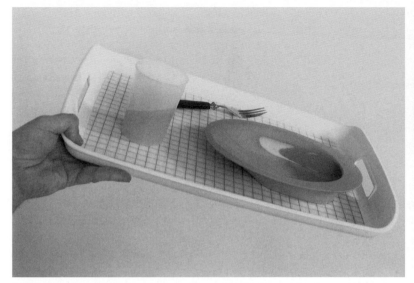

(a)

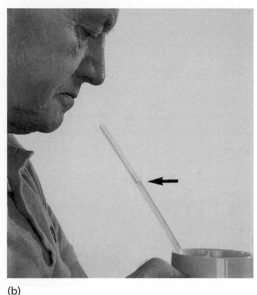

(b)

Fig. 11.36 Simple feeding aids. (a) A combined fork and knife, and a plate with a high side or plate guard facilitates eating one-handed. The non-slip tray helps by fixing the plate and also reduces the risk of spills. (b) This drinking straw has a one-way

valve so that when the user stops sucking the fluid does not fall back into the beaker (*arrow*). This may be useful in patients with facial weakness and poor lip closure but who have a normal swallow.

Table 11.52 Feeding problems and solutions (Fig. 11.36).

> *Cannot cut up food because of poor arm function*
> Solutions: If moderate hand weakness, a large-handled sharp knife may be enough
> Alternatively, a combined knife and spoon or fork may help, but warn the patient to be careful not to cut their mouth
> *Cannot hold bowl or plate still when cutting or spooning*
> Solution: A non-slip mat or tray, or containers with suction pads
> *Cannot push peas onto fork or spoon*
> Solution: Provide a dish with a raised side or rim
> *Dribbling due to facial weakness*
> Solutions: A mug with a spout, or a straw may help. Straws are available with a non-return valve if the patient cannot suck using a conventional one because of facial weakness, but has an intact swallow

identified simply by talking to the patient and/or carer, but often it is useful for a trained observer, usually an occupational therapist, to assess the patient.

Intensive therapy may improve arm function (section 11.21) but, late after stroke, the provision and training in the use of feeding aids is probably more effective. Sometimes very simple problems, which require very simple solutions, are overlooked. For instance, it is important that any dentures are in good working order and in the mouth rather than in a glass of water on the bedside table, that the patient is sitting at a table on a

chair of appropriate height, and that the knife is sharp. Furthermore, the type of food may make the difference between patients being able to feed themselves or not. A hemiplegic patient may be independent eating sandwiches but dependent for eating a steak. Some of the more common feeding problems, and the aids which can help, are shown in Table 11.52 and Fig. 11.36.

11.32.7 Preparing food

Many patients are unable to prepare food for themselves or their family because of a wide variety of post-stroke impairments. Cognitive and visuospatial problems may put patients, and others living in the same building, in danger from lacerations, burns, fires, gas poisoning, explosions and flooding. Again, problems are easily identified by talking to, or observing, the patient in the kitchen. An occupational therapist may be able to teach patients alternative methods of performing certain tasks and for many with physical rather than cognitive problems there is a large variety of kitchen aids available to help with specific difficulties (Table 11.53). Patients with cognitive problems may be helped by things such as electric kettles which turn themselves off and gas detection systems which interrupt the supply automatically, but for those with severe cognitive problems it may be necessary to ban them from the kitchen or to remove cookers.

Where patients cannot prepare food for themselves, it is obviously important to ensure delivery of prepared meals to their homes, or to have a care assistant who

Table 11.53 Problems with food preparation and solutions.

Cannot open cans with one functional hand
Solution: Wall-mounted (electric) tin opener
Cannot open bottles with one functional hand
Solution: A bottle or jar stabilizer to fix the bottles to work surface
Cannot cut up or peel ingredients with one functional hand
Solution: A plate or board with spikes on which to impale the item to be cut

can prepare meals. Often, relatives and social services provide these services.

11.33 Social difficulties

We have already discussed how stroke-related impairments result in disability or dependency in activities of daily living (ADL). However, there is more to life than just ADL. Environmental factors become extremely important in determining the effect of the stroke on a person's role in society and their handicap. This section will address some of the social factors which are often of greatest concern to patients and their carers.

11.33.1 Accommodation

About 50% of the patients who survive a stroke are dependent in ADL (Table 11.45). Some patients with complex or worsening disability may not, if admitted to hospital, be able to return to their own home. A patient's ability to return home depends on the answers to the following questions, among others:

• Is the disability likely to improve or worsen with time?
• Will aids and adaptations reduce dependency?
• What is the patient's accommodation like?
• What level of informal support is available, e.g. family?
• What level of community support is available, e.g. community nursing, home helps?

Any assessment has to identify the needs of the patient to determine whether those needs can be practically provided in the patient's current accommodation, or whether alternative or modified accommodation will be needed. This may involve one or more visits home with the patient and any carer to establish exactly what the practical problems are. If a short visit is not enough, then home visits (with the potential for 'round the clock' supervision) for a few days and nights can be useful to

predict how the patient and carer will cope in the longer term. The layout of the home is obviously important. Are there steps up to the front door which make access difficult? Are the toilet and bathroom upstairs? Is the house cluttered with furniture? Are the carpets deep pile which may cause difficulty for a patient with a foot drop? Some stroke units have predischarge apartments in the hospital which allow the team and the patient to assess under supervision how well the patient copes. This may not be the same as discharge into the community, however.

When to do an accommodation assessment is difficult to predict because it often takes a considerable time to find alternative accommodation, or to make major structural changes to the patient's current home. Thus, if one is going to avoid unnecessary delays in hospital, one has to make a decision before the patient has achieved their optimal functional status. Considerable judgement is required to 'best guess' the patient's final functional level and to identify their accommodation needs well in advance of hospital discharge.

After a thorough assessment, the patient and their family, with help from the team, need to decide where they wish to live, taking into account all the practical issues – including any financial constraints. After all, given unlimited funds, it is almost always possible to maintain even the most severely disabled patient at home. The final decision is often a result of negotiation between the patient, carer and team members. For instance, patients with visuospatial or cognitive problems may not appreciate the likely problems which will face their carers after discharge. For these sorts of reasons it is not always possible to fulfil the wishes of both patient and carer.

Options for alternative accommodation, and the availability of support in the community, vary from place to place, country to country, and from time to time. However, in general, one needs a range of accommodation offering a variety of levels of support and supervision to meet the needs of individual patients.

11.33.2 Employment

About one-third of patients who have a stroke are of employment age. Estmates of the proportion who return to work have varied widely due mainly to methodological factors.[419] Obviously, the nature of previous employment, residual impairments and disabilities, the patient's own wishes, the attitudes and policies of employers, health and safety legislation and insurance issues will determine whether return to employment is feasible.[420] It is also likely that the local arrangements for paying sickness benefit will influence whether patients return to work, and the timing of their return. Of course, many patients who are approaching retirement age may not want to return to work anyway.

Assessment of the patient's ability to return to work is often left to the patient and family, but involvement of members of the team (i.e. occupational therapist, speech and language therapist, physiotherapist and social worker) can be very useful to help explore the possible work options. Some employers have occupational health departments which can provide further specialist advice on their own specific regulations covering return to work, and on any alterations to the working environment or the job itself which would facilitate this.

It is important that patients and their families are counselled about the patient's limitations. They are often under the misconception that patients should rest after a stroke and that physical activity will bring on another stroke.[421] This misconception may have made them rule out, inappropriately, the possibility of return to work.

> Many patients and their carers are under the misconception that exercise, hard work or stress will bring on another stroke. They should be counselled to dispel these myths.

Patients may require specific occupational therapy to improve the physical skills required for particular jobs, and/or retraining to change employment. Patients often complain of marked fatigue (section 11.31.4) so that a return to part-time work, at least initially, is often more successful than struggling to cope with full-time work. And they may find that although they can perform the physical aspects of their work, their concentration may be impaired. In many countries, special schemes are available to provide employment for disabled people.

11.33.3 Leisure

Two-thirds of stroke patients are retired from employment. For them, resumption of a leisure activity is more relevant than work. Restriction in leisure activities may be the result of physical or cognitive impairments but may also be caused by psychological factors and even fear that an activity may bring on a further stroke. Many disabled stroke patients are unable to continue with their normal leisure activities and do not take up new ones which are within their abilities.[422] Reduction in leisure activities will exacerbate social isolation, lower mood and adversely affect relationships with carers. The level of social activities, including leisure, can be measured using the Frenchay activities index; however, the Nottingham leisure questionnaire has been developed specifically for this purpose.[423,424]

Counselling the patient and their carers about the value of maintaining leisure activities and social contacts is useful, and can have dramatic consequences (Fig. 11.37), along with practical help in achieving them. Therapy specifically directed at improving participation in leisure activities, or using leisure goals to improve activities of daily living function, was not effective in a large multicentre trial.[425]

11.33.4 Air travel

We are frequently asked whether a patient can travel on a commercial flight after a stroke. We are not aware of any research into the safety, or otherwise, of doing so. Prolonged immobility on longhaul flights with the attendant risk of venous thromboembolism, and the effect of altitude (most commercial aeroplanes are pressurized to a level equivalent to an altitude of about 7000 feet) on the brain, are two issues which need to be considered. In all patients, but especially those who have had an ischaemic stroke associated with a patent foramen ovale, it may be wise to emphasize simple measures to reduce the risk of venous thromboembolism such as adequate hydration and avoiding prolonged immobility.[426]

In giving advice one also needs to take into account:
- the importance of the flight (e.g. is it to get home or simply part of a holiday?);
- the interval from the stroke which will in part determine the risk of recurrent stroke;
- the ability of the patient to manage everyday activities, such as toileting and feeding, on an aeroplane;
- the availability of an accompanying carer;
- the attitude of the airline and the patient's travel insurer.

Many patients who have a stroke while on holiday are repatriated by air within a week or two without apparent ill effects.

11.33.5 Sex

Although many stroke patients are elderly, they were often sexually active before their stroke. But after stroke, libido, coital frequency and satisfaction are reduced among both patients and their partners.[427] This reduction in activity is due to both physical and psychosocial factors, the latter probably being of greater importance (Table 11.54). Reduced sexual activity may contribute to a worsening emotional relationship with their partner.

A patient and their partner may believe that reduced satisfaction with their sexual relationship is an inevitable consequence of stroke. Although we often feel embarrassed about talking to people about these aspects of their lives, it is important that sexual problems are discussed. Physical difficulties due to the patient's

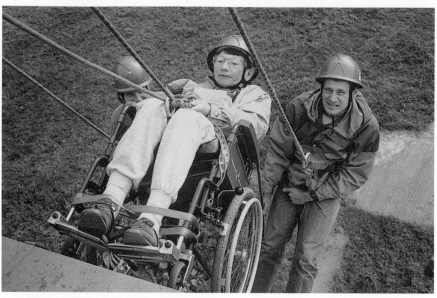

(a)

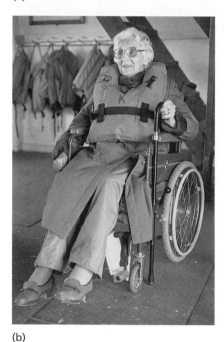

(b)

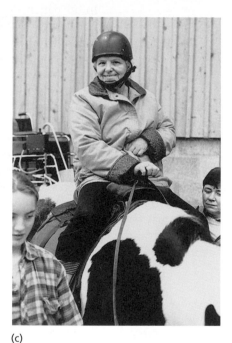

(c)

Fig. 11.37 Leisure activities for patients with mobility problems after stroke: (a) abseiling in a wheelchair; (b) preparing to go canoeing; (c) horse riding. (Photographs by Renzo Mazzolini for the Chest Heart and Stroke Association, Scotland.)

impairments can often be overcome with a little commonsense and a realization that intercourse, with vaginal penetration, is not an absolute requirement. The psychological problems contributing to sexual dysfunction are often the most difficult to sort out. Sometimes patients and their partners simply need to be reassured that sexual activity, like any other physical activity, will not precipitate another stroke. Verbal information may usefully be supplemented by leaflets, supplied by charities and patient organizations, which include advice for patients and carers.

We encourage patients to resume sexual activity as soon as they wish after a stroke. One exception might be a patient with a recent rupture of an aneurysm which has not for some reason been coiled or clipped. One might imagine that the increase in blood pressure associated with orgasm could cause a rebleed.

Unfortunately, strokes can put tremendous strains on a relationship which are more difficult to manage. Where sexual dysfunction is due to medication (Table 11.54), withdrawal and substitution with an alternative drug may be effective. In men with impotence, sildenafil

Table 11.54 Causes of reduced sexual activity and satisfaction after stroke.

> *Psychosocial factors*
> Loss of interest
> Fear of impotence
> Fear of bringing on another stroke
> Emotional changes may adversely affect the relationship
> Inability to discuss problems
> *Physical factors*
> Physical disability may make sexual intercourse difficult or impossible, e.g. indwelling catheter, contractures
> Impotence and reduced libido due to:
> > Drugs (e.g. thiazide diuretics, beta-blockers, tricyclic antidepressants)
> > Comorbidity (e.g. diabetes, peripheral vascular disease)

(Viagra) may be useful although experience of its use after stroke is limited and the manufacturers recommend caution in this situation. Many patients with stroke will be taking nitrates for ischaemic heart disease which precludes the concurrent use of sildenafil. Referral to a sexual dysfunction clinic, or for marital guidance, may be useful if problems persist after attending to the simple and obvious.

11.33.6 Finance

Stroke may place a considerable financial burden on patients and their families. Employment, and therefore income, may be affected.[428] Disability, and the aids and adaptations needed to overcome it, may also be costly. Even when the patient is still in hospital, carers may have difficulty meeting the costs of transport to visit the patient and, if driving, parking when they get there. This is important because the patient's morale may suffer if regular visiting is not possible and this may adversely affect outcome. Of course, in some unenlightened health systems, the patient or family may have to pay directly for their healthcare and financial constraints may even prevent patients from receiving the necessary treatment.

The professionals involved must be alert to any financial problems which affect patients and be ready to offer help as required. In the UK, and other countries, where the level of government support for home care depends on the patient's personal finances, a financial assessment may be necessary for planning care. In the UK, social workers are responsible for these assessments although other agencies may become involved.

Depending on assessment of their needs, and sometimes a financial assessment, patients or carers may be eligible for financial benefits from government, charitable and other sources (e.g. superannuation schemes, insurance policies, etc.).

11.34 Carer problems

Looking after a patient with disability places considerable physical and emotional strains on the carer. Carers worry about the patient's needs and their ability to fulfil them. Caring may well limit the carer's employment and leisure activities and lead to social isolation and loneliness. Carers of disabled stroke patients are often anxious and depressed and have poor physical health.[429] The extent of these difficulties appears to be related to the patient's level of dependency, mood, behaviour and cognitive function. However, the magnitude of the burden of caregiving, as perceived by the carer, may relate to their own physical and emotional state as much as that of the patient. The impact that a stroke has on the family changes over time. Periods which are likely to cause carers particular stress and when extra support may be needed are:

- immediately after the stroke when the carer has to come to terms with what is potentially a life-threatening event and one which may have a major effect on the patient's and potential carer's future life together;
- during a prolonged period of in-patient care; visiting may be difficult because of travelling and also because the patient's behaviour may put emotional pressure on the carer;
- around the period of hospital discharge; suddenly the patient who has been looked after by a team of skilled professionals appears, at least to the carer, to be only the carer's sole responsibility; and
- during the weeks and months following hospital discharge when professional support dwindles (sometimes inappropriately and abruptly), friends stop calling, and the carer becomes physically and emotionally exhausted.

Several stages of adjustment which families typically go through have been identified (Table 11.55). These do not apply to all carers, but it is useful to be aware of them in managing patients and their families.

Although the physical aspects of caring for a person with a disabling stroke are hard, it is often the patient's psychological and resulting behavioural problems which cause most distress to carers. Carers may note a change in personality, the patient may become short-tempered and irritable, depressed or apathetic. Such changes may lead to a deterioration in their relationship which may

Stage 1:	Crisis	Shock
		Confusion
		High anxiety
Stage 2:	Treatment stage	High expectation of recovery
		Denial that disability is permanent
		Periods of grieving
		Fears for the future
		Job
		Mobility
		Lifestyle
		About coping
Stage 3:	Realization of disability	Anger
		Feelings of rejection
		Despair
		Frustration
		Depression
Stage 4:	Adjustment	

Table 11.55 Stages of adjustment amongst families of patients with stroke.[428]

be compounded by a cessation or disturbance of their sexual relationship (section 11.33.5).

Carers often have feelings of guilt which add to their distress. They worry that they contributed to the stroke, perhaps by giving the patient the wrong diet or because of some petty incident which the carer feels should have been avoided. They feel guilty about not visiting enough or for not having the patient home soon enough. After hospital discharge they feel guilty about wanting to carry on with their own lives. They often worry that the patient will fall, have another stroke or even die unless they are in constant attendance. These fears, apart from adding to the distress of carers, may also cause the carers to become overprotective towards the patient, which may prejudice the patient's outcome.

Assessment

It is important that all those involved in managing a stroke patient are aware of the burden that caring for a disabled patient places on the family and other carers. The carer should be invited to discuss *their* problems. This is usually best done when the patient is absent since carers often feel uncomfortable or guilty when talking about *their* own problems if the patient is present. Indeed, carers often need a lot of encouragement to discuss their problems at all. However, they should be encouraged to do so not only for their own sake, but also for the patient's. If they are not coping this will adversely affect the patient.

It is important to assess the carer's physical and mental ability to go on providing the necessary care. If the patient is in hospital, it is often useful to get the carer to help with the patient's nursing care and attend their

therapy sessions. This gives the carer an indication of what caring may involve, it can help the carer and team members identify and hopefully resolve problems before discharge, and it provides a valuable opportunity to 'train' the carer. Pre-discharge visits home for a day or weekend fulfil similar functions. Carers may need physical or simply psychological support. A wide range of assessment tools have been developed to measure the amount of caregiving provided and the subjective burden this places on the caregiver (e.g. caregiver strain index).[430]

Prevention and treatment

Physical support is usually limited while the patient is in hospital, although some carers may need help with finances (section 11.33.6) and visiting. However, physical support is likely to become more important after the patient is discharged home. Examples include:
- providing help with housework to give the carer more time for providing personal care;
- providing a care assistant or district nurse to help with the patient's personal care;
- providing training in practical aspects of caring e.g. transfers, dressing;[431]
- providing a laundry service if the patient has persisting urinary or faecal incontinence;
- arranging for the patient to attend a day hospital or day centre, or arranging 'patient sitting' services to allow the carer to go shopping, have their hair done, or attend some social function; and
- arranging regular respite admissions to a hospital or nursing home to allow the carer to go on holiday, or simply to have a well-earned rest.

Table 11.56 Common questions asked by carers.

Acutely
What is a stroke?
Will they die?
Will they be disabled?
Why did this happen?
Was it my fault?
Will it happen again?
After hospital discharge
How long will they keep improving for?
Will their speech get better?
Why are they not the person I knew before?
Can I leave them alone to go out?
Can they exercise, will it bring on another stroke?
Will I always feel so tired?
Where can I get help with money?
Where can I get help with bathing?
Can I have a rest or holiday, i.e. respite?

Such services may be expensive but they probably prevent or delay the need for long-term institutional care which is even more expensive.

Psychological support: Carers often need help coming to terms with the changes in the person who has had a stroke. They have many questions and sources of concern (Table 11.56). Support is needed while the patient is in hospital and thereafter. It may take a variety of forms:

- an informal talk with the consultant, nurse, therapist or social worker; these are valuable opportunities for carers to ask questions;
- a carers' group where they can ask team members questions, share experiences and provide mutual support;
- formal sessions with a counsellor which may help them come to terms with their problems.[432]

The setting in which support is given needs to be tailored to the individual since, for example, not everybody wants to attend a group. The need for these sorts of services may not be apparent while patients are in hospital, or when they attend an outpatient department. Also, for patients who are not admitted after their stroke, or who remain in hospital for just a few days, the opportunities for the patient and their carer to ask questions and obtain advice are often limited. One approach is to provide a dedicated stroke family support worker who can identify the physical and emotional needs of patients and their families and try to meet them using all available resources. In many places this role is already, at least partially, carried out by social workers and other members of the team, but there are often difficulties in bridging the gap between hospital and community care. Although such support is valued by its recipients, its impact on patient and carer outcomes is unclear (section 17.8.2).

Giving information (section 17.10.1): Carers may know little about stroke, its causes and consequences and have often received misleading information from families and friends.[421] Carers, like patients, vary in the amount, type and format of information they want about stroke. Information-giving therefore needs to be tailored to the individual. Leaflets, audio or video tapes may usefully reinforce verbal transfer of information but more formal evaluation of their relative effectiveness is required. Education programmes appear to increase carers' knowledge and satisfaction with information received but not necessarily their emotional outcome.[432] It is important that patients and carers are given consistent information and advice to avoid confusion. Good communication between potential providers of information is therefore vital.

References

1 Houston JG, Morris AD, Grosset DG, Lees KR, McMillan N, Bone I. Ultrasonic evaluation of movement of the diaphragm after acute cerebral infarction. *J Neurol Neurosurg Psychiatry* 1995; 58(6):738–41.

2 Turkington PM, Bamford J, Wanklyn P, Elliott MW. Prevalence and predictors of upper airway obstruction in the first 24 hours after acute stroke. *Stroke* 2002; 33(8):2037–42.

3 Rowat AM, Dennis MS, Wardlaw JM. Hypoxaemia in acute stroke is frequent and worsens outcome. *Cerebrovascular Diseases* 2006; 21(3):166–72.

4 Tyson SF, Nightingale P. The effects of position on oxygen saturation in acute stroke: a systematic review. *Clin Rehabil* 2004; 18(8):863–71.

5 North JB, Jennett S. Abnormal breathing patterns associated with acute brain damage. *Arch Neurol* 1974; 31(5):338–44.

6 Turkington PM, Bamford J, Wanklyn P, Elliott MW. Effect of upper airway obstruction on blood pressure variability after stroke. *Clin Sci (Lond)* 2004; 107(1):75–9.

7 Bassetti CL, Milanova M, Gugger M. Sleep-disordered breathing and acute ischemic stroke: diagnosis, risk factors, treatment, evolution, and long-term clinical outcome. *Stroke* 2006; 37(4):967–72.

8 Rowat AM, Dennis MS, Wardlaw JM. Central periodic breathing observed on hospital admission is associated with an adverse prognosis in conscious acute stroke patients. *Cerebrovasc Dis* 2006; 21(5–6):340–7.

9 Naughton MT. Pathophysiology and treatment of Cheyne-Stokes respiration. *Thorax* 1998; 53(6):514–18.

10 Cherniack NS, Longobardo G, Evangelista CJ. Causes of Cheyne-Stokes respiration. *Neurocrit Care* 2005; 3(3):271–9.

11 Jensen LA, Onyskiw JE, Prasad NG. Meta-analysis of arterial oxygen saturation monitoring by pulse oximetry in adults. *Heart Lung* 1998; **27**(6):387–408.

12 Roffe C, Sills S, Wilde K, Crome P. Effect of hemiparetic stroke on pulse oximetry readings on the affected side. *Stroke* 2001; **32**(8):1808–10.

13 Ronning OM, Guldvog B. Should stroke victims routinely receive supplemental oxygen? A quasi-randomized controlled trial. *Stroke* 1999; **30**(10):2033–7.

14 Ali K, Sills S, Roffe C. The effect of different doses of oxygen administration on oxygen saturation in patients with stroke. *Neurocrit Care* 2005; **3**(1):24–6.

15 Wessendorf TE, Wang YM, Thilmann AF, Sorgenfrei U, Konietzko N, Teschler H. Treatment of obstructive sleep apnoea with nasal continuous positive airway pressure in stroke. *Eur Respir J* 2001; **18**(4):623–9.

16 White J, Cates C, Wright J. Continuous positive airways pressure for obstructive sleep apnoea. *Cochrane Database Syst Rev* 2002; (2):CD001106.

17 Hsu CY, Vennelle M, Li HY, Engleman HM, Dennis MS, Douglas NJ. Sleep disordered breathing after stroke. A randomized controlled trial of continuous positive airway pressure. *J Neurol Neurosurg Psychiatry* 2006; **77**(10): 1143–9.

18 Foerch C, Kessler KR, Steckel DA, Steinmetz H, Sitzer M. Survival and quality of life outcome after mechanical ventilation in elderly stroke patients. *J Neurol Neurosurg Psychiatry* 2004; **75**(7):988–93.

19 Rabinstein AA, Wijdicks EF. Outcome of survivors of acute stroke who require prolonged ventilatory assistance and tracheostomy. *Cerebrovasc Dis* 2004; **18**(4):325–31.

20 Schielke E, Busch MA, Hildenhagen T, Holtkamp M, Kuchler I, Harms L, Masuhr F. Functional, cognitive and emotional long-term outcome of patients with ischemic stroke requiring mechanical ventilation. *J Neurol* 2005; **252**(6):648–54.

21 Rem JA, Hachinski VC, Boughner DR, Barnett HJ. Value of cardiac monitoring and echocardiography in TIA and stroke patients. *Stroke* 1985; **16**(6):950–6.

22 Sandercock P, Bamford J, Dennis M, Burn J, Slattery J, Jones L *et al.* Atrial fibrillation and stroke: prevalence in different types of stroke and influence on early and long term prognosis (Oxfordshire community stroke project). *Br Med J* 1992; **305**(6867):1460–5.

23 Marini C, De Santis F, Sacco S, Russo T, Olivieri L, Totaro R, Carolei A. Contribution of atrial fibrillation to incidence and outcome of ischemic stroke: results from a population-based study. *Stroke* 2005; **36**(6):1115–19.

24 Sandercock PA, Warlow CP, Jones LN, Starkey IR. Predisposing factors for cerebral infarction: the Oxfordshire Community Stroke Project. *Br Med J* 1989; **298**(6666):75–80.

25 Shafqat S, Kelly PJ, Furie KL. Holter monitoring in the diagnosis of stroke mechanism. *Int Med J* 2004; **34**(6):305–9.

26 Jabaudon D, Sztajzel J, Sievert K, Landis T, Sztajzel R. Usefulness of ambulatory 7-day ECG monitoring for the detection of atrial fibrillation and flutter after acute stroke and transient ischemic attack. *Stroke* 2004; **35**(7):1647–51.

27 Fure B, Bruun WT, Thommessen B. Electrocardiographic and troponin T changes in acute ischaemic stroke. *J Int Med* 2006; **259**(6):592–7.

28 Khechinashvili G, Asplund K. Electrocardiographic changes in patients with acute stroke: a systematic review. *Cerebrovasc Dis* 2002; **14**(2):67–76.

29 Ay H, Arsava EM, Saribas O. Creatine kinase-MB elevation after stroke is not cardiac in origin: comparison with troponin T levels. *Stroke* 2002; **33**(1):286–9.

30 Dimant J, Grob D. Electrocardiographic changes and myocardial damage in patients with acute cerebrovascular accidents. *Stroke* 1977; **8**(4):448–55.

31 James P, Ellis CJ, Whitlock RM, McNeil AR, Henley J, Anderson NE. Relation between troponin T concentration and mortality in patients presenting with an acute stroke: observational study. *Br Med J* 2000; **320**(7248):1502–4.

32 Di Angelantonio E, Fiorelli M, Toni D, Sacchetti ML, Lorenzano S, Falcou A *et al.* Prognostic significance of admission levels of troponin I in patients with acute ischaemic stroke. *J Neurol Neurosurg Psychiatry* 2005; **76**(1):76–81.

33 Mooe T, Olofsson BO, Stegmayr B, Eriksson P. Ischemic stroke. Impact of a recent myocardial infarction. *Stroke* 1999; **30**(5):997–1001.

34 Davenport RJ, Dennis MS, Warlow CP. Gastrointestinal hemorrhage after acute stroke. *Stroke* 1996; **27**(3):421–4.

35 Kitamura T, Ito K. Acute gastric changes in patients with acute stroke. Part 1: with reference to gastroendoscopic findings. *Stroke* 1976; **7**(5):460–3.

36 Dennis MS, Lewis SC, Warlow C. Effect of timing and method of enteral tube feeding for dysphagic stroke patients (FOOD): a multicentre randomised controlled trial. *Lancet* 2005; **365**(9461):764–72.

37 Koch M, Dezi A, Ferrario F, Capurso I. Prevention of nonsteroidal anti-inflammatory drug-induced gastrointestinal mucosal injury: a meta-analysis of randomized controlled clinical trials. *Arch Intern Med* 1996; **156**(20):2321–32.

38 Rostom A, Dube C, Wells G, Tugwell P, Welch V, Jolicoeur E, McGowan J. Prevention of NSAID-induced gastroduodenal ulcers. *Cochrane Database Syst Rev* 2002; (4):CD002296.

39 Wang Y, Zeng C, Wu Z. Proton pump inhibitor and H_2RA pharmacological prevention of stress ulcer bleeding in stroke patients: a systematic review of randomized controlled trials. *Chinese J Evidence-based Med* 2006; **6**(2):107–16.

40 Plum F, Posner JB. Supratentorial lesions causing coma. In: Plum F, Posner JB, eds. *The Diagnosis of Stupor and Coma*. Philadelphia: FA Davis Company, 1980, pp. 134–6.

41 Parvizi J, Damasio AR. Neuroanatomical correlates of brainstem coma. *Brain* 2003; **126**(Pt 7):1524–36.

42 De MA, Melo TP, Crespo M, Ferro JM. Comas in the emergency room of a central hospital. *Acta Med Port* 1992; **5**(8):429–32.

43 Frank JI. Large hemispheric infarction, deterioration, and intracranial pressure. *Neurology* 1995; **45**(7):1286–90.

44 Weir CJ, Bradford AP, Lees KR. The prognostic value of the components of the Glasgow Coma Scale following acute stroke. *Q J Med* 2003; **96**(1):67–74.

45 Wijdicks EF, Kokmen E, O'Brien PC. Measurement of impaired consciousness in the neurological intensive care unit: a new test. *J Neurol Neurosurg Psychiatry* 1998; **64**(1):117–19.

46 Walther SM, Jonasson U, Gill H. Comparison of the Glasgow Coma Scale and the Reaction Level Scale for assessment of cerebral responsiveness in the critically ill. *Intensive Care Med* 2003; **29**(6):933–8.

47 Castillo J. Deteriorating stroke: diagnostic criteria, predictors, mechanisms and treatment. *Cerebrovasc Dis* 1999; **9** Suppl 3:1–8.

48 Scandinavian Stroke Study Group. Multicenter trial of hemodilution in ischemic stroke: background and study protocol. Scandinavian Stroke Study Group. *Stroke* 1985; **16**(5):885–90.

49 Birschel P, Ellul J, Barer D. Progressing stroke: towards an internationally agreed definition. *Cerebrovasc Dis* 2004; **17**(2–3):242–52.

50 Barber M, Stott DJ, Langhorne P. An internationally agreed definition of progressing stroke. *Cerebrovasc Dis* 2004; **18**(3):255–6.

51 Davalos A, Toni D, Iweins F, Lesaffre E, Bastianello S, Castillo J. Neurological deterioration in acute ischemic stroke: potential predictors and associated factors in the European cooperative acute stroke study (ECASS) I. *Stroke* 1999; **30**(12):2631–6.

52 Karepov VG, Gur AY, Bova I, Aronovich BD, Bornstein NM. Stroke-in-evolution: infarct-inherent mechanisms versus systemic causes. *Cerebrovasc Dis* 2006; **21**(1–2):42–6.

53 Barber M, Wright F, Stott DJ, Langhorne P. Predictors of early neurological deterioration after ischaemic stroke: a case-control study. *Gerontology* 2004; **50**(2):102–9.

54 Nakamura K, Saku Y, Ibayashi S, Fujishima M. Progressive motor deficits in lacunar infarction. *Neurology* 1999; **52**(1):29–33.

55 Castillo J, Noya M. [Mechanisms of progression of cerebral infarction]. *Neurologia* 1999; **14**(Suppl 2):2–12.

56 Barber M, Langhorne P, Rumley A, Lowe GD, Stott DJ. Hemostatic function and progressing ischemic stroke: D-dimer predicts early clinical progression. *Stroke* 2004; **35**(6):1421–5.

57 Barber M, Langhorne P, Rumley A, Lowe GD, Stott DJ. D-dimer predicts early clinical progression in ischemic stroke: confirmation using routine clinical assays. *Stroke* 2006; **37**(4):1113–15.

58 Davis M, Hollyman C, McGiven M, Chambers I, Egbuji J, Barer D. Physiological monitoring in acute stroke. *Age Ageing* 1999; **28**(Suppl 1):45.

59 Davenport RJ, Dennis MS, Warlow CP. Improving the recording of the clinical assessment of stroke patients using a clerking pro forma. *Age Ageing* 1995; **24**(1):43–8.

60 Rudd AG, Irwin P, Rutledge Z, Lowe D, Wade D, Morris R, Pearson MG. The national sentinel audit for stroke: a tool for raising standards of care. *J R Coll Physicians Lond* 1999; **33**(5):460–4.

61 Blood pressure in Acute Stroke Collaboration (BASC). Interventions for deliberately altering blood pressure in acute stroke [update of *Cochrane Database Syst Rev* 2000; (2):CD000039; PMID: 10796286]. *Cochrane Database Syst Rev* 2001; (3):CD000039.

62 Harper G, Castleden CM, Potter JF. Factors affecting changes in blood pressure after acute stroke. *Stroke* 1994; **25**(9):1726–9.

63 Abboud H, Labreuche J, Plouin F, Amarenco P, GENIC I. High blood pressure in early acute stroke: a sign of a poor outcome? *J Hypertens* 2006; **24**(2):381–6.

64 Aslanyan S, Weir CJ, Lees KR. Elevated pulse pressure during the acute period of ischemic stroke is associated with poor stroke outcome. *Stroke* 2004; **35**(6):e153–e155.

65 Jensen MB, Yoo B, Clarke WR, Davis PH, Adams HR, Jr. Blood pressure as an independent prognostic factor in acute ischemic stroke. *Can J Neurol Sci* 2006; **33**(1):34–8.

66 Leonardi-Bee J, Bath PM, Phillips SJ, Sandercock PA. Blood pressure and clinical outcomes in the International Stroke Trial. *Stroke* 2002; **33**(5):1315–20.

67 Rodriguez-Garcia JL, Botia E, de La Sierra A, Villanueva MA, Gonzalez-Spinola J. Significance of elevated blood pressure and its management on the short-term outcome of patients with acute ischemic stroke. *Am J Hypertens* 2005; **18**(3):379–84.

68 Willmot M, Leonardi-Bee J, Bath PM. High blood pressure in acute stroke and subsequent outcome: a systematic review. *Hypertension* 2004; **43**(1):18–24.

69 White WB, Anwar YA. Evaluation of the overall efficacy of the Omron office digital blood pressure HEM-907 monitor in adults. *Blood Press Monit* 2001; **6**(2):107–10.

70 Sykes D, Dewar R, Mohanaruban K, Donovan K, Nicklason F, Thomas DM, Fisher D. Measuring blood pressure in the elderly: does atrial fibrillation increase observer variability? *Br Med J* 1990; **300**(6718):162–3.

71 Stewart MJ, Gough K, Padfield PL. The accuracy of automated blood pressure measuring devices in patients with controlled atrial fibrillation. *J Hypertens* 1995; **13**(3):297–300.

72 Panayiotou BN, Harper GD, Fotherby MD, Potter JF, Castleden CM. Interarm blood pressure difference in acute hemiplegia. *J Am Geriatr Soc* 1993; **41**(4):422–3.

73 Bath P, Chalmers J, Powers W, Beilin L, Davis S, Lenfant C *et al.* International Society of Hypertension (ISH): statement on the management of blood pressure in acute stroke. *J Hypertens* 2003; **21**(4):665–72.

74 Horn J, Limburg M. Calcium antagonists for acute ischemic stroke. *Cochrane Database Syst Rev* 2000; (2):CD001928.

75 Eames PJ, Robinson TG, Panerai RB, Potter JF. The systemic haemodynamic and cerebral autoregulatory effects of bendrofluazide in the subacute post-stroke period. *J Hypertens* 2004; **22**(10):2017–24.

76 Eames PJ, Robinson TG, Panerai RB, Potter JF. Bendrofluazide fails to reduce elevated blood pressure

levels in the immediate post-stroke period. *Cerebrovascular Diseases* 2005; **19**(4):253–9.

77 Willmot M, Ghadami A, Whysall B, Clarke W, Wardlaw J, Bath PM. Transdermal glyceryl trinitrate lowers blood pressure and maintains cerebral blood flow in recent stroke [see comment]. *Hypertension* 2006; **47**(6):1209–15.

78 Mistri AK, Robinson TG, Potter JF. Pressor therapy in acute ischemic stroke: systematic review. *Stroke* 2006; **37**(6):1565–71.

79 Camilo O, Goldstein LB. Seizures and epilepsy after ischemic stroke. *Stroke* 2004; **35**(7):1769–75.

80 Burn J, Dennis M, Bamford J, Sandercock P, Wade D, Warlow C. Epileptic seizures after a first stroke: the Oxfordshire Community Stroke Project. *Br Med J* 1997; **315**(7122):1582–7.

81 Kelso ARC, Cock HR. Status epilepticus. *Pract Neurol* 2006; **5**(6):322–33.

82 Marson AG, Williamson PR, Hutton JL, Clough HE, Chadwick DW. Carbamazepine versus valproate monotherapy for epilepsy. *Cochrane Database Syst Rev* 2000; (3):CD001030.

83 Tudur SC, Marson AG, Clough HE, Williamson PR. Carbamazepine versus phenytoin monotherapy for epilepsy. *Cochrane Database Syst Rev* 2002; (2):CD001911.

84 Canhao P, Melo TP, Salgado AV. Nausea and vomiting in acute ischemic stroke. *Cerebrovasc Dis* 1997; **7**:220–5.

85 Ferro JM, Melo TP, Oliveira V, Salgado AV, Crespo M, Canhao P, Pinto AN. A multivariate study of headache associated with ischemic stroke. *Headache* 1995; **35**(6):315–19.

86 Arboix A, Garcia-Trallero O, Garcia-Eroles L, Massons J, Comes E, Targa C. Stroke-related headache: a clinical study in lacunar infarction. *Headache* 2005; **45**(10):1345–52.

87 Mitsias PD, Ramadan NM, Levine SR, Schultz L, Welch KM. Factors determining headache at onset of acute ischemic stroke. *Cephalalgia* 2006; **26**(2):150–7.

88 Tentschert S, Wimmer R, Greisenegger S, Lang W, Lalouschek W. Headache at stroke onset in 2196 patients with ischemic stroke or transient ischemic attack. *Stroke* 2005; **36**(2):e1–3.

89 Kumar A, Dromerick AW. Intractable hiccups during stroke rehabilitation. *Arch Phys Med Rehabil* 1998; **79**(6):697–9.

90 Schiff E, River Y, Oliven A, Odeh M. Acupuncture therapy for persistent hiccups. *Am J Med Sci* 2002; **323**(3):166–8.

91 Moretti R, Torre P, Antonello RM, Ukmar M, Cazzato G, Bava A. Gabapentin as a drug therapy of intractable hiccup because of vascular lesion: a three-year follow-up. *Neurologist* 2004; **10**(2):102–6.

92 Bhalla A, Tallis RC, Pomeroy VM. The effects of positioning after stroke on physiological homeostasis: a review. *Age Ageing* 2005; **34**(4):401–6.

93 Barr J, Stocks J, Wagstaff S, Dey P. Positional interventions for acute stroke patients. (Protocol). *Cochrane Database System Rev* 2004; (4).

94 Drakulovic MB, Torres A, Bauer TT, Nicolas JM, Nogue S, Ferrer M. Supine body position as a risk factor for nosocomial pneumonia in mechanically ventilated patients: a randomised trial. *Lancet* 1999; **354**(9193):1851–8.

95 Rowat AM, Wardlaw JM, Dennis MS, Warlow CP. Patient positioning influences oxygen saturation in the acute phase of stroke. *Cerebrovasc Dis* 2001; **12**(1):66–72.

96 Wojner-Alexander AW, Garami Z, Chernyshev OY, Alexandrov AV. Heads down: flat positioning improves blood flow velocity in acute ischemic stroke. *Neurology* 2005; **64**(8):1354–7.

97 Wojner AW, El-Mitwalli A, Alexandrov AV. Effect of head positioning on intracranial blood flow velocities in acute ischemic stroke: a pilot study. *Crit Care Nurs Q* 2002; **24**(4):57–66.

98 Feldman Z, Kanter MJ, Robertson CS, Contant CF, Hayes C, Sheinberg MA *et al.* Effect of head elevation on intracranial pressure, cerebral perfusion pressure, and cerebral blood flow in head-injured patients. *J Neurosurg* 1992; **76**(2):207–11.

99 Fleuren JF, Nederhand MJ, Hermens HJ. Influence of posture and muscle length on stretch reflex activity in poststroke patients with spasticity. *Arch Phys Med Rehabil* 2006; **87**(7):981–8.

100 Chatterton HJ, Pomeroy VM, Gratton J. Positioning for stroke patients: a survey of physiotherapists' aims and practices. *Disabil Rehabil* 2001; **23**(10):413–21.

101 Jones A, Tilling K, Wilson-Barnett J, Newham DJ, Wolfe CD. Effect of recommended positioning on stroke outcome at six months: a randomized controlled trial. *Clin Rehabil* 2005; **19**(2):138–45.

102 Kammersgaard LP, Jorgensen HS, Rungby JA, Reith J, Nakayama H, Weber UJ *et al.* Admission body temperature predicts long-term mortality after acute stroke: the Copenhagen Stroke Study. *Stroke* 2002; **33**(7):1759–62.

103 Hajat C, Hajat S, Sharma P. Effects of poststroke pyrexia on stroke outcome: a meta-analysis of studies in patients. *Stroke* 2000; **31**(2):410–14.

104 Corbett D, Thornhill J. Temperature modulation (hypothermic and hyperthermic conditions) and its influence on histological and behavioral outcomes following cerebral ischemia. *Brain Pathol* 2000; **10**(1):145–52.

105 Langhorne P, Stott DJ, Robertson L, MacDonald J, Jones L, McAlpine C *et al.* Medical complications after stroke: a multicenter study. *Stroke* 2000; **31**(6):1223–9.

106 Meisel C, Schwab JM, Prass K, Meisel A, Dirnagl U. Central nervous system injury-induced immune deficiency syndrome. *Nature Reviews Neuroscience* 2005; **6**(10):775–86.

107 Schwab JM, Prass K, Meisel A. Secondary immune deficiency after CNS injury: characteristics, pathophysiology and clinical implications. *Neuroform* 2005; **11**(1):5–13.

108 Aslanyan S, Weir CJ, Diener HC, Kaste M, Lees KR. Pneumonia and urinary tract infection after acute ischaemic stroke: a tertiary analysis of the GAIN International trial. *Eur J Neurol* 2004; **11**(1):49–53.

109 Khedr EM, El SO, Khedr T, bdel aziz aY, Awad EM. Assessment of corticodiaphragmatic pathway and pulmonary function in acute ischemic stroke patients. *Eur J Neurol* 2000; **7**(5):509–16.

110 Millns B, Gosney M, Jack CI, Martin MV, Wright AE. Acute stroke predisposes to oral Gram-negative bacilli: a cause of aspiration pneumonia? *Gerontology* 2003; **49**(3):173–6.

111 Leibovitz A, Plotnikov G, Habot B, Rosenberg M, Wolf A, Nagler R *et al.* Saliva secretion and oral flora in prolonged nasogastric tube-fed elderly patients. *Isr Med Assoc J* 2003; **5**(5):329–32.

112 Leibovitz A, Plotnikov G, Habot B, Rosenberg M, Segal R. Pathogenic colonization of oral flora in frail elderly patients fed by nasogastric tube or percutaneous enterogastric tube. *J Gerontol A Biol Sci Med Sci* 2003; **58**(1):52–5.

113 Gosney M, Martin MV, Wright AE. The role of selective decontamination of the digestive tract in acute stroke. *Age Ageing* 2006; **35**(1):42–7.

114 Dromerick AW, Edwards DF. Relation of postvoid residual to urinary tract infection during stroke rehabilitation. *Arch Phys Med Rehab* 2003; **84**(9):1369–72.

115 Niel-Weise BS, van den Broek PJ. Antibiotic policies for short-term catheter bladder drainage in adults. *Cochrane Database Syst Rev* 2005; (3):CD005428.

116 Niel-Weise BS, van den Broek PJ. Urinary catheter policies for short-term bladder drainage in adults. *Cochrane Database Syst Rev* 2005; (3):CD004203.

117 Niel-Weise BS, van den Broek PJ. Urinary catheter policies for long-term bladder drainage. *Cochrane Database Syst Rev* 2005; (1):CD004201.

118 Berger RE. The urine dipstick test useful to rule out infections: a meta-analysis of the accuracy. *J Urol* 2005; **174**(3):941–2.

119 Correia M, Silva M, Veloso M. Cooling therapy for acute stroke. *Cochrane Database Syst Rev* 2000; (2):CD001247.

120 Chamorro A, Horcajada JP, Obach V, Vargas M, Revilla M, Torres F *et al.* The early systemic prophylaxis of infection after stroke study: A randomized clinical trial. *Stroke* 2005; **36**(7):1495–500.

121 Vargas M, Horcajada JP, Obach V, Revilla M, Cervera A, Torres F *et al.* Clinical consequences of infection in patients with acute stroke: is it prime time for further antibiotic trials? *Stroke* 2006; **37**(2):461–5.

122 Davey P, Brown E, Fenelon L, Finch R, Gould I, Holmes A *et al.* Systematic review of antimicrobial drug prescribing in hospitals. *Emerg Infect Dis* 2006; **12**(2):211–16.

123 Kelly J, Rudd A, Lewis RR, Coshall C, Moody A, Hunt BJ. Venous thromboembolism after acute ischemic stroke: a prospective study using magnetic resonance direct thrombus imaging. *Stroke* 2004; **35**(10):2320–5.

124 De Silva DA, Pey HB, Wong MC, Chang HM, Chen CP. Deep vein thrombosis following ischemic stroke among Asians. *Cerebrovasc Dis* 2006; **22**(4):245–50.

125 Warlow C, Ogston D, Douglas AS. Deep venous thrombosis of the legs after strokes. Part I: incidence and predisposing factors. *Br Med J* 1976; **1**(6019):1178–81.

126 Zierler BK. Screening for acute DVT: optimal utilization of the vascular diagnostic laboratory. *Semin Vasc Surg* 2001; **14**(3):206–14.

127 Sachdev U, Teodorescu VJ, Shao M, Russo T, Jacobs TS, Silverberg D *et al.* Incidence and distribution of lower extremity deep vein thrombosis in rehabilitation patients: implications for screening. *Vasc Endovascular Surg* 2006; **40**(3):205–11.

128 Kassai B, Boissel JP, Cucherat M, Sonie S, Shah NR, Leizorovicz A. A systematic review of the accuracy of ultrasound in the diagnosis of deep venous thrombosis in asymptomatic patients. *Thromb Haemost* 2004; **91**(4):655–66.

129 Kelly J, Rudd A, Lewis RR, Coshall C, Parmar K, Moody A, Hunt BJ. Screening for proximal deep vein thrombosis after acute ischemic stroke: a prospective study using clinical factors and plasma D-dimers. *J Thromb Haemost* 2004; **2**(8):1321–6.

130 British Thoracic Society guidelines for the management of suspected acute pulmonary embolism. *Thorax* 2003; **58**(6):470–83.

131 Kelly J, Hunt BJ, Lewis RR, Swaminathan R, Moody A, Seed PT, Rudd A. Dehydration and venous thromboembolism after acute stroke. *Q J Med* 2004; **97**(5):293–6.

132 Asplund K, Israelsson K, Schampi I. Haemodilution for acute ischaemic stroke. *Cochrane Database Syst Rev* 2000; (2):CD000103.

133 Amaragiri SV, Lees TA. Elastic compression stockings for prevention of deep vein thrombosis. *Cochrane Database Syst Rev* 2000; (3):CD001484.

134 Roderick P, Ferris G, Wilson K, Halls H, Jackson D, Collins R, Baigent C. Towards evidence-based guidelines for the prevention of venous thromboembolism: systematic reviews of mechanical methods, oral anticoagulation, dextran and regional anaesthesia as thromboprophylaxis. *Health Technol Assess* 2005; **9**(49):iii–x, 1.

135 Mazzone C, Chiodo GF, Sandercock P, Miccio M, Salvi R. Physical methods for preventing deep vein thrombosis in stroke. *Cochrane Database Syst Rev* 2004; (4):CD001922.

136 Sandercock P, Gubitz G, Foley P, Counsell C. Antiplatelet therapy for acute ischaemic stroke. *Cochrane Database Syst Rev* 2003; (2):CD000029.

137 Gubitz G, Sandercock P, Counsell C. Anticoagulants for acute ischaemic stroke. *Cochrane Database Syst Rev* 2004; (3):CD000024.

138 Lacut K, Bressollette L, Le Gal G, Etienne E, De Tinteniac A, Renault A *et al.* VICTORIAh (Venous Intermittent Compression and Thrombosis Occurrence Related to Intracerebral Acute hemorrhage) Investigators. Prevention of venous thrombosis in patients with acute intracerebral hemorrhage. *Neurology* 2005; **65**(6):865–9.

139 Van Dongen CJ, van den Belt AG, Prins MH, Lensing AW. Fixed dose subcutaneous low molecular weight heparins versus adjusted dose unfractionated heparin for venous

thromboembolism. *Cochrane Database Syst Rev* 2004;
(4):CD001100.

140 Sandercock P, Counsell C, Stobbs SL. Low-molecular-weight heparins or heparinoids versus standard unfractionated heparin for acute ischaemic stroke. *Cochrane Database Syst Rev* 2005; (2):CD000119.

141 Van den Belt AG, Prins MH, Lensing AW, Castro AA, Clark OA, Atallah AN, Burihan E. Fixed dose subcutaneous low molecular weight heparins versus adjusted dose unfractionated heparin for venous thromboembolism. *Cochrane Database Syst Rev* 2000; (2):CD001100.

142 Righini M, Paris S, Le Gal G, Laroche JP, Perrier A, Bounameaux H. Clinical relevance of distal deep vein thrombosis. Review of literature data. *Thromb Haemost* 2006; **95**(1):56–64.

143 Ost D, Tepper J, Mihara H, Lander O, Heinzer R, Fein A. Duration of anticoagulation following venous thromboembolism: a meta-analysis. *J Am Med Assoc* 2005; **294**(6):706–15.

144 Kelly J, Hunt BJ, Lewis RR, Rudd A. Anticoagulation or inferior vena cava filter placement for patients with primary intracerebral hemorrhage developing venous thromboembolism? *Stroke* 2003; **34**(12):2999–3005.

145 Nakayama H, Jorgensen HS, Pedersen PM, Raaschou HO, Olsen TS. Prevalence and risk factors of incontinence after stroke. The Copenhagen Stroke Study. *Stroke* 1997; **28**(1):58–62.

146 Brittain KR, Peet SM, Castleden CM. Stroke and incontinence. *Stroke* 1998; 29(2):524–8.

147 Kolominsky-Rabas PL, Hilz MJ, Neundoerfer B, Heuschmann PU. Impact of urinary incontinence after stroke: results from a prospective population-based stroke register; [see comment]. *Neurourol Urodyn* 2003; **22**(4):322–7.

148 Brittain KR, Castleden CM. Suicide in patients with stroke. Depression may be caused by symptoms affecting lower urinary tract. *Br Med J* 1998; **317**(7164):1016–17.

149 Patel M, Coshall C, Lawrence E, Rudd AG, Wolfe CD. Recovery from poststroke urinary incontinence: associated factors and impact on outcome. *J Am Geriatr Soc* 2001; **49**(9):1229–33.

150 Patel M, Coshall C, Rudd AG, Wolfe CD. Natural history and effects on 2-year outcomes of urinary incontinence after stroke. *Stroke* 2001; **32**(1):122–7.

151 Thomas LH, Barrett J, Cross S, French B, Leathley M, Sutton C, Watkins C. Prevention and treatment of urinary incontinence after stroke in adults. *Cochrane Database Syst Rev* 2005; (3):CD004462.

152 Hay-Smith J, Herbison P, Ellis G, Moore K. Anticholinergic drugs versus placebo for overactive bladder syndrome in adults. *Cochrane Database Syst Rev* 2002; (3):CD003781.

153 Khorsandi M, Ginsberg PC, Harkaway RC. Reassessing the role of urodynamics after cerebrovascular accident. Males versus females. *Urol Int* 1998; **61**(3):142–6.

154 Shirran E, Brazzelli M. Absorbent products for the containment of urinary and/or faecal incontinence in adults. *Cochrane Database Syst Rev* 2000; (2):CD001406.

155 Brosnahan J, Jull A, Tracy C. Types of urethral catheters for management of short-term voiding problems in hospitalised adults. *Cochrane Database Syst Rev* 2004; (1):CD004013.

156 Wu J, Baguley IJ. Urinary retention in a general rehabilitation unit: prevalence, clinical outcome, and the role of screening. *Arch Phys Med Rehabil* 2005; **86**(9):1772–7.

157 Harari D, Coshall C, Rudd AG, Wolfe CD. New-onset fecal incontinence after stroke: prevalence, natural history, risk factors, and impact. *Stroke* 2003; **34**(1):144–50.

158 Coggrave M, Wiesel PH, Norton C. Management of faecal incontinence and constipation in adults with central neurological diseases. *Cochrane Database Syst Rev* 2006; (2):CD002115.

159 Berlowitz DR, Wilking SV. Risk factors for pressure sores. A comparison of cross-sectional and cohort-derived data. *J Am Geriatr Soc* 1989; **37**(11):1043–50.

160 Cullum N, McInnes E, Bell-Syer SE, Legood R. Support surfaces for pressure ulcer prevention. *Cochrane Database Syst Rev* 2004; (3):CD001735.

161 Pancorbo-Hidalgo PL, Garcia-Fernandez FP, Lopez-Medina IM, Varez-Nieto C. Risk assessment scales for pressure ulcer prevention: a systematic review. *J Adv Nurs* 2006; **54**(1):94–110.

162 Allman RM, Walker JM, Hart MK, Laprade CA, Noel LB, Smith CR. Air-fluidized beds or conventional therapy for pressure sores. A randomized trial. *Ann Intern Med* 1987; **107**(5):641–8.

163 McQueen J, MacLennan K, McDiarmid M, Gold S. Educational interventions for healthcare professionals to prevent pressure ulcers. (Protocol). *Cochrane Database of Syst Rev* 2005; (2).

164 Langer G, Schloemer G, Knerr A, Kuss O, Behrens J. Nutritional interventions for preventing and treating pressure ulcers. *Cochrane Database Syst Rev* 2003; (4):CD003216.

165 Cullum N, Deeks J, Sheldon TA, Song F, Fletcher AW. Beds, mattresses and cushions for pressure sore prevention and treatment. *Cochrane Database Syst Rev* 2000; (2):CD001735.

166 Flemming K, Cullum N. Therapeutic ultrasound for pressure sores. *Cochrane Database Syst Rev* 2000; (4):CD001275.

167 Flemming K, Cullum N. Electromagnetic therapy for the treatment of pressure sores. *Cochrane Database Syst Rev* 2001; (1):CD002930.

168 Singh S, Hamdy S. Dysphagia in stroke patients. *Postgrad Med J* 2006; **82**(968):383–91.

169 Mann G, Hankey GJ, Cameron D. Swallowing function after stroke: prognosis and prognostic factors at 6 months. *Stroke* 1999; **30**(4):744–8.

170 Veis SL, Logemann JA. Swallowing disorders in persons with cerebrovascular accident. *Arch Phys Med Rehabil* 1985; **66**(6):372–5.

171 Scottish Intercollegiate Guidelines Network. *Management of Patients with Stroke: Identification and Management of Dysphagia*. SIGN Guideline 78. Scottish Intercollegiate Guidelines Network, 2004.

172 Hinchey JA, Shephard T, Furie K, Smith D, Wang D, Tonn S. Formal dysphagia screening protocols prevent pneumonia. *Stroke* 2005; **36**(9):1972–6.

173 Huang JY, Zhang DY, Yao Y, Xia QX, Fan QQ. Training in swallowing prevents aspiration pneumonia in stroke patients with dysphagia. *J Int Med Res* 2006; **34**(3):303–6.

174 Ramsey D, Smithard D, Donaldson N, Kalra L. Is the gag reflex useful in the management of swallowing problems in acute stroke? *Dysphagia* 2005; **20**(2):105–7.

175 Ramsey D, Smithard D, Kalra L. Silent aspiration: what do we know? *Dysphagia* 2005; **20**(3):218–25.

176 Ramsey DJ, Smithard DG, Kalra L. Early assessments of dysphagia and aspiration risk in acute stroke patients. *Stroke* 2003; **34**(5):1252–7.

177 Addington WR, Stephens RE, Gilliland KA. Assessing the laryngeal cough reflex and the risk of developing pneumonia after stroke: an interhospital comparison. *Stroke* 1999; **30**(6):1203–7.

178 Addington WR, Stephens RE, Gilliland K, Rodriguez M. Assessing the laryngeal cough reflex and the risk of developing pneumonia after stroke. *Arch Phys Med Rehabil* 1999; **80**(2):150–4.

179 Smithard DG, O'Neill PA, Park C, England R, Renwick DS, Wyatt R *et al*. Can bedside assessment reliably exclude aspiration following acute stroke? *Age Ageing* 1998; **27**(2):99–106.

180 Carnaby G, Hankey GJ, Pizzi J. Behavioural intervention for dysphagia in acute stroke: a randomised controlled trial. *Lancet Neurol* 2006; **5**(1):31–7.

181 Dennis M. Dysphagia in acute stroke: a long-awaited trial. *Lancet Neurol* 2006; **5**(1):16–17.

182 Power ML, Fraser CH, Hobson A, Singh S, Tyrrell P, Nicholson DA *et al*. Evaluating oral stimulation as a treatment for dysphagia after stroke. *Dysphagia* 2006; **21**(1):49–55.

183 Berkovic SF, Bladin PF, Darby DG. Metabolic disorders presenting as stroke. *Med J Aust* 1984; **140**(7):421–4.

184 O'Neill PA, McLean KA. Water homeostasis and ageing. *Med Lab Sci* 1992; **49**(4):291–8.

185 Churchill M, Grimm S, Reding M. Risks of diuretic usage following stroke. *Neurorehabil Neural Repair* 2004; **18**(3):161–5.

186 Whelan K. Inadequate fluid intakes in dysphagic acute stroke. *Clin Nutr* 2001; **20**(5):423–8.

187 Bhalla A, Sankaralingam S, Dundas R, Swaminathan R, Wolfe CD, Rudd AG. Influence of raised plasma osmolality on clinical outcome after acute stroke. *Stroke* 2000; **31**(9):2043–8.

188 Gross CR, Lindquist RD, Woolley AC, Granieri R, Allard K, Webster B. Clinical indicators of dehydration severity in elderly patients. *J Emerg Med* 1992; **10**(3):267–74.

189 Kavouras SA. Assessing hydration status. *Curr Opin Clin Nutr Metab Care* 2002; **5**(5):519–24.

190 Challiner YC, Jarrett D, Hayward MJ, al-Jubouri MA, Julious SA. A comparison of intravenous and subcutaneous hydration in elderly acute stroke patients. *Postgrad Med J* 1994; **70**(821):195–7.

191 O'Neill PA, Davies I, Fullerton KJ, Bennett D. Fluid balance in elderly patients following acute stroke. *Age Ageing* 1992; **21**(4):280–5.

192 Joynt RJ, Feibel JH, Sladek CM. Antidiuretic hormone levels in stroke patients. *Ann Neurol* 1981; **9**(2):182–4.

193 Kumar S, Fowler M, Gonzalez-Toledo E, Jaffe SL. Central pontine myelinolysis, an update. *Neurol Res* 2006; **28**(3):360–6.

194 Capes SE, Hunt D, Malmberg K, Pathak P, Gerstein HC. Stress hyperglycemia and prognosis of stroke in nondiabetic and diabetic patients: a systematic overview. *Stroke* 2001; **32**(10):2426–32.

195 Van Kooten F, Hoogerbrugge N, Naarding P, Koudstaal PJ. Hyperglycemia in the acute phase of stroke is not caused by stress. *Stroke* 1993; **24**(8):1129–32.

196 Scott JF, Gray CS, O'Connell JE, Alberti KG. Glucose and insulin therapy in acute stroke: why delay further? *Q J Med* 1998; **91**(7):511–15.

197 Kagansky N, Levy S, Knobler H. The role of hyperglycemia in acute stroke. *Arch Neurol* 2001; **58**(8):1209–12.

198 Garg R, Chaudhuri A, Munschauer F, Dandona P. Hyperglycemia, insulin, and acute ischemic stroke: a mechanistic justification for a trial of insulin infusion therapy. *Stroke* 2006; **37**(1):267–73.

199 Gray CS, Hildreth AJ, Alberti GK, O'Connell JE, Collaboration GIST. Poststroke hyperglycemia: natural history and immediate management. [see comment] [erratum appears in *Stroke* 2004; **35**(5):1229]. *Stroke* 2004; **35**(1):122–6.

200 Gray CS, Hildrett AJ, Sandercoat PA, O'Connell JE, Johnston DE, Cartlidge NEF *et al*., For the GIST Trialists collaboration. Glucose–potassium–insulin infusions in the management of post-stroke hyperglycaemia: the UK Glucose Insulin in Stroke Trial (GIST–UK). *Lancet Neurol* 2007; **6**(5): 397–406.

201 Abarbanell NR. Is prehospital blood glucose measurement necessary in suspected cerebrovascular accident patients? *Am J Emerg Med* 2005; **23**(7):823–7.

202 Sullivan DH, Sun S, Walls RC. Protein-energy undernutrition among elderly hospitalized patients: a prospective study. *J Am Med Assoc* 1999; **281**(21):2013–19.

203 Unosson M, Ek AC, Bjurulf P, von Schenck H, Larsson J. Feeding dependence and nutritional status after acute stroke. *Stroke* 1994; **25**(2):366–71.

204 Choi-Kwon S, Yang YH, Kim EK, Jeon MY, Kim JS. Nutritional status in acute stroke: undernutrition versus overnutrition in different stroke subtypes. *Acta Neurol Scand* 1998; **98**(3):187–92.

205 Smithard DG, O'Neill PA, Parks C, Morris J. Complications and outcome after acute stroke. Does dysphagia matter? *Stroke* 1996; **27**(7):1200–4.

206 Gariballa SE, Parker SG, Taub N, Castleden CM. Influence of nutritional status on clinical outcome after acute stroke. *Am J Clin Nutr* 1998; **68**(2):275–81.

207 Bardutzky J, Georgiadis D, Kollmar R, Schwarz S, Schwab S. Energy demand in patients with stroke who are sedated and receiving mechanical ventilation. *J Neurosurg* 2004; **100**(2):266–71.

208 Chalela JA, Haymore J, Schellinger PD, Kang DW, Warach S. Acute stroke patients are being underfed: a nitrogen balance study. [see comment.] *Neurocrit Care* 2004; **1**(3):331–4.

209 Heckmann JG, Stossel C, Lang CJ, Neundorfer B, Tomandl B, Hummel T. Taste disorders in acute stroke: a prospective observational study on taste disorders in 102 stroke patients. *Stroke* 2005; **36**(8):1690–4.

210 Poor nutritional status on admission predicts poor outcomes after stroke: observational data from the FOOD trial. *Stroke* 2003; **34**(6):1450–6.

211 Martineau J, Bauer JD, Isenring E, Cohen S. Malnutrition determined by the patient-generated subjective global assessment is associated with poor outcomes in acute stroke patients. *Clin Nutr* 2005; **24**(6):1073–7.

212 Dennis MS, Lewis SC, Warlow C. Routine oral nutritional supplementation for stroke patients in hospital (FOOD): a multicentre randomised controlled trial. *Lancet* 2005; **365**(9461):755–63.

213 Thorsdottir I, Jonsson PV, Asgeirsdottir AE, Hjaltadottir I, Bjornsson S, Ramel A. Fast and simple screening for nutritional status in hospitalized, elderly people. *J Hum Nutr Diet* 2005; **18**(1):53–60.

214 Arrowsmith H. A critical evaluation of the use of nutrition screening tools by nurses. *Br J Nurs* 1999; **8**(22):1483–90.

215 Mead GE, Donaldson L, North P, Dennis MS. An informal assessment of nutritional status in acute stroke for use in an international multicentre trial of feeding regimens. *Int J Clin Pract* 1998; **52**(5):316–18.

216 Coombes R. NHS safety agency issues guidance on nasogastric tubes. *Br Med J* 2005; 330:438.

217 Wanklyn P, Cox N, Belfield P. Outcome in patients who require a gastrostomy after stroke. *Age Ageing* 1995; **24**(6):510–14.

218 Norton B, Homer-Ward M, Donnelly MT, Long RG, Holmes GK. A randomised prospective comparison of percutaneous endoscopic gastrostomy and nasogastric tube feeding after acute dysphagic stroke. *Br Med J* 1996; **312**(7022):13–16.

219 James A, Kapur K, Hawthorne AB. Long-term outcome of percutaneous endoscopic gastrostomy feeding in patients with dysphagic stroke. *Age Ageing* 1998; **27**(6):671–6.

220 Skelly R, Terry H, Millar E, Cohen D. Outcomes of percutaneous endoscopic gastrostomy feeding. *Age Ageing* 1999; **28**(4):416.

221 Wijdicks EF, McMahon MM. Percutaneous endoscopic gastrostomy after acute stroke: complications and outcome. *Cerebrovasc Dis* 1999; **9**(2):109–11.

222 Teasell R, Foley N, McRae M, Finestone H. Use of percutaneous gastrojejunostomy feeding tubes in the rehabilitation of stroke patients. *Arch Phys Med Rehabil* 2001; **82**(10):1412–15.

223 Leathley MJ, Gregson JM, Moore AP, Smith TL, Sharma AK, Watkins CL. Predicting spasticity after stroke in those surviving to 12 months. *Clin Rehabil* 2004; **18**(4):438–43.

224 Sommerfeld DK, Eek EU, Svensson AK, Holmqvist LW, Von Arbin MH. Spasticity after stroke: its occurrence and association with motor impairments and activity limitations. *Stroke* 2004; **35**(1):134–9.

225 Welmer AK, von Arbin M, Widen HL, Sommerfeld DK. Spasticity and its association with functioning and health-related quality of life 18 months after stroke. *Cerebrovasc Dis* 2006; **21**(4):247–53.

226 Bhakta BB, Cozens JA, Chamberlain MA, Bamford JM. Quantifying associated reactions in the paretic arm in stroke and their relationship to spasticity. *Clin Rehabil* 2001; **15**(2):195–206.

227 Gregson JM, Leathley MJ, Moore AP, Smith TL, Sharma AK, Watkins CL. Reliability of measurements of muscle tone and muscle power in stroke patients. *Age Ageing* 2000; **29**(3):223–8.

228 Ada L, Goddard E, McCully J, Stavrinos T, Bampton J. Thirty minutes of positioning reduces the development of shoulder external rotation contracture after stroke: a randomized controlled trial. *Arch Phys Med Rehabil* 2005; **86**(2):230–4.

229 Carr EK, Kenney FD. Positioning of the stroke patient: a review of the literature. *Int J Nurs Stud* 1992; **29**(4):355–69.

230 Brown RA, Holdsworth L, Leslie GC, Mutch WJ, Part NJ. The effects of time after stroke and selected therapeutic techniques on quadriceps muscle tone in stroke patients. *Physiother Theory Pract* 1993; **9**:131–42.

231 Cornall C. Self propelling wheelchairs: the effect on spasticity in hemiplegic patients. *Physiother Theory Pract* 1991; **7**:13–21.

232 Barrett JA, Watkins C, Plant R, Dickenson H, Clayton L, Sharma AK *et al.* The COSTAR wheelchair study: a two-centre pilot study of self-propulsion in a wheelchair in early stroke rehabilitation. Collaborative Stroke Audit and Research. *Clin Rehabil* 2001; **15**(1):32–41.

233 Barnes MP. Management of spasticity. *Age Ageing* 1998; **27**(2):239–45.

234 Walton K. Management of patients with spasticity: a practical approach. *Pract Neurol* 2006; **3**:342–53.

235 Gallichio JE. Pharmacologic management of spasticity following stroke. *Phys Ther* 2004; **84**(10):973–81.

236 Bhakta BB, Cozens JA, Chamberlain MA, Bamford JM. Impact of botulinum toxin type A on disability and carer burden due to arm spasticity after stroke: a randomised double blind placebo controlled trial. *J Neurol Neurosurg Psychiatry* 2000; **69**(2):217–21.

237 Botulinum toxin A injections improved wrist and finger spasticity after stroke. *ACP Journal Club* 2003; **138**(1):22.

238 Centre for Reviews and Dissemination. Botulinum toxin type A for the treatment of the upper limb spasticity after stroke: a meta-analysis (Provisional record). *Database Abstr Rev Effects* 2006; **63**:20.

239 Centre for Reviews and Dissemination. Treatment of upper extremity spasticity in stroke patients by focal neuronal or neuromuscular blockade: a systematic review of the literature. *Database Abstr Rev Effects* 2006; (3):26.

240 Centre for Reviews and Dissemination. Intrathecal baclofen for severe spasticity: a meta-analysis. *Database Abstr Rev Effects* 2006; (3):22.

241 Smith MT, Baer GD. Achievement of simple mobility milestones after stroke. *Arch Phys Med Rehabil* 1999; **80**(4):442–7.

242 Medical Research Council. *Aids to the Examination of the Peripheral Nervous System.* Grimsby: Castle Press, 1982.

243 Demeurisse G, Demol O, Robaye E. Motor evaluation in vascular hemiplegia. *Eur Neurol* 1980; **19**(6):382–9.

244 Duncan PW, Goldstein LB, Matchar D, Divine GW, Feussner J. Measurement of motor recovery after stroke. Outcome assessment and sample size requirements. *Stroke* 1992; **23**(8):1084–9.

245 Duncan PW, Goldstein LB, Horner RD, Landsman PB, Samsa GP, Matchar DB. Similar motor recovery of upper and lower extremities after stroke. *Stroke* 1994; **25**(6):1181–8.

246 Sunderland A, Tinson D, Bradley L, Hewer RL. Arm function after stroke. An evaluation of grip strength as a measure of recovery and a prognostic indicator. *J Neurol Neurosurg Psychiatry* 1989; **52**(11):1267–72.

247 Bobath B. *Adult Hemiplegia Evaluation and Treatment.* 2nd ed. London: Heinemann; 1978.

248 Brunnstrom S. *Movement Therapy in Hemiplegia.* New York: Harper & Row, 1970.

249 Flanagan EM. Methods for facilitation and inhibition of motor activity. *Am J Phys Med* 1967; **46**(1):1006–11.

250 Brown DA, Kautz SA. Increased workload enhances force output during pedaling exercise in persons with poststroke hemiplegia. *Stroke* 1998; **29**(3):598–606.

251 Pollock A, Baer G, Pomeroy V, Langhorne P. Physiotherapy treatment approaches for the recovery of postural control and lower limb function following stroke. *Cochrane Database of Systematic Reviews* 2006; (3).

252 Kwakkel G, van Peppen R, Wagenaar RC, Wood DS, Richards C, Ashburn A *et al.* Effects of augmented exercise therapy time after stroke: a meta-analysis. *Stroke* 2004; **35**(11):2529–39.

253 Van Peppen RP, Kwakkel G, Wood-Dauphinee S, Hendriks HJ, Van der Wees PJ, Dekker J. The impact of physical therapy on functional outcomes after stroke: what's the evidence? *Clin Rehabil* 2004; **18**(8):833–62.

254 Lincoln NB, Parry RH, Vass CD. Randomized, controlled trial to evaluate increased intensity of physiotherapy treatment of arm function after stroke. *Stroke* 1999; **30**(3):573–9.

255 Barclay-Goddard R, Stevenson T, Poluha W, Moffatt ME, Taback SP. Force platform feedback for standing balance training after stroke. *Cochrane Database Syst Rev* 2004; (4):CD004129.

256 Heller F. [Postural biofeedback and locomotion reeducation in stroke patients]. *Ann Readapt Med Phys* **48**(4):187–95.

257 Van Peppen RP, Kortsmit M, Lindeman E, Kwakkel G. Effects of visual feedback therapy on postural control in bilateral standing after stroke: a systematic review. *J Rehabil Med* 2006; **38**(1):3–9.

258 Pomeroy VM, King L, Pollock A, Baily-Hallam A, Langhorne P. Electrostimulation for promoting recovery of movement or functional ability after stroke. *Cochrane Database Syst Rev* 2006; (2):CD003241.

259 Wu HM, Tang JL, Lin XP, Lau J, Leung PC, Woo J, Li YP. Acupuncture for stroke rehabilitation. *Cochrane Database of Systematic Reviews* 2006; (3).

260 Robbins SM, Houghton PE, Woodbury MG, Brown JL. The therapeutic effect of functional and transcutaneous electric stimulation on improving gait speed in stroke patients: a meta-analysis. *Arch Phys Med Rehabil* 2006; **87**(6):853–9.

261 Moseley AM, Stark A, Cameron ID, Pollock A. Treadmill training and body weight support for walking after stroke. *Cochrane Database Syst Rev* 2006; (3).

262 Hakkennes S, Keating JL. Constraint-induced movement therapy following stroke: a systematic review of randomised controlled trials. *Aust J Physiother* 2005; **51**(4):221–31.

263 Gladstone DJ, Black SE. Enhancing recovery after stroke with noradrenergic pharmacotherapy: a new frontier? *Can J Neurol Sci* 2000; **27**(2):97–105.

264 Martinsson L, Hardemark HG, Wahlgren NG. Amphetamines for improving stroke recovery: a systematic cochrane review. *Stroke* 2003; **34**(11):2766.

265 Carey LM, Matyas TA. Training of somatosensory discrimination after stroke: facilitation of stimulus generalization. *Am J Phys Med Rehabil* 2005; **84**(6):428–42.

266 Jonsson AC, Lindgren I, Hallstrom B, Norrving B, Lindgren A. Prevalence and intensity of pain after stroke: a population based study focusing on patients' perspectives. *J Neurol Neurosurg Psychiatry* 2006; **77**(5):590–5.

267 Bowsher D. Central pain: clinical and physiological characteristics. *J Neurol Neurosurg Psychiatry* 1996; **61**(1):62–9.

268 Andersen G, Vestergaard K, Ingeman-Nielsen M, Jensen TS. Incidence of central post-stroke pain. *Pain* 1995; **61**(2):187–93.

269 Kimyai-Asadi A, Nousari HC, Kimyai-Asadi T, Milani F. Poststroke pruritus. *Stroke* 1999; **30**(3):692–3.

270 Vestergaard K, Nielsen J, Andersen G, Ingeman-Nielsen M, Arendt-Nielsen L, Jensen TS. Sensory abnormalities in consecutive, unselected patients with central post-stroke pain. *Pain* 1995; **61**(2):177–86.

271 Bowsher D, Leijon G, Thuomas KA. Central poststroke pain: correlation of MRI with clinical pain characteristics and sensory abnormalities. *Neurology* 1998; **51**(5):1352–8.

272 Frese A, Husstedt IW, Ringelstein EB, Evers S. Pharmacologic treatment of central post-stroke pain. *Clin J Pain* 2006; **22**(3):252–60.

273 Wiffen P, Collins S, McQuay H, Carroll D, Jadad A, Moore A. Anticonvulsant drugs for acute and chronic pain [Systematic Review]. *Cochrane Database Syst Rev* 2006; (3).

274 Wiffen PJ, McQuay HJ, Moore RA. Carbamazepine for acute and chronic pain [Systematic Review]. *Cochrane Database Syst Rev* 2006; (3).

275 Ratnasabapathy Y, Broad J, Baskett J, Pledger M, Marshall J, Bonita R. Shoulder pain in people with a

stroke: a population-based study. *Clin Rehabil* 2003; **17**(3):304–11.

276 Gamble GE, Barberan E, Laasch HU, Bowsher D, Tyrrell PJ, Jones AK. Poststroke shoulder pain: a prospective study of the association and risk factors in 152 patients from a consecutive cohort of 205 patients presenting with stroke. *Eur J Pain* 2002; **6**(6):467–74.

277 Turner-Stokes L, Jackson D. Shoulder pain after stroke: a review of the evidence base to inform the development of an integrated care pathway. *Clin Rehabil* 2002; **16**(3):276–98.

278 Pomeroy VM, Frames C, Faragher EB, Hesketh A, Hill E, Watson P, Main CJ. Reliability of a measure of post-stroke shoulder pain in patients with and without aphasia and/or unilateral spatial neglect. *Clin Rehabil* 2000; **14**(6):584–91.

279 Ada L, Foongchomcheay A, Canning C. Supportive devices for preventing and treating subluxation of the shoulder after stroke. *Cochrane Database Syst Rev* 2005; (1):CD003863.

280 Ada L, Foongchomcheay A. Efficacy of electrical stimulation in preventing or reducing subluxation of the shoulder after stroke: a meta-analysis. *Aust J Physiother* 2002; **48**(4):257–67.

281 Price CIM, Pandyan AD. Electrical stimulation for preventing and treating post-stroke shoulder pain. *Cochrane Database of Systematic Reviews* 2006; (3).

282 Green S, Buchbinder R, Glazier R, Forbes A. Interventions for shoulder pain. *Cochrane Database Syst Rev* 2000; (2):CD001156.

283 Green S, Buchbinder R, Glazier R, Forbes A. Systematic review of randomised controlled trials of interventions for painful shoulder: selection criteria, outcome assessment, and efficacy. *Br Med J* 1998; **316**(7128):354–60.

284 Geurts AC, Visschers BA, van Limbeek J, Ribbers GM. Systematic review of aetiology and treatment of post-stroke hand oedema and shoulder-hand syndrome. *Scand J Rehabil Med* 2000; **32**(1):4–10.

285 Boomkamp-Koppen HG, Visser-Meily JM, Post MW, Prevo AJ. Poststroke hand swelling and oedema: prevalence and relationship with impairment and disability. *Clin Rehabil* 2005; **19**(5):552–9.

286 Wanklyn P, Forster A, Young J, Mulley G. Prevalence and associated features of the cold hemiplegic arm. *Stroke* 1995; **26**(10):1867–70.

287 Wang JS, Yang CF, Liaw MY, Wong MK. Suppressed cutaneous endothelial vascular control and hemodynamic changes in paretic extremities with edema in the extremities of patients with hemiplegia. *Arch Phys Med Rehabil* 2002; **83**(7):1017–23.

288 Post MW, Visser-Meily JM, Boomkamp-Koppen HG, Prevo AJ. Assessment of oedema in stroke patients: comparison of visual inspection by therapists and volumetric assessment. *Disabil Rehabil* 2003; **25**(22):1265–70.

289 Roper TA, Redford S, Tallis RC. Intermittent compression for the treatment of the oedematous hand in hemiplegic stroke: a randomized controlled trial. *Age Ageing* 1999; **28**(1):9–13.

290 Nyberg L, Gustafson Y. Patient falls in stroke rehabilitation. A challenge to rehabilitation strategies. *Stroke* 1995; **26**(5):838–42.

291 Teasell R, McRae M, Foley N, Bhardwaj A. The incidence and consequences of falls in stroke patients during inpatient rehabilitation: factors associated with high risk. *Arch Phys Med Rehabil* 2002; **83**(3):329–33.

292 Perennou D, El FA, Masmoudi M, Benaim C, Loigerot M, Didier JP, Pelissier J. [Incidence, circumstances and consequences of falls in patients undergoing rehabilitation after a first stroke]. *Ann Readapt Med Phys* 2005; **48**(3):138–45.

293 Forster A, Young J. Incidence and consequences of falls due to stroke: a systematic inquiry. *Br Med J* 1995; **311**(6997):83–6.

294 Yates JS, Lai SM, Duncan PW, Studenski S. Falls in community-dwelling stroke survivors: an accumulated impairments model. *J Rehabil Res Dev* 2002; **39**(3):385–94.

295 Nyberg L, Gustafson Y. Fall prediction index for patients in stroke rehabilitation. *Stroke* 1997; **28**(4):716–21.

296 Hyndman D, Ashburn A. Stops walking when talking as a predictor of falls in people with stroke living in the community. *J Neurol Neurosurg Psychiatry* 2004; **75**(7):994–7.

297 Watanabe Y. Fear of falling among stroke survivors after discharge from inpatient rehabilitation. *Int J Rehabil Res* 2005; **28**(2):149–52.

298 Dennis MS, Lo KM, McDowall M, West T. Fractures after stroke: frequency, types, and associations. *Stroke* 2002; **33**(3):728–34.

299 Ramnemark A, Nyberg L, Borssen B, Olsson T, Gustafson Y. Fractures after stroke. *Osteoporos Int* 1998; **8**(1):92–5.

300 Melton LJ, III, Brown RD, Jr., Achenbach SJ, O'Fallon WM, Whisnant JP. Long-term fracture risk following ischemic stroke: a population-based study. *Osteoporos Int* 2001; **12**(11):980–6.

301 Whitson HE, Pieper CF, Sanders L, Horner RD, Duncan PW, Lyles KW. Adding injury to insult: fracture risk after stroke in veterans. *J Am Geriatr Soc* 2006; **54**(7):1082–8.

302 Kanis J, Oden A, Johnell O. Acute and long-term increase in fracture risk after hospitalization for stroke. *Stroke* 2001; **32**(3):702–6.

303 Ramnemark A, Nyberg L, Lorentzon R, Olsson T, Gustafson Y. Hemiosteoporosis after severe stroke, independent of changes in body composition and weight. *Stroke* 1999; **30**(4):755–60.

304 Poole KE, Loveridge N, Barker PJ, Halsall DJ, Rose C, Reeve J, Warburton EA. Reduced vitamin D in acute stroke. *Stroke* 2006; **37**(1):243–5.

305 Gillespie LD, Gillespie WJ, Robertson MC, Lamb SE, Cumming RG, Rowe BH. Interventions for preventing falls in elderly people. *Cochrane Database Syst Rev* 2003; (4):CD000340.

306 Lyons RA, Sander LV, Weightman AL, Patterson J, Jones SA, Rolfe B, Kemp A, Johansen A. Modification of the home environment for the reduction of injuries. *Cochrane Database Syst Rev* 2003; (4):CD003600.

307 Parker MJ, Gillespie WJ, Gillespie LD. Hip protectors for preventing hip fractures in older people. *Cochrane Database Syst Rev* 2005; (3):CD001255.

308 Poole KE, Reeve J, Warburton EA. Falls, fractures, and osteoporosis after stroke: time to think about protection? *Stroke* 2002; **33**(5):1432–6.

309 Farquhar CM, Marjoribanks J, Lethaby A, Lamberts Q, Suckling JA. Long term hormone therapy for perimenopausal and postmenopausal women. *Cochrane Database Syst Rev* 2005; (3):CD004143.

310 Lotery AJ, Wiggam MI, Jackson AJ, Refson K, Fullerton KJ, Gilmore DH, Beringer TR. Correctable visual impairment in stroke rehabilitation patients. *Age Ageing* 2000; **29**(3):221–2.

311 Gray CS, French JM, Bates D, Cartlidge NE, Venables GS, James OF. Recovery of visual fields in acute stroke: homonymous hemianopia associated with adverse prognosis. *Age Ageing* 1989; **18**(6):419–21.

312 Nelles G, Esser J, Eckstein A, Tiede A, Gerhard H, Diener HC. Compensatory visual field training for patients with hemianopia after stroke. *Neurosci Lett* 2001 June 29; 306(3):189–92.

313 Loverro J, Reding M. Bed orientation and rehabilitation outcome for patients with stroke and hemianopsia or visual neglect. *J Neurol Rehabil* 1988; **147**:150.

314 Rossi PW, Kheyfets S, Reding MJ. Fresnel prisms improve visual perception in stroke patients with homonymous hemianopia or unilateral visual neglect. *Neurology* 1990; **40**(10):1597–9.

315 Rousseaux M, Bernati T, Saj A, Kozlowski O. Ineffectiveness of prism adaptation on spatial neglect signs. *Stroke* 2006; **37**(2):542–3.

316 Rathore SS, Hinn AR, Cooper LS, Tyroler HA, Rosamond WD. Characterization of incident stroke signs and symptoms: findings from the atherosclerosis risk in communities study. *Stroke* 2002; **33**(11):2718–21.

317 Straube A, Leigh RJ, Bronstein A, Heide W, Riordan-Eva P, Tijssen CC *et al*. EFNS task force: therapy of nystagmus and oscillopsia. *Eur J Neurol* 2004; **11**(2):83–9.

318 Bowen A, McKenna K, Tallis RC. Reasons for variability in the reported rate of occurrence of unilateral spatial neglect after stroke. *Stroke* 1999; **30**(6):1196–202.

319 Stone SP, Halligan PW, Greenwood RJ. The incidence of neglect phenomena and related disorders in patients with an acute right or left hemisphere stroke. *Age Ageing* 1993; **22**(1):46–52.

320 Appelros P, Nydevik I, Karlsson GM, Thorwalls A, Seiger A. Assessing unilateral neglect: shortcomings of standard test methods. *Disabil Rehabil* 2003; **25**(9):473–9.

321 Qiang W, Sonoda S, Suzuki M, Okamoto S, Saitoh E. Reliability and validity of a wheelchair collision test for screening behavioral assessment of unilateral neglect after stroke. *Am J Phys Med Rehabil* 2005; **84**(3):161–6.

322 Menon A, Korner-Bitensky N. Evaluating unilateral spatial neglect post stroke: working your way through the maze of assessment choices. *Top Stroke Rehabil* 2004; **11**(3):41–66.

323 Gillen R, Tennen H, McKee T. Unilateral spatial neglect: relation to rehabilitation outcomes in patients with right hemisphere stroke. *Arch Phys Med Rehabil* 2005; **86**(4):763–7.

324 Appelros P, Karlsson GM, Seiger A, Nydevik I. Prognosis for patients with neglect and anosognosia with special reference to cognitive impairment. *J Rehabil Med* 2003; **35**(6):254–8.

325 Appelros P, Nydevik I, Karlsson GM, Thorwalls A, Seiger A. Recovery from unilateral neglect after right-hemisphere stroke. *Disabil Rehabil* 2004; **26**(8):471–7.

326 Stone SP, Patel P, Greenwood RJ, Halligan PW. Measuring visual neglect in acute stroke and predicting its recovery: the visual neglect recovery index. *J Neurol Neurosurg Psychiatry* 1992; **55**(6):431–6.

327 Bowen A, Lincoln NB, Dewey M. Cognitive rehabilitation for spatial neglect following stroke. *Cochrane Database Syst Rev* 2006; (3).

328 Appelros P, Viitanen M. What causes increased stroke mortality in patients with prestroke dementia? *Cerebrovasc Dis* 2005; **19**(5):323–7.

329 Jorm AF. The Informant Questionnaire on Cognitive Decline in the Elderly (IQCODE): a review. *Int Psychogeriatr* 2004; **16**(3):275–93.

330 Caeiro L, Ferro JM, Albuquerque R, Figueira ML. Delirium in the first days of acute stroke. *J Neurol* 2004; **251**(2):171–8.

331 Santos CO, Caeiro L, Ferro JM, Albuquerque R, Luisa FM. Anger, hostility and aggression in the first days of acute stroke. *Eur J Neurol* 2006; **13**(4):351–8.

332 Arden M, Mayou R, Feldman E, Hawton K. Cognitive impairment in the elderly medically ill: how often is it missed? *Int J Geriatr Psychiatry* 1993; **8**:929–37.

333 Dudas RB, Berrios GE, Hodges JR. The Addenbrooke's Cognitive Examination (ACE) in the differential diagnosis of early dementias versus affective disorder. *Am J Geriatr Psychiatry* 2005; **13**(3):218–26.

334 Larner AJ. An audit of the Addenbrooke's Cognitive Examination (ACE) in clinical practice. *Int J Geriatr Psychiatry* 2005; **20**(6):593–4.

335 Lonergan E, Luxenberg J, Colford J. Haloperidol for agitation in dementia. *Cochrane Database Syst Rev* 2002; (2):CD002852.

336 Ivan CS, Seshadri S, Beiser A, Au R, Kase CS, Kelly-Hayes M, Wolf PA. Dementia after stroke: the Framingham Study. *Stroke* 2004; **35**(6):1264–8.

337 Ballard C, Rowan E, Stephens S, Kalaria R, Kenny RA. Prospective follow-up study between 3 and 15 months after stroke: improvements and decline in cognitive function among dementia-free stroke survivors >75 years of age. *Stroke* 2003; **34**(10):2440–4.

338 Rasquin SM, Lodder J, Ponds RW, Winkens I, Jolles J, Verhey FR. Cognitive functioning after stroke: a one-year follow-up study. *Dement Geriatr Cog Dis* 2004; **18**(2):138–44.

339 Leys D, Henon H, Kowiak-Cordoliani MA, Pasquier F. Poststroke dementia. *Lancet Neurol* 2005; **4**(11):752–9.

340 Barba R, Morin MD, Cemillan C, Delgado C, Domingo J, Del ST. Previous and incident dementia as risk factors for mortality in stroke patients. *Stroke* 2002; **33**(8):1993–8.

341 De Konig I, van Kooten F, Koudstaal PJ, Dippel DW. Diagnostic value of the Rotterdam-CAMCOG in post-stroke dementia. *J Neurol Neurosurg Psychiatry* 2005; **76**(2):263–5.

342 Raven JC. *Guide to Using the Coloured Progressive Matrices.* London: HK Lewis & Co., 1965.

343 Malouf R, Birks J. Donepezil for vascular cognitive impairment. *Cochrane Database Syst Rev* 2004; (1):CD004395.

344 Kimura M, Robinson RG, Kosier JT. Treatment of cognitive impairment after poststroke depression: a double-blind treatment trial. *Stroke* 2000; **31**(7):1482–6.

345 Lincoln NB, Majid MJ, Weyman N. Cognitive rehabilitation for attention deficits following stroke. *Cochrane Database Syst Rev* 2000; (4):CD002842.

346 Majid MJ, Lincoln NB, Weyman N. Cognitive rehabilitation for memory deficits following stroke. *Cochrane Database Syst Rev* 2000; (3):CD002293.

347 Engelter ST, Gostynski M, Papa S, Frei M, Born C, Jdacic-Gross V *et al*. Epidemiology of aphasia attributable to first ischemic stroke: incidence, severity, fluency, etiology, and thrombolysis. *Stroke* 2006; **37**(6):1379–84.

348 Pedersen PM, Vinter K, Olsen TS. Aphasia after stroke: type, severity and prognosis. The Copenhagen aphasia study. *Cerebrovasc Dis* 2004; **17**(1):35–43.

349 Berthier ML. Poststroke aphasia: epidemiology, pathophysiology and treatment. *Drugs Aging* 2005; **22**(2):163–82.

350 Enderby PM, Wood VA, Wade DT, Hewer RL. The Frenchay Aphasia Screening Test: a short, simple test for aphasia appropriate for non-specialists. *Int Rehabil Med* 1987; **8**(4):166–70.

351 Enderby P, Crow E. Frenchay Aphasia Screening Test: validity and comparability. *Disabil Rehabil* 1996; **18**(5):238–40.

352 Greener J, Enderby P, Whurr R. Speech and language therapy for aphasia following stroke. *Cochrane Database Syst Rev* 2006; (3).

353 Roby RR. A meta-analysis of clinical outcomes in the treatment of aphasia. *J Speech Hearing Res* 1998; **41**:172–87.

354 Bakheit AM. Drug treatment of poststroke aphasia. *Exp Rev Neurotherapeutics* 2004; **4**(2):211–17.

355 Greener J, Enderby P, Whurr R. Pharmacological treatment for aphasia following stroke. *Cochrane Database Syst Rev* 2006; (3).

356 Sellars C, Hughes T, Langhorne P. Speech and language therapy for dysarthria due to non-progressive brain damage. *Cochrane Database Syst Rev* 2006; (3).

357 Beekman AT, Penninx BW, Deeg DJ, Ormel J, Smit JH, Braam AW, van Tilburg W. Depression in survivor of stroke: a community-based study of prevalence, risk factors and consequences. *Soc Psychiatry Psychiatr Epidemiol* 1998; **33**(10):463–70.

358 Whyte EM, Mulsant BH, Vanderbilt J, Dodge HH, Ganguli M. Depression after stroke: a prospective epidemiological study. *J Am Geriatr Soc* 2004; **52**(5):774–8.

359 House A. Mood disorders after stroke: a review of the evidence. *Int J Geriatr Psychiatry* 1987; **2**:211–21.

360 Hackett ML, Yapa C, Parag V, Anderson CS. Frequency of depression after stroke: a systematic review of observational studies. *Stroke* 2005; **36**(6):1330–40.

361 Hackett ML, Anderson CS, Auckland Regional Community Stroke (ARCOS) Study Group. Frequency, management, and predictors of abnormal mood after stroke: the Auckland Regional Community Stroke (ARCOS) study, 2002 to 2003. *Stroke* 2006; **37**(8):2123–8.

362 Leppavuori A, Pohjasvaara T, Vataja R, Kaste M, Erkinjuntti T. Generalized anxiety disorders three to four months after ischemic stroke. *Cerebrovasc Dis* 2003; **16**(3):257–64.

363 Dennis M, O'Rourke S, Lewis S, Sharpe M, Warlow C. Emotional outcomes after stroke: factors associated with poor outcome. *J Neurol Neurosurg Psychiatry* 2000; **68**(1):47–52.

364 Dennis M, O'Rourke S, Lewis S, Sharpe M, Warlow C. Emotional outcomes after stroke: factors associated with poor outcome. *J Neurol Neurosurg Psychiatry* 2000; **68**(1):47–52.

365 Hackett ML, Anderson CS. Predictors of depression after stroke: a systematic review of observational studies. *Stroke* 2005; **36**(10):2296–301.

366 Singh A, Black SE, Herrmann N, Leibovitch FS, Ebert PL, Lawrence J, Szalai JP. Functional and neuroanatomic correlations in poststroke depression: the Sunnybrook Stroke Study. *Stroke* 2000; **31**(3):637–44.

367 Yu L, Liu CK, Chen JW, Wang SY, Wu YH, Yu SH. Relationship between post-stroke depression and lesion location: a meta-analysis. *Kaohsiung J Med Sci* 2004; **20**(8):372–80.

368 Bhogal SK, Teasell R, Foley N, Speechley M. Lesion location and poststroke depression: systematic review of the methodological limitations in the literature. *Stroke* 2004; **35**(3):794–802.

369 Singh A, Herrmann N, Black SE. The importance of lesion location in poststroke depression: a critical review. *Can J Psychiatry* 1998; **43**(9):921–7.

370 Carson AJ, MacHale S, Allen K, Lawrie SM, Dennis M, House A, Sharpe M. Depression after stroke and lesion location: a systematic review. *Lancet* 2000; **356**(9224):122–6.

371 Morrison V, Pollard B, Johnston M, MacWalter R. Anxiety and depression 3 years following stroke: demographic, clinical, and psychological predictors. *J Psychosom Res* 2005; **59**(4):209–13.

372 Bruggimann L, Annoni JM, Staub F, von Steinbuchel N, Van der Linden M, Bogousslavsky J. Chronic posttraumatic stress symptoms after nonsevere stroke. *Neurology* 2006; **66**(4):513–16.

373 Ramasubbu R, Patten SB. Effect of depression on stroke morbidity and mortality. *Can J Psychiatry* 2003; **48**(4):250–7.

374 Spalletta G, Ripa A, Caltagirone C. Symptom profile of DSM-IV major and minor depressive disorders in first-ever stroke patients. *Am J Geriatr Psychiatry* 2005; **13**(2):108–15.

375 Watkins C, Daniels L, Jack C, Dickinson H, van Den BM. Accuracy of a single question in screening for depression in a cohort of patients after stroke: comparative study. *Br Med J* 2001; **323**(7322):1159.

376 Aben I, Verhey F, Lousberg R, Lodder J, Honig A. Validity of the Beck depression inventory, hospital anxiety and depression scale, SCL-90, and Hamilton depression rating scale as screening instruments for depression in stroke patients. *Psychosomatics* 2002; **43**(5):386–93.

377 Benaim C, Cailly B, Perennou D, Pelissier J. Validation of the aphasic depression rating scale. *Stroke* 2004; **35**(7):1692–6.

378 Leeds L, Meara RJ, Hobson JP. The utility of the Stroke Aphasia Depression Questionnaire (SADQ) in a stroke rehabilitation unit. *Clin Rehabil* 2004; **18**(2):228–31.

379 Forster A, Smith J, Young J, Knapp P, House A, Wright J. Information provision for stroke patients and their caregivers. *Cochrane Database Syst Rev* 2006; (3).

380 Anderson CS, Hackett ML, House AO. Interventions for preventing depression after stroke. *Cochrane Database Syst Rev* 2006; (3).

381 Hackett ML, Anderson CS, House AO. Management of depression after stroke: a systematic review of pharmacological therapies. *Stroke* 2005; **36**(5):1098–103.

382 Mottram P, Wilson K, Strobl J. Antidepressants for depressed elderly. *Cochrane Database Syst Rev* 2006; (1):CD003491.

383 Cipriani A, Brambilla P, Furukawa T, Geddes J, Gregis M, Hotopf M *et al*. Fluoxetine versus other types of pharmacotherapy for depression. *Cochrane Database Syst Rev* 2005; (4):CD004185.

384 Hackett ML, Anderson CS, House AO. Interventions for treating depression after stroke. *Cochrane Database Syst Rev* 2006; (3).

385 Cole MG, Elie LM, McCusker J, Bellavance F, Mansour A. Feasibility and effectiveness of treatments for post-stroke depression in elderly inpatients: systematic review. *J Geriatr Psychiatry Neurol* 2001; **14**(1):37–41.

386 Murray GB, Shea V, Conn DK. Electroconvulsive therapy for poststroke depression. *J Clin Psychiatry* 1986; **47**(5):258–60.

387 House AO, Hackett ML, Anderson CS, Horrocks JA. Pharmaceutical interventions for emotionalism after stroke. *Cochrane Database Syst Rev* 2006; (3).

388 Calvert T, Knapp P, House A. Psychological associations with emotionalism after stroke. *J Neurol Neurosurg Psychiatry* 1998; **65**(6):928–9.

389 Lincoln NB, Gamlen R, Thomason H. Behavioural mapping of patients on a stroke unit. *Int Disabil Stud* 1989; **11**(4):149–54.

390 Bernhardt J, Dewey H, Thrift A, Donnan G. Inactive and alone: physical activity within the first 14 days of acute stroke unit care. *Stroke* 2004; **35**(4):1005–9.

391 Lincoln NB, Willis D, Philips SA, Juby LC, Berman P. Comparison of rehabilitation practice on hospital wards for stroke patients. *Stroke* 1996; **27**(1):18–23.

392 Choi-Kwon S, Han SW, Kwon SU, Kim JS. Poststroke fatigue: characteristics and related factors. *Cerebrovasc Dis* 2005; **19**(2):84–90.

393 De Groot MH, Phillips SJ, Eskes GA. Fatigue associated with stroke and other neurologic conditions: Implications for stroke rehabilitation. *Arch Phys Med Rehabil* 2003; **84**(11):1714–20.

394 Glader EL, Stegmayr B, Asplund K. Poststroke fatigue: a 2-year follow-up study of stroke patients in Sweden. *Stroke* 2002; **33**(5):1327–33.

395 Outpatient Service Trialists. Therapy-based rehabilitation services for stroke patients at home. *Cochrane Database Syst Rev* 2003; 1.

396 Logan PA, Gladman JR, Drummond AE, Radford KA. A study of interventions and related outcomes in a randomized controlled trial of occupational therapy and leisure therapy for community stroke patients. *Clin Rehabil* 2003; **17**(3):249–55.

397 Collen FM, Wade DT. Residual mobility problems after stroke. *Int Disabil Stud* 1991; **13**(1):12–5.

398 Collen FM, Wade DT, Robb GF, Bradshaw CM. The Rivermead Mobility Index: a further development of the Rivermead Motor Assessment. *Int Disabil Stud* 1991; **13**(2):50–4.

399 Wade DT, Wood VA, Heller A, Maggs J, Langton HR. Walking after stroke. Measurement and recovery over the first 3 months. *Scand J Rehabil Med* 1987; **19**(1):25–30.

400 Green J, Young J, Forster A, Collen F, Wade D. Combined analysis of two randomized trials of community physiotherapy for patients more than one year post stroke. *Clin Rehabil* 2004; **18**(3):249–52.

401 Saunders DH, Greig CA, Young A, Mead GE. Physical fitness training for stroke patients. *Cochrane Database Syst Rev* 2006; (3).

402 Gladman J, Forster A, Young J. Hospital- and home-based rehabilitation after discharge from hospital for stroke patients: analysis of two trials. *Age Ageing* 1995; **24**(1):49–53.

403 Legh-Smith J, Wade DT, Hewer RL. Driving after a stroke. *J R Soc Med* 1986; **79**(4):200–3.

404 Fisk GD, Owsley C, Pulley LV. Driving after stroke: driving exposure, advice, and evaluations. *Arch Phys Med Rehabil* 1997; **78**(12):1338–45.

405 Gommans J, Sye D, MacDonald A. Guideline recommendations for the management of patients admitted with acute stroke: implications of a local audit. *N Z Med J* 2005; **118**(1214):U1435.

406 Samuelsson SM. Physicians' control of driving after stroke attacks. *Tidsskr Den Norske Laegef* 2005; **125**(19):2610–12.

407 Haselkorn JK, Mueller BA, Rivara FA. Characteristics of drivers and driving record after traumatic and nontraumatic brain injury. *Arch Phys Med Rehabil* 1998; **79**(7):738–42.

408 Akinwuntan AE, Feys H, De Weerdt W, Baten G, Arno P, Kiekens C. Prediction of driving after stroke: A prospective study. *Neurorehabilitation & Neural Repair* 2006; **20**(3):417–23.

409 Mazer BL, Korner-Bitensky NA, Sofer S. Predicting ability to drive after stroke. *Arch Phys Med Rehabil* 1998; **79**(7):743–50.

410 Radford KA, Lincoln NB. Concurrent validity of the stroke drivers screening assessment. *Arch Phys Med Rehabil* 2004; **85**(2):324–8.

411 Fox GK, Bowden SC, Smith DS. On-road assessment of driving competence after brain impairment: review of current practice and recommendations for a standardized examination. *Arch Phys Med Rehabil* 1998; **79**(10):1288–96.

412 Akinwuntan AE, DeWeerdt W, Feys H, Baten G, Arno P, Kiekens C. Reliability of a Road Test after Stroke. *Arch Phys Med Rehabil* 2003; **84**(12):1792–6.

413 Akinwuntan AE, De Weerdt W, Feys H, Baten G, Arno P, Kiekens C. The validity of a road test after stroke. *Arch Phys Med Rehabil* 2005; **86**(3):421–6.

414 Akinwuntan AE, De Weerdt W, Feys H, Pauwels J, Baten G, Arno P, Kiekens C. Effect of simulator training on driving after stroke: A randomized controlled trial. *Neurology* 2005; **65**(6):843–50.

415 Chiu CWY, Man DWK. The effect of training older adults with stroke to use home-based assistive devices. *OTJR: Occupation, Participation, & Health* 2006; **24**(3):113–20.

416 Walker CM, Sunderland A, Sharma J, Walker MF. The impact of cognitive impairment on upper body dressing difficulties after stroke: a video analysis of patterns of recovery. *J Neurol Neurosurg Psychiatry* 2004; **75**(1):43–8.

417 Huck J, Bonhotal BH. Fastener systems on apparel for hemiplegic stroke victims. *Appl Ergon* 1997; **28**(4):277–82.

418 Perry L, McLaren S. An exploration of nutrition and eating disabilities in relation to quality of life at 6 months post-stroke. *Health Soc Care Community* 2004; **12**(4):288–97.

419 Wozniak MA, Kittner SJ. Return to work after ischemic stroke: a methodological review. *Neuroepidemiology* 2002; **21**(4):159–66.

420 Vestling M, Tufvesson B, Iwarsson S. Indicators for return to work after stroke and the importance of work for subjective well-being and life satisfaction. *J Rehabil Med* 2003; **35**(3):127–31.

421 Wellwood I, Dennis MS, Warlow CP. Perceptions and knowledge of stroke among surviving patients with stroke and their carers. *Age Ageing* 1994; **23**(4):293–8.

422 Drummond A. Leisure activity after stroke. *Int Disabil Stud* 1990; **12**(4):157–60.

423 Green J, Forster A, Young J. A test-retest reliability study of the Barthel Index, the Rivermead Mobility Index, the Nottingham Extended Activities of Daily Living Scale and the Frenchay Activities Index in stroke patients. *Disabil Rehabil* 2001; **23**(15):670–6.

424 Drummond AE, Parker CJ, Gladman JR, Logan PA. Development and validation of the Nottingham Leisure Questionnaire (NLQ). *Clin Rehabil* 2001; **15**(6):647–56.

425 Parker CJ, Gladman JR, Drummond AE, Dewey ME, Lincoln NB, Barer D *et al.* A multicentre randomized

controlled trial of leisure therapy and conventional occupational therapy after stroke. TOTAL Study Group. Trial of Occupational Therapy and Leisure. *Clin Rehabil* 2001; **15**(1):42–52.

426 Kakkos SK, Geroulakos G. Economy class stroke syndrome: case report and review of the literature. *Eur J Vasc Endovasc Surg* 2004; **27**(3):239–43.

427 Cheung RT. Sexual functioning in Chinese stroke patients with mild or no disability. *Cerebrovasc Dis* 2002; **14**(2):122–8.

428 Holbrook M. Stroke: social and emotional outcome. *J R Coll Physicians Lond* 1982; **16**(2):100–4.

429 Van Exel NJ, Koopmanschap MA, van den BB, Brouwer WB, van den Bos GA. Burden of informal caregiving for stroke patients. Identification of caregivers at risk of adverse health effects. *Cerebrovasc Dis* 2005; **19**(1):11–17.

430 Visser-Meily JM, Post MW, Riphagen II, Lindeman E. Measures used to assess burden among caregivers of stroke patients: a review. *Clin Rehabil* 2004; **18**(6):601–23.

431 Kalra L, Evans A, Perez I, Melbourn A, Patel A, Knapp M, Donaldson N. Training carers of stroke patients: randomised controlled trial. *Br Med J* 2004; **328**(7448):1099.

432 Visser-Meily A, van Heugten C, Post M, Schepers V, Lindeman E. Intervention studies for caregivers of stroke survivors: a critical review. *Patient Educ Couns* 2005; **56**(3):257–67.

433 Hodkinson HM. Evaluation of a mental test score for assessment of mental impairment in the elderly. *Age Ageing* 1972; **1**(4):233–8.

434 Belfield PW. Urinary catheters. In: GP Mulley, ed. *Everyday Aids and Appliances*. London: BMJ Publishers, 1989, pp. 55–9.

435 Smith N. Aids for urinary incontinence. In: GP Mulley, ed. *Everyday Aids and Appliances*. London: BMJ Publishers, 1989, pp. 50–4.

436 Kidd D, Lawson J, Nesbitt R, MacMahon J. Aspiration in acute stroke: a clinical study with videofluoroscopy. *Q J Med* 1993; **86**(12):825–9.

437 Scottish Intercollegiate Guidelines Network. *Management of Patients with Stroke: Identification and Management of Dysphagia*. Edinburgh: Scottish Intercollegiate Guidelines Network, 2004.

438 Ashworth B. Preliminary trial of carisoprodol in multiple sclerosis. *Practitioner* 1964; **192**:540–2.

439 Wade DT. Measurement in neurological rehabilitation. *Curr Opin Neurol Neurosurg* 1992; **5**(5):682–6.

440 Martin J, Meltzer H, Elliot D. *The Prevalence of Disability among Adults*. Office of Population Censuses and Surveys. London: HMSO, 1988.

441 Wanklyn P, Forster A, Young J. Hemiplegic shoulder pain (HSP): natural history and investigation of associated features. *Disabil Rehabil* 1996; **18**(10):497–501.

442 Braus DF, Krauss JK, Strobel J. The shoulder-hand syndrome after stroke: a prospective clinical trial. *Ann Neurol* 1994; **36**(5):728–33.

443 Wilson B, Cockburn J, Halligan P. *Behavioural Inattention Test*. Titchfield, Hants: Thames Valley Test Company, 1987.

444 Folstein MF, Folstein SE, McHugh PR. 'Mini-mental state': a practical method for grading the cognitive state of patients for the clinician. *J Psychiatr Res* 1975; **12**(3):189–98.

445 O'Rourke S, MacHale S, Signorini D, Dennis M. Detecting psychiatric morbidity after stroke: comparison of the GHQ and the HAD Scale. *Stroke* 1998; **29**(5):980–5.

446 Johnson G, Burvill PW, Anderson CS, Jamrozik K, Stewart-Wynne EG, Chakera TM. Screening instruments for depression and anxiety following stroke: experience in the Perth community stroke study. *Acta Psychiatr Scand* 1995; **91**(4):252–7.

447 House A, Dennis M, Hawton K, Warlow C. Methods of identifying mood disorders in stroke patients: experience in the Oxfordshire Community Stroke Project. *Age Ageing* 1989; **18**(6):371–9.

448 Shinar D, Gross CR, Price TR, Banko M, Bolduc PL, Robinson RG. Screening for depression in stroke patients: the reliability and validity of the Center for Epidemiologic Studies Depression Scale. *Stroke* 1986; **17**(2):241–5.

449 Agrell B, Dehlin O. Comparison of six depression rating scales in geriatric stroke patients. *Stroke* 1989; **20**(9):1190–4.

450 Williams LS, Brizendine EJ, Plue L, Bakas T, Tu W, Hendrie H, Kroenke K. Performance of the PHQ-9 as a screening tool for depression after stroke. *Stroke* 2005; **36**(3):635–8.

451 Mulley G. Walking frames. In: G Mulley, ed. *More Everyday Aids and Appliances*. London: BMJ Publishing, 1991, pp. 174–81.

452 Tyson SF, Ashburn A. The influence of walking aids on hemiplegic gait. *Physiother Theory Pract* 1994; **10**:77–86.

453 Lu CL, Yu B, Basford JR, Johnson ME, An KN. Influences of cane length on the stability of stroke patients. *J Rehabil Res Dev* 1997; **34**(1):91–100.

454 Tyson SF. The support taken through walking aids during hemiplegic gait. *Clin Rehabil* 1998; **12**(5):395–401.

455 Tyson S, Thornton H, Downes A. The effect of a hinged ankle-foot orthosis on hemiplegic gait: four single case studies. *Physiother Theory Pract* 1998; **14**:75–85.

456 Beckerman H, Becher J, Lankhorst GJ, Verbeek AL. Walking ability of stroke patients: efficacy of tibial nerve blocking and a polypropylene ankle-foot orthosis. *Arch Phys Med Rehabil* 1996; **77**(11):1144–51.

457 Roberts K, Porter K. How do you size a nasopharyngeal airway. *Resuscitation* 2003; **56**(1):19–23.

458 Roberts K, Whalley H, Bleetman A. The nasopharyngeal airway: dispelling myths and establishing the facts. *Emerg Med J* 2005; **22**(6):394–6.

459 St Clair M. Survey of the uses of the Pegasus Airwave System in the United Kingdom. *J Tiss Viabil* 1992; **2**:9–16.

460 Levine JA, Morris JC. The use of a football helmet to secure a nasogastric tube. *Nutrition* 1995; **11**(3):285.

461 Marson AG, Al-Kharusi AM, Alwaidh M, Appleton R, Baker GA, Chadwick DW, *et al*. The SANAD study of effectiveness of carbamazepine, gabapentin, lamotrigine, oxcarbazepine, or topiramate for treatment of partial epilepsy: an unblinded randomised controlled trial. *Lancet* 2007; **369**:1000–15.

462 Marson AG, Al-Kharusi AM, Alwaidh M, Appleton R, Baker GA, Chadwick DW, *et al*. The SANAD study of effectiveness of valproate, lamotrigine or topiramate for generalised and unclassifiable epilepsy: an unblinded randomised controlled trial. *Lancet* 2007; **369**:1016–26.

12 Specific treatments for acute ischaemic stroke

Focal cerebral ischaemia, caused by acute occlusion of a cerebral blood vessel or sometimes just by low blood flow, initiates a series of events which can lead to irreversible neuronal damage and cell death (i.e. infarction) in the part of the brain supplied or drained by that vessel. Several pathophysiological cascades run in sequence (and in parallel).[1,2] In the vascular system, rapid changes in platelet and coagulation factors, the vessel wall (particularly the endothelium) and in the thrombus itself interact to produce a very dynamic state, not only at the site of vessel occlusion, but also more remotely, in both the macro- and microcirculation.

In brain tissue, changes occur in neurones, glial cells and other structural components in differing degrees and at different times after the onset of ischaemia, which means that cerebral infarction is a dynamic and highly unstable process, not a discrete 'one-off' event. In other words, infarction is *not* an 'all-or-nothing' episode which is instantaneous in onset, maximal in severity at the moment of onset and irreversibly complete within 6 h.[3]

This chapter begins with a review of pathophysiology, particularly aspects which relate to the specific treatments that are described later in the chapter. As far as possible, we base the decision whether or not to use a particular treatment, not merely on its putative physiological effects, but on the evidence from randomized trials in patients which demonstrate the balance of clinical risk and benefit associated with its use. In view of this, the section on each of the specific treatments will assess the strength of evidence available and, where possible, base any recommendations on the results of a systematic review (and meta-analysis) of all the relevant randomized trials of that particular treatment.

12.1 Pathophysiology of acute ischaemic stroke

The pathophysiology of acute ischaemic stroke encompasses two sequential processes: the vascular, haematological or cardiac events that cause the initial reduction in local cerebral blood flow (Chapters 6 and 7) and then the alterations of cellular chemistry that are caused by ischaemia and which lead to necrosis of neurones, glia and other brain cells. This section will discuss cerebral metabolism, regulation of cerebral blood flow, molecular consequences of cerebral ischaemia and how understanding these processes leads to the development of various treatments for acute ischaemic stroke.

12.1.1 Cerebral metabolism

Energy demand and cerebral blood flow

The human brain has a high metabolic demand for energy and, unlike other organs, uses glucose (about 75–100 mg/min, or 125 g/day) as its main substrate for

Stroke: practical management, 3rd edition. C. Warlow, J. van Gijn, M. Dennis, J. Wardlaw, J. Bamford, G. Hankey, P. Sandercock, G. Rinkel, P. Langhorne, C. Sudlow and P. Rothwell. Published 2008 Blackwell Publishing. ISBN 978-1-4051-2766-0.

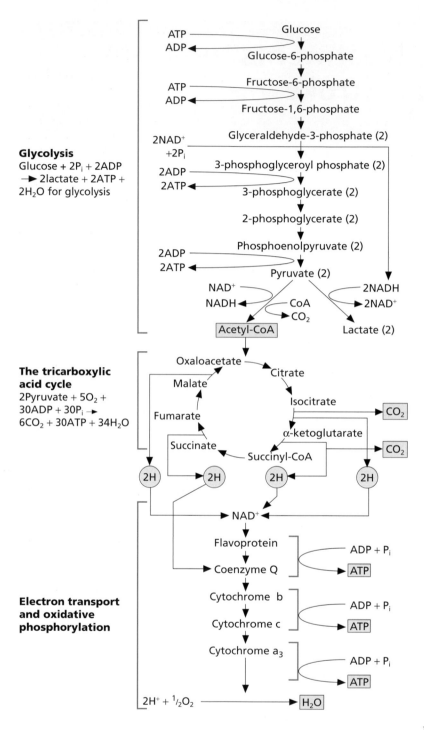

Glycolysis
Glucose + 2P$_i$ + 2ADP
→ 2lactate + 2ATP +
2H$_2$O for glycolysis

The tricarboxylic acid cycle
2Pyruvate + 5O$_2$ +
30ADP + 30P$_i$ →
6CO$_2$ + 30ATP + 34H$_2$O

Electron transport and oxidative phosphorylation

Overall: glucose + 6O$_2$ + 36P$_i$ + 36ADP → 6CO$_2$ + 36ATP + 42H$_2$O

Fig. 12.1 Biochemical pathway of the aerobic metabolism of glucose.

energy metabolism. Glucose is metabolized in the brain entirely via the glycolytic sequence and the tricarboxylic acid cycle (Fig. 12.1).

Each molecule of glucose is broken down in a series of enzymatic steps (glycolysis) into two molecules (2 M) of pyruvate. During these reactions, the oxidized form of

nicotinamide – adenine dinucleotide (NAD+) – is reduced (to NADH) and 2 M each of adenosine diphosphate (ADP) and intracellular phosphorus are converted to 2 M of adenosine triphosphate (ATP). In the *presence* of oxygen, pyruvate is metabolized, first by pyruvate dehydrogenase and then by a series of mitochondrial reactions, to carbon dioxide (CO_2) and water (H_2O) with the formation of 36 M of ATP. This is the maximum ATP yield. In the *absence* of oxygen, this sequence of events is blocked or retarded at the stage of pyruvate oxidation, leading to the reduction of pyruvate to lactate by NADH and lactic dehydrogenase. Anaerobic glycolysis therefore still leads to the formation of ATP, as well as lactate, but the energy yield is relatively small (2 M rather than 36 M of ATP from 1 M of glucose). In addition, lactic acid accumulates within and outside cells (hence, the cell is acidified) and mitochondria lose their ability to sequester calcium, so any calcium entering or released within the cell will raise the intracellular calcium level.[4-6]

Although classical neuroenergetics states that glucose is the exclusive energy substrate of brain cells, and its full oxidation provides all the necessary energy to support brain function, recent data have revealed a more intricate picture in which astrocytes play a central role in metabolic coupling and supplying lactate as an additional energy substrate in register with glutamatergic activity.[7] The basic mechanism involves glutamate-stimulated aerobic glycolysis; the sodium-coupled reuptake of glutamate by astrocytes and the ensuing activation of the Na-K-ATPase triggers glucose uptake and processing via glycolysis, resulting in the release of lactate from astrocytes. Lactate can then contribute to the activity-dependent fuelling of the neuronal energy demands associated with synaptic transmission. An operational model, the 'astrocyte-neurone lactate shuttle', is supported experimentally by a large body of evidence, which provides a molecular and cellular basis for interpreting data obtained from functional brain imaging studies.[8] When neurones are in the presence of both glucose and lactate, they preferentially use lactate as their main oxidative substrate.[9]

> The brain uses glucose as its main source of energy. During aerobic metabolism each molecule of glucose produces 36 molecules of adenosine triphosphate (ATP), but during anaerobic metabolism only two molecules of ATP are produced along with lactic acid.

ATP is the universal currency for energy. Neurones in the brain require a constant supply of ATP to maintain their integrity and to keep the major intracellular cation, potassium ions (K^+), within the cell, and the major extracellular cations, sodium (Na^+) and calcium ions (Ca^{++}), outside the cell. Because the brain is unable to store energy, it requires a constant supply of oxygenated blood containing an adequate glucose concentration to maintain its function and structural integrity.

> The resting brain consumes energy at the same rate as a 20-watt light bulb.

Global cerebral blood flow (CBF), reflecting both grey and white matter compartments, per unit of brain in a healthy young adult, is about 50–55 mL/100 g of brain per minute, with significantly higher values in those below 20 years of age and lower values in those over 60 years.[10] For a brain of average weight (1300–1400 g in a 60–65 kg adult), which is only 2% of total adult body weight, the total CBF at rest is disproportionately large at about 800 mL/min, which is 15–20% of the total cardiac output. At this level of blood flow, whole brain oxygen consumption, usually measured as the cerebral metabolic rate of oxygen ($CMRo_2$), is about 3.3–3.5 mL/100 g of brain per minute, or 45 mL of oxygen per minute, which is 20% of the total oxygen consumption of the body at rest.

12.1.2 Cerebral blood flow regulation

The fraction of oxygen extracted from the blood, the oxygen extraction fraction (OEF), is fairly constant throughout the brain because CBF, cerebral blood volume (CBV) and $CMRo_2$ as well as the cerebral metabolic rate of glucose (CMRglu) are all coupled.[10] In the normal resting brain, measurements of CBF are therefore a reliable reflection of cerebral metabolism ($CMRo_2$). If CBF falls, however (down to 20–25 mL/100 g brain per minute), the OEF increases to maintain the $CMRo_2$ (see below).

Over the past 60 years, the methods for measuring CBF have become more accurate and reliable, and have had a major impact on our understanding of the regulation of CBF and the pathogenesis of cerebral ischaemia.[3,11-17] Positron emission tomography (PET) now enables CBF, $CMRo_2$, OEF and CMRglu all to be measured in various regions of interest in the brain, both in normal people and after stroke.[11,14,18]

Cerebral perfusion pressure (CPP)

Under normal conditions, blood flow through the brain is determined by the CPP and by the cerebrovascular resistance (CVR) imposed by blood viscosity and the size of the intracranial vessels (i.e. flow = pressure/resistance). The CPP represents the difference between arterial pressure forcing blood into the cerebral circulation and the venous pressure. The mean CPP is the mean systemic arterial pressure at the base of the brain in the recumbent position, which approximates to the diastolic blood pressure (about 80 mmHg), plus one-third of the pulse pressure (one-third of about 40 mmHg) minus the intracranial venous pressure (about 10 mmHg), i.e. 80–85 mmHg.

Cerebrovascular resistance

Under normal conditions, when resting CPP is constant, any change in CBF must be caused by a change in CVR, usually as a result of alteration in the diameter of small intracranial arteries or arterioles. Under these circumstances, there is a direct correlation between CBF and the intravascular CBV. CBF and CBV will both increase as vessels dilate and both decrease as vessels constrict. The CBV : CBF ratio remains relatively constant over a wide range of CBF at normal CPP.

When an artery narrows causing CVR to increase, or when CBF increases, the blood flow velocity in that segment of artery increases. Although it may seem paradoxical that a reduction in luminal diameter causes an increase in blood flow velocity, think of using a hose: putting one's finger over the nozzle generates a high-pressure jet of water. The narrower the lumen at the nozzle, the greater the pressure (and velocity of flow) in the stream of water until the lumen is nearly occluded, at which point velocity becomes substantially reduced and the water dribbles out of the hose. This is one of the principles governing the interpretation of blood flow velocities in the major basal arteries by transcranial Doppler ultrasound (section 6.8.9). Mean blood flow velocities within the intracranial arteries vary from 40 to 70 cm/s. As blood flow velocity is proportional to the second power of the vessel radius, it cannot be equated linearly with volume blood flow (mL/s), which is proportional to the fourth power of the vessel radius. If vessel calibre were constant, some assumptions could be made about volume flow from velocity measures, but the calibre of large cerebral arteries varies with changes in blood pressure, partial pressure of arterial carbon dioxide ($PaCO_2$), intracranial pressure and age.

Metabolic rate of cerebral tissue

In the resting brain with normal CPP, CBF is closely matched to the metabolic demands of the tissue. Therefore, grey matter (which has a high metabolic rate) has higher regional CBF than white matter, which has a relatively low metabolic rate. The ratio between CBF and metabolism is fairly uniform in all areas of the brain and, consequently, the OEF and functional extraction of glucose from the blood are much the same in different areas. Normally, regional OEF is about one-third and the regional glucose extraction fraction is about 10%. Similarly, local flow varies directly with local brain function by 10–20%, even though global CBF tends to be

fairly stable under steady state conditions. For example, during voluntary hand movements, the metabolic activity of the contralateral motor cortex increases over a few seconds and is accompanied by rapid vasodilatation of the local cerebral resistance vessels, leading to an increase in CBF and CBV, rather than any increase in the OEF or glucose extraction fraction. Conversely, low regional metabolic activity (as may occur in a cerebral infarct) is associated with reduced metabolic demand and so low CBF. Therefore, low flow does not necessarily mean vessel occlusion but, as in this case, it can mean non-functioning brain. Although this coupling of flow with metabolism and function has been suspected for over a century, the mechanism is unknown; it may be that the metabolically active areas of brain produce vasodilatory metabolites, or the resistance vessels may be under neural regulation, or a combination of both. This is the principle underpinning functional magnetic resonance imaging (fMRI).[19]

> In normal brain, blood flow is closely coupled with metabolic demand. However, if the brain is damaged, blood flow and metabolism become uncoupled and so normal flow no longer necessarily implies normal metabolism and function.

Arterial carbon dioxide tension

Arterial carbon dioxide tension ($PaCO_2$) has a potent effect on CBF;[20] a 1 mmHg rise in $PaCO_2$ within the range of 20–60 mmHg (2.7–8.0 kPa) in normal individuals causes an immediate 3–5% increase in CBF due to dilatation of cerebral resistance vessels. In chronic respiratory failure however, causing CO_2 retention, CBF is normal. Changes in arterial oxygen tension (PaO_2) have a modest inverse effect on CBF, unless the PaO_2 falls below about 50 mmHg (6.7 kPa), when the resultant decline in the oxygen saturation of the blood leads to a fall in CVR and an increase in CBF. Increasing the PaO_2 above the normal level has little effect on CBF.

Whole-blood viscosity

Normally, CBF is inversely related to whole-blood viscosity. As the main determinant of whole-blood viscosity (at normal shear rates) is the haematocrit, it follows that CBF and haematocrit are inversely related. However, this relationship is not because the high haematocrit raises viscosity and thereby slows flow (at least not in normal vessels); rather, the higher oxygen content of high haematocrit blood allows CBF to be lower and yet to maintain normal oxygen delivery to the tissues in accordance with metabolic demands. A practical example is encountered in patients with leukaemia or paraproteinaemia who have very high blood viscosity but normal CBF (or even high CBF if anaemia coexists), because CBF depends more on the oxygen content of the blood (which is normal or low) than the viscosity (which is high). However, at very low shear rates, which might be found in ischaemic brain, for example, because of local vasodilatation, whole-blood viscosity depends more on plasma fibrinogen than haematocrit. In addition, other local factors such as red cell aggregation, platelet aggregation and perhaps increasing red cell fragility as a result of anoxia, all of which increase blood viscosity, may come into play to reduce flow.

Autoregulation

Under normal conditions (i.e. mean systemic arterial blood pressure within 60–160 mmHg), CBF is maintained at a relatively constant level despite changes in the cerebral perfusion pressure (Fig. 12.2). This capacity to maintain a constant CBF is due to the phenomenon of autoregulation.[21-23]

> Autoregulation is the ability of cerebral blood flow to remain constant in the face of changes in mean arterial pressure and cerebral perfusion pressure.

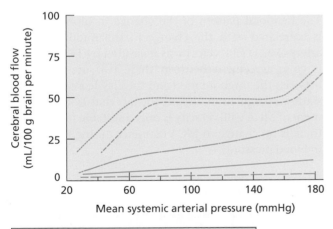

--- Normal brain tissue
--- Normal brain tissue, chronic hypertension
— Mildly ischaemic brain tissue
— Moderately ischaemic brain tissue
- - Severely ischaemic brain tissue

Fig. 12.2 Autoregulation: relationship between mean systemic arterial blood pressure and cerebral blood flow (CBF) in normal brain tissue and in brain ischaemia. Under normal conditions, CBF is maintained at a relatively constant level, independent of the systemic arterial blood pressure, as long as the mean pressure remains between about 60 and 160 mmHg. This capacity to maintain a constant CBF is due to the phenomenon of autoregulation. In chronic hypertension the curve is shifted to the right.

Autoregulation is achieved primarily by varying precapillary resistance; compensatory vasodilatation of pial and intracerebral arterioles occurs when the blood pressure falls, and compensatory vasoconstriction when the blood pressure rises. Whether myogenic, metabolic or neurogenic processes are responsible for this response is unknown.

If mean arterial pressure falls below about 40–50 mmHg, compensatory vasodilatation and therefore cerebral perfusion reserve is exhausted, and CBF parallels the blood pressure (section 6.7.5). Because oxygen delivery to the brain normally far exceeds demand, metabolic activity can still be maintained at a mean blood pressure of around 40–50 mmHg by increasing the oxygen extraction from the blood (Fig. 12.3). This state of increased OEF has been termed 'misery perfusion'.[14] However, when the OEF is maximal, a state of 'ischaemia' exists; flow is inadequate (<20 mL/100 g brain per minute) to meet metabolic demands, cellular metabolism is impaired, and so $CMRo_2$ begins to fall (see below).[24] As neuronal activity ceases, the patient usually develops symptoms of neurological dysfunction (if the whole brain is ischaemic, non-focal symptoms such as faintness, and if only part of the brain is ischaemic, focal symptoms such as hemiparesis).

If the mean arterial pressure rises above the autoregulatory range where compensatory vasoconstriction is maximal (i.e. above about 160 mmHg in normal people), then hyperaemia occurs followed by vasogenic oedema, raised intracranial pressure and the clinical syndrome of hypertensive encephalopathy (section 3.4.5).

Dynamic cerebral autoregulation is not affected by normal ageing,[25] but the autoregulatory curve is 'set' higher in patients with long-standing hypertension. Consequently, hypertensive patients are 'protected' against increasing blood pressure and develop symptoms of ischaemia at higher blood pressure (e.g. mean below about 70 mmHg) than in non-hypertensive patients (e.g. mean below 50 mmHg) (Fig. 12.2).

Autoregulation is impaired in a variety of disease states such as head trauma, diffuse cerebral hypoxia, ischaemic stroke, delayed ischaemia secondary to subarachnoid haemorrhage and in some patients with carotid stenosis or occlusion.[21-23] Autoregulation is also impaired if the $PaCO_2$ is high, presumably because further vasodilatation cannot occur and so the perfusion reserve is exhausted.[26] In some patients who have had transient ischaemic attacks or a mild ischaemic stroke, with subsequently normal angiograms, autoregulation and the cerebrovascular response to $PaCO_2$ may be deranged for several weeks. In all of these situations of impaired autoregulation, CBF varies directly with blood pressure, becoming 'pressure passive', and so predisposing to an increased

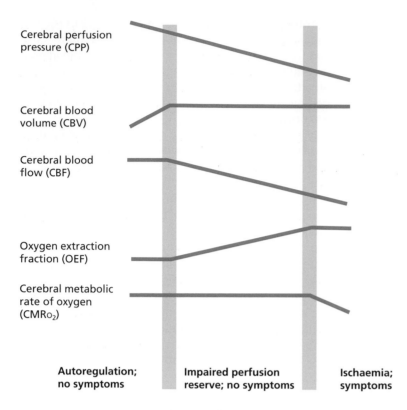

Cerebral perfusion pressure (CPP)

Cerebral blood volume (CBV)

Cerebral blood flow (CBF)

Oxygen extraction fraction (OEF)

Cerebral metabolic rate of oxygen (CMRo$_2$)

Autoregulation; no symptoms   **Impaired perfusion reserve; no symptoms**   **Ischaemia; symptoms**

Fig. 12.3 Schematic representation of the protective responses to a progressive fall in cerebral perfusion pressure (CPP). With falling CPP, intracranial arteries dilate to maintain the cerebral blood flow (CBF) – autoregulation. This results in an increase in cerebral blood volume (CBV). When vasodilatation is maximal, further falls in CPP result in a fall in CBF and therefore a fall in the CBF : CBV ratio, and an increase in the oxygen extraction fraction (OEF) to maintain tissue oxygenation. This represents a state of impaired cerebral perfusion reserve. When the OEF is maximal, further falls in CPP lead to reduction in the cerebral metabolic rate of oxygen (CMRo$_2$) and the symptoms of cerebral ischaemia.

stroke risk, particularly following exposure to hypotensive agents, as occurs perioperatively.

Traditionally, cerebral autoregulation has been measured in animals, and in response to static changes in arterial blood pressure. CBF, or an estimate of CBF such as cerebral blood flow velocity, is measured during a large change in blood pressure, usually induced pharmacologically.[27] However, such techniques are not suitable for patients with stroke, or who are at risk of stroke, because the blood pressure change induced could cause or increase brain ischaemia. Subsequent attempts to safely and non-invasively monitor autoregulation of CBF, or at least the lower limit of autoregulation, have used indirect and dynamic measures such as CBF velocity, as determined by transcranial Doppler (TCD) ultrasound, in response to vasodilatory stimuli such as hypercapnoea (rather than changes in blood pressure).[22] Although these indirect measures generally correlate with direct measures of cerebral autoregulation, they do measure a slightly different physiological response. Other methods of measuring dynamic autoregulation which are non-invasive, and suitable for use in patients at risk of stroke, aim to evaluate the response of CBF or CBF velocity to small physiological changes in arterial blood pressure. These include changes in blood pressure induced by the use of bilateral leg cuffs which are inflated suprasystolically and then suddenly deflated to cause a transient fall in blood pressure, and spontaneous variability in arterial

blood pressure by a servo-controlled plethysmograph.[27] The temporal pattern of the change in blood pressure is correlated with the change in the middle cerebral artery (MCA) CBF velocity as measured by TCD.[26] There is close agreement between these two methods, and between the thigh method and the classic assessment of static autoregulation, despite the fact that TCD measurement of MCA CBF velocity is only a suitable technique if there is no change in MCA diameter during the change in blood pressure.

Cerebral perfusion reserve

The ratio of CBF : CBV (see above) is a measure of cerebral perfusion reserve; a ratio below about 6.0 indicates maximal vasodilatation and CBV, and exhausted reserve, even if the CBF is still normal. If available, PET scanning will show a rising OEF at this stage, to maintain CMRo$_2$ (Fig. 12.4).[10,15,28,29] If PET is unavailable, the mean cerebral transit time (MCTT), which is the reciprocal of CBF : CBV, can be used instead.[30] Other techniques for measuring CBF at rest and after exposure to vasodilatory stimuli (e.g. inhalation of CO$_2$, intravenous administration of acetazolamide, or breath holding), and thus cerebrovascular reserve capacity, include:
- xenon-133 (^{133}Xe) inhalation; ^{133}Xe is a lipophilic radioactive tracer that can be inhaled or injected and easily diffuses through the blood–brain barrier. Probes

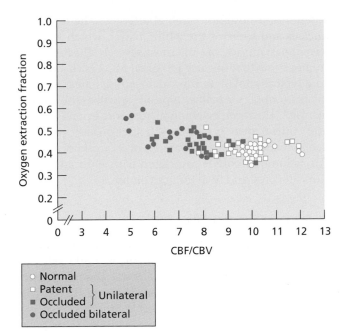

Fig. 12.4 Relationship between oxygen extraction fraction (OEF) and cerebral blood flow (CBF) : cerebral blood volume ratio (CBF : CBV) in each of 82 middle cerebral artery regions from 32 patients with varying degrees of carotid artery stenosis and occlusion and nine normal subjects (with permission from Gibbs *et al.* (1984)[15]). CBF : CBV is a measure of cerebral perfusion reserve. A CBF : CBV ratio below about 6.0 indicates maximal vasodilatation and CBV, and exhausted reserve, even if the CBF is still normal. If cerebral blood flow continues to fall at this stage, OEF rises to maintain CMRo₂.

placed over the scalp can measure perfusion to the cerebral cortex;[19,31]

- stable ('cold') xenon-enhanced computed tomography (CT);[32]
- single-photon emission computed tomography (SPECT) with [133]Xe-, iodine-123 (^{123}I)-labelled isopropyliodo-amphetamine, or technetium-99m (^{99}Tc)-labelled hexamethylpropyleneamine oxime (HMPAO);[19,33]
- perfusion-weighted MRI;[13,16,17,19]
- CT perfusion.[34–37]

Cerebrovascular reactivity can also be evaluated by:

- three-dimensional time-of-flight magnetic resonance angiography; a severely saturated flow signal indicates a higher probability of impaired cerebrovascular reactivity, but is neither sensitive nor specific;[19]
- blood oxygen level-dependent (BOLD) contrast MRI coupled with administration of CO_2;[38–40]
- transcranial Doppler ultrasound (TCD), which measures velocity flow in the MCA as a surrogate for CBF, coupled with administration of CO_2 with or without colour duplex M-mode ultrasound (to estimate extracranial carotid flow volume).[19,32,41]

In clinical practice, cerebral perfusion reserve is generally assessed indirectly by measuring the relative difference between CBF at baseline and then in response to a vasomotor stimulus such as CO_2 (by inhalation or breath holding) or acetazolamide (by intravenous administration), which increase CBF unless the capacity for cerebral dilatation is exhausted. For example, intravenous injection of 1 g of the vasodilating agent acetazolamide (Diamox) produces an increase in CBF of 5–100% within 20–30 min. The lack of such flow augmentation indicates a loss of autoregulation and inadequate cerebrovascular reserve.[36,42]

The completely non-invasive evaluation of cerebrovascular reserve capacity with TCD CO_2 testing is the most widely applied method in clinical practice. Drawbacks of TCD CO_2 testing are an insufficient temporal bone ultrasound window in 10–20% of patients and relatively low diagnostic accuracy.[32] Indeed, all of the indirect methods of measuring perfusion reserve (e.g. SPECT, TCD, MCTT) are inaccurate when the normal relationships between CBF, CBV, OEF and vascular reactivity are distorted, as occurs in ischaemic and infarcted brain.[28]

A common clinical scenario of potentially impaired reserve is a patient with stenosis or occlusion of one or both internal carotid arteries, severe enough (at least 50% diameter stenosis) to produce a fall in CPP distally. If the ophthalmic and leptomeningeal collateral CBF is inadequate, and the oxygen extraction fraction increases, a state of 'misery perfusion' exists.[16,43] Under these circumstances, the brain is vulnerable to any further fall in CPP, as may occur when the patient stands up quickly, when undergoing anaesthesia (e.g. for coronary artery bypass surgery) or starts or increases antihypertensive medication or vasodilators. In patients with symptomatic ICA occlusion, misery perfusion (or severely impaired cerebral vasomotor reactivity as a surrogate) increases the risk of future ipsilateral ischaemic stroke by as much as seven- to eightfold.[15,44,45]

Perfusion imaging with a challenge test (e.g. PET-OEF, Xe/CT perfusion with acetazolamide) may be able to identify patients with enough reduction in cerebral perfusion reserve to benefit from an extracranial to intracranial (EC-IC) bypass to augment the CBF.[28,42,46] However, correlation of the different methods of measuring autoregulatory vasodilatation, secondary to reduced perfusion pressure, is sufficiently variable to have limited the validity of studies associating haemodynamic impairment with stroke risk.[28] An ongoing clinical trial using the OEF as measured with PET scanning will attempt to define the patient population with occlusive vascular disease at high enough risk for stroke that the risk of EC-IC bypass is worth taking for the potential long-term benefit.[46,47]

12.1.3 Pathophysiology of cerebral ischaemia

Thrombosis

Acute cerebral ischaemia usually begins with the occlusion of a cerebral blood vessel, more often on the arterial than venous side of the circulation, usually by thrombus or embolus (Chapter 6). It is rarely due to low flow alone.

When a major artery is suddenly occluded, arterial blood pressure and blood flow fall distal to the occlusion, and the region of brain supplied by that vessel is acutely deprived of its blood supply and is rendered ischaemic. Presumably the pathophysiology of venous infarction is similar, but less has been published about it.

Activated platelets play a critical role in arterial thrombosis (section 6.3.3) and also in mediating an inflammatory response in the brain (see Inflammation below). Activated platelets degranulate and adhere to leucocytes, thus forming platelet–leucocyte coaggregates. They do this by expressing P-selectin on their surface which binds to the leucocyte counter-receptor P-selecting GP ligand-1. This induces leucocyte activation and the release of inflammatory cytokines.[48]

The metabolic and clinical consequences of cerebral ischaemia depend not only on the cascade of events induced by thrombus formation (i.e. biosynthesis of thrombogenic and neurotoxic eicosanoids, inflammation, breakdown of the blood–brain barrier, diffusion of these products into surrounding brain and reduced microvascular flow in the ischaemic penumbra around the initial focus), but also on the site, severity and duration of cerebral ischaemia, the availability of collateral blood flow, other systemic and tissue factors, and the effect of any reperfusion therapies.[49]

Site of cerebral ischaemia

Neurones are the brain cells most vulnerable to ischaemia, followed by oligodendroglia, astrocytes and endothelial cells. However, even within the population of neurones, there are many different types that also vary in their sensitivity to ischaemia, and in some cases the vulnerability varies with the location of the cells. The most vulnerable neurones to mild ischaemia are the pyramidal neurones in the CA1 and CA4 zones of the hippocampus, followed by neurones in the cerebellum, striatum and neocortex.

Acute occlusion of the proximal middle cerebral artery (MCA) reduces distal cerebral perfusion pressure. Cerebral perfusion pressure reductions in the cortical MCA territory are most severe in its centre (perisylvian) region and least in the border zone areas between the MCA and anterior and posterior cerebral arteries.[3] The lentiform nucleus and some of the white matter, which have far fewer anastamoses, are the most severely affected.[3] PET studies show that in early proximal MCA occlusion, the core typically involves the striatocapsular area, whereas the penumbra (see below) typically involves the cortical mantle.[19] However, occasionally the core extends widely into cortical areas as early as 4 h after onset,[19] probably due to inadequate pial collaterals or a carotid occlusion. The volume of core is associated with both admission clinical scores, and final infarct volume.

Availability of collateral blood flow

Occlusion of a cerebral artery reduces but seldom abolishes the delivery of oxygen and glucose to the relevant region of the brain because collateral channels partly maintain blood flow in the ischaemic territory. This incomplete ischaemia is responsible for the spatial and temporal dynamics of cerebral infarction.[24] Some other areas of the brain, including infarcted tissue, may show relative or absolute hyperaemia (called 'luxury perfusion') due to good collateral blood supply, recanalization of the occluded artery, or inflammation or vasodilatation in response to hypercapnia, i.e. flow is in excess of the metabolic demands and so the oxygen extraction fraction is reduced.

Severity of ischaemia: critical flow thresholds

The transition from normal CBF through to cerebral oligaemia, the ischaemic penumbra and frank tissue infarction (see below) occurs, operationally, in phases, depending on the severity and duration of brain ischaemia (Fig. 12.5).

> The key pathophysiological concept is the division of hypoperfused tissue into three operational compartments: tissue that will in principle survive (oligaemia), tissue that may either die or survive (the ischaemic penumbra), and tissue that will inevitably die (core).

Experimental models of focal cerebral ischaemia have identified critical flow thresholds for certain cell functions (Fig. 12.5), notably a threshold for tissue at risk, electrical failure (loss of neuronal electrical activity) and membrane failure (loss of cellular ion homeostasis).[4,5,21]

Initially, small declines in perfusion pressure and CBF (<50 mL/100 g/min) are compensated for by regional vasodilatation to maintain CBF (autoregulation), resulting in a regional increase in CBV (section 12.1.2) (Fig. 12.3). With continued reductions in perfusion pressure (<45 mL/

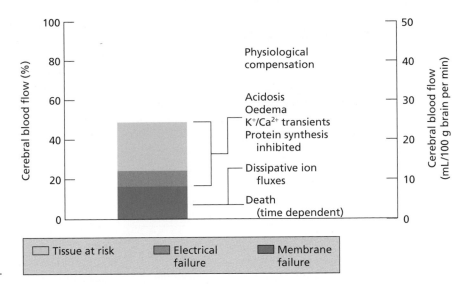

Fig. 12.5 Cerebral blood flow (CBF) thresholds for cell dysfunction and death.

100 g/min), and the dilatation of all vessels to capacity, the oxygen extraction fraction (OEF) and glucose extraction fraction (GEF) are increased to maintain a normal cerebral metabolic rate of oxygen ($CMRo_2$) and glucose (CMRglu).[29] Protein synthesis also becomes inhibited. This is a state of 'misery perfusion' which is characterized by reduced CBF, increased OEF (ranging from the normal value of about 30–40% up to the theoretical maximum of 100%) and relatively preserved or even normal oxygen consumption ($CMRo_2$).[3] The tissue is at risk.

Oligaemia

With further cerebral ischaemia (<35 mL/100 g/min), lack of oxygen inhibits mitochondrial metabolism and activates the inefficient anaerobic metabolism of glucose, causing a local rise in lactate production and so a fall in pH, leading to intra- and extracellular acidosis (Fig. 12.5). The energy-dependent functions of cell membranes to maintain ion homeostasis become progressively impaired; K^+ leaks out of cells into the extracellular space, Na^+ and water enter cells (cytotoxic oedema), and Ca^{++} also moves into cells (where it causes mitochondrial failure and compromises the ability of intracellular membranes to control subsequent ion fluxes, leading to cytotoxicity).[2,6]

Several compensatory mechanisms come into play which sacrifice electrophysiological activity to maintain near-normal ATP concentrations and membrane ion gradients and preserve cell viability, at least temporarily. Hence, the suppression of neuronal electrical activity as seen on the electroencephalogram (EEG) in order to reduce energy use. If moderate ischaemia persists, however (i.e. for several hours), the tissue at risk dies.

Loss of neuronal electrical activity and function

The threshold for *loss of neuronal electrical activity* (i.e. electrical failure) is reached when the CBF falls below about 20–25 mL/100 g of brain per minute.[4,5] At this point, the OEF is maximal, the $CMRo_2$ begins to fall (Fig. 12.3), normal neuronal function of the cerebral cortex is affected, neurotransmitters are released, evoked cerebral responses from the area of focal ischaemia decrease in amplitude and electrical activity in cortical cells begins to fail.[50] With further falls in flow, evoked potentials are lost, the EEG flattens and then becomes isoelectric.

> Reduction of cerebral blood from its mean of around 50 mL/100 g per min to less than 20 mL/100 g per min results in impaired neural function, but preserves tissue integrity; this defines the penumbra.

Loss of cellular ion homeostasis

The threshold for *loss of cellular ion homeostasis* (i.e. membrane failure) and anoxic depolarization is reached when blood flow falls to about 15 mL/100 g of brain per minute.[4,5] The water and electrolyte content of ischaemic tissue changes due to cell pump failure (see below). The critical threshold for the beginning of irreversible cell damage is a CBF of about 10 mL/100 g of brain per minute. For a short period, the neurones may remain viable and recover function if perfusion is restored. Otherwise, rapid efflux of K^+ and influx of Ca^{++} ensue due to failure of the plasma membrane, and there is swelling of the cell and internal organelles, protein degradation and DNA breakup.

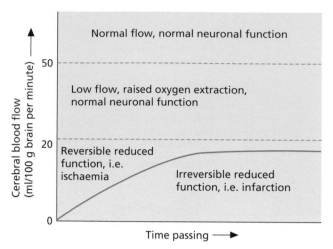

Fig. 12.6 Combined effects of residual cerebral blood flow (CBF) and duration of ischaemia on reversibility of neuronal dysfunction during focal cerebral ischaemia. The solid line delineates the limits of severity and duration of ischaemia that allow survival of any neurones.[50]

Duration of ischaemia

Tissue outcome depends on two factors – the severity of flow reduction (see above) and its duration (Fig. 12.6).[50] The CBF threshold that defines the core increases with time until it reaches the penumbra threshold, at which point all the penumbra has been recruited. Thus, within the penumbra, the lower the CBF, the higher the risk of early infarction. PET studies indicate that substantial penumbra is present in up to 90% of patients within 6 h of onset; this falls to about 50% within 9 h but is still intact in about 30% of patients 18 h after onset.[3] Up to 52% of the ultimate infarct still shows penumbra 16 h after onset.[51]

Two trials suggesting effectiveness of the thrombolytic drug desmoteplase when given 3–9 h after onset of ischaemic stroke (in patients with a DWI-PWI mismatch > 20%), coupled with imaging studies showing a prolonged persistence of substantial volumes of 'at risk', but potentially viable, brain tissue for up to 16–18 h after ischaemic stroke in some patients, suggest that the time window for effective therapeutic intervention may be longer in humans than predicted from animal studies.[3,51–53] Indeed, we have learnt from randomized trials in acute myocardial infarction (MI) that thrombolysis is still effective in reducing case fatality even when given up to 24 h after the onset of chest pain, despite the widely held belief prior to these studies, mainly based on animal models, that thrombolysis could not possibly be effective if given more than a few hours after acute MI.[54]

Cerebral ischaemia is a dynamic process of fluctuating severity over the first few hours and it may not be possible to predict just how long the time window is to allow successful therapeutic intervention in any one individual.[3] Indeed, there is unlikely to be a rigid and universal time window for all patients because there is so much heterogeneity among individuals in the pattern of arterial occlusion and collateral flow, the duration of ischaemia, the size of the ischaemic area, where it is and which cells are involved, and perhaps even the genetic make-up of the patient.[3] The therapeutic time window may also vary for different sites of arterial occlusion and brain ischaemia, and for different interventions. For example, the therapeutic time window for thrombolytics may be shorter than for neuroprotective agents, than for antithrombotic agents; we do not know yet.

> In humans it is not clear how long ischaemic brain can survive and still be salvaged by reperfusion or measures to protect neurones from dying. Consequently, the duration of the 'time window' for effective therapeutic intervention is unknown.

Other systemic and tissue factors

Tissue with small reductions in cerebral blood flow – 20–50 ml/100 g per min, defined as oligaemia, probably maintains its function for a long time and is unlikely to proceed to infarction. However, oligaemia may become penumbral – and hence potentially the core – because of secondary events that reduce cerebral perfusion pressure, such as vasogenic oedema and systemic hypotension, or by factors that aggravate the flow–metabolism mismatch such as hyperglycaemia and pyrexia.[11] This may explain the possible benefits from avoiding physiological complications and maintaining blood pressure early after ischaemic stroke.

Concept of an ischaemic penumbra

The finding of two separate thresholds, one for cessation of electrical signals and the other for loss of ion homeostasis, which are separated by an intermediate zone characterized by cessation of cellular electrical activity but with preservation of their membrane potential, led to the concept of an ischaemic penumbra of brain tissue.[19] The ischaemic penumbra can be defined as an area of severely ischaemic, functionally impaired, but surviving brain tissue which is at risk of infarction but can be saved, and recover, if it is reperfused before it is irreversibly damaged (hence the concept of 'time is brain').[3,11,13,55,56] Otherwise, it will be progressively recruited into the core of the infarct until maximum infarct extension is reached. The ischaemic penumbra is not just a topographic locus, but a dynamic (time × space) process, characterized by an evolving zone of bioenergetic upheaval.[3] This penumbral concept provides an important insight into the nature of tissue survival after stroke and an important target for therapy. Changes in water homeostasis, including shrinkage of the extracellular space and net uptake of water from plasma, also take place in the penumbra.

> As cerebral blood flow falls from its normal mean, around 50 mL/100 g per min, to less than 20 mL/100 g per min, a critical threshold is reached when the electrical activity of neurones is suppressed and neuronal function is impaired. As flow falls further, another threshold is reached when cellular integrity begins to break down. Cells falling in between these two thresholds make up the 'ischaemic penumbra': they may not be functioning, but they are still viable and could either recover function, with early reperfusion or early interruption of the adverse metabolic or neurochemical cascade, or die. Survival of the penumbra is the main determinant of clinical recovery.
>
> Because both the core and the penumbra can contribute to neurological deficits, it is not possible to clinically determine their relative effects; imaging is required.

Imaging the ischaemic penumbra

Imaging studies, with various techniques, have established the clinical importance of penumbral salvage, showing a clear association between the volume of penumbra not progressing to infarction and the improvement in neurological scores of impairments and function.[57] To be accepted as penumbra, the affected tissue must fulfil several well-defined operation criteria (Table 12.1). The main methods of imaging the ischaemic penumbra *in vivo* are by positron emission tomography (PET), magnetic resonance imaging (MRI), CT perfusion and single-

Table 12.1 Currently accepted operational criteria defining the ischaemic penumbra.[19]

> Hypoperfusion < 20 mL/100 g brain per min
> Abnormal neuronal function documented by a correlation with acute clinical deficit
> Physiological and/or biochemical characteristics consistent with cellular dysfunction but not death
> Uncertain fate (i.e. ischaemic brain tissue may die or recover depending on timing and degree of reperfusion)
> Salvage of this tissue is correlated with better clinical recovery

photon emission tomography (SPECT).[12,13,19,34,39,58,59] The parameters they map, the criteria they use to identify the penumbra and their main advantages and limitations are listed in Table 12.2.[19]

Positron emission tomography (PET)

Originally, PET measurements were undertaken with the oxygen-15 steady-state technique. This quantitative imaging maps the main physiological variables involved in tissue ischaemia, namely perfusion (or CBF), and oxygen consumption ($CMRo_2$) together with oxygen extraction ration (OEF) and cerebral blood volume (CBV).[3,11,45] However, because these determinations of flow and energy metabolism required arterial blood sampling and complex logistics, they were difficult to perform in patients with acute stroke and impossible when planning thrombolytic therapy. This led to the development of noninvasive measurement of the extent of the penumbra by means or tracers (that indicate tissue integrity or hypoxia) combined with semiquantitative measures of perfusion.

[^{11}C]Flumazenil (FMZ) is a central benzodiazepine receptor ligand labelled with C-11. It detects neuronal damage in the cortex in the first few hours after ischaemic stroke and is therefore a marker of tissue integrity (but not so much in the white matter and basal ganglia which have low concentrations of benzodiazepine receptors).[60]

[^{18}F]fluoromisonidazole (FMISO) is another tracer and it indicates hypoxic but viable tissue, and can also be used to detect the ischaemic penumbra when the results are directly calibrated by conventional PET measurements.[57] However, because reliable detection of FMISO uptake is delayed (at least 2 h between tracer injection and imaging) its value is limited in guiding treatment decisions in acute ischaemic stroke.

Based on validated thresholds, PET can classify affected tissue as core, penumbra, oligaemia and hyperperfused.[3,19,60] Oligaemia displays mild misery perfusion – i.e. a moderately reduced cerebral blood flow (above the penumbra threshold) and a high oxygen extraction fraction. A high oxygen extraction fraction in itself does not equate with penumbra as this fraction rises as soon as CBF decreases. Early spontaneous hyperperfusion, present in about one-third of patients within 18 h of onset of ischaemic stroke, almost invariably predicts preserved cerebral oxygen metabolism ($CMRo_2$) and tissue integrity, suggesting this as a marker of prior recanalization that salvages the penumbra.[19]

Although PET is arguably still the 'gold standard' for measuring the ischaemic penumbra,[59] particularly given its superior quantification, it is limited by the expensive

Table 12.2 Main physiological imaging techniques, with the parameters they map, the criteria they use to identify the penumbra, and their main advantages and limitations.[19]

Technique	Parameters	Definition of penumbra	Advantages	Limitations
CT				
Perfusion	CBF CBV MTT	Relative CBF < 66%* CBV > 2.5 mL/ 100 g brain	Combined with plain CT, available, fast	Limited brain coverage, insensitive in posterior circulation, indirect visualization of core, iodinated contrast
Xenon (Xe)	CBF	CBF 7–20 mL/ 100 g brain	Quantitative, combined with plain CT	Not fully validated, provides CBF only, pharmacological effects of Xe
MRI				
DWI-PWI	CBF CBV MTT TTP ADC	Relative TPP (or MTT) delay > 4s* and normal DWI	Fast, best sensitivity, no radiation, directly visualizes core	Limited availability, mismatch concept not validated, CBF values not accurate, patient's cooperation required, frequent contraindications
Arterial spin labelling	CBF	Not validated	No contrast needed	Provides CBF only, poor sensitivity to low flows
MRI-based (and PWI)	CBF OEF CMRo$_2$	Not validated	Non-invasive mapping of OEF and CMRo$_2$	Validity unclear
Spectroscopy	NAA Lactate	Elevated lactate and normal NAA	Biochemically characterizes tissue	Not validated, poor resolution
PET				
Multi-tracer ^{15}O	CBF CBV MTT CMRo$_2$ OEF	CBF 7–22 mL/ 100 g brain/min and OEF > 0.70	Quantitative, validated	Complex, time-consuming, not widely available, expensive
[^{11}C]FMZ (+ H$_2$^{15}O)	Tracer binding	Relative binding > 3.4** and CBV < 14 mL/ 100 g brain/min	Based on physiological neuronal integrity	As above and only suitable for cortex, basis not validated
[^{18}F]FMISO	Tracer uptake	Uptake ratio > 1.3*	Produces a direct positive image of viable tissue hypoxia	As above and validation incomplete, long imaging time
SPECT				
[^{99m}Tc]-labelled HMPAO or ECD	CBF	Relative CBF < 65%*	Cheap and relatively available	Provides perfusion only so thresholds uncertain, limited spatial resolution, slow brain kinetics

*relative to mean contralateral hemisphere; **relative to contralateral healthy white matter; ADC, apparent diffusion coefficient; CBF, cerebral blood flow; CBV, cerebral blood volume; DWI, diffusion-weighted imaging; ECD, ethyl-cysteinate dimer; FMISO, fluoromisonidazole; FMZ, flumazenil; HMPAO, hexamethylpropyleneamine oxime; MTT, mean transit time; NAA, N-acetylaspartate; OEF, oxygen extraction fraction; PWI, perfusion-weighted imaging; SPECT, single photon emission computed tomography; TTP, time to peak.

equipment and the complex logistics of a multidisciplinary team.

> PET is able to differentiate between normal, penumbral, and infarcted tissue in the acute stage of ischaemic stroke. However, because of its logistic and practical limitations, its clinical role in acute stroke is limited.

MRI DWI-PWI

A more widely applicable method is the magnetic resonance imaging (MRI) technique of combined diffusion-weighted imaging (DWI) and perfusion-weighted imaging (PWI) as a measure of tissue integrity and cerebral perfusion respectively (section 5.5.2).[12,13,17,19,61–63]

The apparent diffusion coefficient (ADC) on DWI is an 'apparent' or 'relative' measure of the diffusion of free water in one area compared with other areas during the DWI sequence.[61] It is decreased in areas of ischaemic brain which have a critically low CBF.[64,65] A decrease in the ADC is seen as an area of hyperdensity on diffusion-weighted images (due to a restriction in the diffusional movement of water), as soon as 11 min after stroke.[66] Because DWI abnormalities typically evolve into infarction without reperfusion or neuroprotection.[62] It has been suggested that the DWI abnormality corresponds to the ischaemic core, but this is not always the case.[12,63,67]

PWI, on the other hand, provides information on the haemodynamic status of the tissue by using paramagnetic contrast agents, for example, gadolinium-based chelates. On the basis of magnetic resonance perfusion imaging data, maps of relative CBF can be calculated, and these demonstrate impaired perfusion of both the ischaemic core and the surrounding brain regions, thereby complementing the information derived from DWI.[68] During the first few hours of stroke evolution, PWI typically demonstrates regions with abnormal perfusion that are larger than the DWI abnormalities. It has been postulated that this mismatch reflects the ischaemic penumbra (i.e. functionally impaired 'tissue at risk' surrounding the irreversibly damaged ischaemic

core).[17,19,69] Typically, a PWI > DWI lesion is associated with subsequent infarct enlargement but, because PWI is very sensitive in detecting perfusion defects, the PWI/DWI mismatch region may comprise not only tissue at risk but also hypoperfused tissue with CBF values above the critical viability thresholds. Further, the reliability of assessing the degree of diffusion-perfusion mismatch is not established.[70]

The diffusion-perfusion mismatch concept of the ischaemic penumbra (hypoperfusion volume > DWI lesion) has now been modified with the recognition that a portion of hypoperfused brain reflects benign oligaemia, and that the so-called DWI core may in fact be partially salvageable. The validity and reliability of DWI and PWI evidence of mismatch as a marker of the ischaemic penumbra, as compared with PET, has been supported in recent small studies.[63] However, its validity in predicting lesion expansion and response to therapy is uncertain and is being evaluated in ongoing studies.[12,17,19,71–73] Table 12.3 summarizes the evidence base for the DWI-PWI mismatch hypothesis.[19]

T2-based blood oxygen level-dependent (BOLD) MR imaging can visualize deoxyhaemoglobin and may serve as a valid non-invasive indicator of the oxygen extraction fraction and thus the metabolic state of threatened brain tissue.[39]

Table 12.3 Validity of the DWI-PWI mismatch hypothesis to identify the ischaemic penumbra.[19]

Operational criteria (see Table 12.1)	DWI-PWI mismatch
Hypoperfusion < 20 mL/100 g brain per min	Absolute CBF values unreliable with PWI; but TTP > 4 s delay shown to correspond to PET-derived CBF < 20 mL/100 g per min
Abnormal neuronal function documented by a correlation with acute clinical deficit	Volume of DWI lesion and of mismatch significantly correlate with acute-stage stroke severity
Physiological and/or biochemical characteristics	In humans, acutely the ADC starts to decline for CBF consistent with cellular dysfunction but not death, values corresponding to the penumbra threshold. ADC declines represent cytotoxic oedema and consistently correspond to reduced CMRO$_2$ in humans. In the rat, ADC declines shown to correspond with impaired aerobic glycoslysis and ATP production
Uncertain fate	Without early reperfusion, tissue-at-risk progresses to full infarction
Salvage of this tissue is correlated with better clinical recovery	Salvage of tissue-at-risk transfers to better outcome and correlates with clinical recovery

ADC, apparent diffusion coefficient; CBF, cerebral blood flow; CMRo$_2$, cerebral metabolic rate of oxygen; NIHSS, National Institute of Health Stroke Scale; TTP, time to peak.

Meanwhile, other incremental refinements in the definition of the ischaemic penumbra are likely, including measurement of biochemical thresholds with spectroscopy, and imaging of a 'molecular penumbra' by means of measuring gene markers of protein expression.[1]

> Although early studies suggested that various MRI techniques such as perfusion- and diffusion-weighted imaging could differentiate between penumbra and infarct, more recent studies have shown that this may be an oversimplification.

CT perfusion

Measures of CBF and CBV obtained from CT perfusion can be sensitive and specific for infarction, and may have utility for differentiating between infarct and penumbra.[34] Penumbral regions are characterized by a mismatch between CBF (which is reduced) and CBV (which is maintained), whereas infarcted areas show a matched decrease in both parameters.

> Contrast-enhanced CT may be able to delineate infarcted and penumbral tissue in acute stroke.

Reperfusion and brain damage

Reperfusion within the revival times of ischaemic tissues may salvage cells and aid recovery (by restoring oxygen and nutrient delivery to ischaemic brain tissue). However, it may also be detrimental, causing so-called 'reperfusion injury' due to the resupply of glucose (which may increase lactic acidosis), oxygen (which may trigger production of injurious free radicals), water and osmotic equivalents (which may exacerbate vasogenic oedema), and blood-borne cells (such as neutrophils) which may exacerbate ischaemic damage.[74,75]

> Rescue of the penumbra, either by restoration of blood supply or by interruption of the adverse metabolic or neurochemical cascade, is the basis of acute stroke therapy.

As discussed below, leucocytes migrate into the injured region within hours of reperfusion and may cause tissue injury by occluding the microvasculature, generating oxygen-free radicals, releasing cytotoxic enzymes, altering vasomotor reactivity and increasing cytokine and chemo-attractant release.[76] Although, as ever, for every potential benefit of treatment there are potential harms, in humans the empirical evidence suggests that the benefits of reperfusion are greater than the hazards (section 12.5).

12.1.4 Phases and mediators of cell death

With sudden, severe and prolonged reductions in cerebral blood flow (CBF) below about 10 mL/100 g brain per minute, ischaemic necrosis (infarction/cell death) progresses within minutes in the core of the affected region because of low ATP levels and energy stores, ionic disruption and metabolic failure.[77] However, not all brain cells die immediately after stroke. In the ischaemic penumbra that surrounds the anoxic core, cells can be rescued by rapid reperfusion.

Ischaemic brain cells die by the convergence of three main mechanisms: excitotoxicity and ionic imbalance, oxidative stress and apoptotic-like cell death (Fig. 12.7).[77–82]

Excitotoxicity

When the blood supply to a part of the brain is interrupted, neurones deprived of their supply of oxygen and glucose rapidly (within minutes) fail to generate sufficient ATP and energy to maintain ionic gradients across membranes because of failure of the Na^+, K^+-ATPase pump. This causes an increase in extracellular K^+ as well as an influx of Na^+, Cl^- and Ca^{++} into the cells. The initial increase in extracellular K^+ may spread, triggering depolarizations of neurones and reversal of the amino acid transporters. In these conditions, both voltage-operated and receptor-operated calcium channels are recruited, thus provoking an elevation of free cytosolic Ca^{++}. The depolarized presynaptic neurones release the neurotransmitter glutamate into the synaptic cleft. Reuptake of glutamate is impaired, leading to an increase in extracellular concentration of the excitatory amino acid glutamate. Glutamate activates postsynaptic receptors, including the ionotropic N-methyl-D-aspartate (NMDA), 2-amino-3-(3-hydroxy-5-methylisoxazol-4-yl) proprionate (AMPA) and kainate receptors.[83] Upon their activation, these open their associated ion channel to allow the influx of Ca^{++} and Na^+ ions.[2,84] Glutamate-evoked Na^+ increase in astrocytes evokes the transmission of intercellular Na^+ and Ca^{++} metabolic waves and an increase in uptake of glucose.[85]

Under physiological conditions, calcium ions (Ca^{++}) govern a multitude of cellular processes, including cell growth, differentiation and synaptic activity. Consequently, there are energy-dependent homeostatic mechanisms to maintain a low intracellular Ca^{++} concentration (about 100 times lower than its extracellular concentration) so that Ca^{++} signals remain spatially and temporally localized. This permits multiple independent Ca-mediated signalling pathways to occur in the same cell. In excitotoxicity, the excessive synaptic release of glutamate which leads to excessive influx of Ca^{++},

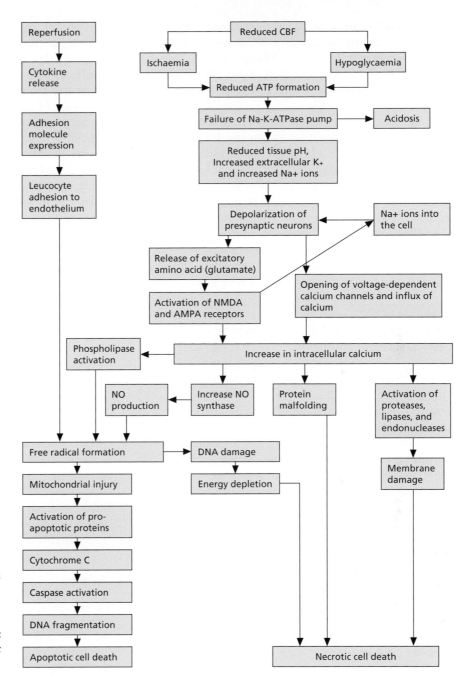

Fig. 12.7 Schematic diagram of some potential mechanisms of ischaemic brain damage and reperfusion injury. CBF, cerebral blood flow; ATP, adenosine triphosphate; AMPA, D-amino-3-hydroxyl-5-ethyl-4-isoxazole propionate; NMDA, N-methyl-D-aspartate; NO, nitric oxide.

together with any Ca^{++} release from intracellular compartments, can overwhelm Ca^{++} regulatory mechanisms and this leads to disregulation of Ca^{++} homeostasis, and ultimately to cell damage and death. The cell damage associated with a non-physiological unregulated rise in intracellular cytoplasmic Ca^{++} is caused mainly by changes in total calcium influx.[6]

The initial calcium load is sequestered, at least in part, by the mitochondria. Mitochondrial injury is associated with failure of mitochondrial functions such as oxidative phosphorylation, and release of reactive oxygen species (see below).[6,84] Mitochondrial calcium accumulation and oxidative stress can then trigger the assembly (opening) of a high-conductance pore in the inner mitochondrial membrane. The mitochondrial permeability transition (MPT) pore leads to a collapse of the electrochemical potential for H^+, thereby arresting ATP production and triggering further production of reactive oxygen species.

An increase in total calcium influx also contributes to cell death by activation of Ca^{++}-ATPase (which results in further consumption of cellular ATP); activation of

Ca^{++}-dependent phospholipases, synthases, proteases and endonucleases (which degrade key cytoskeletal and enzymatic proteins such as phospholipids, proteins and nucleic acids); and alteration of protein phosphorylation, which secondarily affect protein synthesis and genome expression.[2,84,86]

In addition, the augmented intracellular Ca^{++} enhances the increase in extracellular glutamate, thus propagating excitotoxicity.[84] Although Ca^{++} disregulation is paramount to neurodegeneration, the exact mechanism by which Ca^{++} ions actually mediate excitotoxicity is less clear.[2] One hypothesis suggests that Ca^{++}-dependent neurotoxicity occurs following the activation of distinct signalling cascades downstream from key points of Ca^{++} entry at synapses, and that triggers of these cascades are physically colocalized with specific glutamate receptors.[2]

> Calcium influx is mediated directly and predominantly by NMDA receptors, but it is also triggered secondarily by Na$^+$ influx through AMPA-, kainate- and NMDA-receptor-gated channels. The resultant excessive Ca^{++} influx leads to elevated intracellular and intramitochondial Ca^{++} concentrations and lethal metabolic derangements, which include calcium-dependent activation of intracellular enzyme systems, failure of oxidative phosphorylation and the generation of free radicals that further compromise cells by attacking proteins, lipids and nucleic acids.

Oxidative stress (production of free radicals)

A free radical is any atom, group of atoms or molecule with an unpaired electron in its outermost orbital.[80] Free radicals are produced in small quantities by normal cellular processes in all aerobic cells; for example, 'leaks' in mitochondrial electron transport allow oxygen to accept single electrons, forming superoxide (O_2^-). However, they are inherently toxic – they can react with and damage proteins, nucleic acids, lipids and other classes of molecules such as the extracellular matrix glycosaminoglycans (e.g. hyaluronic acid). The sulphur-containing amino acids and the polyunsaturated fatty acids (found in high concentrations in the brain) are particularly vulnerable. Fortunately, cells possess appropriate defence mechanisms in the form of free radical scavengers and enzymes which metabolize free radicals or their precursors.

During severe brain ischaemia, insufficient oxygen is available to accept electrons passed along the mitochondrial electron transport chain, leading to eventual reduction ('electron saturation') of the components of this system. The free radicals which are elevated in cerebral ischaemia include O_2^-, hydroxyl (OH) and nitric oxide (NO). Nitric oxide is generated primarily by neuronal and inducible NO synthases (NOS).[84] Like other free radicals, the free radicals which are elevated in cerebral ischaemia react with and damage proteins, nucleic acids and lipids, particularly the fatty acid component of membrane phospholipids, producing changes in the fluidity and permeability of the cellular membranes (lipid peroxidation).[80,84] The free radicals also cause microvascular dysfunction and disrupt the blood–brain barrier, leading to brain oedema. In addition, the conversion of xanthine dehydrogenase to xanthine oxidase promotes the cellular formation of toxic oxygen free radicals such as the superoxide anion which further breaks down membrane, cytoskeletal and nuclear structures. An important source of oxidative stress-mediated brain damage is the oxidant reactions due to the formation of peroxynitrite, a powerful oxidant that results from the interaction between NO and superoxide. This anion has been shown to cause cell damage by several mechanisms that include lipid peroxidation, tryrosine nitration, sulphydryl oxidation and nitrosylation, and DNA breakage.[84] Neurones undergoing oxidative stress-related injuries typically display a biphasic or sustained pattern of extracellular signal regulated protein kinase (ERK1/2) activation.[87]

With reperfusion, reactive oxygen radicals may be generated as by-products of the reactions of free arachidonic acid (released from membrane phospholipids during ischaemia) to produce prostaglandins and leukotrienes, which perhaps lead to reperfusion injury to the brain and its microvessels.

Apoptosis

Apoptosis is a mode of programmed cell death in which the cell synthesizes proteins and plays an active role in its own demise. It occurs both physiologically and pathologically. For example, during normal human embryonic development, apoptosis results in the loss of the interdigital webs required for normal formation of the fingers and toes. Likewise, tadpoles lose their tails as they develop into frogs. The normal turnover of cells in the intestinal villi is also apoptotic, as is the turnover of normal lymphocytes. Indeed, inhibition of the apoptotic death of lymphocytes may lead to B-cell lymphoma.

Although necrosis is the predominant mechanism of cell death after stroke (mediated by excitotoxicity, as described above), growing evidence indicates that hypoxic/ischaemic cell death also continues to some extent hours to days after the onset of ischaemia, particularly within the peri-infarct zone or ischaemic penumbra, by apoptosis as a consequence of a genetically regulated programme that allows cells to die with minimal inflammation or release of genetic material.

Families of executioner enzymes (e.g. caspases, apoptosis inducing factor[88]) are expressed in neurones and become activated during and after ischaemic stroke. Active caspases kill cells by cleaving critical cell repair and homeostatic proteins as well as cytoskeletal proteins.[82] In other words, they dismantle multiple cell processes in the cytoplasm and nucleus to promote cell death by suicidal mechanisms resembling apoptosis.[81] The c-Jun N-terminal protein kinase (JNK) signalling pathway is implicated in ischaemia-induced neuronal apoptosis.[89] Apoptosis is characterized morphologically by coarse, regularly shaped chromatin condensation, loss of cell volume and extrusion of membrane-bound cytoplasmic fragments (apoptotic bodies), and biochemically by DNA fragmentation in neurones and glia after ischaemic injury. Necrosis may proceed by analogous programmed pathways recently revealed in the nematode *Caenorhabditis elegans*.[90]

Other mediators of ischaemic cell death

Although the original model of excitotoxicity emphasizes calcium influx through glutamate receptor-coupled ion channels, ionic imbalance (and cell death) may also proceed via other routes.[81]

ACIDOSIS

Acidosis arises as a result of energy deprivation by sustained tissue ischaemia. It may contribute to tissue damage and prevent or retard recovery during reoxygenation by several mechanisms: activation of novel classes of acid-sensing ion channels that further perturb sodium and calcium homeostasis,[91] and inhibition of mitochondrial respiration and lactate oxidation.[4,5] Cellular acidosis may also promote intracellular oedema formation by inducing Na^+ and Cl^- accumulation in the cell via coupled Na^+/H^+ and Cl^-/hydrogen carbonate (HCO_3^-) exchange.

PERI-INFARCT DEPOLARIZATION

As stated above, ischaemia-induced failure of the Na^+, K^+-ATPase pump causes an increase in extracellular K^+ which may spread, triggering a propagating wave of neuronal and glial depolarization (cortical spreading depression) associated with depressed neuronal bioelectrical activity, transient loss of membrane ionic gradients, and massive surges in extracellular potassium, neurotransmitters and intracellular calcium (150 times the basal level).[92] After an initial transient hyperaemia (up to

200% of baseline), cortical spreading depression exacerbates cellular injury and augments tissue damage by causing profound oligaemia that persists for up to 3 days, thereby imposing an energy burden of re-establishing ionic equilibrium in hypoxic tissue.[93] Cortical spreading depression also alters blood–brain permeability by activating brain matrix metalloproteinases,[92] and is associated with changes in immediate early genes, growth factors and inflammatory mediators such as interleukin-1β and tumour necrosis factor-α.[92] Proteolysis of the neurovascular matrix by plasminogen activator and metalloproteinases is believed to be linked with haemorrhagic transformation of the brain infarction and brain oedema. However, treatment with matrix metalloproteinase inhibitors has not been shown to protect the brain. Indeed, a recent study suggested that such inhibitors might contribute to brain damage.[94,95]

INFLAMMATION

Cerebral ischaemia triggers an inflammatory reaction, by means of an active gene expression, within hours to days that may last up to several months.[76,96] Important transcription factors are activated and/or synthesized, including NF-κB, hypoxia-inducible factor 1, interferon regulatory factor 1 and STAT3.[97] Several mediators are released or activated, such as adhesion molecules, proteolytic enzymes belonging to the family of metalloproteinases (including matrix metalloproteinases), and inflammatory cytokines.[98,99] Cytokines might activate the expression of inflammation-related genes, such as iNOS and cycloxygenase-2.[98] The result is infiltration of leucocytes into the brain parenchyma, and the activation of resident microglial and astroglial cells.[98,99] The effects of inflammation are both detrimental (e.g. exacerbation of oedema) and potentially beneficial.

ALTERED GENE EXPRESSION

Ischaemia not only decreases protein and mRNA synthesis, but it also induces at least 100 genes (and thus protein synthesis) which include immediate early genes, stress proteins, growth factors, adhesion proteins, cytokines, kinases and genes directly regulating apoptosis.[87,89]

> Cell death occurs by a necrotic pathway characterized by either ischaemic cell change or oedematous cell change. Death also occurs via an apoptotic-like pathway that is characterized by DNA laddering, a dependence on caspase activity, characteristic protein and phospholipid changes, and morphological attributes of apoptosis. Death may also occur by autophagocytosis.

The four major stages of cell death

The cell death process has four major stages:[78]

- The induction stage includes several changes initiated by ischaemia and reperfusion that are very likely to play major roles in cell death. These include inhibition (and subsequent reactivation) of electron transport, decreased ATP, decreased pH, increased cell Ca^{++}, release of glutamate, increased arachidonic acid, and also gene activation leading to cytokine synthesis, synthesis of enzymes involved in free radical production, and accumulation of leucocytes. These changes lead to the activation of five damaging events, termed perpetrators: the damaging actions of free radicals and their product peroxynitrite; the actions of the Ca^{++}-dependent protease calpain; the activity of phospholipases; the activity of poly-ADPribose polymerase (PARP); and the activation of the apoptotic pathway.
- The second stage of cell death involves the long-term changes in macromolecules or key metabolites that are caused by the perpetrators.
- The third stage involves long-term damaging effects of these macromolecular and metabolite changes, and of some of the induction processes, on critical cell functions and structures that lead to the defined end stages of cell damage. These targeted functions and structures include the plasmalemma, the mitochondria, the cytoskeleton, protein synthesis and kinase activities.
- The fourth stage is the progression to the morphological and biochemical end stages of cell death. Of these four stages, the last two are the least well understood. Rather little is known of how the perpetrators affect the structures and functions and whether and how each of these changes contribute to cell death. The key step in ischaemic cell death is adequate activation of the perpetrators.[78]

Implications for future neuroprotective therapies

The neurovascular unit – a conceptual model comprised of cerebral endothelial cells, astrocytes, neurones and the extracellular matrix – provides a framework for understanding the pathophysiology of ischaemic stroke and developing treatments based on an integrative and dynamic view of evolving tissue damage. Drugs which aim to protect the neurovascular unit (neuroprotectants) have been evaluated preclinically and clinically in a large number of trials (section 12.8.1). However, a systematic review of 1026 experimental drug treatments in acute stroke (clinical studies of 114 drugs, animal models of 912 drugs) found that there was no evidence that drugs used clinically were more effective experimentally than

those tested only in animal models.[100] The quality of the studies was highly variable:

- poor trial study design;
- inadequate sample size;
- unreliable outcome evaluation;
- anatomical and aetiological hetereogeneity in the study populations;
- extrapolating results from young rats to old humans with comorbidities;
- dose ceilings imposed by adverse effects of the drug;
- inadequate drug penetration to the site of the lesion;
- possible differences in responsiveness between ischaemic grey and white matter;
- drug delivery after the therapeutic time window had closed;
- publication bias in the basic science literature;
- misleading hypotheses from the basic scientific researchers linking NMDA-receptor-mediated excitotoxicity to hypoxic-ischaemic neuronal death.

All this questions whether the most efficacious drugs have been selected for stroke clinical trials, and suggests that greater rigour in the conduct, reporting and analysis of animal data is required to improve the translation of scientific advances from bench to bedside.[100] Moreover, new approaches and targets for cytoprotection are required.[84,101–105] There seem to be so many pathways leading from ischaemia to neuronal cell death that blocking just one of them is probably fruitless; perhaps this is like ligating a feeding artery to an arteriovenous malformation (there are always others that will take over to keep up its blood supply), or trying to extinguish a large blazing fire with just a small garden hose.

12.1.5 Ischaemic cerebral oedema

Cerebral ischaemia not only causes loss of neuronal function but also cerebral oedema. Within hours of onset, cytotoxic cerebral oedema arises as a result of cell membrane damage allowing intracellular accumulation of water. The grey matter is affected more than the white matter. The CT and MRI scan appearances are of well-circumscribed altered signal density involving the cortex and subcortex (sections 5.4.2 and 5.5.2). Cytotoxic oedema reaches a maximum volume at 2–4 days and then subsides over 1–2 weeks.

Initially, endothelial tight junctions are maintained and the blood–brain barrier remains intact. However, after several days of ischaemia, breakdown of the blood–brain barrier occurs, leading to vasogenic cerebral oedema as plasma constituents enter the brain extracellular space, affecting the white matter more than the grey matter. Blood–brain barrier breakdown may be initiated and regulated by several proinflammatory mediators (oxidative mediators, adhesion molecules, cytokines, chemokines). These mediators not only regulate the magnitude of leucocyte extravasation into brain parenchyma, but also act directly on brain endothelial cells causing loosening of junction complexes between endothelial cells, increasing brain endothelial barrier permeability, and causing vasogenic oedema.[106] The brain scan appearance of vasogenic oedema includes the characteristic finger-like projections of altered signal density in the white matter, which characteristically accompany cerebral tumours. Imaging studies indicate that fluid volume after infarction peaks in 7–10 days and oedema remains detectable for about 1 month.

The effects of cerebral oedema are to compromise blood flow even further by increasing pressure in the extravascular space, thus causing vascular congestion and sometimes haemorrhagic transformation, and to cause mass effect, brain shift and eventually brain herniation (Figs 12.8 and 12.9). The main danger of herniation is that it can initiate vascular and obstructive complications

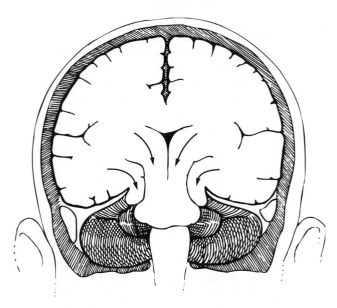

Fig. 12.9 Central transtentorial herniation. Diffuse or multifocal swelling of the cerebral hemispheres (or bilateral subdural or extradural haematomas) compresses and elongates the diencephalon from above. The mammillary bodies are displaced caudally. The cingulate gyrus is not herniated. Modified from Plum F, Posner JB. *The Diagnosis of Stupor and Coma*. Philadelphia, PA: F.A. Davis & Co., 1985.[319]

which aggravate the original expanding lesion by compressing important vessels and tissues and causing even more cerebral ischaemia, congestion and oedema which, in turn, enhance the expanding process. In addition, the herniating brain can compress the aqueduct and subarachnoid spaces and so interfere with cerebrospinal fluid circulation, leading to hydrocephalus and increased cerebrospinal fluid pressure.

There are three anatomical patterns of supratentorial brain shift which can be identified by their end stages: cingulate herniation, central transtentorial herniation and uncal herniation.

Cingulate herniation

Cingulate herniation occurs when the expanding cerebral hemisphere shifts across the intracranial cavity, forcing the ipsilateral cingulate gyrus under the falx cerebri, compressing and displacing the internal cerebral vein and the ipsilateral anterior cerebral artery. This may lead to additional infarction in the territory of the anterior cerebral artery (Fig. 12.8).

Central transtentorial herniation

Central transtentorial herniation of the diencephalon is the end result of displacement of the cerebral

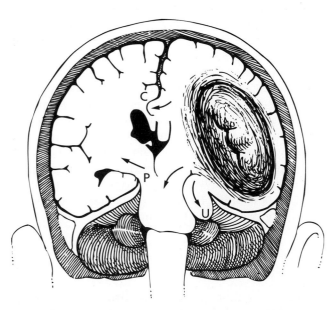

Fig. 12.8 Uncal and cingulate herniation: a mass such as a large cerebral haemorrhage or oedematous infarct displaces the diencephalon and mesencephalon horizontally and caudally. The cingulate gyrus (C) on the side of the lesion herniates under the falx cerebri. The uncus (U) of the ipsilateral temporal lobe herniates under the tentorium cerebelli and becomes grooved and swollen and may compress the ipsilateral oculomotor (third cranial) nerve causing pupillary dilatation (Hutchinson's sign). The cerebral peduncle (P) opposite the supratentorial notch becomes compressed against the edge of the tentorium, leading to grooving (Kernohan's notch)[107] and causes a paresis ipsilateral to the cerebral mass lesion. Central downward displacement also occurs but is less marked than in Fig. 12.9. Modified from Plum F, Posner JB. *The Diagnosis of Stupor and Coma*. Philadelphia, PA: F.A. Davis & Co., 1985.[319]

hemispheres and basal nuclei, compressing and eventually displacing the diencephalon and the adjoining midbrain rostro-caudally through the tentorial notch (Fig. 12.9). The great cerebral vein is compressed, which raises the hydrostatic pressure of the entire deep territory it drains. In addition, downward displacement of the midbrain and pons stretches the medial perforating branches of the basilar artery (the artery cannot shift downward because it is tethered to the circle of Willis), leading to paramedian brainstem ischaemia (and haemorrhage if perfusion continues).

Uncal herniation

Uncal herniation characteristically occurs when expanding lesions in the temporal fossa or temporal lobe shift the inner, basal edge of the uncus and hippocampal gyrus toward the midline so that they bulge over the incisural edge of the tentorium, and push the adjacent midbrain against the opposite incisural edge (Fig. 12.8).[107] The third cranial nerve and the posterior cerebral artery on the side of the expanding temporal lobe are often caught between the overhanging swollen uncus and the free edge of the tentorium or the petroclinoid ligament, leading to a third nerve palsy and occipital and medial temporal lobe infarction and swelling, which further compounds the problem.

Transtentorial herniation is the most common cause of death during the first week after acute stroke, accounting for about 80% of deaths in cerebral infarction and 90% in intracerebral haemorrhage. The risk of death peaks within 24 h for intracerebral haemorrhage, but later at 4–5 days for cerebral infarction as ischaemic cerebral oedema develops. Brainstem compression, with subsequent haemorrhage and infarction within it, accounts for the serious morbidity and mortality associated with herniation.

> Transtentorial herniation is the most common cause of death within the first week of onset of both ischaemic stroke and intracerebral haemorrhage.

12.2 General treatment considerations

The primary aims of the specific treatments considered in this chapter are, broadly speaking, to minimize the volume of brain damaged by ischaemia. The assumption is that, if this can be achieved without excess hazard, neurological impairment, disability and handicap should all correspondingly be reduced in survivors. For patients with a large volume of ischaemic brain, minimizing the volume which infarcts should also reduce the risk of early death, particularly from ischaemic cerebral oedema and transtentorial herniation (section 12.1.5). The pathophysiology of acute cerebral ischaemia is complex (section 12.1.3), and many potential treatments may have more than one mechanism of action; for some, the precise mechanism is unknown. However, the main targets of acute treatment are to restore and then maintain blood flow, and simultaneously keep alive as much ischaemic brain tissue as possible while the blood supply is restored, either spontaneously or therapeutically.

12.2.1 How to evaluate evidence about different treatments

Evidence-based medicine

We try to base our decisions on whether or not to use a particular treatment in clinical practice on the evidence from randomized trials and systematic reviews of randomized trials. This approach is part of what is now known as 'evidence-based medicine', a style of medical practice which Sackett described as 'a life-long process of self-directed learning in which caring for our patients creates the need for clinically important information about diagnosis, prognosis and therapy'.[108] The book by Sackett and co-authors on the subject is short and clear and provides succinct advice on how to find the best evidence, appraise it critically and then apply it in everyday clinical practice (Table 12.4).[108] This section summarizes what the best forms of evidence are (and why) and where up-to-date evidence can be found.

Why are randomized trials the best way to evaluate treatments?

There is now little disagreement that the randomized controlled trial (RCT) is the best way to evaluate most treatments[109] (Table 12.4). Weaker research designs, i.e. case series without any controls, series with retrospective controls, and series with concurrent controls but non-random treatment allocation, may introduce far too many biases into the assessment of treatment effect.[108–110] The Medical Research Council trial of streptomycin for pulmonary tuberculosis, designed by the statistician Sir Austin Bradford Hill, is probably the strongest contender for the title 'first clinical trial to use strictly random allocation', although there is some debate about this claim.[111,112] The trial not only established the benefits of the treatment beyond all reasonable doubt, but also served as the most ethical and equitable way of utilizing

Table 12.4 Methodological questions in the critical assessment of an article evaluating treatment (modified from Sackett).[108,109]

*Was the assignment of patients to treatment really randomized?**
Was the similarity between groups documented?
Was prognostic stratification used in treatment allocation?
Was foreknowledge of the randomly allocated treatment possible?
Were all clinically relevant outcomes reported?
Was case fatality as well as morbidity reported?
Were deaths from all causes reported?
Were quality-of-life assessments conducted?
Was outcome assessment blind to treatment allocation?
Were the study patients recognizably similar to your own?
Were reproducibly defined exclusion criteria stated?
Was the setting primary, secondary or tertiary care?
Was the type of patient included in the study clearly described?
Were both statistical and clinical significance considered?
If statistically significant, was the difference clinically important?
If not statistically significant, was the study big enough to show a clinically important difference if one really exists?
Is the therapeutic manoeuvre feasible in your practice?
Available, affordable, sensible?
Were contamination† and co-intervention avoided?
Was the manoeuvre administered blind?
Was compliance measured?
Were all patients who entered the study accounted for at its conclusion?
(i.e. were drop-outs, withdrawals, non-compliers and those who crossed over handled appropriately in the analysis?)

---

*Methods of allocation such as alternation, use of hospital number or date of birth all provide foreknowledge of the next treatment allocation, and so allow the trial allocation process to be subverted which may lead to selection bias between the two treatment groups.
†In this context, contamination implies that some patients allocated active treatment either did not receive the treatment or were given the treatment which the other treatment group should have received, or some non-trial treatment with similar properties to one of the trial interventions under test.
Note: reports of RCTs should conform to the requirements of the CONSORT statement as far as possible.[127]

the very limited supply of the drug that was available in Britain at the time. It also prevented the treatment 'creeping' into routine clinical practice without being properly evaluated.

> We could answer many of the therapeutic questions posed in this book a great deal faster if a larger proportion of stroke patients were entered in appropriate randomized controlled trials.

Strictly random allocation and proper concealment minimize selection bias.[110,113] If the randomizing clinician can find out what treatment the next patient will be allocated (e.g. by holding a sealed trial allocation envelope up to a bright light), he may be tempted not to enter the patient in the trial. Allocation concealment reduces or avoids this happening.[113] A central telephone randomization system offers complete concealment: the clinician telephones a randomization centre and gives the patient's details, these are then recorded on the central computer during the call, and the computer generates the next treatment allocation only after all the baseline data are checked and entered; the patient is then irrevocably in the trial and selection bias cannot occur.[113] Studies where patients are entered into a trial by selecting a numbered drug pack in the participating hospital, administering the drug/placebo contained in the pack, and then telephoning a central office to notify the trial administrators that a patient has been entered into the trial, are prone to all sorts of bias. In the worst case, the pack could be opened and given but the patient details then not notified to the trial office if there was an early adverse event – the pack could just be recorded as 'opened and discarded'. The pack drug might not have been administered when the hospital said it was, but possibly earlier so as to look better on the records. There is no possibility of balancing the treatment allocation on important key prognostic variables resulting in imbalances between treatment and control arms which could skew the results. Unfortunately, with this system of 'randomization' any of these scenarios is possible, and probably has happened.

It is important to reduce observer bias, if possible, by 'blinding' both the patients and the observers who collect the outcome data.[110,113]

Random error is reduced by recruiting a sufficiently large sample of patients. However, RCTs need to be surprisingly large to provide really reliable evidence on the balance of risk and benefit for a particular treatment.[110] If the measure of outcome is an uncommon but serious event, such as death, and the effect of the treatment on that outcome is only moderate, then the trial may need to recruit several tens of thousands of patients.[110] To recruit such large numbers often involves clinicians in many countries, and hence the trial design needs to be simple, with minimal data collection and audit (though such simplicity is more difficult to achieve in the current over-regulated and bureaucratic research climate).[110,114] The effort of conducting such large RCTs is substantial, and so many of the 'mega trials' have used a factorial design to assess two or three treatments at the same time without loss of statistical efficiency.[110]

> Good trial design seeks to reduce bias and random error in the assessment of treatment effect: strict randomization with concealment reduces selection bias; blinding reduces observer bias; and recruitment of large numbers of patients reduces random error.

Problems with randomized controlled trials in acute stroke from 1956 to the present

Eight years after the streptomycin trial was published in 1948, Dyken and White wrote of the many methodological problems they identified in evaluating treatments for acute stroke; not the least was to know, in an individual patient, whether or not treatment had been effective.[115] They wrote this in the report of the first quasi-randomized study of a medical treatment for acute stroke.[115] Thirty-six patients were alternately (but not randomly) assigned to cortisone or control. Thirteen of the cortisone patients and 10 of the controls died; a trend against treatment, but an inconclusive result. Sadly, a review of the quality of the final reports of RCTs of drug therapies for acute stroke conducted over the next 40 years (i.e. between 1956 and 1996) makes depressing reading.[116] Many trials had weaknesses which included: over-complex eligibility criteria; incomplete descriptions of the methods used (particularly the method of randomization); inadequate sample size; inappropriate measures of outcome; poor standards of execution (i.e. poor trial discipline); an unacceptably high proportion of patients 'lost' to follow-up; inappropriate statistical methods (often with inappropriate subgroup analysis); and failing to account for all patients randomized.[116] On the other hand, trial quality did appear to improve in parallel with an increase in trial size.[116] While this is encouraging, a more recent review of reports of the randomized acute stroke trials completed before 2001 showed that most trials were underpowered, i.e. power <0.90, used inappropriate assumptions for event rates, and were grossly overoptimistic in their expectation of treatment effect.[117] These deficiencies will together have resulted in trials being far too small and reduced their chance of being able to detect real treatment effects.[117]

Most trials in acute stroke to date have been directly sponsored (or financially supported by) the pharmaceutical industry.[118,119] However, of some concern is that research funded by pharmaceutical companies is more likely to report outcomes favouring the sponsor than research funded from other sources.[120,121] Although pharmaceutical company research is certainly not of poorer quality than other research, there is a tendency to delay publishing unfavourable results (or even not to publish them at all).[122,123] The number of industry-sponsored trials in stroke is increasing,[119] so this problem is not going to go away, but there are now guidelines on the relation between sponsors and investigators in stroke trials that may improve the situation.[124]

There is therefore a continuing need to increase the number, size and quality of randomized trials in stroke, to increase non-commercial sources of funding and to improve the quality of the reports of those trials in the literature. Unfortunately, the regulatory hurdles that must now be overcome before a trial is initiated are very great.[114] So much so, that they may stifle this vital form of clinical research, making the ideal of 'most stroke patients get their treatment in the context of a randomized trial' a rather distant dream.[125,126]

Steps to improve the quality of stroke trials and reports of trials in the literature

The CONSORT group have produced guidelines to improve the quality of reports of RCTs.[127] Their statement is available in several languages and has been endorsed by prominent medical journals such as the *Lancet, Annals of Internal Medicine* and *Journal of the American Medical Association*. It comprises a checklist and flow diagram to help improve the quality of reports of RCTs. The checklist includes the items that need to be discussed in the report; the flow diagram provides a clear picture of the progress of all participants in the trial, from the time they are randomized until the end of their involvement. The intent is to make the experimental process clearer, flawed or not, so that users of the data can more appropriately evaluate their validity. The CONSORT website provides evidence to support each aspect of the checklist and is very useful (http://www.consort-statement.org). One can only hope that, in future, stroke triallists will adhere to these guidelines when designing trials and reporting their results.

Describing the effects of treatment in numbers

The effects of a treatment can be expressed in a number of ways. Relative treatment effects can make a treatment appear to have impressive benefits; 'drug X reduced the risk of event Y by a half'. Table 12.5 describes how the most common numerical measures of relative and absolute treatment effects are calculated. The *absolute* benefit is more important for clinical decisions, and is greatly influenced by the frequency of events in the control group. If events are rare in the control group, the absolute benefit – however great the *relative* treatment effect – will be small. In this case, the number-needed-to-treat to prevent one event (NNT) will be correspondingly large, so the treatment may have little clinical value in low-risk patients. For example, in a randomized trial, if fatal pulmonary embolism occurred in 0.5% of stroke

Table 12.5 Describing the numerical results of a clinical trial in different ways.

	Treated	Control
No. originally randomized in this group	1000	1000
No. who were dead at the end of the trial	80(a) (8%)	100(b) (10%)
No. alive at the end of the trial	920(c) (92%)	900(d) (90%)
Relative risk of death (RR) = 8%/10% = 0.80*†		
Relative risk reduction of death (RRR) = (1 − RR) × 100 = (1 − 0.80) × 100 = 20%		
Odds ratio (OR) = (a/c) ÷ (b/d) = ad/bc = 0.78*		
95% Confidence interval of OR = 0.58 − 1.06		
Relative odds reduction = (1 − OR) × 100 = (1 − 0.78) × 100 = 22%†		
Absolute risk of death in control group = 100/1000 = 10%		
Absolute risk of death in treated group = 80/1000 = 8%		
Absolute risk difference in death (ARD) = 10% − 8% = 2%, or 20 deaths avoided or postponed per 1000 patients treated		
Number-needed-to-treat to avoid one event (NNT) = 100/ARD = 100/2 = 50†‡ need to be treated to prevent (or at least postpone) one death		

Notes: The *Cochrane Handbook* is the most up-to-date source of advice on this topic, and is available online through the Cochrane Library.[316]

This table is referred to as a 2 × 2 table. The four 'cells' in the table are labelled a, b, c and d.

*The odds ratio and relative risk both provide an estimate of relative treatment effect. The estimates will be similar if the absolute risk in the control group is low. However, if the absolute risk in the controls is high, then the odds ratio will be larger than the relative risk. For example, in the Cochrane review of the effects of stroke units (compared with general medical wards), about 58% of patients treated on general medical wards were dead or dependent at the end of follow-up, compared with 54% of patients treated on a stroke unit; this gives an odds ratio of 0.80 and a relative odds reduction of 20% in favour of stroke units. When the same results are expressed as relative risks, the relative risk of 0.91 and the relative risk reduction of 9% associated with the benefits of stroke units appear more modest. The odds ratio is easy to calculate, but difficult to understand, the relative risk (and its 95% CI) are harder to calculate, but easier to understand. The *Cochrane Handbook* gives useful advice on the advantages and disadvantages of each measure.[316]

†It is important to calculate the confidence intervals for these estimates of effect. In this example, the upper confidence interval exceeds unity, which is equivalent to 'not significant at the $P < 0.05$ level'. While the effect may not be *statistically* significant, a 20% reduction in the risk of death is potentially *clinically* significant; however, it would require a trial with a much larger sample size of at least 10 000 patients to detect such an effect reliably.[110] To determine reliably whether the effect on death varied between different subgroups would require an even larger trial with several tens of thousands of patients.[110] Formulae to calculate confidence intervals are available in many statistical textbooks. The calculations can be done on a simple calculator or with standard statistical software or with tools available on statistical websites. The book and program published by Altman *et al.* are simple, clear, easy to use and – most importantly – error-free![317]

‡One should not calculate NNTs if the estimate of effect is not statistically significant. If the data from a systematic review of several trials are used to calculate the NNT, interpret the results with caution, since the 'overall' NNT will be very heavily influenced by the event rates in the control groups. It is preferable to take the overall estimate of *relative* treatment effect and apply it to the expected event rate in the group of patients to which the treatment will be applied;[316] a convenient online calculator for this is available at http://www.dcn.ed.ac.uk/csrg/resources.asp

patients allocated to aspirin alone, and in 0.25% of those allocated to the combination of aspirin with a second antithrombotic agent (e.g. low-molecular-weight heparin) the relative risk reduction would be an impressive 50%, but the absolute risk difference would be only 0.25%. In other words, if we treated 1000 patients, only two or three would avoid fatal pulmonary embolism and the NNT to prevent one person having pulmonary embolism would be 400. However, if fatal pulmonary embolism occurred in 5% of controls, and the relative risk reduction was still 50%, the absolute risk difference would be 2.5% and the NNT would be just 40 patients.

What are systematic reviews and why do we need them?

The biomedical literature is so enormous that clinicians are faced with an unmanageably large amount of information to assimilate. For example, the Cochrane Stroke Group's specialized register (published in the *Cochrane Library* issue 3 for 2007) now includes 11 000 reports of stroke trials. The stroke trials literature is growing fast too: on average, about 900 new reports of stroke trials have been added to the register each year for the last few years (Brenda Thomas, personal communication). Faced with such a vast, confusing and rapidly changing array

Table 12.6 Methodological questions in the critical assessment of a systematic review (adapted from Sackett *et al.*, 1991).[109]

> Were the question(s) and methods clearly stated?
> Were the search methods used to locate relevant studies comprehensive?
> Were explicit methods used to determine which articles to include in the review?
> Was the methodological quality of the primary studies assessed?
> Were the selection and assessment of the primary studies reproducible and free from bias?
> Were differences in individual study results adequately explained?
> Were the results of the primary studies combined appropriately?
> Were the reviewers' conclusions supported by the data cited?
>
> Comprehensive details on the design, conduct, analysis and reporting of systematic reviews are available in the *Cochrane Handbook*, which is regularly updated, and also available online.[316]

of information about treatment, what should the busy clinician do? Focus on a few selected reports published in well-known English-language journals? Such selection could easily lead to a biased assessment of the effects of the treatment. Rely on visiting pharmaceutical company representatives and being flown to exotic locations to suffer sponsored symposia? Hopefully not. The best way to minimize bias is to review systematically *all* of the evidence from *all* of the relevant RCTs, both published and unpublished.[108] Briefly, a systematic review:

- defines the question to be answered;
- uses a defined search strategy to identify relevant studies;
- selects studies and extracts data from them using explicit criteria;
- synthesizes the evidence in a quantitative manner whenever possible (i.e. provides an overall estimate of the treatment effect).

The reader should consider the checklist in Table 12.6 when reading a report of a systematic review. For those preparing systematic reviews, the Quality of Reporting of Meta-analyses (QUOROM) Group has defined the criteria for an adequate report of a systematic review.[128]

What is meta-analysis?

Meta-analysis is the numerical technique which derives an overall estimate of the treatment effect from all of the trials included in a systematic (or non-systematic) review. Such overall estimates avoid the selection bias inherent

with choosing estimates derived from subsets of trials, and are more precise than the estimate from any one trial (i.e. less subject to random error) because they are based on more outcome data.

> Meta-analysis is simply the best way to obtain the least biased and most precise estimate of treatment effect from a group of similar trials of the same intervention in the same type of patients and using the same type of outcome measures.

Hazards of inappropriate subgroup analysis in trials (and systematic reviews)

Subgroup analysis is popular with clinical triallists and people who like to generate hypotheses to explain the 'negative' or 'positive' overall results of particular trials. It is, however, a dangerous sport, since even apparently large effects observed in subgroups can merely be due to the play of chance and not to the treatment itself.[110,129] Claims for the benefits of a treatment based on a subgroup analysis of a single trial, or of a meta-analysis, need to be viewed with caution and should be seen as hypothesis generating. To test such subgroup hypotheses reliably, generally requires further very large trials with appropriate and pre-specified hypotheses.[110,129]

Inappropriate subgroup analyses may have disastrous effects. The report of the Canadian aspirin sulphinpyrazone trial concluded that, overall, among people with threatened stroke, aspirin was associated with a significant 30% reduction in the risk of stroke or death.[130] A subgroup analysis suggested that the benefit was confined to males and was not seen in females. As a result, the United States Food and Drug Administration (FDA) licensed aspirin for stroke prevention but only in males, not in females. However, the results of the Antiplatelet Trialists' Collaboration systematic review in 1994 of all of the relevant randomized trials showed that, among high-risk individuals, the benefits of antiplatelet drugs were similar in males and females, so refuting the results of the Canadian trial aspirin subgroup analysis.[131] The FDA did not license aspirin for stroke prevention in women until 1998, so in the years between 1980 and 1998, it seems likely that many women worldwide at high risk of stroke were not treated with aspirin and consequently had strokes which might have otherwise been avoided.

Likewise, undue emphasis on the results of a single positive trial in a meta-analysis may result in misleadingly optimistic conclusions. For example, the most widely cited study of therapeutic thrombolysis in acute ischaemic stroke, the NINDS trial, may have overestimated the benefits of this treatment (section 12.5.2).[132,133]

Translating the results of trials and systematic reviews into improving clinical practice

There are now many books and articles on how to use the results of trials and systematic reviews to improve one's own clinical practice. However, it requires a great deal of time and resources to take the next steps, i.e. to develop and implement evidence-based guidelines or policy documents and then consistently apply them to an entire clinical service over a long period. Many strategies to improve clinicians' performance, ranging from financial incentives, to guidelines, to continuing medical education, have all been suggested. The Cochrane Effective Practice and Organization of Care (EPOC) Group is undertaking systematic reviews to identify which interventions are most likely to achieve an improvement in the clinical practice of healthcare professionals.[134] If we are to spend some of our limited health service resources on getting healthcare professionals to improve their standards of care, it is important that we spend them only on those methods which can bring about a measurable and sustainable change in clinical practice (and do so efficiently and cost-effectively) (Table 17.22). Our efforts to improve standards of care must not be wasted on uncritical application of interventions – such as audit without feedback – that take great effort, but achieve little.[135]

Where we look for up-to-date reports of randomized trials, systematic reviews and clinical practice guidelines

Evidence-based medicine requires one to use up-to-date reports, so, with each year that passes after the publication of this book, more and more of the evidence we have cited will be superseded. However, there are several sources of regularly updated evidence that can fill this 'information gap.'[108] For example, the Cochrane Collaboration Stroke Review Group is coordinating a series of systematic reviews of different forms of healthcare for the treatment and prevention of stroke which are updated as new information becomes available.[136] Its website includes a link to the Cochrane Collaboration website, where abstracts of all the Cochrane systematic reviews are available free of charge (http://www. dcn.ed.ac.uk/csrg).

Where possible therefore we have in this book cited stroke reviews from the *Cochrane Database of Systematic Reviews*, since they are often – but not always – of higher quality and are more frequently updated than many corresponding reviews published in conventional paper journals.[137] Where there is no relevant Cochrane review available, we have searched for a high-quality systematic review. The Cochrane Library includes the *Database of Abstracts of Reviews of Effectiveness* (DARE), a series of quality-assured reviews (and their abstracts) which is a very useful source of such reviews. If we could not find a systematic review, we either resorted to asking a known expert in the field or to a search of the Cochrane Central Register of Controlled Trials (CENTRAL); in the *Cochrane Library* (issue 2 for 2006), CENTRAL contained over 473 000 references to reports of randomized trials and controlled clinical trials.

There are a number of other regularly updated sources of evidence. Some of the ones we often use are:

- The Internet Stroke Center at the University of Washington, St Louis, an independent web resource about stroke care and research which includes an up-to-date register of current stroke trials (http://www.strokecenter.org/);
- *Clinical Evidence* is a compendium of the best available evidence on effective healthcare, published online at http://www.clinicalevidence.com/ceweb/conditions/index.jsp and in various other paper and electronic formats (including a version for your personal digital assistant (PDA) or palmtop organizer);
- The Royal College of Physicians of London (http://www.rcplondon.ac.uk);
- The Scottish Intercollegiate Guidelines Network (http://www.sign.ac.uk/);
- The Cochrane Stroke Group website is building up a list of links to stroke guidelines (http://www.dcn.ed.ac.uk/csrg);
- The National Library for Health (NLH) seeks to make relevant up-to-date information on effective forms of healthcare available to patients and doctors (http://www.library.nhs.uk/).

12.2.2 Organization of acute stroke care

The way acute stroke care is organized within a particular hospital will depend very much on what resources are available and what treatments are planned (Chapter 17). The clinical and radiological diagnosis of acute stroke is dealt with in Chapters 3, 4 and 5. The other aspects of general management in the acute phase are dealt with in Chapters 10, 11 and 17.

12.2.3 Which treatments to use routinely, selectively or not at all

There is strong evidence to support the routine use of aspirin in almost all patients with acute ischaemic stroke (section 12.3). For anticoagulants, the substantial amounts of available data do not support their routine use, but it may be justifiable to use them in a relatively small proportion of patients for specific reasons (section 12.4). Similarly, there is reasonable evidence (based on relatively small trials) that thrombolytic treatment is indicated for the few, very carefully selected cases that meet the very restrictive conditions of the current regulatory approvals; large-scale RCTs will be needed before its place in routine clinical practice worldwide becomes clear (section 12.5). There are many other interventions which have been tested to some extent, but for which the evidence remains inconclusive. The remainder of this chapter explores these broad conclusions in greater detail. Some treatments, such as intravenous thrombolysis, should only be given in the context of a highly organized specialist acute stroke service, whereas others, such as aspirin, could be used very widely, even where healthcare resources are limited.

12.2.4 Variation in treatment worldwide

There are enormous variations in the general management of (and outcome after) acute stroke both between and within different countries.[138–141] There are also large variations in the use of specific agents such as anticoagulants, both as an acute treatment and for secondary prevention.[141] For example, a survey of 36 US academic medical centres showed that 29% of a sample of 497 patients with acute ischaemic stroke were treated with intravenous heparin, but the proportion treated varied enormously between centres; from 'not at all' in seven centres to 88% in one centre.[142] The causes of this variation was explored in a further survey of opinion among 280 neurologists from the United States and 270 neurologists from Canada. US neurologists were significantly more likely than Canadian neurologists to use intravenous heparin for patients with stroke in evolution (51% vs 33%), vertebrobasilar stroke (30% vs 8%), carotid territory stroke (31% vs 4%), and multiple transient ischemic attacks (47% vs 9%).[143] US neurologists more often cited medicolegal factors as a potential influence on the decision-making process than Canadian neurologists.[143] Despite the publication of four clinical trials, which have not shown any long-term benefit from heparin for patients with acute stroke, both US and Canadian neurologists would use intravenous heparin in large numbers for this condition.[143] There is clearly a need to understand why some clinicians persisted in using a treatment which is not supported by reliable evidence (intravenous heparin in acute ischaemic stroke), yet others for many years underused a proven treatment (oral anticoagulants for long-term secondary prevention after ischaemic stroke associated with atrial fibrilla-

tion)[144] (section 16.6.2). Similarly, there is substantial variation in the use of thrombolytic therapy for acute ischaemic stroke in the USA[145,146] and Europe.[147] There are many possible reasons for these variations, but the lack of really reliable evidence from appropriately large RCTs and the lack of widely disseminated systematic reviews of existing trial evidence must play at least some part. For thrombolytic treatment, concern about the risk of bleeding, emergency physicians' perception of lack of evidence of benefit and variation in provision of neurological support in the emergency department are some of the physician-related factors in the variation.[147–149] The barriers to effective delivery of thrombolytic therapy are discussed in section 17.4.4.

> Substantial variation in the use of particular treatments sometimes indicates lack of really reliable evidence on the effects of that treatment; sometimes it merely represents reluctance of doctors or health systems to change. Whatever the cause, major variation in clinical practice or in the delivery of a service is inequitable and ethically indefensible.

12.2.5 Treatment of any specific underlying cause

Although the great majority of ischaemic strokes are in one way or another related to atheroma and its thromboembolic complications (section 6.3), intracranial small vessel disease (section 6.4) and embolism from the heart (section 6.5), a small proportion are due to other, rarer conditions. These unusual causes and their treatment are discussed in Chapter 7. It is important to emphasize that, although conditions like vasculitis are infrequent, failure to recognize and treat them appropriately may lead to a poor outcome or even death. A systematic approach to history taking, examination and investigation will minimize the risk of missing a potentially treatable cause of ischaemic stroke.

12.3 Routine use: aspirin

12.3.1 Rationale

Potential benefits

On the arterial side, aspirin may act in several ways to reduce the volume of brain tissue damaged by ischaemia. It may prevent distal and proximal propagation of arterial thrombus, and may prevent re-embolization and platelet aggregation in the microcirculation. It also reduces the release of thromboxane and other neurotoxic eicosanoids and so may even be neuroprotective.[150,151] In the venous circulation, among patients at high risk (chiefly as a result of general or orthopaedic surgery) antiplatelet drugs significantly reduce the risk of deep venous thrombosis and pulmonary embolism.[152]

Potential risks

However, antiplatelet drugs do have significant anti-haemostatic effects. In a systematic review of the randomized trials, antiplatelet drugs were consistently associated with a small but definite excess of both intracranial and extracranial haemorrhages.[131]

12.3.2 Evidence

Data available

The benefit of aspirin as treatment for acute *myocardial infarction* was first reliably established in 1988.[153] The lack of data about the effects of antiplatelet drugs as a treatment for the acute phase of ischaemic stroke led to two large-scale RCTs of aspirin, the International Stroke Trial (IST)[154] and the Chinese Acute Stroke Trial (CAST),[155] which together randomized over 40 000

patients. In the IST, patients were allocated, in an open factorial design, to treatment policies of: 300 mg aspirin daily, heparin, the combination, or to 'avoid both aspirin and heparin' for 14 days. In the CAST, patients were allocated, in a double-blind design, to 1 month of 160 mg aspirin daily or matching placebo.

There are two main sources of evidence on aspirin in acute ischaemic stroke. The first is a Cochrane systematic review that included all the completed RCTs of any antiplatelet drug in acute stroke and examined their effects on a variety of short- and long-term clinical outcomes.[156] The second is a meta-analysis of individual patient data from CAST and IST that examined the effects of aspirin in particular categories of patient during the scheduled treatment period.[157]

Effects on major outcomes: recurrent stroke, intracranial haemorrhage, death and functional status

The effects of aspirin on various outcomes are summarized in Table 12.7. Aspirin significantly reduces the odds of recurrent ischaemic stroke during the treatment period by 30% (95% CI 20–40%) from 2.3% in controls to 1.6% in treated patients, i.e. avoiding seven events per 1000 patients treated.[157] There is a small excess of symptomatic intracranial haemorrhages with aspirin (including symptomatic transformation of an infarct);

Table 12.7 Effects of aspirin, started within 24 h of an acute ischaemic stroke.[a]

	Events avoided/ caused per 1000 patients
Benefits within the acute treatment period[b]	
Fatal or non-fatal pulmonary embolism	2
Death with no further stroke	4
Death from any cause	5
Fatal or non-fatal recurrent ischaemic stroke	7
Further stroke or death	9
Harms within the acute treatment period[b]	
Fatal or non-fatal intracranial haemorrhage	2
Major extracranial haemorrhage[c]	4
If not receiving heparin	2
If receiving heparin	9
Benefits at final follow-up[b]	
Death from any cause	8
Dead or dependent	13
Full recovery from the stroke	10

[a]Estimates derived from an individual patient data meta-analysis of the CAST and IST trials, and from a Cochrane systematic review;[156,157] the events are not mutually exclusive, so the various events cannot be summed.
[b]The acute treatment period was 14 days in IST and 1 month in CAST, and final follow-up was at 6 months in the IST and 1 month in CAST.[157]
[c]Major was defined as severe enough to require transfusion or to lead to death.

in 0.8% of controls vs 1.0% of treated patients, a non-significant 21% relative increase in odds (95% CI 1% reduction to 49% increase), or an absolute increase of about two per 1000 patients treated.[157] Aspirin significantly reduces the relative odds of death (without further stroke) during the treatment period by 8% (95% CI 1–16%) from 5.4% in controls to 5.0% in treated patients, i.e. avoiding four deaths for every 1000 patients treated.[157] 'Recurrent (further) stroke or death during the treatment period' conveniently summarizes the overall balance of benefit and risk since it encompasses both benefits and harms: recurrent ischaemic stroke, recurrent stroke of unknown type, symptomatic intracranial haemorrhage, symptomatic haemorrhagic transformation of the infarct and death from any cause. We refer to this outcome as 'further stroke or death'. Aspirin significantly reduces the relative odds of this outcome of further stroke or death by 11% (95% CI 5–15%) from 9.1% to 8.2%; for every 1000 patients treated, nine avoid further stroke or death during the treatment period (Fig. 12.10).[157] At the end of follow-up, aspirin avoids about eight deaths for every 1000 patients treated,[156] and also significantly reduces the odds of being dead or dependent by 6% (95% CI 2–8%). The risk difference was 13 extra patients alive and independent for every 1000 patients treated. Aspirin also significantly increases the odds of making a complete recovery by 6% (95% CI 1–11%), an extra 10 patients making a complete recovery for every 1000 patients treated.[156]

Effect on deep venous thrombosis and pulmonary embolism

Aspirin significantly reduced the relative odds of pulmonary embolism (PE) by 29% (95% CI 4–47%), from 0.5% in controls to 0.3% in treated patients, i.e. for every 1000 patients treated, two avoided PE.[157] Though under-ascertainment of events in both groups may mean that the *absolute* benefit has been underestimated, the *proportional* reduction is not likely to be. If the true rate of PE were 3% in the controls, and the same proportional reduction applied, then for every 1000 patients given aspirin, 12 might avoid PE. These benefits are consistent with those seen in the systematic review of aspirin in the prevention of PE in surgical patients[152] and in the Pulmonary Embolism Prevention Trial.[158]

These data therefore strengthen the rationale for the routine use of aspirin in the acute phase of a stroke and continuing it long-term; aspirin is likely to be adequate thromboprophylaxis for patients at low and moderate risk of deep venous thrombosis (DVT) and PE. For patients at high risk of DVT, perhaps because of a history of a previous episode of venous thromboembolism

or the presence of thrombophilia, then the question is 'what to add to aspirin?' Graded compression stockings are one option and low-dose subcutaneous heparin another; both have advantages and disadvantages, which are discussed in detail in section 11.13.

Subgroup analyses

The individual patient data meta-analysis did not identify any group in which the benefits – or the risks – of aspirin were significantly greater than or less than the averages reported above.[157] The recurrence risk among control patients was similar in all 28 subgroups, so the absolute reduction of seven per 1000 did not differ substantially with respect to age, sex, conscious level, atrial fibrillation, CT findings, blood pressure, stroke subtype or concomitant heparin use. There was no good evidence that the 11% reduction in relative odds of death without further stroke was reversed in any subgroup, or that in any subgroup the increase in haemorrhagic stroke was much larger than the average of about two per 1000, and there was no heterogeneity between the reductions in further stroke or death during the scheduled treatment period (Fig. 12.10).

Aspirin in haemorrhagic stroke and in patients without CT or MR brain scans

Among the 9000 patients randomized without a prior CT scan in the IST and CAST, aspirin appeared to be of net benefit, with no unusual excess of haemorrhagic stroke, and among the 800 who had inadvertently been randomized after a haemorrhagic stroke, there was no evidence of net hazard (further stroke or death 67 control vs 63 aspirin).[157,159] The RCT data are broadly reassuring, in that they establish that the patients inadvertently entered in the trials with a haemorrhagic stroke (who then received only one or two doses of aspirin), were not, on average, harmed as a result. However, they do not establish the safety of continued aspirin treatment in patients with intracerebral haemorrhage, nor do they establish the safety of giving aspirin to patients who are not CT scanned at all.

12.3.3 Who to treat

Early aspirin is of benefit for a wide range of patients. The recommendation is therefore that all patients with suspected acute ischaemic stroke – irrespective of lesion location or presumed aetiology (e.g. cardioembolic or not) – receive aspirin unless there is a clear contraindication.[160] However, implementing a hospital policy or guideline of 'immediate aspirin for all patients with acute ischaemic

Fig. 12.10 Aspirin in acute ischaemic stroke: effects on recurrent stroke or death in different subgroups during the scheduled treatment period in the Chinese Acute Stroke Trial (CAST) and International Stroke Trial (IST). Fatal and non-fatal events are included. For each particular subgroup the number of events among aspirin- and no-aspirin-allocated patients, and the odds ratio (dark purple square, with area proportional to the total number of patients with an event) and its 99% confidence interval (horizontal line) are given. A square to the left of the solid vertical line of no treatment difference (odds ratio 1.0) suggests benefit, significant at $2P < 0.01$ only if the whole 99% confidence interval (CI) (horizontal line) is to the left of the solid vertical line. The overall result and its 95% CI is represented by an open diamond. A indicates aspirin; H, heparin. Here and elsewhere, results for those with missing information on particular characteristics are not listed separately (except for computed tomography findings), but numerators and denominators for them can be obtained by subtraction of the subgroup results from the total (e.g. the numbers with no prognostic index calculated were 16/638 aspirin vs 18/638 control). Reproduced from 'Indications for early aspirin use in acute ischemic stroke: a combined analysis of 40 000 randomized patients from the Chinese Acute Stroke Trial and the International Stroke Trial'. *Stroke* 2000; **31**:1240–9 with permission from the authors (Chen *et al.*).[157]

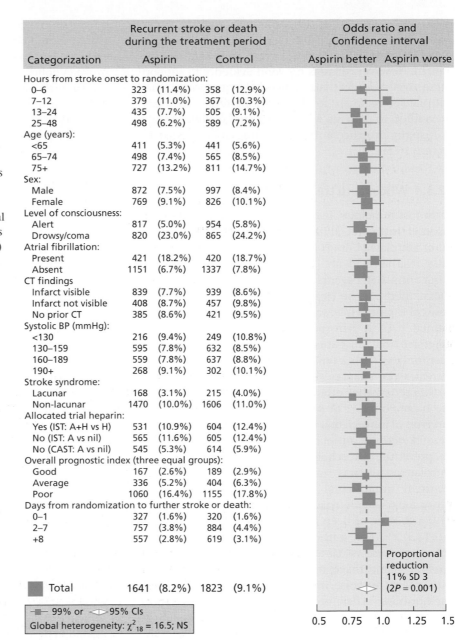

stroke' requires considerable effort; it is of course part of a well-organized stroke service (Chapter 17). Several different strategies may be required to maintain a high level of compliance with the policy (Table 17.22).

Atrial fibrillation

The IST and CAST trials included about 4500 patients who were in atrial fibrillation (AF) at the time of randomization. In these patients, the risk of recurrent stroke in hospital was 2.9% in the controls and 2.0% in patients

allocated to aspirin. The one-third reduction in the relative odds of recurrent ischaemic stroke with aspirin was no different to that seen in patients without AF;[157] all such patients should be started on aspirin.

Patients already on antiplatelet drugs

The priority is to perform a brain CT or magnetic resonance (MR) scan to determine whether the stroke is haemorrhagic or ischaemic. If the scan shows that the stroke was due to haemorrhage, the aspirin should generally be stopped. If the scan shows that the stroke was ischaemic, but there is some petechial haemorrhagic transformation, it is probably reasonable to continue the aspirin. However, there is no good evidence to support these suggestions for management! The question of what antiplatelet regimen to use for long-term secondary prevention in patients who have a stroke while already on aspirin or other antiplatelet drugs is discussed in section 16.5.4.

12.3.4 Who not to treat

From first principles, it is not logical to treat a bleeding disorder (intracerebral haemorrhage) with aspirin or any other antiplatelet drugs (Chapter 12). There is however, little reliable evidence on the effects of aspirin and other antiplatelet agents in such patients. As mentioned above, there was no clear evidence of harm from a few doses of aspirin while waiting for CT scanning to be performed.[157,159] A retrospective observational study has suggested that, in patients who have an intracerebral haemorrhage, being on aspirin at the time of the event increases the chances of haematoma expansion (and, in this series, that often led to surgical evacuation of the haematoma).[161] A prospective cohort study in 207 survivors of intracerebral haemorrhage, of whom 46 (22%) were prescribed antiplatelet agents (most commonly for prevention of ischaemic heart disease), found that antiplatelet use was not significantly associated with recurrent intracerebral haemorrhage; in survivors of either lobar haemorrhage (hazard ratio [HR] 0.8; 95% CI 0.3–2.3) or of deep haemorrhage (HR 1.2; 95% CI 0.1–14.3).[162] The authors concluded that, although antiplatelet use is relatively common following intracerebral haemorrhage, it did not appear to be associated with a large increase in risk of recurrent intracerebral haemorrhage. Therefore, patients with intracerebral haemorrhage who have a very clear and pressing indication to continue aspirin (e.g. unstable angina) and are thought – for whatever reason – to have a low risk of further intracerebral bleeding can probably continue aspirin.[159,162] Furthermore, it is not clear, if aspirin is to be used after intracerebral haemorrhage, whether it is best to stop it for a few days or to just continue without interruption. Patients with a history of definite aspirin sensitivity (e.g. wheeze or skin rash on exposure to aspirin) should not be given aspirin.

12.3.5 When to start

There is no clear evidence of a 'time window' for the benefit of aspirin; the relative benefits among those randomized late (24–48 h after stroke onset) are as great as those randomized early (within the first 0–6 h),[157] so aspirin should be started as soon as a CT or MR scan has excluded intracranial haemorrhage as the cause of the stroke. A policy of 'CT scan immediately and give aspirin if haemorrhage is excluded' is the most cost-effective strategy in this setting.[163] Moreover, if the doctor who admits the patient to hospital writes the prescription for aspirin immediately, the patient is more likely to receive long-term aspirin. If writing the aspirin prescription is left until later, it is easily forgotten. If CT scanning is not immediately available and the clinician is confident, based on the patient's clinical features, that the stroke is unlikely to be haemorrhagic (i.e. there is no history of an 'apoplectic onset' of the stroke with early headache or vomiting, the patient is fully conscious, etc.) (section 5.3.1), then aspirin can be started while the CT or MR scan is being organized. This policy does not appear to reduce the benefits from aspirin.[157]

If the patient is being considered for thrombolysis, it may be necessary to delay the start of aspirin treatment. For thrombolysis with streptokinase, the risk of intracranial haemorrhage is increased if it is given together with aspirin.[133,164] There is no good-quality RCT evidence on whether aspirin increases the risk of bleeding when recombinant tissue plasminogen activator (rt-PA) is the thrombolytic agent, though there is weak evidence from a non-randomized case series suggesting that giving rt-PA in patients already on aspirin is not unduly hazardous.[165] Despite the lack of good RCT evidence about the combination of aspirin and rt-PA, UK and US guidelines recommend, in patients to be treated with rt-PA, that aspirin treatment is only started 24 h after thrombolysis.[166,167]

> Start aspirin immediately even if there is likely to be some delay before a CT or MR scan can be performed and if you think intracranial haemorrhage is an unlikely cause of the stroke. However, delay starting aspirin in patients to be treated with thrombolysis until the day after the treatment has been given.

12.3.6 Agent/dose/route

We use aspirin in a dose of at least 150 mg daily in the acute phase of stroke. The initial dose has to be high (and certainly higher than is required for long-term secondary prevention) to inhibit thromboxane biosynthesis as quickly and completely as possible.[168,169] For patients who can swallow safely (section 11.17), aspirin can be given by mouth; for the remainder, it can be given rectally by suppository,[170] by nasogastric tube, or by intravenous injection (as 100 mg of the lysine salt, infused over 10 min).

12.3.7 Adverse effects

Major extracranial haemorrhage (defined as bleeding serious enough to cause death or require transfusion) is the most frequent serious adverse effect. In the trials, the relative increase in odds was large (68%; 95% CI 34–109%), but the absolute excess was small – four additional major extracranial haemorrhages for every 1000 patients treated.[156] The excess was greater among patients allocated heparin (0.9% heparin alone vs 1.8% allocated aspirin plus heparin; excess nine per 1000) than among other patients (0.5% among those allocated no aspirin and 0.7% allocated aspirin; excess two per 1000).[157] The risk of adverse events with aspirin, both in the short and long term, is best kept to a minimum by avoiding combined treatment with anticoagulants[171] (section 16.6.2 on the use of combined treatment in patients with prosthetic heart valves).

12.4 Selective use: anticoagulants

12.4.1 Rationale

Potential benefits

The rationale for using anticoagulants applies to both the arterial and venous circulations. In large arteries, and in the perforating arteries involved in lacunar infarction, the aim of treatment is to prevent local propagation of any occluding thrombus (or embolus), to tip the balance in favour of spontaneous lysis of the occlusion, and to prevent early re-embolization from any proximal arterial or cardiac sources. In small arteries and the microvessels, anticoagulation might also prevent sludging which may contribute to ischaemia in the penumbral zone around the infarct core. In the venous circulation, anticoagulation should reduce the risk of deep venous thrombosis and pulmonary embolism which are common complications of immobility after stroke (section 11.13).

Potential risks

As a cerebral infarct evolves over the first few days, red cells can leak from microvessels. Minor degrees of leakage appear on CT or MR brain scanning as petechiae, but if bleeding is more extensive, a parenchymal haematoma may form. This pathophysiological process is known as haemorrhagic transformation of cerebral infarction (section 5.7). Any anticoagulant, antiplatelet, thrombolytic or defibrinogenating agent could therefore theoretically increase the tendency to intracranial bleeding and this might offset some, or all, of any benefits.

The clinical impact of haemorrhagic transformation over and above the effects of the original infarct (i.e. the independent contribution of haemorrhagic transformation to the likelihood of a poor outcome) is difficult to assess in an individual patient. Minor degrees of transformation can occur without any clinical deterioration, whereas the development of a large parenchymatous haematoma may be fatal. However, even if a specific category of patient were at especially high risk of symptomatic haemorrhagic transformation, which might be exacerbated by an antihaemostatic agent, this does not necessarily mean that the net balance of risk and benefit will be adverse for that type of patient. By analogy with carotid endarterectomy for carotid stenosis, some patients are at high risk of stroke with surgery, but even higher risk without it, so that the net balance of risk and benefit may be favourable (section 16.11.6), even in high-risk individuals; this may be true for thrombolysis as well (section 12.5).

As well as increasing the risk of haemorrhagic transformation, anticoagulants could both increase the risk of symptomatic intracranial haemorrhage arising de novo (as intracerebral, subarachnoid or subdural bleeding) and the risk of bleeding at other, extracranial sites. The key question is therefore 'do the benefits of anticoagulants in the acute phase of ischaemic stroke treatment outweigh the risks?' Randomized trials provide the best means to assess this balance.

12.4.2 Evidence

Data available

By 2004, 22 RCTs comparing anticoagulants with control had been completed and were available for review.[172] Although the review has not been updated since then, no further RCTs of anticoagulants vs control eligible for inclusion in the review have been published. The trials included in the review tested standard unfractionated heparin, low-molecular-weight heparin, heparinoid, direct thrombin inhibitors and two tested heparin given for just 24 h followed by oral anticoagulation.[172] Most of the data came from trials in which unfractionated heparin was administered by subcutaneous injection in medium (12 500 IU twice daily) or low dose (5000 IU twice daily). In total, the trials included 23 547 patients with acute presumed ischaemic stroke.[172] Most patients had a CT scan to exclude intracerebral haemorrhage before treatment was started. Patients were generally randomized within 48 h of stroke onset, and treatment continued for about 2 weeks. There were fewer trials directly comparing one agent with another.[173] Another review focused on the trials comparing low-molecular-weight heparins or heparinoids with control in acute ischaemic stroke.[174] There have been a smaller number of trials comparing anticoagulants with antiplatelet agents; a review included data from four trials on 16 558 patients comparing either unfractionated heparin or low-molecular-weight heparin with aspirin.[175] Since those reviews were completed, a number of small trials have been published, comparing: intravenous full-dose heparin with aspirin;[176] intravenous full-dose heparin with low-dose heparin;[177] low-molecular-weight heparin with unfractionated heparin;[178,320] different doses of low-molecular-weight heparin;[179] low-molecular-weight

heparin with aspirin;[180] and argatroban, a direct thrombin inhibitor, with control (in which all patients received 81–350 mg aspirin within the first 48 h).[181] In our view, the results of these later studies do not alter the overall conclusions about the effects of anticoagulants in acute ischaemic stroke.

Effects on major outcomes: recurrent stroke, intracranial haemorrhage, death and functional status

The Cochrane review, based on nine trials comparing anticoagulants with control (22 570 patients) showed no evidence of net benefit within the scheduled treatment period (Fig. 12.11) or at the end of follow-up (Fig. 12.12). Although anticoagulants were associated with about

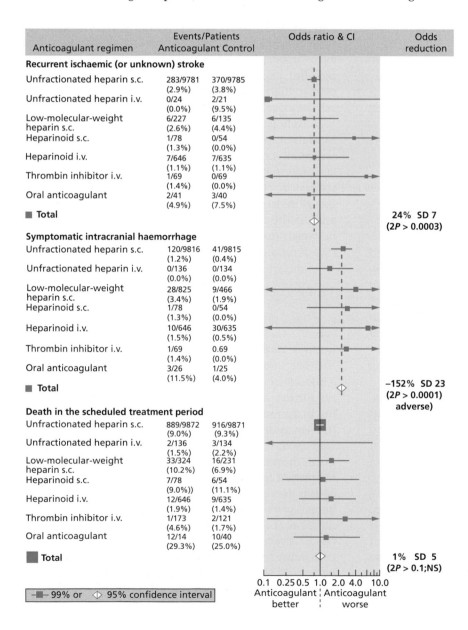

Fig. 12.11 Anticoagulants in acute ischaemic stroke: relative effects within the treatment period. Results of a systematic review of the 21 randomized trials comparing heparin with control groups in patients with acute ischaemic stroke: effects on recurrent ischaemic stroke, symptomatic intracranial haemorrhage and death, all within the scheduled treatment period. The estimate of treatment effect for each heparin regimen is expressed as an odds ratio (solid square) and its 99% confidence interval (horizontal line). The size of the square is proportional to the amount of information available. An odds ratio of 1.0 corresponds to a treatment effect of zero, an odds ratio of less than 1.0 suggests treatment is better than control, and an odds ratio of greater than 1.0 suggests treatment is worse than control. The overall result and its 95% CI is represented by an open diamond. The figures given to the right are relative odds reductions (SD). (Drawn from data from Sandercock, 2003.)[156] NS, not significant; SD, standard deviation; s.c., subcutaneous; i.v., intravenous.

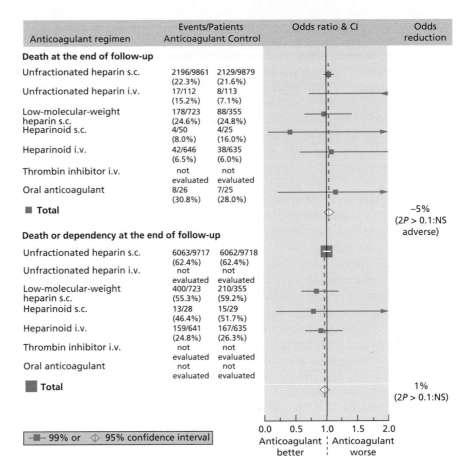

Anticoagulant regimen	Events/Patients Anticoagulant	Control	Odds ratio & CI	Odds reduction
Death at the end of follow-up				
Unfractionated heparin s.c.	2196/9861 (22.3%)	2129/9879 (21.6%)		
Unfractionated heparin i.v.	17/112 (15.2%)	8/113 (7.1%)		
Low-molecular-weight heparin s.c.	178/723 (24.6%)	88/355 (24.8%)		
Heparinoid s.c.	4/50 (8.0%)	4/25 (16.0%)		
Heparinoid i.v.	42/646 (6.5%)	38/635 (6.0%)		
Thrombin inhibitor i.v.	not evaluated	not evaluated		
Oral anticoagulant	8/26 (30.8%)	7/25 (28.0%)		
■ Total				−5% (2P > 0.1:NS adverse)
Death or dependency at the end of follow-up				
Unfractionated heparin s.c.	6063/9717 (62.4%)	6062/9718 (62.4%)		
Unfractionated heparin i.v.	not evaluated	not evaluated		
Low-molecular-weight heparin s.c.	400/723 (55.3%)	210/355 (59.2%)		
Heparinoid s.c.	13/28 (46.4%)	15/29 (51.7%)		
Heparinoid i.v.	159/641 (24.8%)	167/635 (26.3%)		
Thrombin inhibitor i.v.	not evaluated	not evaluated		
Oral anticoagulant	not evaluated	not evaluated		
■ Total				1% (2P > 0.1:NS)

■— 99% or ◇ 95% confidence interval

0.0 0.5 1.0 1.5 2.0
Anticoagulant better | Anticoagulant worse

Fig. 12.12 Anticoagulants in acute ischaemic stroke: relative effects at the end of follow-up. Results of a systematic review of the five randomized trials comparing anticoagulants with control groups in patients with acute ischaemic stroke reporting long-term outcome: effects on death from all causes, and death or dependency. Same conventions as Fig. 12.11. (From Gubitz et al. 'Anticoagulants for acute ischaemic stroke', *Cochrane Database Systematic Reviews* 2004: (3)[172] copyright Cochrane Collaboration, reproduced with permission.)

nine fewer recurrent ischaemic strokes per 1000 patients treated (OR 0.76; 95% CI 0.65–0.88), they were also associated with a similar sized nine per 1000 increase in symptomatic intracranial haemorrhages (OR 2.52; 95% CI 1.92–3.30) (Fig. 12.11). There was no evidence that anticoagulants reduced the odds of death from all causes at the end of follow-up (OR 1.05; 95% CI 0.98–1.12) (Fig. 12.12);[172] if anything, there was a non-significant excess of deaths with anticoagulants. Similarly, there was no evidence that anticoagulants reduced the odds of being dead or dependent at the end of follow-up (OR 0.99; 95% CI 0.93–1.04) (Fig. 12.12).

Bleeding risks with different regimens

In the Cochrane review, each of the regimens tested, when compared with control, appeared to increase the risks of both symptomatic intracranial haemorrhage and extracranial haemorrhage.[172] The relative increase in symptomatic intracranial haemorrhage was consistent across the different regimens, although (because of small numbers) it was only statistically significant for subcutaneous unfractionated heparin (Fig. 12.11). Indirect

comparisons of different dosing regimens showed consistently higher bleeding risks with higher dose regimens. In the IST, patients allocated to subcutaneous unfractionated heparin were randomized to high dose (12 500 IU twice daily) or to low dose (5000 IU twice daily) and the proportions with symptomatic intracranial haemorrhage were 1.8% and 0.7%, respectively – a highly significant 11 per 1000 excess with the higher dose (2P < 0.00001).[154]

As far as extracranial bleeds are concerned, for every 1000 acute ischaemic stroke patients treated with anticoagulants, about nine have a major extracranial haemorrhage. The indirect comparisons of different agents showed that the bleeding risks were higher with higher dose regimens. In the IST, the risk of major extracranial bleeds was 2% among patients allocated high-dose and 0.6% among those allocated low-dose heparin – a highly significant 14 per 1000 excess with the higher dose (2P < 0.00001).

A systematic review of all trials directly comparing high- with low-dose anticoagulants in acute ischaemic stroke supported the finding that the bleeding risks were dose-dependent for both intra-and extracranial bleeds.[182]

The RCTs published since then comparing different doses of low-molecular-weight heparin in acute ischaemic stroke also showed that intracranial bleeding was dose-dependent.[179,183] A recent open RCT comparing full-dose intravenous heparin with low-dose subcutaneous heparin, started within 3 h of stroke onset, also showed a higher risk of intracranial haemorrhages with the higher dose (6.2% vs 1.4%).[177]

Deep venous thrombosis and pulmonary embolism

Data on the effects of anticoagulants on deep venous thrombosis (DVT) are only available for 916 acute stroke patients. There was heterogeneity between the trials, which makes it harder to give a reliable overall estimate of treatment effect. Overall, symptomatic or asymptomatic DVT occurred in 43% of controls and 15% of treated patients, a highly significant 79% reduction in relative odds with anticoagulants (95% CI 61–85%). Thus, for every 1000 patients treated, 280 avoid DVT. Fatal or non-fatal pulmonary embolism (PE) was not systematically sought in the trials. It was reported in only 0.9% of controls and 0.6% of treated patients, a significant 39% reduction in relative odds with anticoagulants (95% CI 17–55%), i.e. for every 1000 patients treated, three avoid PE. It is difficult to judge whether the reductions in DVT or PE are dose-dependent from the indirect comparisons. In the IST, fatal or non-fatal PE occurred in 0.4% of those allocated high dose and 0.7% of those allocated low dose, a non-significant difference.[154] A systematic review of all of the direct randomized comparisons confirmed the greater reduction in PE with higher doses, but the absolute benefit was very small.[182] If we allow for the likely under-ascertainment of pulmonary embolism (section 12.3.2), and assume that the true risk in the controls was 3%, and then apply the same 39% proportional reduction (i.e. from 3% to 1.85%), for every 1000 patients treated about 12 would avoid PE. However, even if the benefit is that large, it will still be substantially offset, since an extra nine patients will have a major extracranial haemorrhage associated with anticoagulants.

Suspected cardioembolic ischaemic stroke

All patients with atrial fibrillation (AF) and ischaemic stroke should have a CT brain scan, since about 5–10% turn out to have intracerebral haemorrhage. A detailed analysis of the 3169 patients in IST with acute ischaemic stroke and AF confirmed that such stroke patients have a higher risk of early death than those in sinus rhythm.[184] This higher death rate was accounted for by the older age and larger infarcts among those with AF but not

by a higher risk of early recurrent ischaemic stroke. In patients with AF, the absolute risk of early recurrent stroke is low (in the IST, about 5% of patients in AF allocated to 'avoid heparin' had a recurrent stroke of ischaemic or unknown type within 14 days), and there was no net advantage to treatment with heparin.[184] The Cochrane review showed no statistically significant difference in the effect of treatment on death or dependence at final follow-up if a cardiac source of embolism was suspected (OR 1.00; 95% CI 0.85–1.18) or not suspected (OR 1.00; 95% CI 0.94–1.06) to be the cause of the stroke.[172] The small Heparin in Acute Embolic Stroke Trial (HAEST) compared a low-molecular-weight heparin with aspirin in 449 patients with acute ischaemic stroke of suspected cardioembolic origin and did not show any advantage to low-molecular-weight heparin.[185] These data do not support the widespread use of either intensive (i.e. full-dose intravenous) unfractionated or low-molecular-weight heparin regimens in the acute phase of ischaemic stroke associated with AF.[160]

> In patients with suspected acute cardioembolic ischaemic stroke, there is no evidence to support the routine use of immediate anticoagulation with heparin, heparinoid or low-molecular-weight heparin. Aspirin is a safe and effective alternative to anticoagulants, which reduces the risk of early recurrent stroke in patients with acute ischaemic stroke and atrial fibrillation.

Progressing hemispheric stroke

By far the most important step is to find out why the stroke is 'progressing'. There are numerous causes besides propagating cerebral arterial thrombosis for a worsening neurological deficit (section 11.5) (Table 11.7). These factors should be identified and – if possible – treated. For patients in whom all other possible causes for progression have been excluded, many textbooks and reviews recommend immediate intravenous heparin. However, there have not been any trials of intravenous heparin specifically in patients with progressing stroke, and neither the trials of intravenous unfractionated heparin nor of intravenous heparinoid in patients with acute ischaemic stroke showed net benefit overall.[172] There is therefore no direct or indirect evidence to support the use of heparin (either intravenous or subcutaneous) in this particular type of patient.[160]

Basilar thrombosis

The IST included over 2000 patients with posterior circulation ischaemic infarcts, and there was no evidence that the effects of treatment in this subgroup were any different to those seen in the trial overall.[154] However, it is likely that only a small proportion had occlusion of the basilar artery. Further trials of anticoagulants in 'vertebrobasilar territory infarcts' are probably not warranted; but a trial focused on patients with proven basilar occlusion might be justified, although trials which seek to recruit a type of patient only rarely encountered in clinical practice are notoriously difficult to do. This lack of evidence led a recent guideline to state that anticoagulants were 'not recommended' for this indication.[160]

Acute stroke in patients with acute myocardial infarction

(See also section 7.10.) The first step in management is to determine whether the stroke was due to intracerebral haemorrhage, either spontaneous or iatrogenic (e.g. caused by thrombolytic or anticoagulant treatment). Some patients may have iatrogenic ischaemic strokes due to particulate emboli reaching the brain as a complication of some invasive cardiological procedure such as coronary angiography or angioplasty. The value of anticoagulants in these latter patients is not clear, as the embolic material is often atheromatous debris from the large arteries rather than fresh thrombus or platelet aggregates. Patients with full-thickness anterior myocardial infarction (MI) have a higher than average risk of developing left ventricular (LV) thrombus (section 7.10). Although two small trials[186,187] showed that medium-dose subcutaneous heparin (12 500 IU twice daily) reduced the frequency of LV thrombus, an overview of the 26 trials of anticoagulants in acute MI (including 73 000 patients) found little evidence of any significant further net clinical benefit (in terms of major clinical events) from adding either subcutaneous or intravenous heparin to the treatment of patients who are given aspirin.[188,189] The value of anticoagulants in a patient with an acute MI complicated by acute ischaemic stroke is therefore unclear.

Oral anticoagulants, given to stroke-free MI survivors for several months, probably reduce the risk of having a first stroke in the longer term, but given the cost and inconvenience of oral anticoagulants and the uncertainty about the optimal intensity of treatment, aspirin is probably the long-term antithrombotic agent of choice in most patients.[189,190] However, 6 months of oral anticoagulants may be worthwhile in patients with MI complicated by acute ischaemic stroke thought to be due to embolism from the left ventricle, especially if congestive heart failure, AF or extensive LV dysfunction are present.[189]

12.4.3 Who to treat

Although there is no indication to use anticoagulants *routinely* in patients with acute ischaemic stroke,[160,166,191] there are still some occasions where they may be appropriate; these are listed in Table 12.8 and discussed below. The use of heparin after thrombolysis to prevent re-occlusion of the opened cerebral artery is discussed in section 12.5.2.

> Heparin, when used for the immediate treatment of patients with acute ischaemic stroke, has risks (haemorrhage in the brain and elsewhere) which exactly cancel out the benefits (fewer recurrent ischaemic strokes and less venous thromboembolism). We therefore do not use this treatment routinely.

Selected patients at high risk of deep venous thrombosis

Factors which increase the risk of deep venous thrombosis (DVT) and pulmonary embolism (PE) after stroke include: hemiplegia or immobility; dehydration; a history of previous episodes of venous thromboembolism; and a known thrombophilia or active cancer.[191] Simple, reliable methods to predict which patients are most likely to develop DVT would be very useful.

Guidelines vary in their recommendations about whether or not heparin should be used for DVT prevention. The Scottish Intercollegiate Guidelines Network recommended aspirin for all patients with ischaemic stroke and that low-dose subcutaneous heparin should only be added to aspirin in patients at high risk of DVT and PE.[191] The Joint American Stroke Association/American Academy of Neurology (ASA/AAN) guideline states 'Subcutaneous unfractionated heparin, low molecular weight heparins, and heparinoids may be considered for DVT prophylaxis in at-risk patients with acute ischaemic stroke, recognising that non-pharmacologic treatments for DVT prevention also exist. A benefit in reducing the incidence of PE has not been demonstrated. The relative benefits of these agents must be weighed against the risk of systemic and intracerebral haemorrhage.'[160]

It is not clear whether low-dose subcutaneous heparin can add useful benefit to aspirin for the prevention of DVT and PE without causing an increase in bleeding complications (Table 12.7 gives an estimate of the increase in risk of extracranial bleeding when subcutaneous heparin is added to aspirin).[154] Other strategies for prevention of DVT and PE (e.g. rehydration, early mobilization, graded compression stockings) and the management of stroke patients who develop symptoms and signs suggestive of DVT or PE after admission are discussed in section 11.13.

Anticoagulants worthwhile

Transient ischaemic attack or mild ischaemic stroke with complete recovery within 1–2 days and in atrial fibrillation (start as soon as possible)

Non-disabling ischaemic stroke, with or without minor (petechial) haemorrhagic transformation and in atrial fibrillation (best time to start unclear)

Anticoagulants probably worthwhile

Acute myocardial infarction within past few weeks and confirmed ischaemic stroke or transient ischaemic attack

Disabling ischaemic stroke and atrial fibrillation

Anticoagulants not worthwhile

Low risk of recurrent cardioembolic stroke without anticoagulants:

    Low-risk cardiac lesion (e.g. hypertrophic cardiomyopathy, minor degree of mitral leaflet prolapse)

    Other, non-cardiac lesion, a more likely cause of the ischaemic stroke

Little to gain from long-term anticoagulation:

    Already severely disabled before the stroke

    Moribund

High risk of cerebral haemorrhage on anticoagulants:

    Infective endocarditis

    Large cerebral infarct with midline shift

    Likely to comply poorly with anticoagulation

    Severe, uncontrolled hypertension

    Major haemorrhagic transformation on brain CT

Absolute or relative contraindication to anticoagulants (Table 12.9)

Table 12.8 Patients with acute ischaemic stroke of suspected cardioembolic origin who should be considered for immediate anticoagulation, and those who should have anticoagulants deferred (or avoided completely).

The choice of method for deep venous thrombosis prophylaxis largely depends on its perceived risk, the likely duration of immobility, and any predisposing factors. For patients with mild strokes who mobilize within a day or so, and have no other predisposing factors for deep venous thrombosis, aspirin is probably adequate. For immobile patients with predisposing factors (and who do not have bad arterial disease or sensory loss in the legs), graded compression stockings may provide additional benefit. If stockings are not acceptable, then low-dose subcutaneous unfractionated heparin in addition to aspirin is an alternative.

Atrial fibrillation

Patients with atrial fibrillation (AF) who have had a stroke or transient ischaemic attack are likely to benefit from long-term oral anticoagulants as secondary prevention, provided there are no contraindications (Table 12.8) (see section 16.6 for further details on the selection of patients with AF most likely to benefit). However, as discussed above, both fixed-dose subcutaneous unfractionated heparin, adjusted-dose intravenous unfractionated heparin and low-molecular-weight heparin are not recommended for the prevention of early recurrent ischaemic stroke in acute ischaemic stroke presumed due to cardioembolic stroke.[160] To help decide whether (and when) to use anticoagulants in the acute phase, one should therefore take into account the factors that are likely to increase the risk of haemorrhagic transformation of the infarct (section 12.4.5), the likely risk of recurrent ischaemic stroke within the first week or so, and the severity of the stroke (sections 12.4.5 and 16.6.6). If anticoagulants are indicated, see section 12.4.5 on when to start and section 12.4.6 for the choice of agent.

12.4.4 Who not to treat

Relative contraindications and cautions about the use of anticoagulants are given in Table 12.9. Any patient with acute stroke due to established intracranial haemorrhage, or who has not had a CT brain scan to exclude intracranial haemorrhage, should not be given anticoagulants. The evidence on the effects of heparin in patients with haemorrhagic stroke is scant but suggests – as one might expect – it may well be associated with some harm, though the confidence interval is wide.[159] Warfarin should not be used during pregnancy (Table 12.9 and section 16.6.3).

Table 12.9 Contraindications to, and cautions with, full-dose anticoagulants (these depend on individual circumstances and are seldom absolute) (adapted from Scottish Intercollegiate Guidelines Network, 1999).[193]

Uncorrected major bleeding disorder
Thrombocytopenia
Haemophilia
Liver failure
Renal failure
Uncontrolled severe hypertension
Systolic blood pressure over 200 mmHg
Diastolic blood pressure over 120 mmHg
Potential bleeding lesions
Active peptic ulcer
Oesophageal varices
Unruptured intracranial aneurysm (especially if large
  and untreated)
Proliferative retinopathy
Recent organ biopsy
Recent trauma or surgery to head, orbit or spine
Confirmed intracranial or intraspinal bleeding
Evidence on MR or CT of previous intracranial bleeding
Recent stroke, but patient has not had brain CT scan or MRI
Recent stroke, with large infarct on brain CT or MRI (i.e.
  high risk of haemorrhagic transformation)
History of heparin-induced thrombocytopenia or thrombosis
(if heparin planned)
If warfarin planned
Pregnancy
Homozygous protein C deficiency (risk of skin necrosis)
History of warfarin-related skin necrosis
Uncooperative/or unreliable patients (long-term therapy)
Risk of falling
Unable to monitor anticoagulation intensity

12.4.5 When to start

The available trial data do not provide reliable evidence on the best time to start anticoagulants. So, in the occasional circumstance where we do feel compelled to use them in acute stroke (section 12.4.3), the decision must be based on the likely risk of events without treatment, and the risk of haemorrhagic transformation with treatment.

In the IST, the frequency of recurrent ischaemic or undefined stroke within 14 days was not significantly different in those with and without AF: 3.9% among those with AF vs 3.3% without.[154,184] Symptomatic haemorrhagic transformation of the infarct occurs most commonly during the first 2 weeks and the risk is highest in patients with large infarcts[192] and in patients given more intensive heparin regimens.[154,177,182] Therefore, in a patient with a major ischaemic stroke and AF, we

would wait at least 1–2 weeks before starting. We would then consider the relative contraindications listed in Table 12.9 and, if necessary, delay the start of anticoagulants further (or abandon the idea altogether). When oral anticoagulants are started in this way (i.e. without aggressive loading doses) some time after the acute event, concomitant heparin (to overcome any transient prothrombotic state associated with the start of warfarin) is probably not needed.[193] In patients with transient ischaemic attack or with an ischaemic stroke which resolves within a day or so, the risk of haemorrhagic transformation is probably negligible; if such a patient has a clear indication for the use of long-term anticoagulants (most commonly AF), we would start treatment immediately.

> In a patient with a disabling acute ischaemic stroke and atrial fibrillation, the risk of stroke recurrence within the first 2 weeks is not high, so we would start aspirin immediately, avoid anticoagulants for the first week or two, or longer if we felt the risk of haemorrhagic transformation of the infarct remained high (e.g. large infarct on CT with mass effect). Patients with transient ischaemic attack or very minor ischaemic stroke and atrial fibrillation can be started on both aspirin and oral anticoagulants immediately. If aspirin is given with anticoagulants, it should be stopped once the international normalized ratio is in the therapeutic range.

12.4.6 Agent/dose/route/adverse effects

Agent

Oral anticoagulants do not act sufficiently fast to have a major effect within the first few hours of onset of an ischaemic stroke. Anticoagulants must be given by injection if they are to achieve a rapid effect. Most of the evidence on heparin in acute stroke comes from trials which used unfractionated heparin.[172] Though other agents have been tested, systematic reviews of the direct and indirect comparisons of different regimens did not provide evidence that any one agent was better than unfractionated subcutaneous heparin.[172,173] In choosing between the different heparin regimens and aspirin, the ASA/AAN guideline states 'Intravenous unfractionated heparin or high-dose low molecular weight heparin or heparinoids are not recommended for any specific subgroup of patients with acute ischaemic stroke that is based on any presumed stroke mechanism or location (e.g., cardioembolic, large vessel atherosclerotic, vertebrobasilar, or 'progressing' stroke) because data are insufficient. Although the low molecular weight heparin, dalteparin, at high doses may be efficacious in patients with AF, it is not more efficacious than aspirin in this setting. Because aspirin is easier to administer, it, rather than dalteparin, is recommended for the various stroke subgroups (Grade A).'[160] The results of the trials published since that guideline[176,178,179,320] have not materially altered those conclusions.

Dose and route

The risk of bleeding with heparin is clearly dose-dependent;[154,179,182,183] the higher the dose, the higher the risk of intracranial and extracranial haemorrhage and there is no evidence to support the use of full-dose adjusted regimens with intravenous unfractionated heparin or heparinoid.[160] The Rapid Anticoagulation Prevents Ischaemic Damage (RAPID) trial in 67 patients with non-lacunar ischaemic stroke within 12 h of onset compared full doses of intravenous unfractionated heparin with aspirin 300 mg daily; showed no evidence of an advantage of full-dose intravenous heparin over aspirin,[176] although a more recent RCT of full-dose intravenous heparin vs low-dose subcutaneous heparin within 3 h of stroke onset suggested net benefit from the higher heparin dose.[177] Hence, since bleeding is dose-related, if anticoagulants are to be used, low-dose subcutaneous regimens are preferable (e.g. 5000 IU unfractionated heparin two or three times daily) since they are simpler, do not require complex monitoring and are associated with lower bleeding risks. The options for the treatment of established deep venous thrombosis and pulmonary embolism are discussed in section 11.13.

Adverse effects

Table 12.10 lists the most important adverse effects and cautions to be considered when using heparin. The most life-threatening risks are of massive intra- or extracranial haemorrhage. Management of severe extracranial haemorrhage consists of stopping any heparin administration; estimation of the clotting time; and reversal with intravenous protamine sulphate in a dose of 1 mg for every 100 IU of heparin infused in the previous hour.[193] Protamine should be given slowly over 10 min and the patient monitored for hypotension and bradycardia. Not more than 40 mg of protamine should be administered in any one injection. For advice on reversal of low-molecular-weight heparin or heparinoids, consult the manufacturer's data sheet. Patients on oral anticoagulants who suffer a head injury or develop any of the neurological symptoms listed in Table 12.11, or who require a diagnostic lumbar puncture, should be investigated and treated as described in Tables 12.11–12.13.[193]

Table 12.10 Adverse effects of heparin.

Local minor complications of subcutaneous heparin at injection site
Discomfort
Bruising
Local complications of intravenous heparin at cannula site (or elsewhere)
Pain at cannula site
Infection at cannula site (sometimes with severe systemic infection)
Reduced patient mobility because of infusion lines and pump
Systemic complications
Intracranial bleeding
Haemorrhagic transformation of cerebral infarct (potentially disabling or fatal)
Intracerebral haemorrhage
Subarachnoid haemorrhage
Subdural haematoma
Extracranial haemorrhage
Subcutaneous (can sometimes be massive)
Visceral (haematemesis, melaena, haematuria)
Thrombocytopenia
Type I: dose and duration related, reversible, mild, usually asymptomatic, not serious and often resolves spontaneously
Type II: idiosyncratic, allergic, severe (may be complicated by arterial and venous thrombosis). Affects 3–11% of patients treated with intravenous heparin and less than 1% of patients treated with subcutaneous heparin
Osteoporosis
Skin necrosis
Alopecia

Reversal of warfarin must be done in consultation with the local haematology specialist (Table 12.13).

12.4.7 Acute stroke in a patient already receiving anticoagulants

Urgent reversal of anticoagulation in patients with intracranial bleeding on anticoagulants

If a patient on oral anticoagulants presents with symptoms suggestive of a stroke or develops any of the neurological symptoms outlined in Table 12.11 (any of which may indicate intracranial bleeding), they must have a *CT or MR scan performed immediately*.[193] If the CT or MR scan shows extradural, subdural, subarachnoid or intracerebral haemorrhage, then anticoagulants should be stopped and *urgently* reversed. If the scan does not show *intracranial* bleeding, consider the possibility that the neurological deficit might be due to a *spinal* haematoma, especially if the neurological deficit spares the face and is associated with neck pain (the diagnosis is best

Table 12.11 Advice on management of problems in patients on anticoagulants.

Indication for immediate CT or MR brain scan if patient has[a]

Significant head injury (i.e. any loss of consciousness or amnesia or the presence of a scalp laceration)

Headache (especially of recent onset, or increasing in severity)

Acute neck pain with neurological deficit in limbs[b]

Drowsiness

Confusion

Onset of focal neurological symptoms or signs

If the scan shows intracranial bleeding

Reverse anticoagulants (Table 12.12)

If scan shows extradural or subdural bleeding or hydrocephalus, consider surgical decompression after reversal

If scan shows only subarachnoid bleeding, consider CT or MR angiography to exclude underlying aneurysm

Is the patient being considered for a diagnostic or therapeutic procedure involving the spine?[c]

Lumbar puncture

Epidural or spinal anaesthesia

Contrast myelography

[a]The CT or MR scan must be performed *as soon after admission as possible.* Delay may reduce the potential benefits of reversing the anticoagulants if intracranial bleeding is found.[196]

[b]In patients with acute neck pain with a neurological deficit in the limbs, but no evidence of intracranial bleeding on the brain scan, MR scanning of the spine may be needed to exclude spinal epidural haematoma.[194]

[c]Lumbar puncture, epidural anaesthesia and myelography in patients on anticoagulants can cause spinal epidural haemorrhage, spinal cord compression and paraplegia. The need for the procedure should be discussed with a neurologist or neurosurgeon before anticoagulants are reversed, since reversal carries a risk of thromboembolism. Alternative investigation (e.g. MR scanning) or alternative methods of anaesthesia may be preferable.

Table 12.12 Strategies for reversal of oral anticoagulation.[193]

Life-threatening haemorrhage (intracranial or major gastrointestinal bleeding)

Stop warfarin prescription *and*

Give intravenous vitamin K1 (5 mg, repeated if necessary) *and either*

Intravenous factor IX complex concentrate (also contains factors II and X) (50 IU/kg body weight) *plus*

Factor VII concentrate (50 IU/kg body weight) (if available) *or*

Recombinant factor VIIa *or*

Fresh frozen plasma (15 mL/kg – approximately 1 L for adult)

Less severe haemorrhage (e.g. haematuria, epistaxis)

Stop warfarin for 1–2 days

Give vitamin K1, 0.5–2 mg intravenously or 5–10 mg orally

High international normalized ratio (INR) but no haemorrhage

Stop warfarin, monitor INR, restart warfarin when INR < 5.0

of PCC, was associated with a better outcome.[196] RCTs of the different options are clearly needed.[195,196] After successful reversal of the haemostatic deficit, further treatment may be needed, depending on the location of the haematoma and any underlying causative lesion, for example: evacuation of a subdural haematoma, clipping or coiling of a ruptured intracranial aneurysm, or evacuation of an intracerebral or spinal haematoma.

Risk of arterial thromboembolism after stopping anticoagulants

Patients with a high risk of arterial thromboembolism (usually because they either have a mechanical prosthetic heart valve or AF) who develop intracranial bleeding while on oral anticoagulants create particular management difficulties.[197–199] There are competing risks to be balanced: of valve thrombosis and re-embolization if anticoagulants are permanently withdrawn, and of further intracranial bleeding if anticoagulants are re-instituted.[197–201] A retrospective non-randomized observational study of 141 patients with a high risk of ischaemic stroke who had an intracranial haemorrhage while taking warfarin examined these competing risks.[198] The indication for anticoagulants fell into one of three categories: prosthetic heart valve in 52 patients, AF in 53 and a recurrent TIA or an ischaemic stroke in 36. The median time off warfarin after the bleed was 10 days. Three patients had an ischaemic stroke within 30 days of stopping warfarin. In the three groups, the Kaplan-Meier estimate of the probability of having an ischaemic stroke within 30 days of stopping warfarin was: prosthetic heart valve 2.9% (95% CI 0–8.0%); AF 2.6% (95% CI 0–7.6%); and TIA or an ischaemic stroke 4.8% (95% CI 0–13.6%)

confirmed by MR scanning of the spine); a spinal epidural haematoma may require neurosurgical treatment.[194]

A narrative review found no reliable evidence from RCTs to select the best method for rapid reversal, but the options are: vitamin K, prothrombin complex concentrates (PCC), recombinant factor VIIa, or fresh frozen plasma (FFP)[195] (section 12.2.4) (Tables 12.12–12.13). There is weak evidence from a retrospective non-randomized observational study in 55 patients with anticoagulant-related intracerebral haemorrhage that haematoma growth within 24 h was significantly lower in patients receiving PCC compared with FFP or vitamin K.[196] There was some evidence that achieving a normal INR within 2 h, generally through the use

Table 12.13 Options for reversal of warfarin therapy.[193]

Method and dosage	Advantages	Disadvantages
Stop warfarin	Simple	May take several days for INR to normalize, particularly with liver disease

Vitamin K1
    0.5–5 mg i.v.
    5–10 mg orally
	Safe if given slowly	2–6 h to take effect
		12–24 h to take effect

Factor IX complex concentrate 50 IU/kg body weight	Acts immediately Small volume Can be given quickly	Exposes patients to blood product which rarely may transmit hepatitis B (but safe from hepatitis C and HIV) Effect is temporary (8–24 h), may need to be repeated Should be combined with vitamin K1 Risk of thromboembolism
Factor VII concentrate 50 IU/kg body weight	Should be given with factor IX complex concentrate	As for factor IX complex
Recombinant factor VIIa	No risk of blood-borne infection	Expense
Fresh frozen plasma 1L for adult	Acts immediately	Large intravenous volume load Allergic reactions Not as efficacious as factor IX complex concentrate Difficult to give repeat infusions because of large volume Virally inactivated plasma is preferred

respectively. Another retrospective review reported that none of the 16 patients with a prosthetic heart valve who had intracranial haemorrhage and then had their warfarin discontinued (for a median of 7 days) suffered a recurrent thromboembolic event while off warfarin.[201] It therefore seems from these very limited data that the risk of recurrent thromboembolism from stopping oral anticoagulants for a week or two after an intracranial haemorrhage is low.

Is it possible to restart anticoagulation after intracranial bleeding, and if so, in whom, and when?

After an intracerebral haemorrhage on anticoagulants, one needs to estimate the risk of recurrent thromboembolism (section 16.6.2 for risk prediction in patients with AF; assessing the risk in patients with mechanical prosthetic heart valves requires expert cardiological advice). In the study of 141 patients by Phan *et al.*, of the 35 who had warfarin therapy restarted, none had recurrence of intracranial bleeding during the same hospital admission.[198] Butler has reported 2-year follow-up data on 13 patients with mechanical prosthetic heart valves who restarted anticoagulation after an intracranial haemorrhage. Of the four patients with intracerebral haemorrhage as the initial bleed, none suffered recurrent intracranial bleeding and two suffered thromboembolic events. On reintroduction of oral anticoagulants, the target INR was lowered in 9 of 13 patients. The authors concluded that careful reintroduction of oral anticoagulation is appropriate in these patients.

However, there are many factors one has to consider in decision-making for an individual patient. Consider the (fairly typical) case of an elderly patient in AF who has been on anticoagulants for a number of years because of a prior ischaemic stroke who presents with an intracerebral haemorrhage. A number of questions immediately spring to mind: was the bleed due to over-anticoagulation (and if so, is there a level of international normalized ratio (INR) which clearly separates 'excessive' from 'acceptable')?; if the INR was in the therapeutic range, how far should investigations to identify the cause be pursued?; and, is the patient still at high risk from recurrent thrombembolism (and if so, should the target INR be lowered)?

If the scan shows infarction, what are the management options?

If the CT or MR is normal or shows infarction with no evidence of any haemorrhage, the reason for the infarction must be sought. Often, the cause is inadequate warfarin dose, but infective endocarditis must be ruled out. If the INR was below target range before – or at the time of onset of – the stroke, more careful supervision to maintain the INR within the target range for that patient should reduce the risk of further ischaemic strokes. If INR control had been poor despite apparent compliance with the prescribed warfarin dose, one must make careful enquiry about recent changes in other prescribed drug treatment, the use of non-prescribed medication (including herbal and complementary therapies) or changes in diet, since all of these can interact with warfarin. However, if a patient suffers a recurrent ischaemic stroke despite an adequate INR, one can consider adding low-dose aspirin; while this may reduce the risk of recurrent stroke, it also increases the risk of intracranial haemorrhage[171,202] (section 16.6.2).

12.5 Selective use: reperfusion with thrombolytic drugs and other methods

12.5.1 Rationale

Potential benefits

Restoration of blood flow, to reperfuse the ischaemic brain as soon as possible after a cerebral vessel has been occluded, should lessen the volume of brain damaged by ischaemia, reduce the likelihood of major cerebral oedema and result in a better clinical outcome (section 12.1.3). Therefore, therapeutic attempts to hasten reperfusion by removing any occluding thrombus with thrombolytic drugs, mechanical methods, ultrasound or a combination of these approaches ought to be helpful.

Potential risks

Thrombolytic drugs will also lyse haemostatic plugs and thus may increase bleeding into the brain in the area of ischaemia, in areas of the brain remote from the ischaemia or in extracranial sites (into the skin, joints, the gastrointestinal or urinary systems). Mechanical methods require intra-arterial instrumentation, which can cause a number of complications, including arterial dissection and rupture.

12.5.2 Evidence

Data available for reperfusion with thrombolytic drugs and mechanical methods

Eighteen RCTs including 5727 patients are included in the most up-to-date systematic review available in the *Cochrane Library*.[133] About half the data relate to trials of intravenous recombinant tissue plasminogen activator (rt-PA) and the remainder to intravenous streptokinase (42%), intravenous urokinase (3%) and intra-arterial recombinant pro-urokinase (5%). Ninety per cent of the data are derived from trials of intravenous thrombolysis with either rt-PA or streptokinase, given within 6 h of onset of confirmed ischaemic stroke. Individual patient data meta-analyses of the rt-PA[203] and streptokinase trials[204] have also been published. Since then a number of small-scale RCTs have been published: a dose-finding study of intravenous tenecteplase;[205] two phase II studies of intravenous desmoteplase;[52,53,206] and, of intra-arterial urokinase in acute posterior circulation stroke.[207] Intravenous glycoprotein (Gp) IIb/IIIa inhibitors are discussed in section 12.6.1. There have not been any large-scale trials of mechanical clot retrieval or ultrasound-assisted reperfusion; the limited data on these interventions are reviewed in section 12.6.3.

Fewer data than for acute myocardial infarction

Over 58 000 patients have been randomized in trials of intravenous thrombolysis vs control in patients with acute myocardial infarction.[208] Compared with this very large amount of data, there are relatively few on the effects of thrombolysis for ischaemic stroke (especially when one recalls the size of the global burden of stroke and that the incidence of acute stroke and acute MI are similar in Western populations). Furthermore, it required a systematic review of these data to establish that, though early treatment was the most effective, for patients with ST elevation or bundle branch block, the 'time window' for worthwhile benefit was up to 12 h (certainly much longer than had originally been thought plausible).[208]

Intracranial haemorrhage

There is a very consistent trend across all the stroke trials for an excess of fatal intracranial haemorrhage with thrombolysis and the proportional excess is similar with all the agents. The absolute excess depends on the risk of haemorrhage in the control group, and this risk was somewhat different between trials. For intravenous rt-PA, the only licensed thrombolytic agent, treatment increases the risk of fatal intracranial haemorrhage about fourfold from 1% in controls to about 4% ($P < 0.00001$), equivalent to 33 extra fatal intracranial haemorrhages per 1000 patients treated (Fig. 12.13). rt-PA increases fatal or non-fatal symptomatic intracranial haemorrhages threefold ($P < 0.00001$).[133] Many of the haemorrhages occur within the ischaemic area, but others occur at sites remote from the ischaemia. These remote bleeds may represent bleeding from an undetected pathological vascular lesion (small arteriovenous malformation, vessel affected by amyloid angiopathy, or a previous microbleed).[209] However, data are also accumulating to suggest that the presence of microbleeds does not materially influence the risk of bleeding with thrombolysis.[210]

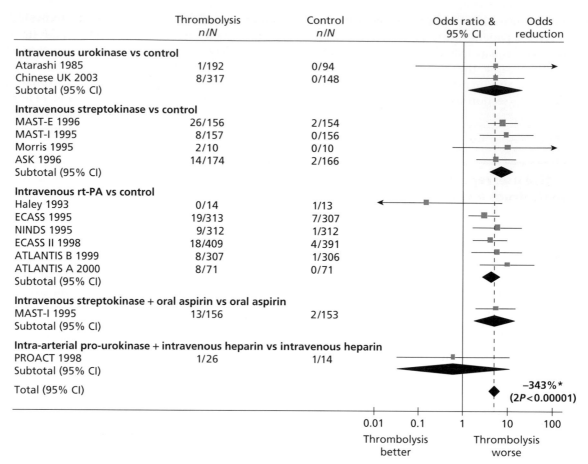

	Thrombolysis n/N	Control n/N	Odds ratio & 95% CI	Odds reduction
Intravenous urokinase vs control				
Atarashi 1985	1/192	0/94		
Chinese UK 2003	8/317	0/148		
Subtotal (95% CI)				
Intravenous streptokinase vs control				
MAST-E 1996	26/156	2/154		
MAST-I 1995	8/157	0/156		
Morris 1995	2/10	0/10		
ASK 1996	14/174	2/166		
Subtotal (95% CI)				
Intravenous rt-PA vs control				
Haley 1993	0/14	1/13		
ECASS 1995	19/313	7/307		
NINDS 1995	9/312	1/312		
ECASS II 1998	18/409	4/391		
ATLANTIS B 1999	8/307	1/306		
ATLANTIS A 2000	8/71	0/71		
Subtotal (95% CI)				
Intravenous streptokinase + oral aspirin vs oral aspirin				
MAST-I 1995	13/156	2/153		
Subtotal (95% CI)				
Intra-arterial pro-urokinase + intravenous heparin vs intravenous heparin				
PROACT 1998	1/26	1/14		
Subtotal (95% CI)				
Total (95% CI)				−343%* (2P<0.00001)

0.01   0.1   1   10   100

Thrombolysis better   Thrombolysis worse

Fig. 12.13 Thrombolysis in acute ischaemic stroke: effects on fatal intracranial haemorrhage. Results of a systematic review of 13 trials. *A negative odds reduction indicates an adverse effect of treatment. Similar conventions as Fig. 12.11 except all the confidence intervals are 95%. (From Wardlaw *et al.* 'Thrombolysis for acute ischaemic stroke', *Cochrane Database of Systematic Reviews* 2003; (3)[133] copyright Cochrane Collaboration, reproduced with permission.)

Massive infarct swelling

Massive swelling of infarction is a common cause of *early* death after acute ischaemic stroke, and is more likely to occur in patients where the occluded artery does not spontaneously reopen (section 5.7). It is reasonable to assume then that reopening the occluded artery might reduce the risk of this event, reduce the risk of death and increase the chance of a good recovery from the stroke. However, an early non-randomized study suggested that rt-PA increased the risk of massive fatal brain swelling.[211] A more recent, but still uncontrolled, case series of patients, all treated with rt-PA, suggested that, while 'malignant' fatal brain oedema was more common that expected, overall 'massive infarct swelling' was less frequent.[212] This outcome has not been extensively studied in the trials to date, but a preliminary analysis of the limited data from four trials suggests rt-PA showed a trend to a non-significant reduction in this outcome by about a fifth (Wardlaw J, personal communication); if confirmed in a large study this could be of substantial clinical significance.

Death

Overall, thrombolysis significantly increased the odds of death within the first 2 weeks, though, by the end of follow-up (3 months in most trials), the difference between the thrombolysis and control was smaller (Fig. 12.14).[133] In the trials of intravenous rt-PA, there was a non-significant 14% increase (95% CI 4% reduction to 37% increase) in the risk of death by the end of follow-up (at around 3 months in most trials).[133] There was statistically significant heterogeneity of treatment effect among the trials of rt-PA which makes the interpretation of this overall estimate difficult.[133] In the individual patient data meta-analysis of the rt-PA trials, the hazard ratio (HR) for death, adjusted for baseline stroke severity, was not significantly different from 1.0 for the 0–90, 91–180 and 181–270 min intervals but for 271–360 min it was

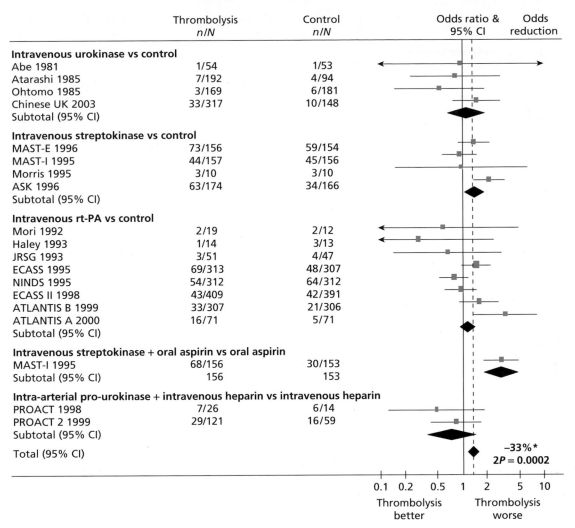

	Thrombolysis n/N	Control n/N
Intravenous urokinase vs control		
Abe 1981	1/54	1/53
Atarashi 1985	7/192	4/94
Ohtomo 1985	3/169	6/181
Chinese UK 2003	33/317	10/148
Subtotal (95% CI)		
Intravenous streptokinase vs control		
MAST-E 1996	73/156	59/154
MAST-I 1995	44/157	45/156
Morris 1995	3/10	3/10
ASK 1996	63/174	34/166
Subtotal (95% CI)		
Intravenous rt-PA vs control		
Mori 1992	2/19	2/12
Haley 1993	1/14	3/13
JRSG 1993	3/51	4/47
ECASS 1995	69/313	48/307
NINDS 1995	54/312	64/312
ECASS II 1998	43/409	42/391
ATLANTIS B 1999	33/307	21/306
ATLANTIS A 2000	16/71	5/71
Subtotal (95% CI)		
Intravenous streptokinase + oral aspirin vs oral aspirin		
MAST-I 1995	68/156	30/153
Subtotal (95% CI)	156	153
Intra-arterial pro-urokinase + intravenous heparin vs intravenous heparin		
PROACT 1998	7/26	6/14
PROACT 2 1999	29/121	16/59
Subtotal (95% CI)		
Total (95% CI)		

Odds ratio & 95% CI   Odds reduction

−33%*
2P = 0.0002

0.1 0.2   0.5   1   2   5   10

Thrombolysis better   Thrombolysis worse

Fig. 12.14 Thrombolysis in acute ischaemic stroke: effects on death at the end of follow-up. Results of a systematic review of 18 trials reporting this outcome. *A negative odds reduction indicates an adverse effect of treatment. Same conventions as Fig. 12.13 (from Wardlaw *et al.* 'Thrombolysis for acute ischaemic stroke', *Cochrane Database of Systematic Reviews* 2003; (3)[133] copyright Cochrane Collaboration, reproduced with permission.)

significant at the 5% level with an HR of 1.45 (1.02–2.07).[203] It is not known reliably whether the survival disadvantage from thrombolysis diminishes or increases with longer-term follow-up, since only one trial with 624 patients has reported follow-up beyond 6 months.[213]

Dead or dependent, or fully recovered at the end of trial follow-up

Despite the excess of deaths from intracranial haemorrhage, patients who survived the treatment were on average less disabled. Most of the trials reported follow-up at 3 months. For patients treated with any agent within 6 h, there was a significant 16% reduction in the risk of death or dependency with thrombolysis (95% CI 5–25%; P = 0.004) (Fig. 12.15). This would be clinically important – if confirmed by further trials – as it is equivalent to about 43 fewer dead or dependent patients per 1000 treated. However, there was heterogeneity of treatment effect between the trials, which makes the overall estimate of effect less reliable. Among the six trials of intravenous rt-PA (2830 patients), thrombolysis reduced the risk of death or dependency by 20% (95% CI 7–31%; P = 0.003) equivalent to 55 fewer patients being dead or dependent. Again, there was significant heterogeneity of treatment effect. The precise definition of dependency did not materially alter these conclusions, i.e. it did not make much difference whether 'dependent' was defined as modified Rankin/Oxford Handicap Score (OHS) 3, 4, 5 or 2, 3, 4, 5 (section 17.12.5). The proportion of

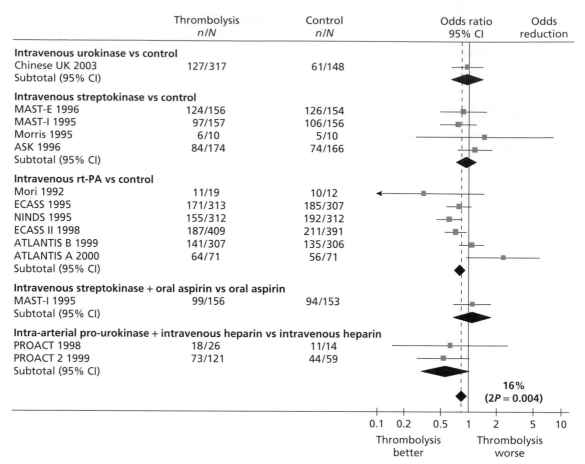

Fig. 12.15 Thrombolysis in acute ischaemic stroke: effects on death or dependency at the end of follow-up. Results of a systematic review of the 13 trials which reported this outcome. Same conventions as Fig. 12.13. (From Wardlaw *et al.*

'Thrombolysis for acute ischaemic stroke', *Cochrane Database of Systematic Reviews* 2003; (3)[133] copyright Cochrane Collaboration, reproduced with permission.)

patients making a complete recovery from their stroke (OHS zero) was also increased with thrombolysis. Only three trials, with a total of 1556 patients, reported follow-up data at 6 months and only one has reported follow-up at 12 months. The benefit seen at 3 months persisted to 12 months in that one trial, but further long-term follow-up data are clearly needed.[213,214]

Subgroups: predicting prognosis is not the same as predicting response to thrombolytic treatment

There is an enormous literature on the clinical and radiological factors that predict outcome after ischaemic stroke[215] though the number of simple, well-validated and robust predictive models that are useful for clinical practice is surprisingly small (section 10.2.7).[215] However, in the context of identifying which patients to treat with thrombolytic therapy, it is important to look for variables that predict a *good response to treatment* rather than those which just predict a good outcome. One needs to be clear whether the treatment effect really is different

in patients with and without the feature in question. In statistical terms, if a variable does influence the size or direction of the treatment effect, there is an 'interaction' between that variable and the treatment effect.[129,216,217] The most common type of interaction is where the treatment is effective in people with and without the variable, and only *the size* of the treatment effect is somewhat different (e.g. a treatment is effective in both men and women, but the benefit is greater in men); this is called a *quantitative interaction*. A less commonly encountered scenario is when the direction of treatment effect is different in the two groups (e.g. harmful or ineffective in men, but beneficial in women); this is called a *qualitative interaction*.[129,216,217] Subgroup analyses looking for such interactions are often very underpowered and multiple underpowered exploratory subgroup analyses are particularly likely to lead to inappropriate interpretations.[110,129,217] This is the case for the RCT evidence for thrombolysis, where there are insufficient data for reliable analyses of the impact of almost all of the different features which have been said to influence the response to treatment. There are also a large number of non-randomized case series purporting to demonstrate factors which modify the response to thrombolysis; but studies with non-randomized controls simply cannot provide an unbiased estimate of interaction with treatment effect.

Subgroups: time since stroke onset

The individual patient data meta-analyses of rt-PA[203] provides evidence that (as in acute myocardial infarction), the earlier treatment is given, the greater the benefit. However, though the curve of decreasing benefit from rt-PA with increasing time to treatment appears smooth, it is somewhat artificial, since there is a significant discontinuity in the underlying data at 90 and 180 min, because of clustering of randomizations at these time points; this clustering reduces the reliability of the analysis.[218] The data for streptokinase show a similar, though not quite statistically significant, trend for decreasing benefit with time.[204] Though there is a statistically significant interaction between treatment benefit with rt-PA and time to treatment, different people draw different conclusions from the data in Fig. 12.16 on exactly what the therapeutic 'window' is (i.e. the time in which there is clear evidence of net benefit): just 90 min; up to 3 h (the regulatory approval in most countries, but only for selected patients); up to 6 h; or, longer than 6 h in some individuals. The interpretation is made more difficult because time is just one of four inextricably linked factors: stroke severity (severe strokes arrive quickest at hospital, mild strokes come later); the appearance of the baseline CT scan (the more severe the stroke, the more likely 'infarction' will be visible on an early scan); the time from onset (the longer the time, the more likely infarction will be visible on CT); and reduction in the benefit from treatment with time. The only way to decide which patients can be treated outside the current very restrictive approved criteria is to obtain further data from further large-scale RCTs.

Subgroups: clinical features to identify who benefits?

The rt-PA study group individual patient data meta-analysis focused on the impact of onset to treatment time on the odds of a favourable outcome with rt-PA.[203] However, the authors also developed a model to examine the influence of the most important prognostic factors that might confound the relationship between the benefit of treatment and time from onset to treatment: age, weight, sex, systolic and diastolic blood pressure (mmHg) at start of treatment, blood glucose concentration at baseline, National Institutes of Health Stroke Scale (NIHSS) score on admission, various items on previous history of vascular events, previous or current atrial fibrillation and whether the patient was on aspirin at the time of the index stroke (but not the influence of baseline CT scan appearances). These analyses suggested that stroke severity did not influence response to treatment and that the likelihood of significant intracerebral haemorrhage was not importantly modified by time to treatment. Beyond those two conclusions, these analyses do not shed light on which patients are most likely to benefit. The RCT data for rt-PA are particularly scanty in older people, since only 42 stroke patients over the age of 80 have been included in randomized trials of the drug.[133,203] While a recent series from Canada has shown that such patients *can* be treated with rt-PA,[219] we would argue that only randomized trial evidence can provide a proper assessment of the balance of risk and benefit in this increasingly large group of patients.

Subgroups: radiological features to identify who benefits?

There has been much debate about whether 'early infarct signs' on a pre-treatment scan should preclude the use of thrombolysis[220,221] (the definition and observer reliability of these signs is discussed in section 5.4.2).[222] A systematic review of the literature published between 1990 and 2003 assessed the evidence. In 15 studies of

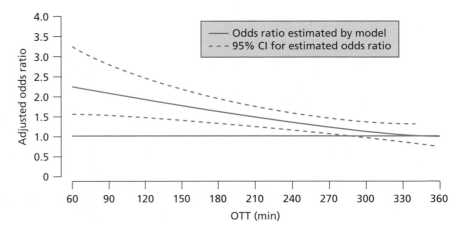

Fig. 12.16 Thrombolysis in acute ischaemic stroke. Model estimating odds ratio for a favourable outcome at 3 months compared with control, by onset to treatment time (OTT) in minutes. Odds ratio adjusted for age, baseline glucose, baseline diastolic pressure, previous hypertension and interaction between age and baseline stroke severity. (From the rt-PA study group 2004 with permission from rt-PA study group[203] and the *Lancet*.)

early infarction signs and outcome (including seven thrombolysis trials) in 3468 patients, any 'early infarction sign' increased the risk of poor outcome regardless of treatment.[222] However, the only two studies that sought an interaction between early infarction signs and thrombolysis found no evidence that thrombolysis, given in the presence of early infarction signs, resulted in worse outcome than that due to early signs alone.[222] A re-analysis of the scans from the NINDS and ECASS-2 studies, applying the Alberta Stroke Program Early CT scale (ASPECTS), found that early ischaemic change was more frequent than originally reported, but there was no evidence that the presence of early ischaemic change modified the response to rt-PA.[223,224] The authors concluded that further work was required to determine whether any early infarction sign should influence decisions concerning thrombolysis. The presence of a perfusion-diffusion 'mismatch' (assessed either with MR or CT) is a much debated radiological criterion[225,226] but unfortunately only one ongoing RCT, the EPITHET study, has an appropriate design to assess the interaction of 'mismatch' with treatment effect, and – since it will include only 120 subjects – it may well lack power to examine the interaction reliably.[227]

Is any one agent better than another?

There are a large amount of data from trials which directly randomized patients with acute myocardial infarction (AMI) to different thrombolytic regimens.[228] A meta-analysis of the 14 trials (total number of randomized subjects 142 907) showed no significant differences in mortality at 30–35 days, but total stroke and haemorrhagic stroke rates were higher for rt-PA than for streptokinase (total stroke, OR 1.29; 95% CI 1.1–1.5; haemorrhagic stroke OR 1.8; 95% CI 1.1–2.9).[228] The authors concluded that in AMI all thrombolytic drugs appeared to be of similar efficacy in reducing mortality, and the differences in stroke favoured streptokinase over newer drugs (tenecteplase, reteplase, rt-PA).[228,229]

Unfortunately, there have not been any comparably large-scale RCTs directly randomizing large numbers of ischaemic stroke patients between streptokinase, rt-PA and urokinase to allow reliable comparison of these agents.[230] The indirect comparisons available are not a reliable way to compare treatment effects but, for what it is worth, they did not provide clear evidence of differences in efficacy between the three agents once the time to treatment was accounted for.[133,229,230]

In summary, systematic reviews of the indirect and the direct randomized comparisons of different intravenous and intra-arterial thrombolytic agents for stroke have not established that any one agent is clearly superior to another (they may be, but we cannot be sure).[133,230] A

number of small-scale RCTs are underway, evaluating: newer thrombolytic agents (tenecteplase, reteplase, microplasmin); intravenous vs intra-arterial thrombolytic therapy; thrombolytic agent combined with intravenous Gp IIb/IIIa inhibitors; supplementing thrombolytic drug therapy with transcranial Doppler ultrasound.[231]

Is any one dose better than another?

For intravenous thrombolytic therapy, there is a suggestion that low-dose urokinase and low-dose rt-PA have a lower risk of symptomatic intracranial haemorrhage, but the comparisons are confounded by a number of factors, such as baseline severity of stroke, race and time to randomization, so no firm recommendation on the 'best' dose can be given.[133,230] rt-PA in dose of 0.9 mg/kg (maximum dose 90 mg) is the most widely tested regime.

Concomitant aspirin or heparin?

In the Multicentre Acute Stroke Trial (MAST-I) there was an interaction between streptokinase and aspirin such that the risk of symptomatic intracranial haemorrhage was significantly higher for the combination of aspirin and streptokinase than for either drug separately.[164,232] In all of the other trials, aspirin was not randomly allocated, so it is very difficult to determine whether any differences in the frequency of symptomatic intracranial haemorrhage were due to concomitant aspirin treatment or to other factors (such as thrombolytic agent, dose, delay, etc.). However, there was a strong tendency for the effect of thrombolysis to be more favourable in trials where antithrombotic therapy was avoided for the first 24 h (and the more antithrombotic therapy that was given, the less favourable the outcome.[133]

The need for concomitant anticoagulants may be different when intra-arterial thrombolysis is used, but there are no trials of intra-arterial thrombolysis which directly randomized patients to 'intravenous heparin' vs 'no intravenous heparin'. In the Prolyse in Acute Cerebral Thromboembolism (PROACT)-I study of intra-arterial pro-urokinase, at the time of angiography, the first 16 patients were given a 100 IU bolus of unfractionated heparin intravenously, followed by an infusion of 1000 IU/h. However, because of the high frequency of intracranial haemorrhage, the heparin dose was reduced for subsequent patients.[233] In the PROACT-II study, all patients received an intravenous bolus of 2000 IU followed by an intravenous infusion of 500 IU/h of unfractionated heparin, and intravenous heparin was given with intra-arterial thrombolysis.[234] Unfortunately these data do not reliably establish whether concomitant aspirin or heparin therapy is necessary with intra-arterial or intravenous thrombolysis, and if so, what the best antithrombotic regimen is.

Blood pressure management

The blood pressure entry criteria and management algorithms that were used in the NINDS thrombolysis trial were included in the ASA Guidelines for stroke patients receiving thrombolysis.[235] However, an independent re-analysis of the NINDS trial identified several problems with blood pressure measurement and management in the study: 112 patients (18%) were found to have identical admission and baseline (randomization) blood pressure readings; 22 patients had missing baseline blood pressure data; an unknown number of patients had high blood pressure treated both before arrival in the emergency department and in the emergency department by non-study physicians; and no data were recorded to indicate whether patients had high blood pressure treated after randomization.[218,236] Based on these observations, the authors concluded that the effect of blood pressure and its management on clinical outcome in acute ischaemic stroke patients treated in the NINDS trial could not be assessed. Consequently, all the blood pressure variables were excluded from the statistical models.[236] Hence, any baseline blood pressure selection or exclusion criteria for thrombolysis, or recommendations on management of blood pressure during thrombolytic treatment, are not based on reliable evidence (in section 11.7 we discuss the general management of high and low blood pressure in acute stroke).

Intra-arterial thrombolysis for acute spontaneous occlusion of a cerebral artery

There have been five small RCTs in which occlusion of the relevant cerebral artery was demonstrated before treatment was given. In two of the trials, angiographic confirmation was available in most patients[237,238] and in the two PROACT trials it was a prerequisite for trial entry.[233,234] The two PROACT trials compared prourokinase plus intravenous heparin vs intravenous heparin alone. The Australian Urokinase Stroke Trial (AUST) comparing intra-arterial thrombolysis plus heparin with heparin alone in basilar artery thrombosis was terminated after only 16 patients were randomized, because of difficulties recruiting.[207] The benefits of intra-arterial thrombolysis appear to be at least as great as with intravenous rt-PA (Fig. 12.15), but the treatment can be given only in a few highly specialized centres, so is only available to a very small proportion of all stroke patients. Treatments which are highly effective, but applicable to only a small proportion of all patients have almost no

effect in reducing the overall burden of stroke (section 18.3). The concomitant heparin treatment used in the PROACT trials was – as might be expected – associated with quite a high risk of symptomatic intracranial haemorrhage in the control groups (14% and 4% of controls in PROACT-1 and -2, respectively), and an even higher rate in the treated patients (15% and 10%, respectively). The Interventional Management of Stroke Study was a non-randomized feasibility study of intravenous followed by intra-arterial thrombolysis (the latter was given only if the target vessel remained occluded); the authors concluded a randomized trial comparing intravenous with intravenous plus intra-arterial thrombolysis was warranted.[239]

Treatment of ischaemic stroke following angiography, interventional radiology or cardiac catheterization

There are many possible causes of stroke after various invasive radiological procedures (sections 6.8.5 and 7.18). The first step – as ever – is an urgent CT to exclude intracranial haemorrhage (since such strokes can be due to haemorrhage).[240] However, if the intra-arterial catheter is left in place (or a sheath has been inserted), or if the cerebral lesion proves to be ischaemic, the radiologist may then inject contrast material to see if an occlusive cerebral arterial lesion can be visualized. Unfortunately, it may be difficult to ascertain whether the vessel has occluded because of local thrombosis, intimal dissection, arterial spasm, emboli dislodged by the catheter from proximal arterial sites or even metallic fragments of the interventional tool itself.[240] And even if the vessel is occluded by emboli, it may not be possible to determine whether the emboli consist of atheromatous debris or fresh thrombus. Nonetheless, interventional cardiologists and radiologists like to intervene, and there are several anecdotal reports of thrombolysis to clear such obstructions. An uncontrolled study in 11 patients who had acute ischaemic strokes during interventional neuroradiological procedures (10 of the 11 were having coils or balloons inserted into inoperable intracranial aneurysms) suggested that thrombolysis within 4 h of symptom onset, with an unspecified intra-arterial dose of urokinase, was not catastrophic.[241] A retrospective review reported the use of intra-arterial rt-PA or urokinase in 21 patients with post-coronary angiography stroke.[242] Without a control group for comparison, it is hard to judge the clinical outcome: however, 48% achieved a modified Rankin Score of 2 or better, but symptomatic intracranial haemorrhage occurred in three (14%), and four (19%) died. A review of case series of thrombolytic treatment for strokes after cardiac catheterization similarly suggested that thrombolytics are often used, but the balance of risk and benefit is unclear.[240] An alternative 'rescue' treatment for peri-procedural stroke due to vessel occlusion by thrombus is to give a Gp IIb/IIIa inhibitor intra-arterially (section 12.6.1).

Treatment of suspected cardioembolic stroke

A small trial comparing rt-PA with controls in 98 patients with suspected cardioembolic ischaemic stroke showed a non-significant trend towards benefit with thrombolysis.[238] There is some suggestion that an embolus obstructing a cerebral artery may be more susceptible to lysis if it is due to embolism from the heart rather than from a lesion in the extracranial arteries.

The need for further large-scale RCTs of intravenous thrombolysis

Although the limited trial data have led to regulatory approval for the use of rt-PA, many questions remain about how this treatment should be used in routine clinical practice. If more patients are to have access to this treatment and if it is to be delivered more equitably, then we need reliable answers to a number of important questions: Is there an upper age limit for treatment? Which patients are most likely to suffer early hazard? Which patients will gain the greatest long-term benefit? How wide is the time window – 3, 4, 5, 6, 7, 8 or even 9 h for some cases? Is the window the same for all ischaemic stroke subtypes? Is there worthwhile net benefit when thrombolysis is given in non-specialist centres?

To answer these questions reliably, we need to design and conduct appropriately large trials.[110,114] Large trials are *essential* because, if the treatment really works as well as we suspect, the time window is longer than just 2 or 3 h, or the selection criteria can be broadened, it should be used more widely. If, on the other hand, large-scale trials show it to be less effective than expected, health services should focus resources on the treatments that yield greater net health gain for the population (e.g. stroke units) (sections 17.6 and 18.4).[243,244]

The rt-PA study group estimated that a randomized controlled trial with about 6000 patients would be needed to confirm or refute the estimates of effect from their pooled analysis.[203] The Third International Stroke Trial (IST-3) began its start-up phase in April 2000. The main UK Medical Research Council phase started in 2005 and will continue until 2009. The trial seeks to randomize 6000 patients with acute ischaemic stroke within 6 h of onset to intravenous rt-PA or control. It has an appropriately streamlined and efficient design, as is appropriate for such a large-scale study.[110,114] Full details of the trial protocol and progress are available at

www.ist3.com. For details of the other current trials see http://www.strokecenter.org/trials/index.aspx.

12.5.3 Who to treat

There is general agreement that thrombolysis for stroke should only be given in centres that have a well-established acute stroke care system, sufficient numbers of appropriately trained staff and adequate facilities. The clinical diagnosis of stroke in the hyperacute phase relevant to clinical triage for thrombolysis is discussed in section 3.3, the imaging strategies to select patients for thrombolysis in sections 5.4 and 5.5, and the organization of the acute stroke service that is needed to support safe and effective thrombolytic treatment (including support via telemedicine) in section 17.5.

If thrombolysis is to be given safely, a great deal of preparation and training are required for staff in the local teams and departments involved in each stage of the chain: emergency call response centre, ambulance service, emergency department, radiology department and the acute stroke unit. Such training needs to be repeated at intervals to allow for staff turnover. And training sessions must be backed up with clearly written simple protocols. Useful materials are available over the Internet on many different websites; this list gives a selection with particular relevance to thrombolysis:

- The IST-3 trial website has a number of resources (monitoring for, and management of complications, training in image interpretation): www.ist3.com
- The NIH website offers a web-based training tool for administering the NIHSS and providing certification of competence: http://www.professionaleducationcentre.americanheart.org
- The Internet Stroke Centre has a variety of educational materials about stroke: http://www.strokecenter.org/prof/index.html

Clinical and radiological selection criteria

The clinical and radiological selection criteria for treatment with intravenous thrombolytic therapy set by the regulatory authorities and laid out in national guidelines vary somewhat between countries. Details of the eligibility criteria for the approved use in Europe are detailed in the summary of product characteristics for rt-PA.[245] The items common to many guidelines are summarized in Table 12.14.

Consent

The risk of fatal intracranial haemorrhage with thrombolysis deters a large number of patients, emergency

Table 12.14 Essential aspects of therapeutic thrombolysis.[a]

Preparation and maintenance of service organization:	History of bleeding disorder (e.g. haemophilia)
Audit existing service, identify delays	History of recent bleeding
Draw up 'fast-track' pathway of care in consultation with all relevant disciplines and departments	Arterial puncture at non-compressible site within past 14 days
Train relevant staff	Major surgery within past 14 days
Inform general public and primary care teams	Previous stroke or serious head injury within past 3 months
Assess patients immediately:	Neurological deficit trivial and likely to recover within next few hours
Ambulance crew perform basic assessment and radio ahead to hospital to warn of arrival	Evidence of accelerated hypertension
Immediate assessment on arrival at hospital by trained 'triage' nurse or paramedic	Blood glucose is < 3 or > 22 mmol/L
Local acute stroke protocol activated including:	*Seek expert advice before giving thrombolysis if any of the following are true:*[c]
Systematic but brief clinical assessment:	Unruptured intracranial aneurysm
Number of hours since onset of stroke symptoms	Menstruation
Focal neurological symptoms and signs	Pregnancy
Vital signs (pulse, blood pressure, respiration, temperature)	*Decision to give thrombolysis or not must be made by senior member of stroke team*
Intravenous cannula inserted and blood samples taken for basic blood tests (blood glucose measurement essential)	*If decision is to give thrombolysis, transfer to place where thrombolysis can be given and monitored closely:*
Immediate transfer to neuroimaging	Establish intravenous (i.v.) infusion if not already done so
Results of preliminary neuroimaging conveyed to stroke team	Estimate weight, draw up infusion with a dose of 0.9 mg/kg rt-PA
Trained stroke physician reviews diagnosis, neuroimaging and other information	Infuse rt-PA i.v.: 10% as a bolus over 1–2 min, remainder over 60 min
Consent/assent sought from patient and/or relative where feasible	Monitor pulse and BP:
Do not give thrombolysis if any of the following are true:[b]	Every 15 min during infusion
Time of stroke onset not clearly known	Every 30 min for next 2 h, then
Neuroimaging shows:	Hourly for 5 h
Acute intracranial haemorrhage	Neurological observations hourly
That the symptomatic infarct is much older than the history suggests	*Postacute management:*
A non-stroke lesion as the cause of the symptoms (e.g. cerebral tumour)	Transfer to stroke unit (if not already there)
On oral anticoagulants and therapeutically anticoagulated (i.e. INR > 1.4)	Start aspirin 160–300 mg daily 24 h after infusion:
	If able to swallow safely, by mouth
	If not able to swallow safely, per rectum or i.v.
	(section 12.3.6)

[a]See www.ist3.com for useful documents, protocols and training resources for thrombolysis in stroke.
[b]This list of contraindications is based on the UK summary of product characteristics, i.e. the European licence for the use of alteplase for stroke. In the IST-3 trial, the protocol states that 'If the patient has had a stroke within the previous 14 days or has had treatment for acute ischaemic stroke with thrombolytic therapy within the past 14 days' this is an absolute contraindication to treatment; patients with a history of an ischaemic stroke more than 2 weeks previously (with or without thrombolytic treatment) may – at the treating physician's discretion – be considered for treatment or inclusion in the trial.
[c]See section 12.5.4 for details.
INR, international normalized ratio; rt-PA, tissue plaminogen activator.

physicians, neurologists and stroke physicians from giving the treatment.[149,246] Although clinicians worry that intracranial bleeding due to treatment may lead to litigation, in practice, failure to administer the treatment in an otherwise eligible patient is the more common reason for litigation, in North America at least.[246] However, when asked, many people (who have not yet had a stroke) would be prepared to accept the short-term risks (of severe haemorrhage or death) in order to have the chance of surviving free of disability.[247,248] A patient's willingness to accept the risks of treatment is often influenced by their own perception of the severity of the stroke. If the patient has neglect or other perceptual difficulties, this can further complicate the consent procedure.[249]

A patient presented with witnessed abrupt onset of complete left hemiplegia, 1 h before arrival at the hospital, had a CT consistent with early ischaemic change in the right cerebral hemisphere, and met all the criteria for thrombolytic treatment within the current approval. However, because she also had anosognosia, she was completely unable to recognize that she had had a stroke, and hence saw no reason to be exposed to the risks associated with thrombolysis. The stroke team felt it inappropriate to treat her against her express wishes.

The scenario above is drawn from a published case report;[249] a comment on the case stated that it would have been reasonable to give the treatment without the patient's consent.[250] This is supported by the fact that the patient in question was left with substantial residual neurological impairment requiring major assistance in all activities of daily living.[249] The risks of thrombolysis are definite and not trivial, so fully informed consent is desirable, whether thrombolysis is to be used in routine clinical practice or in an RCT. But, in practice, getting fully informed consent is often a barrier to early treatment:[251] the patient's acute neurological impairment may impair communication and writing; a close relative or partner may not be available at the critical moment; and the pressure of time may make decision-making difficult for all concerned.[252–257] However, one must seek to achieve whatever degree of consent is required to meet local clinical governance and research practice ethical standards. Simple materials (adaptable for routine clinical or trial use) have been developed with input from patients and lay people, that can facilitate the process of consent (see www.ist3.com).[248,257] However, the rigorous standards for informed consent required in research do not obtain when thrombolysis is used in routine practice. A survey of the documentation of consent for routine clinical use of thrombolysis for stroke in Connecticut hospitals found that a substantial percentage of patients who received rt-PA for stroke had no consent documented.[258] Surrogates often provided consent when the patients had the capacity to give consent; conversely, patients with diminished capacity sometimes provided their own consent.[258]

> There should be no double standards for randomized trials and clinical practice, yet patients given treatments in routine practice are often not given any explanation or information. Many patients refused randomization in the first International Stroke Trial when they were told that aspirin and heparin might cause intracranial bleeding, yet how many tens of thousands of patients with acute stroke have been treated with these two drugs (before and since the large-scale trials began) without being asked for their consent after a full explanation of the risks and benefits? Similar double standards seem to apply to thrombolysis in randomized trials and routine clinical practice.

Treatment

The aim should be to treat – without delay – patients who meet all of the following criteria:

- the time of symptom onset is known with certainty;
- the clinical diagnosis is definitely an acute stroke of sufficient severity to merit the risks of treatment;
- no clear clinical or radiological contraindications are identified;
- consent (or relative's assent) is documented in accordance with local requirements;
- passage through the above system has been fast enough to allow treatment well within 3 h of onset;
- there is a vacant bed and sufficient staff available on the acute stroke unit to monitor the patient during the infusion and the immediate post-treatment period.

Patients who fulfil the above criteria, but do not exactly meet the strict terms of the current approval, and for whom thrombolysis is considered 'promising but unproven' should be considered for inclusion in IST-3 or one of the other relevant RCTs.

> The urgent priorities are to establish, by means of appropriate large-scale randomized trials, whether the balance between early hazard and long-term benefit is still favourable when thrombolysis is used in a wider variety of patients. These data will help decide which categories of patient are most likely to benefit and whether the benefits really persist for more than just a few months.

12.5.4 Who not to treat

The absolute contraindications to thrombolysis are listed in Table 12.14. In addition, there are many relative contraindications reported in the literature, but which are not supported by good evidence. There are case reports of thrombolysis being used for the treatment of acute ischaemic stroke in patients who do have these relative contraindications, including: pregnancy;[259] menstruation;[260] recent surgery;[261] unruptured intracranial aneurysms[262] and anticoagulation with an INR > 1.7.[263,264] We are aware of cases with other contraindications being treated (remote past history of intracranial haemorrhage but current ischaemic stroke, history of ischaemic stroke within past 3 months, etc.); in our view, it would be more informative to consider including patients who have some of these features of uncertain significance in relevant RCTs in order to determine reliably whether or not they should influence patient selection.

The decision about treatment often requires a synthesis of clinical and radiological information. A 70-year-old man who lived alone was brought by ambulance to the emergency department at 9 am, following an emergency call at 8 am. He had aphasia and profound weakness of his right arm. The CT scan showed an area of ischaemia in the left middle cerebral artery territory appropriate to his symptoms. However, the lesion showed marked hypoattenuation and quite well-defined edges, suggesting it had been present for much longer than the 1 h suggested by the ambulance crew. Thrombolysis was not given. The patient's niece later confirmed that her uncle's speech had been 'muddled' when she had telephoned him at 10 pm the evening before, suggesting his ischaemic stroke lesion had been present for at least 11 h by the time he presented to hospital.

At present, age over 80 is a contraindication to treatment within the European approval, whereas it is not in the USA and Canada. The risk of intracranial bleeding with rt-PA rises with age, but so too does the risk of a poor outcome without treatment.[203,265] Hence, given the very limited published RCT data in this age group (just 42 patients), while we accept that such patients *can* be treated,[219] we often prefer to enrol them in IST-3. We do this, because we – and the patients – are usually genuinely uncertain of the balance of risks and benefits.

12.5.5 When to start treatment – as soon as possible!

Since the benefit (but perhaps not the risk) of treatment is very time dependent, the sooner it can be given, the better (whether as part of routine clinical practice, or in a randomized trial). A systems approach is needed to ensure every step in the process of care is completed as efficiently as possible; from the moment the patient develops their stroke symptoms to the safe completion of the treatment in hospital. There are many barriers to the delivery of efficient care, but a variety of interventions to overcome these barriers have been evaluated (section 17.5).[214,251,266]

Many centres have found it useful to create a 'stroke thrombolysis box' (Fig. 12.17). The design and the selection of its contents will vary according to local circumstances, but it should be portable, contain everything needed to carry out a rapid assessment of a potential stroke thrombolysis patient and then initiate therapy (i.e. all the information, printed protocols, drugs, specimen bottles, request forms, intravenous infusion pumps, drug prescription, drug administration charts, clinical monitoring records, etc.). If everything is in one place, valuable time can be saved.

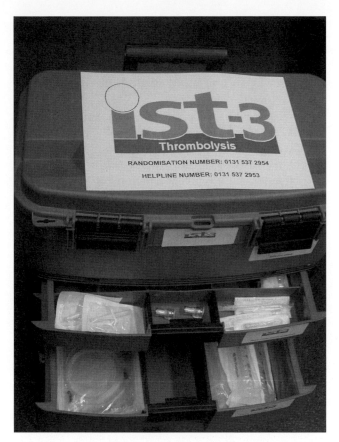

Fig. 12.17 'Thrombolysis box' used on the acute stroke unit at the Western General Hospital, Edinburgh. The top drawer contains the infusion pump and written protocols (on laminated sheets) for nursing management, monitoring, and management of suspected complications. The lower drawers contain the other items required for drug administration. Photograph by Dr I Kane (reproduced with permission).

12.5.6 Agent/dose/route/concomitant treatment

Agent

Intravenous rt-PA is the only agent that has wide regulatory approval for use in stroke. In Europe, at the time of writing, the approval was provisional on two conditions being met:

- Satisfactory evidence of the safety of rt-PA in routine practice. Up to the end of April 2006 clinicians were required to record (in the SITS-MOST registry: http://www.acutestroke.org/) the use of, and the clinical outcome in, patients treated with rt-PA when treated within the terms of the approval. After that date, registering the data has been voluntary.
- Completion of the ECASS-3 RCT.[267]

Dose and route

The approved regimen is 0.9 mg/kg of rt-PA intravenously; 10% of the dose as a bolus over 1 min and the remainder as an infusion over 1 h, and the maximum dose is 90 mg.[133,230]

Intra-arterial thrombolysis does not have regulatory approval, but a variety of regimens have been used: in the PROACT-II trial, patients were given 9 mg of recombinant pro-urokinase intra-arterially;[234] in AUST, intra-arterial urokinase was given in increments of 100 000 IU to a maximum dose of 1 000 000 IU; and, in a recent large case-series, up to 1 000 000 IU of urokinase was given, and if recanalization was not achieved at that dose, gentle mechanical disruption of the clot with the catheter tip was attempted.[268]

Intra-arterial thrombolysis has a number of potential disadvantages: delay in initiation of fibrinolysis while the diagnostic angiogram is performed and the microcatheter positioned (start of the thrombolytic infusion typically occurs 50–90 min later than the start of an intravenous infusion); the procedure is labour- and capital-intensive; and the intervention can only be performed at tertiary and secondary hospitals capable of acute endovascular therapy.[231]

Concomitant antithrombotic treatment

Current US and UK guidelines recommend that antithrombotic therapy with aspirin or heparin should be avoided for at least 24 h after intravenous thrombolysis with rt-PA.[166,167] The situation is less clear for patients who have had intra-arterial thrombolysis. Some centres follow one of the anticoagulant regimes employed in the RCTs of intra-arterial thrombolysis,[207,233,234] whereas others – in the light of the results of the CAST and IST trials – use aspirin instead of heparin as the post-treatment antithrombotic regimen.[268]

Blood pressure management for patients having thrombolytic treatment

The North American Stroke Thrombolysis Guidelines[235] recommended the NINDS trial treatment algorithm,[132] but the more recent version on acute stroke did not make such firm recommendations[167] (section 11.7 for general guidance on blood pressure monitoring and management).

12.5.7 Adverse effects

Intracranial and major extracranial haemorrhage are the most feared adverse effects of thrombolytic treatment.

All treatment protocols should have clear arrangements on how to monitor for, and then treat, these complications if they arise. Examples of the sort of monitoring and management guides (which can be adapted as needed) are available at the IST-3 website (www.ist3.com); they can be laminated and kept in the 'thrombolysis box'. Tables 12.15 and 12.16 outline advice on the management of suspected intracranial or extracranial haemorrhage.

Table 12.15 Advice on management of suspected intracranial bleeding in patients treated with rt-PA.

Suspect intracranial bleeding if
Neurological deterioration
New headache
Fall in conscious level
Acute hypertension
Seizure
Nausea or vomiting
Initial actions
Stop infusion of rt-PA
Arrange an urgent CT scan
Check fibrinogen, PT, APTT, full blood count and send blood for 'group and save'
Support circulation with i.v. fluids if needed
If the scan shows intracranial bleeding
If scan shows extradural or subdural bleeding or hydrocephalus, consider surgical decompression after reversal of any haemostatic defcit
If scan shows only subarachnoid bleeding, consider CT or MR angiography to exclude underlying aneurysm
If the scan shows no intracranial bleeding
If no intracranial bleeding on CT or MR, consider other causes of deterioration
If the patient has a neurological deficit consistent with a spinal location, sparing the face, especially if there is acute neck or back pain, consider MR scan of spine to exclude epidural haematoma

The manufacturers of rt-PA suggest that most patients with severe bleeding can be managed with volume replacement.[245] It is rarely necessary to replace the clotting factors because of the short half-life of the drug and the minimal effect on the systemic coagulation factors. In those who fail to respond, transfusion of cryoprecipitate, fresh frozen plasma and platelets should be considered; the British Society of Haematology guidelines for the use of thrombolysis suggest for severe life-threatening bleeding after rt-PA, that has not responded to initial measures, giving a fibrinolytic inhibitor such as aprotinin or tranexamic acid and replacement of clotting factors depending on the results of a coagulation screen (see also Table 12.16).[318]

Table 12.16 Advice on management of suspected extracranial bleeding in patients treated with rt-PA.

Suspect extracranial bleeding if
Drop in blood pressure
Clinical shock
Evidence of blood loss, e.g. melaena, haematuria
Initial actions
Stop infusion of rt-PA
Use mechanical compression, if possible, to control
    bleeding
Check fibrinogen, PT, APTT, full blood count and send
    blood for 'group and save' or cross-match depending
    on situation
Support circulation with fluids and blood transfusion as
    appropriate
Discuss results with local haematology department
*For severe life-threatening bleeding not responding to fluid
replacement*
Consider giving a fibrinolytic inhibitor (depending on the
    results of a coagulation screen), either:
    500 000 kallikrein inactivator units of aprotinin i.v. over
        10 min followed by 200 000 units over 4 h *or*
    tranexamic acid i.v. 1 g over 15 min repeated every
        8 h as necessary *or*
    fresh frozen plasma *and/or* cryoprecipitate
Delay any surgery until haemostatic deficit corrected

The manufacturers of rt-PA suggest that most patients with severe bleeding can be managed with volume replacement.[245] It is rarely necessary to replace the clotting factors because of the short half-life of the drug and the minimal effect on the systemic coagulation factors. In those who fail to respond, transfusion of cryoprecipitate, fresh frozen plasma and platelets should be considered; the British Society of Haematology guidelines for the use of thrombolysis suggest for severe life-threatening bleeding after rt-PA, that has not responded to initial measures, giving a fibrinolytic inhibitor such as aprotinin or tranexamic acid and replacement of clotting factors depending on the results of a coagulation screen.[318]
[a]The options listed are based on expert opinion and not on reliable RCT evidence; it is prudent to discuss the options with your local haematologist.

If a patient develops intracranial bleeding, early guidelines suggested consideration of surgical evacuation of any intracranial clot.[235] This may not be wise because the STICH trial and a systematic review have not been able to demonstrate net benefit from evacuation of intracerebral haematoma.[269,270] However, if the patient has subdural or extradural bleeding but no major intracerebral haematoma, surgical drainage may be indicated. Surgery for any type of intracranial haemorrhage should be delayed until the haemostatic deficit is fully reversed.

Tissue plasminogen activator can cause anaphylactoid reactions which may require prompt supportive treatment: adrenaline (0.5–1 mL 1 in 1000 i.m. or s.c., but *not* i.v.) – the dose depends on the severity of the reaction, and it may be necessary to repeat the dose; hydrocortisone 200 mg i.v.; chlorpheniramine 10 mg i.v.; salbutamol nebulizer 5 mg; and fluid resuscitation if shocked. It is important to be aware of an uncommon anaphylactoid reaction, orolingual angioneurotic oedema, which occurs in about 2–5% of patients treated with rt-PA, and is more likely if the patient is on an ACE inhibitor.[271,272] It can become life-threatening if the rapid tongue swelling causes upper airway obstruction, which may then require endotracheal intubation.[272]

12.6 Unproven value: other reperfusion strategies

12.6.1 Gp IIb/IIIa inhibitors

Rationale

The platelet glycoprotein (Gp) IIb/IIIa receptor is the final common pathway of platelet aggregation. Agents which block this receptor have antithrombotic and thrombolytic actions; in patients undergoing primary coronary stenting for the treatment of acute myocardial infarction, the Gp IIb/IIIa inhibitor abciximab improved coronary patency before stenting, the success of the stenting procedure, coronary patency at 6 months, left ventricular function and clinical outcomes.[273] A meta-analysis showed that, in patients with acute myocardial infarction, adjunctive abciximab significantly reduced 30-day and long-term mortality in patients treated with primary angioplasty but not in those receiving fibrinolysis.[274] Abciximab and a number of other similar agents are therefore now being tested in acute ischaemic stroke.

Evidence

Abciximab is the agent of this class that has been most widely tested as a treatment for acute ischaemic stroke. A 400-patient phase II study showed promising results,[275] so an 1800 patient efficacy RCT was initiated (AbESTT-2), but it was halted prematurely after 808 patients had been enrolled, because of an unfavourable risk : benefit ratio (largely a higher than anticipated risk of intracranial haemorrhage).[276] In the light of the AbESTT-2 trial results, abciximab is unlikely to become an established treatment for acute stroke.[276] The evidence for the use of tirofiban in acute stroke is more limited.[277] Two Gp IIb/IIIa inhibitors, eptifibatide and tirofiban, are still being evaluated, either alone, or in combination with thrombolytic agents, in ongoing small-scale RCTs, and it is possible that one of these will prove effective in acute stroke.

There are a large number of uncontrolled case series of intra-arterial Gp IIb/IIIa inhibitors (most relating to abciximab or tirofiban) for 'rescue' treatment for the cerebral embolic complications of percutaneous coronary interventions[278] and interventional neuroradiology procedures (e.g. coiling of intracranial aneurysms,[279] carotid angioplasty and stenting[280,281]). A retrospective review of 1373 consecutive patients who underwent neuroendovascular procedures identified 29 (2%) where the procedure was complicated by acute cerebral thromboembolic events and were then treated with abciximab.[282] Angiographic improvement was achieved in 29 (81%) of 36 arteries. Three intracerebral haemorrhages (10%) occurred with abciximab when administered with concurrent mechanical clot disruption; in two of these haemorrhages, recombinant tissue plasminogen activator was also administered.[282] A non-randomized study comparing abciximab with emboli prevention devices suggested the use of emboli prevention devices may be safer.[281]

12.6.2 Defibrinogenation

Rationale

There are several defibrinogenating agents. The most widely tested is ancrod, a serine protease derived from the venom of the Malayan pit viper. It causes a fall in the levels of plasma fibrinogen, plasminogen, plasminogen activator inhibitor and antiplasmin.[283] Large quantities of circulating fibrinogen and fibrin degradation products are generated and tissue plasminogen activator is released from the vascular endothelium. Ancrod also reduces plasma and whole-blood viscosity.[283] Defibrinogenation might therefore improve perfusion in the ischaemic brain and so have a net beneficial effect, provided it is not associated with a substantial excess of major bleeding.

Evidence

A Cochrane systematic review of defibrinogenating agents in acute ischaemic stroke included five trials involving 2926 patients.[284] Four trials tested ancrod and one trial defibrase. The reviewers concluded that, although fibrinogen-depleting agents appeared promising, the data from the ESTAT trial were needed before

more reliable conclusions could be drawn.[284] The ESTAT trial has recently been published. It was a randomized placebo-controlled trial of ancrod which included 1222 patients with an acute ischaemic stroke. The primary outcome was functional success at 3 months (survival, Barthel Index of 95 or 100, or return to prestroke level). Functional success at 3 months did not differ between patients given ancrod (42%) and those given placebo (42%) ($P = 0.94$; OR 0.99, 95% CI 0.76–1.29).[285]

Conclusion

At present, there is not enough evidence to justify the use of defibrinogenating agents in routine clinical practice.

12.6.3 Interventional neuroradiology and ultrasound augmentation of clot lysis

Rationale

For patients with acute ST-segment elevation myocardial infarction (AMI), primary percutaneous transluminal coronary angioplasty (PTCA) is often used as the primary revascularization method in preference to intravenous thrombolytic therapy. A systematic review of the trials comparing PTCA with thrombolysis in AMI, involving 7739 patients, found that primary PTCA was significantly better than thrombolytic therapy at reducing early death, non-fatal reinfarction, stroke, and the combined outcome cluster of death, non-fatal reinfarction and stroke.[286] The advantage to primary PTCA-allocated patients persisted during long-term follow-up, and was independent of both the type of thrombolytic agent used, and whether or not the patient was transferred for primary PTCA.[286]

In centres that regularly perform neuro-interventional procedures in acute ischaemic stroke, if intravenous or intra-arterial thrombolytic drug therapy does not reopen the occluded artery, a number of techniques can now be tried to restore flow, including: direct mechanical balloon angioplasty of the thrombus; mechanical removal of clot; intravascular stenting of the underlying occlusive atherosclerotic lesion; suction thrombectomy; and laser-assisted thrombolysis of emboli.[167,231] Transcranial Doppler ultrasound (with or without supplementary microbubble injection) on its own, or as an adjunct to thrombolytic therapy, may also improve clot lysis.[231,287]

Evidence

The process for approval of the use of devices and procedures for acute stroke treatment is controversial because devices are not subject to the same stringent approval processes as drugs (i.e. there is no requirement for phase III efficacy trials).[288] In acute ischaemic stroke, case series have reported the use of mechanical clot disruption,[289] and the use of the MERCI clot retrieval device.[290] The FDA has approved the MERCI device for the removal of clot from brain arteries on the basis of a non-randomized study,[290] (though not as treatment for acute ischaemic stroke), a decision regarded by some as premature.[288,291] The device is, however, being tested in the MR-RESCUE trial.[292] Future studies will need to evaluate the overall efficacy when compared with intra-arterial or intravenous treatment, overall safety and the major complication rate (e.g. vessel rupture).[288,289,293]

The CLOTBUST RCT has shown that, in patients presenting within 3 h of acute ischaemic stroke onset who were treated with intravenous rt-PA, 2 h of continuous transcranial Doppler ultrasound increased the frequency of cerebral arterial recanalization and this was associated with a trend to better clinical outcomes.[294] Another phase II ultrasound trial, TRUMBI, is ongoing,[287] and CLOTBUST-2, evaluating microbubble-augmented sono-thrombolysis is planned.[231]

Conclusion

Further RCTs of interventional radiology (preferably on a cardiological scale) will be needed to assess its place in routine clinical practice.[288,291,293] As with intra-arterial thrombolysis, the number of centres able to deliver such highly specialized treatments will need to increase dramatically for such trials to become feasible, and enormous investment would be required to minimize the average time to treatment. Ultrasound augmentation of thrombolysis is simpler, and potentially more widely applicable.

12.7 Unproven value: treatment of cerebral oedema and raised intracranial pressure

12.7.1 Corticosteroids

Rationale

Vasogenic cerebral oedema, which tends to develop about 24–48 h or more after stroke onset, particularly in and around large infarcts, may be reduced by corticosteroids (such as dexamethasone) (section 12.1.5). Cytotoxic oedema, that develops almost immediately after the onset of ischaemia, might be reduced by neuroprotective agents which can prevent influx of sodium ions and water into cells (section 12.1.5).

Evidence

There have been at least 17 apparently randomized trials in acute stroke, but unfortunately only seven (involving 453 people) were of sufficient quality to merit inclusion in a Cochrane systematic review.[295] There was no significant difference in the odds of death within 1 year (odds ratio 1.08; 95% CI 0.68–1.72). And nor did treatment appear to improve functional outcome in survivors. The results were inconsistent between individual trials.

Conclusion

These data do not support the routine or selective use of corticosteroids in acute ischaemic stroke. We do not use corticosteroids as a routine treatment for unselected patients with ischaemic stroke, nor do we use them in patients who have massive cerebral oedema complicated by transtentorial herniation. Our only indication is in patients with inflammatory vascular disorders (e.g. giant-cell arteritis, polyarteritis nodosa, systemic lupus erythematosus; section 7.3).

12.7.2 Glycerol and mannitol

Rationale

A 10% solution of glycerol is a hyperosmolar agent which is said to reduce cerebral oedema and possibly increase cerebral blood flow, and mannitol is another osmotically active agent. These treatments aim to reduce intracranial pressure by reducing infarct-related oedema and thereby improve perfusion in and around infarcts.

Evidence

A Cochrane systematic review included 11 randomized trials comparing intravenous glycerol with control (482 glycerol treated patients were compared with 463 control patients).[296] Glycerol was associated with a significant reduction in the odds of death during the scheduled treatment period (OR 0.65; 95% CI 0.44–0.97). However, at the end of the scheduled follow-up period, there was no significant difference in the odds of death (OR 0.98; 95% CI 0.73–1.31). Functional outcome was reported in only two studies and there were non-significantly more patients who had a good outcome at the end of scheduled follow-up in the glycerol group (OR 0.73; 95% CI

0.37–1.42). Haemolysis seemed to be the only relevant adverse effect of glycerol treatment.

A Cochrane systematic review of mannitol in stroke included three small trials with 226 randomized patients. Neither beneficial nor harmful effects of mannitol could be proved.[297] The number of included patients was small, and the follow-up was short. Case fatality, the proportion of dependent patients, and adverse effects were not reported. A similar Cochrane review of mannitol in traumatic head injury found no evidence of benefit in patients with raised intracranial pressure who did not have an operable intracranial haematoma.[298]

Conclusion

These data do not support the routine or selective use of glycerol or mannitol in acute ischaemic stroke, and so we generally do not use them in our own clinical practice (though our colleagues in intensive care may use mannitol in some of our patients with severe elevations of intracranial pressure after ischaemic stroke).

12.7.3 Surgical decompression

Posterior fossa decompression or shunting for massive cerebellar infarcts

Surgical decompression (or ventricular shunting) of massive cerebellar infarcts may improve cerebral perfusion, relieve any obstructive hydrocephalus and so prevent early death. Decompressive surgery has not been evaluated by adequately designed trials, so it is still controversial as to which patients with cerebellar infarction should have decompressive surgery, shunting or medical therapy.

Hemicraniotomy for massive supratentorial infarcts

Decompressive surgical techniques that attempt to relieve high intracranial pressure due to oedema have been described,[299] but their efficacy in reducing case fatality and disability has, until recently, been very uncertain. A Cochrane systematic review did not identify any completed RCTs, five observational studies and some small series and single case reports, so no clear conclusions could be drawn.[300] At least five RCTs have since been initiated: HAMLET, HEADDFIRST, DESTINY, HEMMI and DECIMAL, of which three (HEADDFIRST,[301] DESTINY[302] and DECIMAL[303]) have been completed (recruitment into HAMLET continues). A prospectively pooled analysis of individual data for patients aged between 18 years and 60 years, with space-occupying MCA infarction,

included in DESTINY,[302] DECIMAL[303] and HAMLET[304] and treated within 48 h after stroke onset were pooled for analysis.[321] The protocol for these analyses was designed prospectively when the trials were still recruiting patients and outcomes were defined without knowledge of the results of the individual trials. The primary outcome measure was the score on the modified Rankin scale (mRS) at 1 year dichotomized between favourable (0–4) and unfavourable (5 and death) outcome. A total of 93 patients were included in the pooled analysis. More patients in the decompressive surgery group than in the control group had an mRS ≤ 4 (75% vs 24%; pooled absolute risk reduction 51% [95% CI 34–69]), an mRS ≤ 3 (43% vs 21%; 23% [95% CI 5–41]), and survived (78% vs 29%; 50% [95% CI 33–67]), indicating number-needed-to-treat of two for survival with mRS ≤ 4, four for survival with mRS ≤ 3, and two for survival irrespective of functional outcome. The effect of surgery was highly consistent across the three trials. The authors concluded 'In patients with malignant MCA infarction, decompressive surgery undertaken within 48 h of stroke onset reduces mortality and increases the number of patients with a favourable functional outcome. The decision to perform decompressive surgery should, however, be made on an individual basis in every patient.[321]

Conclusion: decompressive surgery

Even with these results, the decision about whether and when to consider decompressive surgery therefore remains very difficult; leave it too late and you 'miss the boat' and irreversible damage occurs. Operate too soon, and one risks worsening the ischaemic brain insult. We do occasionally refer younger patients with no comorbidity and a 'malignant' course for surgery, and hope to recruit patients in the HAMLET trial.

12.7.4 Hyperventilation

Hyperventilation is used to lower intracranial pressure, but there is no randomized evidence on its effects in patients with stroke available on the Cochrane Controlled Trials Register. A Cochrane review of hyperventilation in severe head injury concluded the data available were inadequate to assess any potential benefit or harm that might result from hyperventilation.[305] We therefore would not recommend hyperventilation to reduce raised intracranial pressure, though we accept that our colleagues in intensive care may sometimes administer hyperventilation to some of our patients with severe elevations of intracranial pressure after ischaemic stroke.

12.8 Unproven value: other interventions

12.8.1 Neuroprotective agents

Rationale

There are many – perhaps too many – points in the patho-physiological cascade between vessel occlusion and irreversible cell death where pharmacological intervention might be beneficial (sections 12.1.3 and 12.1.4), and the pharmaceutical industry has worked through a very large number of compounds for clinical development and testing. There is no generally agreed definition of a neuroprotective drug, but in the context of acute ischaemic stroke, the aim of this class of agents is to limit the volume of brain damaged by ischaemia. There are a number of steps to be taken between first identifying a promising agent during preclinical testing in animals and man before any large-scale clinical trials are mounted.[306,307] And systematic reviews of the available animal data offer the prospect of reducing bias in the assessment of preclinical data.[308–311] Greater attention to achieving these milestones might increase the chances of a successful clinical development and licensing of a neuroprotective drug than hitherto.

Many trials have been completed, but no neuro-protective drug has been licensed for clinical use. The ever-increasing number of compounds withdrawn from clinical development in recent years has been a disappointment. This has certainly tempered the opinions of even the diehard optimists who said, just a few years back, that the neuroprotective drugs would make stroke rehabilitation units redundant. It appeared in early 2006 that an effective agent had been found, when the SAINT-I trial of the agent NXY-059 in 1700 patients with an acute ischaemic stroke showed a significant reduction in post-stroke disabilities (modified Rankin Scale) among patients treated with the study drug ($P = 0.038$).[312] Though the full results of a second phase III trial, SAINT-2, are awaited, a press release in October 2006 stated that 'the SAINT-2 trial did not demonstrate a statistically significant reduction on the primary endpoint of stroke-related disability in patients treated with NXY-059, as assessed versus placebo using the modified Rankin Scale (mRS) ($P = 0.33$, odds ratio 0.94).'[313] These disappointing results led the company to discontinue clinical development of the compound.

Despite these unpromising results, the situation may change, and it is conceivable that one of the neuro-protective compounds currently undergoing trials may gain a licence for use in acute ischaemic stroke in the next few years.

> It is probable that the extremely large reductions in cerebral infarct volumes achieved with neuroprotective agents in experimental animal models will translate into only moderate reductions, if any, in disability when used in humans; neuroprotective therapy is unlikely to prove a panacea for acute stroke.

12.8.2 Haemodilution

Rationale

Haemodilution aims to reduce whole-blood viscosity by an amount that increases cerebral blood flow yet does not reduce cerebral oxygen delivery. The hypothesis is that this should reduce ischaemic damage in and around the infarct. Haemodilution is generally performed by giving an infusion of dextran, hydroxyethyl starch or albumin. Such infusions increase blood volume (hyper-volaemic haemodilution). In patients with acute stroke in whom an increase in total blood volume may be undesirable, haemodilution can be achieved isovolaemic-ally by simultaneously removing several hundred milli-litres of blood. If the optimum haematocrit is achieved, any increase in cerebral oxygen delivery achieved in practice might be neuroprotective and so lessen infarct volume.

Evidence

A Cochrane systematic review of haemodilution started within 72 h of stroke onset included 18 trials (including 2766 patients). Haemodilution did not significantly reduce deaths within the first 4 weeks (OR 1.09; 95% CI 0.86–1.38). Similarly, haemodilution did not influence deaths within 3–6 months (OR 1.01; 95% CI 0.84–1.22), or death and dependency or institutionalization (OR 0.98; 95% CI 0.84–1.15). No statistically significant benefits were documented for any particular type of haemodiluting agent. The overall results of this review were compatible both with modest benefit and moderate harm of haemodilution for acute ischaemic stroke, but it has not been proven to improve survival or functional outcome.[314]

Conclusion

Given this information, we can see no reason to use this treatment in routine clinical practice, although it is used quite widely in Austria and in some parts of Eastern Europe.

12.8.3 Calcium antagonists

Rationale

The influx of calcium through voltage-sensitive channels has a role in neuronal death from ischaemia; this influx can be inhibited by a number of agents, so-called calcium channel blockers or antagonists (section 12.1.4).

Evidence

A systematic review included 29 RCTs (7665 patients).[315] No effect of calcium antagonists on poor outcome at the end of follow-up (relative risk, 1.04; 95% CI 0.98–1.09) or on death at end of follow-up (relative risk, 1.07; 95% CI 0.98–1.17) was found. Indirect comparisons of the effects of intravenous and oral administration showed an increase in the number of patients with poor outcome with intravenous administration. Comparisons of different doses of nimodipine suggested that the highest doses were associated with poorer outcome. Administration within 12 h of onset was associated with an increase in the proportion of patients with poor outcome, but this effect was largely due to the poor results associated with intravenous administration.

Conclusion

The trials do not provide any evidence to support the routine use of oral calcium antagonists in patients presenting within 12 h, or intravenous administration. We do not routinely use calcium antagonists in acute ischaemic stroke patients.

References

1 Sharp FR, Lu A, Tang Y, Millhorn DE. Multiple molecular penumbras after focal cerebral ischemia. *J Cereb Blood Flow Metab* 2000; **20**(7):1011–32.

2 Arundine M, Tymianski M. Molecular mechanisms of calcium-dependent neurodegeneration in excitotoxicity. *Cell Calcium* 2003; **34**(4–5):325–37.

3 Baron JC. Mapping the ischaemic penumbra with PET: implications for acute stroke treatment. *Cerebrovasc Dis* 1999; **9**(4):193–201.

4 Siesjo BK. Pathophysiology and treatment of focal cerebral ischemia. Part I: Pathophysiology. *J Neurosurg* 1992; **77**(2):169–84.

5 Siesjo BK. Pathophysiology and treatment of focal cerebral ischemia. Part II: Mechanisms of damage and treatment. *J Neurosurg* 1992; **77**(3):337–54.

6 Kristian T, Siesjo BK. Calcium in ischemic cell death. *Stroke* 1998; **29**(3):705–18.

7 Pellerin L, Magistretti PJ. Neuroenergetics: calling upon astrocytes to satisfy hungry neurons. *Neuroscientist* 2004; **10**(1):53–62.

8 Magistretti PJ. Neuron-glia metabolic coupling and plasticity. *J Exp Biol* 2006; **209**(Pt 12):2304–11.

9 Bouzier-Sore AK, Voisin P, Canioni P, Magistretti PJ, Pellerin L. Lactate is a preferential oxidative energy substrate over glucose for neurons in culture. *J Cereb Blood Flow Metab* 2003; **23**(11):1298–306.

10 Leenders KL, Perani D, Lammertsma AA, Heather JD, Buckingham P, Healy MJ *et al.* Cerebral blood flow, blood volume and oxygen utilization: normal values and effect of age. *Brain* 1990; **113** (Pt 1):27–47.

11 Baron JC. Mapping the ischaemic penumbra with PET: a new approach. *Brain* 2001; **124**(Pt 1):2–4.

12 Guadagno JV, Warburton EA, Aigbirhio FI, Smielewski P, Fryer TD, Harding S *et al.* Does the acute diffusion-weighted imaging lesion represent penumbra as well as core? A combined quantitative PET/MRI voxel-based study. *J Cereb Blood Flow Metab* 2004; **24**(11):1249–54.

13 Guadagno JV, Donnan GA, Markus R, Gillard JH, Baron JC. Imaging the ischaemic penumbra. *Curr Opin Neurol* 2004; **17**(1):61–7.

14 Baron JC. Stroke research in the modern era: images versus dogmas. *Cerebrovasc Dis* 2005; **20**(3):154–63.

15 Gibbs JM, Wise RJ, Leenders KL, Jones T. Evaluation of cerebral perfusion reserve in patients with carotid-artery occlusion. *Lancet* 1984; **1**(8372):310–14.

16 Warach S, Baron JC. Neuroimaging. *Stroke* 2004; **35**(2):351–3.

17 Warach S, Wardlaw J. Advances in imaging 2005. *Stroke* 2006; **37**(2):297–8.

18 Derdeyn CP. Positron emission tomography imaging of cerebral ischemia. *Neuroimaging Clin N Am* 2005; **15**(2):341–xi.

19 Muir KW, Buchan A, von Kummer R, Rother J, Baron JC. Imaging of acute stroke. *Lancet Neurol* 2006; **5**(9):755–68.

20 Johnston AJ, Steiner LA, Balestreri M, Gupta AK, Menon DK. Hyperoxia and the cerebral hemodynamic responses to moderate hyperventilation. *Acta Anaesthesiol Scand* 2003; **47**(4):391–6.

21 Symon L, Branston NM, Strong AJ. Autoregulation in acute focal ischemia: an experimental study. *Stroke* 1976; **7**(6):547–54.

22 Eames PJ, Blake MJ, Dawson SL, Panerai RB, Potter JF. Dynamic cerebral autoregulation and beat to beat blood pressure control are impaired in acute ischaemic stroke. *J Neurol Neurosurg Psychiatry* 2002; **72**(4):467–72.

23 Dawson SL, Panerai RB, Potter JF. Serial changes in static and dynamic cerebral autoregulation after acute ischaemic stroke. *Cerebrovasc Dis* 2003; **16**(1):69–75.

24 Pulsinelli W. Pathophysiology of acute ischaemic stroke. *Lancet* 1992; **339**(8792):533–6.

25 Yam AT, Lang EW, Lagopoulos J, Yip K, Griffith J, Mudaliar Y *et al*. Cerebral autoregulation and ageing. *J Clin Neurosci* 2005; **12**(6):643–6.

26 Aaslid R, Lindegaard KF, Sorteberg W, Nornes H. Cerebral autoregulation dynamics in humans. *Stroke* 1989; **20**(1):45–52.

27 Panerai RB, Dawson SL, Eames PJ, Potter JF. Cerebral blood flow velocity response to induced and spontaneous sudden changes in arterial blood pressure. *Am J Physiol Heart Circ Physiol* 2001; **280**(5):H2162–H2174.

28 Derdeyn CP, Videen TO, Yundt KD, Fritsch SM, Carpenter DA, Grubb RL *et al*. Variability of cerebral blood volume and oxygen extraction: stages of cerebral haemodynamic impairment revisited. *Brain* 2002; **125**(Pt 3):595–607.

29 Powers WJ. Cerebral hemodynamics in ischemic cerebrovascular disease. *Ann Neurol* 1991; **29**(3):231–40.

30 Schellinger PD, Latour LL, Wu CS, Chalela JA, Warach S. The association between neurological deficit in acute ischemic stroke and mean transit time: comparison of four different perfusion MRI algorithms. *Neuroradiology* 2006; **48**(2):69–77.

31 Muir KW, Santosh C. Imaging of acute stroke and transient ischaemic attack. *J Neurol Neurosurg Psychiatry* 2005; **76** Suppl 3:iii19–iii28.

32 Pindzola RR, Balzer JR, Nemoto EM, Goldstein S, Yonas H. Cerebrovascular reserve in patients with carotid occlusive disease assessed by stable xenon-enhanced CT cerebral blood flow and transcranial Doppler. *Stroke* 2001; **32**(8):1811–17.

33 Mahagne MH, David O, Darcourt J, Migneco O, Dunac A, Chatel M *et al*. Voxel-based mapping of cortical ischemic damage using Tc 99 m L,L-ethyl cysteinate dimer SPECT in acute stroke. *J Neuroimaging* 2004; **14**(1):23–32.

34 Murphy BD, Fox AJ, Lee DH, Sahlas DJ, Black SE, Hogan MJ *et al*. Identification of penumbra and infarct in acute ischemic stroke using computed tomography perfusion-derived blood flow and blood volume measurements. *Stroke* 2006; **37**(7):1771–7.

35 Koroshetz WJ, Lev MH. Contrast computed tomography scan in acute stroke: 'You can't always get what you want but . . . you get what you need'. *Ann Neurol* 2002; **51**(4):415–16.

36 Eastwood JD, Alexander MJ, Petrella JR, Provenzale JM. Dynamic CT perfusion imaging with acetazolamide challenge for the preprocedural evaluation of a patient with symptomatic middle cerebral artery occlusive disease. *Am J Neuroradiol* 2002; **23**(2):285–7.

37 Hellier KD, Hampton JL, Guadagno JV, Higgins NP, Antoun NM, Day DJ *et al*. Perfusion CT helps decision making for thrombolysis when there is no clear time of onset. *J Neurol Neurosurg Psychiatry* 2006; **77**(3):417–19.

38 Ziyeh S, Rick J, Reinhard M, Hetzel A, Mader I, Speck O. Blood oxygen level-dependent MRI of cerebral CO_2 reactivity in severe carotid stenosis and occlusion. *Stroke* 2005; **36**(4):751–6.

39 Geisler BS, Brandhoff F, Fiehler J, Saager C, Speck O, Rother J *et al*. Blood-oxygen-level-dependent MRI allows metabolic description of tissue at risk in acute stroke patients. *Stroke* 2006; **37**(7):1778–84.

40 Roc AC, Wang J, Ances BM, Liebeskind DS, Kasner SE, Detre JA. Altered hemodynamics and regional cerebral blood flow in patients with hemodynamically significant stenoses. *Stroke* 2006; **37**(2):382–7.

41 Markus HS. Transcranial Doppler ultrasound. *J Neurol Neurosurg Psychiatry* 1999; **67**(2):135–7.

42 Derdeyn CP. Is the acetazolamide test valid for quantitative assessment of maximal cerebral autoregulatory vasodilation? *Stroke* 2000; **31**(9):2271–2.

43 Yamauchi H, Kudoh T, Sugimoto K, Takahashi M, Kishibe Y, Okazawa H. Pattern of collaterals, type of infarcts, and haemodynamic impairment in carotid artery occlusion. *J Neurol Neurosurg Psychiatry* 2004; **75**(12):1697–701.

44 Markus H, Cullinane M. Severely impaired cerebrovascular reactivity predicts stroke and TIA risk in patients with carotid artery stenosis and occlusion. *Brain* 2001; **124**(Pt 3):457–67.

45 Baron JC. Using PET to identify carotid occlusion patients at high risk of subsequent stroke: further insights. *J Neurol Neurosurg Psychiatry* 2004; **75**(12):1659–60.

46 Derdeyn CP, Grubb RL, Jr., Powers WJ. PET screening of carotid occlusion. *Adm Radiol J* 2001;**20**(1):20–5.

47 Derdeyn CP, Gage BF, Grubb RL, Jr., Powers WJ. Cost-effectiveness analysis of therapy for symptomatic carotid occlusion: PET screening before selective extracranial-to-intracranial bypass versus medical treatment. *J Nucl Med* 2000; **41**(5):800–7.

48 Htun P, Fateh-Moghadam S, Tomandl B, Handschu R, Klinger K, Stellos K *et al*. Course of platelet activation and platelet-leukocyte interaction in cerebrovascular ischemia. *Stroke* 2006; **37**(9):2283–7.

49 Warach S. Tissue viability thresholds in acute stroke: the 4-factor model. *Stroke* 2001; **32**(11):2460–1.

50 Heiss WD, Rosner G. Functional recovery of cortical neurons as related to degree and duration of ischemia. *Ann Neurol* 1983; **14**(3):294–301.

51 Marchal G, Beaudouin V, Rioux P, de la Sayette V, Le Doze F, Viader F *et al*. Prolonged persistence of substantial volumes of potentially viable brain tissue after stroke: a correlative PET-CT study with voxel-based data analysis. *Stroke* 1996; **27**(4):599–606.

52 Hacke W, Albers G, Al Rawi Y, Bogousslavsky J, Davalos A, Eliasziw M *et al*. The Desmoteplase in Acute Ischemic Stroke Trial (DIAS): a phase II MRI-Based 9-hour window acute stroke thrombolysis trial with intravenous desmoteplase. *Stroke* 2005; **36**:66–73.

53 Furlan AJ, Eyding D, Albers GW, Al-Rawi Y, Lees KR, Rowley HA *et al*. Dose Escalation of Desmoteplase for Acute Ischemic Stroke (DEDAS): evidence of safety and efficacy 3 to 9 hours after stroke onset. *Stroke* 2006; **37**(5):1227–31.

54 Fibrinolytic Therapy Trialists' (FTT) Collaborative Group. Indications for fibrinolytic therapy in suspected acute myocardial infarction: collaborative overview of early mortality and major morbidity results from all randomised trials of more than 1000 patients. *Lancet* 1994; **343**:311–22.

55 Baron JC. How healthy is the acutely reperfused ischemic penumbra? *Cerebrovasc Dis* 2005; **20** (Suppl 2):25–31.

56 Ginsberg MD. Adventures in the pathophysiology of brain ischemia: penumbra, gene expression, neuroprotection: the 2002 Thomas Willis Lecture. *Stroke* 2003; **34**(1):214–23.

57 Markus R, Reutens DC, Kazui S, Read S, Wright P, Pearce DC *et al.* Hypoxic tissue in ischaemic stroke: persistence and clinical consequences of spontaneous survival. *Brain* 2004; **127**(Pt 6):1427–36.

58 Baron JC, Warach S. Imaging. *Stroke* 2005; **36**(2):196–9.

59 Heiss WD. Best measure of ischemic penumbra: positron emission tomography. *Stroke* 2003; **34**(10):2534–5.

60 Heiss WD, Kracht LW, Thiel A, Grond M, Pawlik G. Penumbral probability thresholds of cortical flumazenil binding and blood flow predicting tissue outcome in patients with cerebral ischaemia. *Brain* 2001; **124**(Pt 1):20–9.

61 Latchaw RE, Yonas H, Hunter GJ, Yuh WT, Ueda T, Sorensen AG *et al.* Guidelines and recommendations for perfusion imaging in cerebral ischemia: a scientific statement for healthcare professionals by the writing group on perfusion imaging, from the Council on Cardiovascular Radiology of the American Heart Association. *Stroke* 2003; **34**(4):1084–104.

62 Warach S. Measurement of the ischemic penumbra with MRI: it's about time. *Stroke* 2003; **34**(10):2533–4.

63 Sobesky J, Zaro WO, Lehnhardt FG, Hesselmann V, Neveling M, Jacobs A *et al.* Does the mismatch match the penumbra? Magnetic resonance imaging and positron emission tomography in early ischemic stroke. *Stroke* 2005; **36**(5):980–5.

64 Guadagno JV, Jones PS, Fryer TD, Barret O, Aigbirhio FI, Carpenter TA *et al.* Local relationships between restricted water diffusion and oxygen consumption in the ischemic human brain. *Stroke* 2006; **37**(7):1741–8.

65 Rivers CS, Wardlaw JM. What has diffusion imaging in animals told us about diffusion imaging in patients with ischaemic stroke? *Cerebrovasc Dis* 2005; **19**(5):328–36.

66 Hjort N, Christensen S, Solling C, Ashkanian M, Wu O, Rohl L *et al.* Ischemic injury detected by diffusion imaging 11 minutes after stroke. *Ann Neurol* 2005; **58**(3):462–5.

67 Rivers CS, Wardlaw JM, Armitage PA, Bastin ME, Carpenter TK, Cvoro V *et al.* Do acute diffusion- and perfusion-weighted MRI lesions identify final infarct volume in ischemic stroke? *Stroke* 2006; **37**(1):98–104.

68 Shih LC, Saver JL, Alger JR, Starkman S, Leary MC, Vinuela F *et al.* Perfusion-weighted magnetic resonance imaging thresholds identifying core, irreversibly infarcted tissue. *Stroke* 2003; **34**(6):1425–30.

69 Wardlaw JM, Farrall AJ. Diagnosis of stroke on neuroimaging. *Br Med J* 2004; **328**(7441):655–6.

70 Coutts SB, Simon JE, Tomanek AI, Barber PA, Chan J, Hudon ME *et al.* Reliability of assessing percentage of diffusion-perfusion mismatch. *Stroke* 2003; **34**(7):1681–3.

71 Kidwell CS, Alger JR, Saver JL. Beyond mismatch: evolving paradigms in imaging the ischemic penumbra with multimodal magnetic resonance imaging. *Stroke* 2003; **34**(11):2729–35.

72 Butcher KS, Parsons M, MacGregor L, Barber PA, Chalk J, Bladin C *et al.* Refining the perfusion-diffusion mismatch hypothesis. *Stroke* 2005; **36**(6):1153–9.

73 Kucinski T, Naumann D, Knab R, Schoder V, Wegener S, Fiehler J *et al.* Tissue at risk is overestimated in perfusion-weighted imaging: MR imaging in acute stroke patients without vessel recanalization. *Am J Neuroradiol* 2005; **26**(4):815–19.

74 Coutts SB, Hill MD, Hu WY. Hyperperfusion syndrome: toward a stricter definition. *Neurosurgery* 2003; **53**(5):1053–8.

75 Bright R, Raval AP, Dembner JM, Perez-Pinzon MA, Steinberg GK, Yenari MA *et al.* Protein kinase C delta mediates cerebral reperfusion injury in vivo. *J Neurosci* 2004; **24**(31):6880–8.

76 Price CJ, Warburton EA, Menon DK. Human cellular inflammation in the pathology of acute cerebral ischaemia. *J Neurol Neurosurg Psychiatry* 2003; **74**(11):1476–84.

77 Lo EH, Dalkara T, Moskowitz MA. Mechanisms, challenges and opportunities in stroke. *Nat Rev Neurosci* 2003; **4**(5):399–415.

78 Lipton P. Ischemic cell death in brain neurons. *Physiol Rev* 1999; **79**(4):1431–568.

79 Graham SH, Chen J. Programmed cell death in cerebral ischemia. *J Cereb Blood Flow Metab* 2001; **21**(2):99–109.

80 Chan PH. Reactive oxygen radicals in signaling and damage in the ischemic brain. *J Cereb Blood Flow Metab* 2001; **21**(1):2–14.

81 Lo EH, Moskowitz MA, Jacobs TP. Exciting, radical, suicidal: how brain cells die after stroke. *Stroke* 2005; **36**(2):189–92.

82 Moskowitz MA, Lo EH. Neurogenesis and apoptotic cell death. *Stroke* 2003; **34**(2):324–6.

83 Bergersen LH, Magistretti PJ, Pellerin L. Selective postsynaptic co-localization of MCT2 with AMPA receptor GluR2/3 subunits at excitatory synapses exhibiting AMPA receptor trafficking. *Cereb Cortex* 2005; **15**(4):361–70.

84 Lizasoain I, Cardenas A, Hurtado O, Romera C, Mallolas J, Lorenzo P *et al.* Targets of cytoprotection in acute ischemic stroke: present and future. *Cerebrovasc Dis* 2006; **21** (Suppl 2):1–8.

85 Bernardinelli Y, Magistretti PJ, Chatton JY. Astrocytes generate Na$^+$-mediated metabolic waves. *Proc Natl Acad Sci USA* 2004; **101**(41):14937–42.

86 Aarts MM, Arundine M, Tymianski M. Novel concepts in excitotoxic neurodegeneration after stroke. *Expert Rev Mol Med* 2003; **2003**:1–22.

87 Chu CT, Levinthal DJ, Kulich SM, Chalovich EM, DeFranco DB. Oxidative neuronal injury. The dark side of ERK1/2. *Eur J Biochem* 2004; **271**(11):2060–6.

88 Lipton SA, Bossy-Wetzel E. Dueling activities of AIF in cell death versus survival: DNA binding and redox activity. *Cell* 2002; **111**(2):147–50.

89 Okuno S, Saito A, Hayashi T, Chan PH. The c-Jun N-terminal protein kinase signaling pathway mediates Bax activation and subsequent neuronal apoptosis through

interaction with Bim after transient focal cerebral ischemia. *J Neurosci* 2004; **24**(36):7879–87.

90 Driscoll M, Gerstbrein B. Dying for a cause: invertebrate genetics takes on human neurodegeneration. *Nat Rev Genet* 2003; **4**(3):181–94.

91 Xiong ZG, Zhu XM, Chu XP, Minami M, Hey J, Wei WL *et al.* Neuroprotection in ischemia: blocking calcium-permeable acid-sensing ion channels. *Cell* 2004; **118**(6):687–98.

92 Gursoy-Ozdemir Y, Qiu J, Matsuoka N, Bolay H, Bermpohl D, Jin H *et al.* Cortical spreading depression activates and upregulates MMP-9. *J Clin Invest* 2004; **113**(10):1447–55.

93 Otori T, Greenberg JH, Welsh FA. Cortical spreading depression causes a long-lasting decrease in cerebral blood flow and induces tolerance to permanent focal ischemia in rat brain. *J Cereb Blood Flow Metab* 2003; **23**(1):43–50.

94 Zhao BQ, Wang S, Kim HY, Storrie H, Rosen BR, Mooney DJ *et al.* Role of matrix metalloproteinases in delayed cortical responses after stroke. *Nat Med* 2006; **12**(4):441–5.

95 Zlokovic BV. Remodeling after stroke. *Nat Med* 2006; **12**(4):390–1.

96 Perera MN, Ma HK, Arakawa S, Howells DW, Markus RM, Rowe CC *et al.* Inflammation following stroke. *J Clin Neurosci* 2006; **13**:1–8.

97 Dirnagl U, Iadecola C, Moskowitz MA. Pathobiology of ischaemic stroke: an integrated view. *Trends Neurosci* 1999; **22**(9):391–7.

98 Del Zoppo GJ, Ginis I, Hallenbeck JM, Iadecola C, Wang X, Feuerstein GZ. Inflammation and stroke: putative role for cytokines, adhesion molecules and iNOS in brain response to ischemia. *Brain Pathol* 2000; **10**(1):95–112.

99 Feuerstein GZ, Wang X, Barone FC. Inflammatory gene expression in cerebral ischemia and trauma: potential new therapeutic targets. *Ann N Y Acad Sci* 1997; **825**:179–93.

100 O'Collins VE, Macleod MR, Donnan GA, Horky LL, van der Worp BH, Howells DW. 1026 experimental treatments in acute stroke. *Ann Neurol* 2006; **59**(3):467–77.

101 Wahlgren NG, Ahmed N. Neuroprotection in cerebral ischaemia: facts and fancies: the need for new approaches. *Cerebrovasc Dis* 2004; **17** (Suppl 1):153–66.

102 Fagan SC, Hess DC, Machado LS, Hohnadel EJ, Pollock DM, Ergul A. Tactics for vascular protection after acute ischemic stroke. *Pharmacotherapy* 2005; **25**(3):387–95.

103 Hurtado O, Pradillo JM, Alonso-Escolano D, Lorenzo P, Sobrino T, Castillo J *et al.* Neurorepair versus neuroprotection in stroke. *Cerebrovasc Dis* 2006; **21** (Suppl 2):54–63.

104 Singhal AB, Lo EH, Dalkara T, Moskowitz MA. Advances in stroke neuroprotection: hyperoxia and beyond. *Neuroimaging Clin N Am* 2005; **15**(3):697–xiii.

105 Falcao AL, Reutens DC, Markus R, Koga M, Read SJ, Tochon-Danguy H *et al.* The resistance to ischemia of white and gray matter after stroke. *Ann Neurol* 2004; **56**(5):695–701.

106 Stamatovic SM, Dimitrijevic OB, Keep RF, Andjelkovic AV. Inflammation and brain edema: new insights into the role of chemokines and their receptors. *Acta Neurochir Suppl* 2006; **96**:444–50.

107 Pearce JM. Kernohan's notch. *Eur Neurol* 2006; **55**(4):230–2.

108 Sackett DL, Strauss S, Richardson WS, Rosenberg W, Haynes RB. *Evidence-Based Medicine: How To Practice and Teach EBM.* 2nd edn. Edinburgh: Churchill Livingstone, 2000.

109 Sackett DL, Haynes RB, Guyatt G, Tugwell P. *Clinical Epidemiology. A Basic Science for Clinical Medicine.* Toronto: Little, Brown & Co., 1991.

110 Collins R, MacMahon S. Reliable assessment of the effects of treatment on mortality and major morbidity, I: clinical trials. *Lancet* 2001; **357**(9253):373–80.

111 Medical Research Council. Streptomycin treatment of pulmonary tuberculosis. *Br Med J* 1948; **2**:769–82.

112 Yoshioka A. Use of randomisation in the Medical Research Council's clinical trial of streptomycin in pulmonary tuberculosis in the 1940s. *Br Med J* 2005; **317**:1220–3.

113 Lewis SC, Warlow CP. How to spot bias and other potential problems in randomised controlled trials. *J Neurol Neurosurg Psychiatry* 2004; **75**(2):181–7.

114 Califf RM. Simple principles of clinical trials remain powerful. *J Am Med Assoc* 2005; **293**(4):489–91.

115 Dyken M, White P. Evaluation of cortisone in the treatment of cerebral infarction. *J Am Med Assoc* 1956; **162**:1531–4.

116 Bath FJ, Owen VE, Bath PM. Quality of full and final publications reporting acute stroke trials: a systematic review. *Stroke* 1998; **29**(10):2203–10.

117 Weaver CS, Leonardi-Bee J, Bath-Hextall FJ, Bath PM. Sample size calculations in acute stroke trials: a systematic review of their reporting, characteristics, and relationship with outcome. *Stroke* 2004; **35**(5):1216–24.

118 Dorman PJ, Counsell C, Sandercock P. Reports of randomized trials in acute stroke, 1955 to 1995. What proportions were commercially sponsored? *Stroke* 1999; **30**(10):1995–8.

119 Kidwell CS, Liebeskind DS, Starkman S, Saver JL. Trends in acute ischemic stroke trials through the 20th century. *Stroke* 2001; **32**(6):1349–59.

120 Lexchin J, Bero LA, Djulbegovic B, Clark O. Pharmaceutical industry sponsorship and research outcome and quality: systematic review. *Br Med J* 2003; **326**(7400):1167–70.

121 Bekelman JE, Li Y, Gross CP. Scope and impact of financial conflicts of interest in biomedical research: a systematic review. *J Am Med Assoc* 2003; **289**(4):454–65.

122 Ioannidis JP. Effect of the statistical significance of results on the time to completion and publication of randomized efficacy trials. [see comment]. *J Am Med Assoc* 1998; **279**(4):281–6.

123 Krzyzanowska MK, Pintilie M, Tannock IF. Factors associated with failure to publish large randomized trials presented at an oncology meeting. *J Am Med Assoc* 2003; **290**(4):495–501.

124 Donnan G, Davis SM, Kaste M, International Trial Subcommittee of the International Stroke Liaison Committee ASA. Recommendations for the relationship between sponsors and investigators in the design and conduct of clinical stroke trials. *Stroke* 2003; **34**(4):1041–5.

125 Warlow C. Over-regulation of clinical research: a threat to public health. *Clin Med* 2005; **5**(1):33–8.

126 Warlow C. The Willis Lecture 2003: evaluating treatments for stroke patients too slowly: time to get out of second gear. *Stroke* 2004; **35**(9):2211–19.

127 Moher D, Schulz KF, Altman DG. The CONSORT statement: revised recommendations for improving the quality of reports of parallel-group randomised trials. *Lancet* 2001; **357**(9263):1191–4.

128 Moher D, Cook DJ, Eastwood S, Olkin I, Rennie D, Stroup DF. Improving the quality of reports of meta-analyses of randomised controlled trials: the QUOROM statement. Quality of Reporting of Meta-analyses. *Lancet* 1999; **354**(9193):1896–900.

129 Schulz KF, Grimes DA. Multiplicity in randomised trials II: subgroup and interim analyses. *Lancet* 2005; **365**(9471):1657–61.

130 Gent M, Barnett HJ, Sackett DL, Taylor DW. A randomized trial of aspirin and sulfinpyrazone in patients with threatened stroke. Results and methodologic issues. *Circulation* 1980; **62**(6 Pt 2):V97–105.

131 Antiplatelet Therapy Trialists' Collaboration. Collaborative overview of randomised trials of antiplatelet therapy. I: Prevention of death, myocardial infarction, and stroke by prolonged antiplatelet therapy in various categories of patients. Antiplatelet Trialists' Collaboration. [see comments]. [erratum appears in *Br Med J* 1994; **308**(6943):1540]. *Br Med J* 1994; **308**(6921):81–106.

132 The National Institute of Stroke and Neurological Disorders rt-PA Stroke Study Group. Tissue plasminogen activator for acute ischemic stroke. *N Engl J Med* 1995; **333**(24):1581–7.

133 Wardlaw JM, Zoppo G, Yamaguchi T, Berge E. Thrombolysis for acute ischaemic stroke. [update of *Cochrane Database Syst Rev* 2000; (2):CD000213; PMID: 10796329]. *Cochrane Database Syst Rev* 2003; (3):CD000213.

134 Alderson P, Bero LA, Eccles M, Grilli R, Grimshaw JM, Oxman AD *et al*. Effective Practice and Organisation of Care Group. About the Cochrane Collaboration (Collaborative Review Groups (CRGs)). *Cochrane Library* 2005;(3).

135 Jamtvedt G, Young JM, Kristoffersen DT, Thomson O'Brien MA, Oxman AD. Audit and feedback: effects on professional practice and health care outcomes. [update of *Cochrane Database Syst Rev* 2000; (2):CD000259; PMID: 10796520]. *Cochrane Database Sys Rev* 2003; (3):CD000259.

136 Sandercock P, Fraser H, Thomas B, McInnes A, Dixon S. Cochrane Stroke Group 10 years on: progress to date and future challenges. *Stroke* 2003; **34**(10):2537–9.

137 Jadad AR, Cook DJ, Jones A, Klassen TP, Tugwell P, Moher M *et al*. Methodology and reports of systematic reviews and meta-analyses: a comparison of Cochrane reviews with articles published in paper-based journals. *J Am Med Assoc* 1998; **280**(3):278–80.

138 Asplund K. Stroke care in the UK: is it good enough? *Lancet Neurol* 2002; **1**:341.

139 Asplund K. Stroke in Europe: widening gap between East and West. *Cerebrovasc Dis* 1996; **6**:3–6.

140 Asplund K, Ashburner S, Cargill K, Hux M, Lees K, Drummond M *et al*. Health care resource use and stroke outcome. Multinational comparisons within the GAIN International trial. *Int J Tech Assess Hlth Care* 2003; **19**(2):267–77.

141 Stegmayr B, Asplund K, Hulter-Asberg K, Norrving B, Terent A, Wester PO. Large variations in medical antithrombotic treatment of stroke patients in hospitals. Results from Riks-Stroke, the Swedish National Quality Register. *Stroke* (online) 2004; **35**:E199.

142 Moussouttas MM, Lichtman JH, Krumholtz HM, Cerese J, Brass L. The use of heparin anticoagulation in acute ischemic stroke among academic medical centers. *Stroke* 1999; **30**:265.

143 Al Sadat A, Sunbulli M, Chaturvedi S. Use of intravenous heparin by North American neurologists: do the data matter? *Stroke* 2002; **33**(6):1574–7.

144 Lakshminarayan K, Solid CA, Collins AJ, Anderson DC, Herzog CA. Atrial fibrillation and stroke in the general medicare population: a 10-year perspective (1992 to 2002). *Stroke* 2006; **37**(8):1969–74.

145 Reed SD, Cramer SC, Blough DK, Meyer K, Jarvik JJ. Treatment with tissue plasminogen activator and inpatient mortality rates for patients with ischemic stroke treated in community hospitals. *Stroke* 2001; **32**:1832–40.

146 Johnston SC, Fung LH, Gillum LA, Smith WS, Brass LM, Lichtman JH *et al*. Utilization of intravenous tissue-type plasminogen activator for ischemic stroke at academic medical centers: the influence of ethnicity [see comment]. *Stroke* 2001; **32**(5):1061–8.

147 Heuschmann P, Berger K, Misselwitz B, Hermanek P, Leffmann C, Adelmann M. Frequency of thrombolytic therapy in patients with acute ischemic stroke and the risk of in-hospital mortality. The German Stroke Registers Study Group. *Stroke* 2003; **34**:1106–13.

148 Katzan L, Furlan AJ, Lloyd L, Frank J, Harper D, Hinchey J *et al*. Use of tissue-type plasminogen activator for acute ischemic stroke. The Cleveland Area Experience. *J Am Med Assoc* 2000; **283**:1151–8.

149 Brown D, Barsan W, Lisabeth L, Gallery M, Morgenstern L. Survey of emergency physicians about recombinant tissue plasminogen activator for acute ischemic stroke. *Ann Emerg Med* 2005; **46**(1):56–60.

150 Bednar MM, Gross CE. Antiplatelet therapy in acute cerebral ischemia. [see comment]. *Stroke* 1999; **30**(4):887–93.

151 van Kooten F, Ciabattoni G, Patrono C, Dippel DW, Koudstaal PJ. Platelet activation and lipid peroxidation in patients with acute ischemic stroke. *Stroke* 1997; **28**(8):1557–63.

152 Antiplatelet Therapy Trialists' Collaboration. Collaborative overview of randomised trials of antiplatelet therapy. III: Reduction in venous thrombosis and pulmonary embolism by antiplatelet prophylaxis among surgical and medical patients. Antiplatelet Trialists' Collaboration. *Br Med J* 1994; **308**(6923):235–46.

153 ISIS-2 (Second International Study of Infarct Survival) Collaborative Group. Randomised trial of intravenous

streptokinase, oral aspirin, both, or neither among 17 187 cases of suspected acute myocardial infarction: ISIS-2. [see comment]. *Lancet* 1988; **2**(8607):349–60.

154 Sandercock P, Collins R, Counsell C, Farrell B, Peto R, Slattery J *et al.* The International Stroke Trial (IST): A randomised trial of aspirin, subcutaneous heparin, both, or neither among 19 435 patients with acute ischaemic stroke. *Lancet* 1997; **349**:1569–81.

155 Chen ZM, Collins R, Liu LS, Pan HC, Peto R, Xie JX. CAST: Randomised placebo-controlled trial of early aspirin use in 20 000 patients with acute ischaemic stroke. *Lancet* 1997; **349**:1641–9.

156 Sandercock P, Gubitz G, Foley P, Counsell C. Antiplatelet therapy for acute ischaemic stroke. [see comment] [update of *Cochrane Database Syst Rev* 2000; (2):CD000029; PMID: 10796284]. *Cochrane Database Syst Rev* 2003; (2):CD000029.

157 Chen ZM, Sandercock P, Pan HC, Counsell C, Collins R, Liu LS *et al.* Indications for early aspirin use in acute ischemic stroke : a combined analysis of 40 000 randomized patients from the chinese acute stroke trial and the international stroke trial. *Stroke* 2000; **31**(6):1240–9.

158 Pulmonary Embolism Prevention (PEP) Trial Collaborative Group. Prevention of pulmonary embolism and deep vein thrombosis with low dose aspirin: Pulmonary Embolism Prevention (PEP) trial. [see comment]. *Lancet* 2000; **355**(9212):1295–302.

159 Keir SL, Wardlaw JM, Sandercock PA, Chen Z. Antithrombotic therapy in patients with any form of intracranial haemorrhage: a systematic review of the available controlled studies. *Cerebrovasc Dis* 2002; **14**(3–4):197–206.

160 Coull BM, Williams LS, Goldstein LB, Meschia JF, Heitzman D, Chaturvedi S *et al.* Anticoagulants and antiplatelet agents in acute ischemic stroke: report of the Joint Stroke Guideline Development Committee of the American Academy of Neurology and the American Stroke Association (a division of the American Heart Association). *Stroke* 2002; **33**(7):1934–42.

161 Toyoda K, Okada Y, Minematsu K, Kamouchi M, Fujimoto S, Ibayashi S *et al.* Antiplatelet therapy contributes to acute deterioration of intracerebral hemorrhage. *Neurology* 2005; **65**(7):1000–4.

162 Viswanathan A, Rakich SM, Engel C, Snider R, Rosand J, Greenberg SM *et al.* Antiplatelet use after intracerebral hemorrhage. *Neurology* 2006; **66**(2):206–9.

163 Wardlaw JM, Seymour J, Cairns J, Keir S, Lewis S, Sandercock P. Immediate computed tomography scanning of acute stroke is cost-effective and improves quality of life. *Stroke* 2004; **35**(11):2477–83.

164 MAST-I Group. Randomised controlled trial of streptokinase, aspirin, and combination of both in treatment of acute ischaemic stroke. Multicentre Acute Stroke Trial–Italy (MAST-I) Group. *Lancet* 1995; **346**(8989):1509–14.

165 Schmulling S, Rudolf J, Strotmann-Tack T, Grond M, Schneweis S, Sobesky J *et al.* Acetylsalicylic acid pretreatment, concomitant heparin therapy and the risk

of early intracranial hemorrhage following systemic thrombolysis for acute ischemic stroke. *Cerebrovasc Dis* 2003; **16**(3):183–90.

166 Intercollegiate Stroke Working Party. *National Clinical Guidelines for Stroke.* 2nd edn. Royal College of Physicians of London, 2004.

167 Adams HP, Adams RJ, Brott T, del Zoppo GJ, Furlan AJ, Goldstein LB *et al.* Guidelines for the Early Management of Patients With Ischemic Stroke. A Scientific Statement From the Stroke Council of the American Stroke Association. *Stroke* 2003; **34**, 1056–83.

168 Patrono C. Aspirin as an antiplatelet drug. *N Engl J Med* 1994; **330**(18):1287–94.

169 Patrono C, Ciabattoni G, Davi G. Thromboxane biosynthesis in cardiovascular diseases. *Stroke* 1990; **21**(12 Suppl):IV130–IV133.

170 Hop JW, Rinkel GJ, Algra A, Berkelbach van der Sprenkel JW, van Gijn J. Randomized pilot trial of postoperative aspirin in subarachnoid hemorrhage. *Neurology* 2000; **54**(4):872–8.

171 Hart RG, Tonarelli S, Pearce LA. Avoiding central nervous system bleeding during antithrombotic therapy. Recent data and ideas. *Stroke* 2005; **36**:1588–93.

172 Gubitz G, Sandercock P, Counsell C. Anticoagulants for acute ischaemic stroke. [update of *Cochrane Database Syst Rev* 2000; (2):CD000024; PMID: 10796283]. *Cochrane Database Syst Rev* 2004; (3):CD000024.

173 Sandercock P, Counsell C, Stobbs SL. Low-molecular-weight heparins or heparinoids versus standard unfractionated heparin for acute ischaemic stroke. [update of *Cochrane Database Syst Rev* 2001; (4):CD000119; PMID: 11687069]. *Cochrane Database Syst Rev* 2005; (2):CD000119.

174 Bath PM, Iddenden R, Bath FJ. Low-molecular-weight heparins and heparinoids in acute ischemic stroke: a meta-analysis of randomized controlled trials. *Stroke* 2000; **31**(7):1770–8.

175 Berge E, Sandercock P. Anticoagulants versus antiplatelet agents for acute ischaemic stroke. [see comment]. *Cochrane Database Syst Rev* 2002; (4):CD003242.

176 Chamorro A, Busse O, Obach V, Toni D, Sandercock P, Reverter JC *et al.* The rapid anticoagulation prevents ischemic damage study in acute stroke: final results from the writing committee. *Cerebrovasc Dis* 2005; **19**(6):402–4.

177 Camerlingo M, Salvi P, Belloni G, Gamba T, Cesana BM, Mamoli A. Intravenous heparin started within the first 3 hours after onset of symptoms as a treatment for acute nonlacunar hemispheric cerebral infarctions. *Stroke* 2005; **36**(11):2415–20.

178 Diener HC, Ringelstein EB, von KR, Landgraf H, Koppenhagen K, Harenberg J *et al.* Prophylaxis of thrombotic and embolic events in acute ischemic stroke with the low-molecular-weight heparin certoparin: results of the PROTECT Trial. *Stroke* 2006; **37**:139–44.

179 Diener HC, Ringelstein EB, von Kummer R, Langohr HD, Bewermeyer H, Landgraf H *et al.* Treatment of acute ischemic stroke with the low-molecular-weight heparin certoparin: results of the TOPAS trial. Therapy of Patients

With Acute Stroke (TOPAS) Investigators. *Stroke* 2001; **32**(1):22–9.

180 Wong KS, Chen C, Ng PW, Tsoi TH, Li HL, Fong WC *et al.* Low-molecular-weight heparin compared with aspirin for the treatment of acute ischaemic stroke in Asian patients with large artery occlusive disease: a randomised study. *Lancet Neurol* 2007; **6**:407–13.

181 LaMonte MP, Nash ML, Wang DZ, Woolfenden AR, Schultz J, Hursting MJ *et al.* Argatroban anticoagulation in patients with acute ischemic stroke (ARGIS-1): a randomized, placebo-controlled safety study. *Stroke* 2004; **35**(7):1677–82.

182 Gubitz G, Sandercock P, Counsell C. Immediate anticoagulant therapy for acute ischaemic stroke: a systematic review of seven randomised trials directly comparing different doses of the same anticoagulant. *Stroke* 2000; **31**:308.

183 Bath PM, Lindenstrom E, Boysen G, De Deyn P, Friis P, Leys D *et al.* Tinzaparin in acute ischaemic stroke (TAIST): a randomised aspirin-controlled trial. [see comments]. [erratum appears in *Lancet* 2001; **358**(9289):1276]. *Lancet* 2001; **358**(9283):702–10.

184 Saxena R, Lewis S, Berge E, Sandercock P, Koudstaal PJ. Risk of early death and recurrent stroke and effect of heparin in 3169 patients with acute ischemic stroke and atrial fibrillation in the International Stroke Trial. *Stroke* 2001; **32**(10):2333–7.

185 Berge E, Abdelnoor M, Nakstad PH, Sandset PM. Low molecular-weight heparin versus aspirin in patients with acute ischaemic stroke and atrial fibrillation: a double-blind randomised study. HAEST Study Group. Heparin in Acute Embolic Stroke Trial. [see comments]. *Lancet* 2000; **355**(9211):1205–10.

186 Randomised controlled trial of subcutaneous calcium-heparin in acute myocardial infarction. The SCATI (Studio sulla Calciparina nell'Angina e nella Trombosi Ventricolare nell'Infarto) Group. *Lancet* 1989; **2**(8656):182–6.

187 Turpie AG, Robinson JG, Doyle DJ, Mulji AS, Mishkel GJ, Sealey BJ *et al.* Comparison of high-dose with low-dose subcutaneous heparin to prevent left ventricular mural thrombosis in patients with acute transmural anterior myocardial infarction. *N Engl J Med* 1989; **320**(6):352–7.

188 Collins R, MacMahon S, Flather M, Baigent C, Remvig L, Mortensen S *et al.* Clinical effects of anticoagulant therapy in suspected acute myocardial infarction: systematic overview of randomised trials. [see comment]. *Br Med J* 1996; **313**(7058):652–9.

189 Cairns JA, Theroux P, Lewis HD, Jr., Ezekowitz M, Meade TW. Antithrombotic agents in coronary artery disease. *Chest* 2001; **119**(Suppl 1):228S–52S.

190 Vaitkus PT, Berlin JA, Schwartz JS, Barnathan ES. Stroke complicating acute myocardial infarction. A meta-analysis of risk modification by anticoagulation and thrombolytic therapy. *Arch Intern Med* 1992; **152**(10):2020–4.

191 Scottish Intercollegiate Guidelines Network. *Management of Patients with Stroke. Rehabilitation, Prevention and Management of Complications, and Discharge Planning.* Edinburgh: Royal College of Physicians Edinburgh, 2002.

192 Lindley RI, Wardlaw J, Sandercock P, Rimdusid P, Lewis SC, Signorini D *et al.* Frequency and risk factors for spontaneous hemorrhagic transformation of cerebral infarction. *J Stroke Cerebrovasc Dis* 2004; **13**(6):235–46.

193 Scottish Intercollegiate Guidelines Network. *Antithrombotic Therapy.* Edinburgh: Royal College of Physicians Edinburgh, 1999.

194 Toyonaga M, Hagiwara N, Irie F, Toyoda K, Fujimoto S, Hitotsumatsu T *et al.* [Acute cervical spinal epidural hematoma during antithrombotic therapy: dual warnings against antithrombotic therapy]. *Rinsho Shinkeigaku* 2003; **43**(5):287–90.

195 Steiner T, Rosand J, Diringer M. Intracerebral hemorrhage associated with oral anticoagulant therapy: current practices and unresolved questions. *Stroke* 2006; **37**(1):256–62.

196 Huttner HB, Schellinger PD, Hartmann M, Kohrmann M, Juettler E, Wikner J *et al.* Hematoma growth and outcome in treated neurocritical care patients with intracerebral hemorrhage related to oral anticoagulant therapy: comparison of acute treatment strategies using vitamin k, fresh frozen plasma, and prothrombin complex concentrates. *Stroke* 2006; **37**(6):1465–70.

197 Wijdicks EF, Schievink WI, Brown RD, Mullany CY. Early anticoagulation in patients with prosthetic heart valves and intracerebral hematoma. [comment]. *Neurology* 1999; **52**(3):676–7.

198 Phan TG, Koh M, Wijdicks EFM. Safety of discontinuation of anticoagulation in patients with intracranial hemorrhage at high thromboembolic risk. *Arch Neurol* 2000; **57**(12):1710–13.

199 Phan TG, Wijdicks EF, Phan TG, Wijdicks EF. Management of intracranial bleeding associated with anticoagulation: balancing the risk of further bleeding against thromboembolism from prosthetic heart valves. *J Neurol Neurosurg Psychiatry* 2001; **70**(6):820–1.

200 Eckman MH, Rosand J, Knudsen KA, Singer DE, Greenberg SM. can patients be anticoagulated after intracerebral hemorrhage?: A decision analysis. *Stroke* 2003; **34**(7):1710–16.

201 Butler A, Tait RC, Eckman MH, Singer DE, Rosand J, Knudsen KA *et al.* Restarting oral anticoagulation after intracranial hemorrhage. Response. *Stroke* 2004; **35**(1):5e–6.

202 Little SH, Massel DR. Antiplatelet and anticoagulation for patients with prosthetic heart valves. *Cochrane Database Syst Rev* 2003; (4):CD003464.

203 Hacke W, Donnan G, Fieschi C, Kaste M, von Kummer R, Broderick JP *et al.* Association of outcome with early stroke treatment: pooled analysis of ATLANTIS, ECASS, and NINDS rt-PA stroke trials. *Lancet* 2004; **363**(9411):768–74.

204 Cornu C, Boutitie F, Candelise L, Boissel JP, Donnan G, Hommel M *et al.* Streptokinase in acute ischemic stroke: an individual patient data meta-analysis: The Thrombolysis in Acute Stroke Pooling Project. *Stroke* 2000; **31**(7):1555–60.

205 Haley EC, Lyden P, Johnston KC, Hemmen TM, the TNK in Stroke Investigators. A pilot dose-escalation safety study of

tenecteplase in acute ischemic stroke. *Stroke* 2005; **36**:607–12.

206 Hacke W. The results of the joint analysis of two phase II trials on desmoteplase in acute ischemic stroke with treatment 3 to 9 hours after stroke onset. *Cerebrovasc Dis* 2005; 19 (Suppl 2):69.

207 Macleod MR, Davis SM, Mitchell P, Gerraty R, Hankey G, Fitt G *et al*. Results of a multicentre, randomised controlled trial of intra-arterial urokinase in the treatment of acute posterior circulation ischaemic stroke. *Cerebrovasc Dis* 2005; **20**:12–17.

208 Fibrinolytic Therapy Trialists' Collaborative Group. Indications for fibrinolytic therapy in suspected acute myocardial infarction: collaborative overview of early mortality and major morbidity results from all randomised trials of more than 1000 patients. *Lancet* 1994; **343**:311–22.

209 McCarron MO, Nicoll JA. Cerebral amyloid angiopathy and thrombolysis-related intracerebral haemorrhage. *Lancet Neurol* 2004; **3**(8):484–92.

210 Kakuda W, Thijs VN, Lansberg MG, Bammer R, Wechsler L, Kemp S *et al*. Clinical importance of microbleeds in patients receiving IV thrombolysis. *Neurology* 2005; **65**(8):1175–8.

211 Koudstaal PJ, Stibbe J, Vermeulen M. Fatal ischaemic brain oedema after early thrombolysis with tissue plasminogen activator in acute stroke. *Br Med J* 1988; **297**(6663):1571–4.

212 Rudolf J, Grond M, Stenzel C, Neveling M, Heiss WD. Incidence of space-occupying brain edema following systemic thrombolysis of acute supratentorial ischemia. *Cerebrovasc Dis* 1998; **8**(3):166–71.

213 Kwiatkowski T, Libman RB, Frankel M, Tilley B, Morgenstern L, Lu M *et al*. Effects of tissue plasminogen activator for acute ischemic stroke at one year. *N Engl J Med* 1999; **340**:1781–7.

214 Sandercock P, Berge E, Dennis M, Hand P, Kwan J, Lewis S *et al*. A systematic review of the effectiveness, cost-effectiveness and barriers to the implementation of thrombolytic and neuroprotective treatment in the NHS. *Health Technology Assessment* 2002; **6**(26):1–112.

215 Counsell C, Dennis M. Systematic review of prognostic models in patients with acute stroke. *Cerebrovasc Dis* 2001; **12**:159–70.

216 Altman DG, Bland JM. Interaction revisited: the difference between two estimates. *Br Med J* 2003; **326**(7382):219.

217 Lagakos SW. The challenge of subgroup analyses: reporting without distorting. *N Engl J Med* 2006; **354**(16):1667–9.

218 O'Fallon WM, Asplund K, Goldfrank LR, Hertzberg V, Ingall TJ, Louis TA. Report of the t-PA Review Committee. 2004. http://www.ninds.nih.gov/funding/ review_committees/t-pa_review_committee/ t-pa_committee_report.pdf

219 Simon JE, Sandler DL, Pexman JH, Hill MD, Buchan AM, Calgary Stroke Program. Is intravenous recombinant tissue plasminogen activator (rt-PA) safe for use in patients over 80 years old with acute ischaemic stroke? The Calgary experience. [see comment]. *Age Ageing* 2004; **33**(2):143–9.

220 Von Kummer R. Early major ischemic changes on computed tomography should preclude use of tissue plasminogen activator. *Stroke* 2003; **34**:820–1.

221 Lyden P. Early major ischemic changes on computed tomography should not preclude use of tissue plasminogen activator. *Stroke* 2003; **33**:812–22.

222 Wardlaw JM, Mielke O. Early signs of brain infarction at CT: observer reliability and outcome after thrombolytic treatment: systematic review. *Radiology* 2005; **235**(2):444–53.

223 Demchuk AM, Hill MD, Barber PA, Silver B, Patel SC, Levine SR. Importance of early ischemic computed tomography changes using ASPECTS in NINDS rt-PA Stroke Study. *Stroke* 2005; **36**(10):2110–15.

224 Dzialowski I, Hill MD, Coutts SB, Demchuk AM, Kent DM, Wunderlich O *et al*. Extent of early ischemic changes on computed tomography (CT) before thrombolysis: prognostic value of the Alberta Stroke Program Early CT Score in ECASS II. *Stroke* 2006; **37**(4):973–8.

225 Schellinger PD, Fiebach JB. Perfusion-weighted imaging/diffusion-weighted imaging mismatch on MRI can now be used to select patients for recombinant tissue plasminogen activator beyond 3 hours: pro. [see comment]. *Stroke* 2005; **36**(5):1104–5.

226 Zivin JA. Perfusion-weighted imaging/diffusion-weighted imaging mismatch on MRI can now be used to select patients for recombinant tissue plasminogen activator beyond 3 hours [see comment]. *Stroke* 2005; **36**(5):1105–6.

227 Davis SM. Echoplanar Imaging Thrombolysis Evaluation Trial. EPITHET. http://www strokecenter org/trials/TrialDetail aspx?tid=420, 2005; available from: http://www.astn.org.au/epithet/Epithet_home.htm

228 Dundar Y, Hill R, Dickson R, Walley T. Comparative efficacy of thrombolytics in acute myocardial infarction: a systematic review. *Q J Med* 2003; **96**(2):103–13.

229 Walley T, Dundar Y, Hill R, Dickson R. Superiority and equivalence in thrombolytic drugs: an interpretation. *Q J Med* 2003; **96**(2):155–60.

230 Mielke O, Wardlaw J, Liu M. Thrombolysis (different doses, routes of administration and agents) for acute ischaemic stroke. [update of *Cochrane Database Syst Rev* 2000; (2):CD000514; PMID: 10796381]. *Cochrane Database Syst Rev* 2004; (4):CD000514.

231 Molina CA, Saver JL, Molina CA, Saver JL. Extending reperfusion therapy for acute ischemic stroke: emerging pharmacological, mechanical, and imaging strategies. *Stroke* 2005; **36**(10):2311–20.

232 Ciccone A, Motto C, Aritzu E, Piana A, Candelise L. Risk of aspirin use plus thrombolysis after acute ischaemic stroke: a further MAST-I analysis. MAST-I Collaborative Group. Multicentre Acute Stroke Trial–Italy. *Lancet* 1998; **352**(9131):880.

233 del Zoppo GJ, Higashida R, Furlan AJ, Pessin M, Rowley HA, Gent M *et al*. PROACT: a phase II randomized trial of recombinant pro-urokinase by direct arterial delivery in acute middle cerebral artery stroke. *Stroke* 1998; **29**:4–11.

234 Furlan AJ, Higashida R, Wechsler LR, Gent M, Rowley H, Kase C *et al*. Intra-arterial prourokinase for acute ischemic stroke. The PROACT II Study: a randomized controlled trial. *J Am Med Assoc* 1999; **282**:2003–11.

235 Adams HP, Brott TG, Furlan AJ. Guidelines for thrombolytic therapy in stroke: a supplement to the guidelines for the management of patients with acute ischaemic stroke. A Statement for Healthcare Professionals from a Special Writing Group of the Stroke Council, American Heart Association. *Stroke* 1996; **27**:1711–18.

236 Ingall TJ, O'Fallon WM, Goldfrank LR, Hertzberg V, Louis TA, Christianson TJH. Findings from the reanalysis of the NINDS Tissue Plasminogen Activator for Acute Ischemic Stroke Treatment Trial. *Stroke* 2004; **35**:2418–24.

237 Mori E, Yoneda Y, Tabuchi M, Yoshida T, Ohkawa S, Ohsumi Y *et al*. Intravenous recombinant tissue plasminogen activator in acute carotid artery territory stroke. *Neurology* 1992; **42**:976–82.

238 Yamaguchi T, Hayakawa T, Kiuchi H, Japanese Thrombolysis Study Group. Intravenous tissue plasminogen activator ameliorates the outcome of hyperacute embolic stroke. *Cerebrovasc Dis* 1993; **3**:269–72.

239 IMS study Investigators. Combined intravenous and intra-arterial recanalization for acute ischemic stroke: the Interventional Management of Stroke Study. [see comment]. *Stroke* 2004; **35**(4):904–11.

240 Khatri P, Kasner SE. Ischemic strokes after cardiac catheterization: opportune thrombolysis candidates? *Arch Neurol* 2006; **63**(6):817–21.

241 Berenstein A, Siller K, Setton A, Nelson P, Levin D, Kupersmith MJ. Intra arterial urokinase for acute ischaemic stroke during interventional neuroradiological procedures. *Neurology* 1994; **44** (Suppl 2):A356.

242 Zaidat OO, Slivka AP, Mohammad Y, Graffagnino C, Smith TP, Enterline DS *et al*. Intra-arterial thrombolytic therapy in peri-coronary angiography ischemic stroke. *Stroke* 2005; **36**(5):1089–90.

243 Hankey G, Warlow C. Treatment and secondary prevention of stroke: evidence, costs and effects on individuals and populations. *Lancet* 1999; **354**:1457–63.

244 Gilligan AK, Thrift AG, Sturm JW, Dewey HM, Macdonell RA, Donnan GA. Stroke units, tissue plasminogen activator, aspirin and neuroprotection: which stroke intervention could provide the greatest community benefit? *Cerebrovasc Dis* 2005; **20**(4):239–44.

245 Anonymous. *Summary of product characteristics: Actilyse*. Bracknell, UK: Boehringer Ingelheim, 2003.

246 Weintraub MI. Thrombolysis (tissue plasminogen activator) in stroke: a medicolegal quagmire. *Stroke* 2006; **37**(7):1917–22.

247 Ciccone A, Sterzi R, Crespi V, Defanti CA, Pasetti C, Bioethics and Neurology Study Group of the Italian Neurological Society. Thrombolysis for acute ischemic stroke: the patient's point of view. *Cerebrovasc Dis* 2001; **12**(4):335–40.

248 Koops L, Lindley R. Thrombolysis for acute ischaemic stroke: consumer involvement in the design of new randomised controlled trial. *Br Med J* 2002; **325**:415–17.

249 Katz JM, Segal AZ, Katz JM, Segal AZ. Should thrombolysis be given to a stroke patient refusing therapy due to profound anosognosia? [see comment]. *Neurology* 2004; **63**(12):2440.

250 Worrall BB, Chen DT, Dimberg EL, Worrall BB, Chen DT, Dimberg EL. Should thrombolysis be given to a stroke patient refusing therapy due to profound anosognosia? [comment]. *Neurology* 2005; **65**(3):500.

251 Kwan J, Hand P, Sandercock P. A systematic review of barriers to delivery of thrombolysis for acute stroke. [see comment]. *Age Ageing* 2004; **33**(2):116–21.

252 Ciccone A, Bonito V, Italian Neurological Society's Study Group for Bioethics and Palliative Care in Neurology. Thrombolysis for acute ischemic stroke: the problem of consent. *Neurol Sci* 2001; **22**(5):339–51.

253 Fleck LM, Hayes OW. Ethics and consent to treat issues in acute stroke therapy. *Emerg Med Clin N Am* 2002; **20**(3):703–15.

254 Ciccone A. Consent to thrombolysis in acute ischaemic stroke: from trial to practice. *Lancet Neurol* 2003; **2**:375–8.

255 Bateman BT, Meyers PM, Schumacher HC, Mangla S, Pile-Spellman J. Conducting stroke research with an exception from the requirement for informed consent. *Stroke* 2003; **34**(5):1317–23.

256 Demarquay G, Derex L, Nighoghossian N, Adeleine P, Philippeau F, Honnorat J *et al*. Ethical issues of informed consent in acute stroke: analysis of the modalities of consent in 56 patients enrolled in urgent therapeutic trials. *Cerebrovasc Dis* 2005; **19**(2):65–8.

257 Kane I, Lindley R, Lewis S, Sandercock P. Impact of stroke syndrome and stroke severity on the process of consent in the Third International Stroke Trial. *Cerebrovasc Dis* 2006; **21**(5–6):348–52.

258 Rosenbaum JR, Bravata DM, Concato J, Brass LM, Kim N, Fried TR *et al*. Informed consent for thrombolytic therapy for patients with acute ischemic stroke treated in routine clinical practice. [see comment]. *Stroke* 2004; **35**(9):e353–e355.

259 Johnson DM, Kramer DC, Cohen E, Rochon M, Rosner M, Weinberger J. Thrombolytic therapy for acute stroke in late pregnancy with intra-arterial recombinant tissue plasminogen activator. *Stroke* 2005; **36**(6):e53–e55.

260 Wein TH, Hickenbottom SL, Morgenstern LB, Demchuk AM, Grotta JC. Safety of tissue plasminogen activator for acute stroke in menstruating women. *Stroke* 2002; **33**(10):2506–8.

261 Chalela JA, Katzan I, Liebeskind DS, Rasmussen P, Zaidat O, Suarez JI *et al*. Safety of intra-arterial thrombolysis in the postoperative period. *Stroke* 2001; **32**(6):1365–9.

262 Kane I, Sandercock P, Thomas B. Can patients with unruptured intracranial aneurysms be treated with thrombolysis? A short systematic review. *Cerebrovasc Dis* 2005; **20**(1):51–2.

263 Talkad A, Mathews M, Honings D, Jahnel J, Wang D. Reversal of warfarin-induced anticoagulation with factor VIIa prior to rt-PA in acute stroke. *Neurology* 2005; **64**(8):1480–1.

264 Linfante I, Reddy AS, Andreone V, Caplan LR, Selim M, Hirsch JA. Intra-arterial thrombolysis in patients treated with warfarin. *Cerebrovasc Dis* 2005; 19(2):133–5.

265 Tanne D, Kasner ES, Demchuk AM, Koren-Morag N, Hanson S, Grond M *et al.* Markers of increased risk of intracerebral hemorrhage after intravenous recombinant tissue plasminogen activator therapy for acute ischemic stroke in clinical practice: the multicenter rt-PA acute stroke survey. *Circulation* 2002; 105:1679–85.

266 Kwan J, Hand P, Sandercock P. Improving the efficiency of delivery of thrombolysis for acute stroke: a systematic review. *Q J Med* 2004; 97(5):273–9.

267 Hacke W. Third European Acute Stroke Study (ECASS-III): Placebo controlled trial of alteplase (rt-PA) in acute ischemic hemispheric stroke where thrombolysis is initiated between 3 and 4 hours after stroke onset. http://www strokecenter org/trials/trialDetail aspx?tid=475&search_string=ECASS 2005; available from http://www.strokecenter.org/trials/trialDetail.aspx?tid=475&search_string=ECASS.

268 Arnold M, Schroth G, Nedeltchev K, Loher T, Remonda L, Stepper F *et al.* Intra-arterial thrombolysis in 100 patients with acute stroke due to middle cerebral artery occlusion. *Stroke* 2002; 33(7):1828–33.

269 Fernandes HM, Gregson B, Siddique S, Mendelow AD. Surgery in intracerebral hemorrhage. The uncertainty continues. *Stroke* 2000; 31(10):2511–16.

270 Mendelow AD, Gregson BA, Fernandes HM, Murray GD, Teasdale GM, Hope DT *et al.* Early surgery versus initial conservative treatment in patients with spontaneous supratentorial intracerebral haematomas in the International Surgical Trial in Intracerebral Haemorrhage (STICH): a randomised trial. [see comment]. *Lancet* 2005; 365(9457):387–97.

271 Hill MD, Lye T, Moss H, Barber PA, Demchuk AM, Newcommon NJ *et al.* Hemi-orolingual angioedema and ACE inhibition after alteplase treatment of stroke. Neurology 2003; 60(9):1525–7.

272 Engelter ST, Fluri F, Buitrago-Tellez C, Marsch S, Steck AJ, Ruegg S *et al.* Life-threatening orolingual angioedema during thrombolysis in acute ischemic stroke. *J Neurol* 2005; 252(10):1167–70.

273 Montalescot G, Barragan P, Wittenberg O, Ecollan P, Elhadad S, Villain P *et al.* Platelet glycoprotein IIb/IIIa inhibition with coronary stenting for acute myocardial infarction. *N Engl J Med* 2001; 344(25):1895–903.

274 De Luca G, Suryapranata H, Stone GW, Antoniucci D, Tcheng JE, Neumann FJ *et al.* Abciximab as adjunctive therapy to reperfusion in acute ST-segment elevation myocardial infarction: a meta-analysis of randomized trials. *J Am Med Assoc* 2005; 293(14):1759–65.

275 Abciximab Emergent Stroke Treatment Trial Investigators. Emergency administration of abciximab for treatment of patients with acute ischemic stroke: results of a randomized phase 2 trial. *Stroke* 2005; 36(4):880–90.

276 Ringleb PA. Thrombolytics, anticoagulants, and antiplatelet agents. *Stroke* 2006; 37(2):312–13.

277 Bukow SC, Daffertshofer M, Hennerici MG, Bukow SC, Daffertshofer M, Hennerici MG. Tirofiban for the treatment of ischaemic stroke. *Expert Opin Pharmacother* 2006; 7(1):73–9.

278 Velianou JL, Strauss BH, Kreatsoulas C, Pericak D, Natarajan MK. Evaluation of the role of abciximab (Reopro) as a rescue agent during percutaneous coronary interventions: in-hospital and six-month outcomes. [see comments]. *Cathet Cardiovasc Interv* 2000; 51(2):138–44.

279 Fiorella D, Albuquerque FC, Han P, McDougall CG. Strategies for the management of intraprocedural thromboembolic complications with abciximab (ReoPro). *Neurosurgery* 2004; 54(5):1089–97.

280 Arab D, Yahia AM, Qureshi AI. Use of intravenous abciximab as adjunctive therapy for carotid angioplasty and stent placement. *Int J Cardiovasc Interv* 2003; 5(2):61–6.

281 Chan AW, Yadav JS, Bhatt DL, Bajzer CT, Gum PA, Roffi M *et al.* Comparison of the safety and efficacy of emboli prevention devices versus platelet glycoprotein IIb/IIIa inhibition during carotid stenting. *Am J Cardiol* 2005; 95(6):791–5.

282 Velat GJ, Burry MV, Eskioglu E, Dettorre RR, Firment CS, Mericle RA *et al.* The use of abciximab in the treatment of acute cerebral thromboembolic events during neuroendovascular procedures. *Surg Neurol* 2006; 65(4):352–8.

283 Sherman DG, Atkinson RP, Chippendale T, Levin KA, Ng K, Futrell N *et al.* Intravenous ancrod for treatment of acute ischemic stroke: the STAT study: a randomized controlled trial. Stroke Treatment with Ancrod Trial. *J Am Med Assoc* 2000; 283(18):2395–403.

284 Liu M, Counsell C, Zhao XL, Wardlaw J. Fibrinogen depleting agents for acute ischaemic stroke. [update of *Cochrane Database Syst Rev* 2000; (2):CD000091; PMID: 10796295]. *Cochrane Database Syst Rev* 2003; (3):CD000091.

285 Hennerici MG, Kay R, Bogousslavsky J, Lenzi GL, Verstraete M, Orgogozo JM. Intravenous ancrod for acute ischaemic stroke in the European Stroke Treatment with Ancrod Trial: a randomised controlled trial. *Lancet* 2006; 368(9550):1871–8.

286 Keeley EC, Boura JA, Grines CL. Primary angioplasty versus intravenous thrombolytic therapy for acute myocardial infarction: a quantitative review of 23 randomised trials. [see comment]. *Lancet* 2003; 361(9351):13–20.

287 Daffertshofer M, Hennerici M. Ultrasound in the treatment of ischaemic stroke. *Lancet Neurol* 2003; 2(5):283–90.

288 Furlan AJ, Fisher M. Devices, drugs, and the Food and Drug Administration: increasing implications for ischemic stroke. *Stroke* 2005; 36(2):398–9.

289 Noser EA, Shaltoni HM, Hall CE, Alexandrov AV, Garami Z, Cacayorin ED *et al.* Aggressive mechanical clot disruption: a safe adjunct to thrombolytic therapy in acute stroke? *Stroke* 2005; 36(2):292–6.

290 Smith WS, Sung G, Starkman S, Saver JL, Kidwell CS, Gobin YP *et al.* Safety and efficacy of mechanical embolectomy in acute ischemic stroke: Results of the MERCI trial. *Stroke* 2005; 36(7):1432–8.

291 Becker KJ, Brott TG. Approval of the MERCI clot retriever: a critical view. *Stroke* 2005; **36**(2):400–3.

292 Kidwell CS, Jahan R, Starkman S, Saver J. MR and recanalization of stroke clots using embolectomy (MR RESCUE). *Stroke* 2005; International Stroke Conference 2005. Ongoing Clinical Trials Abstracts.

293 Tomsick TA. Mechanical embolus removal: a new day dawning. [comment]. *Stroke* 2005; **36**(7):1439–40.

294 Alexandrov AV, Molina CA, Grotta JC, Garami Z, Ford SR, varez-Sabin J *et al.* Ultrasound-enhanced systemic thrombolysis for acute ischemic stroke. [see comment]. *NEJM* 2004; **18**; 351:2170–8.

295 Qizilbash N, Lewington SL, Lopez-Arrieta JM, Qizilbash N, Lewington SL, Lopez-Arrieta JM. Corticosteroids for acute ischaemic stroke. [update of *Cochrane Database Syst Rev* 2000; (2):CD000064; PMID: 10796290]. *Cochrane Database Syst Rev* 2002; (2):CD000064.

296 Righetti E, Celani MG, Cantisani T, Sterzi R, Boysen G, Ricci S. Glycerol for acute stroke. [update of *Cochrane Database Syst Rev* 2000; (4):CD000096; PMID: 11034673]. *Cochrane Database Syst Rev* 2004; (2):CD000096.

297 Bereczki D, Liu M, Prado GF, Fekete I. Cochrane report: A systematic review of mannitol therapy for acute ischemic stroke and cerebral parenchymal hemorrhage. [see comment]. *Stroke* 2000; **31**(11):2719–22.

298 Roberts I, Schierhout G, Wakai A. Mannitol for acute traumatic brain injury. [update of *Cochrane Database Syst Rev* 2000; (2):CD001049; PMID: 10796744]. *Cochrane Database Syst Rev* 2003; (2):CD001049.

299 Georgiadis D, Schwarz S, Aschoff A, Schwab S. Hemicraniectomy and moderate hypothermia in patients with severe ischemic stroke. *Stroke* 2002; **33**(6):1584–8.

300 Morley NC, Berge E, Cruz-Flores S, Whittle IR. Surgical decompression for cerebral oedema in acute ischaemic stroke. *Cochrane Database Syst Rev* 2002; (3):CD003435.

301 Frank J. HeaDDFIRST. Hemicraniectomy and Durotomy for Deterioration From Infarction Relating Swelling Trial. 2000; available from http://www.strokecenter.org/trials/TrialDetail.aspx?tid=70.

302 The DESTINY Study Group. DESTINY – DEcompressive Surgery for the Treatment of malignant INfarction of the middle cerebral arterY: Preliminary Results. *Cerebrovasc Dis* 2006; **21** (Suppl 4):59–60.

303 Vahedi K, Vicaut E, Blanquet A, Payen D, Bousser MG. DECIMAL trial: DEcompressive Craniectomy In MALignant Middle Cerebral Artery Infarcts. 2004; available from http://www.strokecenter.org/trials/TrialDetail.aspx?tid=564.

304 Hofmeijer J, Amelink GJ, Algra A, van GJ, Macleod MR, Kappelle LJ *et al.* Hemicraniectomy after middle cerebral artery infarction with life-threatening Edema trial (HAMLET). Protocol for a randomised controlled trial of decompressive surgery in space-occupying hemispheric infarction. *Trials* 2006; **7**:29.

305 Schierhout G, Roberts I. Hyperventilation therapy for acute traumatic brain injury. *Cochrane Database Syst Rev* 2000; (2):CD000566.

306 Fisher M, Stroke Therapy Academic Industry Roundtable. Recommendations for advancing development of acute stroke therapies: Stroke Therapy Academic Industry Roundtable 3. *Stroke* 2003; **34**(6):1539–46.

307 Fisher M. Enhancing the development and approval of acute stroke therapies Stroke Therapy Academic Industry Roundtable. *Stroke* 2005; **36**:1808–13.

308 Sandercock P, Roberts I. Systematic reviews of animal experiments. *Lancet* 2002; **360**(9333):586.

309 Pound P, Ebrahim S, Sandercock P, Bracken MB, Roberts I, Reviewing Animal Trials Systematically (RATS) Group. Where is the evidence that animal research benefits humans? [see comment]. *Br Med J* 2004; **328**(7438):514–17.

310 Macleod MR, O'Collins T, Howells DW, Donnan G. Pooling of animal experimental data reveals influence of study design and publication bias. *Stroke* 2004; **35**(5):1203–8.

311 Macleod MR, Ebrahim S, Roberts I. Surveying the literature from animal experiments: systematic review and meta-analysis are important contributions. [comment]. *Br Med J* 2005; **331**(7508):110.

312 Lees KR, Zivin JA, Ashwood T, Davalos A, Davis SM, Diener HC *et al.* NXY-059 for acute ischemic stroke. *N Engl J Med* 2006; **354**(6):588–600.

313 Renovis Inc. NXY-059 does not meet efficacy endpoints in phase III trial for acute ischemic stroke. 2006; available from: http://www.medicalnewstoday.com/medicalnews.php?newsid=55212.

314 Asplund K. Haemodilution for acute ischaemic stroke. [update of *Cochrane Database Syst Rev* 2000; (2):CD000103; PMID: 10796299]. *Cochrane Database Syst Rev* 2002; (4):CD000103.

315 Horn J, Limburg M. Calcium antagonists for ischemic stroke. A systematic review. *Stroke* 2001; **32**:570–6.

316 *Cochrane Handbook for Systematic Reviews of Interventions* 4.2.5 [updated May 2005]. In: Higgins JPT, Green S, editors. In: *The Cochrane Library*, Issue 3, 2005. Chichester, UK: John Wiley & Sons, Ltd; 2005.

317 Altman DG, Machin D, Bryant TN, Gardner M. *Statistics with Confidence.* 2nd ed. London: BMJ Books; 2000.

318 Ludlam C, Bennett B, Fox KA, Lowe G, Reid A. Guidelines for the use of thrombolytic therapy. Haemostasis and Thrombosis Task Force of the British Committee for Standards in Haematology. *Blood Coag Fibrin* 1995; **6**(3):273–85.

319 Plum F, Posner JB. *The Diagnosis of Stupor and Coma*, Philadelphia, PA: F.A. Davis & Co., 1985.

320 Sherman DG, Albers GW, Bladin C, Fieschi C, Gabbai AA, Kase CS *et al.* The efficacy and safety of enoxaparin versus unfractionated heparin for the prevention of venous thromboembolism after acute ischaemic stroke (PREVAIL Study): an open-label randomised comparison. *Lancet* 2007; **369**:1347–55.

321 Vahedi K, Hofmeijer J, Juettler E, Vicaut E, George B, Algra A *et al.* Early decompressive surgery in malignant infarction of the middle cerebral artery: a pooled analysis of three randomised controlled trials. *Lancet Neurol* 2007; **6**:215–22.

13 Specific treatment of intracerebral haemorrhage

13.1 Pathophysiology

The events following non-traumatic spontaneous intra-cerebral haemorrhage (ICH) have been most intensively studied for the most common type, rupture of one or more deep perforating arteries. These events are surprisingly complex, to begin with because bleeding from a single site often leads adjacent perforators to rupture as well (section 8.2.1). Furthermore, the extravasated blood inevitably causes disruption of white matter tracts and irreversible damage to neurones in the deep nuclei or cortex. The protective encasement of the skull may become a disadvantage with any sudden increase in volume within the intracranial cavity, as with other causes of brain swelling and space-occupying lesions. Apart from the brain tissue destroyed by the haemorrhage itself, the attendant increase in intracranial pressure may threaten other parts of the brain, particularly – but not exclusively – when the intracranial pressure reaches levels of the same order of magnitude as the arterial pressure, bringing the cerebral perfusion pressure close to zero.[1] Direct mechanical compression of the brain tissue surrounding the haemorrhage and, to some extent, vasoconstrictor and pro-inflammatory substances in extravasated blood also lead to impaired blood supply.[2,3] Cellular ischaemia leads to further swelling from oedema,[4,5] which is initially cytotoxic and later vasogenic (section 12.1.5). The zone of ischaemia around the haemorrhage may swell through systemic factors such as hypotension or hypoxia. Often there is also loss of cerebral autoregulation in the vasculature supplying the region of the haemorrhage. Some perifocal ischaemic damage occurs at the time of bleeding and cannot be prevented, but the question to be considered here is whether the vicious cycle of ongoing ischaemia causing steadily increasing pressure can be interrupted in its early stages.

Hydrocephalus may be an additional space-occupying factor.[6] This complication is especially likely to occur with cerebellar haemorrhages, but a large haemorrhage in the region of the basal ganglia may also cause enlargement of the ventricular system, by rupture into the third ventricle, or through dilatation of the opposite lateral ventricle, with midline shift and obstruction of the third ventricle, while the ipsilateral ventricle is compressed.

13.2 Prognosis and predictive models

According to population-based studies the short-term prognosis of patients with ICH is poor, with over 40% dying within the first month.[7,8] Several hospital-based studies have attempted to develop models to predict prognosis based on patients' characteristics on admission, but almost without exception these have not been externally validated (in independent data sets). An accurate prognostic model might theoretically help in treatment decisions, particularly in selecting which patients should benefit from intensive care, and in informing relatives about the chances of recovery.

The most recent systematic review selected 18 hospital-based studies performed before 2004 that met essential criteria (multivariate analysis with logistic regression; no surgical treatment; paper in one of four major European languages); the models proposed in these studies were

Stroke: practical management, 3rd edition. C. Warlow, J. van Gijn, M. Dennis, J. Wardlaw, J. Bamford, G. Hankey, P. Sandercock, G. Rinkel, P. Langhorne, C. Sudlow and P. Rothwell. Published 2008 Blackwell Publishing. ISBN 978-1-4051-2766-0.

then validated against the outcome in 122 other patients with intracerebral haemorrhage admitted to a single centre.[9] Most prediction models proved easy to apply and most could generate a high probability of death or dependency in patients with the combination of factors providing the highest probability of poor outcome (most often the level of consciousness on admission, age, volume of haemorrhage and intraventricular extension). Nevertheless, among the 10 prognostic models that could identity patients with a greater than 90% probability of death or poor outcome, only a small proportion of patients actually had this combination of unfavourable characteristics (5–48%, median 30%). Also the accuracy of the prediction of 30-day case fatality was far from ideal: in these 10 subsets of the validation series the case fatality ranged between 67 and 100% (median 89%);[9] similarly inaccurate was a later predictive model, the so-called Essen ICH score.[10] Early withdrawal of support may then result in a self-fulfilling prophecy without scientific foundation.[11] Clearly characteristics on admission alone, used in the presently available prognostic models, do not allow accurate prediction of outcome in a sufficient proportion of patients to be clinically useful. Single-centre studies published after the systematic review cited above claimed that high levels of D-dimer or troponin, or low levels of cholesterol or triglycerides in serum, are independently associated with poor outcome;[12–14] obviously these findings require confirmation.

> Early characteristics predicting the prognosis for survival of patients with intracerebral haemorrhage are: level of consciousness; age; volume of haemorrhage and intraventricular extension of haemorrhage, but so far predictive models apply to only a small proportion of patients and are not sufficiently accurate for clinical decision making.

One way to improve models to predict poor outcome is to restrict the analysis to specific subgroups of ICH, according to location or presumed cause. This has been attempted for lobar haemorrhages,[15] haemorrhages in the caudate nucleus[16] and pontine haemorrhages,[17] but again there has been no external validation.

Perhaps a more fruitful approach is to move away from characteristics on first admission and to base predictive models more on the clinical course in the first 24 h,[9] if only because expansion of the haemorrhage occurs in a substantial proportion of patients within that period (section 8.2.1); not surprisingly this is an adverse factor.[18] Additional determinants in the early clinical course that probably should be included in the equation are fever[19] and the development of oedema around the haemorrhage.[20]

13.3 Management

13.3.1 Initial management

Admission to a specialized stroke unit is beneficial, as for stroke patients in general.[21] Once the patient's ventilation and circulation have been secured and the diagnosis of intracerebral haemorrhage confirmed by computed tomography (CT) scanning or magnetic resonance imaging (MRI), the next step is often to identify the cause before any specific treatment is initiated (Chapter 8). For example, if surgical evacuation of a life-threatening haemorrhage is considered at all, medical measures may have to be taken first (such as substitution of clotting factors in patients with liver failure or on anticoagulants). Also the surgeon should think twice if amyloid angiopathy is a likely cause (section 13.3.7). Repeat CT scanning is indicated if there is clinical deterioration, which may be caused by rebleeding at the same or sometimes at a distant site, or by hydrocephalus; if there are no structural changes, the search for systemic disorders should be intensified (section 11.5).

Recombinant factor (rF) VIIa is known to decrease the severity of haemorrhage in certain surgical settings, also in patients without clotting abnormalities.[22] A Cochrane review of four phase II randomized clinical trials involving adults aged 18 years or over, within 4 h of ICH found a reduced relative risk of death or dependence on the modified Rankin scale within 90 days of disease onset; 0.79, 95% confidence interval (CI) 0.67–0.93 (Fig. 13.1), but not on the extended Glasgow Outcome Scale; 0.90 (95% CI, 0.81–1.01).[23] There was a statistically significant excess of arterial thromboembolism at 160 µg/kg rFVIIa. In conclusion, adults with acute ICH may benefit from haemostatic therapy with rFVIIa, but the evidence on major clinical outcomes is neither robust nor precise. Claims that this treatment is cost-effective are based on the point estimate of benefit and are therefore premature.[24]

The *blood pressure* is usually increased in patients with ICH, through pre-existing hypertension, a response to a sudden increase in intracranial pressure, or both these factors.[25] There are theoretical arguments in favour of decreasing the blood pressure (in the hope of stopping ongoing bleeding from ruptured small arteries),[26] as well as in favour of increasing it further (in the hope of salvaging marginally perfused areas of brain that are compressed around the haemorrhage). In the absence of even the flimsiest evidence supporting one or other point of view (not surprisingly, a randomized

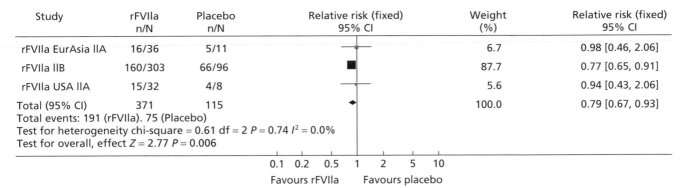

Study	rFVIIa n/N	Placebo n/N	Relative risk (fixed) 95% CI	Weight (%)	Relative risk (fixed) 95% CI
rFVIIa EurAsia IIA	16/36	5/11		6.7	0.98 [0.46, 2.06]
rFVIIa IIB	160/303	66/96		87.7	0.77 [0.65, 0.91]
rFVIIa USA IIA	15/32	4/8		5.6	0.94 [0.43, 2.06]
Total (95% CI)	371	115		100.0	0.79 [0.67, 0.93]

Total events: 191 (rFVIIa). 75 (Placebo)
Test for heterogeneity chi-square = 0.61 df = 2 P = 0.74 I^2 = 0.0%
Test for overall, effect Z = 2.77 P = 0.006

0.1 0.2   0.5   1   2   5   10
Favours rFVIIa   Favours placebo

Fig. 13.1 Meta-analysis of recombinant factor VIIa for intracerebral haemorrhage. Each trial is represented by a horizontal line, the length of which describes the 95% confidence interval around the point estimate of the treatment effect represented by a square, the size of which is proportional to the amount of data in the trial. The diamond represents the overall treatment effect, and its width the 95% confidence interval. The outcome is death or dependency (modified Rankin scale 4–6) at day 90.[23]

trial with 50 patients found no difference in outcome),[27] the only rational course is to leave the blood pressure alone in the acute phase unless it is so high that organ damage develops (especially in the retina and kidney). This is essentially the same for patients with ischaemic stroke (section 11.7.1). This is not to say that the patient should be discharged with a high blood pressure; a single observational study supports the notion that the long-term risk not only of vascular events in general but also of rebleeding may be lowered by adequate long-term blood pressure control.[28]

13.3.2 Reduction of intracranial pressure

Apart from the local effects of the haemorrhage itself and the subsequent perifocal oedema, other factors also contribute to raised intracranial pressure. Frequently, these can be treated more directly than the cerebral lesion itself, so it is important to be aware of them. They include fever, hypoxia, hypertension, seizures and elevations of intrathoracic pressure. A vexing and unsolved question is whether it is useful to measure the intracranial pressure by the introduction of an intraventricular catheter or other device, at least in patients with a decreased level of consciousness. Such an approach can certainly be rationalized.[29] On the other hand, any invasive procedure may cause complications,[30] while the presumed advantages in terms of outcome have not been subjected to controlled studies. For what it is worth, an observational comparison in traumatic brain injury failed to find any advantage of management based on intracranial pressure monitoring.[31] We prefer to err on the side of caution and base management on clinical and radiological features rather than the 'pressure' as measured directly.

Cerebrospinal fluid drainage

Insertion of a catheter in the lateral ventricle may be a definitive treatment in patients with cerebellar haemorrhage and no signs of direct compression of the brainstem (section 13.3.6). But, in patients with supratentorial haemorrhage and hydrocephalus, the benefits of CSF diversion are decidedly uncertain. In a series of 22 patients with supratentorial ICH and hydrocephalus who were treated with ventriculostomy, intracranial pressure was controlled at < 20 mmHg in 20, but only a single patient showed any improvement in not only the degree of hydrocephalus but also in the level of consciousness.[32] Just three patients, with small haemorrhage volumes, survived to 3 months. An alternative strategy is to divert the CSF internally, through callosotomy and fenestration of the septum pellucidum.[33] Controlled studies for all these procedures are woefully lacking.

In patients with extensive intraventricular haemorrhage secondary to deep intraparenchymal or aneurysmal rupture, drainage of CSF is also performed in some centres, in an attempt to improve the dismal prognosis. Systematic reviews of observational studies suggest that this procedure may be helpful, especially when it is combined with instillation of fibrinolytic drugs, but only direct comparisons in a randomized trial can definitively establish the value of these therapeutic measures.[34,35] Later observational studies have not solved the problem.[36,37]

Hyperventilation

There is no doubt that hyperventilation decreases intracranial pressure, but at the same time there is no controlled evidence to allay concerns that the cure may be worse than the disease. The intracranial pressure goes down because hypocapnia (usually down to values of the order of 4 kPa) causes vasoconstriction; in other words, ischaemia by compression is exchanged for ischaemia by vasoconstriction.[38] In head-injured patients, a single and so far the only randomized controlled trial of prolonged hyperventilation not only failed to show any benefit but also raised concerns about potential harm.[39,40] For patients with ICH, no controlled trials of hyperventilation have been done, but the experience with head trauma is not encouraging. Provisionally it seems best to reserve this treatment for bridging a few hours in patients for whom surgical evacuation is planned (sections 13.3.5 and 13.3.6).

Osmotic agents

Osmotic agents include mannitol, glycerol and sorbitol; they are administered by intravenous infusion.[41] Iodide-containing contrast agents used in CT scanning or angiography may inadvertently have the same dehydrating effect.[42] Osmotic agents extract water from the extracellular into the intravascular compartment of the brain. Whether they dehydrate mainly normal instead of damaged brain tissue is a matter of debate.[41] A disturbed blood–brain barrier may facilitate entry of hyperosmotic agents into brain tissue, thereby decreasing the osmotic gradient needed for effective dehydration, but on the other hand it may facilitate movement of fluid from brain tissue to blood. The interval between the infusion and the decrease of intracranial pressure is usually less than 1 h, but the effect of a single dose lasts no more than 4–6 h because the concentration of the solute becomes equilibrated between the intravascular and extracellular compartments. Potential dangers of this treatment include hypotension, hypokalaemia, renal failure from hyperosmolality, haemolysis and congestive heart failure.[43]

Intravenous *mannitol* (20–25% solution) has become the mainstay of osmotic therapy in many centres, despite a long-standing lack of evidence from controlled studies.[44] Recently a clinical trial in India randomized 128 patients with any type of supratentorial haemorrhage within 6 days and found no difference in case fatality at 1 month.[45] The correct dose cannot be predicted, but a safe regimen is to give 0.75–1 g/kg initially, then 0.25–0.5 g/kg every 3–5 h, depending on clinical response and osmolality (the aim being 295–310 mosm/L).[46] A controlled trial of a high dose (1.4 mg/kg) against a standard dose (0.7 mg/kg) of mannitol in 141 preoperative patients with traumatic temporal lobe haemorrhages and ipsilateral pupillary dilatation found better outcome after 6 months in the high-dose group (61% vs 33%),[47] but the relevance of this trial is questionable for patients with spontaneous intracerebral haemorrhages who are managed conservatively. With mannitol infusions, at the very least the central venous pressure should be monitored, and kept between 5 and 12 mmHg, to prevent hypovolaemia.

For intravenous *glycerol*, meta-analysis of one minute trial (eight patients) and one moderately-sized controlled trial in patients with intracerebral haemorrhage failed to find evidence of benefit.[43,48]

Hypertonic saline is apparently 'emerging' in neurosurgical practice as an alternative to other agents,[49] but no controlled studies are available.

Corticosteroids

Corticosteroids reduce peritumoral oedema and at first sight it seems rational to expect a similar effect on oedematous brain tissue around an intracerebral haemorrhage. To date there have been four relevant but small trials, which have been summed up in a Cochrane review.[50] At 1 month after randomization 57 of 92 patients (62%) allocated to glucocorticoid treatment had died, compared with 50 of 94 patients (53%) allocated to the control group; relative risk 1.14 (95% CI, 0.91–1.42). Treatment with glucocorticoids did not reduce poor outcome at 1 month after randomization; relative risk, 0.95 (95% CI, 0.83–1.09; Fig. 13.2). The risk of any adverse effects in the treatment group (13%) was higher than that in the control group patients (8.8%) but the confidence interval was very wide; relative risk, RR 1.48 (95% CI, 0.87–2.51). The most common adverse effects were infections (23%), exacerbation of diabetes mellitus (11%) and gastrointestinal bleeding (5%) but none of them reached a statistically significant difference between the treatment and control groups. Thus, any benefit in terms of neurological function is moderate at best, whereas the adverse effects of corticosteroids in these patients are clearly substantial.[50]

> Mannitol is widely used in patients with intracerebral haemorrhage and a depressed level of consciousness, to decrease intracranial pressure and alleviate the space-occupying effect of the haemorrhage in a deteriorating patient, although this custom is not backed up by randomized trials with clinical status rather than pressure as the outcome variable. With corticosteroids the benefits have so far not been proved to outweigh the disadvantages.

13.3.3 Prevention of deep venous thrombosis and pulmonary embolism

(See also section 11.13.) Patients with ICH have a substantial risk of deep venous thrombosis (DVT):

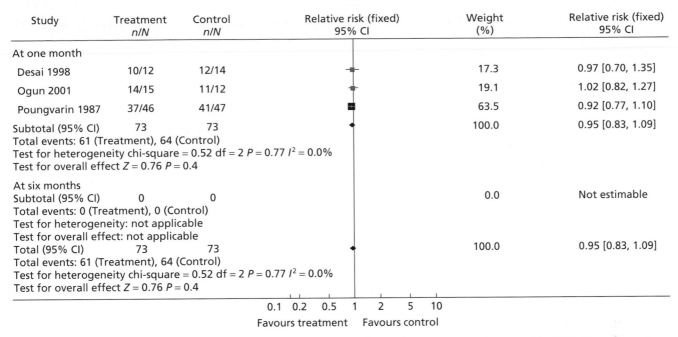

Study	Treatment n/N	Control n/N	Relative risk (fixed) 95% CI	Weight (%)	Relative risk (fixed) 95% CI
At one month					
Desai 1998	10/12	12/14		17.3	0.97 [0.70, 1.35]
Ogun 2001	14/15	11/12		19.1	1.02 [0.82, 1.27]
Poungvarin 1987	37/46	41/47		63.5	0.92 [0.77, 1.10]
Subtotal (95% CI)	73	73		100.0	0.95 [0.83, 1.09]

Total events: 61 (Treatment), 64 (Control)
Test for heterogeneity chi-square = 0.52 df = 2 P = 0.77 I^2 = 0.0%
Test for overall effect Z = 0.76 P = 0.4

At six months					
Subtotal (95% CI)	0	0		0.0	Not estimable

Total events: 0 (Treatment), 0 (Control)
Test for heterogeneity: not applicable
Test for overall effect: not applicable

Total (95% CI)	73	73		100.0	0.95 [0.83, 1.09]

Total events: 61 (Treatment), 64 (Control)
Test for heterogeneity chi-square = 0.52 df = 2 P = 0.77 I^2 = 0.0%
Test for overall effect Z = 0.76 P = 0.4

0.1 0.2 0.5 1 2 5 10
Favours treatment   Favours control

Fig. 13.2 Glucocorticoid treatment vs controls in intracerebral haemorrhage. The same conventions as in Fig. 13.1. The outcome is 'poor outcome at the end of follow up'.[50]

between 30% and 70%, depending on the severity of the stroke and the degree of immobilization, and on how hard one looks for it. The risk of pulmonary embolism has not been studied specifically for patients with haemorrhagic stroke, but extrapolation from what is known for ischaemic stroke or stroke in general the estimate is 1–2% in the first month (section 11.13).[51,52] However, physicians are intuitively cautious in using antithrombotic drugs in patients with intracerebral haemorrhages. On the other hand, drug regimens that prevent clotting as a consequence of venous stasis do not necessarily increase the risk of a small artery in the brain rupturing for a second time. The definitive answer should of course come from clinical trials, not theoretical considerations.

Subcutaneous heparin

Subcutaneous heparin, usually given as 5000 U two or three times a day, reduces the frequency of DVT by 68%, at least after general, orthopaedic and urological surgery.[53] In a small, but so far unique, clinical trial in 46 patients with ICH this regimen was applied 4 days after the onset in the active treatment group and 10 days after the haemorrhage in the control group.[54] In the control group 40% (9 of 23) developed some evidence of pulmonary embolism (as detected by perfusion scintigraphy of the lungs) against 22% (5 of 22) in the treated group. In a subsequent non-randomized study, in 68 patients with ICH, treatment was started on day 2, 4 or 10 after the haemorrhage.[55] For what it is worth, the risk of

pulmonary embolism was significantly lower in the group with treatment started on day 2, without a concomitant increase in rebleeding. But, as the group with early treatment was studied after the two other dosage groups, the results may well have been influenced by factors other than the interval until the initiation of treatment.

Aspirin

Aspirin is effective in reducing the risk of DVT (by approximately 39%) as well as pulmonary embolism in an overview of all trials in the perioperative period and in medical patients at increased risk (section 11.13). In a systematic review of all published trials comparing any antithrombotic agent with control among patients with any form of intracranial haemorrhage, there were two randomized trials in which aspirin had been inadvertently given (for variable periods) to 398 patients with acute ICH (and placebo to 375 patients).[56] The odds ratio (OR) for these ICH patients treated with aspirin was 0.96 (95% CI, 0.62–1.5) for death, and 1.02 (95% CI, 0.5–1.8) for recurrent haemorrhage. These scant data do not support reliable conclusions about the safety or otherwise of antithrombotic agents in patients with acute intracerebral haemorrhage.

Compression stockings and intermittent pneumatic compression

Physical methods are of course likely to be the safest method of thrombosis prevention in patients with ICH, although occasionally they may cause pressure sores (section 11.13). Essentially there are two methods: intermittent pneumatic compression, and graduated compression stockings which vary the pressure from being highest at the ankle and decreasing proximally. A systematic review of 16 trials (totalling more than 2200 patients) of graduated compression stockings in operated or otherwise immobilized patients for a variety of conditions found an odds ratio for deep venous thrombosis of 0.34 (95% CI, 0.25–0.46) if graduated pressure stockings was the only treatment, and of 0.24 (95% CI, 0.15–0.37) if they were used on a background of other prophylactic measures.[57] In stroke patients alone, two small trials (123 patients in all) could not demonstrate any such effect.[58]

A later trial tested intermittent pneumatic compression, specifically in 151 patients with ICH; all were also fitted with graduated elastic stockings.[59] On day 10, DVT (as assessed by compression ultrasonography) was found in 5% of the patients in the group with intermittent compression, against 16% in those with stockings alone, corresponding to a relative risk of 0.29 (95% CI, 0.08–1.00), a marginally significant difference.

Pulmonary embolism was not included in these systematic reviews, but there is no reason to assume that the relationship with DVT is different in patients with ICH. Also a significantly protective effect of compression stockings on the risk of pulmonary emboli has been demonstrated in a large trial of patients who underwent cardiothoracic operations.[60] Thus, unless the disadvantages of heparin are proved to be merely theoretical, application of graduated compression stockings, preferably supplemented with intermittent pneumatic compression, seems to offer the greatest protection and the smallest risk, although the method is fairly labour intensive and the stockings can be uncomfortable after a time. To resolve the existing uncertainties, a multicentre trial of graduated compression stockings has been initiated in the UK (section 11.13).

> Subcutaneous heparin and the application of graduated compression stockings both decrease the risk of deep venous thrombosis in bedridden patients by approximately 70%, and aspirin by approximately 39%, as judged from clinical trials in a variety of postoperative conditions. Because the safety of heparin and aspirin is largely unknown in patients with intracerebral haemorrhage, compression stockings are presently the preferred method of prophylaxis, despite being labour intensive, and despite the lack of direct evidence in patients with primary intracerebral haemorrhage.

13.3.4 Treatment of iatrogenic intracerebral haemorrhage

Anticoagulants

Anticoagulants are associated with an increased risk of intracerebral haemorrhage (section 8.4.1). It seems rational to reverse the deficiency of clotting factors as quickly as possible and to accept the risk of a thrombotic event, especially in view of the frequent progression of clinical deficits that occurs in these patients. Understandably the speed of treatment has never been put to the test in a clinical trial, but observational data confirm that early normalization of clotting status is associated with a relatively low rate of haemorrhage enlargement.[61] In current practice the first step is i.v. 10–20 mg vitamin K, at not more than 5 mg/min, rapidly followed by infusion of prothrombin complex concentrate (PCC), which contains the coagulation factors II, VII, IX and X;[62] every half hour counts in halting progression of the haemorrhage.[63] Infusion of these factors alone restores the coagulation system more rapidly than whole plasma and is safer from the point of view of transmission of virus particles (section 12.4.7).[64–66]

When to resume anticoagulants in patients with a strong indication for this treatment (e.g. those with mechanical heart valves) is a problem many clinicians will recognize. Only anecdotal experience is available, such as a series from the Mayo Clinic in which only one ischaemic stroke occurred in 52 patients with mechanical heart valves in whom anticoagulants were discontinued for a median period of 10 days,[67] in contrast to seven similar patients from Heidelberg in three of whom large brain infarcts occurred within 4 days of normalization of the international normalized ratio (INR).[68] The essential issue in deciding when to restart is probably not when blood has disappeared from the CT scan (that may take weeks or months), but when the ruptured vessel can be assumed to have sufficiently healed. Between 1–2 weeks after the haemorrhage – depending on the stringency of the indication – is probably not a bad guess.[69] No rebleeds were reported with such a regimen, although the numbers were small.[70,71]

Thrombolytic therapy

Thrombolytic therapy after myocardial infarction is complicated by intracerebral haemorrhage in only a small proportion (section 8.4.3), but the case fatality is high. This grim prognosis warrants attempts at intervention, even without the benefits of controlled clinical trials. These measures include control of any hypertension and infusion of coagulation factors; the use of antifibrinolytic drugs is controversial even from a theoretical point of view. Surgical treatment is hazardous, given that amyloid angiopathy is often a contributing factor (section 13.3.7). Life-threatening arrhythmias may occur as a complication of the myocardial infarct for which the treatment was given, often before the onset of the neurological symptoms, and these should of course be promptly treated.[72]

In patients with ischaemic stroke who develop major intracerebral haemorrhage after thrombolytic treatment (section 12.5.2) there is no evidence about what to do. In view of the little we know about operative treatment for intracerebral haemorrhage in general (section 13.3.5) it seems best to leave well alone. The utility of prothrombin complex concentrate or recombinant factor VIIa has not been studied so far.

Aspirin

Aspirin treatment is associated with a small risk of intracerebral haemorrhage (section 8.4.2). It is reasonable to stop the drug once the diagnosis has been made, although no disasters have been documented in instances in which aspirin treatment was continued, or even restarted. At any rate the antiplatelet effect lasts for several days after discontinuation of the drug.[73] In the trials of aspirin for secondary prevention after cerebral ischaemia some patients with small intracerebral haemorrhages must have been inadvertently included before CT scanning established the true diagnosis; there were no obviously untoward effects, but the confidence interval is still wide (section 12.3.3).[74] In patients on regular treatment with aspirin the outcome after ICH is relatively poor,[75] but this is explained by confounding factors; in a large observational study from Germany, the effect disappeared after adjustment for age and premorbid condition.[76]

13.3.5 Surgical treatment of supratentorial haemorrhage

The frequency of surgical intervention for intracerebral haemorrhage varies widely between centres, and even between participants in a clinical trial.[77] There are four possible surgical procedures to treat ICH: simple aspiration, craniotomy with open surgery, endoscopic evacuation, and stereotactic aspiration. Unless specifically indicated otherwise, the assumption is that we are mostly dealing with deep haemorrhages, from degenerative small vessel disease.

Simple aspiration

Aspiration, not accompanied by any other intervention, was attempted mainly in the 1950s but this was subsequently abandoned because only small amounts of clot could be obtained, and because the procedure could precipitate 'blind' rebleeding.[78,79]

Craniotomy

Open surgery was the method for removing haematomas in five trials, one of them (with 131 patients) dating from the pre-CT era. A Cochrane review (last updated in 1999) of this early study and two subsequent trials (totalling 64 randomized patients) in the 1980s showed a non-significant trend towards increased risk of death and dependency among survivors (odds ratio 1.99, 99% CI, 0.92–4.31). Two subsequent but small single-centre randomized trials (54 patients altogether) showed results that were entirely within the range of the overview.[80,81] A pseudo-randomized trial in Houston tested the optimal time for clot evacuation – assuming that the operation was indicated at all; in the experimental group patients were operated within 4 h of symptom onset, patients operated within 12 h forming the control group. The study was stopped early because of rebleeding in the 'ultra-early' group.[82]

The year 2005 saw publication of a landmark trial (STICH) that has substantially added to the modest information from controlled studies so far.[83] A total of 1003 patients were randomized, four times as many as in all previous trials taken together; all had supratentorial haemorrhage. In the group allocated to early operation (craniotomy in 75%) the procedure was scheduled within 24 h, whereas in the other group treatment was initially conservative. A second notable feature was the introduction of a 'sliding dichotomy' for assessing outcome, to take account of the methodological problem that expectations about the result of any treatment are higher when the initial condition of the patient is better.[84] The result was that the cut-off point for 'favourable outcome' depended on three prognostic features at baseline: level of consciousness on the Glasgow Coma Scale, age and volume of the haemorrhage. For 516 patients with a good prognostic profile on admission a favourable outcome included only the categories 'good recovery' and 'moderate disability' on the extended Glasgow outcome scale, whereas for the other half of the study patients with a poorer prognosis 'severe disability' was included in the definition of a favourable outcome.[85]

The analysis of outcome after 6 months failed to show any benefit of craniotomy: of patients randomized to early surgery, 122 (26%) had a favourable outcome compared with 118 (24%) of those randomized to initially conservative treatment; odds ratio 0.89 (95% CI, 0.66–1.19). Separate analysis of 12 prespecified subgroups showed that operation was perhaps beneficial in patients with superficial haemorrhages (1 cm or less from the cortical surface), but of course this may be chance effect. The efficacy of operative treatment did not significantly differ between patients with deep haemorrhages (approximately 60%) and those with lobar haemorrhage.

No systematic review has yet been completed that included this major trial with the five small trials performed previously, but of course such an analysis will not change the current conclusion that – as a routine – craniotomy is not the treatment of choice in patients with intracerebral haemorrhage. A question not addressed by the STICH trial is whether operation improves outcome in patients deteriorating because of haemorrhage expansion. A consecutive series of 26 such patients from the Mayo Clinic (of whom 24 had lobar haemorrhage) reported that no patient regained independence – with or without operation – if corneal and oculocephalic reflexes had been lost, but that approximately one-quarter of the remaining group (6 of 21) did regain independence.[86]

> Given the present state of knowledge routine craniotomy and evacuation of the haemorrhage is not indicated for patients with supratentorial haemorrhage, deep or lobar. No subgroup of patients has yet been reliably identified for whom operation might be beneficial.

Endoscopic evacuation

There are enthusiasts for almost any conceivable type of operation. Endoscopic evacuation of brain haemorrhage by stereotactic methods is no exception.[87,88] The only controlled study so far involved two groups of 50 patients.[89] The authors' interpretation was that surgery had no effect in putaminal and thalamic haemorrhage, but that it was beneficial in subcortical haemorrhages, provided patients are aged 60 years or less and are alert or somnolent. The problem with this analysis is not only that it depends on subgroups, but also no overall analysis was reported and some outcome categories were not reported at all. Recalculation of the results for all patients according to the proportion who were dead or dependent showed an odds ratio of 0.45 in favour of endoscopic operation, but this was not statistically significant (95% CI, 0.19–1.04).[90] In conclusion, stereotactic endoscopic evacuation is a promising technique, but its benefits and specific indications remain to be confirmed by well-conducted and large clinical trials.

Stereotactic aspiration with thrombolysis

Since the 1990s, stereotactic aspiration without endoscopy, mostly combined with instillation of fibrinolytic

agents, has been reported in several observational studies involving hundreds of patients with supratentorial haemorrhage; some of these concentrated on haemorrhages with intraventricular extension.[34] Subsequently two controlled trials of this technique have been performed. A Japanese trial randomized 242 patients with putaminal haemorrhage and a moderately decreased level of consciousness (eyes closed but opened to stimuli) between stereotactic haemorrhage evacuation and conservative treatment. Outcome, assessed by a blinded observer in terms of independence, was better in the surgical group.[91] A smaller trial in the Netherlands (70 patients) combined stereotactic aspiration with liquefaction by means of a plasminogen activating substance; no conclusive differences emerged.[92]

13.3.6 Surgical treatment of infratentorial haemorrhage

Cerebellar haemorrhage

Cerebellar haemorrhages (Figs 8.29 and 13.3) have fairly characteristic clinical features (section 3.3.7), with the exception of massive haemorrhages, which are clinically

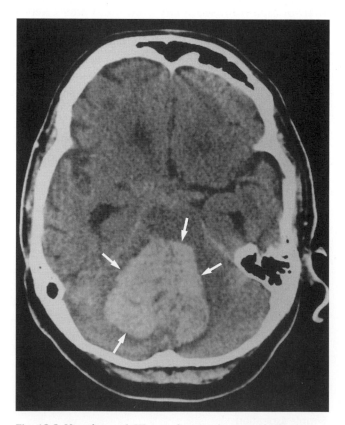

Fig. 13.3 Unenhanced CT scan showing large cerebellar haematoma.

indistinguishable from brainstem strokes, and very small haemorrhages which may simulate a peripheral disorder of the vestibular system.[93] For decades there has been a strong impression that surgical evacuation saves lives in patients with cerebellar haemorrhages who have clinical evidence of progressive brainstem compression.[94] The need for timely surgical treatment in patients who are in danger of progressive brainstem compression is dictated on the one hand by the potentially fatal outcome and on the other hand by the often surprisingly mild sequelae after operation.[95] So strong is this notion, that a clinical trial in this category of patients is as unlikely to be mounted as it would be in acute appendicitis. This is not to say there are no areas of controversy.

First, there is no doubt that some patients can be managed conservatively, but there is uncertainty about the selection criteria.[96,97] In general, an impaired level of consciousness (that is, a Glasgow Coma Scale Score of 13/15 or less) seems a good indication for operative intervention, provided corneal and oculocephalic reflexes have not been lost, in which case the outcome is invariably fatal.[98] Some neurosurgeons advocate surgery with large haemorrhages (>3–4 cm in diameter), even in alert patients, on the basis of experience that delayed deterioration of consciousness may be so rapid that the patient cannot be salvaged at this later stage.[99] Others maintain that such rapid deterioration depends not so much on the absolute size of the haemorrhage as on the degree of effacement of the fourth ventricle and that operative evacuation is indicated in all patients in whom the fourth ventricle is completely obliterated.[100] Since effacement of the fourth ventricle is associated with hydrocephalus and location of the haemorrhage in the midline (vermis), it is not surprising that these features also predispose to secondary deterioration.[101] A rare category of cerebellar haemorrhages are those associated with neurosurgical operations (for any lesion) in the supratentorial compartment, so-called 'remote cerebellar haemorrhages'.[102] The pathogenesis is unclear, while the clinical course is almost invariably self-limiting.

A second contentious issue is that in the past some neurosurgeons have argued that it is not direct compression of the brainstem but obstructive hydrocephalus that is the main problem, and that ventriculostomy is a sufficient measure to prevent a fatal outcome.[103] However, there are two major objections against ventricular shunting as a panacea for cerebellar haemorrhages. The first is the rapid disappearance of pupillary, corneal and oculocephalic reflexes testifying brainstem compression in some patients for whom operation is too late, something not seen with acute hydrocephalus from other causes.[104] The second is the frequent failure of ventricular shunting to improve the level of consciousness.[105] Nevertheless we do not wish to deny that ventriculostomy can be the only effective treatment in some patients with appropriate clinical features of hydrocephalus, i.e. in whom deterioration of consciousness is gradual, with sustained downward gaze and small unreactive pupils but no signs of pontine compression.[100]

> Surgical evacuation of cerebellar haemorrhages can be life-saving, often with surprisingly few neurological sequelae. Sound indications for evacuation are the combination of a depressed level of consciousness with signs of progressive brainstem compression (unless all brainstem reflexes have been lost for more than a few hours, in which case a fatal outcome is inevitable), or haemorrhage diameter is greater than 3–4 cm. If the patient has a depressed level of consciousness and hydrocephalus, without signs of brainstem compression and with a haemorrhage less than 3 cm, ventriculostomy can be carried out as an initial (and perhaps only) procedure.

As with supratentorial haemorrhage, some patients with cerebellar haemorrhage have been successfully treated by stereotactic aspiration, with or without instillation of fibrinolytic drugs.[106] Any advantage of these techniques over the conventional approach with suboccipital craniotomy remains to be proved. The same applies to ventriculostomy by endoscopic perforation of the third ventricle towards the basal cisterns,[107] rather than by the conventional method of a catheter inserted in the lateral ventricle.

Pontine haemorrhage

Pontine haemorrhages (Figs 8.31 and 13.4) are not as invariably fatal as when the diagnosis could only be made at postmortem, but the case fatality is still around 50%.[17,108] The outcome depends to an important extent on the cause, since haemorrhage in the pons from a cavernous malformation is rarely fatal.[109] Cavernous malformations are separately dealt with below (section 13.3.8). The management of patients with 'hypertensive' pontine haemorrhage is usually conservative, but some case reports have documented successful stereotactic aspiration.[110] The natural history may or may not have been influenced by these interventions, and surgical failures in similar cases are likely to receive rather less publicity. There is an extremely narrow margin of uncertainty between patients with poor prognosis because of absent corneal and oculocephalic reflexes and those with small haemorrhages who will do well with conservative management.

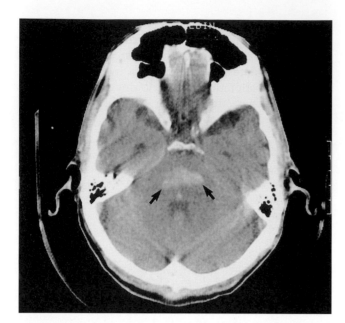

Fig. 13.4 Unenhanced CT brain scan showing a pontine haematoma (*arrows*) in a patient who walked, unsteadily, into (and out of) the outpatient clinic.

13.3.7 Treatment of lobar haemorrhage from (presumed) amyloid angiopathy

In patients with lobar haemorrhage from presumed amyloid angiopathy and an impaired level of consciousness the prognosis is often poor after surgical intervention.[111] Uncontrolled series with a large proportion of survivors after operative treatment fail to answer the question whether the outcome would have been worse without intervention.[112,113] Given these uncertainties and the danger that the operation provokes new haemorrhages from brittle vessels at distant sites,[114] conservative treatment seems the best option unless a deteriorating level of consciousness justifies the risk of operation.

13.3.8 Treatment of cavernous malformations

For cavernous malformations in a cerebral hemisphere or in the cerebellum, any intervention is exceptional, because recurrent haemorrhages from these lesions are usually limited in severity (section 8.2.5). Series with operated patients have been published,[115] but these underline rather than answer the question whether surgical treatment really improves on the natural history. The management of cavernous malformations in the brainstem is also controversial, since the natural history often is rather favourable, regardless of location.[116] Probably pressure from patients themselves accounts for some of the operations.

There is little doubt that (recurrent) haemorrhages from cavernous malformations are less destructive than brainstem haemorrhages from an arterial source.[109] Also the lesions may spontaneously regress.[117] Successes of surgical treatment make it to a publication,[118] but the failure rate can only be guessed at. At any rate incomplete removal can prompt rebleeding.[119]

Stereotactic cobalt-generated radiation ('gamma knife') has been applied to a large number of patients with cavernous malformations; there is no controlled evidence for the efficacy of this treatment and nothing more than a suggestion that seizures or episodes of rebleeding are less likely to occur afterwards.[120,121]

> Cavernous malformations, whether in a cerebral hemisphere or in the brainstem, carry a moderate risk of (re)bleeding, while the functional deficits from such haemorrhages are limited. Surgical treatment or stereotactic radiation is regularly performed but there are no randomized controlled studies.

13.3.9 Treatment of dural arteriovenous fistulae

These malformations are heterogeneous, in that they may or may not be secondary to occlusion of a major sinus and that the abnormal venous drainage from meningeal arteries may be channelled into a dural sinus or into superficial veins on the surface of the brain, cerebellum, or brainstem (section 8.2.8). Accordingly, there is a large variety of methods used to occlude the fistula. Surgical techniques include selective ligation of leptomeningeal draining veins,[122,123] resection of fistulous sinus tracts,[122] and a cranial base approach with extradural bone removal.[124] Endovascular techniques may consist of an approach from the arterial or venous side,[125,126] recanalization and stenting of a venous sinus,[127] or venous embolization via a craniotomy.[128] Finally stereotactic cobalt-generated radiation ('gamma knife') is also used for obliterating arteriovenous fistulae,[129,130] sometimes in conjunction with an endovascular approach.[131]

13.3.10 Treatment of moyamoya syndrome associated with haemorrhage

Gradual stenosis or occlusion of the terminal portions of the internal carotid arteries or proximal middle cerebral arteries, most often the result of an idiopathic proliferative process of the endothelial layer, may lead to the formation of an abnormal collateral network of fragile collaterals, which occasionally rupture (sections 8.2.12 and 7.5). To relieve the pressure on the collaterals by constructing a bypass such as between the superficial temporal artery and the middle cerebral artery is a logical idea,[132] but whether this indeed prevents (re)bleeding remains uncertain. In fact an aneurysm may form and rupture at the site of the arterial bypass.[133]

References

1 Rosand J, Eskey C, Chang Y, Gonzalez RG, Greenberg SM, Koroshetz WJ. Dynamic single-section CT demonstrates reduced cerebral blood flow in acute intracerebral hemorrhage. *Cerebrovasc Dis* 2002; **14**:214–20.

2 Castillo J, Dávalos A, Alvarez-Sabín J *et al*. Molecular signatures of brain injury after intracerebral hemorrhage. *Neurology* 2002; **58**:624–9.

3 Butcher KS, Baird T, MacGregor L, Desmond P, Tress B, Davis S. Perihematomal edema in primary intracerebral hemorrhage is plasma derived. *Stroke* 2004; **35**:1879–85.

4 Gebel JM, Jr., Jauch EC, Brott TG *et al*. Natural history of perihematomal edema in patients with hyperacute spontaneous intracerebral hemorrhage. *Stroke* 2002; **33**:2631–5.

5 Siddique MS, Fernandes HM, Wooldridge TD, Fenwick JD, Slomka P, Mendelow AD. Reversible ischemia around intracerebral hemorrhage: a single-photon emission computerized tomography study. *J Neurosurg* 2002; **96**:736–41.

6 Bhattathiri PS, Gregson B, Prasad KS, Mendelow AD. Intraventricular hemorrhage and hydrocephalus after spontaneous intracerebral hemorrhage: results from the STICH trial. *Acta Neurochir Suppl* 2006; **96**:65–8.

7 Dennis MS. Outcome after brain haemorrhage. *Cerebrovasc Dis* 2003; **16**(Suppl 1):9–13.

8 Flaherty ML, Haverbusch M, Sekar P *et al*. Long-term mortality after intracerebral hemorrhage. *Neurology* 2006; **66**:1182–6.

9 Ariesen MJ, Algra A, Van der Worp HB, Rinkel GJE. Applicability and relevance of models that predict short term outcome after intracerebral haemorrhage. *J Neurol Neurosurg Psychiatry* 2005; **76**:839–44.

10 Weimar C, Benemann J, Diener HC, for the German Stroke Study Collaboration. Development and validation of the Essen Intracerebral Haemorrhage Score. *J Neurol Neurosurg Psychiatry* 2006; **77**:601–5.

11 Becker KJ, Baxter AB, Cohen WA *et al*. Withdrawal of support in intracerebral hemorrhage may lead to self-fulfilling prophecies. *Neurology* 2001; **56**:766–72.

12 Delgado P, Alvarez-Sabin J, Abilleira S *et al*. Plasma d-dimer predicts poor outcome after acute intracerebral hemorrhage. *Neurology* 2006; **67**:94–8.

13 Hays A, Diringer MN. Elevated troponin levels are associated with higher mortality following intracerebral hemorrhage. *Neurology* 2006; **66**:1330–4.

14 Roquer J, Rodriguez CA, Gomis M, Ois A, Munteis E, Bohm P. Serum lipid levels and in-hospital mortality in patients with intracerebral hemorrhage. *Neurology* 2005; **65**:1198–202.

15 Flemming KD, Wijdicks EFM, Li HZ. Can we predict poor outcome at presentation in patients with lobar hemorrhage? *Cerebrovasc Dis* 2001; **11**:183–9.

16 Liliang PC, Liang CL, Lu CH *et al*. Hypertensive caudate hemorrhage prognostic predictor, outcome, and role of external ventricular drainage. *Stroke* 2001; **32**:1195–200.

17 Wijdicks EFM, St. Louis E. Clinical profiles predictive of outcome in pontine hemorrhage. *Neurology* 1997; **49**:1342–6.

18 Davis SM, Broderick J, Hennerici M *et al*. Hematoma growth is a determinant of mortality and poor outcome after intracerebral hemorrhage. *Neurology* 2006; **66**:1175–81.

19 Schwarz S, Häfner K, Aschoff A, Schwab S. Incidence and prognostic significance of fever following intracerebral hemorrhage. *Neurology* 2000; **54**:354–61.

20 Gebel JM, Jr., Jauch EC, Brott TG *et al*. Relative edema volume is a predictor of outcome in patients with hyperacute spontaneous intracerebral hemorrhage. *Stroke* 2002; **33**:2636–41.

21 Ronning OM, Guldvog B, Stavem K. The benefit of an acute stroke unit in patients with intracranial haemorrhage: a controlled trial. *J Neurol Neurosurg Psychiatry* 2001; **70**:631–4.

22 Friederich PW, Henny CP, Messelink EJ *et al*. Effect of recombinant activated factor VII on perioperative blood loss in patients undergoing retropubic prostatectomy: a double-blind placebo-controlled randomised trial. *Lancet* 2003; **361**:201–5.

23 You H, Al-Shahi R. Haemostatic drug therapies for acute primary intracerebral haemorrhage. *Cochrane Database Syst Rev* 2006; CD005951.

24 Earnshaw SR, Joshi AV, Wilson MR, Rosand J. Cost-effectiveness of recombinant activated factor VII in the treatment of intracerebral hemorrhage. *Stroke* 2006; **37**:2751–8.

25 Tomson J, Lip GY. Blood pressure changes in acute haemorrhagic stroke. *Blood Press Monit* 2005; **10**:197–9.

26 Ohwaki K, Yano E, Nagashima H, Hirata M, Nakagomi T, Tamura A. Blood pressure management in acute intracerebral hemorrhage: relationship between elevated blood pressure and hematoma enlargement. *Stroke* 2004; **35**:1364–7.

27 Qureshi AI, Mohammad YM, Yahia AM *et al*. A prospective multicenter study to evaluate the feasibility and safety of aggressive antihypertensive treatment in patients with acute intracerebral hemorrhage. *J Intensive Care Med* 2005; **20**:34–42.

28 Arakawa S, Saku Y, Ibayashi S, Nagao T, Fujishima M. Blood pressure control and recurrence of hypertensive brain hemorrhage. *Stroke* 1998; **29**:1806–9.

29 Broderick JP, Adams HP, Jr., Barsan W *et al*. Guidelines for the management of spontaneous intracerebral hemorrhage: a statement for healthcare professionals from a special writing group of the Stroke Council, American Heart Association. *Stroke* 1999; **30**:905–15.

30 Guyot LL, Dowling C, Diaz FG, Michael DB. Cerebral monitoring devices: analysis of complications. *Acta Neurochir Suppl* 1998; **71**:47–9.

31 Cremer OL, van Dijk GW, van Wensen E *et al*. Effect of intracranial pressure monitoring and targeted intensive care on functional outcome after severe head injury. *Crit Care Med* 2005; **33**:2207–13.

32 Adams RE, Diringer MN. Response to external ventricular drainage in spontaneous intracerebral hemorrhage with hydrocephalus. *Neurology* 1998; **50**:519–23.

33 Holtzman RN, Brust JC, Ainyette IG *et al*. Acute ventricular hemorrhage in adults with hydrocephalus managed by corpus callosotomy and fenestration of the septum pellucidum. Report of three cases. *J Neurosurg* 2001; **95**:111–15.

34 Nieuwkamp DJ, de Gans K, Rinkel GJE, Algra A. Treatment and outcome of severe intraventricular extension in patients with subarachnoid or intracerebral hemorrhage: a systematic review of the literature. *J Neurol* 2000; **247**:117–21.

35 Lapointe M, Haines S. Fibrinolytic therapy for intraventricular hemorrhage in adults. *Cochrane Database Syst Rev* 2002; CD003692.

36 Lee MW, Pang KY, Ho WW, Wong CK. Outcome analysis of intraventricular thrombolytic therapy for intraventricular haemorrhage. *Hong Kong Med J* 2003; **9**:335–40.

37 Fountas KN, Kapsalaki EZ, Parish DC *et al*. Intraventricular administration of rt-PA in patients with intraventricular hemorrhage. *South Med J* 2005; **98**:767–73.

38 Stocchetti N, Maas AI, Chieregato A, van der Plas AA. Hyperventilation in head injury: a review. *Chest* 2005; **127**:1812–27.

39 Muizelaar JP, Marmarou A, Ward JD *et al*. Adverse effects of prolonged hyperventilation in patients with severe head injury: a randomized clinical trial. *J Neurosurg* 1991; **75**:731–9.

40 Schierhout G, Roberts I. Hyperventilation therapy for acute traumatic brain injury. *Cochrane Database Syst Rev* 2000; CD000566.

41 Nau R. Osmotherapy for elevated intracranial pressure: a critical reappraisal. *Clin Pharmacokinet* 2000; **38**:23–40.

42 Bettmann MA. Frequently asked questions: iodinated contrast agents. *Radiographics* 2004; **24**(Suppl 1):S3–10.

43 Yu YL, Kumana CR, Lauder IJ *et al*. Treatment of acute cerebral hemorrhage with intravenous glycerol. A double-blind, placebo-controlled, randomized trial. *Stroke* 1992; **23**:967–71.

44 Bereczki D, Liu M, do Prado GF, Fekete I. Mannitol for acute stroke. *Cochrane Database Syst Rev* 2001; CD001153.

45 Misra UK, Kalita J, Ranjan P, Mandal SK. Mannitol in intracerebral hemorrhage: a randomized controlled study. *J Neurol Sci* 2005; **234**:41–5.

46 Dziedzic T, Szczudlik A, Klimkowicz A, Rog TM, Slowik A. Is mannitol safe for patients with intracerebral hemorrhages? Renal considerations. *Clin Neurol Neurosurg* 2003; **105**:87–9.

47 Cruz J, Minoja G, Okuchi K. Major clinical and physiological benefits of early high doses of mannitol for intraparenchymal temporal lobe hemorrhages with abnormal pupillary widening: a randomized trial. *Neurosurgery* 2002; **51**:628–37.

48 Righetti E, Celani MG, Cantisani T, Sterzi R, Boysen G, Ricci S. Glycerol for acute stroke. *Cochrane Database Syst Rev* 2004; CD000096.

49 Ogden AT, Mayer SA, Connolly ES, Jr. Hyperosmolar agents in neurosurgical practice: the evolving role of hypertonic saline. *Neurosurgery* 2005; **57**:207–15.

50 Feigin VL, Anderson N, Rinkel GJ, Algra A, van Gijn J, Bennett DA. Corticosteroids for aneurysmal subarachnoid haemorrhage and primary intracerebral haemorrhage. *Cochrane Database Syst Rev* 2005; CD004583.

51 Davenport RJ, Dennis MS, Wellwood I, Warlow CP. Complications after acute stroke. *Stroke* 1996; **27**:415–20.

52 Kelly J, Hunt BJ, Lewis RR, Rudd A. Anticoagulation or inferior vena cava filter placement for patients with primary intracerebral hemorrhage developing venous thromboembolism? *Stroke* 2003; **34**:2999–3005.

53 Collins R, Scrimgeour A, Yusuf S, Peto R. Reduction in fatal pulmonary embolism and venous thrombosis by perioperative administration of subcutaneous heparin. Overview of results of randomized trials in general, orthopedic, and urologic surgery. *N Engl J Med* 1988; **318**:1162–73.

54 Dickmann U, Voth E, Schicha H, Henze T, Prange H, Emrich D. Heparin therapy, deep-vein thrombosis and pulmonary embolism after intracerebral hemorrhage. *Klin Wochenschr* 1988; **66**:1182–3.

55 Boeer A, Voth E, Henze T, Prange HW. Early heparin therapy in patients with spontaneous intracerebral haemorrhage. *J Neurol Neurosurg Psychiatry* 1991; **54**:466–7.

56 Keir SL, Lewis SC, Wardlaw JM, Sandercock PA, on behalf of IST and CAST collaborative groups. Effect of aspirin or heparin inadvertently given to patients with hemorrhagic stroke. *Stroke* 2000; **31**:314.

57 Amaragiri SV, Lees TA. Elastic compression stockings for prevention of deep vein thrombosis. *Cochrane Database Syst Rev* 2000; CD001484.

58 Mazzone C, Chiodo GF, Sandercock P, Miccio M, Salvi R. Physical methods for preventing deep vein thrombosis in stroke. *Cochrane Database Syst Rev* 2004; CD001922.

59 Lacut K, Bressollette L, Le Gal G *et al*. Prevention of venous thrombosis in patients with acute intracerebral hemorrhage. *Neurology* 2005; **65**:865–9.

60 Ramos R, Salem BI, De Pawlikowski MP, Coordes C, Eisenberg S, Leidenfrost R. The efficacy of pneumatic compression stockings in the prevention of pulmonary embolism after cardiac surgery. *Chest* 1996; **109**:82–5.

61 Yasaka M, Minematsu K, Naritomi H, Sakata T, Yamaguchi T. Predisposing factors for enlargement

of intracerebral hemorrhage in patients treated with warfarin. *Thromb Haemost* 2003; **89**:278–83.

62 Steiner T, Rosand J, Diringer M. Intracerebral hemorrhage associated with oral anticoagulant therapy: current practices and unresolved questions. *Stroke* 2006; **37**:256–62.

63 Goldstein JN, Thomas SH, Frontiero V *et al.* Timing of fresh frozen plasma administration and rapid correction of coagulopathy in warfarin-related intracerebral hemorrhage. *Stroke* 2006; **37**:151–5.

64 Makris M, Greaves M, Phillips WS, Kitchen S, Rosendaal FR, Preston FE. Emergency oral anticoagulant reversal: the relative efficacy of infusions of fresh frozen plasma and clotting factor concentrate on correction of the coagulopathy. *Thromb Haemost* 1997; **77**:477–80.

65 Butler AC, Tait RC. Management of oral anticoagulant-induced intracranial haemorrhage. *Blood Rev* 1998; **12**:35–44.

66 Huttner HB, Schellinger PD, Hartmann M *et al.* Hematoma growth and outcome in treated neurocritical care patients with intracerebral hemorrhage related to oral anticoagulant therapy: comparison of acute treatment strategies using vitamin K, fresh frozen plasma, and prothrombin complex concentrates. *Stroke* 2006; **37**:1465–70.

67 Phan TG, Koh M, Wijdicks EFM. Safety of discontinuation of anticoagulation in patients with intracranial hemorrhage at high thromboembolic risk. *Arch Neurol* 2000; **57**:1710–13.

68 Bertram M, Bonsanto M, Hacke W, Schwab S. Managing the therapeutic dilemma: patients with spontaneous intracerebral hemorrhage and urgent need for anticoagulation. *J Neurol* 2000; **247**:209–14.

69 Estol CJ, Kase CS. Need for continued use of anticoagulants after intracerebral hemorrhage. *Curr Treat Options Cardiovasc Med* 2003; **5**:201–9.

70 Wijdicks EFM, Schievink WI, Brown RD, Mullany CJ. The dilemma of discontinuation of anticoagulation therapy for patients with intracranial hemorrhage and mechanical heart valves. *Neurosurgery* 1998; **42**:769–73.

71 Leker RR, Abramsky O. Early anticoagulation in patients with prosthetic heart valves and intracerebral hematoma. *Neurology* 1998; **50**:1489–91.

72 Sloan MA, Price TR, Petito CK *et al.* Clinical features and pathogenesis of intracerebral hemorrhage after rt-PA and heparin therapy for acute myocardial infarction: The Thrombolysis in Myocardial Infarction (TIMI) II pilot and randomized clinical trial combined experience. *Neurology* 1995; **45**:649–58.

73 Patrono C. Aspirin as an antiplatelet drug. *N Engl J Med* 1994; **330**:1287–94.

74 Keir SL, Wardlaw JM, Sandercock PAG, Chen ZM. Antithrombotic therapy in patients with any form of intracranial haemorrhage: a systematic review of the available controlled studies. *Cerebrovasc Dis* 2002; **14**:197–206.

75 Saloheimo P, Ahonen M, Juvela S, Pyhtinen J, Savolainen ER, Hillbom M. Regular aspirin-use preceding the onset of

primary intracerebral hemorrhage is an independent predictor for death. *Stroke* 2006; **37**:129–33.

76 Foerch C, Sitzer M, Steinmetz H, Neumann-Haefelin T. Pretreatment with antiplatelet agents is not independently associated with unfavorable outcome in intracerebral hemorrhage. *Stroke* 2006; **37**:2165–7.

77 Gregson BA, Mendelow AD. International variations in surgical practice for spontaneous intracerebral hemorrhage. *Stroke* 2003; **34**:2593–7.

78 McKissock W, Richardson A, Walsh L. Primary intracerebral haematoma: results of surgical treatment in 244 consecutive cases. *Lancet* 1959; **ii**:683–6.

79 Mitsuno T, Kanaya H, Shirakata S, Ohsawa K, Ishikawa Y. Surgical treatment of hypertensive intracerebral hemorrhage. *J Neurosurg* 1966; **24**:70–6.

80 Morgenstern LB, Frankowski RF, Shedden P, Pasteur W, Grotta JC. Surgical treatment for intracerebral hemorrhage (STICH): a single-center, randomized clinical trial. *Neurology* 1998; **51**:1359–63.

81 Zuccarello M, Brott T, Derex L *et al.* Early surgical treatment for supratentorial intracerebral hemorrhage: a randomized feasibility study. *Stroke* 1999; **30**:1833–9.

82 Morgenstern LB, Demchuk AM, Kim DH, Frankowski RF, Grotta JC. Rebleeding leads to poor outcome in ultra-early craniotomy for intracerebral hemorrhage. *Neurology* 2001; **56**:1294–9.

83 Mendelow AD, Gregson BA, Fernandes HM *et al.* Early surgery versus initial conservative treatment in patients with spontaneous supratentorial intracerebral haematomas in the International Surgical Trial in Intracerebral Haemorrhage (STICH): a randomised trial. *Lancet* 2005; **365**:387–97.

84 Murray GD, Barer D, Choi S *et al.* Design and analysis of phase III trials with ordered outcome scales: the concept of the sliding dichotomy. *J Neurotrauma* 2005; **22**:511–17.

85 Mendelow AD, Teasdale GM, Barer D, Fernandes HM, Murray GD, Gregson BA. Outcome assignment in the International Surgical Trial of Intracerebral Haemorrhage. *Acta Neurochir (Wien)* 2003; **145**:679–81.

86 Rabinstein AA, Atkinson JL, Wijdicks EFM. Emergency craniotomy in patients worsening due to expanded cerebral hematoma: to what purpose? *Neurology* 2002; **58**:1367–72.

87 Qiu Y, Lin Y, Tian X, Luo Q. Hypertensive intracranial hematomas: endoscopic-assisted keyhole evacuation and application of patent viewing dissector. *Chin Med J (Engl)* 2003; **116**:195–9.

88 Nishihara T, Nagata K, Tanaka S *et al.* Newly developed endoscopic instruments for the removal of intracerebral hematoma. *Neurocrit Care* 2005; **2**:67–74.

89 Auer LM, Deinsberger W, Niederkorn K *et al.* Endoscopic surgery versus medical treatment for spontaneous intracerebral hematoma: a randomized study. *J Neurosurg* 1989; **70**:530–5.

90 Hankey GJ, Hon C. Surgery for primary intracerebral hemorrhage: Is it safe and effective? A systematic review of case series and randomized trials. *Stroke* 1997; **28**:2126–32.

91 Hattori N, Katayama Y, Maya Y, Gatherer A. Impact of stereotactic hematoma evacuation on activities of daily living during the chronic period following spontaneous putaminal hemorrhage: a randomized study. *J Neurosurg* 2004; **101**:417–20.

92 Teernstra OP, Evers SM, Lodder J, Leffers P, Franke CL, Blaauw G. Stereotactic treatment of intracerebral hematoma by means of a plasminogen activator: a multicenter randomized controlled trial (SICHPA). *Stroke* 2003; **34**:968–74.

93 Jensen MB, St Louis EK. Management of acute cerebellar stroke. *Arch Neurol* 2005; **62**:537–44.

94 Fisher CM, Picard EH, Polak A, Dalal P, Ojemann R. Acute hypertensive cerebellar hemorrhage. *J Nerv Ment Dis* 1965; **140**:38–57.

95 Cohen ZR, Ram Z, Knoller N, Peles E, Hadani M. Management and outcome of non-traumatic cerebellar haemorrhage. *Cerebrovasc Dis* 2002; **14**:207–13.

96 Wijdicks EFM, Louis EKS, Atkinson JD, Li HZ. Clinician's biases toward surgery in cerebellar hematomas: an analysis of decision-making in 94 patients. *Cerebrovasc Dis* 2000; **10**:93–6.

97 Wessels PH, Ter Berg JWM, Spincemaille GH, Dippel DWJ. Treatment of cerebellar hematoma in the Netherlands: a questionnaire survey. *Cerebrovasc Dis* 2001; **11**:190–4.

98 St Louis EK, Wijdicks EFM, Li HZ, Atkinson JD. Predictors of poor outcome in patients with a spontaneous cerebellar hematoma. *Can J Neurol Sci* 2000; **27**:32–6.

99 Kobayashi S, Sato A, Kageyama Y, Nakamura H, Watanabe Y, Yamaura A. Treatment of hypertensive cerebellar hemorrhage: surgical or conservative management? *Neurosurgery* 1994; **34**:246–50.

100 Kirollos RW, Tyagi AK, Ross SA, Van Hille PT, Marks PV. Management of spontaneous cerebellar hematomas: a prospective treatment protocol. *Neurosurgery* 2001; **49**:1378–86.

101 St Louis EK, Wijdicks EFM, Li HZ. Predicting neurologic deterioration in patients with cerebellar hematomas. *Neurology* 1998; **51**:1364–9.

102 Amini A, Osborn AG, McCall TD, Couldwell WT. Remote cerebellar hemorrhage. *Am J Neuroradiol* 2006; **27**:387–90.

103 Shenkin HA, Zavala H. Cerebellar strokes: mortality, surgical indications, and results of ventricular drainage. *Lancet* 1982; **ii**:429–31.

104 Van Gijn J, Hijdra A, Wijdicks EFM, Vermeulen M, van Crevel H. Acute hydrocephalus after aneurysmal subarachnoid hemorrhage. *J Neurosurg* 1985; **63**:355–62.

105 Mathew P, Teasdale G, Bannan A, Oluoch-Olunya D. Neurosurgical management of cerebellar haematoma and infarct. *J Neurol Neurosurg Psychiatry* 1995; **59**:287–92.

106 Mohadjer M, Eggert R, May J, Mayfrank L. CT-guided stereotactic fibrinolysis of spontaneous and hypertensive cerebellar hemorrhage: long-term results. *J Neurosurg* 1990; **73**:217–22.

107 Roux FE, Boetto S, Tremoulet M. Third ventriculocisternostomy in cerebellar haematomas. *Acta Neurochir (Wien)* 2002; **144**:337–42.

108 Balci K, Asil T, Kerimoglu M, Celik Y, Utku U. Clinical and neuroradiological predictors of mortality in patients with primary pontine hemorrhage. *Clin Neurol Neurosurg* 2005; **108**:36–9.

109 Rabinstein AA, Tisch SH, McClelland RL, Wijdicks EFM. Cause is the main predictor of outcome in patients with pontine hemorrhage. *Cerebrovasc Dis* 2004; **17**:66–71.

110 Shitamichi M, Nakamura J, Sasaki T, Suematsu K, Tokuda S. Computed tomography guided stereotactic aspiration of pontine hemorrhages. *Stereotact Funct Neurosurg* 1990; **54–55**:453–6.

111 McCarron MO, Nicoll JA, Love S, Ironside JW. Surgical intervention, biopsy and APOE genotype in cerebral amyloid angiopathy-related haemorrhage. *Br J Neurosurg* 1999; **13**:462–7.

112 Greene GM, Godersky JC, Biller J, Hart MN, Adams HP, Jr. Surgical experience with cerebral amyloid angiopathy. *Stroke* 1990; **21**:1545–9.

113 Izumihara A, Ishihara T, Iwamoto N, Yamashita K, Ito H. Postoperative outcome of 37 patients with lobar intracerebral hemorrhage related to cerebral amyloid angiopathy. *Stroke* 1999; **30**:29–33.

114 Brisman MH, Bederson JB, Sen CN, Germano IM, Moore F, Post KD. Intracerebral hemorrhage occurring remote from the craniotomy site. *Neurosurgery* 1996; **39**:1114–21.

115 Zotta D, Di RA, Scogna A, Ricci A, Ricci G, Galzio RJ. Supratentorial cavernomas in eloquent brain areas: application of neuronavigation and functional MRI in operative planning. *J Neurosurg Sci* 2005; **49**:13–9.

116 Kupersmith MJ, Kalish H, Epstein F *et al*. Natural history of brainstem cavernous malformations. *Neurosurgery* 2001; **48**:47–53.

117 Yasui T, Komiyama M, Iwai Y *et al*. A brainstem cavernoma demonstrating a dramatic, spontaneous decrease in size during follow-up: case report and review of the literature. *Surg Neurol* 2005; **63**:170–3.

118 Ferroli P, Sinisi M, Franzini A, Giombini S, Solero CL, Broggi G. Brainstem cavernomas: long-term results of microsurgical resection in 52 patients. *Neurosurgery* 2005; **56**:1203–12.

119 Kikuta K, Nozaki K, Takahashi JA, Miyamoto S, Kikuchi H, Hashimoto N. Postoperative evaluation of microsurgical resection for cavernous malformations of the brainstem. *J Neurosurg* 2004; **101**:607–12.

120 Régis J, Bartolomei F, Kida Y *et al*. Radiosurgery for epilepsy associated with cavernous malformation: retrospective study in 49 patients. *Neurosurgery* 2000; **47**:1091–7.

121 Liu KD, Chung WY, Wu HM *et al*. Gamma knife surgery for cavernous hemangiomas: an analysis of 125 patients. *J Neurosurg* 2005; **102**(Suppl):81–6.

122 Collice M, D'Aliberti G, Arena O, Solaini C, Fontana RA, Talamonti C. Surgical treatment of intracranial dural arteriovenous fistulae: role of venous drainage. *Neurosurgery* 2000; **47**:56–66.

123 Van Dijk JM, TerBrugge KG, Willinsky RA, Wallace MC. Selective disconnection of cortical venous reflux as

treatment for cranial dural arteriovenous fistulas. *J Neurosurg* 2004; **101**:31–5.

124 Kattner DA, Roth TC, Giannotta SL. Cranial base approaches for the surgical treatment of aggressive posterior fossa dural arteriovenous fistulae with leptomeningeal drainage: report of four technical cases. *Neurosurgery* 2002; **50**:1156–60.

125 Klisch J, Huppertz HJ, Spetzger U, Hetzel A, Seeger W, Schumacher M. Transvenous treatment of carotid cavernous and dural arteriovenous fistulae: results for 31 patients and review of the literature. *Neurosurgery* 2003; **53**:836–56.

126 Tomak PR, Cloft HJ, Kaga A, Cawley CM, Dion J, Barrow DL. Evolution of the management of tentorial dural arteriovenous malformations. *Neurosurgery* 2003; **52**:750–60.

127 Murphy KJ, Gailloud P, Venbrux A, Deramond H, Hanley D, Rigamonti D. Endovascular treatment of a grade IV transverse sinus dural arteriovenous fistula by sinus recanalization, angioplasty, and stent placement: technical case report. *Neurosurgery* 2000; **46**:497–500.

128 Houdart E, Saint-Maurice JP, Chapot R *et al.* Transcranial approach for venous embolization of dural arteriovenous fistulas. *J Neurosurg* 2002; **97**:280–6.

129 O'Leary S, Hodgson TJ, Coley SC, Kemeny AA, Radatz MW. Intracranial dural arteriovenous malformations: results of stereotactic radiosurgery in 17 patients. *Clin Oncol (R Coll Radiol)* 2002; **14**:97–102.

130 Pan DH, Chung WY, Guo WY *et al.* Stereotactic radiosurgery for the treatment of dural arteriovenous fistulas involving the transverse-sigmoid sinus. *J Neurosurg* 2002; **96**:823–9.

131 Friedman JA, Pollock BE, Nichols DA, Gorman DA, Foote RL, Stafford SL. Results of combined stereotactic radiosurgery and transarterial embolization for dural arteriovenous fistulas of the transverse and sigmoid sinuses. *J Neurosurg* 2001; **94**:886–91.

132 Kawaguchi S, Okuno S, Sakaki T. Effect of direct arterial bypass on the prevention of future stroke in patients with the hemorrhagic variety of moyamoya disease. *J Neurosurg* 2000; **93**:397–401.

133 Nishimoto T, Yuki K, Sasaki T, Murakami T, Kodama Y, Kurisu K. A ruptured middle cerebral artery aneurysm originating from the site of anastomosis 20 years after extracranial-intracranial bypass for moyamoya disease: case report. *Surg Neurol* 2005; **64**:261–5.

14 Specific treatment of aneurysmal subarachnoid haemorrhage

14.1 General principles

The essence of managing patients with subarachnoid haemorrhage (SAH) from a ruptured aneurysm is deceptively simple: make the diagnosis, locate the aneurysm and occlude it. But, although occlusion of the ruptured aneurysm by an interventional radiologist or neurosurgeon is an important part, it is by no means the only part in the management. Treating patients with aneurysmal SAH requires taking care of acutely ill patients threatened by many more complications than only rebleeding, and should be done by a dedicated, multidisciplinary team.

This chapter deals with the treatment of patients with a (suspected) aneurysmal cause of their SAH. Those with perimesencephalic non-aneurysmal haemorrhage are not threatened by complications except for the rare patient who develops a symptomatic hydrocephalus within the first 1 or 2 days after the onset. We usually discharge patients with a perimesencephalic haemorrhage after 2 or 3 days, and do not give medications other than analgesics. In contrast, patients with an aneurysmal pattern of haemorrhage, even without an aneurysm (or other cause) detected, are admitted for at least 14 days and treated similarly to patients who have had an aneurysm detected.

The case fatality after aneurysmal SAH is still as high as 50%,[1] if one takes into account the 10–15% who die before receiving medical attention.[2] And of the 50% who survive the initial weeks after the haemorrhage, again half are left with permanent deficits in high-level (neuropsychological) functioning, resulting in impairment in their social role.[3] To a large extent this poor outcome is caused by the many complications other than rebleeding that beset the course of the disease: delayed cerebral ischaemia, hydrocephalus, a variety of systemic disorders,[4] and complications of the aneurysm treatment itself.[5] However, despite the considerable proportion of patients who die from the impact of the first haemorrhage and the many complications that can occur, the prognosis for patients with SAH has gradually improved over the last decades.[1,6]

Patients should always be transferred as quickly as possible to a centre where a multidisciplinary team is available 24 hours a day, 7 days a week, and where enough patients are managed to maintain and improve standards of care.[7] The need for referral applies especially to

Stroke: practical management, 3rd edition. C. Warlow, J. van Gijn, M. Dennis, J. Wardlaw, J. Bamford, G. Hankey, P. Sandercock, G. Rinkel, P. Langhorne, C. Sudlow and P. Rothwell. Published 2008 Blackwell Publishing. ISBN 978-1-4051-2766-0.

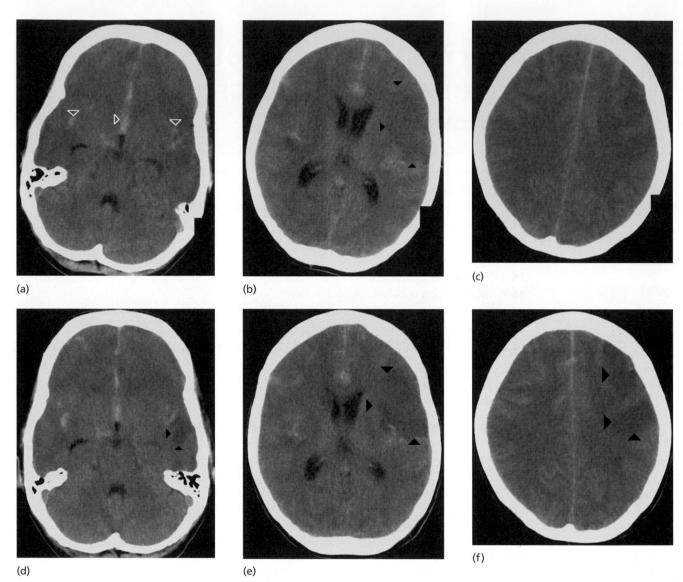

(a)

(b)

(c)

(d)

(e)

(f)

Fig. 14.1 CT scans of a patient with extensive initial ischaemia. This 50-year-old woman suddenly lost consciousness, and remained comatose. (a, b, c) CT scan on admission showing subarachnoid blood in the frontal interhemispheric fissure and sylvian fissures (*white arrowheads*), and areas with poorly demarcated white and grey matter (*black arrowheads*), but no other abnormalities that explain the coma. (d, e, f) CT scan 12 h later showing extensive areas of infarction (*black arrowheads*).

patients who are designated as 'poor grade cases';[8] these may be the very patients who need urgent intervention because of, for example, early rebleeding, progressive brain shift from a haematoma, acute hydrocephalus or hypovolaemia. For the first 2 weeks after the haemorrhage, patients should be managed in an intensive or medium care unit. The neurologist can play a central role in the team, which should consist of neurosurgeons, interventional neuroradiologists, neuro-intensivists, rehabilitation physicians, neuropsychologists, and a dedicated team of nurses, physiotherapists, speech therapists and occupational therapists. The neurologist is well suited and available for assessing the patient's general medical and neurological condition on a frequent basis, and can act immediately if there is any clinical deterioration. Moreover, the neurologist can use his or her experience from working in a stroke unit in the management of SAH patients.

14.2 Treatable causes of poor clinical condition on admission and their management

A decreased level of consciousness, with the initial haemorrhage or after early rebleeding, may be caused by neurological complications such as an intracerebral haematoma, extensive intraventricular haemorrhage, subdural haematoma or hydrocephalus,[8] and by cardiopulmonary complications. Only by exclusion should it be assumed that the cause is global brain damage as a result of the high pressure after aneurysmal rupture,

resulting in impaired or absent cerebral blood flow and subsequent ischaemia (Fig. 14.1).

14.2.1 Early rebleeding

In the first few hours after the initial haemorrhage, up to 15% of patients have a sudden episode of clinical deterioration that suggests rebleeding (Fig. 14.2).[9–11] Because such episodes often occur before the first CT scan, or even before admission to hospital, a definite diagnosis is difficult and the true frequency of rebleeding on the first day is invariably underestimated. If respiratory or cardiac arrest occurs at the time of (suspected) rebleeding during transportation to hospital or early after arrival at the

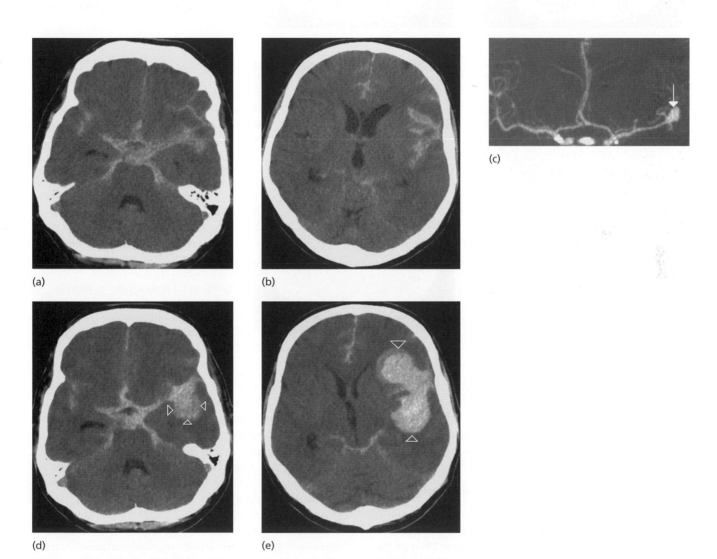

(a)　(b)　(c)

(d)　(e)

Fig. 14.2 CT scans of a patient with early rebleeding. (a,b) CT scan on admission showing large amounts of subarachnoid blood in the basal cisterns and left sylvian fissure. (c) CT angiogram on admission showing an aneurysm of the left middle cerebral artery (*arrow*). Shortly after the initial scan the patient suddenly lost consciousness. (d, e) Repeated CT scan after the clinical deterioration confirmed rebleeding with more extravasated blood (*arrowheads*).

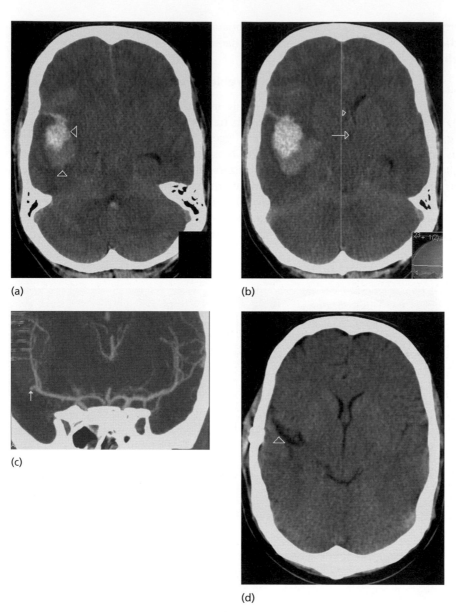

(a)

(b)

(c)

(d)

Fig. 14.3 CT scans of a patient with a poor clinical condition on admission from intracerebral extension of the haemorrhage. (a) CT scan on admission showing intracerebral extension of the haemorrhage (*arrowheads*) and (b) shift of the lateral (*arrowhead*) and third ventricle (*arrow*) across the midline. (c) CT angiogram showing an aneurysm of the right middle cerebral artery (*arrow*). The patient was operated upon immediately with clipping of the aneurysm and evacuation of the haematoma.
(d) Repeat CT scan 3 months after the haemorrhage showing only a small loss of parenchyma (*arrowhead*); the patient had regained independence for activities of daily living.

emergency department, the patient should be resuscitated and ventilated, because survival without brain damage is still possible (section 14.6.2).[12,13] After resuscitation, it will usually become clear within a matter of hours whether there is persisting brainstem dysfunction.

14.2.2 Intracerebral extension of the haemorrhage

Intracerebral extension of the haemorrhage occurs in about one-third of patients with ruptured aneurysms[14] and, not surprisingly, the outcome is worse than in patients with purely subarachnoid blood.[15] When the most likely cause of deterioration in the level of consciousness is a large temporal lobe haemorrhage, usually from a ruptured aneurysm of the middle cerebral artery, immediate

evacuation should be considered (Figs 14.3 and 14.4). The traditional intervention is evacuation of the haematoma with simultaneous clipping of the aneurysm if it can be identified, usually only by MR angiography or CT angiography rather than by catheter angiography; this course of action is backed up by a small randomized study, in which 11 of 15 patients in the operated group survived, against 3 of 15 in the conservatively treated group (relative risk 0.27; 95% CI 0.09–0.74).[16] Nowadays of course this approach may be modified to immediate occlusion of the aneurysm by endovascular coiling, followed by evacuation of the haematoma.[17] Another option is immediate aneurysm occlusion followed by an extensive hemicraniectomy that allows external expansion of the brain.[18]

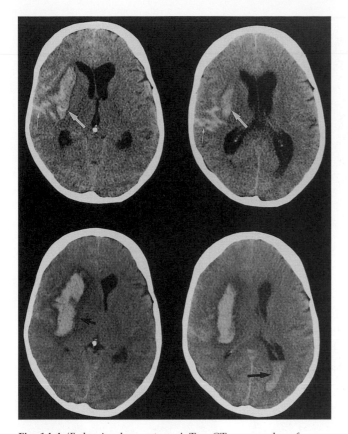

Fig. 14.4 'Enlarging haematoma'. *Top*: CT scan on day of subarachnoid haemorrhage from a ruptured aneurysm of the right middle cerebral artery, in a 51-year-old man on anticoagulant treatment because of myocardial infarction with mitral valve regurgitation. Haematoma in the right sylvian fissure (*thin arrow*) and in the subinsular cortex (*thick arrow*); at the time of the scan anticoagulation had already been reversed by infusion of a concentrate of coagulation factors. *Bottom*: CT scan 5 days after the haemorrhage, showing a marked increase of the space-occupying effect, with compression of the right lateral ventricle and the third ventricle. The increased mass effect results not only from a newly formed rim of oedema around the haematoma (*short arrow*), but also from an increase in size of the haematoma itself. There had been no new neurological signs or other clinical features indicating rebleeding. The newly formed collection of blood in the posterior horn of the left lateral ventricle (*long arrow*) is often seen in the absence of rebleeding (sedimentation effect).

14.2.3 Acute subdural haematoma

In about 2% of patients an acute subdural haematoma complicates rupture of an intracranial aneurysm, usually at the origin of the posterior communicating artery (Fig. 14.5),[19,20] more often with recurrent aneurysmal rupture than a first bleed.[21] Sometimes there is no associated haemorrhage in the subarachnoid space to indicate a ruptured aneurysm as the underlying cause.[22–24]

Subdural haematomas secondary to a ruptured aneurysm may be life threatening, in which case immediate evacuation seems called for, despite the lack of controlled studies.[8,25]

14.2.4 Acute hydrocephalus and intraventricular haemorrhage

Gradual obtundation within 24 h of haemorrhage, sometimes accompanied by slow pupillary responses to light and downward deviation of the eyes, is fairly characteristic of acute hydrocephalus;[26,27] and some patients lapse into coma from hydrocephalus within a few hours of the haemorrhage. If the diagnosis is confirmed by brain CT, then a lumbar puncture or early ventricular drainage may be needed,[28,29] although some patients improve spontaneously in the first 24 h. This is an area badly in need of randomized trials.

Acute hydrocephalus with a large amount of intraventricular blood is often associated with a poor clinical condition from the outset (Fig. 14.6). In patients with ruptured aneurysms, i.e. an arterial source of bleeding, an intraventricular haemorrhage volume of 20 mL or more is invariably lethal.[30] An indirect comparison of observational studies suggests that an external ventricular catheter is not very helpful, but that a strategy where drainage is combined with fibrinolysis through the drain results in a good outcome in half the patients.[31] This needs to be confirmed in randomized controlled trials.[32] Surgical evacuation of a 'packed' intraventricular haemorrhage, especially in the fourth ventricle, is pointless according to some,[33] while others disagree.[34] At any rate, ventriculostomy is certainly indicated in patients with acute symptomatic hydrocephalus caused by a small clot plugging the proximal aqueduct.[35]

14.2.5 Cardiopulmonary complications

Pulmonary oedema and cardiac dysfunction, which can aggravate the pulmonary oedema,[36] may develop within hours of the haemorrhage, even in patients who are admitted in good clinical condition (Fig. 14.7). A rapid decline in consciousness associated with hypoxaemia and hypotension occurs in the emergency department or soon after admission.[37] According to a systematic review, pulmonary oedema and echocardiographic abnormalities occur in 4% of patients admitted in good clinical condition,[38] but because these complications are related to the clinical condition, in patients admitted in coma pulmonary oedema is found in one-third and echocardiographic abnormalities in one-half.[37] The cardiopulmonary dysfunction can last for weeks, but even after prolonged intensive care treatment good recovery can still occur.[37]

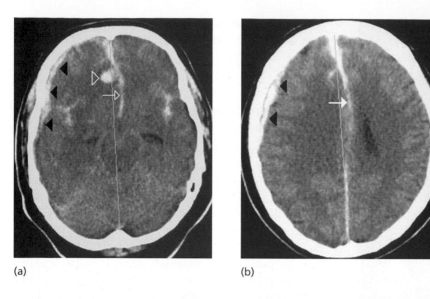

(a)   (b)

Fig. 14.5 CT scans of a patient with a poor clinical condition on admission from a subdural haematoma. (a, b) Subarachnoid haemorrhage in the frontal interhemispheric fissure and the sylvian fissures with shift of the anterior interhemispheric fissure over the midline (*arrow*). The intracerebral extension (*white open arrowhead*) is too small to explain this midline shift. There is a large subdural haematoma (*black arrowheads*).

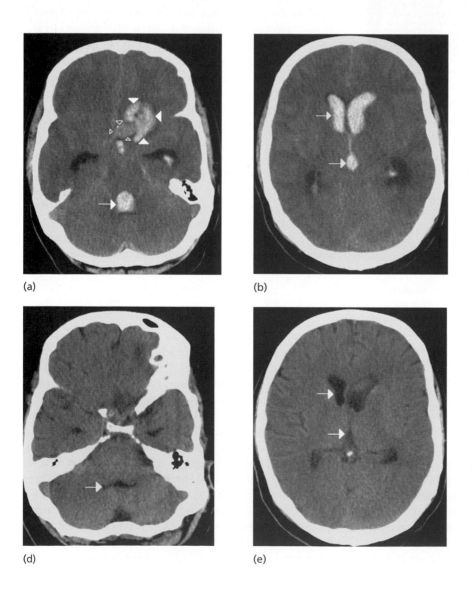

(a)   (b)

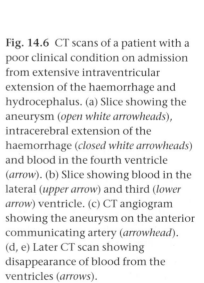

(c)

(d)   (e)

Fig. 14.6 CT scans of a patient with a poor clinical condition on admission from extensive intraventricular extension of the haemorrhage and hydrocephalus. (a) Slice showing the aneurysm (*open white arrowheads*), intracerebral extension of the haemorrhage (*closed white arrowheads*) and blood in the fourth ventricle (*arrow*). (b) Slice showing blood in the lateral (*upper arrow*) and third (*lower arrow*) ventricle. (c) CT angiogram showing the aneurysm on the anterior communicating artery (*arrowhead*). (d, e) Later CT scan showing disappearance of blood from the ventricles (*arrows*).

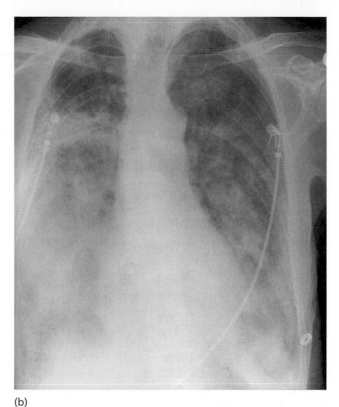

(b)

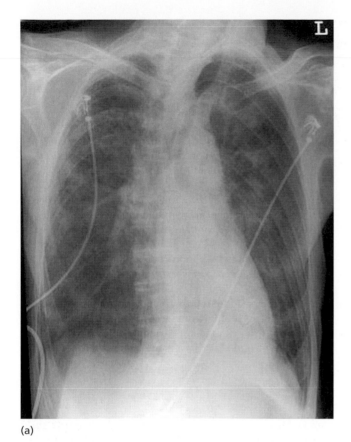

(a)

Fig. 14.7 A 70-year-old man admitted with a subarachnoid haemorrhage. On admission blood pressure was 100/50 and the pulse 50/min. He opened his eyes when spoken to, obeyed simple commands and was disoriented. Within hours he developed shortness of breath and lapsed into coma. (a) Chest X-ray on admission. (b) Chest X-ray several hours later showing pulmonary oedema (more prominent on the right side).

14.3 General care

14.3.1 Blood pressure

Aggressive treatment of high blood pressure carries a definite risk of ischaemia in brain areas with loss of autoregulation. The rational approach is therefore to advise against treating hypertension following aneurysmal rupture. The empirical evidence from clinical trials is sparse, but tends to support the avoidance of antihypertensive drugs. An observational study from the 1980s, in which all events had been documented by serial CT scanning, compared patients who had been treated for SAH-induced hypertension with normotensive controls; the rate of rebleeding was lower but the rate of cerebral infarction was higher than in untreated controls, despite the blood pressures being, on average, higher than in the controls.[39] This suggests that hypertension after SAH is a compensatory phenomenon, at least to some extent, and one that should not be interfered with. In keeping with this notion, a further observational study from the same centre (Rotterdam) suggested that the combined strategy of avoiding antihypertensive medication and increasing fluid intake decreases the risk of cerebral infarction.[40]

It seems best to reserve antihypertensive therapy for patients with extreme elevations of blood pressure (mean arterial pressure [(systolic blood pressure + 2 × diastolic blood pressure)/3] of 130 mmHg or over), and for those with signs of rapidly progressive end organ deterioration, such as proteinuria. An effective treatment is esmolol, an ultra-short acting, cardioselective beta-blocking drug (as a 0.5–1 mg/kg intravenous loading dose over 1 min, followed by an infusion starting at 50 µg/kg per min and increasing up to 300 µg/kg per min as necessary), or labetalol hydrochloride, a combined α_1- and non-selective β-adrenergic receptor blocker (as an intravenous loading dose of 20 mg, followed by repeated incremental doses of 20–80 mg by intravenous bolus every 10 min until the desired level of blood pressure is achieved).[41] It is reasonable to aim for a 25% decrease in mean arterial pressure below the initial baseline. For monitoring the blood pressure in these situations an arterial line is almost mandatory. In practice, however, there is rarely any need for antihypertensive therapy. In many patients surges of high blood pressure can be attenuated by adequate pain management.

> Hypertension in the acute phase of subarachnoid haemorrhage can be left untreated unless the blood pressure is extremely high, or there are signs of end-organ damage.

14.3.2 Fluids and electrolytes

Fluid management after subarachnoid haemorrhage (SAH) should aim to prevent a reduction in plasma volume, because this may contribute to the development of cerebral ischaemia (section 14.7). However, the arguments for a liberal (some might say aggressive) regimen of fluid administration are indirect:

- Approximately one-third of SAH patients decrease their plasma volume by more than 10% between the second and tenth day after the haemorrhage; this is associated with a negative sodium balance; in other words, there is loss of sodium as well as of water – so-called 'cerebral salt wasting'.[42,43]
- Fluid restriction in patients with hyponatraemia, applied in the past because it was erroneously attributed to water retention via inappropriate secretion of antidiuretic hormone, associated with an increased risk of cerebral ischaemia.[44]
- Two cohort studies with historical controls suggested that a daily intake of at least 3 L of saline (against 1.5–2.0 L in the past) was associated with a lower risk of delayed cerebral ischaemia and a better overall outcome.[40,45] The interpretation of these two studies is difficult not only because of their observational nature, but also because the liberal administration of saline in the second period was accompanied by avoidance of antihypertensive drugs as well.

Despite the incomplete evidence, it seems reasonable to prevent hypovolaemia. We aim for normovolaemia by giving 2.5–3.5 L/day of isotonic saline, unless contraindicated by signs of impending cardiac failure (see below). The amount of intravenous saline should be reduced if the patient is also receiving nutritional solution via the enteral route. In patients with fever, from whatever cause (section 14.3.3), fluid intake should be gradually increased.[46]

Fluid requirements may be guided by recording the central venous pressure (the directly measured value should be above 8 mmHg), especially in patients with hyponatraemia or a negative fluid balance who are at risk

of developing heart failure, but frequent calculation of fluid balance (four times a day until approximately day 10) is the main way to estimate how much fluid should be given to keep the patient normovolaemic. Pulmonary artery catheters have been advocated on the basis of historical controls,[47] but in a retrospective series of 184 patients with SAH they were associated with complications such as catheter-related sepsis (13%), congestive heart failure (2%), subclavian venous thrombosis (1%) and pneumothorax (1%).[48] Moreover, their usefulness in critically ill patients in general has become uncertain.[49,50] The lack of evidence for prophylactic hypervolaemia instead of aiming for normovolaemia is discussed in section 14.5.7.

> We recommend a high fluid intake of 2.5–3.5 L per day of isotonic saline in patients with aneurysmal subarachnoid haemorrhage, to compensate for 'cerebral salt wasting' and to prevent hypovolaemia which predisposes to cerebral ischaemia.

14.3.3 Analgesics and general nursing care

Headache

Headache can sometimes be managed with just mild analgesics such as paracetamol (acetaminophen); salicylates are best avoided because of their antihaemostatic effect which is unwanted in patients who may have to undergo neurosurgical clipping of the aneurysm or external ventricular drainage; also aspirin administered after aneurysm occlusion probably does not protect against delayed cerebral ischaemia (section 14.5.4). In practice, the pain is usually so severe that codeine needs to be added, which will not mask neurological signs. Sometimes, pain can be alleviated with anxiolytic drugs such as midazolam (5 mg via an infusion pump). Often a synthetic opiate such as tramadol is needed to obtain relief (for doses see Table 14.1). As a last resort, severe headache can be treated with piritramide. Constipation is a common problem with all opiates.

> In patients with a decreased level of consciousness headache may present as restlessness. The 'analgesic staircase' consists of frequent doses of paracetamol, then codeine if necessary, tramadol or, as a last resort, piritramide.

For as long as the aneurysm has not been occluded the patient should be kept on complete bed rest, traditionally flat and with as few external stimuli as possible, on the assumption that any form of excitement increases the risk of rebleeding.

Table 14.1 Recommendations for nursing and general management of patients with subarachnoid haemorrhage.

Nursing
Continuous observation (Glasgow Coma Scale, temperature, ECG monitoring, pupils, any focal deficits)

Nutrition
Oral route
Only with intact cough and swallowing reflexes
Keep stools soft by adequate fluid intake and by restriction of milk content; if necessary add laxatives
Nasogastric tube
Deflate endotracheal cuff (if present) on insertion
Confirm proper placement by X-ray
Begin with small test feeds of 5% dextrose
Prevent aspiration by feeding in sitting position and by checking gastric residue every hour
Tablets should be crushed and flushed down
Total parenteral nutrition should only be used as a last resort

Blood pressure
Do not treat hypertension unless the mean arterial pressure is ≥ 130 mmHg or there is clinical or laboratory evidence of progressive end organ damage

Fluids and electrolytes
Intravenous line mandatory
Give at least 3 L/day (isotonic saline, 0.9%)
Insert an indwelling bladder catheter
Compensate for a negative fluid balance and for fever
Monitor electrolytes (and white blood cell count) at least every other day

Pain
Start with paracetamol (acetaminophen) 500 mg every 3–4 h; avoid aspirin
Midazolam can be used if pain is accompanied by anxiety (5 mg via infusion pump)
For severe pain, use codeine (30–60 mg every 4 h, as needed), tramadol (50–100 mg every 4 h, as needed) or, as a last resort, piritramide 0.2–0.3 mg/kg body weight i.m. (maximum 80 mg per 24 h, in four doses).

Prevention of deep venous thrombosis and pulmonary embolism
Compression stockings or intermittent compression by pneumatic devices, or both before aneurysm occlusion. Low molecular heparin if the aneurysm has been treated.

Monitoring conscious level

Continuous assessment of the consciousness level is essential, preferably recorded with the Glasgow Coma Scale (section 3.3.2), although it should be remembered that with inexperienced observers errors of more than one point may occur.[51,52] Any change in the level of consciousness may signify early cerebral ischaemia, rebleeding, hydrocephalus or a systemic medical complication. The nurses should be familiar with the peak times of occurrence of rebleeding and cerebral ischaemia, and they should be able to detect the early signs of delirium, which is seldom caused by SAH per se but more often by the combined effects of isolation, sleep deprivation, narcotic drugs and alcohol withdrawal.

Constipation

Coughing and straining must be rigorously prevented because of the attendant surges in arterial blood pressure.

Stool softeners should be prescribed routinely. Enemas are contraindicated because they markedly increase intra-abdominal pressure and secondarily intracranial pressure.

The bladder

A catheter is almost always needed for accurate calculation of fluid balance, except in men who are alert and have perfect bladder control. Condom devices leak or slip off too often to be of any use in these critically ill patients. Intermittent catheterization may substantially decrease the risk of urinary infections but the procedure is too stressful for patients with SAH (and requires more time from the nursing staff than most hospital budgets allow).

Confusion

In confused patients specific causes of confusion should be excluded, such as pain, hypoxia, alcohol withdrawal, infection or a blocked urinary catheter.

Venous access

A reliable intravenous route should be maintained for emergency administration of plasma expanders or anti-epileptic drugs. Oral administration of antacids is said to be sufficient to protect against stress bleeding; proton pump inhibitors should be considered only in mechanically ventilated patients or in patients with a previous history of ulcers.

Fever

The body temperature should be measured frequently, up to four times a day, depending on the time since the SAH, and the level of consciousness. After the first few hours mild fever (up to 38.5°C) often occurs, probably as the result of the inflammatory reaction in the subarachnoid space,[53] in which case the pulse is characteristically normal.[54] Infection should be suspected if the temperature exceeds 38.5°C, if the pulse is elevated as well, or if the patient has vomited. An elevated white cell count is not helpful in distinguishing infection from non-infective causes of pyrexia.[46]

Venous thromboembolism

Deep venous thrombosis (DVT) is not as common after SAH as in patients with ischaemic stroke, presumably because the patients are restless, generally younger and, most important, seldom have a paralysed leg; in a large and prospective series DVT was clinically diagnosed in only 4%.[55] DVT can be prevented by subcutaneous low-dose heparin or heparinoids (section 11.13), but the obvious fear is that anticoagulation will not be confined to the venous system. In a placebo-controlled trial of the low-molecular-weight heparinoid enoxaparin given after aneurysm occlusion, intracranial bleeding complications occurred more often in the treatment group, while there was no influence on overall outcome or the risk of delayed ischaemia.[56] In the absence of proof of effectiveness, many physicians prefer to err on the side of caution and do not recommend prophylactic heparin or the low-molecular-weight heparinoids.

Graduated compression stockings reduce the risk of DVT in patients undergoing general surgical, neurosurgical or orthopaedic procedures (section 11.13).[57] Therefore, because low-molecular-weight heparinoids increase the risk of intracranial bleeding,[56] graduated compression stockings are the preferred form of DVT prevention in SAH patients – although admittedly this advice lacks support from a randomized trial in this specific situation. However, because compression stockings must be individually fitted to be efficacious, some favour pneumatic devices that apply intermittent venous compression to the legs; a study specifically performed in patients with SAH but with non-randomized controls suggested DVT can be successfully prevented in this way.[58] And in a randomized trial, but in patients with intracerebral haemorrhage, the combination of stockings and intermittent pneumatic compression resulted in a smaller risk of DVT than prevention by stockings alone (relative risk 0.29; 95% CI 0.08–1.00); there is no reason to assume that this effect would be any different in patients with SAH.[59] The devices are well tolerated by patients and can be managed easily by the nursing staff but one problem is that their success depends on a repair service that keeps them running. It has been argued that impedance plethysmography or duplex Doppler sonography should be performed to exclude clinically occult thrombosis before any kind of compression is applied to the calves, but no systematic studies have answered the question whether the danger of dislodging emboli to the lungs is imaginary or not.

Antiepilpetic drugs

The prophylactic use of anti-epileptic drugs is controversial. Seizures in the first few weeks after aneurysmal rupture occur in about 10% (6–16%) of patients, and may be easily confused with rebleeding.[60-62] The majority occur soon after the initial haemorrhage.[63] Predictive factors for epileptic seizures have not been consistently identified. Intracranial surgery,[64] and probably also intracerebral extension of the haemorrhage, increase the risk, but a randomized trial of anti-epileptic drugs after supratentorial craniotomy for benign lesions (not only aneurysms) in 276 patients failed to show benefit in terms of seizure rate or case fatality, although the confidence intervals were wide.[65] Currently, we adhere to the principle of '*in dubio abstine*' (abstain when in doubt) because the possible disadvantage of a serious drug reaction may well outweigh any benefits.

Our recommendations for the general management of patients with SAH are summarized in Table 14.1. Before considering the diagnosis and prevention of all the possible complications we will discuss the *prevention* of the two most common causes of clinical deterioration: rebleeding and cerebral ischaemia.

14.4 Prevention of rebleeding

14.4.1 Risk of rebleeding

In the first few hours after admission for the initial haemorrhage, up to 15% of patients experience a sudden episode of clinical deterioration that suggests rebleeding (section 14.2.1). In patients who survive the first day, the risk of rebleeding is more or less evenly distributed over the next 4 weeks.[66] After the first day, the cumulative risk within the first 3 weeks, and without measures to prevent it, is about 40%.[67] Between 4 weeks and 6 months after the haemorrhage the risk of rebleeding gradually declines, from the initial level of 1–2%/day to a constant level of about 3%/year[68] (section 14.10.2).

> The risk of rebleeding after rupture of an intracranial aneurysm, without medical, endovascular or surgical intervention, is about 40% in the first 3 weeks, i.e. 1–2% per day.

After rebleeding the prognosis is poor; 80% of patients die or remain disabled.[4] Indeed, given its frequency and morbidity, rebleeding is still a major cause of poor outcome, even in centres aiming at early occlusion of the aneurysm.[45,69,70] Unfortunately, there are few prognostic factors that predict an increased risk of rebleeding. Some studies suggest that it occurs more often in patients with a previous bout of sudden headache,[71] with a decreased level of consciousness,[72] or with larger aneurysms[72–74] but none of these factors reliably identify the patients at highest risk. And even if high-risk groups could be identified, there would still be almost as many rebleeds because most occur in the larger number of patients at moderate risk – the prevention paradox again (section 18.5.1).[75]

> Rebleeding of a ruptured aneurysm cannot be predicted reliably.

14.4.2 Endovascular occlusion

Over the last decade, endovascular occlusion of aneurysms has largely replaced surgical occlusion as the intervention of choice for the prevention of rebleeding, at least in centres where this expertise is available. The technique consists of packing the aneurysm with platinum coils, nowadays with a system for controlled detachment.[76] This was initially mainly used for posterior circulation aneurysms (Fig. 14.8), and then later for aneurysms on the anterior circulation (Figs 14.9 and 14.10). The procedure is generally performed under general anaesthesia, though not invariably.[77]

Remarkably soon after its introduction in the early 1990s coiling was compared with neurosurgical clipping in randomized trials. A systematic review of these trials (one large and two small trials, of which one was still unpublished) included a total of 2272 patients (Fig. 14.11).[78] Most of the patients were in good clinical condition and had an aneurysm of the anterior circulation. After 1 year of follow-up, the relative risk of a poor outcome (death or dependency) for coiling vs clipping was 0.76 (95% CI 0.67–0.88). The absolute risk reduction of a poor outcome was 7% (95% CI 4–11%). For anterior circulation aneurysms the relative risk of a poor outcome was 0.78 (95% CI 0.68–0.90) and the absolute risk reduction was 7% (95% CI 3–10%). For posterior circulation

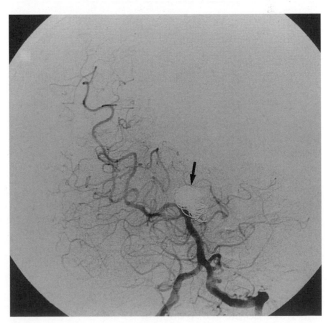

(a)

(b)

Fig. 14.8 (a) Catheter angiogram showing aneurysm at the tip of the basilar artery (arrow). (b) Repeat angiogram after the aneurysm has been occluded by detachable coils, through an endovascular approach.

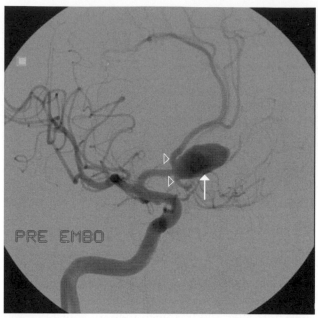

(a)

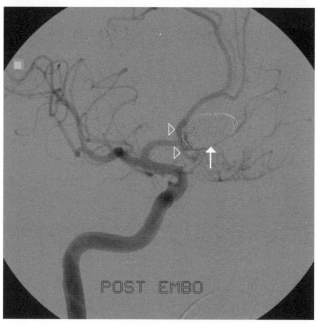

(b)

Fig. 14.9 Endovascular occlusion of an aneurysm on the anterior communicating artery. Same patient as in Fig. 14.6. (a) Catheter angiogram before occlusion showing the aneurysm (*arrow*) and branching vessels (*arrowheads*). (b) Catheter angiogram after occlusion showing the coils mass in the aneurysm (*arrow*) and the still patent branching vessels (*arrowheads*).

aneurysms the relative risk was 0.41 (95% CI 0.19–0.92) and the absolute risk reduction 27% (95% CI 6–48%). Also the cognitive impairment after 1 year tends to be less after coiling than after clipping.[79]

Several qualifications are needed to avoid the impression that these results fully define the relative merits of endovascular and surgical occlusion of aneurysms:

- First, aneurysms in some locations are more suitable for occlusion by one rather than the other technique. Basilar artery aneurysms and many other types of posterior circulation aneurysms are relatively easy to coil,[80] whereas surgical treatment is often very difficult and complicated. Conversely, aneurysms at the trifurcation of the middle cerebral artery are often difficult to coil without interfering with major arterial branches. These preferences are reflected in the under-representation of posterior circulation aneurysms and aneurysms of the middle cerebral artery among the 2143 patients randomized in by far the largest trial, the international ISAT study.[81]

- Second, patients over 70 years old were under-represented in the ISAT trial, reflecting a preference for coiling – or perhaps for no treatment – in many aged patients with SAH. However, it is not an unrealistic guess that the relative advantages of coiling over surgical treatment are even greater in patients over the age of 70 than in younger patients, given that the risk of complications from treatment of unruptured aneurysms in older patients is much higher for operation than for coiling.[5] SAH patients older than 70 or 75 years of age have in general a poor prognosis, but several observational studies suggest that they can still benefit from endovascular or surgical occlusion of the aneurysm, especially if admitted in a good condition; without treatment the most important cause of a poor outcome is recurrent haemorrhage.[82]

- A third and last concern is the durability of the occlusion with coils, given that the early rebleeding rate after surgical occlusion is very low (section 14.10.2). Ideally, after coiling, any remaining aneursymal lumen becomes occluded by a process of reactive thrombosis, but early or late rebleeding does nevertheless occur – even after a technically competent procedure. In a consecutive series of 431 patients, six (1.4%) rebled within 30 days after coiling; in four of these patients the aneurysm had been completely occluded during the procedure.[83] All six patients died after rebleeding. Risk factors for rebleeding in this series were a haematoma in the vicinity of the aneurysm, anterior communicating aneurysms, and small aneurysm size. In the ISAT trial the rate of rebleeding from the target aneurysm between the procedure and the end of the first year was somewhat higher after coiling than clipping (2.6% vs 1.0%), but the initial 7.4% absolute gain in the avoidance of death or dependence was maintained at 1 year, while the early survival advantage was still seen to 7 years.[64] Most episodes of rebleeding occurred in

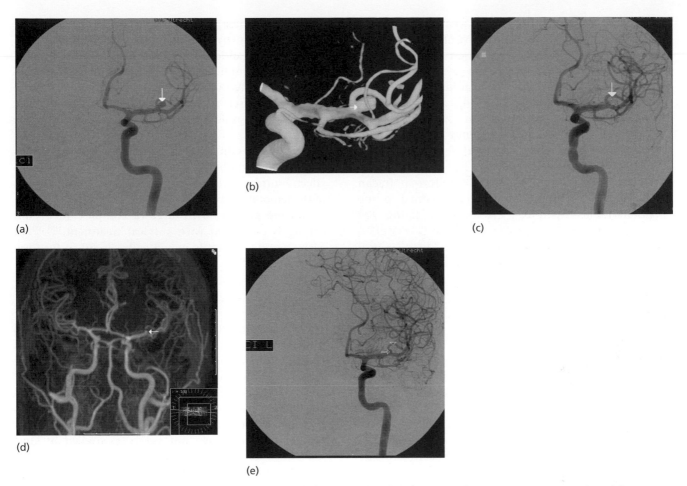

Fig. 14.10 Endovascular occlusion of an aneurysm on the left middle cerebral artery. (a) Catheter angiogram before occlusion showing the aneurysm (*arrow*). (b) Three-dimensional reconstruction showing detailed delineation of the aneurysm with relatively wide neck (*arrow*). (c) Catheter angiogram after occlusion showing the coils mass in the aneurysm (*arrow*). (d) MRA after 6 months suggests some reopening of the neck of the aneurysm (*arrow*). (e) Catheter angiogram after 6 months confirming the reopening of the neck (*arrow*). The fundus of the aneurysm is still occluded by the coils mass (*arrowhead*). On further follow-up angiograms the reopening remained the same and no further treatment was performed.

Study or sub-category	coil n/N	clip n/N	RR (fixed) 95% CI	Weight (%)	RR (fixed) 95% CI
Brilstra 2000b	3/8	4/8		1.16	0.75 [0.24, 2.33]
Koivisto 2000	11/52	14/57		3.88	0.86 [0.43, 1.72]
ISAT	250/1063	326/1055		94.96	0.76 [0.66, 0.88]
Total (95% CI)	1123	1120		100.00	0.76 [0.67, 0.88]

Total events: 264 (coil), 344 (clip)
Test for heterogeneity Chi^2 = 0.12, df = 2 (P = 0.94), I^2 = 0%
Test for overall effect: Z = 3.83 (P = 0.0001)

0.1　0.2　0.5　1　2　5　10
Favours coiling　　Favours clipping

Fig. 14.11 Forest plot of Cochrane review of endovascular coiling vs surgical clipping in patients with aneurysmal subarachnoid haemorrhage (SAH). Outcome, death or dependency at 12 months after SAH. RR, relative risk.

the first 30 days, with either procedure. Rebleeding after the first month occurred in five of a cohort of 381 patients (1.3%) with a mean period of follow-up of 4 years.[84] More data on the risk of late rebleeding after coiling will follow in the near future, but in any event this must be weighed against the risk of late rebleeding after surgical treatment, which is around 3% after 10 years.[85,86] In a multicentre study that compared rebleeding after the initial year after coiling or clipping, rebleeding rates were low in both cohorts after a relatively short period of follow-up (mean 4.4 years).[87] Rebleeding after 1 year occurred in one patient treated with coil embolization during 904 person-years of follow-up (annual rate 0.11%; 95% CI 0–0.63%) and in no patients treated with surgical clipping during 2666 person-years (annual rate 0%; 95% CI 0–0.14%).

When to coil

The optimal timing of coiling has not been studied, but given the risk of rebleeding in the first few days, the general opinion is 'the sooner the better'.[88] If endovascular occlusion is not possible in the first few days, there is probably no need to avoid the period between day 4 and 12 which is regarded as unfavourable for surgical intervention (section 14.4.3), since delayed cerebral ischaemia is relatively unlikely to be precipitated by endovascular occlusion.[89]

The complications of coiling

Bearing in mind that coiling is not a technically feasible option in every patient,[90] a problem that can be reduced by the use of three-dimensional angiography,[91] and despite its many advantages over surgical treatment, coiling is not without its hazards. In a large consecutive series from a single centre, procedural complications occurred in 40 of 681 patients (5.9%; 95% CI 4.2–7.9%), leading to death in 18 (procedural mortality, 2.6%; 95% CI 1.6–4.2%) and to disability in another 22 patients (procedural morbidity, 3.2%; 95% CI 2.0–4.9%).[92] The most frequent complication was thromboembolism, which occurred in 4.7% of patients; intraprocedural re-rupture occurred in 1.2% of patients (Fig. 14.12). If rebleeding occurs during coiling the bleeding is much more difficult to control than during surgical exploration, which explains the high case fatality of 40%.[93] Risk factors for procedural complications are small aneurysm size and the use of a temporary occlusion balloon.[92,93] To reduce the risk of thromboembolism, most interventional radiologists start heparin during treatment and advise continuing for at least 1–2 days. Some advise even

3 months of therapy with antiplatelet drugs but this is supported only by comparisons with historical controls,[94] not by randomized trials.[95]

Another complication is that one or more coils may become dislodged and herniate or embolize into the parent vessel, which again may lead to ischaemic brain damage, unless a surgical approach retrieves the fragment.[96,97]

Finally, rare complications include secondary infection of the thrombosed aneurysm,[98] worsening of mass effect,[99] intracranial artery dissection, and false aneurysms of the femoral artery.

In some patients with large or complex aneurysms coiling is combined with surgical treatment,[100,101] or with stenting.[102] Stents may also be useful in fusiform aneurysms.[103,104]

Follow-up

There is still uncertainty about how long patients need to be followed up with imaging beyond the period of 6 months that is fairly standard, and also about the most suitable radiological technique. Conventional catheter angiography is time-consuming and carries a small but definite risk. MR angiography is feasible and gives good-quality images,[105–108] but its test characteristics and effectiveness have not yet been studied in large series of patients.

A final area of uncertainty is the need for a second procedure for aneurysm necks that have recanalized by impaction of the coils, by re-coiling[109] or surgical occlusion.[110] Since rebleeding can occur after incomplete aneurysm occlusion and re-coiling has a low risk of complications,[109] currently most teams recommend re-coiling, but the risk : benefit ratio of this strategy has not yet been properly assessed.

New developments are radioactive platinum coils and hydrogel-coated coils,[111,112] but their usefulness has not yet been properly evaluated.

14.4.3 Surgical occlusion

Surgical occlusion of ruptured aneurysms has now become the second choice, at least for most patients and most aneurysms. A statistical modelling exercise that weighed the prevention of rebleeding against the complications of the operation at current standards estimated an absolute reduction in the risk of a poor outcome of almost 10% and a relative risk reduction of 0.81 for surgical occlusion vs no occlusion.[67] In fact, no proper randomized trial has ever been done in modern times; the only randomized trial that compared surgical with conservative treatment in SAH patients,

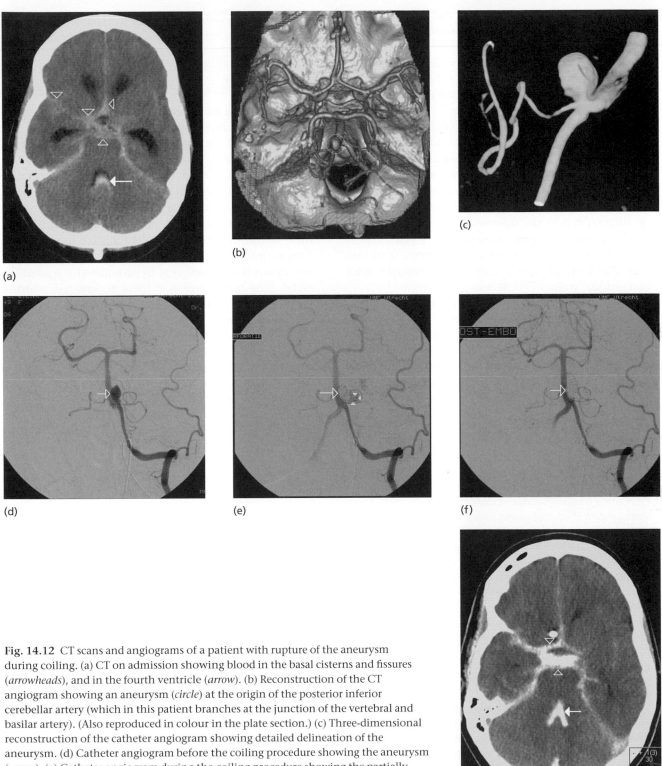

Fig. 14.12 CT scans and angiograms of a patient with rupture of the aneurysm during coiling. (a) CT on admission showing blood in the basal cisterns and fissures (*arrowheads*), and in the fourth ventricle (*arrow*). (b) Reconstruction of the CT angiogram showing an aneurysm (*circle*) at the origin of the posterior inferior cerebellar artery (which in this patient branches at the junction of the vertebral and basilar artery). (Also reproduced in colour in the plate section.) (c) Three-dimensional reconstruction of the catheter angiogram showing detailed delineation of the aneurysm. (d) Catheter angiogram before the coiling procedure showing the aneurysm (*arrow*). (e) Catheter angiogram during the coiling procedure showing the partially coiled aneurysm (*arrow*) and extravasation of contrast (*arrowheads*). (f) Catheter angiogram after occlusion showing the coils mass in the aneurysm (*arrow*). (g) CT scan after the procedure showing contrast material in the basal cisterns (*arrowheads*) and fourth ventricle (*arrow*).

performed in the 1950s in London, tested carotid ligation, not aneurysm clipping, and was restricted to patients who had survived the first 12 days.[113,114]

Nowadays, aneurysms are usually clipped early, i.e. within 3 days of the initial bleed – if possible within 24 h – and this policy is no longer restricted to patients admitted in good clinical condition.[70] The main rationale for early surgery is, of course, optimal prevention of early rebleeding. The only randomized trial of the timing of operation, performed in Finland, allocated 216 patients to one of three groups: operation within 3 days, after 7 days, or in the intermediate period.[115] The outcome tended to be better after early than intermediate or late surgery, but as the difference was not statistically significant a disadvantage of early surgery could not be excluded.[115,116] The same result – no difference in outcome after early or late operation – also emerged from observational studies.[117–119]

Some believe that early operation also helps prevent ischaemia, because the clots that surround blood vessels in the subarachnoid space can be washed away and no longer contribute their assumed effect in the development of vasospasm, but there is little evidence to support this notion (section 14.5.8). Another theoretical advantage of early aneurysm clipping is that if cerebral ischaemia does develop hypertensive and hypervolaemic treatment can be given without the danger of rebleeding (section 14.7.2).

> Although early aneurysm operation is now the usual practice when surgical clipping is indicated, this policy is vulnerable to challenge and reversal because it has not been supported by any randomized controlled trial.

Neurosurgical and anaesthetic techniques have undergone considerable evolution other than through the introduction of the operating microscope. For example, three-dimensional angiography facilitates accurate placing of the occlusive clip.[120] Mild intra-operative hypothermia confers no benefit.[121] Although this is not a textbook about technical details of operative treatment, it is useful for physicians to know something about these developments and Table 14.2 lists some of them. A most unusual complication of operative treatment of aneurysms is a delayed type hypersensitivity against the metal alloy presenting as intense generalized pruritus, which may necessitate removal of the clip.[122]

It should not be assumed that surgical treatment is always definitive; rebleeding from the treated aneurysm can occur even in the first year after rupture, and also later during follow-up at which time haemorrhages from newly developed aneurysms at the site of the original aneurysm or at other sites, or from small unruptured incidental aneurysms that were left untreated at time of the subarachnoid haemorrhage, may begin to be seen (section 14.10.2).[123]

Vessel reconstruction, with fusiform aneurysms or giant aneurysms
Permanent occlusion of parent vessel[319–321]
Temporary occlusion of parent vessel[322,323]
'Trapping' without revascularization[320]
Opening the aneurysm for thrombectomy, followed by reconstruction of the
　　artery[319,324]
Excision of aneurysm, with end-to-end anastomosis of parent artery[319,325]
Excision of aneurysm, with large-artery bypass, supratentorially,[326,327] or
　　infratentorially[321,328]
Combination with endovascular techniques
Intra-operative angiography, to verify clip placement[329,330]
Incomplete clipping, followed by endovascular coiling[331,332]
Combination with endoscopy, to verify clip placement[333]
Combination with intra-operative MR angiography, to verify clip placement[334]
Special clips
Clips with different shapes and physical properties[335]
Titanium clips, which do not cause artifacts on MR imaging[336]
Approaches to aneurysms in specific locations
Distal part of posterior inferior cerebellar artery: skull-base and far-lateral
　　transcondylar approach[321]
Non-branching site of intracranial internal carotid artery ('blister-like aneurysms'):
　　clipping or wrapping,[337] or suturing followed by an encircling clip,[338] or balloon
　　occlusion followed by trapping[339]
Middle cerebral artery: side-to-side anastomosis after unplanned occlusion of a
　　major branch[340]

Table 14.2 Special neurosurgical techniques used for occlusion of aneurysms.

14.4.4 Pharmacological treatment

Antifibrinolytic drugs

Because fibrinolytic activity in the cerebrospinal fluid is thought to break down clots sealing the tear in the aneurysm sac, it is logical to suppose that rebleeding might be prevented by antifibrinolytic drugs which cross the blood–brain barrier rapidly after SAH.[124] The two most commonly used are tranexamic acid (TEA; 1 g intravenously or 1.5 g orally, four to six times daily), or epsilon-aminocaproic acid (EACA; 3–4.5 g 3-hourly intravenously or orally). Both agents are structurally similar to lysine and so block the lysine binding sites by which the plasminogen molecules bind to complementary sites on fibrin. It is assumed that it takes 36 h to achieve complete inhibition of fibrinolysis in the cerebrospinal fluid.

Ten randomized trials of antifibrinolytic drugs in SAH have so far been performed. The most recent Cochrane review included nine of them, involving 1399 patients. Treatment did not significantly influence death from all causes (OR 0.99; 95% CI 0.79–1.24) or poor outcome (death, vegetative state or severe disability; OR 1.12; 95% CI 0.88–1.43). On the other hand, there were striking differences in specific event rates: antifibrinolytic treatment reduced the risk of rebleeding at the end of follow-up, with some heterogeneity between the trials (OR 0.55; 95% CI 0.42–0.71), but increased the risk of cerebral ischaemia (OR 1.39; 95% CI 1.07–1.82) with considerable heterogeneity between the most recent study, in which specific treatments to prevent cerebral ischemia were used,[125] and the four older studies. However, even in the trial where antifibrinolytic agents were tested in the presence of nimodipine and a strategy avoiding hypovolaemia, the drug still did not improve overall outcome.[125] The tenth and most recent trial was performed in Sweden and included 505 patients; but again the overall outcome did not appreciably improve in patients treated with TEA, despite an impressive reduction in rebleeding.[126]

> Antifibrinolytic drugs prevent rebleeding after aneurysmal rupture, but because they increase the risk of cerebral ischaemia they have no useful effect on overall outcome.

How antifibrinolytic treatment precipitates cerebral ischaemia is still unclear. Possible explanations include increased blood viscosity, the development of microthrombi, delayed clearance of blood clots around the arteries at the base of the brain, and the development of hydrocephalus through delayed resorption of blood. In brief, antifibrinolytic drugs work, but they do not help.

But this is not necessarily the end of the story if measures could be found to prevent the attendant ischaemia.

Recombinant factor VIIa

Theoretically, this activated coagulation factor might prevent rebleeding. Unfortunately, although an open-label, dose escalation safety study showed no evidence of ischaemic complications in the first nine patients, it was suspended when the tenth patient developed middle cerebral artery branch occlusion contralateral to the aneurysm.[127]

14.5 Prevention of delayed cerebral ischaemia

14.5.1 Pathogenesis and risk factors

Unlike ischaemic stroke as a result of disease of the extra- or intracranial arteries, cerebral ischaemia or infarction after subarachnoid haemorrhage (SAH) is not usually confined to the territory of a single cerebral artery or one of its branches.[128] Vasospasm is often implicated as the cause because its peak frequency from day 5 to 14 coincides with that of delayed ischaemia, and also because it is often generalized, in keeping with the multifocal or diffuse nature of the clinical manifestations and of the ischaemic lesions found on brain CT and at autopsy. Nevertheless, we have strong objections to the widespread use of the term 'vasospasm' as a synonym for delayed cerebral ischaemia, not so much out of fastidiousness on our part, but because the exchange of one term for the other impedes understanding and, even worse, progress. The eventual goal of treatment in this area is preventing cerebral ischaemia, not preventing arterial narrowing.

There are at least five reasons why vasospasm is not synonymous with delayed cerebral ischaemia:

- First, arterial narrowing does not necessarily signify contraction of smooth muscle in the arterial wall, but may represent necrosis and secondary oedema,[129–131] or intimal proliferation.[132,133]
- Second, arterial narrowing can be asymptomatic even if severe.[134–136]
- Third, interpretation of the severity or even the presence of arterial narrowing on an angiogram is subject to considerable variation between observers.[137]
- Fourth, strategies that reduce vasospasm may not be beneficial (endothelin receptor antagonists; section

14.5.6) and strategies that reduce the risk of cerebral ischaemia may do so without influencing vasospasm (calcium antagonists; section 14.5.2).

- Last, arterial narrowing is only one of the many factors involved in the pathogenesis of cerebral ischaemia in patients with ruptured aneurysms. One-third of patients with vasospasm do not develop cerebral ischaemia and one-third of patients with cerebral ischaemia have no vasospasm (Fig. 14.13).[138]

Many of the predictive factors for delayed cerebral ischaemia (Table 14.3) are interrelated or depend on

intermediate factors, and these interactions are complex and poorly understood. Also one should bear in mind that a sizeable proportion of patients who eventually develop delayed ischaemia have none of these risk factors.[138] An often quoted study postulated a close relationship between the location of subarachnoid blood and the 'thickness' of the clot on the one hand with the occurrence of vasospasm and delayed cerebral ischaemia on the other, but these observations were based on only 41 patients.[139] Moreover, the method of assessing local amounts of subarachnoid blood (called the Fisher scale,

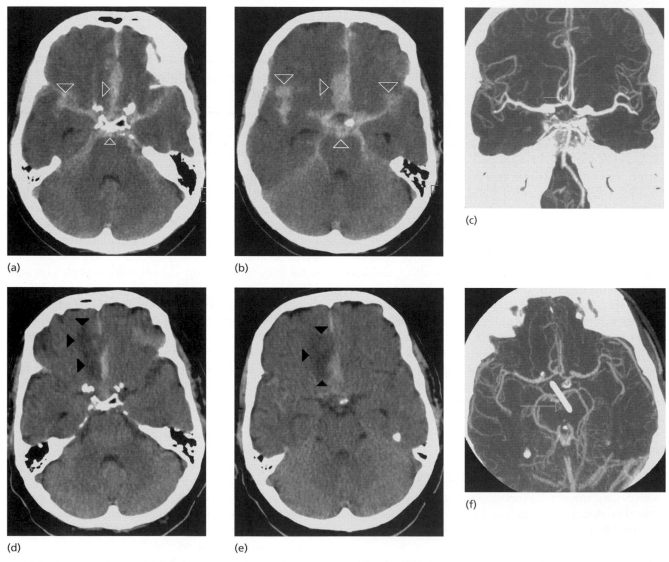

(a)   (b)   (c)   (d)   (e)   (f)

Fig. 14.13 CT scans and CT angiograms of a patient who deteriorated 5 days after the onset of subarachnoid haemorrhage. The cause of the deterioration was secondary ischaemia; CT angiograms show unchanged diameter of the intracranial vessels of the circle of Willis. (a, b) CT scan on admission showing diffuse subarachnoid blood in the basal cisterns and fissures (*white arrowheads*). (c) CT angiogram on admission with normal size of intracranial vessels and an aneurysm of the anterior communicating artery (*arrow*). (d, e) Repeat CT scan after the clinical deterioration showing areas of infarction in the territory of the right anterior cerebral artery (*black arrowheads*). (f) CT angiogram after the deterioration shows unchanged diameter of the intracranial vessels. An intraventricular drain has been inserted (*arrow*).

Table 14.3 Factors at baseline and during the clinical course that have been associated with delayed cerebral ischaemia after subarachnoid haemorrhage.

At baseline:
Cerebral arterial narrowing on initial angiogram[139,341]
but also:
Previous cigarette smoking?[342]
Previous cocaine use[343]
Loss of consciousness > 1 h at onset[142,148]
Amount of subarachnoid blood on early CT scanning[142,344–347]
Location of ruptured aneurysm on the anterior communicating artery or internal carotid artery,[346] or on the anterior choroidal artery[348]
Acute hydrocephalus[26,143,193,349]
Perfusion deficit on initial CT scan[147]
4G-allele in the 4G/5G-promotor polymorphism in the plasminogen activator inhibitor-1 (PAI-1) gene[350]
During the clinical course:
Hyponatraemia and hypovolaemia[42–44]
Treatment with antihypertensive drugs[39]
Hypotension during anaesthesia[351]
Treatment with antifibrinolytic drugs[352]
Emboli on transcranial Doppler monitoring after surgical clipping,[353] but not confirmed in another study[354]
Early ischaemic lesions on MR scanning[355]
Impaired cerebral autoregulation[136,356]

after the last author), has wide inter-observer variation.[140] Not surprisingly, therefore, in a comparison with a method of assessing the amount of blood in each of the cisterns and fissures separately in a semi-quantitative manner, this Fisher scale performed worse: it did not predict delayed cerebral ischaemia and poor clinical outcome, whereas the semi-quantitative scale did.[141] Although there is little doubt that the overall amount of subarachnoid blood as determined on CT scan is a powerful predictor of delayed cerebral ischaemia, larger series have failed to show any relationship between the anatomical distribution or even the side of infarction and the site of the extravasated blood in the subarachnoid space,[128,142] or at best in half the patients.[143] Another awkward fact – often conveniently overlooked – is that delayed cerebral ischaemia is rare after SAH from arteriovenous malformations despite arterial narrowing in some cases,[144] and also after bleeding from traumatic brain injury,[145] while it does not occur at all in perimesencephalic non-aneurysmal SAH, even after matching for the amount of extravasated blood.[146] It seems that subarachnoid blood is not a sufficient factor for the development of delayed cerebral ischaemia – the source has to be a ruptured artery. This suggestion is further supported by the finding that a generalized

perfusion deficit at the time of bleeding is an independent risk factor for the development of delayed cerebral ischaemia.[147]

Cerebral ischaemia after subarachnoid haemorrhage occurs only if the source is a ruptured aneurysm; whether or not it develops is strongly related to the total amount of subarachnoid blood, much less to the distribution of the extravasated blood.

The search for chemicals that might be mediators for arterial narrowing and the development of delayed cerebral ischaemia has been intensified as several new candidate molecules have been recognized (Table 14.4). However, the multitude of these isolated and often conflicting findings attests to the paltriness of our current insights into the chain of molecular events between aneurysmal rupture and delayed cerebral ischaemia. At any rate, the relationship between the amount of extravasated blood and the development of delayed cerebral ischaemia is not sufficiently explained by the simplistic notion that toxic substances are released from clots around the large arteries at the base of the brain. Because loss of consciousness at the time of the haemorrhage is an important and independent predictive factor for

Table 14.4 Intermediate substances implicated in the pathogenesis of delayed cerebral ischaemia. For many, the relation with delayed cerebral ischaemia could not be confirmed in other studies.

nitric oxide[357]
endothelin[358–362]
protein C kinase[358]
lipid peroxides[363]
free fatty acids[364]
soluble intercellular adhesion molecule-1 (ICAM-1)[365,366]
P-selectin and L-selectin[367]
sP-selectin[368]
E-selectin[369]
von Willebrand factor[370,371]
D-dimer[349,372]
prothrombin fragments I and II, thrombin-antithrombin III complex[372]
plasminogen activator inhibitor-1[372,373]
vascular endothelial growth factor[370]
inflammatory cytokines[374,375]
matrix metalloproteinase-9[370]
brain natriuretic peptide[376]
transferrin[377]
adrenomedullin (protective)[378]
tissue oxygen pressure[379,380]
lactate in CSF[381,382]
excitatory amino acids[382]

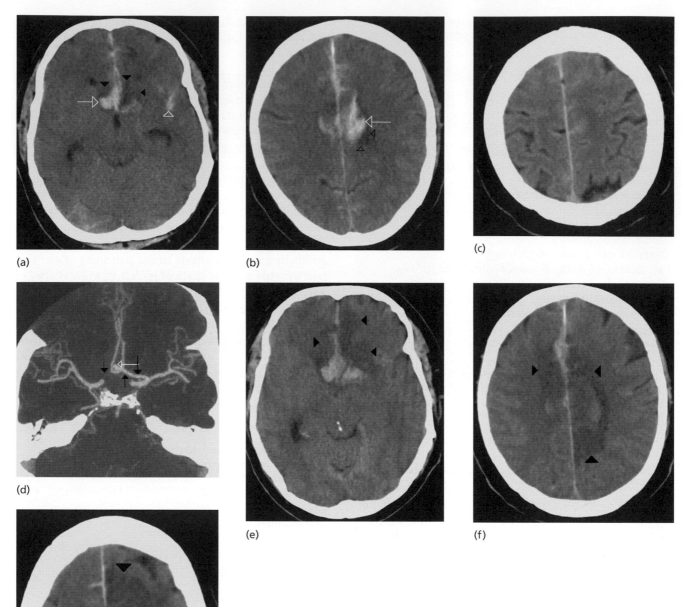

Fig. 14.14 CT scans of a patient with subarachnoid haemorrhage from an anterior communicating artery aneurysm with long-lasting loss of consciousness after the haemorrhage. During the following days his clinical condition improved, but on the sixth day his level of consciousness decreased again. (a, b, c) CT on admission showing intracerebral extension of the haemorrhage (*arrows*) and blood in the left sylvian fissure (*arrowhead*). There are already some areas of hypodensity (*black arrowheads*). (d) CT angiogram on admission showing an aneurysm on the anterior communicating artery (*white open arrow*). The left A1 part of the anterior communicating artery is present (*black arrows*), but on the right side this artery is missing (*arrow*). (e, f, g) CT scans after the clinical deterioration showing large areas of infarction in the territories of both anterior cerebral arteries (*black arrowheads*).

delayed cerebral ischaemia,[142,148] it is conceivable that global ischaemia during this brief period, along with a massive increase in intracranial pressure, may sensitize neurones to marginal perfusion associated with later complications, such as arterial narrowing and hypovolaemia (Fig. 14.14).

Practical measures that may help to prevent ischaemia are first of all avoidance of antihypertensive drugs (section 14.3.1) and an adequate intake of fluid and sodium, although the evidence for these recommendations is rather slender (section 14.3.2). Other interventions will be discussed below.

14.5.2 Calcium antagonists

A Cochrane review has assessed the trials of calcium antagonists in patients with aneurysmal SAH:[149] nimodipine (eight trials, 1574 patients), nicardipine (two trials, 954 patients), AT877 (one trial, 276 patients) and magnesium (one trial, 40 patients). Overall, calcium antagonists reduced the risk of poor outcome: relative risk (RR) 0.82 (95% CI 0.72–0.93); the absolute risk reduction was 5.1%, and the corresponding number of patients needed to treat to prevent a single poor outcome event was 20. For oral nimodipine alone the RR was 0.70 (0.58–0.84). The RR of death on treatment with calcium antagonists was 0.90 (95% CI 0.76–1.07), of clinical signs of delayed cerebral ischaemia 0.67 (95% CI 0.60–0.76), and of CT or MR confirmed infarction 0.80 (95% CI 0.71–0.89). In brief, the risk reduction for 'poor outcome' is statistically robust, but depends mainly on trials with oral nimodipine, and especially on a single large trial;[150] the evidence for nicardipine and AT877 was inconclusive (Fig. 14.15).

The intermediate factors through which nimodipine exerts its beneficial effect after aneurysmal SAH remain uncertain. Calcium entry-blocking drugs were tested for this indication because they inhibit the contractile properties of smooth muscle cells, particularly in cerebral arteries. Paradoxically, but not inconsistent with their effect on delayed cerebral ischaemia, several studies of nimodipine found there was no difference between treated patients and controls in the frequency of arterial narrowing on a repeat angiogram.[150–152] Therefore, at least with nimodipine, the protective effect on neurones seems to be more important than any reduction in vasospasm (section 14.5.1).

The practical implication is that the regimen in the dominant nimodipine trial (60 mg orally every 4 h, for 3 weeks) is currently regarded as the standard treatment in patients with aneurysmal SAH. But, given the uncertain effect on case fatality and the possibility that the results of the meta-analysis might be affected by unpublished negative trials, the benefits of nimodipine cannot be regarded as being beyond all reasonable doubt.

> Oral nimodipine probably reduces the risk of a poor outcome after subarachnoid haemorrhage by about one-third.

If the patient is unable to swallow, the nimodipine tablets should be crushed and washed down a nasogastric tube with normal saline. Intravenous administration is advocated by the manufacturer and is more expensive, but there is no evidence to support this.[149] Moreover, intravenous administration of nicardipine does not improve outcome.[149] The lack of effectiveness of calcium antagonists via the intravenous route is probably explained by the resulting hypotension,[153] which may even be a problem if nimodipine is given orally. Therefore, if no other cause for hypotension is found, the dose of nimodipine should be at first halved (to 30 mg every 4 h) and subsequently discontinued if the blood pressure continues to fall or the patient remains hypotensive.

14.5.3 Magnesium sulphate

Hypomagnesaemia occurs in more than 50% of patients with SAH and is associated with delayed cerebral ischaemia and poor outcome.[154] Magnesium reduces infarct volume after experimental SAH in rats[155] and its putative modes of action are inhibition of the release of excitatory amino acids and blockade of the N-methyl-D-aspartate-glutamate receptor. It is also a non-competitive antagonist of voltage-dependent calcium channels and dilates cerebral arteries.

Two randomized controlled trials have studied intravenous magnesium sulphate in addition to nimodipine. The smallest included only 60 patients and was inevitably inconclusive.[156] The larger trial included 283 patients but was still intended as a preliminary (phase II) study with delayed cerebral ischaemia and not overall clinical outcome as the primary measure of effectiveness.[157] Magnesium sulphate reduced delayed cerebral ischaemia by 34% (hazard ratio 0.66; 95% CI 0.38–1.14). After 3 months, the risk reduction for poor outcome was 23% (risk ratio 0.77; 95% CI 0.54–1.09). At that time, 18 patients in the treatment group and six in the placebo group had an excellent outcome (risk ratio 3.4; 95% CI 1.3–8.9). A phase III trial has subsequently been launched with poor outcome as the primary measure of outcome (http://www.controlled-trials.com/mrct/trial/MAGNESIUM/2061/132459.html). Just one trial has compared intravenous nimodipine with magnesium sulphate, and found no difference in delayed cerebral ischaemia, but the trial was too small (104 patients) to draw sound conclusions.[158]

14.5.4 Aspirin and other antithrombotic agents

Several studies have found that platelets are activated from day 3 after subarachnoid haemorrhage, mostly

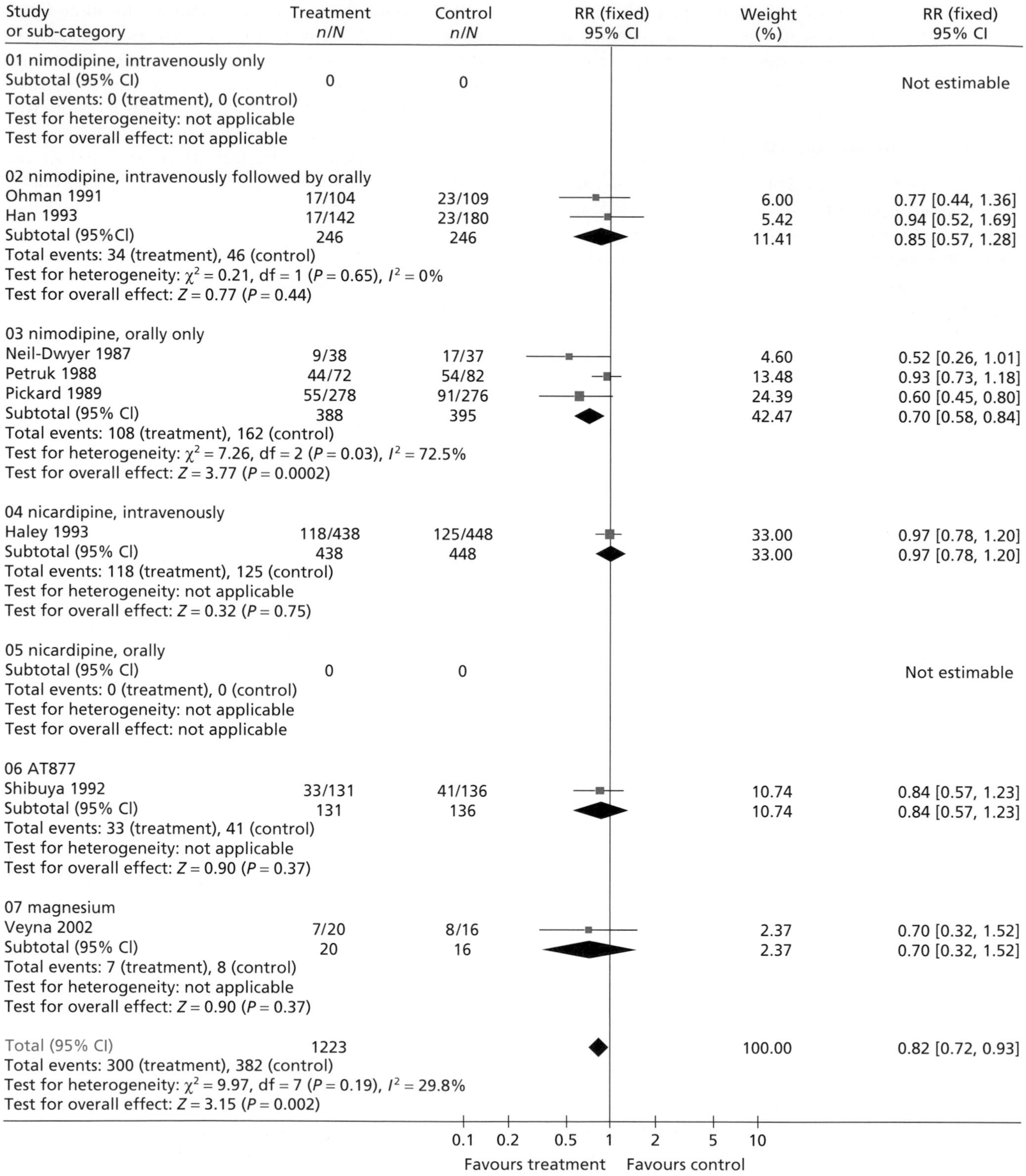

Study or sub-category	Treatment n/N	Control n/N	RR (fixed) 95% CI	Weight (%)	RR (fixed) 95% CI
01 nimodipine, intravenously only					
Subtotal (95% CI)	0	0			Not estimable
Total events: 0 (treatment), 0 (control)					
Test for heterogeneity: not applicable					
Test for overall effect: not applicable					
02 nimodipine, intravenously followed by orally					
Ohman 1991	17/104	23/109		6.00	0.77 [0.44, 1.36]
Han 1993	17/142	23/180		5.42	0.94 [0.52, 1.69]
Subtotal (95%CI)	246	246		11.41	0.85 [0.57, 1.28]
Total events: 34 (treatment), 46 (control)					
Test for heterogeneity: $\chi^2 = 0.21$, df = 1 ($P = 0.65$), $I^2 = 0\%$					
Test for overall effect: $Z = 0.77$ ($P = 0.44$)					
03 nimodipine, orally only					
Neil-Dwyer 1987	9/38	17/37		4.60	0.52 [0.26, 1.01]
Petruk 1988	44/72	54/82		13.48	0.93 [0.73, 1.18]
Pickard 1989	55/278	91/276		24.39	0.60 [0.45, 0.80]
Subtotal (95% CI)	388	395		42.47	0.70 [0.58, 0.84]
Total events: 108 (treatment), 162 (control)					
Test for heterogeneity: $\chi^2 = 7.26$, df = 2 ($P = 0.03$), $I^2 = 72.5\%$					
Test for overall effect: $Z = 3.77$ ($P = 0.0002$)					
04 nicardipine, intravenously					
Haley 1993	118/438	125/448		33.00	0.97 [0.78, 1.20]
Subtotal (95% CI)	438	448		33.00	0.97 [0.78, 1.20]
Total events: 118 (treatment), 125 (control)					
Test for heterogeneity: not applicable					
Test for overall effect: $Z = 0.32$ ($P = 0.75$)					
05 nicardipine, orally					
Subtotal (95% CI)	0	0			Not estimable
Total events: 0 (treatment), 0 (control)					
Test for heterogeneity: not applicable					
Test for overall effect: not applicable					
06 AT877					
Shibuya 1992	33/131	41/136		10.74	0.84 [0.57, 1.23]
Subtotal (95% CI)	131	136		10.74	0.84 [0.57, 1.23]
Total events: 33 (treatment), 41 (control)					
Test for heterogeneity: not applicable					
Test for overall effect: $Z = 0.90$ ($P = 0.37$)					
07 magnesium					
Veyna 2002	7/20	8/16		2.37	0.70 [0.32, 1.52]
Subtotal (95% CI)	20	16		2.37	0.70 [0.32, 1.52]
Total events: 7 (treatment), 8 (control)					
Test for heterogeneity: not applicable					
Test for overall effect: $Z = 0.90$ ($P = 0.37$)					
Total (95% CI)	1223			100.00	0.82 [0.72, 0.93]
Total events: 300 (treatment), 382 (control)					
Test for heterogeneity: $\chi^2 = 9.97$, df = 7 ($P = 0.19$), $I^2 = 29.8\%$					
Test for overall effect: $Z = 3.15$ ($P = 0.002$)					

0.1   0.2   0.5   1   2   5   10

Favours treatment   Favours control

Fig. 14.15 Forest plot of the Cochrane review on the effectiveness of calcium antagonists on death and dependency, 3–6 months after subarachnoid haemorrhage.[149] The results are shown separately for each drug and route of administration. RR, relative risk; CI, confidence interval.

inferred from increased levels of thromboxane B2, the stable metabolite of thromboxane A2, which promotes platelet aggregation and vasoconstriction (section 16.5.3).[159,160] The question then is whether interventions aimed at counteracting platelet activation are therapeutically useful. A retrospective analysis of 242 patients who had survived the first 4 days after SAH showed that patients who had used salicylates before their haemorrhage had a significantly decreased risk of delayed cerebral ischaemia, with or without permanent deficits (relative risk 0.40; 95% CI 0.18–0.93).[161] The first randomized clinical trial was reported as early as 1982 but it failed to show any benefit from aspirin;[162] however, the number of patients was small,[53] unoperated patients were also included, and all were treated with tranexamic acid which increases the risk of ischaemia (section 14.4.4). A further study of aspirin after early operation in 50 patients confirmed that this treatment was feasible and probably safe.[163] The efficacy, however, could not be confirmed in a randomized trial of aspirin given after occlusion of the aneurysm that aimed to include 200 patients; this was prematurely stopped after the second interim analysis because by then the chances of a positive effect were negligible. At the final analysis, aspirin did not reduce the risk of delayed ischaemia (hazard ratio (HR) 1.83; 95% CI 0.8–3.9) nor that of poor outcome (HR 0.79; 95% CI 0.4–1.6).[95]

Three other antiplatelet drugs have been tested in patients with SAH: dipyridamole;[164] the thromboxane A2 synthetase inhibitor, cataclot;[165] and the experimental antiplatelet agent OKY-46.[166] Ischaemic neurological deficits were reduced in one[166] but not in the other trial that assessed this outcome event.[165] In a systematic overview of these three trials and the three published aspirin trials, the risk of delayed cerebral ischaemia (reported in only four of the five trials) was decreased, but not to a statistically significant level (relative risk 0.81; 95% CI 0.6–1.1). For the three aspirin studies alone, the relative risk for delayed cerebral ischaemia was 1.34 (95% CI 0.8–2.3). Poor clinical outcome was not significantly different between patients treated with antiplatelet drugs and controls (relative risk 0.86; 95% CI 0.6–1.3) (Dorhout Mees *et al.*, unpublished data).

A low-molecular-weight heparinoid, enoxoparin has been tested in a trial of 170 patients but it did not improve outcome and was associated with intracranial haemorrhage in 4 of 85 patients in the experimental group.[56]

14.5.5 Statins

HMG-CoA reductase inhibitors, or statins, are primarily used to lower LDL-cholesterol levels but they also have anti-inflammatory, immunomodulatory, antithrombotic and vascular effects. It has often been claimed that these 'pleiotropic effects' contribute to the reduction in vascular events such as myocardial infarction beyond that expected from LDL-cholesterol reduction alone, although this has not been confirmed by a meta-regression analysis of the randomized trials.[167] In patients with SAH, two randomized trials have been performed so far. One included only 39 patients and found that 80 mg simvastatin given within 48 h of the onset reduced 'vasospasm' (undefined),[168] and the other enrolled 80 patients and found that 40 mg pravastatin given within 72 h reduced angiographic vasospasm and impairment of autoregulatory responses as well as vasospasm-related ischaemic complications.[169] On the other hand, an observational study found that previous use of statins increased the risk of angiographic vasospasm though not that of associated ischaemic complications.[170] In conclusion, the evidence for a beneficial effect of statins after SAH is still very meagre.

14.5.6 Other drugs

Tirilazad mesylate, a 21-aminosteroid free radical scavenger, has not consistently improved outcome in four randomized controlled trials, with a total of more than 3500 patients.[171–174] Although, in one single subgroup (the one with the highest dosage) a beneficial effect on overall outcome was seen,[171] this could not be reproduced in the corresponding subgroup from a parallel trial,[172] nor in two subsequent trials.[173,174] In these last two trials, only women were included and they were treated with even higher dosages than in the preceding trials, because in the first two trials women had appeared to respond less than men. A paper reporting that patients on the study drug in a small subgroup from New Zealand had less fatigue and better neuropsychological performance than controls suggests desperation rather than conviction among the investigators and the sponsoring company.[175]

A single trial with another hydroxyl radical scavenger, N′-propylenedinicotinamide (nicaraven), in 162 patients, showed a decrease in delayed cerebral ischaemia but not in poor clinical outcome at 3 months after SAH.[176] Curiously enough, the reverse was found in a trial of 286 patients with ebselen, a seleno-organic compound with antioxidant activity through a glutathione peroxidase-like action.[177] A formal overview of all the evidence for free radical scavengers is not yet available, but the case for these drugs seems weak.

Nizofenone, an anionic channel blocker believed to inhibit glutamate release, was studied in a randomized trial of 100 patients, of whom only 90 were included in the analysis;[178] angiographic vasospasm and poor outcome were not affected, and an effect on poor outcome was found only in an on-treatment analysis in the subgroup of patients with vasospasm.

The endothelin$_{A/B}$ receptor antagonist TAK-044 was tested in a multicentre phase II trial in 420 patients;[179] there was a non-significant risk reduction of 0.8 in delayed ischaemic deficits (95% CI 0.61–1.06).

14.5.7 Increasing the plasma volume

The usefulness of circulatory volume expansion to prevent delayed cerebral ischaemia after SAH has been assessed in a recent Cochrane review.[180] Only one truly randomized and one quasi-randomized trial with comparable baseline characteristics for both groups could be included in the analyses. Volume expansion did not improve outcome (relative risk [RR] 1.0; 95% CI 0.5–2.2), nor delayed cerebral ischaemia (RR 1.1; 95% CI 0.5–2.2), but tended to increase the complications (RR 1.8; 95% CI 0.9–3.7). In another quasi-randomized trial, not included in the analyses, outcome was assessed only on the day of operation (7–10 days after SAH). In the period before operation, treatment resulted in a reduction of secondary ischaemia (RR 0.33; 95% CI 0.11–0.99) and case fatality (RR 0.20; 95% CI 0.07–1.2). In conclusion, volume expansion has been studied properly in only two trials of patients with aneurysmal SAH, with very small numbers, and so far there is no sound evidence to support this therapy.

Because of its mineralocorticoid activity (reabsorption of sodium in the distal tubules of the kidney) fludrocortisone might, in theory, prevent a negative sodium balance, hypovolaemia and so ischaemic complications.[181] A randomized study in 91 patients with SAH showed that although fludrocortisone acetate did reduce natriuresis in the first 6 days after the haemorrhage, there was no definite effect on plasma volume depletion or on ischaemic complications, although any beneficial effects may have been masked because patients in the control group were often treated with plasma expanders after they had developed clinical signs of ischaemia.[182] These results were confirmed by a smaller trial in 30 patients.[183] Finally, hydrocortisone was also shown in a small trial of 28 patients to prevent hyponatraemia and a drop in central venous pressure.[184] The evidence from these studies is insufficiently conclusive to warrant routine fludrocortisone for all patients with SAH.

> Although it is reasonable to prevent a decrease in plasma volume, there is no good evidence to support prevention of cerebral ischaemia after SAH through increasing plasma volume by infusion of albumin or colloids, or by the administration of fludrocortisone.

14.5.8 Cisternal drainage and intracisternal fibrinolysis

On the assumption that vasospasm increases the risk of delayed cerebral ischaemia and that extravasated blood induces vasospasm, removal of the subarachnoid blood by drainage or fibrinolysis has been suggested and then studied in several trials. For example, in a non-randomized comparison, patients treated with lumbar drainage of CSF had cerebral infarction less often and more often returned home than patients with no lumbar drainage.[185] Because no randomized trials have been performed yet, this strategy cannot be recommended for routine clinical practice. An even more aggressive way to remove subarachnoid blood is intracisternal fibrinolysis. A meta-analysis of this treatment strategy included nine trials of which only one was randomized.[186] Pooled results demonstrated beneficial effects of treatment but the conclusions for practice are obviously very limited by the predominance of non-randomized studies. An open, randomized, controlled trial not yet included in the meta-analysis tested fibrinolysis in 110 patients treated with endovascular coiling.[187] Urokinase was administered into the cisterna magna through a microcatheter inserted via a lumbar puncture. There was a statistically significant improvement in the primary outcome of clinical vasospasm, defined as clinical deterioration combined with evidence of vasospasm on angiography, but case fatality was not reduced even though patients in the treated group more often had a good clinical outcome. Larger studies with overall clinical outcome as the primary measurement of outcome are needed before this treatment can be implemented in clinical practice.

14.6 Management of rebleeding

14.6.1 Diagnosis

Loss of consciousness was the cardinal feature of rebleeding in a prospective series of 39 patients with CT-proven rebleeding: of the 36 patients who were awake at the time, 35 lost consciousness, with preceding headache in one-third; in the remaining patient a sudden increase in headache was the only symptom.[188] Serial CT scanning uncovered rebleeding in two of the three remaining patients, in whom the level of consciousness was already minimal. No 'silent rebleeding' was found in awake patients. In patients with a first episode of subarachnoid

Table 14.5 Specific causes of *sudden* deterioration in patients with aneurysmal subarachnoid haemorrhage.[383]

> Rebleeding (two-thirds) (section 14.6.1)
> Epileptic seizure (section 14.3.3)
> Delayed cerebral ischaemia, with atypical, sudden onset (section 14.7)
> Ventricular fibrillation (section 14.9.3)

haemorrhage, loss of consciousness is less common, occurring in slightly less than half.[55] That unconsciousness occurs more often with rebleeding than with a first rupture confirms that rebleeding has a more severe impact on the brain, and so a higher risk of a poor outcome (80%).[4] In fatal episodes of rebleeding most patients immediately lose their brainstem reflexes at the same time as consciousness, but without initial apnoea.

However, rebleeding is not the only cause of a sudden deterioration of consciousness in a patient with a ruptured aneurysm; other complications underlie about one-third of such episodes (Table 14.5). Therefore, once the respiratory and circulatory state of the patient has sufficiently stabilized, it is mandatory to confirm the diagnosis of rebleeding by repeat brain CT.

14.6.2 To resuscitate or not?

Whether patients with rebleeding should be resuscitated and ventilated if respiratory arrest occurs is not academic; in the series of 39 patients with CT-confirmed rebleeding, 14 had initial respiratory abnormalities that called for assisted ventilation. Spontaneous respiration returned within 1 h in eight of these 14 patients, and in three more between 1 and 24 h.[188] In another study of episodes of respiratory arrest but in which first bleeds were also included, whether the patient would or would not regain spontaneous respiration could not be predicted from the anatomical site of haemorrhage on CT, the initial presence or absence of brainstem reflexes, or the type of respiratory disorder.[12] Many patients with initial apnoea who were successfully resuscitated later died from subsequent complications, but survival without brain damage is clearly possible – even after respiratory arrest.

Rebleeding can also cause cardiac arrest, but again in this situation resuscitation is worthwhile. Cardiac function usually recovers within minutes and some patients can have a good overall outcome. Out of 11 patients with 14 episodes of well-documented cardiac arrest, six survived and three of them became independent for activities of daily living.[13] After resuscitation, it will usually become clear within a matter of hours whether the patient will indeed survive the episode or whether dysfunction of the brainstem will persist. There are no grounds to fear that resuscitation will only result in prolongation of a vegetative state and, in patients who do progress to a state of brain death, the resuscitation procedure at least allows organ donation to be considered, with some benefits to others.

> Sudden apnoea or cardiac arrest in a patient with subarachnoid haemorrhage usually signifies rebleeding. With full resuscitative measures cardiac function usually recovers within minutes and spontaneous respiration will rapidly return in approximately 50% of the cases, followed within hours by return of consciousness and of brainstem reflexes if these had been lost at the same time. If spontaneous respiration does not return, then organ donation should be considered.

14.6.3 Emergency occlusion of the aneurysm

A large haematoma that causes brain shift without gross intraventricular haemorrhage is infrequent after rebleeding, occurring in around 10% of patients.[189] In these rare cases, emergency evacuation of the haematoma after aneurysm occlusion may be indicated, as after first rupture (section 14.2.2). A more common reason for urgent aneurysm occlusion after rebleeding is the concern that, among the survivors, 50–75% will have further episodes of rebleeding if the aneurysm is left untreated.[9,188] This implies that emergency clipping or coiling of the aneurysm should be seriously considered in patients who regain consciousness after rebleeding. Of course, the risk of the operation is increased after rebleeding but the risks of a wait-and-see policy at that stage seem even more intimidating. The management of rebleeding is summarized in Table 14.6.

Table 14.6 Management of rebleeding.

> If cardiac or respiratory arrest, resuscitate and ventilate; cardiac resuscitation is usually successful and within hours either spontaneous respiration will return or all brainstem functions will be lost
> Repeat CT brain scan to confirm diagnosis
> Consider emergency clipping or coiling of aneurysm after recovery, because many patients will have further episodes of rebleeding, with a high case fatality
> Large intracerebral haematomas can be evacuated at the same time

Table 14.7 Causes of *gradual* deterioration after subarachnoid haemorrhage.

Oedema surrounding intracerebral haematoma
Delayed cerebral ischaemia (section 14.7.1)
Hydrocephalus (section 14.8.1)
Unsuspected rebleeding (section 14.6.1)
Systemic complication (section 14.9)
Hyponatraemia
Disturbance of heart rhythm
Hypoxia from pulmonary oedema or chest infection
Hypotension
Infection

14.7 Management of delayed cerebral ischaemia

14.7.1 Diagnosis

The diagnosis of delayed cerebral ischaemia after SAH is far less straightforward than diagnosing ischaemic stroke, not only in daily practice, but also in research. To compound the problem, in many papers delayed cerebral ischaemia is poorly defined or not even defined at all.[190] This difficulty in recognising reliably delayed cerebral ischaemia is disturbing because it is only one of several other causes of gradual deterioration in patients after SAH (Table 14.7).

The clinical manifestations of delayed cerebral ischaemia evolve gradually, over several hours, and usually between day 4 and 12 after the haemorrhage. In 25% of the patients ischaemia causes hemispheric focal deficits, in another 25% a decrease in the level of consciousness, and in the remaining 50% these two features develop at the same time.[128] The diagnosis should be based not only on this clinical picture, but also on the results of laboratory investigations and a repeat brain CT to exclude other intracranial causes of subacute deterioration, such as oedema surrounding an intracerebral haematoma, dilatation of the ventricular system or unsuspected rebleeding. Positive evidence of ischaemia is shown by CT in about 80% of patients after exclusion of these other causes, at least after a few days from the onset of the clinical signs of delayed cerebral ischaemia.[128] The disadvantage of CT scanning is that it confirms cerebral ischaemia only some time after the clinical deterioration, which is too late for interventions that may be applied early after the onset of the ischaemia. However, currently CT scanning is the only method to confirm delayed cerebral ischaemia. One advantage of CT scanning is that it provides information about the

extent and location of the ischaemia. A recent study distinguished two patterns of infarction: single cortical infarcts, typically near the ruptured aneurysm, and multiple widespread lesions including subcortical locations and often unrelated to the site of aneurysm rupture.[143]

MRI is more sensitive in detecting early changes in the water content of the brain, especially with diffusion-weighted imaging,[191] but the acquisition time needed to obtain good images is often too long for ill and restless patients. Single-photon emission CT (SPECT) scanning may be helpful but hypoperfusion may also result from oedema around a resolving haematoma or, in the basal parts of the brain, from hydrocephalus.[192,193]

Transcranial Doppler sonography (TCD) may suggest impending cerebral ischaemia by the increased blood flow velocity from arterial narrowing, but there is considerable overlap with patients who do not develop ischaemia. A systematic review of studies in which TCD findings were compared with vascular imaging found that only for the middle cerebral artery was there good specificity (99%; 95% CI 98–100%) and moderate sensitivity (67%; 95% CI 48–87%).[194] For other arteries, TCD was neither accurate nor useful. However, most of these data are of low methodological quality, bias cannot be ruled out and the data reporting was often uncritical. Furthermore, demonstration of arterial narrowing does not prove in itself that clinical deterioration has been caused by ischaemia. Factors such as intracranial pressure, arterial blood pressure and respiration may all influence the form of the velocity wave.

Multi-slice CT angiography provides results that are in good agreement with those of catheter angiography,[195,196] but the question still remains how useful is it to obtain information about arterial narrowing, given the imperfect correlation with the occurrence of brain ischaemia. In a study where vasospasm was diagnosed by TCD and catheter angiography, its presence was associated with delayed cerebral ischaemia in only two-thirds of patients (positive predictive value 0.67) and its absence with no delayed cerebral ischaemia in a similar proportion (negative predictive value 0.72).[138]

Because delayed cerebral ischaemia is difficult to diagnose from the outset, many physicians rely on TCD or angiographic studies to rule in or out the presence of vasospasm. However, since the negative and positive predictive values of vasospasm for cerebral ischaemia are moderate at best, knowing whether there is or is not vasospasm is not very helpful. In fact, ordering a transcranial Doppler (or even worse catheter angiography) in a patient suspected of delayed cerebral ischaemia is comparable to ordering a duplex of the carotid artery to confirm by the presence or absence of carotid artery stenosis a transient ischaemic attack as the cause of an episode of unclear neurological symptoms.

14.7.2 Induced hypertension and volume expansion

Since the 1960s, induced hypertension has been used to combat ischaemic deficits in patients with SAH. Particularly remarkable was the report of a patient in whom postoperative aphasia and right hemiparesis fluctuated with the level of the blood pressure.[197] Later, induced hypertension was often combined with volume expansion, but again only in uncontrolled case series, of which just one had an acceptable definition of outcome events.[198] Another case series argued that hypertensive and hypervolaemic therapy was unlikely to be successful in patients with a Glasgow Coma Score of 11 or less, as well as with hydrocephalus.[199] However, on the basis of these and other case reports and series many physicians have used induced hypertension and hypervolaemia and seen their patients improve, but randomized controlled trials are sadly missing.

If raising the blood pressure and increasing plasma volume can indeed reverse ischaemic deficits – which remains to be proven beyond doubt – the most plausible explanation is a defect of cerebral autoregulation that makes the perfusion of the injured brain passively dependent on the systemic blood pressure. To add haemodilution to hypertensive and hypervolaemic treatment (the so-called 'triple-H' regimen) is not only of uncertain benefit, but even controversial.[200]

The risks of deliberately increasing the arterial pressure and plasma volume include rebleeding of untreated aneurysms additional to the ruptured aneurysm, although this procedure did not in fact cause haemorrhages in a series of 40 patients with 73 unsecured additional aneurysms.[201] Other complications are increased cerebral oedema, haemorrhagic transformation in areas of infarction,[202] reversible leucencephalopathy,[203] myocardial infarction and congestive heart failure. Certainly the circulatory system should be closely monitored, though arterial lines and pulmonary artery catheters carry their own risks: infection, pneumothorax, haemothorax, ventricular arrhythmia and pulmonary infarction.[48–50]

A currently recommended regimen (Table 14.8), although not supported by rigorously controlled trials, is to start with plasma volume expansion with Hetastarch or another colloid solution (5% albumin does not increase plasma volume).[204] The aim is to raise the central venous filling pressure to approximately 8–12 mmHg. If there is no clinical improvement, one might consider raising the blood pressure with dopamine or dobutamine by 20–40 mmHg above pre-treatment

Table 14.8 Management of cerebral ischaemia.

Immediately give 500 mL of colloid solution i.v.
Consider subclavian vein catheter and maintain central venous pressure between 8 and 12 mmHg
Consider increasing mean arterial pressure by 20–40 mmHg above baseline values
Correct any hypoxaemia
Maintain fluid intake with at least 3 L of normal saline (0.9%) per 24 h
Correct hyponatraemia if severe (Table 14.10)

values. These procedures should be carried out only in an intensive care unit with facilities for specialized care and close monitoring.

14.7.3 Transluminal angioplasty and vasodilating drugs

Only a few centres have reported on endovascular treatment of 'symptomatic vasospasm' after SAH, claiming sustained improvement in more than half the cases, but these series were uncontrolled and there must be publication bias.[205] Some of these studies reported results only for arteries, and not – more relevantly – for patients. Vessel rupture is precipitated by this procedure in about 1%, even after the aneurysm has been occluded, and other complications such as hyperperfusion injury in 4%.[205] In another uncontrolled series of patients treated with transluminal angioplasty, papaverine injection or both, overall clinical outcome was poor despite successful arterial dilatation. Half the patients died or remained disabled, and half the survivors had permanent deficits from cerebral infarction.[206] In view of the risks, the high costs and the lack of controlled trials, transluminal angioplasty should still be regarded as a strictly experimental procedure.[207]

The same caution applies to uncontrolled reports of improvement of ischaemic deficits after intra-arterial infusion of drugs through super-selective catheterization. Papaverine has gained undeserved popularity,[208] the more so because not all impressions are positive.[209,210] Intra-arterial milrinone, verapamil or nicardipine dilate vessels but whether they improve clinical outcome is very uncertain.[211–213]

Calcitonin gene-related peptide (CGRP) is a potent vasodilator in the carotid vascular bed, but a randomized, multicentre, single-blind clinical trial in 62 patients with ischaemic complications after SAH failed to show any benefit in terms of overall clinical outcome: the relative risk of a poor outcome in CGRP-treated patients was 0.88 (95% CI 0.60–1.28).[214]

14.8   Management of acute hydrocephalus

14.8.1 Diagnosis

About 20% of unselected patients admitted within 3 days of SAH develop acute hydrocephalus, defined as a bicaudate index above the 95th percentile for age (Fig. 14.16).[26,215,216] Predisposing factors are frank intraventricular haemorrhage (Fig. 14.17),[26,217,218] extensive haemorrhage in the perimesencephalic cisterns in the tentorial hiatus (Fig. 14.18)[217,219] and – in only a single study – increasing age.[218] Fenestration of the lamina terminalis as part of any surgical treatment may reduce the risk of hydrocephalus according to observational studies,[220,221] but the increasing application of

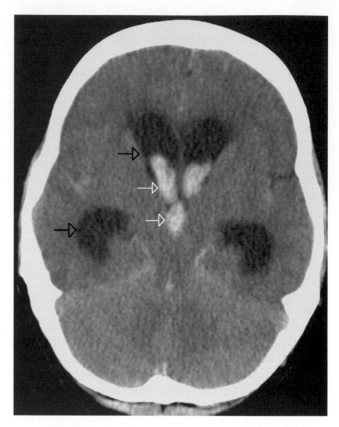

Fig. 14.17 CT scan of a patient with hydrocephalus from intraventricular extension of the haemorrhage. The lateral (*upper black arrow*) and temporal horns (*lower black arrow*) are enlarged; there is blood in the lateral (*upper white arrow*) and third (*lower white arrow*) ventricles.

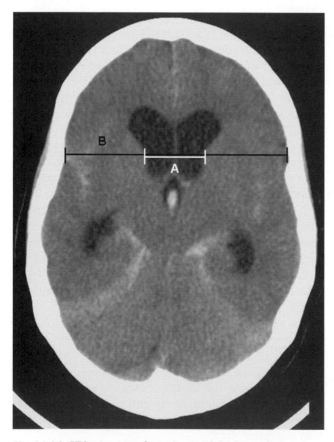

Fig. 14.16 CT brain scan of a patient with hydrocephalus (same patient as in Fig. 14.12) showing the bicaudate index (A/B), a simple and linear method for measuring the size of the ventricular system. A is the width of the frontal horns between the parallel walls of the caudate nuclei, at the level of the foramina of Monro, B the diameter of the brain at the same level. The 95th percentile for the bicaudate index is 0.16 at age 30 years or under, 0.18 at 50 years, 0.19 at 60 years, 0.21 at 80 years, and 0.25 at 100 years.

endovascular techniques for aneurysm occlusion will make this procedure less feasible.

The typical presentation of acute hydrocephalus is that of a patient who is alert immediately after the initial haemorrhage, but who in the next few hours becomes increasingly drowsy, to the point that he or she only moans and localizes to pain. Nonetheless only half of all patients with acute hydrocephalus present in this way.[26] In the others consciousness is impaired from the onset, or the course is unknown because the patient was alone at the time of haemorrhage. If the patient is admitted very early and secondary deterioration occurs because of hydrocephalus, serial investigation by CT may show that the level of consciousness correlates more or less inversely with the width of the lateral ventricles.[27] But when different patients are compared within one series, the relationship between the level of consciousness and the degree of ventricular dilatation is rather erratic.[26,215]

Ocular signs do not always accompany the obtundation as a result of acute hydrocephalus; they help to corroborate but not to exclude the diagnosis. In a prospective study in which 30 of 34 patients with acute

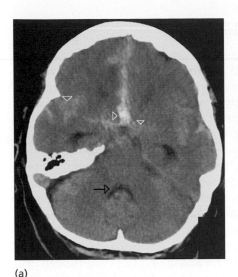
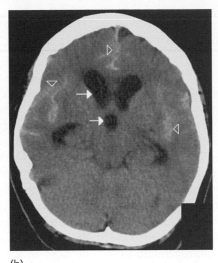
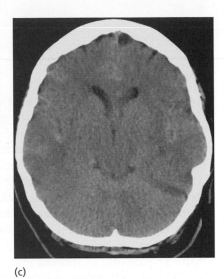

(a)   (b)   (c)

Fig. 14.18 CT scans of a patient with hydrocephalus from diffuse subarachnoid blood without intraventricular extension of the haemorrhage. The hydrocephalus was treated with lumbar punctures. (a, b) CT scan on admission showing diffuse subarachnoid blood (*white arrowheads*) and no blood in the fourth ventricle (*black arrow*). The lateral and third ventricles are enlarged (*white arrows*). (c) Later CT scan showing disappearance of the hydrocephalus.

hydrocephalus had an impaired level of consciousness, nine of these 30 had small, non-reactive pupils, and four of these nine also showed persistent downward deviation of the eyes, with otherwise intact brainstem reflexes.[26] These eye signs reflect dilatation of the proximal part of the aqueduct, which causes dysfunction of the pretectal area.[222] All nine patients with non-reactive pupils had a relative ventricular size of more than 1.20 and were in coma, i.e. they did not open their eyes, obey commands or utter words.

> Repeat CT scanning is required to diagnose or exclude hydrocephalus in a patient with subarachnoid haemorrhage who deteriorates within hours or days of the initial event, with or without eye signs of hydrocephalus (small, unreactive pupils and downward deviation of gaze). Patients with intraventricular blood or with extensive haemorrhage in the perimesencephalic cisterns are particularly likley to develop acute hydrocephalus.

14.8.2 Possible interventions

Possible interventions are listed in Table 14.9.

Wait-and-see

A policy of wait-and-see for 24 h is eminently justified in patients with dilated ventricles who are alert because only about one-third of them will become symptomatic in the next few days.[215] Postponing interventions for a day can also be rewarding if the level of consciousness

Table 14.9 Management of acute hydrocephalus

> Consider diagnosis if level of consciousness gradually deteriorates, particularly on the first day after the bleed
> Repeat the CT brain scan and compare the bicaudate index with that on any previous scan
> Spontaneous improvement occurs within 24 h in 50% of patients (except those with massive intraventricular haemorrhage); take action if patient further deteriorates or fails to improve within 24 h
> Lumbar punctures are reasonably safe if there is no brain shift, and effective in about 50% of the patients who have no intraventricular obstruction
> External drainage of the ventricles is very effective in restoring the level of consciousness, but may increase the risk of rebleeding (consider emergency clipping or coiling at the same time), and does increase the risk of infection (this may to some degree be prevented by prophylactic antibiotics, subcutaneous tunnelling, or both)

is decreased because spontaneous improvement within this period has been documented in approximately half of the patients (7 of 13) with acute hydrocephalus who were only drowsy, and in almost half (19 of 43) who had a Glasgow Coma Score of 12/14 or worse but no massive intraventricular haemorrhage.[215] It is not always easy to make a definitive decision on the need for surgical measures even after 1 day has elapsed because patients may temporarily improve to some extent but then reach a plateau or again deteriorate; such fluctuations are encountered in about one-third of patients with symptomatic hydrocephalus.[215] Any further deterioration in the level of consciousness warrants active intervention.

Lumbar puncture

Lumbar puncture was suggested as a therapeutic measure a long time ago,[223] but formal studies are scarce. In a prospective but uncontrolled study, 17 patients were treated in this way because they had acute hydrocephalus with neither a haematoma nor gross intraventricular haemorrhage.[28] Between one and seven lumbar punctures per patient were performed in the first 10 days, the number depending on the rate of improvement; each time a maximum of 20 mL of cerebrospinal fluid was removed, the aim being a closing pressure of 15 cmH$_2$O. Of the 17 patients, 12 showed initial improvement: of these 12, six fully recovered, two showed incomplete improvement but fully recovered after insertion of an internal shunt, and four patients died of other complications several days after the lumbar punctures had been started. Of the five remaining patients in whom lumbar puncture had no effect, two recovered after an internal shunt and three died of other complications.

Whether the risk of rebleeding is increased by lumbar punctures or drainage is uncertain. In a study of the risk of rebleeding after lumbar puncture, a series of patients with SAH and hydrocephalus treated with one or more lumbar punctures within 4 days after the haemorrhage and before aneurysm occlusion was compared with control patients with untreated hydrocephalus and with control patients without ventricular enlargement. Patients and controls were matched for interval since SAH, use of tranexamic acid, clinical condition on admission, and age. In the group treated with one or more lumbar punctures, rebleeding occurred in one of 21 patients (5%), in three of 21 controls (14%) with untreated hydrocephalus and in none of the 21 controls without hydrocephalus. Thus, this study did not confirm an increased risk of rebleeding after lumbar puncture, but because of the small number of patients it could not rule this out.[224] Until randomized controlled trials are available, and we think these are still needed and ethically justifiable, the tentative conclusion is that lumbar puncture seems a safe and reasonably effective way of treating those forms of acute hydrocephalus that are not obviously caused by intraventricular obstruction.

> In patients deteriorating from acute hydrocephalus after subarachnoid haemorrhage it is worth trying lumbar punctures if spontaneous improvement does not occur within 24 h, and if the probable site of obstruction is in the subarachnoid space, not in the ventricular system.

External ventricular drainage

External drainage of the cerebral ventricles by a catheter inserted through a burr hole is, in many centres, the most common method of treating acute hydrocephalus; the improvement is usually rapid and sometimes dramatic.[26,215] Internal drainage, to the right atrium or peritoneal cavity, is rarely considered in the first few days because the blood in the cerebrospinal fluid will almost inevitably block the shunt system. However, a major concern is that the abrupt lowering of the intracranial pressure could precipitate rebleeding due to decreased transmural pressure, or removal of clot sealing the ruptured aneurysm. Therefore, the pressure of the cerebrospinal fluid after external ventricular drainage should be kept between 15 and 25 mmHg,[225] although this does not abolish the risk of rebleeding.[215] Aneurysm pulsatilty and size increase after ventricular drainage, which further supports the notion of an increased risk of rebleeding.[226] Indeed, several studies have suggested a significantly increased risk of rebleeding in patients with external ventricular drainage, compared with patients without it.[227] However, many variables that could affect the rebleeding rate, such as the timing of surgery, the timing and duration of drainage, the size of the aneurysm, as well as the severity of the initial haemorrhage, do not seem to have been adequately explored in most of these studies.[227] In a recent study, the risk of rebleeding after external ventricular drainage within 4 days after the haemorrhage and before aneurysm occlusion was compared with control patients with untreated hydrocephalus, and with control patients without ventricular enlargement. Patients and controls were matched for interval since SAH, duration of exposure, use of tranexamic acid, clinical condition on admission, and age. Rebleeding occurred in seven of 34 patients treated with external ventricular drainage (21%), in seven of 34 controls (21%) with untreated hydrocephalus, and in six of 34 controls (18%) without hydrocephalus.[224] Thus, this study did not confirm an increased risk, but because of the small number of patients it could not rule it out.[224]

Ventriculitis is a frequent complication of external drainage, especially if it is continued for more than a few days.[215] But regular exchange of the intraventricular catheter, in a randomized controlled study, did not decrease the risk of infection.[228] Likewise, a review of studies, all retrospective, before that trial was published found prophylactic catheter exchange did not modify the risk of developing later infection.[229] Some advocate very rigid antiseptic techniques and prophylactic antibiotics,[230] but without proper evidence. Implementation of a protocol for insertion and for handling the drain in the intensive care unit with strict surveillance of adhering to the protocol may be helpful; in one single-centre study it reduced the rate of infections compared with the period before the protocol.[231] Long subcutaneous tunnelling has also been recommended, but infection has only been compared with risks reported in the literature,[232] or with the risk of percutaneous drainage via Rickham reservoirs in a hospital where neurosurgeons could choose between these two methods.[233]

External lumbar drainage probably carries a lower risk of infection than ventricular drainage,[234] although not all studies agree;[235] obviously lumbar drainage cannot be used in patients with large intracerebral haematomas or extensive intraventricular haemorrhage. As with lumbar punctures and external ventricular drainage, external lumbar drainage may increase the risk of rebleeding,[236] but there are no data from randomized trials.

To shorten the period for which ventricular catheterization is necessary, test occlusion is often applied. But gradual weaning by sequential increases in the pressure of the external ventricular drainage system over 4 days preceding drain closure conferred no advantage, according to a randomized study of 81 patients.[237]

14.9 Management of systemic complications

Neurologists and neurosurgeons are regularly confronted by non-neurological complications in patients with aneurysmal subarachnoid haemorrhage: fever, anaemia, hypertension and hypotension, hyperglycaemia, hypernatraemia and hyponatraemia, hypomagnesaemia, cardiac failure and arrhythmias, and pulmonary oedema and pneumonia. More than half the patients have one or more of these complications and they are an important contributor to poor outcome.[238–240] The importance of medical complications is further underlined by the finding that grading scales in which they are taken into account are more accurate predictors of outcome than scales made up only of neurological characteristics.[241]

14.9.1 Hyponatraemia and other electrolyte disturbances

Both hyper- and, more often, hyponatraemia can occur after SAH,[242] although not all studies agree.[240] Hypernatraemia has been independently associated with poor outcome in some studies,[242] but not in others.[240] Hyponatraemia is associated with hypovolaemia and

thereby with the development of delayed cerebral ischaemia. After the syndrome of inappropriate secretion of antidiuretic hormone (SIADH) had been initially described in the 1950s,[243] hyponatraemia in SAH was incorrectly attributed to this syndrome. In SIADH there is a continuing secretion of ADH, inappropriate to changes of plasma volume and osmolality. The extracellular volume *increases* and the expansion of the intravascular component of this volume causes a *dilutional hyponatraemia*. Natriuresis takes place because the volume expansion increases the glomerular filtration rate and inhibits the secretion of aldosterone. Balance studies have shown that the degree of natriuresis is relatively small and approximately equals intake. The high concentration of urinary sodium in SIADH can be simply explained by the fact that the sodium intake must be excreted in a smaller volume of urine.

By contrast, hyponatraemia after SAH results from excessive natriuresis, or *cerebral salt wasting*.[244] Serial measurement of plasma volume shows that this is decreased in most patients who developed hyponatraemia, and is preceded by a negative sodium balance in all instances.[42] Plasma volume considerably decreases, even in some patients with normal sodium levels, usually as a result of excessive natriuresis. Serum ADH levels are increased or normal on admission, but decrease by the time hyponatraemia occurs.

Predisposing factors for the development of hyponatraemia are hydrocephalus, particularly enlargement of the third ventricle,[245] and ruptured aneurysms of the anterior communicating artery.[246] Mechanical pressure on the hypothalamus can perhaps disturb sodium and water homeostasis. Four substances have been identified that are related to natriuresis and may act as intermediary factors: a digoxin-like substance,[247] atrial natriuretic factor,[248–252] brain natriuretic peptide[252–255] and dendroaspis natriuretic peptide.[256]

The frequency of hyponatraemia depends on the cut-off point; if defined as a sodium level of 134 mmol or less on at least two consecutive days, it occurs in about one-third of patients.[182] It develops most commonly between the second and tenth day. Severe hyponatraemia (120–124 mmol/L) occurs in 4%.[42]

Correction of hyponatraemia in SAH is in practice a problem of correcting volume depletion (Table 14.10). Acute symptomatic hyponatraemia is rare and requires urgent treatment with hypertonic saline (1.8% or even 3%). However, over-rapid infusion of sodium may precipitate myelinolysis in the pons and the white matter of the cerebral hemispheres.[257] If possible, correction should not be faster than 8 mmol/L/day.[258,259] A mild degree of hyponatraemia (125–134 mmol/L) is usually well tolerated, self-limiting and need not be treated

Table 14.10 Management of hyponatraemia.

Almost invariably caused by sodium *depletion*, not by sodium dilution
Associated hypovolaemia increases the risk of delayed cerebral ischaemia
Give isotonic saline (with or without plasma expander) or a mixture of glucose and saline; no free water
If necessary, add fludrocortisone acetate, 400 mg/day in two doses, orally or intravenously
Keep central venous pressure between 8 and 12 mmHg, or pulmonary capillary wedge pressure between 14 and 18 mmHg

in itself. Hyponatraemia in patients with evidence of a negative fluid balance or excessive natriuresis is corrected with saline (0.9%; sodium concentration 150 mmol/L).

> Hyponatraemia after subarachnoid haemorrhage usually reflects cerebral salt wasting (sodium depletion) and not secretion of antidiuretic hormone (sodium dilution). Because hyponatraemia may lead to hypovolaemia, it should not be treated with fluid restriction.

Hypomagnesaemia is found in half the patients on admission, or during the clinical course.[154] On admission it is related to poor clinical condition and large amounts of extravasated blood, but not with the later occurrence of delayed cerebral ischaemia or poor outcome, at least not independently. By contrast, hypomagnesaemia developing between day 2 and 12 after SAH is independently associated with the development of delayed cerebral ischaemia.[154] Why hypomagnesemia occurs after SAH is unclear; renal excretion of magnesium is an unlikely explanation because hypomagnesaemia occurs within hours of the haemorrhage.

Hypomagnesaemia has been linked to cardiac arrhythmias,[260] and in cases of acute arrhythmia 4–8 mmol as an intravenous load in 5–10 min, followed by 25 mmol per day is recommended.[260] The aim is to keep the magnesium concentration above 0.4 mmol/L. Infusion of 64 mmol per day results in concentrations between 1.0 and 2.0 mmol/L,[261] and is associated with a reduced risk of developing delayed cerebral ischaemia,[157] but whether this regimen results in improved overall outcome is not yet clear (section 14.5.3).

Low serum potassium occurs in approximately half the patients with SAH, and is associated with an increased risk of severe Q–Tc prolongation.[262] But whether hypokalaemia is associated with overall outcome is unsettled. The influence of serum potassium on delayed cerebral ischemia and outcome has been investigated in only a single retrospective study without consecutive data collection in operated patients between 1971 and 1987; potassium levels were not related to delayed cerebral ischemia or death.[263]

14.9.2 Hyperglycaemia

Hyperglycaemia defined as a plasma concentration of > 11.1 mmol/L is found in one-third of the patients during their clinical course, and is associated with a poor clinical condition on admission.[240] From admission through day 10, glucose levels remain higher in patients with a poor outcome compared with those with a good clinical outcome.[264] Hyperglycaemia is independently associated with poor outcome.[264,265] Whether correction of hyperglycaemia results in improved outcome is an unresolved issue.

14.9.3 Disorders of cardiac rhythm and function

Aneurysmal rupture is commonly associated with cardiac arrhythmias, ischaemia-like electrocardiographic (ECG) abnormalities, and sometimes with cardiac arrest.[13] It is therefore not surprising that patients are sometimes initially misdiagnosed as having acute myocardial infarction and admitted to coronary care units. Cardiogenic shock may also occur, usually in combination with pulmonary oedema (section 14.9.4). The probable explanation is sustained sympathetic stimulation, associated with massive excretion of catecholamines,[266,267] and also of cortisol and ADH.[267] This may result in structural damage to the myocardium, according to echocardiographic evidence,[268] raised troponin I levels,[269–272] and histological features at postmortem – contraction bands, focal myocardial necrosis and subendocardial ischaemia.[273] Secretion of B-type natriuretic peptide is probably a consequence of myocardial damage.[274] Low magnesium levels may play an intermediary role.[275]

The most common ECG abnormalities in SAH (Fig. 14.19) are ST depression and elevation, T-wave changes, pathological Q waves and bundle branch block.[276] Life-threatening arrhythmias such as ventricular fibrillation and 'torsade de pointe' may occur,[277,278] but in under 5% of patients.[12,13,279] A striking finding in a large series of patients investigated by serial ECGs was that every patient had at least one abnormal ECG.[280] Virtually all ECG abnormalities changed to other abnormalities, in no consistent order, and then disappeared, in an observation period of 10 days.

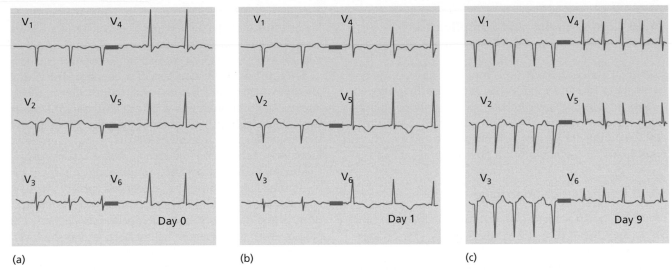

(a)   (b)   (c)

Fig. 14.19 ECG abnormalities in a 74-year-old woman with subarachnoid haemorrhage. (a) Day 0: ischaemic ST segment, prominent U wave and prolonged Q–Tc interval. (b) Day 1: sinus bradycardia, ischaemic ST segment, ischaemic T wave, prolonged Q–Tc interval and signs of left ventricular hypertrophy. (c) Day 9: sinus tachycardia, transient pathological Q wave and ischaemic ST segment.

A prolonged Q–T interval often represents delayed ventricular repolarization and predisposes to ventricular arrhythmias, but in patients with SAH it is more important as an indicator of severe intracranial disease than of potentially serious cardiac complications.[280,281] Rhythm disturbances have some association with lesions of the insular cortex,[282] more often with right- than with left-sided haemorrhages,[3,283] an association that is not limited to ruptured aneurysms.[284]

> Abnormalities of heart rhythm after subarachnoid haemorrhage mostly represent 'smoke' rather than 'fire' and rarely need to be treated.

Generally, severe ventricular arrhythmias are brief. Beta-blockade has been proposed as preventive treatment aimed at lowering the sympathetic tone. In patients with head injury a double-blind, randomized study found that beta-blockers reduced catecholamine-induced cardiac necrosis, but not in-hospital case fatality.[285] In patients with SAH, routine administration of beta-blockers is not warranted until there is evidence of improved overall outcome; the net benefits may be disappointing because beta-blockers lower blood pressure.

Left ventricular dysfunction also occurs, most often in the initial days after the SAH.[286] In a review of four studies of consecutive series of patients examined by echocardiography, irrespective of clinical condition or ECG findings, left ventricular dysfunction was found in 12% of patients.[287] These patients had an increased risk of delayed cerebral ischaemia and poor outcome.

14.9.4 Pulmonary oedema

Pulmonary oedema occurs to some degree in approximately one-third of patients with SAH[36,288] but the fulminant variety is much rarer (2% in the largest series to date).[289] The onset is usually rapid, within hours of the SAH. What triggers pulmonary oedema is unclear. Raised intracranial pressure can lead to a massive sympathetic discharge, mediated by the anterior hypothalamus – the same location that is held responsible for electrolyte disturbances (section 14.9.1). This would lead to increased permeability of endothelial cells in the pulmonary capillary bed. Any cardiac failure may aggravate the pulmonary oedema.[36]

The typical clinical picture consists of unexpected dyspnoea, cyanosis and the production of pink and frothy sputum. Many patients are pale, sweat excessively and are hypertensive. A chest X-ray usually demonstrates impressive pulmonary oedema (Fig. 14.7) which may disappear in a matter of hours following positive end-expiratory pressure ventilation. A problem is that liberal administration of fluids is beneficial for brain perfusion but may delay recovery of pulmonary oedema and hence impair brain oxygenation, and that positive end-expiratory pressure ventilation increases intracranial pressure.

If there is associated left ventricular failure, clinically manifested by sudden hypotension following initially elevated blood pressure, transient lactic acidosis and mild elevation of the creatine kinase MB fraction,[37,290] inotropic agents are indicated (intravenous dobutamine, 5–15 μg/kg/min).[291]

14.10 Late sequelae and complications

In general, functional outcome improves significantly between 4 months and 18 months after SAH with improved quality of life.[292] Nevertheless, specific late complications require attention. Therefore, we favour a multidisciplinary clinic for patients who have had an SAH where neurologists and rehabilitation physicians are at hand.

14.10.1 Vitreous haemorrhages

Preretinal haemorrhages associated with SAH (section 3.7.1) may break into the vitreous cavity (Terson syndrome). This has been documented in 13% of patients in prospective studies;[293] the rates were three times as high in patients who had lost consciousness at some stage.[294] These haemorrhages occur in one or both eyes, usually at the time of the initial haemorrhage, but sometimes several days later, and then mostly in association with rebleeding. It may, however, take days or weeks before the patient is sufficiently alert to complain about blurred vision. In most cases, the vitreous haemorrhage clears spontaneously in a matter of weeks to months. If not, vitrectomy may be indicated to improve vision.[295] Operation is unnecessary if preretinal haemorrhages have not involved the vitreous body.[296]

14.10.2 New episodes of subarachnoid haemorrhage

When the ruptured aneurysm is left untreated, the rate of rebleeding after the first 6 months have passed is 3.5% per year during the first decade, but of course this situation is now increasingly unusual.[297] However, even in patients with successfully occluded ruptured aneurysms new episodes of bleeding do occur – from de novo aneurysms, incidental aneurysms that were left untreated at the time of the initial haemorrhage, or from regrowth of the aneurysm that caused the first bleed. From the patient's perspective the source of a new episode is not very relevant, but from a management perspective it is. In a study of 30 patients with late rebleeding (after an average period of more than 7 years) the ruptured aneurysm had developed at a new location in somewhat more than half the cases, it had regrown at the previous aneurysm site in about a quarter, and in the rest the source of bleeding was an additional aneurysm that had been overlooked at the time of the first episode.[298]

In the surgical arm of the ISAT trial rebleeding from the clipped aneurysm occurred in 1% of the operated patients within the first year.[64] A long-term study in Japan estimated the rebleeding rate after initially successful clipping was 2.2% after 10 years and 9% after 20 years,[85] while in a Dutch cohort the rate of new episodes of SAH (from newly developed aneurysms, incidental aneurysms that were left untreated and from regrowth aneurysms combined) was 3.2% after 10 years.[86] Despite this relatively high risk of new episodes of SAH after successful surgical treatment of the initial episode, a modelling study estimated that repeated screening and treatment of newly detected aneurysms could not be recommended, because the prevented episodes of new episodes of SAH would be outweighed by the complications of the diagnostic and therapeutic procedures. For patients with an increased risk of both aneurysm development and aneurysm rupture, screening was beneficial in this model, but at present we cannot identify who these patients are (section 15.2.5).

After endovascular occlusion of the aneurysm, there is still little information about the rate of rebleeding in the long term (section 14.4.2).

14.10.3 Late hydrocephalus

Permanent shunting for hydrocephalus persisting for 2–4 weeks after the initial haemorrhage is needed in approximately 20% of patients, according to two neurosurgical series.[299,300] Aneurysm site (anterior communicating artery complex or posterior circulation) is an established risk factor for late hydrocephalus.[301,302] Putative risk factors, identified only in single studies, are age,[303] intraventricular haemorrhage[301] and the clearance rate of subarachnoid blood.[304] The risk of chronic hydrocephalus is no lower after endovascular treatment than after surgical clipping.[305–307] If fenestration of the lamina terminalis is performed, as part of the microsurgical procedure for aneurysm repair, late hydrocephalus is a rare event.[308]

14.10.4 Epilepsy

New-onset epilepsy (two or more unprovoked seizures) in the first year after discharge from hospital was reported in 17 of 242 patients (7%) from Columbia University, New York, while an additional 10 patients (4%) had a single seizure.[309] In a British cohort late epilepsy occurred in 4.9% in the first year after the haemorrhage (23 of 872 patients).[310] Unfortunately neither cohort recorded a possible relationship with seizures at the time of the haemorrhage or during hospital stay; this is important because in a small cohort of 95 patients from Detroit all eight with epileptic seizures after discharge fell into this category.[311] Putative risk factors (identified in single studies only) include focal lesions such as subdural haematoma and cerebral infarction,[309,312] as well as disability on discharge,[310] which of course is largely a consequence of structural brain damage. De novo epileptic seizures are relatively rare after coiling.[64,313]

14.10.5 Cognitive dysfunction and psychosocial impact

It is important to appreciate just who should be asked if a patient has 'recovered'. The patients rate their own outcome worse than the treating physician, but better than their spouses.[314] Even patients who seem to make a good functional recovery and who are independent in activities of daily living often can have psychosocial and cognitive deficits in the first year after the SAH.[3,315,316] Although improvement still occurs between 4 and 18 months after the SAH, many patients and their partners still experience reduced quality of life 1–2 years after the haemorrhage.[317] The psychosocial impact at even longer follow-up is considerable. In a survey of 610 patients who were interviewed about 9 years after their SAH, a quarter of the employed patients had stopped working and another quarter worked shorter hours or had a position with less responsibility.[318] On average, patients returned to work about 9 months after discharge (range 0–96). A total of 60% of the patients reported changes in personality, most commonly increased irritability (37%) or emotionality (29%). The patients had a statistically significant higher depression score than the reference population, and only 25% reported a complete recovery without any psychosocial or neurological problems.

References

1 Hop JW, Rinkel GJE, Algra A, van Gijn J. Case-fatality rates and functional outcome after subarachnoid hemorrhage: a systematic review. *Stroke* 1997; **28**(3):660–4.

2 Huang J, Van Gelder JM. The probability of sudden death from rupture of intracranial aneurysms: a meta-analysis. *Neurosurgery* 2002; **51**:1101–5.

3 Hackett ML, Anderson CS, for the ACROSS Group. Health outcomes 1 year after subarachnoid hemorrhage: an international population-based study. *Neurology* 2000; **55**:658–62.

4 Roos YBWEM, de Haan RJ, Beenen LFM, Groen RJM, Albrecht KW, Vermeulen M. Complications and outcome in patients with aneurysmal subarachnoid haemorrhage: a prospective hospital based cohort study in the Netherlands. *J Neurol Neurosurg Psychiatry* 2000; **68**:337–41.

5 Wiebers DO, Whisnant JP, Huston J, III, Meissner I, Brown RD, Jr., Piepgras DG *et al.* Unruptured intracranial aneurysms: natural history, clinical outcome, and risks of surgical and endovascular treatment. *Lancet* 2003; **362**:103–10.

6 Stegmayr B, Eriksson M, Asplund K. Declining mortality from subarachnoid hemorrhage: changes in incidence and case fatality from 1985 through 2000. *Stroke* 2004; **35**:2059–63.

7 Bardach NS, Zhao SJ, Gress DR, Lawton MT, Johnston SC. Association between subarachnoid hemorrhage outcomes and number of cases treated at California hospitals. *Stroke* 2002; **33**:1851–6.

8 Sasaki T, Sato M, Oinuma M, Sakuma J, Suzuki K, Matsumoto M *et al.* Management of poor-grade patients with aneurysmal subarachnoid hemorrhage in the acute stage: importance of close monitoring for neurological grade changes. *Surg Neurol* 2004; **62**:531–5.

9 Inagawa T, Kamiya K, Ogasawara H, Yano T. Rebleeding of ruptured intracranial aneurysms in the acute stage. *Surg Neurol* 1987; **28**(2):93–9.

10 Fujii Y, Takeuchi S, Sasaki O, Minakawa T, Koike T, Tanaka R. Ultra-early rebleeding in spontaneous subarachnoid hemorrhage. *J Neurosurg* 1996; **84**:35–42.

11 Ohkuma H, Tsurutani H, Suzuki S. Incidence and significance of early aneurysmal rebleeding before neurosurgical or neurological management. *Stroke* 2001; **32**:1176–80.

12 Hijdra A, Vermeulen M, van Gijn J, van Crevel H. Respiratory arrest in subarachnoid hemorrhage. *Neurology* 1984; **34**(11):1501–3.

13 Toussaint LG, III, Friedman JA, Wijdicks EFM, Piepgras DG, Pichelmann MA, McIver JI *et al.* Survival of cardiac arrest after aneurysmal subarachnoid hemorrhage. *Neurosurgery* 2005; **57**:25–31.

14 Van Gijn J, van Dongen KJ. The time course of aneurysmal haemorrhage on computed tomograms. *Neuroradiology* 1982; **23**(3):153–6.

15 Hauerberg J, Eskesen V, Rosenorn J. The prognostic significance of intracerebral haematoma as shown on CT scanning after aneurysmal subarachnoid haemorrhage. *Br J Neurosurg* 1994; **8**(3):333–9.

16 Heiskanen O, Poranen A, Kuurne T, Valtonen S, Kaste M. Acute surgery for intracerebral haematomas caused by rupture of an intracranial arterial aneurysm: a prospective randomized study. *Acta Neurochir (Wien)* 1988; **90**(3–4):81–3.

17 Niemann DB, Wills AD, Maartens NF, Kerr RS, Byrne JV, Molyneux AJ. Treatment of intracerebral hematomas caused by aneurysm rupture: coil placement followed by clot evacuation. *J Neurosurg* 2003; **99**:843–7.

18 Smith ER, Carter BS, Ogilvy CS. Proposed use of prophylactic decompressive craniectomy in poor-grade aneurysmal subarachnoid hemorrhage patients presenting with associated large sylvian hematomas. *Neurosurgery* 2002; **51**:117–24.

19 Inamasu J, Saito R, Nakamura Y, Ichikizaki K, Suga S, Kawase T *et al.* Acute subdural hematoma caused by ruptured cerebral aneurysms: diagnostic and therapeutic pitfalls. *Resuscitation* 2002; **52**:71–6.

20 Gelabert-Gonzalez M, Iglesias-Pais M, Fernandez-Villa J. Acute subdural haematoma due to ruptured intracranial aneurysms. *Neurosurg Rev* 2004; **27**:259–62.

21 Linn FHH, Rinkel GJE, Algra A, van Gijn J. The notion of 'warning leaks' in subarachnoid haemorrhage: are such patients in fact admitted with a rebleed? *J Neurol Neurosurg Psychiatry* 2000; **68**:332–6.

22 Nonaka Y, Kusumoto M, Mori K, Maeda M. Pure acute subdural haematoma without subarachnoid haemorrhage caused by rupture of internal carotid artery aneurysm. *Acta Neurochir (Wien)* 2000; **142**:941–4.

23 Krishnaney AA, Rasmussen PA, Masaryk T. Bilateral tentorial subdural hematoma without subarachnoid hemorrhage secondary to anterior communicating artery aneurysm rupture: a case report and review of the literature. *Am J Neuroradiol* 2004; **25**:1006–7.

24 Koerbel A, Ernemann U, Freudenstein D. Acute subdural haematoma without subarachnoid haemorrhage caused by rupture of an internal carotid artery bifurcation aneurysm: case report and review of literature. *Br J Radiol* 2005; **78**:646–50.

25 O'Sullivan MG, Whyman M, Steers JW, Whittle IR, Miller JD. Acute subdural haematoma secondary to ruptured intracranial aneurysm: diagnosis and management. *Br J Neurosurg* 1994; **8**(4):439–45.

26 Van Gijn J, Hijdra A, Wijdicks EFM, Vermeulen M, van Crevel H. Acute hydrocephalus after aneurysmal subarachnoid hemorrhage. *J Neurosurg* 1985; **63**(3):355–62.

27 Rinkel GJE, Wijdicks EFM, Ramos LMP, van Gijn J. Progression of acute hydrocephalus in subarachnoid haemorrhage: a case report documented by serial CT scanning. *J Neurol Neurosurg Psychiatry* 1990; **53**(4):354–5.

28 Hasan D, Lindsay KW, Vermeulen M. Treatment of acute hydrocephalus after subarachnoid hemorrhage with serial lumbar puncture. *Stroke* 1991; **22**(2):190–4.

29 Suzuki M, Otawara Y, Doi M, Ogasawara K, Ogawa A. Neurological grades of patients with poor-grade subarachnoid hemorrhage improve after short-term pretreatment. *Neurosurgery* 2000; **47**:1098–104.

30 Roos YBWEM, Hasan D, Vermeulen M. Outcome in patients with large intraventricular haemorrhages: a volumetric study. *J Neurol Neurosurg Psychiatry* 1995; **58**:622–4.

31 Nieuwkamp DJ, de Gans K, Rinkel GJE, Algra A. Treatment and outcome of severe intraventricular extension in patients with subarachnoid or intracerebral hemorrhage: a systematic review of the literature. *J Neurol* 2000; **247**:117–21.

32 Naff NJ, Carhuapoma JR, Williams MA, Bhardwaj A, Ulatowski JA, Bederson J *et al.* Treatment of intraventricular hemorrhage with urokinase: effects on 30-day survival. *Stroke* 2000; **31**:841–7.

33 Shimoda M, Oda S, Shibata M, Tominaga J, Kittaka M, Tsugane R. Results of early surgical evacuation of packed

34 Lagares A, Putman CM, Ogilvy CS. Posterior fossa decompression and clot evacuation for fourth ventricle hemorrhage after aneurysmal rupture: case report. *Neurosurgery* 2001; **49**:208–11.

35 Yoshimoto Y, Ochiai C, Kawamata K, Endo M, Nagai M. Aqueductal blood clot as a cause of acute hydrocephalus in subarachnoid hemorrhage. *Am J Neuroradiol* 1996; **17**:1183–6.

36 McLaughlin N, Bojanowski MW, Girard F, Denault A. Pulmonary edema and cardiac dysfunction following subarachnoid hemorrhage. *Can J Neurol Sci* 2005; **32**:178–85.

37 Parr MJ, Finfer SR, Morgan MK. Reversible cardiogenic shock complicating subarachnoid haemorrhage. *Br Med J* 1996; 313(7058):681–3.

38 Macrea LM, Tramer MR, Walder B. Spontaneous subarachnoid hemorrhage and serious cardiopulmonary dysfunction: a systematic review. *Resuscitation* 2005; **65**:139–48.

39 Wijdicks EFM, Vermeulen M, Murray GD, Hijdra A, van Gijn J. The effects of treating hypertension following aneurysmal subarachnoid hemorrhage. *Clin Neurol Neurosurg* 1990; **92**(2):111–17.

40 Hasan D, Vermeulen M, Wijdicks EFM, Hijdra A, van Gijn J. Effect of fluid intake and antihypertensive treatment on cerebral ischemia after subarachnoid hemorrhage. *Stroke* 1989; **20**(11):1511–15.

41 Varon J, Marik PE. Clinical review: the management of hypertensive crises. *Crit Care* 2003; **7**:374–84.

42 Wijdicks EFM, Vermeulen M, ten Haaf JA, Hijdra A, Bakker WH, van Gijn J. Volume depletion and natriuresis in patients with a ruptured intracranial aneurysm. *Ann Neurol* 1985; **18**(2):211–16.

43 Hasan D, Wijdicks EFM, Vermeulen M. Hyponatremia is associated with cerebral ischemia in patients with aneurysmal subarachnoid hemorrhage. *Ann Neurol* 1990; **27**(1):106–8.

44 Wijdicks EFM, Vermeulen M, Hijdra A, van Gijn J. Hyponatremia and cerebral infarction in patients with ruptured intracranial aneurysms: is fluid restriction harmful? *Ann Neurol* 1985; **17**(2):137–40.

45 Vermeij FH, Hasan D, Bijvoet HWC, Avezaat CJJ. Impact of medical treatment on the outcome of patients after aneurysmal subarachnoid hemorrhage. *Stroke* 1998; **29**:924–30.

46 Oliveira-Filho J, Ezzeddine MA, Segal AZ, Buonanno FS, Chang Y, Ogilvy CS *et al.* Fever in subarachnoid hemorrhage: relationship to vasospasm and outcome. *Neurology* 2001; **56**:1299–304.

47 Kim DH, Haney CL, Van Ginhoven G. Reduction of pulmonary edema after SAH with a pulmonary artery catheter-guided hemodynamic management protocol. *Neurocrit Care* 2005; **3**:11–15.

48 Rosenwasser RH, Jallo JI, Getch CC, Liebman KE. Complications of Swan-Ganz catheterization for

intraventricular hemorrhage from aneurysm rupture in patients with poor-grade subarachnoid hemorrhage. *J Neurosurg* 1999; **91**:408–14.

hemodynamic monitoring in patients with subarachnoid hemorrhage. *Neurosurgery* 1995; **37**:872–5.

49 Harvey S, Harrison DA, Singer M, Ashcroft J, Jones CM, Elbourne D *et al.* Assessment of the clinical effectiveness of pulmonary artery catheters in management of patients in intensive care (PAC-Man): a randomised controlled trial. *Lancet* 2005; **366**:472–7.

50 Shah MR, Hasselblad V, Stevenson LW, Binanay C, O'Connor CM, Sopko G *et al.* Impact of the pulmonary artery catheter in critically ill patients: meta-analysis of randomized clinical trials. *J Am Med Assoc* 2005; **294**:1664–70.

51 Rowley G, Fielding K. Reliability and accuracy of the Glasgow Coma Scale with experienced and inexperienced users. *Lancet* 1991; **337**(8740):535–8.

52 Gill MR, Reiley DG, Green SM. Interrater reliability of Glasgow Coma Scale scores in the emergency department. *Ann Emerg Med* 2004; **43**:215–23.

53 Takagi K, Tsuchiya Y, Okinaga K, Hirata M, Nakagomi T, Tamura A. Natural hypothermia immediately after transient global cerebral ischemia induced by spontaneous subarachnoid hemorrhage. *J Neurosurg* 2003; **98**:50–56.

54 Rousseaux P, Scherpereel R, Bernard MH, Graftieaux JP, Guyot JF. Fever and cerebral vasospasm in intracranial aneurysms. *Surg Neurol* 1980; **14**:459–65.

55 Vermeulen M, Lindsay KW, Murray GD, Cheah F, Hijdra A, Muizelaar JP *et al.* Antifibrinolytic treatment in subarachnoid hemorrhage. *N Engl J Med* 1984; **311**(7):432–7.

56 Siironen J, Juvela S, Varis J, Porras M, Poussa K, Ilveskero S *et al.* No effect of enoxaparin on outcome of aneurysmal subarachnoid hemorrhage: a randomized, double-blind, placebo-controlled clinical trial. *J Neurosurg* 2003; **99**:953–9.

57 Amaragiri SV, Lees TA. Elastic compression stockings for prevention of deep vein thrombosis. *Cochrane Database Syst Rev* 2000; CD001484.

58 Black PM, Crowell RM, Abbott WM. External pneumatic calf compression reduces deep venous thrombosis in patients with ruptured intracranial aneurysms. *Neurosurgery* 1986; **18**(1):25–8.

59 Lacut K, Bressollette L, Le Gal G, Etienne E, De Tinteniac A, Renault A *et al.* Prevention of venous thrombosis in patients with acute intracerebral hemorrhage. *Neurology* 2005; **65**:865–9.

60 Hart RG, Byer JA, Slaughter JR, Hewett JE, Easton JD. Occurrence and implications of seizures in subarachnoid hemorrhage due to ruptured intracranial aneurysms. *Neurosurgery* 1981; **8**(4):417–21.

61 Hasan D, Schonck RS, Avezaat CJ, Tanghe HL, van Gijn J, van der Lugt PJ. Epileptic seizures after subarachnoid hemorrhage. *Ann Neurol* 1993; **33**(3):286–91.

62 Pinto AN, Canhao P, Ferro JM. Seizures at the onset of subarachnoid haemorrhage. *J Neurol* 1996; **243**(2):161–4.

63 Butzkueven H, Evans AH, Pitman A, Leopold C, Jolley DJ, Kaye AH *et al.* Onset seizures independently predict poor outcome after subarachnoid hemorrhage. *Neurology* 2000; **55**:1315–20.

64 Molyneux AJ, Kerr RS, Yu LM, Clarke M, Sneade M, Yarnold JA *et al.* International subarachnoid aneurysm trial (ISAT) of neurosurgical clipping versus endovascular coiling in 2143 patients with ruptured intracranial aneurysms: a randomised comparison of effects on survival, dependency, seizures, rebleeding, subgroups, and aneurysm occlusion. *Lancet* 2005; **366**:809–17.

65 Foy PM, Chadwick DW, Rajgopalan N, Johnson AL, Shaw MD. Do prophylactic anticonvulsant drugs alter the pattern of seizures after craniotomy? *J Neurol Neurosurg Psychiatry* 1992; **55**(9):753–7.

66 Brilstra EH, Rinkel GJE, Algra A, van Gijn J. Rebleeding, secondary ischemia, and timing of operation in patients with subarachnoid hemorrhage. *Neurology* 2000; **55**:1656–60.

67 Brilstra EH, Algra A, Rinkel GJE, Tulleken CAF, van Gijn J. Effectiveness of neurosurgical clip application in patients with aneurysmal subarachnoid hemorrhage. *J Neurosurg* 2002; **97**:1036–41.

68 Jane JA, Kassell NF, Torner JC, Winn HR. The natural history of aneurysms and arteriovenous malformations. *J Neurosurg* 1985; **62**(3):321–3.

69 Roos YBWEM, Beenen LF, Groen RJ, Albrecht KW, Vermeulen M. Timing of surgery in patients with aneurysmal subarachnoid haemorrhage: rebleeding is still the major cause of poor outcome in neurosurgical units that aim at early surgery. *J Neurol Neurosurg Psychiatry* 1997; **63**:490–3.

70 Laidlaw JD, Siu KH. Ultra-early surgery for aneurysmal subarachnoid hemorrhage: outcomes for a consecutive series of 391 patients not selected by grade or age. *J Neurosurg* 2002; **97**:250–8.

71 Beck J, Raabe A, Szelenyi A, Berkefeld J, Gerlach R, Setzer M *et al.* Sentinel headache and the risk of rebleeding after aneurysmal subarachnoid hemorrhage. *Stroke* 2006; **37**:2733–2737.

72 Naidech AM, Janjua N, Kreiter KT, Ostapkovich ND, Fitzsimmons BF, Parra A *et al.* Predictors and impact of aneurysm rebleeding after subarachnoid hemorrhage. *Arch Neurol* 2005; **62**:410–16.

73 Inagawa T, Hirano A. Ruptured intracranial aneurysms: an autopsy study of 133 patients. *Surg Neurol* 1990; **33**(2):117–23.

74 Pleizier CM, Ruigrok YM, Rinkel GJE. Relation between age and number of aneurysms in patients with subarachnoid haemorrhage. *Cerebrovasc Dis* 2002; **14**:51–3.

75 Rose G. *The Strategy of Preventive Medicine.* Oxford: Oxford Medical Publications, 1992.

76 Guglielmi G, Vinuela F, Duckwiler G, Dion J, Lylyk P, Berenstein A *et al.* Endovascular treatment of posterior circulation aneurysms by electrothrombosis using electrically detachable coils. *J Neurosurg* 1992; **77**(4):515–24.

77 Qureshi AI, Suri MFK, Khan J, Kim SH, Fessler RD, Ringer AJ *et al.* Endovascular treatment of intracranial aneurysms by using Guglielmi detachable coils in awake patients: safety and feasibility. *J Neurosurg* 2001; **94**:880–5.

78 Van der Schaaf IC, Algra A, Wermer MJH, Molyneux A, Clarke M, van Gijn J *et al.* Endovascular coiling versus neurosurgical clipping for patients with aneurysmal subarachnoid haemorrhage. *Cochrane Database Syst Rev* 2005; (4) CD003085.

79 Hadjivassiliou M, Tooth CL, Romanowski CAJ, Byrne J, Battersby RDE, Oxbury S *et al.* Aneurysmal SAH: cognitive outcome and structural damage after clipping or coiling. *Neurology* 2001; **56**:1672–7.

80 Lozier AP, Connolly ES, Jr., Lavine SD, Solomon RA. Guglielmi detachable coil embolization of posterior circulation aneurysms: a systematic review of the literature. *Stroke* 2002; **33**:2509–18.

81 Molyneux A, Kerr R, Stratton I, Sandercock P, Clarke M, Shrimpton J *et al.* International Subarachnoid Aneurysm Trial (ISAT) of neurosurgical clipping versus endovascular coiling in 2143 patients with ruptured intracranial aneurysms: a randomised trial. *Lancet* 2002; **360**:1267–74.

82 Nieuwkamp DJ, Rinkel GJE, Silva R, Greebe P, Schokking DA, Ferro JM. Subarachnoid haemorrhage in patients older than 75 years: clinical course, treatment and outcome. *J Neurol Neurosurg Psychiatry* 2006; **77**:933–7.

83 Sluzewski M, Van Rooij WJ. Early rebleeding after coiling of ruptured cerebral aneurysms: incidence, morbidity, and risk factors. *Am J Neuroradiol* 2005; **26**:1739–43.

84 Sluzewski M, Van Rooij WJ, Beute GN, Nijssen PC. Late rebleeding of ruptured intracranial aneurysms treated with detachable coils. *Am J Neuroradiol* 2005; **26**:2542–9.

85 Tsutsumi K, Ueki K, Usui M, Kwak S, Kirino T. Risk of recurrent subarachnoid hemorrhage after complete obliteration of cerebral aneurysms. *Stroke* 1998; **29**:2511–13.

86 Wermer MJH, Greebe P, Algra A, Rinkel GJE. Incidence of recurrent subarachnoid hemorrhage after clipping for ruptured intracranial aneurysms. *Stroke* 2005; **36**:2394–9.

87 CARAT Investigators. Rates of delayed rebleeding from intracranial aneurysms are low after surgical and endovascular treatment. *Stroke* 2006; **37**:1437–42.

88 Baltsavias GS, Byrne JV, Halsey J, Coley SC, Sohn MJ, Molyneux AJ. Effects of timing of coil embolization after aneurysmal subarachnoid hemorrhage on procedural morbidity and outcomes. *Neurosurgery* 2000; **47**:1320–9.

89 Rabinstein AA, Pichelmann MA, Friedman JA, Piepgras DG, Nichols DA, McIver JI *et al.* Symptomatic vasospasm and outcomes following aneurysmal subarachnoid hemorrhage: a comparison between surgical repair and endovascular coil occlusion. *J Neurosurg* 2003; **98**:319–25.

90 Shanno GB, Armonda RA, Benitez RP, Rosenwasser RH. Assessment of acutely unsuccessful attempts at detachable coiling in intracranial aneurysms. *Neurosurgery* 2001; **48**:1066–72.

91 Albuquerque FC, Spetzler RF, Zabramski JM, McDougall CG. Effects of three-dimensional angiography on the coiling of cerebral aneurysms. *Neurosurgery* 2002; **51**:597–605.

92 Van Rooij WJ, Sluzewski M, Beute GN, Nijssen PC. Procedural complications of coiling of ruptured intracranial aneurysms: incidence and risk factors in a consecutive series of 681 patients. *Am J Neuroradiol* 2006; **27**:1498–501.

93 Sluzewski M, Bosch JA, Van Rooij WJ, Nijssen PCG, Wijnalda D. Rupture of intracranial aneurysms during treatment with Guglielmi detachable coils: incidence, outcome, and risk factors. *J Neurosurg* 2001; **94**:238–40.

94 Ries T, Buhk JH, Kucinski T, Goebell E, Gryska U, Zeumer H *et al.* Intravenous administration of acetylsalicylic acid during endovascular treatment of cerebral aneurysms reduces the rate of thromboembolic events. *Stroke* 2006; **37**:1816–21.

95 Van den Bergh WM, Algra A, Dorhout Mees SM, van Kooten F, Dirven CM, van Gijn J *et al.* Randomized controlled trial of acetylsalicylic acid in aneurysmal subarachnoid hemorrhage. The MASH Study. *Stroke* 2006; **37**:2326–30.

96 Spetzger U, Reul J, Thron A, Warnke JP, Gilsbach JM. Microsurgical embolectomy and removal of a migrated coil from the middle cerebral artery. *Cerebrovasc Dis* 1997; **7**:226–31.

97 Raftopoulos C, Goffette P, Billa RF, Mathurin P. Transvascular coil hooking procedure to retrieve an unraveled Guglielmi detachable coil: Technical note. *Neurosurgery* 2002; **50**:912–14.

98 Kirollos RW, Bosma JJD, Radhakrishnan J, Pigott TDJ. Endovascularly treated cerebral aneurysm using Guglielmi detachable coils acting as a nidus for brain abscess formation secondary to *Salmonella* bacteremia: case report. *Neurosurgery* 2002; **51**:234–7.

99 Russell SM, Nelson PK, Jafar JJ. Neurological deterioration after coil embolization of a giant basilar apex aneurysm with resolution following parent artery clip ligation: case report and review of the literature. *J Neurosurg* 2002; **97**:705–8.

100 Hacein-Bey L, Connolly ES, Jr., Mayer SA, Young WL, Pile-Spellman J, Solomon RA. Complex intracranial aneurysms: Combined operative and endovascular approaches. *Neurosurgery* 1998; **43**:1304–12.

101 Lawton MT, Quinone-Hinojosa A, Sanai N, Malek JY, Dowd CF. Combined microsurgical and endovascular management of complex intracranial aneurysms. *Neurosurgery* 2003; **52**:263–74.

102 Lanzino G, Wakhloo AK, Fessler RD, Hartney ML, Guterman LR, Hopkins LN. Efficacy and current limitations of intravascular stents for intracranial internal carotid, vertebral, and basilar artery aneurysms. *J Neurosurg* 1999; **91**:538–46.

103 Higashida RT, Smith W, Gress D, Urwin R, Dowd CF, Balousek PA *et al.* Intravascular stent and endovascular coil placement for a ruptured fusiform aneurysm of the basilar artery: case report and review of the literature. *J Neurosurg* 1997; **87**:944–9.

104 Hoh BL, Putman CM, Budzik RF, Carter BS, Ogilvy CS. Combined surgical and endovascular techniques of flow alteration to treat fusiform and complex wide-necked intracranial aneurysms that are unsuitable for clipping or coil embolization. *J Neurosurg* 2001; **95**:24–35.

105 Boulin A, Pierot L. Follow-up of intracranial aneurysms treated with detachable coils: Comparison of gadolinium-enhanced 3D time-of-flight MR angiography and digital subtraction angiography. *Radiology* 2001; **219**:108–13.

106 Majoie CB, Sprengers ME, Van Rooij WJ, Lavini C, Sluzewski M, van Rijn JC *et al*. MR angiography at 3T versus digital subtraction angiography in the follow-up of intracranial aneurysms treated with detachable coils. *Am J Neuroradiol* 2005; **26**:1349–56.

107 Gauvrit JY, Leclerc X, Caron S, Taschner CA, Lejeune JP, Pruvo JP. Intracranial aneurysms treated with Guglielmi detachable coils: imaging follow-up with contrast-enhanced MR angiography. Stroke 2006; **37**:1033–7.

108 Pierot L, Delcour C, Bouquigny F, Breidt D, Feuillet B, Lanoix O *et al*. Follow-up of intracranial aneurysms selectively treated with coils: prospective evaluation of contrast-enhanced MR angiography. *Am J Neuroradiol* 2006; **27**:744–9.

109 Slob MJ, Sluzewski M, Van Rooij WJ, Roks G, Rinkel GJE. Additional coiling of previously coiled cerebral aneurysms: clinical and angiographic results. *Am J Neuroradiol* 2004; **25**:1373–6.

110 Zhang YJ, Barrow DL, Cawley CM, Dion JE. Neurosurgical management of intracranial aneurysms previously treated with endovascular therapy. *Neurosurgery* 2003; **52**:283–93.

111 Raymond J, Roy D, Leblanc P, Roorda S, Janicki C, Normandeau L *et al*. Endovascular treatment of intracranial aneurysms with radioactive coils: initial clinical experience. *Stroke* 2003; **34**:2801–6.

112 Gaba RC, Ansari SA, Roy SS, Marden FA, Viana MA, Malisch TW. Embolization of intracranial aneurysms with hydrogel-coated coils versus inert platinum coils: effects on packing density, coil length and quantity, procedure performance, cost, length of hospital stay, and durability of therapy. *Stroke* 2006; **37**:1443–50.

113 McKissock W, Richardson A, Walsh L. 'Posterior-communicating aneurysms': a controlled trial of conservative and surgical treatment of ruptured aneurysms of the internal carotid artery at or near the point of origin of the posterior communicating artery. *Lancet* 1960; **i**:1203–6.

114 McKissock W, Richardson A, Walsh L. Anterior communicating aneurysms: a trial of conservative and surgical treatment. *Lancet* 1965; **i**:873–6.

115 Öhman J, Heiskanen O. Timing of operation for ruptured supratentorial aneurysms: a prospective randomized study. *J Neurosurg* 1989; **70**(1):55–60.

116 Whitfield PC, Kirkpatrick PJ. Timing of surgery for aneurysmal subarachnoid haemorrhage. *Cochrane Database Syst Rev* 2001; CD001697.

117 De Gans K, Nieuwkamp DJ, Rinkel GJE, Algra A. Timing of aneurysm surgery in subarachnoid hemorrhage: A systematic review of the literature. *Neurosurgery* 2002; **50**:336–40.

118 Ross N, Hutchinson PJ, Seeley H, Kirkpatrick PJ. Timing of surgery for supratentorial aneurysmal subarachnoid haemorrhage: report of a prospective study. *J Neurol Neurosurg Psychiatry* 2002; **72**:480–4.

119 Nieuwkamp DJ, de GK, Algra A, Albrecht KW, Boomstra S, Brouwers PJ *et al*. Timing of aneurysm surgery in subarachnoid haemorrhage: an observational study in The Netherlands. *Acta Neurochir (Wien)* 2005; **147**:815–21.

120 Tanoue S, Kiyosue H, Kenai H, Nakamura T, Yamashita M, Mori H. Three-dimensional reconstructed images after rotational angiography in the evaluation of intracranial aneurysms: Surgical correlation. *Neurosurgery* 2000; **47**:866–71.

121 Todd MM, Hindman BJ, Clarke WR, Torner JC. Mild intraoperative hypothermia during surgery for intracranial aneurysm. *N Engl J Med* 2005; **352**:135–45.

122 Ross IB, Warrington RJ, Halliday WC. Cell-mediated allergy to a cerebral aneurysm clip: case report. *Neurosurgery* 1998; **43**:1209–11.

123 Wermer MJH, Van der Schaaf IC, Velthuis BK, Algra A, Buskens E, Rinkel GJE. Follow-up screening after subarachnoid haemorrhage: frequency and determinants of new aneurysms and enlargement of existing aneurysms. *Brain* 2005; **128**:2421–9.

124 Fodstad H, Pilbrant A, Schannong M, Stromberg S. Determination of tranexamic acid (AMCA) and fibrin/fibrinogen degradation products in cerebrospinal fluid after aneurysmal subarachnoid haemorrhage. *Acta Neurochir (Wien)* 1981; **58**(1–2):1–13.

125 Roos YBWEM, for the STAR Study Group. Antifibrinolytic treatment in subarachnoid hemorrhage: a randomized placebo-controlled trial. *Neurology* 2000; **54**:77–82.

126 Hillman J, Fridriksson S, Nilsson O, Yu Z, Saveland H, Jakobsson KE. Immediate administration of tranexamic acid and reduced incidence of early rebleeding after aneurysmal subarachnoid hemorrhage: a prospective randomized study. *J Neurosurg* 2002; **97**:771–8.

127 Pickard JD, Kirkpatrick PJ, Melsen T, Andreasen RB, Gelling L, Fryer T *et al*. Potential role of NovoSeven(R) in the prevention of rebleeding following aneurysmal subarachnoid haemorrhage. *Blood Coagul Fibrinolysis* 2000; **11**:S117–S120.

128 Hijdra A, van Gijn J, Stefanko S, van Dongen KJ, Vermeulen M, van Crevel H. Delayed cerebral ischemia after aneurysmal subarachnoid hemorrhage: clinicoanatomic correlations. *Neurology* 1986; **36**(3):329–33.

129 Conway LW, McDonald LW. Structural changes of the intradural arteries following subarachnoid hemorrhage. *J Neurosurg* 1972; **37**:715–23.

130 Hughes JT, Schianchi PM. Cerebral artery spasm: a histological study at necropsy of the blood vessels in cases of subarachnoid hemorrhage. *J Neurosurg* 1978; **48**:515–25.

131 Smith RR, Clower BR, Peeler DF, Jr., Yoshioka J. The angiopathy of subarachnoid hemorrhage: angiographic and morphologic correlates. *Stroke* 1983; **14**(2):240–5.

132 Findlay JM, Weir BK, Kanamaru K, Espinosa F. Arterial wall changes in cerebral vasospasm. *Neurosurgery* 1989; **25**(5):736–45.

133 Borel CO, McKee A, Parra A, Haglund MA, Solan A, Prabhakar V *et al*. Possible role for vascular cell proliferation in cerebral vasospasm after subarachnoid hemorrhage. *Stroke* 2003; **34**:427–32.

134 Millikan CH. Cerebral vasospasm and ruptured intracranial aneurysm. *Arch Neurol* 1975; **32**(7):433–49.

135 Fisher CM, Roberson GH, Ojemann RG. Cerebral vasospasm with ruptured saccular aneurysm: the clinical manifestations. *Neurosurgery* 1977; **1**(3):245–8.

136 Lam JMK, Smielewski P, Czosnyka M, Pickard JD, Kirkpatrick PJ. Predicting delayed ischemic deficits after aneurysmal subarachnoid hemorrhage using a transient hyperemic response test of cerebral autoregulation. *Neurosurgery* 2000; **47**:819–25.

137 Eskesen V, Karle A, Kruse A, Kruse Larsen C, Praestholm J, Schmidt K. Observer variability in assessment of angiographic vasospasm after aneurysmal subarachnoid haemorrhage. *Acta Neurochir (Wien)* 1987; **87**(1–2):54–57.

138 Rabinstein AA, Friedman JA, Weigand SD, McClelland RL, Fulgham JR, Manno EM *et al*. Predictors of cerebral infarction in aneurysmal subarachnoid hemorrhage. *Stroke* 2004; **35**:1862–6.

139 Kistler JP, Crowell RM, Davis KR, Heros R, Ojemann RG, Zervas T *et al*. The relation of cerebral vasospasm to the extent and location of subarachnoid blood visualized by CT scan: a prospective study. *Neurology* 1983; **33**(4):424–36.

140 Svensson E, Starmark JE, Ekholm S, Von Essen C, Johansson A. Analysis of interobserver disagreement in the assessment of subarachnoid blood and acute hydrocephalus on CT scans. *Neurol Res* 1996; **18**:487–94.

141 Van Norden AG, van Dijk GW, van Huizen MD, Algra A, Rinkel GJE. Interobserver agreement and predictive value for outcome of two rating scales for the amount of extravasated blood after aneurysmal subarachnoid haemorrhage. *J Neurol* 2006; **253**:1217–20.

142 Brouwers PJAM, Wijdicks EFM, van Gijn J. Infarction after aneurysm rupture does not depend on distribution or clearance rate of blood. *Stroke* 1992; **23**(3):374–9.

143 Rabinstein AA, Weigand S, Atkinson JL, Wijdicks EFM. Patterns of cerebral infarction in aneurysmal subarachnoid hemorrhage. *Stroke* 2005; **36**:992–7.

144 Maeda K, Kurita H, Nakamura T, Usui M, Tsutsumi K, Morimoto T *et al*. Occurrence of severe vasospasm following intraventricular hemorrhage from an arteriovenous malformation: report of two cases. *J Neurosurg* 1997; **87**:436–9.

145 Servadei F, Murray GD, Teasdale GM, Dearden M, Iannotti F, Lapierre F *et al*. Traumatic subarachnoid hemorrhage: demographic and clinical study of 750 patients from the European Brain Injury Consortium survey of head injuries. *Neurosurgery* 2002; **50**:261–7.

146 Rinkel GJE, Wijdicks EFM, Vermeulen M, Hasan D, Brouwers PJAM, van Gijn J. The clinical course of perimesencephalic nonaneurysmal subarachnoid hemorrhage. *Ann Neurol* 1991; **29**(5):463–8.

147 Van der Schaaf I, Wermer MJ, van der GY, Velthuis BK, van de Kraats CIB, Rinkel GJE. Prognostic value of cerebral perfusion-computed tomography in the acute stage after subarachnoid hemorrhage for the development of delayed cerebral ischemia. *Stroke* 2006; **37**:409–13.

148 Hop JW, Rinkel GJE, Algra A, van Gijn J. Initial loss of consciousness and risk of delayed cerebral ischemia after aneurysmal subarachnoid hemorrhage. *Stroke* 1999; **30**:2268–71.

149 Rinkel GJE, Feigin VL, Algra A, Van den Bergh WM, Vermeulen M, van Gijn J. Calcium antagonists for aneurysmal subarachnoid haemorrhage. *Cochrane Database Syst Rev* 2005; CD000277.

150 Pickard JD, Murray GD, Illingworth R, Shaw MD, Teasdale GM, Foy PM *et al*. Effect of oral nimodipine on cerebral infarction and outcome after subarachnoid haemorrhage: British aneurysm nimodipine trial. *Br Med J* 1989; **298**(6674):636–42.

151 Philippon J, Grob R, Dagreou F, Guggiari M, Rivierez M, Viars P. Prevention of vasospasm in subarachnoid haemorrhage: a controlled study with nimodipine. *Acta Neurochir (Wien)* 1986; **82**(3–4):110–14.

152 Petruk KC, West M, Mohr G, Weir BK, Benoit BG, Gentili F *et al*. Nimodipine treatment in poor-grade aneurysm patients: results of a multicenter double-blind placebo-controlled trial. *J Neurosurg* 1988; **68**(4):505–17.

153 Ahmed N, Nasman P, Wahlgren NG. Effect of intravenous nimodipine on blood pressure and outcome after acute stroke. *Stroke* 2000; **31**:1250–5.

154 Van den Bergh WM, Algra A, Van der Sprenkel JWB, Tulleken CAF, Rinkel GJE. Hypomagnesemia after aneurysmal subarachnoid hemorrhage. *Neurosurgery* 2003; **52**:276–81.

155 Van den Bergh WM, Zuur JK, Kamerling NA, Van Asseldonk JHT, Rinkel GJE, Tulleken CAF *et al*. Role of magnesium in the reduction of ischemic depolarization and lesion volume after experimental subarachnoid hemorrhage. *J Neurosurg* 2002; **97**:416–22.

156 Wong GK, Chan MT, Boet R, Poon WS, Gin T. Intravenous magnesium sulfate after aneurysmal subarachnoid hemorrhage: a prospective randomized pilot study. *J Neurosurg Anesthesiol* 2006; **18**:142–8.

157 Van den Bergh WM, on behalf of the MASH study group. Magnesium sulfate in aneurysmal subarachnoid hemorrhage: a randomized controlled trial. *Stroke* 2005; **36**:1011–15.

158 Schmid-Elsässer R, Kunz M, Zausinger S, Prueckner S, Briegel J, Steiger HJ. Intravenous magnesium versus nimodipine in the treatment of patients with aneurysmal subarachnoid hemorrhage: a randomized study. *Neurosurgery* 2006; **58**:1054–65.

159 Juvela S, Kaste M, Hillbom M. Platelet thromboxane release after subarachnoid hemorrhage and surgery. *Stroke* 1990; **21**(4):566–71.

160 Ohkuma H, Suzuki S, Kimura M, Sobata E. Role of platelet function in symptomatic cerebral vasospasm following aneurysmal subarachnoid hemorrhage. *Stroke* 1991; **22**:854–9.

161 Juvela S. Aspirin and delayed cerebral ischemia after aneurysmal subarachnoid hemorrhage. *J Neurosurg* 1995; **82**:945–52.

162 Mendelow AD, Stockdill G, Steers AJ, Hayes J, Gillingham FJ. Double-blind trial of aspirin in patient receiving tranexamic acid for subarachnoid hemorrhage. *Acta Neurochir (Wien)* 1982; **62**(3–4):195–202.

163 Hop JW, Rinkel GJE, Algra A, Berkelbach van der Sprenkel JW, van Gijn J. Randomized pilot trial of postoperative aspirin in subarachnoid hemorrhage. *Neurology* 2000; **54**:872–8.

164 Shaw MD, Foy PM, Conway M, Pickard JD, Maloney P, Spillane JA *et al*. Dipyridamole and postoperative ischemic deficits in aneurysmal subarachnoid hemorrhage. *J Neurosurg* 1985; **63**:699–703.

165 Tokiyoshi K, Ohnishi T, Nii Y. Efficacy and toxicity of thromboxane synthetase inhibitor for cerebral vasospasm after subarachnoid hemorrhage. *Surg Neurol* 1991; **36**:112–18.

166 Suzuki S, Sano K, Handa H, Asano T, Tamura A, Yonekawa Y *et al*. Clinical study of OKY-046, a thromboxane synthetase inhibitor, in prevention of cerebral vasospasms and delayed cerebral ischaemic symptoms after subarachnoid haemorrhage due to aneurysmal rupture: a randomized double-blind study. *Neurol Res* 1989; **11**:79–88.

167 Robinson JG, Smith B, Maheshwari N, Schrott H. Pleiotropic effects of statins: benefit beyond cholesterol reduction? A meta-regression analysis. *J Am Coll Cardiol* 2005; **46**:1855–62.

168 Lynch JR, Wang H, McGirt MJ, Floyd J, Friedman AH, Coon AL *et al*. Simvastatin reduces vasospasm after aneurysmal subarachnoid hemorrhage: results of a pilot randomized clinical trial. *Stroke* 2005; **36**:2024–6.

169 Tseng MY, Czosnyka M, Richards H, Pickard JD, Kirkpatrick PJ. Effects of acute treatment with pravastatin on cerebral vasospasm, autoregulation, and delayed ischemic deficits after aneurysmal subarachnoid hemorrhage: a phase II randomized placebo-controlled trial. *Stroke* 2005; **36**:1627–32.

170 Singhal AB, Topcuoglu MA, Dorer DJ, Ogilvy CS, Carter BS, Koroshetz WJ. SSRI and statin use increases the risk for vasospasm after subarachnoid hemorrhage. *Neurology* 2005; **64**:1008–13.

171 Kassell NF, Haley EC, Jr., Apperson-Hansen C, Stat M, Alves WM, Dorsch NW *et al*. Randomized, double-blind, vehicle-controlled trial of tirilazad mesylate in patients with aneurysmal subarachnoid hemorrhage: a cooperative study in Europe, Australia, and New Zealand. *J Neurosurg* 1996; **84**:221–8.

172 Haley EC, Jr., Kassell NF, Apperson-Hansen C, Maile MH, Alves WM. A randomized, double-blind, vehicle-controlled trial of tirilazad mesylate in patients with aneurysmal subarachnoid hemorrhage: a cooperative study in North America. *J Neurosurg* 1997; **86**(3):467–74.

173 Lanzino G, Kassell NF, Dorsch NWC, Pasqualin A, Brandt L, Schmiedek P *et al*. Double-blind, randomized, vehicle-controlled study of high-dose tirilazad mesylate in women with aneurysmal subarachnoid hemorrhage. Part I. A cooperative study in Europe, Australia, New Zealand, and South Africa. *J Neurosurg* 1999; **90**:1011–17.

174 Lanzino G, Kassell NF. Double-blind, randomized, vehicle-controlled study of high-dose tirilazad mesylate in women with aneurysmal subarachnoid hemorrhage. Part II. A cooperative study in North America. *J Neurosurg* 1999; **90**:1018–24.

175 Ogden JA, Mee EW, Utley T. Too little, too late: Does tirilazad mesylate reduce fatigue after subarachnoid hemorrhage? *Neurosurgery* 1998; **43**:782–7.

176 Asano T, Takakura K, Sano K, Kikuchi H, Nagai H, Saito I *et al*. Effects of a hydroxyl radical scavenger on delayed ischemic neurological deficits following aneurysmal subarachnoid hemorrhage: results of a multicenter, placebo-controlled double-blind trial. *J Neurosurg* 1996; **84**:792–803.

177 Saito I, Asano T, Sano K, Takakura K, Abe H, Yoshimoto T *et al*. Neuroprotective effect of an antioxidant, ebselen, in patients with delayed neurological deficits after aneurysmal subarachnoid hemorrhage. *Neurosurgery* 1998; **42**:269–77.

178 Saito I, Asano T, Ochiai C, Takakura K, Tamura A, Sano K. A double-blind clinical evaluation of the effect of Nizofenone (Y-9179) on delayed ischemic neurological deficits following aneurysmal rupture. *Neurol Res* 1983; **5**:29–47.

179 Shaw MDM, Vermeulen M, Murray GD, Pickard JD, Bell BA, Teasdale GM. Efficacy and safety of the endothelin$_{A/B}$ receptor antagonist TAK-044 in treating subarachnoid hemorrhage: a report by the Steering Committee on behalf of the UK/Netherlands/Eire TAK-044 Subarachnoid Haemorrhage Study Group. *J Neurosurg* 2000; **93**:992–7.

180 Rinkel GJE, Feigin VL, Algra A, van Gijn J. Circulatory volume expansion therapy for aneurysmal subarachnoid haemorrhage. *Cochrane Database Syst Rev* 2004; CD000483.

181 Wijdicks EFM, Vermeulen M, van Brummelen P, van Gijn J. The effect of fludrocortisone acetate on plasma volume and natriuresis in patients with aneurysmal subarachnoid hemorrhage. *Clin Neurol Neurosurg* 1988; **90**(3):209–14.

182 Hasan D, Lindsay KW, Wijdicks EFM, Murray GD, Brouwers PJAM, Bakker WH *et al*. Effect of fludrocortisone acetate in patients with subarachnoid hemorrhage. *Stroke* 1989; **20**(9):1156–61.

183 Mori T, Katayama Y, Kawamata T, Hirayama T. Improved efficiency of hypervolemic therapy with inhibition of natriuresis by fludrocortisone in patients with aneurysmal subarachnoid hemorrhage. *J Neurosurg* 1999; **91**:947–52.

184 Moro N, Katayama Y, Kojima J, Mori T, Kawamata T. Prophylactic management of excessive natriuresis with hydrocortisone for efficient hypervolemic therapy after subarachnoid hemorrhage. *Stroke* 2003; **34**:2807–11.

185 Klimo P, Jr., Kestle JR, MacDonald JD, Schmidt RH. Marked reduction of cerebral vasospasm with lumbar drainage of cerebrospinal fluid after subarachnoid hemorrhage. *J Neurosurg* 2004; **100**:215–24.

186 Amin-Hanjani S, Ogilvy CS, Barker FG. Does intracisternal thrombolysis prevent vasospasm after aneurysmal

subarachnoid hemorrhage? A meta-analysis. *Neurosurgery* 2004; **54**:326–34.

187 Hamada J, Kai Y, Morioka M, Yano S, Mizuno T, Hirano T *et al*. Effect on cerebral vasospasm of coil embolization followed by microcatheter intrathecal urokinase infusion into the cisterna magna: a prospective randomized study. *Stroke* 2003; **34**:2549–54.

188 Hijdra A, Vermeulen M, van Gijn J, van Crevel H. Rerupture of intracranial aneurysms: a clinicoanatomic study. *J Neurosurg* 1987; **67**(1):29–33.

189 Hijdra A, Braakman R, van Gijn J, Vermeulen M, van Crevel H. Aneurysmal subarachnoid hemorrhage: complications and outcome in a hospital population. *Stroke* 1987; **18**(6):1061–7.

190 Van der Schaaf IC, Ruigrok YM, Rinkel GJE, Algra A, van Gijn J. Study design and outcome measures in studies on aneurysmal subarachnoid hemorrhage. *Stroke* 2002; **33**:2043–6.

191 Phan TG, Huston J, III, Campeau NG, Wijdicks EFM, Atkinson JL, Fulgham JR. Value of diffusion-weighted imaging in patients with a nonlocalizing examination and vasospasm from subarachnoid hemorrhage. *Cerebrovasc Dis* 2003; **15**:177–81.

192 Davis S, Andrews J, Lichtenstein M, Kaye A, Tress B, Rossiter S *et al*. A single-photon emission computed tomography study of hypoperfusion after subarachnoid hemorrhage. *Stroke* 1990; **21**(2):252–9.

193 Hasan D, van Peski J, Loeve I, Krenning EP, Vermeulen M. Single photon emission computed tomography in patients with acute hydrocephalus or with cerebral ischaemia after subarachnoid haemorrhage. *J Neurol Neurosurg Psychiatry* 1991; **54**(6):490–3.

194 Lysakowski C, Walder B, Costanza MC, Tramér MR. Transcranial Doppler versus angiography in patients with vasospasm due to a ruptured cerebral aneurysm: a systematic review. *Stroke* 2001; **32**:2292–8.

195 Otawara Y, Ogasawara K, Ogawa A, Sasaki M, Takahashi K. Evaluation of vasospasm after subarachnoid hemorrhage by use of multislice computed tomographic angiography. *Neurosurgery* 2002; **51**:939–42.

196 Yoon DY, Choi CS, Kim KH, Cho BM. Multidetector-row CT angiography of cerebral vasospasm after aneurysmal subarachnoid hemorrhage: comparison of volume-rendered images and digital subtraction angiography. *Am J Neuroradiol* 2006; **27**:370–7.

197 Kosnik EJ, Hunt WE. Postoperative hypertension in the management of patients with intracranial arterial aneurysms. *J Neurosurg* 1976; **45**(2):148–54.

198 Kassell NF, Peerless SJ, Durward QJ, Beck DW, Drake CG, Adams HP, Jr. Treatment of ischemic deficits from vasospasm with intravascular volume expansion and induced arterial hypertension. *Neurosurgery* 1982; **11**(3):337–43.

199 Qureshi AI, Suarez JI, Bhardwaj A, Yahia AM, Tamargo RJ, Ulatowski JA. Early predictors of outcome in patients receiving hypervolemic and hypertensive therapy for symptomatic vasospasm after subarachnoid hemorrhage. *Crit Care Med* 2000; **28**:824–9.

200 Sen J, Belli A, Albon H, Morgan L, Petzold A, Kitchen N. Triple-H therapy in the management of aneurysmal subarachnoid haemorrhage. *Lancet Neurol* 2003; **2**:614–21.

201 Hoh BL, Carter BS, Ogilvy CS. Risk of hemorrhage from unsecured, unruptured aneurysms during and after hypertensive hypervolemic therapy. *Neurosurgery* 2002; **50**:1207–11.

202 Amin-Hanjani S, Schwartz RB, Sathi S, Stieg PE. Hypertensive encephalopathy as a complication of hyperdynamic therapy for vasospasm: report of two cases. *Neurosurgery* 1999; **44**:1113–16.

203 Wartenberg KE, Parra A. CT and CT-perfusion findings of reversible leukoencephalopathy during triple-H therapy for symptomatic subarachnoid hemorrhage-related vasospasm. *J Neuroimaging* 2006; **16**:170–5.

204 Mayer SA, Solomon RA, Fink ME, Lennihan L, Stern L, Beckford A *et al*. Effect of 5% albumin solution on sodium balance and blood volume after subarachnoid hemorrhage. *Neurosurgery* 1998; **42**:759–67.

205 Hoh BL, Ogilvy CS. Endovascular treatment of cerebral vasospasm: transluminal balloon angioplasty, intra-arterial papaverine, and intra-arterial nicardipine. *Neurosurg Clin N Am* 2005; **16**:501–16, vi.

206 Rabinstein AA, Friedman JA, Nichols DA, Pichelmann MA, McClelland RL, Manno EM *et al*. Predictors of outcome after endovascular treatment of cerebral vasospasm. *Am J Neuroradiol* 2004; **25**:1778–82.

207 Polin RS, Coenen VA, Hansen CA, Shin P, Baskaya MK, Nanda A *et al*. Efficacy of transluminal angioplasty for the management of symptomatic cerebral vasospasm following aneurysmal subarachnoid hemorrhage. *J Neurosurg* 2000; **92**:284–90.

208 Fandino J, Kaku Y, Schuknecht B, Valavanis A, Yonekawa Y. Improvement of cerebral oxygenation patterns and metabolic validation of super-selective intraarterial infusion of papaverine for the treatment of cerebral vasospasm. *J Neurosurg* 1998; **89**:93–100.

209 Polin RS, Hansen CA, German P, Chadduck JB, Kassell NF. Intra-arterially administered papaverine for the treatment of symptomatic cerebral vasospasm. *Neurosurgery* 1998; **42**:1256–64.

210 Smith WS, Dowd CF, Johnston SC, Ko NU, DeArmond SJ, Dillon WP *et al*. Neurotoxicity of intra-arterial papaverine preserved with chlorobutanol used for the treatment of cerebral vasospasm after aneurysmal subarachnoid hemorrhage. *Stroke* 2004; **35**:2518–22.

211 Arakawa Y, Kikuta K, Hojo M, Goto Y, Ishii A, Yamagata S. Milrinone for the treatment of cerebral vasospasm after subarachnoid hemorrhage: report of seven cases. *Neurosurgery* 2001; **48**:723–8.

212 Feng L, Fitzsimmons BF, Young WL, Berman MF, Lin E, Aagaard BD *et al*. Intraarterially administered verapamil as adjunct therapy for cerebral vasospasm: safety and 2-year experience. *Am J Neuroradiol* 2002; **23**:1284–10.

213 Badjatia N, Topcuoglu MA, Pryor JC, Rabinov JD, Ogilvy CS, Carter BS *et al*. Preliminary experience with intra-arterial nicardipine as a treatment for cerebral vasospasm. *Am J Neuroradiol* 2004; **25**:819–26.

214 European CGRP in Subarachnoid Haemorrhage Study Group. Effect of calcitonin-gene-related peptide in patients with delayed postoperative cerebral ischaemia after aneurysmal subarachnoid haemorrhage. *Lancet* 1992; **339**(8797):831–4.

215 Hasan D, Vermeulen M, Wijdicks EFM, Hijdra A, van Gijn J. Management problems in acute hydrocephalus after subarachnoid hemorrhage. *Stroke* 1989; **20**(6):747–53.

216 Milhorat TH. Acute hydrocephalus after aneurysmal subarachnoid hemorrhage. *Neurosurgery* 1987; **20**(1):15–20.

217 Hasan D, Tanghe HL. Distribution of cisternal blood in patients with acute hydrocephalus after subarachnoid hemorrhage. *Ann Neurol* 1992; **31**(4):374–8.

218 Dorai Z, Hynan LS, Kopitnik TA, Samson D. Factors related to hydrocephalus after aneurysmal subarachnoid hemorrhage. *Neurosurgery* 2003; **52**:763–9.

219 Rinkel GJE, Wijdicks EFM, Vermeulen M, Tans JTJ, Hasan D, van Gijn J. Acute hydrocephalus in nonaneurysmal perimesencephalic hemorrhage: evidence of CSF block at the tentorial hiatus. *Neurology* 1992; **42**(9):1805–7.

220 Komotar RJ, Olivi A, Rigamonti D, Tamargo RJ. Microsurgical fenestration of the lamina terminalis reduces the incidence of shuntdependent hydrocephalus after aneurysmal subarachnoid hemorrhage. *Neurosurgery* 2002; **51**:1403–12.

221 Andaluz N, Zuccarello M. Fenestration of the lamina terminalis as a valuable adjunct in aneurysm surgery. *Neurosurgery* 2004; **55**:1050–9.

222 Swash M. Periaqueductal dysfunction (the sylvian aqueduct syndrome): a sign of hydrocephalus? *J Neurol Neurosurg Psychiatry* 1974; **37**(1):21–6.

223 Kolluri VR, Sengupta RP. Symptomatic hydrocephalus following aneurysmal subarachnoid hemorrhage. *Surg Neurol* 1984; **21**(4):402–4.

224 Hellingman CA, Van den Bergh WM, Beijer I, van Dijk GW, Algra A, van Gijn J *et al*. Risk of rebleeding after treatment of acute hydrocephalus in patients with aneurysmal subarachnoid hemorrhage. *Stroke* 2007; **38**(1):96–9.

225 Pickard JD. Early posthaemorrhagic hydrocephalus. *Br Med J* 1984; **289**(6445):569–70.

226 Wardlaw JM, Cannon J, Statham PFX, Price R. Does the size of intracranial aneurysms change with intracranial pressure? Observations based on color 'power' transcranial Doppler ultrasound. *J Neurosurg* 1998; **88**:846–50.

227 Fountas KN, Kapsalaki EZ, Machinis T, Karampelas I, Smisson HF, Robinson JS. Review of the literature regarding the relationship of rebleeding and external ventricular drainage in patients with subarachnoid hemorrhage of aneurysmal origin. *Neurosurg Rev* 2005; **29**:14–18.

228 Wong GKC, Poon WS, Wai S, Yu LM, Lyon D, Lam JMK. Failure of regular external ventricular drain exchange to reduce cerebrospinal fluid infection: result of a randomised controlled trial. *J Neurol Neurosurg Psychiatry* 2002; **73**:759–61.

229 Lozier AP, Sciacca RR, Romagnoli MF, Connolly ES, Jr. Ventriculostomy-related infections: a critical review of the literature. *Neurosurgery* 2002; **51**:170–81.

230 Choksey MS, Malik IA. Zero tolerance to shunt infections: can it be achieved? *J Neurol Neurosurg Psychiatry* 2004; **75**:87–91.

231 Korinek AM, Reina M, Boch AL, Rivera AO, De BD, Puybasset L. Prevention of external ventricular drain-related ventriculitis. *Acta Neurochir (Wien)* 2005; **147**:39–45.

232 Khanna RK, Rosenblum ML, Rock JP, Malik GM. Prolonged external ventricular drainage with percutaneous long-tunnel ventriculostomies. *J Neurosurg* 1995; **83**:791–4.

233 Kim DK, Uttley D, Bell BA, Marsh HT, Moore AJ. Comparison of rates of infection of two methods of emergency ventricular drainage. *J Neurol Neurosurg Psychiatry* 1995; **58**:444–6.

234 Coplin WM, Avellino AM, Kim DK, Winn HR, Grady MS. Bacterial meningitis associated with lumbar drains: a retrospective cohort study. *J Neurol Neurosurg Psychiatry* 1999; **67**:468–73.

235 Schade RP, Schinkel J, Visser LG, van Dijk JM, Voormolen JH, Kuijper EJ. Bacterial meningitis caused by the use of ventricular or lumbar cerebrospinal fluid catheters. *J Neurosurg* 2005; **102**:229–34.

236 Ruijs AC, Dirven CM, Algra A, Beijer I, Vandertop WP, Rinkel G. The risk of rebleeding after external lumbar drainage in patients with untreated ruptured cerebral aneurysms. *Acta Neurochir (Wien)* 2005; **147**:1157–62.

237 Klopfenstein JD, Kim LJ, Feiz-Erfan I, Hott JS, Goslar P, Zabramski JM *et al*. Comparison of rapid and gradual weaning from external ventricular drainage in patients with aneurysmal subarachnoid hemorrhage: a prospective randomized trial. *J Neurosurg* 2004; **100**:225–9.

238 Solenski NJ, Haley EC, Jr., Kassell NF, Kongable G, Germanson T, Truskowski L *et al*. Medical complications of aneurysmal subarachnoid hemorrhage: a report of the multicenter, cooperative aneurysm study. *Crit Care Med* 1995; **23**:1007–17.

239 Gruber A, Reinprecht A, Görzer H, Fridrich P, Czech T, Illievich UM *et al*. Pulmonary function and radiographic abnormalities related to neurological outcome after aneurysmal subarachnoid hemorrhage. *J Neurosurg* 1998; **88**:28–37.

240 Wartenberg KE, Schmidt JM, Claassen J, Temes RE, Frontera JA, Ostapkovich N *et al*. Impact of medical complications on outcome after subarachnoid hemorrhage. *Crit Care Med* 2006; **34**:617–23.

241 Schuiling WJ, de Weerd AW, Dennesen PJ, Algra A, Rinkel GJE. The simplified acute physiology score to predict outcome in patients with subarachnoid hemorrhage. *Neurosurgery* 2005; **57**:230–6.

242 Qureshi AI, Suri MFK, Sung GY, Straw RN, Yahia AM, Saad M *et al*. Prognostic significance of hypernatremia and hyponatremia among patients with aneurysmal subarachnoid hemorrhage. *Neurosurgery* 2002; **50**:749–55.

243 Bartter FC, Schwartz WB. The syndrome of inappropriate secretion of antdiuretic hormone. *Am J Med* 1967; **42**:790–806.

244 Harrigan MR. Cerebral salt wasting syndrome: a review. *Neurosurgery* 1996; **38**:152–60.

245 Wijdicks EFM, van Dongen KJ, van Gijn J, Hijdra A, Vermeulen M. Enlargement of the third ventricle and hyponatraemia in aneurysmal subarachnoid haemorrhage. *J Neurol Neurosurg Psychiatry* 1988; **51**(4):516–20.

246 Sayama T, Inamura T, Matsushima T, Inoha S, Inoue T, Fukui M. High incidence of hyponatremia in patients with ruptured anterior communicating artery aneurysms. *Neurol Res* 2000; **22**:151–5.

247 Wijdicks EFM, Vermeulen M, van Brummelen P, den Boer NC, van Gijn J. Digoxin-like immunoreactive substance in patients with aneurysmal subarachnoid haemorrhage. *Br Med J* 1987; **294**(6574):729–32.

248 Diringer M, Ladenson PW, Stern BJ, Schleimer J, Hanley DF. Plasma atrial natriuretic factor and subarachnoid hemorrhage. *Stroke* 1988; **19**(9):1119–24.

249 Rosenfeld JV, Barnett GH, Sila CA, Little JR, Bravo EL, Beck GJ. The effect of subarachnoid hemorrhage on blood and CSF atrial natriuretic factor. *J Neurosurg* 1989; **71**(1):32–7.

250 Wijdicks EFM, Ropper AH, Hunnicutt EJ, Richardson GS, Nathanson JA. Atrial natriuretic factor and salt wasting after aneurysmal subarachnoid hemorrhage. *Stroke* 1991; **22**(12):1519–24.

251 Isotani E, Suzuki R, Tomita K, Hokari M, Monma S, Marumo F *et al.* Alterations in plasma concentrations of natriuretic peptides and antidiuretic hormone after subarachnoid hemorrhage. *Stroke* 1994; **25**:2198–203.

252 Wijdicks EFM, Schievink WI, Burnett JC, Jr. Natriuretic peptide system and endothelin in aneurysmal subarachnoid hemorrhage. *J Neurosurg* 1997; **87**:275–80.

253 Berendes E, Walter M, Cullen P, Prien T, Van Aken H, Horsthemke J *et al.* Secretion of brain natriuretic peptide in patients with aneurysmal subarachnoid haemorrhage. *Lancet* 1997; **349**:245–9.

254 Tomida M, Muraki M, Uemura K, Yamasaki K. Plasma concentrations of brain natriuretic peptide in patients with subarachnoid hemorrhage. *Stroke* 1998; **29**:1584–7.

255 McGirt MJ, Blessing R, Nimjee SM, Friedman AH, Alexander MJ, Laskowitz DT *et al.* Correlation of serum brain natriuretic peptide with hyponatremia and delayed ischemic neurological deficits after subarachnoid hemorrhage. *Neurosurgery* 2004; **54**:1369–73.

256 Khurana VG, Wijdicks EFM, Heublein DM, McClelland RL, Meyer FB, Piepgras DG *et al.* A pilot study of dendroaspis natriuretic peptide in aneurysmal subarachnoid hemorrhage. *Neurosurgery* 2004; **55**:69–75.

257 Martin RJ. Central pontine and extrapontine myelinolysis: the osmotic demyelination syndromes. *J Neurol Neurosurg Psychiatry* 2004; **75** (Suppl 3):iii22–iii28.

258 Adrogué HJ, Madias NE. Hyponatremia. *N Engl J Med* 2000; **342**:1581–9.

259 Adrogué HJ. Consequences of inadequate management of hyponatremia. *Am J Nephrol* 2005; **25**:240–9.

260 Weisinger JR, Bellorin-Font E. Magnesium and phosphorus. *Lancet* 1998; **352**:391–396.

261 van Norden AG, Van den Bergh WM, Rinkel GJE. Dose evaluation for long-term magnesium treatment in aneurysmal subarachnoid haemorrhage. *J Clin Pharm Ther* 2005; **30**:439–42.

262 Fukui S, Katoh H, Tsuzuki N, Ishihara S, Otani N, Ooigawa H *et al.* Multivariate analysis of risk factors for QT prolongation following subarachnoid hemorrhage. *Crit Care* 2003; **7**:R7–R12.

263 Disney L, Weir B, Grace M, Roberts P. Trends in blood pressure, osmolality and electrolytes after subarachnoid hemorrhage from aneurysms. *Can J Neurol Sci* 1989; **16**:299–304.

264 Dorhout Mees SM, van Dijk GW, Algra A, Kempink DR, Rinkel GJE. Glucose levels and outcome after subarachnoid hemorrhage. *Neurology* 2003; **61**:1132–3.

265 Frontera JA, Fernandez A, Claassen J, Schmidt M, Schumacher HC, Wartenberg K *et al.* Hyperglycemia after SAH: predictors, associated complications, and impact on outcome. *Stroke* 2006; **37**:199 203.

266 Naredi S, Lambert G, Edén E, Zäll S, Runnerstam M, Rydenhag B *et al.* Increased sympathetic nervous activity in patients with nontraumatic subarachnoid hemorrhage. *Stroke* 2000; **31**:901–6.

267 Espiner EA, Leikis R, Ferch RD, MacFarlane MR, Bonkowski JA, Frampton CM *et al.* The neuro-cardio-endocrine response to acute subarachnoid haemorrhage. *Clin Endocrinol (Oxf)* 2002; **56**:629–35.

268 Mayer SA, Lin J, Homma S, Solomon RA, Lennihan L, Sherman D *et al.* Myocardial injury and left ventricular performance after subarachnoid hemorrhage. *Stroke* 1999; **30**:780–6.

269 Parekh N, Venkatesh B, Cross D, Leditschke A, Atherton J, Miles W *et al.* Cardiac troponin I predicts myocardial dysfunction in aneurysmal subarachnoid hemorrhage. *J Am Coll Cardiol* 2000; **36**:1328–35.

270 Tung P, Kopelnik A, Banki N, Ong K, Ko N, Lawton MT *et al.* Predictors of neurocardiogenic injury after subarachnoid hemorrhage. *Stroke* 2004; **35**:548–51.

271 Schuiling WJ, Dennesen PJ, Tans JT, Kingma LM, Algra A, Rinkel GJE. Troponin I in predicting cardiac or pulmonary complications and outcome in subarachnoid haemorrhage. *J Neurol Neurosurg Psychiatry* 2005; **76**:1565–9.

272 Naidech AM, Kreiter KT, Janjua N, Ostapkovich ND, Parra A, Commichau C *et al.* Cardiac troponin elevation, cardiovascular morbidity, and outcome after subarachnoid hemorrhage. *Circulation* 2005; **112**:2851–6.

273 Greenhoot JH, Reichenbach DD. Cardiac injury and subarachnoid hemorrhage: a clinical, pathological and physiological correlation. *J Neurosurg* 1969; **30**:521–31.

274 Tung PP, Olmsted E, Kopelnik A, Banki NM, Drew BJ, Ko N *et al.* Plasma B-type natriuretic peptide levels are associated with early cardiac dysfunction after subarachnoid hemorrhage. *Stroke* 2005; **36**:1567–9.

275 Van den Bergh WM, Algra A, Rinkel GJE. Electrocardiographic abnormalities and serum

magnesium in patients with subarachnoid hemorrhage. *Stroke* 2004; **35**:644–8.

276 Khechinashvili G, Asplund K. Electrocardiographic changes in patients with acute stroke: a systematic review. *Cerebrovasc Dis* 2002; **14**:67–76.

277 Carruth JE, Silverman ME. Torsade de pointe atypical ventricular tachycardia complicating subarachnoid hemorrhage. *Chest* 1980; **78**(6):886–8.

278 Hess EP, Boie ET, White RD. Survival of a neurologically intact patient with subarachnoid hemorrhage and cardiopulmonary arrest. *Mayo Clin Proc* 2005; **80**:1073–6.

279 Andreoli A, di Pasquale G, Pinelli G, Grazi P, Tognetti F, Testa C. Subarachnoid hemorrhage: frequency and severity of cardiac arrhythmias: a survey of 70 cases studied in the acute phase. *Stroke* 1987; **18**(3):558–64.

280 Brouwers PJAM, Wijdicks EFM, Hasan D, Vermeulen M, Wever EF, Frericks H et al. Serial electrocardiographic recording in aneurysmal subarachnoid hemorrhage. *Stroke* 1989; **20**(9):1162–7.

281 Manninen PH, Ayra B, Gelb AW, Pelz D. Association between electrocardiographic abnormalities and intracranial blood in patients following acute subarachnoid hemorrhage. *J Neurosurg Anesthesiol* 1995; **7**(1):12–16.

282 Svigelj V, Grad A, Tekavcic I, Kiauta T. Cardiac arrhythmia associated with reversible damage to insula in a patient with subarachnoid hemorrhage. *Stroke* 1994; **25**(5):1053–5.

283 Hirashima Y, Takashima S, Matsumura N, Kurimoto M, Origasa H, Endo S. Right sylvian fissure subarachnoid hemorrhage has electrocardiographic consequences. *Stroke* 2001; **32**:2278–81.

284 Cheung RT, Hachinski V. The insula and cerebrogenic sudden death. *Arch Neurol* 2000; **57**:1685–8.

285 Cruickshank JM, Neil-Dwyer G, Degaute JP, Hayes Y, Kuurne T, Kytta J et al. Reduction of stress/catecholamine-induced cardiac necrosis by beta 1-selective blockade. *Lancet* 1987; **2**(8559):585–9.

286 Banki N, Kopelnik A, Tung P, Lawton MT, Gress D, Drew B et al. Prospective analysis of prevalence, distribution, and rate of recovery of left ventricular systolic dysfunction in patients with subarachnoid hemorrhage. *J Neurosurg* 2006; **105**:15–20.

287 Schuiling WJ, Dennesen PJ, Rinkel GJE. Extracerebral organ dysfunction in the acute stage after aneurysmal subarachnoid hemorrhage. *Neurocrit Care* 2005; **3**:1–10.

288 Vespa PM, Bleck TP. Neurogenic pulmonary edema and other mechanisms of impaired oxygenation after aneurysmal subarachnoid hemorrhage. *Neurocrit Care* 2004; **1**:157–70.

289 Friedman JA, Pichelmann MA, Piepgras DG, McIver JI, Toussaint LG, III, McClelland RL et al. Pulmonary complications of aneurysmal subarachnoid hemorrhage. *Neurosurgery* 2003; **52**:1025–31.

290 Mayer SA, Fink ME, Homma S, Sherman D, LiMandri G, Lennihan L et al. Cardiac injury associated with neurogenic pulmonary edema following subarachnoid hemorrhage. *Neurology* 1994; **44**(5):815–20.

291 Deehan SC, Grant IS. Haemodynamic changes in neurogenic pulmonary oedema: effect of dobutamine. *Intensive Care Med* 1996; **22**:672–6.

292 Hop JW, Rinkel GJE, Algra A, van Gijn J. Changes in functional outcome and quality of life in patients and caregivers after aneurysmal subarachnoid hemorrhage. *J Neurosurg* 2001; **95**:957–63.

293 McCarron MO, Alberts MJ, McCarron P. A systematic review of Terson's syndrome: frequency and prognosis after subarachnoid haemorrhage. *J Neurol Neurosurg Psychiatry* 2004; **75**:491–3.

294 Frizzell RT, Kuhn F, Morris R, Quinn C, Fisher WS, III. Screening for ocular hemorrhages in patients with ruptured cerebral aneurysms: a prospective study of 99 patients. *Neurosurgery* 1997; **41**:529–33.

295 Kuhn F, Morris R, Witherspoon CD, Mester V. Terson syndrome: results of vitrectomy and the significance of vitreous hemorrhage in patients with subarachnoid hemorrhage. *Ophthalmology* 1998; **105**:472–7.

296 Stiebel-Kalish H, Turtel LS, Kupersmith MJ. The natural history of nontraumatic subarachnoid hemorrhage-related intraocular hemorrhages. *Retina* 2004; **24**:36–40.

297 Winn HR, Richardson AE, Jane JA. The long-term prognosis in untreated cerebral aneurysms: I. The incidence of late hemorrhage in cerebral aneurysm: a 10-year evaluation of 364 patients. *Ann Neurol* 1977; **1**(4):358–70.

298 Wermer MJH, Rinkel GJE, Greebe P, Albrecht KW, Dirven CM, Tulleken CAF. Late recurrence of subarachnoid hemorrhage after treatment for ruptured aneurysms: patient characteristics and outcomes. *Neurosurgery* 2005; **56**:197–204.

299 Vale FL, Bradley EL, Fisher WS, III. The relationship of subarachnoid hemorrhage and the need for postoperative shunting. *J Neurosurg* 1997; **86**(3):462–6.

300 Gruber A, Reinprecht A, Bavinzski G, Czech T, Richling B. Chronic shunt-dependent hydrocephalus after early surgical and early endovascular treatment of ruptured intracranial aneurysms. *Neurosurgery* 1999; **44**:503–9.

301 Tapaninaho A, Hernesniemi J, Vapalahti M, Niskanen M, Kari A, Luukkonen M et al. Shunt-dependent hydrocephalus after subarachnoid haemorrhage and aneurysm surgery: timing of surgery is not a risk factor. *Acta Neurochir (Wien)* 1993; **123**(3–4):118–24.

302 Pietila TA, Heimberger KC, Palleske H, Brock M. Influence of aneurysm location on the development of chronic hydrocephalus following SAH. *Acta Neurochir (Wien)* 1995; **137**:70–3.

303 Yoshioka H, Inagawa T, Tokuda Y, Inokuchi F. Chronic hydrocephalus in elderly patients following subarachnoid hemorrhage. *Surg Neurol* 2000; **53**:119–24.

304 Hirashima Y, Hamada H, Hayashi N, Kuwayama N, Origasa H, Endo S. Independent predictors of late hydrocephalus in patients with aneurysmal subarachnoid hemorrhage: analysis by multivariate logistic regression model. *Cerebrovasc Dis* 2003; **16**:205–10.

305 Bavinzski G, Killer M, Gruber A, Reinprecht A, Gross CE, Richling B. Treatment of basilar artery bifurcation

aneurysms by using Guglielmi detachable coils: a 6-year experience. *J Neurosurg* 1999; **90**:843–52.

306 Sethi H, Moore A, Dervin J, Clifton A, MacSweeney JE. Hydrocephalus: comparison of clipping and embolization in aneurysm treatment. *J Neurosurg* 2000; **92**:991–4.

307 Dehdashti AR, Rilliet B, Rufenacht DA, de Tribolet N. Shunt-dependent hydrocephalus after rupture of intracranial aneurysms: a prospective study of the influence of treatment modality. *J Neurosurg* 2004; 101:402–7.

308 Tomasello F, D'Avella D, De Divitiis O. Does lamina terminalis fenestration reduce the incidence of chronic hydrocephalus after subarachnoid hemorrhage? *Neurosurgery* 1999; **45**:827–31.

309 Claassen J, Peery S, Kreiter KT, Hirsch LJ, Du EY, Connolly ES *et al*. Predictors and clinical impact of epilepsy after subarachnoid hemorrhage. *Neurology* 2003; **60**:208–14.

310 Buczacki SJ, Kirkpatrick PJ, Seeley HM, Hutchinson PJ. Late epilepsy following open surgery for aneurysmal subarachnoid haemorrhage. *J Neurol Neurosurg Psychiatry* 2004; **75**:1620–2.

311 Rhoney DH, Tipps LB, Murry KR, Basham MC, Michael DB, Coplin WM. Anticonvulsant prophylaxis and timing of seizures after aneurysmal subarachnoid hemorrhage. *Neurology* 2000; **55**:258–65.

312 Olafsson E, Gudmundsson G, Hauser WA. Risk of epilepsy in long-term survivors of surgery for aneurysmal subarachnoid hemorrhage: a population-based study in Iceland. *Epilepsia* 2000; **41**:1201–5.

313 Byrne JV, Boardman P, Ioannidis I, Adcock J, Traill Z. Seizures after aneurysmal subarachnoid hemorrhage treated with coil embolization. *Neurosurgery* 2003; **52**:545–50.

314 Buchanan KM, Elias LJ, Goplen GB. Differing perspectives on outcome after subarachnoid hemorrhage: the patient, the relative, the neurosurgeon. *Neurosurgery* 2000; **46**:831–8.

315 Mayer SA, Kreiter KT, Copeland D, Bernardini GL, Bates JE, Peery S *et al*. Global and domain-specific cognitive impairment and outcome after subarachnoid hemorrhage. *Neurology* 2002; **59**:1750–8.

316 Powell J, Kitchen N, Heslin J, Greenwood R. Psychosocial outcomes at three and nine months after good neurological recovery from aneurysmal subarachnoid haemorrhage: predictors and prognosis. *J Neurol Neurosurg Psychiatry* 2002; **72**:772–81.

317 Powell J, Kitchen N, Heslin J, Greenwood R. Psychosocial outcomes at 18 months after good neurological recovery from aneurysmal subarachnoid haemorrhage. *J Neurol Neurosurg Psychiatry* 2004; **75**:1119–24.

318 Wermer MJ, Kool H, Albrecht KW, Rinkel GJE, for the ASTRA study group. Long-term effects of subarachnoid hemorrhage on employment, relationships, personality and mood. *Neurosurgery* 2007; **60**(1):91–7, discussion 97–8.

319 Anson JA, Lawton MT, Spetzler RF. Characteristics and surgical treatment of dolichoectatic and fusiform aneurysms. *J Neurosurg* 1996; **84**:185–93.

320 Drake CG, Peerless SJ. Giant fusiform intracranial aneurysms: review of 120 patients treated surgically from 1965 to 1992. *J Neurosurg* 1997; **87**:141–62.

321 Lewis SB, Chang DWJ, Peace DA, LaFrentz PJ, Day AL. Distal posterior inferior cerebellar artery aneurysms: clinical features and management. *J Neurosurg* 2002; **97**:756–66.

322 Ogilvy CS, Carter BS, Kaplan S, Rich C, Crowell RM. Temporary vessel occlusion for aneurysm surgery: Risk factors for stroke in patients protected by induced hypothermia and hypertension and intravenous mannitol administration. *J Neurosurg* 1996; **84**:785–91.

323 Piepgras DG, Khurana VG, Whisnant JP. Ruptured giant intracranial aneurysms. Part II. A retrospective analysis of timing and outcome of surgical treatment. *J Neurosurg* 1998; **88**:430–5.

324 Sinson G, Philips MF, Flamm ES. Intraoperative endovascular surgery for cerebral aneurysms. *J Neurosurg* 1996; **84**:63–70.

325 Chang HS, Fukushima T, Miyazaki S, Tamagawa T. Fusiform posterior cerebral artery aneurysm treated with excision and end-to-end anastomosis: case report. *J Neurosurg* 1986; **64**(3):501–4.

326 Brilstra EH, Rinkel GJE, Klijn CJM, van der Zwan A, Algra A, Lo RTH *et al*. Excimer laser-assisted bypass in aneurysm treatment: short-term outcomes. *J Neurosurg* 2002; **97**:1029–15.

327 Sekhar LN, Duff JM, Kalavakonda C, Olding M. Cerebral revascularization using radial artery grafts for the treatment of complex intracranial aneurysms: techniques and outcomes for 17 patients. *Neurosurgery* 2001; **49**:646–58.

328 Hamada J, Todaka T, Yano S, Kai Y, Morioka M, Ushio Y. Vertebral artery-posterior inferior cerebellar artery bypass with a superficial temporal artery graft to treat aneurysms involving the posterior inferior cerebellar artery. *J Neurosurg* 2002; **96**:867–71.

329 Derdeyn CP, Moran CJ, Cross DT, III, Sherburn EW, Dacey RG, Jr. Intracranial aneurysm: anatomic factors that predict the usefulness of intraoperative angiography. *Radiology* 1997; **205**:335–9.

330 Tang G, Cawley CM, Dion JE, Barrow DL. Intraoperative angiography during aneurysm surgery: a prospective evaluation of efficacy. *J Neurosurg* 2002; **96**:993–9.

331 Forsting M, Albert FK, Jansen O, Von Kummer R, Aschoff A, Kunze S *et al*. Coil placement after clipping: Endovascular treatment of incompletely clipped cerebral aneurysms: report of two cases. *J Neurosurg* 1996; **85**:966–9.

332 Rabinstein AA, Nichols DA. Endovascular coil embolization of cerebral aneurysm remnants after incomplete surgical obliteration. *Stroke* 2002; **33**:1809–15.

333 Kalavakonda C, Sekhar LN, Ramachandran P, Hechl P. Endoscope-assisted microsurgery for intracranial aneurysms. *Neurosurgery* 2002; **51**:1119–26.

334 Sutherland GR, Kaibara T, Wallace C, Tomanek B, Richter M. Intraoperative assessment of aneurysm clipping using magnetic resonance angiography and diffusion-weighted

imaging: technical case report. *Neurosurgery* 2002; **50**:893–7.

335 Ooka K, Shibuya M, Suzuki Y. A comparative study of intracranial aneurysm clips: Closing and opening forces and physical endurance. *Neurosurgery* 1997; **40**:318–23.

336 Lawton MT, Heiserman JE, Prendergast VC, Zabramski JM, Spetzler RF. Titanium aneurysm clips. 3. Clinical application in 16 patients with subarachnoid hemorrhage. *Neurosurgery* 1996; **38**:1170–5.

337 Ogawa A, Suzuki M, Ogasawara K. Aneurysms at nonbranching sites in the supraclinoid portion of the internal carotid artery: Internal carotid artery trunk aneurysms. *Neurosurgery* 2000; **47**:578–83.

338 Yanaka K, Meguro K, Nose T. Repair of a tear at the base of a blister-like aneurysm with suturing and an encircling clip: technical note. *Neurosurgery* 2002; **50**:218–21.

339 Pelz DM, Ferguson GG, Lownie SP, Kachur E. Combined endovascular/neurosurgical therapy of blister-like distal internal carotid aneurysms. *Can J Neurol* Sci 2003; **30**:49–53.

340 Steiger HJ, Ito S, Schmid-Elsässer R, Uhl E. M2/M2 side-to-side rescue anastomosis for accidental M2 trunk occlusion during middle cerebral artery aneurysm clipping: technical note. *Neurosurgery* 2001; **49**:743–7.

341 Baldwin ME, Macdonald RL, Huo D, Novakovia RL, Goldenberg FD, Frank JI *et al.* Early vasospasm on admission angiography in patients with aneurysmal subarachnoid hemorrhage is a predictor for in-hospital complications and poor outcome. *Stroke* 2004; **35**:2506–11.

342 Lasner TM, Weil RJ, Riina HA, King JT, Zager EL, Raps EC *et al.* Cigarette smoking-induced increase in the risk of symptomatic vasospasm after aneurysmal subarachnoid hemorrhage. *J Neurosurg* 1997; **87**:381–4.

343 Conway JE, Tamargo RJ. Cocaine use is an independent risk factor for cerebral vasospasm after aneurysmal subarachnoid hemorrhage. *Stroke* 2001; **32**:2338–43.

344 Hijdra A, van Gijn J, Nagelkerke NJ, Vermeulen M, van Crevel H. Prediction of delayed cerebral ischemia, rebleeding, and outcome after aneurysmal subarachnoid hemorrhage. *Stroke* 1988; **19**(10):1250–6.

345 Öhman J, Servo A, Heiskanen O. Risks factors for cerebral infarction in good-grade patients after aneurysmal subarachnoid hemorrhage and surgery: a prospective study. *J Neurosurg* 1991; **74**(1):14–20.

346 Qureshi AI, Sung GY, Razumovsky AY, Lane K, Straw RN, Ulatowski JA. Early identification of patients at risk for symptomatic vasospasm after aneurysmal subarachnoid hemorrhage. *Crit Care Med* 2000; **28**:984–90.

347 Friedman JA, Goerss SJ, Meyer FB, Piepgras DG, Pichelmann MA, McIver JI *et al.* Volumetric quantification of Fisher Grade 3 aneurysmal subarachnoid hemorrhage: a novel method to predict symptomatic vasospasm on admission computerized tomography scans. *J Neurosurg* 2002; **97**:401–7.

348 Friedman JA, Pichelmann MA, Piepgras DG, Atkinson JLD, Maher CO, Meyer FB *et al.* Ischemic complications of surgery for anterior choroidal artery aneurysms. *J Neurosurg* 2001; **94**:565–72.

349 Fujii Y, Takeuchi S, Sasaki O, Minakawa T, Koike T, Tanaka R. Serial changes of hemostasis in aneurysmal subarachnoid hemorrhage with special reference to delayed ischemic neurological deficits. *J Neurosurg* 1997; **86**(4):594–602.

350 Vergouwen MD, Frijns CJ, Roos YB, Rinkel GJE, Baas F, Vermeulen M. Plasminogen activator inhibitor-1 4G allele in the 4G/5G promoter polymorphism increases the occurrence of cerebral ischemia after aneurysmal subarachnoid hemorrhage. *Stroke* 2004; **35**:1280–3.

351 Chang HS, Hongo K, Nakagawa H. Adverse effects of limited hypotensive anesthesia on the outcome of patients with subarachnoid hemorrhage. *J Neurosurg* 2000; **92**:971–5.

352 Roos YBWEM, Rinkel GJE, Vermeulen M, Algra A, van Gijn J. Antifibrinolytic treatment in aneurysmal subarachnoid haemorrhage. *Cochrane Database Syst Rev* 2003; (2):CD001245.

353 Giller CA, Giller AM, Landreneau F. Detection of emboli after surgery for intracerebral aneurysms. *Neurosurgery* 1998; **42**:490–3.

354 Romano JG, Forteza AM, Concha M, Koch S, Heros RC, Morcos JJ *et al.* Detection of microemboli by transcranial Doppler ultrasonography in aneurysmal subarachnoid hemorrhage. *Neurosurgery* 2002; **50**:1026–30.

355 Dreier JP, Sakowitz OW, Harder A, Zimmer C, Dirnagl U, Valdueza JM *et al.* Focal laminar cortical MR signal abnormalities after subarachnoid hemorrhage. *Ann Neurol* 2002; **52**:825–9.

356 Lang EW, Diehl RR, Mehdorn HM. Cerebral autoregulation testing after aneurysmal subarachnoid hemorrhage: the phase relationship between arterial blood pressure and cerebral blood flow velocity. *Crit Care Med* 2001; **29**:158–63.

357 Khaldi A, Zauner A, Reinert M, Woodward JJ, Bullock MR. Measurement of nitric oxide and brain tissue oxygen tension in patients after severe subarachnoid hemorrhage. *Neurosurgery* 2001; **49**:33–8.

358 Sobey CG, Faraci FM. Subarachnoid haemorrhage: What happens to the cerebral arteries? *Clin Exp Pharmacol Physiol* 1998; **25**:867–76.

359 Fassbender K, Hodapp B, Rossol S, Bertsch T, Schmeck J, Schütt S *et al.* Endothelin-1 in subarachnoid hemorrhage: an acute-phase reactant produced by cerebrospinal fluid leukocytes. *Stroke* 2000; **31**:2971–5.

360 Juvela S. Plasma endothelin concentrations after aneurysmal subarachnoid hemorrhage. *J Neurosurg* 2000; **92**:390–400.

361 Mascia L, Fedorko L, Stewart DJ, Mohamed F, Terbrugge K, Ranieri VM *et al.* Temporal relationship between endothelin-1 concentrations and cerebral vasospasm in patients with aneurysmal subarachnoid hemorrhage. *Stroke* 2001; **32**:1185–9.

362 Juvela S. Plasma endothelin and big endothelin concentrations and serum endothelin-converting enzyme activity following aneurysmal subarachnoid hemorrhage. *J Neurosurg* 2002; **97**:1287–93.

363 Kamezaki T, Yanaka K, Nagase S, Fujita K, Kato N, Nose T. Increased levels of lipid peroxides as predictive of symptomatic vasospasm and poor outcome after aneurysmal subarachnoid hemorrhage. *J Neurosurg* 2002; **97**:1302–5.

364 Pilitsis JG, Coplin WM, O'Regan MH, Wellwood JM, Diaz FG, Fairfax MR *et al.* Free fatty acids in human cerebrospinal fluid following subarachnoid hemorrhage and their potential role in vasospasm: a preliminary observation. *J Neurosurg* 2002; **97**:272–9.

365 Mack WJ, Mocco J, Hoh DJ, Huang J, Choudhri TF, Kreiter KT *et al.* Outcome prediction with serum intercellular adhesion molecule-1 levels after aneurysmal subarachnoid hemorrhage. *J Neurosurg* 2002; **96**:71–5.

366 Mocco J, Mack WJ, Kim GH, Lozier AP, Laufer I, Kreiter KT *et al.* Rise in serum soluble intercellular adhesion molecule-1 levels with vasospasm following aneurysmal subarachnoid hemorrhage. *J Neurosurg* 2002; **97**:537–41.

367 Nissen JJ, Mantle D, Gregson B, Mendelow AD. Serum concentration of adhesion molecules in patients with delayed ischaemic neurological deficit after aneurysmal subarachnoid haemorrhage: the immunoglobulin and selectin superfamilies. *J Neurol Neurosurg Psychiatry* 2001; **71**:329–33.

368 Frijns CJM, Kasius KM, Algra A, Fijnheer R, Rinkel GJE. Endothelial cell activation markers and delayed cerebral ischaemia in subarachnoid haemorrhage. *J Neurol Neurosurg Psychiatry* 2006; **77**:863–7.

369 Polin RS, Bavbek M, Shaffrey ME, Billups K, Bogaev CA, Kassell NF *et al.* Detection of soluble E-selectin, ICAM-1, VCAM-1, and L-selectin in the cerebrospinal fluid of patients after subarachnoid hemorrhage. *J Neurosurg* 1998; **89**:559–67.

370 McGirt MJ, Lynch JR, Blessing R, Warner DS, Friedman AH, Laskowitz DT. Serum von Willebrand factor, matrix metalloproteinase-9, and vascular endothelial growth factor levels predict the onset of cerebral vasospasm after aneurysmal subarachnoid hemorrhage. *Neurosurgery* 2002; **51**:1128–34.

371 Frijns CJ, Fijnheer R, Algra A, van Mourik JA, van Gijn J, Rinkel GJ. Early circulating levels of endothelial cell activation markers in aneurysmal subarachnoid haemorrhage: associations with cerebral ischaemic events and outcome. *J Neurol Neurosurg Psychiatry* 2006; **77**:77–83.

372 Peltonen S, Juvela S, Kaste M, Lassila R. Hemostasis and fibrinolysis activation after subarachnoid hemorrhage. *J Neurosurg* 1997; **87**:207–14.

373 Ikeda K, Asakura H, Futami K, Yamashita J. Coagulative and fibrinolytic activation in cerebrospinal fluid and plasma after subarachnoid hemorrhage. *Neurosurgery* 1997; **41**:344–9.

374 Gaetani P, Tartara F, Pignatti P, Tancioni F, Baena RRY, De Benedetti F. Cisternal CSF levels of cytokines after subarachnoid hemorrhage. *Neurol Res* 1998; **20**:337–42.

375 Fassbender K, Hodapp B, Rossol S, Bertsch T, Schmeck J, Schütt S *et al.* Inflammatory cytokines in subarachnoid haemorrhage: association with abnormal blood flow velocities in basal cerebral arteries. *J Neurol Neurosurg Psychiatry* 2001; **70**:534–7.

376 Sviri GE, Feinsod M, Soustiel JF. Brain natriuretic peptide and cerebral vasospasm in subarachnoid hemorrhage: clinical and TCD correlations. *Stroke* 2000; **31**:118–22.

377 Takenaka KV, Sakai N, Murase S, Kuroda T, Okumura A, Sawada M. Elevated transferrin concentration in cerebral spinal fluid after subarachnoid hemorrhage. *Neurol Res* 2000; **22**:797–801.

378 Wijdicks EFM, Heublein DM, Burnett JC, Jr. Increase and uncoupling of adrenomedullin from the natriuretic peptide system in aneurysmal subarachnoid hemorrhage. *J Neurosurg* 2001; **94**:252–6.

379 Hoffman WE, Wheeler P, Edelman G, Charbel FT, Torres NJ, Ausman JI. Hypoxic brain tissue following subarachnoid hemorrhage. *Anesthesiology* 2000; **92**:442–6.

380 Kett-White R, Hutchinson PJ, Al Rawi PG, Gupta AK, Pickard JD, Kirkpatrick PJ. Adverse cerebral events detected after subarachnoid hemorrhage using brain oxygen and microdialysis probes. *Neurosurgery* 2002; **50**:1213–21.

381 Schulz MK, Wang LP, Tange M, Bjerre P. Cerebral microdialysis monitoring: determination of normal and ischemic cerebral metabolisms in patients with aneurysmal subarachnoid hemorrhage. *J Neurosurg* 2000; **93**:808–14.

382 Staub F, Graf R, Gabel P, Köchling M, Klug N, Heiss WD. Multiple interstitial substances measured by microdialysis in patients with subarachnoid hemorrhage. *Neurosurgery* 2000; **47**:1106–14.

383 Vermeulen M, van Gijn J, Hijdra A, van Crevel H. Causes of acute deterioration in patients with a ruptured intracranial aneurysm: a prospective study with serial CT scanning. *J Neurosurg* 1984; **60**(5):935–9.

15 Specific interventions to prevent intracranial haemorrhage

15.1 Introduction

This chapter will deal with patients who have not yet had a stroke but who do have a vascular lesion that might give rise to a stroke in the future, mostly unruptured intracranial aneurysms or arteriovenous malformations (AVMs). Sometimes these lesions warrant preventive intervention, but in many situations uncertainty abounds,[1] and in many other situations intervention will probably do more harm than good.[2] A general point to be made about the management of these lesions is that there is no hurry. Most of these patients are in perfect health and it is important to carefully balance the risks and benefits of all treatment options and to take time to counsel the 'patient'. *Primum non nocere* is a pivotal guideline when a lesion is found by chance, or as the result of an 'excludogram' in patients with innocuous types of headache or dizziness, or – even worse – as the result of whole-body MR scans for personal health checks. Doing no harm also includes refraining from descriptions of these lesions as 'a time bomb in your head' before referring the unfortunate patient to a neuro-interventional centre. For many of these patients no intervention is the best option, but having to live with an untreated aneurysm or AVM imposes a threat on quality of life, of which anxiety is an important component and may need managing in its own right.[3] Careful counselling and weighing the pros and cons is even more important when screening for aneurysms or AVMs is considered. Screenees often have unrealistic risk perceptions,[4] and screening for intracranial aneurysms is associated with considerable psychosocial effects, both positive and negative.[5]

> Incidentally found aneurysms or arteriovenous malformations can give rise to subarachnoid or intracerebral haemorrhage, but in many situations preventive treatment will either do more harm than good, or is of uncertain benefit.

Other intracranial vascular malformations such as cavernous malformations (section 8.2.5), cranial dural arteriovenous fistulae (section 8.2.8.), and venous angiomas (section 8.2.6) are not discussed in this chapter. Their management is seldom guided by their risk of causing a stroke (section 13.3.8). And abnormalities such as venous angiomas are better left untreated, in part because they have an important function in venous drainage.

15.2 Saccular intracranial aneurysms

15.2.1 Prevalence of aneurysms

Intracranial saccular aneurysms are almost never found in neonates, and they are rare in children (section 9.1.1). Their frequency in the general adult population depends on the definition of their size and the diligence with which the search for unruptured aneurysms has been performed. In our systematic overview of studies reporting the prevalence of intracranial aneurysms in patients

Stroke: practical management, 3rd edition. C. Warlow, J. van Gijn, M. Dennis, J. Wardlaw, J. Bamford, G. Hankey, P. Sandercock, G. Rinkel, P. Langhorne, C. Sudlow and P. Rothwell. Published 2008 Blackwell Publishing. ISBN 978-1-4051-2766-0.

Frequency	%	(95% CI)
Retrospective autopsy studies	0.4	(0.4–0.5)
Prospective autopsy studies	3.6	(3.1–4.1)
Retrospective angiography studies	3.7	(3.0–4.4)
Prospective angiography studies	6.0	(5.3–6.8)
Age	%	
< 20	0.01	(0.00–0.03)
20–39	1.3	(0.8–2.1)
40–59	1.8	(1.4–2.2)
60–80	2.3	(1.9–2.6)
> 80	2.1	(1.5–3.0)
Adult without risk factors	2.3	(1.7–3.1)
Risk factors	*Relative risk*	*(95% CI)*
Women	1.3	(0.9–2.0)
Atherosclerotic diseases	2.3	(1.7–3.1)
One or more affected relatives	4.0	(2.7–6.0)
Autosomal dominant polycystic kidney disease	4.4	(2.7–7.3)
Sizes of aneurysms	%	
< 6 mm	72	(68–77)
6–10 mm	21	(17–25)
11–20 mm	6	(4–10)
> 20 mm	2	(0.1–3)
Sites of aneurysms	%	*(95% CI)*
Anterior communicating artery	24	(20–27)
Middle cerebral artery	30	(26–34)
Internal carotid artery	42	(37–46)
Posterior circulation	10	(7.7–13)

Table 15.1 Prevalence of, risk factors for, and site of unruptured intracranial aneurysms.[6]

studied for reasons other than subarachnoid haemorrhage (SAH), 23 studies were identified, totalling 56 304 patients.[6] The prevalence was lowest in retrospective autopsy studies and highest in prospective angiography studies (Table 15.1). The angiography studies were somewhat biased towards overestimation, because in around 15% of the patients the indication was a planned operation for a suspected pituitary tumour, polycystic kidney disease or a family history of SAH, conditions in which the frequency of aneurysms is higher than average. For adults without specific risk factors for aneurysms, the prevalence was 2.3% (95% CI 1.7–3.1%); most of the aneurysms were small and located in the anterior circulation. In the general population, the prevalence of *known* aneurysms in Olmsted County, Minnesota, was estimated at 0.83%,[7] which implies that even in that highly investigated region only about one out of four aneurysms is detected.

The prevalence of aneurysms is higher in women than in men and tends to increase with increasing age; other risk factors are the presence of carotid artery stenosis or ischaemic heart disease (not unexpected because these conditions share common risk factors with aneurysms such as smoking, hypertension and excessive use of alcohol (section 9.1.1), having one or more affected relatives with SAH, autosomal dominant polycystic kidney disease (ADPKD), and a previous episode of SAH.

> Around 2% of the adult population have one or more intracranial aneurysms. Most are very small and located in the anterior circulation. The risk of having an intracranial aneurysm is higher in women, in people with a family history of intracranial aneurysms, and in patients with autosomal dominant polycystic kidney disease or a history of aneurysmal subarachnoid haemorrhage.

Family history

The chance of having an aneurysm and the lifetime risk of subarachnoid haemorrhage depend on the number of affected first-degree relatives, defined as parents, siblings and children (Table 15.2).[6,8] The lifetime risk of SAH in individuals with two or more affected first-degree relatives is unknown because there are so few families with this history, and because members of these families tend to seek screening for aneurysms and treatment of those detected. The chance of an aneurysm depends not only on the number of affected relatives but also on the nature of the relationship. If the affected relatives are

Table 15.2 Risk of having an aneurysm, and lifetime risk of subarachnoid haemorrhage, according to the number of affected first-degree relatives.

Number affected first-degree relatives	Risk of aneurysm % (95% CI)	Risk of subarachnoid haemorrhage % (95% CI)
None	2.3 (1.7–3.1)	0.6 (0.6–0.7)
1	4.0 (2.6–5.8)	3.3 (1.0–11)
2 or more	8.0 (3.9–14)	No data

siblings, the risk of having an aneurysm is higher than if they are parents or children.[6,8,9] No other characteristics of the patient who presents for screening or their relatives have been identified that affect the risk of an aneurysm. After negative screening, new aneurysms may develop. People with two or more affected relatives and with normal magnetic resonance angiography have a 7% risk of developing an aneurysm within 5 years of screening.[10]

Aneurysms are more commonly large and multiple in familial than in sporadic SAH.[11] However, because only 10% of cases of SAH are associated with a family history, large and multiple aneurysms are actually more commonly seen in sporadic than in familial SAH. Patients with familial SAH tend to be younger than sporadic cases, and in families with two generations affected the age at onset is earlier in the later than the previous generation.[12–14]

Autosomal dominant polycystic kidney disease

SAH from a ruptured aneurysm is common in patients with autosomal dominant polycystic kidney disease (ADPKD),[15] and causes a large proportion of deaths in these patients (section 9.1.1). In a series of 101 autopsies, of which 89 included assessment of the brain, 17 had had a recent SAH from a ruptured aneurysm.[16] Although selection bias may have occurred, the proportion of deaths from ruptured aneurysms was much higher than in the general population.[6] There are some differences in the features of aneurysms between patients with and without ADPKD:

- The most common site of aneurysm in ADPKD patients is the middle cerebral artery, whereas it is the internal carotid artery in the general population.[6,17]
- Aneurysms in ADPKD patients are more often larger than 10 mm (in 25%) than in patients without ADPKD (in 10%).[17]
- A positive family history, defined as a first-degree or second-degree relative with SAH or intracranial aneurysm, is found in 40% of ADPKD compared with 10% of those without ADPKD.[8]

In ADPKD patients, the large proportion of aneurysms of the middle cerebral artery, the large proportion of large aneurysms and the younger age at onset of SAH[17] more closely matches patients with familial than sporadic SAH.[11,12]

Intracranial aneurysms are found in about 10% of patients with ADPKD.[6] But apart from a family history for SAH, no clinical characteristics have been identified that increase the risk of aneurysm in these patients.[18] Although the position of the mutation in *PKD1* is predictive of development of intracranial aneurysms,[19] currently this mutation detection is not yet available in clinical practice. Aneurysms commonly develop in these patients in the absence of hypertension,[17,20] which indicates that blood pressure is not an essential factor in the development of their aneurysms. Patients with ADPKD are at risk of new episodes of SAH from newly developed aneurysms,[21] but at present there are no precise estimates of this risk. Only three studies, each with no more than 20 patients and with various periods of follow-up, have been published thus far. The risk of aneurysm development ranged from 1 in 17 patients (6%) after 7 years to 5 of 20 patients (25%) after 15 years.[22–24] The size of the newly developed aneurysms ranged from 2 to 7 mm.

Development of new aneurysms

The continuing development of aneurysms during life and the presence of multiple aneurysms in up to 30% of patients with SAH suggest that patients who have been successfully treated for one aneurysm are at risk of developing another one. A few series have reported on the risk of developing recurrent (at the same site as the previously clipped aneurysm) or de novo (at another site) aneurysm. This risk of finding a new aneurysm increases, not unexpectedly, with the increasing interval after the initial SAH from around 2% after 4 years, to 10% after 10 years, to more than 15% after 15 years.[25–29] Around 20% of the newly found aneurysms are located at the site of the original aneurysm, and the other 80% at other sites (Figs 15.1 and 15.2). Approximately one-third of the detected aneurysms are truly de novo, the remaining two-thirds were in fact already visible in retrospect.[29] Risk factors for de novo aneurysm formation are multiple aneurysms at the time of the SAH (Hazard ratio (HR) 3.2; 95% CI 1.2–8.6), current smoking (HR 3.8; 95% CI 1.5–9.4) and hypertension (HR 2.3; 95% CI 1.1–4.9).[27,28] All this suggests that having one or more intracranial aneurysms should not be considered as a single event but

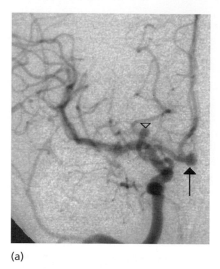
(a)

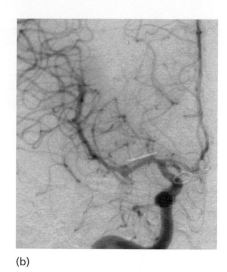
(b)

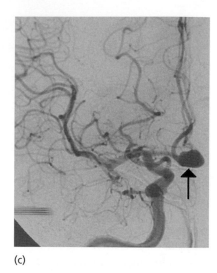
(c)

Fig. 15.1 Regrowth of an aneurysm at the site of the initial aneurysm. (a) Preoperative catheter angiogram from 1992 of a patient with a subarachnoid haemorrhage, presumably from the anterior communicating artery aneurysm (*arrow*). There is an additional aneurysm distal on the posterior communicating artery (*arrowhead*). (b) Postoperative angiogram from 1992 showing complete obliteration of both aneurysms by clips. (c) Angiogram from 2003 showing regrowth of the aneurysm on the anterior communicating artery (*arrow*). (Adapted from Werner *et al.*[29] with permission from Oxford Journals.)

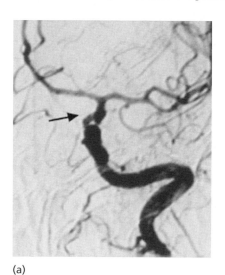
(a)

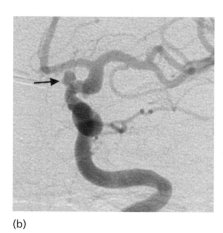
(b)

Fig. 15.2 Development of a new aneurysm at a different site from the initial aneurysm. (a) Preoperative catheter angiogram from 1993 of the left carotid artery of a patient with a subarachnoid haemorrhage from a ruptured aneurysm of the anterior communicating artery (not shown). There is no aneurysm on the carotid artery (*arrow*). (b) Angiogram from 2001 showing a new aneurysm on the left carotid artery (*arrow*). (Reproduced with permission from Werner *et al.*[10] © 2003 *Stroke.*)

rather as a continuous process – aneurysms can and do develop de novo, and they grow.

In addition to recurrent or de novo aneurysms, patients who have survived an SAH may have had additional aneurysms that were small and therefore missed during angiography, or were thought to be too small to be harmful and therefore left untreated. These aneurysms can grow, which increases the risk of rupture. The enlargement increases with longer periods of follow-up from 25% after 9 years to 45% after 19 years.[28,29]

These new and enlarged aneurysms clearly put patients who have survived an SAH at some increased risk

of another SAH. The risk estimates vary between 3% in 10 years to 9% in 20 years after successful clipping of a ruptured aneurysm.[30,31] In the first 10 years after SAH the incidence of SAH is about 20 times higher than the risk in an age- and sex-matched cohort in the general population (section 14.10.2).[31] These estimates include all causes of SAH, including re-rupture of the initially treated aneurysm. Since endovascular-treated aneurysms have a higher risk of re-rupture at least in the initial year after the SAH,[32] patients with endovascular-treated aneurysms probably have an even higher risk of recurrent SAH than the estimates given here, but precise estimates are not available yet.

Intracranial aneurysms are not congenital lesions, but develop during life. Patients who have survived an episode of subarachnoid haemorrhage are at risk of having a new episode from new aneurysms, from already existing but enlarging aneurysms, and from recurrence of the treated aneurysm.

15.2.2 Risk of rupture of unruptured intracranial aneurysms

In our systematic review of all the follow-up studies on the risk of SAH from unruptured aneurysms between 1965 and 1995, the overall risk of rupture was 1.9% per annum.[6] The absolute risk for aneurysms equal to or less than 10 mm diameter (i.e. the most common type) was 0.7% per annum. Subsequent to this systematic overview, the first report from the International Study of Unruptured Intracranial Aneurysms (ISUIA) study group was published, in which a retrospective cohort of 1449 patients with 1937 intracranial aneurysms greater than 2 mm diameter had been followed up for an average of 8.3 years.[33] Half the patients had one or more incidental aneurysms (no history of SAH from a different aneurysm), the other half had an aneurysm additional to a ruptured aneurysm that had been successfully repaired. In the former group, the cumulative rate of rupture of aneurysms that were less than 10 mm in diameter at diagnosis was less than 0.05% per year; in the latter group, it was approximately 10 times higher (0.5% per year). The size and location of the aneurysm were independent predictors of rupture: the relative risk was 11.6 for aneurysms greater than 10 mm, 13.7 for posterior circulation aneurysms and 8.0 for posterior communicating artery aneurysms. Of course, the retrospective design used for case finding in this study may have led to important sources of bias. For example, the risk of rupture may have been underestimated because one inclusion criterion was a complete set of angiograms being available, and yet it is conceivable that the films of patients who had died in the meantime, e.g. from aneurysmal rupture, may have been removed from the hospital records.

The later report from the ISUIA study group describes the largest ever *prospectively* studied cohort of patients with unruptured aneurysms, 1692 patients of whom 1077 had incidental aneurysms and 615 additional aneurysms.[2] The period of follow-up was relatively short, a mean of 4.1 years, during which 534 patients (32%) in the intention-not-to-treat arm nevertheless had their aneurysm occluded, and another 193 (11%) died for reasons other than aneurysmal rupture. This case fatality is rather high, which suggests that in many patients the decision to withhold treatment was based on patient characteristics (e.g. reduced life expectancy) rather than aneurysm characteristics. The risk of rupture for the remaining patients was presented as 5 years cumulative risks (Table 15.3), and not as mean rupture rates per year, which is a strength of the paper.

However, despite the merits of being the largest prospective study on risk of rupture of unruptured intracranial aneurysms, the ISUIA report has several important weaknesses:

- First, the dichotomy for small vs large aneurysms was set at 7 mm and not at 10 mm as in previous reports from this group, but this dichotomy was not pre-specified in the study protocol.
- Second, aneurysms of the posterior communicating artery were included with posterior circulation aneurysms and not with anterior circulation aneurysms. This classification of posterior communicating aneurysms (which arise from the internal carotid artery and are therefore technically on the anterior circulation) is different from all other studies, and again was not pre-specified in the study protocol. Subsequently this approach has been criticized by a review of 11 papers (including the two ISUIA reports) that contained sufficient data to calculate rupture rates for anatomical subgroups;[34] bleeding rates for aneurysms of the posterior communicating artery (0.46% per year) were

Table 15.3 Five-year cumulative risk of rupture of an unruptured intracranial aneurysm according to the prospective ISUIA report.[2]

Size	ACA/MCA/ICA	Post communicating/ post circulation
< 7 mm no previous SAH	0% (95% CI unknown)	2.5% (95% CI unknown)
< 7 mm but previous SAH	1.5% (95% CI unknown)	3.4% (95% CI unknown)
7–12 mm	2.6% (95% CI unknown)	14.5% (95% CI unknown)
13–24 mm	14.5% (95% CI unknown)	18.4% (95% CI unknown)
> 24 mm	40% (95% CI unknown)	50% (95% CI unknown)

SAH, subarachnoid haemorrhage; ACA, anterior cerebral artery (includes anterior communicating artery); MCA, middle cerebral artery; ICA, internal carotid artery.

similar to those of aneurysms on the remaining sites on the anterior circulation (0.49% per year) but much lower than those for aneurysms of the posterior circulation (1.8% per year).

- A third criticism is that only 51 aneurysms ruptured during follow-up which precludes a sound analysis of risk factors for rupture.
- Fourth, the confidence intervals are not given, and cannot be calculated from the data presented in the paper, probably they are very wide for lack of numbers. For example for patients with aneurysms < 7 mm on the anterior circulation the number at risk decreased from 535 at 1 year of follow-up to only 35 at 6 years.

The uncertainty around the estimates is one reason why longer follow-up of these patients is crucial. The second reason is that real data on 5 or 10 years and preferably even longer periods of follow-up are likely to be more accurate than extrapolations of risks from short-term follow-up into yearly risks of rupture that are considered to be constant during the remaining life expectancy of patients. Existing decision models on aneurysm management (implicitly) incorporate a constant, time-independent risk of rupture. It is however likely that aneurysms exhibit fast growth in short periods of time,[35,36] and that the risk of rupture is confined to these episodes. It is therefore over-simplistic to calculate a mean rupture rate per annum from the observed but short period of follow-up and extrapolate that rupture rate to the remaining life expectancy. Very long-term follow-up in patients with unruptured aneurysms is essential before firm conclusions can be made. This long-term follow-up can also take into account the risk of SAH from newly developed aneurysms.[37] Patients of course are more interested in the risk of rupture in the following 20 or 30 years than in the next 5 years alone. Happily the ISUIA investigators are now continuing their follow-up.

In the 2007 update of our systematic review of follow-up studies on the risk of SAH from unruptured aneurysms we included 19 studies with a total of 4705 patients.[38] The overall risk of rupture of untreated aneurysms in the studies with a mean follow-up < 5 years was 1.2% (95% CI 1.0–1.5), in those with a mean follow-up between 5 and 10 years 0.6% (0.5–0.7%) and in the studies with a mean follow-up of greater than 10 years 1.3% (0.9–1.8%) per patient-year. The lack of an increase in risk of rupture with increasing duration of follow-up might be explained by the different study populations have inherently different risks of rupture. Pooled analysis of individual data, taking also into account risk factors other than duration of follow-up, are needed to better estimate the relation between duration of follow-up and risk of rupture. Patient characteristics that had in univariable analysis a statistically significant association with an increased risk of rupture were age > 60, female gender and Japanese or Finnish descent (Table 15.4). In addition, although smoking increased the risk of rupture, this was not statistically significant. There were not enough data to evaluate the effects of excessive alcohol use or a family history of SAH. Circumstantial evidence, however, suggests that aneurysms in patients with a

Variable	Patient years of follow-up	No. with subarachnoid haemorrhage	Relative risk (95% CI)
Age			
< 20 years	—	—	—
20–29 years	848	12	(0.5–2.2)
40–59 years	1830	24	1.0
60–79 years	709	19	2.0 (1.1–3.7)
> 80 years	12	0	—
Gender			
Men	2255	32	1.0
Women	2885	65	1.6 (1.1–2.4)
Hypertension			
No	2357	35	1.0
Yes	572	9	1.1 (0.5–2.2)
Smoking			
No	1404	13	1.0
Yes	1304	20	1.7 (0.8–3.3)
Population			
Non-Japanese/Finnish	20422	111	1.0
Japanese or Finnish	6093	113	3.4 (2.6–4.4)

Relative risk of 1.0 indicates the reference category.

Table 15.4 Relative risk of rupture of an unruptured intracranial aneurysm according to patient characteristics.[38]

Table 15.5 Relative risk of rupture of an unruptured intracranial aneurysm according to aneurysm characteristics.[38]

Variable	Patient years of follow-up	No. with subarachnoid haemorrhage	Relative risk (95% CI)
Site of aneurysm			
ACA	1083	19	1.4 (0.8–2.3)
ICA*	3558	46	1.0
MCA	2734	33	0.9 (0.6–1.5)
Posterior circulation**	791	26	2.5 (1.6–4.1)
Cavernous sinus	2159	2	0.1 (0–0.3)
Size of aneurysm			
< 5 mm	1939	10	1.0
5–10 mm	1187	14	2.3 (1.0–5.2)
> 10 mm	3670	55	2.9 (1.5–5.7)
> 12 mm	1089	42	7.5 (3.8–14.9)
giant (>15 mm)	293	18	11.9 (5.5–25.8)
Type of aneurysm			
Incidental	3315	50	1.0
Additional	3158	46	1.0 (0.7–1.4)
Symptomatic	472	31	4.4 (2.8–6.8)

*includes posterior communicating artery; **posterior circulation = vertebral artery, basilar artery and posterior cerebral artery; ACA, anterior cerebral artery (includes anterior communicating artery); ICA, internal carotid artery; MCA, middle cerebral artery.

Relative risk of 1.0 indicates the reference category.

family history of SAH are at higher risk of rupture; individuals with one affected relative carry a 5.5-fold greater lifetime risk for SAH than the general population (Table 15.2). Nevertheless, the chance of finding an aneurysm by screening an individual with one affected relative is only 1.7 times higher than the general population. A possible explanation is that familial intracranial aneurysms have a higher risk of rupture. An alternative explanation is that individuals with a family history of SAH are more likely to develop a new aneurysm than those without.

Aneurysm characteristics that were related to an increased risk of rupture were site at the posterior circulation, size > 5 mm and symptoms caused by the aneurysm other than SAH (Table 15.5). We could not confirm a higher risk of rupture in additional compared with incidental aneurysms but this should not be considered as proof of absence of a difference. A potential explanation is that the additional aneurysms were smaller than the incidental aneurysms; a higher risk for additional aneurysms may therefore have been masked by their smaller size with inherently lower rupture risk.

The published data from the parent papers did not allow any multivariable analysis. Thus, we could not assess the independent contribution of patient and aneurysm characteristics to the risk of aneurysm rupture. After all, it is likely that some of the characteristics are not independent, for example although we found high rate ratios for both large and for symptomatic aneurysms, it is unlikely that these factors are independent because larger aneurysms have a greater tendency to cause compression problems than smaller ones. Due to this lack of multivariable analyses, there is still considerable uncertainty for the calculation of aneurysmal rupture risk in an individual. Pooled analysis of individual data are needed to identify independent risk factors for aneurysm rupture, and follow-up time should be taken into account since the growth of aneurysms is probably not constant over time. Only then will we have more reliable risk estimates for individual patients.

> Small aneurysms are less likely to rupture than large aneurysms. Other risk factors for rupture are age, female gender and the site of the aneurysm. However, there are still many uncertainties about the absolute risks of rupture, especially for periods longer than 5 years after detection of the aneurysm.

The importance of aneurysm size for the risk of rupture puzzles many physicians and surgeons, because most ruptured aneurysms they encounter in clinical practice are smaller than 10 mm, or even smaller than 5 mm.[39,40] The most likely explanation for this paradox is that the vast majority of aneurysms are small, and that even a minute fraction of those that do rupture will still outnumber a large proportion of the much smaller group of patients with larger aneurysms that rupture (in the same way as most children with Down syndrome are born to young mothers, even though the risk increases with age). This 'prevention paradox' means that screening the population for people at highest risk (large aneurysms) will do little to change the burden of the disease (i.e. ruptured aneurysms) because most patients who actually have an SAH have ruptured a small aneurysm.[41]

15.2.3 Treatment options

Neurosurgical clipping and endovascular coiling are not without risks. Those of neurosurgical clipping have been studied most intensively, because this treatment has been available the longest.

Neurosurgical clipping

A systematic review of studies on complications of neurosurgical clipping for unruptured aneurysms published between 1966 and 1996 included 61 studies, on 2460 patients, with at least 2568 aneurysms.[42] Of these aneurysms one-quarter were larger than 25 mm and one-third located on the posterior circulation, which implies a bias towards 'dangerous' and 'difficult-to-treat' aneurysms. Overall case fatality was 2.6% (95% CI 2.0–3.3%); permanent morbidity occurred in another 10.9% (95% CI 9.6–12.2%). Postoperative mortality and morbidity were significantly lower in more recent years, for non-giant aneurysms and for aneurysms on the anterior circulation.

The most recent report of the ISUIA investigators included 1917 prospectively identified patients who underwent neurosurgical clipping of an unruptured aneurysm.[2] Poor outcome from surgical treatment was defined as death or a Rankin score of 3, 4 or 5 (indicating dependence in the sense that help was required for activities of daily living), a score less than 24 on the mini-mental state examination, or a score less than 27 on a telephone interview for cognitive status (both indicating a serious cognitive abnormality). The proportion of patients with a poor outcome ranged between 5% and 40% according to their age and site and size of the aneurysm (Table 15.6). Of note is that both the review and the ISUIA report describe the data from many centres in many countries, with unspecified but probably varying degrees of treatment team expertise. Reports from single centres with a lot of experience describe complication rates as low as 2% in patients with aneurysms smaller than 10 mm,[43–45] but assessment

of outcome in these studies was less rigorous than in the ISUIA study. Nevertheless, the experience of the neurosurgeon seems to be an important factor in the risk of complications.[44,46]

Endovascular coiling

A systematic review of success and complications of occlusion by means of coils included 30 studies with 1379 patients published before 2003.[47] The overall case fatality was 0.6% (95% CI 0.2–1%) and the permanent morbidity was 7% (95% CI 5.3–8.7%). The bleeding risk of treated aneurysms was 0.9% per year (95% CI 0.4–1.4%), but rebleeding occurred only in incompletely coiled aneurysms larger than 10 mm. For the subset of patients with aneurysms larger than 10 mm the bleeding risk was 3.5% per year (95% CI 0.8–6.2%). Unfortunately, most of the studies included in the review were weak, so weak that the pre-specified subgroup analysis of good quality studies could not be performed because none of the included studies satisfied the predefined criteria for high quality. An important and promising observation was that the complication rate was significantly lower in recent studies compared with the older studies.

Data from the ISUIA investigators were published after the inclusion period of the systematic review, but are comparable (Table 15.6).[2] An advantage of the ISUIA report over the systematic review is that the ISUIA investigators were able to assess complication rates according to site and size of the aneurysms, and the age of the patients. As was the case with neurosurgical clipping, the risk of complications increased with increasing size of aneurysm. A difference compared with clipping is that while the risk of complications rises considerably after the age of 50 for clipping it remains stable for coiling. Only after the age of 70 does the complication rate increase for coiling.[2]

Similar to neurosurgical clipping, the systematic review and the ISUIA report describe data from many centres in many countries, with varying degrees of expertise in treatment, whereas single-centre reports describe lower complication rates. For example, an observational study from the Netherlands reported on 48 patients with 58 incidental aneurysms and no previous SAH; the case fatality was zero and morbidity was 2%, even though half the aneurysms were larger than 10 mm.[48] However, such single-centre reports are subject to several sources of bias, and are likely to give an underestimate of the actual complication risks.[49,50] Interestingly, as well as clinically obvious complications, almost half the patients develop new lesions on MR imaging during endovascular treatment of aneurysms.[51]

Table 15.6 Risk of complications (%) of treatment of unruptured intracranial aneurysms according to site and size of the aneurysm and age of the patient in the prospective ISUIA 2003 report.[2]

Site, size, age	Surgical clipping (n = 1917)		Endovascular coiling (n = 451)	
	%	(95% CI)	%	(95% CI)
Anterior / < 50 yrs				
< 13 mm	5.7	(4.3–7.1)	7.1	(0.1–15)
13–24 mm	4.3	(0.1–8.6)	4.6	(0.1–15)
> 24 mm	23	(2–42)	15	(0.1–44)
Anterior / > 50 yrs				
< 13 mm	11	(7.9–14)	6.3	(1.3–11)
13–24 mm	24	(18–30)	8.3	(2.1–15)
> 24 mm	31	(19–43)	13	(1.3–25)
Posterior / < 50 yrs				
< 13 mm	11	(1.6–20)	11	(0.1–28)
13–24 mm	29	(4.7–53)	17	(0.1–57)
> 24 mm	44	(unknown)*	no data	
Posterior / > 50 yrs				
< 13 mm	12	(3.2–21)	7.9	(0.1–19)
13–24 mm	43		23	(5.5–41)
> 24 mm	no data	(unknown)*	40	(unknown)*

*The confidence intervals are recalculated from bars in a figure; for this confidence interval the bar extended to the upper limit of the figure.

There are no *randomized* comparisons between clipping and coiling for unruptured aneurysms. An indirect prospective comparison between only 19 patients treated by coiling and 32 treated by clipping revealed that in the short term, operation of patients with an unruptured aneurysm had a considerable impact on their functional health and quality of life. After 1 year, improvement had occurred but recovery was incomplete.[52] Coiling did not affect functional health and quality of life, but one of the patients treated by coiling had a haemorrhage from the coiled aneurysm during follow-up. In a retrospective cohort study from the USA using inpatient data from 1996 to 2000, no difference between clipping and coiling was found for case fatality and discharge to long-term care.[53] On the basis of a four-level discharge status outcome scale, coiled patients had a significantly better discharge disposition. Moreover, length of stay was longer and charges were higher for clipped than for coiled patients. In another study from the US of patients who were in retrospect eligible for both clipping and coiling, those who had actually been treated by clipping had a longer stay in hospital, more often were dependent on help for activities of daily living, and more often reported persistent new symptoms or disability after treatment.[54] Thus, for patients with unruptured aneurysms, coiling seems to be associated with fewer complications than clipping. Because long-term follow-up data are not yet available, it is not known if these two treatments prevent SAH to the same extent.

> Neurosurgical clipping and endovascular coiling of unruptured aneurysms both carry a definite risk of death or permanent disability, even for small aneurysms. The risk increases for larger aneurysms and with increasing age, although the risk starts to increase at an earlier age for clipping than for coiling. Indirect comparisons suggest that the impact on health is less severe for coiling than for clipping, especially in the short term.

15.2.4 Management of patients with unruptured aneurysms

Every time a cerebral aneurysm is a surprise finding on an imaging study performed for another purpose, there is a practical dilemma: is the risk of preventive clipping or coiling of the aneurysm at that time outweighed by the risk of death or disability from rupture of the untreated aneurysm at some time later in life, if it ruptures at all? Two pivotal factors in this balance of risks are the size and site of the aneurysm, but these factors are not necessarily helpful because both the risk of rupture and the risk of treatment complications are greater for large aneurysms and for aneurysms on the posterior circulation. Age is the most discriminating factor, because at a young age the benefit of treatment – which is long term – is large, provided life expectancy is not reduced for other reasons, and the risk of treatment relatively small. With increasing age, the benefit decreases (because life expectancy decreases) while the risk of complications of preventive treatment increases. Further factors that should be taken into account are the type of aneurysm (incidental, additional or symptomatic; section 15.2.2), family history and comorbidity.

Patients with a positive family history may have an increased risk of rupture, but definitely have a different risk perception than someone with no experience of an SAH in their family. If someone has already lost one or more relatives from SAH (in most instances from rupture of a small aneurysm) it will be very difficult for him or her to accept that their own aneurysm has a negligible risk of rupture, even if it is small.

Comorbidity reduces life expectancy (and thereby the benefit of preventive treatment) and often also increases the risk of complications. For example, for a 64-year-old patient with a minor ischaemic stroke and 50% stenosis of the symptomatic carotid artery, the chance of dying from ischaemic cardio- or cerebral vascular disease in the next 10 years is probably much higher than the risk of dying from SAH from the incidental 9-mm aneurysm on the left MCA detected during work-up after the stoke. Moreover, the carotid stenosis increases the risk of complications from preventive treatment.

For balancing the risks and benefits, decision analysis can be helpful, but most of the decision models developed thus far are over-simplistic. An important drawback is that these models (implicitly) presume a constant, time-independent risk of rupture, whereas a 'chaotic' or 'periodic' growth process with inherent short-lasting episodes of high risk of rupture is much more likely.[36] This means that the rupture risks found during a certain period of time cannot be extrapolated to the patient's remaining lifetime. A further problem is that the risk of preventive treatment for the aneurysm in question and for the neurosurgeon or radiologist in particular should be known. In many instances the overall risk of the procedure will be no more than an educated guess (probably underestimated by the surgeon or radiologist and over-estimated by the neurologist). Also, the remaining life expectancy often will be another educated guess, especially because for many patients the aneurysm will have been detected during the work-up for another disease, which may have its own impact on life expectancy. Thus, before decision models can be used in clinical practice, they have to be refined.

Despite all these uncertainties, in some situations giving balanced advice is not that difficult. In a young person with an aneurysm larger than 10 mm at the top of the basilar artery that is easily accessible for the radiologist (who has ample experience and a good track record for the procedure), most physicians would advise preventive treatment. Another 'easy' example is the 75-year-old man

with diabetes, a recent myocardial infarction, a more than 70% (asymptomatic) carotid artery stenosis and a 4-mm ipsilateral middle cerebral artery aneurysm. Most physicians would advise to leave the aneurysm untreated, although one of us saw such a patient die from SAH the very day after the advice 'not to treat'. A third example, which starts easy, is the young (say 35 years old) patient with a 3-mm aneurysm on the anterior communicating artery and no further risk factors. Most of us would advise not treating the aneurysm. The difficulty in this example is whether or not to perform follow-up imaging to assess aneurysmal growth. The yield of annual follow-up is small. In a prospective study of 93 patients with 125 small aneurysms CTA or MRA was performed after an interval of 1 year;[55] in three patients (3.2%) an aneurysm enlarged slightly (0.5 to 1.5 mm), but for none did the enlargement lead to a decision to treat. In the meantime, two of the 93 patients (2.2%) had an SAH: one from an aneurysm at the clip site of a previous operation that ruptured without enlargement, and the other from a newly developed dissecting aneurysm. The number of enlarged aneurysms was too small for sound analysis of risk factors, but patients with enlarged aneurysm more often had a positive family history of SAH or a previous episode of stroke, were younger, more often had multiple aneurysms and more often were current smokers than patients without enlargement.[55] Since one of every four aneurysms increases in size over 10 years and one of every two aneurysms over 20 years (section 15.2.1) further studies are clearly needed to assess the optimal screening interval.

In some other circumstances the decision whether or not to treat is made simple by the patient, for example the patient with a 6-mm aneurysm of the posterior communicating artery who has already lost three relatives from SAH. Most such patients will ask for treatment regardless of the actual balance of risks and benefits. In all other circumstances the best way to deal with the problem is to spend a lot of time in the outpatient clinic discussing the risks, benefits and most importantly the uncertainties of each option. In this way the patient can come to an informed decision.

> Small unruptured aneurysms in patients with no other risk factors should probably be left alone; large but easily accessible aneurysms in young patients should probably be offered treatment. In most other situations the physician should discuss in depth the risks, benefits and uncertainties of each strategy. The eventual decision is left to the patient and thus influenced by the patient's own perception of risk.

Whatever the final decision regarding treatment, it is crucial to stress that patients should stop smoking (or should not start smoking) and have their blood pressure checked regularly and hypertension treated, since active smoking and hypertension are strong risk factors for growth and rupture of aneurysms.[28,29,56]

> All patients should be offered advice on risk factor modification regardless of what decision is taken about occlusion of the aneurysm.

15.2.5 Screening for aneurysms

The eventual goal of screening is not to detect or to treat an aneurysm, but to increase the number of quality years of life. Therefore, before intracranial vessels are imaged, the risks and benefits of screening should be weighed up. This process includes calculation of the risks of the diagnostic procedures and any treatment, and the gain in life expectancy by preventive treatment of aneurysms detected by screening. But the assessment of risks should also include the amount of anxiety before screening, the reassurance that can be given with a negative result, and the anxiety that can be caused by finding an aneurysm – e.g. if a 3-mm aneurysm is found and is left untreated but followed up regularly,[3] or if an unrelated abnormality is found. Invitation for screening in itself does not lead to increased anxiety or depression,[4] but actual screening for familial aneurysms is associated with considerable psychosocial effects, both positive and negative.[5] Despite these effects, only a small minority of screenees regret being screened,[5] and most are motivated for follow-up screening.[10] Finally, we should like to emphasize that even screening, repeated screening and preventive treatment cannot prevent all episodes of SAH. In rare instances, aneurysms can develop and rupture within the regular screening interval of 5 years.[57]

No clinical trials have been done on screening for aneurysms in patients at increased risk, and presumably such trials will not be done in the near future because the follow-up needs to be 20 years or longer in a large sample of patients. As for decisions on the management of unruptured aneurysms, decisions on screening must be made from calculations and assumptions, including assumptions on perceived quality of life. This requires extensive counselling in the outpatient clinic. During this counselling the physician should provide clear and detailed information because relatives substantially underestimate the risk of harbouring an aneurysm and of aneurysmal rupture.[4]

Imaging techniques for screening

Screening has become possible by the advent of non- or minimally invasive imaging techniques for intracranial vessels. The test characteristics of CT angiography (CTA) and magnetic resonance angiography (MRA) are similar.[58] Both have a substantial risk of missing very small aneurysms,[59] but these are the lesions that are typically not treated if detected. MRA can be used to screen for familial aneurysms,[60] and has the advantages over CTA that contrast injection is not needed and there is no radiation exposure. In patients who have previously had an aneurysm clipped, the clips cause extensive artifact with MRA,[61] and older intracranial aneurysm clips are usually a contraindication – for them CTA is the preferred assessment technique (Fig. 15.3).[62] MRA is the best option in patients who have been coiled, because coils produce little artifact with this technique (Fig. 15.4).[63]

Indications for screening

Screening should be considered in individuals with two or more affected first-degree relatives, and in patients with autosomal dominant polycystic kidney disease (ADPKD). Because aneurysms are very rare before the age of 20, screening is typically started after this age. If a first screen is negative, repeated screening should be discussed. In a study of individuals with a positive family history and negative initial screening, we found a new aneurysm at repeat screening 5 years later in 7%.[10] If the life expectancy of the patient is short, because of advanced age or comorbidity, screening should not be advised. The maximum age for screening is 60–70 years of age, depending on the individual's health status. Screening should also be considered in identical twins if SAH has occurred in one of the pair, although no systematic studies in twins have been done. Thus far, at least 13 pairs of identical twins with aneurysms in both have been reported.[64] In many twin pairs, the aneurysms are at the same site and SAH tends to occur at around the same age,[65] but in some twin pairs SAH occurs decades apart.[66] At least two twin pairs have been reported with SAH in one, but no aneurysm in the other at the time of screening;[67] such discordant identical twins may have been under-reported.

In individuals with only one affected first-degree relative, screening is not very efficient or effective. To prevent one episode of fatal SAH, 300 at-risk people must be screened. The general advice is, therefore, not to screen individuals with only one affected relative; exceptions can be made for siblings with one affected relative who are younger than 40 years and who are highly anxious about SAH, and therefore already have impaired quality of life. Patients with Ehlers-Danlos syndrome type IV are typically advised against screening, because the fragility of the vessel wall substantially increases the risks of

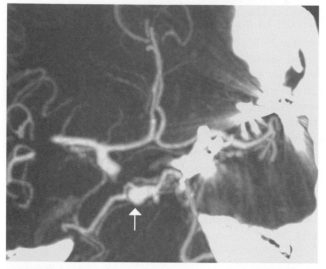

(a)

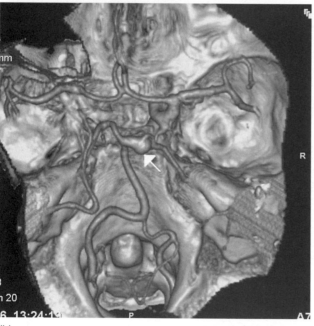

(b)

Fig. 15.3 Follow-up CT angiogram in a patient with a ruptured posterior communicating artery aneurysm treated by neurosurgical clipping. (a) CT angiography shows clip artifacts at the site of the left posterior communicating artery aneurysm, and an aneurysm at the basilar artery tip (*arrow*). (b) Reconstruction of the CT angiogram confirms the basilar artery tip aneurysm (*arrow*) and provides better detail of the anatomy. (Note that this reconstruction is a view from above, thus the right side of the patient is on the right.) (Also reproduced in colour in the plate section.)

treatment.[68] Because an increased risk of SAH has not been confirmed for patients with neurofibromatosis or Marfan syndrome, there is no indication for screening these patients.

Although patients with no family history and no ADPKD who have survived an episode of SAH are at increased risk for a new episode from a new aneurysm or from recurrence of the treated aneurysm,[31] according to a Markov decision model, screening of all such patients cannot be recommended (Wermer *et al.*/ASTRA study group, unpublished data). Although screening prevented almost half of the recurrent SAHs and slightly increased life expectancy, it reduced quality of life and increased costs. In patients with a more than a twofold risk of both aneurysm formation and aneurysm rupture, screening was cost-saving but did not increase quality of life. Only if the risks of aneurysm formation and aneurysm rupture were at least 4.5 times increased, did screening both reduce costs and increase quality of life. Thus, screening seems beneficial only in individuals with previous SAH who have a considerably increased risk of aneurysm formation and of aneurysm rupture. Unfortunately we cannot yet identify who these patients are. Risk factors for recurrent SAH are smoking, multiple aneurysms at the time of the SAH, and young age at time of the initial SAH.[31] However, a recurrent SAH is the result of both the formation of a new aneurysm *and* its rupture. If only one of these risks is increased, screening 5 years after the SAH is not beneficial because even if the risk of aneurysm formation is strongly increased, if the risk of rupture is low, many 'safe' aneurysms will be detected and treated at the costs of complications and resources. Also, if the risk of rupture is increased but the risk of formation is low, aneurysms will be present for only a short period of time, and therefore difficult to detect. Because we have insufficient data on these risk factors for formation and rupture separately, we are for the time being reluctant to screen patients after an SAH, and consider it only in patients (especially women) with an initial episode at a very young age and with multiple aneurysms.

Advice on counselling

Counselling when considering screening is time-consuming, but commonly two or more siblings or other relatives can be counselled at one consultation, and many relatives prefer to come together. When seeing people with a possible family history of SAH, we draw a family tree to start off with. If the individuals report that relatives have had a stroke or SAH, we try to get as much information as possible. Often medical records of relatives who have died are difficult to retrieve, because they have been destroyed or because – perversely – the hospital will only provide copies of records with written informed consent of the patient, even after death. However, in a study in the Netherlands the information recalled by a relative has a positive predictive value for

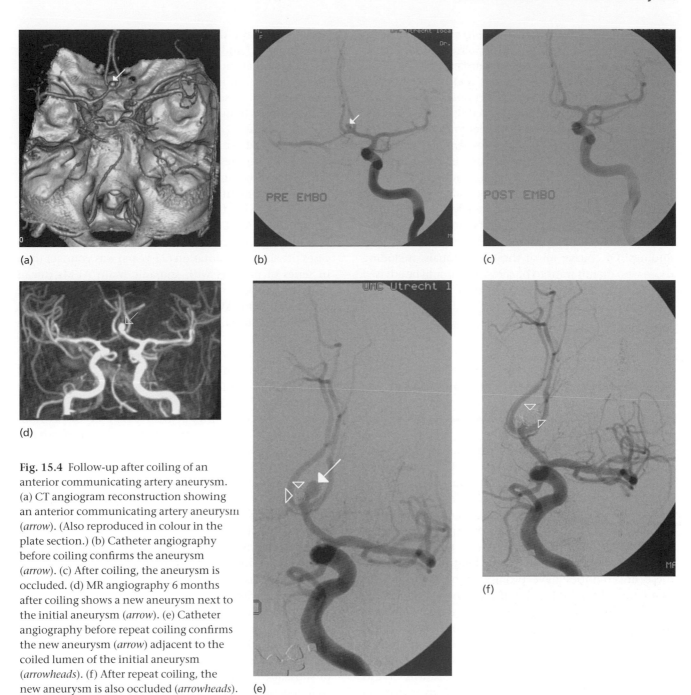

(a)

(b)

(c)

(d)

Fig. 15.4 Follow-up after coiling of an anterior communicating artery aneurysm. (a) CT angiogram reconstruction showing an anterior communicating artery aneurysm (*arrow*). (Also reproduced in colour in the plate section.) (b) Catheter angiography before coiling confirms the aneurysm (*arrow*). (c) After coiling, the aneurysm is occluded. (d) MR angiography 6 months after coiling shows a new aneurysm next to the initial aneurysm (*arrow*). (e) Catheter angiography before repeat coiling confirms the new aneurysm (*arrow*) adjacent to the coiled lumen of the initial aneurysm (*arrowheads*). (f) After repeat coiling, the new aneurysm is also occluded (*arrowheads*).

(e)

(f)

SAH of about 70%, which makes it a sufficiently useful tool for clinical practice.[69] During the next part of the consultation, we explain the procedure and the risks of screening – the chance of having an aneurysm, of an aneurysm rupturing, of treatment, and of finding a very small aneurysm that will not be treated but followed up. We also discuss the implications for driving and flying licences and life insurance (which differ by country), and the yield of repeated screening if the initial screening is negative. In general our advice is to repeat screening every 5 years, and every 2 or 3 years in the rare families in whom rupture of newly developed aneurysms has occurred within 5 years of screening. Individuals with two or more affected first-degree relatives are mostly very willing to undergo repeated screening. In one study, more than 80% returned 5 years after the initial screening, having been given the advice to undergo repeated screening.[10] At the end of the initial consultation, we leave the decision about screening to the patient: to go for screening; to make a second appointment for further discussion or information (sometimes siblings come together, but without their spouses, and eventually want to make a final decision with their spouses); or to make no further appointment. Audio recording the consultation and giving the tape to the patient might be helpful, but we do not have personal experience with this method of informing individuals. If the screening candidate wishes to be screened, another important decision that has to be made beforehand is what to do about unrelated findings. Some people do not wish to be informed about arachnoid cysts, non-specific white matter lesions of unknown relevance, or other incidental findings. Of course, all of these individuals, including those who do not want to be screened, should be advised against smoking and to have their blood pressure checked regularly.

15.3 Arteriovenous malformations of the brain

The section on incidental intracranial aneurysms described many uncertainties and unanswered questions. For incidental brain arteriovenous malformations (AVMs) the situation is even worse. Uncertainty about the risk of haemorrhage and of treatment is fuelled by the presence of three treatment modalities (and combinations of these modalities) as well as the option of no intervention. But there is some light in the darkness: these uncertainties have prompted the launch of an international trial on the management of unruptured brain AVMs (www.arubastudy.org). This trial will compare the strategy 'no intervention' with intervention (if the brain AVM is potentially treatable), the type of intervention being left to the treating team. Clearly, this trial will not answer all the questions, but at least will serve as a starting point for evidence-based treatment advice and for further studies, depending on the outcome.

15.3.1 Frequency and presentation of brain arteriovenous malformations

Brain AVMs are much rarer than intracranial aneurysms (section 8.2.4). Their prevalence ranges between 15 and 19 per 100 000 adults,[70] the overall detection rate is about 1 per 100 000 adults per year,[71–73] and the incidence of haemorrhage from a brain AVM around 0.5 per 100 000 adults per year.[71,73] Compared with intracranial aneurysms, brain AVMs are seldom multiple (around 4% of patients),[74,75] and there are no known risk factors. There are no data that modifiable risk factors such as smoking and hypertension increase the risk of brain AVMs, and also there are no sound data to support a familial preponderance of brain AVMs. In a recent systematic review of the literature, only 53 patients from 25 families were identified (van Beijnum, unpublished data). This number of families is so small that it may be chance rather than a common familial factor that is important in the development of brain AVMs. The characteristics of the patients with familial brain AVMs were in general similar to those of patients with sporadic brain AVMs. The only difference was that in the reported familial cases the age at presentation (27 years) was younger than in series of patients with sporadic brain AVMs (mean difference 8 years) (van Beijnum, unpublished data). Although brain AVMs are thought to be congenital lesions,[76] rare instances of development during life have been reported.[77,78] The good news for patients is that in rare instances AVMs disappear spontaneously.[79]

In around half of all patients in whom a brain AVM is detected, the reason for detection is an intracranial haemorrhage,[80] although recent data suggest that this proportion is declining, at least where access to non-invasive brain imaging is so easy that non-haemorrhagic presentations are more often detected.[1] Other reasons for detection are epilepsy, focal neurological deficits and as an incidental finding in patients investigated for other reasons or non-specific complaints. In applicants for military flying duties, brain AVMs are found by chance in around 0.1%.[81]

Initial presentation with haemorrhage is considered the main determinant of future haemorrhage.[82] In contrast to previously held beliefs, recurrent bleeding episodes tend to occur with highest frequency in the first few months after the initial bleed. The rate of subsequent haemorrhage has been reported as high as 33% in the first year after presentation with haemorrhage, decreasing to 11% per annum in subsequent years.[83] Over the years, the risk of subsequent haemorrhage tends to become similar to that of patients who presented in other ways.[84]

The high rate of subsequent bleeding, at least in the initial years after presentation with haemorrhage, favours obliteration of the AVM, if technically feasible. Moreover, although there is not the immediate hurry as there is in patients with a ruptured aneurysm to treat the lesions within the first 1 or 2 days, the aim should be to treat the lesion within the first few weeks after the haemorrhage, if the patient's condition allows it. The greatest uncertainty arises when an unruptured brain AVM is detected. The remainder of this section will focus on this issue.

15.3.2 Natural history of brain arteriovenous malformations

Little is known of the natural history of brain AVMs. The knowledge we have is biased, and based on wrong outcome measures and erroneous assumptions. First, bias is introduced because natural history has been studied in patients who received no treatment, and the main reason for not treating these patients was that the AVM was (very) difficult to treat. The natural history of brain AVMs that are difficult to treat may well differ from that of patients with 'easily' treatable AVMs. Second, most studies on natural history have taken 'haemorrhage' as the measure of outcome, and yet haemorrhage may not always lead to disability; indeed, several studies suggest that haemorrhage from brain AVMs is less detrimental than intracerebral haemorrhage in general.[85] Also, recurrent haemorrhage from an AVM often does not result in increased morbidity.[84,85] Third, follow-up in most studies has been relatively short,[86] and the haemorrhage rates found within this short period of follow-up have been recalculated as 'yearly rates of rupture', even though haemorrhage rates decrease over time after an initial haemorrhage.[84]

Studies comparing brain AVM characteristics between patients who presented with haemorrhage and patients who presented with other symptoms or no symptoms at all, concur in finding deep venous drainage, a single draining vein, venous stenosis and high pressure in the feeding artery more often in patients with haemorrhage than in other patients.[86] The proof that these same factors determine the occurrence of haemorrhage *in the future* in patients with *unruptured* brain AVMs has to come from prospective follow-up studies. In the prospectively followed series of untreated patients from the Columbia AVM Databank exclusive deep venous drainage was indeed associated with increased risk of haemorrhage, other risk factors being increasing age and deep AVM location.[82] On the basis of these data, for patients without previous haemorrhage, annual haemorrhage rates have been estimated as 0.9% for patients with no risk factors, 2.4% for those with deep drainage and 3.1% for those with deep location of the haemorrhage.[1] However, as pointed out above, extrapolating observed haemorrhage rates to constant future haemorrhage rates is probably unrealistic.

> The long-term risk of haemorrhage and more importantly of death or disability from brain arteriovenous malformations is unknown. For patients without previous rupture and no risk factors (deep venous drainage) these risks are probably very low.

15.3.3 Treatment options for brain arteriovenous malformations

The available options for treatment are: medical management only (e.g. of epilepsy or headaches), surgical excision, endovascular embolization, stereotactic radiotherapy (often described as radiosurgery) and combinations of these treatment modalities. There are no randomized trials or non-randomized comparisons for these strategies, even though they have been used for more than a decade.[78,79] We are left with several observational studies of these strategies, and not even a systematic overview. Methodological weaknesses abound. Many of the studies are retrospective, and most of them used occurrence of haemorrhage and not measures of morbidity, disability or dependence as the outcome measurement.[78] Such an outcome measurement excludes complications from treatment other than haemorrhage. For stereotactic radiotherapy of brain AVMs in the brainstem, non-haemorrhagic complications have been reported in up to 7% of patients.[80] Even recent studies published in high-ranking journals have used reduction in haemorrhage rate after the start of the therapy as the outcome measure,[81] but such a reduction might very well reflect the natural course; without a randomized comparison with an untreated group, no conclusions can be drawn from these studies. Comparing results between treatment strategies from observational studies is further hampered by heterogeneity of patients and by different treatment goals. Patients so often cannot be compared because they were selected for the particular intervention because of certain characteristics of the AVM (which often makes these patients ineligible for other interventions). Also, surgical intervention usually aims at total excision of the AVM, whereas endovascular treatment may be offered to diminish the size of an AVM so that it becomes treatable by surgery or stereotactic radiotherapy.

Neurosurgical excision

The most important determinants for neurosurgical management are the size and location of the malformation, along with the type of venous drainage. For example, a small and superficial AVM in the occipital lobe is much more easily accessible than an anomaly involving almost an entire hemisphere, with feeders from all the major arteries and with extensive drainage into the deep venous system. For these reasons, Spetzler and Martin have proposed a grading system for AVMs that takes account of these three key features (Table 15.7).[87] Of course, it is more useful to describe the three features separately than to rely on the sum score alone; in the process of summation important information gets lost.

Table 15.7 Grading system for arteriovenous malformations, according to Spetzler and Martin (1986).[87]

Graded feature	Points assigned
Size of arteriovenous malformation	
small (<3 cm)	1
medium (3–6 cm)	2
large (>6 cm)	3
Location	
non-eloquent area	0
eloquent area	1
Pattern of venous drainage	
superficial only	0
deep (any part)	1

Grade = [size] + [eloquence] + [venous drainage], i.e. [1, 2 or 3] + [0 or 1] + [0 or 1].

A cautionary note is appropriate about the dangers of making too facile a distinction between 'eloquent' and so-called 'silent' areas of the brain. Operation in specialized areas of the cerebral cortex may result in easily recognizable deficits such as hemiparesis, aphasia or a visual field defect, but this does not mean that less specialized areas of the brain are functionally unimportant; they play an important role in complex mental processes, which are at least as important as elementary functions. Surgical excision of, say, the right temporal lobe will not result in impairments that are obvious when the patient is making a brief visit to a hospital clinic. But a conversation with the patient's partner will drastically cure any previous belief on the part of the surgeon that 'silent' areas of the brain can be excised without any consequences for the patient's mood or personality. To illustrate this point with a comparison: if the function of the intact brain is symbolized by a beautiful painting, lesions in 'eloquent' brain areas can be compared with holes or blots in the picture, whereas lesions in 'silent' areas correspond with darkening of the varnish and fading of the colours.

The term 'silent area of the brain' should be interpreted as an area with a general rather than a specific function (such as language or movements), not as an area that is redundant.

Neurosurgical management is the treatment that has been available for longest and many series have reported on the success rate, management morbidity and case fatality. In a systematic review (published in French), data on 2452 patients were included.[88] It is important to keep in mind that is impossible to segregate the results of the studies according to whether the brain AVM was ruptured or not – another criticism of the treatment literature, in addition to its uncontrolled, non-randomized nature. Morbidity was found in all studies, and varied between 1.5% and 19%; overall postoperative mortality was 3.3%. The risk of complications was related to increasing Spetzler-Martin grade, and to the size and site of the AVM. For AVMs smaller than 3 cm a 4.6% morbidity (from 1.5% to 9.7%) and a zero mortality were reported. Total excision of the AVM was reported in 97% of patients on average, with a range from 91% to 100%. Thus, neurosurgical intervention is a successful strategy, at least for patients selected for this treatment, and has a reasonably low risk of complications for patients with small AVMs. Series published after this review reported similar results.[89]

Endovascular embolization

The aim of endovascular therapy is to obliterate the feeding arteries and the vessels at the site of the nidus by use of embolic agents, such as N-butylcyanoacrylate, polyvinyl alcohol particles, detachable coils, or Onyx liquid polymer. The results from the different agents in terms of occlusion of the AVM do not seem to differ significantly.[90] Endovascular embolization is most often used to reduce the size of the AVM to make it amenable for neurosurgical treatment, or for stereotactic radiotherapy. Often, multiple procedures are necessary to reach this goal. In those series where surgical excision is preceded by endovascular treatment, the morbidity related to this pre-surgical embolization ranges from 4% to 8.9%.[88,91] In a study on combined endovascular and neurosurgical intervention with prospective assessment of complications by an independent physician, disabling treatment-related complications occurred in 5% (95% CI 1–9%) of the patients, and non-disabling new deficits in another 42% (95% CI 33–51%), while none of the patients died.[92] Risk factors for complications were non-haemorrhagic presentation, deep venous drainage, AVM location in an 'eloquent' brain region and large AVM size. As is the case for the series describing the neurosurgical treatment of AVMs, it is difficult to disentangle the results of endovascular treatment according to whether the brain AVM had ruptured or not.

Endovascular embolization as the only therapy results in complete obliteration of the AVM in only 10–40% of the patients, depending on their selection.[93–95] In large series from experienced centres reporting on complications from endovascular therapy in general (including embolization before neurosurgery or stereotactic radiotherapy) case fatality varies from 1% to 3%, and morbidity from 2% to 6%.[94,95]

Stereotactic radiotherapy (radiosurgery)

Focused radiation is an increasingly important option in the management of brain AVMs that are considered inaccessible to surgical treatment, i.e. lesions in the deep regions of a cerebral hemisphere, in the brainstem or in important primary projection areas such as for language or for motor control of the dominant hand. But lesions of more than 3.0–3.5 cm in size are not suitable for stereotactic radiotherapy, because the dose to normal tissues would be excessive, so for larger brain AVMs embolization is often used to reduce their size first.

The rationale for radiation treatment is that it damages and eventually occludes the blood vessels constituting the AVM.[96] This takes place in the long term, after months or years, which is an important drawback, because in the meantime there is still a risk of haemorrhage.[97] This risk of haemorrhage may even be increased within this 'obliteration period',[98] although this suggestion is not confirmed in all relevant studies.[99] In a prospective study, presentation of the AVM with haemorrhage was a risk factor for haemorrhage after stereotactic radiotherapy.[100] In this study haemorrhage occurred in 3.8% (95% CI 2.0–6.7%) of patients with no haemorrhage and in 8.6% (95% CI 6.1–11.6%) of patients with a haemorrhage before starting the therapy. Haemorrhage resulted in death in 7% and morbidity in almost 50% of patients. Patients with angiographic disappearance of the AVM after stereotactic radiotherapy are considered to be 'cured', but even in them new haemorrhages can sometimes occur. In a series of 236 patients with angiographic evidence of obliteration of the AVM after stereotactic radiotherapy, the cumulative risk of haemorrhage for the initial 10 years after treatment was 2.2%.[101]

Other complications from stereotactic radiotherapy are radiation injury of the brain parenchyma (6.5%), radiation-induced cranial nerve palsies (1%) and new or worsened seizures (1%).[102] In one out of four patients these complications were disabling and 2% of patients died from the complications. Unfortunately, the study did not describe risk factors for developing these complications. In half the patients, the symptoms resolved over time.[102] Radiation injury of the brain parenchyma may result in the formation of cysts that can appear as long as 2–7 years later.[103] These cysts may need to be treated with a permanent shunt or with total excision.[103] In summary, if any intervention at all is needed for an AVM, the technique of focused radiation is not much

safer and is probably less effective than surgical resection, certainly in the short term.

15.3.4 Management of patients with unruptured arteriovenous malformations

Ideally, patients with unruptured brain AVMs for whom treatment is considered should be entered into a randomized controlled trial. Currently, one such trial is running (www.arubastudy.org) and, if possible, patients should be referred to a centre that is participating in this trial (or future trials). If this is not possible, the pros and cons of all treatment options should be discussed with the patient, and based upon these uncertainties a decision has to be made. An important factor in this decision is the patient's psychological attitude towards living with an unoperated lesion in the brain that may unexpectedly bleed. In general, knowledge of having such a lesion results in a decreased quality of life,[3] but some patients show admirable *sangfroid* in coping with this knowledge. For others, however, their life may turn out to be so dominated by the perceived danger that they insist on intervention even when the balance of risks would seem to argue against such a course of action. If treatment is opted for, it seems that open surgery is best for superficial and small AVMs. For larger lesions, endovascular embolization preceding neurosurgery or stereotactic radiotherapy seems a reasonable approach. Stereotactic radiotherapy is probably a good option for AVMs that are inaccessible to surgery such as small and deep lesions, fed by small blood vessels.

Given the absence of a clear familial preponderance of brain AVMs, there is no indication for screening relatives of patients with an AVM, probably not even if several relatives are affected. In some relatives brain AVMs have been detected by means of screening,[104–106] but in other families screening did not yield any new AVM.[107–109] Screening of close relatives of all patients with an AVM is bound to have a low yield. Furthermore, this would be very expensive. Another reason to withhold screening is that the clinical consequences of finding an asymptomatic AVM are still uncertain.

Migraine is sometimes suggested as an indication for screening for an AVM, but in patients with migraine the chance of finding one is well below 1%.[110] Moreover, in view of the dilemmas with regard to invasive treatment, it is far from certain that a patient with migraine benefits from the knowledge that there is an underlying AVM. Another disadvantage of ordering imaging studies in all migraineurs with stereotyped attacks is the cost, discomfort and risk of the negative investigations in the vast majority.

References

1 Stapf C, Mohr JP, Choi JH, Hartmann A, Mast H. Invasive treatment of unruptured brain arteriovenous malformations is experimental therapy. *Curr Opin Neurol* 2006; **19**(1):63–8.

2 Wiebers DO, Whisnant JP, Huston J, III, Meissner I, Brown RDJ, Piepgras DG *et al*. Unruptured intracranial aneurysms: natural history, clinical outcome, and risks of surgical and endovascular treatment. *Lancet* 2003; **362**(9378):103–10.

3 Van der Schaaf IC, Brilstra EH, Rinkel GJE, Bossuyt PMM, van Gijn J. Quality of life, anxiety, and depression in patients with an untreated intracranial aneurysm or arteriovenous malformation. *Stroke* 2002; **33**(2):440–3.

4 Bossuyt PM, Raaymakers TWM, Bonsel GJ, Rinkel GJE. Screening families for intracranial aneurysms: Anxiety, perceived risk, and informed choice. *Prev Med* 2005; **41**:795–9.

5 Wermer MJ, van der Schaaf IC, Van Nunen P, Bossuyt PM, Anderson CS, Rinkel GJE. Psychosocial impact of screening for intracranial aneurysms in relatives with familial subarachnoid hemorrhage. *Stroke* 2005; **36**(4):836–40.

6 Rinkel GJE, Djibuti M, Algra A, van Gijn J. Prevalence and risk of rupture of intracranial aneurysms: a systematic review. *Stroke* 1998; **29**(1):251–6.

7 Menghini VV, Brown RD, Jr., Sicks JD, O'Fallon WM, Wiebers DO. Incidence and prevalence of intracranial aneurysms and hemorrhage in Olmsted County, Minnesota, 1965 to 1995. *Neurology* 1998; **51**(2):405–11.

8 Bromberg JEC, Rinkel GJE, Algra A, Greebe P, van Duyn CM, Hasan D *et al*. Subarachnoid haemorrhage in first and second degree relatives of patients with subarachnoid haemorrhage. *Br Med J* 1995; **311**:288–9.

9 Raaymakers TWM, MARS study group. Aneurysms in relatives of patients with subarachnoid hemorrhage. Frequency and risk factors. *Neurology* 1999; **53**(5):982–8.

10 Wermer MJ, Rinkel GJE, van Gijn J. Repeated screening for intracranial aneurysms in familial subarachnoid hemorrhage. *Stroke* 2003; **34**:2788–91.

11 Ruigrok YM, Rinkel GJE, Algra A, Raaymakers TWM, van Gijn J. Characteristics of intracranial aneurysms in patients with familial subarachnoid hemorrhage. *Neurology* 2004; **62**:891–4.

12 Bromberg JEC, Rinkel GJE, Algra A, van Duyn CM, Greebe P, Ramos LMP *et al*. Familial subarachnoid hemorrhage: distinctive features and patterns of inheritance. *Ann Neurol* 1995; **38**(6):929–34.

13 Ruigrok YM, Rinkel GJE, Wijmenga C, van Gijn J. Anticipation and phenotype in familial intracranial aneurysms. *J Neurol Neurosurg Psychiatry* 2004; **75**:1436–42.

14 Struycken PM, Pals G, Limburg M, Pronk JC, Wijmenga C, Pearson PL *et al*. Anticipation in familial intracranial aneurysms in consecutive generations. *Eur J Hum Genet* 2003; **11**:737–43.

15 Belz MM, Hughes RL, Kaehny WD, Johnson AM, Fick-Brosnahan GM, Earnest MP *et al*. Familial clustering of ruptured intracranial aneurysms in autosomal dominant polycystic kidney disease. *Am J Kidney Dis* 2001; **38**(4):770–6.

16 Schievink WI, Torres VE, Piepgras DG, Wiebers DO. Saccular intracranial aneurysms in autosomal dominant polycystic kidney disease. *J Am Soc Nephrol* 1992; **3**(1):88–95.

17 Gieteling EW, Rinkel GJE. Characteristics of intracranial aneurysms and subarachnoid haemorrhage in patients with polycystic kidney disease. *J Neurol* 2003; **250**(4):418–23.

18 Huston J, III, Torres VE, Sulivan PP, Offord KP, Wiebers DO. Value of magnetic resonance angiography for the detection of intracranial aneurysms in autosomal dominant polycystic kidney disease. *J Am Soc Nephrol* 1993; **3**:1871–7.

19 Rossetti S, Chauveau D, Kubly V, Slezak JM, Saggar-Malik AK, Pei Y *et al*. Association of mutation position in polycystic kidney disease 1 (PKD1) gene and development of a vascular phenotype. *Lancet* 2003; **361**:2196–201.

20 Chauveau D, Pirson Y, Verellen-Dumoulin C, Macnicol A, Gonzalo A, Grunfeld JP. Intracranial aneurysms in autosomal dominant polycystic kidney disease. *Kidney Int* 1994; **45**(4):1140–6.

21 Chauveau D, Sirieix ME, Schillinger F, Legendre C, Grünfeld JP. Recurrent rupture of intracranial aneurysms in autosomal dominant polycystic kidney disease. *Br Med J* 1990; **301**:966–7.

22 Nakajima F, Shibahara N, Arai M, Gohji K, Ueda H, Katsuoka Y. Intracranial aneurysms and autosomal dominant polycystic kidney disease: followup study by magnetic resonance angiography. *J Urol* 2000; **164**(2):311–13.

23 Belz MM, Fick-Brosnahan GM, Hughes RL, Rubinstein D, Chapman AB, Johnson AM *et al*. Recurrence of intracranial aneurysms in autosomal-dominant polycystic kidney disease. *Kidney Int* 2003; **63**:1824–30.

24 Gibbs GF, Huston J, III, Qian Q, Kubly V, Harris PC, Brown RD, Jr. *et al*. Follow-up of intracranial aneurysms in autosomal-dominant polycystic kidney disease. *Kidney Int* 2004; **65**:1621–7.

25 Akyuz M, Tuncer R, Yilmaz S, Sindel T. Angiographic follow-up after surgical treatment of intracranial aneurysms. *Acta Neurochir (Wien)* 2004; **146**:245–50.

26 David CA, Vishteh AG, Spetzler RF, Lemole M, Lawton MT, Partovi S. Late angiographic follow-up review of surgically treated aneurysms. *J Neurosurg* 1999; **91**(3):396–401.

27 Tsutsumi K, Ueki K, Morita A, Usui M, Kirino T. Risk of aneurysm recurrence in patients with clipped cerebral aneurysms. Results of long-term follow-up angiography. *Stroke* 2001; **32**(5):1191–4.

28 Juvela S, Poussa K, Porras M. Factors affecting formation and growth of intracranial aneurysms: a long-term follow-up study. *Stroke* 2001; **32**(2):485–91.

29 Wermer MJ, van der Schaaf IC, Velthuis BK, Algra A, Buskens E, Rinkel GJE. Follow-up screening after subarachnoid haemorrhage: frequency and determinants

of new aneurysms and enlargement of existing aneurysms. *Brain* 2005; **128**:2421–9.

30 Tsutsumi K, Ueki K, Usui M, Kwak S, Kirino T. Risk of recurrent subarachnoid hemorrhage after complete obliteration of cerebral aneurysms. *Stroke* 1998; **29**:2511–13.

31 Wermer MJ, Greebe P, Algra A, Rinkel GJE. Incidence of recurrent subarachnoid hemorrhage after clipping for ruptured intracranial aneurysms. *Stroke* 2005; **36**(11):2394–9.

32 Molyneux AJ, Kerr RS, Yu LM, Clarke M, Sneade M, Yarnold JA *et al.* International subarachnoid aneurysm trial (ISAT) of neurosurgical clipping versus endovascular coiling in 2143 patients with ruptured intracranial aneurysms: a randomised comparison of effects on survival, dependency, seizures, rebleeding, subgroups, and aneurysm occlusion. *Lancet* 2005; **366**(9488):809–17.

33 The International Study of Unruptured Intracranial Aneurysms Investigators. Unruptured intracranial aneurysms: risk of rupture and risks of surgical intervention. *N Engl J Med* 1998; **339**:1725–33.

34 Clarke G, Mendelow AD, Mitchell P. Predicting the risk of rupture of intracranial aneurysms based on anatomical location. *Acta Neurochir (Wien)* 2005; **147**:259–63.

35 Kailasnath P, Chaloupka JC, Dickey PS. A multiplicative statistical model predicts the size distribution of unruptured intracranial aneurysms. *Neurol Res* 1998; **20**(5):421–6.

36 Mitchell P, Jakubowski J. Estimate of the maximum time interval between formation of cerebral aneurysm and rupture. *J Neurol Neurosurg Psychiatry* 2000; **69**(6):760–7.

37 Tsutsumi K, Ueki K, Usui M, Kwak S, Kirino T. Risk of subarachnoid hemorrhage after surgical treatment of unruptured cerebral aneurysms. *Stroke* 1999; **30**(6):1181–4.

38 Wermer MJ, van der Schaaf IC, Algra A, Rinkel GJE. Risk of rupture of unruptured intracranial aneurysms in relation to patient and aneurysm characteristics: an updated meta-analysis. *Stroke.* 2007 Apr; **38**(4):1404–10.

39 Jane JA, Kassell NF, Torner JC, Winn HR. The natural history of aneurysms and arteriovenous malformations. *J Neurosurg* 1985; **62**:321–3.

40 Juvela S, Porras M, Heiskanen O. Natural history of unruptured intracranial aneurysms: a long-term follow-up study. *J Neurosurg* 1993; **79**(2):174–82.

41 Rose G. *The Strategy of Preventive Medicine.* Oxford: Oxford Medical Publications, 1992.

42 Raaymakers TWM, Rinkel GJE, Limburg M, Algra A. Mortality and morbidity of surgery for unruptured intracranial aneurysms: a meta-analysis. *Stroke* 1998; **29**(8):1531–8.

43 Solomon RA, Fink ME, Pile-Spellman J. Surgical management of unruptured intracranial aneurysms. *J Neurosurg* 1994; **80**:440–6.

44 Chyatte D, Porterfield R. Functional outcome after repair of unruptured intracranial aneurysms. *J Neurosurg* 2001; **94**(3):417–21.

45 Matsumoto K, Akagi K, Abekura M, Nakajima Y, Yoshiminie T. Investigation of the surgically treated and untreated unruptured cerebral aneurysms of the anterior circulation. *Surg Neurol* 2003; **60**:516–22.

46 Solomon RA, Mayer SA, Tarmey JJ. Relationship between the volume of craniotomies for cerebral aneurysm performed at New York state hospitals and in-hospital mortality. *Stroke* 1996; **27**(1):13–17.

47 Lanterna LA, Tredici G, Dimitrov BD, Biroli F. Treatment of unruptured cerebral aneurysms by embolization with guglielmi detachable coils: case-fatality, morbidity, and effectiveness in preventing bleeding – a systematic review of the literature. *Neurosurgery* 2004; **55**(4):767–75.

48 Van Rooij WJ, de Gast A, Sluzewski M, Nijssen PC, Beute GN. Coiling of truly incidental intracranial aneurysms. *Am J Neuroradiol* 2006; **27**(2):293–6.

49 Rothwell PM, Slattery J, Warlow CP. A systematic review of the risks of stroke and death due to endarterectomy for symptomatic carotid stenosis. *Stroke* 1996; **27**(2):260–5.

50 Lee T, Baytion M, Sciacca R, Mohr JP, Pile-Spellman J. Aggregate analysis of the literature for unruptured intracranial aneurysm treatment. *Am J Neuroradiol* 2005; **26**(8):1902–8.

51 Grunwald IQ, Papanagiotou P, Politi M, Struffert T, Roth C, Reith W. Endovascular treatment of unruptured intracranial aneurysms: occurrence of thromboembolic events. *Neurosurgery* 2006; **58**(4):612–18.

52 Brilstra EH, Rinkel GJE, van der Graaf Y, Sluzewski M, Groen RJ, Lo RT *et al.* Quality of life after treatment of unruptured intracranial aneurysms by neurosurgical clipping or by embolisation with coils. a prospective, observational study. *Cerebrovasc Dis* 2004; **17**:44–52.

53 Barker FG. Age-dependent differences in short-term outcome after surgical or endovascular treatment of unruptured intracranial aneurysms in the United States, 1996–2000. *Neurosurg* 2004; **54**:18–30.

54 Johnston SC, Wilson CB, Halbach VV, Higashida RT, Dowd CF, McDermott MW *et al.* Endovascular and surgical treatment of unruptured cerebral aneurysms: comparison of risks. *Ann Neurol* 2000; **48**:11–19.

55 Wermer MJ, van der Schaaf IC, Velthuis BK, Majoie CB, Albrecht KW, Rinkel GJE. Yield of short-term follow-up CT/MR angiography for small aneurysms detected at screening. *Stroke* 2006; **37**(2):414–18.

56 Juvela S, Porras M, Poussa K. Natural history of unruptured intracranial aneurysms: probability of and risk factors for aneurysm rupture. *J Neurosurg* 2000; **93**:379–87.

57 Schievink WI, Limburg M, Dreissen JJ, Peeters FL, ter Berg HW. Screening for unruptured familial intracranial aneurysms: subarachnoid hemorrhage 2 years after angiography negative for aneurysms. *Neurosurgery* 1991; **29**:434–7.

58 White PM, Teasdale EM, Wardlaw JM, Easton V. Intracranial aneurysms: CT angiography and MR angiography for detection prospective blinded comparison in a large patient cohort. *Radiology* 2001; **219**(3):739–49.

59 Wardlaw JM, White PM. The detection and management of unruptured intracranial aneurysms. *Brain* 2000; **123**(Pt 2):205–21.

60 Raaymakers TWM, Buys PC, Verbeeten B, Jr., Ramos LMP, Witkamp TD, Hulsmans FJ *et al*. MR angiography as a screening tool for intracranial aneurysms: feasibility, test characteristics, and interobserver agreement. *Am J Roentgenol* 1999; **173**(6):1469–75.

61 Gonner F, Lovblad KO, Heid O, Remonda L, Guzman R, Barth A *et al*. Magnetic resonance angiography with ultrashort echo times reduces the artefact of aneurysm clips. *Neuroradiology* 2002; **44**:755–8.

62 Van der Schaaf IC, Velthuis BK, Wermer MJ, Frenkel NJ, Majoie CB, Witkamp TD *et al*. Multislice computed tomography angiography screening for new aneurysms in patients with previously clip-treated intracranial aneurysms: Feasibility, positive predictive value, and interobserver agreement. *J Neurosurg* 2006; **105**(5):682–8.

63 Majoie CB, Sprengers ME, Van Rooij WJ, Lavini C, Sluzewski M, van Rijn JC *et al*. MR angiography at 3T versus digital subtraction angiography in the follow-up of intracranial aneurysms treated with detachable coils. *Am J Neuroradiol* 2005; **26**(6):1349–56.

64 Ohno S, Ikeda Y, Onitsuka T, Nakajima S, Uchino H, Haraoka J *et al*. [Cerebral aneurysms in identical twins]. *No Shinkei Geka* 2004; **32**:875–9.

65 Puchner MJ, Lohmann F, Valdueza JM, Siepmann G, Freckmann N. Monozygotic twins not identical with respect to the existence of intracranial aneurysms: a case report. *Surg Neurol* 1994; **41**:284–9.

66 Hager P, Steiger HJ. Identical cerebral aneurysms in siblings: report of two families. *J Clin Neurosci* 2004; **11**:80–4.

67 Astradsson A, Astrup J. An intracranial aneurysm in one identical twin, but no aneurysm in the other. *Br J Neurosurg* 2001; **15**:168–71.

68 Schievink WI, Link MJ, Piepgras DG, Spetzler RF. Intracranial aneurysm surgery in Ehlers-Danlos syndrome type IV. *Neurosurg* 2002; **51**(3):607–13.

69 Bromberg JEC, Rinkel GJE, Algra A, Greebe P, Beldman T, van Gijn J. Validation of family history in subarachnoid hemorrhage. *Stroke* 1996; **27**(4):630–2.

70 Al Shahi R, Fang JS, Lewis SC, Warlow CP. Prevalence of adults with brain arteriovenous malformations: a community based study in Scotland using capture-recapture analysis. *J Neurol Neurosurg Psychiatry* 2002; **73**(5):547–51.

71 Stapf C, Labovitz DL, Sciacca RR, Mast H, Mohr JP, Sacco RL. Incidence of adult brain arteriovenous malformation hemorrhage in a prospective population-based stroke survey. *Cerebrovasc Dis* 2002; **13**(1):43–6.

72 Al Shahi R, Bhattacharya JJ, Currie DG, Papanastassiou V, Ritchie V, Roberts RC *et al*. Prospective, population-based detection of intracranial vascular malformations in adults: the Scottish Intracranial Vascular Malformation Study (SIVMS). *Stroke* 2003; **34**(5):1163–9.

73 Stapf C, Mast H, Sciacca RR, Berenstein A, Nelson PK, Gobin YP *et al*. The New York Islands AVM Study: design, study progress, and initial results. *Stroke* 2003; **34**(5):e29–e33.

74 Salcman M, Scholtz H, Numaguchi Y. Multiple intracerebral arteriovenous malformations: report of three cases and review of the literature. *Surg Neurol* 1992; **38**(2):121–8.

75 Willinsky RA, Lasjaunias P, TerBrugge K, Burrows P. Multiple cerebral arteriovenous malformations (AVMs): review of our experience from 203 patients with cerebral vascular lesions. *Neuroradiology* 1990; **32**(3):207–10.

76 Fleetwood IG, Steinberg GK. Arteriovenous malformations. *Lancet* 2002; **359**(9309):863–73.

77 Bulsara KR, Alexander MJ, Villavicencio AT, Graffagnino C. De novo cerebral arteriovenous malformation: case report. *Neurosurg* 2002; **50**(5):1137–41.

78 Gonzalez LF, Bristol RE, Porter RW, Spetzler RF. De novo presentation of an arteriovenous malformation. Case report and review of the literature. *J Neurosurg* 2005; **102**(4):726–9.

79 Buis DR, van den BR, Lycklama G, van der Worp HB, Dirven CM, Vandertop WP. Spontaneous regression of brain arteriovenous malformations: a clinical study and a systematic review of the literature. *J Neurol* 2004; **251**(11):1375–82.

80 Brown RD, Wiebers DO, Torner JC, O'Fallon WM. Incidence and prevalence of intracranial vascular malformation in Omsted County, Minnesota, 1965 to 1992. *Neurology* 1996; **46**:949–52.

81 Weber F, Knopf H. Incidental findings in magnetic resonance imaging of the brains of healthy young men. *J Neurol Sci* 2006; **240**(1–2):81–4.

82 Stapf C, Mast H, Sciacca RR, Choi JH, Khaw AV, Connolly ES *et al*. Predictors of hemorrhage in patients with untreated brain arteriovenous malformation. *Neurology* 2006; **66**(9):1350–5.

83 Mast H, Young WL, Koennecke HC, Sciacca RR, Osipov A, Pile-Spellman J *et al*. Risk of spontaneous haemorrhage after diagnosis of cerebral arteriovenous malformation. *Lancet* 1997; **350**(9084):1065–8.

84 Halim AX, Johnston SC, Singh V, McCulloch CE, Bennett JP, Achrol AS *et al*. Longitudinal risk of intracranial hemorrhage in patients with arteriovenous malformation of the brain within a defined population. *Stroke* 2004; **35**:1697–702.

85 Choi JH, Mast H, Sciacca RR, Hartmann A, Khaw AV, Mohr JP *et al*. Clinical outcome after first and recurrent hemorrhage in patients with untreated brain arteriovenous malformation. *Stroke* 2006; **37**:1243–7.

86 Al Shahi R, Warlow C. A systematic review of the frequency and prognosis of arteriovenous malformations of the brain in adults. *Brain* 2001; **124**(10):1900–26.

87 Spetzler RF, Martin NA. A proposed grading system for arteriovenous malformations. *J Neurosurg* 1986; **65**(4):476–83.

88 Castel JP, Kantor G. [Postoperative morbidity and mortality after microsurgical exclusion of cerebral arteriovenous malformations. Current data and analysis of recent literature]. *Neurochirurgie* 2001; **47**(2–3 Pt 2):369–83.

89 Morgan MK, Rochford AM, Tsahtsarlis A, Little N, Faulder KC. Surgical risks associated with the management of

Grade I and II brain arteriovenous malformations. *Neurosurgery* 2004; **54**(4):832–7.

90 Al Shahi R, Warlow C. Arteriovenous malformations of the brain: ready to randomise? *J Neurol Neurosurg Psychiatry* 2005; **76**(10):1327–9.

91 Taylor CL, Dutton K, Rappard G, Pride GL, Replogle R, Purdy PD *et al.* Complications of preoperative embolization of cerebral arteriovenous malformations. *J Neurosurg* 2004; **100**(5):810–12.

92 Hartmann A, Mast H, Mohr JP, Pile-Spellman J, Connolly ES, Sciacca RR *et al.* Determinants of staged endovascular and surgical treatment outcome of brain arteriovenous malformations. *Stroke* 2005; **36**(11):2431–5.

93 Wikholm G, Lundqvist C, Svendsen P. The Goteborg cohort of embolized cerebral arteriovenous malformations: a 6-year follow-up. *Neurosurgery* 2001; **49**(4):799–805.

94 Hartmann A, Pile-Spellman J, Stapf C, Sciacca RR, Faulstich A, Mohr JP *et al.* Risk of endovascular treatment of brain arteriovenous malformations. *Stroke* 2002; **33**(7):1816–20.

95 Haw CS, TerBrugge K, Willinsky R, Tomlinson G. Complications of embolization of arteriovenous malformations of the brain. *J Neurosurg* 2006; **104**(2):226–32.

96 Ogilvy CS. Radiation therapy for arteriovenous malformations: a review. *Neurosurgery* 1990; **26**(5):725–35.

97 Friedman WA, Bova FJ, Bollampally S, Bradshaw P. Analysis of factors predictive of success or complications in arteriovenous malformation radiosurgery. *Neurosurgery* 2003; **52**(2):296–307.

98 Pollock BE. Stereotactic radiosurgery for arteriovenous malformations. *Neurosurg Clin N Am* 1999; **10**(2):281–90.

99 Maruyama K, Kawahara N, Shin M, Tago M, Kishimoto J, Kurita H *et al.* The risk of hemorrhage after radiosurgery for cerebral arteriovenous malformations. *N Engl J Med* 2005; **352**(2):146–53.

100 Nataf F, Ghossoub M, Schlienger M, Moussa R, Meder JF, Roux FX. Bleeding after radiosurgery for cerebral arteriovenous malformations. *Neurosurgery* 2004; **55**(2):298–305.

101 Shin M, Kawahara N, Maruyama K, Tago M, Ueki K, Kirino T. Risk of hemorrhage from an arteriovenous malformation confirmed to have been obliterated on angiography after stereotactic radiosurgery. *J Neurosurg* 2005; **102**(5):842–6.

102 Flickinger JC, Kondziolka D, Lunsford LD, Pollock BE, Yamamoto M, Gorman DA *et al.* A multi-institutional analysis of complication outcomes after arteriovenous malformation radiosurgery. *Int J Radiat Oncol Biol Phys* 1999; **44**(1):67–74.

103 Pollock BE, Brown RD, Jr. Management of cysts arising after radiosurgery to treat intracranial arteriovenous malformations. *Neurosurgery* 2001; **49**(2):259–64.

104 Boyd MC, Steinbok P, Paty DW. Familial arteriovenous malformations. Report of four cases in one family. *J Neurosurg* 1985; **62**(4):597–9.

105 Larsen PD, Hellbusch LC, Lefkowitz DM, Schaefer GB. Cerebral arteriovenous malformation in three successive generations. *Pediatr Neurol* 1997; **17**(1):74–6.

106 Snead OC, III, Acker JD, Morawetz R. Familial arteriovenous malformation. *Ann Neurol* 1979; **5**(6):585–7.

107 Herzig R, Burval S, Vladyka V, Janouskova L, Krivanek P, Krupka B *et al.* Familial occurrence of cerebral arteriovenous malformation in sisters: case report and review of the literature. *Eur J Neurol* 2000; **7**(1):95–100.

108 Kamiryo T, Nelson PK, Bose A, Zalzal P, Jafar JJ. Familial arteriovenous malformations in siblings. *Surg Neurol* 2000; **53**(3):255–9.

109 Goto S, Abe M, Tsuji T, Tabuchi K. Familial arteriovenous malformations of the brain: two case reports. *Neurol Med Chir (Tokyo)* 1994; **34**(4):221–4.

110 Frishberg BM. Neuroimaging in presumed primary headache disorders. *Semin Neurol* 1997; **17**(4):373–82.

Preventing recurrent stroke and other serious vascular events

16.1 General approach to preventing recurrent stroke and other serious vascular events

16.1.1 What are we trying to prevent?

This chapter deals with the long-term prevention of recurrent vascular events among patients with a prior ischaemic stroke, transient ischaemic attack (TIA) or intracerebral haemorrhage. Specific treatment of acute ischaemic stroke, intracerebral haemorrhage and sub-arachnoid haemorhage, treatment of the rare causes of stroke, and specific strategies for the prevention of intra-cranial haemorrhage are covered in Chapters 7, 12–15.

Patients with stroke and TIA are not just at high risk of stroke, but also of myocardial infarction, lower limb ischaemia, and cognitive impairment due to vascular disease of the brain. Doctors caring for patients with stroke therefore need to pay attention to the heart and peripheral vascular tree not just in their clinical examination but also when deciding on treatments for secondary prevention. Indeed, many trials and systematic reviews of drug and lifestyle interventions for prevention after stroke or TIA have focused primarily on the prevention of 'serious vascular events', usually defined as the combination of stroke, myocardial infarction and death from vascular causes. We too will focus largely on this outcome cluster, since it captures most serious recurrent vascular events from which patients with stroke or TIA are at risk. However, it omits the serious consequences of lower limb ischaemia (such as gangrene or amputation) and the cognitive impairment and

Stroke: practical management, 3rd edition. C. Warlow, J. van Gijn, M. Dennis, J. Wardlaw, J. Bamford, G. Hankey, P. Sandercock, G. Rinkel, P. Langhorne, C. Sudlow and P. Rothwell. Published 2008 Blackwell Publishing. ISBN 978-1-4051-2766-0.

consequent disability resulting from vascular dementia (section 11.29.2). Reducing the risk of these additional outcomes is clearly also very important, and a number of the more recent trials of interventions that primarily aim to prevent recurrent stroke and other serious vascular events (such as blood pressure reduction and cholesterol reduction) have sought or are seeking to determine whether the intervention also reduces the frequency and severity of cognitive impairment due to cerebrovascular disease (see relevant section on each of the specific interventions).

Although primary prevention of stroke is not the main subject of this chapter, we have included here a discussion of the evidence for using various interventions for people with no prior history of stroke or TIA, and sometimes for those with no history of vascular disease at all, since it makes sense to discuss this alongside the evidence for these same interventions in secondary prevention.

16.1.2 Evidence from randomized trials and systematic reviews

As in the other chapters of this book, we will try to base our treatment recommendations on the best available evidence, using information from randomized controlled trials (RCTs) and systematic reviews of these wherever possible (section 12.2.1). Sometimes, however, no relevant RCTs are available and we have to make treatment decisions and recommendations by extrapolating the evidence from RCTs conducted in other patient groups (but not those with a stroke or TIA), or by relying on other sources such as observational studies, clinical reasoning, pathophysiology, common sense or anecdotal experience.

16.1.3 Relative and absolute effects of treatment

It is important to emphasize that the decision whether or not to use a particular preventive treatment should be based on the *absolute* rather than *relative* benefit of that treatment (and, likewise, on the absolute rather than relative increase in any serious risks) (section 12.2.1 and Table 12.5). For example, for patients whose absolute risk of stroke in the next year is 2%, a treatment which reduces the relative risk of stroke by 50% will reduce the absolute risk to 1%, yielding an absolute benefit of 1%, or 10 strokes avoided per 1000 patients treated, so 100 (1000/10) patients have to be treated for 1 year to prevent one stroke. On the other hand, if the same treatment is given to patients whose untreated risk of stroke in the next year is five times higher, 10%, the same relative risk reduction will reduce the absolute risk to 5%, an absolute reduction of 5%, or 50 strokes avoided per 1000

patients treated. Only 20 (1000/50) of these high-risk patients have to be treated for 1 year to prevent one stroke.

The relative effect of a particular treatment on a particular outcome is usually consistent across subgoups of patients at different levels of untreated absolute risk. This is not invariably the case, particularly when the outcome under consideration is a composite one, made up of several different component outcomes, and especially if the risk of some of these is increased and of others is decreased by treatment. It usually holds true, however, if the benefits and risks of treatment are considered separately.[1] Thus, if we know the relative effect of a treatment on an outcome, we can calculate the absolute benefit for any particular patient, so long as we know (or can estimate) what their untreated risk of the outcome is. Similarly, if we consider adverse effects of treatment, if we know both the relative increased risk from treatment and our patient's untreated risk, we can calculate the absolute excess risk of any important adverse effect. It is the balance of absolute benefit on the one hand, and absolute risk of adverse effects on the other, that will determine the absolute net benefit of treatment in a particular patient or group of patients. The size of this net benefit will then help to determine whether or not taking the treatment is worthwhile. To make sensible treatment decisions, it is therefore essential to know something of the likely prognosis for our patients (section 16.2). Other factors, such as the costs of treatment, whether or not the treatment is available, and the patient's attitudes and preferences will also contribute to the decision-making process.

16.2 Prognosis and prediction of future vascular events

The prognosis for early death and disability after stroke has been discussed in section 10.2. This section describes the early and long-term prognosis of patients with transient ischaemic attacks (TIAs) and stroke for important future vascular events that might be prevented by appropriate treatment strategies, particularly recurrent stroke but also myocardial infarction and death. As highlighted in section 10.2, much of the information we have about the prognosis of these patients comes from following large cohorts of patients over time. The most informative studies of prognosis are those adhering to the criteria set out in Table 10.2. But, because the prognosis of an individual patient may vary considerably from the average prognosis of all patients (because of their different underlying causes of the TIA/stroke and different comorbidities, etc. – see below), we also discuss ways in which the risk of particular individual patients might be more accurately predicted, allowing us to answer the question 'What is the risk of another important vascular event for *this* patient?' and thereby to be able to identify the appropriate goals and treatments for an individual patient.

16.2.1 Prognosis early after transient ischaemic attack and mild ischaemic stroke

High early risk of stroke after a transient ischaemic attack or mild ischaemic stroke

About 20% of patients with stroke have a preceding transient ischaemic attack (TIA), and a similar proportion of major ischaemic strokes are preceded by minor ones. These 'warning' events provide an opportunity for prevention, and evidence is accumulating for the beneficial effects of various interventions very early after a TIA or mild (i.e. non-disabling) ischaemic stroke (sections 16.3 to 16.6 and chapter 12). Patients with TIA and mild ischaemic stroke are not only similar in terms of age, sex and prevalence of coexistent vascular diseases and risk factors, but they also have a similar (albeit not identical) early and long-term prognosis for recurrent stroke and other vascular events and will therefore be considered together.[2–6]

Recent studies have shown that the very early risk of stroke after a TIA or mild ischaemic stroke is much higher than previously thought.[7,8] Two emergency-department-based studies of TIA in California and Alberta reported cumulative risks of stroke at 30 days of about 7% and at 90 days of about 10%.[9,10] In one of the studies, almost half of the 90-day strokes occurred within the first 2 days.[10] Two prospective, community-based cohort studies in Oxfordshire, UK, one in the 1980s and the other in 2002–2004, found even higher cumulative stroke risks from the date of onset of first-ever TIA of about 8% at 7 days, 12% at 30 days and 17% at 90 days. The cumulative risks of recurrent stroke early after a mild ischaemic stroke in the 2002–2004 Oxfordshire study were similar: 12% at 7 days, 15% at 30 days and 18% at 90 days (Fig. 16.1, Table 16.1). These risk estimates were hardly affected by excluding patients who had a TIA or mild ischaemic stroke during the study period but did not seek medical attention until they had a subsequent stroke.[2] A further population-based study in patients with a TIA in the USA found very similar risks to those reported in Oxfordshire.[11] Four studies which reported the timing of preceding TIAs in a total of about 2500 patients with stroke found that 23% gave a history

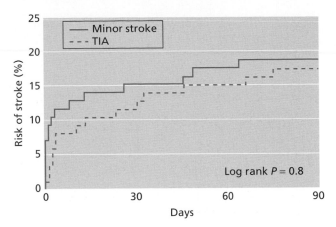

Fig. 16.1 Cumulative early risk of stroke after a transient ischaemic attack (TIA) or mild ischaemic stroke in the Oxford Vascular Study. (Reprinted from Coull *et al.*[2] © 2004 with permission of BMJ Publishing Group.)

of prior TIA, of which 17% occurred on the day of the stroke and 43% within the previous week (Fig. 16.2).[12] The implication of all these studies is that the risk of stroke early after a TIA or mild ischaemic stroke is very high, suggesting that assessment and preventive interventions should start very quickly indeed.[7]

> The early risk of stroke after a transient ischaemic attack or mild ischaemic stroke is very high. Cumulative risks are up to about 10% at 1 week, 14% at 1 month, and 18% at 3 months, so assessment and preventive interventions must start very quickly.

Predicting the early risk of stroke after a TIA or mild ischaemic stroke in individual patients

Two of the above studies have shown that the clinical features of a TIA provide substantial prognostic information, and the authors have produced simple risk scores to allow doctors more accurately to assess the likely risk of early stroke for individual patients. In the California emergency department cohort, increasing age, longer symptom duration, motor weakness, speech impairment and diabetes independently increased the risk of stroke at 90 days.[10] In the Oxfordshire community-based cohorts, the independent predictors of stroke risk at 7 days were the same, with the addition of increased blood pressure.[13] Both groups developed simple scoring systems suitable for everyday clinical practice, and both scores have subsequently been validated and shown to perform well in several independent population-based, clinic-based and emergency-department-based data sets.[14] A further score, based on the variables included in the California and Oxfordshire ABCD scores, the ABCD²

	Hospital-referred	Community-based
After TIA or mild ischaemic stroke		
Death		
Average annual risk	5%	8%
Stroke		
In 1st week	—	10%
In 1st month	7%	14%
In 1st 3 months	10%	18%
In 1st year	15%	at least 20%
In each subsequent year†	3%	6%
Myocardial infarction		
Average annual risk	2%	2%
After any ischaemic stroke		
Death		
In 1st month	—	10–20%
In 1st year	—	25%
In each subsequent year	—	7%
Stroke		
In 1st year	—	at least 10–15%
In each subsequent year	—	4–5%
Myocardial infarction		
Average annual risk	2%	2%
After intracerebral haemorrhage		
Death		
In 1st month	—	42%
Average annual risk thereafter	—	8%
Stroke		
Average annual risk	4%	6%
Myocardial infarction	—	—

Table 16.1 Approximate absolute average risks of death, stroke, and myocardial infarction after transient ischaemic attack (TIA) or mild ischaemic stroke, any ischaemic stroke, and intracerebral haemorrhage.*

*Data from: Johnston *et al.*, 2000;[10] Hill *et al.*, 2004;[9] Coull *et al.*, 2004;[2] Hankey and Warlow, 1994;[19] Touzé *et al.*, 2005;[20] van Wijk *et al.*, 2005;[5] Feigin *et al.*, 2003;[26] Dennis *et al.*, 1993;[27] Petty *et al.*, 1998;[29] Hardie *et al.*, 2003;[28] Dennis *et al.*, 2003;[55] Counsell *et al.*, 1995;[57] Bailey *et al.*, 2001.[60]

†Risks from Hankey and Warlow, 1994,[19] adjusted downwards slightly to allow for overestimation caused by inclusion of higher-risk period in first year.

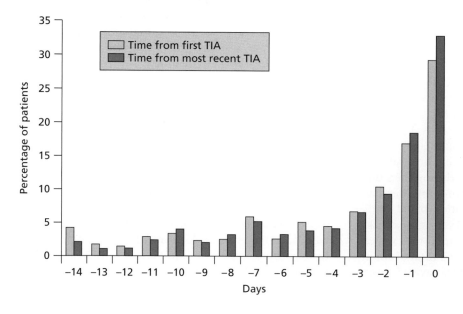

Fig. 16.2 Distribution of time from preceding transient ischaemic attack to stroke for patients who reported a transient ischaemic attack (TIA) within the previous 14 days of a stroke. (From Rothwell and Warlow, 2005.[12]) (Figs 16.2, 16.3, 16.6–16.8 & 16.12 reprinted with permission from Lippincott, Williams & Wilkins.)

Table 16.2 Independent risk factors and scoring systems for early stroke risk after transient ischaemic attack (TIA) derived from an emergency department cohort of patients with TIA in the USA (California score), a population-based study of TIA in the UK (Oxfordshire ABCD score), and a combination of both cohorts (ABCD^2 score).*

Risk factor	Points for score
California score (stroke risk at 90 days)	
Age ≥ 60 years	1
Clinical features	
Unilateral weakness	1
Speech disturbance	1
Duration of symptoms ≥ 10 minutes	1
Diabetes	1
Oxfordshire 'ABCD' score (stroke risk at 7 days)	
Age ≥ 60 years	1
Blood pressure	
Systolic > 140 and/or diastolic ≥ 90 mmHg	1
Clinical features	
Unilateral weakness	2
Speech disturbance without weakness	1
Other	0
Duration of symptoms	
≥ 60 min	2
10–59 min	1
< 10 min	0
Combined ABCD^2 score (stroke risk at 2 days)	
Age ≥ 60 years	1
Blood pressure	
Systolic > 140 and/or diastolic ≥ 90 mmHg	1
Clinical features	
Unilateral weakness	2
Speech disturbance without weakness	1
Other	0
Duration of symptoms	
≥ 60 min	2
10–59 min	1
< 10 min	0
Diabetes	1

*Data from Johnston *et al.*, 2000;[10] Rothwell *et al.*, 2005;[13] Johnston *et al.*, 2007.[14]

score, was found to be slightly better at predicting risk at 2 days and also performed well at 7 and 90 days (Tables 16.2 and 16.3).[14] In fact, these scores may predict subsequent stroke risk simply because patients with higher scores are more likely to have actually had a TIA than those with lower scores. However they work, any one of them is a potentially very useful tool for identifying groups of patients with a diagnosis of TIA who are at particularly high risk, and who merit immediate evaluation, further investigation, possibly admission to hospital, and urgent intervention with preventive strategies.[14]

Other clinical features may also help in the prediction of early stroke risk, allowing these scoring systems to be further refined. For example, the early risk of stroke after transient or permanent monocular blindness due to ischaemia is lower than after cerebral TIAs, and a systematic review and meta-analysis of cohort studies demonstrated that the early risk after vertebrobasilar territory TIAs is probably higher than after carotid territory events.[15] The early risk also depends on the vascular pathology. A recent meta-analysis of 1700 patients with a first-ever stroke in four population-based studies showed that the risks of recurrent stroke were highest in those with large artery atherothrombotic strokes and lowest in those with lacunar ischaemic stroke due to small vessel disease (Fig. 16.3).[16] However, these ischaemic stroke subtype differences may well be less marked in patients with TIA, partly because it is more difficult to categorize TIA patients than strokes and so bias is introduced, and also because some patients with lacunar TIAs have a very high risk of subsequent stroke, the so-called 'capsular warning syndrome'.[17] The presence of infarction on a CT or diffusion-weighted MR brain scan increases the risk of stroke after a TIA or mild ischaemic stroke, while detection of cerebral microemboli might predict risk in patients with large artery atherothrombotic disease.[7,17,18] Novel biomarkers may also help in risk prediction. Further research is needed to assess whether these various characteristics add independent prognostic value to the existing – and remarkably good – predictive models.[7]

Table 16.3 Stroke risks at 2, 7 and 90 days after transient ischaemic attack in patients at low, moderate and high risk according to the ABCD^2 score. Data are from a total of 4799 patients in the California and Oxfordshire derivation cohorts and four California and Oxfordshire validation cohorts.*

Risk level	ABCD^2 score	Patients (*n*)	Risk at 2 days (no. strokes)	Risk at 7 days (no. strokes)	Risk at 90 days (no. strokes)
Low	0–3	1628	1.0% (17)	1.2% (19)	3.1% (50)
Moderate	4–5	2159	4.1% (89)	5.9% (128)	9.8% (211)
High	6–7	1012	8.1% (82)	11.7% (118)	17.8% (180)

*Data from Johnston *et al.*, 2007.[14]

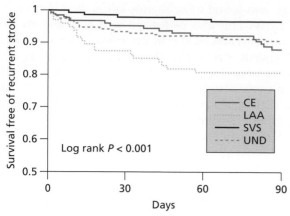

Actuarial recurrent stroke risks (95% CI)

	At 7 days	At 1 month	At 3 months
SVS	0%	2.0% (0–4.2)	3.4% (0.5–6.3)
CE	2.5% (0.1–4.9)	4.6% (1.3–7.9)	11.9% (6.4–17.4)
UND	2.3% (0.5–4.1)	6.5% (3.6–9.6)	9.3% (5.6–13.0)
LAA	4.0% (0.2–7.8)	12.6% (5.9–19.3)	19.2% (11.2–27.2)

Fig. 16.3 Three-month survival free of recurrent stroke by Trial of ORG 10172 in Acute Stroke Treatment (TOAST) sub type for patients in the Oxford Vascular Study and the Oxfordshire Community Stroke Project. CE, cardioembolic; LAA, large-artery atherosclerosis; SVS, small-vessel stroke; UND, undetermined. The corresponding actuarial risks of recurrent stroke in each subtype are given below the figure with 95% confidence intervals. (From Lovett *et al.*, 2004.[16])

> Simple clinical features of a transient ischaemic attack (such as patient age, blood pressure, neurological deficit and duration of symptoms) can help predict which patients are at highest risk of stroke in the first few days, weeks and months after onset.

16.2.2 Longer-term prognosis after transient ischaemic attack or mild ischaemic stroke

While many studies of prognosis after a transient ischaemic attack (TIA) or mild ischaemic stroke underestimated the very early risk of stroke, they still provide very useful information on the longer-term prognosis. Data from studies that more or less fulfil the criteria for an ideal prognostic study (Table 10.2) have shown approximate average annual risks over the first 5 years as follows (Table 16.1):[19]

- *Death*: about 8% per year in community-based studies (about 1.4 times greater than individuals of the same age and sex without a TIA), and about 5% per year in hospital-referred cohorts. About 40% of deaths after

TIA are due to ischaemic heart disease, 25% to stroke, 5% to other vascular events such as ruptured aortic aneurysm and 30% to non-vascular disorders.

- *Stroke*: about 7% per year in community-based studies (about 7 times greater than individuals of the same age and sex without a TIA), and about 4% per year in hospital-referred cohorts. Most of these strokes are ischaemic and about two-thirds are major disabling strokes.
- *Myocardial infarction*: about 2% per year in community and hospital-referred cohort studies.[20]
- *Vascular events (stroke, myocardial infarction or vascular death)*: about 10% per year in community-based studies and about 8% per year in hospital-referred cohorts.

For stroke, we know that the early risk is particularly high (section 16.2.1). Of the studies that have provided reliable data on early risk (section 16.2.1), only one hospital-based TIA cohort study reported results beyond the first few months, and found a risk of stroke of about 15% at 1 year. This may have been an underestimate, since strokes in the first 24 h were excluded and follow-up depended on administrative data alone.[9] The first-year stroke risk in community-based studies is bound to be higher than this and probably in excess of 20%, since by 3 months the risk is already 17–18% (section 16.2.1).[2] Therefore, the average annual risks given above substantially underestimate the risks of stroke (and so of vascular events) in the first year and, by incorporating some of the early high risk, slightly overestimate the risks of these outcomes from year 2 onwards.

Prospective follow-up data for about 10 years have recently been published for a cohort of around 2500 patients recruited within 3 months of a mild ischaemic stroke or TIA into a factorial randomized trial of different aspirin doses and of atenolol vs placebo (the Dutch TIA trial). The average annual risks of a death, stroke and other vascular events in the first few years were slightly lower than those reported above for hospital-referred cohorts.[5] This is consistent with previous observations, and reflects the slightly lower age and generally rather better prognosis of patients recruited into trials.[21] The longer-term follow-up in this study showed that the relatively high early annual stroke risk fell over the first few years to around 1–2% after the fourth year, annual mortality increased gradually with time from less than 4% to 7–8% by the tenth year of follow-up, and the annual risk of a vascular event fell from about 7% to about 3.5% over the first 3 years and then rose steadily thereafter to around 7% by year 10 (Fig. 16.4).[5] A long-term follow-up study of 290 patients with a previous TIA, who had originally been recruited into either a community-based or hospital-based cohort in Oxfordshire and had survived free of stroke for a median of 3.8 years from their most

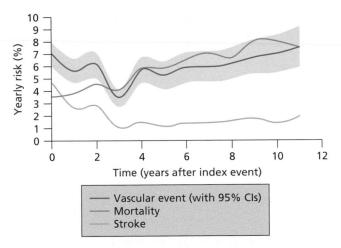

Fig. 16.4 Annual risks of death, stroke and vascular events over time in a cohort of transient ischaemic attack and mild ischaemic stroke patients recruited into a randomized trial. (Reprinted from van Wijk *et al. Lancet*[5] © 2005 with permission from Elsevier)

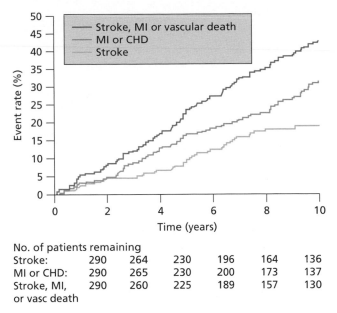

No. of patients remaining						
Stroke:	290	264	230	196	164	136
MI or CHD:	290	265	230	200	173	137
Stroke, MI, or vasc death	290	260	225	189	157	130

Fig. 16.5 Kaplan–Meier event rates for any stroke, any myocardial infarction (MI) or death from coronary heart disease (CHD), and any stroke, myocardial infarction, or vascular death among patients with a prior transient ischaemic attack (from the Oxfordshire Community Stroke Project and a contemporaneous hospital-referred series of TIA patients) and a median of 3.8 years between their most recent transient ischaemic attack and the start of follow-up. (From Clark *et al.*[22] © 2005 BMJ Publishing Group.)

recent TIA and were therefore selected to be at low stroke risk, found constant risks up to 10 years of about 2% per year for stroke, 3% per year for myocardial infarction or death attributable to coronary heart disease and 4% per year for vascular events (Fig. 16.5).[22]

The message from these studies is that, although the very high early risk of stroke after TIA or mild ischaemic stroke falls to a constant, lower rate after the first few months, the annual risks of myocardial infarction and of all vascular events remain constant, or even increase, with long-term follow-up. The implication is that, after preventive efforts are started early, they need to be sustained in the long term.

> After a transient ischaemic attack or mild ischaemic stroke, the very high early risk of stroke falls to a constant lower rate after the first few months, while the annual risks of myocardial infarction and of all vascular events remain constant, or even increase, with long-term follow-up. Preventive efforts must therefore be started early and sustained long term.

Predicting long-term prognosis after transient ischaemic attack or mild ischaemic stroke in individual patients

Several large cohort studies have identified independent predictors of the long-term risks of vascular outcomes after transient ischaemic attack (TIA) or mild ischaemic stroke, and three predictive models have been developed and validated in independent data sets to allow more refined estimates of the risks in individual patients.[1,23–25] The predictive variables used in these three models are shown in Table 16.4. The predicted risks can be calculated using information in the original publications; online versions of two of the models are available (Table 16.4) allowing rapid calculation of predicted risk; and for the model specifically developed to predict the risk of ipsilateral ischaemic stroke in patients with recently symptomatic carotid stenosis being considered for surgery, a simplified version using a set of coloured charts is available (section 16.11.8 and Fig. 16.46), similar to those used for prediction of cardiovascular risk in primary care (section 18.5.1).

Although the variables included in these predictive models vary, because of differences between studies in the variables available for modelling, the types of patients included, the outcomes predicted and the precise statistical methods used, it is striking that the variables are largely those available from the clinical history, with just a few from clinical examination and investigations. Modelling of long-term risk of stroke, death and vascular events in the Dutch TIA trial also showed the predictive power of the history alone. Simply documenting the patient's age, sex, history of myocardial infarction, diabetes, hypertension and peripheral artery disease provided almost as much information about the risk of a

Table 16.4 Variables used in prediction models for long-term outcome after transient ischaemic attack (TIA) or mild ischaemic stroke.*

Derivation cohort	Test cohorts	Outcomes predicted	Predictive variables increasing risk in model	Website for online version
469 patients with hospital-referred TIAs	1653 TIA patients in the UK-TIA trial 107 TIA patients in the Oxfordshire Community Stroke Project	5-year risks of: – stroke – coronary events – vascular events (stroke, MI or vascular death)	Increasing age Male sex Cerebral *vs* only ocular TIAs Carotid and vertebrobasilar TIAs Increasing number of TIAs in preceding 3 months Peripheral vascular disease Left ventricular hypertrophy (ECG) Residual neurological signs (Ischaemic heart disease – only in coronary events model)	www.dcn.ed.ac.uk/model/models.asp
525 female patients with TIA or mild ischaemic stroke in the WEST trial	2449 patients in the UK-TIA trial 6431 prior ischaemic stroke patients in the CAPRIE trial 340 ischaemic stroke and TIA patients in the population-based NoMaSS study	2-year risk of stroke or death	Congestive heart failure Diabetes mellitus Prior stroke Age > 70 years Stroke (not TIA) Severe hypertension Coronary artery disease	—
1211 medically treated patients with recent TIA or mild ischaemic stroke and 0–99% ipsilateral carotid stenosis in the ESCT trial†	759 medically treated patients with recent TIA or mild ischaemic stroke and 50–99% ipsilateral carotid stenosis in the NASCET trial†	5-year risk of ipsilateral carotid territory ischaemic stroke	Increasing ipsilateral carotid stenosis or near occlusion‡ Male sex Increasing age Time since last event (risk decreases with time) Nature of presenting event (major stroke vs minor stroke vs multiple TIAs vs single TIAs vs ocular attacks only) Diabetes mellitus Previous myocardial infarction Peripheral vascular disease Treated hypertension Irregular/ulcerated plaque (on carotid angiography)	www.stroke.ox.ac.uk

*Data from: Hankey *et al.*, 1992[23]; Hankey *et al.*, 1993[24]; Kernan *et al.*, 2000[25]; Rothwell *et al.*, 2005.[1]

†% stenosis measured using the NASCET criteria.

‡Near occlusion reduces risk compared with increasing stenosis above 50%.

TIA, transient ischaemic attack; MI, myocardial infarction; ECG, electrocardiogram; WEST, Women's Estrogen to prevent Stroke Trial; UK-TIA, United Kingdom Transient Ischaemic Attack trial; CAPRIE, Clopidogrel versus Aspirin in Patients at Risk of Ischaemic Events trial; NoMaSS, Northern Manhattan Stroke Study; ECST, European carotid Surgery Trial; NASCET, North American Symptomatic Carotid Endarterectomy Trial.

future event as adding the results of the examination findings and diagnostic procedures such as CT scan and ECG.[5] Thus, as discussed for very early risk prediction (section 16.2.1), to further improve existing models of risk prediction, we need to know whether extra variables, such as cerebral microemboli, brain imaging findings, and so on, have *additional* predictive value.

> Simple clinical features can help predict an individual patient's long-term risk of stroke and other vascular events after a transient ischaemic attack or mild ischaemic stroke.

16.2.3 Prognosis after all severities of ischaemic stroke

The prognosis for death and disability in the first few months after acute ischaemic stroke has been discussed in section 10.2. Older cohort studies of the *long-term* prognosis after stroke generally reported results for all types of stroke combined, often because brain imaging was not performed on a large proportion of the patients so that the pathological type of stroke (ischaemic or haemorrhagic) could not be assigned accurately. Because most strokes are ischaemic in type, the results of these studies mainly reflect the prognosis of ischaemic stroke. However, several studies in which a much larger proportion of patients had brain imaging early enough after their stroke to allow a pathological diagnosis have reported outcome up to several years after stroke, and some of these have also reported data on ischaemic stroke subtypes.

Death after any ischaemic stroke

Community-based studies of first-ever strokes from 1990 onwards have reported a risk of dying in the first month after ischaemic stroke of 10–20%[26] (Table 16.1). Predictors and causes of early case fatality have been discussed in section 10.2. About one-quarter of ischaemic stroke patients in community-based studies in white patients were dead within 1 year of their stroke, about half by 5 years, and over three-quarters by 10 years. The risk of dying is highest in the first year, and thereafter falls to about 6–7% per year, similar to the long-term annual risk of death after a TIA (Fig. 16.6 and Table 16.1) (section 16.2.2).[27–29] Although deaths related to the index stroke are commonest in the first month, in the longer term deaths from recurrent stroke, cardiac disease and non-vascular causes become increasingly important (Fig. 16.7).[27,28,30–32]

Early after ischaemic stroke, the risk of death is highest in those with cardioembolic stroke and lowest in those

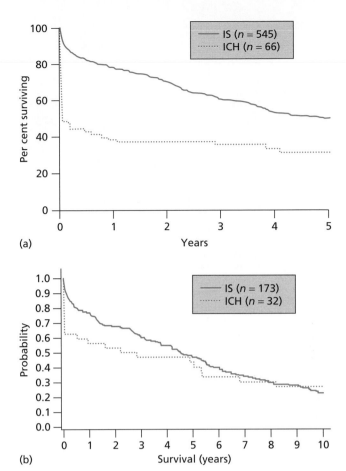

Fig. 16.6 Kaplan-Meier curves showing probability of survival over long-term follow-up stratified by the pathology of first-ever stroke in (a) the Oxfordshire Community Stroke Project, UK and (b) the Perth Community Stroke Study, Australia; IS, ischaematic stroke; ICH, intracerebral haemorrhage. (From Dennis *et al.*, 1993[27] and Hardie *et al.*, 2003.[28])

with lacunar stroke. Most of this difference between ischaemic subtypes occurs in the first month, probably as a result of larger infarct size and higher stroke recurrence risk among the non-lacunar subtypes. Beyond the first month, the difference in risk of dying between ischaemic subtypes attenuates, but the early difference means that the risk of being dead by 5 years is about 80% after cardioembolic stroke, about 50% after ischaemic stroke of uncertain cause, and about one-third after large artery (atherothrombotic) or lacunar stroke, although these risks are generally lower in hospital-based series (Figs 16.8 and 16.9).[30,33–35]

Increasing age, initial infarct severity (of which ischaemic subtype is one important indicator), stroke recurrence, cardiovascular and respiratory comorbidities, and seizures appear to be independent predictors of death at any time after ischaemic stroke.[31]

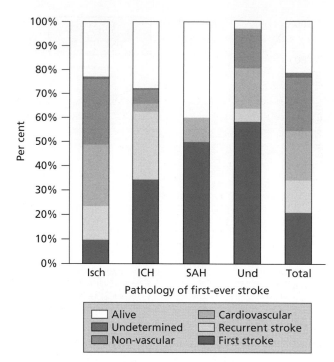

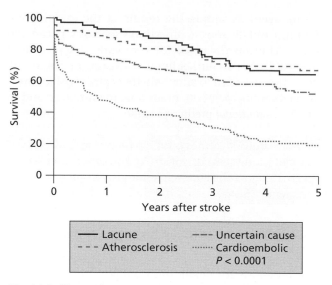

Fig. 16.8 Observed percentage surviving (Kaplan-Meier estimates) after incident ischaemic stroke among 442 residents of Rochester, Minnesota, 1985–1989, by ischaemic stroke subtype. (From Petty *et al.*, 2000.[35])

Fig. 16.7 Histogram showing cause of death and survival patterns over 10 years stratified by the pathology of first-ever stroke. Data are from the Perth Community Stroke Study, Australia. Isch, ischaemic stroke; ICH, intraceberal haemorrhage; SAH, subarachnoid haemorrhage; Und, unknown pathology. (From Hardie *et al.*, 2003.[28])

Recurrent stroke after any ischaemic stroke

As discussed for TIA and mild ischaemic stroke, varying definitions of recurrent stroke in different studies mean that many underestimate the recurrence risk in the first

year after any ischaemic stroke, but all studies still show a much higher risk during the first year (mainly confined to the first month) and an average annual risk of about 4–5% per year thereafter, similar to the longer-term risk after a TIA or mild ischaemic stroke (Table 16.1). As we saw above (section 16.2.2), the early recurrence risk is substantially higher after large artery atherothrombotic ischaemic stroke than lacunar stroke, with cardioembolic stroke and other types of ischaemic stroke intermediate between these two. In the longer term, however, this difference attenuates (Figs 16.3 and 16.9). The

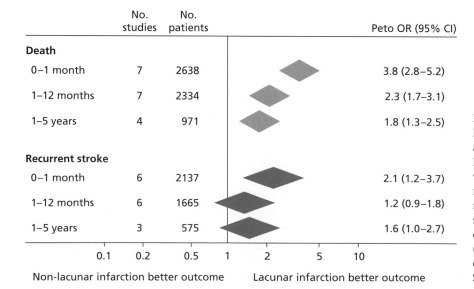

Fig. 16.9 Pooled odds ratios (OR) (non-lacunar vs lacunar ischaemic stroke) from a meta-analysis of community and hospital-based inception cohort studies with available data on death and recurrent stroke at 1 month, 1–12 months, and 1–5 years after ischaemic stroke. The pooled ORs are represented by diamonds, with 95% confidence intervals (CI) represented by the width of the diamonds. (Data from Jackson and Sudlow, 2005.[33])

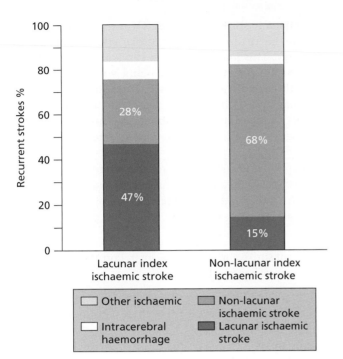

Fig. 16.10 Pooled data from prospective studies of recurrent stroke subtypes following lacunar and non-lacunar ischaemic stroke at baseline. Total number of recurrent strokes among lacunar patients = 279, and among non-lacunar patients = 117. Other ischaemic = unclassified ischaemic recurrences; ICH, intracerebral haemorrhage. (Reprinted from Jackson and Sudlow[33] © 2005 with permission of Oxford University Press.)

particularly high risk early after larger artery atherothrombotic stroke may be due to the presence of unstable atherosclerotic plaque causing artery-to-artery embolism, with the risk falling when the plaque endothelializes or 'stabilizes' in some other way.[36]

At least three-quarters of recurrent strokes after an ischaemic stroke are ischaemic again. However, the true figure may be as high as 90% or more, since in most studies the proportion of recurrent strokes of uncertain pathological type was rather high, and most of these were probably ischaemic.[35,37–40] There is also some evidence that recurrent ischaemic strokes tend to be of the same subtype as the index stroke (Fig. 16.10).[33,41,42] However, potential biases mean that the data should be interpreted cautiously. Distinguishing between genuine stroke recurrence and other causes of neurological worsening, especially when the symptoms and or signs are similar to those from the index stroke, can be very difficult, definitions of stroke recurrence vary between studies, and assigning a precise pathological type and subtype is also very challenging.[8] Of course, modern brain imaging techniques, in particular diffusion-weighted magnetic resonance imaging (DW-MRI) (section 5.5.2), are very helpful, but very few studies of recurrent stroke

so far have used MRI, and none DWI. Furthermore, even when state-of-the-art imaging is readily available, patients with recurrent stroke may not be admitted to hospital, or may be to too unwell for – or have other contraindications to – MR scanning.[33]

Relatively few studies have assessed independent predictors of recurrent stroke in the long term after any ischaemic stroke, but several have assessed these after any stroke (i.e. of all pathological types). The most consistent predictor is age, with previous stroke, initial stroke severity, stroke subtype, ischaemic heart disease, atrial fibrillation, increased blood pressure, diabetes and smoking also emerging in several studies.[30,37,38,40,43–47] We are not aware of any validated models for predicting recurrent stroke or other vascular outcomes in individual patients after any ischaemic stroke, although earlier we have discussed prediction models for patients with TIA or mild ischaemic stroke (section 16.2.2).

There have been a number of studies specifically assessing risk of recurrent stroke after ischaemic stroke in young patients (under 50 years). The numbers of recurrences have generally been very small, making their estimates imprecise, but all have found much lower risks of recurrence than in older patients, particularly in those with no identified cause or risk factors for ischaemic stroke.[48–54] Therefore, secondary preventive interventions may not be appropriate for this group of very low-risk young patients, but the identification of precisely which young patients in this low-risk group should or should not receive preventive treatments needs more precise information than is currently available. Probably the only way to achieve this would be by pooled analysis of individual patient data sets from many different centres, since single-centre studies will never be able to accrue sufficient numbers of patients and outcome events for precise estimates.

Myocardial infarction after any ischaemic stroke

The risk of myocardial infarction after any ischaemic stroke is about 2% per year, the same as after a TIA or mild ischaemic stroke (Table 16.1).[20] There is no clear evidence of an initially high early risk as there is for recurrent stroke. Within the first month after ischaemic stroke, the risk of recurrent stroke is at least 2.5 times that of myocardial infarction, but thereafter the ratio falls to about two times. However, although recurrent strokes occur more commonly than cardiac events over the long term after an ischaemic stroke, cardiac mortality is about two times higher than stroke mortality from about 1 month onwards.[32] There is very little information on whether the risk of myocardial infarction after ischaemic stroke varies by ischaemic stroke subtype. What little information there is suggests that cardiac deaths occur with approximately equal frequency among the different ischaemic stroke subtypes, but even in a meta-analysis of data from all the available studies, numbers of events were limited, making the results imprecise.[33]

> After transient ischaemic attacks and ischaemic stroke it is important to recognize the risk of non-stroke vascular events such as myocardial infarction; indeed, coronary heart disease is a more likely cause of death than stroke in the long term.

> Like patients with a TIA or mild ischaemic stroke, patients with any ischaemic stroke remain at elevated risk of recurrent stroke and other serious vascular events for at least 10 years after their initial event, and so prevention efforts must also be sustained long term.

16.2.4 Prognosis after intracerebral haemorrhage

The prognosis for death and disability in the first few months after intracerebral haemorrhage (ICH) has been discussed in section 10.2. Here, we consider what is known about vascular events and death, both early on and in the long term after ICH.

Death after intracerebral haemorrhage

Community-based studies have shown a much higher early case fatality after ICH than after ischaemic stroke, with a pooled estimate of 42% dying within 1 month (Table 16.1). The relatively low incidence of ICH, which comprises between 10 and 20% of all first-ever strokes, at least in white populations where the incidence has been best studied, combined with the high early case fatality, means that the number of patients available for long-term follow-up in single centres is relatively small, making estimates from individual studies imprecise.[55] In addition, increasing use of brain imaging earlier after stroke is probably leading to an increased proportion of mild haemorrhages being diagnosed (section 5.2), so changing the nature of the cohorts being followed up.[56]

Factors associated with a high early case fatality are older age, clinical severity of the initial stroke, the size of the haematoma, the presence of intraventricular blood and anticoagulant treatment. Some of these, such as haematoma size, intraventricular blood and clinical severity, are correlated with each other and may not be independent outcome predictors.[55]

After the first month, the average annual risk of death is about 8% per year, similar to the long-term risk after an ischaemic stroke (Fig. 16.6). Over the long term, the survival curves for ischaemic stroke and ICH appear to converge. This may be due to a survival effect, with the longer-term survivors of ICH being younger and fitter than those with an index ischaemic stroke.[27,28,55,57,58] The main causes of death in 1-month survivors are the initial or a recurrent stroke (about one-third) and cardiac or other vascular causes (about one-quarter).[59]

> The risk of death in the first month after intracerebral haemorrhage, as currently diagnosed, is at least twice that for ischaemic stroke. Thereafter, the long-term risk of death appears similar to ischaemic stroke.

Recurrent stroke and myocardial infarction after intracerebral haemorrhage

A systematic review of studies reporting recurrent stroke after ICH analysed data from three community-based populations (including a total of 146 patients) and seven hospital-based cohorts (including a total of 1734 patients). Pooled recurrent stroke rates were 6.2% per year in the community-based studies and 4% per year in the hospital-based studies, similar to the recurrence rates after an ischaemic stroke (section 16.2.3). However, while most recurrences after ischaemic stroke are ischaemic again, over half (59%) of recurrences after ICH were haemorrhagic again, 26% were ischaemic and 15% were of uncertain pathology.[60]

> The long-term risk of recurrent stroke after intracerebral haemorrhage seems similar to that for ischaemic stroke (excluding the very high early risk after ischaemic stroke).

Unsurprisingly, the risk of recurrence seems to depend on the underlying cause of the initial haemorrhage. In younger patients, the commonest cause of ICH is an intracranial vascular malformation, and the specific recurrence risk is discussed in section 15.3. In studies which distinguished between deep and lobar haemorrhage, recurrence was about twice as frequent in the former group.[60] This may reflect the different predominant underlying causes in these different locations, with a preponderance of cerebral amyloid angiopathy thought to underly many lobar haemorrhages in older patients, and intracranial small vessel disease thought to be the vascular pathology causing most deep haemorrhages. Haemorrhages due to cerebral amyloid angiopathy are said to be particularly likely to recur.

Possession of an apolipoprotein E ε4 or ε2 allele may predispose to cerebral amyloid angiopathy and lobar ICH, and one study has demonstrated an increased risk of recurrent ICH in patients with lobar haemorrhage who are carriers of either the ε4 or ε2 allele.[61] Several observational studies have also shown that uncontrolled hypertension is a risk factor for recurrence after ICH, and randomized trials of blood pressure reduction among patients with a history of stroke, including those with ICH, support this (section 16.3.2).[62–67]

There are really no reliable data about the risk of myocardial infarction long term specifically after ICH, and no validated prognostic models for predicting stroke, myocardial infarction or vascular death. Since the numbers of individuals available for study in single-centre cohorts is small, pooling of data from cohort studies of ICH collecting similar baseline data and using similar definitions is probably the only feasible way of obtaining more precise data on independent predictors of prognosis after ICH.

> Up to 90% of recurrent strokes after an ischaemic stroke are ischaemic again, while around 60% of recurrent strokes after intracerebral haemorrhage are haemorrhagic again.

16.3 Pharmacological blood pressure reduction

16.3.1 Relationship between blood pressure and stroke in observational studies

Raised blood pressure is the most important causal and treatable risk factor for stroke (section 6.6.3). Systematic reviews of prospective observational studies in healthy, middle-aged adults, with appropriate adjustment for regression dilution bias, have demonstrated a continuous log linear relationship between usual systolic and diastolic blood pressure and stroke risk. For every 10 mmHg reduction in usual systolic and 5 mmHg reduction in usual diastolic blood pressure, the relative risk of stroke decreases by about one-third.[68–71] This relationship is not so steep in the elderly, but their higher absolute risk of stroke means that their absolute reduction in stroke risk for a given absolute decrease in blood pressure is still substantially greater than in younger people. The relationship is similar in Asian and white populations, and for ischaemic and haemorrhagic stroke. Unfortunately, there were neither sufficient numbers of events nor enough detail on stroke subtypes in these large overviews of prospective observational studies to allow comparisons between blood pressure and different subtypes of ischaemic or haemorrhagic stroke.[68–71] However, methodologically rigorous studies comparing the frequency of prior hypertension in patients with different subtypes of ischaemic stroke do not support the common assertion that lacunar ischaemic stroke is more strongly associated with raised blood pressure than other ischaemic stroke subtypes.[72,73] Similarly, data from the most methodologically sound studies comparing the frequency of prior hypertension in patients with deep vs lobar locations of intracerebral haemorrhage provide little – if any – evidence to support the often stated view that hypertension is associated particularly with deep intracerebral haemorrhage (section 8.2.1).[74]

Some studies of the association between blood pressure *after* a stroke and subsequent stroke risk have suggested that the risk of stroke recurrence may be higher at both high and low blood pressures, giving a U- or J-shaped relationship.[75,76] However, the higher recurrence risk at the two ends of the blood pressure distribution may not be because of a *causal* effect of blood pressure but because of so-called 'reverse causality', i.e. severe strokes may be independently associated both with a very high or low post-stroke blood pressure as well as with a higher risk of recurrence. In fact, in patients with a previous mild ischaemic stroke or TIA included in a randomized trial of antiplatelet treatment, the relationship between the risk of stroke and both systolic and diastolic blood pressure was similar to that observed in healthy populations, with lower blood pressures conferring a lower risk of stroke throughout the observed range of blood pressures. Each 10 mmHg decrease in usual systolic pressure and 5 mmHg decrease in usual diastolic pressure was associated with about a one-third decrease in stroke risk (Fig. 16.11).[77]

However, the relationship between blood pressure and stroke risk may be different in patients with severe disease of the extracranial arteries in the neck, since cerebral perfusion (and autoregulation of cerebral blood flow) may be so severely impaired that it is directly dependent on systemic blood pressure. Data from patients with a history of recent mild ischaemic stroke or TIA and stenosis of at least one carotid artery who were randomized to medical treatment in two large carotid surgery trials showed that, although the risk of stroke increased with blood pressure in most patients with symptomatic carotid artery disease, it was not so steep as in other patients with prior stroke or TIA, despite appropriate correction for regression dilution bias (Fig. 16.12). And, importantly, the relationship was reversed in patients with bilateral severe carotid stenosis, so that in this small group of patients lower blood pressure was associated with an increasing risk of stroke (Fig. 16.12c).[78]

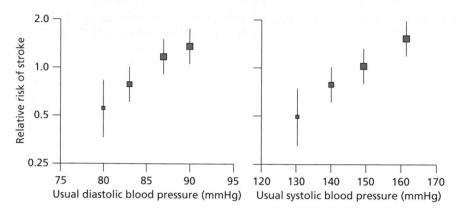

Fig. 16.11 Relative risk of stroke by approximate usual diastolic and systolic blood pressure among 2435 patients with a history of transient ischaemic attack or mild ischaemic stroke in the UK-TIA aspirin trial. Solid squares represent stroke risk in each category relative to the risk in the whole study population. The sizes of the squares are proportional to the number of events in each category. The vertical lines indicate the 95% confidence intervals. (From Rodgers *et al.*[77] © 1996 BMJ Publishing Group.)

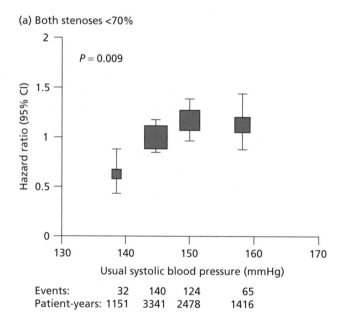

(a) Both stenoses <70%

P = 0.009

Events:	32	140	124	65
Patient-years:	1151	3341	2478	1416

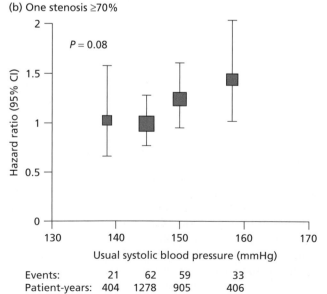

(b) One stenosis ≥70%

P = 0.08

Events:	21	62	59	33
Patient-years:	404	1278	905	406

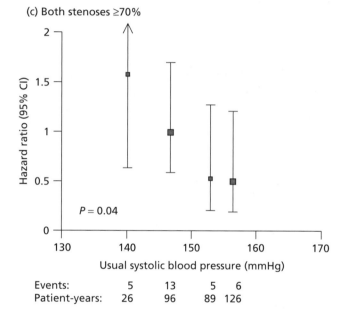

(c) Both stenoses ≥70%

P = 0.04

Events:	5	13	5	6
Patient-years:	26	96	89	126

Fig. 16.12 Relationships between usual systolic blood pressure and stroke risk in patients from the North American Symptomatic Carotid Endarterectomy Trial (NASCET) and European Carotid Surgery Trial (ECST), stratified according to severity of carotid disease. Please refer to Fig. 16.11 for conventions. (From Rothwell *et al.*, 2003.[78])

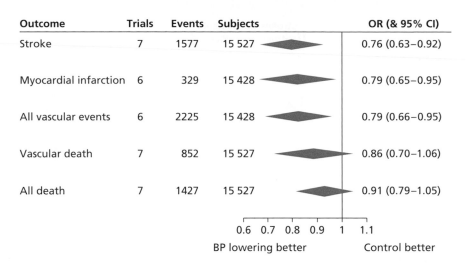

Fig. 16.13 Effects on vascular outcomes in a systematic review of seven randomized trials of pharmacological blood-pressure-lowering treatment in patients with a prior stroke or transient ischaemic attack. Mean duration of trials was 3 years and mean blood pressure reduction (treatment minus control) was 8/4 mmHg. Odds ratios (ORs) are shown as diamonds (with 95% confidence intervals = width of diamonds). (Data from Rashid *et al.*, 2003.[67])

Outcome	Trials	Events	Subjects	OR (& 95% CI)
Stroke	7	1577	15 527	0.76 (0.63–0.92)
Myocardial infarction	6	329	15 428	0.79 (0.65–0.95)
All vascular events	6	2225	15 428	0.79 (0.66–0.95)
Vascular death	7	852	15 527	0.86 (0.70–1.06)
All death	7	1427	15 527	0.91 (0.79–1.05)

0.6 0.7 0.8 0.9 1 1.1

BP lowering better   Control better

16.3.2 Randomized trials of blood-pressure-lowering drugs

There have now been seven randomized controlled trials (RCTs) of pharmacological blood pressure reduction in around 15 500 patients with a prior stroke (more than 2 weeks from onset) or TIA. More than three-quarters of these patients were included in just two of the trials, the worldwide perindopril protection against recurrent stoke study (PROGRESS) and the Chinese post-stroke antihypertensive treatment study (PATS).[79,80] A meta-analysis of all seven trials found that treatment for about 3 years reduced blood pressure by a mean of 8 mmHg systolic/4 mmHg diastolic and produced highly statistically significant reductions in the risks of stroke, myocardial infarction, and total vascular events (i.e. stroke, myocardial infarction or vascular death), although reductions in vascular and in all-cause mortality did not reach statistical significance (Fig. 16.13). The average control group 3-year risks of stroke, myocardial infarction and vascular events were 12%, 4% and 16% respectively. Applying to these absolute risks the odds reductions of about one-quarter for stroke and about one-fifth for both myocardial infarction and vascular events shows us that treating 1000 patients similar to those in the trials for about 3 years would lead to the avoidance or delay of about 34 vascular events, of which 25 would be strokes and nine would be myocardial infarctions.[67]

Further analyses showed that the relative benefits of treatment were similar irrespective of baseline blood pressure (hypertensive or not) and the type of qualifying cerebrovascular event (ischaemic stroke, haemorrhagic stroke or TIA) (Fig. 16.14).[80,81] Furthermore, PROGRESS demonstrated that the reduction in stroke started early and continued throughout several years of follow-up,

and found similar relative risk reductions for disabling and non-disabling strokes, and for the different major pathological types (ischaemic, haemorrhagic or unknown) and ischaemic subtypes of stroke outcome (Fig. 16.15).[80,81] Substudies exploring other important outcomes in the PROGRESS trial found that blood pressure lowering was also associated with significantly reduced disability and cognitive decline, although both of these benefits appeared to be mediated through the reduction in recurrent stroke. Treating 1000 patients for 4 years resulted in 30 avoiding long-term disability and 20 avoiding cognitive decline.[82,83]

> People with a prior stroke or transient ischaemic attack benefit from drug treatment to reduce blood pressure, whether 'hypertensive' or 'normotensive' and irrespective of whether their cerebrovascular event was ischaemic or haemorrhagic. Treating 1000 such people for about 3 years to reduce the blood pressure by about 8/4 mmHg will result in the avoidance of about 34 serious vascular events (25 strokes, nine myocardial infarctions), and will reduce the risk of long-term disability and cognitive decline.

16.3.3 Which antihypertensive drug or drugs?

Data from RCTs can be used in two ways to compare the effects of different classes of antihypertensive drugs. First, the relative effects of the various different drug classes vs no antihypertensive treatment can be compared. Such *indirect* comparisons are rather similar to comparing two football teams (let's say France and Italy) by comparing their scores against a third team (say Germany). There tend to be plenty of relevant football

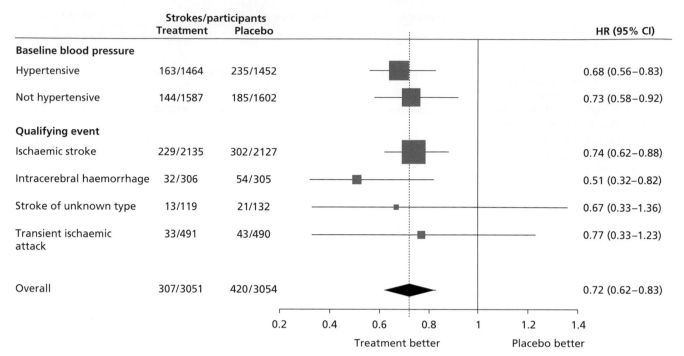

	Strokes/participants			HR (95% CI)
	Treatment	Placebo		
Baseline blood pressure				
Hypertensive	163/1464	235/1452		0.68 (0.56–0.83)
Not hypertensive	144/1587	185/1602		0.73 (0.58–0.92)
Qualifying event				
Ischaemic stroke	229/2135	302/2127		0.74 (0.62–0.88)
Intracerebral haemorrhage	32/306	54/305		0.51 (0.32–0.82)
Stroke of unknown type	13/119	21/132		0.67 (0.33–1.36)
Transient ischaemic attack	33/491	43/490		0.77 (0.33–1.23)
Overall	307/3051	420/3054		0.72 (0.62–0.83)

0.2 0.4 0.6 0.8 1 1.2 1.4

Treatment better   Placebo better

Fig. 16.14 Effects of blood-pressure lowering in the PROGRESS trial on stroke risk among patients with and without hypertension at baseline (systolic ≥ 160 mmHg or diastolic ≥ 90 mmHg), and among patients with different types of qualifying cerebrovascular event. Hazard ratios (HRs) are shown as squares with size proportional to number of events, along with 95% confidence intervals (horizontal lines). The result for all patients is shown as a diamond (with 95% confidence interval = width of diamond). (Data from PROGRESS Collaborative Group, 2001[80] and Chapman *et al.*, 2004.[81])

	Number of events			HR (95% CI)
	Treatment	Placebo		
Stroke type	n = 3051	n = 3054		
Fatal or disabling	123	181		0.67 (0.54–0.85)
Not fatal or disabling	201	262		0.76 (0.63–0.91)
Ischaemic	246	319		0.76 (0.65–0.90)
Lacunar	64	83		0.77 (0.56–1.07)
Cardioembolic	20	26		0.77 (0.43–1.38)
Large artery	32	53		0.61 (0.39–0.95)
Unknown ischaemic	150	184		0.81 (0.65–1.00)
Haemorrhagic	37	74		0.50 (0.33–0.74)
Unknown pathological type	42	51		0.82 (0.55–1.24)
Total stroke	307	420		0.72 (0.62–0.83)

0.3   0.8   1.3

Favours treatment   Favours placebo

Fig. 16.15 Effects of blood-pressure lowering on strokes of different type occurring during follow-up in the PROGRESS trial. Hazard ratios (HRs) are shown as squares with size proportional to number of events, along with 95% confidence intervals (horizontal lines). The result for all types of stroke combined is shown as a diamond (with 95% confidence interval = width of diamond). (Data from PROGRESS Collaborative Group, 2001[80] and Chapman *et al.*, 2004.[81])

matches (analogous to RCTs) available for such comparisons. However, they are not as reliable as *direct* comparisons, a match between France and Italy or an RCT that directly compares two antihypertensive drugs.

Evidence from randomized trials in patients with a previous cerebrovascular event

The number of RCTs among people with a history of cerebrovascular disease (and more importantly the limited number of people included in those trials) for making either indirect or direct comparisons is rather small.

Indirect comparisons in the systematic review of seven trials comparing antihypertensive treatment vs no treatment found larger effects on stroke and on vascular events for those regimens producing greater reductions in blood pressure (diuretics alone, or diuretics combined with angiotensin-converting enzyme (ACE) inhibitors), with smaller and non-statistically significant effects for those regimens producing smaller reductions in blood pressure (beta-blockers or ACE inhibitors alone). A meta-regression analysis of these seven trials found a direct relationship between the size of the reductions in stroke and in vascular events and increasing reductions in blood pressure.[67] The largest trial (PROGRESS) assessed the effects of the ACE inhibitor, perindopril, either with or without the addition of the thiazide diuretic, indapamide, vs placebo. Combination therapy produced larger reductions in blood pressure and – not surprisingly – stroke risk than did single drug therapy with perindopril alone, consistent with the effects on stroke predicted from the observed relationship between blood pressure and stroke in patients with a prior ischaemic stroke or TIA (Figs 16.11 and 16.16).[77,84]

Only one RCT (the MOSES study) has *directly* compared one drug regimen with another in patients with a history of stroke or TIA. After 2–4 years, blood pressure had fallen by a mean of 13/6 mmHg in the eprosartan (angiotensin II receptor blocker) group and 16/7 mmHg in the nitrendipine (calcium channel blocker) group. There was an apparent advantage of eprosartan, with significant relative reductions of about one-fifth in the primary outcome of death and all cardiovascular and cerebrovascular events, including TIAs, and of about one-quarter in cerebrovascular events.[85] However, these results are difficult to interpret because: they were not based on an intention-to-treat analysis; they relied very heavily on the relatively 'soft' outcome of TIAs which made up two-thirds of the cerebrovascular outcome events; and patients could have more than one event counted so that the results could have been unduly influenced by multiple events occurring in just a few patients. Sufficient data to carry out a more appropriate

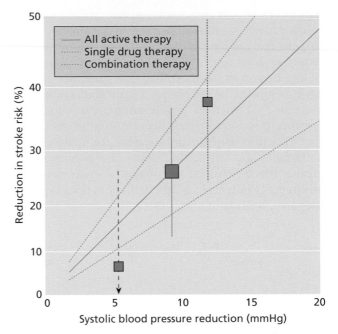

Fig. 16.16 Predicted and observed effects of blood-pressure lowering among patients with ischaemic stroke or transient ischaemic attacks. Predicted reduction in stroke risk with 95% confidence interval is indicated by diagonal lines, from the UK-TIA aspirin study.[77] Observed effects of treatment from the PROGRESS trial on stroke risk and 95% confidence intervals are indicated by boxes and vertical lines. Box sizes are proportional to the number of strokes. All estimates of reductions in stroke risk are plotted on a logarithmic scale. (From MacMahon *et al.*[84] © 2004 BMJ Publishing Group)

intention-to-treat analysis allowing only one event per patient were not given.

Evidence from randomized trials in all types of patients

A larger amount of data is available from RCTs of antihypertensive drugs in other types of patients – those with hypertension, coronary heart disease, diabetes, and so on. Because the early systematic reviews showed that the effects of blood pressure reduction were similar regardless of the particular types of patients included (including those with cerebrovascular disease), these data are likely to be helpful in guiding treatment decisions for patients with a prior stroke or TIA.[86–88]

Over the last decade or so, since these early systematic reviews emerged, many more RCTs have been completed, some comparing various different antihypertensive regimens with no treatment in different types of patients, and others directly comparing different drug regimens. Many systematic reviews of these newer trials have now been done. Although their results vary slightly, depending on exactly which trials were included and how the data were analysed, one consistent message emerges: the relative benefits of blood pressure reduction on major vascular outcomes directly depend on the blood pressure reduction achieved.[67,71,89,90] Although there have been claims from time to time that one particular class of agent is superior or inferior for a particular condition or outcome,[91–94] when all the relevant trials are considered together, it is overwhelmingly the size of the blood pressure reduction rather than the specific regimen used that determines the effect: the greater the reduction, the greater the benefit. Of the major vascular outcomes assessed, the only one for which this does not seem to be the case is heart failure (Fig. 16.17).[90]

> It is the size of the blood pressure reduction achieved rather than the specific drug or drugs used that is the major determinant of the reduction in risk of future stroke and other major vascular events.

The most recent systematic review from the Blood Pressure Lowering Treatment Trialists' Collaboration (BPLTTC) included up-to-date direct comparisons between the effects of various different drug classes on major vascular outcomes, and to these should be added the results of a subsequent, large RCT, the Anglo Scandinavian Cardiac Outcomes Trial – Blood Pressure Lowering Arm (ASCOT-BPLA), which compared newer

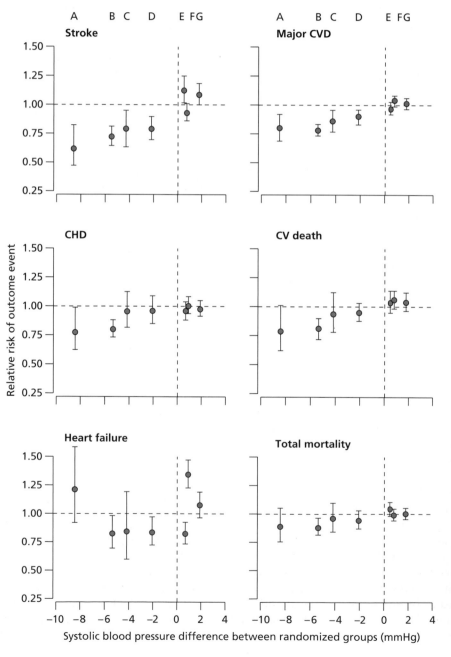

Fig. 16.17 Randomized trials of blood-pressure-lowering drugs vs placebo or open control and of one blood-pressure-lowering regimen vs another in all types of patients, including those with a prior stroke or transient ischaemic attack: associations of blood-pressure differences between treatment groups with risks of major vascular outcomes and death. The circles are plotted at the point estimate of effect for the relative risk for every event type and the mean follow-up blood pressure in the first listed group compared with the second listed group. Vertical lines are 95% confidence intervals. CHD, coronary heart disease; CVD, cardiovascular event; CV death, cardiovascular death. (A) Calcium antagonist vs placebo. (B) ACE inhibitor vs placebo. (C) more intensive vs less intensive blood-pressure lowering. (D) Angiotensin receptor blocker vs control. (E) ACE inhibitor vs calcium antagonist. (F) Calcium antagonist vs diuretic or beta-blocker. (G) ACE inhibitor vs diuretic and beta-blocker. (Reprinted from Blood Pressure Lowering Treatment Trialists' Collaboration, *Lancet*[90] © 2003 with permission from Elsevier.)

with older antihypertensive regimens (amlodipine with perindopril as required vs atenolol with bendroflumethiazide as required) in over 19 000 patients with hypertension.[95] Taking all the evidence from these comparisons together, there seems to be little to make one choose one drug class over another (Fig. 16.18).

Following the results from several individual RCTs, it has been claimed that particular drug classes, in particular ACE inhibitors and angiotensin II blockers, have additional cardio- and renal protective effects beyond their effects on the blood pressure.[96–98] However, in one very large trial where this appeared to be the case, the apparently small blood-pressure reduction achieved by the ACE inhibitor, ramipril, which was nonetheless associated with substantial clinical benefit, may have been due to the timing of office blood-pressure measurements.[99] In addition, a recent systematic review that assessed the effects of ACE inhibitors and angiotensin II blockers on renal outcomes found no clear evidence that the renoprotective actions of these drugs went beyond what might be expected from their blood-pressure-lowering effects.[100] There does, however, appear to be some evidence emerging that beta-blockers may be somewhat less effective than other antihypertensive drug classes, particularly for the outcome of stroke.[101] It remains unclear whether or not this is due to less effective lowering of the blood pressure, or some other reason. Recent evidence also suggests that beta-blockers may be less favourable than alternative antihypertensive drugs with respect to other outcomes, such as new-onset diabetes.[95,102] Furthermore, a systematic review that included a meta-analysis of randomized trials directly comparing beta-blockers with thiazide diuretics found that beta-blockers were associated with a significantly higher rate of withdrawal of treatment due to adverse effects.[103]

A further issue is whether a single drug or a combination of drugs is most appropriate. Useful guidance comes from a meta-analysis of 354 RCTs of thiazides, beta-blockers, ACE inhibitors, angiotensin II receptor blockers and calcium channel antagonists in fixed dose, including around 56 000 patients. Standard doses of each drug class produced similar reductions in blood pressure of around 9/5.5 mmHg. The effects of different drug classes were additive. However, doubling the dose of any particular drug produced less than twice the blood-pressure-lowering effect while halving the dose produced more than half the blood-pressure-lowering effect. The frequency of adverse effects for each drug was strongly related to dose, but the frequency of symptoms from adverse effects with two drugs in combination was less than additive. The conclusion drawn was that combination low-dose drug treatment increases efficacy and reduces adverse effects, such that using three drugs at half standard dose could reduce blood pressure by 20/11

mmHg, potentially reducing the risk of stroke by almost two-thirds and ischaemic heart disease events by almost one-half.[104]

Conclusion

So, how can one use all this evidence to help with the choice of antihypertensive treatment in clinical practice? We try to be guided, where possible, by RCTs conducted among the types of patients we are treating, i.e. those with a prior stroke or TIA, calling on the evidence from trials among other types of patients where necessary. The largest trials in stroke and TIA patients found convincing benefit from a thiazide diuretic (indapamide was used in the trials but there is no clear evidence to suggest superiority of one particular thiazide over another), with further benefit from the combination of a thiazide and ACE inhibitor (perindopril was used in the relevant trial, but it seems likely that any ACE inhibitor at equivalent dose would produce similar effects).[67,79,80] Therefore, we generally recommend starting with a thiazide, in no more than the standard dose (i.e. 2.5 mg daily of bendrofluazide or equivalent), and adding an ACE inhibitor if necessary to achieve the desired blood-pressure-lowering effect. Further drugs of other classes can be added (again, generally we do not recommend exceeding the standard dose) if needed. We tend not to use beta-blockers for first- or second-line treatment in most cases, unless there is some other reason for the patient to be on a beta-blocker. Our emphasis is generally on getting the blood pressure down, and if thiazides or ACE inhibitors are not tolerated because of adverse effects, or are contraindicated for some other reason, then we substitute another class of drug or drugs.

> In the absence of specific indications or contraindications, the most appropriate blood-pressure-lowering treatment for patients who have had a stroke or transient ischaemic attack is to start with a thiazide, and then add an ACE inhibitor if necessary, and then – again if necessary – drugs from other classes to achieve the desired blood-pressure-lowering effect and to avoid adverse effects.

16.3.4 How low to go and who not to treat

We have seen that the larger the reduction in blood pressure, the greater the benefits, suggesting that the lower one can get the blood pressure the better. Up to a point. Eventually, if the blood pressure is lowered far enough, patients develop symptoms due to low blood pressure, particularly when standing, and the absolute blood pressure level at which this occurs varies between individuals. It would clearly not be sensible to increase

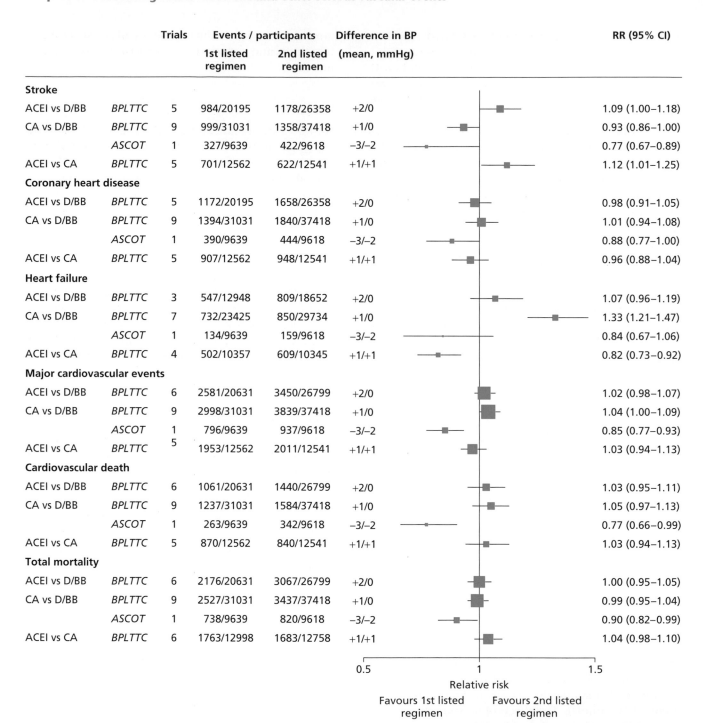

	Trials	Events / participants		Difference in BP		RR (95% CI)
		1st listed regimen	2nd listed regimen	(mean, mmHg)		
Stroke						
ACEI vs D/BB	BPLTTC	5	984/20195	1178/26358	+2/0	1.09 (1.00–1.18)
CA vs D/BB	BPLTTC	9	999/31031	1358/37418	+1/0	0.93 (0.86–1.00)
	ASCOT	1	327/9639	422/9618	−3/−2	0.77 (0.67–0.89)
ACEI vs CA	BPLTTC	5	701/12562	622/12541	+1/+1	1.12 (1.01–1.25)
Coronary heart disease						
ACEI vs D/BB	BPLTTC	5	1172/20195	1658/26358	+2/0	0.98 (0.91–1.05)
CA vs D/BB	BPLTTC	9	1394/31031	1840/37418	+1/0	1.01 (0.94–1.08)
	ASCOT	1	390/9639	444/9618	−3/−2	0.88 (0.77–1.00)
ACEI vs CA	BPLTTC	5	907/12562	948/12541	+1/+1	0.96 (0.88–1.04)
Heart failure						
ACEI vs D/BB	BPLTTC	3	547/12948	809/18652	+2/0	1.07 (0.96–1.19)
CA vs D/BB	BPLTTC	7	732/23425	850/29734	+1/0	1.33 (1.21–1.47)
	ASCOT	1	134/9639	159/9618	−3/−2	0.84 (0.67–1.06)
ACEI vs CA	BPLTTC	4	502/10357	609/10345	+1/+1	0.82 (0.73–0.92)
Major cardiovascular events						
ACEI vs D/BB	BPLTTC	6	2581/20631	3450/26799	+2/0	1.02 (0.98–1.07)
CA vs D/BB	BPLTTC	9	2998/31031	3839/37418	+1/0	1.04 (1.00–1.09)
	ASCOT	1	796/9639	937/9618	−3/−2	0.85 (0.77–0.93)
ACEI vs CA	BPLTTC	5	1953/12562	2011/12541	+1/+1	1.03 (0.94–1.13)
Cardiovascular death						
ACEI vs D/BB	BPLTTC	6	1061/20631	1440/26799	+2/0	1.03 (0.95–1.11)
CA vs D/BB	BPLTTC	9	1237/31031	1584/37418	+1/0	1.05 (0.97–1.13)
	ASCOT	1	263/9639	342/9618	−3/−2	0.77 (0.66–0.99)
ACEI vs CA	BPLTTC	5	870/12562	840/12541	+1/+1	1.03 (0.94–1.13)
Total mortality						
ACEI vs D/BB	BPLTTC	6	2176/20631	3067/26799	+2/0	1.00 (0.95–1.05)
CA vs D/BB	BPLTTC	9	2527/31031	3437/37418	+1/0	0.99 (0.95–1.04)
	ASCOT	1	738/9639	820/9618	−3/−2	0.90 (0.82–0.99)
ACEI vs CA	BPLTTC	6	1763/12998	1683/12758	+1/+1	1.04 (0.98–1.10)

0.5   1   1.5

Relative risk

Favours 1st listed   Favours 2nd listed
regimen   regimen

Fig. 16.18 Randomized trials directly comparing different blood-pressure-lowering regimens in all types of patients, including those with a prior stroke or transient ischaemic attack: comparisons of effects on major vascular outcomes of regimens based on different drug classes. Results (given as relative risks, RR) for each comparison are represented by a square, the size of which is proportional to the number of events. Horizontal lines represent 95% confidence intervals. ACEI, ACE inhibitor; CA, calcium antagonist D/BB diuretic or beta-blocker; BPLTTC, Blood Pressure Lowering Treatment Trialists' Collaboration meta-analysis; ASCOT, Anglo Scandinavian Cardiac Outcomes Trial. Positive values for mean difference in blood pressure indicate a higher mean follow-up blood pressure in the first listed group (ACEI and CA) than in the second listed group (D/BB and CA). (Data from Blood Pressure Lowering Treatment Trialists' Collaboration, 2003[90] and Dahlöf et al., 2005.[95])

antihypertensive treatment beyond this point, and even if one did, adherence by the patient to the suggested treatment would – in all likelihood and quite understandably – be poor. Furthermore, the observational data do not tell us much about what happens to the relationship between blood pressure and stroke or recurrent stroke below pressures of around 120/70 mmHg (section 6.6.3, Fig. 6.17 and Fig. 16.11) (it cannot be log linear for ever-decreasing blood pressures because a blood pressure of 0/0 mmHg is incompatible with life!). In the largest trial of blood-pressure lowering among patients with a prior stroke or TIA (PROGRESS), the mean blood pressure at baseline was 147/86 mmHg and only around 10–20% of patients had baseline blood pressures of less than 120–130/70 mmHg.[105] Although benefits from blood-pressure lowering in PROGRESS occurred irrespective of baseline blood pressure, results were not presented separately for those in the bottom quintile. Taking this together with what we know from observational studies, we do not feel that there is clear evidence for further blood pressure reductions for those whose blood pressure is already consistently about 120–130/70 mmHg or lower. For patients with higher blood pressures than this, we would generally recommend treating to reduce the blood pressure to a target of around 120–130/70 mmHg, so long as the necessary medication can be tolerated.

One important caveat is that there are doubts about whether or not the blood pressure should be lowered in patients with severe atherosclerotic stenotic disease of the extracranial arteries. There is no specific guidance from randomized trials, but observational data suggest that the relationship between usual blood pressure and stroke risk may be reversed in people with severe bilateral carotid stenoses (section 16.3.1). Because of this, we currently recommend proceeding particularly cautiously in patients known to have more than one severely stenosed extracranial neck artery, and we tend to avoid lowering the blood pressure below around 140 mmHg systolic in such patients.

> We generally recommend lowering blood pressure about as far as 120–130/70 mmHg, but tend to avoid lowering the systolic blood pressure below around 140 mmHg in patients with known severe stenosis of more than one extracranial neck artery.

16.3.5 When to start antihypertensive treatment after an acute stroke

The RCTs that support routine blood-pressure lowering after a prior stroke or TIA generally recruited patients at least 2 weeks or more after their most recent event,

sometimes up to several years afterwards.[67] Observational data suggest that both high and low blood pressures early after acute stroke are independently associated with poor outcome, but there is a lack of evidence from RCTs about whether or not the potential benefits of lowering blood pressure in the first week or two after a stroke outweigh the potential risks. Neither is there clear evidence about whether or not continuing antihypertensive medication taken prior to an acute stroke is of net benefit (section 11.7.1).[106,107] We therefore encourage recruitment of patients with acute stroke into ongoing RCTs assessing blood-pressure lowering early after stroke (section 11.7.1). Patients with malignant hypertension should have carefully monitored, urgent blood-pressure reduction. For other patients who cannot, for whatever reason, be randomized into one of the ongoing trials, our usual management until further evidence becomes available is to delay the routine introduction of blood-pressure-lowering drugs for a week or two, or at least until the post-stroke blood pressure has stabilized, although for TIA and very mild stroke patients we generally start treatment more or less at once. If a patient already on an antihypertensive drug is admitted with a stroke, we continue the treatment, provided they can swallow it safely or receive it via nasogastric tube, unless the blood pressure is below about 120–130/70 mmHg or we are aware of severe extracranial neck artery stenoses, which would lead us to stop antihypertensive treatment. Sometimes, patients whose blood pressure has fallen to satisfactory levels by the time of hospital discharge have raised blood pressures at a post-discharge clinic visit. While this may be spurious due to the 'white coat' effect (i.e. the stress of seeing a doctor), it does highlight the need to check the blood pressure in stroke survivors on more than one occasion after discharge from hospital.

> It is unclear how soon raised blood pressure should be lowered after acute stroke and we encourage recruitment of suitable patients into ongoing randomized trials addressing this issue.

16.4 Pharmacological cholesterol reduction

16.4.1 Relationship between cholesterol and stroke in observational studies

Prospective studies have shown a strong relationship between usual blood cholesterol and risk of ischaemic heart disease; a decrease in total cholesterol concentration of 0.6 mmol/L is associated with a relative reduction in ischaemic heart disease of around 50% at age 40, 40% at age 50, 30% at age 60 and 20% at age 70.[108] By contrast, an overview of prospective studies found no overall association between cholesterol and stroke risk, although they generally recorded only fatal strokes, of which about half each were ischaemic and haemorrhagic (section 6.6.6).[109] Subsequent overviews were able to analyse data for ischaemic and haemorrhagic stroke separately and found that for every 1.0 mmol/L decrease in LDL cholesterol concentration there was a 15% relative reduction in ischaemic stroke risk and a 19% relative increase in haemorrhagic stroke risk (section 6.6.6).[68,110] These opposing effects might explain why there was no overall relationship for all types of stroke combined when mainly fatal strokes were considered.[109]

16.4.2 Randomized trials of cholesterol-lowering drugs

Randomized controlled trials (RCTs) and systematic reviews of non-statin cholesterol-lowering treatments, in particular fibrates, found significant reductions in ischaemic heart disease but not in stroke.[111–116] However, the development of the far more potent cholesterol-lowering drugs, the 3-hydroxy-3-methylglutaryl coenzyme A (HMG-CoA) reductase inhibitors (statins) made possible substantially larger reductions in total – and in particular LDL – cholesterol concentrations. A meta-analysis by the Cholesterol Treatment Trialists Collaborators of large RCTs of statins available by 2004 included over 90 000 participants, of whom about half had a history of ischaemic heart disease, about 15% had some other vascular disease (including several thousand with a prior stroke or TIA), either with or without ischaemic heart disease, and about half had no history of vascular disease. Participants were generally middle-aged and elderly. Mean baseline LDL cholesterol concentration was 3.8 mmol/L. Treatment with a statin for about 5 years, leading to a reduction in LDL cholesterol of about 1.0 mmol/L, produced highly statistically significant relative reductions of about one-fifth in major vascular events (non-fatal myocardial infarction, coronary heart disease death, coronary revascularization, or stroke) and in the separate outcomes of major coronary events, coronary revascularizations and stroke (Fig. 16.19). There were also significant reductions in vascular and all-cause mortality. The reduction in stroke risk was amost entirely due to a one-fifth reduction in ischaemic or unknown type of stroke, with no significant effect on haemorrhagic stroke (although the wide confidence interval was consistent with either a reduction or an increase in haemorrhagic stroke risk, since the

number of haemorrhagic stroke events was relatively small) (Fig. 16.19). The relative reduction in major vascular events and its component outcomes was similar irrespective of age and gender, previous history of coronary heart disease, diabetes or hypertension, and baseline concentrations of total, LDL or HDL cholesterol, or of triglycerides. Meta-regression analyses found that larger reductions in LDL cholesterol led to larger reductions in risk of major vascular events and its component outcomes, suggesting that adherence to a statin regimen producing a 1.5 mmol/L reduction in LDL cholesterol would lead to a reduction of about one-third in the relative risk of major vascular events (Fig. 16.20). The full benefits of cholesterol lowering with a statin emerged over the first 2–3 years of treatment and continued for each year that treatment was continued thereafter.[117]

The largest of the RCTs in this meta-analysis, the Heart Protection Study (HPS), included over 20 000 people with a history of ischaemic heart disease, other arterial occlusive disease including stroke or diabetes, randomized to treatment for 5 years with simvastatin 40 mg daily or placebo.[118] In subgroup analyses, the relative reductions in major vascular events in aggregate (stroke, major coronary event or revascularization), major coronary events and revascularizations with treatment were similar and separately statistically significant in those with and without a history of cerebrovascular disease. But, there appeared to be no effect on stroke in those with a history of cerebrovascular disease, compared with a one-quarter reduction in stroke in those with no such history. However, given the large number of subgroup analyses, and the fact that, while several subgroup analyses based on the primary outcome of major vascular events were prespecified, subgroup analyses based on the outcome of stroke were not, this apparent difference may have been due to the play of chance.

In a subsequent RCT, the Stroke Prevention by Aggressive Reduction in Cholesterol Levels (SPARCL) trial, not included in the meta-analysis, patients with a recent stroke (almost all ischaemic) or TIA and no known coronary heart disease were randomly assigned to either atorvastatin 80 mg daily or placebo for about 5 years. Key features and results for the stroke and TIA patients in the HPS and the SPARCL trial are shown in Table 16.5. Like HPS, SPARCL found significant reductions in coronary heart disease and major vascular events. Reassuringly, in contrast to HPS, it also found a significant relative reduction in stroke of about 15%. The difference between HPS and SPARCL in the effects on stroke in patients with a history of stroke or TIA could be explained by chance, different treatment regimens (larger reduction in LDL cholesterol achieved in SPARCL), the recruitment of patients earlier after their event in SPARCL, or a different

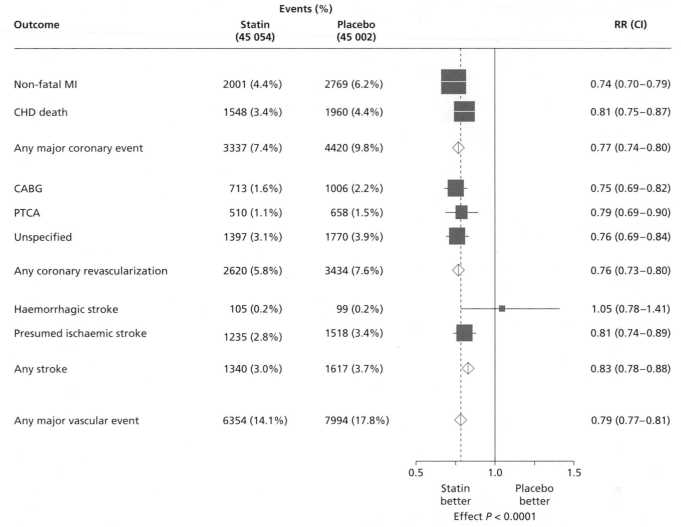

Outcome	Events (%)		RR (CI)
	Statin (45 054)	**Placebo (45 002)**	
Non-fatal MI	2001 (4.4%)	2769 (6.2%)	0.74 (0.70–0.79)
CHD death	1548 (3.4%)	1960 (4.4%)	0.81 (0.75–0.87)
Any major coronary event	3337 (7.4%)	4420 (9.8%)	0.77 (0.74–0.80)
CABG	713 (1.6%)	1006 (2.2%)	0.75 (0.69–0.82)
PTCA	510 (1.1%)	658 (1.5%)	0.79 (0.69–0.90)
Unspecified	1397 (3.1%)	1770 (3.9%)	0.76 (0.69–0.84)
Any coronary revascularization	2620 (5.8%)	3434 (7.6%)	0.76 (0.73–0.80)
Haemorrhagic stroke	105 (0.2%)	99 (0.2%)	1.05 (0.78–1.41)
Presumed ischaemic stroke	1235 (2.8%)	1518 (3.4%)	0.81 (0.74–0.89)
Any stroke	1340 (3.0%)	1617 (3.7%)	0.83 (0.78–0.88)
Any major vascular event	6354 (14.1%)	7994 (17.8%)	0.79 (0.77–0.81)

0.5 1.0 1.5

Statin   Placebo
better   better
Effect $P < 0.0001$

Fig. 16.19 Meta-analysis of randomized trials of a statin vs placebo: relative reductions in major vascular events per mmol LDL cholesterol reduction. Squares represent relative risks (RR) for individual categories, with the size of each square proportional to the amount of statistical information in that category. Horizontal lines are 99% confidence intervals. Diamonds represent relative risks for totals and subtotals, together with their 95% confidence intervals (width of diamonds). Relative risks (RR) are weighted to represent reduction in rate per 1.0 mmol/L LDL cholesterol reduction. CHD, coronary heart disease; CABG, coronary artery bypass graft; MI, myocardial infarction; PTCA, percutaneous transluminal angioplasty. (Reprinted from Cholesterol Treatment Trialists' Collaborators Group, *Lancet*[117] © 2005 with permission from Elsevier.)

balance between ischaemic and haemorrhagic stroke outcomes (but this is difficult to assess since 25% of stroke outcomes in HPS vs only a few % in SPARCL were of unknown pathological type). Both trials found similar relative reductions of about 20% in ischaemic stroke, and a 70% or more increased relative risk of haemorrhagic stroke, although the latter estimates were uncertain because of small numbers of events and so wide confidence intervals. Both trials found relative reductions with a statin of about 20% in major vascular events, although they used slightly different definitions for this outcome, with 5-year absolute reductions of about 50 and 70 vascular events per 1000 patients allocated statin treatment in HPS and SPARCL, respectively (Table 16.5).[119,120]

> There is very good evidence for routinely considering the use of prolonged statin treatment to lower cholesterol levels in all patients at high risk of any type of major vascular event, including those with a prior ischaemic stroke or transient ischaemic attack, and irrespective of the baseline cholesterol concentration. Treating 1000 people with a prior ischaemic stroke or transient ischaemic attack for 5 years with a statin will lead to the avoidance of over 50 major vascular events.

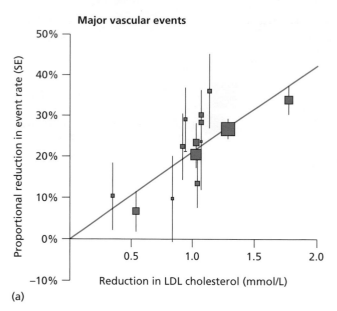

(a)

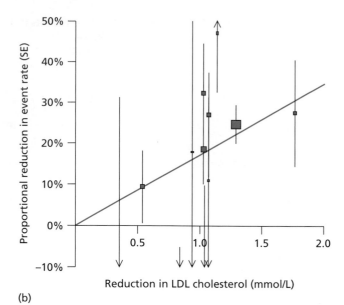

(b)

Fig. 16.20 Relation between relative reduction in incidence of (a) major vascular events and (b) stroke vs mean absolute LDL cholesterol reduction at one year. Each square represents a single randomized trial of a statin vs placebo plotted against mean absolute LDL cholesterol reduction at 1 year, with vertical lines above and below corresponding to one standard error of the unweighted event rate reduction. Trials are plotted in order of the magnitude of the difference in LDL cholesterol at 1 year. For each outcome, the regression line (which is forced to pass through the origin) represents the weighted event rate reduction per mmol/L LDL cholesterol reduction. (Reprinted from Cholesterol Treatment Trialists' Collaborators Group, *Lancet*[117] © 2005 with permission from Elsevier.)

16.4.3 Other benefits of cholesterol reduction with a statin

There have been several RCTs evaluating the effect of statins on the progression of carotid atheroma; meta-analysis found that with each 10% reduction in LDL cholesterol there was a 0.7% reduction in carotid intima media thickness annually.[121] Although it is plausible that cholesterol reduction may prevent vascular dementia as well as ischaemic stroke, the Heart Protection Study found no difference between simvastatin and placebo in the proportions of participants developing cognitive impairment,[118] and other RCTs have not reported on this outcome. There is some evidence that the effects of statins may be mediated through their anti-inflammatory properties as well as cholesterol lowering. Substudies within two trials of more vs less intensive lipid-lowering statin regimens in patients with ischaemic heart disease showed that more intensive regimens reduced C-reactive protein levels as well as LDL cholesterol, and that these effects were independently associated with better clinical outcomes.[122,123]

16.4.4 Adverse effects of cholesterol-lowering treatments

Earlier fears that cholesterol lowering may be associated with an increased risk of suicide and cancer have now been allayed by large systematic reviews of RCTs.[110,117] However, there are some other rare but clinically important adverse effects of statins: rhabdomyolysis, liver failure from hepatitis, and peripheral neuropathy.

Muscle problems

However, neither systematic reviews of RCTs nor the subsequent SPARCL trial have found any significant excess of rhabdomyolysis with a statin vs placebo (nine patients allocated a statin vs six allocated placebo in the systematic review; two allocated atorvastatin vs three placebo in SPARCL).[117,120] Neither was there any significant excess of raised serum creatine kinase activity.[110,120] A cohort study in the US found that the incidence of rhabdomyolysis in those taking simvastatin, pravastatin or atorvastatin monotherapy was < 0.5 per 10 000 person-years compared with none in those unexposed to statins or fibrates. The incidence was higher in those taking cerivastatin or a fibrate, and was increased substantially by combined statin-fibrate use, such that the combination of cerivastatin and a fibrate conferred a risk of about 1 in 10 treated people per year.[124] Cerivastatin was not one of the statins assessed in the RCTs included in the systematic reviews and has now been withdrawn from the market.[125] The risk of rhabdomyolysis is also increased when statins metabolized by cytochrome

Table 16.5 Randomized trials of cholesterol reduction with a statin in patients with a previous stroke or transient ischaemic attack (TIA).

Trial	SPARCL[120]	HPS[118,119]
Population recruited	Adults > 18 years with stroke or TIA within the last 1–6 months, and no known ischaemic heart disease. Those with haemorrhagic stroke only included if considered at high risk of ischaemic stroke or ischaemic heart disease Baseline LDL cholesterol 2.6–4.9 mmol/L	Adults aged 40–80 years with history of ischaemic stroke or TIA, ischaemic heart disease, peripheral arterial disease, diabetes, or hypertension Baseline total cholesterol > 3.5 mmol/L
Treatments compared	Atorvastatin 80 mg daily vs placebo	Simvastatin 40 mg daily vs placebo
Total number of participants	4731	20 536
Number of participants with prior stroke or TIA	4731	3280
Baseline characteristics*		
Mean time from stroke/TIA to randomization	3 months	4 years
Mean age (years)	63	66
Male : female (%)	60 : 40	75 : 25
Mean baseline total/LDL cholesterol (mmol/L)	5.5/3.4	5.9/3.4
Mean follow-up (years)*	4.9	4.8
Mean difference in LDL cholesterol between treatment groups (placebo-statin, mmol/L)†	1.4	1

Effects on various outcomes† (number and % with each outcome and relative risk for statin vs placebo)

	Atorvastatin (n = 2365)	Placebo (n = 2366)	RR (95% CI)	Simvastatin (n = 1645)	Placebo (n = 1635)	RR (95% CI)
Any stroke	265 (11%)	311 (13%)	0.85 (0.73 to 0.99)	169 (10%)	170 (10%)	0.99 (0.81 to 1.21)
Ischaemic stroke	218 (9%)	274 (12%)	0.80 (0.67 to 0.94)	100 (6%)	122 (7%)	0.81 (0.63 to 1.05)
Haemorrhagic stroke	55 (2%)	33 (1%)	1.7 (1.1 to 2.6)	21 (1%)	11 (0.7%)	1.9 (0.9 to 3.9)
Major coronary events‡	81 (3%)	120 (5%)	0.68 (0.51 to 0.89)	171 (10%)	218 (13%)	0.78 (0.65 to 0.94)
Major vascular events§	530 (22%)	687 (29%)	0.77 (0.74 to 0.86)	406 (25%)	488 (30%)	0.83 (0.74 to 0.93)

SPARCL Stroke Prevention by Aggressive Reduction of Cholesterol Levels study. HPS Heart Protection Study. RR relative risk.
*Of patients with prior stroke or TIA.
†In patients with prior stroke or TIA.
‡Non-fatal myocardial infarction or coronary death.
§Stroke, major coronary event, revascularization, emergency hospitalization for coronary ischaemia, or clinically significant peripheral arterial disease in the SPARCL trial; stroke, major coronary event or revascularization in the HPS.

P450 (simvastatin and atorvastatin) are combined with inhibitors of this enzyme (such as 'azole' antifungal agents, HIV protease inhibitors, amiodarone, verapamil, diltiazem and grapefruit juice), and it is important always to consider this possibility when prescribing them.[126]

Liver problems

The US Food and Drug Administration reported a rate of liver failure attributable to statins of one per million person-years of use, but there were no cases of liver failure reported in the RCTs, and a very small excess (0.2%)

of raised liver enzymes in those allocated a statin compared with placebo.[110,118,120]

Peripheral neuropathy

Case–control studies have found users of statins to have an increased risk of developing polyneuropathy of at least 2.5 times the background population risk, with a substantial increase in this risk after prolonged treatment. Assuming the background population risk of idiopathic polyneuropathy to be about one per 10 000 person-years, this implies an excess absolute risk of at least 2.5 per 10 000 person-years. However, no significant excess of peripheral neuropathy was reported in the largest of the statin trials.[127,128]

These data are generally very reassuring. With the exception of the SPARCL trial, the large trials assessed statin doses equivalent to simvastatin 40 mg or less, but safety data from trials comparing intensive vs moderate cholesterol-lowering statin regimens are also generally reassuring about higher statin doses as well (section 16.4.6). However, it is important to remember that the RCTs generally screened for and excluded individuals with raised liver enzymes, raised creatinine kinase or impaired renal function, and the largest trial had a several-week pre-randomization run-in period that included a period of active treatment, designed to identify and exclude those unlikely to continue to take allocated treatment for several years. Their results on adverse effects should be interpreted in this context, since patients developing early adverse effects or considered to be at risk of adverse effects were not randomized.[118]

> Cholesterol-lowering treatments do not increase the risks of cancer or suicide, and serious adverse effects of statin monotherapy (such as rhabdomyolysis or liver failure) are extremely rare. However, the combination of a statin with a fibrate substantially increases the risk of rhabdomyolysis and should be avoided or used only with extreme caution.

16.4.5 Who to treat and who not to treat

The specific evidence for patients with a prior stroke or TIA from the HPS and the SPARCL trial, and the systematic reviews of RCTs of a statin vs placebo in a wide range of individuals at increased risk of major vascular events, suggests that cholesterol lowering with a statin should be considered in everyone with a history of an ischaemic cerebrovascular event.

Although subgroup analyses suggest that the effects of lowering cholesterol are similar regardless of the baseline cholesterol or LDL cholesterol level, participants in

HPS had a non-fasting baseline cholesterol level of > 3.5 mmol/L, and those in SPARCL an LDL-cholesterol of > 2.6 mmol/L.[118,120] Since these are the trials from which most of the direct evidence comes, we do not recommend statins for patients whose untreated cholesterol or LDL cholesterol levels are below these levels, but in our experience of clinical practice in European populations this is rare. Neither do we recommend routine prescription of a statin for patients with a history of intracerebral haemorrhage (ICH) but no ischaemic vascular events, since only very few such patients were included in the RCTs. Furthermore, these patients are at higher risk of a subsequent ICH than those with a prior ischaemic cerebrovascular event (section 16.2.4), and there may be an increased risk of haemorrhagic stroke with statin treatment (section 16.4.2). For patients with a history of ICH who are *also* considered to be at particularly high risk of future ischaemic stroke or coronary events, it is probably reasonable to prescribe a statin. There must have been patients like this in the RCTs of statins, although they have not been separately enumerated, and direct evidence in this group of patients is not available.

The mean age of the participants in the statin trials was about 60, and there were relatively few very elderly (over 80 years). However, subgroup analyses found no evidence that the relative effects of treatment were influenced by age.[117] Furthermore, an observational study of statin use in routine clinical practice in Scotland found that, although the patients treated with statins in the population under study were older on average than the trial participants, their overall effects were similar to those found in the trials.[129] Thus, old age per se should not be a barrier to treatment with a statin, but the possible problems of polypharmacy should always be considered, especially in older patients (section 16.18.2).

16.4.6 How low to go and which statin regimen to use

The *indirect evidence* evidence from the RCTs suggests that greater benefits are conferred by larger reductions in LDL cholesterol (section 16.4.2 and Fig. 16.20). Furthermore, recent RCTs *directly* comparing intensive with moderate lipid-lowering statin regimens suggest that more intensive regimens achieve significantly greater reductions in LDL cholesterol, reduce progression of coronary artery atherosclerosis, and reduce the risks of major vascular events including stroke.[130–133] The two largest of these trials between them included almost 20 000 patients and found no significant difference between atorvastatin 80 mg daily and atorvastatin 10 mg or simvastatin 20 mg daily in the risks of death, cancer, violent or traumatic death, rhabdomyolysis or myopathy. In both trials there was a small (no more than 1%) absolute increase in the risk of persistently raised transaminases with the higher dose of atorvastatin but no cases of liver failure were reported.[131,133] One of the trials found a slight excess of myalgia and gastrointestinal symptoms with the higher dose of atorvastatin.[133] The ongoing Study of the Effectiveness of Additional Reductions in Cholesterol and Homocysteine (SEARCH) trial of 12 000 patients with ischaemic heart disease randomized to 80 mg vs 20 mg daily simvastatin for 5 years will provide additional evidence on this issue (see http://www.ctsu.ox.ac.uk/projects/search/index_html).

At present our recommended statin regimen is either the HPS regimen of simvastatin 40 mg daily or the SPARCL regimen of atorvastatin 80 mg daily. In keeping with the indirect and direct comparisons between different statin regimens, we would expect atorvastatin 80 mg to produce a larger relative reduction in cholesterol, LDL cholesterol and clinical outcomes than simvastatin 40 mg. However, since more intensive lipid lowering may be associated with a slightly increased risk of adverse effects (see above), one might prefer to use atorvastatin 80 mg daily in patients at particularly high risk of further ischaemic vascular events, in whom the absolute benefit of increasing the intensity of cholesterol-lowering treatment will be greatest. Cost may also influence the decision since, at least in the UK, atorvastatin is currently substantially more expensive than simvastatin. Sometimes, patients who are unable to tolerate one particular statin can tolerate another, and it is reasonable to use alternative statins to simvastatin or atorvastatin if necessary. Approximate equivalent doses to simvastatin 40 mg (in terms of LDL cholesterol lowering effect) of other statins are shown in Table 16.6. [110]

16.4.7 When to start

There is no specific evidence from RCTs for the use of statins in the *very* early period after an ischaemic stroke or TIA. However, impressive reductions in ischaemic vascular events, including stroke, have been reported with the use of statins within the first few days of an acute coronary syndrome, suggesting that early use after cerebrovascular events may also be beneficial.[134] Furthermore, there is no reason to suppose that the potential adverse effects of statin treatment should be any greater early after an ischaemic stroke or TIA, while the high absolute risk of recurrence at this time should make the absolute benefits of treatment greater. An ongoing RCT of simvastatin 40 mg daily in patients who have had a TIA or minor ischaemic stroke within the previous

Table 16.6 Approximate equivalent doses to simvastatin 40 mg daily (in terms of LDL cholesterol lowering effect) of various other statins. (Data from Law *et al.*, 2003.[110])

Statin regimen	Absolute (%) reduction in LDL cholesterol in mmol/L*
Simvastatin 40 mg daily	1.8 (37%)
Rosuvastatin 5 mg daily	1.8 (38%)
Atorvastatin 10 mg daily	1.8 (37%)
Lovastatin 40 mg daily	1.8 (37%)
Fluvastatin 80 mg daily	1.6 (33%)
Pravastatin 80 mg daily	1.6 (33%)

*Standardized to pre-treatment serum LDL cholesterol concentration of 4.8 mmol/L. Summary estimates from 164 randomized placebo-controlled trials of statin vs placebo in 38 000 people.

24 h should provide some evidence on this issue (see http://www.strokecenter.org/trials/TrialDetail.aspx?tid=483).[7] In the meantime, we tend to start treatment with a statin as soon as the diagnosis is made of an ischaemic stroke or TIA with a baseline total cholesterol of > 3.5 mmol/L or LDL cholesterol > 2.6 mmol/L.

> All patients with a prior ischaemic stroke or transient ischaemic attack and a pre-treatment total cholesterol level of > 3.5 mmol/L or LDL cholesterol level of > 2.6 mmol/L should be considered for treatment with a statin. Both simvastatin 40 mg daily and atorvastin 80 mg daily have been shown to be beneficial in these patients. We generally start treatment as soon as the diagnosis has been confidently made.

16.4.8 The role of non-statin lipid-lowering drugs

Because the evidence for statins is more extensive and compelling than for other lipid-lowering drugs, these should generally be the first choice of lipid-lowering agent. For patients with very abnormal lipid profiles (very high cholesterol, triglycerides, or both) which respond insufficiently to maximum statin dose, other lipid-lowering drugs such as anion-exchange resins (which prevent reabsorption of bile acids, so increasing clearance of LDL cholesterol), ezetimibe (which inhibits the intestinal absorption of cholesterol), or – with great caution because of the increased risk of rhabdomyolysis – fibrates (which act mainly by decreasing triglyceride concentration) may be used in addition. This is generally best done under the supervision of a lipid specialist. For patients unable to tolerate a statin, and despite the lack of evidence from RCTs for a reduction in stroke, and the absence of large RCTs spefically in patients with a prior stroke or TIA, it seems reasonable to use an alternative drug to try to lower the LDL cholesterol concentration to some extent, since this seems very likely to reduce the risk of future vascular events.

16.5 Antiplatelet drugs

Platelets are involved in the pathophysiology not just of acute thrombosis in arteries and veins, but probably also in the process of atherogenesis itself (section 6.3). Antiplatelet drugs should, in theory, therefore reduce the risk not only of ischaemic stroke but also of myocardial infarction and other serious thrombotic events in both arteries and veins, such as intracranial venous thrombosis and pulmonary emboli. Their most important potential adverse effect is bleeding, most importantly intracranial haemorrhage because it is so frequently fatal or disabling, and serious extracranial haemorrhage (mainly from the gastrointestinal tract) leading to hospital admission and sometimes requiring blood transfusion or surgery. Therefore, probably the best outcome to assess the overall benefits of antiplatelet treatment is the composite outcome of 'stroke, myocardial infarction and vascular death' (whichever occurs first), which we will refer to as 'serious vascular events'. This outcome includes not only the serious ischaemic events which antiplatelet treatment should prevent, but also the most important potential adverse effects, all intracranial as well as fatal extracranial haemorrhages. Because the number of events is greater, this composite outcome also provides more statistical power, and therefore precision, in estimating treatment effect than any of the individual components. However, if the number of outcome events is sufficient, it is not unreasonable to explore treatment effects on individual outcomes, such as stroke or myocardial infarction separately.[135] There is also increasing interest in whether aspirin might reduce the risk of progressive cognitive impairment and vascular dementia in high-risk subjects.[136]

The most comprehensive evidence for the role of antiplatelet treatment in the prevention of serious vascular events in patients at high risk of vascular disease (including those with a previous ischaemic stroke or TIA) is the most recent systematic review of RCTs by the Antithrombotic Trialists' Collaboration (ATT).[137] Several large, relevant randomized trials have been completed since then, and these will also be considered below.

16.5.1 Antiplatelet treatment for long-term secondary prevention of serious vascular events

Evidence from RCTs of immediate antiplatelet treatment (mainly aspirin 160–300 mg daily) in over 40 000 patients with acute ischaemic stroke, mainly randomized within 48 h of onset into one of two large trials, has shown a clear net benefit.[137–139] This has been discussed in detail in section 12.3.

Benefits in a wide range of high-risk patients

The ATT overview included more than 140 000 patients at high risk of vascular disease in 195 RCTs comparing an antiplatelet regimen (mostly aspirin) with placebo or open control; antiplatelet treatment produced a highly significant relative reduction of about one-quarter in the risk of a serious vascular event among all types of high-risk patient, excluding those with acute ischaemic stroke for whom the relative reduction was somewhat smaller. The relative effects of were similar, regardless of whether the patients had a prior ischaemic stroke or TIA, a prior or acute myocardial infarction, stable or unstable angina, peripheral arterial disease, atrial fibrillation or some other high-risk condition (Fig. 16.21).[137] In addition, previous analyses found that the relative reduction in vascular events was similar in males and females, diabetics and non-diabetics, older patients and younger patients, and in patients with and without hypertension.[140]

Benefits in patients with a previous ischaemic stroke or TIA

Among the 20 000 or so patients with a prior ischaemic stroke or TIA, included in 21 RCTs, antiplatelet treatment produced a relative reduction of 22% in the odds of a serious vascular event (Fig. 16.21). This corresponded to the avoidance or delay of 36 serious vascular events (25 non-fatal strokes, six non-fatal myocardial infarctions and seven vascular deaths) per 1000 patients treated for about 3 years. Antiplatelet treatment was also associated with a reduction in all-cause mortality of about 15 per 1000 patients (Fig. 16.22).[137]

Risks in patients with a previous ischaemic stroke or TIA

In the ATT overview, antiplatelet treatment produced about a one-fifth proportional increase in the risk of intracranial haemorrhage, and about half of these events were fatal. However, the absolute excess risk among patients with a prior ischaemic stroke or TIA was less than one per 1000 patients over about 3 years of treatment. This excess risk is accounted for in the estimate of effect on all serious vascular events (see above).

Category of trial	No. of trials with data	No. (%) of vascular events		Observed–expected	Variance	Odds ratio (CI) Antiplatelet : control	% Odds reduction (SE)
		Allocated antiplatelet	Adjusted control				
Previous myocardial infarction	12	1345/9984 (13.5)	1708/10 022 (17.0)	–159.8	567.6		25 (4)
Acute myocardial infarction	15	1007/9658 (10.4)	1370/9644 (14.2)	–181.5	519.2		30 (4)
Previous stroke/transient ischaemic attack	21	2045/11 493 (17.8)	2464/11 527 (21.4)	–152.1	625.8		22 (4)
Acute stroke	7	1670/20 418 (8.2)	1858/20 403 (9.1)	–94.6	795.3		11 (3)
Other high risk	140	1638/20 359 (8.0)	2102/20 543 (10.2)	–222.3	737.0		26 (3)
Subtotal: all except acute stroke	188	6035/51 494 (11.7)	7644/51 736 (14.8)	–715.7	2449.6		25 (2)
All trials	**195**	**7705/71 912 (10.7)**	**9502/72 139 (13.2)**	**–810.3**	**3244.9**		**22 (2)**

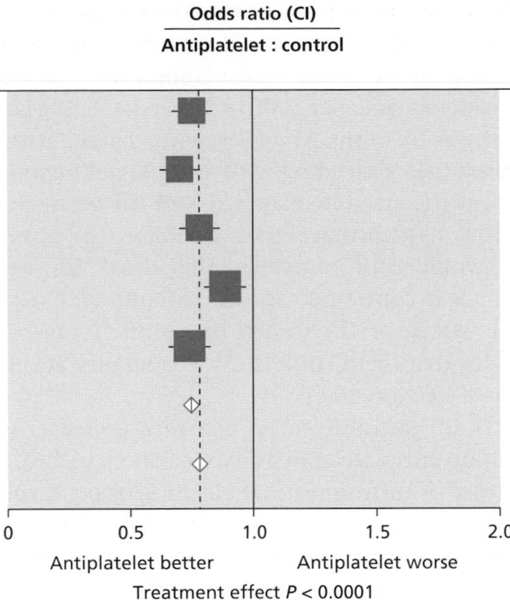

Heterogeneity of odds reductions between:
Five categories of trial: $\chi^2 = 21.4$, df = 4; $P = 0.0003$
Acute stroke v other: $\chi^2 = 18.0$, df = 1; $P = 0.00002$

Odds ratio scale: 0, 0.5, 1.0, 1.5, 2.0
Antiplatelet better — Antiplatelet worse
Treatment effect $P < 0.0001$

Fig. 16.21 Meta-analysis of randomized trials of antiplatelet drugs vs placebo or open control, showing proportional effects on vascular events (myocardial infarction, stroke, or vascular death) in five main high-risk categories. Stratified ratio of odds of an event in treatment groups to that in control groups is plotted for each group of trials (purple square) along with its 99% confidence interval (horizontal line) (CI). Meta-analysis of results for all trials (and 95% confidence interval) is represented by open diamonds. Adjusted control totals have been calculated after converting any unevenly randomized trials to even ones by counting control groups more than once, but other statistical calculations are based on actual numbers from individual trials. SE, standard error. (From Antithrombotic Trialists' Collaboration[137] © 2002 BMJ Publishing Group.)

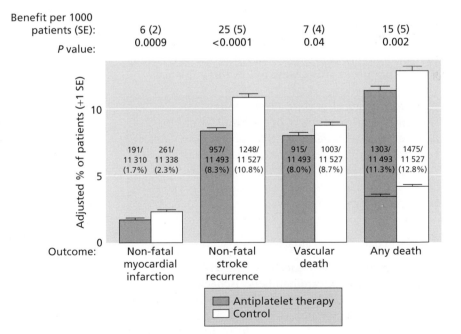

Benefit per 1000 patients (SE):
Non-fatal myocardial infarction: 6 (2); Non-fatal stroke recurrence: 25 (5); Vascular death: 7 (4); Any death: 15 (5)

P value: 0.0009; <0.0001; 0.04; 0.002

Non-fatal myocardial infarction: 191/11 310 (1.7%) vs 261/11 338 (2.3%)
Non-fatal stroke recurrence: 957/11 493 (8.3%) vs 1248/11 527 (10.8%)
Vascular death: 915/11 493 (8.0%) vs 1003/11 527 (8.7%)
Any death: 1303/11 493 (11.3%) vs 1475/11 527 (12.8%)

■ Antiplatelet therapy
□ Control

Fig. 16.22 Meta-analysis showing absolute effects of antiplatelet drugs on various outcomes in patients with previous stroke or transient ischaemic attack (21 randomized trials, mean treatment duration 3 years). Adjusted control totals have been calculated after converting any unevenly randomized trials to even ones by counting control groups more than once. In the 'any death' column, non-vascular deaths are represented by the lower horizontal line (and may be calculated by subtracting vascular deaths from any deaths). (From Antithrombotic Trialists' Collaboration, 2002.[137]) SE, standard error.

Antiplatelet treatment was also associated with about a 60% excess relative risk of serious extracranial haemorrhage (mainly from the gastrointestinal tract) corresponding to an absolute excess risk of about five per 1000 patients with a prior ischaemic stroke or TIA treated for about 3 years. About one in five serious extracranial haemorrhages was fatal and so included in the composite outcome of serious vascular events.[137] Thus, the relatively large absolute reduction in serious vascular events (36 per 1000 in 3 years) clearly outweighs the much smaller excess risk (about four non-fatal extra-cranial haemorrhages per 1000 in 3 years). Of note is that most of the RCTs in the ATT overview excluded patients at increased risk of bleeding with antiplatelet treatment. But, even if the absolute excess risk of intracranial and extracranial haemorrhage were doubled, the absolute benefits would still outweigh the risks. So, unless there are clear contraindications, patients with a prior ischaemic stroke or TIA should be routinely prescribed antiplatelet treatment, unless anticoagulants are more appropriate (section 16.6).

The risk of gastrointestinal bleeding increases with combination antiplatelet treatment (section 16.5.5), age, prior history of gastrointestinal bleeding or peptic ulcer, and concurrent use of non-steroidal anti-inflammatory drugs or cyclo-oxygenase-2 inhibitors.[141,142] Infection with *Helicobacter pylori* also increases the bleeding risk, but this is greatly reduced when the infection is cleared.[143] It has been suggested that the risk of bleeding should be minimized by the use of a proton-pump inhibitor and *Helicobacter pylori* eradication in all patients receiving aspirin who have risk factors for gastrointestinal bleeding (including all those receiving dual antiplatelet treatment).[142] However, this advice is not based on evidence from randomized trials with clinically meaningful outcomes and, while it is always worth considering gastric protection in patients considered to be at high risk of gastrointestinal bleeding, especially those with a history of relevant upper gastrointestinal symptoms or bleeding, we may not necessarily always follow this guidance.

> Unless there are clear contraindications to antithrombotic treatment, or clear indications for anticoagulants, patients at high risk of serious vascular events, including those with a prior ischaemic stroke or transient ischaemic attacks, should receive long-term antiplatelet treatment, since the benefits greatly outweigh the risks.

Benefits in patients with atrial fibrillation

Atrial fibrillation (AF) increases the risk of vascular events, particularly cardioembolic ischaemic stroke in patients who have already had an ischaemic stroke or TIA, and systemic emboli (section 16.6.2). Seven RCTs have assessed the effects of antiplatelet treatment (mainly aspirin, in a daily dose varying between 75 mg and 325 mg) in over 4000 AF patients. There have been several systematic reviews, varying slightly in their inclusion criteria but including the same large trials, with similar findings: antiplatelet treatment just significantly reduced the risks of both serious vascular events

and stroke, consistent with the overall results for high-risk patients in the ATT overview.[137,144–146] There was no statistically significant increase in the risk of major bleeding but numbers were small.[144–146]

There was no significant heterogeneity between the results of individual trials or between trials including patients with and without a history of previous ischaemic stroke or TIA (Fig. 16.23). Because patients in AF with ischaemic stroke or TIA are at much higher risk of subsequent stroke than those with no such history, this higher absolute risk translates into a higher absolute risk reduction. Thus, for every 1000 patients treated with aspirin for a year, about 25 subsequent strokes will be avoided among those with a prior ischaemic stroke or TIA, while about 15 will be avoided among those with no prior ischaemic stroke or TIA. [144]

However, patients with AF and a history of ischaemic stroke or TIA generally have a sufficiently high risk of recurrence to justify the use of oral anticoagulants (section 16.6.2). But, for patients with contraindications to warfarin, aspirin is a safe – albeit less effective – alternative. The effects of anticoagulants compared with control and with antiplatelet treatment are discussed in section 16.6.2. Restoration and maintenance of sinus rhythm as a further means of avoiding the need for anticoagulation is discussed in section 16.10.1.

Benefits in patients with other cardioembolic risk conditions

The ATT overview analyses suggested that patients with a potential cardiac source of embolism other than AF – including mitral valve (leaflet) prolapse, isolated aortic stenosis, mitral annulus calcification, cardiac failure and bioprosthetic heart valve – may also benefit from antiplatelet drugs.[137] For these patients, if there is a history of systemic embolism (or TIA or ischaemic stroke), or if AF is present, anticoagulants are often preferable to antiplatelet drugs. However, if anticoagulants are contraindicated, or the risk of embolism is low, then antiplatelet drugs are likely to be beneficial. Examples of situations where the risks and inconvenience of anticoagulants probably outweigh their benefits, making antiplatelet treatment a more appropriate choice, include patients with mitral leaflet prolapse who have had an ischaemic stroke or TIA with no other obvious cause, patients with aortic valve disease and no other indication for anticoagulation, and long-term preventive treatment in patients with a bioprosthetic heart valve who do not have AF.[147]

People without symptomatic vascular disease

Although the benefits of aspirin (or some other antiplatelet regimen) have been unequivocally demonstrated

Fig. 16.23 Meta-analysis of randomized trials of aspirin vs control, showing proportional effects of aspirin on stroke in patients with atrial fibrillation, with and without a history of ischaemic stroke or transient ischaemic attack (TIA). Odds ratios (OR) for aspirin vs control for each trial are shown as squares, with area proportional to statistical weight, and 95% confidence intervals (CI) are represented by horizontal lines. Meta-analysis of results for subgroups of trials and overall (and 95% confidence interval) are represented by diamonds. AFASAK, Copenhagen Atrial Fibrillation, Aspirin, and Anticoagulation study; SPAF, Stroke Prevention in Atrial Fibrillation study; LASAF, Low-dose Aspirin, Stroke and Atrial Fibrillation pilot study; JAST, Japan Atrial Fibrillation Stroke Trial; EAFT, European Atrial Fibrillation Trial; ESPS-2, second European Stroke Prevention Study; UK-TIA, United Kingdom-Transient Ischaemic Attack trial. (Data from Hart *et al.*, 1999[144] and Sato *et al.*, 2006.[145])

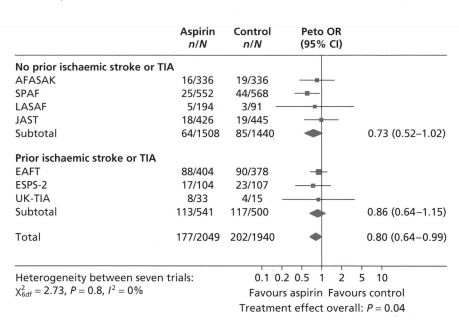

to outweigh the risks in high-risk patients with clinically evident vascular disease, predicting the benefits and hazards of aspirin in someone without known arterial disease is far less straightforward. There have been six RCTs in the primary prevention of vascular events in a total of almost 100 000 asymptomatic individuals. Although a meta-analysis of these demonstrated a statistically significant 12% relative reduction in vascular events, the risk of a serious vascular event in the untreated groups was only five or six per 1000 per year, despite a deliberate policy in several of the trials to recruit high-risk asymptomatic individuals. The absolute reduction in risk was therefore small, only about three or four vascular events per 1000 people treated for about 6 years (i.e. less than one event prevented per 1000 per year). Against this, one must consider the increased risk of major bleeding, which, although small, was similar in magnitude to the absolute benefit. Further uncertainty arises from the fact that the apparent reduction in vascular events appeared to be due to a reduction in stroke risk in women, with no effect on myocardial infarction, and a reduction in myocardial infarction risk in men, with no effect on stroke.[148] This contrasts with the consistent effects in men and women and in other subgroups in high-risk patients, and the explanation for the discrepancy is uncertain.[137,148,149]

Thus, the unselective use of aspirin in individuals without symptomatic vascular disease could cause harm to healthy individuals, and we do not recommend this.[150] However, aspirin may be appropriate for *some* asymptomatic individuals estimated to be at substantially increased risk of vascular events; for example, most people with asymptomatic carotid stenosis, many of whom have many other vascular risk factors and/or symptoms of vascular disease elsewhere in the arterial tree. For the most part, further evidence from ongoing RCTs is needed to allow the reliable identification of apparently healthy people who would gain net benefit from aspirin (see http://www.ctsu.ox.ac.uk/ascend/; http://www.show.scot.nhs.uk/cso/ [CSO Annual Report 2002–2003]).[151]

Effects on dementia and cognitive function

By reducing the incidence of stroke, antiplatelet treatment should reduce the frequency and severity of vascular dementia, although there is no direct evidence from RCTs.[136] However, a systematic review of *observational* studies suggested that aspirin and other non-steroidal anti-inflammatory drugs could reduce Alzheimer's disease.[152] In addition, a small substudy from the Thrombosis Prevention Trial of aspirin, warfarin or both in the primary prevention of vascular events reported that men at risk of vascular events who were allocated antithrombotic therapy had greater verbal fluency and mental flexibility.[153] A planned trial of low-dose aspirin in asymptomatic elderly people and a substudy in the ongoing Aspirin for Asymptomatic Atherosclerosis trial will examine both cognitive decline and dementia (see http://www.show.scot.nhs.uk/cso/ [CSO Annual Report 2002–2003]).[151]

16.5.2 Who not to treat

Patients with recent gastrointestinal bleeding (haematemesis or melaena), with symptoms suggestive of active peptic ulceration, or with other recent major bleeding should probably not receive antiplatelet drugs. Those with a definite allergy to aspirin or another antiplatelet drug should obviously avoid it and use an alternative wherever possible. And those with neutropenia or thrombocytopenia should avoid the thienopyridine antiplatelet drugs (see section 16.5.5).

Since antiplatelet drugs increase the risk of intracranial haemorrhage, it seems illogical to give them to somebody with a spontaneous or traumatic intracerebral haemorrhage (ICH). Although a systematic review of RCTs suggested there was no definite harm from giving antithrombotic treatment to patients with intracerebral haemorrhage, the data were very limited, and we therefore avoid it in patients with an acute ICH.[154] Although patients with an ICH have about twice the risk of further ICH than of ischaemic stroke (section 16.2.4), some may have a clear indication for aspirin, such as ischaemic heart disease or a previous ischaemic stroke. In an obser-

vational study of survivors of ICH, antiplatelet treatment was prescribed in 22%, most commonly for the prevention of ischaemic heart disease. Reassuringly, this was not associated with an increased risk of further ICH, although the numbers of events were very small, making the estimates of risk imprecise.[155]

Despite the lack of direct evidence from RCTs, it seems reasonable to us to use antiplatelet treatment for secondary prevention in patients who have had an ICH but only if they are at high risk of future *ischaemic* vascular events.[156] Again based on our assessment of the likely balance of risks and benefits, rather than direct evidence, we tend to avoid early aspirin in patients with acute ischaemic stroke with haemorrhagic transformation visible on brain imaging, but we would certainly recommend that such patients are discharged on an antiplatelet drug for long-term secondary prevention.

16.5.3 Aspirin

Aspirin was by far the most widely studied antiplatelet drug in the ATT overview. It irreversibly inhibits the enzyme cyclo-oxygenase, therefore inhibiting the production from arachidonic acid of prostaglandin H_2, which is metabolized in platelets to the platelet agonist, thromboxane A_2 (Fig. 16.24). [157]

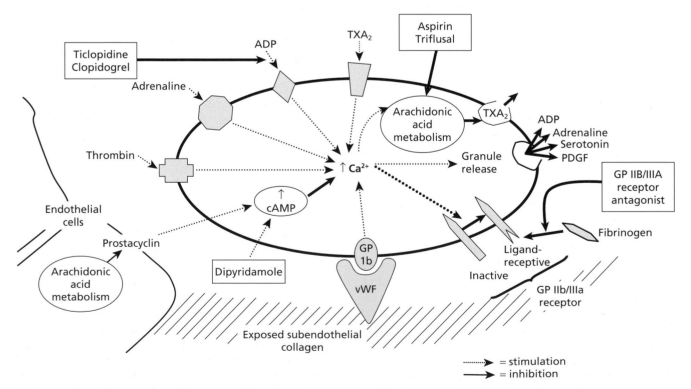

Fig. 16.24 Intra-platelet metabolic pathways and sites of action of various antiplatelet drugs. GP, glycoprotein; PDGF, platelet derived growth factor; vWF, von Willebrand factor; cAMP, cyclic adenosine monophosphate; ADP, adenosine diphosphate; TXA_2, thromboxane A_2.

Benefits

Among almost 60 000 high-risk patients, excluding those with acute ischaemic stroke, aspirin alone reduced the odds of a serious vascular event by about one-quarter. Almost 10 000 of these patients (in 11 randomized trials) had a prior ischaemic stroke or TIA. In these patients, aspirin highly significantly reduced the relative odds of a serious vascular event by 17%, corresponding to an absolute risk reduction of 30 per 1000 over about 3 years (i.e. similar to the result for antiplatelet treatment in general – see section 16.5.1).

BENEFITS OF DIFFERENT DOSES OF ASPIRIN

Controversy has surrounded the most appropriate dose of aspirin, with arguments for daily doses as low as 30 mg to as high as 1500 mg.[158–160] There are theoretical reasons to suggest that lower doses might in fact provide greater net benefit than higher doses:

- First, although not of proven relevance in humans, it has been argued that lower doses should inhibit the production of thromboxane A_2 by platelets, without much affecting the production of prostacyclin (a platelet anti-aggregant and vasodilator) by endothelial cells, which, unlike platelets, have the biosynthetic machinery to regenerate supplies of cyclo-oxygenase. A single oral dose of 100 mg is enough to almost completely suppress thromboxane A_2 production in humans. Because of the irreversible nature of aspirin's inhibition of platelet cyclo-oxygenase, daily doses as low as 30–50 mg have a cumulative inhibitory effect and result in virtually complete suppression of thromboxane A_2 biosynthesis after 7–10 days.[157,161]
- Second, because inhibition of cyclo-oxygenase by aspirin also inhibits the production of prostaglandins that protect the gastrointestinal mucosa, lower doses of aspirin might produce a smaller excess of bleeding, at least from the gastrointestinal tract.
- Third, even if the risk of major haemorrhage does not depend on the dose of aspirin, any reduction in minor adverse effects with lower doses would improve tolerability and compliance, and so effectiveness, particularly with long-term treatment.

The most reliable evidence for the relative effect of different doses of aspirin comes from *direct* randomized comparisons between daily doses of 75–325 mg and 500–1500 mg in 3197 high-risk patients in the ATT overview (about half of whom had a history of ischaemic stroke or TIA) (Fig. 16.25a), and an additional RCT in 2849 patients undergoing carotid endarterectomy; these doses were similarly effective in prevention of serious vascular events.[137,162] Direct comparisons between daily doses of > 75 mg and < 75 mg in 3750 patients in the ATT overview found no significant difference in the effects on vascular events (Fig. 16.25a);[137] most of these patients were included in an RCT comparing 283 mg vs 30 mg daily in patients with a recent TIA or minor ischaemic stroke.[163] However, because the confidence intervals were very wide, the possibility of a small (yet clinically important) difference in effectiveness between these doses of > 75 mg and < 75 mg cannot be excluded on the basis of these direct comparisons.

Indirect comparisons of the effects of different doses compared with control are less reliable but the number of outcome events was much higher. Trials comparing daily aspirin doses of 500–1500 mg, 160–325 mg, 75–150 mg and < 75 mg with control in high-risk patients (excluding those with acute ischaemic stroke) in the ATT overview revealed similar relative reductions in serious vascular events for the three higher daily dose ranges, but a somewhat smaller effect with < 75 mg daily (Fig. 16.25b).[137] Another meta-analysis based on indirect comparisons between the effects of different daily aspirin doses on stroke found no definite evidence of differences between doses.[164]

Considering all the available evidence from direct and indirect comparisons in high-risk patients, it seems reasonable to conclude that aspirin at a dose of 75–150 mg daily is as effective as higher doses. Doses below 75 mg daily may be as effective, but this remains somewhat uncertain.

Risks of different doses of aspirin

A meta-analysis of trials in which participants were randomized to aspirin or control treatment found that aspirin produced a small increased risk of intracranial haemorrhage of about one per 1000 patients treated for 3 years (i.e. similar to the risk of antiplatelet treatment in general; section 16.5.1). There was no clear variation in risk with the dose.[165] In RCTs directly comparing different daily doses, there were no significant differences in the risk of intracranial haemorrhage but the numbers of events were very small and the confidence intervals wide.[137] In contrast, observational studies have suggested that the risk may be dose-related, but their methodological limitations prevent firm conclusions from being drawn.[166,167]

In the ATT overview, aspirin produced a small increased risk of major extracranial haemorrhage, similar to the risk for antiplatelet treatment in general (section 16.5.1). Both indirect and direct comparisons found similar risks of major extracranial haemorrhage with different daily doses.[137] Another meta-analysis found the relative excess risk of gastrointestinal bleeding with aspirin to be about 70%, with no definite variation in

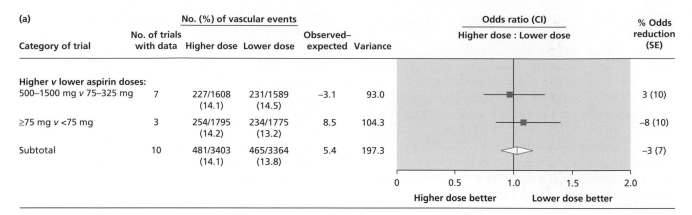

Fig. 16.25 (a) Meta-analysis of randomized trials of one dose of aspirin vs another, showing direct comparisons of proportional effects of different daily aspirin doses on vascular events in high-risk patients. Stratified ratio of odds of an event in higher dose group to that in lower dose group is plotted for each group of trials (purple square with area proportional to statistical weight) along with its 99% confidence interval (CI) (horizontal line). Meta-analysis of results for all trials (and 95% confidence interval) is represented by an open diamond. (From Antithrombotic Trialists' Collaboration, 2002.[137]) (b) Meta-analysis of randomized trials of aspirin vs control, showing indirect comparisons of proportional effects of different daily aspirin doses on vascular events in high-risk patients (excluding those with acute stroke). Stratified ratio of odds of an event in aspirin groups to that in control groups is plotted for each group of trials (purple square with area proportional to statistical weight) along with its 99% CI (horizontal line). Meta-analysis of results for all trials (and 95% CI) is represented by an open diamond. Adjusted control totals have been calculated after converting any unevenly randomized trials to even ones by counting control groups more than once, but statistical calculations are based on actual numbers from individual trials. Some trials contributed to more than one comparison. SE, standard error. (From Antithrombotic Trialists' Collaboration, 2002.[137])

risk between doses or different formulations.[168] On the other hand, RCTs directly comparing different doses showed a trend towards more gastrointestinal haemorrhages with high (500–1500 mg) vs medium (75–325 mg) daily doses, but no difference between 283 and 30 mg daily (Table 16.7).[137] An overview of 15 observational studies, including over 10 000 cases of upper gastrointestinal bleeding or perforation requiring hospital admission, found the relative risk with aspirin to be almost twofold, similar to that found in the RCTs. Studies that examined the effects of different doses of aspirin found greater risks for daily doses > 300 mg than for lower doses. The studies that reported data on aspirin formulation found similar relative risks for enteric coated and plain preparations.[170]

Randomized trials directly comparing different aspirin doses indicate that high dose (500–1500 mg daily) aspirin significantly increases the odds of upper gastrointestinal

Table 16.7(a) Direct randomized comparisons between the effects of different daily doses of aspirin on gastrointestinal haemorrhage.

Trials with data (*n*)	Events/patients		Higher vs lower dose	
	Higher dose (%)	Lower dose (%)	Odds ratio (95% CI)	2*p*
High vs medium				
2[†]	58/2224 (2.6%)	41/2201 (1.9%)	1.4 (0.9 to 2.1)	0.09
Medium vs low				
1[‡]	30/1576 (1.9%)	25/1555 (1.6%)	1.2 (0.7 to 2.0)	NS

Table 16.7(b) Direct randomized comparisons between the effects of different daily doses of aspirin on upper gastrointestinal symptoms.

Trials with data	Events/patients		Higher vs lower dose	
	Higher dose (%)	Lower dose (%)	Odds ratio (95% CI)	2*p*
High vs medium				
2[†]	583/2224 (26.2%)	483/2201 (21.8%)	1.3 (1.1 to 1.5)	0.0007
Medium vs low				
1[‡]	179/1576 (11.4%)	164/1555 (10.6%)	1.1 (0.9 to 1.4)	NS

[†]UK-TIA Study Group, 1991;[169] Taylor *et al.*, 1999[162] (ACE trial).
[‡]Dutch TIA Trial Study Group, 1991.[163]
High-dose aspirin = 500–1500 mg daily (1200 mg in UK-TIA trial;[69] 650 mg or 1300 mg in ACE trial).
Medium-dose aspirin = 75–325 mg daily (300 mg in UK-TIA trial;[169] 81 mg or 325 mg in ACE trial;[162] 283 mg in Dutch TIA trial[163]).
Low-dose aspirin = < 75 mg daily (30 mg in Dutch TIA trial[163]).
NS not significant (*P* > 0.1). CI, confidence interval.

symptoms compared with medium dose (75–325 mg daily), and that medium dose (283 mg daily) is associated with a trend towards an increased odds of these symptoms compared with low dose (30 mg daily)[137] (Table 16.7).

> Aspirin 75–150 mg daily is probably the most appropriate dose for long-term secondary prevention of serious vascular events to maximize benefits and to minimize adverse effects.

16.5.4 What to do with aspirin treatment 'failures'

Because aspirin only prevents about one-quarter of vascular events that would otherwise occur, inevitably some patients will have events despite taking aspirin with or without other secondary preventive treatments. This may not necessarily represent a 'failure' of treatment, since patients who do have further events while on aspirin might have had more or earlier events without aspirin. Nonetheless, there is increasing interest in the possibility of inter-individual variation in the response to aspirin, and a large number of laboratory measures of so-called 'aspirin resistance' are now available. These tests are not currently useful in clinical practice, since they have not been standardized and, although several studies have suggested an association between aspirin resistance and risk of subsequent vascular events, methodological problems limit the reliability of their results.[171] Non-platelet sources of thromboxane A_2 (particularly in inflammatory states) or altered thromboxane metabolism (e.g. in smokers) can alter thromboxane measurements in laboratory tests of aspirin resistance. Furthermore, although these laboratory measures may predict an increased risk of vascular events, it is not clear whether or not aspirin can still reduce this risk:

There are a number of potential reasons why patients may continue to have events while taking aspirin.[171]

- *Poor adherence*. Up to 40% of patients with vascular disease do not adhere to their aspirin treatment, making this a common and often neglected reason for aspirin 'failure'.[171] Poor adherence may be as much of an issue with other secondary preventive medication, and this also needs to be explored.[172]

- *Incorrect clinical diagnosis.* In patients with repeated events despite the implementation of all reasonable secondary preventive measures, including regular aspirin, it is always worth revisiting the diagnosis. Sometimes the actual cause of recurrent events (e.g. focal seizures, migraine) only comes to light with follow-up, the occurrence of further episodes, and the emergence of additional pieces of key information from the patient or others (sections 3.4 and 3.5).

- *Non-atherothromboembolic pathology*, such as arterial dissection, arteritis, or infective endocarditis. Not all vascular events are due to atherothromboembolism (section 6.2 and chapter 7),[173] and furthermore the complex pathophysiology of atherothrombotic and embolic processes means that we would not expect aspirin to prevent all ischaemic events.

- *Inadequate aspirin dose.* The evidence (section 16.5.3) from RCTs suggests that a daily dose of 75 mg daily is as effective as higher doses. However, this is based on meta-analyses of data from large numbers of patients and does not necessarily apply to each individual. It is uncertain whether individual patients' dose requirements vary. Once other possible causes of treatment failure have been excluded, one reasonable, although non-evidence-based, strategy is to increase the dose of aspirin above 75–150 mg daily.

- *Interference from other drugs.* There is some evidence that gastric acid suppression with a proton-pump inhibitor may impair aspirin absorption, and that concurrent intake of non-steroidal anti-inflammatory drugs (NSAIDs) such as ibuprofen may inhibit binding of aspirin to platelet cyclo-oxygenase-1. However, data are conflicting and further studies are needed to assess these possibilities further.

- *Genetically determined reduced effect of aspirin.* Polymorphisms in the genes encoding cyclo-oxygenase and other proteins that are involved in platelet pathways can modify the antiplatelet effects of aspirin, and may account for inter-individual differences in laboratory measures of aspirin resistance, and possibly in clinically evident aspirin treatment 'failures'.

- *Increased turnover of platelets*, for example in infection, inflammation or following surgery, may reduce the effectiveness of aspirin.

Apart from increasing the dose of aspirin, other strategies used by some clinicians are to add another antiplatelet drug, such as modified release dipyridamole, to aspirin (if the patient is not already taking it), or even to replace aspirin with an alternative such as clopidogrel

(the evidence for alternative regimens is discussed in section 16.5.5). However, there have been no RCTs of alternative antiplatelet strategies among the specific group of patients who have events while taking aspirin. Neither is there any evidence that, for patients in sinus rhythm, oral anticoagulants alone, or in combination with aspirin, offer any definite net advantage over aspirin alone, and they can do harm (section 16.6.1). We would, however, consider the addition of clopidogrel to aspirin, or the substitution of antiplatelet treatment with heparin, sometimes followed by warfarin, in patients who are having very frequent TIAs on aspirin alone (sections 16.5.5 and 16.6.2).

In patients who have further events while taking aspirin, it is important to check that the patient really is having atherothromboembolic episodes and, if so, that they are actually taking their aspirin and sticking to other secondary preventive strategies. It is reasonable to consider the addition of modified dipyridamole 200 mg twice daily if the patient is not already taking this, but there is no randomized evidence to support increasing the aspirin dose.

16.5.5 Alternative antiplatelet regimens to aspirin

Aspirin acts on only one of a number of pathways leading to platelet activation and so thrombosis. Antiplatelet drugs acting through different pathways might therefore be more effective than aspirin if given as alternatives to, or combined with, aspirin (Fig. 16.24). However, any differences in effects on clinical outcomes between two antiplatelet regimens are likely to be small and so to detect such differences reliably, randomized comparisons would need to include very large numbers (i.e. tens of thousands) of patients. In the ATT overview, indirect comparisons provided no clear evidence of any differences in effects on serious vascular events,[137] and in the direct comparisons the numbers of patients were generally too small to exclude a difference. However, several recent large trials have provided further information about alternative antiplatelet regimens.

Thienopyridines vs aspirin

The thienopyridine antiplatelet drugs (ticlopidine and clopidogrel) prevent adenosine diphosphate (ADP) binding to its receptor on platelets, so reducing ADP-dependent activation of the glycoprotein IIb-IIIa complex which is the major receptor for fibrinogen on the platelet surface (Fig. 16.24).[161]

A systematic review of RCTs of a thienopyridine vs aspirin in high-risk patients identified 10 relevant trials

Fig. 16.26 Meta-analysis of randomized trials of a thienopyridine antiplatelet drug (ticlopidine or clopidogrel) vs aspirin in high vascular risk patients. Outcome is vascular events. Odds ratios (OR) for thienopyridine vs aspirin for each trial shown as squares, with area proportional to statistical weight, and 95% confidence intervals (CI) are represented by horizontal lines. Pooled odds ratio (and 95% CI) represented by diamond. AAASPS, African American Antiplatelet Stroke Prevention Study; CAPRIE, Clopidogrel versus Aspirin to Prevent Recurrent Ischemic Events; STAMI, Study of Ticlopidine versus Aspirin after Myocardial Infarction; TASS, Ticlopidine Aspirin Stroke Study. (Data of from Sudlow *et al.*, in press.[174])

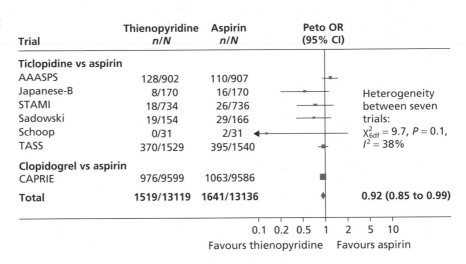

Trial	Thienopyridine n/N	Aspirin n/N	Peto OR (95% CI)
Ticlopidine vs aspirin			
AAASPS	128/902	110/907	
Japanese-B	8/170	16/170	
STAMI	18/734	26/736	
Sadowski	19/154	29/166	
Schoop	0/31	2/31	
TASS	370/1529	395/1540	
Clopidogrel vs aspirin			
CAPRIE	976/9599	1063/9586	
Total	**1519/13119**	**1641/13136**	**0.92 (0.85 to 0.99)**

Heterogeneity between seven trials: $\chi^2_{6df} = 9.7$, $P = 0.1$, $I^2 = 38\%$

Favours thienopyridine   Favours aspirin

in 26 865 patients (Fig. 16.26). Aspirin was compared with clopidogrel in one trial of 19 185 patients with ischaemic stroke, myocardial infarction or peripheral arterial disease, and with ticlopidine in the remaining nine trials in a total of 7633 patients, most of whom had a recent TIA or mild ischaemic stroke. The thienopyridines modestly and just significantly reduced the odds of a serious vascular event compared with aspirin (OR 0.92; 95% CI 0.85–0.99; 10 events avoided per 1000 patients treated, 95% CI 0–20 events per 1000), but the wide confidence interval included the possibility of no additional benefit. The result was similar, although not statistically significant, when only trials that randomized patients on the basis of their history of ischaemic stroke or TIA were considered.[174] There have been several subsequent attempts to identify subgroups of patients likely to gain particular benefit from a thienopyridine (particularly clopidogrel) instead of aspirin, but in the face of an overall result of such marginal statistical significance, apparent differences in treatment effects between subgroups are highly likely to occur through the play of chance alone, and such analyses should be regarded with extreme caution.[175,176]

In terms of adverse effects, the systematic review found no significant difference between the thienopyridines and aspirin in intracranial or major extracranial haemorrhage. On the other hand, compared with aspirin, the thienopyridines were associated with a lower risk of gastrointestinal upset and haemorrhage. However, ticlopidine approximately doubled and clopidogrel increased by about one-third the risks of both skin rash and diarrhoea compared with aspirin. Ticlopidine, but not clopidogrel, was associated with an excess of neutropenia compared with aspirin, but there was no

significant difference between the thienopyridines and aspirin in the risk of thrombocytopenia.[174] Ticlopidine has been associated with thrombocytopenia in observational studies, and both ticlopidine and clopidogrel have also been associated in post-marketing surveillance studies with thrombotic thrombocytopenic purpura, although this is very rare.[177–182] The few trials which have compared the two thienopyridines directly have suggested better safety and tolerability with clopidogrel vs ticlopidine,[183–185] which makes clopidogrel the thienopyridine of choice on safety grounds.

Although, in the systematic review, the thienopyridines had a significantly lower rate of gastrointestinal upset and haemorrhage compared with aspirin, the most commonly used dose of aspirin in the trials of 325 mg was higher than the currently recommended daily dose of 75–150 mg, which is associated with less gastrointestinal adverse effects, and may compare more favourably with the thienopyridines.[174]

In summary, clopidogrel appears to be as effective as aspirin (and possibly somewhat more so), and is probably as safe, although it has a different adverse effect profile. The high cost of clopidogrel and the uncertainty of any additional benefit compared to aspirin make it unreasonable to suggest that it should replace aspirin as the first-choice antiplatelet drug for all patients at high vascular risk. It has been suggested that clopidogrel should be an alternative to aspirin in patients who are intolerant of or are allergic to aspirin. However we have no direct evidence of the relative effectiveness of thienopyridines compared with aspirin in this particular subgroup of patients as they were excluded from the RCTs. Furthermore, in an RCT in patients who developed peptic ulcer bleeding while taking aspirin to reduce vascular events, those who were assigned aspirin plus esomeprazole (a proton-pump inhibitor) had a statistically significant reduction in the cumulative incidence of recurrent ulcer bleeding in comparison to those treated with clopidogrel only. The combination of clopidogrel with a proton-pump inhibitor was not assessed.[186] Thus, while clopidogrel still seems a reasonable alternative antiplatelet drug for patients who are genuinely allergic to aspirin, in patients who experience gastrointestinal problems with aspirin, current evidence provides more support for adding a proton-pump inhibitor than for replacing aspirin with clopidogrel.

> Clopidogrel appears to be as effective and as safe as aspirin, but is much more expensive. It is a reasonable alternative antiplatelet drug for patients with a history of ischaemic stroke or transient ischaemic attack, or for others at high risk of vascular events, who are genuinely allergic to aspirin. For patients unable to tolerate aspirin because of upper gastrointestinal symptoms, the addition of a proton-pump inhibitor is probably safer than changing to clopidogrel.

Thienopyridines plus aspirin vs aspirin

Because the thienopyridines act through a different mechanism to that of aspirin, their effects might be expected to be additive, making the combination of aspirin with a thienopyridine a theoretically attractive one, so long as any excess bleeding risks do not outweigh additional benefit. When the ATT antiplatelet trials database was completed in 1997, there was just one small RCT of aspirin plus a thienopyridine (ticlopidine) vs aspirin alone in about 1000 patients undergoing coronary artery stenting, and the results were inconclusive.[137,187] Since then, several RCTs have assessed adding clopidogrel to aspirin in over 60 000 patients with acute coronary syndromes (with or without ST segment elevation) and/or those undergoing percutaneous coronary intervention. In this high-risk setting, the combination has shown definite reductions in serious vascular events compared with aspirin alone, although this is at the expense of a small increased risk of major (but not intracranial or life-threatening) haemorrhage.[188–191]

However, the same benefits of the combination of clopidogrel and aspirin have not been seen in long-term secondary prevention. The Clopidogrel for High Atherothrombotic Risk and Ischemic Stabilization, Management and Avoidance (CHARISMA) randomized trial recruited over 15 000 patients with symptoms of ischaemic heart disease, ischaemic stroke, TIA, or peripheral arterial disease within the previous 5 years, or multiple atherothrombotic risk factors. There was no statistically

significant difference between treatment groups in the rate of serious vascular events, but the risk of moderate to severe bleeding was increased with combination treatment. There was a suggestion that patients with previous symptoms of vascular disease might achieve net benefit with combination treatment while asymptomatic patients with multiple risk factors might be harmed.[192] However, this subgroup effect was one of many tested and could well have arisen purely by chance, and so cannot be regarded as anything more than hypothesis generating. Another RCT, the Management of Athero-Thrombosis with Clopidogrel in High-risk patients (MATCH) trial, compared clopidogrel plus aspirin with clopidogrel alone in over 7000 high-risk patients with a recent (within 3 months) ischaemic stroke or TIA and found no significant effect on the combined outcome of ischaemic stroke, myocardial infarction, vascular death, or rehospitalization for acute ischaemia, but there was an increased risk of life-threatening bleeding with the combination compared with clopidogrel alone.[193]

Thus, there is currently no clear evidence to support the use of clopidogrel plus aspirin (rather than single antiplatelet therapy, for which the first choice is aspirin alone – see above) in patients with a prior ischaemic stroke or TIA, or other patients with stable previously symptomatic vascular disease. There are, however, some indications that the combination of clopidogrel and aspirin may ultimately prove to be of net benefit very early after ischaemic stroke or TIA, when the risk of recurrence is highest. In the MATCH trial, subgroup analyses suggested the possibility of net benefit from combination treatment in patients randomized within a week of symptom onset, and the overall negative result of MATCH may reflect the inclusion of a large proportion of patients with lacunar ischaemic events, who may benefit less from intensive antiplatelet treatment but be at higher risk of intracerebral bleeding compared to those with large artery disease.[193] In addition, an RCT of clopidogrel plus aspirin vs aspirin alone in patients with recently symptomatic carotid stenosis and ongoing asymptomatic emboli detected by transcranial Doppler ultrasound found that the combination was more effective than aspirin alone in reducing asymptomatic emboli.[18,194] Further RCTs assessing clopidogrel plus aspirin vs aspirin alone very early after a minor ischaemic stroke or TIA are either ongoing or planned (see http://www.strokecenter.org/trials/TrialDetail.aspx?tid=483).[7]

> There is currently no clear evidence from randomized trials to support the use of the combination of clopidogrel plus aspirin to prevent vascular events in patients with ischaemic stroke or transient ischaemic attacks.

Dipyridamole vs aspirin

Dipyridamole is a pyrimidopyridine derivative with both antiplatelet and vasodilator properties, whose mechanism of action on platelets remains a subject of controversy. Several possible antiplatelet actions have been observed *in vitro*, including inhibition of platelet phosphodiesterase, direct stimulation of the release of prostacyclin from endothelial cells, and inhibition of adenosine uptake by platelets. All of these putative mechanisms increase intraplatelet cyclic AMP, which inhibits the mobilization of free calcium, central to platelet activation (Fig. 16.24). However, although dipyridamole is widely accepted to be an antiplatelet drug, none of these actions has been demonstrated *in vivo* at the doses used in clinical practice.[161] It is also a vasodilator, which is why it is used in diagnostic stress echocardiography and thallium imaging, and during rapid intravenous administration in these procedures it tends to cause hypotension.[195] However, in a randomized comparison of aspirin vs aspirin plus 400 mg of oral dipyridamole daily in about 600 patients with recent cerebral ischaemia it did not appear to affect the blood pressure over the long term.[196]

The ATT meta-analysis of direct randomized comparisons between dipyridamole alone and aspirin alone in a total of about 3500 high-risk patients found no significant difference in the effect on serious vascular events (OR dipyridamole vs aspirin 1.02; 95% CI 0.85–1.21).[137] Since the largest body of evidence for the use of any single antiplatelet drug is for aspirin (Fig. 16.25b), and the wide confidence interval includes the possibility that dipyridamole is less effective than aspirin, this implies that dipyridamole alone should not generally be considered as an alternative to aspirin.

> Dipyridamole alone should not generally be considered as an alternative to aspirin for secondary prevention of serious vascular events in high-risk patients, including those with a history of ischaemic stroke or transient ischaemic attack.

Dipyridamole plus aspirin vs aspirin

Dipyridamole plus aspirin was compared with aspirin alone in 25 RCTs in high-risk patients in the ATT overview. Overall, the combination produced a non-significant reduction in serious vascular events. When the separate components of the composite outcome were assessed, the combination appeared to be particularly effective in reducing non-fatal stroke, but not non-fatal myocardial infarction or vascular death.[137]

This non-fatal stroke result was derived mainly from one large study, the second European Stroke Prevention Study (ESPS-2), in which about 6000 patients with a previous ischaemic stroke or TIA were randomly assigned in a factorial design to aspirin 50 mg daily, modified-release dipyridamole 400 mg daily, both or neither.[197] Dipyridamole plus aspirin significantly reduced the relative risk of vascular events by about one-fifth compared with aspirin alone, due to a significant reduction in stroke, with no detectable effect on either myocardial infarction or vascular death (although numbers of non-stroke outcomes were small (Fig. 16.27).[137,198] Until further evidence emerged, it remained unclear whether the favourable results for stroke were explained by chance (since the number of patients and relevant outcome events was relatively small), the dose of aspirin (since 50 mg might be less effective than 75 mg or more daily – see above) or the particular dose and preparation of dipyridamole used.[195] Analyses that included only trials with ischaemic stroke and TIA patients, or that considered only ESPS-2 (the only study to use the modified-release preparation of dipyridamole), suggested that the combination reduced vascular events compared with aspirin alone,[197,199] but since these results were dominated by the stroke outcomes in ESPS-2, they too were subject to the possible effects of chance and the very low dose of aspirin.

A further RCT, the European/Australasian Stroke Prevention in Reversible Ischaemia Trial (ESPRIT) has now compared aspirin (median daily dose 75 mg) plus dipyridamole (mainly modified release, 200 mg twice daily) vs aspirin alone in around 3000 patients with a prior ischaemic stroke or TIA of presumed arterial origin (patients with atrial fibrillation were excluded).[198] Like ESPS-2, the combination produced a statistically significant one-fifth relative reduction in vascular events, arising from reductions in *each* of ischaemic stroke, cardiac events and vascular death (although none of these separate outcomes was independently statistically significant) (Fig. 16.27). ESPRIT also showed that benefits continued to accrue for up to 5 years, and there were no significant differences in the relative effects of treatment according to several characteristics, including age, gender, history of ischaemic heart disease and aspirin dose.[198]

An up-to-date meta-analysis of all RCTs comparing the combination of aspirin plus dipyridamole with aspirin alone in patients with a prior ischaemic stroke or TIA largely reflects the results of ESPS-2 and ESPRIT, shows a significant one-fifth relative reduction in vascular events (Fig. 16.27). In ESPRIT, the annual risk of vascular events in the aspirin-only arm was 5%, falling to 4% in the aspirin plus dipyridamole arm, and so adding modified-release dipyridamole 200 mg twice daily to aspirin at this

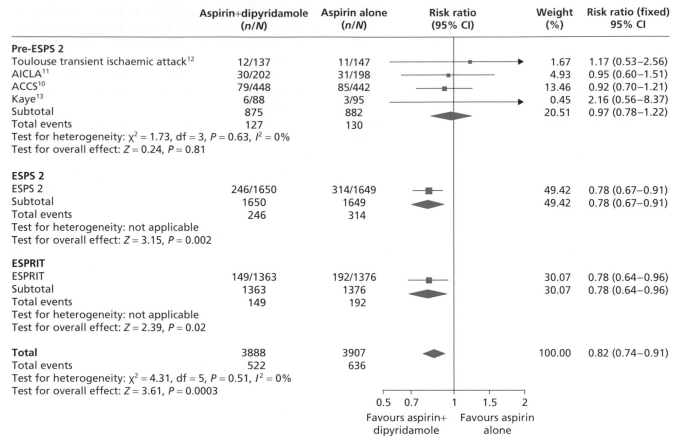

	Aspirin+dipyridamole (n/N)	Aspirin alone (n/N)	Risk ratio (95% CI)	Weight (%)	Risk ratio (fixed) 95% CI
Pre-ESPS 2					
Toulouse transient ischaemic attack[12]	12/137	11/147		1.67	1.17 (0.53–2.56)
AICLA[11]	30/202	31/198		4.93	0.95 (0.60–1.51)
ACCS[10]	79/448	85/442		13.46	0.92 (0.70–1.21)
Kaye[13]	6/88	3/95		0.45	2.16 (0.56–8.37)
Subtotal	875	882		20.51	0.97 (0.78–1.22)
Total events	127	130			
Test for heterogeneity: $\chi^2 = 1.73$, df = 3, $P = 0.63$, $I^2 = 0\%$					
Test for overall effect: $Z = 0.24$, $P = 0.81$					
ESPS 2					
ESPS 2	246/1650	314/1649		49.42	0.78 (0.67–0.91)
Subtotal	1650	1649		49.42	0.78 (0.67–0.91)
Total events	246	314			
Test for heterogeneity: not applicable					
Test for overall effect: $Z = 3.15$, $P = 0.002$					
ESPRIT					
ESPRIT	149/1363	192/1376		30.07	0.78 (0.64–0.96)
Subtotal	1363	1376		30.07	0.78 (0.64–0.96)
Total events	149	192			
Test for heterogeneity: not applicable					
Test for overall effect: $Z = 2.39$, $P = 0.02$					
Total	3888	3907		100.00	0.82 (0.74–0.91)
Total events	522	636			
Test for heterogeneity: $\chi^2 = 4.31$, df = 5, $P = 0.51$, $I^2 = 0\%$					
Test for overall effect: $Z = 3.61$, $P = 0.0003$					

0.5 0.7 1 1.5 2

Favours aspirin+ dipyridamole   Favours aspirin alone

Fig. 16.27 Meta-analysis of randomized trials of aspirin + dipyridamole vs aspirin alone in patients with a prior ischaemic stroke or TIA. Outcome = vascular events (stroke, myocardial infarction or vascular death). Purple squares represent trial-specific risk ratios with the area of each square proportional to the statistical weight of that study, and horizontal lines denoting 95% confidence intervals (CI). Pooled risk ratios are shown as diamonds whose width denotes the 95% CI. ESPS 2, Second European Stroke Prevention Study; ESPRIT, European/Australian Stroke Prevention in Reversible Ischaemia Trial. (Reprinted from The ESPRIT Study Group, *Lancet*[198] © 2006 with permission from Elsevier.)

level of risk should prevent about 10 vascular events per 1000 patients treated per year (i.e. 100 patients would have to be treated for 1 year to prevent one event).[198]

> The addition of dipyridamole (modified-release formulation, 200 mg twice daily) to aspirin produces about a one-fifth reduction in the relative risk of vascular events in patients with a prior ischaemic stroke or transient ischaemic attack, corresponding to an average absolute reduction of about one event per 100 treated per year (in patients already receiving other proven secondary prevention treatments).

Although a combined preparation of 200 mg modified-release dipyridamole and 25 mg aspirin, designed to be taken twice daily, is available, most of the authors of this book are more comfortable with continuing a daily aspirin dose of 75–150 mg and adding 200 mg twice daily of modified-release dipyridamole separately (section 16.5.3).

Neither ESPS-2 nor ESPRIT found any excess major bleeding in patients allocated the combination compared with aspirin alone. However, both reported an excess of premature cessations of treatment in the combination treatment arm, mainly due to adverse effects, particularly dipyridamole-induced headache, which may occur in up to one-third of people receiving dipyridamole but this usually settles in 1–2 weeks and might be reduced by dipyridamole dose titration.[197,198,200]

Since rapid intravenous injection of dipyridamole reduces blood pressure (see above), there have been anxieties about its use in patients with ischaemic heart disease.[195] However, in ESPRIT, long-term oral dipyridamole did not affect blood pressure, and the benefits of adding dipyridamole to aspirin were similar in those with and without ischaemic heart disease.[196,198]

Patients should be warned of the risk of dipyridamole-related headache, which may occur in up to one-third of people receiving dipyridamole, but it usually settles in 1–2 weeks.

Triflusal vs aspirin

Triflusal is structurally related to aspirin and exerts its antitplatelet effect mainly through inhibition of platelet cyclo-oxygenase (Fig. 16.24), but it is also thought to act on several other targets involved in platelet aggregation, and to increase nitric oxide synthesis, so giving it vasodilatory potential.[201] A systematic review of RCTs of aspirin vs triflusal in high-risk patients identified five trials including a total of 5219 patients, more than half of whom had a history of ischaemic stroke or TIA. For serious vascular events in aggregate, there was no significant difference between the two drugs (OR 1.04; 95% CI 0.87–1.23), although the wide 95% confidence interval could not exclude a clinically important difference in favour of one or other drug. Aspirin was associated with a higher risk of major and minor haemorrhages and a lower risk of non-haemorrhagic gastrointestinal adverse events compared with triflusal.[201] Although the lower risk of bleeding makes triflusal a potentially attractive alternative, it remains unclear whether it is definitely as effective as aspirin, and this will only be established by further, very large trials.

Glycoprotein IIb/IIIa receptor antagonists plus aspirin vs aspirin

While all the antiplatelet drugs discussed so far inhibit one of several possible pathways of platelet activation, the glycoprotein (GP) IIb/IIIa receptor antagonists prevent the binding of fibrinogen to the GP IIb/IIIa receptor, and so inhibit the final common pathway of platelet aggregation (Fig. 16.24). The GP IIb/IIIa receptor antagonists include monoclonal antibodies against the receptor, naturally occurring peptides isolated from snake venoms, synthetic peptides, and peptidomimetic and non-peptide molecules that compete with fibrinogen and other ligands for occupancy of the platelet receptor.[161]

RCTs in over 20 000 patients have demonstrated that the addition to standard antithrombotic therapy of a short intravenous infusion of a GP IIb/IIIa receptor antagonist immediately prior to percutaneous coronary intervention reduces the risk of subsequent ischaemic complications, albeit at the cost of a higher risk of major extracranial bleeding. RCTs have also assessed intravenous IIb/IIIa GP antagonists in over 30 000 patients with acute coronary syndromes without persistent ECG ST-segment elevation not undergoing percutaneous intervention, and in smaller numbers of patients with ST-segment acute myocardial infarction receiving thrombolytic therapy. The balance of risks and benefits in these two groups of patients remains unclear.[161,202,203] And pilot studies suggest that the intravenous GP IIb/IIIa receptor antagonists may have a role in the early treatment of acute ischaemic stroke, but far more data will be needed before the balance between benefits and risks can be determined reliably (section 12.6.1).[204]

Not surprisingly, the success of short-term high-grade blockade of the GP IIb/IIIa receptor with intravenous agents led to the development of oral GP IIb/IIIa receptor antagonists, in the hope that these may be beneficial in the long-term prevention of ischaemic vascular events in high-risk patients. Five large-scale RCTs involving over 40 000 patients, mainly with ischaemic heart disease but also including several hundred patients with prior ischaemic stroke, followed up for between 3 and 24 months, have now assessed these drugs. The results were very disappointing. There was no reduction in risk of recurrent ischaemic vascular events, but there was an increased risk of major haemorrhage and of death, which could not be entirely attributed to haemorrhage. The explanation for these results remains elusive, but may be related to the lower level of inhibition of the GP IIb/IIa receptor compared with the > 80% inhibition achieved with short-term intravenous administration. This may lead to paradoxical prothrombotic and proinflammatory effects of the orally administered drugs.[161,205,206]

16.5.6 How long should antiplatelet treatment continue?

It is difficult to determine from the available RCTs how long treatment should continue, because there are no large directly randomized comparisons between different durations of treatment, few trials have assessed the effects of antiplatelet treatment for longer than 2 or 3 years, and none have assessed the effects of stopping treatment after a period of freedom from vascular events. In their earlier analyses, the ATT (then the Antiplatelet Trialists' Collaboration) made indirect comparisons between the effects of treatment during sequential years of follow-up. Although there was an apparent pattern of greater effect during the earlier years, this may be explained by decreasing adherence to treatment over time, as well as bias in the comparisons in later years produced by the longer delay of vascular events in high-risk patients in the active treatment group. Therefore, without direct evidence to the contrary, it seems sensible to continue treatment indefinitely in patients who remain at high risk of a serious vascular event, unless some contraindication develops.[140]

16.6 Anticoagulants

Both platelets and fibrin are important components of thrombi. Thus, inhibitors of the coagulation cascade, whose final step is the conversion of fibrinogen to fibrin, should reduce thrombotic and thromboembolic events. Anticoagulants first became available for clinical use in the 1950s and have been extensively used in patients with ischaemic stroke and TIA ever since, despite limited evidence from RCTs. As for antiplatelet drugs, the main risk of anticoagulation is major haemorrhage. Thus, as for antiplatelet treatment, the most appropriate outcome for assessing the balance of benefits and risks of anti-coagulants is usually the combination of serious vascular events: stroke, myocardial infacrtion or vascular death. Given that the net benefits of antiplatelet treatment have been reliably demonstrated in a wide range of high-risk patients, including those with a prior ischaemic stroke or transient ischaemic attack (TIA) (section 16.5.1), the main question of clinical relevance today is: are there any patients for whom anticoagulants given alone or combined with antiplatelet treatment confer greater net benefit than antiplatelet treatment alone?

16.6.1 Anticoagulants for long-term prevention of vascular events in patients with a prior non-cardioembolic ischaemic stroke or TIA

Anticoagulants vs control

A systematic review of all randomized controlled trials (RCTs) of all types of anticoagulants given early after acute ischaemic stroke found that, although they reduced the risk of *early* recurrent ischaemic stroke and pulmonary embolism, they increased the risk of intracranial and major extracranial haemorrhage, with no net benefit in terms of death or death and dependency at the end of follow-up.[207] This evidence has been discussed in detail in section 12.4. Of more relevance here are the 11 RCTs comparing *long-term* treatment with an anticoagulant vs control in around 2500 patients in sinus rhythm with a previous presumed non-cardioembolic ischaemic stroke or TIA, followed up for about 2 years. These trials gener-ally assessed an oral anticoagulant, either a coumarin, such as warfarin, or phenindione. Their methodological quality was generally poor; in particular, nine were com-pleted in the 1960s and 1970s and so pre-dated routine CT scanning and the international normalized ratio (INR) to monitor anticoagulation. A meta-analysis of these trials found no significant difference between anticoagulants and control in the outcomes of serious

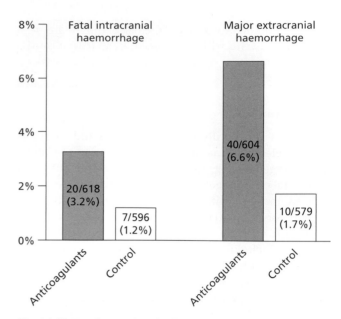

Fig. 16.28 Randomized trials of anticoagulants vs control in patients with a prior presumed non-cardioembolic ischaemic stroke or transient ischaemic attack. Percentage of patients randomized experiencing fatal intracranial haemorrhage and major extracranial haemorrhage during about 2 years of follow-up. (Data from Sandercock *et al.*, 2003.[208])

vascular events, death and dependency, death, or recurrent ischaemic stroke. However, anticoagulants statistically significantly increased fatal intracranial haemorrhages more than twofold, and fatal extracranial haemorrhages more than threefold, equivalent to anti-coagulants causing about 11 additional fatal intracranial haemorrhages and 25 additional major extracranial haemorrhages per year for every 1000 patients treated (Fig. 16.28).[208]

Anticoagulants vs antiplatelet treatment

Six RCTs have compared various different intensities of oral anticoagulation (mainly warfarin) with antiplatelet treatment (mainly aspirin) in over 5000 patients with non-cardioembolic ischaemic stroke or TIA followed for 1–2 years.[209–211] Over 90% of these patients were included in one of the four largest trials, and the results for outcomes that were recorded in all (or at least three) of these are shown in Fig. 16.29. The target INRs in the warfarin arms of the three trials were low (INR 1.4–2.8), medium (INR 2.0–3.0) and high (INR 3.0–4.5).[210–213] In none of the trials was there any evidence of net benefit from anticoagulants, but there was a statistically signific-antly increased risk of major haemorrhage and of death with both moderate and high-intensity anticoagulants. The excess risk of major haemorrhage appeared to be

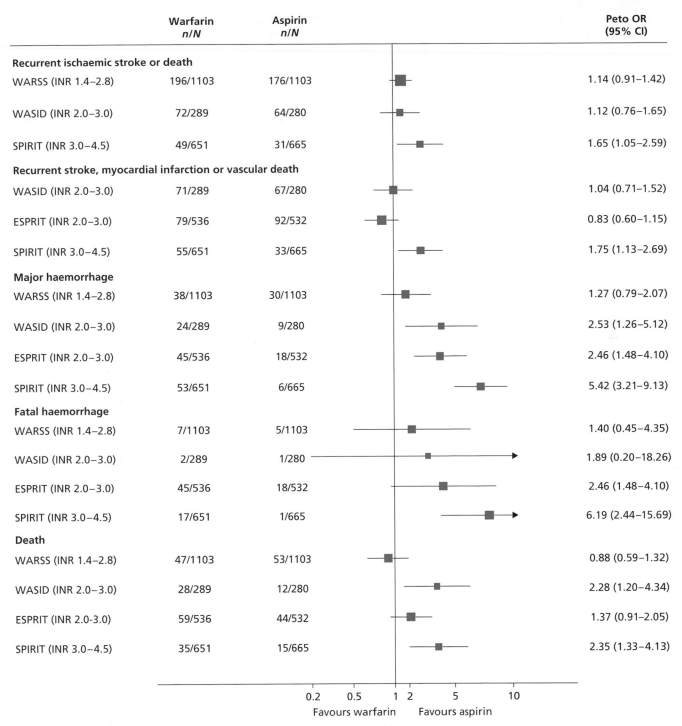

Fig. 16.29 Meta-analysis showing various outcomes from large randomized trials of warfarin vs aspirin in patients with a prior presumed non-cardioembolic ischaemic stroke or transient ischaemic attack. Odds ratios (OR) for each outcome are shown for the individual trials as squares, whose size is proportional to the statistical weight of the trial for the outcome, with horizontal lines denoting 95% confidence intervals (CI). INR, international normalized ratio. WARSS, Warfarin Aspirin Recurrent Stroke Study; WASID, Warfarin-Aspirin Symptomatic Intracranial Disease trial; ESPRIT, European/Australasian Stroke Prevention in Reversible Ischaemia Trial; SPIRIT, Stroke Prevention In Reversible Ischemia Trial. (Data from The Stroke Prevention In Reversible Ischemia Trial [SPIRIT] Study Group, 1997;[212] Mohr *et al.*, 2001;[213] Chimowitz *et al.*, 2005;[210] The ESPRIT Study Group, 2007.[211])

dose-related (Fig. 16.29). Although the Warfarin Aspirin Recurrent Stroke Study (WARSS) trial of low-intensity anticoagulation vs aspirin found no significant difference between treatments in major haemorrhage, there was a significant 60% increase in the relative odds of minor haemorrhage.[213] Further analyses of data from patients in the Stroke Prevention in Reversible Ischemia Trial (SPIRIT) and patients with non-disabling cerebral ischaemia with atrial fibrillation in the European Atrial Fibrillation Trial (EAFT) found that intensity of anticoagulation, cerebral ischaemia of arterial rather than cardioembolic origin, presence of leukoaraiosis on the pre-treatment brain scan, and age over 65 years were independent predictors of increased risk of anticoagulant-related major haemorrhage.[214]

There is therefore no intensity of anticoagulation at which the beneficial effect of reducing ischaemic events suggested by some of the trials exceeds the increased risk of major haemorrhage in patients with non-cardioembolic ischaemic stroke or TIA.[211,213]

> Anticoagulants should not be used for the long-term prevention of recurrent stroke and other vascular events after a presumed non-cardioembolic ischaemic stroke or transient ischaemic attack, because they increase the risk of haemorrhage compared with either control or aspirin without any clear evidence of net benefit.

16.6.2 Anticoagulants for long-term prevention of vascular events in patients with a prior ischaemic stroke or TIA in atrial fibrillation

Atrial fibrillation (AF) is an important risk factor for stroke, mainly ischaemic cardioembolic stroke, increasing risk about fivefold (section 6.5.1).[215,216] However, the absolute risk of stroke varies 20-fold among AF patients depending on their age, risk factors and history of vascular disease. A history of stroke or TIA is the most consistent and powerful independent predictor of stroke, increasing the absolute risk to around 10% per year in patients receiving aspirin but no anticoagulants. Other consistent independent predictors of stroke risk are age (increasing risk by about 1.5 times per decade) and raised blood pressure. Diabetes and female gender may also independently increase the risk of stroke. Many other potential predictors have been studied but the results have not been consistent. Various risk stratification schemes have now been developed to allow patients with AF to be grouped into those with low, moderate, high or very high risk of subsequent stroke (Table 16.8). Along with the evidence from RCTs (see below and section 16.5.1), and an assessment of the patient's likely

Table 16.8 Risk stratification scheme for patients in atrial fibrillation. (Adapted from Hart and Halperin, 1999[218] and Gage et al., 2004.[217])

Very high risk (~12% per year untreated risk of stroke)
Previous ischaemic stroke or transient ischaemic attack
High risk (~5 to 8% per year untreated risk of stroke)
Age > 65 years and hypertension, diabetes, heart failure, left ventricular dysfunction
High-risk cardiac disease, e.g. valvular heart disease or recent myocardial infarction
Moderate risk (~3 to 5% per year untreated risk of stroke)
Age > 65 years with no other risk factors
Age < 65 years and hypertension or diabetes
Low risk (~1% per year untreated risk of stroke)
Age < 65 years and no other risk factors

risk of adverse effects of treatment, these help to inform the best choice of antithrombotic treatment for individual patients.[217,218]

Our recommendations (below) for treatment of patients with AF apply also to patients with paroxysmal atrial fibrillation or atrial flutter, because the available evidence suggests that they have similarly increased risks of stroke.[219]

Oral anticoagulants vs control

Systematic reviews of RCTs of adjusted-dose warfarin (with an average achieved INR of around 2.5) vs control in almost 3000 patients with AF have shown that oral anticoagulation produces a clear and consistent reduction in the risk of stroke of around two-thirds, and of all serious vascular events of around one-half (Fig. 16.30). The relative reductions were similar in those with and without a previous history of ischaemic stroke or TIA. However, control group patients with a history of ischaemic stroke or TIA had an absolute stroke risk of 12% per year, compared with < 5% per year in those without such a history, so the absolute reduction in stroke risk in the secondary prevention trials was much higher than in the primary prevention trials (>8% vs about 3% per year). Excess risks of major haemorrhage were small, about 2 per thousand per year for intracranial haemorrhage and about 3 per thousand per year for major extracranial haemorrhage.[144,220,221]

Because the RCTs excluded large numbers of patients with a variety of contraindications to anticoagulants (e.g. those with a history of gastrointestinal bleeding, at risk of falls, likely poor adherence to treatment, alcoholism, etc.), concerns have persisted about the generalizability of the results to everyday clinical practice. Reassuringly, observational studies of AF patients in non-trial clinical settings have confirmed their relative

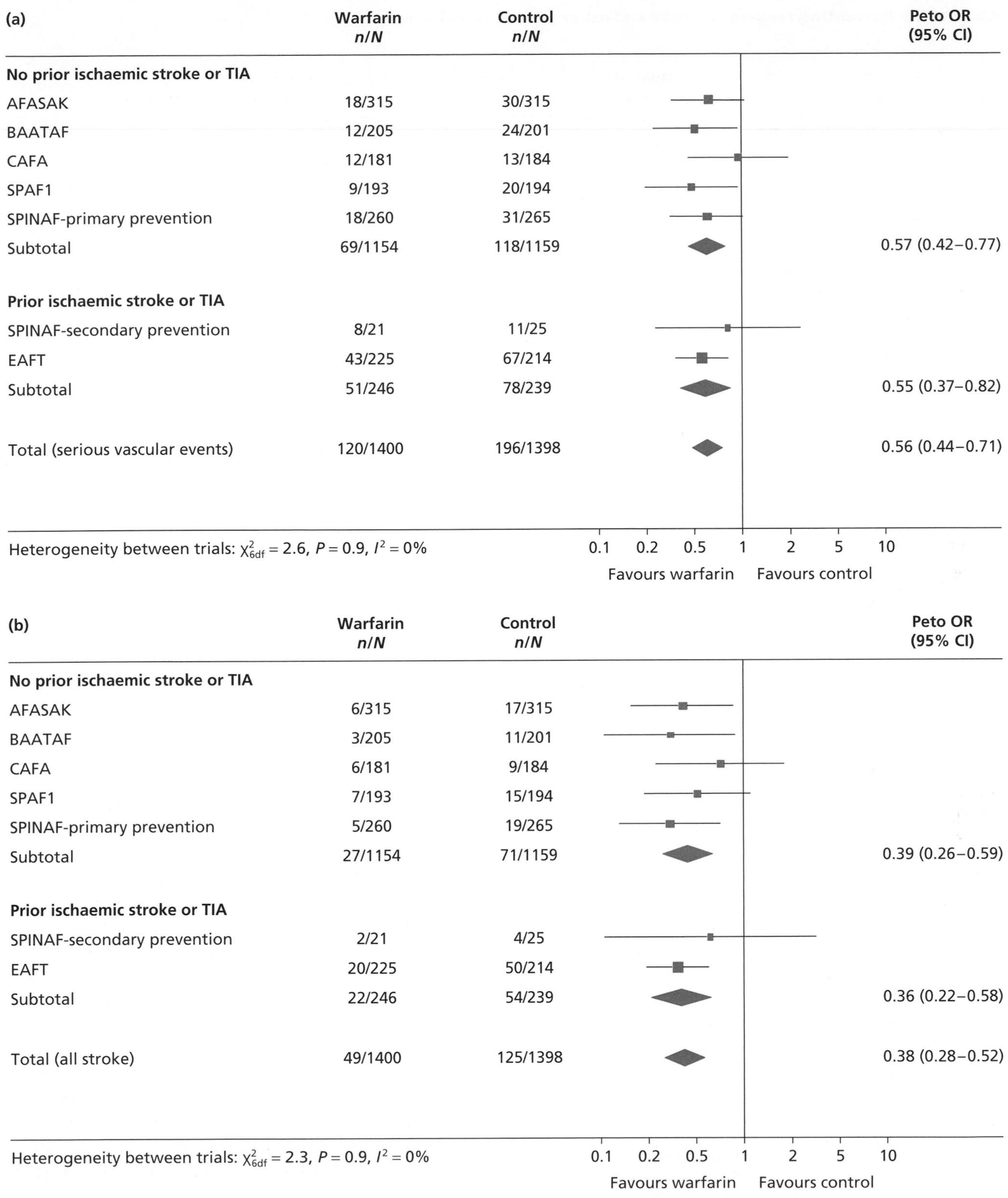

(a)

	Warfarin n/N	Control n/N		Peto OR (95% CI)
No prior ischaemic stroke or TIA				
AFASAK	18/315	30/315		
BAATAF	12/205	24/201		
CAFA	12/181	13/184		
SPAF1	9/193	20/194		
SPINAF-primary prevention	18/260	31/265		
Subtotal	69/1154	118/1159		0.57 (0.42–0.77)
Prior ischaemic stroke or TIA				
SPINAF-secondary prevention	8/21	11/25		
EAFT	43/225	67/214		
Subtotal	51/246	78/239		0.55 (0.37–0.82)
Total (serious vascular events)	120/1400	196/1398		0.56 (0.44–0.71)

Heterogeneity between trials: $\chi^2_{6df} = 2.6$, $P = 0.9$, $I^2 = 0\%$

0.1 0.2 0.5 1 2 5 10
Favours warfarin   Favours control

(b)

	Warfarin n/N	Control n/N		Peto OR (95% CI)
No prior ischaemic stroke or TIA				
AFASAK	6/315	17/315		
BAATAF	3/205	11/201		
CAFA	6/181	9/184		
SPAF1	7/193	15/194		
SPINAF-primary prevention	5/260	19/265		
Subtotal	27/1154	71/1159		0.39 (0.26–0.59)
Prior ischaemic stroke or TIA				
SPINAF-secondary prevention	2/21	4/25		
EAFT	20/225	50/214		
Subtotal	22/246	54/239		0.36 (0.22–0.58)
Total (all stroke)	49/1400	125/1398		0.38 (0.28–0.52)

Heterogeneity between trials: $\chi^2_{6df} = 2.3$, $P = 0.9$, $I^2 = 0\%$

0.1 0.2 0.5 1 2 5 10
Favours warfarin   Favours control

Fig. 16.30 Meta-analysis showing effects on (a) serious vascular events and (b) all stroke (ischaemic and haemorrhagic) in randomized trials of adjusted-dose warfarin vs control in patients with non-rheumatic atrial fibrillation, with and without a history of ischaemic stroke or transient ischaemic attack (TIA). Odds ratios (OR) for each trial are shown as squares, whose size is proportional to the statistical weight of the trial for the relevant outcome, with horizontal lines denoting 95% confidence intervals (CI). Pooled results for subgroups and overall are shown as diamonds (with 95% CI). AFASAK, Copenhagen Atrial Fibrillation, Aspirin and Anticoagulation Study; BAATAF, Boston Area Anticoagulation Trial for Atrial Fibrillation; CAFA, Canadian Atrial Fibrillation Anticoagulation Study; SPAF, Stroke Prevention in Atrial Fibrillation Study; SPINAF, Stroke Prevention in Non-rheumatic Atrial Fibrillation; EAFT, European Atrial Fibrillation Trial. (Data from Hart et al., 1999;[144] Aguilar and Hart, 2005;[220] Saxena and Koudstaal, 2004.[221])

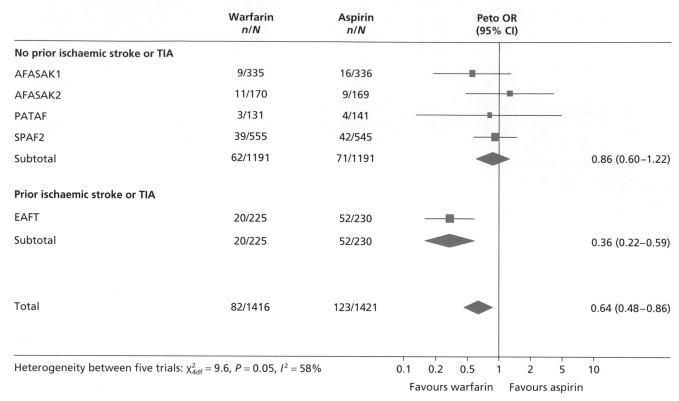

	Warfarin n/N	Aspirin n/N	Peto OR (95% CI)
No prior ischaemic stroke or TIA			
AFASAK1	9/335	16/336	
AFASAK2	11/170	9/169	
PATAF	3/131	4/141	
SPAF2	39/555	42/545	
Subtotal	62/1191	71/1191	0.86 (0.60–1.22)
Prior ischaemic stroke or TIA			
EAFT	20/225	52/230	
Subtotal	20/225	52/230	0.36 (0.22–0.59)
Total	82/1416	123/1421	0.64 (0.48–0.86)

Heterogeneity between five trials: $\chi^2_{4df} = 9.6$, $P = 0.05$, $I^2 = 58\%$

0.1 0.2 0.5 1 2 5 10

Favours warfarin   Favours aspirin

Fig. 16.31 Meta-analysis showing effects on stroke in randomized trials of warfarin vs aspirin in patients with non-rheumatic atrial fibrillation, with and without a history of ischaemic stroke or transient ischaemic attack (TIA). Odds ratios (OR) for each trial are shown as squares, whose size is proportional to the statistical weight of the trial for the relevant outcome, with horizontal lines denoting 95% confidence intervals (CI). Pooled results for subgroups and overall are shown as diamonds (with 95% CI). AFASAK 1 and 2, first and second Copenhagen Atrial Fibrillation, Aspirin and Anticoagulation Studies; PATAF, Primary Prevention of Arterial Thromboembolism in Nonrheumatic Atrial Fibrillation Study; SPAF 2, second Stroke Prevention in Atrial Fibrillation Study; EAFT, European Atrial Fibrillation Trial. (Data from Hart *et al.*, 1999;[144] van Walraven *et al.*, 2002;[225] Saxena and Koudstaal, 2004.[221])

effectiveness, and have generally shown rates of major haemorrhage similar to the RCTs.[222,223] However, high-quality monitoring and management of anticoagulation are required to maintain the net benefit and low rate of adverse effects. Of note is the fact that the very elderly, who face the highest risk of both stroke and haemorrhagic complications, were not well represented in the RCTs, and so further studies in such patients are required to better assess the balance of risks and benefits of oral anticoagulants.[219,224]

Oral anticoagulants vs antiplatelet treatment

Adjusted-dose warfarin (with an average achieved INR of around 2.5) has been directly compared with aspirin in five trials among about 3000 patients with AF, one of them among patients with a prior ischaemic stroke or TIA. One further RCT compared adjusted-dose warfarin with the antiplatelet drug, indobufen, a reversible inhibitor of cyclo-oxygenase.

The pooled results (whether or not the indobufen study is included) suggest that oral anticoagulants are more effective at preventing stroke than aspirin or other antiplatelet treatment, with a relative risk reduction of about one-third, overall (Fig. 16.31).[144,221,225] There was statistically significant heterogeneity between the results of the individual trials, and the relative benefits of treatment appeared somewhat greater in those with a prior ischaemic stroke or TIA. Because of their substantially higher risk of stroke on aspirin (see above), the absolute reduction in stroke risk with adjusted-dose warfarin vs aspirin was much higher for patients with a history of prior ischaemic stroke or TIA vs those without such a history (7% per year vs 0.4% per year). The risk of any major haemorrhage (extracranial or intracranial) was increased by about twofold, an absolute increase of about 1% per year, and appeared not to vary substantially between groups with different levels of baseline risk of stroke. Mortality was similar in the warfarin and aspirin or antiplatelet treatment groups.[144,218,221,225]

The superiority of adjusted-dose warfarin over antiplatelet treatment is strengthened by the results of the Atrial Fibrillation Clopidogrel Trial with Irbesartan for prevention of Vascular Events-W (ACTIVE-W trial). This trial randomized 6700 patients with AF and one other risk factor to either warfarin with a target INR of 2–3 or the combination of clopidogrel and aspirin. About 1000 participants had a history of stroke or TIA. The trial was stopped early when an interim analysis showed clear superiority of adjusted-dose warfarin, with highly significant relative reductions of one-third in stroke and in the primary outcome of stroke, systemic embolism, myocardial infarction or vascular death.[226]

In the types of patients who were randomized in these trials and in the trials of anticoagulants vs control (see above), it is clear that the benefits of adjusted-dose warfarin with a target INR of around 2.5 far outweigh the risks in patients with a history of an ischaemic stroke or TIA, so long as there are no contraindications to anticoagulants. Unfortunately, many patients do have such contraindications; factors that may make clinicians reluctant to prescribe long-term anticoagulants include uncontrolled hypertension, recent gastrointestinal bleeding, alcoholic liver disease, confusion or dementia, tendency to falls, difficulties with access to an anticoagulant clinic, and extensive leukoaraiosis on the brain scan.[227] These factors increase the likelihood of over-anticoagulation and major bleeding.[224] For these patients, aspirin is a reasonable alternative

antithrombotic treatment, albeit less effective (section 16.5.3).

> Patients with a prior ischaemic stroke or transient ischaemic attack and atrial fibrillation are at very high risk of subsequent stroke. They should generally be treated with oral anticoagulants or, if anticoagulation is contraindicated, with aspirin (or some other antiplatelet regimen if aspirin cannot be used for some reason).

For patients *without* a history of ischaemic stroke or TIA, the balance of benefits of warfarin on the one hand, and the inconvenience of monitoring and risks of major bleeding on the other, need to be considered on an individual patient basis. There are several risk stratification schemes to help with this process. They vary somewhat, but all use a combination of clinical variables (age, blood pressure, diabetes, and sometimes heart failure, other cardiac disease, and echocardiographic findings) to assign the patient to low, moderate, high or very high-risk groups (Table 16.8). Table 16.9 shows the estimated annual risks of stroke in untreated patients in these groups along with the estimated absolute reductions in risk of stroke and increases in risk of major extracranial bleeding with adjusted-dose warfarin or aspirin for patients in the various baseline risk categories:

- In low-risk patients (under 65 years without any risk factors other than AF) the absolute benefits and risks of

Table 16.9 Approximate size of main treatment benefits and harms according to risk of stroke in patients with atrial fibrillation. (Adapted from Hart *et al.*, 1999[144] and Hart and Halperin, 1999.[218])

	Stroke in patients without a prior ischaemic stroke or transient ischaemic attack			Stroke in patients with a prior ischaemic stroke or transient ischaemic attack	Major extracranial haemorrhage[§]
Untreated risk (% per year)	Low risk 1%	Moderate risk 3 to 5%	High risk 5 to 8%	Very high risk 12%	0.6%
Events avoided (↓) or produced (↑) per 1000 patients treated per year with:					
Adjusted dose warfarin vs no treatment[†]	↓6 (NNT 167)	↓18 to 30 (NNT 33 to 55)	↓30 to 48 (NNT 21 to 33)	↓72 (NNT 14)	↑3 (NNH 333)
Aspirin vs no treatment[‡]	↓2 (NNT 500)	↓6 to 10 (NNT 100 to 167)	↓10 to 16 (NNT 62 to 100)	↓24 (NNT 42)	↑1 (NNH 1000)
Adjusted dose warfarin vs aspirin[¶]	↓4 (NNT 250)	↓12 to 20 (NNT 50 to 83)	↓20 to 32 (NNT 31 to 50)	↓48 (NNT 21)	↑2 (NNH 500)

[†]Relative risk reduction for stroke = 60%.
[‡]Relative risk reduction for stroke = 20%.
[¶]Relative risk reduction for stroke = 40%.
[§]Based on estimates from relevant systematic reviews of randomized trials. Bleeding risks may be higher in patients outside clinical trials, particularly the elderly.
NNT, number-needed-to-treat (number treated to avoid one stroke).
NNH, number-needed-to-harm (number treated to produce one major extracranial bleed).

warfarin are very finely balanced, and aspirin seems a better option because of its lower risk and ease of use.

- For patients without a history of ischaemic stroke or TIA but at high risk (over the age of 65 years and with at least one other risk factor) or for those with a history of prior ischaemic stroke or TIA, the absolute reduction in stroke with warfarin (compared with either control or with aspirin) is substantial, and outweighs the absolute bleeding risks, making anticoagulants the appropriate choice of antithrombotic treatment in most cases, provided there are no contraindications.
- For patients at moderate risk (over the age of 65 years, or under 65 with risk factors other than AF), either adjusted-dose warfarin or aspirin may be justified, depending on the patient's preferences, the inconvenience of anticoagulant intensity monitoring, and likely risk of bleeding complications, which may exceed the average risks derived from clinical trials shown in Table 16.9, particularly in the elderly. An ongoing RCT should provide further information on the balance of risks and benefits of anticoagulation in the elderly.[228]

> The risks of stroke and of anticoagulant-related bleeding should be assessed for individuals with atrial fibrillation. In the absence of contraindications, anticoagulants are appropriate for those at high risk of stroke, while aspirin is appropriate for those at low risk. Either anticoagulants or aspirin may be appropriate for moderate-risk individuals, depending on the balance of risks and benefits, and patient preference.

Different anticoagulant intensities

Several RCTs have assessed very low intensities and/or fixed doses of anticoagulants in an attempt to reduce the risk of bleeding and the inconvenience of regular monitoring for adjusted-dose anticoagulation. Two have compared adjusted-dose warfarin (with an average achieved INR of about 2.5) with aspirin plus low, fixed doses of warfarin (1–3 mg, mean achieved INR about 1.3) in about 1400 patients with AF, over one-third of whom had a history of stroke or TIA. The first and largest of these trials recruited patients at high risk of stroke, and was stopped early after an interim analysis found large reductions in relative and absolute risk for adjusted-dose warfarin, without a significant difference in the risk of major bleeding. The second trial was also stopped early in response to the results of the first, and found no difference between treatment arms. A further three RCTs have compared adjusted-dose warfarin (target INRs of 2–3.5) with low or fixed doses of warfarin alone (mean achieved INR 1.1–1.4) in almost 900 patients without a prior

stroke or TIA. No significant difference was found between treatments but there was a non-significant reduction in stroke with adjusted-dose warfarin, in keeping with the results of the trials comparing adjusted-dose warfarin with aspirin plus low-intensity warfarin.[144,219]

Data from observational studies support those from the RCTs, and suggest that a target INR of about 2.5 is optimal. Below about 2.0, the risk of ischaemic stroke increases and strokes that do occur are more likely to be severe or fatal, while above about 3.0 there is an increased risk of major bleeding. Patients over 75 years old are at greater risk of major bleeding on oral anticoagulants, but are also at increased risk of stroke, and there is currently no evidence to suggest that the target INR should be lower in them.[219,224,229–231]

The addition of antiplatelet treatment to anticoagulants

Two RCTs have assessed adding antiplatelet treatment to adjusted-dose warfarin with a slightly lower than standard INR range compared with standard adjusted-dose warfarin.

One small trial in 157 AF patients at high risk of stroke compared the oral anticoagulant fluindione (target INR 2.0–2.6) alone or combined with aspirin 100 mg daily. It was stopped early because of an increased rate of major haemorrhage in the combination group, and the number of events accrued was too small to assess the effect on stroke or other vascular events.[232]

The second study comprised two parallel RCTs, one comparing oral anticoagulants (mean achieved INR 2) plus the antiplatelet drug triflusal 600 mg daily vs oral anticoagulants alone (mean achieved INR 2.5) in around 500 high-risk patients with AF and rheumatic mitral stenosis or a history of embolism, and the other comparing triflusal alone vs oral anticoagulants (mean achieved INR 2.5) alone vs triflusal plus oral anticoagulants (mean achieved INR 2) in around 700 intermediate-risk patients with AF and aged over 60 years, with hypertension or heart failure. The primary outcome of vascular death and non-fatal stroke or systemic embolism was significantly reduced in the combination treatment arm compared with anticoagulants alone in both high- and intermediate-risk groups. Rates of severe bleeding were slightly lower in the combination treatment group compared with anticoagulants alone but numbers of events were small and the difference was not significant.[233] This result raises the possibility that the combination of oral anticoagulation with an INR of about 2 with antiplatelet treatment may be more effective and safer than oral anticoagulants alone with an INR of about 2.5.[219] Further trials are needed to explore this possibility further.

A systematic review of six RCTs comparing aspirin combined with warfarin vs the same intensity of warfarin alone in almost 4000 patients with ischaemic heart disease or prosthetic heart valves found that the addition of aspirin approximately doubled the risk of intracranial haemorrhage.[234] For most categories of patients, and especially those already at high risk of bleeding with anticoagulants, the combination should be avoided. However, in some categories of patients at particularly high risk of thromboembolism (e.g. those with mechanical prosthetic valves), the greater antithrombotic benefit of the combination may outweigh the extra bleeding risk.[137,147,187]

> The combination of oral anticoagulation (target INR 2.5) with aspirin or another antiplatelet drug should generally be avoided because of the increased risk of major bleeding. However, the greater benefit of the combination may outweigh the bleeding risk in some patients at particularly high risk of thromboembolism (e.g. those with mechanical heart valves).

Alternative anticoagulants to warfarin

Warfarin and other vitamin K antagonists are associated with an increased risk of major bleeding, and require regular, careful monitoring of anticoagulation intensity (through measurement of the INR) with appropriate adjustment of the dose as required. This represents a significant burden of cost and time, both for health services and for patients. Indeed, several studies have shown that warfarin is taken by only one- to two-thirds of appropriate patients with AF, at least in part because physicians tend to be influenced more by major adverse bleeding associated with warfarin in their patients than by ischaemic strokes in those with AF not taking warfarin.[235]

The development of an oral anticoagulant that is as effective as warfarin, and as safe or safer, and without the requirement for regular monitoring, would be a significant advance. The orally administered anticoagulant, ximelagatran, showed considerable promise in this regard. It is a prodrug form of the direct thrombin inhibitor, melagatran, which is rapidly absorbed in the small intestine and then bioconverted to its active form. Importantly, its anticoagulant effect is predictable at a fixed dose, and there have been no reported drug or food interactions, making monitoring of anticoagulation intensity unnecessary.

There have been a number of RCTs comparing it with either low-molecular-weight heparin, adjusted-dose warfarin, or both in a total of around 14 000 patients in several different settings: prevention of venous thromboembolism after orthopaedic surgery, treatment of patients with venous thromboembolism, acute myocardial infarction, and atrial fibrillation. These generally found either increased or similar effectiveness and similar or reduced bleeding risks with ximelagatran.[236] Pooled results of the two large RCTs comparing ximelagatran with adjusted-dose warfarin (target INR 2–3) in 7300 patients with non-valvular AF and at least one additional risk factor for stroke found no significant difference between treatments in the risk of the primary outcome of stroke or systemic embolism (although the confidence interval included the possibility of a clinically important difference in either direction), and significantly less major bleeding in the ximelagatran group.[237]

Unfortunately, there have been concerns about the potential hepatotoxicity of ximelagatran, with the RCTs showing about a 6% absolute excess of asymptomatic elevations in transaminases after 1–2 months, and two deaths in the ximelagatran group in one of the AF trials, one from hepatitis with necrosis and the other from gastrointestinal haemorrhage in a patient with markedly elevated transaminases.[236,237] Despite these concerns, ximelagatran received marketing approval from France in December 2003, and then from the European Medicines Agency in May 2004 for short-term use in the prevention of venous thromboembolic events after orthopaedic surgery, but the United States Food and Drug Administration withheld marketing approval in October 2004. In February 2006, AstraZeneca withdrew ximelagatran from the market and terminated its development, because of further concerns about hepatotoxicity arising during a trial of ximelagatran in extended venous thromboembolism prophylaxis up to 35 days after orthopaedic surgery (http://www.astrazeneca.com/archivelist/).

Thus, the search is still on for an alternative to warfarin and other vitamin K antagonists, which for the time being are the only available oral anticoagulants of proven effectiveness. Other anticoagulant molecules are in development and there are planned or ongoing trials of long-acting subcutaneous heparinoids, and of oral factor Xa antagonists and direct thrombin inhibitors (see http://www.clinicaltrials.gov/ct/show/NCT00070655, http://www.clinicaltrials.gov/ct/show/NCT00412984, http://www.clinicaltrials.gov/ct/show/NCT00262600).[219]

Anticoagulants for patients with repeated transient ischaemic attacks or ischaemic strokes despite optimum antiplatelet drug therapy

In our experience, this situation is relatively uncommon. The first step should be to verify again that the attacks are truly ischaemic in nature and are not due to structural brain disease of some sort, low-flow ischaemic events, epilepsy, migraine, psychogenic disorder, etc. (sections 3.4, 3.5 and 6.7.5). If the diagnosis is correct, these admittedly rare patients are often very worried, as are their doctors. Of course, those with carotid ischaemic events and severe carotid stenosis should be considered for endarterectomy, but sometimes this is not possible or practical (section 16.11.6), and very occasionally the attacks continue after what appears to be a technically adequate operation. Two or three months of moderate-intensity oral anticoagulants (INR 2–3) may perhaps reduce the frequency and severity of the TIAs, which is comforting for the patient and reduces anxiety all round. Sometimes, if the attacks are very frequent, it may be necessary to admit the patients to hospital for unfractionated or low-molecular-weight heparin in the first instance. We do this in the full knowledge that this treatment is not based on evidence from RCTs and may not reduce the risk of stroke or vascular death; it is purely given for symptom control. It is often possible, after a few weeks, to withdraw the anticoagulants gradually and replace them with aspirin or some other antiplatelet regimen. In such cases, the unstable atheromatous plaque that was causing the frequent attacks (we presume) has perhaps 'healed' and become covered with endothelium (section 6.3.5).

16.6.3 Anticoagulants for patients with mechanical prosthetic heart valves

Patients with mechanical prosthetic heart valves are at very high risk of embolism, and require anticoagulation whether or not they have a history of ischaemic stroke or other embolic problems. For some types of mechanical prosthetic valve, and in patients who have additional risk factors, such as a history of embolism, atrial fibrillation or cardiac failure, a higher target INR of 3 (range 2.5–3.5) combined with low-dose aspirin is warranted.[147] The management of acute stroke in patients with prosthetic mechanical valves already on anticoagulants has been discussed in sections 12.4.7 and 13.3.4.

The management of ischaemic stroke and other thromboembolic events among pregnant women with mechanical prosthetic heart valves is controversial because evidence is limited, and this is discussed in detail elsewhere.[238] In brief, since oral anticoagulants increase the risk of fetal abnormalities, they should be avoided during the first trimester. Also, because they increase the risk of fetal bleeding during delivery, they should also be avoided in the weeks before delivery. Options for anticoagulation in these patients during pregnancy include low-molecular-weight heparin throughout pregnancy, very carefully monitored adjusted-dose unfractionated heparin throughout pregnancy, or unfractionated or low-molecular-weight heparin until the 13th week and then change to warfarin until the middle of the third trimester before restarting heparin for the later weeks of pregnancy until after delivery. In very high-risk cases, the addition of low-dose aspirin may be warranted.[238]

16.6.4 Risks of bleeding with oral anticoagulants

The main determinants of the risk of bleeding with warfarin and other vitamin K antagonists are:[224]

- *Intensity of anticoagulation*: the risk is higher at INR above 3 compared with INR of 2–3. Variation in the intensity of anticoagulation (i.e. poor control of the INR) also increases the risk of bleeding independent of the mean INR.

- *Underlying patient characteristics*: most consistently increasing age, history of gastrointestinal bleeding and (for intracranial haemorrhage) history of stroke, especially if brain imaging shows leukoaraiosis. Other characteristics less consistently associated with increased risk are a history of hypertension, alcoholism, falls, dementia, liver disease and malignancy.

- *Length of treatment*: the risk of bleeding is higher early in the course of treatment and falls with time.

- *Concomitant medications*: there is a long list of drugs which should either be avoided or used with caution, with increased monitoring of the INR in patients taking warfarin or another vitamin K antagonist because they may increase the risk of bleeding or embolic events through a variety of different types of interaction (Table 16.10).[239] The possibility that any new drug might interact with warfarin should always be considered and checked in a reliable source (e.g. the *British National Formulary*) before it is started or stopped. It is also worth bearing in mind that herbal medicines and some food and drink items (for example cranberry juice) may interact with warfarin.[240]

A number of models to aid with prediction of risk of anticoagulant-related bleeding have been developed. These should not be used in isolation but in conjunction with assessments of each individual patient's functional status, risk of ischaemic events and personal preferences. Other factors, such as microhaemorrhages on an MR brain scan and genotype (e.g. apolipoprotein E genotype may modify the risk of cerebral amyloid angiopathy and so of intracerebral haemorrhage, and polymorphisms in the genes encoding cytochrome P450 enzymes and epoxide reductase complex 1 may identify patients with altered anticoagulant metabolism at increased risk of bleeding during the initiation of anticoagulants), may prove useful in the future to refine clinical risk prediction,

Table 16.10 Drugs which interact with oral anticoagulants (adapted from the Scottish Intercollegiate Guidelines Network, 1999, see http://www.sign.ac.uk/pdf/sign36.pdf).

Avoid	
Aspirin	Except where combination specifically indicated
Analgesics	Co-proxamol
	Ketorolac (postoperative)
Antifungals	Miconazole
Diabetes	Glucagon
Non-steroidal anti-inflammatory	Azapropazone
	Phenylbutazone
Others	Enteral feeds containing vitamin K
Adjust dose	
Ulcer healing	Cimetidine
	Omeprazole
Anti-arrhythmics	Amiodarone
	Propafenone
Lipid-lowering	Fibrates
Anti-epileptics	Carbamazepine
	Phenobarbitone
	Phenytoin
	Primidone
Alcohol dependency	Disulfiram
Antibiotics/antifungals	Aztreonam
	Cephamandole
	Chloramphenicol
	Ciprofloxacin
	Co-trimoxazole
	Erythromycin
	Griseofulvin
	Metronidazole
	Ofloxacin
	Rifampicin
	Sulphonamides
Thyroid	Carbimazole
	Thiouracils
	Thyroxine
Non-steroidal anti-inflammatory	Diflunisal
Gout	Allopurinol
	Sulphinpyrazone
Others	Aminoglutethimide
	Barbiturates
	Cyclosporin
	Mercaptopurine
	Oral contraceptives
Monitor international normalized ratio	
Gastrointestinal motility	Cisapride
Anti-arrhythmics	Quinidine
Lipid-lowering	Cholestyramine
	Statins
Antidepressants	Serotonin uptake antagonists
Antibiotics/antifungals	Check product data sheet, if not listed under 'adjust dose' above
Diabetes	Tolbutamide
Non-steroidal anti-inflammatory	Check product data sheet, if not listed under 'avoid' or 'adjust dose' above
Others	Anabolic steroids
	Corticosteroids
	Hormone antagonists
	Ifosfamide
	Influenza vaccine
	Rawachol
	Sucralfate

but further studies are needed to establish their value in this context.[224,241–243]

> The risk of anticoagulant-induced bleeding depends on the intensity of anticoagulation, age, various other patient characteristics, time since anticoagulation started, and concomitant medications. The optimum balance between benefits and risks for most patients in atrial fibrillation is probably achieved with an INR of 2.5 (target range 2–3).

16.6.5 Who not to treat

In general, the main contraindication to oral anti-coagulation is a high risk of bleeding (section 16.6.4). However, many of the characteristics (e.g. age) which increase the risk of bleeding also increase the risk of thromboembolism and there has to be a trade-off be-tween risks and benefits in individual patients. So for patients in atrial fibrillation at low risk of stroke the risks of anticoagulation are probably too high and they are more appropriately treated with aspirin (section 16.5.1). Patients with active infective endocarditis have a high risk of intracerebral haemorrhage, and should not be treated with anticoagulants even though they have a serious embolic risk.[244]

If possible, we always obtain a brain CT (or MR) scan to exclude intracranial haemorrhage before starting anti-coagulants, because anticoagulation of patients with intracranial bleeding is presumably unwise, at least in the short term, if not in the long term. Brain CT needs to be performed within the first few days of stroke before any evidence of intracranial haemorrhage has disap-peared, but for patients presenting later, MR scanning with appropriate sequences is necessary to detect pre-vious intracerebral haemorrhage (section 5.5.1). As was discussed above for antiplatelet treatment (section 16.5.2), there are sometimes compelling reasons for long-term anticoagulants in patients with a history of intracranial haemorrhage, and in such cases the poten-tial benefits and hazards have to be considered on an individual basis. For example, patients with atrial fibril-lation, particularly those with rheumatic valve disease or a mechanical heart valve at high risk of subsequent ischaemic events, may warrant long-term anticoagulants despite a prior history of intracerebral haemorrhage.[156]

It is not clear whether or not the presence of haemor-rhagic transformation of a cerebral infarct is an absolute contraindication to the use of anticoagulants. If we felt the patient had a clear indication for immediate anti-coagulation, we would not delay if the scan showed a minor degree of haemorrhagic transformation (e.g. a few petechiae). On the other hand, if there were confluent haemorrhage or a parenchymatous haematoma, we would prefer to wait a week or two at least.

16.6.6 Practicalities of long-term anticoagulation

Starting anticoagulants

If oral anticoagulants are to be used for long-term sec-ondary prevention, a baseline full blood count, platelet count, INR and liver function tests should be done – and the results known – before treatment is started.

On the rare occasions when there is an urgent need for immediate anticoagulation, intravenous unfractionated heparin or low-molecular-weight heparin can be given, since oral anticoagulants take several days to become effective. Most hospitals have their own local guidelines for the administration (and monitoring in the case of intravenous unfractionated heparin) of these drugs, and these should be followed.

After taking the first few doses of oral anticoagulants without concomitant heparin, some patients may develop a transient pro-coagulant state. Therefore, in non-urgent situations, for patients with protein S or protein C deficiency or another thrombophilic condi-tion, it is prudent to begin heparin therapy before or at the same time as warfarin to protect against this and then to withdraw the heparin once a therapeutic INR has been reached.[239]

There is room for flexibility in selecting a starting dose of warfarin. A dose of 10 mg is often preferred for many patients, but several studies have suggested a starting dose of 5 mg or less in the elderly, or patients with liver disease, congestive heart failure or at increased risk of bleeding. The starting dose generally needs to be given daily for 1–2 days until the INR is in the thera-peutic range, with subsequent dosing based on the INR response. Suitable dosing schedules are available for guiding this process.[239]

Monitoring anticoagulants

In hospitalized patients, daily monitoring is appropriate until a therapeutic INR has been achieved and main-tained for at least two consecutive days, followed by two to three times weekly for 1–2 weeks, and then less often, depending on the stability of the INR. Once the INR is stable, the frequency of monitoring can be reduced to once every few weeks. The American College of Chest Physicians suggests no more than 4 weeks between tests, while the British Society for Haematology's guidelines suggest 12 weeks, although more frequent monitoring may be required in patients with an unstable INR, for whatever reason.[239,245]

Different models of anticoagulation management

Since the risk of bleeding and of embolic complications is increased by instability in the anticoagulation intensity, careful management of anticoagulation is crucial to maintain the benefits and reduce the risks. The key principles are that management of anticoagulation should be well organized and coordinated, incorporating patient education, systematic INR testing, tracking, follow-up, and effective communication of results and dosing decisions to the patient. There are a number of different ways of achieving this, some of which may be effectively combined, including anticoagulation clinics based in hospitals or in the community, INR testing in general practice with dosing advice from specialist departments in the hospital, patient self-testing with dosing advice from the hospital or patient self-management of dosing decisions, and computer software programs to aid in dose adjustment.[239] There is evidence from a systematic review of RCTs that, compared with standard monitoring, patient self-monitoring or self-management improves outcomes, with fewer thromboembolic events, lower mortality and a higher proportion of INR values in range, although no clear reduction in haemorrhage risk. However, self-management is only feasible for patients who are capable of self-monitoring and self-adjusting therapy, and so requires their identification and education.[246] Otherwise there is little clear evidence from RCTs to suggest the superiority of one method of managing anticoagulation over another.[239] The best choice is likely to depend on the patient, their doctor and local health services.

16.6.7 How long should treatment continue?

As with antiplatelet treatment (section 16.5.6), most of the trials have tested only a few years of anticoagulants and none have directly compared different treatment durations. Thus, it is not known whether the balance of risk and benefit alters with prolonged therapy, particularly as the patient becomes older and so at higher risk of bleeding. If a patient has a serious haemorrhage, not due to over-anticoagulation, then the reason for giving anticoagulants should be reviewed, and the risk of thromboembolism reassessed. Since occult pathological lesions in the gastrointestinal tract and genitourinary system often present with bleeding, investigation of such patients (even if apparently over-anticoagulated) is usually justified.[224] Further research is clearly required to determine the optimum duration of treatment. In the meantime, if we consider that a patient remains at high risk (whatever their age), no bleeding events have occurred, and no factors that might increase the risk of

bleeding have developed (e.g. tendency to falls or dementia), most of us would keep the patient on anticoagulants indefinitely.

16.7 Lifestyle modification

16.7.1 Smoking cessation

Risks of smoking

In 2000, smoking was estimated to have caused almost 5 million premature deaths worldwide, about half in developed and half in developing countries, and about 80% of these in men. The leading causes of smoking-related death were vascular disease (including ischaemic heart disease and stroke), chronic obstructive pulmonary disease, and lung cancer.[247] Results from 40 years of prospective observations on over 30 000 male British doctors demonstrated that almost half of all regular cigarette smokers will eventually be killed by their habit.[248] Smoking is clearly a risk factor for ischaemic stroke (section 6.6.4) and for subarachnoid haemorrhage (section 9.1.1), although its effect on the risk of intracerebral haemorrhage is less clear.[249-252]

Benefits of stopping

Because of the clearly established adverse effects of all forms of tobacco consumption (cigarettes, pipes, cigars and chewing tobacco) and the overwhelming indications for stopping, there have, unsurprisingly, been no successful RCTs of 'continue smoking' vs 'stop smoking'. However, observational studies show substantial early and long-term health benefits of stopping smoking for smokers of all ages. The excess mortality falls soon after stopping and continues to do so for at least 10–15 years. Stopping smoking before the age of about 35 years leads to the avoidance of almost all the subsequent excess mortality, but stopping later in life still confers substantial benefit.[248] Stopping smoking halves the risk of mortality due to ischaemic heart disease within a year, and the risk of stroke declines substantially within 2–5 years.[253-256]

Best methods to aid smoking cessation

Systematic reviews have demonstrated the effectiveness of a variety of interventions to help people stop

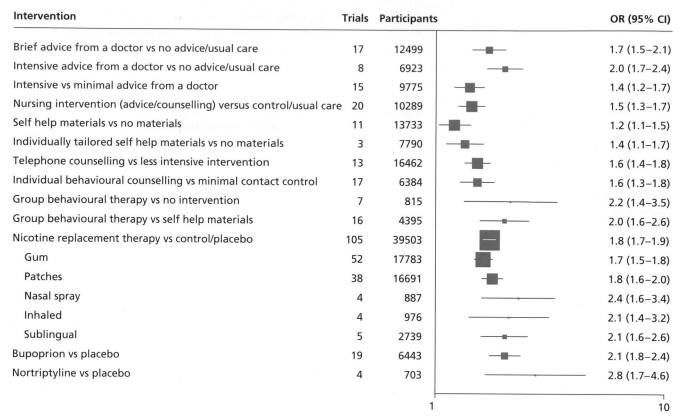

Intervention	Trials	Participants		OR (95% CI)
Brief advice from a doctor vs no advice/usual care	17	12499		1.7 (1.5–2.1)
Intensive advice from a doctor vs no advice/usual care	8	6923		2.0 (1.7–2.4)
Intensive vs minimal advice from a doctor	15	9775		1.4 (1.2–1.7)
Nursing intervention (advice/counselling) versus control/usual care	20	10289		1.5 (1.3–1.7)
Self help materials vs no materials	11	13733		1.2 (1.1–1.5)
Individually tailored self help materials vs no materials	3	7790		1.4 (1.1–1.7)
Telephone counselling vs less intensive intervention	13	16462		1.6 (1.4–1.8)
Individual behavioural counselling vs minimal contact control	17	6384		1.6 (1.3–1.8)
Group behavioural therapy vs no intervention	7	815		2.2 (1.4–3.5)
Group behavioural therapy vs self help materials	16	4395		2.0 (1.6–2.6)
Nicotine replacement therapy vs control/placebo	105	39503		1.8 (1.7–1.9)
Gum	52	17783		1.7 (1.5–1.8)
Patches	38	16691		1.8 (1.6–2.0)
Nasal spray	4	887		2.4 (1.6–3.4)
Inhaled	4	976		2.1 (1.4–3.2)
Sublingual	5	2739		2.1 (1.6–2.6)
Bupoprion vs placebo	19	6443		2.1 (1.8–2.4)
Nortriptyline vs placebo	4	703		2.8 (1.7–4.6)

1　　　　　　　　　　　　　　10

Fig. 16.32 Meta-analyses of randomized trials of various interventions for smoking cessation showing effects on abstinence from smoking. Squares represent summary odds ratios (OR) for the various interventions shown, with the size of each square proportional to the amount of statistical information for that intervention. Horizontal lines are 95% confidence intervals (CI). (Data from Lancaster and Stead, 2004;[257] Rice and Stead, 2004;[259] Lancaster and Stead, 2005;[258;261] Stead and Lancaster, 2005;[260] Stead et al., 2003;[262] Silagy et al., 2004;[264] Hughes et al., 2004.[265])

smoking, and in general these increase quit rates by about 1.5 to 2-fold (Fig. 16.32). Advice from doctors, structured interventions from nurses, and individual and group counselling are all effective.[257–260] Generic self-help materials and telephone counselling are no better than brief advice but are more effective than doing nothing, and personalized self-help materials are better than standard materials.[261,262] Simple advice to give up smoking is one of the most cost-effective interventions in the whole of medicine.[263]

All forms of nicotine replacement therapy are similarly effective, and remain effective when given in combination with various types of support, such as advice or counselling.[264] There are no known serious adverse effects, but all can cause local irritation, of the nose, mouth or skin, depending on the route of administration.

The antidepressants bupropion and nortriptyline also increase quit rates. Bupropion can cause dry mouth and insomnia, but the only serious adverse effect is seizures, for which the risk is about one in 1000. The drug is therefore contraindicated in those with a history of current or previous epilepsy, and should be used with caution in people who may have a lowered seizure threshold, which includes patients with a history of cerebrovascular disease (section 11.8). It should not be used with a monoamine oxidase inhibitor.[265]

> All smokers, including those with a history of stroke or transient ischaemic attack, should be advised to stop, and interventions such as counselling, nicotine replacement or bupropion should be used if needed to help them achieve this.

16.7.2 Avoiding excess alcohol

Observational studies suggest that, compared with no alcohol consumption, light to moderate alcohol consumption (about 1–3 units per day) reduces the risk of death, ischaemic heart disease and stroke, while excessive alcohol consumption increases the risk of these outcomes, giving rise to J-shaped associations (sections 6.6.13 and

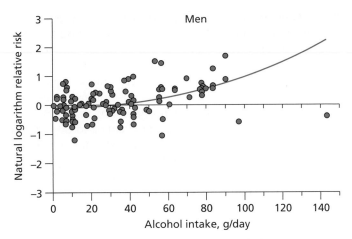

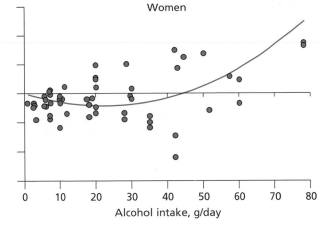

Fig. 16.33 Log relative risk of stroke versus alcohol consumption for men and women. Scatterplot of results of individual studies in a meta-analysis, and meta-regression curve. (Reprinted from Reynolds *et al.*[269] © 2003 with permission from the American Medical Association.)

8.5.2) (Fig. 16.33).[266–269] Several studies have compared the effects of beer, wine and spirits, and, in general, the effects of different types of alcohol are very similar.[270–273]

On the basis of the observational evidence, it is therefore sensible to advise avoiding heavy alcohol intake for everyone, including patients who have had a stroke or TIA, but it is conceivable that a couple of drinks a day may provide net protection against further vascular events. However, since it is difficult to completely exclude residual confounding in the observational studies, and since there is an association between the mean level of alcohol consumption and the prevalence of heavy drinking at the population level, it does not seem sensible to encourage the use of alcohol for vascular prevention as a public health measure.[274–276]

> Everyone, including those who have had a stroke or transient ischaemic attack, should avoid heavy drinking, but a couple of units of alcohol per day may protect against future vascular events.

16.7.3 Dietary modification

Dietary advice to reduce blood pressure by modifying salt intake, and potassium

Observational data suggest an association between dietary salt (sodium) consumption and blood pressure, and public health recommendations in most developed countries are to reduce salt intake by about half, from approximately 10 g down to 5 g/day. Modest reductions of this size can be achieved with relatively simple dietary modifications (not adding salt at the table or in cooking, and avoiding salty foods). A systematic review of RCTs found that these modest reductions for at least 4 weeks among hypertensive people reduced blood pressure by about 5 mmHg systolic/3 mmHg diastolic, while among normotensive individuals they reduced blood pressure by about 2 mmHg systolic/1 mmHg diastolic; there was a correlation between the reduction in urinary sodium excretion and the reduction in blood pressure.[277] Older people with higher blood pressures are likely to achieve greater absolute reductions in blood pressure with dietary modification. In another systematic review of RCTs assessing the longer-term effects of dietary salt restriction on blood pressure in about 3500 people, followed up for between 6 months and 7 years, very few vascular outcomes were recorded with no significant differences detected. Salt intake was reduced by an average of only about 2 g/day, and so blood pressure fell by only 1.1 mmHg systolic/0.5 mmHg diastolic. This shows that long-term maintenance of low salt intake is difficult for individuals, even with a great deal of support, advice and encouragement. Nevertheless, this small reduction in salt intake did cause a small but significant fall in blood pressure, which, on a population basis, should lead to a worthwhile reduction in vascular events, including strokes. The review also found that people on antihypertensive medication were able to stop their medication more often on a reduced sodium diet as compared with controls, while maintaining similar blood-pressure control.[278] Subsequently, a long-term follow-up study of outcomes 10–15 years after two of the trials included found no significant reduction in all-cause mortality, but did find, among the 2400 people for whom morbidity data were available (77% of those originally randomized), a just statistically significant one-quarter relative reduction in myocardial infarction, stroke, coronary revascularization or cardiovascular death.[279] Given the marginal statistical significance and rather large proportion of participants lost to follow-up, this is not a conclusive result, but nonetheless considerably strengthens the evidence that a lower dietary salt intake reduces the risk of vascular events.

> Reducing dietary salt intake reduces blood pressure, particularly in older people with high blood pressure, perhaps resulting in long-term reduction in vascular events. It may also help those on antihypertensive medication to stop their treatment without a rise in blood pressure. However, it is difficult for people to stick to a low salt diet.

Observational epidemiological studies have shown an association between increased potassium and reductions in blood pressure, and in stroke risk.[280] A systematic review of RCTs of increased dietary potassium found that short-term increases equivalent to about five bananas per day reduced blood pressure by about 3 mmHg systolic/ 2 mmHg diastolic, and appeared more effective in those with higher sodium intake, suggesting that potassium supplementation may be helpful for blood pressure reduction in people who are unable to reduce their intake of sodium.[281] The best way to increase dietary potassium is to increase consumption of fresh fruit and vegetables.[280]

Dietary advice to reduce cholesterol

A meta-analysis of metabolic ward studies of diets designed to reduce cholesterol levels in healthy volunteers found that dietary change could reduce blood cholesterol concentrations by about 0.8 mmol/L (i.e. by 10–15%). Achieving this involved replacing 60% of saturated fats with other fats and avoiding about 60% of dietary cholesterol in a typical British diet.[282] In the real world, rather than under carefully controlled conditions, reductions of this size are not achievable. Several systematic reviews of RCTs in free-living subjects found that dietary advice produced total cholesterol reductions of only around 5% (about 0.3 mmol/L with a baseline cholesterol of 6.3 mmol/L), and more intensive diets were somewhat more effective than less intensive ones. Difficulties in complying with the prescribed dietary change explain the difference between the real world and the ward-based studies.[283,284]

Thus, although some useful reduction in cholesterol levels can be achieved with dietary advice, it is important to be realistic about the reductions in vascular events that are likely to result. A systematic review of the effects on vascular outcomes found 27 trials in which the dietary interventions included provision of the majority of food for trial participants over several years, advice about diets with dietary fat restriction or modification, and provision of a combination of dietary advice and supplementation. Meta-analysis showed a trend towards a reduction in vascular mortality, and a marginally significant reduction in fatal and non-fatal vascular events (including myocardial infarction, angina, stroke, heart failure, peripheral vascular events and unplanned cardiovascular interventions) (rate ratio 0.84; 95% CI 0.72–0.99).[285] No significant harms are likely to result from dietary advice, however, so despite small effects at the individual level, it seems very reasonable to recommend cholesterol-lowering dietary advice for all stroke and TIA patients.

> It seems sensible to advise all patients with a prior stroke or transient ischaemic attack to reduce their dietary intake of saturated fat, since this produces moderate reductions in cholesterol levels, which are probably associated with small reductions in subsequent vascular events.

Weight reduction

In observational studies increasing body mass index (BMI) above 21–22 is associated with an increased risk of ischaemic heart disease, hypertension, stroke, diabetes, cancer and osteoarthritis (section 6.6.10). The effects on ischaemic heart disease and stroke are mediated mainly through effects on blood pressure, diabetes and changes in lipid profile rather than raised BMI per se.[286,287] A systematic review of RCTs of various non-surgical interventions for weight loss in overweight and obese people found that both dietary and drug interventions led to modest reductions in weight and, as anticipated, favourable effects on vascular risk factors. The most widely studied dietary intervention was a low-fat or reduced calorie diet, producing reductions at 1 year of about 5 kg in weight, along with small reductions in total cholesterol, diastolic and systolic blood pressure, and fasting plasma glucose. The drugs orlistat and sibutramine both led to weight reductions of 3–4 kg at 1 year. Exercise programmes and behaviour therapy produced additional weight loss when combined with dietary interventions, but there was no clear evidence to suggest that individual therapy was more effective than group or family therapy. However, limited sample sizes and follow-up duration mean that there is no reliable evidence about the effects of any of these interventions on vascular outcomes or mortality.[288] Another systematic review of RCTs in morbidly obese people (BMI > 40) found that surgical interventions, compared with conventional treatment, led to long-term weight loss of 23–37 kg, as well as improved quality of life and reduced comorbidity, and that gastric bypass was the most effective surgical procedure.[289]

The Mediterranean diet

Observational epidemiological studies have shown that increased consumption of fruit and vegetables, increased fish consumption (particularly oily fish, which is rich in omega 3 fatty acids), and increased dietary fibre are all associated with a reduced risk of stroke and ischaemic heart disease.[290–296] These apparently protective dietary components are combined with low saturated fat intake in the so-called 'Mediterranean diet', which is characterized by a high intake of fruit, vegetables and cereals, a moderate to high intake of fish, a low intake of saturated lipids but high intake of unsaturated lipids (particularly olive oil), a low to moderate intake of dairy products, a low intake of meat and a modest intake of alcohol, mainly as wine. This Mediterranean diet is associated in observational studies with reduced mortality from all causes, vascular disease and cancer.[297,298] However, there is no evidence from either observational studies or from RCTs that dietary or supplemental omega 3 fats alter total mortality, combined vascular events, stroke or cancer in people with, or at high risk of, vascular disease or in the general population.[299,300] One small RCT of the Mediterranean diet in 605 ischaemic heart disease patients did find that all-cause mortality, myocardial infarction and cancer risks were more than halved but the small numbers of outcome events and early stopping of the study mean that these results may well be overoptimistic.[301] And the very promising results of another RCT of a similar diet, the Indo-Mediterranean diet, have been called into question.[302–304] A systematic review of RCTs of dietary advice (encouraging reduced consumption of at least one of fat, saturated fatty acids, cholesterol, or sodium, or increased consumption of at least one of fruit, vegetables, polyunsaturated fatty acids, monounsaturated fatty acids, fish, fibre or potassium) found modest benefits on dietary intake and several vascular risk factors, but longer-term effects on vascular outcomes are unknown.[305]

> Obese individuals should be encouraged to lose weight using dietary – or if necessary pharmacological or surgical – interventions, and all patients should receive general advice about a healthy diet, low in saturated fat, with plenty of fish, fibre, fruit and vegetables. These interventions have beneficial effects on vascular risk factors, and seem likely to produce small reductions in vascular outcomes, although there is no clear evidence that they do.

16.7.4 Exercise

Observational studies have shown that physical activity is associated with a lower risk of myocardial infarction and stroke, but most were done in middle-aged people without a history of vascular disease, limiting their applicability to other groups (section 6.6.9).[306,307] A systematic review of RCTs found that aerobic exercise reduces blood pressure, but any effects on vascular outcomes are uncertain.[307,308] Cardiac rehabilitation programmes (of which exercise is just a part) reduce the frequency of death and major cardiac events after myocardial infarction.[309] However, the effects of exercise programmes alone after myocardial infarction or stroke on the occurrence of further vascular events are unknown. It therefore seems reasonable to encourage patients to return to normal physical activities as much as possible after a stroke, but there is no evidence that exercise programmes reduce the risk of recurrent stroke or other vascular events. However, exercise may bring other benefits; for example, a programme of muscle strengthening and balance retraining reduces the risk of falls in elderly people.[310]

16.8 Dietary supplements: B vitamins and antioxidants

16.8.1 Folic acid and other B vitamins

Systematic reviews of observational studies have suggested an association between raised plasma homocysteine concentrations and both ischaemic heart disease and stroke.[311,312] While this does not necessarily imply a cause-and-effect relationship, these findings are supported by the association with ischaemic heart disease and stroke of the common functional polymorphism C677T in the gene encoding methyltetrahydrofolate reductase (MTHFR), an enzyme involved in homocysteine metabolism, showing that the observed increases in risk of both stroke and ischaemic heart disease in individuals with the TT genotype is close to that predicted from the increase in homocysteine concentration conferred by this variant.[312–315] However, the apparent association could be due to another nearby gene in linkage disequilibrium with the MTHFR gene, to confounding by different ethnic composition of cases and controls (population stratification), or to publication bias (positive studies are more likely to be published and so included in systematic reviews than negative ones) (section 6.6.8).[316,317]

If the association between homocysteine concentrations and vascular disease is causal, then lowering homocysteine concentrations should reduce the risk of stroke and ischaemic heart disease. Such lowering is relatively easy to achieve, and RCTs of 0.5–5 mg folic acid daily (with about 0.5 mg vitamin B_{12} to minimize the potential for neurological complications due to B_{12} deficiency) do lower homocysteine concentrations by about one-quarter to one-third (e.g. from about 12 to 8–9 μmol/L).[318] Four large RCTs of folic acid supplements in the prevention of vascular events in high-risk patients have now been completed:

- The Vitamin Intervention for Stroke Prevention (VISP) trial randomly allocated patients with a previous ischaemic stroke to high vs low doses of folate, vitamin B_6 and vitamin B_{12} and followed them for a mean of 20 months. Compared with low dose, high-dose vitamins reduced homocysteine concentrations by 2 μmol/L, but did not affect recurrent ischaemic stroke, ischaemic heart disease or death.[319]

- In the second Cambridge Heart Antioxidant Study (CHAOS-2) (which has so far only been published in abstract form), patients with ischaemic heart disease received folic acid or placebo for almost 2 years. There was a 13% reduction in homocysteine concentration in the folic acid group, but no reduction in vascular outcomes.[320]

- The Norwegian Vitamin Study (NORVIT) randomized patients who had survived an acute myocardial infarction in a factorial design to folic acid and vitamin B_{12}, folic acid, vitamin B_{12} and vitamin B_6, vitamin B_6, or placebo, and followed them for 3.5 years. Treatment with folic acid and vitamin B_{12} reduced homocysteine levels by almost one-third (over 4 μmol/L), but again had no significant effect on recurrent myocardial infarction, stroke or death.[321]

- Finally, in the Heart Outcomes Prevention Evaluation (HOPE) 2 trial, patients with vascular disease or diabetes were randomized to daily treatment with folic acid, vitamin B_6 and vitamin B_{12} or placebo for an average of 5 years. The difference in mean plasma homocysteine levels between active treatment and placebo groups was 3.2 μmol/L. Active treatment significantly reduced the relative risk of stroke by about one-quarter, but did not reduce vascular death, myocardial infarction, or major cardiovascular events combined.[322]

A meta-analysis of RCTs of folic acid supplementation, including these four large trials along with several smaller ones among a total of 17 000 participants with pre-existing vascular disease, found no evidence of a reduction in all-cause mortality or vascular outcomes.[323] Although these results appear disappointing, they are still compatible with a beneficial effect of folate supplementation, since only a relatively small number of outcome events occurred in these four trials, and in CHAOS-2 and VISP both the treatment duration and the difference in homocysteine concentrations achieved between groups were limited.

At least eight further large trials in a variety of secondary prevention settings are still under way, between them including over 37 000 participants and expected to generate almost 8000 vascular events. In combination, these trials should have adequate power to detect moderate effects of homocysteine lowering on vascular outcomes, and to assess whether the effects vary among different populations.[324] Two of the ongoing studies are among or include patients with a history of ischaemic stroke or TIA, and together will include a total of around 9000 such patients.[325,326]

Thus, the currently available evidence does not rule out a beneficial role for folate supplementation in prevention of serious vascular outcomes. However, since there are possible hazards (e.g. of breast and prostate cancer),[327] even of something as benign-sounding as vitamin supplements, for now we must await the evidence that will emerge from the ongoing RCTs.

> At present there is no evidence from randomized trials to support the routine use of homocysteine lowering with folate supplements to prevent vascular events, either in primary prevention or after a stroke or transient ischaemic attack.

16.8.2 Antioxidants

Laboratory studies suggest that antioxidants protect against atherosclerosis by limiting the oxidation of low-density lipoprotein in the arterial wall.[328,329] In keeping with this, observational epidemiological studies have found an association between low intake and low levels of antioxidants (mainly beta-carotene, vitamin C and vitamin E) and risk of stroke and ischaemic heart disease (section 6.6.12).[296,330] This suggests that dietary antioxidant supplements might reduce the risk of ischaemic stroke and other vascular outcomes. A number of dietary constituents have antioxidant properties, including certain minerals (e.g. selenium, copper, zinc, manganese), vitamins (C, E), pro-vitamins (beta-carotene) and flavonoids. However, tens of thousands of individuals have now been randomized in several trials assessing the effects of antioxidant supplements (mainly vitamins E and C and beta-carotene) on vascular outcomes, both in primary and secondary prevention settings. Systematic reviews have found no evidence of benefit, even with follow-up for over 7 years.[331–333] In fact, beta-carotene appeared to be associated with increased vascular mortality.[333] Thus, there is no indication to use antioxidant supplements for secondary prevention after stroke.

> Randomized trials do not support the use of antioxidant supplements after a stroke or transient ischaemic attack.

16.9 Management of diabetes mellitus and glucose intolerance

Diabetes mellitus and glucose intolerance are important risk factors for ischaemic stroke and other vascular diseases; patients with type 2 diabetes have an annual risk of stroke, MI or vascular death of about 6%[334–337] (section 6.6.5). There is good evidence that blood-pressure-lowering drugs, statins to reduce cholesterol, and antiplatelet treatment produce similar relative benefits in people with and without diabetes, so it is clearly appropriate to use these treatments after stroke, regardless of whether or not the patient has diabetes.[117,140,338]

But does tight diabetes control affect the risk of stroke or myocardial infarction? Randomized trials (the United Kingdom Prospective Diabetes Study [UKPDS] and another smaller trial) found that intensive blood-glucose control (aiming for a fasting plasma glucose level of less than 6 mmol/L) with either a sulphonylurea or insulin in patients with type 2 diabetes substantially decreased the risk of *micro*vascular complications (retinopathy and renal damage), but increased the risk of hypoglycaemic episodes and weight gain, and did not appear to reduce macrovascular disease (i.e. stroke and myocardial infarction).[339,340] The UKPDS also found that blood glucose control with metformin in overweight patients reduced microvascular complications, as well as reducing risk of death, myocardial infarction and stroke (the latter non-significantly), with less excess risk of weight gain and hypoglycaemia than with sulphonylureas or insulin.[341] More recently, a randomized placebo-controlled trial of the new hypoglycaemic drug, pioglitazone, including over 5000 patients with type 2 diabetes and a history of stroke, ischaemic heart disease or peripheral arterial disease, found that treatment reduced the risk of death, myocardial infarction or stroke, such that treatment of 1000 subjects like those in the trial for 3 years would result in the avoidance or delay of 21 myocardial infarctions, strokes or deaths. Active treatment also reduced the need to start insulin. However, this benefit was at the expense of an in-creased risk of hypoglycaemic episodes, weight gain and heart failure, although there was no overall difference in the risk of serious adverse events between treatment groups.[342] Thus, since careful control of glycaemia in diabetes improves outcome in terms of microvascular – and perhaps macrovascular – complications, detecting and treating undiagnosed diabetes and ensuring adequate treatment for known diabetes in patients who have had a stroke or TIA is appropriate. In overweight patients, metformin is probably the most appropriate first choice, but otherwise there remain some uncertainties about the best way of achieving glycaemic control. Management of diabetes is probably best coordinated in a dedicated diabetes clinic, where one is available. The management of hyperglycaemia and diabetes in the acute phase of stroke is discussed in section 11.18.3.

> Good glycaemic control in patients with diabetes reduces the risk of microvascular – and perhaps macrovascular – complications.

16.10 Treatment of specific underlying causes

Specific treatment of rare causes of stroke has been discussed in Chapter 7. Here, we outline the specific treatment of some of the commoner causes of stroke.

16.10.1 Atrial fibrillation: rate control vs attempted cardioversion to sinus rhythm

Patients in atrial fibrillation (AF) can in theory be managed either by attempted electrical or pharmacological cardioversion to sinus rhythm or by rate control along with long-term antithrombotic (anticoagulant or antiplatelet) treatment to reduce the risk of embolism. The advantages of cardioversion are that successful restoration of sinus rhythm should improve left ventricular ejection fraction and maximal exercise capacity, and it may reduce the risk of embolic complications so obviating the need for long-term anticoagulation with its attendant inconvenience and risks. However, it is not certain that restoration of sinus rhythm does reduce embolic risk. In addition, about three-quarters of patients spontaneously revert to AF within 1 year of electrical cardioversion, and this occurs in one-quarter to one-half of those initially restored to sinus rhythm using drugs. Finally, neither the procedure of electrical cardioversion nor the drugs used for pharmacological cardioversion are free of risk.[343,344]

A systematic review of electrical cardioversion followed by anti-arrhythmic drugs to maintain sinus rhythm, generally with oral anticoagulants for a few weeks before and after the electrical cardioversion, vs rate control with digoxin, a beta-blocker or a calcium-channel antagonist, plus oral long-term anti-coagulants identified three RCTs. There was no significant difference in death, stroke and TIA, or peripheral embolism. Physical aspects of quality of life were significantly better in the rhythm control group, perhaps because of the larger proportion in sinus rhythm, but since quality of life was only reported for a little over half of the total number of patients, this result may not be reliable.[344] Another systematic review of pharmacological cardioversion vs rate control identified two RCTs that had been published in full, between them including about 4300 subjects with a mean age of 70 years, with almost 95% of the subjects included in just one trial.[343] In this trial, the rhythm control group received the treating physician's drug of choice (most often amiodarone or sotalol, with over half receiving digoxin, a beta-blocker or a calcium-channel antagonist as initial therapy), electrical cardioversion as necessary (this occurred in about one-third of subjects), and anticoagulation was encouraged (and received by 70% throughout the course of the trial). The rate control group received digoxin, beta-blockers, or calcium-channel antagonists, and anticoagulation was mandatory (and received by 85% throughout the course of the trial). Follow-up was for a mean of 3.5 years. Again there was no significant difference between treatment groups in death, ischaemic stroke, systemic embolism, intracranial haemorrhage or extracranial haemorrhage. More patients needed hospitalization, and a slight excess of malignant dysrhythmias occurred during follow-up in the rhythm control compared with the rate control group.[345]

Therefore, the available evidence does not suggest any definite advantage of either electrical or pharmacological cardioversion over rate control with long-term anticoagulation, and suggests some excess risks of pharmacological rhythm control. However, these results only apply to patients eligible for anticoagulants, and do not guide us in choosing the most appropriate treatment strategy for patients in whom anticoagulants are clearly contraindicated. At present, we tend to opt for a policy of rate control plus antiplatelet treatment (usually aspirin) in these patients. Furthermore, the results cannot be generalized to younger patients with new-onset atrial fibrillation.

> In older patients with atrial fibrillation, a strategy of rate control (plus anticoagulation if possible, and antiplatelet treatment if not) is a highly acceptable primary strategy.

16.10.2 Patent foramen ovale and atrial septal aneurysm

A patent foramen ovale (PFO) is present in about one-third of the general population and is associated with an atrial septal aneurysm (ASA) in about 20% of cases.[346] A meta-analysis of case–control studies found that, among younger (<55 years approx.) subjects, having a PFO was associated with an approximately threefold excess risk of ischaemic stroke, having an ASA was associated with about a sixfold risk, and having both was associated with about a 16-fold risk. The relative risks were higher when only cryptogenic ischaemic stroke was considered, but there was no definite excess risk of ischaemic stroke in older subjects with a PFO, ASA or both.[347] It is however uncertain whether these associations are causal. If they are, the mechanism could be paradoxical embolism of thrombus from the venous to the arterial circulation, embolization of thrombi formed locally within the PFO or an associated ASA, or atrial fibrillation associated with the PFO, ASA or both. And, even if there is a causal link in some cases, because of its high background prevalence, PFO must coexist by chance in many young adults with ischaemic stroke, and may well be an innocent bystander in most older patients in whom it is detected (section 6.5.12).[346,348]

Only two studies of the risk of recurrent stroke in patients with vs without a PFO and/or ASA have been published at the time of writing. One recruited almost 600 consecutive adult patients ≤ 55 years old with a recent cryptogenic ischaemic stroke. Of these, 24 patients had a stroke during a mean follow-up of about 3 years, and there was about a fourfold increased risk of recurrent stroke among those with both PFO and ASA: the average annual rates of stroke were 1.1% in those with no septal disorder, 0.6% in those with an isolated PFO and 4% in those with both PFO and ASA.[349] The second study (the Patent foramen ovale In Cryptogenic Stroke Study [PICSS]) followed 601 patients with a recent ischaemic stroke who had been randomized in the Warfarin-Aspirin Recurrent Stroke Study. The patients had a mean age of 59, 250 had cryptogenic stroke, and 203 had a PFO. During about 2 years of follow-up there were 71 recurrent strokes and 21 deaths. There was no apparent increase in the risk of recurrent stroke or death with a PFO, regardless of its size or association with ASA, in either the whole study population or in the cryptogenic subgroup. However, this may have been because of the older age of the subjects and the addition of 'noise' to the outcome measure by including deaths as well as recurrent strokes.[350]

The most appropriate treatment strategy for secondary prevention in stroke patients with PFO and/or ASA

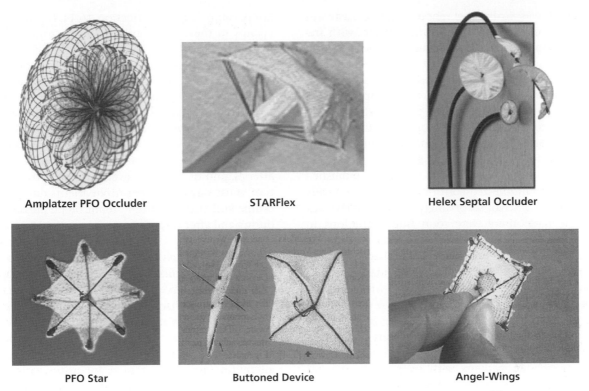

Amplatzer PFO Occluder   **STARFlex**   **Helex Septal Occluder**

PFO Star   **Buttoned Device**   **Angel-Wings**

Fig. 16.34 Various devices used for percutaneous catheter-based patent foramen ovale closure. (From Meier[351] © 2005 BMJ Publishing Group.)

remains very uncertain. Therapeutic options include antiplatelet treatment, oral anticoagulants, or closure of the foramen, generally percutaneously with one of several possible devices (Fig. 16.34) or occasionally with open heart surgery.[351] Although percutaneous closure may appear an attractive, definitive treatment, it is of course not without its risks, which include early device migration (requiring surgical intervention) and periprocedural cardiac tamponade and, in the longer term, device malalignment and significant shunt.[352] A systematic review of observational studies of percutaneous transcatheter closure estimated an incidence of major complications of 1.5% and of minor complications of 7.9%.[353] Since it is usually the best centres who publish their results, these figures probably represent minimum estimates.

In the PICSS, there was no significant difference in the effects of warfarin compared with aspirin on the primary outcome of stroke or death among patients with a PFO, but there was a trend towards a benefit from warfarin over aspirin in those with or without a PFO in the cryptogenic subgroup, albeit at the expense of a significantly higher risk of minor haemorrhage.

Otherwise, there is no available evidence from RCTs on which to base treatment recommendations and, unsurprisingly, experts vary in their views.[346,348,354,355]

However, most agree that there is no good evidence to recommend PFO closure in older patients. In view of the uncertainty, our own practice in younger patients is to discuss with them the possibility of randomization in a trial assessing the effects of treatment with aspirin, warfarin or percutaneous closure (see http://www.clinicaltrials.gov/show/NCT00166257).

16.11 Endarterectomy for symptomatic carotid stenosis

16.11.1 Introduction

Soon after the introduction of catheter angiography and the rediscovery that atherothrombotic stenosis at the origin of the internal carotid artery (ICA) could cause ischaemic stroke (which had actually been suggested many decades earlier, section 2.5), surgeons began to devise methods to remove or bypass the arterial lesion.[356] After early surgical attempts in China and Argentina, the first successful endarterectomy was done by DeBakey in 1953, but not reported until more than 20 years later.[357-359]

However, it was really the report of Felix Eastcott's successful carotid reconstruction in a patient with frequent 'low-flow' transient ischaemic attacks (TIAs) at St Mary's Hospital in London that gave the impetus to what was to become, in North America at least, an epidemic of carotid endarterectomies for asymptomatic as well as symptomatic stenosis.[360–362] ICA occlusion generally came to be regarded as inoperable and surgical attempts to correct carotid coils, kinks and fibromuscular dysplasia are not supported by any good evidence.

Innumerable surgical case series were soon published and two early randomized controlled trials (RCTs) were inconclusive.[363,364] Not surprisingly, in view of the lack of reliable data, there were soon huge variations in surgery rates between countries, and even within the same country.[365,366] Physicians therefore began to question publicly the utility of carotid endarterectomy, inappropriate use of surgery was documented, and the number of operations – perhaps as a consequence – began to fall.[361,362,365,367,368] Eventually, in the early 1980s, these pressures persuaded surgeons and physicians to mount RCTs large enough to be conclusive, and the first results in patients with *symptomatic* stenosis began to appear in the early 1990s.[369–371] Surgery clearly did prevent stroke in patients with recently symptomatic severe ICA stenosis, but at a price: the risk of stroke as a consequence of surgery, the risk of other complications of surgery, the cost of surgery, and the risk and cost of the investigations to select suitable patients (sections 16.11.3, 16.11.4, 6.8.5 and 6.8.13). By then carotid endarterectomy was rapidly becoming one of the most studied surgical procedures ever, leading to economic analyses (section 16.11.6), an estimate of the public health impact of surgery (section 18.4.1), and comparisons of risk between institutions and even individual surgeons (section 16.11.3). After the RCTs, not surprisingly, surgery rates started rising again and there is now concern in North America that much of this rise is to do with operating on *asymptomatic* stenosis and on patients with non-specific symptoms (section 16.12).[362,372,373] Paradoxically, there is also concern at unmet needs, at least in the UK.[374,375] Nowadays, the challenge has become to decide exactly which individuals should be offered surgery (sections 16.11.6–16.11.8).

16.11.2 The carotid endarterectomy operation

The carotid bifurcation is exposed, gently mobilized, and slings placed around the internal, external and common carotid arteries (Fig. 16.35). During this exposure, embolic material may be inadvertently dislodged from the arterial lumen, and nerves which lie close to the

artery can be damaged (section 16.11.4). After applying clamps to these three arteries, away from any atheromatous plaque as far as possible, the bifurcation is opened through a longitudinal incision, the entire stenotic lesion cored out, the distal intimal margin secured, the arteriotomy closed and the clamps released to restore blood flow to the brain. Most patients should already be on antiplatelet drugs before surgery and these should be continued afterwards because the patients are still at high risk of ischaemic stroke in the territory of other arteries, and of coronary events (section 16.2). In addition, most surgeons heparinize patients during the procedure itself. Controlling systemic blood pressure before, during and after surgery is crucial to avoid hypotension, which will make any cerebral ischaemia worse, and hypertension which may cause cerebral oedema or even intracerebral haemorrhage (section 16.11.3). Operative damage to the nerve to the carotid sinus, or changes in the carotid sinus itself, may make control of postoperative blood pressure more of a problem, but in the long term has little if any effect.[376] This then is the operation at its simplest, and for over 50 years surgeons have been attempting to make it safer by using various modifications on the basic technique.

One particular variation, eversion endarterectomy, is becoming increasingly popular.[377–381] A systematic review of five RCTs compared eversion vs conventional endarterectomy either with primary closure or patch angioplasty.[380] Overall, there were no significant differences in the risks of perioperative stroke, stroke or death, or local complication rates, but the absolute risks were rather low (risk of stroke or death was 1.7% with eversion vs 2.6% with conventional endarterectomy).

Cerebral protection (shunting)

In theory, it should be possible to prevent low cerebral blood flow during carotid clamping, and so perhaps an ischaemic stroke, by inserting a temporary intraluminal shunt from the common carotid artery (CCA) to the internal carotid artery (ICA) distal to the operation site. Some surgeons routinely shunt for this reason, and to allow more time to teach trainees, but there are problems:

- insertion may be difficult, particularly with small-calibre arteries, and the shunt can dissect the arterial wall or dislodge atherothrombotic material which embolizes to the brain;
- clot may form in the shunt and embolize, or even occlude the shunt completely;
- the shunt may kink and then obstruct, or obstruct if the end abuts against the arterial wall;
- the shunt can transmit emboli from thrombus in the CCA damaged during shunt insertion;

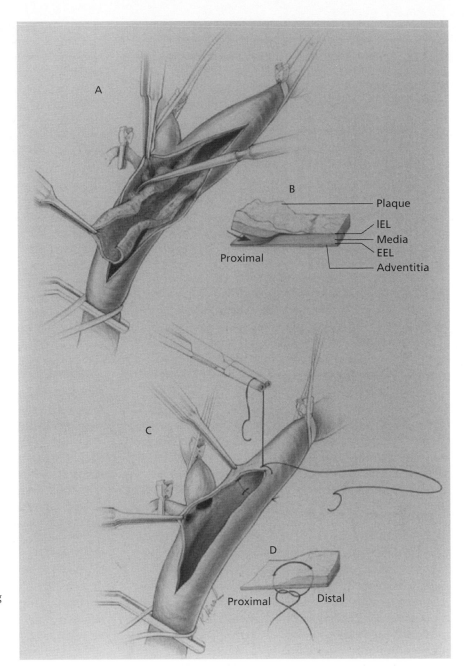

Fig. 16.35 Illustration of a standard carotid endarterectomy. At A the atherothrombotic plaque is being cored out, the plane of dissection usually being between the media and external elastic lamina (EEL) at B. At C the artery is being closed with particular attention to tacking down the distal intimal flap at D. IEL, internal elastic lamina. (Reprinted from Zarins and Gewertz[571] © 1987 with permission from Elsevier.)

- the shunt itself may make the operation technically more difficult, and longer, and the more extensive surgical exposure required increases the chance of nerve damage, postoperative haematoma and infection.

A compromise is to selectively shunt only patients *likely* to develop, or who actually are experiencing, cerebral ischaemia as a result of low flow. However, numerous efforts to identify the patients who need shunting have been inconclusive and there is considerable variation in routine practice.[382–386] Some believe that a shunt should be used if there is contralateral ICA occlusion, or if the patient has had a recent ischaemic stroke. Others shunt patients who have a low ICA 'stump' pressure (measured distal to the ICA clamp), perhaps indicating poor collateral blood flow to the ipsilateral cerebral hemisphere. Collateralization itself can possibly be predicted preoperatively with transcranial Doppler techniques.[387] Intraoperative monitoring of the electroencephalogram, sensory evoked potentials, regional cerebral blood flow, middle cerebral artery blood flow and emboli detection with transcranial Doppler, jugular venous oxygen saturation, cerebrovascular haemoglobin oxygen saturation with near-infrared spectroscopy, and the neurological state of the patient if operated under regional anaesthesia, may all provide early warning that cerebral ischaemia is occurring; inserting a shunt may then prevent a stroke due to low flow, but presumably not due to embolism. However, there is no good evidence that any of these approaches helps to reduce the operative risk and randomized trials of different shunting policies have been too small and too few to provide reliable answers.[388] As a result, there is no standard policy for either operative monitoring or the use of shunts, and surgeons rely on their own experience, common sense and whatever monitoring technique they have available and are comfortable with.

> There is no standard method to predict reliably which patients will have an ischaemic stroke during carotid clamping. It is therefore difficult to select patients who should be protected by a shunt during carotid endarterectomy, which is why there is so much variation in practice.

Restenosis and patch angioplasty

After carotid endarterectomy the long-term risk of ischaemic stroke ipsilateral to the operated artery is so low that recurrent stenosis cannot be of any great clinical concern, at least in the sense of causing stroke (section 16.11.5).[389] This is fortunate because if stenosis does recur then a second endarterectomy is more difficult and more risky,[390] and angioplasty or stenting may be preferable, although there is no randomized evidence for either procedure in symptomatic or asymptomatic restenosis.[391] In fact, the reported frequency of restenosis has varied enormously depending on whether the study was prospective or retrospective, the completeness and length of follow-up, the sensitivity and specificity of the imaging method used, and the definition of restenosis.[392] Sometimes, a restenosis is not even a restenosis at all but a residual stenosis from a technically inadequate carotid endarterectomy. Certainly, recurrent atherothrombotic stenosis can occur, but usually not for some years, while early restenosis (within a year or so) is more likely to be due to neointimal hyperplasia.[393] On balance, therefore, there is no point in repeated clinical or ultrasonographic follow-up just to detect asymptomatic restenosis, but if the operated artery becomes symptomatic again, and the stenosis has recurred, then repeat endarterectomy or stenting is probably reasonable.

Many surgeons routinely use a patch of autologous vein, or synthetic material, to close the artery, enlarge the lumen and so (they hope) reduce the risk of restenosis and, more importantly, of stroke. Patching increases the surgery time, there are two suture lines rather than one and there are complications, albeit rarely: the centre of a vein patch can become necrotic and rupture to cause a life-threatening neck haematoma, perhaps less often if the vein is harvested from the thigh than the ankle; aneurysmal bulging and dilatation of the carotid bifurcation; and synthetic grafts can become infected. Also, it may be impossible to find enough leg vein left over after any earlier coronary artery surgery, and removing what vein there is can cause local haematoma, infection, ulceration and discomfort. Randomized trials are clearly necessary therefore to determine the balance of risk and benefit.

The most recent meta-analysis of RCTs of primary closure, vein patch or synthetic patch included data from 1281 operations in several relatively poor-quality trials.[394] Follow-up varied from as early as hospital discharge to 5 years. Carotid patch angioplasty was associated with a relative reduction in the risk of stroke or death during the perioperative period (OR 0.40; 95% CI 0.2–0.8), in perioperative arterial occlusion (OR 0.12; 95% CI 0.06–0.4), and in restenosis (OR 0.22; 95% CI 0.1–0.3) during long-term follow-up in five trials. However, the trials were relatively small, all relevant data were not always available, and there was significant loss to follow-up. Very few local complications, including haemorrhage, infection, cranial nerve palsies and pseudo-aneurysm formation, were recorded with either patch or primary closure. Nevertheless, the evidence suggests that carotid patch angioplasty does more good than harm.

Some surgeons who use carotid patching favour a patch made from an autologous vein, while others prefer to use synthetic materials. The most recent meta-analysis of seven RCTs of different types of patch included data on 1480 operations and concluded that the differences between different types of patch material were small. More data will be required to establish whether there are any real differences.[395]

General vs regional anaesthesia

Surgery has traditionally been performed most often under general anaesthesia, but regional anaesthesia is becoming more widespread. Both approaches have their supporters and detractors. With general anaesthesia, the patient lies perfectly still and there is good control over the cardiovascular system, but there are likely to be more cardiac and pulmonary complications. With regional anaesthesia, there is much less shunt use because it is immediately obvious when a shunt is needed to restore blood flow distal to the carotid clamps, elaborate intraoperative monitoring is unnecessary and hospital stay may be shorter. On the other hand, some patients will not tolerate the procedure and a quick change to general anaesthesia may be required. A systematic review of randomized and non-randomized studies has provided some useful information.[396] Meta-analysis of the non-randomized studies showed that regional anaesthesia was associated with significant reductions in the odds of death, stroke, stroke or death, myocardial infarction, and pulmonary complications within 30 days of the operation, but these non-randomized data are potentially biased and so unreliable. Meta-analysis of the fewer and generally small randomized studies showed that regional anaesthesia was associated with a significant reduction in local haemorrhage (OR 0.31; 95% CI 0.12–0.79) within 30 days of the operation, but there was only a borderline statistically significant trend towards a reduced risk of operative death and no evidence of any reduction in operative stroke. There is clearly insufficient evidence from RCTs to inform clinical practice, but a large multicentre trial (GALA) has now randomized over 3000 patients and will report its findings in late 2008 (http://www.dcn.ed.ac.uk/gala).

Early technical failure

Just occasionally the carotid artery occludes immediately or a few days after surgery, as a result of thrombosis, dissection of the arterial wall or excessive kinking at the operation site. This does not necessarily cause stroke if the collateral blood supply to the brain is sufficient. Both thrombosis and dissection are thought to be largely due to poor operative technique, particularly if the distal intimal flap has been left unsecured or there is a ridge of arterial tissue due to faulty suturing. Residual disease is another cause of thrombosis. Therefore, before closing the skin, some surgeons check the endarterectomy site with conventional ultrasonography, angiography, angioscopy or intravascular ultrasound and, if necessary, reopen the artery to improve the anatomical result. Whether this has much effect on surgical or later stroke risk is unknown.

16.11.3 Perioperative stroke

The most feared complication of carotid endarterectomy is stroke, the very thing the operation is designed to prevent (Table 16.11).[397–399] The reported risk ranges from an implausibly low 1% or less, to an unacceptably high 20% or more.[400] This variation may be explained by differences in: the definition of stroke; whether all or only some strokes are included; the accuracy of stroke diagnosis; the completeness of the clinical details;

Table 16.11 Complications of carotid endarterectomy.

Ischaemic stroke or transient ischaemic attack (almost always ipsilateral to the operated artery) due to:
Embolism from the operation site during surgery
Embolism from the operation site after surgery
Carotid dissection
Perioperative internal carotid artery occlusion
Low cerebral blood flow during surgery
Perioperative systemic hypotension
Haemorrhagic stroke (almost always ipsilateral to the operated artery) due to:
Perioperative hypertension
Postendarterectomy cerebral hyperperfusion
Antithrombotic drugs
Death due to:
Stroke
Myocardial infarction
Pulmonary embolism
Rupture of arterial operation site
Cardiovascular and respiratory complications:
Myocardial infarction
Angina
Hypotension/hypertension
Cardiac arrhythmia
Cardiac failure
Chest infection
Local complications:
Cranial and peripheral nerve injury (recurrent and superior laryngeal, vagal, hypoglossal, marginal mandibular branch of facial, spinal accessory, greater auricular, transverse cervical nerves)
Wound infection
Neck haematoma
Aneurysmal dilatation at operation site
Patch disruption and haemorrhage
Malignant tumour in the scar
Chyle fistula
Others:
Deep venous thrombosis and pulmonary embolism
Transhemispheric cerebral oedema
Headache
Focal epileptic seizures
Facial (parotid) pain
Pain at vein donor site after vein patch angioplasty

whether the study was retrospective or prospective; whether the diagnosis of stroke was based on patient observation or just medical record review; variation in case mix, surgical and anaesthetic skills; whether the rate is per patient or per operated artery; chance and random variation; and publication bias.[401,402] No more than 20% of perioperative strokes are likely to be fatal, being mostly either total or partial anterior circulation infarcts with 30-day case fatalities of about 40% and 5%, respectively (Table 10.3). Therefore, reports of less than four times as many non-fatal as fatal strokes are almost certainly undercounting mild strokes, a tendency which may be due to surgeons reporting their own results without the 'help' of any neurologists.[403]

Despite the obvious implications for service planning, it has been all but impossible to sort out whether there is any systematic difference in risk between surgeons, or institutions. This is largely due to the problems of adjusting for case mix, as well as chance effects due to the inevitably rather small numbers operated on by each surgeon or even in each institution.[404] One might anticipate that 'practice makes perfect' and there is at least some case-mix-adjusted evidence that high-volume surgeons have lower operative risks than low-volume surgeons.[405,406] But, whatever anyone claims, and even though the size of any stroke risk depends on the study quoted, there is no doubt that there is a risk of stroke and death, realistically somewhere between 3% and 10%, depending on various factors (section 16.11.7).

There are several causes for perioperative stroke but these are difficult to identify when it occurs during general anaesthesia, or even afterwards. In an emergency situation on a surgical ward, it may be impossible to get one or more of a neurologist, brain CT scan, carotid ultrasound and angiogram quickly enough to allow any useful corrective action (see below). Clinical details are often so poorly recorded that, in retrospect, it can be impossible to establish a cause. Also, despite attempts to do so, it is difficult to be sure whether *any* stroke, let alone a perioperative stroke, is due to embolism or low flow (section 6.7.5).[407–410]

Embolism from the operation site

This is probably the most common cause of stroke *during* surgery. Atherothrombotic debris may be released while the carotid bifurcation is being mobilized, as the carotid clamps are applied, when any shunt is inserted, and when the clamps are removed. Indeed, air bubbles or particulate emboli during surgery are very commonly detected by transcranial Doppler ultrasound, although most seem to be of little clinical consequence.[411,412] *Postoperative* ischaemic stroke is usually due to embolism from residual but disrupted atheromatous plaque; thrombus forming on the endarterectomized surface or on suture lines, or more probably on a loose distal intimal flap where the lesion has been carelessly snapped off; thrombus complicating damaged arterial wall as a result of the clamps; and thrombus complicating arterial dissection starting at a loose intimal flap of the internal carotid artery (ICA) or as a result of shunt damage to the arterial wall. A high rate of postoperative microembolic signals on transcranial Doppler monitoring may predict

ischaemic stroke, but the number of strokes is very small so it is difficult to be sure.[413]

Acute internal carotid artery occlusion

This is caused by occlusive thrombosis or dissection, usually a result of technical failure during surgery (see above). It may not cause stroke if the collateral blood supply is adequate.

Low-flow ischaemic stroke

Clearly, temporary reduction in ICA blood flow during carotid clamping may cause ipsilateral ischaemic stroke if the collateral supply from the contralateral ICA and vertebrobasilar system, through the circle of Willis, is inadequate, particularly if there is already maximal cerebral vasodilatation (i.e. cerebrovascular reserve is exhausted). Rarely, systemic hypotension may cause ischaemic stroke and low-flow infarction contralateral to surgery, but probably only if the contralateral ICA is occluded.

Haemorrhagic stroke and cerebral hyperperfusion

Intracranial haemorrhage accounts for about 5% of perioperative strokes.[399,414] This can occur during surgery or up to about 1 week later, almost always ipsilateral to the operated artery. It may be due to the increase in perfusion pressure and cerebral blood flow that occurs after removal of a severe ICA stenosis, particularly if cerebral autoregulation is defective as a consequence of a recent cerebral infarct.[415] Antithrombotic drugs and uncontrolled hypertension may also play a part.[414,416–419]

Interestingly, transient cerebral hyperperfusion, ipsilateral but sometimes bilateral, lasting some days is quite common after carotid endarterectomy, particularly if the lesion was severely stenosing and cerebrovascular reserve is already poor with impaired autoregulation.[420] This may be the cause of the occasional case of ipsilateral transhemispheric cerebral oedema, intracerebral haemorrhage, focal epileptic seizures and headache which can all occur a few days after surgery. Clearly this syndrome is different from ischaemic stroke due to low flow or embolism, and is distinguished by the slower onset, as well as by brain and arterial imaging.[420–426] To complicate matters, a very similar clinical syndrome has been described as a result of cerebral vasoconstriction.[427]

> Stroke complicating carotid endarterectomy is most commonly due to embolism from the operation site during or soon after surgery. Ischaemic stroke due to interruption of carotid blood flow during surgery is less common and intracerebral haemorrhage is very rare.

Management of perioperative stroke

Unless the operation was performed under regional anaesthesia, or cerebral ischaemia was not already suspected by intraoperative monitoring, the first clue that a patient has had an intraoperative stroke is usually delay or failure to awaken from general anaesthesia. It is then vital to determine, within minutes if possible, whether the cause is thrombosis at the operation site, because this is amenable to correction. If transcranial Doppler monitoring had been used during the operation, a change in the middle cerebral artery velocity signal may have suggested a problem at the endarterectomy site (any confusion with intracerebral haemorrhage distorting the Doppler signal is most unlikely). Ideally, a rapid bedside duplex scan should be done and the neck immediately reopened if ICA occlusion is suspected, even taking the very low risk that there is actually an intracerebral haemorrhage. Passage of a Fogarty catheter, restoration of flow, and correction of any technical fault which caused the thrombosis can, in some circumstances, be followed by complete neurological recovery. The later after operation a stroke occurs the less likely that return to the operating theatre is either practical or effective, but how late is too late is a guess. If the operated ICA is still patent, then the next question is whether the stroke is due to intracerebral haemorrhage. A brain CT scan is therefore needed and further management is the same as for spontaneous stroke, and it would help to involve a neurologist or stroke physician at the earliest possible stage.

16.11.4 Other complications

Carotid endarterectomy is associated with a wide variety of potential complications other than stroke (Table 16.11).[397,399]

Death within a few days of surgery occurs in about 1–2% of patients and is generally due to stroke, myocardial infarction or some other complication of the frequently associated coronary heart disease or, rarely, to pulmonary embolism.[401] Higher risks can be found in 'administrative data sets' which may be a more realistic reflection of routine practice than large RCTs, but any comparisons are confounded by variation in case mix, particularly the proportion of patients with asymptomatic stenosis who have a lower case fatality.[390,428,429]

Cardiovascular and respiratory complications. Myocardial infarction during, or in the early days after surgery, occurs in 1–2% of patients, more often if there is symptomatic coronary heart disease, and particularly if myocardial infarction has occurred in the previous few months or if the patient has unstable angina.[399]

Perioperative myocardial infarction can be painless so clues to the diagnosis are unexplained hypotension, tachycardia and dysrhythmias. Congestive cardiac failure, angina and cardiac dysrhythmias are also occasional concerns.[370,399,430–432] Postoperative hypertension and hypotension may be a problem, perhaps due to operative interference with the carotid baroreceptors, but it is transient. Postoperative chest infection occurs in less than 1%.

Cranial and peripheral nerve injuries as a result of traction, pressure or transection occur in up to 20% of cases, the frequency partly depending on how hard one looks (Fig. 16.36). Fortunately, these injuries are not necessarily symptomatic, and are seldom of any long-term consequence:[433]

- Damage to the recurrent and superior laryngeal branches of the vagus nerve, or more likely the vagus itself, causes change of voice quality, hoarseness, difficulty coughing and sometimes dyspnoea on exertion due to vocal cord paralysis. If a simultaneous or staged bilateral carotid endarterectomy is done, and causes bilateral vocal cord paralysis, then airway obstruction can occur.
- Hypoglossal nerve injury causes ipsilateral weakness of the tongue which can lead to temporary or even permanent dysarthria, difficulty with mastication or dysphagia. Again, bilateral damage causes much more serious speech and swallowing problems, and sometimes even upper airway obstruction.
- Damage to the marginal mandibular branch of the facial nerve causes rather trivial weakness at the corner of the mouth.
- Spinal accessory nerve injury is rare and causes pain and stiffness in the shoulder and neck, along with weakness of the sternomastoid and trapezius muscles.
- A high incision can cut the greater auricular nerve to cause numbness over the ear lobe and angle of the jaw, which may persist and be irritating for the patient.
- Damage to the transverse cervical nerves is almost inevitable and causes numbness around the scar area which is seldom a problem.

Clearly, permanent disability from a nerve injury can be as bad as a mild stroke and needs to be taken into account when considering the risks and benefits of surgery.[433–436]

> Permanent disability from surgical injury to a nerve in the neck is very rare but can be as bad or worse than many operative strokes, and must be taken into account when assessing the risk of surgery.

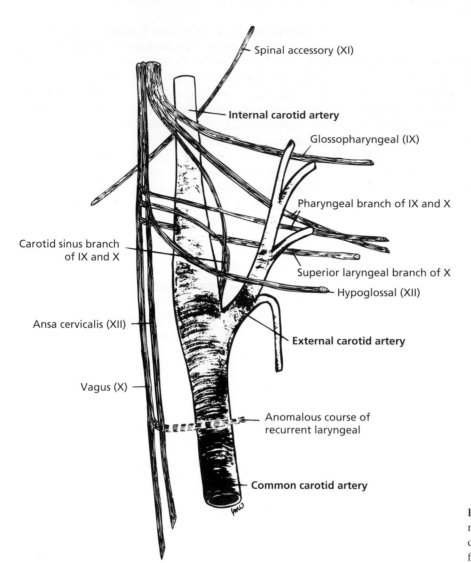

Spinal accessory (XI)

Internal carotid artery

Glossopharyngeal (IX)

Pharyngeal branch of IX and X

Carotid sinus branch
of IX and X

Superior laryngeal branch of X

Hypoglossal (XII)

Ansa cervicalis (XII)

External carotid artery

Vagus (X)

Anomalous course of
recurrent laryngeal

Common carotid artery

Fig. 16.36 Diagram of the nerves in the neck which may be damaged during carotid endarterectomy. (With permission from Schroeder and Levi, 1999.[572])

Therefore, if a patient has symptoms referable to *both* severely stenosed carotid arteries, requiring bilateral carotid endarterectomy, it is probably safer to do the operations a few weeks apart rather than under the same anaesthetic, mostly because of the dangers of bilateral hypoglossal or vagal nerve damage.

> Before a staged second carotid endarterectomy it is always wise to inspect the tongue and vocal cords to ensure there has been no subclinical unilateral nerve damage from the first operation because, if so, the second operation should be postponed.

Local wound complications include: infection; haematoma or, rarely, major haemorrhage, due to leakage or rupture of the arteriotomy or patch which can be life threatening if it causes tracheal compression; aneurysm

formation weeks or years later; and malignant tumour in the scar – all are rare.[399,437,438] Although surgeons often notice the haemostatic defect caused by preoperative aspirin, this probably does not increase the need for reoperation for bleeding.[439] Very rarely the thoracic duct can be damaged and cause a chyle fistula.

Headache ipsilateral to the operation may herald cerebral hyperperfusion but may also be due to something akin to cluster headache due to subtle damage to the sympathetic plexus around the carotid artery.[420,426,440,441] Very rarely, *focal epileptic seizures* occur as well as headache.[442,443] Of course, seizures may occasionally complicate perioperative stroke, just like any other stroke (sections 6.7.6 and 11.8).

Facial pain ipsilateral to surgery and related to eating is most unusual and may in some way be due to disturbed innervation of the parotid gland.[444]

16.11.5 Evidence of benefit

As a result of the large RCTs, it is now quite clear that endarterectomy of recently symptomatic *severe* carotid stenosis almost completely abolishes the high risk of ischaemic stroke ipsilateral to the operated artery over the subsequent 2 or 3 years. Moreover, this effect is durable over at least 10 years.[369–371,445–447] Indeed, the ipsilateral stroke risk becomes so low that presumably both embolic and low-flow strokes are being prevented (Fig. 16.37b). Because so few strokes in these patients are anything other than ipsilateral and ischaemic (Fig. 16.37c),

and taking account of the early risk of surgical death or stroke (Fig. 16.37a), the balance of surgical risk and long-term benefit is – on average – in favour of surgery combined with best medical treatment compared with best medical treatment alone (i.e. treatment of hypertension, statins, stopping smoking, antithrombotic drugs, etc.) (Fig. 16.37d).

On average, there is clearly an advantage to surgery when the symptomatic stenosis exceeds 80% diameter reduction of the arterial lumen using the European Carotid Surgery Trial (ECST) method, which is about the same as 70% using the North American Symptomatic

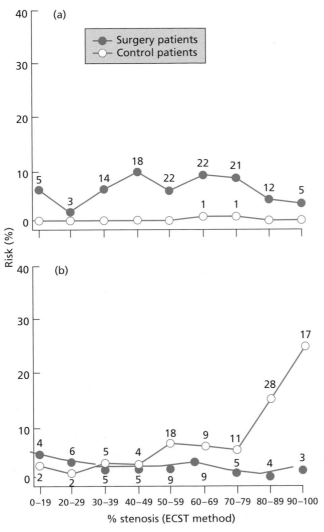

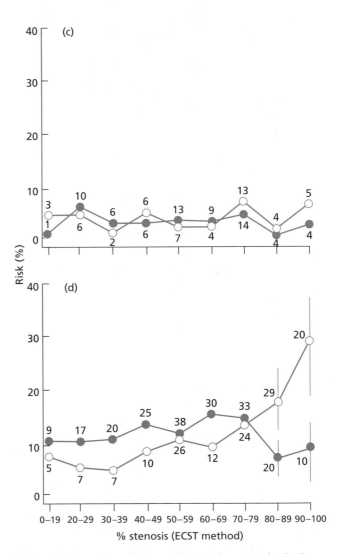

Fig. 16.37 Risk (%) of various outcome events at 3 years in the surgery vs no surgery control group by severity of carotid diameter stenosis in the European Carotid Surgery Trial (ECST). (a) The surgical risk: risk of stroke lasting more than 7 days and all deaths within 30 days of trial surgery. (b) The surgical benefit: risk of ipsilateral ischaemic stroke lasting more than 7 days. (c) The 'noise': risk of all other strokes lasting more than 7 days. (d) The net benefit by combining the surgical risk, the surgical benefit and the noise: risk of any stroke lasting more than 7 days and the risk of a stroke lasting more than 7 days or death as a result of surgery. Vertical lines are 95% confidence intervals. (Reprinted from European Carotid Surgery Trialists' Collaborative Group, *Lancet*[445] © 1998 with permission from Elsevier.)

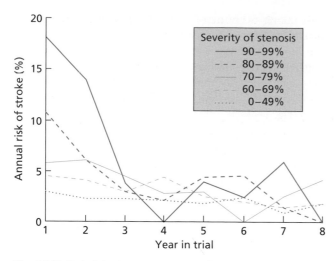

Fig. 16.38 Risk (%) of any stroke lasting more than 7 days (first or subsequent) in the no-surgery patients in the European Carotid Surgery Trial by severity of carotid diameter stenosis and in each of the 8 years following randomization. (With permission from European Carotid Surgery Trialists' Collaborative Group, 1998.[445])

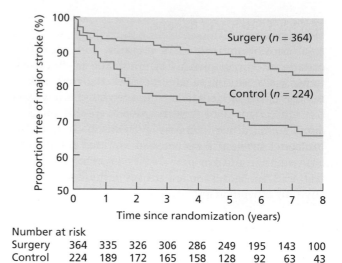

Number at risk								
Surgery	364	335	326	306	286	249	195	143	100
Control	224	189	172	165	158	128	92	63	43

Fig. 16.39 Kaplan–Meier survival curves to show survival free of stroke lasting more than 7 days (non-stroke deaths occurring more than 30 days after surgery are censored) in the surgery and no-surgery control patients with 80–99% diameter stenosis of the symptomatic carotid artery in the European Carotid Surgery Trial. (With permission from European Carotid Surgery Trialists' Collaborative Group, 1998.[445])

Carotid Endarterectomy Trial (NASCET) method (Fig. 6.27). The risk of surgery is much the same at all degrees of stenosis and so, because the unoperated risk of stroke in patients with less than 60% (ECST) stenosis is so low, the risk of surgery is not worthwhile for them (Fig. 16.37); presumably, most of these patients who have had TIAs and some will go on to have strokes in the future, due not just to embolism from the mildly diseased carotid bifurcation but to undiscovered (by imaging) atherothrombosis elsewhere, or cardiac sources of embolism, or to intracranial small vessel disease. For patients with between 60% and 80% (ECST) stenosis there is still some uncertainty left because there may be a few patients at high enough risk of stroke who would gain from surgery, if only we knew who they were (section 16.11.8).

The high risk of stroke with *unoperated* severe stenosis rapidly attenuates in the first 2 years after presentation, and within 3 years it is the same as in patients with mild stenosis (Fig. 16.38). This can also be inferred from inspection of the survival curves of unoperated and operated patients which become parallel after about 2 years (Fig. 16.39). Where the curves cross at about 6 months, the risk of stroke is equal in surgical and non-surgical patients but, because the surgical strokes have occurred earlier and may have caused persisting disability, the surgery group is not advantaged until 6 months after this point when the two groups have a similar number of 'stroke-disability' years.

> After successful surgery for recently symptomatic severe carotid stenosis, the high risk of ischaemic stroke ipsilateral to the operated artery is almost completely removed. For patients with recently symptomatic mild and moderate stenosis the unoperated risk of stroke is not high enough to make the immediate risk of surgery worthwhile.

Because the risk of stroke in moderate stenosis patients remains low for several years (Fig. 16.38), there is no point in duplex follow-up in case the stenosis becomes more severe. No doubt severe stenosis does sometimes develop but, unless there are further symptoms, the stenosis by this time is essentially asymptomatic and carries such a low risk of stroke that there is no overall advantage for surgery (section 16.12). It is preferable to ask the patient to return if there are any further cerebrovascular symptoms and, if the stenosis is *then* 80% (ECST) or more, it is reasonable to consider carotid endarterectomy.

Cognitive performance

Carotid endarterectomy may improve cognitive performance, perhaps by increasing cerebral blood flow or by reducing the frequency of subclinical emboli which declines after surgery.[448,449] On the other hand, subtle cognitive difficulties short of an obvious stroke may complicate the procedure itself, and there is some evidence that previous carotid endarterectomy is associated with more rapid cognitive decline in the longer term.[450–453] Unfortunately, studies addressing this issue have been beset with such methodological difficulties that no conclusions can be drawn.[454] Indeed, it is difficult to imagine that this balance of cognitive benefit and risk will ever be resolved because further RCTs will probably never be done, at least not in symptomatic stenosis patients.

Cerebral reactivity

It is conceivable that patients with impaired cerebral reactivity and raised oxygen extraction fraction are at particular risk of stroke without surgery, and that this impairment can be corrected by carotid endarterectomy, but the studies have been too small to be sure.[455–462] Also, we do not know what proportion of strokes in patients with recently symptomatic severe carotid stenosis are actually due to impaired cerebral reactivity, either as a direct result of low flow or perhaps indirectly as a result of an inadequate collateral circulation to compensate for acute arterial occlusion if it should occur. Nor do we know whether the risk of surgery is higher in these patients and so whether on balance carotid endarterectomy will indeed reduce stroke risk any more than in those without impaired reactivity. Finally, there is a great variety of techniques for measuring cerebrovascular reactivity which do not necessarily correlate with each other (section 6.8.9).

16.11.6 Selection of patients for carotid endarterectomy

Patients find carotid endarterectomy not only inconvenient and frightening, but there are a number of usually trivial and temporary problems such as nerve palsies, and there is always some risk of stroke and occasionally of death. On average, patients even with severe stenosis are unlikely to gain more than a year or two of stroke-free life.[445] Clearly, therefore, several essential conditions must be fulfilled (Table 16.12) before recommending surgery.

If the surgical risk of stroke is, say, 7% in routine clinical practice rather than the more optimistic estimates of some surgeons, if the unoperated risk of stroke is 20% after 2 years which is on average the case for severe stenosis, and if successful surgery reduces this risk of stroke to zero which is not far from the truth, then doing about 15 operations would cause one stroke and avoid three. The net gain would be two strokes avoided. If one only considers disabling strokes, comprising about half

Table 16.12 Conditions to be fulfilled before recommending patients for carotid endarterectomy.

A patient with one or more carotid distribution* transient ischaemic attacks or non-disabling ischaemic strokes in the previous few months and who has, therefore, everything or almost everything to lose from a major hemisphere stroke. Vascular risk factors should be under control (sections 16.3, 16.4 and 16.9) and most patients should be taking antiplatelet drugs (section 16.5).

Duplex sonography shows severe carotid bifurcation disease of the symptomatic artery (likely to be at least 70% stenosis by European Carotid Surgery Trial measurement on catheter angiography).

The patient is prepared to consider and accept the early risk and inconvenience of surgery for long-term benefit.

The patient is fit for surgery: no recent myocardial infarction; angina controlled; no cardiac failure; hypertension controlled; reasonable lung function; and biologically not too aged.

If catheter angiography is still being used, the institution has an experienced neuroradiology team with a low complication rate, preferably kept under prospective and independent audit.

The institution has an experienced surgical and anaesthetic team with a low surgical complication rate, preferably kept under prospective and independent audit.

*For distinction between carotid and vertebrobasilar distribution attacks, see Table 4.3.

the total number, then the 'number-needed-to-operate' doubles. Clearly, to reduce this number of patients that have to be operated on to prevent one having a stroke, and therefore to maximize cost-effectiveness and the chance of an individual patient being benefited, we need to know more exactly who is at highest risk of surgical stroke, and who will survive to be at highest risk of ipsilateral ischaemic stroke if surgery is not done.

It is essential that safe surgery is offered to those patients who have most to gain (i.e. those at highest risk of ipsilateral ischaemic stroke without surgery) and who are most likely to survive for a number of years to enjoy that gain. Ideally we must focus surgery on the small number of patients who *will* have a stroke without it, not on the larger number of patients who *might* have a stroke, because in the latter group there would be a lot of unnecessary operations. After all, even with more than 90% stenosis, seven out of 10 patients will *not* have a stroke in 3 years (Fig. 16.37b).

Furthermore, the cost of identifying suitable patients for carotid surgery is high, with more than 30% of the cost attributed to the initial consultation at the neurovascular clinics. The cost of preventing one stroke by surgery in the UK in 1997–98 was in the region of

£100 000 ($200 000) if all the costs incurred in the workup of a cohort for potential surgery are included.[463] Even excluding the cost of working up the very large number of TIA and stroke patients to find the 5–10% or so suitable for surgery, surgery is still not cheap: about $10 000 (£5000) in a recent systematic review.[464]

16.11.7 Who is at high (or low) risk of surgery?

Perioperative stroke risk (and the risk of the few non-stroke deaths which are usually cardiac in origin) is presumably related to the skill of the surgeon; the skill of the anaesthetist; aspects of the surgical technique; patient's age and sex; the nature of the presenting event, coexisting pathology, such as coronary heart disease; the state of the brain and any ischaemic damage; and the state of the arterial supply to the brain.

Surgeon and surgical factors

Although surgical and anaesthetic skill must be important, the risk of surgery is not necessarily related to the number of operations done by each surgeon. In any event, the risk is difficult to quantify accurately, particularly

when the risk of surgical stroke is so low and when most surgeons operate on a relatively small number of patients every year.[404] A surgeon doing as many as one operation per week might not expect to have more than five stroke complications in 2 years, i.e. 5%, but with a 95% confidence interval of about 2–11%. In the next 2 years his or her complication rate might, just by chance alone, be as good as 2% or as bad as 11%. Variation in surgical technique – the use of shunts, patches, etc. – is mostly of uncertain benefit with respect to perioperative stroke risk (section 16.11.2). Interestingly, although considerable effort has been made to improve surgical and anaesthetic techniques over the years, there has been no evidence of any systematic reduction in the operative risks of stroke or death over the last 25 years.[400]

The presenting event

The operative risk of stroke and death is not only lower for patients with asymptomatic stenosis than for those with symptomatic stenosis, but the risk also depends on the nature of the presenting symptoms (Table 16.13).[390,428] For example, the operative risk in patients with ocular events is about the same as for patients

Table 16.13 A systematic review of the studies reporting the operative risks of stroke or death due to carotid endarterectomy according to the nature of the presenting event and stratified according to year of publication (Bond *et al.*, 2003[390]).

Presenting	Time period	Number of studies	Number of operations	Absolute risk of stroke or death (%) (95% CI)
Symptomatic	< 1995	57	17 597	5.0 (4.4–5.5)
	≥ 1995	38	18 885	5.1 (4.7–5.6)
	Total	95	36 482	5.1 (4.6–5.6)
Urgent	< 1995	9	143	16.8 (8.0–25.5)
	≥ 1995	4	65	24.6 (17.6–31.6)
	Total	12	208	19.2 (10.7–27.8)
Stroke	< 1995	27	3 071	7.3 (6.1–8.5)
	≥ 1995	23	4 563	7.0 (6.2–7.9)
	Total	50	7 634	7.1 (6.1–8.1)
Cerebral transient ischaemic attack	< 1995	11	4 279	4.6 (3.9–5.2)
	≥ 1995	13	3 648	6.9 (6.2–7.5)
	Total	24	8 138	5.5 (4.7–6.3)
Ocular event	< 1995	9	1 050	3.0 (2.5–3.4)
	≥ 1995	9	734	2.7 (1.9–3.3)
	Total	18	1 784	2.8 (2.2–3.4)
Non-specific	< 1995	16	1 275	4.2 (3.2–5.3)
	≥ 1995	8	476	4.3 (3.4–5.2)
	Total	24	1 751	4.2 (3.2–5.2)
Asymptomatic	< 1995	29	3 197	3.4 (2.5–4.4)
	≥ 1995	28	10 088	3.0 (2.5–3.5)
	Total	60	14 399	2.8 (2.4–3.2)
Redo surgery	< 1995	3	215	3.8 (2.7–4.9)
	≥ 1995	9	699	4.4 (3.1–5.8)
	Total	12	914	4.4 (2.4–6.4)

with asymptomatic stenosis, less than those with stroke and cerebral TIA. Therefore, given that the operative risk of stroke depends so much on the clinical indication, audits of risk must be stratified by the nature of any presenting symptoms and patients should be informed of the risk that relates to their own presenting event.

Sex and age

In the RCTs for both symptomatic and asymptomatic carotid stenosis the benefit was less in women than in men, due partly to a higher operative risk in women, and there was little effect of increasing age.[465,466] Although these trial-based observations might not be generalizable to routine clinical practice, in a systematic review of all publications reporting relevant data females had a higher risk of operative stroke and death than males (OR 1.31; 95% CI 1.17–1.47), but no increase in operative mortality (OR 1.05; 95% CI 0.81–0.86).[467]

In the same systematic review, compared with younger patients, operative mortality was higher in older people, for example at ≥ 75 years the odds ratio was 1.36 (95% CI 1.07–1.68). In contrast, however, operative risk of non-fatal stroke alone was not increased. Consequently, the overall perioperative risk of stroke and death was only slightly increased at age ≥ 75 years (OR 1.18; 95% CI 0.94–1.44).

Thus, the effects of age and sex on the operative risk in published case series are broadly consistent with those observed in the trials. Operative risk of stroke is increased in women, and operative mortality but not the risk of stroke is increased in patients aged ≥ 75 years.

Other patient factors

Very few serious attempts have been made to sort out which other patient-related factors affect perioperative stroke risk, and then which factors are independent from each other so they can be used in combination to predict surgical risk in individuals.[398,405,409,468–471] Risk factors almost certainly include hypertension, peripheral vascular disease, contralateral internal carotid occlusion, and stenosis of the ipsilateral external carotid artery and carotid siphon.[472] Operating on the left carotid artery being more risky than on the right clearly needs confirmation and, if true, might be to do with the easier detection of verbal than non-verbal cognitive deficits, or with the surgical feeling that it is more difficult operating on the left side.[398,405,446]

The *independent* surgical risk factors for patients in the pooled analysis of data from ECST and NASCET were female sex, presenting event, diabetes, ulcerated plaque and previous stroke.[466] Other predictors in the ECST that

were not available from NASCET included systolic blood pressure and peripheral vascular disease.[399]

> Perioperative stroke risk depends not just on the skill of the surgeon and anaesthetist, but also on various patient-related factors such as age, female sex, the nature of the presenting event, peripheral vascular disease, contralateral internal carotid artery occlusion and hypertension.

Timing of surgery

The optimal timing of surgery has been a highly controversial topic.[473,474] However, it is increasingly clear that surgery should be performed as soon as it is reasonably safe to do so, given the very high early risk of stroke during the first few days and weeks after the presenting TIA or stroke in patients with symptomatic carotid stenosis.[16,475] Of course any increased operative risk of early surgery must be balanced against the substantial risk of stroke prior to delayed surgery.[475,476] If the operative risk were unrelated to the timing of surgery then urgent surgery would be indicated. In fact, the pooled analyses of data from the RCTs of endarterectomy for symptomatic carotid stenosis showed that benefit from surgery was greatest in patients randomized early after their last ischaemic event and fell rapidly with increasing delay;[466] for patients with ≥ 50% stenosis, the number-needed-to-operate to prevent one ipsilateral stroke in 5 years was only five for patients randomized within 2 weeks vs 125 for patients randomized at more than 12 weeks. This trend was due, in part, to the fact that the operative risk in the trials was not increased in patients operated on within 1 week of their last event.[465,466] A systematic review of all published surgical case series also found that there was no difference between early (first 3–4 weeks) and later surgery in stable patients (OR 1.13; 95% CI 0.79–1.62).[390] Thus, for neurologically *stable* patients with TIA and minor stroke, benefit from endarterectomy is greatest if performed within 1 week of the event.

However, in the same systematic review, *emergency* carotid endarterectomy for patients with evolving symptoms (stroke in evolution, crescendo TIAs, 'urgent cases') had a high operative risk of stroke and death (19%) which was much greater than that for surgery in patients with stable symptoms in the same studies (OR 3.9; 95% CI 2.7–5.7).[390,477] There is therefore still some uncertainty about the balance of risk and benefit of surgery within perhaps 24–72 h of the presenting event, particularly in patients with stroke, and an RCT of early vs delayed surgery during this time scale would be ethical.[475,478,479]

Unfortunately, delays to surgery in routine clinical practice in many countries can currently be measured in months and so the question of by how many hours should surgery be delayed is of somewhat theoretical interest in these healthcare systems.[477,480–482]

Audit and monitoring of surgical results

It is completely impossible to compare surgical morbidity between surgeons or institutions, or in the same place at different times, or before and after the introduction of a particular change in the technique, without adjusting adequately for case mix – in other words, for the patient's inherent surgical risk. In addition, large enough numbers have to be collected to avoid random error.[404] This level of sophistication has never been achieved, and nor probably have adequate methods of routine data collection to support it, in normal clinical practice. It is clearly important, however, to have some idea of the risk of surgery in one's own hospital (*and* of any preceding catheter angiography, section 6.8.5) in the sort of patients that are usually operated on. Risks reported in the literature are irrelevant because they are not necessarily generalizable to one's own institution.

> Valid comparison of surgical stroke risk between different surgeons or institutions, or in the same place at different times, is impossible without both adjustment for case mix and many hundreds of patients in each comparison group. Such a worthy ideal has never been, and may never be, achieved.

16.11.8 Who benefits most from surgery for symptomatic carotid stenosis?

Not *all* patients with even extremely severe symptomatic stenosis go on to have an ipsilateral ischaemic stroke, far from it. In the ECST, although about 30% with 90–99% stenosis had a stroke in 3 years, 70% did not and these 70% could only have been harmed by surgery, never helped (Fig. 16.37b). Both the ECST and NASCET have shown very clearly the importance of increasing severity of carotid stenosis ipsilateral to the cerebral or ocular symptoms in the prediction of ischaemic stroke in the same arterial distribution, although even this relationship is not straightforward in that if the ICA 'collapses' distal to an extreme stenosis the risk of stroke is substantially reduced.[483,484] *Angiographically* demonstrated 'ulceration' or 'irregularity' increases the stroke risk even more, but it is unclear whether this can be translated to the appearances on ultrasound.[485,486] These and other determinants of benefit are discussed below. To complicate matters further one also must avoid offering surgery to patients unlikely to survive long enough to enjoy any benefit of stroke prevention and so for whom the immediate surgical risks would not be worthwhile; these include the very elderly and patients with advanced cancer. It would also seem sensible to avoid surgery in patients with severe symptomatic cardiac disease who are likely to die a cardiac death within a year or two.

> The risk of ischaemic stroke ipsilateral to symptomatic carotid stenosis increases as the stenosis becomes more severe, particularly when it is more than about 80% (ECST method) of the vessel diameter. On the other hand, the risk of perioperative stroke is largely independent of the amount of stenosis. Therefore, on average, the more severe the stenosis, the more a patient has to gain from successful carotid endarterectomy. In practice, the risk of surgery is unacceptable if the stenosis is less than about 70–80% (ECST), but the exact break-even point must depend on other factors which predict stroke without surgery, such as ischaemia in the brain rather than the eye.

Which range of stenosis?

To target carotid endarterectomy appropriately, it is first necessary to determine as precisely as possible how the overall average benefit from surgery relates to the degree of carotid stenosis. Although the analyses of each of the main trials of endarterectomy for symptomatic carotid stenosis were stratified by the severity of stenosis of the symptomatic carotid artery, different methods of measurement on the pre-randomization angiograms were used; the NASCET method underestimates stenosis as compared with the ECST method.[487] Stenoses of 70–99% in the NASCET were equivalent to 82–99% in the ECST, and stenoses of 70–99% in the ECST were 55–99% in the NASCET.[488] Not surprisingly, the reported results of the two trials for each grade of stenosis were quantitatively different. Given this apparent disparity, the ECST group re-measured their angiograms so they were comparable with the NASCET.[488] This then allowed a pooled analysis of data from the ECST, NASCET and VA#309 trials, which included over 95% of patients with symptomatic carotid stenosis ever randomized to endarterectomy vs medical treatment.[447]

This pooled analysis showed that there was no statistically significant heterogeneity between the trials in the effect of the randomized treatment allocation on the relative risks of any of the main outcomes in any of the stenosis groups. Data were therefore merged on 6092 patients with 35 000 patient-years of follow-up.[447] The overall operative mortality was 1.1% (95% CI 0.8–1.5), and the operative risk of stroke or death was 7.1%

(95% CI 6.3–8.1). The effect of surgery on the main trial outcomes is shown by stenosis group in Fig. 16.40. Endarterectomy reduced the 5-year absolute risk of *any stroke or death* in patients with [NASCET]50–69% stenosis (absolute risk reduction of 7.8%; 95% CI 3.1–12.5) and was highly beneficial in patients with [NASCET]70–99% stenosis (absolute risk reduction of 15.3%; 95% CI 9.8–20.7), but was of no benefit in patients with near occlusion. The confidence intervals around the estimates of treatment effect in the near occlusions were wide, but the difference in the effect of surgery between this group and patients with ≥ 70% stenosis without near occlusion was statistically highly significant for each of the outcomes. Qualitatively similar results were seen for disabling stroke.

These results show that with the exception of near occlusions, the degree of stenosis above which surgery is beneficial is [NASCET]50% (equivalent to about [ECST]65% stenosis). Given the confusion generated by the use of different methods of measurement of stenosis in the original trials, it has been suggested that the NASCET method be adopted as the standard in future.[447] Although there are some arguments in favour of the continued use of catheter angiography in the selection of patients for endarterectomy,[489,490] if non-invasive techniques are used to select patients for surgery, then they must be properly validated against catheter angiography within individual centres.[491] More work is also required to assess the accuracy of non-invasive methods of carotid imaging in detecting near occlusion.[492,493]

What about near occlusions?

Near occlusions (Fig. 16.41) were identified in the NASCET, because it is not possible to measure the degree of stenosis using the NASCET method when the post-stenotic ICA is narrowed or collapsed due to markedly reduced post-stenotic blood flow. Patients with 'abnormal post-stenotic narrowing' of the ICA were also identified in the ECST.[483] In both trials, these patients had a paradoxically low risk of stroke on medical treatment, most likely due to the presence of a good collateral circulation, which is visible on catheter angiography in the vast majority of the patients with narrowing of the ICA distal to a severe stenosis (Fig. 16.41). The benefit from surgery in near occlusions in the NASCET had been minimal, and both the re-analysis of the ECST and the pooled analysis suggested no benefit at all in this group in terms of preventing stroke (Fig. 16.40).[447,488] However, in the re-analysis of the ECST, endarterectomy did reduce the risk of recurrent TIA and so some patients may wish to undergo surgery, particularly if they experience recurrent TIAs, even though endarterectomy does not prevent stroke.[488]

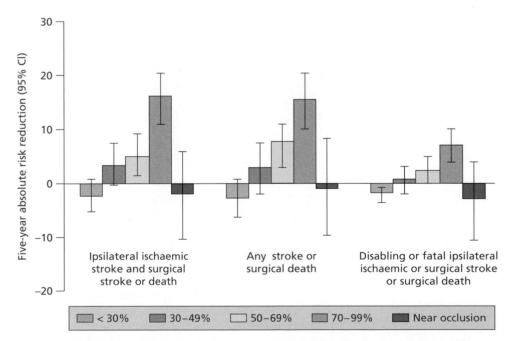

Fig. 16.40 The effect of carotid endarterectomy on the 5-year absolute risks of each of the main trial outcomes by severity of stenosis, in an analysis of pooled data from the three main randomized trials of endarterectomy vs medical treatment alone for recently symptomatic carotid stenosis. (Reprinted from Rothwell *et al.*, *Lancet*[447] © 2003 with permission from Elsevier.)

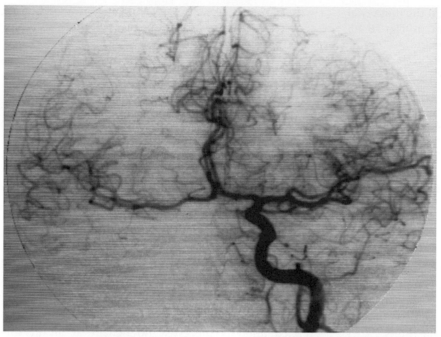

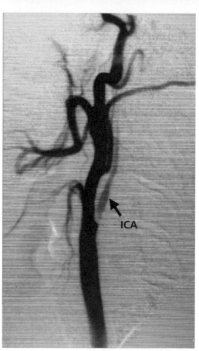

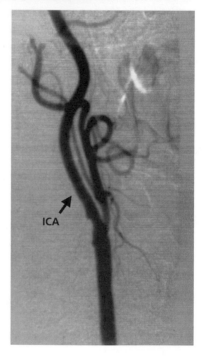

Fig. 16.41 Selective catheter angiograms of both carotid circulations in a patient with a recently symptomatic carotid 'near-occlusion' (*left*), and a mild stenosis at the contralateral carotid bifurcation (*right*). The near-occluded internal carotid artery (ICA) is markedly narrowed, and flow of contrast into the distal ICA is delayed. After selective injection of contrast into the contralateral carotid artery significant collateral flow can be seen across the anterior communicating artery with filling of the middle cerebral artery of the symptomatic hemisphere (*top*).

Which subgroups benefit most?

The overall trial results are of only limited help to patients and clinicians in making decisions about surgery. Although endarterectomy reduces the relative risk of stroke by about 30% over the next 3 years in patients with a recently symptomatic severe stenosis, only 20% of such patients have a stroke on medical treatment alone. The operation is of no value in the other 80% who, despite having a symptomatic stenosis, are destined to remain stroke-free without surgery and can only be harmed by surgery. It would, therefore, be useful to be able to identify in advance, and operate on, only those patients with a high risk of stroke on medical treatment alone, but a relatively low operative risk. The degree of stenosis is a major determinant of benefit from endarterectomy, but there are several other clinical and angiographic characteristics that might influence the risks and benefits of surgery as discussed above.

NASCET published 11 reports of different univariate subgroup analyses, which are summarized elsewhere.[1] Although interesting, the results are difficult to interpret because several of the subgroups contained only a few tens of patients, with some of the estimates of the effect of surgery based on only one or two outcome events in each treatment group, the 95% confidence intervals around the absolute risk reductions in each subgroup have generally not been given, and there were no formal tests of the interaction between the subgroup variable and the treatment effect. It is, therefore, impossible to be certain whether differences in the effect of surgery between subgroups were real or due to chance. Subgroup analyses of pooled data from ECST and NASCET have greater power to determine subgroup–treatment interactions reliably and there are several clinically important interactions: sex, age, and time from the last

symptomatic event to randomization all modified the effectiveness of surgery (Fig. 16.42).[466] For patients with ≥ 50% stenosis, the number needed to operate to prevent one ipsilateral stroke in five years was:

- nine for men vs 36 for women;
- five for age ≥ 75 vs 18 for age < 65 years;
- five for patients randomized within 2 weeks after their last ischaemic event vs 125 for patients randomized > 12 weeks.

These observations were consistent across the 50–69% and ≥ 70% stenosis groups and similar trends were present in both ECST and NASCET. The fall-off in the absolute benefit of surgery with time since last event (Fig. 16.43) is particularly important in terms of auditing the performance of stroke prevention services in routine clinical practice.

Women had a lower risk of ipsilateral ischaemic stroke on medical treatment and a higher operative risk in comparison to men. For recently symptomatic carotid stenosis, surgery is very clearly beneficial in women with

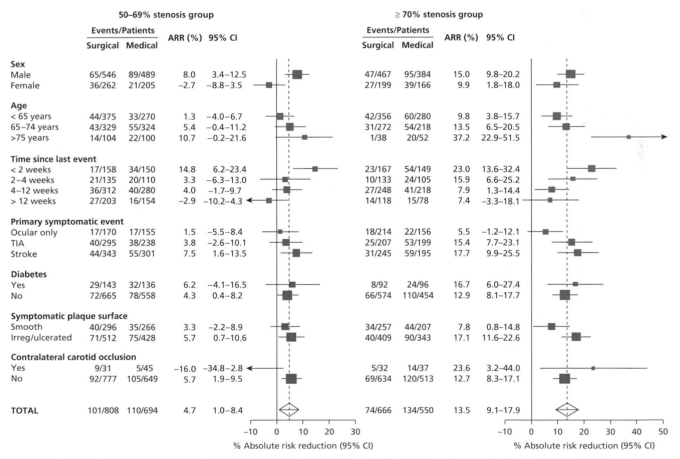

Fig. 16.42 Absolute reduction with surgery in the 5-year risk of ipsilateral carotid territory ischaemic stroke and any stroke or death within 30 days after surgery according to predefined subgroup variables in: patients with 50–69% stenosis; patients with ≥ 70% stenosis. The size of the purple boxes is proportional to the amount of data represented by each box and the horizontal lines represent 95% confidence intervals. (Derived from Rothwell *et al.*, 2004.[466]) CI, confidence interval; ARR, absolute risk reduction.

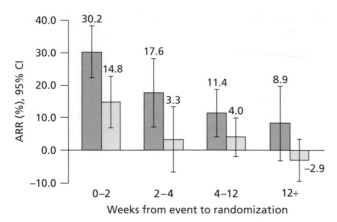

Fig. 16.43 Absolute risk reduction (ARR) with surgery in the 5-year risk of ipsilateral carotid territory ischaemic stroke and any stroke or death within 30 days after surgery in patients with 50–69% stenosis (light purple bars) and ≥ 70% stenosis (purple bars) without near-occlusion, stratified by the time from last symptomatic event to randomization (Rothwell et al., 2004[466]). The numbers above the bars indicate the actual absolute risk reduction. CI, confidence interval.

≥ 70% stenosis, but not in women with 50–69% stenosis (Fig. 16.42). In contrast, surgery reduced the 5-year absolute risk of stroke by 8.0% in men with 50–69% stenosis. These same patterns were also shown in both of the large published trials of endarterectomy for asymptomatic carotid stenosis.[494]

Benefit from surgery increased with age in the pooled analysis, particularly in patients aged over 75 years (Fig. 16.42). Although patients randomized in trials generally have a good prognosis and there is some evidence of an increased operative mortality in elderly patients in routine clinical practice, as discussed above there is no increase in the operative risk of stroke and death in older age groups. There is therefore no justification for withholding surgery in patients aged over 75 years who are deemed to be medically fit. The evidence suggests that benefit is likely to be greatest in this group because of their high risk of stroke without surgery.

Finally, benefit from surgery is probably greatest in patients with stroke, intermediate in those with cerebral TIA and lowest in those with ocular events (Fig. 16.42). There was also a trend in the trials towards greater benefit in patients with irregular plaque than a smooth plaque.

Which individuals benefit most?

Although there are some clinically useful subgroup observations in the pooled analysis of the trials, univariate subgroup analysis is often of only limited use in clinical practice. Individual patients frequently have several important risk factors, each of which interacts in

a way that cannot be described using univariate subgroup analysis, and all of which should be taken into account to determine the likely balance of risk and benefit from surgery.[495] For example, what would be the likely benefit from surgery in a 78-year-old (increased benefit) female (reduced benefit) with 70% stenosis who presented within 2 weeks (increased benefit) of an ocular ischaemic event (reduced benefit) and who was found to have an ulcerated carotid plaque (increased benefit)? One way to weigh the often-conflicting effects of the important characteristics of an individual patient on the likely benefit from treatment is to base decisions on the predicted absolute risks of a poor outcome with each treatment option, using prognostic models.

One such model for prediction of the risk of stroke on medical treatment in patients with recently symptomatic carotid stenosis has been derived from the ECST (Table 16.14).[1,495] The model was validated using data from the NASCET and showed very good agreement between predicted and observed medical risk, reliably distinguishing between individuals with a 10% risk of ipsilateral ischaemic stroke after 5 years of follow-up and those with a risk of over 40% (Fig. 16.44). Importantly, Fig. 16.44 also shows that the operative risk of stroke or death in patients who were randomized to surgery in NASCET was unrelated to the medical risk. Thus,

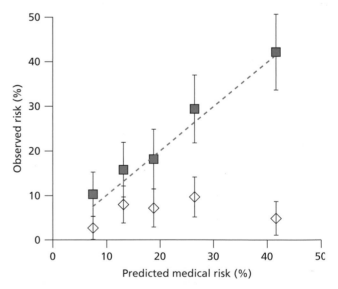

Fig. 16.44 Validation of the ECST model (Table 16.14) for the 5-year risk of stroke on medical treatment in patients with 50–99% stenosis in NASCET (Rothwell et al., 2005[1]). Predicted medical risk is plotted against observed risk of stroke in patients randomized to medical treatment in NASCET (squares) and against the observed operative risk of stroke or death in patients randomized to surgical treatment (diamonds). Groups are quintiles of predicted risk. Error bars represent 95% confidence intervals.

Table 16.14 A predictive model for the 5-year risk of ipsilateral ischaemic stroke on medical treatment in patients with recently symptomatic carotid stenosis (Rothwell *et al.*, 2005[1]). Hazard ratios derived from the model are used for the scoring system. The score for the 5-year risk of stroke is the product of the individual scores for each of the risk factors present. The score is converted into a risk using the graphic in Fig. 16.45. An example is shown.

MODEL			SCORING SYSTEM		EXAMPLE
Risk factor	Hazard ratio (95%CI)	*P*-value	Risk factor	Score	
Stenosis (per 10%)	1.18 (1.10–1.25)	<0.0001	Stenosis (%)		
			50–59	2.4	2.4
			60–69	2.8	
			70–79	3.3	
			80–89	3.9	
			90–99	4.6	
Near occlusion	0.49 (0.19–1.24)	0.1309	Near occlusion	0.5	No
Male sex	1.19 (0.81–1.75)	0.3687	Male sex	1.2	No
Age (per 10 years)	1.12 (0.89–1.39)	0.3343	Age (years)		
			31–40	1.1	
			41–50	1.2	
			51–60	1.3	
			61–70	1.5	1.5
			71–80	1.6	
			81–90	1.8	
Time since last event (per 7 days)	0.96 (0.93–0.99)	0.0039	Time since last event (days)		
			0–13	8.7	8.7
			14–28	8.0	
			29–89	6.3	
			90–365	2.3	
Presenting event		0.0067	Presenting event		
Ocular	1.000		Ocular	1.0	
Single transient ischaemic attack	1.41 (0.75–2.66)		Single transient ischaemic attack	1.4	
Multiple transient ischaemic attacks	2.05 (1.16–3.60)		Multiple transient ischaemic attacks	2.0	
Minor stroke	1.82 (0.99–3.34)		Minor stroke	1.8	
Major stroke	2.54 (1.48–4.35)		Major stroke	2.5	2.5
Diabetes	1.35 (0.86–2.11)	0.1881	Diabetes	1.4	1.4
Previous myocardial infarction	1.57 (1.01–2.45)	0.0471	Previous myocardial infarction	1.6	No
Peripheral vascular disease	1.18 (0.78–1.77)	0.4368	Peripheral vascular disease	1.2	No
Treated hypertension	1.24 (0.88–1.75)	0.2137	Treated hypertension	1.2	1.2
Irregular/ulcerated plaque	2.03 (1.31–3.14)	0.0015	Irregular/ulcerated plaque	2.0	2.0
TOTAL RISK SCORE					263
PREDICTED MEDICAL RISK USING NOMOGRAM (Fig. 16.45)					37%

In cases of near-occlusion, enter degree of stenosis as 85%. Presenting event is coded as the most severe ipsilateral symptomatic event in the last 6 months (severity is as ordered above, i.e. ocular events are least severe and major stroke is most severe). Major stroke is defined as stroke with symptoms persisting for at least 7 days. Treated hypertension includes previously treated or newly diagnosed.

when the operative risk and the small additional residual risk of stroke following successful endarterectomy were taken into account, benefit from endarterectomy at 5 years varied significantly across the quintiles, with no benefit in patients in the lower three quintiles of predicted medical risk (absolute risk reduction 0–2%), moderate benefit in the fourth quintile (absolute risk reduction 12%), and substantial benefit in the highest quintile (absolute risk reduction 32%).

Prediction of risk using models requires a computer, a pocket calculator with an *exponential* function, or internet access (the ECST model is at www.stroke.ox.ac.uk). As an alternative, a simplified risk score based on the hazard ratios derived from the relevant risk model can be derived (Table 16.14). As is shown in the example, the total risk score is the product of the scores for each risk factor. Figure 16.45 shows a plot of the total risk score against the 5-year predicted risk of ipsilateral carotid territory ischaemic stroke derived from the full model, and is used as a nomogram for the conversion of the score into a risk prediction.

Alternatively, risk tables allow a relatively small number of important variables to be considered and have the major advantage that they do not require the calculation of any score by the clinician or patient. Figure 16.46 shows a risk table for the 5-year risk of ipsilateral ischaemic stroke in patients with recently symptomatic carotid stenosis on medical treatment derived from the ECST model.

One potential problem with the ECST risk model is that it might overestimate risk in current patients because of improvements in medical treatment, such as the increased use of statins. However, this poses more problems for generalizability of the overall trial results than for the risk modelling approach. For example, it would take only a relatively modest improvement in the effectiveness of medical treatment to erode the overall benefit of endarterectomy in patients with 50–69% stenosis. In contrast, very major improvements in medical treatment would be required to significantly reduce the benefit from surgery in patients in the high predicted-risk quintile in Fig. 16.44. Thus, the likelihood that ancillary treatments have improved, and are likely to continue to improve, is an argument in favour of a risk-based approach to targeting treatment. However, it would be reasonable in a patient on treatment with a statin, for example, to reduce the risks derived from the risk model by 20% in relative terms (Fig 16.45).

Other prognostic tools, such as measurements of cerebral reactivity and emboli load on transcranial Doppler (section 6.8.9) are not widely used in clinical practice and it is unclear to what extent they are likely to add to the predictive value of the ECST model.[18,496,497]

16.11.9 Management of patients with other potential causes of stroke as well as carotid stenosis

An occasional patient with a lacunar ischaemic stroke or transient ischaemic attack (TIA) may have ipsilateral severe carotid stenosis (section 6.4). The question then arises whether the stenosis is 'symptomatic' (i.e. a small deep lacunar infarct has, unusually, been caused by artery-to-artery embolism or low flow) or 'asymptomatic' (i.e. the stenosis is a coincidental bystander and the infarct was really due to intracranial small vessel disease). The observational studies mostly show that severe stenosis is about equally rare in the symptomatic and contralateral carotid arteries of patients with lacunar stroke, which rather supports the notion of the stenosis being coincidental,[498] but this doesn't mean that surgery wouldn't still be beneficial. In fact, the published data from RCTs show that endarterectomy is beneficial for patients with severe stenosis ipsilateral to a lacunar TIA or stroke, although not for patients with moderate stenosis.[499,500]

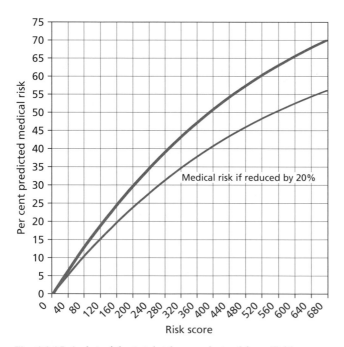

Fig. 16.45 A plot of the total risk score derived from Table 16.14 against the 5-year predicted risk of ipsilateral carotid territory ischaemic stroke derived from the full model in the table in patients in the ECST (*thick line*). This should be used as a nomogram for the conversion of the score into a prediction of the percentage risk (Rothwell *et al.*, 2005[1]). The thin line represents a 20% reduction in risk as might be seen with more intensive medical treatment than was available in the ECST in the late 1980s and 1990s.

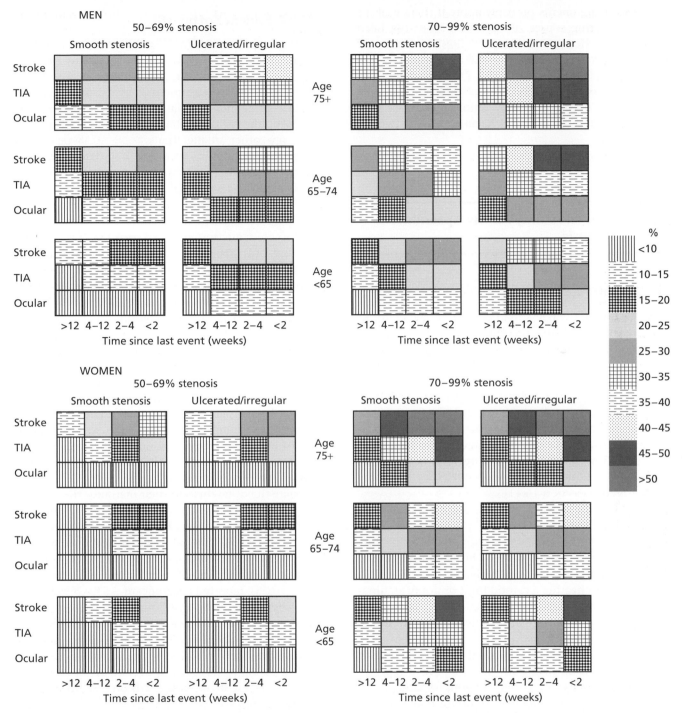

Fig. 16.46 A table of the 5-year predicted absolute risk of ipsilateral carotid territory ischaemic stroke on medical treatment in ECST patients with recently symptomatic carotid stenosis derived from a Cox model based on six clinically important patient characteristics. TIA, transient ischaemic attack. (Figs 16.44–16.46 reprinted from Rothwell *et al.*, *Lancet*[1] © 2005 with permission from Elsevier.)

The same arguments probably apply if there is also a major coexisting source of embolism from the heart (such as non-rheumatic atrial fibrillation), in which case the patient may reasonably be offered surgery as well as anticoagulation (section 16.6.2). With the more widespread use of MR DWI it is, of course, more often possible now to infer the likely aetiology of stroke from the distribution of acute ischaemic lesions (section 5.5.2).

16.12 Endarterectomy for asymptomatic carotid stenosis

16.12.1 Introduction

As far as one can tell, less than 20% of ischaemic stroke patients have had any preceding transient ischaemic attacks (TIAs), even when the stroke is likely to have been due to the embolic or low-flow consequences of severe carotid stenosis. Until the moment of stroke, any stenosis in the other 80% of the patients had been 'asymptomatic'. It follows that if these asymptomatic stenoses could be detected before the stroke, then unheralded (by TIA) stroke might be preventable by carotid endarterectomy, particularly as surgery is beneficial in patients whose stenosis has revealed itself by becoming 'symptomatic' (section 16.11).

Asymptomatic carotid stenosis may be identified under at least four circumstances:

- during screening programmes of apparently healthy people when a carotid bruit is heard and/or carotid ultrasound is being used routinely;
- as a result of hearing a carotid bruit or doing an ultrasound examination during the course of working up patients with angina, claudication or non-focal neurological symptoms;
- when bilateral carotid imaging is done in patients with unilateral carotid symptoms (i.e. the patient is symptomatic but one carotid artery is asymptomatic);
- when patients are being worked up for major surgery below the neck and a carotid bruit is heard or an ultrasound reveals carotid stenosis.

When asymptomatic carotid stenosis does come to attention, four questions arise: What is the risk of operating on it? What is the risk (of stroke) if the stenosis is left unoperated? Does surgery reduce the risk of stroke? What is the balance of immediate surgical risk vs long-term benefit?

16.12.2 Evidence of benefit

Whether the benefits of carotid endarterectomy in patients with asymptomatic stenosis justify the risks and cost is still unclear, particularly in an era of improved medical treatments.[501,502] Until relatively recently, guidelines were largely based on the results of the Asymptomatic Carotid Atherosclerosis Study (ACAS) and a few other smaller trials.[502,503] ACAS reported a 47% relative reduction in the risk of ipsilateral stroke or perioperative death in the surgical arm, but a 5-year risk of ipsilateral stroke without the operation of only 11%, even though the patients had moderate or severe stenosis. Therefore, even in this optimal trial environment, the absolute reduction in risk of stroke with endarterectomy was only about 1% per year. Of some concern is that the remarkably low operative risks in ACAS may not be matched in routine clinical practice because ACAS only accepted surgeons with an excellent safety record, rejecting 40% of the initial applicants and subsequently barring from further participation some surgeons who had adverse operative outcomes during the trial.[504]

Before joining the later, and more pragmatic Asymptomatic Carotid Surgery Trial (ACST), the surgeons had to provide evidence of an operative risk of 6% or less for their last 50 patients having an endarterectomy for asymptomatic stenosis, but none were excluded on the basis of his/her operative risk during the trial.[505] Selection of patients was based on the 'uncertainty principle', with very few exclusion criteria.

Despite the differences in their methods, the absolute reductions in 5-year risk of stroke with surgery were similar in the two trials: 5.3% (95% CI 3.0–7.8%) in ACST vs 5.1% (95% CI 0.9–9.1%) in ACAS. In addition, whereas ACAS had reported only a non-significant 2.7% reduction in the absolute risk of disabling or fatal stroke with surgery, ACST reported a significant 2.5% (95% CI 0.8–4.3%) absolute reduction, although the number-needed-to-operate to prevent one disabling or fatal stroke after 5 years remains about 40. The main difference between the trials was in the 30-day operative risks of death of 0.14% in ACAS vs 1.11% in ACST, and in the combined operative risk of stroke and death of 1.5% in ACAS vs 3.0% in ACST.

16.12.3 Selection of patients for carotid endarterectomy

As discussed earlier, the decision to perform carotid endarterectomy should not be taken lightly, given the inevitable anxiety and risks faced by patients undergoing surgery. Applying the same arithmetical approach used for symptomatic stenosis (section 16.11.6), if the surgical risk of stroke is say 4% in routine clinical practice, if the unoperated risk of stroke is 10% after 5 years on intensive medical treatment, and if successful surgery reduces this risk of stroke to almost zero, then doing about 100 operations would cause four strokes and avoid up to 10, the numbers-needed-to-operate to prevent one stroke would be 17, about 34 for disabling stroke. Therefore to reduce the number-needed-to-operate and increase the chance of an individual patient being benefited, it is essential that we know who is at highest risk of surgical stroke, and who will survive to be at highest risk of ipsilateral ischaemic stroke without surgery. Furthermore, given the high cost of surgery even for symptomatic carotid stenosis, we need to be aware of the health-economic and public health issues related to surgery for asymptomatic stenosis.[463,464]

16.12.4 Risk of carotid endarterectomy for asymptomatic carotid stenosis

There are a large number of case series with very different reported surgical stroke risks for the same reasons as in symptomatic carotid stenosis (section 16.11.3). Although the risk is about half that for symptomatic carotid stenosis, there is still *some* risk.[428,506] Indeed, the risk may not necessarily be very low in, for example, patients with angina whose carotid stenosis was discovered during preparation for coronary artery surgery, or in patients who have already had an endarterectomy on one side and are at risk of bilateral vagal or hypoglossal nerve palsies if both sides are operated on (section 16.11.4).

As for symptomatic stenosis, the risk of surgery cannot be generalized from the literature to one's own institution, that risk should be known locally. Even judging from the literature, a systematic review found much higher risks than in ACAS.[506] The overall risk of stroke and death was 3.0% in 28 studies published post-ACAS. The risk in 12 studies in which outcome was assessed by a neurologist (4.6%) was three times higher than in ACAS. Operative mortality (1.1%) was eight times higher than in ACAS. In studies that reported outcome after endarterectomy for symptomatic and asymptomatic stenosis in the same institution, operative mortality was no lower for asymptomatic stenosis (OR 0.80; 95% CI 0.6–1.1). Thus, published risks of stroke and death due to surgery for asymptomatic stenosis are considerably higher than in ACAS, particularly if outcome had been assessed by a neurologist. And even after community-wide performance measurement and feedback, the overall risk for stroke or death after endarterectomy for asymptomatic stenosis in 10 US states was still 3.8%.[507]

16.12.5 Who benefits most from surgery for asymptomatic carotid stenosis?

Given the surgical risk (which to some extent must depend on the type of patient under consideration as well as surgical skill), the added risk of any preceding catheter angiography unless non-invasive vascular imaging is deemed sufficiently accurate, and what appears to be a remarkably low risk of stroke in unoperated patients (even when they have major surgery below the neck), there is clearly no reason to recommend *routine* carotid endarterectomy for asymptomatic stenosis. It follows that deliberately screening apparently healthy people for carotid stenosis is also unwise. What is needed is a prognostic model to pick out those very few patients whose asymptomatic stenosis is particularly likely to cause stroke, and then operate only on them.

> Although carotid endarterectomy may even halve the risk of stroke in patients with asymptomatic severe stenosis, the absolute unoperated risk of stroke is usually so low in these patients that surgery is rarely worthwhile.

Which range of stenosis?

Although the risk of ipsilateral ischaemic stroke on medical treatment increases with degree of carotid stenosis (Fig. 16.47), in contrast to trials of endarterectomy in patients with symptomatic carotid stenosis, neither ACST nor ACAS showed increasing benefit from surgery with increasing stenosis within the 60–99% range. There are several possible explanations for this:

- First, ultrasound may be less accurate than catheter angiography in measuring the degree of stenosis. In ACAS, only patients randomized to surgery underwent catheter angiography, and in ACST all imaging was by ultrasound without any centralized audit.[508] The importance of the precise method used to measure stenosis was highlighted in a study of patients in the no-surgery arm of the ECST which demonstrated that angiographic measures of stenosis were most reliable in predicting recurrent stroke when selective carotid contrast injections had been given, biplane views were available and when the mean of measurements made by two independent observers was used.[509]
- Second, patients with carotid near-occlusion, which is not readily detectable on ultrasound, were not identified in the asymptomatic stenosis trials. In the ECST, for example, only when near-occlusions were removed was the increased benefit of surgery with increasing stenosis between 70% and 99% clearly

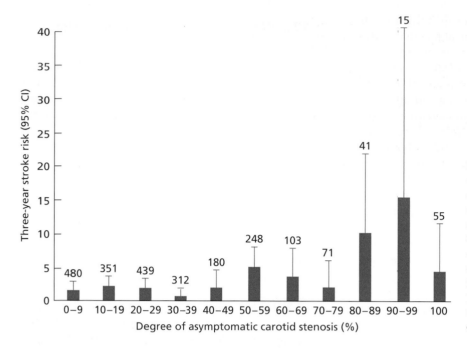

Fig. 16.47 Kaplan–Meier 3-year estimates (with 95% confidence intervals) of the risk of stroke lasting more than 7 days in the distribution of the *asymptomatic* carotid artery in patients in the European Carotid Surgery Trial by deciles of diameter carotid stenosis. The number above each error bar refers to the number of patients in each stenosis group. (Reprinted from European Carotid Surgery Trialists' Collaborative Group, *Lancet*[573] © 2005 with permission from Elsevier.)

apparent.[447] This issue is further complicated by the findings of recent study in which increasing asymptomatic stenosis on ultrasound was positively associated with the risk of ipsilateral hemispheric ischaemic events when stenosis was measured using the ECST criteria, but not when NASCET criteria were used.[510]

- Third, the rate of stenosis progression may determine the risk of stroke in patients with asymptomatic stenosis, which is potentially important considering the longer time frame over which strokes occur compared with symptomatic stenosis. In the ECST, there was a strong association between the risk of ipsilateral stroke and the degree of carotid stenosis only for strokes that occurred during the first year after randomization, and no relationship was seen between initial stenosis and strokes occurring more than 2 years later.[445,483] While this could have been partly due to plaque 'healing', it is conceivable that in some patients the stenosis had progressed and the rate of this progression, rather than the degree of stenosis at baseline, was the important determinant of stroke risk.

Which subgroups benefit most?

Although some subgroup analyses were reported in ACAS, the trial had insufficient power to reliably analyse subgroup–treatment effect interactions. Because of its larger sample size, ACST had greater power, although no analyses were pre-specified in the protocol, and the reduction in risk of non-perioperative stroke (i.e. the benefit) and the perioperative risk (i.e. the harm) were

reported separately.[505] The *overall* balance of hazard and benefit, which is of most importance to patients and clinicians, was not reported, although data could be extracted from the web-tables that accompanied the ACST report. In a meta-analysis of the effect of endarterectomy on the 5-year risk of any stroke and perioperative death in ACAS and ACST (Fig. 16.48) the benefit from surgery was greater in men than in women, and it was uncertain whether there was any worthwhile benefit in women at all, although some benefit may emerge with longer follow-up which is ongoing in ACST.[494] In patients with symptomatic 70–99% stenosis, the surgical complication risk is higher in the presence of contralateral occlusion, although the evidence still favours endarterectomy in these patients.[466] However, a post-hoc analysis from ACAS found that patients with contralateral occlusion derived no long-term benefit from endarterectomy, largely due to a lower long-term risk on medical treatment but this analysis was under-powered (163 patients) and there was no confirmation of this effect in ACST.[505,511]

Which individuals benefit most?

Given the small absolute reductions in the risk of stroke in ACST and ACAS, and the lack of a definite effect in women, there is an urgent need to identify exactly which individual patients are at highest risk of stroke and which individuals are at such low risk that the risks of surgery cannot be justified. At present, it does not seem justifiable to operate on patients 'just because they have asymptomatic severe stenosis', the number-needed-to-operate

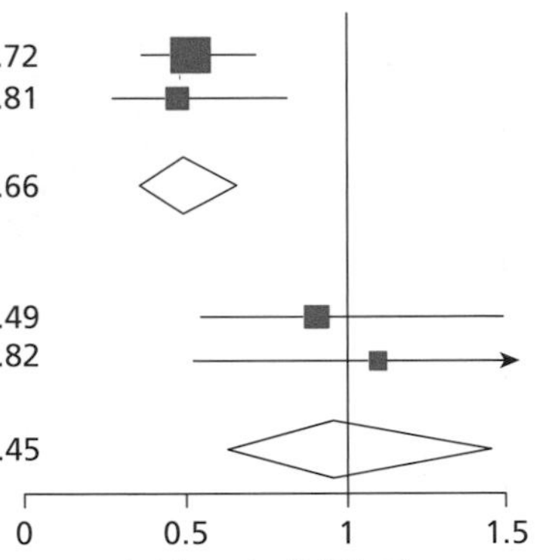

Fig. 16.48 The effect of endarterectomy for asymptomatic carotid stenosis on the risk of any stroke or operative death by sex in the Asymptomatic Carotid Surgery Trial (ACST) and the Asymptomatic Carotid Atherosclerosis Study (ACAS). Each trial result is represented by a purple box whose size is proportional to the statistical weight for that outcome, and horizontal lines representing 95% confidence intervals. The pooled results are represented by diamonds whose widths represent the 95% confidence intervals. (From Rothwell, 2004[494]).

Subgroup	Events/Patients Surgical	Events/Patients Medical	OR	95% CI
Males				
ACST	51/1021	97/1023	0.50	0.35–0.72
ACAS	18/544	38/547	0.46	0.26–0.81
TOTAL	69/1565	135/1570	0.49	0.36–0.66
Females				
ACST	31/539	34/537	0.90	0.55–1.49
ACAS	15/281	14/287	1.10	0.52–1.82
TOTAL	46/820	48/824	0.96	0.63–1.45

Odds ratio (95% CI) 0   0.5   1   1.5

to prevent one stroke is far too high, and the advantage for any individual patient is far too low. A risk modelling approach similar to that used in symptomatic carotid stenosis is required, perhaps combining patient clinical features with the results of potentially prognostic investigations, such as transcranial Doppler-detected emboli, impaired cerebral reactivity, the nature of the stenotic plaque on imaging and the rate of plaque progression. Rates of micro-embolic signals detected on transcranial Doppler ultrasound scanning might well provide prognostically useful information but so far the results of studies are mixed.[18,512,513] Further data will soon be available from the ongoing ACES study.[514]

Several observational studies have suggested that increased plaque echolucency (a marker of plaque lipid and haemorrhage content) on ultrasound is associated with higher risks of stroke and TIA distal to a carotid stenosis.[515] However, most were in patients with symptomatic stenosis and included TIA in the primary outcome. In a recent cohort study of asymptomatic stenosis patients, the cumulative stroke rate was 2% per year in patients with plaques which were uniformly or partly echolucent and 0.14% per year in the remaining patients.[516] However, plaque echolucency on ultrasound was not associated with benefit from surgery in ACST and further research is required to clarify the significance of plaque lipid content in patients with asymptomatic stenosis.[505]

Other methods of plaque imaging might also turn out to be of prognostic value. In a study of 154 patients with asymptomatic carotid stenosis imaged with multi-contrast-weighted MRI, thin or ruptured fibrous cap, intra-plaque haemorrhage, and large lipid core were all associated with ipsilateral TIA and stroke on follow-up.[517] With gadolinium enhancement, the fibrous cap can be visualized more easily on MRI which may allow accurate quantification of fibrous cap thickness.[518] There is also good evidence that inflammation has a causal role in carotid plaque instability.[519,520] MR visualization of plaque macrophages after their uptake of ultra-small particles of iron oxide (USPIO) is now possible.[521,522] However, large prospective studies are required to determine whether any of these imaging characteristics predict the risk of stroke well enough to help select asymptomatic stenosis patients for endarterectomy.

16.13 Carotid angioplasty and stenting

Endovascular treatment was first used for the limb arteries in the 1960s, and subsequently in the renal and coronary arteries,[523] but was introduced more cautiously for treatment of carotid stenosis in the early 1990s because of the likely high risk of stroke due to embolization of atheromatous debris during the procedure. However, the argument goes that if endarterectomy of a recently symptomatic severe carotid stenosis more-or-less abolishes the risk of ipsilateral ischaemic stroke, then percutaneous transluminal balloon angioplasty (Fig. 16.49), particularly with stenting (Fig. 16.50) to maintain arterial patency, could do so as well.[524] Indeed, the endovascular approach has now become widely used when carotid pathology makes endarterectomy difficult (e.g. high bifurcation or post-radiation stenosis), although it is not always feasible because of contrast allergy, difficult vascular anatomy or lumen thrombus.

Of course, angioplasty and stenting is usually less unpleasant and less invasive than carotid endarterectomy, and generally more convenient and quicker. Not requiring

(a)

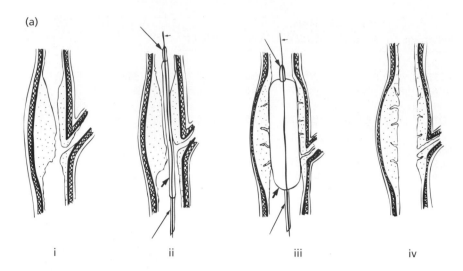

i   ii   iii   iv

(b)

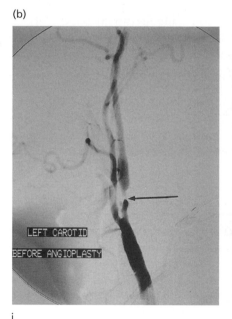

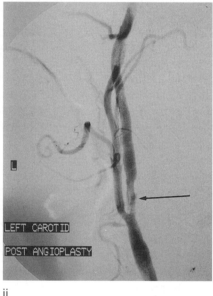

i   ii

Fig. 16.49 Percutaneous transluminal balloon angioplasty of the carotid artery. (a) Diagram to show the principle of angioplasty: (i) the carotid bifurcation with a severe atherothrombotic stenosis; (ii) the guidewire (*small short arrow*) with the deflated (*short thick arrow*) balloon catheter (*long arrows*) is passed across the stenosis; (iii) the balloon is inflated (in some systems the guidewire may be withdrawn prior to inflation, in others it is left in) and the plaque is pushed outwards, so stretching the arterial wall and cracking the plaque; (iv) after the balloon is deflated and removed, the lumen has been widened, the arterial wall remains stretched and the plaque remains. (b) Catheter carotid angiogram to show stenosis: (i) before (*arrow*) and (ii) after (*arrow*) angioplasty; the tight stenosis has been converted to a more normal (looking) lumen.

general anaesthesia, there may be less perioperative hypertension although cerebral haemorrhage and hyperperfusion have been reported.[525,526] It is unlikely to cause nerve injuries, wound infection, venous thromboembolism or myocardial infarction, and hospital stay may be shorter, but there are potential disadvantages:

- The angioplasty balloon may dislodge atherothrombotic debris which then embolizes to the brain or eye, although protection devices might help to reduce the risk of stroke due to periprocedural embolization.
- The procedure may cause arterial wall dissection at the time or afterwards, and embolization might occur due to thrombus formation on the damaged plaque.
- The angioplasty balloon may obstruct carotid blood flow for long enough to cause low-flow ischaemic stroke.

- Dilatation of the balloon may cause bradycardia or hypotension due to carotid sinus stimulation, or aneurysm formation and even arterial rupture due to over-distension of the arterial wall.
- Rarely the stent may erode through the arterial wall, or fracture.
- In the longer-term, restenosis might be more problematic after stenting than after endarterectomy.
- Haematoma and aneurysm formation may occur at the site of arterial cannulation in the groin.

Data on the complications after carotid angioplasty/stenting are available from published case series and registries, but as for endarterectomy, these studies tend to underestimate risks. Formal randomized comparisons of endarterectomy and angioplasty/stenting are therefore required to reliably determine the overall balance of risks

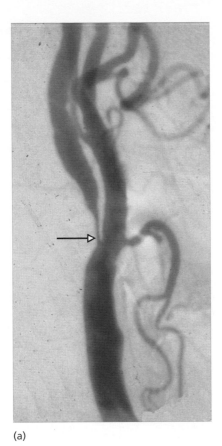
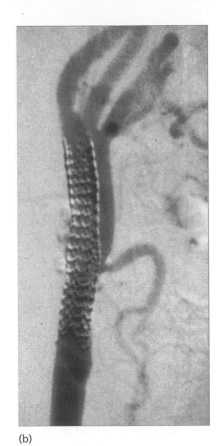

Fig. 16.50 Selective catheter angiogram before (a) and after (b) stenting; before stenting there is severe stenosis of the internal carotid artery (*arrow*) and afterwards the mesh of the stainless steel stent can be seen spanning the carotid bifurcation (modern stents are not so easily seen). (Courtesy of Professor Martin Brown, London.)

(a)　　　　　　　(b)

and benefits. Prior to 2006 only five relatively small RCTs had been reported, the largest of which suggested that the procedural stroke risk was similar to carotid endarterectomy (albeit with wide confidence intervals) and that there are few strokes in the long-term (with even wider confidence intervals).[527–531] Taken together, the five trials suggested that angioplasty/stenting might have a *higher* procedural risk of stroke or death than endarterectomy (OR 1.33; 95% CI 0.86–2.04) and a *higher* risk of restenosis.[532]

However, improvements in endovascular techniques and cerebral protection might have reduced the procedural risks,[533] and so several larger trials have been done, two of which reported their initial results in 2006. The SPACE Trial is the largest trial of carotid stenting vs endarterectomy to date, doubling the number of randomized patients. It was intended to study 1900 patients with 50–99% recently symptomatic carotid stenosis, but randomization was stopped early, partly due to a shortage of funding. The procedural 30-day risk of stroke or death was non-significantly higher in the angioplasty/stenting group with 37 (6.3%) strokes and deaths among 584 patients randomized to surgery vs 41 (6.8%) in 599 patients randomized to stenting. The Endarterectomy versus Angioplasty in Patients With Symptomatic Severe

carotid Stenosis (EVA-3S) was also of angioplasty/stenting vs endarterectomy for 60–99% recently symptomatic carotid stenosis.[534] The trial stopped early after a high 30-day procedural risk was found after angioplasty/stenting, and there were also more local complications after angioplasty/stenting. The results of further follow-up are awaited and two other large trials are currently ongoing.[535–537]

Any advantage for angioplasty/stenting might be further eroded if the GALA trial (www.galatrial.com) finds that endarterectomy under regional rather than general anaestheia is associated with less stroke risk, because the angioplasty/stenting trials have mainly used the comparison with endarterectomy under general anaesthetic.

Taking all the currently available randomized evidence from the trials comparing carotid endarterectomy with angioplasty/stenting, the endovascular approach appears to have a higher procedural risk of stroke or death (Fig. 16.51), but there is still sufficient uncertainty to justify continuing the remaining ongoing trials. Pending their results, carotid stenting should be confined to RCTs or to cases in which endarterectomy is technically difficult. Whichever procedure is used, early intervention and selection of patients based on predicted risk of stroke

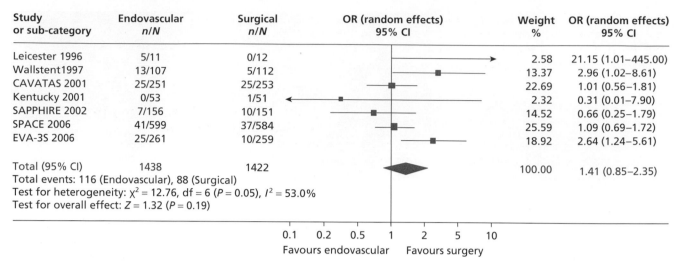

Study or sub-category	Endovascular n/N	Surgical n/N	OR (random effects) 95% CI	Weight %	OR (random effects) 95% CI
Leicester 1996	5/11	0/12		2.58	21.15 (1.01–445.00)
Wallstent1997	13/107	5/112		13.37	2.96 (1.02–8.61)
CAVATAS 2001	25/251	25/253		22.69	1.01 (0.56–1.81)
Kentucky 2001	0/53	1/51		2.32	0.31 (0.01–7.90)
SAPPHIRE 2002	7/156	10/151		14.52	0.66 (0.25–1.79)
SPACE 2006	41/599	37/584		25.59	1.09 (0.69–1.72)
EVA-3S 2006	25/261	10/259		18.92	2.64 (1.24–5.61)
Total (95% CI)	1438	1422		100.00	1.41 (0.85–2.35)

Total events: 116 (Endovascular), 88 (Surgical)
Test for heterogeneity: $\chi^2 = 12.76$, df = 6 ($P = 0.05$), $I^2 = 53.0\%$
Test for overall effect: $Z = 1.32$ ($P = 0.19$)

0.1　0.2　0.5　1　2　5　10
Favours endovascular　　Favours surgery

Fig. 16. 51 Meta-analysis of the randomized controlled trials of endovascular treatment vs endarterectomy for carotid stenosis, outcome of stroke or death within 30 days of the procedure. Each trial result is represented by a purple box whose size is proportional to the statistical weight for that outcome and a horizontal line representing the 95% confidence interval (CI). OR, odds ratio (random effects model). (Courtesy of Roland Featherstone, London.)

without the intervention remain the keys to effective stroke prevention.

> At present, there is no evidence to support the routine use of carotid angioplasty stenting outside well-conducted randomized trials.

16.14 Carotid endarterectomy before, during or after coronary artery surgery?

If patients with recently symptomatic carotid stenosis also have symptomatic coronary heart disease requiring surgery, it is unclear whether coronary bypass should be done before the carotid endarterectomy (and risk a stroke during the procedure), after the carotid endarterectomy (and risk cardiac complications during carotid endarterectomy) or simultaneously under the same general anaesthetic (and risk both stroke and cardiac complications all at once).[538–540] The apparently high risk of the last option may well be unacceptable, although a very small quasi-randomized trial suggests otherwise.[541,542]

Although endarterectomy or stenting for carotid stenosis are increasingly recommended before coronary surgery, there is little evidence to support this practice. A systematic review of published case series found that the risk of stroke during the first few weeks after coronary artery bypass grafting (CABG) was about 2% and had

remained unchanged from 1970 to 2000; nine out of ten screened CABG patients had no significant carotid disease. Stroke risk was about 3% in predominantly asymptomatic patients with unilateral 50–99% carotid stenosis, 5% in those with bilateral 50–99% stenoses and 7–11% in those with carotid occlusion. Significant predictive factors for post-CABG stroke included carotid bruit, prior stroke/transient ischaemic attack and severe carotid stenosis/occlusion. However, half those who had a perioperative stroke did not have significant carotid disease, and 60% of territorial infarctions on CT scan/autopsy could not be attributed to carotid disease alone.[543] Thus, although carotid disease is one important aetiological factor in post-CABG stroke, even assuming that prophylactic carotid endarterectomy carried no additional risk, it could only ever prevent about 40% of procedural strokes at most.

A subsequent systematic review aimed to determine the overall cardiovascular risk for patients with coronary and carotid artery disease undergoing simultaneous CABG and carotid endarterectomy, endarterectomy then CABG, and CABG then endarterectomy. Mortality was highest in patients undergoing simultaneous operations (4.6%), as was the risk of death or stroke (8.7%) and lowest following endarterectomy then CABG (6.1%). The risk of death/stroke or myocardial infarction was 11.5% following simultaneous procedures.[544]

In summary, the available data suggest that only about 40% of strokes complicating CABG can be attributable to carotid artery disease. The risk of death or stroke following staged or simultaneous carotid surgery is high, and a large RCT is necessary to determine whether a policy of prophylactic carotid endarterectomy reduces the risk of stroke after cardiac surgery. In the meantime, the available data do not support a policy of routine intervention for carotid stenosis in patients undergoing CABG.[545]

> At present routine extra-to-intracranial bypass surgery cannot be recommended.

16.15 Extra-to-intracranial bypass surgery

About 10% of patients with minor carotid ischaemic events have occlusion of the internal carotid artery (ICA), or stenosis of the ICA well distal to the bifurcation, or middle cerebral artery (MCA) occlusion or stenosis. All these lesions are inoperable, or out of reach of the vascular surgeon, if not of the angioplasty enthusiast's balloon. However, these lesions can be bypassed by anastomosing a branch of the external carotid artery (usually the superficial temporal) via a skull burr hole to a cortical branch of the MCA. It was anticipated that this 'surgical collateral' would improve the blood supply in the distal MCA bed and so reduce the risk of stroke, and reduce the severity of any stroke that did occur. However, there are several reasons why the procedure might not work:[546–550]

- The artery feeding the anastomosis can take months to dilate into an effective collateral channel.
- Many patients have good collateral flow already from orbital collaterals or via the circle of Willis.
- Not all strokes distal to ICA/MCA occlusion or inaccessible stenosis are due to low flow (section 6.3.4).
- The risk of stroke in patients with ICA occlusion is not that high compared with severe and recently symptomatic ICA stenosis (less than 10%/year) and, anyway, not all of these strokes are ipsilateral to the occlusion.
- Neither resting cerebral blood flow nor cerebral reactivity are necessarily depressed in these patients.
- The risk of surgery may outweigh the benefit, if any.

The risk–benefit relationship has been evaluated in only one completed randomized trial and this failed to show any benefit from routine surgery (EC–IC Bypass Study Group 1985).[551] However, it has been argued that patients with impaired cerebrovascular reactivity, or with maximal oxygen extraction, were not identified and perhaps it is *these* patients who *might* be benefited by surgery.[552,553] But to show whether stroke is prevented, and not just that pathophysiology is improved, would require another RCT in this specific subgroup, not a series of anecdotes, however persuasive. Such a trial is now ongoing.[554]

16.16 Surgery and angioplasty for vertebrobasilar ischaemia

There is no good evidence that surgery improves the prognosis for patients with vertebrobasilar ischaemia. There is, however, no shortage of ingenious, if technically demanding, techniques which are far from risk-free:

- Endarterectomy of severe carotid stenosis to improve collateral blood flow, via the circle of Willis, to the basilar artery distal to severe vertebral or basilar artery stenosis or occlusion.
- Resection and anastomosis, resection and reimplantation, bypass or endarterectomy of proximal vertebral artery stenosis.
- Release of the vertebral artery from compressive fibrous bands or osteophytes.
- Various extra-to-intracranial procedures to bypass vertebral artery stenosis or occlusion.

There are no RCTs of surgical procedures for posterior circulation disease; data are only available from case series. For proximal vertebral reconstruction, perioperative mortality is 0–4%, and the risk of stroke or death 2.5–25%.[555] For distal vertebral reconstruction 2–8% mortality has been reported.

Several case series have described angioplasty and stenting of symptomatic vertebral and basilar stenosis.[556] A recent review of more than 600 cases published up to 2005 provides useful information.[555] In the early studies, proximal lesions were treated primarily with angioplasty but this was associated with restenosis in 15–31% of cases after 15–30 months of follow-up. More recently stenting has been used for the proximal vertebral system, especially lesions at the origin. Several series have reported low periprocedural or post-interventional stroke risks; pooling data, there was a perioperative stroke risk of 1.3% and of death of 0.3%. However, restenosis during about 14 months of follow-up still occurred in about one-quarter of the patients, albeit usually asymptomatic. The complication risk of distal vertebrobasilar lesions treated with angioplasty and stenting is higher: 7.1% for stroke and 3.7% for death after angioplasty, and 10.6% for stroke and 3.2% for death after stenting, suggesting that complication rates do not differ much between angioplasty and stenting in the distal vertebrobasilar system.[555] The only RCT of stenting for vertebral artery disease was far too small to be informative.[557] Therefore, there are no robust data on the safety and efficacy of vertebral artery stenting.

Subclavian (and innominate) steal (section 6.8.6), although commonly detected with ultrasonography, very rarely causes neurological symptoms and does not seem to lead on to ischaemic stroke. However, incapacitatingly frequent vertebrobasilar TIAs in the presence of demonstrated unilateral or bilateral retrograde vertebral artery flow distal to severe subclavian or innominate disease may sometimes be relieved by: endarterectomy or angioplasty of the subclavian artery; carotid-to-subclavian or femoral-to-subclavian bypass; transposition of the subclavian artery to the common carotid artery (CCA); transposition of the vertebral artery to the CCA; and axillary-to-axillary artery bypass grafting. All these procedures carry a risk and it is not clear which is the most sensible. Irrespective of the neurological situation, some kind of vascular surgical procedure may be needed if the hand and arm become ischaemic distal to subclavian or innominate artery disease.

16.17 Other surgical procedures

Aortic arch atheroma is now increasingly diagnosed by transoesophageal echocardiography in patients with transient ischaemic attacks or ischaemic stroke, but so far there are no surgical, or indeed medical, treatment options over and above controlling vascular risk factors and antiplatelet drugs. One trial has been started, the ARCH trial, which is an open-label, multicentre, randomized, controlled trial of warfarin (target INR = 2.0–3.0) vs 75–325 mg of aspirin plus 75 mg clopidogrel per day in patients with an ischaemic stroke within 6 months, and an aortic arch atheromatous plaque that is either mobile or greater than 4 mm thick.

Innominate or proximal common carotid artery stenosis or occlusion is quite often seen on angiograms in symptomatic patients but, unless very severe, does not influence the decision about endarterectomy for any internal carotid artery stenosis. Although it is possible to bypass such lesions it is highly doubtful whether this reduces the risk of stroke unless, perhaps, several major neck vessels are involved and the patient has low-flow cerebral or ocular symptoms (section 6.7.5). This very rare situation can be due to atheroma, Takayasu's disease or aortic dissection. Clearly, close consultation between physicians and vascular surgeons is needed to sort out, on an individual patient basis, what to do for the best.

Coronary artery bypass surgery (or angioplasty) may of course be indicated for patients presenting with cerebrovascular events who *also* happen to have cardiac symptoms. But, because asymptomatic coronary artery disease is so often associated with symptomatic cerebrovascular disease (section 6.8.10), would coronary intervention also be worthwhile even if there were no cardiac symptoms or signs? Given the high risk of cardiac events which might be reduced in the long term (section 16.2), this is a perfectly reasonable question, but one which could only be answered by an RCT, perhaps first in patients who are thought to be at particularly high risk of myocardial infarction on the basis of clinical features, or non-invasive cardiac investigation.

16.18 Putting secondary prevention into practice

16.18.1 Involving patients and carers in treatment decisions

What influences adherence to treatment?

Involving patients (and, where appropriate, their carers) in decisions about their treatment is an important part of healthcare. Patients need to understand what has happened to them, and why various treatment options are being recommended for them. Adherence to medication, especially long-term preventive treatments, is known to be poor outside the setting of a clinical trial,[558–560] but seems likely to be improved if patients understand what each treatment is for, and how they will personally benefit. However, a study of patients who had survived a myocardial infarction and of subjects free of cardiovascular disease suggested that patients' expectations of the absolute benefits of medications are usually higher than the actual benefit, so that giving accurate information about the likely benefits of a particular treatment, although clearly important, may not necessarily increase uptake and long-term adherence.[561]

Rates of, and influences on, adherence to long-term preventive medication among patients who have had a stroke or transient ischaemic attack (TIA) have not been studied much.[562] Randomized trials of interventions to improve adherence to long-term medication have had mixed results, and the most successful methods have generally been complex and of limited effectiveness in terms of improved adherence and clinical outcomes.[558,563] Furthermore, as far as we are aware there have been no randomized trials of interventions to improve adherence specifically among patients who have had a stroke or TIA, and limited numbers of trials (and trial subjects) in the elderly.

Communicating benefits and risks

Communicating with patients who have had a stroke or TIA can be particularly challenging. Disability resulting from a stroke may directly (e.g. due to dysphasia) or indirectly (e.g. due to pain, visual field defects, incontinence, inattention or neglect, etc.) affect the process of communication with the patient, as may the hearing and visual impairment and other age-related problems that frequently affect elderly patients. It is usually helpful if a relative, friend or carer can also be present during any discussions with doctors or other health professionals. Information leaflets using simple language are often helpful, and give the patient or carer something to refer to later. Guidance about websites that provide the most helpful, accurate and up-to-date information for patients and carers can also be important. Making sure that other health professionals involved know what has been said is also crucial, to ensure consistency and avoid confusion.

Because doctors' treatment recommendations should be based on weighing up the estimated absolute benefits and harms of any treatment (section 16.1.3), we must also attempt to communicate the same type of information about treatment options to patients and/or carers. We should be aware that we may inappropriately influence patients' decisions or behaviour by providing information about treatment benefits in terms of relative risk reductions (e.g. 'Adding this new tablet dipyridamole to your aspirin will reduce your risk of another stroke, a heart attack or dying by 20%') rather than absolute risk reductions (e.g. 'If 100 people like you took this new tablet dipyridamole as well as their aspirin, then each year one less of these people would have a stroke, a heart attack or die'). We should always try to tailor our means of presenting information on benefits and harms to the level of understanding, needs and wishes of the patient or carer. Quoting benefits and risks in terms of natural frequencies rather than percentages (e.g. 'one in ten people will develop x', rather than '10% of people will develop x' or 'the risk of x is 10%') and using diagrams or pictures can make the concepts easier to understand.[561,564,565] Finally, we must be aware that patients' and carers' interpretation of and response to this sort of information depends on how much they trust the doctor or other healthcare professional imparting it, other sources of information they may have access to (other healthcare professionals, friends, the media, and so on),

their background knowledge about health-related matters, and a host of social and psychological factors.[566,567]

16.18.2 Which interventions for which patients?

Many preventive interventions have been discussed in this chapter and an overall summary of which interventions should be considered for which patients is given in Fig. 16.52. Clearly, the introduction of each treatment should be considered in terms of both the balance of benefit and risk as well as the individual preferences of the particular patient, taking into account their age, comorbidities, and – for medications – all drugs already being taken and the possible effects of any medication changes on adherence, drug interactions and adverse effects.[568]

Incremental effectiveness

Another important consideration is the incremental effectiveness of each of several new treatments added. The order in which various treatments are added will depend on the mode and timing of the patient's presentation. For illustrative purposes, let us imagine a 75-year-old woman presenting to her family doctor 2 days after onset of an acute, non-disabling stroke. She is a non-smoker, drinks no more than 5 units of alcohol per week, and her only past medical history is of a hip replacement and her only medication is occasional paracetamol. The family doctor assumes the stroke to be ischaemic, prescribes aspirin 300 mg immediately followed by 75 mg daily, takes blood for full blood count, erythrocyte sedimentatation rate (ESR), renal function, cholesterol, and glucose, and refers the patient to a rapid access stroke specialist outpatient clinic at the local hospital for confirmation of the clinical diagnosis and further investigation as appropriate. The specialist assesses the patient 5 days later, and agrees with the clinical diagnosis, noting that the patient has a regular pulse with a rate of 80 beats per minute, a blood pressure of 140/83, a clinically normal heart, and that the stroke almost certainly affected the carotid (anterior circulation) territory. That day, a 12-lead electrocardiograph confirms sinus rhythm, a CT brain scan confirms that the stroke was ischaemic and Doppler ultrasound of the carotid arteries reveals minor atheroma in both carotid bulbs but no significant stenoses. The results of the blood tests show a normal full blood count, ESR and renal function, random blood glucose of 5 mmol/L, and cholesterol of 5.2 mmol/L. The specialist recommends the addition of a statin (simvastatin 40 mg daily), and modified release dipyridamole, warning of the possibility of headache with the latter medication, usually settling within 1–2 weeks.

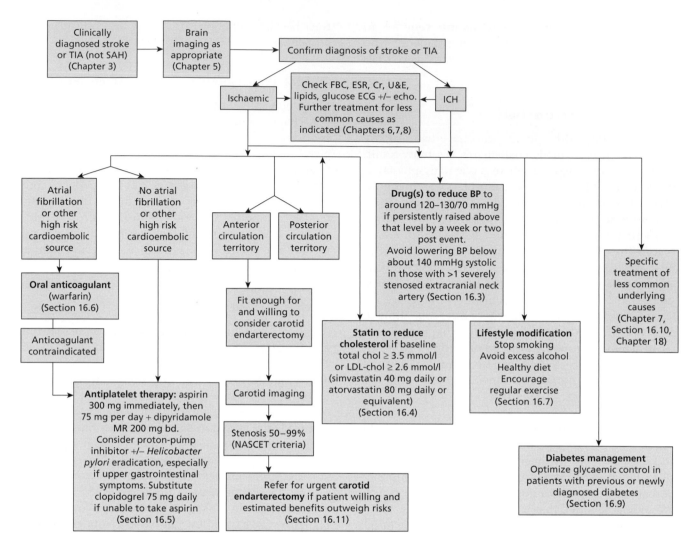

Fig. 16.52 Summary of long-term preventive interventions to be considered after a stroke or transient ischaemic attack. NB: Statins to reduce cholesterol, and antithrombotic treatment, may occasionally be appropriate for patients with intracerebral haemorrhage at particularly high risk of future ischaemic events (sections 16.4.5, 16.5.2, 16.6.5). TIA, transient ischaemic attack; SAH, subarachnoid haemorrhage; ICH, intracerebral haemorrhage; MR, modified release; FBC, full blood count; ESR, erythrocyte sedimentation rate; Cr, creatinine; U&E, urea and electrolytes; ECG, electrocardiogram; echo, echocardiogram; NASCET, North American Symptomatic Carotid Endarterectomy Trial.

The specialist also asks the family doctor to monitor the blood pressure regularly and introduce blood-pressure-lowering medication if the pressure is persistently above 120–130 mmHg systolic/70 mmHg diastolic. A thiazide diuretic plus an ACE inhibitor if needed are the suggested first-line treatments. Finally, the specialist gives some written information about stroke, incorporating advice about lifestyle.

Table 16.15 shows the order and timing of introduction of medications in this patient's case, and the estimated benefits for each during the first year and annually thereafter, assuming adherence at the levels achieved in the randomized trials of these treatments.

Because the risk of a vascular event (mainly recurrent stroke) is highest early after stroke, the earlier preventive medications are started the greater the absolute benefit in the first year. However, as we have seen in earlier sections of this chapter, clear evidence for starting preventive medications immediately after stroke is present for some, but not all, of the various available options. In addition, if several medications are started at the same time and the patient subsequently experiences a suspected adverse effect, it can be difficult to sort out which medication is at fault and should be discontinued. Hence a staged introduction of secondary preventive medications may be best in many circumstances, but with as

Table 16.15 Illustration of *incremental* benefit to an individual patient from reducing the risk of a vascular event by adding, in turn, long-term preventive medications after stroke or transient ischaemic attack (see section 16.18.2 for details of clinical case).

Treatment	From treatment start to end of first year				Annually from end of first year			
	Approx risk with no treatment*	Approx risk on all previous treatments†	RRR‡	ARR¶	Approx risk with no treatment*	Approx risk on all previous treatments†	RRR‡	ARR¶
Aspirin from day 2	18%	18.0%	20%	3.6%	7%	7.0%	20%	1.4%
Statin from day 7§	13%	10.4%	20%	2.1%	7%	5.6%	20%	1.1%
MR dipyridamole from day 7	13%	8.3%	20%	1.7%	7%	4.5%	20%	0.9%
Thiazide and ACE-inhibitor from day 14**	11%	5.6%	20%	1.1%	7%	3.6%	20%	0.7%
All treatments				8.5%††				4.1%‡‡

RRR, relative risk reduction; ARR, absolute risk reduction.

*Rough estimate of untreated (i.e. no treatment at all) risks from section 16.2 and Table 16.1 (note: in the first few days after the stroke/TIA this risk is falling rapidly from 18% at day 2 to 11% at day 14 until the end of the first year).

†Calculated by applying a 20% reduction to completely untreated risk for each treatment already being taken.

‡Assuming that: RRR for vascular events about the same (20%) for all treatments (actual range of point estimates is about 18–22%; see sections 16.3 to 16.5); treatment benefit accrues at a similar rate in the first and subsequent years (may not necessarily be the case – e.g. benefits from cholesterol lowering may not be fully realized until second or third year of treatment – see section 16.4); adherence similar to that in randomized trials.

¶20% of approx risk after earlier treatments started.

§Reducing LDL-cholesterol by ~ 1 mmol/L.

**Reducing BP by ~ 8 mmHg systolic/4 mmHg diastolic.

††Number-needed-to-treat to prevent or delay one vascular event at 1 year = 100/8.5 = 12, i.e. the patient has a 1 in 12 chance of benefiting from combined drug treatment in the first year.

‡‡Number-needed-to-treat to prevent or delay one vascular event annually after the first year = 100/4.1 = 24, i.e. the patient has a 1 in 24 chance of benefiting from combined drug treatment annually after the first year.

little delay as possible between the introduction of each additional medication to ensure that they are added as early after the presenting event as is feasible, to maximize the benefit to the patient.

> A staged introduction of secondary preventive medications may be best, but with as little delay as possible between the introduction of each additional medication to ensure that they are added as early after the presenting event as is feasible.

What about a Polypill?

In the rather straightforward example above, the patient was taking only paracetamol before her stroke, but several weeks later she is also taking aspirin 75 mg daily, simvastatin 40 mg daily, modified-release dipyridamole 200 mg daily, bendrofluazide 2.5 mg daily and perindopril 4 mg daily – that is, five additional drugs and six additional tablets per day. For a cognitively intact, non-disabled patient, this is already quite an undertaking, and the difficulties will be more substantial for disabled, cognitively impaired patients. Increased complexity of medication regimens is unsurprisingly one predictor of reduced adherence.[558] Although many patients would consider the benefits of each individual drug insufficient to make it worth taking regularly, if they genuinely understood them,[561] the combined benefit of all of these drugs is more substantial, making the combined package a much better option. This makes the proposal of a so-called 'Polypill', a single combined tablet containing all the components proven to reduce risk of vascular events, a potentially highly attractive one.

The original Polypill proposal was for a single combined pill for anyone with a history of vascular disease and for anyone over 55 years old, regardless of a history of vascular disease. However, commentators raised a range of potential problems and criticisms of such an approach.[569] The proposed combined pill contained aspirin for antiplatelet effect, folic acid to lower plasma homocysteine, three different drugs in low dose to reduce blood pressure, and a statin to reduce cholesterol.[570] One immediately apparent problem is that this particular combination does not reflect the current state of the evidence (discussed throughout this chapter) for preventive interventions in patients with stroke or TIA. For example, there is currently no evidence from randomized trials to support routine homocysteine lowering with folate supplements to prevent vascular events, either in primary prevention or after a stroke or TIA. And even a combined pill whose components reflected the current evidence would surely soon run into practical difficulties, in that the components of the pill would need to be varied for different patients to ensure tolerability and to allow tailoring of treatment to a particular patient's clinical history and needs. For example, a patient with a recent intracerebral haemorrhage would require a very different pill composition from a patient with a recent ischaemic stroke, and oral anticoagulants would be preferred over antiplatelet treatment for many patients with atrial fibrillation. At the very least, evidence from randomized trials of the effectiveness of a combined pill approach in various different primary and secondary prevention settings would be needed before it could be considered for use in routine clinical practice.

> A combined Polypill would soon run into practical difficulties because the components would need to be varied for different patients to ensure tolerability and to allow tailoring of treatment to a particular patient's clinical history and needs.

References

1 Rothwell PM, Mehta Z, Howard SC, Gutnikov SA, Warlow CP. Treating individuals 3: from subgroups to individuals: general principles and the example of carotid endarterectomy. *Lancet* 2005; **365**(9455):256–65.

2 Coull AJ, Lovett JK, Rothwell PM. Population based study of early risk of stroke after transient ischaemic attack or minor stroke: implications for public education and organisation of services. *Br Med J* 2004; **328**(7435):326.

3 Dennis MS, Bamford JM, Sandercock PA, Warlow CP. A comparison of risk factors and prognosis for transient ischemic attacks and minor ischemic strokes. The Oxfordshire Community Stroke Project. *Stroke* 1989; **20**(11):1494–9.

4 Koudstaal PJ, van Gijn J, Frenken CW, Hijdra A, Lodder J, Vermeulen M *et al*. TIA, RIND, minor stroke: a continuum, or different subgroups? Dutch TIA Study Group. *J Neurol Neurosurg Psychiatry* 1992; **55**(2):95–7.

5 Van Wijk I, Kappelle LJ, van Gijn J, Koudstaal PJ, Franke CL, Vermeulen M *et al*. Long-term survival and vascular event risk after transient ischaemic attack or minor ischaemic stroke: a cohort study. *Lancet* 2005; **365**(9477):2098–104.

6 Wiebers DO, Whisnant JP, O'Fallon WM. Reversible ischemic neurologic deficit (RIND) in a community: Rochester, Minnesota, 1955–1974. *Neurology* 1982; **32**(5):459–65.

7 Rothwell PM, Buchan A, Johnston SC. Recent advances in management of transient ischaemic attacks and minor ischaemic strokes. *Lancet Neurol* 2006; **5**(4):323–31.

8 Coull AJ, Rothwell PM. Underestimation of the early risk of recurrent stroke: evidence of the need for a standard definition. *Stroke* 2004; **35**(8):1925–9.

9 Hill MD, Yiannakoulias N, Jeerakathil T, Tu JV, Svenson LW, Schopflocher DP. The high risk of stroke immediately after transient ischemic attack: a population-based study. *Neurology* 2004; **62**(11):2015–20.

10 Johnston SC, Gress DR, Browner WS, Sidney S. Short-term prognosis after emergency department diagnosis of TIA. *J Am Med Assoc* 2000; **284**(22):2901–6.

11 Kleindorfer D, Panagos P, Pancioli A, Khoury J, Kissela B, Woo D *et al*. Incidence and short-term prognosis of transient ischemic attack in a population-based study. *Stroke* 2005; **36**(4):720–3.

12 Rothwell PM, Warlow CP. Timing of TIAs preceding stroke: time window for prevention is very short. *Neurology* 2005; **64**(5):817–20.

13 Rothwell PM, Giles MF, Flossmann E, Lovelock CE, Redgrave JN, Warlow CP *et al*. A simple score (ABCD) to identify individuals at high early risk of stroke after transient ischaemic attack. *Lancet* 2005; **366**(9479):29–36.

14 Johnston SC, Rothwell PM, Nguyen-Huynh MN, Giles MF, Elkins JS, Bernstein AL *et al*. Validation and refinement of scores to predict very early stroke risk after transient ischaemic attack. *Lancet* 2007; **369**(9558):283–92.

15 Flossmann E, Rothwell PM. Prognosis of vertebrobasilar transient ischaemic attack and minor stroke. *Brain* 2003; **126**(9):1940–54.

16 Lovett JK, Coull AJ, Rothwell PM. Early risk of recurrence by subtype of ischemic stroke in population-based incidence studies. *Neurology* 2004; **62**(4):569–73.

17 Donnan GA, O'Malley HM, Quang L, Hurley S, Bladin PF. The capsular warning syndrome: pathogenesis and clinical features. *Neurology* 1993; **43**(5):957–62.

18 Markus HS, MacKinnon A. Asymptomatic embolization detected by Doppler ultrasound predicts stroke risk in symptomatic carotid artery stenosis. *Stroke* 2005; **36**(5):971–5.

19 Hankey GJ, Warlow CP. *Transient Ischaemic Attacks of the Brain and Eye*. London: W B Saunders; 1994.

20 Touze E, Varenne O, Chatellier G, Peyrard S, Rothwell PM, Mas JL. Risk of myocardial infarction and vascular death after transient ischemic attack and ischemic stroke: a systematic review and meta-analysis. *Stroke* 2005; **36**(12):2748–55.

21 Hankey GJ, Dennis MS, Slattery JM, Warlow CP. Why is the outcome of transient ischaemic attacks different in different groups of patients? *Br Med J* 1993; **306**(6885):1107–11.

22 Clark TG, Murphy MF, Rothwell PM. Long term risks of stroke, myocardial infarction, and vascular death in 'low risk' patients with a non-recent transient ischaemic attack. *J Neurol Neurosurg Psychiatry* 2003; **74**(5):577–80.

23 Hankey GJ, Slattery JM, Warlow CP. Transient ischaemic attacks: which patients are at high (and low) risk of serious vascular events? *J Neurol Neurosurg Psychiatry* 1992; **55**(8):640–52.

24 Hankey GJ, Slattery JM, Warlow CP. Can the long term outcome of individual patients with transient ischaemic attacks be predicted accurately? *J Neurol Neurosurg Psychiatry* 1993; **56**(7):752–9.

25 Kernan WN, Viscoli CM, Brass LM, Makuch RW, Sarrel PM, Roberts RS *et al.* The stroke prognosis instrument II (SPI–II): A clinical prediction instrument for patients with transient ischemia and nondisabling ischemic stroke. *Stroke* 2000; **31**(2):456–62.

26 Feigin VL, Lawes CM, Bennett DA, Anderson CS. Stroke epidemiology: a review of population-based studies of incidence, prevalence, and case-fatality in the late 20th century. *Lancet Neurol* 2003; **2**(1):43–53.

27 Dennis MS, Burn JP, Sandercock PA, Bamford JM, Wade DT, Warlow CP. Long-term survival after first-ever stroke: the Oxfordshire Community Stroke Project. *Stroke* 1993; **24**(6):796–800.

28 Hardie K, Hankey GJ, Jamrozik K, Broadhurst RJ, Anderson C. Ten-year survival after first-ever stroke in the Perth Community Stroke Study. *Stroke* 2003; **34**(8):1842–6.

29 Petty GW, Brown RD, Jr., Whisnant JP, Sicks JD, O'Fallon WM, Wiebers DO. Survival and recurrence after first cerebral infarction: a population-based study in Rochester, Minnesota, 1975 through 1989. *Neurology* 1998; **50**(1):208–16.

30 Eriksson SE, Olsson JE. Survival and recurrent strokes in patients with different subtypes of stroke: a fourteen-year follow-up study. *Cerebrovasc Dis* 2001; **12**(3):171–80.

31 Vernino S, Brown RD, Jr., Sejvar JJ, Sicks JD, Petty GW, O'Fallon WM. Cause-specific mortality after first cerebral infarction: a population-based study. *Stroke* 2003; **34**(8):1828–32.

32 Dhamoon MS, Sciacca RR, Rundek T, Sacco RL, Elkind MS. Recurrent stroke and cardiac risks after first ischemic stroke: the Northern Manhattan Study. *Neurology* 2006; **66**(5):641–6.

33 Jackson C, Sudlow C. Comparing risks of death and recurrent vascular events between lacunar and non-lacunar infarction. *Brain* 2005; **128**(11):2507–17.

34 Norrving B. Long-term prognosis after lacunar infarction. *Lancet Neurol* 2003; **2**(4):238–45.

35 Petty GW, Brown RD, Jr., Whisnant JP, Sicks JD, O'Fallon WM, Wiebers DO. Ischemic stroke subtypes: a population-based study of functional outcome, survival, and recurrence. *Stroke* 2000; **31**(5):1062–8.

36 Bamford J, Sandercock P, Dennis M, Burn J, Warlow C. Classification and natural history of clinically identifiable subtypes of cerebral infarction. *Lancet* 1991; **337**(8756):1521–6.

37 Burn J, Dennis M, Bamford J, Sandercock P, Wade D, Warlow C. Long-term risk of recurrent stroke after a first-ever stroke. The Oxfordshire Community Stroke Project. *Stroke* 1994; **25**(2):333–7.

38 Hankey GJ, Jamrozik K, Broadhurst RJ, Forbes S, Burvill PW, Anderson CS *et al.* Long-term risk of first recurrent stroke in the Perth Community Stroke Study. *Stroke* 1998; **29**(12):2491–500.

39 Hata J, Tanizaki Y, Kiyohara Y, Kato I, Kubo M, Tanaka K *et al.* Ten year recurrence after first ever stroke in a Japanese community: the Hisayama study. *J Neurol Neurosurg Psychiatry* 2005; **76**(3):368–72.

40 Hillen T, Coshall C, Tilling K, Rudd AG, McGovern R, Wolfe CD. Cause of stroke recurrence is multifactorial: patterns, risk factors, and outcomes of stroke recurrence in the South London Stroke Register. *Stroke* 2003; **34**(6):1457–63.

41 Kappelle LJ, van Latum JC, van Swieten JC, Algra A, Koudstaal PJ, van Gijn J. Recurrent stroke after transient ischaemic attack or minor ischaemic stroke: does the distinction between small and large vessel disease remain true to type? Dutch TIA Trial Study Group. *J Neurol Neurosurg Psychiatry* 1995; **59**(2):127–31.

42 Yamamoto H, Bogousslavsky J. Mechanisms of second and further strokes. *J Neurol Neurosurg Psychiatry* 1998; **64**(6):771–6.

43 Appelros P, Nydevik I, Viitanen M. Poor outcome after first-ever stroke: predictors for death, dependency, and recurrent stroke within the first year. *Stroke* 2003; **34**(1):122–6.

44 Hier DB, Foulkes MA, Swiontoniowski M, Sacco RL, Gorelick PB, Mohr JP *et al.* Stroke recurrence within 2 years after ischemic infarction. *Stroke* 1991; **22**(2):155–61.

45 Lai SM, Alter M, Friday G, Sobel E. A multifactorial analysis of risk factors for recurrence of ischemic stroke. *Stroke* 1994; **25**(5):958–62.

46 Sacco RL, Shi T, Zamanillo MC, Kargman DE. Predictors of mortality and recurrence after hospitalized cerebral infarction in an urban community: the Northern Manhattan Stroke Study. *Neurology* 1994; **44**(4):626–34.

47 Viitanen M, Eriksson S, Asplund K. Risk of recurrent stroke, myocardial infarction and epilepsy during long-term follow-up after stroke. *Eur Neurol* 1988; **28**(4):227–31.

48 Ferro JM, Crespo M. Prognosis after transient ischemic attack and ischemic stroke in young adults. *Stroke* 1994; **25**(8):1611–16.

49 Kappelle LJ, Adams HP, Jr., Heffner ML, Torner JC, Gomez F, Biller J. Prognosis of young adults with ischemic stroke: a long-term follow-up study assessing recurrent vascular events and functional outcome in the Iowa Registry of Stroke in Young Adults. *Stroke* 1994; **25**(7):1360–5.

50 Kittner SJ, Stern BJ, Wozniak M, Buchholz DW, Earley CJ, Feeser BR *et al.* Cerebral infarction in young adults: the Baltimore-Washington Cooperative Young Stroke Study. *Neurology* 1998; **50**(4):890–4.

51 Leys D, Bandu L, Henon H, Lucas C, Mounier-Vehier F, Rondepierre P *et al.* Clinical outcome in 287 consecutive

young adults (15 to 45 years) with ischemic stroke. *Neurology* 2002; **59**(1):26–33.

52 Marini C, Totaro R, Carolei A. Long-term prognosis of cerebral ischemia in young adults. National Research Council Study Group on Stroke in the Young. *Stroke* 1999; **30**(11):2320–5.

53 Naess H, Waje-Andreassen U, Thomassen L, Nyland H, Myhr KM. Do all young ischemic stroke patients need long-term secondary preventive medication? *Neurology* 2005; **65**(4):609–11.

54 Nedeltchev K, der Maur TA, Georgiadis D, Arnold M, Caso V, Mattle HP *et al.* Ischaemic stroke in young adults: predictors of outcome and recurrence. *J Neurol Neurosurg Psychiatry* 2005; **76**(2):191–5.

55 Dennis MS. Outcome after brain haemorrhage. *Cerebrovasc Dis* 2003; **16**(Suppl 1):9–13.

56 Keir SL, Wardlaw JM, Warlow CP. Stroke epidemiology studies have underestimated the frequency of intracerebral haemorrhage: a systematic review of imaging in epidemiological studies. *J Neurol* 2002; **249**(9):1226–31.

57 Counsell C, Boonyakarnkul S, Dennis M. Primary intracerebral haemorrhage in the Oxfordshire Community Stroke Project. *Cerebrovasc Dis* 1995; **5**:26–34.

58 Flaherty ML, Haverbusch M, Sekar P, Kissela B, Kleindorfer D, Moomaw CJ *et al.* Long-term mortality after intracerebral hemorrhage. *Neurology* 2006; **66**(8):1182–6.

59 Fogelholm R, Murros K, Rissanen A, Avikainen S. Long term survival after primary intracerebral haemorrhage: a retrospective population based study. *J Neurol Neurosurg Psychiatry* 2005; **76**(11):1534–8.

60 Bailey RD, Hart RG, Benavente O, Pearce LA. Recurrent brain hemorrhage is more frequent than ischemic stroke after intracranial hemorrhage. *Neurology* 2001; **56**(6):773–7.

61 O'Donnell HC, Rosand J, Knudsen KA, Furie KL, Segal AZ, Chiu RI *et al.* Apolipoprotein E genotype and the risk of recurrent lobar intracerebral hemorrhage. *N Engl J Med* 2000; **342**(4):240–5.

62 Arakawa S, Saku Y, Ibayashi S, Nagao T, Fujishima M. Blood pressure control and recurrence of hypertensive brain hemorrhage. *Stroke* 1998; **29**(9):1806–9.

63 Bae H, Jeong D, Doh J, Lee K, Yun I, Byun B. Recurrence of bleeding in patients with hypertensive intracerebral hemorrhage. *Cerebrovasc Dis* 1999; **9**(2):102–8.

64 Gonzalez-Duarte A, Cantu C, Ruiz-Sandoval JL, Barinagarrementeria F. Recurrent primary cerebral hemorrhage: frequency, mechanisms, and prognosis. *Stroke* 1998; **29**(9):1802–5.

65 Neau JP, Ingrand P, Couderq C, Rosier MP, Bailbe M, Dumas P *et al.* Recurrent intracerebral hemorrhage. *Neurology* 1997; **49**(1):106–13.

66 Passero S, Burgalassi L, D'Andrea P, Battistini N. Recurrence of bleeding in patients with primary intracerebral hemorrhage. *Stroke* 1995; **26**(7):1189–92.

67 Rashid P, Leonardi-Bee J, Bath P. Blood pressure reduction and secondary prevention of stroke and other vascular events: a systematic review. *Stroke* 2003; **34**(11):2741–8.

68 Eastern Stroke and Coronary Heart Disease Collaborative Research Group. Blood pressure, cholesterol, and stroke in eastern Asia. *Lancet* 1998; **352**(9143):1801–7.

69 Prospective Studies Collaboration. Age-specific relevance of usual blood pressure to vascular mortality: a meta-analysis of individual data for one million adults in 61 prospective studies. *Lancet* 2002; **360**(9349):1903–13.

70 Lawes CM, Rodgers A, Bennett DA, Parag V, Suh I, Ueshima H *et al.* Blood pressure and cardiovascular disease in the Asia Pacific region. Asia Pacific Cohort Studies Collaboration. *J Hypertens* 2003; **21**(4):707–16.

71 Lawes CM, Bennett DA, Feigin VL, Rodgers A. Blood pressure and stroke: an overview of published reviews. *Stroke* 2004; **35**(4):1024.

72 Schulz UG, Rothwell PM. Differences in vascular risk factors between etiological subtypes of ischemic stroke: importance of population-based studies. *Stroke* 2003; **34**(8):2050–9.

73 Jackson C, Sudlow C. Are lacunar strokes really different? A systematic review of differences in risk factor profiles between lacunar and nonlacunar infarcts. *Stroke* 2005; **36**(4):891–901.

74 Jackson CA, Sudlow CL. Is hypertension a more frequent risk factor for deep than for lobar supratentorial intracerebral haemorrhage? *J Neurol Neurosurg Psychiatry* 2006; **77**(11):1244–52.

75 Irie K, Yamaguchi T, Minematsu K, Omae T. The J-curve phenomenon in stroke recurrence. *Stroke* 1993; **24**(12):1844–9.

76 Leonardi-Bee J, Bath PM, Phillips SJ, Sandercock PA. Blood pressure and clinical outcomes in the International Stroke Trial. *Stroke* 2002; **33**(5):1315–20.

77 Rodgers A, MacMahon S, Gamble G, Slattery J, Sandercock P, Warlow C. Blood pressure and risk of stroke in patients with cerebrovascular disease. The United Kingdom Transient Ischaemic Attack Collaborative Group. *Br Med J* 1996; **313**(7050):147.

78 Rothwell PM, Howard SC, Spence JD. Relationship between blood pressure and stroke risk in patients with symptomatic carotid occlusive disease. *Stroke* 2003; **34**(11):2583–90.

79 PATS Collaborating Group. Post-stroke antihypertensive treatment study. A preliminary result. *Chin Med J (Engl)* 1995; **108**(9):710–17.

80 PROGRESS Collaborative Group. Randomised trial of a perindopril-based blood-pressure-lowering regimen among 6,105 individuals with previous stroke or transient ischaemic attack. *Lancet* 2001; **358**(9287):1033–41.

81 Chapman N, Huxley R, Anderson C, Bousser MG, Chalmers J, Colman S *et al.* Effects of a perindopril-based blood pressure-lowering regimen on the risk of recurrent stroke according to stroke subtype and medical history: the PROGRESS Trial. *Stroke* 2004; **35**(1):116–21.

82 Fransen M, Anderson C, Chalmers J, Chapman N, Davis S, MacMahon S *et al.* Effects of a perindopril-based blood pressure-lowering regimen on disability and dependency in 6105 patients with cerebrovascular disease: a randomized controlled trial. *Stroke* 2003; **34**(10):2333–8.

83 Tzourio C, Anderson C, Chapman N, Woodward M, Neal B, MacMahon S et al. Effects of blood pressure lowering with perindopril and indapamide therapy on dementia and cognitive decline in patients with cerebrovascular disease. *Arch Intern Med* 2003; **163**(9):1069–75.

84 MacMahon S, Neal B, Rodgers A, Chalmers J. The PROGRESS trial three years later: time for more action, less distraction. *Br Med J* 2004; **329**(7472):970–1.

85 Schrader J, Luders S, Kulschewski A, Hammersen F, Plate K, Berger J et al. Morbidity and mortality after stroke, eprosartan compared with nitrendipine for secondary prevention: principal results of a prospective randomized controlled study (MOSES). *Stroke* 2005; **36**(6):1218–26.

86 PROGRESS Management Committee. Perindopril Protection Against Recurrent Stroke Study. Blood pressure lowering for the secondary prevention of stroke: rationale and design for PROGRESS. *J Hypertens Suppl* 1996; **14**(2):S41–S45.

87 Collins R, MacMahon S. Blood pressure, antihypertensive drug treatment and the risks of stroke and of coronary heart disease. *Br Med Bull* 1994; **50**(2):272–98.

88 MacMahon S, Rodgers A. Blood pressure, antihypertensive treatment and stroke risk. *J Hypertens Suppl* 1994; **12**(10):S5–S14.

89 Staessen JA, Li Y, Thijs L, Wang JG. Blood pressure reduction and cardiovascular prevention: an update including the 2003–2004 secondary prevention trials. *Hypertens Res* 2005; **28**(5):385–407.

90 Blood Pressure Lowering Treatment Trialists' Collaboration. Effects of different blood-pressure-lowering regimens on major cardiovascular events: results of prospectively-designed overviews of randomised trials. *Lancet* 2003; **362**(9395):1527–35.

91 Angeli F, Verdecchia P, Reboldi GP, Gattobigio R, Bentivoglio M, Staessen JA et al. Calcium channel blockade to prevent stroke in hypertension: a meta-analysis of 13 studies with 103,793 subjects. *Am J Hypertens* 2004; **17**(9):817–22.

92 McDonald MA, Simpson SH, Ezekowitz JA, Gyenes G, Tsuyuki RT. Angiotensin receptor blockers and risk of myocardial infarction: systematic review. *Br Med J* 2005; **331**(7521):873.

93 Pahor M, Psaty BM, Alderman MH, Applegate WB, Williamson JD, Cavazzini C et al. Health outcomes associated with calcium antagonists compared with other first-line antihypertensive therapies: a meta-analysis of randomised controlled trials. *Lancet* 2000; **356**(9246):1949–54.

94 Verma S, Strauss M. Angiotensin receptor blockers and myocardial infarction. *Br Med J* 2004; **329**(7477):1248–9.

95 Dahlof B, Sever PS, Poulter NR, Wedel H, Beevers DG, Caulfield M et al. Prevention of cardiovascular events with an antihypertensive regimen of amlodipine adding perindopril as required versus atenolol adding bendroflumethiazide as required, in the Anglo-Scandinavian Cardiac Outcomes Trial-Blood Pressure Lowering Arm (ASCOT-BPLA): a multicentre randomised controlled trial. *Lancet* 2005; **366**(9489):895–906.

96 Poulter NR, Wedel H, Dahlof B, Sever PS, Beevers DG, Caulfield M et al. Role of blood pressure and other variables in the differential cardiovascular event rates noted in the Anglo-Scandinavian Cardiac Outcomes Trial-Blood Pressure Lowering Arm (ASCOT-BPLA). *Lancet* 2005; **366**(9489):907–13.

97 Sleight P, Yusuf S, Pogue J, Tsuyuki R, Diaz R, Probstfield J. Blood-pressure reduction and cardiovascular risk in HOPE study. *Lancet* 2001; **358**(9299):2130–1.

98 Weber MA, Julius S, Kjeldsen SE, Brunner HR, Ekman S, Hansson L et al. Blood pressure dependent and independent effects of antihypertensive treatment on clinical events in the VALUE Trial. *Lancet* 2004; **363**(9426):2049–51.

99 Svensson P, de Faire U, Sleight P, Yusuf S, Ostergren J. Comparative effects of ramipril on ambulatory and office blood pressures: a HOPE Substudy. *Hypertension* 2001; **38**(6):E28–E32.

100 Casas JP, Chua W, Loukogeorgakis S, Vallance P, Smeeth L, Hingorani AD et al. Effect of inhibitors of the renin-angiotensin system and other antihypertensive drugs on renal outcomes: systematic review and meta-analysis. *Lancet* 2005; **366**(9502):2026–33.

101 Lindholm LH, Carlberg B, Samuelsson O. Should beta blockers remain first choice in the treatment of primary hypertension? A meta-analysis. *Lancet* 2005; **366**(9496):1545–53.

102 Kaplan NM, Opie LH. Controversies in hypertension. *Lancet* 2006; **367**(9505):168–76.

103 Wright JM, Lee CH, Chambers GK. Systematic review of antihypertensive therapies: does the evidence assist in choosing a first-line drug? *Can Med Assoc J* 1999; **161**(1):25–32.

104 Law MR, Wald NJ, Morris JK, Jordan RE. Value of low dose combination treatment with blood pressure lowering drugs: analysis of 354 randomised trials. *Br Med J* 2003; **326**(7404):1427.

105 PROGRESS Management Committee Perindopril protection against recurrent stroke study: characteristics of study population at baseline. *J Hypertens* 1999; **17**(11):1647–55.

106 Blood Pressure in Acute Stroke Collaboration (BASC). Interventions for deliberately altering blood pressure in acute stroke. *Cochrane Database Syst Rev* 2001; (3):CD000039.

107 Bath P. High blood pressure as risk factor and prognostic predictor in acute ischaemic stroke: when and how to treat it? *Cerebrovasc Dis* 2004; **17**(Suppl 1):51–7.

108 Law MR, Wald NJ, Thompson SG, Law MR, Wald NJ, Morris JK et al. By how much and how quickly does reduction in serum cholesterol concentration lower risk of ischaemic heart disease? Value of low dose combination treatment with blood pressure lowering drugs: analysis of 354 randomised trials. *Br Med J* 1994; **308**(6925):367–72.

109 Prospective studies collaboration. Cholesterol, diastolic blood pressure, and stroke: 13,000 strokes in 450,000 people in 45 prospective cohorts. *Lancet* 1995; **346**(8991–8992):1647–53.

110 Law MR, Wald NJ, Rudnicka AR. Quantifying effect of statins on low density lipoprotein cholesterol, ischaemic heart disease, and stroke: systematic review and meta-analysis. *Br Med J* 2003; **326**(7404):1423.

111 Di Mascio R, Marchioli R, Tognoni G. Cholesterol reduction and stroke occurrence: an overview of randomized clinical trials. *Cerebrovasc Dis* 2000; **10**(2):85–92.

112 Hebert PR, Gaziano JM, Hennekens CH. An overview of trials of cholesterol lowering and risk of stroke. *Arch Intern Med* 1995; **155**(1):50–5.

113 Meade T, Zuhrie R, Cook C, Cooper J. Bezafibrate in men with lower extremity arterial disease: randomised controlled trial. *Br Med J* 2002; **325**(7373):1139.

114 Rubins HB, Robins SJ, Collins D, Fye CL, Anderson JW, Elam MB *et al.* Gemfibrozil for the secondary prevention of coronary heart disease in men with low levels of high-density lipoprotein cholesterol. Veterans Affairs High-Density Lipoprotein Cholesterol Intervention Trial Study Group. *N Engl J Med* 1999; **341**(6):410–18.

115 The BIP Study Group. Secondary prevention by raising HDL cholesterol and reducing triglycerides in patients with coronary artery disease: the Bezafibrate Infarction Prevention (BIP) study. *Circulation* 2000; **102**(1):21–7.

116 Keech A, Simes RJ, Barter P, Best J, Scott R, Taskinen MR *et al.* Effects of long-term fenofibrate therapy on cardiovascular events in 9795 people with type 2 diabetes mellitus (the FIELD study): randomised controlled trial. *Lancet* 2005; **366**(9500):1849–61.

117 Cholesterol Treatment Trialists' Collaborators (CTT). Efficacy and safety of cholesterol-lowering treatment: prospective meta-analysis of data from 90,056 participants in 14 randomised trials of statins. *Lancet* 2005; **366**(9493):1267–78.

118 Heart Protection Study Collaborative Group. MRC/BHF Heart Protection Study of cholesterol lowering with simvastatin in 20,536 high-risk individuals: a randomised placebo-controlled trial. *Lancet* 2002; **360**(9326):7–22.

119 Heart Protection Study Collaborative Group. Effects of cholesterol-lowering with simvastatin on stroke and other major vascular events in 20536 people with cerebrovascular disease or other high-risk conditions. *Lancet* 2004; **363**(9411):757–67.

120 The Stroke Prevention by Aggressive Reduction in Cholesterol Levels (SPARCL) Investigators. High-dose atorvastatin after stroke or transient ischemic attack. *N Engl J Med* 2006; **355**(6):549–59.

121 Amarenco P, Labreuche J, Lavallee P, Touboul PJ. Statins in stroke prevention and carotid atherosclerosis: systematic review and up-to-date meta-analysis. *Stroke* 2004; **35**(12):2902–9.

122 Nissen SE, Tuzcu EM, Schoenhagen P, Crowe T, Sasiela WJ, Tsai J *et al.* Statin therapy, LDL cholesterol, C-reactive protein, and coronary artery disease. *N Engl J Med* 2005; **352**(1):29–38.

123 Ridker PM, Cannon CP, Morrow D, Rifai N, Rose LM, McCabe CH *et al.* C-reactive protein levels and outcomes after statin therapy. *N Engl J Med* 2005; **352**(1):20–8.

124 Graham DJ, Staffa JA, Shatin D, Andrade SE, Schech SD, La Grenade L *et al.* Incidence of hospitalized rhabdomyolysis in patients treated with lipid-lowering drugs. *J Am Med Assoc* 2004; **292**(21):2585–90.

125 Furberg CD, Pitt B. Withdrawal of cerivastatin from the world market. *Curr Control Trials Cardiovasc Med* 2001; **2**(5):205–7.

126 UK Committee on Safety of Medicines. Statins and cytochrome P450 interactions. *Curr Probl Pharmacovigilance* 2004; **30**:1–12.

127 Gaist D, Garcia Rodriguez LA, Huerta C, Hallas J, Sindrup SH. Are users of lipid-lowering drugs at increased risk of peripheral neuropathy? *Eur J Clin Pharmacol* 2001; **56**(12):931–3.

128 Gaist D, Jeppesen U, Andersen M, Garcia Rodriguez LA, Hallas J, Sindrup SH. Statins and risk of polyneuropathy: a case-control study. *Neurology* 2002; **58**(9):1333–7.

129 Wei L, Ebrahim S, Bartlett C, Davey PD, Sullivan FM, MacDonald TM. Statin use in the secondary prevention of coronary heart disease in primary care: cohort study and comparison of inclusion and outcome with patients in randomised trials. *Br Med J* 2005; **330**(7495):821.

130 Cannon CP, Braunwald E, McCabe CH, Rader DJ, Rouleau JL, Belder R *et al.* Intensive versus moderate lipid lowering with statins after acute coronary syndromes. *N Engl J Med* 2004; **350**(15):1495–504.

131 LaRosa JC, Grundy SM, Waters DD, Shear C, Barter P, Fruchart JC *et al.* Intensive lipid lowering with atorvastatin in patients with stable coronary disease. *N Engl J Med* 2005; **352**(14):1425–35.

132 Nissen SE, Tuzcu EM, Schoenhagen P, Brown BG, Ganz P, Vogel RA *et al.* Effect of intensive compared with moderate lipid-lowering therapy on progression of coronary atherosclerosis: a randomized controlled trial. *J Am Med Assoc* 2004; **291**(9):1071–80.

133 Pedersen TR, Faergeman O, Kastelein JJ, Olsson AG, Tikkanen MJ, Holme I *et al.* High-dose atorvastatin vs usual-dose simvastatin for secondary prevention after myocardial infarction: the IDEAL study: a randomized controlled trial. *J Am Med Assoc* 2005; **294**(19):2437–45.

134 Schwartz GG, Olsson AG, Ezekowitz MD, Ganz P, Oliver MF, Waters D *et al.* Effects of atorvastatin on early recurrent ischemic events in acute coronary syndromes: the MIRACL study: a randomized controlled trial. *J Am Med Assoc* 2001; **285**(13):1711–18.

135 Sudlow C, Hankey G. Antiplatelet drugs in the secondary prevention of stroke. *Pract Neurol* 2002; **2**:12–25.

136 Williams PS, Rands G, Orrel M, Spector A. Aspirin for vascular dementia. *Cochrane Database Syst Rev* 2000; (4):CD001296.

137 Antithrombotic Trialists' Collaboration. Collaborative meta-analysis of randomised trials of antiplatelet therapy for prevention of death, myocardial infarction, and stroke in high risk patients. *Br Med J* 2002; **324**(7329):71–86.

138 Chen ZM, Sandercock P, Pan HC, Counsell C, Collins R, Liu LS *et al.* Indications for early aspirin use in acute

ischemic stroke : A combined analysis of 40 000 randomized patients from the chinese acute stroke trial and the international stroke trial. On behalf of the CAST and IST collaborative groups. *Stroke* 2000; **31**(6):1240–9.

139 Sandercock P, Gubitz G, Foley P, Counsell C. Antiplatelet therapy for acute ischaemic stroke. *Cochrane Database Syst Rev* 2003; (2):CD000029.

140 Antiplatelet Trialists' Collaboration. Collaborative overview of randomised trials of antiplatelet therapy – I: Prevention of death, myocardial infarction, and stroke by prolonged antiplatelet therapy in various categories of patients. *Br Med J* 1994; **308**(6921):81–106.

141 Hallas J, Dall M, Andries A, Andersen BS, Aalykke C, Hansen JM *et al.* Use of single and combined antithrombotic therapy and risk of serious upper gastrointestinal bleeding: population based case–control study. *Br Med J* 2006; **333**(7571):726.

142 Sung JJ. Combining aspirin with antithrombotic agents. *Br Med J* 2006; **333**(7571):712–13.

143 Chan FK, Chung SC, Suen BY, Lee YT, Leung WK, Leung VK *et al.* Preventing recurrent upper gastrointestinal bleeding in patients with *Helicobacter pylori* infection who are taking low-dose aspirin or naproxen. *N Engl J Med* 2001; **344**(13):967–73.

144 Hart RG, Benavente O, McBride R, Pearce LA. Antithrombotic therapy to prevent stroke in patients with atrial fibrillation: a meta-analysis. *Ann Intern Med* 1999; **131**(7):492–501.

145 Sato H, Ishikawa K, Kitabatake A, Ogawa S, Maruyama Y, Yokota Y *et al.* Low-dose aspirin for prevention of stroke in low-risk patients with atrial fibrillation: Japan Atrial Fibrillation Stroke Trial. *Stroke* 2006; **37**(2):447–51.

146 Segal JB, McNamara RL, Miller MR, Powe NR, Goodman SN, Robinson KA *et al.* Anticoagulants or antiplatelet therapy for non-rheumatic atrial fibrillation and flutter. *Cochrane Database Syst Rev* 2001; (1):CD001938.

147 Salem DN, Stein PD, Al Ahmad A, Bussey HI, Horstkotte D, Miller N *et al.* Antithrombotic therapy in valvular heart disease – native and prosthetic: the Seventh ACCP Conference on Antithrombotic and Thrombolytic Therapy. *Chest* 2004; **126**(3 Suppl):457S–482S.

148 Berger JS, Roncaglioni MC, Avanzini F, Pangrazzi I, Tognoni G, Brown DL. Aspirin for the primary prevention of cardiovascular events in women and men: a sex-specific meta-analysis of randomized controlled trials. *J Am Med Assoc* 2006; **295**(3):306–13.

149 Becker DM, Segal J, Vaidya D, Yanek LR, Herrera-Galeano JE, Bray PF *et al.* Sex differences in platelet reactivity and response to low-dose aspirin therapy. *J Am Med Assoc* 2006; **295**(12):1420–7.

150 Baigent C. Aspirin for everyone older than 50? Against. *Br Med J* 2005; **330**(7505):1442–3.

151 Nelson M, Reid C, Beilin L, Donnan G, Johnston C, Krum H *et al.* Rationale for a trial of low-dose aspirin for the primary prevention of major adverse cardiovascular events and vascular dementia in the elderly: Aspirin in Reducing Events in the Elderly (ASPREE). *Drugs Aging* 2003; **20**(12):897–903.

152 Szekely CA, Thorne JE, Zandi PP, Ek M, Messias E, Breitner JC *et al.* Nonsteroidal anti-inflammatory drugs for the prevention of Alzheimer's disease: a systematic review. *Neuroepidemiology* 2004; **23**(4):159–69.

153 Richards M, Meade TW, Peart S, Brennan PJ, Mann AH. Is there any evidence for a protective effect of antithrombotic medication on cognitive function in men at risk of cardiovascular disease? Some preliminary findings. *J Neurol Neurosurg Psychiatry* 1997; **62**(3):269–72.

154 Keir SL, Wardlaw JM, Sandercock PA, Chen Z. Antithrombotic therapy in patients with any form of intracranial haemorrhage: a systematic review of the available controlled studies. *Cerebrovasc Dis* 2002; **14**(3–4):197–206.

155 Viswanathan A, Rakich SM, Engel C, Snider R, Rosand J, Greenberg SM *et al.* Antiplatelet use after intracerebral hemorrhage. *Neurology* 2006; **66**(2):206–9.

156 Wani M, Nga E, Navaratnasingham R. Should a patient with primary intracerebral haemorrhage receive antiplatelet or anticoagulant therapy? *Br Med J* 2005; **331**(7514):439–42.

157 Patrono C. Aspirin as an antiplatelet drug. *N Engl J Med* 1994; **330**(18):1287–94.

158 Barnett HJ, Kaste M, Meldrum H, Eliasziw M. Aspirin dose in stroke prevention: beautiful hypotheses slain by ugly facts. *Stroke* 1996; **27**(4):588–92.

159 Patrono C, Roth GJ. Aspirin in ischemic cerebrovascular disease. How strong is the case for a different dosing regimen? *Stroke* 1996; **27**(4):756–60.

160 Van Gijn J. Low doses of aspirin in stroke prevention. *Lancet* 1999; **353**(9171):2172–3.

161 Patrono C, Coller B, FitzGerald GA, Hirsh J, Roth G. Platelet-active drugs: the relationships among dose, effectiveness, and side effects: the Seventh ACCP Conference on Antithrombotic and Thrombolytic Therapy. *Chest* 2004; **126**(3 Suppl):234S–264S.

162 Taylor DW, Barnett HJ, Haynes RB, Ferguson GG, Sackett DL, Thorpe KE *et al.* Low-dose and high-dose acetylsalicylic acid for patients undergoing carotid endarterectomy: a randomised controlled trial. ASA and Carotid Endarterectomy (ACE) Trial Collaborators. *Lancet* 1999; **353**(9171):2179–84.

163 The Dutch TIA Trial Study Group. A comparison of two doses of aspirin (30 mg vs. 283 mg a day) in patients after a transient ischemic attack or minor ischemic stroke. *N Engl J Med* 1991; **325**(18):1261–6.

164 Johnson ES, Lanes SF, Wentworth CE, III, Satterfield MH, Abebe BL, Dicker LW. A metaregression analysis of the dose-response effect of aspirin on stroke. *Arch Intern Med* 1999; **159**(11):1248–53.

165 He J, Whelton PK, Vu B, Klag MJ. Aspirin and risk of hemorrhagic stroke: a meta-analysis of randomized controlled trials. *J Am Med Assoc* 1998; **280**(22):1930–5.

166 Thrift AG, McNeil JJ, Forbes A, Donnan GA. Risk of primary intracerebral haemorrhage associated with aspirin and non-steroidal anti-inflammatory drugs: case–control study. *Br Med J* 1999; **318**(7186):759–64.

167 Iso H, Hennekens CH, Stampfer MJ, Rexrode KM, Colditz GA, Speizer FE *et al*. Prospective study of aspirin use and risk of stroke in women. *Stroke* 1999; **30**(9):1764–71.

168 Derry S, Loke YK. Risk of gastrointestinal haemorrhage with long term use of aspirin: meta-analysis. *Br Med J* 2000; **321**(7270):1183–7.

169 Farrell B, Godwin J, Richards S, Warlow C. The United Kingdom transient ischaemic attack (UK-TIA) aspirin trial: final results. *J Neuro Neurosurg Psychiatry* 1991; **54**:1044–54.

170 Garcia Rodriguez LA, Hernandez-Diaz S, de Abajo FJ. Association between aspirin and upper gastrointestinal complications: systematic review of epidemiologic studies. *Br J Clin Pharmacol* 2001; **52**(5):563–71.

171 Hankey GJ, Eikelboom JW. Aspirin resistance. *Lancet* 2006; **367**(9510):606–17.

172 Applegate WB. Elderly patients' adherence to statin therapy. *J Am Med Assoc* 2002; **288**(4):495–7.

173 Warlow C, Sudlow C, Dennis M, Wardlaw J, Sandercock P. Stroke. *Lancet* 2003; **362**(9391):1211–24.

174 Sudlow C, Mason G, Hankey G. Thienopyridine derivatives (ticlopidine, clopidogrel) versus aspirin for preventing stroke and other serious vascular events in high vascular risk patients. *Cochrane Database Syst Rev.* In press 2007.

175 Bhatt DL, Chew DP, Hirsch AT, Ringleb PA, Hacke W, Topol EJ. Superiority of clopidogrel versus aspirin in patients with prior cardiac surgery. *Circulation* 2001; **103**(3):363–8.

176 Ringleb PA, Bhatt DL, Hirsch AT, Topol EJ, Hacke W. Benefit of clopidogrel over aspirin is amplified in patients with a history of ischemic events. *Stroke* 2004; **35**(2):528–32.

177 Bennett CL, Weinberg PD, Rozenberg-Ben-Dror K, Yarnold PR, Kwaan HC, Green D. Thrombotic thrombocytopenic purpura associated with ticlopidine: a review of 60 cases. *Ann Intern Med* 1998; **128**(7):541–4.

178 Bennett CL, Davidson CJ, Raisch DW, Weinberg PD, Bennett RH, Feldman MD. Thrombotic thrombocytopenic purpura associated with ticlopidine in the setting of coronary artery stents and stroke prevention. *Arch Intern Med* 1999; **159**(21):2524–8.

179 Bennett CL, Connors JM, Carwile JM, Moake JL, Bell WR, Tarantolo SR *et al*. Thrombotic thrombocytopaenic purpura associated with clopidagrel. *N Engl J Med* 2000; **342**:1773–7.

180 Moloney BA. *An Analysis of the Side Effects of Ticlopidine.* New York: Springer, 1993.

181 Torok TJ, Holman RC, Chorba TL. Increasing mortality from thrombotic thrombocytopenic purpura in the United States: analysis of national mortality data, 1968–1991. *Am J Hematol* 1995; **50**(2):84–90.

182 Zakarija A, Bandarenko N, Pandey DK, Auerbach A, Raisch DW, Kim B *et al*. Clopidogrel-associated TTP: an update of pharmacovigilance efforts conducted by independent researchers, pharmaceutical suppliers, and the Food and Drug Administration. *Stroke* 2004; **35**(2):533–7.

183 Bertrand ME, Rupprecht HJ, Urban P, Gershlick AH. Double-blind study of the safety of clopidogrel with and without a loading dose in combination with aspirin compared with ticlopidine in combination with aspirin after coronary stenting : the clopidogrel aspirin stent international cooperative study (CLASSICS). *Circulation* 2000; **102**(6):624–9.

184 Muller C, Buttner HJ, Petersen J, Roskamm H. A randomized comparison of clopidogrel and aspirin versus ticlopidine and aspirin after the placement of coronary-artery stents. *Circulation* 2000; **101**(6):590–3.

185 Taniuchi M, Kurz HI, Lasala JM. Randomized comparison of ticlopidine and clopidogrel after intracoronary stent implantation in a broad patient population. *Circulation* 2001; **104**(5):539–43.

186 Chan FK, Ching JY, Hung LC, Wong VW, Leung VK, Kung NN *et al*. Clopidogrel versus aspirin and esomeprazole to prevent recurrent ulcer bleeding. *N Engl J Med* 2005; **352**(3):238–44.

187 Leon MB, Baim DS, Popma JJ, Gordon PC, Cutlip DE, Ho KK *et al*. A clinical trial comparing three antithrombotic-drug regimens after coronary-artery stenting. Stent Anticoagulation Restenosis Study Investigators. *N Engl J Med* 1998; **339**(23):1665–71.

188 Chen ZM, Jiang LX, Chen YP, Xie JX, Pan HC, Peto R *et al*. Addition of clopidogrel to aspirin in 45,852 patients with acute myocardial infarction: randomised placebo-controlled trial. *Lancet* 2005; **366**(9497):1607–21.

189 Sabatine MS, Cannon CP, Gibson CM, Lopez-Sendon JL, Montalescot G, Theroux P *et al*. Addition of clopidogrel to aspirin and fibrinolytic therapy for myocardial infarction with ST-segment elevation. *N Engl J Med* 2005; **352**(12):1179–89.

190 Steinhubl SR, Berger PB, Mann JT, III, Fry ET, DeLago A, Wilmer C *et al*. Early and sustained dual oral antiplatelet therapy following percutaneous coronary intervention: a randomized controlled trial. *J Am Med Assoc* 2002; **288**(19):2411–20.

191 Yusuf S, Zhao F, Mehta SR, Chrolavicius S, Tognoni G, Fox KK. Effects of clopidogrel in addition to aspirin in patients with acute coronary syndromes without ST-segment elevation. *N Engl J Med* 2001; **345**(7):494–502.

192 Bhatt DL, Fox KA, Hacke W, Berger PB, Black HR, Boden WE *et al*. Clopidogrel and aspirin versus aspirin alone for the prevention of atherothrombotic events. *N Engl J Med* 2006; **354**(16):1706–17.

193 Diener HC, Bogousslavsky J, Brass LM, Cimminiello C, Csiba L, Kaste M *et al*. Aspirin and clopidogrel compared with clopidogrel alone after recent ischaemic stroke or transient ischaemic attack in high-risk patients (MATCH): randomised, double-blind, placebo-controlled trial. *Lancet* 2004; **364**(9431):331–7.

194 Markus HS, Droste DW, Kaps M, Larrue V, Lees KR, Siebler M *et al*. Dual antiplatelet therapy with clopidogrel and aspirin in symptomatic carotid stenosis evaluated using doppler embolic signal detection: the Clopidogrel and Aspirin for Reduction of Emboli in Symptomatic Carotid Stenosis (CARESS) trial. *Circulation* 2005; **111**(17):2233–40.

195 Sudlow C. What is the role of dipyridamole in long-term secondary prevention after an ischemic stroke or transient ischemic attack? *Can Med Assoc J* 2005; **173**(9):1024–6.

196 De Schryver EL. Dipyridamole in stroke prevention: effect of dipyridamole on blood pressure. *Stroke* 2003; **34**(10):2339–42.

197 Diener HC, Cunha L, Forbes C, Sivenius J, Smets P, Lowenthal A. European Stroke Prevention Study. 2. Dipyridamole and acetylsalicylic acid in the secondary prevention of stroke. *J Neurol Sci* 1996; **143**(1–2):1–13.

198 The ESPRIT Study Group. Aspirin plus dipyridamole versus aspirin alone after cerebral ischaemia of arterial origin (ESPRIT): randomised controlled trial. *Lancet* 2006; **367**(9523):1665–73.

199 Leonardi-Bee J, Bath PM, Bousser MG, Davalos A, Diener HC, Guiraud-Chaumeil B *et al*. Dipyridamole for preventing recurrent ischemic stroke and other vascular events: a meta-analysis of individual patient data from randomized controlled trials. *Stroke* 2005; **36**(1):162–8.

200 Lindgren A, Husted S, Staaf G, Ziegler B. Dipyridamole and headache: a pilot study of initial dose titration. *J Neurol Sci* 2004; **223**(2):179–84.

201 Costa J, Ferro JM, Matias-Guiu J, Alvarez-Sabin J, Torres F. Triflusal for preventing serious vascular events in people at high risk. *Cochrane Database Syst Rev* 2005; (3):CD004296.

202 Boersma E, Harrington RA, Moliterno DJ, White H, Theroux P, Van de WF *et al*. Platelet glycoprotein IIb/IIIa inhibitors in acute coronary syndromes: a meta-analysis of all major randomised clinical trials. *Lancet* 2002; **359**(9302):189–98.

203 Robinson M, Ginnelly L, Sculpher M, Jones L, Riemsma, Palmer S *et al*. A systematic review update of the clinical effectiveness and cost-effectiveness of glycoprotein IIb/IIIa antagonists. *Health Technol Assess* 2002; **6**(25):1–160.

204 Molina CA, Saver JL. Extending reperfusion therapy for acute ischemic stroke: emerging pharmacological, mechanical, and imaging strategies. *Stroke* 2005; **36**(10):2311–20.

205 Chew DP, Bhatt DL, Sapp S, Topol EJ. Increased mortality with oral platelet glycoprotein IIb/IIIa antagonists: a meta-analysis of phase III multicenter randomized trials. *Circulation* 2001; **103**(2):201–6.

206 Topol EJ, Easton D, Harrington RA, Amarenco P, Califf RM, Graffagnino C *et al*. Randomized, double-blind, placebo-controlled, international trial of the oral IIb/IIIa antagonist lotrafiban in coronary and cerebrovascular disease. *Circulation* 2003; **108**(4):399–406.

207 Gubitz G, Sandercock P, Counsell C. Anticoagulants for acute ischaemic stroke. *Cochrane Database Syst Rev* 2004; (3):CD000024.

208 Sandercock P, Mielke O, Liu M, Counsell C. Anticoagulants for preventing recurrence following presumed non-cardioembolic ischaemic stroke or transient ischaemic attack. *Cochrane Database Syst Rev* 2003; (1):CD000248.

209 Algra A, De Shryver ELLM, van Gijn J. Oral anticoagulants versus antiplatelet therapy for preventing further vascular events after transient ischaemic attack or minor stroke of presumed arterial origin. *Cochrane Database Syst Rev* 2001; (4).

210 Chimowitz MI, Lynn MJ, Howlett-Smith H, Stern BJ, Hertzberg VS, Frankel MR *et al*. Comparison of warfarin and aspirin for symptomatic intracranial arterial stenosis. *N Engl J Med* 2005; **352**(13):1305–16.

211 The ESPRIT Study Group. Medium intensity oral anticoagulants versus aspirin after cerebral ischaemia of arterial origin (ESPRIT): a randomised controlled trial. *Lancet Neurol* 2007; **6**(2):115–24.

212 The Stroke Prevention in Reversible Ischemia Trial (SPIRIT) Study Group. A randomized trial of anticoagulants versus aspirin after cerebral ischemia of presumed arterial origin. *Ann Neurol* 1997; **42**(6):857–65.

213 Mohr JP, Thompson JL, Lazar RM, Levin B, Sacco RL, Furie KL *et al*. A comparison of warfarin and aspirin for the prevention of recurrent ischemic stroke. *N Engl J Med* 2001; **345**(20):1444–51.

214 Gorter JW. Major bleeding during anticoagulation after cerebral ischemia: patterns and risk factors. Stroke Prevention In Reversible Ischemia Trial (SPIRIT). European Atrial Fibrillation Trial (EAFT) study groups. *Neurology* 1999; **53**(6):1319–27.

215 Hart RG, Pearce LA, Miller VT, Anderson DC, Rothrock JF, Albers GW *et al*. Cardioembolic vs. noncardioembolic strokes in atrial fibrillation: frequency and effect of antithrombotic agents in the stroke prevention in atrial fibrillation studies. *Cerebrovasc Dis* 2000; **10**(1):39–43.

216 Wolf PA, Abbott RD, Kannel WB. Atrial fibrillation as an independent risk factor for stroke: the Framingham Study. *Stroke* 1991; **22**(8):983–8.

217 Gage BF, van Walraven C, Pearce L, Hart RG, Koudstaal PJ, Boode BS *et al*. Selecting patients with atrial fibrillation for anticoagulation: stroke risk stratification in patients taking aspirin. *Circulation* 2004; **110**(16):2287–92.

218 Hart RG, Halperin JL. Atrial fibrillation and thromboembolism: a decade of progress in stroke prevention. *Ann Intern Med* 1999; **131**(9):688–95.

219 Singer DE, Albers GW, Dalen JE, Go AS, Halperin JL, Manning WJ. Antithrombotic therapy in atrial fibrillation: the Seventh ACCP Conference on Antithrombotic and Thrombolytic Therapy. *Chest* 2004; **126**(3 Suppl):429S–456S.

220 Aguilar MI, Hart R. Oral anticoagulants for preventing stroke in patients with non-valvular atrial fibrillation and no previous history of stroke or transient ischemic attacks. *Cochrane Database Syst Rev* 2005; (3):CD001927.

221 Saxena R, Koudstaal PJ. Anticoagulants for preventing stroke in patients with nonrheumatic atrial fibrillation and a history of stroke or transient ischaemic attack. *Cochrane Database Syst Rev* 2004; (2):CD000185.

222 Evans A, Kalra L. Are the results of randomized controlled trials on anticoagulation in patients with atrial fibrillation generalizable to clinical practice? *Arch Intern Med* 2001; **161**(11):1443–7.

223 Go AS, Hylek EM, Chang Y, Phillips KA, Henault LE, Capra AM *et al*. Anticoagulation therapy for stroke prevention in atrial fibrillation: how well do randomized trials translate into clinical practice? *J Am Med Assoc* 2003; **290**(20):2685–92.

224 Levine MN, Raskob G, Beyth RJ, Kearon C, Schulman S. Hemorrhagic complications of anticoagulant treatment:

the Seventh ACCP Conference on Antithrombotic and Thrombolytic Therapy. *Chest* 2004; **126**(3 Suppl):287S–310S.

225 Van Walraven C, Hart RG, Singer DE, Laupacis A, Connolly S, Petersen P *et al.* Oral anticoagulants vs aspirin in nonvalvular atrial fibrillation: an individual patient meta-analysis. *J Am Med Assoc* 2002; **288**(19):2441–8.

226 Connolly S, Pogue J, Hart R, Pfeffer M, Hohnloser S, Chrolavicius S *et al.* Clopidogrel plus aspirin versus oral anticoagulation for atrial fibrillation in the Atrial fibrillation Clopidogrel Trial with Irbesartan for prevention of Vascular Events (ACTIVE W): a randomised controlled trial. *Lancet* 2006; **367**(9526):1903–12.

227 Hylek EM, D'Antonio J, Evans-Molina C, Shea C, Henault LE, Regan S. Translating the results of randomized trials into clinical practice: the challenge of warfarin candidacy among hospitalized elderly patients with atrial fibrillation. *Stroke* 2006; **37**(4):1075–80.

228 Mant JW, Richards SH, Hobbs FD, Fitzmaurice D, Lip GY, Murray E *et al.* Protocol for Birmingham Atrial Fibrillation Treatment of the Aged study (BAFTA): a randomised controlled trial of warfarin versus aspirin for stroke prevention in the management of atrial fibrillation in an elderly primary care population [ISRCTN89345269]. *BMC Cardiovasc Disord* 2003; **3**:9.

229 The European Atrial Fibrillation Trial Study Group. Optimal oral anticoagulant therapy in patients with nonrheumatic atrial fibrillation and recent cerebral ischemia. *N Engl J Med* 1995; **333**(1):5–10.

230 Hylek EM, Skates SJ, Sheehan MA, Singer DE. An analysis of the lowest effective intensity of prophylactic anticoagulation for patients with nonrheumatic atrial fibrillation. *N Engl J Med* 1996; **335**(8):540–6.

231 Hylek EM, Go AS, Chang Y, Jensvold NG, Henault LE, Selby JV *et al.* Effect of intensity of oral anticoagulation on stroke severity and mortality in atrial fibrillation. *N Engl J Med* 2003; **349**(11):1019–26.

232 Lechat P, Lardoux H, Mallet A, Sanchez P, Derumeaux G, Lecompte T *et al.* Anticoagulant (fluindione)-aspirin combination in patients with high-risk atrial fibrillation. A randomized trial (Fluindione, Fibrillation Auriculaire, Aspirin et Contraste Spontane; FFAACS). *Cerebrovasc Dis* 2001; **12**(3):245–52.

233 Perez-Gomez F, Alegria E, Berjon J, Iriarte JA, Zumalde J, Salvador A *et al.* Comparative effects of antiplatelet, anticoagulant, or combined therapy in patients with valvular and nonvalvular atrial fibrillation: a randomized multicenter study. *J Am Coll Cardiol* 2004; **44**(8):1557–66.

234 Hart RG, Benavente O. Increased risk of intracranial hemorrhage when aspirin is added to warfarin: a meta-analysis. *Stroke* 1999; **30**:258.

235 Choudhry NK, Anderson GM, Laupacis A, Ross-Degnan D, Normand SL, Soumerai SB. Impact of adverse events on prescribing warfarin in patients with atrial fibrillation: matched pair analysis. *Br Med J* 2006; **332**(7534):141–5.

236 Gurewich V. Ximelagatran: promises and concerns. *J Am Med Assoc* 2005; **293**(6):736–9.

237 Hankey GJ, Klijn CJ, Eikelboom JW. Ximelagatran or warfarin for stroke prevention in patients with atrial fibrillation? *Stroke* 2004; **35**(2):389–91.

238 Bates SM, Greer IA, Hirsh J, Ginsberg JS. Use of antithrombotic agents during pregnancy: the Seventh ACCP Conference on Antithrombotic and Thrombolytic Therapy. *Chest* 2004; **126**(3 Suppl):627S–644S.

239 Ansell J, Hirsh J, Poller L, Bussey H, Jacobson A, Hylek E. The pharmacology and management of the vitamin K antagonists: the Seventh ACCP Conference on Antithrombotic and Thrombolytic Therapy. *Chest* 2004; **126**(3 Suppl):204S–233S.

240 Anon. Interaction between warfarin and cranberry juice: new advice. *Curr Probl Pharmacovigilance* 2004; 30:10.

241 Rieder MJ, Reiner AP, Gage BF, Nickerson DA, Eby CS, McLeod HL *et al.* Effect of VKORC1 haplotypes on transcriptional regulation and warfarin dose. *N Engl J Med* 2005; **352**(22):2285–93.

242 Viswanathan A, Chabriat H. Cerebral microhemorrhage. *Stroke* 2006; **37**(2):550–5.

243 Cordonnier C, Al-Shahi SR, Wardlaw J. Spontaneous brain microbleeds: systematic review, subgroup analyses and standards for study design and reporting. *Brain* 2007, doi:10.1093/brain/aw1387.

244 Hart RG, Boop BS, Anderson DC. Oral anticoagulants and intracranial hemorrhage: facts and hypotheses. *Stroke* 1995; **26**(8):1471–7.

245 Blann AD, Fitzmaurice DA, Lip GY. Anticoagulation in hospitals and general practice. *Br Med J* 2003; **326**(7381):153–6.

246 Heneghan C, Alonso-Coello P, Garcia-Alamino JM, Perera R, Meats E, Glasziou P. Self-monitoring of oral anticoagulation: a systematic review and meta-analysis. *Lancet* 2006; **367**(9508):404–11.

247 Ezzati M, Lopez AD. Estimates of global mortality attributable to smoking in 2000. *Lancet* 2003; **362**(9387):847–52.

248 Doll R, Peto R, Wheatley K, Gray R, Sutherland I. Mortality in relation to smoking: 40 years' observations on male British doctors. *Br Med J* 1994; **309**(6959):901–11.

249 Donnan GA, You R, Thrift A, McNeil JJ. Smoking as a risk factor for stroke. *Cerebrovasc Dis* 1993; **3**(129):138.

250 Hankey GJ. Smoking and risk of stroke. *J Cardiovasc Risk* 1999; **6**(4):207–11.

251 Shinton R, Beevers G. Meta-analysis of relation between cigarette smoking and stroke. *Br Med J* 1989; **298**(6676):789–94.

252 Vessey M, Painter R, Yeates D. Mortality in relation to oral contraceptive use and cigarette smoking. *Lancet* 2003; **362**(9379):185–91.

253 Kawachi I, Colditz GA, Stampfer MJ, Willett WC, Manson JE, Rosner B *et al.* Smoking cessation and decreased risk of stroke in women. *J Am Med Assoc* 1993; **269**(2):232–6.

254 Wannamethee SG, Shaper AG, Whincup PH, Walker M. Smoking cessation and the risk of stroke in middle-aged men. *J Am Med Assoc* 1995; **274**(2):155–60.

255 Wilson K, Gibson N, Willan A, Cook D. Effect of smoking cessation on mortality after myocardial infarction: meta-

analysis of cohort studies. *Arch Intern Med* 2000; **160**(7):939–44.

256 Wolf PA, D'Agostino RB, Kannel WB, Bonita R, Belanger AJ. Cigarette smoking as a risk factor for stroke. The Framingham Study. *J Am Med Assoc* 1988; **259**(7):1025–29.

257 Lancaster T, Stead L. Physician advice for smoking cessation. *Cochrane Database Syst Rev* 2004; (4):CD000165.

258 Lancaster T, Stead LF. Individual behavioural counselling for smoking cessation. *Cochrane Database Syst Rev* 2005; (2):CD001292.

259 Rice VH, Stead LF. Nursing interventions for smoking cessation. *Cochrane Database Syst Rev* 2004; (1):CD001188.

260 Stead LF, Lancaster T. Group behaviour therapy programmes for smoking cessation. *Cochrane Database Syst Rev* 2002; (3):CD001007.

261 Lancaster T, Stead LF. Self-help interventions for smoking cessation. *Cochrane Database Syst Rev* 2005; (3):CD001118.

262 Stead LF, Lancaster T, Perera R. Telephone counselling for smoking cessation. *Cochrane Database Syst Rev* 2003; (1):CD002850.

263 Coleman T. ABC of smoking cessation. Use of simple advice and behavioural support. *Br Med J* 2004; **328**(7436):397–9.

264 Silagy C, Lancaster T, Stead L, Mant D, Fowler G. Nicotine replacement therapy for smoking cessation. *Cochrane Database Syst Rev* 2004; (3):CD000146.

265 Hughes J, Stead L, Lancaster T. Antidepressants for smoking cessation. *Cochrane Database Syst Rev* 2004; (4):CD000031.

266 Corrao G, Rubbiati L, Bagnardi V, Zambon A, Poikolainen K. Alcohol and coronary heart disease: a meta-analysis. *Addiction* 2000; **95**(10):1505–23.

267 Doll R. One for the heart. *Br Med J* 1997; **315**(7123):1664–8.

268 Elkind MS, Sciacca R, Boden-Albala B, Rundek T, Paik MC, Sacco RL. Moderate alcohol consumption reduces risk of ischemic stroke: the Northern Manhattan Study. *Stroke* 2006; **37**(1):13–19.

269 Reynolds K, Lewis B, Nolen JD, Kinney GL, Sathya B, He J. Alcohol consumption and risk of stroke: a meta-analysis. *J Am Med Assoc* 2003; **289**(5):579–88.

270 Di Castelnuovo A, Rotondo S, Iacoviello L, Donati MB, De Gaetano G. Meta-analysis of wine and beer consumption in relation to vascular risk. *Circulation* 2002; **105**(24):2836–44.

271 Gaziano JM, Hennekens CH, Godfried SL, Sesso HD, Glynn RJ, Breslow JL et al. Type of alcoholic beverage and risk of myocardial infarction. *Am J Cardiol* 1999; **83**(1):52–7.

272 Rimm EB, Klatsky A, Grobbee D, Stampfer MJ. Review of moderate alcohol consumption and reduced risk of coronary heart disease: is the effect due to beer, wine, or spirits. *Br Med J* 1996; **312**(7033):731–6.

273 Rimm EB, Stampfer MJ. Wine, beer, and spirits: are they really horses of a different color? *Circulation* 2002; **105**(24):2806–7.

274 Naimi TS, Brown DW, Brewer RD, Giles WH, Mensah G, Serdula MK et al. Cardiovascular risk factors and confounders among nondrinking and moderate-drinking US adults. *Am J Prev Med* 2005; **28**(4):369–73.

275 Marmot MG. Commentary: reflections on alcohol and coronary heart disease. *Int J Epidemiol* 2001; **30**(4):729–34.

276 Jackson R, Broad J, Connor J, Wells S. Alcohol and ischaemic heart disease: probably no free lunch. *Lancet* 2005; **366**(9501):1911–12.

277 He FJ, MacGregor GA. Effect of longer-term modest salt reduction on blood pressure. *Cochrane Database Syst Rev* 2004; (3):CD004937.

278 Hooper L, Bartlett C, Davey SG, Ebrahim S. Advice to reduce dietary salt for prevention of cardiovascular disease. *Cochrane Database Syst Rev* 2004; (1):CD003656.

279 Cook NR, Cutler JA, Obarzanek E, Buring JE, Rexrode KM, Kumanyika SK et al. Long term effects of dietary sodium reduction on cardiovascular disease outcomes: observational follow-up of the trials of hypertension prevention (TOHP). *Br Med J* 2007; **334**(7599):885.

280 He FJ, MacGregor GA. Fortnightly review: beneficial effects of potassium. *Br Med J* 2001; **323**(7311):497–501.

281 Whelton PK, He J, Cutler JA, Brancati FL, Appel LJ, Follmann D et al. Effects of oral potassium on blood pressure. Meta-analysis of randomized controlled clinical trials. *J Am Med Assoc* 1997; **277**(20):1624–32.

282 Clarke R, Frost C, Collins R, Appleby P, Peto R. Dietary lipids and blood cholesterol: quantitative meta-analysis of metabolic ward studies. *Br Med J* 1997; **314**(7074):112–17.

283 Ebrahim SDSG. *Health Promotion in Older People for the Prevention of Coronary Heart Disease and Stroke*. Health Promotion effectiveness series. (1). London: Health Education Authority, 1996.

284 Tang JL, Armitage JM, Lancaster T, Silagy CA, Fowler GH, Neil HA. Systematic review of dietary intervention trials to lower blood total cholesterol in free-living subjects. *Br Med J* 1998; **316**(7139):1213–20.

285 Hooper L, Summerbell CD, Higgins JP, Thompson RL, Clements G, Capps N et al. Reduced or modified dietary fat for prevention of cardiovascular disease. *Cochrane Database Syst Rev* 2000; (2):CD002137.

286 Haslam DW, James WP. Obesity. *Lancet* 2005; **366**(9492):1197–209.

287 Shaper AG, Wannamethee SG, Walker M. Body weight: implications for the prevention of coronary heart disease, stroke, and diabetes mellitus in a cohort study of middle aged men. *Br Med J* 1997; **314**(7090):1311–17.

288 Avenell A, Broom J, Brown TJ, Poobalan A, Aucott L, Stearns SC et al. Systematic review of the long-term effects and economic consequences of treatments for obesity and implications for health improvement. *Health Technol Assess* 2004; **8**(21):iii–182.

289 Clegg AJ, Colquitt J, Sidhu MK, Royle P, Loveman E, Walker A. The clinical effectiveness and cost-effectiveness of surgery for people with morbid obesity: a systematic review and economic evaluation. *Health Technol Assess* 2002; **6**(12):1–153.

290 Din JN, Newby DE, Flapan AD. Omega 3 fatty acids and cardiovascular disease: fishing for a natural treatment. *Br Med J* 2004; **328**(7430):30–5.

291 He FJ, Nowson CA, MacGregor GA. Fruit and vegetable consumption and stroke: meta-analysis of cohort studies. *Lancet* 2006; **367**(9507):320–6.

292 Kelly S, Frost G, Whittaker V, Summerbell C. Low glycaemic index diets for coronary heart disease. *Cochrane Database Syst Rev* 2004; (4):CD004467.

293 Marckmann P, Gronbaek M. Fish consumption and coronary heart disease mortality: a systematic review of prospective cohort studies. *Eur J Clin Nutr* 1999; **53**(8):585–90.

294 Mozaffarian D, Longstreth WT, Jr., Lemaitre RN, Manolio TA, Kuller LH, Burke GL *et al.* Fish consumption and stroke risk in elderly individuals: the cardiovascular health study. *Arch Intern Med* 2005; **165**(2):200–6.

295 Ness AR, Powles JW. Fruit and vegetables, and cardiovascular disease: a review. *Int J Epidemiol* 1997; **26**(1):1–13.

296 Ness AR, Powles JW. The role of diet, fruit and vegetables and antioxidants in the aetiology of stroke. *J Cardiovasc Risk* 1999; **6**(4):229–34.

297 Knoops KT, de Groot LC, Kromhout D, Perrin AE, Moreiras-Varela O, Menotti A *et al.* Mediterranean diet, lifestyle factors, and 10-year mortality in elderly European men and women: the HALE project. *J Am Med Assoc* 2004; **292**(12):1433–9.

298 Trichopoulou A, Orfanos P, Norat T, Bueno-de-Mesquita B, Ocke MC, Peeters PH *et al.* Modified Mediterranean diet and survival: EPIC-elderly prospective cohort study. *Br Med J* 2005; **330**(7498):991.

299 Hooper L, Thompson RL, Harrison RA, Summerbell CD, Moore H, Worthington HV *et al.* Omega 3 fatty acids for prevention and treatment of cardiovascular disease. *Cochrane Database Syst Rev* 2004; (4):CD003177.

300 Hooper L, Thompson RL, Harrison RA, Summerbell CD, Ness AR, Moore HJ *et al.* Risks and benefits of omega 3 fats for mortality, cardiovascular disease, and cancer: systematic review. *Br Med J* 2006; **332**(7544):752–60.

301 De Lorgeril M, Salen P, Martin JL, Monjaud I, Boucher P, Mamelle N. Mediterranean dietary pattern in a randomized trial: prolonged survival and possible reduced cancer rate. *Arch Intern Med* 1998; **158**(11):1181–7.

302 Mann J. The Indo-Mediterranean diet revisited. *Lancet* 2005; **366**(9483):353–4.

303 Singh RB, Dubnov G, Niaz MA, Ghosh S, Singh R, Rastogi SS *et al.* Effect of an Indo-Mediterranean diet on progression of coronary artery disease in high risk patients (Indo-Mediterranean Diet Heart Study): a randomised single-blind trial. *Lancet* 2002; **360**(9344):1455–61.

304 White C. Suspected research fraud: difficulties of getting at the truth. *Br Med J* 2005; **331**(7511):281–8.

305 Brunner EJ, Thorogood M, Rees K, Hewitt G. Dietary advice for reducing cardiovascular risk. *Cochrane Database Syst Rev* 2005; (4):CD002128.

306 Wendel-Vos GC, Schuit AJ, Feskens EJ, Boshuizen HC, Verschuren WM, Saris WH *et al.* Physical activity and stroke: a meta-analysis of observational data. *Int J Epidemiol* 2004; **33**(4):787–98.

307 Murphy M, Foster C, Nicholas JJ, Pignone M. Cardiovascular disorders. Primary prevention. *Clin Evid* 2003; **10**:154–87.

308 Whelton SP, Chin A, Xin X, He J. Effect of aerobic exercise on blood pressure: a meta-analysis of randomized, controlled trials. *Ann Intern Med* 2002; **136**(7):493–503.

309 Taylor RS, Brown A, Ebrahim S, Jolliffe J, Noorani H, Rees K *et al.* Exercise-based rehabilitation for patients with coronary heart disease: systematic review and meta-analysis of randomized controlled trials. *Am J Med* 2004; **116**(10):682–92.

310 Gillespie LD, Gillespie WJ, Robertson MC, Lamb SE, Cumming RG, Rowe BH. Interventions for preventing falls in elderly people. *Cochrane Database Syst Rev* 2003; (4):CD000340.

311 Homocysteine Studies Collaboration Homocysteine and risk of ischemic heart disease and stroke: a meta-analysis. *J Am Med Assoc* 2002; **288**(16):2015–22.

312 Wald DS, Law M, Morris JK. Homocysteine and cardiovascular disease: evidence on causality from a meta-analysis. *Br Med J* 2002; **325**(7374):1202.

313 Casas JP, Bautista LE, Smeeth L, Sharma P, Hingorani AD. Homocysteine and stroke: evidence on a causal link from mendelian randomisation. *Lancet* 2005; **365**(9455):224–32.

314 Cronin S, Furie KL, Kelly PJ. Dose-related association of MTHFR 677T allele with risk of ischemic stroke: evidence from a cumulative meta-analysis. *Stroke* 2005; **36**(7):1581–7.

315 Klerk M, Verhoef P, Clarke R, Blom HJ, Kok FJ, Schouten EG. MTHFR 677C–>T polymorphism and risk of coronary heart disease: a meta-analysis. *J Am Med Assoc* 2002; **288**(16):2023–31.

316 Hankey GJ, Eikelboom JW. Homocysteine and stroke. *Lancet* 2005; **365**(9455):194–196.

317 Lewis SJ, Ebrahim S, Davey SG. Meta-analysis of MTHFR 677C–>T polymorphism and coronary heart disease: does totality of evidence support causal role for homocysteine and preventive potential of folate? *Br Med J* 2005; **331**(7524):1053.

318 Lowering blood homocysteine with folic acid based supplements: meta-analysis of randomised trials. Homocysteine Lowering Trialists' Collaboration. *Br Med J* 1998; **316**(7135):894–8.

319 Toole JF, Malinow MR, Chambless LE, Spence JD, Pettigrew LC, Howard VJ *et al.* Lowering homocysteine in patients with ischemic stroke to prevent recurrent stroke, myocardial infarction, and death: the Vitamin Intervention for Stroke Prevention (VISP) randomized controlled trial. *J Am Med Assoc* 2004; **291**(5):565–75.

320 Baker F, Picton D, Blackwood S. Blinded comparison of folic acid and placebo in patients with ischemic heart disease: an outcome trial. *Circulation* 2002; **106**(Suppl 11):741.

321 Bonaa KH, Njolstad I, Ueland PM, Schirmer H, Tverdal A, Steigen T *et al.* Homocysteine lowering and cardiovascular events after acute myocardial infarction. *N Engl J Med* 2006; **354**(15):1578–88.

322 Lonn E, Yusuf S, Arnold MJ, Sheridan P, Pogue J, Micks M *et al.* Homocysteine lowering with folic acid and B vitamins in vascular disease. *N Engl J Med* 2006; **354**(15):1567–77.

323 Bazzano LA, Reynolds K, Holder KN, He J. Effect of folic acid supplementation on risk of cardiovascular diseases: a meta-analysis of randomized controlled trials. *J Am Med Assoc* 2006; **296**(22):2720–6.

324 B-Vitamin Treatment Trialists' Collaboration. Homocysteine-lowering trials for prevention of cardiovascular events: a review of the design and power of the large randomized trials. *Am Heart J* 2006; **151**(2):282–7.

325 The VITATOPS Trial Study Group. The VITATOPS (Vitamins to Prevent Stroke) Trial: rationale and design of an international, large, simple, randomised trial of homocysteine-lowering multivitamin therapy in patients with recent transient ischaemic attack or stroke. *Cerebrovasc Dis* 2002; **13**(2):120–6.

326 Galan P, de Bree A, Mennen L, Potier de Courcy G, Preziozi P, Bertrais S *et al.* Background and rationale of the SU.FOL.OM3 study: double-blind randomized placebo-controlled secondary prevention trial to test the impact of supplementation with folate, vitamin B6 and B12 and/or omega-3 fatty acids on the prevention of recurrent ischemic events in subjects with atherosclerosis in the coronary or cerebral arteries. *J Nutr Health Aging* 2003; **7**(6):428–35.

327 Davey SG, Ebrahim S. Folate supplementation and cardiovascular disease. *Lancet* 2005; **366**(9498):1679–81.

328 Brown BG, Crowley J. Is there any hope for vitamin E? *J Am Med Assoc* 2005; **293**(11):1387–90.

329 Witzlum JL. The oxidation hypothesis of atherosclerosis. *Lancet* 1994; **344**(8925):793–5.

330 Jha P, Flather M, Lonn E, Farkouh M, Yusuf S. The antioxidant vitamins and cardiovascular disease. A critical review of epidemiologic and clinical trial data. *Ann Intern Med* 1995; **123**(11):860–72.

331 Eidelman RS, Hollar D, Hebert PR, Lamas GA, Hennekens CH. Randomized trials of vitamin E in the treatment and prevention of cardiovascular disease. *Arch Intern Med* 2004; **164**(14):1552–6.

332 Lonn E, Bosch J, Yusuf S, Sheridan P, Pogue J, Arnold JM *et al.* Effects of long-term vitamin E supplementation on cardiovascular events and cancer: a randomized controlled trial. *J Am Med Assoc* 2005; **293**(11):1338–47.

333 Vivekananthan DP, Penn MS, Sapp SK, Hsu A, Topol EJ. Use of antioxidant vitamins for the prevention of cardiovascular disease: meta-analysis of randomised trials. *Lancet* 2003; **361**(9374):2017–23.

334 Kanters SD, Banga JD, Stolk RP, Algra A. Incidence and determinants of mortality and cardiovascular events in diabetes mellitus: a meta-analysis. *Vasc Med* 1999; **4**(2):67–75.

335 Lawes CM, Parag V, Bennett DA, Suh I, Lam TH, Whitlock G *et al.* Blood glucose and risk of cardiovascular disease in the Asia Pacific region. *Diabetes Care* 2004; **27**(12):2836–42.

336 Tanne D, Koren-Morag N, Goldbourt U. Fasting plasma glucose and risk of incident ischemic stroke or transient ischemic attacks: a prospective cohort study. *Stroke* 2004; **35**(10):2351–5.

337 Tuomilehto J, Rastenyte D. Diabetes and glucose intolerance as risk factors for stroke. *J Cardiovasc Risk* 1999; **6**(4):241–9.

338 Sigal R, Malcolm J, Arnaout A. Prevention of cardiovascular events in diabetes. *Clin Evid* 2006; **15**:623–45.

339 UK Prospective Diabetes Study (UKPDS) Group. Intensive blood-glucose control with sulphonylureas or insulin compared with conventional treatment and risk of complications in patients with type 2 diabetes (UKPDS 33). *Lancet* 1998; **352**(9131):837–53.

340 Abraira C, Colwell J, Nuttall F, Sawin CT, Henderson W, Comstock JP *et al.* Cardiovascular events and correlates in the Veterans Affairs Diabetes Feasibility Trial. Veterans Affairs Cooperative Study on Glycemic Control and Complications in Type II Diabetes. *Arch Intern Med* 1997; **157**(2):181–8.

341 UK Prospective Diabetes Study (UKPDS) Group. Effect of intensive blood-glucose control with metformin on complications in overweight patients with type 2 diabetes (UKPDS 34). *Lancet* 1998; **352**(9131):854–65.

342 Dormandy JA, Charbonnel B, Eckland DJ, Erdmann E, Massi-Benedetti M, Moules IK *et al.* Secondary prevention of macrovascular events in patients with type 2 diabetes in the PROactive Study (PROspective pioglitAzone Clinical Trial In macroVascular Events): a randomised controlled trial. *Lancet* 2005; **366**(9493):1279–89.

343 Cordina J, Mead G. Pharmacological cardioversion for atrial fibrillation and flutter. *Cochrane Database Syst Rev* 2005; (2):CD003713.

344 Mead GE, Elder AT, Flapan AD, Kelman A. Electrical cardioversion for atrial fibrillation and flutter. *Cochrane Database Syst Rev* 2005; (3):CD002903.

345 Wyse DG, Waldo AL, DiMarco JP, Domanski MJ, Rosenberg Y, Schron EB *et al.* A comparison of rate control and rhythm control in patients with atrial fibrillation. *N Engl J Med* 2002; **347**(23):1825–33.

346 Mas J-L. Patent forman ovale and stroke. *Pract Neurol* 2003; **3**:4–11.

347 Overell JR, Bone I, Lees KR. Interatrial septal abnormalities and stroke: a meta-analysis of case–control studies. *Neurology* 2000; **55**(8):1172–9.

348 Amarenco P. Patent foramen ovale and the risk of stroke: smoking gun guilty by association? *Heart* 2005; **91**(4):441–3.

349 Mas JL, Arquizan C, Lamy C, Zuber M, Cabanes L, Derumeaux G *et al.* Recurrent cerebrovascular events associated with patent foramen ovale, atrial septal aneurysm, or both. *N Engl J Med* 2001; **345**(24):1740–6.

350 Homma S, Sacco RL, Di Tullio MR, Sciacca RR, Mohr JP. Effect of medical treatment in stroke patients with patent foramen ovale: patent foramen ovale in Cryptogenic Stroke Study. *Circulation* 2002; **105**(22):2625–31.

351 Meier B. Closure of patent foramen ovale: technique, pitfalls, complications, and follow up. *Heart* 2005; **91**(4):444–8.

352 Martin F, Sanchez PL, Doherty E, Colon-Hernandez PJ, Delgado G, Inglessis I *et al.* Percutaneous transcatheter closure of patent foramen ovale in patients with paradoxical embolism. *Circulation* 2002; **106**(9):1121–6.

353 Khairy P, O'Donnell CP, Landzberg MJ. Transcatheter closure versus medical therapy of patent foramen ovale and presumed paradoxical thromboemboli: a systematic review. *Ann Intern Med* 2003; **139**(9):753–60.

354 Flachskampf FA, Daniel WG. Closure of patent foramen ovale: is the case really closed as well? *Heart* 2005; **91**(4):449–50.

355 Wu LA, Malouf JF, Dearani JA, Hagler DJ, Reeder GS, Petty GW *et al.* Patent foramen ovale in cryptogenic stroke: current understanding and management options. *Arch Intern Med* 2004; **164**(9):950–6.

356 Thompson JE. The evolution of surgery for the treatment and prevention of stroke. The Willis Lecture. *Stroke* 1996; **27**(8):1427–34.

357 Chao WH, Kwan ST, Lyman RS, Loucks HH. Thrombosis of the left internal carotid artery. *Arch Surg* 1938; **37**:100–11.

358 Carrea R, Molins M, Murphy G. Surgical treatment of spontaneous thrombosis of the internal carotid artery in the neck. Carotid-carotideal anastomosis. Report of a case. *Acta Neurologica Latin America* 1955; **1**:71–8.

359 DeBakey ME. Successful carotid endarterectomy for cerebrovascular insufficiency. Nineteen-year follow-up. *J Am Med Assoc* 1975; **233**(10):1083–5.

360 Eastcott HH, Pickering GW, Rob CG. Reconstruction of internal carotid artery in a patient with intermittent attacks of hemiplegia. *Lancet* 1954; **267**(6846):994–6.

361 Pokras R, Dyken ML. Dramatic changes in the performance of endarterectomy for diseases of the extracranial arteries of the head. *Stroke* 1988; **19**(10):1289–90.

362 Tu JV, Hannan EL, Anderson GM, Iron K, Wu K, Vranizan K *et al.* The fall and rise of carotid endarterectomy in the United States and Canada. *N Engl J Med* 1998; **339**(20):1441–7.

363 Fields WS, Maslenikov V, Meyer JS, Hass WK, Remington RD, Macdonald M. Joint study of extracranial arterial occlusion. V. Progress report of prognosis following surgery or nonsurgical treatment for transient cerebral ischemic attacks and cervical carotid artery lesions. *J Am Med Assoc* 1970; **211**(12):1993–2003.

364 Shaw DA, Venables GS, Cartlidge NE, Bates D, Dickinson PH. Carotid endarterectomy in patients with transient cerebral ischaemia. *J Neurol Sci* 1984; **64**(1):45–53.

365 Warlow C. Carotid endarterectomy: does it work? *Stroke* 1984; **15**(6):1068–76.

366 UK-TIA Study Group. Variation in the use of angiography and carotid endarterectomy by neurologists in the UK-TIA aspirin trial. *Br Med J (Clin Res Ed)* 1983; **286**(6364):514–17.

367 Barnett H, Meldrum H. Status of carotid endarterectomy. *Curr Opin Neurol* 1994; **7**(1):54–9.

368 Winslow CM, Solomon DH, Chassin MR, Kosecoff J, Merrick NJ, Brook RH. The appropriateness of carotid endarterectomy. *N Engl J Med* 1988; **318**(12):721–7.

369 European Carotid Surgery Trialists' Collaborative Group. MRC European Carotid Surgery Trial: interim results for symptomatic patients with severe (70–99%) or with mild (0–29%) carotid stenosis. *Lancet* 1991; **337**(8752):1235–43.

370 North American Symptomatic Carotid Endarterectomy Trial Collaborators. Beneficial effect of carotid endarterectomy in symptomatic patients with high-grade carotid stenosis. *N Engl J Med* 1991; **325**(7):445–53.

371 Mayberg MR, Wilson SE, Yatsu F, Weiss DG, Messina L, Hershey LA *et al.* Carotid endarterectomy and prevention of cerebral ischemia in symptomatic carotid stenosis. Veterans Affairs Cooperative Studies Program 309 Trialist Group. *J Am Med Assoc* 1991; **266**(23):3289–94.

372 Cebul RD, Snow RJ, Pine R, Hertzer NR, Norris DG. Indications, outcomes, and provider volumes for carotid endarterectomy. *J Am Med Assoc* 1998; **279**(16):1282–7.

373 Matsen SL, Chang DC, Perler BA, Roseborough GS, Williams GM. Trends in the in-hospital stroke rate following carotid endarterectomy in California and Maryland. *J Vasc Surg* 2006; **44**(3):488–95.

374 Ferris G, Roderick P, Smithies A, George S, Gabbay J, Couper N *et al.* An epidemiological needs assessment of carotid endarterectomy in an English health region. Is the need being met? *Br Med J* 1998; **317**(7156):447–51.

375 Fairhead JF, Rothwell PM. Underinvestigation and undertreatment of carotid disease in elderly patients with transient ischaemic attack and stroke: comparative population based study. *Br Med J* 2006; **333**(7567):525–7.

376 Eliasziw M, Spence JD, Barnett HJ. Carotid endarterectomy does not affect long-term blood pressure: observations from the NASCET. North American Symptomatic Carotid Endarterectomy Trial. *Cerebrovasc Dis* 1998; **8**(1):20–4.

377 Loftus CM, Quest DO. Technical controversies in carotid artery surgery. *Neurosurgery* 1987; **20**(3):490–5.

378 Darling RC, III, Paty PS, Shah DM, Chang BB, Leather RP. Eversion endarterectomy of the internal carotid artery: technique and results in 449 procedures. *Surgery* 1996; **120**(4):635–9.

379 Cao P, Giordano G, De Rango P, Zannetti S, Chiesa R, Coppi G *et al.* A randomized study on eversion versus standard carotid endarterectomy: study design and preliminary results: the Everest Trial. *J Vasc Surg* 1998; **27**(4):595–605.

380 Cao PG, De Rango P, Zannetti S, Giordano G, Ricci S, Celani MG. Eversion versus conventional carotid endarterectomy for preventing stroke. *Cochrane Database Syst Rev* 2000;(4):CD001921.

381 Brothers TE. Initial experience with eversion carotid endarterectomy: absence of a learning curve for the first 100 patients. *J Vasc Surg* 2005; **42**:429–34.

382 Ferguson GG. Carotid endarterectomy. To shunt or not to shunt? *Arch Neurol* 1986; **43**(6):615–17.

383 Ojemann RG, Heros RC. Carotid endarterectomy. To shunt or not to shunt? *Arch Neurol* 1986; **43**(6):617–18.

384 Naylor AR, Bell PR, Ruckley CV. Monitoring and cerebral protection during carotid endarterectomy. *Br J Surg* 1992; **79**(8):735–41.

385 Belardi P, Lucertini G, Ermirio D. Stump pressure and transcranial Doppler for predicting shunting in carotid

endarterectomy. *Eur J Vasc Endovasc Surg* 2003; **25**(2):164–7.

386 Bond R, Warlow CP, Naylor AR, Rothwell PM. Variation in surgical and anaesthetic technique and associations with operative risk in the European carotid surgery trial: implications for trials of ancillary techniques. *Eur J Vasc Endovasc Surg* 2002; **23**(2):117–26.

387 Schneider PA, Ringelstein EB, Rossman ME, Dilley RB, Sobel DF, Otis SM *et al.* Importance of cerebral collateral pathways during carotid endarterectomy. *Stroke* 1988; **19**(11):1328–34.

388 Bond R, Rerkasem K, Counsell C, Salinas R, Naylor R, Warlow CP *et al.* Routine or selective carotid artery shunting for carotid endarterectomy (and different methods of monitoring in selective shunting). *Cochrane Database Syst Rev* 2002; (2):CD000190.

389 Cunningham EJ, Bond R, Mehta Z, Mayberg MR, Warlow CP, Rothwell PM. Long-term durability of carotid endarterectomy for symptomatic stenosis and risk factors for late postoperative stroke. *Stroke* 2002; **33**(11):2658–63.

390 Bond R, Rerkasem K, Rothwell PM. Systematic review of the risks of carotid endarterectomy in relation to the clinical indication for and timing of surgery. *Stroke* 2003; **34**(9):2290–301.

391 Yadav JS, Roubin GS, King P, Iyer S, Vitek J. Angioplasty and stenting for restenosis after carotid endarterectomy. Initial experience. *Stroke* 1996; **27**(11):2075–9.

392 Frericks H, Kievit J, van Baalen JM, van Bockel JH. Carotid recurrent stenosis and risk of ipsilateral stroke: a systematic review of the literature. *Stroke* 1998; **29**(1):244–50.

393 Hunter GC, Palmaz JC, Hayashi HH, Raviola CA, Vogt PJ, Guernsey JM. The etiology of symptoms in patients with recurrent carotid stenosis. *Arch Surg* 1987; **122**(3):311–15.

394 Bond R, Rerkasem K, Aburahma AF, Naylor AR, Rothwell PM. Patch angioplasty versus primary closure for carotid endarterectomy. *Cochrane Database Syst Rev* 2004; (2):CD000160.

395 Bond R, Rerkasem K, Naylor R, Rothwell PM. Patches of different types for carotid patch angioplasty. *Cochrane Database Syst Rev* 2004; (2):CD000071.

396 Rerkasem K, Bond R, Rothwell PM. Local versus general anaesthesia for carotid endarterectomy. *Cochrane Database Syst Rev* 2004; (2):CD000126.

397 Naylor AR, Ruckley CV. Complications after carotid surgery. In: Campbell B, ed. *Complications in Arterial Surgery*. Oxford: Butterworth-Heinemann, 1996, pp. 73–88.

398 Ferguson GG, Eliasziw M, Barr HW, Clagett GP, Barnes RW, Wallace MC *et al.* The North American Symptomatic Carotid Endarterectomy Trial: surgical results in 1415 patients. *Stroke* 1999; **30**(9):1751–8.

399 Bond R, Narayan SK, Rothwell PM, Warlow CP. Clinical and radiographic risk factors for operative stroke and death in the European carotid surgery trial. *Eur J Vasc Endovasc Surg* 2002; **23**(2):108–16.

400 Bond R, Rerkasem K, Shearman CP, Rothwell PM. Time trends in the published risks of stroke and death due to endarterectomy for symptomatic carotid stenosis. *Cerebrovasc Dis* 2004; **18**(1):37–46.

401 Rothwell PM, Slattery J, Warlow CP. A systematic review of the risks of stroke and death due to endarterectomy for symptomatic carotid stenosis. *Stroke* 1996; **27**(2):260–5.

402 Campbell WB. Can reported carotid surgical results be misleading? In: Greenhalgh RM, Hollier LH, eds. *Surgery for Stroke*. London: W B Saunders, 1993, pp. 331–7.

403 Rothwell P, Warlow C. Is self-audit reliable? *Lancet* 1995; **346**(8990):1623.

404 Rothwell PM, Warlow CP. Interpretation of operative risks of individual surgeons. European Carotid Surgery Trialists' Collaborative Group. *Lancet* 1999; **353**(9161):1325.

405 Kucey DS, Bowyer B, Iron K, Austin P, Anderson G, Tu JV. Determinants of outcome after carotid endarterectomy. *J Vasc Surg* 1998; **28**(6):1051–8.

406 Killeen SD, Andrews EJ, Redmond HP, Fulton GJ. Provider volume and outcomes for abdominal aortic aneurysm repair, carotid endarterectomy, and lower extremity revascularization procedures. *J Vasc Surg* 2007; **45**(3):615–26.

407 Steed DL, Peitzman AB, Grundy BL, Webster MW. Causes of stroke in carotid endarterectomy. *Surgery* 1982; **92**(4):634–41.

408 Krul JM, van Gijn J, Ackerstaff RG, Eikelboom BC, Theodorides T, Vermeulen FE. Site and pathogenesis of infarcts associated with carotid endarterectomy. *Stroke* 1989; **20**(3):324–8.

409 Riles TS, Imparato AM, Jacobowitz GR, Lamparello PJ, Giangola G, Adelman MA *et al.* The cause of perioperative stroke after carotid endarterectomy. *J Vasc Surg* 1994; **19**(2):206–14.

410 Spencer MP. Transcranial Doppler monitoring and causes of stroke from carotid endarterectomy. *Stroke* 1997; **28**(4):685–91.

411 Gaunt ME, Naylor AR, Sayers RD, Ratliff DA, Bell PR. Sources of air embolization during carotid surgery: the role of transcranial Doppler ultrasonography. *Br J Surg* 1993; **80**(9):1121.

412 Jansen C, Ramos LM, van Heesewijk JP, Moll FL, van Gijn J, Ackerstaff RG. Impact of microembolism and hemodynamic changes in the brain during carotid endarterectomy. *Stroke* 1994; **25**(5):992–7.

413 Levi CR, O'Malley HM, Fell G, Roberts AK, Hoare MC, Royle JP *et al.* Transcranial Doppler detected cerebral microembolism following carotid endarterectomy: high microembolic signal loads predict postoperative cerebral ischaemia. *Brain* 1997; **120**(Pt 4):621–9.

414 Wilson PV, Ammar AD. The incidence of ischemic stroke versus intracerebral hemorrhage after carotid endarterectomy: a review of 2452 cases. *Ann Vasc Surg* 2005; **19**(1):1–4.

415 Ouriel K, Shortell CK, Illig KA, Greenberg RK, Green RM. Intracerebral hemorrhage after carotid endarterectomy: incidence, contribution to neurologic morbidity, and predictive factors. *J Vasc Surg* 1999; **29**(1):82–7.

416 Solomon RA, Loftus CM, Quest DO, Correll JW. Incidence and etiology of intracerebral hemorrhage following carotid endarterectomy. *J Neurosurg* 1986; **64**(1):29–34.

417 Hafner DH, Smith RB, III, King OW, Perdue GD, Stewart MT, Rosenthal D *et al.* Massive intracerebral hemorrhage following carotid endarterectomy. *Arch Surg* 1987; **122**(3):305–7.

418 Piepgras DG, Morgan MK, Sundt TM, Jr., Yanagihara T, Mussman LM. Intracerebral hemorrhage after carotid endarterectomy. *J Neurosurg* 1988; **68**(4):532–6.

419 Jansen C, Sprengers AM, Moll FL, Vermeulen FE, Hamerlijnck RP, van Gijn J *et al.* Prediction of intracerebral haemorrhage after carotid endarterectomy by clinical criteria and intraoperative transcranial Doppler monitoring. *Eur J Vasc Surg* 1994; **8**(3):303–8.

420 Adhiyaman V, Alexander S. Cerebral hyperperfusion syndrome following carotid endarterectomy. *Q J Med* 2007; **100**(4):239–44.

421 Andrews BT, Levy ML, Dillon W, Weinstein PR. Unilateral normal perfusion pressure breakthrough after carotid endarterectomy: case report. *Neurosurgery* 1987; **21**(4):568–71.

422 Schroeder T, Sillesen H, Sorensen O, Engell HC. Cerebral hyperperfusion following carotid endarterectomy. *J Neurosurg* 1987; **66**(6):824–9.

423 Naylor AR, Whyman MR, Wildsmith JA, McClure JH, Jenkins AM, Merrick MV *et al.* Factors influencing the hyperaemic response after carotid endarterectomy. *Br J Surg* 1993; **80**(12):1523–7.

424 Chambers BR, Smidt V, Koh P. Hyperfusion post-endarterectomy. *Cerebrovasc Dis* 1994; **4**:32–7.

425 Breen JC, Caplan LR, Dewitt LD, Belkin M, Mackey WC, O'Donnell TP. Brain edema after carotid surgery. *Neurology* 1996; **46**(1):175–81.

426 Van Mook WN, Rennenberg RJ, Schurink GW, van Oostenbrugge RJ, Mess WH, Hofman PA *et al.* Cerebral hyperperfusion syndrome. *Lancet Neurol* 2005; **4**(12):877–88.

427 Lopez-Valdes E, Chang HM, Pessin MS, Caplan LR. Cerebral vasoconstriction after carotid surgery. *Neurology* 1997; **49**(1):303–4.

428 Rothwell PM, Slattery J, Warlow CP. A systematic comparison of the risks of stroke and death due to carotid endarterectomy for symptomatic and asymptomatic stenosis. *Stroke* 1996; **27**(2):266–9.

429 Wennberg DE, Lucas FL, Birkmeyer JD, Bredenberg CE, Fisher ES. Variation in carotid endarterectomy mortality in the Medicare population: trial hospitals, volume, and patient characteristics. *J Am Med Assoc* 1998; **279**(16):1278–81.

430 Riles TS, Kopelman I, Imparato AM. Myocardial infarction following carotid endarterectomy: a review of 683 operations. *Surgery* 1979; **85**(3):249–52.

431 Urbinati S, Di PG, Andreoli A, Lusa AM, Carini G, Grazi P *et al.* Preoperative noninvasive coronary risk stratification in candidates for carotid endarterectomy. *Stroke* 1994; **25**(10):2022–7.

432 Paciaroni M, Eliasziw M, Kappelle LJ, Finan JW, Ferguson GG, Barnett HJ. Medical complications associated with carotid endarterectomy. North American Symptomatic Carotid Endarterectomy Trial (NASCET). *Stroke* 1999; **30**(9):1759–63.

433 Cunningham EJ, Bond R, Mayberg MR, Warlow CP, Rothwell PM. Risk of persistent cranial nerve injury after carotid endarterectomy. *J Neurosurg* 2004; **101**(3):445–8.

434 Gutrecht JA, Jones HR, Jr. Bilateral hypoglossal nerve injury after bilateral carotid endarterectomy. *Stroke* 1988; **19**(2):261–2.

435 Maniglia AJ, Han DP. Cranial nerve injuries following carotid endarterectomy: an analysis of 336 procedures. *Head Neck* 1991; **13**(2):121–4.

436 Sweeney PJ, Wilbourn AJ. Spinal accessory (11th) nerve palsy following carotid endarterectomy. *Neurology* 1992; **42**(3 Pt 1):674–5.

437 Graver LM, Mulcare RJ. Pseudoaneurysm after carotid endarterectomy. *J Cardiovasc Surg (Torino)* 1986; **27**(3):294–7.

438 Martin-Negrier ML, Belleannee G, Vital C, Orgogozo JM. Primitive malignant fibrous histiocytoma of the neck with carotid occlusion and multiple cerebral ischemic lesions. *Stroke* 1996; **27**(3):536–7.

439 Lindblad B, Persson NH, Takolander R, Bergqvist D. Does low-dose acetylsalicylic acid prevent stroke after carotid surgery? A double-blind, placebo-controlled randomized trial. *Stroke* 1993; **24**(8):1125–8.

440 De Marinis M, Zaccaria A, Faraglia V, Fiorani P, Maira G, Agnoli A. Post-endarterectomy headache and the role of the oculosympathetic system. *J Neurol Neurosurg Psychiatry* 1991; **54**(4):314–17.

441 Ille O, Woimant F, Pruna A, Corabianu O, Idatte JM, Haguenau M. Hypertensive encephalopathy after bilateral carotid endarterectomy. *Stroke* 1995; **26**(3):488–91.

442 Youkey JR, Clagett GP, Jaffin JH, Parisi JE, Rich NM. Focal motor seizures complicating carotid endarterectomy. *Arch Surg* 1984; **119**(9):1080–4.

443 Naylor AR, Evans J, Thompson MM, London NJ, Abbott RJ, Cherryman G *et al.* Seizures after carotid endarterectomy: hyperperfusion, dysautoregulation or hypertensive encephalopathy? *Eur J Vasc Endovasc Surg* 2003; **26**(1):39–44.

444 Truax BT. Gustatory pain: a complication of carotid endarterectomy. *Neurology* 1989; **39**(9):1258–60.

445 European Carotid Surgery Trialists' Collaborative Group. Randomised trial of endarterectomy for recently symptomatic carotid stenosis: final results of the MRC European Carotid Surgery Trial (ECST). *Lancet* 1998; **351**(9113):1379–87.

446 Barnett HJ, Taylor DW, Eliasziw M, Fox AJ, Ferguson GG, Haynes RB *et al.* Benefit of carotid endarterectomy in patients with symptomatic moderate or severe stenosis. North American Symptomatic Carotid Endarterectomy Trial Collaborators. *N Engl J Med* 1998; **339**(20):1415–25.

447 Rothwell PM, Eliasziw M, Gutnikov SA, Fox AJ, Taylor DW, Mayberg MR *et al.* Analysis of pooled data from the randomised controlled trials of endarterectomy for symptomatic carotid stenosis. *Lancet* 2003; **361**(9352):107–16.

448 Markus HS, Thomson ND, Brown MM. Asymptomatic cerebral embolic signals in symptomatic and

asymptomatic carotid artery disease. *Brain* 1995; **118**(Pt 4):1005–11.

449 Van Zuilen EV, Moll FL, Vermeulen FE, Mauser HW, van Gijn J, Ackerstaff RG. Detection of cerebral microemboli by means of transcranial Doppler monitoring before and after carotid endarterectomy. *Stroke* 1995; **26**(2):210–13.

450 Lloyd AJ, Hayes PD, London NJ, Bell PR, Naylor AR. Does carotid endarterectomy lead to a decline in cognitive function or health related quality of life? *J Clin Exp Neuropsychol* 2004; **26**(6):817–25.

451 Bossema ER, Brand N, Moll FL, Ackerstaff RG, van Doornen LJ. Perioperative microembolism is not associated with cognitive outcome three months after carotid endarterectomy. *Eur J Vasc Endovasc Surg* 2005; **29**(3):262–8.

452 Lal BK. Cognitive function after carotid artery revascularization. *Vasc Endovascular Surg* 2007; **41**(1):5–13.

453 Bo M, Massaia M, Speme S, Cappa G, Strumia K, Cerrato P *et al*. Risk of cognitive decline in older patients after carotid endarterectomy: an observational study. *J Am Geriatr Soc* 2006; **54**(6):932–6.

454 Lunn S, Crawley F, Harrison MJ, Brown MM, Newman SP. Impact of carotid endarterectomy upon cognitive functioning. A systematic review of the literature. *Cerebrovasc Dis* 1999; **9**(2):74–81.

455 Schroeder T. Hemodynamic significance of internal carotid artery disease. *Acta Neurol Scand* 1988; **77**(5):353–72.

456 Naylor AR, Merrick MV, Sandercock PA, Gillespie I, Allen P, Griffin TM *et al*. Serial imaging of the carotid bifurcation and cerebrovascular reserve after carotid endarterectomy. *Br J Surg* 1993; **80**(10):1278–82.

457 Yonas H, Smith HA, Durham SR, Pentheny SL, Johnson DW. Increased stroke risk predicted by compromised cerebral blood flow reactivity. *J Neurosurg* 1993; **79**(4):483–9.

458 Hartl WH, Janssen I, Furst H. Effect of carotid endarterectomy on patterns of cerebrovascular reactivity in patients with unilateral carotid artery stenosis. *Stroke* 1994; **25**(10):1952–7.

459 Yamauchi H, Fukuyama H, Nagahama Y, Nabatame H, Nakamura K, Yamamoto Y *et al*. Evidence of misery perfusion and risk for recurrent stroke in major cerebral arterial occlusive diseases from PET. *J Neurol Neurosurg Psychiatry* 1996; **61**(1):18–25.

460 Visser GH, van Huffelen AC, Wieneke GH, Eikelboom BC. Bilateral increase in CO2 reactivity after unilateral carotid endarterectomy. *Stroke* 1997; **28**(5):899–905.

461 Silvestrini M, Vernieri F, Pasqualetti P, Matteis M, Passarelli F, Troisi E *et al*. Impaired cerebral vasoreactivity and risk of stroke in patients with asymptomatic carotid artery stenosis. *J Am Med Assoc* 2000; **283**(16):2122–7.

462 Markus H, Cullinane M. Severely impaired cerebrovascular reactivity predicts stroke and TIA risk in patients with carotid artery stenosis and occlusion. *Brain* 2001; **124**(Pt 3):457–67.

463 Benade MM, Warlow CP. Cost of identifying patients for carotid endarterectomy. *Stroke* 2002; **33**(2):435–9.

464 Benade MM, Warlow CP. Costs and benefits of carotid endarterectomy and associated preoperative arterial imaging: a systematic review of health economic literature. *Stroke* 2002; **33**(2):629–38.

465 Rothwell PM, Eliasziw M, Gutnikov SA, Warlow CP, Barnett HJ. Sex difference in the effect of time from symptoms to surgery on benefit from carotid endarterectomy for transient ischemic attack and nondisabling stroke. *Stroke* 2004; **35**(12):2855–61.

466 Rothwell PM, Eliasziw M, Gutnikov SA, Warlow CP, Barnett HJ. Endarterectomy for symptomatic carotid stenosis in relation to clinical subgroups and timing of surgery. *Lancet* 2004; **363**(9413):915–24.

467 Bond R, Rerkasem K, Cuffe R, Rothwell PM. A systematic review of the associations between age and sex and the operative risks of carotid endarterectomy. *Cerebrovasc Dis* 2005; **20**(2):69–77.

468 Sundt TM, Sandok BA, Whisnant JP. Carotid endarterectomy. Complications and preoperative assessment of risk. *Mayo Clin Proc* 1975; **50**(6):301–6.

469 McCrory DC, Goldstein LB, Samsa GP, Oddone EZ, Landsman PB, Moore WS *et al*. Predicting complications of carotid endarterectomy. *Stroke* 1993; **24**(9):1285–91.

470 Goldstein LB, McCrory DC, Landsman PB, Samsa GP, Ancukiewicz M, Oddone EZ *et al*. Multicenter review of preoperative risk factors for carotid endarterectomy in patients with ipsilateral symptoms. *Stroke* 1994; **25**(6):1116–21.

471 Golledge J, Cuming R, Beattie DK, Davies AH, Greenhalgh RM. Influence of patient-related variables on the outcome of carotid endarterectomy. *J Vasc Surg* 1996; **24**(1):120–6.

472 Rothwell PM, Slattery J, Warlow CP. Clinical and angiographic predictors of stroke and death from carotid endarterectomy: systematic review. *Br Med J* 1997; **315**(7122):1571–7.

473 Pritz MB. Timing of carotid endarterectomy after stroke. *Stroke* 1997; **28**(12):2563–67.

474 Eckstein HH, Schumacher H, Klemm K, Laubach H, Kraus T, Ringleb P *et al*. Emergency carotid endarterectomy. *Cerebrovasc Dis* 1999; **9**(5):270–81.

475 Fairhead JF, Rothwell PM. The need for urgency in identification and treatment of symptomatic carotid stenosis is already established. *Cerebrovasc Dis* 2005; **19**(6):355–8.

476 Blaser T, Hofmann K, Buerger T, Effenberger O, Wallesch CW, Goertler M. Risk of stroke, transient ischemic attack, and vessel occlusion before endarterectomy in patients with symptomatic severe carotid stenosis. *Stroke* 2002; **33**(4):1057–62.

477 Fairhead JF, Mehta Z, Rothwell PM. Population-based study of delays in carotid imaging and surgery and the risk of recurrent stroke. *Neurology* 2005; **65**(3):371–5.

478 Welsh S, Mead G, Chant H, Picton A, O'Neill PA, McCollum CN. Early carotid surgery in acute stroke: a multicentre randomised pilot study. *Cerebrovasc Dis* 2004; **18**(3):200–5.

479 Rantner B, Pavelka M, Posch L, Schmidauer C, Fraedrich G. Carotid endarterectomy after ischemic stroke: is there a justification for delayed surgery? *Eur J Vasc Endovasc Surg* 2005; **30**(1):36–40.

480 Rodgers H, Oliver SE, Dobson R, Thomson RG. A regional collaborative audit of the practice and outcome of carotid endarterectomy in the United Kingdom. Northern Regional Carotid Endarterectomy Audit Group. *Eur J Vasc Endovasc Surg* 2000; **19**(4):362–9.

481 Turnbull RG, Taylor DC, Hsiang YN, Salvian AJ, Nanji S, O'Hanley G *et al*. Assessment of patient waiting times for vascular surgery. *Can J Surg* 2000; **43**(2):105–11.

482 Pell JP, Slack R, Dennis M, Welch G. Improvements in carotid endarterectomy in Scotland: results of a national prospective survey. *Scott Med J* 2004; **49**(2):53–6.

483 Rothwell PM, Warlow CP. Low risk of ischemic stroke in patients with reduced internal carotid artery lumen diameter distal to severe symptomatic carotid stenosis: cerebral protection due to low poststenotic flow? On behalf of the European Carotid Surgery Trialists' Collaborative Group. *Stroke* 2000; **31**(3):622–30.

484 Morgenstern LB, Fox AJ, Sharpe BL, Eliasziw M, Barnett HJ, Grotta JC. The risks and benefits of carotid endarterectomy in patients with near occlusion of the carotid artery. North American Symptomatic Carotid Endarterectomy Trial (NASCET) Group. *Neurology* 1997; **48**(4):911–15.

485 Eliasziw M, Streifler JY, Fox AJ, Hachinski VC, Ferguson GG, Barnett HJ. Significance of plaque ulceration in symptomatic patients with high-grade carotid stenosis. North American Symptomatic Carotid Endarterectomy Trial. *Stroke* 1994; **25**(2):304–8.

486 Rothwell PM, Gibson R, Warlow CP. Interrelation between plaque surface morphology and degree of stenosis on carotid angiograms and the risk of ischemic stroke in patients with symptomatic carotid stenosis. On behalf of the European Carotid Surgery Trialists' Collaborative Group. *Stroke* 2000; **31**(3):615–21.

487 Rothwell PM, Gibson RJ, Slattery J, Sellar RJ, Warlow CP. Equivalence of measurements of carotid stenosis: a comparison of three methods on 1001 angiograms. European Carotid Surgery Trialists' Collaborative Group. *Stroke* 1994; **25**(12):2435–9.

488 Rothwell PM, Gutnikov SA, Warlow CP. Reanalysis of the final results of the European Carotid Surgery Trial. *Stroke* 2003; **34**(2):514–23.

489 Johnston DC, Goldstein LB. Clinical carotid endarterectomy decision making: noninvasive vascular imaging versus angiography. *Neurology* 2001; **56**(8):1009–15.

490 Norris JW, Rothwell PM. Noninvasive carotid imaging to select patients for endarterectomy: is it really safer than conventional angiography? *Neurology* 2001; **56**(8):990–1.

491 Rothwell PM, Pendlebury ST, Wardlaw J, Warlow CP. Critical appraisal of the design and reporting of studies of imaging and measurement of carotid stenosis. *Stroke* 2000; **31**(6):1444–50.

492 Ascher E, Markevich N, Hingorani A, Kallakuri S. Pseudo-occlusions of the internal carotid artery: a rationale for treatment on the basis of a modified carotid duplex scan protocol. *J Vasc Surg* 2002; **35**(2):340–5.

493 Berman SS, Devine JJ, Erdoes LS, Hunter GC. Distinguishing carotid artery pseudo-occlusion with color-flow Doppler. *Stroke* 1995; **26**(3):434–8.

494 Rothwell PM. ACST: which subgroups will benefit most from carotid endarterectomy? *Lancet* 2004; **364**(9440):1122–3.

495 Rothwell PM, Warlow CP. Prediction of benefit from carotid endarterectomy in individual patients: a risk-modelling study. European Carotid Surgery Trialists' Collaborative Group. *Lancet* 1999; **353**(9170):2105–10.

496 Mackinnon AD, Aaslid R, Markus HS. Ambulatory transcranial Doppler cerebral embolic signal detection in symptomatic and asymptomatic carotid stenosis. *Stroke* 2005; **36**(8):1726–30.

497 Molloy J, Markus HS. Asymptomatic embolization predicts stroke and TIA risk in patients with carotid artery stenosis. *Stroke* 1999; **30**(7):1440–3.

498 Mead GE, Lewis SC, Wardlaw JM, Dennis MS, Warlow CP. Severe ipsilateral carotid stenosis and middle cerebral artery disease in lacunar ischaemic stroke: innocent bystanders? *J Neurol* 2002; **249**(3):266–71.

499 Boiten J, Rothwell P, Slattery J, Warlow C, for the European Carotid Surgery Trialists' Collaborative Group. Lacunar stroke in the European Carotid Surgery Trial: risk factos, distribution of carotid stenosis, effect of surgery and type of recurrent stroke. *Cerebrovasc Dis* 1996; **6**:281–7.

500 Inzitari D, Eliasziw M, Sharpe BL, Fox AJ, Barnett HJ. Risk factors and outcome of patients with carotid artery stenosis presenting with lacunar stroke. North American Symptomatic Carotid Endarterectomy Trial Group. *Neurology* 2000; **54**(3):660–6.

501 Chaturvedi S, Bruno A, Feasby T, Holloway R, Benavente O, Cohen SN *et al*. Carotid endarterectomy: an evidence-based review. Report of the Therapeutics and Technology Assessment Subcommittee of the American Academy of Neurology. *Neurology* 2005; **65**(6):794–801.

502 Chambers BR, Donnan GA. Carotid endarterectomy for asymptomatic carotid stenosis. *Cochrane Database Syst Rev* 2005; (4):CD001923.

503 Executive Committee for the Asymptomatic Carotid Atherosclerosis Study. Endarterectomy for asymptomatic carotid artery stenosis. *J Am Med Assoc* 1995; **273**(18):1421–8.

504 Moore WS, Young B, Baker WH, Robertson JT, Toole JF, Vescera CL *et al*. Surgical results: a justification of the surgeon selection process for the ACAS trial. The ACAS Investigators. *J Vasc Surg* 1996; **23**(2):323–8.

505 MRC Asymptomatic Carotid Surgery Trial (ACST) Collaborative Group. Halliday A, Mansfield A, Marro J, Peto C, Peto R, Potter J *et al*. Prevention of disabling and fatal strokes by successful carotid endarterectomy in patients without recent neurological symptoms: randomised controlled trial. *Lancet* 2004; **363**(9420):1491–502.

506 Bond R, Rerkasem K, Rothwell P. High morbidity due to endarterectomy for asymptomatic carotid stenosis. *Cerebrovasc Dis* 2003; **16**(Suppl 4):65.

507 Kresowik TF, Bratzler DW, Kresowik RA, Hendel ME, Grund SL, Brown KR *et al.* Multistate improvement in process and outcomes of carotid endarterectomy. *J Vasc Surg* 2004; **39**(2):372–80.

508 Halliday AW, Thomas D, Mansfield A. The Asymptomatic Carotid Surgery Trial (ACST). Rationale and design. Steering Committee. *Eur J Vasc Surg* 1994; **8**(6):703–10.

509 Cuffe RL, Rothwell PM. Effect of nonoptimal imaging on the relationship between the measured degree of symptomatic carotid stenosis and risk of ischemic stroke. *Stroke* 2006; **37**(7):1785–91.

510 Nicolaides AN, Kakkos SK, Griffin M, Sabetai M, Dhanjil S, Tegos T *et al.* Severity of asymptomatic carotid stenosis and risk of ipsilateral hemispheric ischaemic events: results from the ACSRS study. *Eur J Vasc Endovasc Surg* 2005; **30**(3):275–84.

511 Baker WH, Howard VJ, Howard G, Toole JF. Effect of contralateral occlusion on long-term efficacy of endarterectomy in the asymptomatic carotid atherosclerosis study (ACAS). ACAS Investigators. *Stroke* 2000; **31**(10):2330–4.

512 Spence JD, Tamayo A, Lownie SP, Ng WP, Ferguson GG. Absence of microemboli on transcranial Doppler identifies low-risk patients with asymptomatic carotid stenosis. *Stroke* 2005; **36**(11):2373–8.

513 Abbott AL, Chambers BR, Stork JL, Levi CR, Bladin CF, Donnan GA. Embolic signals and prediction of ipsilateral stroke or transient ischemic attack in asymptomatic carotid stenosis: a multicenter prospective cohort study. *Stroke* 2005; **36**(6):1128–33.

514 Markus H, Cullinane M. Asymptomatic Carotid Emboli (ACES) Study. *Cerebrovasc Dis* 2000; **10**(Suppl 1):3.

515 Gronholdt ML. Ultrasound and lipoproteins as predictors of lipid-rich, rupture-prone plaques in the carotid artery. *Arterioscler Thromb Vasc Biol* 1999; **19**(1):2–13.

516 Nicolaides AN, Kakkos SK, Griffin M, Sabetai M, Dhanjil S, Thomas DJ *et al.* Effect of image normalization on carotid plaque classification and the risk of ipsilateral hemispheric ischemic events: results from the asymptomatic carotid stenosis and risk of stroke study. *Vascular* 2005; **13**(4):211–21.

517 Takaya N, Yuan C, Chu B, Saam T, Underhill H, Cai J *et al.* Association between carotid plaque characteristics and subsequent ischemic cerebrovascular events: a prospective assessment with MRI: initial results. *Stroke* 2006; **37**(3):818–23.

518 Cai J, Hatsukami TS, Ferguson MS, Kerwin WS, Saam T, Chu B *et al.* In vivo quantitative measurement of intact fibrous cap and lipid-rich necrotic core size in atherosclerotic carotid plaque: comparison of high-resolution, contrast-enhanced magnetic resonance imaging and histology. *Circulation* 2005; **112**(22):3437–44.

519 Van der Wal AC, Becker AE, van der Loos CM, Das PK. Site of intimal rupture or erosion of thrombosed coronary atherosclerotic plaques is characterized by an inflammatory process irrespective of the dominant plaque morphology. *Circulation* 1994; **89**(1):36–44.

520 Redgrave JN, Lovett JK, Gallagher PJ, Rothwell PM. Histological assessment of 526 symptomatic carotid plaques in relation to the nature and timing of ischemic symptoms: the Oxford plaque study. *Circulation* 2006; **113**(19):2320–8.

521 Trivedi RA, King-Im JM, Graves MJ, Cross JJ, Horsley J, Goddard MJ *et al.* In vivo detection of macrophages in human carotid atheroma: temporal dependence of ultrasmall superparamagnetic particles of iron oxide-enhanced MRI. *Stroke* 2004; **35**(7):1631–5.

522 Tang T, Howarth SP, Miller SR, Trivedi R, Graves MJ, King-Im JU *et al.* Assessment of inflammatory burden contralateral to the symptomatic carotid stenosis using high-resolution ultrasmall, superparamagnetic iron oxide-enhanced MRI. *Stroke* 2006; **37**(9):2266–70.

523 Dotter CT, Judkins MP, Rosch J. Nonoperative treatment of arterial occlusive disease: a radiologically facilitated technique. *Radiol Clin North Am* 1967; **5**(3):531–42.

524 Mathur A, Roubin GS, Iyer SS, Piamsonboon C, Liu MW, Gomez CR *et al.* Predictors of stroke complicating carotid artery stenting. *Circulation* 1998; **97**(13):1239–45.

525 McCabe DJ, Brown MM, Clifton A. Fatal cerebral reperfusion hemorrhage after carotid stenting. *Stroke* 1999; **30**(11):2483–6.

526 Qureshi AI, Luft AR, Sharma M, Janardhan V, Lopes DK, Khan J *et al.* Frequency and determinants of postprocedural hemodynamic instability after carotid angioplasty and stenting. *Stroke* 1999; **30**(10):2086–93.

527 CAVATAS Investigators. Endovascular versus surgical treatment in patients with carotid stenosis in the Carotid and Vertebral Artery Transluminal Angioplasty Study (CAVATAS): a randomised trial. *Lancet* 2001; **357**:1729–37.

528 Naylor AR, Bolia A, Abbott RJ, Pye IF, Smith J, Lennard N *et al.* Randomized study of carotid angioplasty and stenting versus carotid endarterectomy: a stopped trial. *J Vasc Surg* 1998; **28**(2):326–34.

529 Alberts MJ, for the Publications Committee of the WALLSTENT. Results of a multicentre prospective randomised trial of carotid artery stenting vs carotid endarterectomy. *Stroke* 2001; **32**:325.

530 Brooks WH, McClure RR, Jones MR, Coleman TC, Breathitt L. Carotid angioplasty and stenting versus carotid endarterectomy: randomized trial in a community hospital. *J Am Coll Cardiol* 2001; **38**(6):1589–95.

531 Yadav JS, Wholey MH, Kuntz RE, Fayad P, Katzen BT, Mishkel GJ *et al.* Protected carotid-artery stenting versus endarterectomy in high-risk patients. *N Engl J Med* 2004; **351**(15):1493–501.

532 Coward LJ, Featherstone RL, Brown MM. Safety and eficacy of endovascular treatment of carotid artery stenosis compared with carotid endarterectomy: a Cochrane systematic review of the randomized evidence. *Stroke* 2005; **36**(4):905–11.

533 Reimers B, Corvaja N, Moshiri S, Sacca S, Albiero R, Di Mario C *et al.* Cerebral protection with filter devices during carotid artery stenting. *Circulation* 2001; **104**(1):12–15.

534 Mas JL, Chatellier G, Beyssen B, Branchereau A, Moulin T, Becquemin JP *et al.* Endarterectomy versus stenting in patients with symptomatic severe carotid stenosis. *N Engl J Med* 2006; **355**(16):1660–71.

535 Featherstone RL, Brown MM, Coward LJ. International carotid stenting study: protocol for a randomised clinical trial comparing carotid stenting with endarterectomy in symptomatic carotid artery stenosis. *Cerebrovasc Dis* 2004; **18**(1):69–74.

536 CARESS Steering Committee. Carotid Revascularization Using Endarterectomy or Stenting Systems (CaRESS) phase I clinical trial: 1-year results. *J Vasc Surg* 2005; **42**(2):213–19.

537 Major ongoing stroke trials. *Stroke* 2006; **37**(10):e36–e44.

538 Graor RA, Hetzer NR. Management of coexistent carotid artery and coronary artery disease. *Stroke* 1988; **19**(11):1441–4.

539 Akins CW. The case for concomitant carotid and coronary artery surgery. *Br Heart J* 1995; **74**(2):97–8.

540 Davenport RJ, Dennis MS, Sandercock PA, Warlow CP, Starkey IR, Ruckley CV *et al.* How should a patient presenting with unstable angina and a recent stroke be managed? *Br Med J* 1995; **310**(6992):1449–52.

541 Hertzer NR, Loop FD, Beven EG, O'Hara PJ, Krajewski LP. Surgical staging for simultaneous coronary and carotid disease: a study including prospective randomization. *J Vasc Surg* 1989; **9**(3):455–63.

542 Borger MA, Fremes SE, Weisel RD, Cohen G, Rao V, Lindsay TF *et al.* Coronary bypass and carotid endarterectomy: does a combined approach increase risk? a meta-analysis. *Ann Thorac Surg* 1999; **68**(1):14–20.

543 Naylor AR, Mehta Z, Rothwell PM, Bell PR. Carotid artery disease and stroke during coronary artery bypass: a critical review of the literature. *Eur J Vasc Endovasc Surg* 2002; **23**(4):283–94.

544 Naylor AR, Cuffe RL, Rothwell PM, Bell PR. A systematic review of outcomes following staged and synchronous carotid endarterectomy and coronary artery bypass. *Eur J Vasc Endovasc Surg* 2003; **25**(5):380–9.

545 Naylor AR. A critical review of the role of carotid disease and the outcomes of staged and synchronous carotid surgery. *Semin Cardiothorac Vasc Anesth* 2004; **8**(1):37–42.

546 Latchaw RE, Ausman JI, Lee MC. Superficial temporal-middle cerebral artery bypass. A detailed analysis of multiple pre- and postoperative angiograms in 40 consecutive patients. *J Neurosurg* 1979; **51**(4):455–65.

547 Hankey GJ, Warlow C. Prognosis of symptomatic carotid artery occlusion: an overview. *Cerebrovasc Dis* 1991; **1**:245–56.

548 Karnik R, Valentin A, Ammerer HP, Donath P, Slany J. Evaluation of vasomotor reactivity by transcranial Doppler and acetazolamide test before and after extracranial-intracranial bypass in patients with internal carotid artery occlusion. *Stroke* 1992; **23**(6):812–17.

549 Klijn CJ, Kappelle LJ, Tulleken CA, van Gijn J. Symptomatic carotid artery occlusion. A reappraisal of hemodynamic factors. *Stroke* 1997; **28**(10):2084–93.

550 Powers WJ, Derdeyn CP, Fritsch SM, Carpenter DA, Yundt KD, Videen TO *et al.* Benign prognosis of never-symptomatic carotid occlusion. *Neurology* 2000; **54**(4):878–82.

551 EC-IC Bypass Study Group. Failure of extracranial-intracranial arterial bypass to reduce the risk of ischaemic stroke: results of an international randomised trial. *N Engl J Med* 1985; **313**:1191–200.

552 Warlow CP. Extracranial to intracranial bypass and the prevention of stroke. *J Neurol* 1986; **233**(3):129–30.

553 Derdeyn CP, Grubb RL, Jr., Powers WJ. Indications for cerebral revascularization for patients with atherosclerotic carotid occlusion. *Skull Base* 2005; **15**(1):7–14.

554 Grubb RL, Jr., Powers WJ, Derdeyn CP, Adams HP, Jr., Clarke WR. The Carotid Occlusion Surgery Study. *Neurosurg Focus* 2003; **14**(3):e9.

555 Eberhardt O, Naegele T, Raygrotzki S, Weller M, Ernemann U. Stenting of vertebrobasilar arteries in symptomatic atherosclerotic disease and acute occlusion: case series and review of the literature. *J Vasc Surg* 2006; **43**(6):1145–54.

556 Cloud GC, Crawley F, Clifton A, McCabe DJ, Brown MM, Markus HS. Vertebral artery origin angioplasty and primary stenting: safety and restenosis rates in a prospective series. *J Neurol Neurosurg Psychiatry* 2003; **74**(5):586–90.

557 Coward LJ, Featherstone RL, Brown MM. Percutaneous transluminal angioplasty and stenting for vertebral artery stenosis. *Cochrane Database Syst Rev* 2005; (2):CD000516.

558 Osterberg L, Blaschke T. Adherence to medication. *N Engl J Med* 2005; **353**(5):487–97.

559 Benner JS, Glynn RJ, Mogun H, Neumann PJ, Weinstein MC, Avorn J. Long-term persistence in use of statin therapy in elderly patients. *J Am Med Assoc* 2002; **288**(4):455–61.

560 Jackevicius CA, Mamdani M, Tu JV. Adherence with statin therapy in elderly patients with and without acute coronary syndromes. *J Am Med Assoc* 2002; **288**(4):462–7.

561 Trewby PN, Reddy AV, Trewby CS, Ashton VJ, Brennan G, Inglis J. Are preventive drugs preventive enough? A study of patients' expectation of benefit from preventive drugs. *Clin Med* 2002; **2**(6):527–33.

562 Hamman GF, Weimar C, Glahn J, Busse O, Diener HC. Adherence to secondary stroke prevention strategies: results from the German Stroke Data Bank. *Cerebrovasc Dis* 2003; **15**(4):282–8.

563 Haynes RB, Yao X, Degani A, Kripalani S, Garg A, McDonald HP. Interventions to enhance medication adherence. *Cochrane Database Syst Rev* 2005; (4):CD000011.

564 Gigerenzer G, Edwards A. Simple tools for understanding risks: from innumeracy to insight. *Br Med J* 2003; **327**(7417):741–4.

565 Edwards A, Elwyn G, Mulley A. Explaining risks: turning numerical data into meaningful pictures. *Br Med J* 2002; **324**(7341):827–30.

566 Alaszewski A, Horlick-Jones T. How can doctors communicate information about risk more effectively? *Br Med J* 2003; **327**(7417):728–31.

567 Fuller R, Dudley N, Blacktop J. Avoidance hierarchies and preferences for anticoagulation: semi-qualitative analysis of older patients' views about stroke prevention and the use of warfarin. *Age Ageing* 2004; **33**(6):608–11.

568 Zhan C, Correa-de-Araujo R, Bierman AS, Sangl J, Miller MR, Wickizer SW *et al*. Suboptimal prescribing in elderly outpatients: potentially harmful drug-drug and drug-disease combinations. *J Am Geriatr Soc* 2005; **53**(2):262–7.

569 White C. 'Polypill' to fight cardiovascular disease. Summary of rapid responses. *Br Med J* 2003; **327**:809.

570 Wald NJ, Law MR. A strategy to reduce cardiovascular disease by more than 80%. *Br Med J* 2003; **326**(7404):1419.

571 Zarins CK, Gewertz BL. *Atlas of Vascular Surgery*. New York: Churchill Livingstone, 1987.

572 Schroeder T, Levi N. What steps can I take to minimise inadvertent cranial nerve injury. In: Naylor AR, Mackey AE, eds. *Carotid Artery Surgery: A Problem Based Approach*. London: Saunders, 1999.

573 The European Carotid Surgery Trialists Collaborative Group. Risk of stroke in the distribution of an asymptomatic carotid artery. *Lancet* 1995; **345**(8944):209–12.

17 The organization of stroke services

17.1 Introduction

17.1.1 The impact of stroke

Governments, and in particular those responsible for providing healthcare, have become increasingly aware of the impact that stroke has on the health of the population and the cost to the community. In the UK, stroke patients account for about 6% of hospital costs and almost 5% of National Health Service costs[1] (www.nao.org.uk/stroke). Studies from other countries (e.g. Sweden, US, Canada, Netherlands and Japan) suggest that the financial burden may be even greater than in the UK, possibly because of greater expenditure on all health services.[2–11] Moreover, demographic changes are likely to cause increasing mortality and morbidity in the developing world.[12]

Stroke: practical management, 3rd edition. C. Warlow, J. van Gijn, M. Dennis, J. Wardlaw, J. Bamford, G. Hankey, P. Sandercock, G. Rinkel, P. Langhorne, C. Sudlow and P. Rothwell. Published 2008 Blackwell Publishing. ISBN 978-1-4051-2766-0.

Relatively little attention was paid to stroke in the UK until the publication of the King's Fund Consensus Conference[13] in 1988. This highlighted the many deficiencies in the services provided for stroke patients, concluding that 'services were often haphazard and poorly tailored to the patient's needs'. Since then, in the UK, stroke has moved up the political agenda, and was identified as a key chapter in the *National Service Framework for Older People in England and Wales* (www.dh.gov.uk/PolicyAndGuidance/HealthAndSocial CareTopics/OlderPeoplesServices) and the Coronary Heart Disease and Stroke strategy in Scotland (www. scotland.gov.uk/library5/health/chds). There has been a similar and continuing emphasis on stroke in many other countries. These changes have led to a tremendous surge of interest in stroke in general, and in stroke services in particular. Over the last few years, an increasing amount of research has been done to determine the best and most cost-effective ways of providing care for stroke patients.

This chapter will cover the organization of services for people who have had a transient ischaemic attack or stroke. Inevitably, the discussion will tend to reflect the UK – and to some extent other North European and

Australian – models of care, but we hope it will have relevance for services elsewhere.

17.1.2 Aims of stroke services

The overall aim of stroke services is to deliver the care required by patients and their families in the most efficient, effective, equitable and humane manner possible. Such services may not necessarily be stroke-specific; they could be part of those for internal medicine, care of the elderly, neurology, rehabilitation or continuing care.

Good organization is probably the most important factor in determining service effectiveness. When considering exactly how stroke services should best be organized, it is useful to consider the main objectives when caring for patients with stroke and transient ischaemic attack (TIA) (Table 17.1 and Fig. 17.1). In addition, given the lack of evidence for many of our interventions, services should facilitate research and education. We have not included primary prevention among the components of care, although this is potentially the most effective method of reducing stroke-related death, disability and handicap, at least in the long term (Chapter 18). Primary stroke prevention has so much in common with the prevention of other vascular diseases that it makes more sense to link these preventive services together, especially as their success is likely to depend more on political and social change than on health services.

Table 17.1 Key components for managing stroke and transient ischaemic attack.

Public awareness to recognize warning signs and seek help promptly (section 17.5.1)
Prompt and accurate assessment and diagnosis (including transportation) (Chapter 3)
Specific acute medical and surgical treatment (Chapters 11, 12, 13, 14 and 15)
Identification and assessment of patients' problems (chapter 11)
Secondary prevention of further vascular events (Chapter 16)
General care, including interventions to resolve problems (includes many aspects of rehabilitation) (Chapter 11)
Provision of information and advice (section 17.10.1)
Terminal care for patients who are unlikely to survive (section 10.4)
Hospital discharge and reintegration into the community (section 17.7)
Continuing or long-term care for severely disabled patients (section 17.8)
Follow-up to detect and manage late-onset problems (section 17.9)

17.1.3 Establishing the effectiveness of stroke services

In an ideal world our decisions about the delivery of stroke services would always be informed by robust evidence from randomized trials and priority given to those aspects of care that have been proven to be effective. However, we must recognize that carrying out randomized trials of complex interventions such as stroke services is challenging[14] and these trials are often few in number and difficult to interpret. There is no reason why most of the important methodological principles (www.cochrane.org/resources/handbook) of robust clinical trials (random treatment allocation, concealment of treatment allocation, blinding of follow-up, intention-to-treat analyses) should not apply to those of stroke services. However, randomized trials of complex interventions such as stroke services offer some unique challenges. In particular it is often difficult to develop and describe the intervention adequately, to blind the trial participants to their treatment and to rule out confounding from other aspects of care. Therefore even if a service is shown to work well in one setting, specific local factors may have influenced the results. For these reasons we have approached the evaluation of stroke services in the following way:

- Has the service component been shown to work in a specific circumstance (in one randomized trial)?
- Has it been shown to work in several settings (systematic review of clinical trials)?
- Do we know if the benefits justify the costs (economic analyses)?

The Stroke Review Group of the Cochrane Collaboration is an excellent source of this type of information, providing an increasing number of systematic reviews (http://www.dcn.ed.ac.uk/csrg).

It is important that those who are responsible for planning services should be aware of all the available evidence concerning the effectiveness of interventions, and the methods of delivering these interventions to the appropriate patients. However, often we will not have any reliable evidence from randomized trials to guide our decisions simply because of the methodological challenges outlined above. Planners should be aware that lack of evidence of benefit is not the same as evidence of lack of benefit. If there are reliable data concerning the cost of interventions, and various other aspects of the service, this may allow healthcare planners to make more informed choices about which services should be provided. At the same time, they should not deny patients services which are generally accepted as being effective just because of lack of randomized trial evidence.

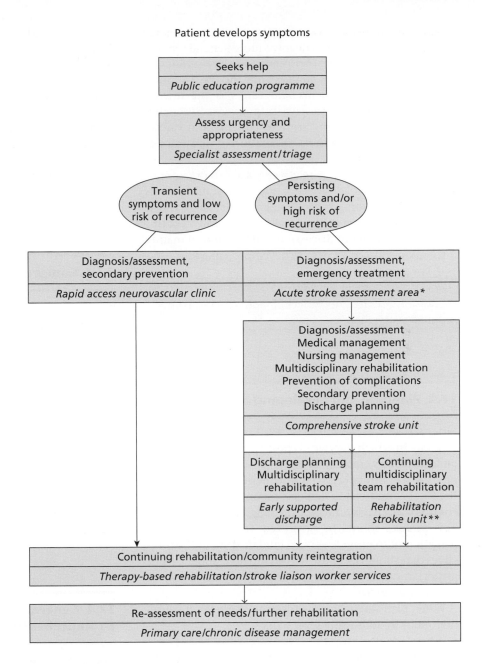

Patient develops symptoms

| Seeks help |
| *Public education programme* |

| Assess urgency and appropriateness |
| *Specialist assessment/triage* |

Transient symptoms and low risk of recurrence

Persisting symptoms and/or high risk of recurrence

| Diagnosis/assessment, secondary prevention |
| *Rapid access neurovascular clinic* |

| Diagnosis/assessment, emergency treatment |
| *Acute stroke assessment area** |

| Diagnosis/assessment |
| Medical management |
| Nursing management |
| Multidisciplinary rehabilitation |
| Prevention of complications |
| Secondary prevention |
| Discharge planning |
| *Comprehensive stroke unit* |

| Discharge planning Multidisciplinary rehabilitation | Continuing multidisciplinary team rehabilitation |
| *Early supported discharge* | *Rehabilitation stroke unit*** |

| Continuing rehabilitation/community reintegration |
| *Therapy-based rehabilitation/stroke liaison worker services* |

| Re-assessment of needs/further rehabilitation |
| *Primary care/chronic disease management* |

Fig. 17.1 A diagram illustrating the components, functions and interrelationships of a hospital-based stroke service that is integrated with community services. The upper box indicates the objectives of the services and the lower (purple) boxes (*in italics*) a proposed solution. We believe that elements of the rehabilitation process are important even on the day of the stroke onset. *Could be in stroke unit or stroke centre. **Could continue in comprehensive stroke unit.

> Clinical trials of services can be complex and challenging – remember that lack of evidence of benefit is not the same as evidence of lack of benefit.

17.1.4 Pressures that may shape stroke services

Several factors other than evidence of effectiveness or cost-effectiveness may shape stroke service delivery and constrain the options available to clinicians and service planners. These can include:

- *Local healthcare culture and economy*: the traditional approach to providing healthcare, and the way it is funded or reimbursed, will influence the way services

are delivered. Developing a stroke service in the US or Germany would present different challenges from doing so in Scandinavia, the Netherlands or the UK. There are likely to be particular challenges in the former Soviet bloc countries and the developing world where many basic assumptions about the availability of healthcare resources may simply not apply.

- *Needs of different patient groups*: stroke presents a complex challenge to service planners in that most patients require a similar general service but a small number (for instance those with subarachnoid haemorrhage or those eligible for intravenous thrombolysis) may require more specialist services. There is frequently a tension between the need to centralize specialist services for the few and the need to devolve more general services for the majority to local hospitals and communities.

- *Views of patients and families*: one of the common complaints from patients and carers is the discontinuity of services they receive (http://www.chss.org.uk/pdf/research/Improving_services_patients_and_carers_views.pdf), resulting in fragmentation of care and dissatisfaction with services.
- *Resources available*: it is relatively easier to organize or reorganize a stroke service if the basic staffing levels and investigation services are already available, albeit distributed around the hospital or community. For this reason much of our discussion will be relevant mainly to well-resourced services in developed countries.

> Local stroke services must be tailored to local conditions; there is no perfect blueprint that can be applied everywhere.

17.2 Planning and developing a stroke service

The way in which a service is best provided will depend on local history, geography, needs, resources, people and politics. Any stroke service must therefore be tailored to the local conditions to achieve maximum effectiveness. For this reason, it is difficult to be dogmatic about exactly how services should be organized. In this chapter we will attempt to provide general guidance about the principles that should be of use to the clinician, public health physician or health service manager (administrator) in planning a service.

When planning or reviewing stroke services, it is useful to start by addressing several questions:

- Where do we want to be (sections 17.5–17.9)? What is the evidence for the effectiveness (and cost-effectiveness) of the components of both the existing and planned stroke service?
- Where are we now (sections 17.11)? What are the needs of the population to be served by the stroke service and what are the *current* resources, people and facilities committed to the management of patients with TIAs and stroke?
- How will we get to where we want to be (section 17.12)? What are the major gaps in the present provision of services (i.e. unmet needs and failure to provide effective interventions)? What resources, people and facilities will be required to meet the needs of the population? Assuming that resources are limited, to what extent

can the needs of the population realistically be met? How should these resources best be organized?

- How do we know if we have succeeded (section 17.12)? How can the performance of the stroke services be monitored and maintained?

In this chapter we will begin (sections 17.3–17.10) with a review of the effectiveness (and where possible cost-effectiveness) of components of stroke services. In the second part (sections 17.11–17.16) we will discuss practical approaches to planning, developing, monitoring and maintaining a stroke service.

17.3 Comprehensive stroke service

We have used the term 'comprehensive stroke service' to mean a stroke service that covers most of the needs of patients with stroke or transient ischaemic attack (TIA) and which is integrated in a way that provides a continuous patient journey – 'a seamless service' (Table 17.2 and Fig. 17.1). In doing so it should provide all of the functions outlined in Table 17.1. Figure 17.1 outlines what we believe to be important components of a comprehensive stroke service, and in this chapter we will discuss the evidence and rationale for some of those suggestions.

> A comprehensive stroke service should provide for most of the needs of most patients and do so within a 'seamless service'.

17.4 General principles when discussing a comprehensive stroke service

When proposing various approaches to service delivery – and suggesting particular components of a comprehensive stroke service – we have tried to employ some general principles:

- Basic needs first – stroke services should first ensure they provide basic care (from medical, nursing and therapy staff) for all stroke patients and their families.
- Evidence-based options – priority should be given to those aspects of care that are generally accepted as being, or have been proven to be, effective. The Stroke Review Group of the Cochrane Collaboration is an excellent source of this type of information (http://www.dcn.ed.ac.uk/csrg).

Table 17.2 Key objectives and service solutions for managing patients with stroke and transient ischaemic attack.

Objectives	Proposed service options	Cross-reference
Public awareness to recognize warning symptoms and seek help promptly	Public education campaigns	section 17.5.1
Prompt and accurate assessment and diagnosis	Transport (ambulance and helicopter) protocols	sections 17.5.2, 17.5.3, 17.5.4
	Emergency department and hospital protocols	section 17.5.6, 17.5.7
	Designated stroke centres	
	Telemedicine networks	
	Rapid access TIA clinics	
Specific acute medical and surgical treatment	Designated stroke centres	sections 17.5.5, 17.5.6, 17.6
	Telemedicine networks	chapters 12, 13, 14
	Stroke units	
Identification and assessment of patients' problems	Designated stroke centres	sections 17.5.5, 17.5.6, 17.6
	Telemedicine networks	
	Stroke units	
Secondary prevention of further vascular events	Stroke units	sections 17.5.5, 17.5.6, 17.6
	Designated stroke centres	chapter 16
	Rapid access TIA clinics	
General care, including interventions to resolve problems (includes many aspects of rehabilitation)	Stroke units	section 17.6
		chapter 10
Terminal care for patients who are unlikely to survive	Stroke units	section 17.6
		section 10.4
Hospital discharge and reintegration into the community	Early supported discharge services	section 17.7
	Discharge planning	
Continuing or long-term care for severely disabled patients	Therapy-based rehabilitation services	section 17.8
	Stroke liaison worker services	
Follow-up to detect and manage late-onset problems	Chronic disease management	section 17.9
	Outpatient clinics	

- Patient and carer views – surveys of the views of patients and carers have frequently highlighted a wish that care is coordinated and provided by expert staff. A survey of user views in Scotland (http://www.chss.org.uk/pdf/research/Improving_services_patients_and_carers_views.pdf) highlighted five main themes:
  - care should be provided in designated stroke units;
  - staff should be trained in the physical and emotional needs of stroke patients;
  - comprehensive information should be available to all patients and carers;
  - trained liaison staff should help with patients returning home;
  - there should be access to 'someone to talk to' (someone who understands the challenges that patients and their carers face).
- Awareness of alternatives – where possible we have tried to acknowledge that there may be valid alternative approaches to achieving the same objective. However, frequently there is no research evidence to help make such decisions about the best service option.

- Level of development – most of our discussion reflects experience from developed western economies. It is at present difficult to give specific advice for other healthcare settings although many of the general principles above will apply.

17.4.1 Why refer stroke and transient ischaemic attack patients to hospital?

Before discussing each service component in turn we also need to consider why we have emphasized a system of hospital-based rather than community-based services (at least during the earlier phase of the illness).

The vast majority of patients who have a stroke or TIA have it in the community and not in hospital. Community-based incidence studies have shown wide variations in hospital admission rates for stroke, varying from 55% in Oxfordshire, UK, in the 1980s to over 95% in Sweden and Germany in the 1990s.[15–17] The main reason for admission to hospital in the past was for nursing care rather than diagnosis and treatment.[15] However, the need for early imaging to establish whether a stroke is ischaemic or haemorrhagic has now become accepted and immediate imaging appears to be the most cost-effective option.[18] The potential for early intervention to limit brain damage and prevent stroke recurrence[19–21] is increasingly being recognized (Chapters 12, 16). Finally there are a small number of comparisons (in clinical trials) of a conventional policy of admitting most patients to hospital with a policy of avoiding admission by providing a rapid-response service in the community to support patients in their own homes. Although the evidence is limited,[22,23] major practical problems were identified with the policy of hospital avoidance[23,24] and clinical outcomes were best in those admitted directly to a stroke unit.

Transient events, transient ischaemic attacks (TIAs) and episodes that may be confused with them (Table 17.3)

Table 17.3 Some of the non-cerebrovascular problems referred to one of our neurovascular clinics by general practitioners over a period of 5 years. There were, of course, countless patients with transient symptoms in whom no definite diagnosis could be made.

General medical problems
Cardiac syncope (dysrhythmias, aortic stenosis)
Vasovagal syncope
Cough syncope
Postural hypotension
Hyperventilation
Sleep apnoea
Hypoglycaemia
Neurological problems
Migraine (both with and without headache)
Epilepsy
Transient global amnesia
Glioma
Meningioma
Cerebral metastases
Subdural haematoma
Lymphocytic meningitis
Peripheral neuropathy
Guillain–Barré syndrome
Cervical myelopathy
Brachial neuritis
Mononeuropathies
Herpes zoster neuropathy
Bell's palsy
Syringobulbia
Myasthenia gravis
Multiple sclerosis
Motor neurone disease
Creutzfelt–Jakob disease
Psychiatric problems
Somatization disorder
Ophthalmic problems
Retinal vein occlusion
Glaucoma

are less reliably diagnosed than strokes and more often require input from a specialist, especially when the diagnosis is crucial to future decision-making – for example, in distinguishing between carotid and posterior circulation TIAs in a patient with severe carotid stenosis (section 4.3.1) (Table 4.3). Thus, referral to hospital for assessment, even if only as an outpatient, is the accepted norm for such patients.

17.4.2 Who may not need hospital admission?

In view of the above discussions, can we identify a group of individuals who do not need hospital admission after stroke or TIA? In the absence of direct evidence from randomized trials comparing different policies of care, we can only base our decisions on a logical rationale. Hospital admission appears to be valuable for rapid diagnosis and assessment, prompt acute treatment and secondary prevention plus effective early multidisciplinary rehabilitation.[25] We would therefore suggest that the following groups may be able to be managed without hospital admission:

- For people with a TIA who are at low risk of early recurrence, early assessment at a one-stop neurovascular outpatient clinic[61,62] could be justified providing we can reliably identify them (section 16.2).
- People with a stroke who are at low risk of early recurrence or other complications such as neurological deterioration (section 16.2); once again this requires accurate identification of low-risk individuals. In practice, predicting neurological deterioration and other complications is difficult so this group is likely to include only those individuals who have delayed referral for several days and so are past the higher-risk period for developing problems.
- People who refuse hospital admission; rapid assessment at a one-stop neurovascular clinic may be very appropriate for this group.

17.4.3 Why is rapid specialist assessment and treatment necessary?

Rapid specialist assessment of patients experiencing symptoms of acute stroke or TIA can only really be justified if that assessment improves patient outcomes (including 'softer' outcomes such as reassurance and advice). The arguments in favour of rapid assessment have been made for both acute stroke and TIA patients:

- Thrombolysis for acute stroke has been licensed for several years in US and has had a restricted licence in Europe since 2003. However, thrombolysis has not had the impact many of its supporters would have expected. First, it is a complex intervention requiring intensive use of resources and personnel with a narrow therapeutic window. Current product licences restrict its use to within 3 h of symptom onset. This requires very rapid specialist assessment ensuring accurate diagnosis of ischaemic stroke prior to the initiation of treatment. In doing so, one needs to demonstrate the absence of haemorrhage on brain scanning, good blood pressure control, National Institute of Health stroke scale (NIHSS) score of greater than 4, and an exclusion of patients at high risk of bleeding with thrombolytic therapy. Treatment must be given within 3 h of symptom onset and the earlier that treatment is given the better the outcome (section 12.5). Initial enthusiasm in the US resulted in a large number of centres commencing acute treatment with recombinant tissue plasminogen activator (rt-PA). However, this demonstrated the very significant hazards of thrombolysis when implementation is poorly controlled. Haemorrhage rates as high as 16% were experienced and this high risk was closely correlated with violations of treatment protocols.[26] The implementation of a stroke quality improvement programme was associated with a reduced rate of protocol deviation and symptomatic intracranial haemorrhage. As a result of these experiences, pressure groups such as the Brain Attack Coalition have proposed criteria for designation of stroke centres that are permitted to provide treatment with rt-PA.[27]

- Patients with intracerebral haemorrhage may benefit from early treatment with recombinant factor VII,[28] although, at the time of writing, the treatment is not licensed for this use (section 13.3.1).

- Recent epidemiological studies suggest that similar issues may arise with the rapid diagnosis and treatment of patients with TIA or mild stroke.[29,30] The risk of very early recurrence of cerebrovascular events appears to be much greater than was previously thought (approximately 10% in the first week and up to 20% in the first month; section 16.2.1) emphasizing the importance of very early diagnostic assessment and prevention. More recently, systems of identifying very high-risk individuals have been reported based on the presenting clinical features[21,31] or MRI findings.[32] The underlying assumption is that identifying individuals at high risk of recurrent stroke or TIA will lead to effective prevention of these recurrent events. Although this remains uncertain for drug treatments, there is good evidence that very early carotid endarterectomy (within 2 weeks) is not associated with an increased operative risk and results in improved stroke prevention (section 16.11.8).[33,34] Furthermore there is no convincing argument for delaying the implementation of other secondary prevention treatments beyond the first few days post-stroke. Randomized trials of very early secondary prevention are currently under way.

17.4.4 Barriers to rapid assessment and treatment

If we accept that rapid specialist assessment and treatment is worthwhile – at least for a proportion of stroke and TIA patients – we then need to consider how best to achieve this (Table 17.4). A recent systematic review of 54 observational studies examining the barriers to

Table 17.4 Potential barriers to rapid specialist assessment and treatment, and interventions aiming to overcome them.

	Potential barriers	Proposed solutions which have been associated with some improvements in observational studies	
recognition	Failure of the patient or family to recognize symptoms of stroke or to seek urgent help	Public education programmes (section 17.5.1)	Centralized Brain Attack Centre initiatives (designated stroke centres) (section 17.5.5)
react	Failure of public and primary care medical services to recognize stroke as an emergency	Education programmes for the public and primary care services (section 17.5.1)	
response	Failure of ambulance and emergency medical services to treat stroke as a medical emergency	Training of paramedics and emergency medical services; rapid transport systems (section 17.5.2)	
reveal	Delays in diagnostic assessment (particularly brain imaging)	Training of emergency department staff and redesign of hospital systems (section 17.5.3)	Telemedicine networks (to facilitate remote specialist assessment and management) (section 17.5.6)
reperfusion	Delays in delivery of acute drug therapy (where appropriate) including physician's uncertainty	Centralization of expertise (designated stroke centre) (section 17.5.5)	

delivery of thrombolysis in acute stroke is also relevant when considering the barriers to more comprehensive stroke assessment and treatment, including transient ischaemic attacks.[35]

Barriers included:

- failure of the patient or family to recognize symptoms of stroke or to seek urgent help;
- initially seeking help from the general practitioner rather than calling an ambulance;
- paramedical and emergency department staff triage stroke as non-urgent;
- delays in obtaining brain imaging;
- inefficient processes of in-hospital emergency stroke care;
- difficulties in obtaining consent for treatment (thrombolysis);
- physician uncertainty of administering treatment (thrombolysis).

These potential barriers operate right across the initial patient pathway and a range of solutions is likely to be required if acute treatments are to be provided efficiently and equitably.

17.5 Interventions to improve access to early specialist assessment and treatment

When considering the necessary components to overcome the barriers to early assessment and treatment, researchers have developed a checklist (based on the 'five Rs') to describe the key stages:

- recognition of symptoms;
- reaction to the acute illness;
- response of emergency services;
- revealing the diagnosis;
- reperfusion therapy.

We can use this scheme to consider the potential solutions to these barriers. When you take this approach (Table 17.4), it is striking that there is often no really reliable evidence for particular components of the early patient journey, and that many of the interventions that have been tested have overlapping roles.

17.5.1 Public education programmes

One of the most consistently reported prehospital barriers to acute stroke assessment and treatment is that patients or families have a poor knowledge of stroke. Poor awareness of stroke symptoms[36] and a failure to recognize their seriousness[37] often delays the request for urgent medical help.[38] Even with adequate knowledge the public has to be convinced that it is appropriate to call emergency services, not primary care services which so often leads to delays in management (see below). A number of suggestions have been made for public education programmes to increase the knowledge of stroke symptoms[39,40] in the hope that they would reduce delays and so improve treatment rates with thrombolysis, and any other new emerging acute stroke treatments. However, experience in acute myocardial infarction has raised concerns about the effectiveness of media campaigns.[41] Furthermore, even where people have appropriate knowledge this may not translate into action; patients in the Asymptomatic Carotid Atherosclerosis Study[42] showed delays in reporting stroke symptoms despite receiving targeted education. Finally, the symptoms transmitted to the public in education campaigns are non-specific and identification and immediate action by the public could result in a large increase in the number of non-stroke patients reporting to emergency departments.

Only one controlled clinical trial[43] has evaluated a community education programme by comparing two communities. In the 'intervention community' the programme targeted 'at risk' members of the public, emergency medical services, emergency department physicians, neurologists and primary care providers, a higher priority for the transport of acute stroke patients by the emergency medical services. The control community did not receive these interventions. The proportion of eligible patients treated with rt-PA appeared to be greater in the intervention community and there was also a non-significant increase in the proportion of patients presenting within 2 h of symptom onset (Table 17.5). There were also reductions in within-hospital delays and in the reluctance of physicians to give rt-PA. The observed gains were relatively modest and we still need more robust evidence from properly randomized trials. Although public education programmes are likely to be important, they may have only a relatively modest impact on speedy referral rates.

17.5.2 Transport protocols (prehospital assessment and transport)

The next stage in the chain of referral is the rapid response of ambulance and emergency medical services to treat stroke as a medical emergency. There are no randomized trials of this approach but observational studies have described the use of rapid recognition instruments[44,45] to allow paramedical staff to triage patients with suspected stroke. These instruments appear to have acceptable diagnostic accuracy but the their impact on

Table 17.5 Interventions aiming to facilitate rapid access to specialist assessment and treatment in acute stroke.

Intervention:	Education programmes for the public and primary care services	Training of paramedics and emergency medical services; rapid transport systems	Training of emergency department staff and redesign of hospital systems	Designated stroke centres (public education, rapid transport, emergency department training, hospital system redesign)	Telemedicine networks (networks between sites including local staff training)
Country:	USA	UK, USA	USA, Germany	USA, Canada, Germany	USA, Germany
Main observations:	Increase in proportion of people presenting early with symptoms of suspected stroke	Acceptable diagnostic accuracy of ambulance staff in identifying stroke patients	Reduction in hospital delays and door-to-needle times	Reduced delays both prehospital and within hospital	Telemedicine approach feasible and acceptable Modest increases in consultation time (of 6–14 min)
Absolute increase in rt-PA use*:	5%	NA	9%	4–17%	2–20%
Post-intervention rt-PA use	6%	21% (in selected helicopter transport patients)	11%	4–22%	2–25%
References:	43	45,183,184	185	185,186	55,56

Summary of the findings of a range of studies describing changes in the chain of referral and treatment of acute stroke patients. None of these were randomized controlled trials.
*% delivery after intervention minus % delivery before.
rt-PA recombinant tissue plasminogen activator; NA, no data available.

patient outcomes is unknown. Furthermore, the implementation and evaluation of ambulance protocols has often been included in an assessment of wider service changes (e.g. implementation of public education programmes and establishment of stroke centres).

Helicopter transport appears to be a feasible transport option (Table 17.5) and there are claims that it can be cost-effective.[46] However, it is notable that even in reports of helicopter transport of highly selected patients only a minority transported this way actually received rt-PA.

17.5.3 Emergency department protocols

Many enthusiasts have advocated hospital acute 'stroke teams' to increase the proportion of patients who are eligible to receive thrombolytic therapy. Once again, there are no randomized trials of such strategies, although several observational studies have been described (Table 17.5). In general, these studies indicate that the protocols were associated with reduced time delays within the emergency department, particularly if backed up with educational programmes and rapid access to appropriate expert advice. However, it is also clear that

these are complex systems and frequently other changes were also made (e.g. moving CT scanning and near-patient biochemistry testing to within the emergency department) which may have influenced the outcome.

17.5.4 Coordination of services

One of the major challenges with any of the initiatives outlined above is how to coordinate them within the broader picture of delivering stroke care, in particular, the need to be able to access expert advice and diagnostic imaging within a very short time. In general, two approaches appear to have been applied to try and tackle this problem:

- designated stroke centres, a centralized approach where patients are transported to a single centre ('hub' model);
- telemedicine networks emphasizing a network of expert advice usually delivered from some form of specialized centre using teleconferencing technology ('hub and spoke' model).

We shall consider in turn the rationale and evidence for these different approaches.

17.5.5 Designated stroke centres

Following reports from the USA that without careful control of thrombolytic management, there is a high risk of protocol violations and treatment complications,[26] stroke quality improvement programmes have been developed. These were associated with a fall in protocol deviations from 50% to 19% and in symptomatic haemorrhage from 16% to 6%. As a result of this and other experience, the Brain Attack Coalition (a group with representatives from major professional and advocacy organizations involved in stroke care in the US) suggested criteria for the designation of stroke centres:[27,47]

- acute stroke teams;
- stroke units or teams;
- written care protocols;
- integrated emergency response systems;
- support services (in particular, the availability and interpretation of CT scans and rapid laboratory testing).

However, critics[48] have commented that the establishment of stroke units was not given emphasis in the Brain Attack Coalition recommendations. Stroke units, for which there exists substantial randomized trial evidence and which are seen as central to the Helsingborg Declaration (with the target that organized stroke unit care should be available for all patients by the year 2005), were not considered an absolute requirement for primary stroke centres. By contrast, acute stroke teams, which lack evidence of effectiveness,[49] were included among the key elements. In hospital surveys in the US,[50,51] stroke units were established in only a minority of centres. Similarly, limited access to stroke units was also seen in Canada and Australia.[52,53] Because stroke unit care is applicable to all patients, the overall impact on outcome is likely to be considerably greater than that of tissue plasminogen activator – there is much more to acute stroke care than thrombolysis.

There are no randomized or controlled clinical trials evaluating designated stroke centres. However, four prospective observational studies (Table 17.5) have reported improvements associated with establishing a stroke centre. The establishment of such centres was complex but included:

- forming a 'brain attack' team;
- establishing a care pathway (based on the five 'Rs' recognition, reaction, response, reveal and reperfusion; Table 17.4);
- establishing a protected bed in a stroke unit;
- establishing public education campaigns;
- raising the priority of stroke with emergency medical services;
- ambulances bypassing other hospitals to get to a stroke centre.

No data are available on whether patient outcomes were improved by such changes but across these studies there was a reduction in symptom onset to treatment time and a modest increase in the delivery of rt-PA (Table 17.5). There do not appear to be any analysis of the impact of such changes on other aspects of stroke care such as access to rehabilitation services and number of patient transfers.

In summary, designated stroke centres have gained ground in North America and Germany where the healthcare system appears to be conducive to such systems of care. In particular, stroke centres appear to have become more established where there are more fragmented care pathways (different providers delivering acute care and rehabilitation) with relatively short lengths of stay. There should be concern about the unnecessary transfer of unstable patients to stroke centres,[54] since the majority will not receive the intended treatment (thrombolysis) and the stroke centre model (at least in the US) does not emphasize the best evidence for service delivery through stroke units.[48] This, among other pressures, has raised interest in alternative ways of delivering expert assessment and diagnosis. The most prevalent of these appears to be telemedicine services.

> Because stroke unit care is applicable to all patients, the overall impact on outcome is likely to be considerably greater than that of tissue plasminogen activator – there is much more to acute stroke care than thrombolysis.

17.5.6 Telemedicine services (networks)

Telemedicine has been broadly defined as 'the use of telecommunication technology to provide medical information and services'.[55,56] In relation to stroke it can be defined as 'the process by which electronic visual and audio communications are used to provide diagnostic and consultation support to practitioners at distant sites, to assist in or directly deliver medical care to patients, and to enhance the skills and knowledge of distant medical care providers'. Telemedicine consultation has been incorporated into a variety of aspects of modern healthcare but only relatively recently into acute stroke services. Some of the stated advantages[57] of such systems over traditional telephone consultations are:

- assisting in neurological assessment;
- identification of neurological deterioration and provision of immediate feedback on treatment;
- identification of patients who do not require rt-PA;
- to assess risk and benefit questions directly with the family without time delay;
- direct supervision of specialist procedures such as delivery of rt-PA;

- to monitor haemodynamic status and neurological examination prior to transport to a stroke centre;
- ability of the stroke specialist to direct advice to the transport team on the therapeutic needs of the patient.

Proponents of telemedicine for acute stroke have pointed out that over half of hospitals in the US are located in rural areas and there is currently a shortage of neurologists and radiologists to provide expert advice across the whole country.[58] In addition, surveys of neurologists in the US have shown less than half felt comfortable about giving intravenous rt-PA.[58] Telemedicine also fits well within the concept of establishing primary and comprehensive stroke centres that provide a network of coverage to related sites. Lastly, telemedicine may allow other sites within a network to participate in clinical trials; from consenting to follow-up, all the components for a quality stroke trial can potentially be achieved through telemedicine. Many of the reported barriers are essentially man-made (for example, reimbursement for services and the availability of suitable equipment).

There are no completed randomized trials of telemedicine services in acute stroke to provide any reliable evidence about their impact on patient outcomes. However, several key questions have been addressed using other study designs.[55,56] These indicate (Table 17.5) that telemedicine services in acute stroke appear to be:

- Practical; experience from the US and Germany[55,56] has demonstrated the feasibility of establishing telemedicine networks. These systems usually used some form of teleconferencing facility linked to a stroke centre. Technical failures were uncommon (0–4% of consultations).
- Reliable; if telemedicine services are to be useful they must offer reliable diagnostic evaluation of both clinical features and brain imaging. The interrater reliability of assessing neurological status (using the NIH Stroke Scale, the Scandinavian Stroke Scale, or the European Stroke Scale) was as good as with face-to-face assessment.[55] Two studies[59,60] reported complete agreement between telemedicine assessment of CT scan and conventional neuroradiology from the point of view of eligibility for thrombolysis and major exclusions.
- Feasible and acceptable; on average telemedicine consultations were about 10 min longer than conventional bedside consultations. Although this appears to be more than offset by reductions in the need for transfers to other hospitals, there were no explicit comparisons. Patient and clinician satisfaction with the telemedicine service was reported to be good.[55,56]
- Associated with improved delivery of rt-PA; the proportion of patients receiving rt-PA increased in association with telemedicine services.

Telemedicine (teleconsultation) services appear to offer a promising approach to improve access to acute assessment and treatment, particularly where the healthcare economy does not favour stroke centres, where populations are dispersed, and where local hospital stroke services can provide good post-acute stroke care (but not rapid assessment and treatment). A final point is that telemedicine services may allow workable medical on-call rotas to be developed by allowing a large group of experienced stroke specialists – who may be based in different hospitals – to cover a region.

17.5.7 Transient ischaemic attack services

Most of the debate has focused on services for patients with stroke. However, substantial numbers of patients have a transient ischaemic attack (TIA) and have made a full clinical recovery before they seek help. The risk of stroke after a TIA, or of recurrent stroke after a first stroke, is very high in the early period and tails off later (section 16.2.1). Thus, one has most to gain from starting secondary prevention as early as possible. Also, since the accurate diagnosis of TIA depends on a good history, it makes sense to assess patients as soon after the event as possible. Traditionally, services have varied between countries.

In the US it is relatively common for TIA patients to be seen in the emergency room. In Scandinavia and Germany they are often admitted to hospital. In the UK the move has been towards early specialist assessment in outpatient clinics, so-called 'one-stop' neurovascular, TIA or stroke clinics which are characterized by:

- rapid access to a specialist opinion on TIAs, minor strokes and episodes that may mimic them;
- streamlined access to the necessary investigations (which requires close liaison with the radiology department);
- close links with surgeons who can offer timely carotid endarterectomy.

These clinics ought to minimize unnecessary hospital admission and delay in accessing specialist opinion, investigation and treatment. However, they attract patients with a wide range of other neurological conditions (Table 17.3), so the clinician must have neurological training, or at least easy access to sound neurological advice.[61,62]

> Rapid-access 'one-stop' neurovascular clinics should provide rapid clinical assessment of patients who may have had a transient ischaemic attack or minor stroke, with streamlined and cost-effective investigations and early intervention to reduce the risk of a serious vascular event.

However, the recognition that TIA patients may have a 20% risk of early stroke occurrence within the first 2 weeks, with the majority in the first day,[30] has raised concerns about delays in assessment and diagnosis even where rapid-access clinics are available. In addition, the effectiveness of carotid endarterectomy is greatest if carried out within 2 weeks of symptom onset.[34] These developments challenge us to diagnose and treat TIA and minor stroke far more quickly. In general, three approaches appear feasible (although none have been tested in clinical trials).

- *Outpatient management*: with a daily stroke clinic, it is possible to see most TIA and minor stroke patients within 48 h of symptom onset.[34] However, this is resource-intensive[63] and presents challenges for the organization of investigations.
- *Assessment within emergency departments*: if the emergency departments have rapid access to investigations, including ultrasound and CT scanning, then it may be possible to provide a rapid turnaround of investigation and early secondary prevention. This approach, which appears to be common in the US,[64] carries the risk of inappropriate investigation and treatment if non-specialist staff are planning patient care.
- *Hospital admission*: in some countries (e.g. Scandinavia) hospital admission for TIA is an established approach, however it is not common elsewhere (including the UK). Recently a scoring system has been developed which may identify individuals at highest risk of early recurrence.[31,65] If a subgroup of TIA and minor stroke patients really are at extremely high risk of early recurrence, then a short period of hospital admission would be justified provided we can provide rapid assessment and effective treatment. Although there are some uncertainties about whether current treatments prevent *early* recurrence, most would argue that a very high early risk of recurrence (e.g. greater than 20% in the first week) would warrant hospital admission. Indeed, to deny admission to similar high-risk individuals with an acute coronary syndrome would be considered unacceptable.

The next few years are likely to see a greatly increased move towards rapid assessment and treatment of TIA and minor stroke patients and the solutions adopted will vary depending on the region. However, it is crucial that we have good evidence about what forms of early assessment and treatment effectively reduce early recurrence.

17.6 Organized inpatient (stroke unit) care

The types of stroke services that hospitals traditionally provided have varied from place to place reflecting local interests and politics. However, there is now widespread acceptance that hospital-based stroke services should be *organized* within stroke units.[66,67] Much of the evidence for this comes from a systematic review of clinical trials that compared the outcome for stroke patients cared for in a specialist stroke unit with those cared for in general wards. Patients managed in stroke units are more likely to survive, return home and regain independence (Table 17.6). Stroke units may also improve patients' quality of life, and improvements in outcome may persist for several years.[68]

Table 17.6 Summary of patient outcomes in the stroke unit trials.

	Stroke unit[a]	Conventional care[a]	Odds ratio[b] (95% CI)	Absolute risk difference[c] (95% CI)	Difference in number of outcomes per 1000 admitted[d]
Home (independent)	45%	40%	1.25 (1.12, 1.40)	0.05 (0.02, 0.07)	50
Home (dependent)	17%	15%	1.16 (0.88, 1.53)	0.01 (−0.01, 0.03)	10
Institutional care	14%	16%	0.84 (0.72, 0.98)	−0.02 (0.00, 0.04)	−20
Dead	23%	28%	0.80 (0.70, 0.91)	−0.04 (−0.02, −0.06)	−40

[a]The proportion (%) of patients with various outcomes at the end of scheduled follow-up (median 1 year) in the randomized trials of stroke unit care vs conventional care.
[b]The odds ratio for that outcome (95% confidence interval).
[c]The proportion of outcomes achieved (+) or avoided (−) with stroke unit care.
[d]The number of outcomes achieved (+) or avoided (−) for every 1000 patients cared for in a stroke unit, assuming the absolute risk of an outcome in the population is similar to that in the trials.
Figures based on data from 31 trials (6900 patients).[68]

> Stroke patients managed in a stroke unit are more likely to survive, return home and regain independence than those managed in a general medical or even in a neurology ward.

These trials were testing much more heterogeneous interventions than is usual in drug trials, where the intervention is precisely defined in terms of the chemical, the dose and the timing. Because of this heterogeneity of the intervention – but not of the results – it is sometimes difficult to generalize from the stroke unit overview, and some important questions remain when applying the results to everyday clinical practice.

17.6.1 What is stroke unit care?

Although comprehensive stroke unit care is a complex and multi-faceted intervention, the key components are reasonably well described[69] (Table 17.7):

Table 17.7 Outline of comprehensive stroke unit care.

- *Ward base*: effective stroke units have usually been based in a discrete ward with dedicated nursing staff. Mobile stroke teams do not appear to improve patient outcomes.[70]
- *Specialist staffing*: they have been staffed by medical, nursing and therapy staff with a specialist interest and expertise in stroke and/or rehabilitation.
- *Multidisciplinary team working*: they have always included good multidisciplinary communication (defined as a formal meeting of all staff once per week to plan the management of individual patients).
- *Education and training*: they have incorporated programmes of education and training for staff and provision of information for patients and carers.

Although many stroke units were not described in detail, several consistent features of the process of care have been described[66,69] (Table 17.7). This typically did not depend on high-tech facilities but did implement a systematic approach to care that incorporated:

Structure
Geographically discrete ward
Medical staff with specialist interest in stroke and rehabilitation
Nursing staff with specialist interest in stroke and rehabilitation
Multidisciplinary staffing (nursing, medical, physiotherapy, occupational therapy, speech therapy, social work)
Coordination of care
Regular multidisciplinary team meetings (formal meeting of all staff once weekly, informal meetings 2–3× per week)
Close linking of nursing and multidisciplinary team care
Educational programmes for staff
Assessment and monitoring
Rapid admission to stroke unit
Medical history and examination
Routine investigations (biochemistry, haematology, ECG, CT scanning)
Further selective investigations (carotid ultrasound, echocardiogram, MR scanning)
Nursing assessments (vital signs, general care needs, swallow test, fluid balance, pressure areas, neurological monitoring)
Therapy assessments of impairments and disability
Early management
Careful management of food and fluids
Pyrexia management, paracetamol for pyrexia, antibiotic for suspected infection
Hypoxia management, oxygen if hypoxia, drowsiness or cardiorespiratory disease
Glycaemic management, insulin for hyperglycaemia
Early mobilization, up to sit, stand and walk as soon as possible
Careful positioning and handling
Pressure area care
Avoid urinary catheterization if possible
Ongoing multidisciplinary rehabilitation
Early goal setting
Early involvement of carers in rehabilitation
Provision of information to patients and carers
Discharge planning
Early assessment of discharge needs
Discharge plan involving patient and carers

- Careful assessment and monitoring – of medical, nursing and therapy needs.
- Early active management – incorporating management of food and fluids, control of pyrexia, hypoxia, hyperglycaemia, early mobilization, careful positioning and handling, and avoidance of urinary catheterization.
- Ongoing multidisciplinary rehabilitation – with early goal setting, early involvement of carers in rehabilitation, and provision of information to patients and carers. This also included early planning of discharge needs.

Many of these processes of care will come as no surprise to those experienced in stroke care but recent audits support concerns that many are not routinely provided.[71]

Beyond describing the basic components of stroke unit care, it is difficult to determine whether the effectiveness of the stroke units is due to the total package of care, or to particular components. Some of the individual components can be evaluated in randomized trials (e.g. guidelines for prevention of deep venous thrombosis, early mobilization, intensive physiotherapy), and these trials can be reviewed systematically to provide reliable data, but some of the less well-defined components and any possible synergy between them is much less amenable to such assessment. For example, better communication between health professionals, stroke patients and their carers, which is so often inadequate and a major source of dissatisfaction in non-specialized wards, may in part explain the success of stroke units, but this would be difficult, if not impossible, to prove.[72,73]

17.6.2 Types of stroke unit

Although the basic principles of stroke unit care are reasonably well described they have been delivered in a variety of ways, and the term 'stroke unit' means different things to different people. So it is important to define our terms (Table 17.8). Inevitably, the question arises as to which type of unit is most effective. This is very difficult to answer with confidence and attempts to do so[74] are prone to bias. They do indicate (Table 17.9) that effective stroke units have usually provided organized multidisciplinary care for a reasonable period of time. We shall discuss this in more detail.

> Effective models of organized inpatient (stroke unit) care are able to provide specialist multidisciplinary care for most of the inpatient pathway of care.

Acute stroke units

'Acute' refers to the policy of rapid admission of the stroke patient to the stroke unit. Admitting all acute

Table 17.8 Classification of organized inpatient (stroke unit) care.

Type	Philosophy of care	Patient group	MDT base	Timing of admission	Timing of discharge from a stroke unit	Type of care
Acute (intensive) stroke unit	Acute care; life support	Stroke	Ward	Acute (hours)	Early (3–7 days)	Acute medical & nursing care (with high staffing levels)
Acute (semi-intensive) stroke unit	Acute care; close monitoring	Stroke	Ward	Acute (hours)	Early (3–7 days)	Acute medical & nursing care Monitoring & management of physiological variables
Comprehensive stroke unit	Acute care and multidisciplinary rehabilitation	Stroke	Ward	Acute (hours)	Later (days – weeks) some referral to specialist rehabilitation	Acute medical & nursing care Non-intensive management of physiological variables Early active multidisciplinary rehabilitation
Rehabilitation stroke unit	Multidisciplinary rehabilitation	Stroke	Ward	Delayed (days)	Later (weeks)	Multidisciplinary rehabilitation
Mixed rehabilitation unit	Multidisciplinary rehabilitation	Stroke & other disabling illness	Ward	Early (hours–days)	Later (weeks)	Multidisciplinary rehabilitation
Mobile stroke team	Acute care and/or multidisciplinary rehabilitation	Stroke	Mobile (no ward) base	Early (hours–days)	Later (weeks)	Acute medical care and/or multidisciplinary rehabilitation; no specialist nursing input

This table summarizes, in broad terms, the characteristics of different types of stroke unit. MDT multidisciplinary team.

Table 17.9 Effectiveness of different types of stroke unit: summary of direct and indirect comparisons of different models of stroke unit care.

Type of stroke unit evaluated	Number of comparisons (subjects)	Control service comparator in trials	Estimated odds ratio for death or dependency (95% CI) compared with a general ward	Statistical significance
Acute (intensive) stroke unit	None	No data	No data	No data
Acute (semi-intensive) stroke unit	3 (530)	Mixed rehabilitation unit, comprehensive stroke unit	0.77 (0.53–1.12)	P = 0.17
Comprehensive stroke unit	10 (3010)	General ward, mobile stroke team	0.89 (0.79–0.99)	P = 0.03
Rehabilitation stroke unit	7 (870)	General ward, mixed rehabilitation unit	0.85 (0.77–0.93)	P = 0.0007
Mixed rehabilitation unit	9 (1170)	General ward, rehabilitation stroke unit	0.87 (0.79–0.96)	P = 0.007
Mobile stroke team	5 (1000)	General ward, comprehensive stroke unit	0.98 (0.91–1.10)	P = 0.5

The results of a series of comparisons of different types of stroke unit care.[74] This approach attempts to provide a standard measure of stroke unit effect where trials have used different control groups. Data analysis used methods[185] of combining direct comparisons (trials that directly compare a stroke unit vs general ward) with indirect comparisons (e.g. the effect of a stroke unit vs general ward is inferred from trials of stroke unit vs mobile team and mobile team vs general ward). Data are presented as the summary estimate of the odds ratio (95% confidence interval) for death or dependency of stroke unit vs general ward. Please note that these estimates are based in part on indirect comparisons of treatments and are potentially subject to bias (e.g. from different patient groups being recruited into different trials).

stroke patients directly into a unit makes the introduction of assessment protocols easier, allows expertise to be focused, and will certainly facilitate the large randomized trials of acute interventions that are needed to identify effective treatments.[75] It also facilitates a policy of active early mobilization (section 11.11), hydration (section 11.18), control of temperature (section 11.12), avoidance of hypoxia (section 11.2) and large changes in blood pressure (section 11.7). Although there are no reliable data from randomized trials demonstrating that any one of these interventions improves outcomes, they are supported by a reasonable theoretical rationale and some observational data.[76–79]

In some centres, particularly in North America and Germany, there has been a vogue for admitting stroke patients to ward areas with facilities for intensive monitoring of physiological functions (cardiac, respiratory and neurological). Interventions are introduced to correct these abnormalities (e.g. raised intracranial pressure, systemic hypertension), in the belief that this will improve outcome.[80] Broadly speaking two approaches have been described:

- Intensive care units which can offer all monitoring (including intracranial monitoring) and life support options (e.g. respiratory support). There have been several non-randomized studies of stroke intensive care units,[81–84] but there is no good evidence that these improve patient outcome. The approach has come under more scrutiny recently, presumably because it inevitably requires extra resources due to the high staffing levels and expensive equipment. Also, there is currently little evidence from randomized trials that the various individual interventions employed are effective. Thus, although stroke intensive care units may help, we need randomized trials to evaluate them.

- Semi-intensive units are similar to coronary care units where monitoring and intervention focus on physiological variables but not life support. There have been three small clinical trials of semi-intensive units that have rather inconclusive findings. One[85] indicated no benefit over care in a less intensive setting while two others[86] have indicated a potential benefit. As mentioned above, there is limited evidence for the individual elements of monitoring and intervention although one trial[79] has indicated that intensive monitoring can reduce early neurological deterioration after stroke.

Comprehensive stroke units

Perhaps the most successfully implemented model has been the comprehensive stroke unit, which admits patients acutely and then provides at least a few weeks

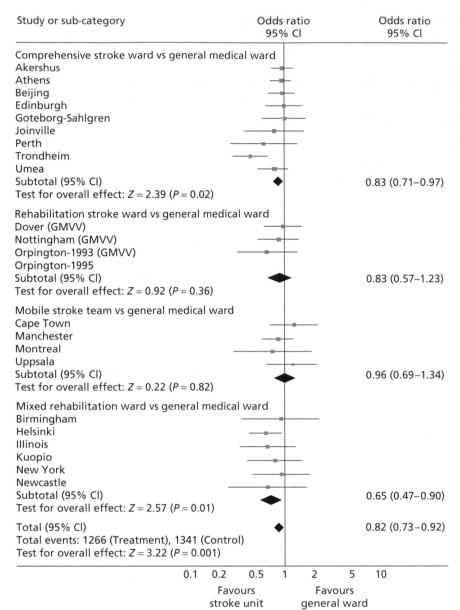

Study or sub-category	Odds ratio 95% CI	Odds ratio 95% CI
Comprehensive stroke ward vs general medical ward		
Akershus		
Athens		
Beijing		
Edinburgh		
Goteborg-Sahlgren		
Joinville		
Perth		
Trondheim		
Umea		
Subtotal (95% CI)		0.83 (0.71–0.97)
Test for overall effect: Z = 2.39 (P = 0.02)		
Rehabilitation stroke ward vs general medical ward		
Dover (GMVV)		
Nottingham (GMVV)		
Orpington-1993 (GMVV)		
Orpington-1995		
Subtotal (95% CI)		0.83 (0.57–1.23)
Test for overall effect: Z = 0.92 (P = 0.36)		
Mobile stroke team vs general medical ward		
Cape Town		
Manchester		
Montreal		
Uppsala		
Subtotal (95% CI)		0.96 (0.69–1.34)
Test for overall effect: Z = 0.22 (P = 0.82)		
Mixed rehabilitation ward vs general medical ward		
Birmingham		
Helsinki		
Illinois		
Kuopio		
New York		
Newcastle		
Subtotal (95% CI)		0.65 (0.47–0.90)
Test for overall effect: Z = 2.57 (P = 0.01)		
Total (95% CI)		0.82 (0.73–0.92)
Total events: 1266 (Treatment), 1341 (Control)		
Test for overall effect: Z = 3.22 (P = 0.001)		

0.1   0.2   0.5   1   2   5   10

Favours   Favours
stroke unit   general ward

Fig. 17.2 The results of a systematic review of randomized trials testing the effectiveness of stroke unit care compared with a general medical ward. The result of each individual trial, expressed as the odds ratio, is represented by a purple box with a horizontal line indicating the 95% confidence interval. The block size is proportional to the amount of information in the trial. An odds ratio to the left of the vertical line indicates that the odds of the outcome (in this case events refer to death or dependency between 6 and 12 months after randomization) is less with stroke unit care than care in general wards. Estimates based on an overview of all the trials are represented by solid diamonds. Reproduced with permission from the Stroke Unit Trialists' Collaboration.[88]

of rehabilitation. Such a model, which is widespread in Norway and Sweden, is supported by the largest group of clinical trials included in the systematic review (Fig. 17.2) and results from a national stroke register in Sweden.[87] Although we believe that rehabilitation should start on the day of the stroke, such units do present some practical challenges. For example, very sick stroke patients might require care that would disrupt a rehabilitation unit, at a time when they are unlikely to benefit from a rehabilitation environment. However, models that separate acute assessment and rehabilitation areas may disorientate some patients (and their families) and can compromise continuity of care. The comprehensive unit approach appears to be well suited to

medium-sized hospitals where one team can manage most stroke patients within one unit. In practice, although these units provide most care for most patients, referral of some patients with ongoing complex rehabilitation needs to other rehabilitation services is common.

Rehabilitation stroke units

Several trials have indicated benefit from rehabilitation units that admit patients a few days after stroke onset and continue rehabilitation for several weeks. These trials have inevitably examined a more selected patient group who are stable enough for that environment and have ongoing rehabilitation needs.

Mixed rehabilitation units

The meta-analysis of organized inpatient (stroke unit) care predominantly included trials comparing organized care within stroke-specific units with care in general wards (general medicine or general neurology). However, some trials explored the impact of organizing stroke care within generic rehabilitation services (e.g. geriatric medicine or neurological rehabilitation services); patients achieve better outcomes in mixed rehabilitation units than in general wards without multidisciplinary team care.[88] Comparisons with stroke-specific units indicate a trend towards better outcomes in stroke-specific units (Table 17.9) but there are insufficient data to determine whether stroke-specific units are clearly more effective.

Mixed rehabilitation units may have a role in smaller hospitals or very specialized services (e.g. young adult rehabilitation) where there may be too few stroke patients to make stroke-specific services viable. However, stroke-specific services certainly allow more specialization among the team members, which enhances the educational and research potential of the service. Training of junior doctors and other staff, which might suffer if all the stroke patients were managed by a single team, can be protected and probably improved by organizing rotation of staff through the unit. Moreover, stroke specialists are more likely to be enthusiastic about teaching students and staff about strokes than generalists or those with another specialist interest.

Mobile stroke teams

Overall the trials in the meta-analysis indicated that a stroke team working across several general wards may improve aspects of the processes of care (e.g. access to specialist assessments) but cannot achieve patient outcomes as good as those of a team based in a stroke unit.[24,49,70] Probably the most important advantage of having the patients in one location is that the nursing staff can play a greater role in the rehabilitation process. When patients are scattered, it is more difficult to incorporate the essential role of nurses. Also, stroke patients managed in acute general areas have to compete for nursing time with patients who may be perceived to have more urgent needs (e.g. chest pain). Stroke patients may, for example, need regular toileting to maintain continence and thus dignity. These aspects of care are very important, but can be seen as less urgent. A geographically defined stroke unit removes this competition for nursing time, and allows the nurses to take on a new role – not just as carers, but also as facilitators of patient independence – and to continue therapy (directed by specialist therapists) throughout the 24-h period. The main role for stroke teams is probably to provide outreach care for those unable to get into the stroke unit, and to prioritize admission to the stroke unit.

> The main advantage of caring for stroke patients in one place is that nurses can play a major role in the rehabilitation process.

17.6.3 Who should be admitted to the stroke unit?

Stratification of patients within the meta-analysis by stroke severity showed that patients with mild, moderate and severe strokes are all likely to benefit from stroke unit care.[88,89] In terms of absolute outcomes more severe patients have the greatest survival advantage from stroke unit care but milder patients gained more in terms of regaining independence. Data from non-randomized, and thus potentially biased, comparisons of outcomes following admission to a stroke unit or general care support the notion that stroke unit care benefits unselected stroke patients.[87,90–92] Of course, bed shortages may force staff to make triage decisions. Many of the serious early complications of stroke (including early neurological deterioration) are more common with severe stroke and may respond to stroke unit care. Milder stroke patients (e.g. those who are mobile) probably have less to lose from not being admitted to a stroke unit.

There is little evidence that patients of particular ages gain more or less from care in a stroke unit.[88,93] There are good reasons to believe that older stroke patients may be at higher risk of some complications, and therefore have more to gain from admission to a stroke unit. Although we think that *needs* rather than *age* should dictate where and by whom patients are managed, local conditions will often dictate which service is the best option. For example, where an age-related geriatric service (e.g. one that admits any patient who is over 75 years old, whatever the problem) already provides effective stroke rehabilitation, there may be a case for adding a new rehabilitation service for younger stroke patients rather than dismantling the current service. Professionals and patients' families are often concerned that younger patients' morale will suffer if they are treated in a ward with mainly older patients, although this concern is by no means universal.

17.6.4 How long should patients remain in the unit?

Some units, particularly those that admit patients acutely, define maximum lengths of stay. It seems to us that the only reason to do this is to allow admission of new cases.

If the unit is of sufficient size for the population's needs, works flexibly and is efficient in discharging patients, then a defined maximum length of stay should not be needed. If one does insist on a maximum length of stay, one must ensure that there are facilities and staff elsewhere to deliver appropriate continuing care (e.g. 'slower-stream' rehabilitation facilities;[93] and that patients are not left to languish on an acute medical ward. One might argue that patients who are no longer improving, but are having to wait for placement in the community or an institution, should not be kept in a stroke unit. However, for some individuals the unit may offer the best environment to maintain any functional improvement already gained. Moves under these circumstances should only be considered where beds are limited and patients who are judged likely to gain more from the unit environment are waiting to be admitted.

17.6.5 How large should a stroke unit be?

Age-specific and sex-specific stroke incidence data and details of the hospital catchment population, along with hospital activity data, should allow an estimate of the number of patients who are likely to require admission to hospital each year (section 17.11.3). Unfortunately, there may be variations due simply to chance or the season of the year. Although consistent seasonal differences in the *incidence* of stroke have not been demonstrated in community-based studies, at least in temperate regions, there is an excess of hospital admissions and stroke deaths during the winter.[94,95] Of course, this may simply reflect referral bias and a higher case fatality during cold weather. Whatever the explanation for any seasonal variation, it does cause difficulties when planning stroke services. Prior to the development of a stroke unit, a survey in one of our own medical units, which admitted between 200 and 250 stroke patients each year, demonstrated that the number of stroke inpatients on any one day varied between 9 and 35 over a year. Therefore, whatever organization one sets up to manage these patients, it must be flexible enough to cope with large fluctuations in their numbers. The unit should be able to accommodate different proportions of men and women, as the proportions are bound to fluctuate. The inevitable limit on the number of beds may be managed by ensuring that the stroke unit is part of a larger area, into which it can expand with demand and then contract again. Such arrangements also mean that, at times, non-stroke patients are cared for in the stroke unit. Inevitably, there are times when resources are not adequate to meet all the needs of the patients, and it is then important for the team to support its members in the difficult task of prioritizing – in other words rationing – care.

A survey in one of our own medical units, which admits between 200 and 250 stroke patients each year, demonstrated that the number of stroke inpatients on any one day varied between 9 and 35 over a year. Therefore, stroke services must be flexible enough to cope with large fluctuations in the numbers and types of patients referred.

17.6.6 Who should staff and run the stroke unit?

The units included in the systematic review were run by geriatricians, neurologists, general (internal) physicians and rehabilitationists. Indirect comparisons of the benefits of units run by different specialist groups did not show any significant differences.[66,88] We believe that whoever is responsible should have the necessary knowledge, training and above all enthusiasm to take on the task. The most appropriate professional group will vary from place to place. For example, in the Netherlands, practically all acute stroke patients are managed by neurologists, while in the UK most are managed, at least initially, by general physicians and geriatricians.[71,96] British neurologists may have the knowledge and training to diagnose and investigate stroke patients, but unfortunately most do not have the time or interest, support staff, access to beds, or training in rehabilitation to run a comprehensive stroke service without help from other specialists. In the UK, geriatricians are often in the best position to take a leading role, although most need extra training in neurology and the active participation of their local neurologist – who can very usefully contribute to diagnosis and management of patients, especially those with unusual causes of stroke, patients with 'funny turns' and the many and varied neurological problems that arise in inpatient and outpatient stroke care (Table 17.3). The advent of thrombolysis requires additional training, expertise and support in assessment of the 'brain attack' patient and interpreting acute imaging. In the UK training for stroke specialists is being implemented and an increasing number of hospitals are appointing specialist stroke physicians (from a variety of specialist backgrounds) to coordinate stroke services.

17.6.7 Planning a stroke unit development

The good evidence for the effectiveness of stroke units means that in many countries their development is supported by national initiatives. However, the development of such units is often resisted by those who perceive them as a threat. Some points are worth considering in local discussions.

- Stroke units generally make more efficient use of existing staff and beds, and so may eventually even increase the resources available to other specialties.
- De-skilling of their junior medical, nursing and paramedical staff can be overcome by rotating staff and students through the unit.
- Adopting an evolutionary approach to developing the service may be encounter less resistance – for example, one might introduce a stroke assessment protocol before trying to set up an acute assessment area, or a stroke team working on the general medical wards before trying to set up a geographically defined stroke unit. Stroke units are not just a research intervention, they have been implemented in a range of settings with improvements in outcome.[71,87,91,92]
- One can try to influence the local organizations that fund healthcare (i.e. health authorities and general or family practitioners in the UK; health insurers in other countries) to exert pressure for change, since they are generally keen to fund services for which there is scientific evidence of efficacy (curiously, and irritatingly for those of us concerned with stroke, neither coronary care units nor regional oncology services have been nearly as well evaluated as stroke units, and yet their utility is said to be 'obvious' and they are widely encouraged).

> Curiously, and irritatingly for those of us concerned with stroke, neither coronary care units nor regional oncology services have been nearly as well evaluated as stroke units, and yet their utility is said to be 'obvious' and they are widely encouraged.

There are likely to be significant pressures (other than evidence of effectiveness) that will influence local service delivery, since its structure must be tailored to local needs, resources, geography, people and politics. One needs to consider what is the best way to deliver comprehensive stroke care within the constraints of the local circumstances. We suggest three factors come into play:

- evidence that a particular model of stroke unit is effective (Table 17.9);
- the ability of the stroke unit model to deliver all aspects of care required;
- the ability of the stroke unit to provide for the broadest group of stroke patients (i.e. meet the needs of the stroke population).

The following list of options outline some common solutions:

- *Comprehensive stroke unit*: where possible, the comprehensive stroke unit, which combines both acute care and rehabilitation for the majority of patients, is probably the preferred option. This could include the delivery of thrombolysis or take over the care of patients following thrombolysis in an emergency department setting. This option has a good evidence base to support it and would be most appropriate for small to medium-sized hospitals (e.g. 100–300 stroke patients per year).
- *Acute stroke unit and rehabilitation stroke unit*: in larger hospitals, it may be difficult to provide all stroke unit beds in one place. In this circumstance, a combination of acute stroke unit and rehabilitation stroke unit has often been adopted. In theory this should provide comprehensive stroke unit care but is largely untested in clinical trials. If this model is adopted, we suggest that the components of comprehensive stroke unit care must be provided throughout the patient journey (e.g. early mobilization and early multidisciplinary planning applies in the acute stroke unit, patients in the rehabilitation stroke unit should have access to acute medical care). In addition, the patient and family should experience a continuous process of care rather than discontinuity between components of the service.
- *Mixed rehabilitation unit*: in smaller hospitals with dispersed populations (e.g. less than 100 stroke admissions per year), it may be appropriate to have protocols of delivery of acute care in general wards and to provide rehabilitation services in a mixed rehabilitation setting. Telemedicine services (section 17.5.6) may offer options for accessing expert advice from larger stroke centres.

In a stroke unit development it is important to compare the characteristics of your planned service with those in the stroke unit trials to ensure you are delivering care that is, as far as possible, evidence-based (Tables 17.8 and 17.9).

17.7 Transfer from hospital to community

One of the main areas of concern to patients, and more particularly to carers, is the organization (or rather the lack of organization) of hospital discharge.[72,97] One can well understand their concern. One day patients are being cared for in hospital by a team of professionals, and the next they are at home and the responsibility of the carers. A number of things can be attempted to try and reduce the stress of the transition from hospital to home:

- Provide adequate information (section 17.10.1) and train the carers while the patient is in hospital, for example invite the carers to therapy sessions and involve them in the patient's care on the unit. Unfortunately, trials of information provision and patient education do not provide clear evidence to guide practice.

- Predischarge home visits with the patient and one or more members of the team to ensure that the home environment is tailored to the patient's needs. Also, informal visits home, initially for a day and then graduating to overnight and weekend stays, allow the patient and carer to gain confidence, identify potential problems and help maintain morale. Although this is a well-established approach we could not identify any clinical trials of such policies.
- Predischarge case conferences allow the patient and carer to meet with the hospital-based team and any professionals who are to be involved in their care in the community. Once again this is a well-established approach for which we could not identify any clinical trials.
- Clear guidelines about who to contact in the event of problems. General (family) practitioners, or one of their team, are the ideal points of contact, but they can only fulfil this role if adequately briefed before the patient's discharge. It follows that detailed records of the patient's problems, and the plans for support in the community, must be relayed to those expected to monitor the home situation.
- A programme of training carers to manage their new role has been tested in one moderately large randomized trial.[98] This involved training by stroke unit staff about stroke plus practical caring skills. The brief programme also continued after discharge. This approach was surprisingly effective – trained carers reported less caregiver burden, anxiety or depression and had a higher quality of life, while patients in the carer training group experienced less anxiety and depression and a better quality of life. The intervention was also

cost-effective, reducing the overall cost of caring[99] and is the subject of further research.

In some circumstances, it may be appropriate to further break down the boundary between hospital and home by organizing for the patient to attend a day hospital or outpatient department regularly to be reviewed medically, or to receive further rehabilitation input.

17.7.1 Early supported discharge services

Partly in response to the well-reported limitations of conventional hospital discharge arrangements, a number of services have been developed to try and improve the transition between hospital and community, in particular, early supported discharge services, which aim to accelerate discharge home from hospital but provide more continuity of rehabilitation in the home setting. To date, 12 randomized trials have tested this approach to care in a variety of settings around the world.[70,100] Most were based around a small multidisciplinary team of physiotherapy, occupational therapy, nursing and assistant staff – with input from medical, speech and language therapy and social work staff. The teams were either hospital-based (and went out to the patient's home) or community-based (and came into hospital to recruit patients). All incorporated regular multidisciplinary team meetings to plan patient care. A typical pathway of care is shown in Table 17.10.

Typically these services input for up to 3 months but in some cases this might be shorter with handover to other community services.[70]

Even compared with high-quality care from a hospital-based stroke unit, an early supported discharge team

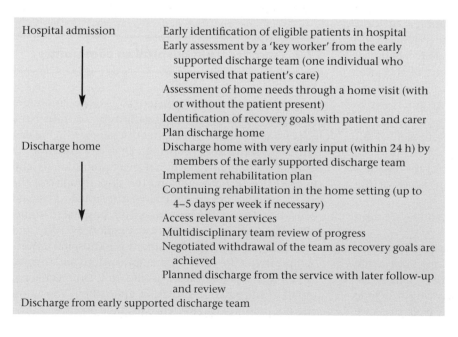

Hospital admission	Early identification of eligible patients in hospital
	Early assessment by a 'key worker' from the early supported discharge team (one individual who supervised that patient's care)
	Assessment of home needs through a home visit (with or without the patient present)
	Identification of recovery goals with patient and carer
	Plan discharge home
Discharge home	Discharge home with very early input (within 24 h) by members of the early supported discharge team
	Implement rehabilitation plan
	Continuing rehabilitation in the home setting (up to 4–5 days per week if necessary)
	Access relevant services
	Multidisciplinary team review of progress
	Negotiated withdrawal of the team as recovery goals are achieved
	Planned discharge from the service with later follow-up and review
Discharge from early supported discharge team	

Table 17.10 Illustrative pathway of care with early supported discharge service.

Fig. 17.3 The results of a systematic review of randomized trials testing the effectiveness of early supported discharge (ESD) services compared with conventional discharge services. The result of each individual trial, expressed as the odds ratio, is represented by a purple box with a horizontal line indicating the 95% confidence interval. The box size is proportional to the amount of information in the trial. An odds ratio to the left of the vertical line indicates that the odds of the outcome (in this case events refer to death or dependency between 6 and 12 months after randomization) is less with the ESD service than with conventional care. The estimates based on an overview of all the trials are represented by diamonds. Reproduced with permission from the Early Supported Discharge Trialists.[100]

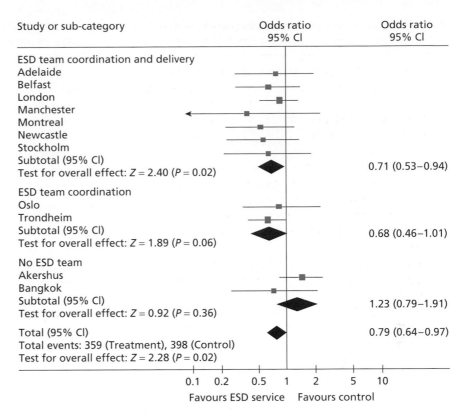

could not only accelerate discharge home (with an average reduction in length of stay of 7 days), but could also result in the patient having a greater chance of remaining at home and regaining independence (Fig. 17.3). Overall, for every 100 patients randomized to early supported discharge services, an extra five (95% CI 1–9) remained at home and an extra five (95% CI 1–10) were independent at 6–12 months after the stroke. Good results were most likely with a well-resourced, coordinated multidisciplinary supported discharge team and if patients were recruited with mild to moderate stroke severity (i.e. those who achieve a Barthel Index of at least 10/20 in the first week – equivalent to rapidly regaining standing balance). There is a suggestion that such services may not work as well in more dispersed rural populations[101] but this requires confirmation.

Economic analyses[100] indicate that the potential saving in hospital costs (reduced hospital bed-days) is greater than the additional costs of community rehabilitation. In practice it is often difficult to release such costs, but at the very least early supported discharge services appear to offer a way of both improving patient care and optimizing the use of a limited number of hospital beds. In addition to the 'harder' outcomes above, it is also noteworthy that patient and carers allocated to early supported discharge services were more likely to report satisfaction with their services.[70] Early supported

discharge services appear to be an essential component of a truly comprehensive stroke service and should particularly target patients with mild to moderately severe strokes.

> Early supported discharge services – based on a specialist multidisciplinary team – can help accelerate discharge home and improve the longer-term recovery of selected stroke patients without incurring excessive costs.

17.8 Continuing rehabilitation and reintegration back to normal life

Even where stroke patients have received good care in hospital and around the discharge period, they may still have difficulty maintaining independence and reintegration back to normal life (Table 17.11). At this stage of the patient journey, services are often very variable and may be completely non-existent. This probably reflects the diversity of approaches in different countries but also a limited evidence base to suggest that effective interventions really can improve recovery. In general terms two broad approaches have been tested at this late stage:

Table 17.11 Common problems that arise late after a stroke, often when the patient is no longer in hospital.

> *Patient*
> Deteriorating function due to:
> – inactivity
> – progressing comorbidities
> – lack of continuing rehabilitation input?
> – depression or anxiety, even agoraphobia (section 11.31)
> – overprotection from the carer
> Social isolation
> Financial difficulties (section 11.33.6)
> Sexual dysfunction (section 11.33.5)
> Undetected rise in blood pressure
> Central post-stroke pain (section 11.23)
> *Carer* (section 11.34)
> Physical ill-health due to the strain of caring
> Depression or anxiety
> Poor relationship with patient because of personality change
> Social isolation because unable to get out to meet people
> Financial difficulties

- Therapy-based rehabilitation services (provided by physiotherapy, occupational therapy or multidisciplinary staff and primarily aiming to increase activities in daily living). In practice this might include a range of task-related interventions aiming to improve mobility, activities of daily living or specific tasks such as dressing.

- Stroke liaison worker services (provided by stroke nurses, family support workers or specialist social workers and primarily aiming to improve participation in normal living and quality of life). In practice these have included a mix of interventions which could deliver a programme of rehabilitation (e.g.[102]) or respond to identified problems.[103]

There is considerable variation within these broad approaches but they do provide a framework for considering the evidence.

17.8.1 Therapy-based rehabilitation services

In a systematic review[104] of therapy-based rehabilitation services, most of the trials assessed input in the patient's home by an occupational therapist although the review also included physiotherapy or multidisciplinary team services (such as community teams and day hospital services). Therapy-based rehabilitation services (when compared with no routine intervention) helped prevent stroke patients deteriorating in their ability to carry out activities of daily living (ADL) (Fig. 17.4) and improved ADL scores. Therefore, even relatively late after stroke onset (several months) patients may gain from input from a therapist. What is less clear is the absolute benefit likely to be achieved and the cost-effectiveness of these services. However they do indicate that within a

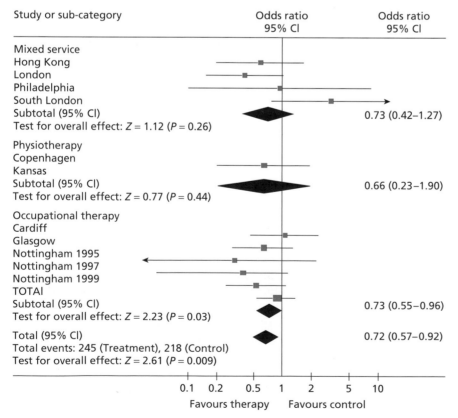

Fig 17.4 The results of a systematic review of randomized trials testing the effectiveness of therapy-based rehabilitation (provided to patients living at home) compared with conventional services (usually no routine input). The result of each individual trial, expressed as the odds ratio, is represented by a purple box with a horizontal line indicating the 95% confidence interval. The block size is proportional to the amount of information in the trial. An odds ratio to the left of the vertical line indicates that the odds of the outcome (in this case events refer to poor outcomes – death, deterioration in activities of daily living or dependency between 6 and 12 months after randomization) is less with the therapy service than with conventional care. Estimate based on an overview of all the trials are represented by diamonds at the bottom of the figure. Reproduced with permission from the Outpatient Therapy Trialists.[104]

comprehensive stroke service, some system of review and further intervention by therapists are valuable.

> A comprehensive stroke service should include systems that can review the stroke patient's progress and provide further intervention by therapists if required.

The discussion above does not indicate how such therapy services should be delivered (e.g. in the patient's home, outpatient clinic, day hospital). The effectiveness of domiciliary physiotherapy and of physiotherapy provided in a day hospital have been compared in randomized trials.[105–109] Together they demonstrate only small differences in outcome.[110] The relative costs of providing care in these settings varied between the studies, with no clear conclusion.

17.8.2 Stroke liaison worker services

The generic title of 'stroke liaison worker' can be defined as 'someone who provides emotional and social support and information to stroke patients and their families and liaises with services with the aim of reducing aspects of handicap and improving quality of life for patients with stroke and/or their carers'.[111] These services (which have also been termed 'specialist nurse support', 'stroke family care worker' and 'stroke family support organizer') often involve approaching patients and families during hospital admission, when they can provide information and education about stroke. They are also available for input after discharge home, particularly to identify problems or unmet needs and to develop customized solutions.[112] At least 15 randomized trials have tested out this type of service in the UK, Australia, the US and the Netherlands. Their impact on patient outcomes is unclear[102,111,113,114] but they do appear to be valued by patients and carers.

In summary, in a comprehensive stroke service there should be systems to allow review of stroke patients' progress and to provide therapy input if required. There may be a number of ways to deliver such services (domiciliary, outpatient clinic, day hospital).

17.9 Longer-term follow-up and chronic disease management

Stroke has now been recognized as one of the diseases which requires ongoing management – so-called chronic disease management. The rationale is to provide a system for managing the various needs, in particular prevention of disease and management of disability.

The best setting in which to provide such chronic disease management is likely to depend on the local healthcare system. In countries such as the UK and the Netherlands with a well-developed primary care service, it may be appropriate for much of this continuing care to be provided by the patient's own general family practitioner. In countries without developed primary care services this may need to be done through a hospital outpatient clinic. Whatever system is in place, it is important that it provides not only secondary prevention but an opportunity for reassessment, and identification and treatment of problems that may become apparent only after several weeks or months (Table 17.11). A follow-up checklist should ensure that late problems are not overlooked (Table 17.12).

Some patients make little progress in the first few months after the stroke (perhaps due to intercurrent illness) and are discharged to a supported environment, but then unexpectedly begin to improve. Ideally, such patients should be identified and re-enter a rehabilitation programme, but few services are sufficiently well organized or adequately resourced to offer this.

> Secondary prevention, which will be lifelong, can be provided in a hospital-based clinic, but is managed more conveniently (for the patient) in the primary healthcare sector.

Table 17.12 A stroke follow-up checklist.

Impairments	Ask about weakness, balance, speech, pain
Disabilities	Do you need help with any everyday activities?
Aids and adaptations	Do you need any aids? Have they been delivered yet? Are you using them? Are they in good working order?
Support services	Are they in place? Are they appropriate and adequate?
New problems	Any new problems since last seen?
Aspirations	Anything you want to do but cannot do?
Work	Are you back to work?
Driving	Are you driving a car?
Carer	Do you have a carer? How is your carer coping?
Prevention	Check blood pressure, cholesterol, diabetic control, smoking, diet, exercise, adherence with medication

17.10 Generic issues in stroke service delivery

17.10.1 Information for patients and carers

One generic theme in the management of stroke – which is relevant throughout the patient pathway – is communication of information. Studies of the attitudes of patients and their carers to medical services in general, and stroke services in particular, have demonstrated that one of the greatest sources of dissatisfaction is with communication.[72,97] Patients and carers may receive very little information about the nature of stroke, its cause, management and likely prognosis.[25,115] Even where information is provided, it may be in a form that is difficult to understand or retain.

Patients' and carers' perceptions of the stroke service are likely to depend not just on the degree of recovery, but also on the quality of communication. Although it is easy to show that many patients receive little information, one must also remember that for some it may be enough. Some patients do not want a lot of information, preferring to trust in the professionals' judgement.[115,116]

It is therefore important to tailor the provision of information to the individual's needs and wishes. These complexities may in part explain the mixed results from clinical trials of information and education interventions.[109] There is some evidence that information combined with educational sessions improves knowledge and is more effective than providing information only. Information provision alone seems to have no measurable effect on mood, perceived health status or quality of life for patients or carers. The impact on satisfaction is inconsistent.

In the absence of good evidence to guide us we aim to provide information using a number of different media, including:

- a notice board on the stroke unit (Fig. 17.5);
- an information pack containing appropriate leaflets;
- audio and video tapes;
- individual interviews with patients and carers by members of the team;
- patient and carer groups.

However, there is probably no substitute for one of the team sitting down with the patient and family on one or more occasions to explain the situation and answer any specific questions. This can then be backed up with

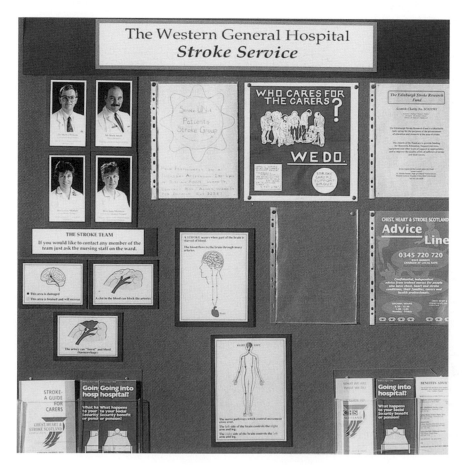

Fig. 17.5 A notice board at the entrance to a stroke unit. Typically it introduces the members of the stroke team, indicating how they might be contacted. It presents, in simple terms, what a stroke is and how it can affect the patient. We also include useful pamphlets and information relating to patient and carer groups.

Table 17.13 Tips on improving communication with carers of hospitalized stroke patients.

Provide a notice board at the entrance to the unit introducing staff and informing relatives about how to contact members of the team
Hold ward rounds during visiting times
Hold a regular 'open access' clinic where carers can meet the consultant
Invite carers to participate in patient care (including therapy sessions)
Set up a carers' group
Document the content of any discussions with relatives in the notes and report these at team meetings to ensure consistency
Arrange predischarge case conferences or family meetings
Back up verbal communication with written or audio material

written material. One approach, which has been used in other areas (e.g. oncology), is to record the interview and give the recording to the patient or family so they can review what has been said as and when they wish.[117] This might overcome the problem of patients and families only taking in a small proportion of the information given to them. Like all other areas of stroke care, a service needs to establish a system ensuring that input – in this case the provision of information – is tailored to the individual needs of patients and carers (Table 17.13).

17.10.2 Integration of services

Inevitably, most stroke patients require both community-based and hospital-based resources at some stage in their illness. They may even need more than one hospital-based service. It is therefore important to consider how these can be integrated to ensure that patients are appropriately placed at each stage of their illness and that transfers between each part of the service are as seamless as possible. Figure 17.1 illustrates how the components of a stroke service might fit together.

Many places have the necessary facilities and skills to provide an excellent service to patients with stroke. More often, the problem lies with the organization and integration of these facilities. The key areas where problems may arise are:

- Transfer from community to hospital; section 17.4 summarizes many initiatives to improve such transfers. Agreed protocols between primary and secondary care are essential.
- Transfer to specialist hospital services (e.g. neurosurgery and neuroradiology); these facilities should be readily available, because urgent neurosurgery can

occasionally be life-saving and produce a good functional outcome (sections 12.7.3, 13.3.5, 13.3.6). Neuroradiological interventions are now a key component of subarachnoid haemorrhage management (section 14.6). Inevitably, many smaller hospitals do not have these facilities. However, for the 1–2% of stroke patients who are at risk of deteriorating rapidly with a surgically remediable complication (e.g. acute hydrocephalus), a management plan should be available. This should include a policy to ensure the early identification and safe transfer of suitable patients to a neurosurgical centre.

- Transfer for continuing rehabilitation; where patients have been admitted to one service for acute care but have to be referred to a separate institution for rehabilitation, needless delays can result. In such circumstances, one will often read in the case notes 'waiting for rehabilitation' when, of course, rehabilitation should have started on the day of the stroke (section 11.11). Thus, one needs to organize services so that the patient's needs are matched by the care provided at all stages of his or her illness.

- Transfer from hospital to community: these challenges were considered in section 17.7.

> Many problems can arise when patients are transferred from one service to another. Remember rehabilitation is a journey, not a destination.

17.10.3 The hazards of transfer

Where patients have to be transferred between institutions (or teams) to receive the appropriate care, there is a very real danger that continuity of care will suffer. A consistent approach to patients and their families will not be achieved without excellent communication between the professionals involved. Patients' medical records should follow them through the system, and ideally at least one health professional should be involved in a patient's care from admission to discharge, and perhaps even beyond.

17.11 Planning, developing and maintaining a stroke service

In the remaining sections of this chapter, we will focus on the practical aspects of planning, developing, establishing, monitoring and maintaining a stroke service.

The exact manner in which the service is best provided will depend on local history, geography, needs, resources, people and politics. Any stroke service must therefore be tailored to the local conditions to achieve maximum effectiveness. Therefore it is difficult to be dogmatic about exactly how services should be organized.

17.11.1 Determining the needs of the population

If the aim of the service is to provide care for all those in the population who require it, not just those who can afford to pay for it, then the first factor to consider is the incidence of stroke and transient ischaemic attack in that population. This provides the basis for a 'needs assessment' which is fundamental to determining *how much* stroke service should be provided.

Incidence of acute stroke and transient ischaemic attack

Despite the huge burden that cerebrovascular disease places on communities throughout the world, there are less reliable data on its burden than one might expect. Although a large number of 'incidence' studies have appeared in the literature over the past 40 years, most have had methodological weaknesses that make their results, at least in part, unreliable. The criteria for an 'ideal' study are listed in Table 17.14. Table 17.5 gives the age-specific incidence of stroke provided by some more-or-less 'ideal' studies, most of which were based on white populations because little reliable information is available elsewhere.

> There are quite good data on the incidence of stroke and TIA in many white populations, some data on Oriental populations, but little reliable data for other parts of Asia, South America or Africa.

17.11.2 Possible approaches to assessing need

Because of the dearth of reliable data on *stroke incidence* (i.e. the number of first-ever-in-a-lifetime cases of stroke occurring in the population over a defined time period), those planning stroke services may decide to base their estimates of need on routinely collected mortality data (i.e. the number of deaths attributed to stroke in the population over a defined time period). They should, however, be aware of the potential problems of adopting this policy.

Mortality statistics

These depend on the collation of data from death certificates. They are thus dependent on the accuracy of death certification, which even in countries with quite high postmortem rates is known to be poor (section

Table 17.14 Criteria for an 'ideal' stroke and transient ischaemic attack (TIA) incidence study.[122,186]

A large, stable well-defined study population; the number and sex of the people in the population should be available in at least 10-year age intervals during the study. This usually requires a recent census.

Complete ascertainment of all patients with either stroke or TIA occurring in that population, whether referred to hospital or not. This requires multiple overlapping methods to detect cases, including contacting primary health teams, review of hospital admissions, imaging records and death certificates.

Accurate assessment of the cross-boundary flows in both directions.

First-ever-in-a-lifetime strokes and TIAs should be distinguished from recurrent strokes and TIAs.

Prospective assessment of all suspected cases so that standard diagnostic criteria (WHO definition) can be applied rigorously soon after the patient presents to medical attention (so-called 'hot pursuit').

Studies should register patients with 'TIAs' as well as strokes to ensure that mild strokes, which may be misclassified as TIAs by referring doctors in routine clinical practice, are not under-represented.

Brain imaging to determine the pathological type of stroke. This should be performed early enough after stroke onset to reliably distinguish ischaemic from haemorrhagic stroke.

Case ascertainment over whole years to avoid bias due to any seasonal fluctuations in incidence.

Standard methods of data presentation – i.e. not more than 5 years of data averaged together, incidence for men and women presented separately, incidence in those of over 85 years old if possible, incidence presented as mid-decade age bands (e.g. 55–64 years) but 5-year bands available, 95% confidence intervals.

18.2.1). The accuracy of mortality statistics also depends on the accuracy of the population denominators used and thus on the reliability and timing of the most recent census. Furthermore, mortality statistics only include the deaths attributed to stroke (and not the number of stroke episodes), and are not in themselves of much value in estimating the need for health services. Although they are bound to reflect, at least indirectly, the incidence of stroke in the population, the case fatality may differ from place to place, and so there will not be a uniform relationship between stroke mortality and incidence. There is some evidence that case fatality is falling, while incidence is not (section 18.2).

Hospital admission or discharge statistics

These are an alternative source of information which may reflect the incidence of stroke. Outpatient attendances

Table 17.15 Annual age-specific incidence of stroke per 100 000 population in the 1980s and 1990s. (Adapted from Feigin, 2005[12] and Sudlow & Warlow, 1997.[187])

Place and mid-year of study	Age (years)					
	0–44	45–54	55–64	65–74	75–84	≥85
Northern Europe						
Norway, Innherred (1995)	12†	40	217	741	1820	3039
Sweden, Soderhamn (1990)	12	67	313	976	2056	2995
Denmark, Frederiksberg (1989)	4	104	306	712	1298	1599
Finland, Espoo-Kaunianen (1990)		125	306	618		
UK, London (1996)	21	87	221	516	891	1892
UK, Oxfordshire (1984)	9	57	291	690	1428	2009
UK, Teesside (1996)	11	89	297	611	1247	2099
UK, Scottish Borders (1999)	13	131	255	659	1587	2400
Eastern Europe and Russia						
Poland, Warsaw‡ (1991)	14	76	268	408	901§	1355¶
Ukraine, Uzhgorod (2000)	10	400	750	1500	2600	750
Georgia, Tbilisi (2002)	12	78	360	721	1029	1030
Russia, Novosibirsk (1992)	28	246	496	1060	1554	1513
Central and Southern Europe						
France, Dijon (1987)	10	62	119	410	979	1641
Germany, Erlangen (1995)	16	105	196	508	1226	2117
Greece, Arcadia (1994)	14	82	218	568	1220	2661
Italy, Aosta (1989)	13	82	255	707	1607	3237
Italy, Belluno (1993)	10	114	242	720	1317	3413
Italy, Umbria (1988)	5	115	280	541	1458	2180
Italy, Calabria (1996)	10	69	149	570	1454	2040
Portugal, Porto (1999)		162	337	681	1092	1685
Australia and New Zealand						
Australia, Perth (1989)	17	98	207	511	1679	2369
New Zealand, Auckland (1991)	18*	82	253	647	1267	1967
Australia, Melbourne (1996)		105	213	535	1290	2900
North America						
US, Rochester (1988)	9	62	269	642	1272	2111
South America and West Indies						
French West Indies, Martinique (1999)		124	272	630	1196	1820
Barbados, West Indies (2002)	11	94	219	578	963	2208
Chile, Iquiqie (2000)	8	100	308	462	1037	1089
Eastern Asia						
Japan, Oyabe (1989)		153	308	781	1940	4385

*Age group 15–44 years.
†Age group 15–44 years.
‡Subarachnoid haemorrhage excluded.
§Age group 75–79 years.
¶Age group ≥ 80 years.

are seldom recorded. Again, inaccuracies in diagnostic codes may limit their usefulness.[118,119] Also, data may be distorted by double counting, which frequently occurs when patients are transferred from an acute centre to a rehabilitation or continuing care facility. Stroke incidence estimated from hospital discharge data has been found to be much higher than that derived from a population-based stroke register.[120] But the biggest problem is that these data only include those patients who are admitted to hospital with a stroke. They are therefore a better measure of the hospital service that is currently provided than of the population's needs. The relationship between stroke incidence and hospitalization can only be known with certainty where a reliable stroke incidence study has been performed to determine the proportion of stroke patients who attend hospital. Where hospital admission rates have been determined, they vary considerably between places – 55% to over 95% in developed countries, while there is no information from Asia and Africa.[15,16,34,121] There is also relatively little information about changes in admission rates with time.[121] The rate of hospital admission, or even the attendance at an outpatient clinic, depends on several factors that are independent of population need and may be difficult to predict.

Stroke prevalence is another measure of the frequency of stroke that some suggest is useful in planning services. Prevalence is the number of people who have ever had a stroke living in the population at any one point in time. Prevalence data could be useful in determining the needs for long-term support services in the community. However, we would argue that the greater the time that elapses after an acute stroke or transient ischaemic attack (TIA), the less important disease-specific services become. If one is interested in determining the need for long-term support services, it is more useful to estimate the prevalence of disability due to *all* causes, rather than just that related to stroke. In addition, stroke prevalence can never reflect the true burden of stroke, because the patients who die soon after a stroke are not represented. There are also a number of important methodological difficulties with measuring the prevalence of stroke and TIA, not least the need to make accurate diagnoses sometimes years after the actual event and to survey thousands of people. Where this has been done the prevalence usually ranges from 5 to 10 per 1000 population.[122] As a quicker alternative, one can estimate the prevalence of stroke from its incidence and case fatality using the 'bath principle' (Fig. 17.6). Where this has been done for a predominantly white population in New Zealand, the prevalence was estimated to be 8 per 1000 population (9 in men, 7 in women) aged 15 years and older.[123] Of the prevalent cases, around 55% had not made a complete recovery from their stroke, and 21% needed help with self-care activities.

> Stroke prevalence is difficult to measure directly, and of limited use for planning stroke services.

17.11.3 A practical approach to needs assessment

The vast majority of health service planners are not fortunate enough to have had a recent, methodologically sound, stroke incidence study in the population they serve. Rather than carrying out their own incidence study, which is time-consuming and expensive, we recommend the following approach for determining local

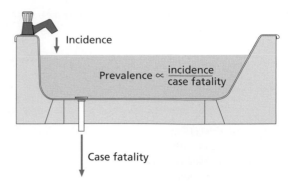

Fig. 17.6 A bath with water running in (representing incident cases), the water level (representing prevalence) and water going down the plug hole (representing deaths in prevalent cases). The prevalence is directly proportional to the incidence and inversely proportional to the case fatality among prevalent cases, although the mathematical relationship is quite complex.

needs, which uses both local data and information from incidence studies from other areas (Table 17.16). If one looks at the estimates of incidence from the most reliable studies (Table 17.14), it is surprising how little variation there is in the incidence of stroke (Table 17.15). However, these estimates are based mainly on white populations, and the incidence may vary in different ethnic groups. For instance, in both New York and London, the incidence of stroke is significantly higher in blacks than in whites[124,125] – although this has been attributed to case-finding artifact.[126] Also, the incidence of stroke among people of Pacific origin in New Zealand is higher than in those of European origin.[123] However, the incidence of stroke among ethnic groups may not be the same as the incidence in the same ethnic group living in the original population from which they came, and it may be that differences between ethnic groups in the same country may be more to do with socioeconomic circumstances than race.

One should start with the age-specific and sex-specific stroke incidence in the population that is closest to the local one in terms of geography, ethnic composition and culture. These rates can then be applied to the local population numbers to obtain an age-specific and sex-standardized incidence. A comparison of routinely collected data from the area in which the stroke incidence study was performed with equivalent data from one's own vicinity may give further evidence of the relevance of the incidence data. The cause-specific mortality data are likely to be the most reliable and easily obtained. One can then judge whether the incidence locally is likely to be greater or less than that in the available incidence study.

An alternative approach might be to use local hospital admission or discharge data and to adjust them to take

Table 17.16 A step-by-step guide to estimating approximately the number of strokes in a local population of interest.

Step 1	Obtain the most accurate census data for the population of interest for each sex and age band.
Step 2	Identify the 'ideal' incidence study that is likely to have been done in a similar population to the one of interest (e.g. geography, race).
Step 3	Multiply each age-specific and sex-specific incidence by the number of people of that age and sex in the population of interest – e.g. if the incidence in men 65–74 years old is 690 per 100 000 and there are 11 000 men in this age band in the population of interest, one would expect about 76 men (i.e. $690 \times 11\,000/100\,000$) between 65 and 74 years of age to have a stroke each year in the population of interest.
Step 4	Sum the numbers of patients of each sex in each age band expected to have stroke to obtain the total number expected in the population.
Step 5	Consider making an adjustment for any marked differences in, for example, the cause-specific mortality between the population of interest and the population in which the incidence study was done.
Step 6	If one is interested in transient ischaemic attacks, then their incidence is usually about 30% that of stroke (section 18.4).
Step 7	The number of recurrent strokes is of the order of 30% of first-ever-in-a-lifetime strokes, so that to estimate the total number of strokes likely to occur in the population of interest, the number of incident strokes should be inflated by 30%.

If interested in the total numbers of patients who could be referred to your service with suspected stroke or TIA then add the additional number of referred patients who may be expected to have a non-stroke diagnosis (possibly 50% for TIAs and 30% for acute stroke).[44,188]

account of the likely proportion of stroke patients admitted. This will be more reliable for stroke than for TIAs. One could estimate this proportion admitted by surveying the local primary health teams and asking them to report the proportion of patients with acute stroke who they refer to hospital. This may be reliable enough if they report that they refer virtually all cases (as in Sweden), but if the proportion is smaller, their estimate may be misleading.[16] Also, hospital discharge data may be inaccurate for a number of reasons:[118,119]

- inaccuracy of routine clinical diagnosis, especially of TIAs;
- lack of CT brain scans to confirm the stroke diagnosis and exclude other diagnoses;
- use of vague terms, e.g. 'acute hemiparesis', 'cerebrovascular disease' in medical records and discharge summaries from which routine codes may be derived;
- coding errors;
- failure to distinguish acute stroke admissions from those due to complications of an earlier stroke;
- failure to code strokes occurring in hospital, or in the context of another diagnosis.

Table 17.17 gives the likelihood that a patient allocated one of the cerebrovascular codes on discharge from one of five Scottish hospitals had actually had an acute stroke. It was also reported from Norway[120] that certain diagnostic codes were more likely to identify true strokes

than others. Therefore, if one plans to use hospital discharge data, one would be wise to be selective in one's choice of discharge codes.

The crude incidence of stroke tells one how common the problem is, but in itself is not sufficient to determine the health service needs of the population. Before one can plan a service, one needs to have estimates of the following.

Age-and sex-specific incidence. Younger patients require different facilities from older ones, e.g. retraining for employment. Older women more often live alone, and may require more formal support in the community.

Type-specific incidence (that is transient ischaemic attack, ischaemic stroke, primary intracerebral haemorrhage and subarachnoid haemorrhage). These data may be useful in more detailed planning of the population's needs. Patients with TIA and minor ischaemic stroke require prompt diagnosis, investigation and initiation and supervision of secondary prevention but not prolonged inpatient care, rehabilitation or community support services. Patients with subarachnoid haemorrhage require emergency hospitalization and neuro-radiological and neurosurgical facilities (Chapter 14). Haemorrhagic strokes have a higher early case fatality, so although they may require more care in the very early stages, the longer-term burden of severe disability may be less than for patients with ischaemic stroke. The

Code	All hospital admissions	Emergency admissions only
	Positive predictive value for acute stroke (%)	
Subarachnoid haemorrhage	85–88	88–93
Intracranial haemorrhage	87–91	92–94
Non-traumatic intracranial haemorrhage	58–75	63–75
Stenosis/occlusion of a precerebral artery	1	0
Ischaemic stroke	83–93	86–95
Transient ischaemic attack	5	6
Stroke unspecified	78–87	82–88
Cerebrovascular disease, unspecified	25–28	31
Cerebrovascular disease sequelae	0	0

Table 17.17 Positive predictive values of cerebrovascular disease codes (ICD 9 or 10) for a diagnosis of stroke.

The proportion of patients who were allocated a cerebrovascular code (ICD 9 or 10) on discharge from five Scottish hospitals and who actually had had an acute stroke. The values are higher for emergency admissions. This study did not attempt to identify patients who had a stroke but received a non-stroke code.

estimates of the relative frequency of the pathological type of stroke are remarkably similar in most of the published incidence studies, which come from predominantly white populations (Fig. 17.7). Although the proportion of patients who are haemorrhagic is probably higher in Oriental populations, it is difficult to be certain, because of limited information. The proportion of strokes due to subarachnoid haemorrhage and primary intracerebral haemorrhage is greater in the young than the old.

The prognosis of stroke and its subtypes. From the type-specific incidence and case fatality, one can estimate the likely requirements for assessment and diagnostic services, acute care, rehabilitation and terminal care services, long-term care, community support and secondary prevention. The prognosis of stroke and its subtypes has been discussed elsewhere (section 10.2.3). Information on stroke severity and comorbidity would be invaluable, since these will be major determinants of patients' health service use. However, such data are unlikely to be routinely available unless a stroke register has been kept.

Changes over time. When one is planning a stroke service, one has to take account of any changes that may occur in the future, because one's service will need to alter to take these into account. Trends in stroke mortality and incidence are discussed later, and there is evidence that the incidence, and maybe even the severity, of stroke is falling in many western populations. Apart from the changing incidence, one also has to take into account changing demographics. In most developed countries, older people account for an increasing proportion of the population. Therefore, for a disease such as stroke in which the incidence is much higher in older people, the total number of strokes will increase unless offset by a falling incidence. However, one has to remember that case fatality is higher in older patients and in those with prior disability, and therefore fewer of these older stroke patients will survive to require long-term care. Changes in clinical practice are likely to force rapid and quite unpredictable alterations in the shape of clinical services for stroke. The changes in management of stroke have, until now, been small and gradual, but with recent increases in research efforts, major changes are more likely and the needs of the population could alter rapidly and unpredictably. The introduction of coiling rather than clipping of ruptured intracranial aneurysms after the ISAT trial (section 14.4.2) has resulted in large, sudden and difficult-to-manage changes in services; patients once admitted under neurosurgeons and operated on may now be admitted under neurologists and treated by radiologists. People's expectations of healthcare, often driven by media reports of medical successes and failures, may also force changes in services that go beyond the evidence of effectiveness.

17.11.4 Assuming that resources are limited, to what extent will the needs of the population be met?

Having obtained an estimate of one's local age-specific, sex-specific and type-specific incidence and outcome of

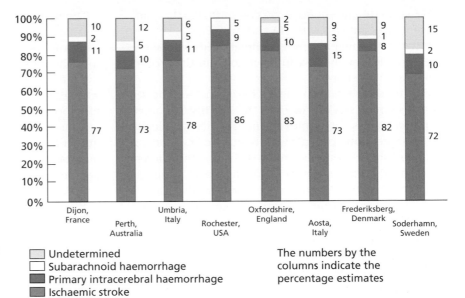

Fig. 17.7 Histogram showing the proportions of patients aged between 45 and 84 years with a first-ever-in-a-lifetime stroke due to ischaemia, primary intracerebral haemorrhage, subarachnoid haemorrhage and uncertain, in more or less 'ideal' incidence studies. Only studies where a computed tomography (CT) brain scan was done in more than 70%, and including patients with subarachnoid haemorrhage, are covered.

stroke and TIA, one is still a long way from determining the needs of the population. After all, this estimate does not indicate the actual resources these people will require, and of course at some stage somebody has to make a political decision about how completely the population's needs are to be met. Inevitably, where there are limited resources for health services, choices have to be made about allocating resources between areas (e.g. should one build a new hospital or a new school?). Having been given limited resources, however, it is important that those planning stroke services should use them in as an efficient a manner as possible and should prioritize (i.e. ration) to make sure that sufficient funds are available for whatever are perceived to be the most important aspects of the service. These decisions are usually taken by politicians but, because they depend on information about the effectiveness of components of the stroke services, it is essential for the politicians to receive sound medical advice.

The perceived pressures to develop particular components of stroke services and the way in which these services develop are likely to reflect a number of factors apart from the effectiveness of the service offered:

- *Local healthcare culture and economy.* The types of services provided for stroke patients vary greatly between the developed economies. In the US and Germany services often focus around centralized neurological centres or stroke centres where selected patients receive acute care but not ongoing rehabilitation. There is evidence that access to these services[127] may be reduced for certain patient groups such as the elderly. In contrast the Scandinavian countries have tended to approach stroke services with a more devolved delivery offering

similar services in all parts of the country. In the UK, stroke services are tending to evolve out of existing rehabilitation facilities, which were traditionally provided by geriatric medicine or general medicine services.

- *The needs of the patient population.* Within stroke care, as within healthcare in general, there is frequently a tension between the need to centralize services for individuals with very specialist needs (for example, subarachnoid haemorrhage) and the aspiration to provide as much high-quality care as close to the individual's home as possible.

- *Patients' wishes.* Once again there is a tension between pressures to centralize and fragment care, for example, between acute and rehabilitation services and to provide continuity throughout the patient journey which is usually valued by patients and carers.

- *Costs and resources.* There are increasing pressures to control the costs of healthcare services and this is particularly relevant when considering emergency cover by senior medical staff. Once again centralized services meet these challenges by having large groups of staff, or at least networks of staff, who are available to be on call.

17.11.5 Planning a stroke service

Having established the aims of the service, the needs of the population and the degree to which one expects to fulfil these, one can then plan the development of services. Usually, one starts with the existing services, even if these are inadequate and chaotic. It is then useful to consider the following two questions prior to making any changes:

- What are the current resources committed to the management of patients with TIA and stroke?
- What are the major gaps (i.e. unmet needs and failure to provide cost-effective interventions) in the present provision of services?

One needs to establish the strengths and weaknesses of the current services in order to identify the most important areas for improvement. Priority should be given to providing patients with basic care (e.g. nursing to provide for basic needs) and to delivering those interventions that are of proven effectiveness. Although information about current services may already be available, it is likely that in addition to routinely collected data, it will be useful to carry out a survey to determine:

- How many and what sort of patients are currently being managed (i.e. demographic and clinical data)?
- Where are they being managed (i.e. in the hospital or community, in accident and emergency departments, neurology, internal medicine or geriatric medicine)?
- By whom are they being managed (i.e. general or family practitioner, neurologist, general physician)?
- How are they being managed (i.e. the process of care)?
- What resources are currently being used?

A community-based register that identified all patients in the population who had a stroke or TIA would be an ideal but expensive and impractical way of answering these questions. A hospital-based stroke register is a practical alternative that can help to answer most of the questions, although clearly it cannot provide detailed information about patients who are not referred to hospital. A register is an invaluable tool for monitoring the performance of services as well as planning them.

> Set up a hospital-based stroke register to get some idea of the current state of the local stroke service – however fragmented and chaotic it is.

The simplest, quickest and most practical approach is to carry out a survey of the current services against certain standards. Those working within a service are often fully aware of its deficiencies, and their knowledge should not be ignored (although sadly it often is). This will only work where there is a willingness by the important parties to acknowledge deficiencies and to change practice. This approach can identify areas of strength and weakness, and may determine which area to concentrate on first (e.g. Sentinel Audit[128]).

> An honest, objective appraisal of services against some agreed standards by those involved in providing them, perhaps facilitated by an independent observer, may be the best stimulus for service development.

The immediate priorities for improving a service will also depend on how easily or cheaply particular problems can be solved. For instance, poor standards of medical assessment may be improved by the introduction of a protocol and education for junior medical staff with little implication for resources, while the provision of an occupational therapy department where there isn't one has major resource implications. Planning a stroke unit is likely to be less challenging in a well-resourced hospital setting where reorganization of staff and work patterns is needed. However the obstacles are formidable if the key staff members are not available at all, and even if they are many staff do not like being reorganized without very good reason, much explanation and proper support.

17.12 Evaluating and monitoring stroke services

We believe that the most reliable way of determining the relative effectiveness of interventions is an appropriately designed randomized trial where feasible, or a systematic review if more than one trial is available. This of course is not an option in the evaluation of a local stroke service rather than stroke services in general, so we have to rely on less robust methodologies.

Non-randomized comparisons of the process of care, or of patient and carer outcomes achieved by services, are the only practical methods of evaluation. If one is setting up a new service in a hospital, the process, or outcomes, can be compared with those in a nearby hospital without a new service. Alternatively, one could measure the process and outcomes achieved by the existing service and then measure whether these are improved after the new service has been established (i.e. a before-and-after study). However, such evaluations can be misleading. They may demonstrate improvements (or worsening), or differences in the process or outcome of care, but they cannot provide reliable data to indicate that any changes are actually due to the new service. One cannot rely on such non-randomized evaluations to influence practice elsewhere, but they may fulfil important *local* functions. One could reasonably argue that, as long as the new service is not much more expensive to run, it does not matter whether any improvements observed can be attributed directly to that service. Obviously, if the new service was very costly, one would want reassurance that the improvements had not occurred spontaneously. But if a non-randomized evaluation demonstrates either no improvement or even a worse outcome, it is difficult to know how to respond. Were the changes due to the new service, in which case it ought to be modified, or were they due to some unforeseen confounding factor?

There are several other methodological problems, which can affect randomized as well as non-randomized comparisons, and which need to be considered:

- small numbers of patients; so that any change observed may be accounted for by the play of chance or missing a real and worthwhile change because too few patients were studied;
- observer bias in assessing the process or outcome; often, the observers have an interest in the result of the evaluation, which may influence their judgements.

So what aspects of a service can we measure? The simplest way to monitor the service is to measure the amount and nature of work being carried out. Unfortunately, politicians and those who fund healthcare place too much emphasis on the volume rather than quality of service. A stroke service may include some components (e.g. processes) for which there is little doubt of their effectiveness (e.g. aspirin for cerebral infarct, low-risk carotid surgery). When assessing performance, it is therefore most important to monitor how well the service delivers those components whose effectiveness is established.

In assessing the quality of care (or 'clinical audit', as it tends to be called) one should consider three aspects of the service:[128] the structure, or facilities available; the process of care; and the outcomes for those treated.

Structure

From all that has been said above, it should be fairly obvious that a stroke service needs certain essential facilities to provide all the components necessary to care for patients with stroke and TIA (Tables 17.1 and 17.2). This makes the setting of standards and the measurement of performance for structure relatively straightforward. Some basic standards (incorporated into Scottish service standards; http://www.nhshealthquality.org/nhsqis/1288.html) for structure might include:

- an identified individual who is responsible for the organization of stroke services;
- early access to a stroke unit;
- multidisciplinary staffing of the stroke unit (section 17.6);
- early access to outpatient assessment by a specialist for patients who do not need admission to hospital (i.e. a 'one-stop' neurovascular outpatient clinic);
- prompt access to CT scanning;

- prompt access to non-invasive vascular imaging, and carotid surgery if necessary (section 16.11);
- continuing care facilities, both community-based and institutional.

However, care has to be taken in defining these standards. For example, what does 'prompt access' really mean, what is a specialist, what does a stroke unit consist of? One could very quickly fulfil a requirement for a stroke unit by simply relabelling a general medical ward, but of course one is unlikely to accrue the benefits of stroke unit care.

7.12.2 Process

Some aspects of the process of care are easily monitored, e.g. waiting times for appointments. It may be relatively easy to define a standard (for example, patients with TIAs and ischaemic strokes should be given aspirin to reduce the risk of further vascular events, unless there are contraindications), but for other procedures for which there is less scientific justification, it is more difficult. The lack of scientific justification can, and frequently is, overcome by using the combined views of recognized experts, i.e. a consensus. However, what appears to be a fairly straightforward standard cannot be applied sensibly to every patient because – for example – they cannot comply with the assessment. The UK National Sentinel Audit of Stroke[71] addressed this problem by having a 'no but . . .' clause attached to each standard (Fig. 17.8). This is essential for the process of care to be compared in different groups of patients.

Another difficulty is that, by directly observing the care, one is likely to alter its delivery (the so-called Hawthorne effect). Also, such an approach is likely to be very costly if performed on all stroke admissions. The alternative is to audit the records of care, but this immediately raises the question of the validity of the medical record, i.e. whether the records reflect the actual care provided. However, most people would agree that good records probably do reflect good care given, and that this is a reasonable method of measuring the process of care. The other methodological problems involved in audits of case notes are summarized in Table 17.18.

> Monitoring the process of care by case note review raises a number of important methodological problems that must be addressed if one's assessment is to be useful and valid.

Although one may be measuring the performance against some 'ideal' standard, one is likely to want to compare the performance in the same service over time, or to compare performances between services. To do this

Patient assessment

2.1.0 First 24 hours
        Neurological assessment in the first 24 hours
2.1.1 (a) Have the following been specifically recorded in the first 24 hours?

	Yes	No	No but
(i) Conscious level (eg Glasgow Coma Scale, alert / oriented)	☐	☐	☐
(ii) Eye movements (eg Cranials 3, 4 and 6 intact, doll's eye response if unconscious)	☐	☐	☐
(iii) Limb movements (response to pain if conscious)	☐	☐	☐

(b) If patient is noted to be conscious, are the following recorded?
Answer No, but if....... impaired level of consciousness is documented

	Yes	No	No but
(i) Screening for swallowing disorders (not gag reflex)	☐	☐	☐
(ii) Communication	☐	☐	☐
(iii) Trunk control or gait	☐	☐	☐

(c) If patient is alert and able to communicate, is there a formal assessment of:
Answer No. but if..... impaired level of consciousness/communication is documented.

	Yes	No	No but
(i) Formal mental test (eg mental test score)	☐	☐	☐
(ii) Visual fields	☐	☐	☐
(iii) Visual inattention	☐	☐	☐
(iv) Sensory testing	☐	☐	☐

Fig. 17.8 One of the sections from the National Sentinel Audit of Stroke. This one relates to the recording of the neurological examination. The interval (e.g. 24 h) since admission at which these data should be recorded, and the circumstances in which it is acceptable for the information not to be recorded, are given in each section.[132]

Table 17.18 Important methodological issues in the audit of case notes.

Patient selection bias
The case notes audited should be a representative sample of all those treated (either a consecutive series or a random sample). Beware the missing notes because so often these patients are more 'interesting' to somebody, perhaps because they had a rare form of stroke, or died.

Case note retrieval bias
Poor-quality case notes or those of dead patients may be more difficult to retrieve, which might bias the audit in a favourable direction. A high proportion retrieved is an important step in reducing bias.[189]

Lack of precision
A sufficiently large number of case notes should be audited to provide a precise estimate of performance and to allow precise comparisons to be made with other centres, or with audits performed at different times in the same centre.

Observer bias
Auditors may have an interest in the result of the audit, which may influence their assessment of performance; blinded, or at least impartial, observers should be employed if possible.

Poor inter-observer reliability of measure
If the measure of performance is not reliable, then it will be more difficult to demonstrate real differences between centres. Also, if there is a consistent difference in the way an audit measure is applied by different auditors, this may produce invalid comparisons.

Differences in case mix
A standard that is applicable to one patient may not apply to another. It is important that standards should be adjusted for differences in case mix.

meaningfully, one has to have a valid and reliable measure of performance, one needs to audit enough cases to produce statistically robust results, and one must be able to take into account differences in case mix between services or changes over time. The *Stroke Audit Package* was originally developed by the Royal College of Physicians to overcome these methodological problems and enable valid comparisons to be made.[129] But because this package only addressed a limited number of the more medical aspects of care, the Royal College of Physicians of London therefore also developed the National Sentinel Audit, which includes other important aspects of care delivered by different members of the multidisciplinary team.[130]

17.12.3 Outcome

The term 'outcome' is used in different ways and so causes confusion. Clinicians use the term to refer to the clinical outcome of the patient or carer. Outcomes therefore include survival, functional status, complications, or less easily defined concepts such as quality of life. Others, particularly those with a management background, use the term 'outcome' to refer to any result of an intervention, e.g. reduced waiting times or readmission rates. In this section, we use 'outcome' to refer to the *clinical* outcome of patients (i.e. physical, functional, cognitive, emotional, etc.).

Since the main aim of stroke services is to optimize the outcome for patients and carers, the measurement of outcome is obviously the most relevant criterion by which to judge the performance of a service. This recognition has prompted the development of outcome analyses such as *Dr Foster's notes* (drfoster.co.uk). Unfortunately, the use of outcomes to reflect the quality of care is the most challenging area of stroke audit, and there are many well-known difficulties to be overcome.[131–136] Until they are, those involved in providing and monitoring health services must be extremely careful not to misinterpret outcome data.

The observed outcome in a group of patients treated by a particular service will be determined by four factors:
- the quality and effectiveness of the care provided;
- the method of measurement of outcome (e.g. who is measuring it, and how?);
- chance (or random error);
- case mix (or mix of prognostic factors at baseline).

17.12.4 The quality and effectiveness of care

This is the aspect we hope outcomes will reflect. However, it is important to remember that most interventions have only small or moderate-sized effects, which may be difficult to detect even in large randomized trials. For example, a wildly implausible 50% relative reduction in the death rate from 30% to 15% after the opening of a stroke unit would require a sample of 200 patients both before and after its introduction to eliminate the effects of chance, and in itself contribute nothing to the elimination of biases of various sorts. The impact of stroke unit care is far less than this (Table 17.6).

There are several examples of studies of stroke unit services[71,91] where treatment in a hospital with a stroke unit was associated with improved outcomes even after adjusting for case mix. However, they were based on large patient samples of several thousands, and smaller studies have often failed to show a clear link between process and outcome.[137]

17.12.5 The method of measurement of outcome

Many attempts to monitor the quality of service by measuring patient outcomes have relied on mortality data, presumably because they are often routinely available, reasonably objective and may indicate where there are major problems. Unfortunately, mortality is unlikely to be influenced by many components of care (discharge planning being one obvious example). Some outcome measures that may better reflect the quality of care are shown in Table 17.19. They measure outcome at different

Table 17.19 Aspects of outcome that may be relevant in assessing stroke services, and some tools for measuring these outcomes.

Outcome	Promising measurement tools
Survival	Case fatality during a defined time period, e.g. at 30 days or 6 months after stroke onset
Complications	Proportion of patients developing pressure ulcers or fractures; there are difficulties in defining these and reliably recording them; paradoxically, better services may identify more and record them more often
Residual impairments	Probably not very useful, and not easily collected after hospital discharge
Mobility	10-m walking speed
Arm function	Nine-hole peg test
Psychological outcome	Hospital anxiety and depression scale
	General health questionnaire
	Many of the most disabled patients will not be capable of responding to measures of psychological outcome
Disability	Barthel Index
	Functional Independence Measure (FIM)
	Three simple questions (Fig. 17.9)
	Oxford Handicap Scale (also known as the Modified Rankin Scale) – should be measured at a defined point after the stroke, e.g. 6 months; easily collected after hospital discharge
Handicap	London Handicap Scale[190] – a difficult area with no well-tested measures; the Oxford Handicap Scale does not really address handicap in isolation
Patient or carer satisfaction	Hospsat and Homesat[99] – is this an outcome or process measure?
General health or health-related quality of life	Nottingham Health Profile
	Short Form 36
	Euroqol – potentially interesting because it could allow comparisons with other disease states; however, many stroke patients cannot complete the questionnaires because of cognitive problems

Validity, different types include:
- Criterion validity, when the measure is related to an accepted 'gold standard'.
- Construct validity, where the measure is related to existing measures of similar aspects of outcome.
- Content (or face) validity, which relies on expert agreement that the measure is a reasonable reflection of what it is supposed to be measuring.

There can be considerable difficulties in demonstrating the validity of a particular measure.[192]

Reliability

This is the reproducibility of a measurement, most commonly between observers (inter-observer reliability) and over time (intra-observer or test-retest reliability).

Relevance

The scale should measure some aspect of outcome that is relevant to the patient or carer as well as to the doctor. Thus, the size of a cerebral infarct on a CT brain scan is of little relevance, while patients' ability to look after themselves is very important to the patient and carer.

Practicality

Scales vary in their complexity and the time taken to complete an assessment. Studies of long-term outcome involving hundreds of patients need very simple measures which can be completed by postal or telephone questionnaire, while smaller studies in hospital can afford to use more complex measures.

Sensitivity

A scale should distinguish between patients who have different outcomes or detect important changes in a particular patient. Usually, more sensitive scales are more complex and unfortunately less reliable.

Communicability

Ideally, the measure will mean something to other health professionals or even patients. It is more useful to know that a patient feels 'fine' than to be told that their score on a particular stroke scale was 23 out of 100, for example.

Table 17.20 Important features of scales for the measurement of outcome after stroke.

levels of disease – pathology, impairment, activity, participation and quality of life. It is important that they should have acceptable validity (i.e. they measure what they are intended to measure) and reliability (i.e. they are reproducible in different settings and when used by different people).

A number of different types of scale have been developed and used to measure outcome after stroke and there are a number of features that one should look for in choosing an outcome measure (Table 17.20).[138] One can loosely categorize the measures of outcome after stroke under the following headings.

Stroke scales

So-called 'stroke scales' (e.g. the Scandinavian Stroke Scale, Canadian Stroke Scale, National Institute of Health Stroke Scale) were largely developed to describe the severity of acute stroke and to monitor changes in the patient's condition.[139,140] Most concentrate on the type and severity of the neurological impairments. They have been criticized for lacking relevance for patients, being complex and therefore impractical, and for summing 'apples and pears'.[138] They rely on a clinical examination, although reduced scales can be completed from case notes.[141] We do not think they are particularly useful in evaluating stroke services. They might be used as a measure of case mix.

> 'Far better an approximate answer to the right question, which is often vague, than an exact answer to the wrong question, which can always be made precise'.[142]

Functional scales (activity)

These include measures of disability or dependence in activities of daily living (ADL), such as the Barthel Index, the Nottingham ADL Scale and the Functional Independence Measure (FIM).[143,144] Under this heading one could also include the so-called extended ADL (EADL) scales such as the Frenchay Activities Index and the Nottingham Extended ADL Scale[145–147] which identify whether patients are participating in more complex activities such as shopping, leisure or work. These scales appear to measure relevant aspects of outcome, although some demonstrate ceiling effects (e.g. the Barthel Index) and may not pick up problems in particular areas, e.g. communication. Indeed, one can score maximum points on the Barthel and yet be blind, deaf and mute. The scales are in general 'ordinal', so that care must be taken in choosing the appropriate statistical method to describe or compare groups of patients. Some of these scales are simple enough to incorporate into a postal or telephone questionnaire, and may therefore be used in large studies of long-term outcome.[148]

Handicap (participation)

Handicap, or its more acceptable converse, participation, is difficult to define and therefore difficult to measure, but is undoubtedly of relevance to stroke patients and their carers. The Oxford Handicap Scale (Table 17.19), which is a modification of the Rankin Scale, sounds from its name as if it measures handicap, but it really measures a combination of symptoms, dependency and change in lifestyle.[149,150] However, it has been widely used, is relevant and simple enough to be used reliably over the telephone, and is therefore useful in large studies.[151] Precision of assessment can be improved by using a structured interview.[152]

Quality of life

Like handicap, quality of life is difficult to define and thus measure. A large number of generic measures (otherwise known as multidimensional measures) have been developed that attempt to measure outcomes in relation to various aspects, including physical function, psychological function, pain and social function. They include the Short Form 36, Nottingham Health Profile, EuroQol, Sickness Impact Profile, Stroke Impact Scale and the Assessment of Quality of Life (AQoL) instrument.[153,154] Most provide a profile of outcome rather than an overall measure, and group comparisons are therefore complex. However, the EuroQol and AQoL provide a single measure of 'utility', and researchers have made some headway in deriving summary scores for the other measures. Because they are generic (i.e. can be used across many different health states) they offer health economists and others the opportunity to compare the utility of different health outcomes in different diseases. Some are long and complex (e.g. the Sickness Impact Profile) and are not suited to large-scale studies in which face-to-face administration is not practical. Also, they all rely on patients' views of their health status, which limits their use in patients with severe communication and cognitive difficulties. It is unclear how valid the carers' responses on behalf of the patient are to these questionnaires.[155]

> Like motherhood, quality of life is much admired, difficult to define and even more difficult to measure.

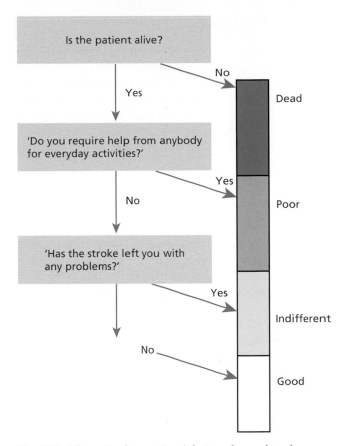

Fig. 17.9 'Three simple questions' that can be used to place stroke patients into four different outcome categories.[160]

Three simple questions

We have used 'three simple questions' to categorize patients into those with poor, fair and good outcomes after stroke (Fig. 17.9).[103,156] This approach appears to be reasonably valid and reliable, and is certainly practical when the outcome of very large numbers of patients needs to be measured. Further work is required to establish the optimal wording of the simple questions and to test them in different languages and settings.[157]

Patient satisfaction

Many healthcare systems are being influenced by market forces and the idea that patients are consumers. This has placed increasing importance on the satisfaction of our 'clients' (i.e. patients) with their healthcare. Many health service managers regard patient satisfaction as being an important outcome, although some consider satisfaction to be a measure of process; measures of patient and carer satisfaction with hospital and home care have been developed.[97]

Patient and carer satisfaction appears to reflect the process of care and the patients' outcomes. Improvements in satisfaction have been observed in trials of occupational therapy[158] and early supported discharge services.[70] As one would expect, those with poorer physical outcomes and depression are likely to report less satisfaction with care.[159] However, patients – and particularly women and the elderly – appear to have low expectations and are often satisfied with what professionals would regard as poor treatment.[72,159]

When should we measure outcome?

Outcomes some months after the stroke are probably most relevant to patients, but are more difficult and expensive to measure than at an earlier stage. Many services monitor the patient's functional status at the time of hospital discharge, and this information is easily and cheaply collected. However, because patients usually improve for several months after a stroke, the longer they stay in hospital the better their outcome at discharge. Furthermore, patients tend to be discharged at much the same level of disability. Thus, such measures are easily manipulated and difficult to interpret. It is far more relevant to measure the outcome at a fixed interval after the stroke, but after discharge this will inevitably be more time-consuming and expensive. However, some of the simpler measures can be completed by telephone or postal questionnaire.[148,151,160] Some measures (e.g. EuroQol), which seem ideally suited for use as postal questionnaires, include visual analogue scales, but these appear to be particularly unreliable in stroke patients.[161]

How to score dead patients?

Because many patients die after stroke, outcome measurements can only be applied to the survivors. If these measures are averaged, and groups of patients compared, then there may be a serious problem of interpretation if there are more survivors in one group than in the other. Some attempt to get round this by giving the worst score to the dead patients and then including them in the analysis but, depending on the scale used, this is not necessarily valid. One solution is to measure the proportion of patients who are 'dead or disabled/handicapped', but this may sacrifice sensitivity. However, in studies including large numbers, such dichotomized outcomes may be adequate.[162]

17.12.6 Chance (or random error)

With small numbers, the imprecision of the estimate of performance may prevent useful comparisons being

made. Thus, it is important to measure outcomes in a large, representative sample of patients or carers. This has implications for the type of measure of outcome used, since it must be simple and practical to administer to large numbers, exactly as in large randomized trials. Therefore, to obtain precise estimates of outcome may take several years for a hospital to accumulate enough data to provide precise estimates – for example, of its case fatality. Thus, there is likely to be a considerable delay between a change in the quality of care and any statistically significant change in measured outcomes. Figure 17.10 shows the case fatality in five Scottish hospitals with and without adjustment for important case mix variables. This illustrates that even with several hundred patients, the 95% confidence interval around the estimates of case fatality are surprisingly wide. We suggest that power calculations should be performed (as for randomized trials) before instigating any audit to demonstrate changes in the outcomes following modification of a service.

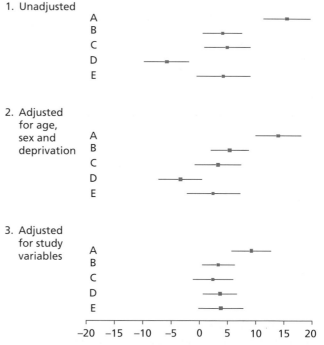

Fig. 17.10 Number of deaths above or below that predicted per 100 stroke patients admitted (*w* score) to each of five Scottish hospitals (A through E) at 6 months. Plots are shown for (1) unadjusted case fatality; (2) after adjustment for age, sex and deprivation; and (3) after adjustment for the study prognostic variables (age; whether the patient lived alone before the stroke and was independent in simple activities of daily living; and, on admission, whether the patient could speak and was orientated in time and place, could lift both arms against gravity, and could walk without the help of another person). Used with permission from Weir *et al.*, 2001.[136]

When planning an audit, estimate the likely number of cases that will need to be included in order to identify a difference reliably (i.e. do a power calculation).

Although the evidence that institutions with greater throughput have better outcomes is conflicting (e.g. for carotid endarterectomy), one argument for stipulating a minimum patient volume per year is to ensure that measures of performance can be reasonably precise. If one's local surgeon performed 50 operations in the previous year, with only two deaths or perioperative strokes, this is a very acceptable 4% complication rate. However, the 95% confidence interval extends up to a very unacceptable 14%. It is therefore very difficult to know with any certainty whether one's local surgeon has results that make carotid endarterectomy worthwhile.

If outcomes are measured in a relatively small number of patients or carers, bad outcomes may reflect bad luck rather than bad care, while conversely, good outcomes may reflect good luck rather than good care.

17.12.7 Case mix

The most important determinant of outcome is probably not the *quality* or even the *effectiveness* of care, but the type of patient treated. The patient's age, pre-stroke status, comorbidities and the severity of the stroke are bound to have an overwhelming effect on the outcome, and may well obscure any real effect that our treatments may have. That is why large randomized trials are required to demonstrate modest treatment effects.

Case mix can vary considerably in different services and in the same service over time, which means that raw outcome data simply cannot be used to reflect the quality or effectiveness of care; they have to be adjusted for differences in case mix. Unfortunately, this assumes that we know how to adjust for case mix in stroke, which is not the case. Good case mix descriptors include those factors that are highly predictive of outcome. But as we have already seen, our ability to predict outcome after stroke, even in terms of survival, is relatively poor (section 10.2.7). Also, we can only correct for those prognostic factors that we can identify and measure reliably. After all, we rely on randomized controlled trials to provide evidence of the effectiveness of interventions simply because randomization ensures that the different treatment groups are balanced for recognized, unrecognized and unmeasurable prognostic factors and that the treatment allocation is not biased. In the report comparing outcomes after stroke in Scottish hospitals, the only prognostic factors that were routinely collected, and could therefore be adjusted for, were age, sex and social deprivation.[136]

If more powerful predictive factors such as those identified in the Oxfordshire Community Stroke Project (Fig. 17.10) are taken into account, most of the variation between hospitals with respect to case fatality disappears and can be accounted for by chance alone.[136,163] Unfortunately, these variables are not routinely available to allow such adjustment. If variations in outcome remain, it is impossible to know whether they are due to failure to completely adjust for case mix, or some aspect of the care given.[84] In accounting for random variation, one must also recognize the imprecision of any statistical model used, which will depend on the size of the cohort from which the model was derived.

The problems of adjusting for case mix are even greater if one considers other relevant outcomes such as quality of life, where we know almost nothing about the factors that predict this. Before we use outcomes to reflect the effectiveness and quality of care, and to alter services as a consequence, we have to develop reliable methods of interpreting them. It will be interesting to see whether this will ever be possible.

Crude measures of patient outcome do not necessarily reflect the quality or effectiveness of the care provided. Even adjusting for case mix may not solve this problem.

Rather than attempting to interpret measures of outcome at a particular interval after the stroke, the change in the patient's condition can be used as an 'outcome'. For example, some research groups have used the functional independence measure (FIM) to assess patients on admission to and discharge from a treatment programme. Any change in the FIM might be considered, at least in part, to be a measure of the effectiveness of the treatment programme, although most of the improvement may actually be spontaneous. The change in FIM can be divided by some measure of the amount of treatment provided, e.g. length of stay, to give an idea of 'efficiency'. Unfortunately, differences in case mix such as age, severity and location of the brain lesion and other medical problems, as well as the interval since the stroke, are likely to influence the rate of change in the FIM. To interpret the change in the FIM as a reflection of effectiveness or efficiency would therefore still require a measure of case mix.[164] Another problem is that measures such as the FIM are not 'interval' scales (Table 17.19). A change of 10 points at one end of the scale is therefore not equivalent to a 10-point change at the other. This makes changes in score difficult to interpret.

17.12.8 A practical approach

Given the limitations of using structure, process or outcome measurement, it is probably best not to rely on any one method, but to use a combination. This has the advantage of reflecting most aspects of the service. Also, if one relies on only a small number of performance indicators, it can have a number of adverse effects on health services. Effort and resources may be directed at improving one service or one aspect of a service, to the detriment of other areas (so-called 'measure fixation').

Clinicians and managers whose income or reputations depend on the indicators may alter their practice (e.g. refuse to treat sicker patients) or manipulate data to enhance their apparent performance (i.e. gaming). For instance, by altering the coding of factors used to adjust for case mix (e.g. stroke severity), one can increase the expected mortality for one's patients and thus improve one's apparent performance (i.e. the observed/expected mortality ratio). One of the best examples of such gaming was following the publication of institution-specific and surgeon-specific death rates for cardiac surgery in New York.[165] The reported proportion of patients with comorbidities, such as renal failure and chronic obstructive pulmonary disease, which were used to adjust outcomes for case mix, increased several-fold over 2 years. It is highly unlikely that the type of patient had changed. The surgeons were simply *reporting* more comorbidity.

Whatever measures are used it is important that the audit covers all stroke patients, not just those admitted to a stroke unit. We suggest the following approach to assessing the quality of stroke services, although this will inevitably change as our understanding improves:

- Perform a structural audit to ensure that services include access to the facilities shown in Table 17.7.
- Assess the process of care by performing a regular audit of a representative sample of case notes using a well-tested and reliable audit instrument that will allow comparisons to be made with other units, or in the same unit over time, e.g. the National Sentinel Audit of Stroke.[71] The results should identify where the problems lie.[134] Also, by setting challenging targets one could use this approach to drive forward improvements in services.
- Collect any outcome data that purchasers or commissioners of the stroke service require – but these should be kept simple, to minimize the cost and because they are likely to be easier to interpret. However, any interpretation will require more complex data about the patients who the service treats. The case mix and outcome data together could form the basis for a minimum data set; our suggestions are outlined in Table 17.21 and include those variables that we have found useful in predicting outcomes after stroke (sec-

Table 17.21 Minimum data set for stroke. This reflects known factors that influence the outcome after stroke and also data that may be routinely available to health service workers.

Case mix data
Age
Sex
Marital status, or living alone before the stroke
Pre-stroke function, i.e. was the patient independent in
   activities of daily living?
Stroke severity:
   Conscious level (normal or reduced?)
   Can the patient talk?
   Is the patient orientated in time, place and person?
   Severity of weakness – can he or she lift an affected limb
      against gravity?
   Can he or she walk independently?
   Urinary incontinence during first week after the stroke?
Process
Number of physicians responsible for stroke care–a lower
   number suggests more specialization
Proportion of patients discussed by a multidisciplinary team
Proportion of patients managed on a stroke unit
Proportion of patients having CT or magnetic resonance scans
Proportion of patients with ischaemic stroke on aspirin at
   discharge
Proportion of patients with ischaemic stroke and atrial
   fibrillation on anticoagulants at discharge
Carotid imaging for appropriate patients
Delays to accessing the above items
Outcomes
Survival at 30 days
Independence/dependence in activities of daily living at
   6 months
Complications, e.g. pressure ulcers
Place of residence at 6 months

tion 10.2.7). These items include some demographic data, which are usually collected routinely (e.g. age, marital status) and which are likely to relate to outcome. Pre-stroke function, which will also reflect comorbidity, relates closely to functional outcome, and, to a lesser extent, increases the risk of death. Other possible indicators of stroke severity are level of consciousness, urinary incontinence, severity of motor weakness, or the proportion of patients with total anterior circulation syndromes (section 10.2).

Poor outcomes may at best reflect poor care, but do not – unlike audits of process – identify the areas in which the service needs to be improved.

- Monitor the frequency of complications after stroke. Although this is unlikely to provide any quantitative information about the quality of care, the data might be used to identify problems. For example, a high or rising proportion of patients with pressure sores may indicate inadequate numbers of nurses, poor-quality nursing care or delays in discharging dependent patients. Unfortunately, there are considerable problems in defining complications and in providing reliable diagnostic criteria to allow monitoring.[22,166,167] A system of critical incident recording might focus on these and other problems and provide a simple indicator that the service may be performing poorly.

- Provide an environment in which the identification of problems is encouraged and not penalized. One suspects that informal judgements that 'there may be a problem with quality' made by those working within a service, or using a service, are as sensitive a method of identifying major problems as any of those discussed above. This approach will only be effective if those working within a service are objective and honest and if the system does not punish healthcare workers, but encourages everyone constantly to provide better services.

- Develop a system to provide an external and independent review of services by professionals from another centre. This can usefully identify problems that need to be resolved.

> It is essential that politicians and health service managers understand the difficulties in interpreting measures of process and outcome, and their limitations. They must not make important decisions about the distribution of resources on the basis of simplistic analyses of crude data. However, large discrepancies in the apparent performance of different stroke services should trigger a detailed enquiry into the possible explanation. Also, it is important not to use the results of a non-randomized evaluation of a local stroke service to guide service development elsewhere.

17.13 Stroke guidelines

In recent years, huge numbers of guidelines have been written about how to manage stroke patients.[19–21,168] These are intended to describe best practice in the most common clinical situations, and not necessarily how every individual patient should be treated. They provide useful standards against which at least the process of care can be monitored. In the past, guidelines have been based on incomplete and thus potentially biased and misleading assessments of the evidence for the effectiveness of interventions. However, the methodology for guideline development is becoming increasingly rigorous, with recommendations being based on systematic reviews of the literature. There are standards against which one can assess the quality of a clinical guideline

Table 17.22 Factors associated with a greater chance of improving practice in accordance with guidelines.

> *Consistently effective interventions*
> Educational outreach visits (for prescribing in North America)
> Patient-specific reminders (manual or computerized)
> Multifaceted interventions (a combination that includes two or more of the following: audit and feedback, reminders, local consensus processes, or marketing)
> Interactive educational meetings (participation of healthcare providers in workshops that include discussion or practice)
> *Interventions of uncertain effectiveness*
> Audit and feedback (or any summary of clinical performance)
> The use of local opinion leaders (practitioners identified by their colleagues as influential)
> Local consensus processes (inclusion of participating practitioners in discussions to ensure they agree that the chosen clinical problem is important and the approach to managing the problem is appropriate)
> Patient-mediated interventions (any intervention aimed at changing the performance of healthcare providers for which specific information was sought from or given to patients)
> *Interventions that have little or no effect*
> Educational materials (distribution of recommendations for clinical care, including clinical practice guidelines, audio-visual materials and electronic publications)
> Educational meetings (such as lectures)

Adapted from Davis *et al.*, 2006.[192]

(Scottish Intercollegiate Guidelines Network No. 50; http://www.show.scot.nhs.uk/sign/home.htm).

If guidelines are to improve clinical practice, it is important that they are effectively implemented. Several factors have been identified (Table 17.22) that may improve practice in accordance with guidelines.[169,192]

> When one has to decide whether to implement clinical guidelines, it is important to assess the methodological rigour with which they were developed. Failure to do so could lead to the adoption of ineffective or even harmful practices.

17.14 Integrated care pathways

Clearly, a multifaceted approach must be taken to ensure that stroke patients are managed in line with guidelines unless there is a valid reason to deviate from them in an individual patient. One approach that is increasingly used in stroke units is the integrated care pathway, which often facilitates local activities that are very likely to increase adherence to guidelines (for an example, see http://www.dcn.ed.ac.uk/spgm).

The development of integrated care pathways usually requires local scrutiny of available guidelines and discussion of how patients should be managed, and introducing them involves local educational sessions. They usually incorporate patient-specific reminders, i.e. guidance on how to manage common problems. They are often a focus of local audits, which measure the degree of compliance with the pathways and the reasons for any deviations, and feed these back to the staff in the unit. There is no robust evidence from randomized trials that integrated care pathways lead to better patient outcomes, although they may at least improve documentation.[170,171]

17.15 Impact of a comprehensive stroke service

When making the case for establishing and maintaining a comprehensive stroke service, it is worth considering the potential impact that such changes may bring. The following arguments justify establishing and maintaining a comprehensive stroke service:

- *Clinical standards and guidelines.* Many countries now have standards or guidelines that require service components to be in place (e.g. stroke units) – see Table 17.7.
- *Quality of care.* Many clinical standards cannot be adequately met without having a coordinated service in place (e.g. coordinated multidisciplinary team care).
- *Patient outcomes.* Table 17.23 outlines an estimate of the potential impact of a comprehensive stroke service using data from systematic reviews of randomized trials. The figures are approximate, and assume that your patient population is similar to those in the clinical trials. However, they do reveal the potential impact in clinical outcomes. The stroke unit component of these estimates is also supported by epidemiological observations that implementing stroke unit care improves stroke recovery.[71,87,91]
- *Cost-effectiveness.* Research into the cost-effectiveness of stroke services indicates that not only may they be cost-neutral but they may actually save money to society in general. For this reason it is worth considering in more detail the cost-effectiveness of stroke services.

17.16 Cost-effectiveness of stroke services

Because of its high frequency in most populations, the resulting severe disability and the need for prolonged institutional care, stroke places a very considerable

Table 17.23 Potential impact of different components of a comprehensive stroke service (based on a hypothetical population of 1000 cerebrovascular patients; 300 with transient ischaemic attack (TIA) and 700 with stroke).

Component	Absolute gain per 1000 patients treated		Proportion of the population eligible for treatment	Actual health gain in the stroke population (per 1000 patients)		Assumptions
	Survivors	Independent survivors		Survivors	Independent survivors	
Thrombolysis (rt-PA within 3 h)	0	100	10%	0	7	10% of stroke population are eligible
Very rapid access TIA service	(1)	(40)	30%	(<1)	(12)	20% of early recurrent (disabling) stroke are preventable
Comprehensive stroke unit	30	50	70%	21	35	Most stroke patients are eligible
Early supported discharge service	5	50	30%	1	15	About half of the stroke patients are eligible
Therapy-based rehabilitation service	0	(10)	30%	0	(3)	About half of the stroke patients are eligible
Total	—	—	—	22	72	

The data presented are calculated from systematic reviews of services[87,100,104,193] or from projections of other data (figures in parentheses).

financial burden on most societies (section 17.1.1). Therefore, when planning stroke services it is important not only to aim for maximum effectiveness, in terms of achieving the best possible outcomes for the patients and their families, but also to do this as efficiently as possible. As we have seen, there is little reliable information about the effectiveness of many interventions, but there is even less about the relative costs of treatment. One can use several different types of economic analysis to relate the effect of treatment and its associated costs (Table 17.24). Ideally, data for both the effectiveness and the costs of treatment should come from the same study, but are rarely available. More often, we have to use data from a variety of sources. Also, any conclusions from economic analyses are likely to be very sensitive to the assumptions made and to whether both direct and indirect costs are estimated.

Hospital care accounts for most of the direct costs associated with acute stroke, at least in countries with sophisticated healthcare systems.[6–8,172] Figure 17.11 shows the relative size of the components of the cost of hospital care for acute stroke patients in one of our institutions. It appears that at least in the British model of care, and probably in other models as well, most of the direct hospital costs are accounted for by nursing salaries and hospital overheads, with relatively little being spent on investigation or specific treatments.[3,7,8,173,174] Even in the US, where patients stay in an acute hospital for only a few days, assessment, investigations and treatment account for less than half of the costs, and the length of

Table 17.24 Some terms used in health economics.

Types of economic analysis

Cost minimization refers to situations in which the health outcomes are similar in different treatment groups and the analysis aims to identify which group is associated with lower costs, i.e. what is the most efficient way of achieving a particular goal

Cost-effectiveness aims to relate improvement in health outcome using natural units (e.g. life-years gained, recurrent strokes avoided) to the cost of achieving those outcomes

Cost utility analyses relate improvement in health outcome expressed in terms of non-financial value of the gain in health outcome (e.g. quality-adjusted life-years, health-years equivalents)

Cost–benefit analyses simply relate to the overall cost in financial terms of competing strategies; for example, the benefits from a treatment are expressed in the reduction in expenditure that would result

Types of direct costs

Health service costs: staff time, medical supplies, hotel services, use of capital equipment (including depreciation, interest paid) and overheads, e.g. heating, lighting; some costs are fixed (i.e. independ of activity), while others are variable (e.g. dependent on number of patients treated)

Costs borne by patients and relatives: transport to visit, cost of home care

Costs borne by other agencies and society generally: social services providing home care or nursing home care

Types of indirect costs

Loss of income for patient or family members

Loss of production for society

'Cost' of psychological distress or pain suffered

These costs are impossible to put a financial value on, except in the law courts

Other terms

Discounting puts greater value on costs or savings now compared with the same costs or savings that might accrue in the future

Marginal costs refer to the extra costs incurred in providing more service. The cost per extra operation may be quite different from the average cost per operation overall

Charges that may be levied by an organization providing healthcare, which may include profit or which may be subsidizing another service, are distinct from costs

Sensitivity analyses are used to take account of uncertainty about the costs and effectiveness of treatments. The components of the evaluation are varied to examine any effect on the conclusion of the economic analysis

Information from several review articles.[194–197]

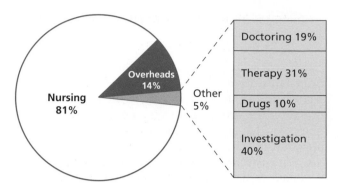

Fig. 17.11 The proportion of direct hospital costs attributable to different aspects of care provided in Edinburgh, Scotland. These data relate to a period before stroke services were organized. The development of a stroke team and unit may have altered the proportions, although probably not by very much.[174]

stay is the most important predictor of hospital costs.[175] Thus, the cost to the health service of managing a patient with stroke is highly dependent on the length of hospital stay – assuming that the intensity of nursing input remains constant.[176]

> Because most of the cost of stroke care in hospital is accounted for by nursing services and overheads, it does not make sense to waste time arguing about even quite large changes in the cost of investigations and treatments.

Interventions that promote more rapid or complete recovery may be very cost-effective, as long as they are not themselves very expensive. An analysis of the cost-effectiveness of stroke unit care suggested that better patient outcomes could be achieved with at worst moderate increases in costs (and at best small decreases in cost), and that stroke unit care was more cost-effective than that in general medical settings.[177] Thus, it seems likely that by providing better-coordinated stroke care in units, the cost of managing a patient with stroke in hospital can be reduced.

Attempts to restrict or rationalize the use of investigations or drug therapies can only have a marginal effect on the overall hospital costs. Several non-randomized studies from the US have shown that the introduction of care pathways for stroke patients can reduce hospital costs (or charges), mainly by reducing length of stay.[173,178–180] A policy of accelerated discharge appears to reduce the per capita costs considerably, although – depending on funding arrangements – this is likely to be transferred onto another budget, e.g. community care and families.[70] In fact, the evidence available from randomized trials suggests that early supported discharge

schemes are marginally cheaper overall than more prolonged hospital-based rehabilitation (section 17.7.1).

A practical approach to monitoring the cost-effectiveness of a stroke service might include collecting data about the total length of stay in hospital (i.e. in both the acute and rehabilitation units) since this appears to be – at least in some countries – a reasonable reflection of direct hospital costs.[6–8,174] However, note would have to be taken of any major changes in nursing costs or those related to investigations and treatment. The length of stay needs to be interpreted in the light of data about the destination on discharge and the patient's functional status. It is easy to reduce the length of stay by discharging patients into nursing homes instead of to their own homes, and by discharging more severely dependent patients into the community, but this adds to the costs (financial, physical and emotional) to the family and social services. Except for billing purposes, setting up systems for collecting detailed data about exactly what investigations, drugs and therapy patients receive would be time-consuming and expensive, and would probably provide little extra information about the overall cost of care. Reducing the length of stay by just 1 day would probably pay for all of the average patient's basic investigations and drugs.

> An organized stroke service is likely to be cheaper than a disorganized one, and it could release resources for other areas.

Please note that all references taken from *The Cochrane Library* are given a current date as this database is updated on a quarterly basis. Please refer to the current *Cochrane Library* article for the latest review. Information from the evidence website www.effectivestrokecare.org was used extensively in this review. Please refer to it for the latest version. The same applies to the *British Medical Journal* 'Clinical Evidence' series which is updated every six months.

References

1 Isard PA, Forbes JF. The cost of stroke to the National Health Service in Scotland. *Cerebrovasc Dis* 1992; **2**:47–50.
2 Persson U, Silverberg R, Lindgren Bea. Direct costs of stroke for a Swedish population. *Int J Technol Assess Health Care* 1990; **6**:125–37.
3 Smurawska LT, Alexandrov AV, Bladin CF, Norris JW. Cost of acute stroke care in Toronto, Canada. *Stroke* 1994; **25**(8):1628–31.

4 Taylor TN, Davis PH, Torner JC, Holmes J, Meyer JW, Jacobson MF. Lifetime cost of stroke in the United States. *Stroke* 1996; **27**:1459–66.

5 Evers SMAA, Engel GL, Ament AJHA. Cost of stroke in the Netherlands from a societal perspective. *Stroke* 1997; **28**:1375–81.

6 Caro JJ, Huybrechts KF, Duchesne I. Management patterns and costs of acute ischemic stroke: an international study. *Stroke* 2000; **31**:582–90.

7 Grieve R, Hutton J, Bhalla A, Rastenyte D, Ryglewicz D, Sarti C *et al.* A comparison of the costs and survival of hospital-admitted stroke patients across Europe. *Stroke* 2001; **32**(7):1684–91.

8 Yoneda Y, Uehara T, Yamasaki H, Kita Y, Tabuchi M, Mori E. Hospital-based study of the care and cost of acute ischemic stroke in Japan. *Stroke* 2003; **34**:718–24.

9 Dewey HM, Thrift AG, Mihalopoulos C, Carter R, Macdonell RAL, NcNeil JJ *et al.* Cost of stroke in Australia from a societal perspective: results from the North East Melbourne Stroke Incidence Study (NEMESIS). *Stroke* 2001; **32**:409–16.

10 Dewey HM, Thrift AG, Mihalopoulos C, Carter R, Macdonell RAL, NcNeil JJ *et al.* Lifetime cost of stroke subtypes in Australia: findings from the North East Melbourne Stroke Incidence Study (NEMESIS). *Stroke* 2003; **34**:2502–7.

11 Ghatneckar O, Persson U, Glader EL, Terent A. Cost of stroke in Sweden: an incidence estimate. *Int J Technol Assess Health Care* 2004; **20**(3):375–80.

12 Feigin VL. Stroke epidemiology in the developing world. *Lancet* 2005; **265**:2160–1.

13 King's Fund Consensus Conference. Treatment of stroke. *Br Med J* 1988; **297**(126):128.

14 Campbell M, Fitzpatrick R, Haines A, Kinmonth AL, Sandercock P, Spiegelhalter D *et al.* Framework for design and evaluation of complex interventions to improve health. *Br Med J* 2000; **321**:694–6.

15 Bamford J, Sandercock P, Warlow C, Gray M. Why are patients with acute stroke admitted to hospital? *Br Med J* 1986; **292**:1369–72.

16 Asplund K, Bonita R, Kuulasmaa K. Multi-national comparisons of stroke epidiology: evaluation of case ascertainment in the WHO MONICA stroke study. *Stroke* 1995; **26**:355–60.

17 Kolominsky-Rabas PL, Sarti C, Heuschmann PU *et al.* A prospective community-based study of stroke in Germany – the Erlangen Stroke Project (ESPro): incidence and case fatality at 1, 3 and 12 months. *Stroke* 1998; **29**:2501–6.

18 Wardlaw JM, Seymour J, Cairns J, Keir S, Lewis S, Sandercock P. Immediate computed tomography scanning of acute stroke is cost-effective and improves quality of life. *Stroke* 2004; **35**(11):2477–83.

19 Royal College of Physicians. *National Clinical Guidelines for Stroke.* London: Royal College of Physicians, 2000.

20 Brainin M, Olsen TS, Chammorro A, Diener HC, Ferro J, Hennerici MG *et al.* Organisation of stroke care: education, referral, emergency management and imaging, stroke units and rehabilitation. European Stroke Initiative. *Cerebrovasc Dis* 2004; **17**(2):1–14.

21 Johnston SC, Nguyen-Huynh MN, Schwarz ME, Fuller K, Williams CE, Josephson SA *et al.* National Stroke Association guidelines for the management of transient ischemic attacks. *Ann Neurol* 2006; **60**(3):301–13.

22 Langhorne P, Stott DJ, Robertson L, MacDonald J, Jones L, McAlpine C *et al.* Medical complications after stroke: a multi-centre study. *Stroke* 2000; **31**:1223–9.

23 Kalra L, Evans E, Perez I, Knapp M, Donaldson N, Swift C. Alternative strategies for stroke care: a prospective randomised controlled trial. *Lancet* 2000; **356**:894–9.

24 Evans A, Perez I, Melbourn A, teadman, J, Kalra L. Alternative strategies in stroke: randomised controlled trial of three strategies of stroke management and rehabilitation. *Cerebrovasc Dis* 2000; (Suppl 2):60.

25 Rodgers H, Bond S, Curless R. Inadequacies in the provision of information to stroke patients and their families. *Age Ageing* 2001; **20**:129–33.

26 Katzan IL, Furlan AJ, Lloyd LE, Frank JI, Harper DL, Hinchey JA *et al.* Use of tissue-type plasminogen actibator for acute ischemic stroke: the Cleveland area experience. *J Am Med Assoc* 2000; **283**(9):1151–8.

27 Alberts MJ. Recommendations for comprehensive stroke centres: a consensus statement from the brain attach coalition (report). *Stroke* 2005; **36**(7):1597–616.

28 Mayer SA, Brun NC, Begtrup K, Broderick J, Davis S, Diringer MN *et al.* Recombinant activated factor VII for acute intracerebral hemorrhage. *N Engl J Med* 2005; **352**(8):777–85.

29 Lovett JK, Dennis MS, Sandercock P, Bamford J, Warlow CP, Rothwell PM. Very early risk of stroke after a first transient ischemic attack. *Stroke* 2003; **34**:138–40.

30 Coull AJ, Lovett JK, Rothwell PM. Population-based study of early risk of stroke after transient ischaemic attack or minor stroke: implications for public education and organisation of services. *Br Med J* 2004; **328**(7435):326.

31 Rothwell PM, Giles MF, Flossmann E, Lovelock CE, Redgrave JN, Warlow CP *et al.* A simple score (ABCD) to identify individuals at high early risk of stroke after transient ischaemic sttach. *Lancet* 2005; **366**(9479):29–36.

32 Coutts SB, Simon JE, Eliasziw M, Sohn CH, Hill MD, Barber PA *et al.* Triaging transient ischaemic attack and minor stroke patients using acute magnetic resonance imaging. *Ann Neurol* 2005; **57**(6):848–54.

33 Fairhead JF, Rothwell PM. The need for urgency in identification and treatment of symptomatic carotid stenosis is already established. *Cerebrovasc Dis* 2005; **19**:355–8.

34 Rothwell PM, Coull AJ, Giles MF, Howard SC, Silver LE, Bull LM *et al.* Change in stroke incidence, mortality, case-fatality, severity and risk factors in Oxfordshire, UK from 1981 to 2004 (Oxford Vascular Study). *Lancet* 2004; **363**(9425):1925–33.

35 Kwan J, Hand P, Sandercock P. A systematic review of barriers to delivery of thrombolysis for acute stroke. *Age Ageing* 2004; **33**:116–21.

36 Schneider AT, Pancioli AM, Khoury JC, Rademacher E, Tuchfarber A, Miller R *et al.* Trends in community knowledge of the warning signs and risk factors for stroke. *J Am Med Assoc* 2003; **289**(3): 343–6.

37 Williams LS, Bruno A, rouch D, Marriott DJ. Stroke patients' knowledge of stroke. Influence on time topresentation. *Stroke* 1997; **28**(5):912–15.

38 Gorelick PB, Sacco RL, Smith DB, Alberts M, Mustone-Alexander L, Rader D *et al.* Prevention of a first stroke: a review of guidelines and a multidisciplinary consensus statement from the National Stroke Association. *J Am Med Assoc* 1999; **281**(12):1112–20.

39 Brice JH, G Riswell JK, Delbridge TR, Key CB. Stroke: from recognition by the public to management by emergency medical services. *Prehosp Emerg Care* 2002; **6**(1):99–106.

40 Carrozzella J, Jauch EC. Emergency stroke management: a new era. *Nurs Clin North Am* 2002; **37**(1):35–57.

41 Smith MA, Doliszny KM, Shahar E, McGovern PG, Arnett DK, Luepker RV. Delayed hospital arrival for acute stroke: The Minnesota Stroke Survey. *Ann Int Med* 1998; **129**(3):190–6.

42 Castaldo JE, Nelson JJ, Reed JF3, Longenecker JE, Toole JF. The delay in reporting symptoms of carotid artery stenosis in an at-risk population. The Asymptomatic Carotid Atherosclerosis experience: a statement of concern regarding watchful waiting. *Arch Neurol* 1997; **54**(10):1267–71.

43 Morgenstern LB, Bartholomew LK, Grotta JC, Staub L, King M, Chan W. Sustained benefit of a community and professional intervention to increase acute stroke therapy. *Arch Intern Med* 2003; **163**(18):2198–202.

44 Nor AM, Davis J, Sen B, Shipsey D, Louw SJ, Dyker AG *et al.* The Recognition of Stroke in the Emergency Room (ROSIER) scale: development and validation of a stroke recognition instrument. *Lancet Neurol* 2005; **4**(11):727–34.

45 Kidwell CS, Starkman S, Eckstein M, Weems K, Saver JL. Identifying stroke in the field. Prospective validation of the Los Angeles Prehospital Stroke Screen (LAPSS). *Stroke* 2000; **31**:71–6.

46 Silbergleit Re, Scott PA, Lowell MJ. Cost-effectiveness of helicopter transport of stroke patients for thrombolysis. *Acad Emerg Med* 2003; **10**(9):966–72.

47 Alberts MA, Hademenos G, Latchaw RE, Jagoda A, Marler JR, Mayberg MR *et al.* Recommendation for the establishment of primary stroke centres. *J Am Med Assoc* 2006; **283**:3102–9.

48 Norrving B. Organised stroke care: the core of effective stroke care provision. *Stroke* 2005; **36**(7):1616–18.

49 Langhorne P, Dey P, Woodman M, Kalra L, Wood-Dauphinee S, Patel N *et al.* Is stroke unit care portable? A systematic review of the clinical trials. *Age Ageing* 2006; **34**:324–30.

50 Knapp, Kidwell CS, Shephard T, Tonn S, Sawyer B, Murdock M *et al.* A survey of physician attitudes and hospital resources. *Neurology* 2003; **60**:1452–6.

51 Douglas VC, Tong DC, Gillum RF, Zhao S, Brass LM, Dostal JJSC. Do the Brain Attack Coalition's criteria for stroke centers improve care for ischemic stroke? *Neurology* 2005; **64**:422–7.

52 Kapral MK, Laupacis A, Phillips SJ, Silver FL, Hill MD, Fang J *et al.* Stroke care delivery in institutions participating in the Registry of the Canadian Stroke Network. *Stroke* 2006; **35**:1756–62.

53 Cadilhac DA, Ibrahim J, Pearce DC, Oqden KJ, McNeill J, Davis SM, Donnan GA, SCOPES Study Group. Multicenter comparison of processes of care between stroke units and conventional care wards in Australia. *Stroke* 2004; **35**(5):1035–40.

54 Weir NU, Buchan AM. A study of the workload and effectiveness of a comprehensive acute stroke service. *J Neurol Neurosurg Psychiatry* 2005; **76**(6): 863–5.

55 Wu O, Langhorne P. The role of telemedicine in acute stroke: a systematic review. *Int J Stroke* 2006; **1**:201–7.

56 Hess DC, Wang S, Gross H, Nichols FT, Hall CE, Adams RJ. Telestroke: extending stroke expertise into underserved areas. *Lancet Neurol* 2006; **5**(3):275–8.

57 Lamonte MP, Bahouth MN, Hu P, Yarbrough KL, Gunawardane R, Crarey P *et al.* Telemedicine for acute stroke: triumphs and pitfalls. *Stroke* 2003; **34**(3):725–28.

58 Wang DZ. Telemedicine: the solution to provide rural stroke coverage and the answer to the shortage of stroke neurologists and radiologists. *Stroke* 2003; **34**(12):2957.

59 Johnston KC, Worrall BB. Teleradiology Assessment of Computerized Tomographs Online Reliability Study (TRACTORS) for acute stroke evaluation. *Telemed J e-Health* 2003; **3**:227–33.

60 Schwamm LH, Pancioli A, Acker JE 3rd, Goldstein LB, Zorowitz RD, Shephard TJ *et al.*; American Stroke Association's Task Force on the Development of Stroke Systems. Recommendations for the establishment of stroke systems of care: recommendations from the American Stroke Association's Task Force on the Development of Stroke Systems. *Stroke* 2005; **36**(3):690–703.

61 Martin PJ, Young G, Enevoldson TP, Humphrey PRD. Overdiagnosis of TIA and minor stroke: experience at a regional neurovascular clinic. *Q J Med* 1997; **90**:759–63.

62 Karunaratne PM, Norris CA, Syme PD. Analysis of six months referrals to a 'one-stop' neurovascular clinic in a district general hospital: implications for purchasers of a stroke service. *Health Bull* 1999; **57**:17–26.

63 Widjaja E, Salam SN, Griffiths PD, Kamara D, Doyle C, Venables GS. Is the rapid assessment clinic rapid enough in assessing transient ischaemic attack and minor stroke? *J Neurol Neurosurg Psychiatry* 2005; **76**(1):145–6.

64 Johnston SC, Gress DR, Browner WS, Sidney S. Short-term prognosis after emergency department diagnosis of TIA. *J Am Med Assoc* 2000; **284**:2901–6.

65 Rothwell PM, Buchan A, Johnston SC. Recent advances in managementof transient ischaemic attacks and minor ischaemic strokes. *Lancet Neurol* 2006; **5**(4):323–31.

66 Stroke Unit Trialists' Collaboration, Langhorne P. Collaborative systematic review of the randomised trials of organised inpatient (stroke unit) care after stroke. *Br Med J* 1997; **314**:1151–9.

67 Stroke Unit Trialists' Collaboration. Organised inpatient (stroke unit) care after stroke (Cochrane Review). *Cochrane Library Update Software*, Oxford, 2000; (3).

68 Stroke Unit Trialists' Collaboration. Organised inpatient (stroke unit) care for stroke. The *Cochrane Database Syst Rev* 2006; (3).

69 Langhorne P, Pollock A, in conjunction with the Stroke Unit Trialists Collaboration. What are the components of effective stroke unit care? *Age Ageing* 2002; 31(5):365–71.

70 Langhorne P, Taylor G, Murray G, Dennis M, Anderson C, Bautz-Holter E *et al*. Early supported discharge services for srokepatients: an individual patient data meta-analysis. *Lancet* 2005; **365**:501–6.

71 Rudd AG, Hoffman A, Irwin P, Lowe D, Pearson MG. Stroke unit care and outcome: results from the 2001 National Sentinel Audit of Stroke. *Stroke* 2005; **36**:103–6.

72 Wellwood I, Dennis M, Warlow C. Patients' and carers' satisfaction with acute stroke management. *Age Ageing* 1995; **24**:519–24.

73 O'Mahoney PG, Rodger H, Thompson RS, Dobson R, James OFW. Satisfaction with information and advice received by stroke patients. *Clin Rehab* 1997; **11**:68–72.

74 Langhorne P on behalf of the Stroke Unit Trialists' Collaboration. The effect of different types of organised inpatient (stroke unit) care: an updated systematic review and meta-analysis. *Cerebrovasc Dis* 2005; **19**(2):1–17.

75 Bath PMW, Soo J, Butterworth RJ, Kerr JE. Do acute stroke units improve care? *Cerebrovasc Dis* 1996; **6**:346–9.

76 Indredavik B, Bakke F, Slordahl SA, Rokseth R, Haaheim L. Treatment in a combined acute and rehabilitation stroke unit. *Stroke* 1999; **30**:917–23.

77 Langhorne P. Measures to improve recovery in the acute phase of stroke. *Cerebrovasc Dis* 1999; **9**(Suppl 15):2–5.

78 Langhorne P, Li Pak Tong B, Stott DJ. Association between physiological homeostasis and early recovery after stroke. *Stroke* 2000; **31**:2518–19.

79 Davis M, Hollymann C, McGiven M, Chambers I, Egbuji JBD. Physiological monitoring in acute stroke. *Age Ageing* 1999; **28**(Suppl 1):45.

80 Hacke W, Schwab S, De Georgia M. Intensive care of acute ischemic stroke. *Cerebrovasc Dis* 1994; **4**:385–92.

81 Kennedy FB, Pozen TJ, Gableman EH, Tuthill JE, Zaentz SD. Stroke intensive care: an appraisal. *Am Heart J* 1970; **80**:188–96.

82 Drake WE, Hamilton MJ, Carlsson M, Kand F, Blumenkrantz J. Acute stroke management and patient outcome:the value of neurovascular care units (NCU). *Stroke* 1973; **4**:933–45.

83 Pitner SE, Mance CJ. An evaluation of stroke intensive care: results in a municipal hospital. *Stroke* 1973; **4**:737–41.

84 Wolfe CD, Tilling K, Beech R, Rudd AG. Variations in case fatality and dependency from stroke in western and central Europe. The European BIOMED Study of Stroke Care Group. *Stroke* 1999; **30**(2):350–6.

85 Ilmavirta M, Frey H, Erila T, Fogelholm R. Does treatment in a non-intensive care stroke unit improve the outcome of ischemic stroke? *Det 7 Nordiska Motet om Cereborvasculara Sjukdomar*, Jyvaskyla, Finland, 1993.

86 Cavallini A, Micieli G, Marcheselli S, Quaglini S. Role of monitoring in management of acute ischemic stroke patients. *Stroke* 2006; **34**:2599–603.

87 Stegmayr B, Asplund K, Hulter-Asberg K. Stroke units in their natural habitat: can results of randomised trials be reproduced in routine clinical practice? *Stroke* 1999; **30**:709–14.

88 Stroke Unit Trialists' Collaboration. Organised inpatient (Stroke Unit) care after stroke (Cochrane Review). *Cochrane Database Syst Rev* 2002; **1**:CD000197

89 Stroke Unit Trialists' Collaboration, Langhorne P. How do stroke units improve patient outcomes? A collaborative systematic review of the randomised trials. *Stroke* 1997; **28**:2139–44.

90 Jorgensen HS, Nakayama H, Raaschou HO, Larsen K, Hubbe P, Olsen TS. The effect of a stroke unit: reductions in mortality, discharge rate to nursing home, length of hospital stay, and cost: a community-based study. *Stroke* 1995; **26**(7):1178–82.

91 Glader EL, Stegmayr B, Johansson L, Hulter-Asberg KO, Wester PO. Differences in long-term outcome between patients treated in stroke units and in general wards: a 2-year follow-up of stroke patients in Sweden. *Stroke* 2001; **32**(9):2124–30.

92 Seenan P, Langhorne P, Long M. Stroke units in their natural habitat: a systematic review of observational studies of routine stroke unit care. *Cerebrovasc Dis* 2006; **21**(4):120.

93 Indredavik B, Bakke F, Solberg R, Rokseth R, Haahein LL, Holme I. Benefit of stroke unit: a randomised controlled trial. *Stroke* 1991; **22**:1026–31.

94 Kelly-Hayes M, Wolf PA, Kase CS, Brand FN, McGuirk JM, D'Agostino RB. Temporal patterns of stroke onset: the Framingham study. *Stroke* 1995; **26**:1343–7.

95 Rothwell PM, Wroe SJ, Slattery J, Warlow CP. Is stroke incidence related to season or temperature? *Lancet* 1996; **347**:934–6.

96 Ebrahim S, Redfern J. *Stroke Care: A Matter of Chance – a National Survey of Stroke Services*. London: The Stroke Association, 1999.

97 Pound P, Gompretz P, Ebrahim S. Patients' satisfaction with stroke services. *Clin Rehab* 1994; **8**:7–17.

98 Kalra L, Evans A, Perez I, Melbourn A, Patel A, Knapp M *et al*. Training carers of stroke patients: randomised controlled trial. *Br Med J* 2004; **328**(7448):1099.

99 Patel A, Knapp M, Perez I, Evans A, Kalra L. Alternative strategies for stroke care: cost-effectiveness and cost-utility analyses from a prospective randomised controlled trial. *Stroke* 2004; **35**(1):196–203.

100 Early Supported Discharge Trialists. Services for reducing duration of hospital care for acute stroke patients (Cochrane Review). *Cochrane Database Syst Rev* 2005; **2**:CD000443.

101 Askim T, Rohweder G, Lydersen S, Indredavik B. *Clin Rehab* 2004; **18**:238–48.

102 Forster A, Young J. Specialist nurse support for patients with stroke in the community: a randomised controlled trial. *Br Med J* 1996; **312**:1642–6.

103 Dennis M. Commentary: Why we didn't ask patients for their consent. *Br Med J* 1997; **314**:1077.

104 The Outpatient Service Trialists. Therapy-based rehabilitation services for stroke patients at home. *Cochrane Database Syst Rev* 2003; **1**:CD002925.

105 Young J, Forster A. The Bradford community stroke trial: results at six months. *Br Med J* 1992; **304**:1085–9.

106 Gladman JRF, Lincoln NB, Barer DH. A randomised controlled trial of domiciliary and hospital-based rehabilitation for stroke patients after discharge from hospital. *J Neurol Neurosurg Psychiatry* 1993; **56**:960–6.

107 Gladman JRF, Lincoln NB. Follow-up of a controlled trial of domiciliar stroke rehabilitation (DOMINO Study). *Age Ageing* 1994; **23**:9–13.

108 Baskett JJ, Broad JB, Reekie G, Hocking C, Green G. Shared responsibility for ongoing rehabilitation: a new approach to home-based therapy after stroke. *Clin Rehab* 1999; **13**(1):23–33.

109 Forster A, Young J, Smith J, Knapp P, House A, Knight J. Information provision for stroke patients and their caregivers (protocol for a Cochrane Review). *Cochrane Library Update Software*: Oxford, 2000.

110 Gladman J, Forster A, Young J. Hospital- and home-based rehabilitation after discharge from hospital for stroke patients: analysis of two trials. *Age Ageing* 1995; **24**:49–53.

111 Ellis G, Rodger J, McAlpine C, Langhorne P. The impact of stroke nurse specialist input on risk factor modification: a randomised controlled trial. *Age Ageing* 2005; **34**(4):389–92.

112 Tilling K, Cochall C, McKevitt C, Daneski K, Wolfe C. A family support organiser for stroke patients and their carers: a randomised controlled trial. *Cerebrovasc Dis* 2005; **2**:85–91.

113 Lincoln NB, Francis VM, Lilley SA, Sharma JC, Summerfield M. Evaluation of a stroke family support organiser: a randomised controlled trial. *Stroke* 2003; **34**:116–21.

114 Mant J, Carter J, Wade DT, Winner S. Family support for stroke: a randomised controlled trial. *Lancet* 2000; **356**(9232):808–13.

115 Wellwood I, Dennis MS, Warlow CP. Perceptions and knowledge of stroke among surviving patients with stroke and their carers. *Age Ageing* 1994; **23**:293–8.

116 Anderson S, Marlett NJ. Communication in stroke: the overlooked rehabilitation tool. *Age Ageing* 2004; **33**(5):440–3.

117 Scott JT, Entwistle VA, Sowden AJ, Watt I. Provision of recordings or summaries of consultations to people with cancer. *Cochrane Library Updated Software*: Oxford, 2000.

118 Leibson CL, Naessens JM, Brown RD, Whisnant JP. Accuracy of hospital discharge abstracts for identifying stroke. *Stroke* 1994; **25**:2348–55.

119 Davenport RJ, Dennis MS, Warlow CP. The accuracy of Scottish Morbidity Record (SMR1) data for identifying hospitalised stroke patients. *Health Bull* 1996; **54**:402–6.

120 Ellekjaer H, Holmen J, Kruger O, Terent A. Identification of incident stroke in Norway: hospital discharge data compared with a population-based stroke register. *Stroke* 1999; **30**:56–60.

121 Carter K, Anderson C, Hacket M, Feigin V, Barber PA, Broad JB *et al.* Trends in ethnic disparities in stroke incidence in Auckland, New Zealand, during 1981 to 2003. *Stroke* 2006; **37**(1):56–62.

122 Feigin VL, Carter K. Stroke incidence studies one step closer tothe elusive gold standard? *Stroke* 2004; **35**(9):2045–7.

123 Bonita R, Solomon N, Broad JB. Prevalence of stroke and stroke-related disability: estimates from the Auckland Stroke Studies. *Stroke* 1997; **28**:1898–902.

124 Sacco RL, Boden-Albala B, Gan R, Chen X, Kargman DE, Shea S. Stroke incidence among white, black and Hispanic residents of an urban community: the North Manhattan stroke study. *Am J Epidemiol* 1998; **147**:259–68.

125 Wolfe CD, Corbin DO, Smeeton NC, Gay GH, Rudd AG, Hennis AJ, Wilkes RJ, Fraser HS. Estimation of the risk of stroke in black populations in Barbados and South London. *Stroke* 2006; **37**:1986–90.

126 Sudlow C. Survival after stroke in south London. *Br Med J* 2005; **331**(7514):414–15.

127 Richard C, Dodel MD, Haacke C, Zamzow K, Pawelzik S, Spottke A *et al.* Resource utilisation and costs of stroke unit care in Germany. *Value Health* 2004; **7**(2):144.

128 Donabedian A. The quality of care: how can it be assessed? *J Am Med Assoc* 1988; **260**:19–26.

129 Hancock RJY, Oddy M, Saweirs WM, Court B. The RCP stroke audit package in practice. *J R Coll Phys Lond* 1997; **31**:74–8.

130 Rudd AG, Irwin P, Rutledge Z. The National Sentinel Audit for stroke: a tool for raising standards of care. *J R Coll Phys Lond* 1999; **33**:460–4.

131 Gompertz P, Pound P, Briffa J, Ebrahim S. How useful are non-random comparisons of outcomes and quality of care in purchasing hospital stroke services? *Age Ageing* 1995; **24**:137–41.

132 Dennis M. Stroke services: the good, the bad and the . . . *J R Coll Phys Lond* 2000; **34**:92–6.

133 Goldstein H, Spiegelhalter DJ. League tables and their limitations: statistical issues in comparisons of institutional performance. *J R Stat Soc* 1996; **159**:385–443.

134 Davies HTA, Crombie IK. Interpreting health outcomes. *J Eval Clin Pract* 1997; **3**:187–99.

135 Thomas JW, Hofer TP. Research evidence on the validity of risk-adjusted mortality rate as a measure of hospital quality of care. *Med Care Res Rev* 1998; **55**:371–404.

136 Weir N, Dennis MS, Scottish Stroke Outcomes Study Group. Towards a national system for monitoring the quality of hospital-based stroke services. *Stroke* 2001; **32**(6):1415–21.

137 McNaughton H, McPherson K, Taylor W, Weatherall M. Relationship between process and outcome in stroke care. *Stroke* 2003; **34**:713–17.

138 Van Gijn J, Warlow CP. Down with stroke scales. *Cerebrovasc Dis* 1992; **2**:239–47.

139 Cote R, Battista RN, Wolfson C, Boucher J, Adam J, Hachinski V. The Canadian Neurological Scale: validation and reliability assessment. *Neurology* 1989; **39**:638–43.

140 Brott T, Adams HP, Olinger CP, Marler JR, Barsan WG, Biller J *et al.* Measurements of acute cerebral infarction: a clinical examination scale. *Stroke* 1989; **20**:864–870.

141 Barber M, Fail M, Shields M, Stott DJ, Langhorne P. Validity and reliability of estimating the Scandinavian stroke scale score from medical records. *Cerebrovasc Dis* 2004; **17**:224–7.

142 Tukey JW. The future of data analysis. *Ann Math Stat* 1962; **33**:1–67.

143 Mahoney FI, Barthel DW. Functional evaluation: the Barthel index. *Maryland State Med J* 1965; **14**:61–5.

144 Ebrahim S, Nouri FM, Barer D. Measuring disability after stroke. *J Epidemiol Commun Health* 1985; **39**:86–9.

145 Holbrook M, Skilbeck CE. An activities index for use with stroke patients. *Age Ageing* 1983; **12**:166–70.

146 Nouri FM, Lincoln NB. An extended activities of daily living scale for stroke patients. *Clin Rehab* 1987; **4**:301–5.

147 Schuling J, Greidanus J, Meyboom de Jong B. Measuring functional status of stroke patients with the Sickness Impact Profile. *Disabil Rehabil* 1993; **15**:19–23.

148 Shinar D, Gross CR, Bronstein KS. Reliability of the activities of daily living scale and its use in telephone interview. *Arch Phys Med Rehab* 1987; **68**:723–8.

149 Rankin J. Cerebral vascular accidents in patients over the age of 60: II. Prognosis. *Scott Med J* 1957; **2**:200–15.

150 Bamford J, Sandercock P, Warlow CP, Slattery J. Inter-observer agreement for the assessment of handicap in stroke patients (letter). *Stroke* 1989; **20**:828.

151 Candelise L, Pinardi G, Aritzu E, Musicco M. Telephone interview for stroke outcome assessment. *Cerebrovasc Dis* 1994; **4**:341–3.

152 Wilson JTL, Hareendran A, Grant M, Baird T, Schulz UGR, Muir KW *et al.* Improving the assessment of outcomes in stroke: use of a structured interview to assign grades on the modified Rankin scale. *Stroke* 2002; **33**:2243–6.

153 Buck D, Jacoby A, Massey A, Ford G. Evaluation of measures used to assess quality of life after stroke. *Stroke* 2000; **31**:2004–10.

154 Hawthorne G, Richardson J, Day NA. A comparison of the Assessment of Qualitfy of Life (AQol) with four other generic utility instruments. *Ann Med* 2001; **33**:358–70.

155 Dorman PJ, Waddell F, Slattery J, Dennis M. Are proxy assessments of health status after stroke with the Euroqol questionnaire feasible, accurate and unbiased? *Stroke* 1997; **28**:1883–7.

156 Dennis M, O'Rourke S, Slattery J, Staniforth T, Warlow C. Evaluation of a stroke family care worker: results of a randomised controlled trial. *Br Med J* 1997; **314**:1071–6.

157 McKevitt C, Dundas R, Wolfe C, European BIOMED II Study of Stroke Care Group. Two simple questions to assess outcome after stroke: a European study. *Stroke* 2001; **32**(3):681–6.

158 Gilbertson L, Langhorne P. Home-based occupational therapy: stroke patients' satisfaction with occupational performance and service provision. *Br J Occup Ther* 2000; **63**:464–8.

159 Pound P, Sabin C, Ebrahim S. Observing the process of care: a stroke unit, elderly care unit and general medical ward compared. *Age Ageing* 1999; **28**:433–40.

160 Lindley RI, Waddell F, Livingstone Mea. Can simple questions assess outcome after stroke? *Cerebrovasc Dis* 1994; **4**:314–24.

161 Price CIM, Curless RH, Rodgers H. Can stroke patients use visual analogue scales? *Stroke* 1999; **30**:1357–61.

162 Peto R. Monitoring cancer patients in clinical trials need not be precise. In: Symington T, Williams AE, McVie JG, eds. *Cancer: Assessment and Monitoring.* Edinburgh: Churchill Livingstone, 1980, pp. 377–81.

163 Weir N, The Scottish Stroke Outcomes Group. Stroke league tables: are they likely to reflect differences in quality? *Cerebrovasc Dis* 1999; **9**(Suppl 1):115.

164 Alexander MP. Stroke rehabilitation outcome: a potential use of predictive variables to establish levels of care. *Stroke* 1994; **25**:128–34.

165 Green J, Wintfield N. Report cards on cardiac surgeons: assessing New York State's approach. *N Engl J Med* 1995; **332**:1229–32.

166 Kalra L, Eade J. Role of stroke rehabilitation units in managing severe disability after stroke. *Stroke* 1995; **26**:2031–4.

167 Davenport RJ, Dennis MS, Wellwood I, Warlow CP. Complications after acute stroke. *Stroke* 1996; **27**:415–20.

168 Scottish Intercollegiate Guidelines Network (SIGN). *The Management of Patients with Stroke 1: Assessment, Investigation, Immediate Management and Secondary Prevention.* Edinburgh: SIGN, 1997.

169 Bero LA, Grilli R, Grimshaw JM, Harvey E, Oxman AD, Thomson MA. Closing the gap between research and practice: an overview of systematic reviews of interventions to promote the implementation of research findings. The Cochrane Effective Practice and Organization of Care Review Group. *Br Med J* 1998; **317**(7156):465–8.

170 Sulch D, Kalra L. Integrated care pathways in stroke management. *Age Ageing* 2000; **29**:349–52.

171 Kwan J, Sandercock P. In-hospital care pathways for stroke. *Cochrane Database Syst Rev* 2004; (4):CD002924.

172 Terent A, Marke LA, Asplund K, Norrving B, Jonsson E, Wester P-O. Costs of stroke in Sweden: a national perspective. *Stroke* 1994; **25**:2363–9.

173 Bowen J, Yaste C. Effect of a stroke protocol on hospital costs of stroke patients. *Neurology* 1994; **44**:1961–4.

174 Dennis M, Wellwood I, McGregor E, Dent J, Forbes J. What are the major components of the cost of caring for stroke patients in hospital in the UK? *Cerebrovasc Dis* 1995; **5**:243.

175 Diringer MN, Edwards DF, Mattson DT. Predictors of acute hospital costs for treatment of ischemic stroke in an academic center. *Stroke* 1999; **30**:724–8.

176 Holloway RG, Witter DM, Lawton KB, Lipscomb J, Samsa G. Inpatient costs of specific cerebrovascular events at five academic medical centers. *Neurology* 1996; **46**:854–60.

177 Major K, Walker A. Economics of stroke unit care. In: Langhorne P, Dennis M, eds. *Stroke Units: An Evidence Based Approach.* London: BMJ Books, 1998, pp. 56–65.

178 Odderson IR, McKenna BS. A model for management of patients with stroke during the acute phase: outcome and economic implications. *Stroke* 1993; **24**:1823–7.

179 Wentworth DA, Atkinson RP. Implementation of an acute stroke program decreases hospitalisation costs and length of stay. *Stroke* 1996; **27**:1040–3.

180 Mamoli A, Censori B, Casto L, Sileo C, Cesana B, Camerlingo M. An analysis of the costs of ischemic stroke in an Italian stroke unit. *Neurology* 1999; **53**:112–16.

181 Harbison JH, Hossain O, Jenkinson D, Davis J, Louw SJ, Ford GA. Diagnostic accuracy of stroke referrals from primary care, emergency room physicians and ambulance staff using the Face Arm Speech Test. *Stroke* 2003; **34**:71–6.

182 Silliman SL, Quinn B, Huggett V, Merino JG. Use of a field-to-stroke center helicopter transport program to extend thrombolytic therapy to rural residents. *Stroke* 2003; **34**(3):729–33.

183 Kwan J, Hand P, Sandercock P. Improving the efficiency of delivery of thrombolysis for acute stroke: a systematic review. *Q J Med* 2004; **97**(5):273–9.

184 Wojner-Alexandrov A, Alexandrov AV, Rodriguez DP, Grotta JC. Houston paramedic & emergency stroke treatment and outcomes study (HoPSTO). *Stroke* 2005; **36**:1512.

185 Song F, Altman DG, Glenny AM, Deeks JJ. Validity of indirect comparison for estimating efficacy of competing interventions: empirical evidence from published meta-analyses. *Br Med J* 2003; **326**(7387):472.

186 Rothwell PM, Coull AJ, Giles MF, Howard SC, Silver LE, Bull LM *et al.* Change in stroke incidence, mortality, case-fatality, severity and risk factors in Oxfordshire, UK, from 1981–2004. *Lancet* 2004; **363**(9425):1920 (comment), 1925–33.

187 Sudlow CLM, Warlow CP. Comparable studies of the incidence of stroke and its pathological types: results from an international collaboration. *Stroke* 1997; **28**:491–9.

188 Hand PJ, Kwan J, Lindley RJ, Dennis MS, Wardlow JM. Distinguishing between stroke and mimic at the bedside: the brain attack study. *Stroke* 2006; **37**(3):769–75.

189 Vickers N, Pollock A. Incompleteness and retrieval of case note in a case note audit of colorectal cancer. *Qual Health Care* 1993; **2**:170–4.

190 Harwood RH, Gompretz P, Ebrahim S. Handicap one year after stroke: validity of a new scale. *J Neurol Neurosurg Psychiatry* 1994; **57**:825–9.

191 Lyden PD, Lau GT. A critical appraisal for stroke evaluaton and rating scales. *Stroke* 1991; **22**:1345–52.

192 Davis D, O'Brien MA, Freemantle N, Wolf FM, Mazmanian P, Taylor-Vaisey A. Impact of formal continuing medical education: do conferences, workshops, rounds, and other traditional continuing education activities change physician behavior or health care outcomes?. *J Am Med Assoc* 1999; **282**(9):867–74.

193 Wardlaw JM, Warlow CP, Counsell C. Systematic review of evidence on thrombolytic therapy for acute ischaemic stroke. *Lancet* 1997; **350**:607–14.

194 Robinson R. Economic evaluation and health care: what does it mean? *Br Med J* 2006; **307**:670–3.

195 Robinson R. Economic evaluation and health care: costs and cost-minimisation analysis. *Br Med J* 2006; **307**:670–3.

196 Robinson R. Economic evaluation and health care: cost-effectiveness analysis. *Br Med J* 2006; **307**:793–5.

197 Drummond MF, Jefferson, The BMJ Economic Evaluation Working Party. Guidelines for authors and peer reviewers of economic submissions to the BMJ. *Br Med J* 1996; **313**:275–83.

18 Reducing the impact of stroke and improving the public health

18.1 Introduction

The huge burden of stroke on patients, their families and friends, and society is constantly and appropriately being emphasized.[1,2] The Global Burden of Disease study has attempted to quantify the contribution to worldwide disability and mortality of over 100 diseases and injuries and selected risk factors; cerebrovascular disease is a major and increasingly important player. Stroke is the second commonest cause of death worldwide after ischaemic heart disease, causing over 5 million deaths (that is, almost 10% of all deaths) in 2001.[3] Strikingly, while most stroke research occurs in high-income countries, 85% of stroke deaths occur in low- and middle-income countries. And, despite being a disease mainly of older people, stroke is still a globally important cause of premature death (Fig. 18.1). In addition, it is a leading cause of disability worldwide, ranking second in high-income countries and fifth in low- and middle-income countries.[3] On a more local level, in the UK, it is the most common life-threatening neurological condition, the most important single cause of severe disability in people living in their own homes, and it accounts for about 6% of National Health Service and Social Services expenditure.[2,4]

In descending order of interest to most clinicians but, as we shall see, not in order of likely impact on the public health, there are four complementary strategies to reduce stroke burden (Fig. 18.2):

- treating first-ever-in-a-lifetime and recurrent acute strokes to reduce case fatality and maximize independence and quality of life in the survivors (section 18.3);
- reducing the risk of stroke after transient ischaemic attack (TIA), and of recurrent stroke after a first-ever-in-a-lifetime stroke (secondary prevention) (section 18.4);
- seeking out and treating people at particularly high risk of stroke to reduce their risk (the 'high-risk' strategy for primary prevention) (section 18.5);
- reducing the average level of causative risk factors in the whole population (the 'mass' strategy for primary prevention) (section 18.5).

However, we must first consider how the burden of stroke can be measured and monitored routinely over time so that goals to reduce it can be set, and then worked towards by implementing the four strategies. Second, we must compare their effectiveness, practicability and cost where we can.

> Stroke is the second commonest cause of death worldwide, a leading cause of premature death and disability globally, and a major source of health and social service expenditure in high-income countries.

Stroke: practical management, 3rd edition. C. Warlow, J. van Gijn, M. Dennis, J. Wardlaw, J. Bamford, G. Hankey, P. Sandercock, G. Rinkel, P. Langhorne, C. Sudlow and P. Rothwell. Published 2008 Blackwell Publishing. ISBN 978-1-4051-2766-0.

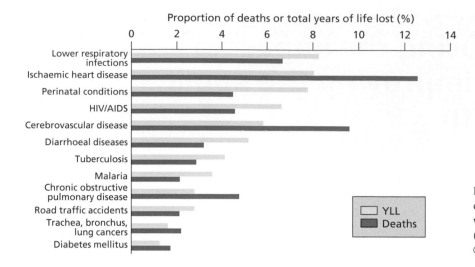

Proportion of deaths or total years of life lost (%)

Fig. 18.1 Leading causes of premature death (years of life lost) and of deaths worldwide, 2001. YLL years of life lost. (Reprinted from Lopez *et al. Lancet*[3] © 2006 with permission from Elsevier.)

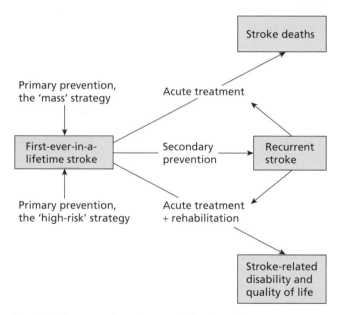

Fig. 18.2 Strategies for reducing the burden of stroke.

18.2 Measuring and monitoring changes in the impact of stroke

No country in the world has a routine method of monitoring stroke *incidence*; it is too difficult to measure at one point in time, let alone at several (section 18.2.2). Hospital discharge rates are unreliable: admitted patients generally have more severe strokes, and the proportion of strokes admitted is mostly unknown and could change unpredictably and unmeasurably with time as a result of bed availability, new treatments and variation in admission policy (section 17.11.2).[5] Moreover, many

routine coding systems double-count patients as they move from one service to another within the same hospital. Nor is there a routine method for monitoring stroke *case fatality* or *outcome* in survivors, and certainly not for monitoring the *cost* of stroke. Stroke *prevalence* depends on both incidence and case fatality. Therefore, any change would be impossible to interpret without also measuring one of its two components. In any event, prevalence is tedious and time-consuming to measure; it is probably inaccurate because distant and mild strokes are forgotten and the evidence for any past stroke may not be very good. Different screening methods can yield very different estimates of prevalence in the same population and the answers to screening questions may be affected by cultural factors, or differ at different time periods in the same culture (section 17.11.2).[6] Therefore, unless population-based incidence studies can be repeated, or sustained over time with rigorous standardization of their methods, which has seldom been achieved, often the only realistic way to assess the success of strategies for reducing stroke burden is by monitoring stroke *mortality* (section 18.6). So, how reliable are routine stroke mortality statistics, what do they mean, and is stroke mortality changing?

18.2.1 Stroke mortality

Mortality statistics provide the most widely available data for measuring the burden of stroke, comparing different countries, and monitoring changes over time. But, even this method tends to be woefully inaccurate – if measured at all – in almost all developing countries, and leaves much to be desired even in developed countries. Routine mortality data are limited by the inaccuracies of death certificates and the lack of reliable information about different pathological types of stroke. Furthermore, they depend on both the incidence of and survival from stroke, and tell us nothing about strokes that are disabling but not fatal (such as lacunar strokes).

Stroke mortality appears to vary widely between those countries for which routine death certificate data are available. For example, in the late 1990s, age-standardized mortality from cerebrovascular diseases in Russia was between five and seven times higher than in North America, France and Switzerland[7] (Fig. 18.3). Age-standardized stroke mortality declined from the mid-1960s to the late 1990s in North and South America, Western European countries, Australasia, and – particularly dramatically up to the early 1980s – in Japan.

However, in Eastern European countries, stroke mortality did not fall but instead tended to increase over the decades (Fig. 18.4). These trends have generally paralleled changes in ischaemic heart disease mortality, making it more likely that they are real.[7,8] Any observed differences in trends between stroke and ischaemic heart disease mortality may be explained by the pathological heterogeneity of stroke, since when ratios of ischaemic to haemorrhagic stroke from autopsy studies were used to estimate secular trends in ischaemic and haemorrhagic stroke mortality throughout the 20th century in England and Wales, the trends in *ischaemic* stroke and *ischaemic* heart disease mortality were almost identical,

(a)

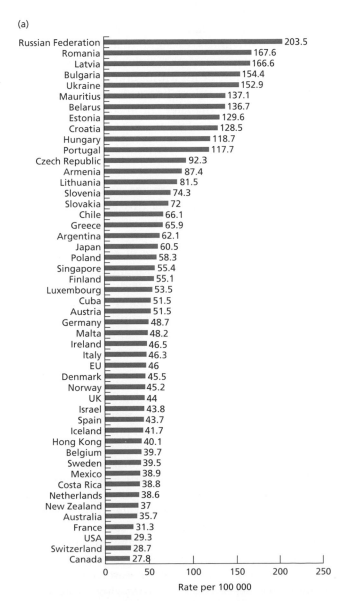

(b)

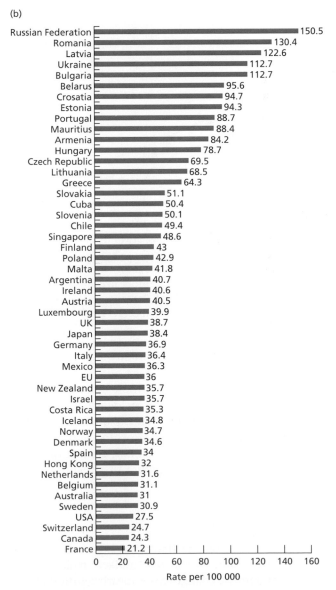

Fig. 18.3 Age-standardized (world population) annual death certification rates from cerebrovascular diseases in (a) men and (b) women in 48 countries and the European Union (EU), 1995 to 1998. (From Levi *et al.*[7] © 2002 BMJ Publishing Group.)

(a)

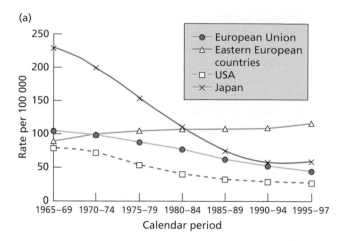

(b)

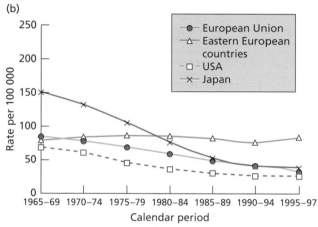

Fig. 18.4 Trends in age-standardized (world population) annual death certification rates from cerebrovascular diseases in (a) men and (b) women in all age groups from the European Union (as it was in 2002), eastern European countries (Bulgaria, Czech Republic, Hungary, Poland, Romania and Slovakia), the USA and Japan, 1965 to 1997. (From Levi et al.[7] © 2002 BMJ Publishing Group.)

while haemorrhagic stroke mortality had a somewhat different trend.[9]

It is commonly assumed that these mortality changes are explained by changes in the incidence of stroke. But, there are several other potential explanations: changes in death certification practice, errors in age standardization, changes in diagnostic accuracy, competing causes of death, changes in the mixture of stroke types and changes in case fatality.

Changes in death certification practice

The decline in stroke mortality has been so consistent in so many countries that it is unlikely to be entirely due to a systematic change in how death certificates have been completed and then coded. However, there are many ambiguous situations, leading to wide variation in

classification of cause of death in patients who die after a stroke.[10] For example, when a patient who remains bedridden after a stroke dies of pneumonia 6 months later, the underlying cause of death may be coded either as pneumonia, with stroke not even mentioned on the death certificate, or as stroke. The documented inaccuracy of death certification of stroke is of particular concern in the elderly, in whom most strokes occur, although this may be less of a problem when patients with suspected stroke are admitted to hospitals with CT scanning facilities.[11–13] Some of the apparently steep decline in stroke mortality in the years since the Second World War in Japan may be attributed to inaccurate death certification, with coding of sudden deaths as due to stroke.[14] We now know that most sudden deaths are caused by complications of coronary heart disease, especially arrhythmias,[15,16] and that, of the various pathological types of stroke, only subarachnoid haemorrhage can cause death within minutes of onset (section 14.1). However, this coding artifact is unlikely to be the explanation for the later fall in stroke mortality in Japan, or in other parts of the world.

Errors in age standardization

Stroke mortality increases with age, and so if mortality is measured in age-band strata that are too wide, any change in the distribution of the age of people within a single stratum could lead to apparent rather than real changes in stroke mortality. After all, even across a mere 10-year age difference, stroke mortality can more than double.[17] This problem is particularly pertinent in the oldest age stratum with an open upper end (e.g. 85 years plus), because this stratum might contain people of very different ages, whose proportions may change with time.

Changes in diagnostic accuracy

The clinical diagnosis of stroke vs not-stroke as a cause of death should be reasonably secure in countries with good healthcare even though postmortem rates to confirm the diagnosis have declined precipitously.[18,19] It is thus unlikely that inaccurate diagnosis completely explains changing mortality, particularly in patients under 75 years old where the diagnosis is rather easier and, rightly or wrongly, more likely to be attempted carefully than in the very elderly. Of course, for *epidemiological* purposes, the World Health Organization clinical definition of stroke[20] must be adhered to rigidly and at present we can see no compelling reason for any modification that depends on brain imaging. A definition based on imaging would inevitably change with time as imaging technology becomes more widely available, and improves (section 3.2). In developing countries, and indeed in cultures where postmortem is culturally unacceptable, the technique of 'verbal autopsy' may be better than nothing but there is no standard methodology. Furthermore, verbal autopsy requires questioning of all relevant family, carers, witnesses, medical and other staff as soon after death as possible, as well as local validation against some reasonable 'gold standard', and this has seldom been achieved.[21–24]

Competing causes of death

It has been argued that stroke mortality is declining because those likely to die of stroke are now dying earlier of ischaemic heart disease, or some other non-stroke cause. However, this is unlikely because, in countries with available data on both, stroke and ischaemic heart disease mortality have similar trends.[7] In fact, because myocardial infarction and ischaemic stroke share the same risk factors, and so the same sort of people have both, it is conceivable that more effective treatment after acute myocardial infarction, and so longer survival, might leave *more* people at high risk of stroke and so *increase* stroke mortality.[25]

Changes in the mixture of stroke types

Certain types of stroke are far more likely to cause death than others. For example, the 30-day case fatality after lacunar infarction is less than 5%, whereas after total anterior circulation infarction it is about 40% (Table 10.3). If, therefore, the proportion of strokes due to lacunar infarction is increasing, and the proportion due to total anterior circulation infarction is decreasing, then stroke mortality would fall even if overall stroke incidence remained constant. This kind of detail of stroke subtype is simply not available or accurate in routine mortality statistics, and even in incidence studies it is difficult to achieve.

Changes in case fatality

A reduction in case fatality might have the effect of reducing stroke mortality (but not incidence) because patients surviving their acute stroke would then be more likely to die of a non-stroke event, such as myocardial infarction, than of the stroke itself. Some population-based stroke studies have found reductions in early (usually about 1 month) case fatality over the past 20–30 years, while others found no change.[26–30] Where it is present, improved survival could be due to:
- a change in the relative proportion of various stroke types (e.g. a higher proportion of lacunar strokes, see

above), although there is no clear evidence for this changing with time;
- improvements in drug treatment of acute stroke; although only aspirin is known to reduce the risk of death after acute ischaemic stroke, the large trials demonstrating this were not published until the late 1990s (section 12.3.2), and even if it were appropriately used in all eligible patients, it would still only produce a 3% reduction in all stroke deaths at the population level (section 18.3);
- the introduction of stroke units, which, if widely and appropriately used, could reduce stroke deaths at the population level by about 10%, but this is only a relatively recent innovation and stroke service audit data suggest that current levels of stroke unit availability and use are far from optimal[31] (section 18.3); or
- strokes may have been getting milder, although studies that have examined this issue suggest that this is not in fact the case.[30]

In summary therefore, there are several more-or-less plausible reasons for changes in stroke mortality, which are not determined by changes in incidence. A fall (or rise) in stroke mortality does not necessarily mean that there has been a fall (or rise) in incidence. Unfortunately, stroke incidence is laborious and expensive to measure at one point in time (section 17.11.1), and even more so at several points in time (section 18.2.2), and nowhere is this routine practice. While it might be more cost-effective to improve on all the possible biases and inaccuracies of routinely collected mortality statistics and then use them as an (imperfect) surrogate for stroke incidence, there will be continuing concern about their accuracy and comparability between different countries and different time periods. In addition, it is far from certain that stroke mortality reflects stroke incidence, particularly when changes in mortality have generally been much more dramatic than changes in incidence (section 18.2.2).

> Stroke mortality varies widely (up to seven-fold) between those countries with available data. Stroke mortality has fallen over the last few decades in many countries, but it is unclear whether this is due to a fall in stroke incidence, lower case fatality, some artifact of the collection and analysis of routine mortality data, or a combination of all of these.

18.2.2 Stroke incidence and case fatality

Geographic variation

Measuring stroke incidence accurately is not technically difficult but requires considerably more resources than

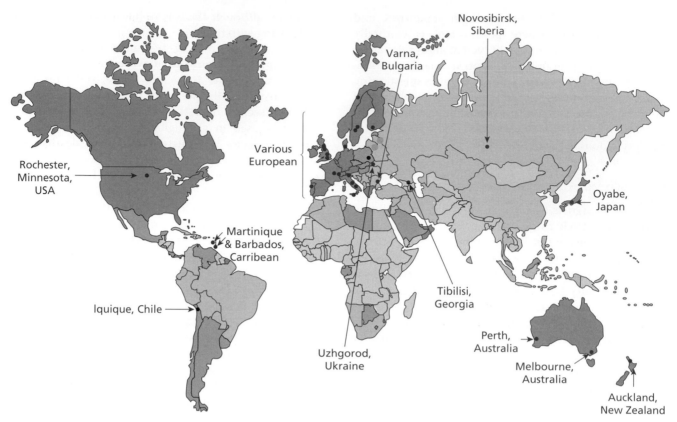

Fig. 18.5 Community-based, methodologically 'ideal' stroke incidence studies around the world.

are available in routine clinical and public health practice, and it is time-consuming. As a consequence, few stroke incidence studies conducted over the last 20 years or so meet an ideal – or even a more-or-less ideal – standard, when set against explicit methodological criteria; and those that do come mainly from predominantly white populations in high-income countries (Table 17.15, Fig. 18.5).[26,30,32–39] The exceptions are Oyabe in Japan, Novosibirsk in Siberia, Russia, Varna in Bulgaria, Uzhgorod in Ukraine, Tbilisi in Georgia, Martinique and Barbados in the Caribbean, and Iquique in Chile.[36–38,40–44]

While in general there is little difference between studies in overall age-adjusted stroke incidence, or in the proportions of the main pathological types of stroke, the Japanese, Russian, Bulgarian and Ukrainian studies all found age-adjusted incidence that was about two to three times higher than the lowest incidences which were in Perth (Australia), Auckland (New Zealand) and Dijon (France). (It is unclear whether or not the Ukrainian study included only first-ever-in-a-lifetime strokes or whether recurrences were included, so the apparently very high incidence in this study may be a methodological artifact.) In the case of Russia, Bulgaria and Ukraine, these higher incidences are paralleled but exceeded by

higher mortality rates (five to seven times higher than in France),[7] while stroke mortality is higher in Japan by the same amount as stroke incidence (about twofold). The reasons for the discrepancies between stroke incidence and mortality are likely to be a combination of the causes outlined in section 18.2.1 above.

None of the four studies with high overall adjusted stroke incidence had enough patients CT scanned to allow reliable comparisons of different pathological types of stroke. The Caribbean, Georgian and Chilean studies found similar overall stroke incidence to the white high-income populations. Furthermore, in Iquique (Chile) and Barbados, where most patients had a CT scan (>90%), the distribution of pathological types was also similar to that in white high-income populations.

There is a lack of population-based data on the incidence of stroke and its pathological types from large areas of the world, particularly developing countries (Fig. 18.5). Thus, while it has been suggested that the proportion of strokes due to intracerebral haemorrhage is higher in China, India and Africa than it is in mainly white populations in high-income countries, this could be due to methodological artifact, since few incidence studies with adequate brain imaging have been performed in developing countries, and those that have been done were generally hospital-based and so prone to hospital admission bias.[24,45]

> Where it has been studied reliably (mainly in high-income white populations), stroke incidence does not vary as much between countries as stroke mortality. Incidence appears higher in Japan, Russia, Bulgaria and Ukraine, but reliable stroke incidence studies are simply not available from many parts of the world, including China, India and Africa.

Ethnic variation

Variation in stroke incidence between countries, if real rather than due to methodological artifact, could be due to variations in environmental factors operating at the level of the population (e.g. climate, air pollution, environmental tobacco smoke) or the individual (e.g. smoking, blood pressure, diet), or differences in stroke risk between different ethnic groups, which may or may not be due to genetic factors. Rather few population-based stroke incidence studies have been able to compare stroke incidence between different ethnic groups within the same population, so reducing the population level environmental variation.

Two population-based stroke registers in US cities and one in south London in the UK have found the age- and sex-adjusted incidence of stroke in black people to be about twice that in white people.[46–48] One of these – the south London study – fulfilled proposed methodological criteria for an ideal stroke incidence study, and found that the higher stroke incidence in black people persisted after adjusting for socioeconomic group.[48] Much of the remaining difference could be due to ethnic differences in vascular risk factors, and population-based studies in south London and in the US have shown that such differences exist.[49–51] The south London study also found a slightly higher proportion of intracerebral haemorrhage and of lacunar ischaemic stroke among black compared with white stroke patients. In addition, it found survival after stroke to be better among black than white patients, even after adjusting for known confounders.[52] Although both a higher stroke incidence and better survival might be explained by better case-finding (and so identification of more mild cases) among blacks (at least in the UK, where black people may be more likely to use the free and more easily monitored National Health Service), this seems unlikely to explain all of the difference. Further work is needed to explore the reasons for these intriguing ethnic differences in stroke incidence and survival.[53]

A recent 'ideal' population-based study in Auckland, New Zealand, compared the incidence of stroke and its main pathological types among those of European origin, Maori/Pacific people and Asian and other ethnicities. The age-adjusted incidence of all types of stroke was almost twice as high in Maori/Pacific people and about one-third higher in Asian and other ethnicities than in European New Zealanders. This was accounted for by a higher incidence both of ischaemic stroke (relative risk 1.7 for Maori/Pacific people and 1.3 for Asian/other ethnicities) and intracerebral haemorrhage (relative risk 2.7 for Maori/Pacific people and 2.3 for Asian/other ethnicities), with no significant difference for either subarachnoid haemorrhage or strokes of undetermined type. Chance, and ethnic differences in vascular risk factors and socioeconomic status, could be at least partly responsible for the differences observed, and further work is needed to establish the true explanation.[54]

> Few studies have reliably compared stroke incidence between different ethnic groups in the same population. Those that have show a higher incidence in non-white, and generally lower income, ethnic groups than in whites, but it is uncertain whether these differences are due to different socioeconomic status, vascular risk factor patterns, genetic factors, or a combination of these.

Time trends

Rather few stroke incidence studies have been repeated, or continued for long enough, to provide reliable time trend information. Of the few population-based studies that have assessed stroke incidence trends in a given population, most showed a decline in stroke incidence through to the late 1970s or early 1980s. Thereafter, from the 1980s to the late 1990s, stroke incidence has stabilized or even increased slightly in some studies, while in others the decline in incidence has continued. Once again, the studies of incidence trends were mainly in white high-income countries, with a relative lack of information from other parts of the world.[26,28–30,55–60]

The most dramatic results came from Oxfordshire in the UK where there was a reduction between 1981 and 2004 in age- and sex-adjusted stroke incidence of almost one-third. Unlike most previous studies of stroke incidence trends, data were available on trends for the main pathological types of stroke. The overall decline was due to a decrease of about one-half in intracerebral haemorrhage, and of about one-quarter in ischaemic stroke, with no change in subarachnoid haemorrhage.[30] This latter finding extended the findings of a previous systematic review, which suggested that the incidence of aneurysmal subarachnoid haemorrhage remained stable between 1960 and the early 1990s.[61]

So, if stroke incidence is falling, at least in affluent areas of the world, why is this? In the Oxfordshire study, there were also substantial reductions in premorbid vascular risk factors, with major increases in premorbid treatment with vascular preventive drugs, suggesting that improvements in primary preventive strategies could be at least partly responsible for the observed decline in stroke incidence.[30] In the Auckland study, where the decline in stroke incidence was much less dramatic, changes in vascular risk factors were difficult to interpret, since the frequency of some fell while others increased.[60] In the WHO-MONICA study, repeated population surveys of vascular risk factors and continuous monitoring of stroke events were conducted in people up to the age of 64 over a period of 7–13 years in 15 populations in nine countries. Variations in stroke trends between populations could be partly – but not wholly – explained by changes in known vascular risk factors.[62] The identification and treatment of transient ischaemic attacks cannot have had much impact on stroke incidence, largely because only a small proportion of strokes are preceded by TIAs[30,63] (section 18.4.1).

Of course, because most populations are ageing, the *number* of stroke patients may increase even if the *incidence* in each age band decreases. Using current estimates of stroke incidence and population projections based on demographic information, calculations show that the number of strokes in all European Union and European Free Trade Association countries will increase from 1.1 million per year in 2000 to 1.5 million per year in 2025 without any change in stroke incidence for each age group. If the age-adjusted incidence increases by 2% per 5 years, then there will be 1.65 million strokes by 2025, and even if incidence falls by 2% per 5 years, the absolute number of stroke events will still increase to 1.35 million.[64] However, the number of *dependent* stroke survivors will not necessarily increase as much because elderly dependent people are more likely to die early as a consequence of stroke than young independent people.[65] We need far more dramatic falls in stroke incidence (so far only recorded in the Oxfordshire, UK study) if absolute numbers of strokes are to fall because of the increasing numbers of older people in the population.

In general, therefore, as we saw for mortality and incidence variation between different countries, the dramatic decline in mortality over time seen in many parts of the world has not been accompanied by as steep a decline in incidence, and therefore cannot be entirely explained by falling incidence (section 18.2.1). However, the Oxfordshire stroke incidence data are very encouraging, and do suggest that primary prevention efforts may be starting to pay off.[30]

> In the few places where it has been measured reasonably reliably, stroke incidence mainly declined up to the early 1980s. Thereafter, incidence has stayed about the same or even increased slightly in some places, while in others the downward trend has continued, perhaps due to improved primary prevention.

We must now consider the four strategies which *might* reduce stroke burden in the future, whether such strategies could be implemented, and how the effects, if any, should be monitored.

18.3 Likely effect and costs of acute stroke treatment on stroke burden in the population

18.3.1 Effects

Enormous efforts are being devoted to developing and testing promising new treatments for acute stroke and at long last there has been some progress, at least for ischaemic stroke (Chapter 12). Also, reorganizing haphazard stroke care into stroke units is not just an effective strategy to reduce case fatality and dependency, but greatly facilitates randomized trials of new treatments (section 17.6.2). But what impact might the present treatment of acute stroke be having on the overall burden of stroke? To assess this, we have used previously described methods combined with the most recent available data.[66]

Only three interventions have been shown in randomized trials to reduce either death or the combined outcome of death or dependency after acute ischaemic stroke or intracerebral haemorrhage: organized stroke unit care, aspirin given within 48 h of onset of acute ischaemic stroke, and intravenous thrombolysis given with the first few hours of onset of acute ischaemic stroke. Clearly, treating acute stroke will have no effect on stroke incidence, except that some patients otherwise destined to have a stroke might only have a transient ischaemic attack if they are successfully treated with intravenous thrombolysis within a few hours of onset. Acute treatments for subarachnoid haemorrhage are not considered here, since this accounts for only a small proportion of all stroke patients.

If we imagine a notional European population of 1 million people then, using incidence estimates from the recently conducted Oxford Vascular Study in the UK, we might expect 1600 people to have a first-ever-in-a-lifetime

Table 18.1 Estimated number of cerebrovascular events occurring each year in a notional European population of 1 million people.*

Event type	Incident	Recurrent
Transient ischaemic attack	660	440
Ischaemic stroke	1410	600
Intracerebral haemorrhage	120	30
Subarachnoid haemorrhage	70	30
Any stroke	1600	660

*Data are taken from the Oxford Vascular Study, a recent population-based study of the incidence of acute vascular events, including stroke and transient ischaemic attack (Rothwell *et al.*, 2005[70]).

stroke and 660 a recurrent stroke each year (Table 18.1). If we assume that the untreated outcomes in terms of death or death and dependency of these 2260 stroke patients are similar to those observed in the Oxfordshire Community Stroke Project, then by 3 months after stroke we would expect 520 (23%) to have died and 1240 (55%) to be either dead or dependent, while at 1 year we would expect 700 (31%) to have died but the same total number (i.e. 1240) to be dead or dependent (see footnotes to Table 18.2, Table 10.3 and Figs 10.4 and 10.6). If, very optimistically, we assume that 80% of these 2260 stroke patients can be admitted to – and receive organized care in – a stroke unit, then the number of stroke deaths avoided at 1 year will be 108 out of 700, i.e. 15% (Table 18.2a). The effect of giving early aspirin to the 85% of the patients whose stroke is ischaemic and who have no contraindication to or intolerance of aspirin would be to reduce stroke deaths at 3 months by 15 out of 520, i.e. 3% (Table 18.2a). The number of patients who are either dead or dependent from 3 months to 1 year could be reduced by 24 out of 1240 (2%) with optimum use of intravenous thrombolysis (giving i.v. thrombolyis within 3 h of onset to an optimistic 10% of all acute ischaemic stroke patients), by 29 (2%) with optimum use of aspirin for acute ischaemic stroke, and by 72 (6%) with optimal provision of stroke unit care (Table 18.2b). Thus, the impact of treatment for acute stroke on the number of stroke deaths, or on the number of people with stroke-related death or dependency in the population, even making optimistic assumptions about treatment delivery, is only small. This is because some patients die before treatment can be started; all the available treatments are of limited effectiveness, and most have risks as well as benefits; and many treatments are contraindicated in various types of patients.

The treatment of acute stroke cannot influence stroke incidence, and will have rather little impact on stroke-related morbidity and mortality in the population, either because the effect of treatment is weak (like aspirin) or because treatment is only suitable for a small proportion of patients (like thrombolysis).

18.3.2 Costs

Detailed cost-effectiveness analyses can give healthcare providers very valuable information on the relative health gains from various interventions or strategies. However, such detailed analyses are beyond the scope of this chapter. Table 18.3 shows the direct drug costs (for the individual, the population, and per death or death or dependency avoided annually) of the acute stroke drug treatments discussed above, and demonstrates that the current cost per poor outcome avoided is far less for aspirin than it is for intravenous thrombolysis. Costs have been taken from the *British National Formulary* (see http://www.bnf.org/bnf/bnf/current/index.htm).[67] The costs of stroke unit care may be slightly greater or slightly less than the alternative of routine general medical care, and so we have assumed stroke units to be cost-neutral. Since they reduce death and disability, however, they are highly likely to be cost-effective.

18.4 Likely effects and costs of long-term treatment after transient ischaemic attack and stroke on stroke occurrence: secondary stroke prevention

18.4.1 Effects

Transient ischaemic attack (TIA) and stroke patients are at high risk of subsequent stroke (section 16.2). Of course, TIAs are essentially ischaemic strokes which, by definition, have recovered within 24 h and so treating TIAs is really secondary stroke prevention. If the very early high-risk period is included, then on average about 20% of patients with a TIA or (mainly ischaemic) stroke will have a recurrent stroke within 1 year, and then about 5% per year thereafter (section 16.2 and Table 16.1). For many of these individual patients, a combination of secondary preventive interventions (including lifestyle changes such as quitting smoking, antiplatelet, cholesterol-lowering and blood-pressure-lowering drugs and, in some cases, carotid endarterectomy) (chapter 16) can and should be used to reduce risk of recurrent stroke

Table 18.2 The estimated effect on the population of interventions for acute stroke on (a) death and (b) death or dependency in a notional European population of 1 million people and 2260 patients with an incident or recurrent acute stroke each year.

(a) Death

Intervention	Relative risk reduction (%)	% dead without intervention	% dead with intervention	Absolute risk reduction (%)	Number of deaths avoided per 1000 treated	Number of patients to be treated to prevent one death	Number in target population (% of all 2260 strokes)	Number (%) of all stroke deaths avoided in population of 1 million§
Stroke unit*	18	31	25	6	60	17	1808 (80%)	108/700 (15%)
Aspirin†	6	13	12.2	0.8	8	125	1910 (85%)	15/520 (3%)

(b) Death or dependency

Intervention	Relative risk reduction (%)	% dead/ dependent without intervention	% dead/ dependent with intervention	Absolute risk reduction (%)	Number of deaths/ dependents avoided per 1000 treated	Number of patients to be treated to prevent one death/ dependency	Number in target population (% of all 2260 strokes)	Number (%) of all stroke deaths/ dependents avoided in population of 1 million§
Stroke unit*	8	55	51	4	40	25	1808 (80%)	72/1240 (6%)
Aspirin†	3	50	48.5	1.5	15	67	1910 (85%)	29/1240 (2%)
Thrombolysis‡	17	60.3	49.7	10.6	106	9	226 (10%)	24/1240 (2%)

*Data on the relative effects of stroke units on death and death or dependency at 1 year are taken from the most recent Cochrane systematic review (Stroke Unit Trialists' Collaboration, 2006, table 17.6). Estimates of 1-year outcomes without stroke unit care are taken from the Oxfordshire Community Stroke Project (OCSP), a population-based study of the incidence of and outcome after stroke in the 1980s (Chapter 10, Table 10.3 and Figs 10.4 and 10.6): % of all 2260 patients dead at 1 year = 31%, and dead/dependent at 1 year = 55%.

†Data on the relative effects of aspirin on death and death or dependency at ~3 months are taken from the most recent Cochrane systematic review (Sandercock *et al.*, 2003, section 12.3.2). Estimates of 3-month outcomes without aspirin are taken from the OCSP (Chapter 10, Table 10.3 and Figs 10.4 and 10.6): % of ischaemic stroke patients dead at 3 months = 13%, and dead/dependent at 3 months = 50%.

‡Data on the relative effects of thrombolysis on death or dependency at 3 months are taken from the most recent Cochrane systematic review, using data available for intravenous treatment within 3 h of onset (the time window for which treatment is currently licensed). The effects of treatment are likely to be overestimates, because they are dominated by one trial, in which there were problems with the randomization process (Wardlaw *et al.*, 2003, section 12.5.2). Estimates of 3-month outcomes without thrombolysis are taken from the systematic review, since patients eligible for treatment with thrombolysis are not typical of ischaemic stroke patients in the community in general, making the randomized trial data more likely to be representative than that for unselected ischaemic stroke patients from the OCSP.

§Estimates of outcomes for all 2260 stroke patients are taken from the OCSP (Chapter 10, Table 10.3 and Figs 10.4 and 10.6): number (%) of all 2260 stroke patients dead at 3 months = 520 (23%); dead or dependent at 3 months = 1240 (55%); dead at 1 year = 700 (31%); dead or dependent at 1 year = 1240 (55%).

(and of other vascular events). But what impact might these interventions have on stroke occurrence at the population level?

We can calculate the approximate number of prevalent TIA and stroke patients in our notional European population of 1 million people by using available information on incidence and survival, as shown in Table 18.4. Our secondary preventive efforts will be targeted at the 13 000 prevalent stroke and TIA patients in the population, of whom about 1000 (8%) each year will have a stroke that is potentially preventable by secondary preventive efforts.

Table 18.4 shows how much we might expect to reduce strokes in the population by the optimal use of the various secondary preventive interventions whose benefits are proven by robust evidence from randomized trials

Table 18.3 Costs of effective drug treatments for acute stroke.

Treatment	Cost per patient with acute stroke*	Annual cost of treating all eligible patients in population of 1 million[†]	Cost per poor outcome avoided[‡]	
			Death	Death or disability
Aspirin for 2 weeks after acute ischaemic stroke	£0.50	£955	£62.50	£33.50
I.V. thrombolysis for very early acute ischaemic stroke (rt-PA)	£480	£108 480	–	£4320

*Costs are given in UK £ sterling and taken from the *British National Formulary*, March 2007.[67] These are estimated drug costs only, and so are a minimum since we have not included the costs of administration, adverse effects, or monitoring.
†Calculated using data on numbers of eligible patients given in Table 18.2.
‡Calculated using data on number-needed-to-treat given in Table 18.2.

(chapter 16), and again we have drawn on previously established methods and the most recent available data to make the necessary calculations.[66] All the patients with an ischaemic stroke (around 90% of the strokes) and all those with a TIA should be considered for long-term antiplatelet treatment (section 16.5.1). If we make the optimistic assumption that, after excluding patients with a contraindication to aspirin and those with atrial fibrillation for whom oral anticoagulants are not contraindicated, we can treat around 85% of patients with an ischaemic stroke or TIA (i.e. about 77% of all prevalent stroke and TIA patients) with aspirin, then at best we could prevent 180 (8%) of the 2260 strokes occurring each year (Table 18.4). Assuming that we can treat around 85% of prevalent stroke and TIA patients with a statin to reduce cholesterol (those with an ischaemic event and with a pretreatment cholesterol of ≥ 3.5 mmol/L or LDL-cholesterol of ≥ 2.6 mmol/L), we could prevent 166 (7%) of the strokes occurring each year (Table 18.4). A total of perhaps around 20% of all the prevalent stroke and TIA patients will be ineligible for routine blood pressure reduction because they have had a subarachnoid haemorrhage (the secondary preventive blood-pressure-lowering randomized trials in patients with cerebrovascular disease included those with TIA, ischaemic stroke and intracerebral – but generally not subarachnoid – haemorrhage – section 16.3.2), already have a blood pressure below around 120–130/70, or cannot tolerate any blood-pressure-lowering medication (section 16.3.4). At the most optimistic, we might therefore treat 80% of the prevalent patients, and would expect, at best, to avoid 146 (6%) of the 2260 strokes occurring each year (Table 18.4). A small proportion of patients who have started aspirin will have a contraindication to an additional antiplatelet drug, so we might expect to be able to treat about 65% of all prevalent stroke and TIA patients with modified-release dipyridamole in addition to aspirin, so avoiding about 94 (4%) of all strokes occurring annually (Table 18.4). For oral anticoagulants, potentially eligible patients are those with a prior ischaemic event who have atrial fibrillation or some other high-risk cardiac source of emboli. These probably comprise up to about 20% of prevalent ischaemic stroke/TIA patients, but an optimistic maximum of 50% of these (about 1000 patients) are likely to be free of contraindications to anticoagulation.[68,69] Assuming we do treat these 1000 patients with oral anticoagulants, then we could avoid 73 (3%) of all the strokes occurring each year (Table 18.4). Finally, each year only a very small proportion of patients with a new ischaemic stroke or TIA will be eligible for carotid endarterectomy, since they must be fit enough and willing for surgical intervention and have severe recently symptomatic carotid stenosis. In the recent OXVASC community-based study of stroke and TIA in Oxfordshire, 95% of patients with a TIA or non-disabling ischaemic stroke (i.e. the majority who might be eligible for carotid endarterectomy) had carotid imaging. Over a 3-year period, 40 out of a total of 918 patients with an incident or recurrent stroke or TIA (4%) had severe carotid stenosis with relevant symptoms in the last 6 months.[70,71] If we make the optimistic assumption that 80% of these are fit enough and willing to have surgery and can be operated on within 2 weeks of their symptom onset, then we could prevent an average of 4 (0.2%) of the 2260 strokes occurring each year in the population (Table 18.4).

So, with optimistic assumptions, each of the secondary preventive treatments discussed above might reduce the

Table 18.4 The estimated effect on strokes occurring in the population of interventions for prevention of recurrent stroke (and other vascular events) among 13 000 stroke and TIA patients prevalent in a notional European population of 1 million people.*

Intervention	Relative risk reduction (%)	% recurrent stroke per year without intervention	% recurrent stroke per year with intervention	Absolute risk reduction (%)	Number of strokes avoided per 1000 treated per year	Number of patients to be treated to prevent one stroke per year	Number in target population (% of all 13 000 prevalent TIA/stroke patients)	Number (%) of all 2260 strokes avoided each year in population of 1 million
Aspirin[†]	20	9.0	7.2	1.8	18	56	10 000 (77%)	180/2260 (8%)
Statins to reduce cholesterol[‡]	17	9.0	7.5	1.5	15	67	11 050 (85%)	166/2260 (7%)
Drugs to reduce blood pressure[§]	23	6.0	4.6	1.4	14	71	10 400 (80%)	146/2260 (6%)
Modified release dipyridamole added to aspirin[¶]	22	4.8	3.7	1.1	11	91	8500 (65%)	94/2260 (4%)
Anticoagulants[¥]	61	12	4.7	7.3	73	14	1000 (8%)	73/2260 (3%)
Carotid endarterectomy[$]	59	6.0	2.5	3.5	35	29	117 (1%)	4/2260 (0.2%)

*The prevalence of stroke and TIA is assumed to be given by the incidence multiplied by the time (in years) taken for half of the incident cases to die. Every year there are 1600 incident strokes (Table 18.1), of whom about half will die within 5 years (section 16.2), so that the number of prevalent stroke patients in the population at any one point in time is about 8000. Each year, there are also 660 incident TIAs, of whom about half will die in 7–8 years (based on 5-year follow-up data from the Oxfordshire Community Stroke Project, adjusted for later increases in mortality as documented in long-term follow-up of a cohort of patients with a TIA or mild ischaemic stroke recruited into a randomized trial) (Dennis et al., 1990;[104] van Wijk et al., 2005[105]), so that the number of prevalent TIA patients in the population at any one point in time is about 5000.

Three thousand three hundred and sixty of the 13 000 prevalent patients have had an incident or recurrent stroke or TIA within the last year (see Table 18.1 above). The risk of recurrent stroke in the first year after a TIA or stroke is about 20% (section 16.2). We assume that, for all eligible stroke patients, aspirin and a statin are started immediately, while blood pressure reduction, dipyridamole and anticoagulants are started on average 1–2 weeks after the TIA or stroke. For these slightly later treatments, the 'treatable' risk in the first year decreases to about 10% (since we miss the very early high risk period). The annual stroke recurrence risk in the remaining 9640 patients is about 5% per year. For aspirin and statin treatment, this means that the overall average annual untreated risk for all 13 000 patients is about 9% (equivalent to 20% of 3360 + 5% of 9640), and for blood pressure reduction the overall average annual untreated risk for all 13 000 patients is about 6% (equivalent to 10% of 3360 + 5% of 9640). Since the average annual untreated risk from 1–2 weeks post event is about 6%, but the proven benefits of dipyridamole are in addition to those of aspirin, we assume that aspirin has already been started, reducing the risk without dipyridamole by 20% to 4.8%. For anticoagulants, mainly for patients with atrial fibrillation, the untreated average annual risk is estimated at about 12% (the control group risk in randomized trials of oral anticoagulants vs control for long-term prevention in patients with atrial fibrillation and a history of ischaemic stroke or TIA – section 16.6.2).

†Relative risk reduction based on only the aspirin vs control trials in the Antithrombotic Trialists' overview of antiplatelet therapy, assuming the effect on stroke among patients with prior ischaemic stroke or TIA to be similar to that found for all patients at high risk of vascular disease (Antithrombotic Trialists' Collaboration, 2002[106]).

‡Relative risk reduction taken from systematic review of statins to reduce cholesterol, assuming the effect on stroke of a 1 mmol reduction in LDL cholesterol among patients with prior ischaemic stroke or TIA to be similar to that found overall (Cholesterol Treatment Trialists' Collaboration, 2005[87]).

§Relative risk reduction for reduction in blood pressure of 8 mmHg systolic/4 mmHg diastolic taken from a systematic review of blood pressure lowering after prior stroke or TIA (Rashid et al., 2003[107]).

¶Relative risk reduction based on a meta-analysis of randomized trials of aspirin + dipyridamole vs aspirin alone in patients with a prior ischaemic stroke or TIA (The ESPRIT Study Group, 2006[108]).

¥Relative risk reduction based on a meta-analysis of randomized trials of warfarin vs control in patients with atrial fibrillation (section 16.6.2 and Fig. 16.30b).

$Relative risk reduction based on meta-analysis of two large randomized trials of carotid endarterectomy for recently symptomatic severe stenosis. This is the reduction in any ipsilateral ischaemic stroke and any stroke or death within 30 days of surgery for patents operated on within 2 weeks of symptom onset. The relative and absolute risk reductions are assumed to remain constant over the 5-year follow-up period in order to obtain a notional average annual risk reduction. The average annual risk without intervention is that of the control group within the subgroup of patients operated on within 2 weeks of symptom onset in the meta-analysis (30% over 5 years, about 6% per year) (Rothwell et al., 2004[109]).

number of strokes occurring each year in the population by up to a few per cent. These effects may be additive but the figures shown do not, except in the case of adding dipyridamole to aspirin, account for decreasing increment in absolute benefit, since each new treatment is, in reality, given to patients whose baseline risk is lowered by taking whichever treatment(s) they have already started (section 16.18.2). We saw above that about 1000 (less than half) of the 2260 strokes occurring each year in our population of 1 million people occur in those with a prior stroke or TIA and so are potentially preventable by secondary preventive strategies (Table 18.4). Thus, although treatment for a relatively small number of high-risk patients who have already had a stroke or TIA will be reasonably effective for many (but not all) in terms of reduced stroke risk, it will have little impact on stroke in the population because most strokes occur in lower-risk individuals who have not already had a stroke or TIA (the so-called 'prevention paradox' – section 18.5.3). Furthermore, as Table 18.4 shows, treatment is always much less than 100% effective and not without risk, and each treatment is only appropriate for a variable proportion of all prevalent stroke and TIA patients. The optimistic assumptions used in Table 18.4 include

assuming that treatment adherence is as good as in the randomized trials and that the treatments are used for all eligible patients in a timely way. In real clinical practice, effective drugs and surgery are not applied optimally,[72,73] and patients prescribed long-term medications only take about 50% of their pills.[74] However, it is worth bearing in mind that the secondary preventive treatments discussed will also have a small impact on non-stroke vascular events (such as ischaemic heart disease) in addition to their modest effects on stroke at the population level.

> Prevention of stroke after a stroke or transient ischaemic attack is an example of the 'high-risk' prevention strategy and will have little effect on stroke incidence, even though the individual patient may have much to gain.

18.4.2 Costs

Table 18.5 shows the direct costs of the various secondary preventive interventions listed in Table 18.4 and discussed in section 18.4.1 above. As in section 18.3.2, we have estimated drug costs from the *British National Formulary*,[67] and these are a minimum because the costs of monitoring,

Table 18.5 Costs of interventions for long-term secondary prevention of stroke.

Intervention*	Cost per patient (per year)[†]	Annual cost of treating all eligible patients in population of 1 million[‡]	Cost per stroke prevented[¶]
Aspirin	£16	£160 000	£896
Simvastatin 40 mg daily	£44	£486 200	£2 948
Atorvastatin 10 mg daily	£235	£2 396 750	£15 745
Indapamide 2.5 mg daily and perindopril 4 mg daily	£32 + £133 = £164	£1 705 600	£11 644
Bendrofluazide 2.5 mg daily and lisinopril 10 mg daily	£15 + £20 = £35	£364 000	£2 485
Modified release dipyridamole added to aspirin	£118	£1 003 000	£10 738
Anticoagulants	£54[§]	£54 000	£756
Carotid endarterectomy	£4 350[¥]	£508 950	£126 150

*Effects on blood pressure and cholesterol of the two alternative regimens for blood pressure and cholesterol reduction shown are assumed to be approximately equivalent (section 16.3.3 and Table 16.6).

†Drug costs are given in UK £ sterling and taken from the *British National Formulary*, March 2007.[67] These are estimated drug costs only, and so are a minimum since we have not included the costs of administration, adverse effects, or monitoring.

‡Calculated using data on numbers of eligible patients given in Table 18.4.

¶Calculated using data on number-needed-to-treat given in Table 18.4.

§Allowing for any combination of 1, 3 and 5 mg tablets each day.

¥From Benade and Warlow, 2002,[75] with cost inflation to 2006 (Wardlaw *et al.*, 2006[76]). Only the costs of the endarterectomy procedure are given here, and costs of investigative workup are not included.

adverse effects and so on are not included. The cost of carotid endarterectomy (the procedure itself only) is taken from a recent UK-based prospective costing study and inflated to 2006.[75,76] Thus, these are only approximate, UK-specific estimates, but nonetheless they give a fairly good idea of the relative costs per stroke avoided of the various different interventions. Aspirin and warfarin appear by far the cheapest per stroke avoided, although the non-inclusion of monitoring and adverse effects costs will lead to a substantial exaggeration of the apparent cost-effectiveness of warfarin here. For blood pressure and cholesterol reduction, Table 18.5 also shows the rather dramatic effects of choosing one specific drug regimen rather than another of approximately equivalent efficacy. It is clear that the average cost of carotid endarterectomy per stroke avoided is high. Quite apart from its risks, this is a good reason to consider restricting carotid endarterectomy to those patients at highest risk without surgery (sections 16.11.6, 16.11.7 and 16.11.8).

18.5 Primary stroke prevention: targeted high-risk strategy or population-level 'mass' strategy?

A recent assessment of the global burden of disease attributable to 20 selected leading, potentially modifiable risk factors showed that, above certain theoretical minimum values, high blood pressure, high cholesterol, overweight, low fruit and vegetable intake, physical inactivity, smoking and alcohol consumption together account for over two-thirds of both disease burden (in terms of healthy life expectancy) and mortality due to stroke. Even higher proportions of disease burden and mortality from ischaemic heart disease could be explained by the same seven risk factors (Table 18.6).[77] The implication is that, if we were able to reduce the level of these risk factors to the theoretical minimum in the entire population, then we could substantially reduce the population-wide burden of stroke, ischaemic heart disease and several other major diseases. Even though the reduction of all of these risk factors to their theoretical minimum seems unlikely to be possible, there is clearly great potential for reducing the global burden of stroke and other vascular diseases by intervening to reduce known risks.

Public health epidemiologists generally agree that the strategies of identifying and treating those at highest risk in the population, as well as adopting population-wide strategies to reduce the average level of risk factors in the whole population (the third and fourth strategies outlined in section 18.1 above) are complementary, and that both will be necessary if we are to effectively reduce the burden of stroke and other vascular diseases through altering the known important risk factors.[78–80] However, debate continues about the relative acceptability, feasibility, effectiveness and cost-effectiveness of the two approaches.

Table 18.6 Contributions to global disease burden* and mortality due to stroke and ischaemic heart disease of seven major risk factors (data from Ezzati *et al.*, 2003[77]).

Risk factor	Theoretical minimum	Individual risk factor contributions to:†		Joint risk factor contributions to:‡			
		Stroke disease burden*	IHD disease burden*	Stroke disease burden*	Stroke mortality	IHD disease burden*	IHD mortality
High blood pressure	Systolic 115 mmHg	62%	49%	70–76%	65–73%	83–89%	78–85%
High cholesterol	3.8 mmol/L	18%	56%				
High BMI	21 kg/m²	13%	21%				
Low fruit and vegetable intake	600 g/day for adults	11%	31%				
Physical inactivity	2.5 hours per week of moderate-intensity activity	7%	22%				
Smoking	None	12%	12%				
Alcohol	None	4%	2%				

*Expressed in disability-adjusted life years (DALYs). BMI, body mass index; IHD, ischaemic heart disease.
†Per cent reduction in disease burden that would occur if exposure to risk factor reduced to theoretical minimum.
‡Per cent reduction in disease burden or mortality that would occur if exposure to all seven risk factors reduced to theoretical minimum.

> Seven potentially modifiable risk factors (high blood pressure, high cholesterol, overweight, low fruit and vegetable intake, physical inactivity, smoking and alcohol consumption) together account for over two-thirds of morbidity and mortality due to stroke and ischaemic heart disease.

18.5.1 The targeted high-risk strategy

Opportunistic identification or widespread systematic screening?

It seems intuitively appropriate to identify for specific risk-reducing interventions those individuals who have not yet had symptoms of vascular disease, but are at highest risk. However, it is not universally agreed whether such individuals should be identified through opportunistic identification and/or through widespread, systematic screening of apparently healthy people. The latter will depend both on a combination of an individual's interpretation of any symptoms, background knowledge, and healthcare-seeking behaviour, as well as on the quality, availability and accessibility of healthcare services, and the attitudes and behaviour of healthcare professionals. Both of these in turn will depend on cultural, geographic and socioeconomic factors.

Opportunistic identification of people considered to be at increased risk of vascular disease may occur because: they are being assessed medically for some other reason (e.g. identification of high blood pressure or asymptomatic diabetes when registering with a new family doctor, undergoing preoperative assessment prior to surgery, or having an occupational health check); they choose to attend a healthcare professional for a health check; or they develop or have a risk factor which can cause symptoms leading to their presentation to healthcare services (e.g. atrial fibrillation presenting with palpitations or breathlessness, diabetes presenting with thirst, polyuria and weight loss, and so on).

To justify a widespread systematic screening programme, there should be evidence that the screening procedure identifies people who genuinely have the risk factor or risk factors in question, that there is a possibility of intervening to reduce risk, that such intervention is of net benefit to individuals, that appropriate resources are available to provide the intervention, and that the whole screening programme (including, importantly, the costs of treating those identified) is cost-effective. The psychological, behavioural and quality-of-life impact of identifying, labelling and treating apparently healthy, previously asymptomatic people as being at high risk needs to be carefully considered and weighed against the potential benefits.[81] These considerations must surely become increasingly important as the level of risk or of a particular risk factor leading to identification, labelling and treatment is reduced.

> The targeted high-risk strategy for prevention of stroke (and other vascular diseases) requires the identification and treatment of those at high risk. The potential consequences of 'medicalizing' apparently healthy, asymptomatic people need to be weighed against any potential benefits of treatment.

Single risk factors vs risk scores to estimate overall absolute risk

A further crucial point is that identifying people on the basis of single risk factors will not reliably identify those at highest risk. It is combinations of risk factors that are important in determining overall risk. The concept that a large number of people at low and moderate risk may give rise to more cases of disease than a small number of people at high risk, described by the British epidemiologist Geoffrey Rose and illustrated in Fig. 18.6,[82] occurs particularly when single risk factors (or poorly predictive risk scores or models) are used to allocate people to low- or high-risk categories,[78,83] and also depends on the level of the risk factor (and so associated average risk at levels above and below it) above which risk is considered to be high. As an example, Table 18.7 shows the expected number of cases of stroke arising in a notional population of 10 000 men aged 40–49 over a 24-year period for different levels of systolic blood pressure.[84] Over half of all the strokes occur in the 72% of men with systolic blood pressures between 120 and 159 mmHg. If the level for high blood pressure and high risk is set at 180 mmHg, then only 22% of cases of stroke arise in those at high risk as defined by blood pressure. But, if high blood pressure is considered to be > 140 mmHg, then over two-thirds (68%) of stroke cases arise in those at high risk.

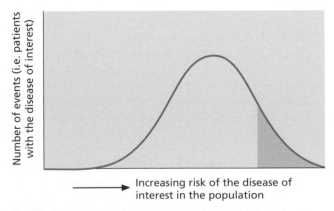

Fig. 18.6 Most cases of a disease occur in people at moderate risk; rather few (*shaded*) occur in people at the very highest risk in the right-hand tail of a normal distribution.

Systolic blood pressure (mmHg)	Prevalence (%)	Incidence of stroke per 100 men during 24 years follow-up	Expected number of cases of stroke occurring over 24 years in a population of 10 000 men aged 40–49 at baseline (% of total)*
< 120	16	1.7	27 (4.7)
120–139	43	3.6	155 (27)
140–159	29	5.6	162 (28.3)
160–179	8	12.8	102 (17.8)
180+	4	31.8	127 (22.2)
Total	100		573 (100)

*Calculated by multiplying column 2 by column 3.

Table 18.7 Systolic blood pressure and the risk of stroke in men aged 40–49 years. The prevalence of various levels of blood pressure and the incidence and expected number of cases of stroke arising in each blood pressure stratum over 24 years, using Framingham Study data (from Table 2.3 in Ebrahim and Harwood, 1999[84]).

Specific levels of risk factors (e.g. of blood pressure and cholesterol) are of little clinical relevance when considered in isolation from a person's overall estimated risk of future vascular disease. For practically any risk factor that can be measured as a continuous variable (blood pressure and cholesterol are good examples), risk of vascular disease increases continuously with increase in the level of the risk factor within the range of values observed in most populations (section 6.6.3), so the notion that some people have or do not have, say, hypertension or hypercholesterolaemia is an artificial one based on arbitrary cut-off values.[85] Indeed, since an individual's absolute risk of a future vascular event is determined by the combined effect of all vascular risk factors present, differences in risk can vary more than 20-fold in patients with the same blood pressure or cholesterol levels.[86] Figure 18.7 shows how risk of future vascular disease is increased by successively adding risk factors in individuals with different systolic blood pressure (Fig. 18.7a) or blood cholesterol concentration (Fig. 18.7b), and how someone with a blood pressure or cholesterol concentration at the lower end of the spectrum and several other risk factors may have a higher overall risk than someone with a much higher blood pressure or cholesterol concentration but no other risk factors.[86]

There is now increasing evidence from observational studies and randomized trials, in particular of blood pressure and cholesterol lowering, both in primary and secondary prevention settings, that we should be thinking less in terms of reducing levels of these risk factors down to specific targets in individuals whose risk factor level is above a particular arbitrary cut-off value (these are still the focus of many treatment guidelines), but more in terms of reducing these risk factors as much as possible (at least down to the lower end of the ranges studied in the trials and observational studies) in those at highest absolute risk of future vascular events.[85,87,88] Both observational and randomized trial data suggest that the greater the absolute amount by which either blood pressure or

cholesterol are lowered, the greater the relative benefit on clinically meaningful outcomes (sections 16.3 and 16.4).[85]

Several risk prediction scores, based on models derived from population-based cohort studies (mainly the Framingham cohort study) in which risk factors were measured and subjects followed up over many years for the subsequent occurrence of vascular events, are now widely available for estimating individual risk, mainly in primary care settings. These scores are presented for use as paper or hand-held calculator-based equations, colour charts, or online calculators, and allow clinicians to integrate information on a number of different recognized risk factors (including age, gender, blood pressure, cholesterol, atrial fibrillation, diabetes, obesity, smoking and family history) to estimate an individual's risk of various vascular events over the next 5–10 years.[86,89] Integrated risk factor scoring systems such as these seem intuitively likely to be useful, certainly better than single risk factor identification methods, and they are increasingly used in risk factor treatment guidelines and in primary care settings, but they are not without their limitations:

- The currently available scores tend to be focused on ischaemic heart disease, although a few either include stroke or are specific for stroke[86,89] (see http://www.bhsoc.org/Cardiovascular_Risk_Charts_and_Calculators.stm, http://www.riskscore.org.uk/). In patients without a history of a vascular event, those that estimate together the combined risk of all potentially important future vascular events (including stroke as well as ischaemic heart disease) are likely to be the most helpful in identifying people at the highest overall vascular risk.
- The predictive accuracy of the existing risk scores is suboptimal. Validation studies of Framingham-based risk scores suggest that vascular risk in low-risk populations is likely to be overestimated, potentially resulting in unnecessary treatment of many people, while that in high-risk populations is likely to be underestimated.[89]

Fig. 18.7 Absolute risk of cardiovascular disease (CVD) over 5 years by (a) systolic blood pressure (SBP) and (b) blood total cholesterol (TC) at specific levels of other risk factors, added consecutively. (Reprinted from Jackson *et al. Lancet*[86] © 2005 with permission from Elsevier.) (a) Reference category is a non-diabetic, non-smoker female aged 50 with total cholesterol of 4.0 mmol/L and HDL of 1.6 mmol/L. In each category, risks are given for systolic blood pressure levels of 110, 120, 130, 140, 150, 160, 170 and 180 mmHg (each level represented by a different shade), and additional risk factors going from left to right are added consecutively (e.g. the diabetes category represents a diabetic, 50-year-old male cigarette smoker with a total cholesterol of 7 mmol/L and HDL of 1 mmol/L). TC total cholesterol.
(b) Reference category is a non-diabetic, non-smoker female aged 50 with systolic blood pressure of 110 mmHg and HDL of 1.6 mmol/L. In each category, risks are given for cholesterol concentrations of 4.0, 4.5, 5.0, 5.5, 6.0, 6.5, 7.0, 7.5 and 8.0 mmol/L (each level represented by a different shade) and additional risk factors going from left to right are added consecutively (e.g. the HDL = 1 mmol/L category represents a 50-year-old, non-diabetic, female cigarette smoker with systolic BP 170 mmHg and HDL of 1 mmol/L).

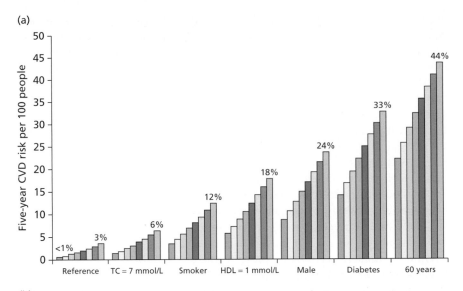

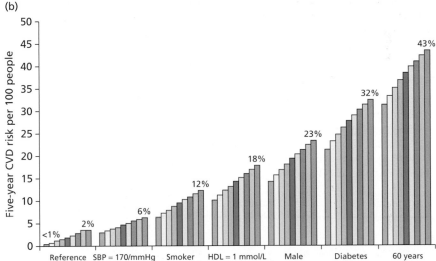

The vascular risk scores may perform particularly poorly in populations with different risk factor patterns or different average levels of risk (for example Africans or Asians) from the predominantly white populations in which they were developed.[86,89,90] In general, risk prediction scores should be developed in populations with reasonably similar risk profiles and event rates to those to which they are to be applied, or at the very least should be calibrated to fit the target population.[86,90,91] The scores may also be further refined and improved by incorporating additional, newer risk factors such as the level of C-reactive protein.[86] However, it has been argued that refining risk prediction any further with measurement and incorporation of other risk factors may not justify the additional complexity and cost.[85,92]

- There is no strong evidence from randomized trials that assigning cardiovascular risk on the basis of a risk prediction score improves outcomes in primary prevention settings. However, very few such trials have been done and they were generally rather small.[89]

> Properly validated risk scores using combinations of risk factors predict risk of stroke and other vascular diseases more accurately then single risk factors.

18.5.2 Potential impact of the targeted high-risk strategy

Assuming it is considered acceptable and feasible to identify asymptomatic people at high risk of stroke and other vascular events, what interventions could be used to reduce their future risk and what might the impact be?

Lowering blood pressure and cholesterol

Drugs to reduce blood pressure and cholesterol have been considered in several recent modelling exercises to assess the potential impact of the targeted high-risk strategy on the occurrence at population level of stroke and other vascular events combined.[79,80] There is good evidence that reductions in blood pressure and blood cholesterol levels (regardless of the baseline level) decrease risk of stroke and other vascular events across the spectrum of risk, in both primary and secondary prevention settings. The largest reductions both in levels of these risk factors and in the vascular diseases associated with them are produced by drugs (as opposed to non-pharmacological interventions) (sections 16.3 and 16.4), which could therefore be considered appropriate for people at high risk, in whom any serious adverse effects are likely to be rare compared with absolute reductions in vascular events.

The potential effects of blood pressure and cholesterol lowering in high-risk individuals, identified either by a single risk factor-based threshold, or by estimating absolute risk using combinations of risk factors, are shown for one particular model in Table 18.8. This model considers the impact of interventions for individuals identified as being at high risk from a population of middle-aged men in the UK without vascular disease at baseline followed up for 10 years. The outcome assessed is the combination of fatal or non-fatal myocardial infarction and stroke ('major cardiovascular events'),

and the model assumes that the relative risk of this outcome could be reduced by 30% and 22% by cholesterol lowering with a statin and blood-pressure-lowering medication respectively.[80] Greater relative risk reductions could be achieved by combining cholesterol and blood-pressure-lowering drugs, perhaps also with other risk-lowering interventions, and in this model the effects of a combined intervention (consisting of a statin, several different blood-pressure-lowering drugs and aspirin), assumed to achieve a relative risk reduction of 68%, were also assessed. Since there are uncertainties about the net effects of the aspirin component of this particular combination (see below and section 16.5.1), we refer to this in Table 18.8 simply as a notional 'combined intervention' and use it only to illustrate what the impact on vascular disease in the population might be of combining interventions to achieve a relative risk reduction of this size.

Two clear patterns emerge from the data shown in Table 18.8. First, the proportion of strokes and myocardial infarctions avoided in the population increases as the proportion of individuals treated increases (so including more and more people in the mid-range of the risk distribution). This is true for either the single risk factor or combined risk factor threshold-setting methods. Second, the larger the relative risk reduction achieved by

Table 18.8 Potential impact on incidence of fatal or non-fatal myocardial infarction or stroke of treating individuals identified to be at high risk with drugs to reduce blood pressure and/or cholesterol (adapted from Emberson *et al.*, 2004[80]).*

Criterion for treatment	Treatment	Relative risk reduction in fatal or non-fatal myocardial infarction or stroke	Predicted % reduction in incidence of fatal or non-fatal myocardial infarction or stroke		
Single risk factor approach			*Treat top 10%*	*Treat top 20%*	*Treat top 30%*
Cholesterol level	Statin	30%	6%	9%	12%
Systolic BP	BP lowering drugs(s)	22%	6%	8%	10%
Cholesterol level	Combined intervention†	68%	13%	21%	28%
Systolic BP	Combined intervention†	68%	18%	25%	31%
Combined risk factor estimated absolute risk approach			*Treat at ≥*	*Treat at ≥*	*Treat at ≥*
(Framingham 10-year coronary heart disease risk)			*30% risk*	*20% risk‡*	*15% risk§*
	Statin	30%	5%	15%	21%
	BP lowering drugs(s)	22%	4%	11%	16%
	Combined intervention†	68%	11%	34%	49%

*Population for this model: 5997 middle-aged men in the British Regional Heart Survey with no history of stroke or coronary heart disease and not taking drugs to reduce blood pressure or cholesterol at baseline, followed for 10 years. Four hundred and fifty men had a major cardiovascular disease event during follow-up.
†See text.
‡Would mean treating one-quarter of the population.
§Would mean treating half of the population.
BP, blood pressure.

the intervention, the larger the predicted percentage reduction in strokes and myocardial infarctions. However, although the numbers of these events could be almost halved by a combined intervention reducing relative risk by 68% given to all those with an estimated 10-year coronary heart disease risk of ≥ 15%, this would entail treating half of the total population with multiple preventive treatments.[80] This would be both expensive and probably unacceptable in most populations. In addition, the model optimistically assumes that drug prescription and adherence rates for those identified as being at high risk are as high as those observed in the relevant randomized trials, but these would be highly unlikely to be achieved if this strategy were to be applied in a real population.

Aspirin

One proposed combined intervention (the so-called Polypill) for the targeted high-risk strategy included aspirin and folic acid with cholesterol and blood-pressure-lowering medication. Estimating the effects of the Polypill using data from randomized trials and observational studies demonstrated that it could reduce the relative risks of myocardial infarction and stroke by 88% and 80% respectively.[92] Others have proposed including aspirin with cholesterol and blood-pressure-lowering medication in suggested combined interventions.[79,80] But the benefits of aspirin in all of these cases were based on the assumption that the relative reductions in vascular events are similar at all levels of baseline risk and can be extrapolated from randomized trials among patients with a history of symptomatic vascular disease.[79,80,92] However, this does not seem to be the case, since the relative reduction in vascular events produced by aspirin is smaller in those without than in those with a history of vascular disease, and the absolute risks and benefits appear to be much more finely balanced (section 16.5.1). In our view, therefore, further evidence on the balance of benefits and risks of aspirin in different types of individuals in primary prevention settings is needed before its use in such settings can be recommended.

Folic acid supplementation

Furthermore, although observational studies would suggest that folic acid supplementation to reduce serum homocysteine levels may be an appropriate strategy for primary and secondary prevention, in neither setting is there sufficient evidence from randomized trials to support its use, although further evidence will emerge in due course from ongoing trials (section 16.8.1).

Lifestyle modification

Targeted advice to avoid smoking and excess alcohol, eat a healthy diet and take regular exercise (section 16.7) all seem likely to increase the benefit from a notional combined intervention (see above) that might be used in individuals identified to be at high risk. This sort of intervention would be generally acceptable, and the costs would be small if these people were in any case being identified for drug treatment.

Antithrombotic drugs for people with atrial fibrillation

There is good evidence from randomized trials for the use of antithrombotic drugs (either anticoagulants or aspirin, depending on the absolute risks of stroke, bleeding risks, and contraindications to anticoagulants) in people with atrial fibrillation, with similar relative effects on stroke in both primary and secondary prevention populations (section 16.6.2 and Fig. 16.30). Table 18.9 gives a very rough idea of the numbers and proportion of all strokes occurring in a notional European population of 1 million people that could be avoided by giving antithrombotic treatment to people with atrial fibrillation and no history of prior stroke or transient ischaemic attack in the general population. We assume that a reliable means exists of identifying these people, with estimates of treatment effects taken from the relevant randomized trials and systematic reviews (Table 16.9). The simple model shown suggests that about 7% of all strokes occurring in the population could be avoided. A more sophisticated model would take account of variation in prevalence of atrial fibrillation with age (about 2.3% in those over 40 years, and 6–7% in those over 65 years),[93,94] and could also use information on age structure and the distributions of other risk factors (such as diabetes and blood pressure) in the population to estimate the numbers of people with atrial fibrillation in the low, moderate and high-risk strata (shown in Tables 16.8 and 16.9) and to assign and estimate effects of the ideal antithrombotic treatment (warfarin or aspirin). This would make the model more accurate, but much more complex and difficult both to produce and to understand.

Carotid endarterectomy for people with asymptomatic carotid stenosis

Randomized trials also suggest that subsequent strokes are reduced in people with asymptomatic carotid stenosis who undergo carotid endarterectomy. However, the unoperated annual risk of stroke in such people is very low (about 2% on average), the absolute reduction in

Table 18.9 The estimated effect of antithrombotic treatment among patients with atrial fibrillation (AF) on strokes occurring in a notional European population of 1 million people.

Age (years)	Number in population*	% with AF†	Number with AF	Average annual untreated risk of stroke for all in AF‡	Number (%) treated with anticoagulants§	Number of strokes avoided annually by treatment with anticoagulants¶	Number (%) treated with aspirin§	Number of strokes avoided annually by treatment with aspirin¥	Number of strokes avoided annually by antithrombotic treatment	% of all 2260 strokes avoided each year in population of 1 million$
> 40	430 000	2.3%	9890	4%	9890 (50%)	119	3956 (40%)	32	151	151 (7%)

*Estimated by applying Segi's standard European population structure to population of 1 million.
†From Feinberg *et al.*, 1995.[93]
‡Approximate average from low, medium and high-risk strata from Tables 16.8 and 16.9.
§Assuming 50% of all those in AF eligible and willing to take warfarin, 10% have contraindication to any antithrombotic treatment and 40% take aspirin.
¶Assuming warfarin produces relative reduction in stroke risk of 60% (Table 16.9).
¥Assuming aspirin produces relative reduction in stroke risk of 20% (Table 16.9).
$From Table 18.1.

stroke risk estimated by the randomized trials was only about 1% per year, and the small net benefit observed took several years to become apparent because of the upfront risk of surgery. In addition, the average surgical risk of stroke or death in the trials was almost certainly lower than in routine clinical practice, so in the real world the balance of benefits and risks might be less favourable than in the trials. It is not yet clear for which subgroups the unoperated risk is high enough and the surgical risk low enough for surgery to be clearly beneficial (section 16.12).

Moreover, because the population prevalence of asymptomatic carotid stenosis severe enough to warrant consideration for surgery is low (about 1% in those aged 50–59 years rising to about 10% in those aged over 80 years, at least in predominantly white populations in high-income countries),[95–98] and no non-invasive screening test is perfect, screening is likely to identify far more false-positive than true-positive stenoses, which could actually lead to more harm than good if inappropriate surgery followed.[99,100]

At present, therefore, routine carotid endarterectomy for asymptomatic carotid stenosis cannot be justified and calls for widespread carotid artery screening go beyond the evidence currently available.

> Substantial reductions in the incidence of stroke and other vascular diseases are only likely to be achievable with the 'targeted' high-risk approach if multiple interventions (including drugs) to reduce risk factors are used widely in a large proportion of the population.

18.5.3 The mass population strategy

In recent years epidemiologists have begun to calculate what the effect might be of not just truncating the right-hand tail of the risk distribution (Fig. 18.6) by treating the high-risk individuals, but of shifting the entire distribution slightly to the left (the 'mass' prevention strategy) (Fig. 18.8). This would not only reduce the mean value of a continuously varying risk factor (such as blood pressure or plasma cholesterol level) but also the number of patients at particularly high risk who are labelled as 'diseased' and so requiring treatment. But what matters just as much if not more, is not the few events prevented by reducing the small number of high-risk individuals, but the greater number of events avoided in the much larger number of people at moderate risk. A small left shift in the distribution of multiple risk factors might be achievable by a 'mass' public health

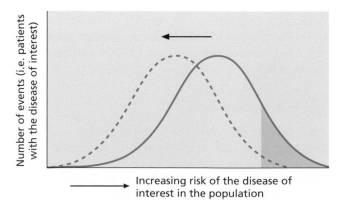

Fig. 18.8 The 'mass' strategy of disease prevention involves a small left shift in the risk distribution.

strategy, usually involving relatively risk-free lifestyle changes, aimed at the *whole* population where everyone reduces their risk by just a little bit: a slightly lower blood pressure and cholesterol in everyone as well as fewer with very high blood pressure or cholesterol levels, fewer cigarettes smoked by all smokers as well as more quitters, somewhat more exercise all round as well as fewer couch potatoes and more marathon runners, a little less alcohol for all as well as fewer alcoholics, a touch of weight reduction for all as well as fewer morbidly obese.

The types of interventions that are applicable at the population level might include, for example:

- public health campaigns and legislation to reduce dietary salt intake (and so reduce the mean population blood pressure)[79] and promote other aspects of a healthy diet, helping to reduce the mean population weight, mean cholesterol level and prevalence of diabetes (section 16.7);
- legislation to prevent smoking in public places, so discouraging smokers and reducing exposure to passive smoking;
- encouraging more exercise through promotional campaigns and provision of cycle tracks, attractive sports facilities, and so on.

All these interventions depend on education, reduction in poverty, peer pressure, role models, advertising, the media and political action and very little on action at the individual doctor level. Moreover, the political will must come not just from government health departments, but also (and perhaps more importantly) from departments of finance, education, housing, welfare, agriculture, transport, the environment, and so on – that is, from across the whole of government. It is certainly not the case that any improvement or deterioration in

public health is inevitably to do with the Department of Health. These interventions are no more invasive or prescriptive than providing a clean water supply or mass immunization, both of which are clearly in the domain of public health services. But, one has to accept the 'prevention paradox' that a preventive strategy that brings large benefits to the community offers little to each participating individual.[82]

> The mass strategy for prevention of stroke and other vascular diseases requires a small leftward shift in the entire distribution of relevant risk factors such as blood pressure. This may have a surprisingly large impact on the incidence of stroke and other vascular diseases although each individual will gain very little.

18.5.4 Potential impact of the mass population strategy compared with the targeted high-risk strategy

The mass population strategy cannot be evaluated by a randomized controlled trial, not because the outcome is unmeasurable or because the sample size would have to be too big or it would take too long to demonstrate an effect, but because the strategy requires everybody to be 'treated' and it would simply be impracticable to apply the 'treatment' to a random 50% of the population. But the effects and costs can be estimated using more or less sophisticated modelling techniques, and this allows theoretical comparisons to be made with the targeted high-risk strategy.

For example, reducing the population mean systolic blood pressure by just 1–2% could reduce the incidence of stroke by about 16% (Table 18.10).[84] Such blood pressure

Table 18.10 The estimated effect on stroke incidence of a reduction in the population mean systolic blood pressure by 1 to 2% in men aged 40–49 years, using Framingham Study data (from Table 2.5 in Ebrahim and Harwood, 1999[84]).

Systolic blood pressure (mm Hg)	Prevalence (%)		Incidence of stroke per 100 men during 24-year follow-up	Expected number of cases of stroke occurring over 24 years in a population of 10 000 men aged 40–49 at baseline	
	Before blood pressure reduction	After blood pressure reduction		Before blood pressure reduction	After blood pressure reduction
< 120	16	23	1.7	27	39
120–139	43	43	3.6	155	155
140–159	29	26	5.6	162	146
160–179	8	6	12.8	102	77
> 180	4	2	31.8	127	64
Total	100			573	481

i.e. a proportional reduction of (573–481)/573 = 16% in stroke numbers (and incidence).

reductions should be achievable through legislation leading to population-wide reductions in salt intake of around 15%,[79] and indeed substantially larger reductions in mean population blood pressure may be possible.[80]

Modelling exercises to compare the potential effects on the burden of stroke and vascular disease of the targeted high-risk and mass population strategies depend on the assumptions made about the effects of various interventions, the age, sex and risk factor profile of the population, and the thresholds set for intervention in the targeted high-risk strategy. Calculating and comparing cost-effectiveness involves further assumptions about the costs of these interventions. A complex – but elegant and informative – global analysis of the reduction in morbidity and mortality from ischaemic heart disease and stroke (expressed as disability-adjusted life years) for 14 World Health Organization epidemiological subregions of the world assessed and compared the effects and cost-effectiveness of various population-level (mass population strategy) and individual (targeted high-risk strategy) health interventions aimed at reducing the risks associated with raised cholesterol and blood pressure.[79] The effect sizes of the various interventions were based on systematic reviews and meta-analyses of randomized trials and observational studies. The population-level interventions assessed were:

- voluntary agreements or legislation on salt content to ensure labelling and stepwise decreases in salt content of processed foods (assumed to achieve reductions in dietary salt content of 15–30% and in blood pressure of 1–5% depending on age, sex and world subregion);
- health education through the mass media (focusing on cholesterol concentration and body mass index and assumed to achieve a 2% reduction in blood cholesterol concentrations);
- and a combination of these.

The individual health interventions assessed were drugs to reduce blood pressure and cholesterol, and a combination of these with aspirin, similar to those assessed by others and described above (section 18.5.2) and shown in Table 18.8. For the individual health interventions (targeted high-risk strategy), different cholesterol and blood pressure threshold levels as well as various different absolute risk thresholds were evaluated. Combinations of the targeted high-risk and mass population strategies were also assessed.[79]

The results of this modelling exercise for one of the European subregions are shown graphically in Fig. 18.9. Unsurprisingly, the cost-effectiveness (i.e. the cost per DALY averted) was lowest for the population mass strategy interventions. However, perhaps rather counter-intuitively, the potential to reduce the burden of disease was larger for the targeted high-risk approaches, albeit at

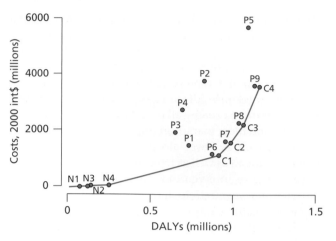

Fig. 18.9 Yearly costs (2000 int$ = international dollars, base year 2000 – vertical axis) and effectiveness (DALYs, disability-adjusted life years averted – horizontal axis) of various interventions to reduce the burden of stroke and ischaemic heart disease in the World Health Organization EurA subregion of Europe. (From Murray *et al.*, 2003.[79])

Interventions N1 to N4 are population-level interventions to reduce salt intake through voluntary agreements with industry (N1) or legislation (N2), health education through the mass media focusing on cholesterol concentrations and body mass index (N3) and a combination of N2 and N3 (N4).

Interventions P1 to P9 are individual interventions based on drugs to lower blood pressure at systolic blood pressure thresholds of 160 or 140 mmHg (P1 and P2), drugs to reduce cholesterol concentration thresholds of 6.2 and 5.7 mmol/L (P3 and P4), a combination of P2 and P3 (P5), and a combined drug treatment strategy (statin, diuretic, beta-blocker and aspirin) based on thresholds of absolute 10-year risk of ischaemic heart disease or stroke of 35% (P6), 25% (P7), 15% (P8) and 5% (P9).

Interventions C1 to C4 are combined population and individual interventions (combination of N4 with P6 to P9).

The slope of the line connecting the origin to each point is the cost per DALY averted. The steeper the slope, the more expensive the intervention is per DALY averted (less cost-effective). The solid lines join the least expensive interventions for increasing effectiveness in terms of DALYs averted and show the best sequential choices of interventions to be made with increasing resources. Costs are reported in international dollars, a hypothetical currency where one dollar has the same purchasing power as one US dollar regardless of location.

a higher cost per DALY averted. This may relate – at least in part – to the effect size estimates. The population level effect sizes were assumed to be rather modest (which may be realistic) while the effects of cholesterol and blood pressure lowering were assumed to be the same as those achieved in randomized trials of cholesterol and blood-pressure-lowering drugs (which, given doubts about acceptability and adherence, is probably not realistic). However, moving between different world subregions and varying the range of values used for effects and costs in an uncertainty analysis did not change the general pattern of the results. This modelling exercise suggests that, in parts of the world where resources are scarce, public health policy should focus on investing in the mass population strategies first, with additional resources used for individually targeted combination interventions for high-risk individuals on the basis of estimated absolute risk of vascular disease, shifting the threshold for intervention to lower levels of risk as more resources become available.[79]

Additional interventions not included in the modelling exercise above could of course enhance the mass population strategy. For example, small reductions in smoking population-wide could have a surprising impact on stroke burden and cost, as well as on other vascular diseases and a host of other common smoking-related diseases.[101,102]

A further argument in favour of the mass population strategy is that it focuses on the determinants of risk factor distributions rather than simply the treatment of risk factors. Population approaches may be more likely to reduce the development of vascular disease, while a high-risk strategy without priority given to population approaches would ensure a steady supply of middle-aged people requiring drug treatment.[80]

> Common sense as well as modelling exercises suggest that the mass population strategy is almost certainly more cost-effective than the targeted high-risk approach. A combination of both probably achieves the best population health for the available resources.

Are there any risks of the mass population strategy?

Because moving the distribution of a risk factor to the left may increase the number of individuals at very low risk of the disease in question, one would need to be reasonably confident that these same individuals or society in general would not be systematically disadvantaged in some way, for example by an increased risk of depression or fatigue at very low blood pressures,[103] of intracranial haemorrhage at very low cholesterol levels (section 6.6.6) or of hypothermia in the very thin and elderly. For the most part, however, the risk factor levels below which significant problems might possibly arise are beyond the values likely to be reached by risk factor reductions, certainly in societies adopting 'western' lifestyles.[85]

Because being simple goes against the grain of societies which believe in a quick technological or mystical fix for illness, or which may crave short-term results in the marketplace, and in societies which exalt the individual over the community, the mass population prevention strategy may be very difficult to implement. However,

the argument in favour of this strategy for not just stroke prevention, but for health promotion and the prevention of disease in general, is persuasive, if not compelling.[82]

18.6 Goals, strategies and measuring success (or failure)

Setting targets or goals in any human endeavour is surely reasonable provided they are not so easily achieved that no effort is required, nor so difficult that demoralization sets in. This certainly applies to stroke rehabilitation (section 10.3.3) and could be applied to reducing the burden of stroke and other vascular diseases in the whole community. The difficulty is deciding which target to select. It has to be at the level of the whole community, or a random sample of it, to avoid selection bias; it has to be simple so that it is measurable in very large numbers of people at reasonable cost; it has to be robust so that it can be measured reliably at various points in time; it must be valid and so measure something meaningful; and it almost certainly has to be measurable in routine practice to ensure complete coverage for the foreseeable future. At present, the *only* measure which comes anywhere near fulfilling these criteria is stroke mortality, despite its imperfections (section 18.2). However, one can reasonably hope, and even expect, that an intervention which reduces stroke incidence and disability would also have *some* impact on stroke mortality, although this impact could well be attenuated by the fact that not all types of stroke are fatal, mortality statistics are inaccurate, and so on.

> At present, mortality statistics are, despite their imperfections, the only routinely available method to measure the success or failure of stroke prevention programmes.

In the meantime it is surely important to develop some routine method of measuring stroke incidence, as well as of outcome and survival, at the level of the whole community, not just in hospitalized patients. This must be practicable, and inexpensive, which will be difficult and take time to achieve. At the very least, one might think that routine measurement of stroke outcome is required to inform healthcare decisions, for how else can one system or provider of care be compared with another? But maybe even this is too fraught with difficulties to be useful, and measuring process of care is probably more meaningful (section 17.12.2).

As to which stroke prevention strategy to choose, it seems sensible to pursue all of them while accepting that each one on its own is unlikely to have a dramatic effect. It would be impossible to deny an effective treatment to an individual if the benefits outweighed the risks, and the cost was acceptable, either to the individual or to a third-party payer. It would be inconceivable not to continue to search for and evaluate treatments for acute stroke. And it would be unforgivable to ignore the theoretical attractions of the 'mass' strategy for stroke prevention.

Finally, almost any strategy for stroke prevention must be intimately linked with almost any strategy for the prevention of other vascular diseases (mainly coronary heart disease and peripheral vascular disease), because they are largely caused by the same underlying degenerative vascular disorders. So, stroke prevention should not be considered in isolation, but as part of a general strategy for the prevention of all forms of vascular disease, including stroke.

> Stroke prevention must not be seen in isolation, but as part of a programme to prevent the clinical manifestations of all forms of degenerative vascular disease.

References

1 Warlow CP. Epidemiology of stroke. *Lancet* 1998; **352** Suppl 3:SIII1–SIII4.

2 Rothwell PM. The high cost of not funding stroke research: a comparison with heart disease and cancer. *Lancet* 2001; **357**(9268):1612–16.

3 Lopez AD, Mathers CD, Ezzati M, Jamison DT, Murray CJ. Global and regional burden of disease and risk factors, 2001: systematic analysis of population health data. *Lancet* 2006; **367**(9524):1747–57.

4 Martin J, Meltzer H, Elliot D. *The Prevalence of Disability Among Adults*. London: HMSO, 1988.

5 Giroud M, Lemesle M, Quantin C, Vourch M, Becker F, Milan C *et al*. A hospital-based and a population-based stroke registry yield different results: the experience in Dijon, France. *Neuroepidemiology* 1997; **16**(1):15–21.

6 Di Carlo A, Candelise L, Gandolfo C, Grigoletto F, Volonnino G, Baldereschi M *et al*. Influence of different screening procedures on the stroke prevalence estimates: the Italian Longitudinal Study on Aging. *Cerebrovasc Dis* 1999; **9**(4):231–7.

7 Levi F, Lucchini F, Negri E, La Vecchia C. Trends in mortality from cardiovascular and cerebrovascular diseases in Europe and other areas of the world. *Heart* 2002; **88**(2):119–24.

8 Sarti C, Rastenyte D, Cepaitis Z, Tuomilehto J. International trends in mortality from stroke, 1968 to 1994. *Stroke* 2000; **31**(7):1588–601.

9 Lawlor DA, Smith GD, Leon DA, Sterne JA, Ebrahim S. Secular trends in mortality by stroke subtype in the 20th century: a retrospective analysis. *Lancet* 2002; **360**(9348):1818–23.

10 Halkes PH, van Gijn J, Kappelle LJ, Koudstaal PJ, Algra A. Classification of cause of death after stroke in clinical research. *Stroke* 2006; **37**(6):1521–4.

11 Corwin LE, Wolf PA, Kannel WB, McNamara PM. Accuracy of death certification of stroke: the Framingham Study. *Stroke* 1982; **13**(6):818–21.

12 Hasuo Y, Ueda K, Kiyohara Y, Wada J, Kawano H, Kato I *et al*. Accuracy of diagnosis on death certificates for underlying causes of death in a long-term autopsy-based population study in Hisayama, Japan; with special reference to cardiovascular diseases. *J Clin Epidemiol* 1989; **42**(6):577–84.

13 Iso H, Jacobs DR, Jr, Goldman L. Accuracy of death certificate diagnosis of intracranial hemorrhage and nonhemorrhagic stroke. The Minnesota Heart Survey. *Am J Epidemiol* 1990; **132**(5):993–8.

14 Netsky MG, Miyaji T. Prevalence of cerebral hemorrhage and thrombosis in Japan: study of the major causes of death. *J Chronic Dis* 1976; **29**(11):711–21.

15 Phillips LH, Whisnant JP, Reagan TJ. Sudden death from stroke. *Stroke* 1977; **8**(3):392–5.

16 Thomas AC, Knapman PA, Krikler DM, Davies MJ. Community study of the causes of 'natural' sudden death. *Br Med J* 1988; **297**(6661):1453–6.

17 Bonita R, Beaglehole R. Explaining stroke mortality trends. *Lancet* 1993; **341**(8859):1510–11.

18 Lanska DJ. Decline in autopsies for deaths attributed to cerebrovascular disease. *Stroke* 1993; **24**(1):71–5.

19 Roulson J, Benbow EW, Hasleton PS. Discrepancies between clinical and autopsy diagnosis and the value of post mortem histology; a meta-analysis and review. *Histopathology* 2005; **47**(6):551–9.

20 Hatano S. Experience from a multicentre stroke register: a preliminary report. *Bull World Health Organ* 1976; **54**(5):541–53.

21 Chandramohan D, Maude GH, Rodrigues LC, Hayes RJ. Verbal autopsies for adult deaths: issues in their development and validation. *Int J Epidemiol* 1994; **23**(2):213–22.

22 Kaufman JS, Asuzu MC, Rotimi CN, Johnson OO, Owoaje EE, Cooper RS. The absence of adult mortality data for sub-Saharan Africa: a practical solution. *Bull World Health Organ* 1997; **75**(5):389–95.

23 Walker RW, McLarty DG, Kitange HM, Whiting D, Masuki G, Mtasiwa DM *et al*. Stroke mortality in urban and rural Tanzania. Adult Morbidity and Mortality Project. *Lancet* 2000; **355**(9216):1684–7.

24 Connor MD, Walker R, Modi G, Warlow CP. Burden of stroke in black populations in sub-Saharan Africa. *Lancet Neurol* 2007; **6**(3):269–78.

25 Bonneux L, Looman CW, Barendregt JJ, Van der Maas PJ. Regression analysis of recent changes in cardiovascular morbidity and mortality in The Netherlands. *Br Med J* 1997; **314**(7083):789–92.

26 Feigin VL, Lawes CM, Bennett DA, Anderson CS. Stroke epidemiology: a review of population-based studies of incidence, prevalence, and case-fatality in the late 20th century. *Lancet Neurol* 2003; **2**(1):43–53.

27 Sarti C, Stegmayr B, Tolonen H, Mahonen M, Tuomilehto J, Asplund K. Are changes in mortality from stroke caused by changes in stroke event rates or case fatality? Results from the WHO MONICA Project. *Stroke* 2003; **34**(8):1833–40.

28 Terent A. Trends in stroke incidence and 10-year survival in Soderhamn, Sweden, 1975–2001. *Stroke* 2003; **34**(6):1353–8.

29 Pessah-Rasmussen H, Engstrom G, Jerntorp I, Janzon L. Increasing stroke incidence and decreasing case fatality, 1989–1998: a study from the stroke register in Malmo, Sweden. *Stroke* 2003; **34**(4):913–18.

30 Rothwell PM, Coull AJ, Giles MF, Howard SC, Silver LE, Bull LM *et al*. Change in stroke incidence, mortality, case-fatality, severity, and risk factors in Oxfordshire, UK from 1981 to 2004 (Oxford Vascular Study). *Lancet* 2004; **363**(9425):1925–33.

31 Rudd AG, Hoffman A, Irwin P, Lowe D, Pearson MG. Stroke unit care and outcome: results from the 2001 National Sentinel Audit of Stroke (England, Wales, and Northern Ireland). *Stroke* 2005; **36**(1):103–6.

32 Sudlow CL, Warlow CP. Comparable studies of the incidence of stroke and its pathological types: results from an international collaboration. International Stroke Incidence Collaboration. *Stroke* 1997; **28**(3):491–9.

33 Appelros P, Nydevik I, Seiger A, Terent A. High incidence rates of stroke in Orebro, Sweden: Further support for regional incidence differences within Scandinavia. *Cerebrovasc Dis* 2002; **14**(3–4):161–8.

34 Di Carlo A, Inzitari D, Galati F, Baldereschi M, Giunta V, Grillo G *et al*. A prospective community-based study of stroke in Southern Italy: the Vibo Valentia incidence of stroke study (VISS). Methodology, incidence and case fatality at 28 days, 3 and 12 months. *Cerebrovasc Dis* 2003; **16**(4):410–17.

35 Correia M, Silva MR, Matos I, Magalhaes R, Lopes JC, Ferro JM *et al*. Prospective community-based study of stroke in Northern Portugal: incidence and case fatality in rural and urban populations. *Stroke* 2004; **35**(9):2048–53.

36 Corbin DO, Poddar V, Hennis A, Gaskin A, Rambarat C, Wilks R *et al*. Incidence and case fatality rates of first-ever stroke in a black Caribbean population: the Barbados Register of Strokes. *Stroke* 2004; **35**(6):1254–8.

37 Tsiskaridze A, Djibuti M, van MG, Lomidze G, Apridonidze S, Gauarashvili I *et al*. Stroke incidence and 30-day case-fatality in a suburb of Tbilisi: results of the first prospective population-based study in Georgia. *Stroke* 2004; **35**(11):2523–8.

38 Lavados PM, Sacks C, Prina L, Escobar A, Tossi C, Araya F *et al*. Incidence, 30-day case-fatality rate, and prognosis of stroke in Iquique, Chile: a 2-year community-based prospective study (PISCIS project). *Lancet* 2005; **365**(9478):2206–15.

39 Syme PD, Byrne AW, Chen R, Devenny R, Forbes JF. Community-based stroke incidence in a Scottish population: the Scottish Borders Stroke Study. *Stroke* 2005; **36**(9):1837–43.

40 Morikawa Y, Nakagawa H, Naruse Y, Nishijo M, Miura K, Tabata M *et al*. Trends in stroke incidence and acute case fatality in a Japanese rural area : the Oyabe study. *Stroke* 2000; **31**(7):1583–7.

41 Feigin VL, Wiebers DO, Whisnant JP, O'Fallon WM. Stroke incidence and 30-day case-fatality rates in Novosibirsk, Russia, 1982 through 1992. *Stroke* 1995; **26**(6):924–9.

42 Powles J, Kirov P, Feschieva N, Stanoev M, Atanasova V. Stroke in urban and rural populations in north-east Bulgaria: incidence and case fatality findings from a 'hot pursuit' study. *BMC Public Health* 2002; **2**:24.

43 Mihalka L, Smolanka V, Bulecza B, Mulesa S, Bereczki D. A population study of stroke in West Ukraine: incidence, stroke services, and 30-day case fatality. *Stroke* 2001; **32**(10):2227–31.

44 Smadja D, Cabre P, May F, Fanon JL, Rene-Corail P, Riocreux C *et al*. ERMANCIA: Epidemiology of Stroke in Martinique, French West Indies: Part I: methodology, incidence, and 30-day case fatality rate. *Stroke* 2001; **32**(12):2741–7.

45 Liu M, Wu B, Wang WZ, Lee LM, Zhang SH, Kong LZ. Stroke in China: epidemiology, prevention, and management strategies. *Lancet Neurol* 2007; **6**(5):456–64.

46 Sacco RL, Boden-Albala B, Gan R, Chen X, Kargman DE, Shea S *et al*. Stroke incidence among white, black, and Hispanic residents of an urban community: the Northern Manhattan Stroke Study. *Am J Epidemiol* 1998; **147**(3):259–68.

47 Kissela B, Schneider A, Kleindorfer D, Khoury J, Miller R, Alwell K *et al*. Stroke in a biracial population: the excess burden of stroke among blacks. *Stroke* 2004; **35**(2):426–31.

48 Wolfe CD, Rudd AG, Howard R, Coshall C, Stewart J, Lawrence E *et al*. Incidence and case fatality rates of stroke subtypes in a multiethnic population: the South London Stroke Register. *J Neurol Neurosurg Psychiatry* 2002; **72**(2):211–16.

49 Hajat C, Tilling K, Stewart JA, Lemic-Stojcevic N, Wolfe CD. Ethnic differences in risk factors for ischemic stroke: a European case-control study. *Stroke* 2004; **35**(7):1562–7.

50 McGruder HF, Malarcher AM, Antoine TL, Greenlund KJ, Croft JB. Racial and ethnic disparities in cardiovascular risk factors among stroke survivors: United States 1999 to 2001. *Stroke* 2004; **35**(7):1557–61.

51 Feigin VL, Rodgers A. Ethnic disparities in risk factors for stroke: what are the implications? *Stroke* 2004; **35**(7):1568–9.

52 Wolfe CD, Smeeton NC, Coshall C, Tilling K, Rudd AG. Survival differences after stroke in a multiethnic population: follow-up study with the South London stroke register. *Br Med J* 2005; **331**(7514):431.

53 Sudlow C. Survival after stroke in south London. *Br Med J* 2005; **331**(7514):414–15.

54 Feigin V, Carter K, Hackett M, Barber PA, McNaughton H, Dyall L *et al*. Ethnic disparities in incidence of stroke subtypes: Auckland Regional Community Stroke Study, 2002–2003. *Lancet Neurol* 2006; **5**(2):130–9.

55 Hong Y, Bots ML, Pan X, Hofman A, Grobbee DE, Chen H. Stroke incidence and mortality in rural and urban Shanghai from 1984 through 1991. Findings from a community-based registry. *Stroke* 1994; **25**(6):1165–9.

56 Lemesle M, Milan C, Faivre J, Moreau T, Giroud M, Dumas R. Incidence trends of ischemic stroke and transient ischemic attacks in a well-defined French population from 1985 through 1994. *Stroke* 1999; **30**(2):371–7.

57 Jorgensen HS, Plesner AM, Hubbe P, Larsen K. Marked increase of stroke incidence in men between 1972 and 1990 in Frederiksberg, Denmark. *Stroke* 1992; **23**(12):1701–4.

58 Kubo M, Kiyohara Y, Kato I, Tanizaki Y, Arima H, Tanaka K *et al*. Trends in the incidence, mortality, and survival rate of cardiovascular disease in a Japanese community: the Hisayama study. *Stroke* 2003; **34**(10):2349–54.

59 Sivenius J, Tuomilehto J, Immonen-Raiha P, Kaarisalo M, Sarti C, Torppa J *et al*. Continuous 15-year decrease in incidence and mortality of stroke in Finland: the FINSTROKE study. *Stroke* 2004; **35**(2):420–5.

60 Anderson CS, Carter KN, Hackett ML, Feigin V, Barber PA, Broad JB *et al*. Trends in stroke incidence in Auckland, New Zealand, during 1981 to 2003. *Stroke* 2005; **36**(10):2087–93.

61 Linn FH, Rinkel GJ, Algra A, van Gijn J. Incidence of subarachnoid hemorrhage: role of region, year, and rate of computed tomography: a meta-analysis. *Stroke* 1996; **27**(4):625–9.

62 Tolonen H, Mahonen M, Asplund K, Rastenyte D, Kuulasmaa K, Vanuzzo D *et al*. Do trends in population levels of blood pressure and other cardiovascular risk factors explain trends in stroke event rates? Comparisons of 15 populations in 9 countries within the WHO MONICA Stroke Project. World Health Organization Monitoring of Trends and Determinants in Cardiovascular Disease. *Stroke* 2002; **33**(10):2367–75.

63 Rothwell PM, Warlow CP. Timing of TIAs preceding stroke: time window for prevention is very short. *Neurology* 2005; **64**(5):817–20.

64 Truelsen T, Piechowski-Jozwiak B, Bonita R, Mathers C, Bogousslavsky J, Boysen G. Stroke incidence and prevalence in Europe: a review of available data. *Eur J Neurol* 2006; **13**(6):581–98.

65 Malmgren R, Bamford J, Warlow C, Sandercock P, Slattery J. Projecting the number of patients with first ever strokes and patients newly handicapped by stroke in England and Wales. *Br Med J* 1989; **298**(6674):656–60.

66 Hankey GJ, Warlow CP. Treatment and secondary prevention of stroke: evidence, costs, and effects on individuals and populations. *Lancet* 1999; **354**(9188):1457–63.

67 Mehta DK. *British National Formulary*. 53rd edn. London: BMJ Publishing Group Ltd and RPS Publishing, 2007.

68 Hylek EM, D'Antonio J, Evans-Molina C, Shea C, Henault LE, Regan S. Translating the results of randomized trials into clinical practice: the challenge of warfarin candidacy among hospitalized elderly patients with atrial fibrillation. *Stroke* 2006; **37**(4):1075–80.

69 Somerfield J, Barber PA, Anderson NE, Kumar A, Spriggs D, Charleston A *et al*. Not all patients with atrial fibrillation-associated ischemic stroke can be started on anticoagulant therapy. *Stroke* 2006; **37**(5):1217–20.

70 Rothwell PM, Coull AJ, Silver LE, Fairhead JF, Giles MF, Lovelock CE *et al*. Population-based study of event-rate, incidence, case fatality, and mortality for all acute vascular events in all arterial territories (Oxford Vascular Study). *Lancet* 2005; **366**(9499):1773–83.

71 Fairhead JF, Rothwell PM. Underinvestigation and undertreatment of carotid disease in elderly patients with transient ischaemic attack and stroke: comparative population based study. *Br Med J* 2006; **333**(7567):525–7.

72 Rudd AG, Lowe D, Hoffman A, Irwin P, Pearson M. Secondary prevention for stroke in the United Kingdom: results from the National Sentinel Audit of Stroke. *Age Ageing* 2004; **33**(3):280–6.

73 Ovbiagele B, Saver JL, Fredieu A, Suzuki S, McNair N, Dandekar A *et al*. PROTECT: a coordinated stroke treatment program to prevent recurrent thromboembolic events. *Neurology* 2004; **63**(7):1217–22.

74 Osterberg L, Blaschke T. Adherence to medication. *N Engl J Med* 2005; **353**(5):487–97.

75 Benade MM, Warlow CP. Cost of identifying patients for carotid endarterectomy. *Stroke* 2002; **33**(2):435–9.

76 Wardlaw JM, Chappell FM, Stevenson M, De Nigris E, Thomas S, Gillard J *et al*. Accurate, practical and cost-effective assessment of carotid stenosis in the UK. *Health Technology Assessment* 2006; **10**(30):1–200.

77 Ezzati M, Hoorn SV, Rodgers A, Lopez AD, Mathers CD, Murray CJ. Estimates of global and regional potential health gains from reducing multiple major risk factors. *Lancet* 2003; **362**(9380):271–80.

78 Jackson R, Lynch J, Harper S. Preventing coronary heart disease. *Br Med J* 2006; **332**(7542):617–18.

79 Murray CJ, Lauer JA, Hutubessy RC, Niessen L, Tomijima N, Rodgers A *et al*. Effectiveness and costs of interventions to lower systolic blood pressure and cholesterol: a global and regional analysis on reduction of cardiovascular-disease risk. *Lancet* 2003; **361**(9359):717–25.

80 Emberson J, Whincup P, Morris R, Walker M, Ebrahim S. Evaluating the impact of population and high-risk strategies for the primary prevention of cardiovascular disease. *Eur Heart J* 2004; **25**(6):484–91.

81 Marteau TM, Kinmonth AL. Screening for cardiovascular risk: public health imperative or matter for individual informed choice? *Br Med J* 2002; **325**(7355):78–80.

82 Rose G. *The Strategy of Preventive Medicine*. New York: Oxford University Press, 1992.

83 Rothwell PM, Mehta Z, Howard SC, Gutnikov SA, Warlow CP. Treating individuals 3: from subgroups to

individuals: general principles and the example of carotid endarterectomy. *Lancet* 2005; **365**(9455):256–65.

84 Ebrahim S, Harwood R. *Stroke: Epidemiology, Evidence and Clinical Practice.* 2nd edn. New York: Oxford University Press, 1999.

85 Law MR, Wald NJ. Risk factor thresholds: their existence under scrutiny. *Br Med J* 2002; **324**(7353):1570–6.

86 Jackson R, Lawes CM, Bennett DA, Milne RJ, Rodgers A. Treatment with drugs to lower blood pressure and blood cholesterol based on an individual's absolute cardiovascular risk. *Lancet* 2005; **365**(9457):434–41.

87 Cholesterol Treatment Trialists' Collaborators. Efficacy and safety of cholesterol-lowering treatment: prospective meta-analysis of data from 90,056 participants in 14 randomised trials of statins. *Lancet* 2005; **366**(9493):1267–78.

88 MacMahon S, Neal B, Rodgers A. Hypertension: time to move on. *Lancet* 2005; **365**(9464):1108–9.

89 Brindle P, Beswick A, Fahey T, Ebrahim S. Accuracy and impact of risk assessment in the primary prevention of cardiovascular disease: a systematic review. *Heart* 2006; **92**(12):1752–9.

90 Brindle P, May M, Gill P, Cappuccio F, D'Agostino R, Sr., Fischbacher C *et al.* Primary prevention of cardiovascular disease: a web-based risk score for seven British black and minority ethnic groups. *Heart* 2006; **92**(11):1595–602.

91 D'Agostino RB, Sr., Grundy S, Sullivan LM, Wilson P. Validation of the Framingham coronary heart disease prediction scores: results of a multiple ethnic groups investigation. *J Am Med Assoc* 2001; **286**(2):180–7.

92 Wald NJ, Law MR. A strategy to reduce cardiovascular disease by more than 80%. *Br Med J* 2003; **326**(7404):1419.

93 Feinberg WM, Blackshear JL, Laupacis A, Kronmal R, Hart RG. Prevalence, age distribution, and gender of patients with atrial fibrillation: analysis and implications. *Arch Intern Med* 1995; **155**(5):469–73.

94 Hobbs FDR, Fitzmaurice DA, Jowett S, Mant J, Bryan S, Raftery J *et al.* A randomised controlled trial and cost-effectiveness study of systematic screening (targeted and total population screening) versus routine practice for the detection of atrial fibrillation in people aged 65 and over. The SAFE study. *Health Technology Assessment* 2005; **9**(40):1–90.

95 Ricci S, Flamini FO, Celani MG, Marini M, Antonini D, Bartolini S *et al.* Prevalence of internal carotid-artery stenosis in subjects older than 49 years: a population study. *Cerebrovasc Dis* 1991; **1**:16–19.

96 O'Leary DH, Anderson KM, Wolf PA, Evans JC, Poehlman HW. Cholesterol and carotid atherosclerosis

in older persons: the Framingham Study. *Ann Epidemiol* 1992; **2**(1–2):147–53.

97 Willeit J, Kiechl S. Prevalence and risk factors of asymptomatic extracranial carotid artery atherosclerosis: a population-based study. *Arterioscler Thrombosis* 1993; **13**:661–8.

98 Prati P, Vanuzzo D, Casaroli M, Di Chiara A, De Biasi F, Feruglio GA *et al.* Prevalence and determinants of carotid atherosclerosis in a general population. *Stroke* 1992; **23**(12):1705–11.

99 Lee TT, Solomon NA, Heidenreich PA, Oehlert J, Garber AM. Cost-effectiveness of screening for carotid stenosis in asymptomatic persons. *Ann Intern Med* 1997; **126**(5):337–46.

100 Whitty CJ, Sudlow CL, Warlow CP. Investigating individual subjects and screening populations for asymptomatic carotid stenosis can be harmful. *J Neurol Neurosurg Psychiatry* 1998; **64**(5):619–23.

101 Lightwood JM, Glantz SA. Short-term economic and health benefits of smoking cessation: myocardial infarction and stroke. *Circulation* 1997; **96**(4):1089–96.

102 Ezzati M, Lopez AD. Estimates of global mortality attributable to smoking in 2000. *Lancet* 2003; **362**(9387):847–52.

103 Barrett-Connor E, Palinkas LA. Low blood pressure and depression in older men: a population based study. *Br Med J* 1994; **308**(6926):446–9.

104 Dennis M, Bamford J, Sandercock P, Warlow C. Prognosis of transient ischemic attacks in the Oxfordshire Community Stroke Project. *Stroke* 1990; **21**(6):848–53.

105 Van Wijk I, Kappelle LJ, van Gijn J, Koudstaal PJ, Franke CL, Vermeulen M *et al.* Long-term survival and vascular event risk after transient ischaemic attack or minor ischaemic stroke: a cohort study. *Lancet* 2005; **365**(9477):2098–104.

106 Antithrombotic Trialists' Collaboration. Collaborative meta-analysis of randomised trials of antiplatelet therapy for prevention of death, myocardial infarction, and stroke in high risk patients. *Br Med J* 2002; **324**(7329):71–86.

107 Rashid P, Leonardi-Bee J, Bath P. Blood pressure reduction and secondary prevention of stroke and other vascular events: a systematic review. *Stroke* 2003; **34**(11):2741–8.

108 The ESPRIT Study Group. Aspirin plus dipyridamole versus aspirin alone after cerebral ischaemia of arterial origin (ESPRIT): randomised controlled trial. *Lancet* 2006; **367**(9523):1665–73.

109 Rothwell PM, Eliasziw M, Gutnikov SA, Warlow CP, Barnett HJ. Endarterectomy for symptomatic carotid stenosis in relation to clinical subgroups and timing of surgery. *Lancet* 2004; **363**(9413):915–24.

Index

Page numbers in *italics* represent figures, those in **bold** represent tables.